THE NEUROSCIENCES

FOURTH STUDY PROGRAM

THE

FOURTH STUDY

The MIT Press

CAMBRIDGE, MASSACHUSETTS, AND

LONDON, ENGLAND

NEUROSCIENCES

PROGRAM Francis O. Schmitt and
Frederic G. Worden *Editors-in-Chief*

Associate Editors: George Adelman

Barry H. Smith

Contributing Editors: Floyd E. Bloom

John E. Dowling

Gerald M. Edelman

Gordon G. Hammes

Leslie L. Iversen

Rodolfo R. Llinás

Gordon M. Shepherd

Hans Thoenen

This book was set in VIP Baskerville by DEKR Corporation and was printed
and bound by The Murray Printing Company in the United States of America.

ISSN 0094-4866
ISBN 0-262-19162-8

INTRODUCTION

THE IDIOM of the Intensive Study Program (ISP) has been evolved by the Neurosciences Research Program (NRP) as a mechanism for the collaborative examination in depth of various areas of neuroscience by authorities in each aspect of the subjects and by Fellows who have been carefully selected for their research promise and for their special interest in the subjects under study. Three previous volumes have presented the papers, appropriately interrelated and edited, from the ISPs held in 1966, 1969, and 1972.

This Fourth Study Program differs in several respects from the preceding three. Instead of dealing with neuroscience on a broad front, this ISP was organized to focus attention on a new phase of neuroscience research that will be based on novel concepts of the functional organization of the central nervous system. These include certain unconventional ideas of information processing in the brain by means of electrotonic currents, which characterize the functioning of neuronal local circuits, and a new view of the functional organization of the cerebral cortex. Both concepts are likely to prove crucial in investigations of the mechanisms of higher brain function.

The purpose of this ISP was achieved by an intensive examination of brain functions in terms of three types of circuitry: structural, electrical, and chemical.

The scope and aims of the fourth ISP were articulated in an initial series of six keynote lectures, followed by the main body of some sixty lectures. Forming a bridge to future studies of higher brain function, the ISP ends with the exposition of a hypothesis about the functioning of the brain as a whole, featuring a group-selectional process with reentrant signaling in contrast to the conventional instructional model whereby information from the outer world, communicated via sensory mechanisms, informs and instructs the brain in an ongoing stream of experience. Mechanisms of consciousness and other cognitive processes seem amenable to effective investigation along such lines.

The new data and ideas discussed at the ISP lead to a more dynamic concept of brain functioning. One senses a new intellectual ferment not unlike the one that triggered the great advance in molecular genetics when genes were first defined as sequences of codonic nucleotides. Dimly perceived is a concept of a unit of function, termed the brain's module by Mountcastle in his keynote lecture. This functional unit, still only nebulously characterized, may well consist of columns or slabs, each containing some hundreds or thousands of neurons interacting both electrotonically in local circuits and in more conventional spike-conducted modes.

The ISP points the direction along which further research might prove of historic importance, namely the study of the functional organization of the brain as viewed in the new perspectives. It also suggests a need for new technical and conceptual developments capable of dealing with the dynamic multimodal interrelations of hundreds of cells within the local circuitry of individual cortical columnar units.

The ISP was held at the University of Colorado at Boulder from 20 June to 1 July 1977. Following the introductory keynote speakers, the sixty lectures constituting the main body of the ISP were delivered in morning and afternoon sessions over nine working days. The individual sections were organized, chaired, and the manuscripts later edited, by: Gordon M. Shepherd (neuronal local circuits), John E. Dowling (retinal function), Rodolfo L. Llinás (bioelectric aspects of neuronal information processing), Gerald M. Edelman (membranes, cellular ultrastructure, and molecular circuitry), Gordon G. Hammes (chemical regulation, phosphorylation, and ion transport), Hans Thoenen (regulation of gene expression in the nervous system), Leslie L. Iversen (modulators and effectors of neuronal signaling), and Floyd E. Bloom (interaction of multineuronal systems). We thank these section chairmen for their constructive and very effective efforts before and during the event and for their perceptive editing of the manuscripts in their sections after the event.

To this ISP, as to each of the three preceding ones, fifty postdoctoral Fellows were invited. They were selected from a large list of highly qualified candidates nominated by prominent neuroscientists around the world. We are deeply indebted to Dana L. Farnsworth, Seymour S. Kety, Irwin W. Sizer, William H. Sweet, and Richard J. Wurtman, who served on the ISP Fellowship Selection Committee.

The strong interest in neuroscience of NRP's sponsoring institution, the Massachusetts Institute of Technology, was expressed in closing remarks by the Chairman of its Corporation, Dr. Howard W. Johnson. For his encouraging words and for his attendance during the ISP, we express our deep appreciation.

A special thanks is due to Parvati Dev and Bruce L. Brandt of the NRP Center Staff who, over a period of months, worked hard to provide essential scientific planning and research assistance to the editors in the development of the ISP.

The logistical planning and smooth operation of the fourth ISP, as of the preceding three, were due to the commitment, administrative ability, and sagacity of Katheryn Cusick, Associate Director of NRP. Closely cooperating with her, William E. Wright marshaled the supporting staff and facilities of the University of Colorado's Bureau of Conferences and Institutes.

The federal agencies and philanthropic foundations that provided the financial support that made the ISP possible are listed on page viii. We express to them the very great appreciation of NRP and of all participants privileged to attend the ISP.

To the Associates and Staff of NRP we extend sincere thanks for their advice and their labors during the months of planning as well as for their willing professional assistance during the course of the ISP.

FRANCIS O. SCHMITT and FREDERIC G. WORDEN

Boston, Massachusetts
1 June 1978

Acknowledgment of Sponsorship and Support

The Neurosciences Research Program, a research center of the Massachusetts Institute of Technology, is an interdisciplinary, interuniversity organization with the primary goal of facilitating the investigation of how the nervous system mediates behavior including the mental processes of man. To this end, the NRP, as one of its activities, conducts scientific meetings to explore crucial problems in the neurosciences. The NRP is supported in part by U.S. Public Health Service, National Institutes of Health Contract No. NO1-NS-6-2343, National Institute of Mental Health Grant No. NIH-5-RO1-MH23132-07, National Science Foundation Grant No. 78-09115-BNS, The Arthur Vining Davis Foundation, William T. Grant Foundation, van Ameringen Foundation, Inc., Vingo Trust, and the Neurosciences Research Foundation, Inc. Grateful acknowledgment for direct support of the Intensive Study Program is made to the following: National Institutes of Health Contract No. 278-77-009 (ER), National Science Foundation, International Business Machine Corp., Vollmer Foundation, Inc., Surdna Foundation, Inc., The Teagle Foundation, Inc., The National Foundation–March of Dimes, and the Camille and Henry Dreyfus Foundation, Inc.

CONTENTS

ELEMENTS OF RETINAL FUNCTION

SPIKELESS AND ELECTROTONIC INFORMATION PROCESSING

HIGH-SENSITIVITY TRANSDUCTION

MEMBRANE DYNAMICS AND CELLULAR INTERACTION

CHEMICAL REGULATION AND TRANSDUCTION

PHOSPHORYLATION AND ION TRANSPORT

REGULATION OF GENE EXPRESSION IN THE NERVOUS SYSTEM

MODULATORS AND EFFECTORS OF NEURONAL INTERACTION

A THEORY OF HIGHER BRAIN FUNCTION

THE NEUROSCIENCES

FOURTH STUDY PROGRAM

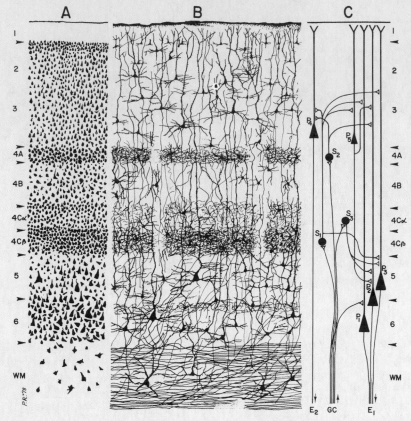

A   B   C

I
2
3
4A
4B
4Cα
4Cβ
5
6
WM

P.R.'78

E_2 GC E_1

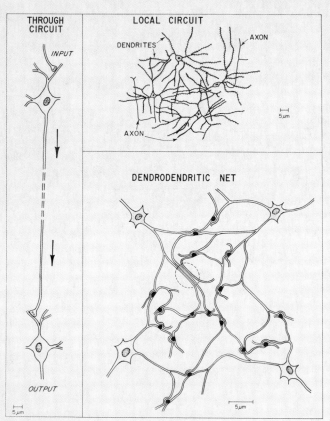

THROUGH CIRCUIT

INPUT

OUTPUT

5 μm

LOCAL CIRCUIT

DENDRITES   AXON

AXON

5 μm

DENDRODENDRITIC NET

5 μm

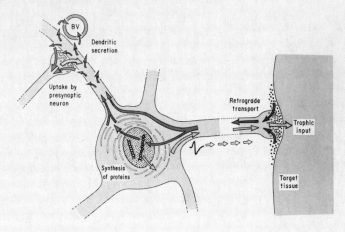

BV

Dendritic secretion

Uptake by presynaptic neuron

Synthesis of proteins

Retrograde transport

Trophic input

Target tissue

KEYNOTE PAPERS

Like the three motifs of this Intensive Study Program, these illustrations reflect the study of brain circuitry at three levels of neuronal circuitry. The upper diagram shows the laminar and cortical structural organization of the cerebral cortex (taken from Rakic, this volume). The lower left diagram depicts the electrical circuitry of through circuits and local circuits. The lower right diagram shows chemical circuitry involving the fast transport of substances in both directions through neurons and across synaptic junctions; such circuitry leads to trophic and regulatory control of the neurons' immediate microenvironment.

1 The Role of Structural, Electrical, and Chemical Circuitry in Brain Function

FRANCIS O. SCHMITT

NEUROSCIENCE, the multidisciplinary study of the central nervous system and behavior, has expanded greatly during the last two decades both in numbers of investigators and in subjects being investigated at all levels of complexity, from that of molecules, brain cells, and neuronal circuitry to that of behavior. New discoveries and conceptual advances enliven the meetings of national and international societies of neuroscience. Highly sophisticated concepts of the function of various partial systems of the brain have been developed on the basis of ingenious experimental designs in anatomy, physiology, and other aspects of neuroscience. These advances are valuable not only in their own right but also as a foundation for a scientifically significant attempt to understand the most complex system known to science, the human brain, as well as to make progress in achieving the highest ultimate aim of neuroscience, to understand human selfhood and psyche.

Many theories of higher brain function (learning, memory, perception, self-awareness, consciousness) have been proposed, but these lack both cogency with respect to established anatomical and physiological facts and, in general, biophysical and biochemical plausibility. In such theories heavy reliance is usually placed on processes subserved by spike action potential waves traveling in hard-wired neuronal circuits of Golgi Type I neurons. Such circuits consist of neurons whose cell bodies are large enough to permit easy impalement by microelectrodes and which possess long axons that connect processing centers in various regions of the brain and spinal cord.

Such theories, based on studies of the properties of partial systems, are subject to the component–systems dilemma that bedevils all attempts at biological

generalization: they fail to explain how distributive global functional capabilities emerge from complex interactions of functional units, such as neurons or neuronal circuits. No detailed, self-consistent theory has yet been proposed that specifies and functionally characterizes the operational repertoires at each level of complexity and that defines the postulated information-processing mechanism explicitly.

The fourth Intensive Study Program (ISP) held under the auspices of the Neurosciences Research Program (NRP) at Boulder, Colorado, in June 1977 was designed to accelerate the emergence of a new phase in neuroscience based on new information about brain structure and on unconventional concepts that have merged primarily in the last decade (see Schmitt, Dev, and Smith, 1976). It was hoped that the ISP would pinpoint the most promising direction in the search for an understanding of basic mechanisms of higher brain functions.

The ISP examined in depth the basic componentry of the brain and its mode of functioning in terms of structural, electrical, and chemical circuits. Particular emphasis was placed on two areas. The first deals with the broad subject of neuronal local circuits or "microcircuits," as Shepherd (1978) has recently called them. Local circuits as described by Rakic (1975) comprise short-axon Golgi Type II neurons interacting within defined locales primarily by dendrodendritic synaptic interaction; they are activated by graded electrotonic currents rather than by spike action potentials. In the ISP, local circuits were interpreted much more broadly as local integrative processes at the level of molecules, subcellular components, or neuronal nets.

The second area of emphasis involved particular local circuits that occur in the cerebral cortex; these are of utmost importance in the search for an explanation of mechanisms of higher functions. To understand the cerebral cortex, the nervous tissue of

FRANCIS O. SCHMITT   Neurosciences Research Program, Jamaica Plain, MA 02130

greatest complexity, and its organization, we must clearly start by reducing it to simple concepts and principles of operation. Much was made of ubiquitous local assemblies of neurons, such as Szentágothai's "modules" and Mountcastle's "columns" and "minicolumns," that consist of hundreds or thousands of neurons whose organization and operational logic form the structural and functional basis of the cerebral cortex.

The ISP opened with a series of six keynote lectures that defined the scope and aims of the study program. The main body of lectures, some sixty in all, dealt with circuitry at three levels: structural, bioelectrical, and biochemical. They were delivered in morning and afternoon sessions over nine days. The final session was devoted to the presentation of a hypothesis by Gerald Edelman that we hope will serve as a bridge to the next major period of neuroscience, which may be expected to concentrate on cortical properties and higher brain function. In the remainder of this paper I shall deal in turn with the keynote lectures, the major areas of concern of the main body of lectures, and the bearing of the ISP upon the evolution of neuroscience.

The keynote lectures

In his keynote lecture, V. B. Mountcastle suggests that an understanding of the unique structure and function of the cerebral cortex is a requisite for any fruitful theory of higher brain function. He proposes that higher functions depend on the ensemble actions of very large populations of cortical neurons that are organized into complex interacting systems. The discussion focuses on the fantastically large numbers of neurons in the neocortex of the forebrain, which are organized in multiply replicated local neuronal circuits or ensembles constituting columns, composed, in turn, of closely linked subsets or "minicolumns" which are postulated to be the developmental units of cortical structure. The true functional unit of the cortex remains to be accurately defined. The hypercolumns of Hubel and Wiesel (1977), specified with respect to ocular dominance and directionality vectors, play a valuable role in clarifying the issue, but the clear definition of the cortical functional unit remains to be determined by further investigations of physiology, morphology, and developmental neurobiology.

Columns, which may comprise hundreds to thousands of neurons, are composed of both Golgi Type I neurons in conventional synaptic patterns and local circuits of Golgi Type II neurons as described by Rakic (1975) and Shepherd (1978). Their relative fractions and the types of interaction that occur between conventional projection circuits and local circuits are not known.

The shapes of the columns vary among the various areas of the cortex according to the number and mode of packing of the constituent minicolumns and of their interconnections. The neocortex is pictured as being organized according to much more uniform principles than had hitherto been supposed: the onrush of cortical enlargement in primate evolution occurred more by replication of basically similar columns than by the development of new neuronal types or different modes of intrinsic organization. The neocortex, which receives afferent input upon the cortical columns, has outputs to almost every major entity of the CNS, forming massive reentrant systems with many points of entry and exit. Intracolumnar and intercolumnar connections are precisely positioned; the cortex is composed of a repetitive, pervasive, columnar internal organization that is everywhere the same. The columns and minicolumns constitute distributed systems serving distributive functions.

The uninitiated reader may well be surprised by two aspects of Mountcastle's description: first, the apparent constancy of the number of neurons contained within relatively small columnar domains (see Rockel, Hiorns, and Powell, 1974); and, second, the fact that the 600 million minicolumns of the human neocortex contain on the order of 50 billion nerve cells. It has been only about a decade since most textbooks put the total population of the *entire brain* at 10 billion neurons.

In his keynote lecture, T. H. Bullock points out that, although a large fraction of the ISP is concerned with local circuits as defined by Rakic (1975), the range of the word "local" is really much broader, including integrative operations at the molecular, intracellular, and intercellular levels (see also Shepherd's [1978] usage of the word "microcircuit"). A comparative electrophysiologist, Bullock identifies some 23 functional variables on which different anatomically defined neuronal units can achieve "local" integrative actions. The word "local" may thus apply to molecular and subcellular levels as well as to neuronal circuits and brain regions.

In a companion keynote paper to Bullock's, F. E. Bloom considers chemical integrative mechanisms primarily at the synaptic level, citing three dimensions or domains of neuronal specification from which the integrative logic of neuronal interaction may be derived. He lists an impressive array of chemically derived responses to nonspiking, small graded potentials that may be effective in information processing, such as alteration of local ion pools due to ion pumping, alteration of metabolic pools, and transmitter synthesized by genetic evocation of necessary enzymes and organelles. Calcium ions, prostaglandins, and adenosine are listed as having important intracellular and intercellular integrative functions; these biodynamically active chemical agents and the protein substrates through which they express their actions represent "a microcosm of cross-integrating and self-regulating chemical systems rivaling any other known set of partially coupled reactions."

Bloom employs a three-dimensional map to compare properties ascribable to neural systems to which specific chemical mediation can be assigned. Space, time, and energy are the parameters or "domains of neuronal operations" in which he characterizes the integrative actions of various transmitters and other neuroactive substances. Thus, complete functional understanding requires, in addition to chemical identification, a consideration of temporal contexts and operational logic. Knowledge of such chemical integrative processes may eventually lead to the formulation of basic principles according to which neurons intercommunicate and produce harmonious functioning of the whole organism.

W. M. Cowan, in his keynote paper, provides a masterly review of neuronal circuitry at the cellular and structural level. He is concerned particularly with factors involved in the developmental control of four parameters: neuronal number, location, morphology, and connectivity.

Clearly it would be a great help in our efforts to understand the structural organization of the primate brain if we could trace the temporal and spatial development of the brain and specify the selectional and control mechanisms, genetic and epigenetic, that operate at each stage in neurogenesis.

Most of Cowan's review is based on Golgi Type I large-cell neurons that project to distant targets simply because less information is available concerning the much more numerous Golgi Type II, short-axon local circuit neurons with which this ISP is concerned. Wherever the facts are available, Cowan does compare and contrast the two types of systems, particularly with respect to time of development, genetic control, and patterns of axonal connectivity.

Werner Reichardt, whose experimental background includes many years of multidisciplinary analysis of the behavior of the house fly, presented the final keynote talk. He provides a valuable heuristic approach in which quantitative analysis of behav-

ior defines the functional constraints of a complex central nervous system; this is in sharp contrast to research in which neural processes are investigated without behaviorally based guidelines.

The experimental logic of Reichardt and his colleagues is reductionistic: by a quantitative study of the fly's behavior, fundamental laws are deduced concerning phenomena at cellular and molecular levels. The converse is of course not true: behavior is not deducible from a knowledge of the properties of the cellular and molecular components.

Reichardt's analysis and explanation of behavior covers three levels: (1) the phenomenological level, encompassing the input-output behavior of the system as well as its logical organization in terms of computations performed by nervous interaction upon the visual input; (2) the level of functional principles of the subsystems; and (3) the "lowest" level, concerned with individual components and detailed neuronal circuitry (studies at this level employ electron-microscopic, bioelectric, and many sophisticated biophysical and biochemical procedures). Reichardt concludes that the complex orientation behavior of the fly is based on the cooperative interplay of only three different types of neuronal interaction.

Major concerns of the ISP

The sixty lectures that constituted the main body of the ISP deal with circuitry at three levels: structural, bioelectrical, and biochemical. The following is offered as a brief synoptic characterization not of individual lectures but of some of the major concepts dealt with in the course of the study program.

NEURONAL LOCAL CIRCUITS: STRUCTURE AND FUNCTION Bearing in mind the ambiguity of the adjective "local" and the noun "circuit," we start by inquiring into the fundamental logic of neuronal circuits composed characteristically of short-axon, Golgi Type II neurons. The axons of such neurons are sometimes bushy, but they remain in the local area, seldom extending into projection tracts of the white matter. Interneuronal linkage is therefore primarily dendrodendritic (D-D), although it may also be dendrosomatic, somatodendritic, somatoaxonic, and even dendroaxonic and axoaxonic. The functionally most challenging picture is that of a matrix enclosing small, Golgi Type II neurons interpenetrated by neurites, primarily dendritic processes connected by D-D synapses (Figure 1). The shortness of the axons and the multiple synaptic interaction between extensively developed dendritic trees favor the formation of local

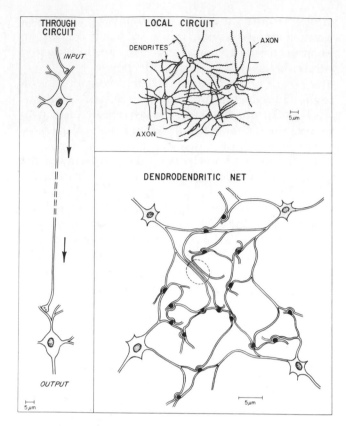

FIGURE 1 Comparison between through-projection circuit of Golgi Type I neurons (left) and neuronal local circuits composed of dendrodendritic networks of Golgi Type II short-axon neurons (right).

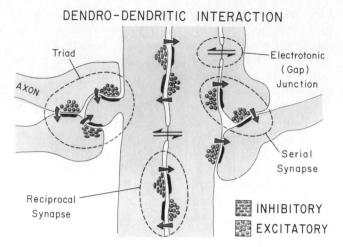

FIGURE 2 Unconventional synapses in which dendrites may be both pre- and postsynaptic to each other, forming reciprocal dendrodendritic synapses. A triad, in which an axon synapses with two mutually synapsing dendrites, is shown on the left. A serial synapse, in which a dendrite is postsynaptic to one dendrite and presynaptic to another dendrite, thus interconnecting a series of dendrites, is shown on the right. Two low-resistance electrotonic ("gap") junctions are also shown.

groups or ensembles within a large dendritic network. It seems probable that, although such D-D nets may extend over distances vastly greater than the size of the constituent cells, the extent of the ensembles or "local circuits" is to some extent self-limited, making possible the transfer of information not only within and between neighboring ensembles but also to remote nets, the transfer occurring primarily by graded electrotonic currents although spiking through-projection neurons may also participate.

Electron-microscopic examination of neuronal local circuits has revealed the existence of several unconventional modes of synaptic connectivity (Figure 2). These include reciprocal electrotonic ("gap") junctions, mixed chemical and electrical junctions, and other forms of D-D synapses, including triads and serial synapses.

Electrotonic junctions represent a fascinating form of interneuronal coupling previously thought to be rare, particularly in the mammalian brain, but now known to comprise a "substantial minority" among

junctional and synaptic types in the CNS (Bennett, 1974). That direct electrical coupling between cells occurs via electrotonic junctions is shown by the fact that low-resistance electrical coupling is found in those tissues in which electrotonic junctions can be demonstrated electron-microscopically (Sotelo, 1975; see also the papers of Korn and of Gilula, this volume).

The full significance of electrical coupling is still unknown (see Bennett and Goodenough, 1978). Synchronization of firing, as it occurs in the fish electric organ, is one obvious function. However, it is possible that, in local ensembles of neuronal circuits, electrical coupling gives rise not only to certain obvious metastable states, such as oscillatory behavior, but also to more sophisticated, yet unexplored communicational functions. How electrotonic junctions modify chemical synaptic action in mixed electrical-chemical junctions is not known.

The biophysics of electrotonic junctions offers a challenging field for study. Hundreds of individual conducting channels occur in single junctions or plaques, as seen in freeze-etch electron micrographs. The diameter of an individual channel, determined by x-ray diffraction studies, is about 2 nm (Caspar et al., 1977; Makowski et al., 1977). This is but a few times greater than the Debye length of the inorganic ions carrying the current. There may thus be strong electrical interaction between the ions and the negatively charged proteinaceous molecules that make up the channel wall, and this may well influence electrical properties such as the conductivity and the electrical capacity of the aqueous channels. Conversely, there may be a transductive coupling between the ionic current and the protein subunits composing channel walls. Such a transductive process might gate or regulate the ionic flow through the channels, hence constituting a mechanism for information processing, particularly if the channel protein is capable of altering its tertiary or quaternary molecular conformation in response to biochemical alterations imposed by cellular metabolism.

Not without possible significance regarding the role of local circuitry is the fact that the number of neurons that interact exclusively by local synaptic circuitry increases systematically with phylogenetic advance, reaching a clear-cut maximum both in absolute numbers and in ratio of Golgi Type I to Golgi Type II neurons in the human brain.

The distribution of local (micro) circuits in different regions of the mammalian brain is discussed by Schmitt, Dev, and Smith (1976) and by Shepherd (1978), who points out that much of the information flowing into the cerebral cortex is processed by microcircuits at the thalamic level.

Important in the ontogenesis of the brain is the fact that local circuit neurons develop relatively late. The possible role in plasticity and directional or selectional design that emerges from the large pool of modifiable Golgi II neurons has been discussed by Jacobson (1970, 1975) and by Cowan (this volume).

The olfactory bulb and the retina as prototypes of neuronal local circuits   The two brain tissues that best illustrate neuronal local circuits are the olfactory bulb and the retina (Figure 3). Each was dealt with extensively during the ISP.

The olfactory bulb illustrates how a local circuit neuron, the axonless amacrine granule cell, can, by D-D interaction via graded electrotonic potentials, modulate the through-projection mitral cells (Rall and Shepherd, 1968; Rall, 1970; Shepherd, 1970). The periglomerular neurons play a similar modulatory role.

The retina, an ontogenetically externalized bit of central nervous tissue, comprises five major cell types in addition to the recently discovered interplexiform neurons. There are no through-projection neurons in the retina, and all bioelectrical interaction peripheral to the ganglion cells is transacted without spike impulses. Spikes may be propagated under certain conditions in the processes of the amacrine cells, but such spikes are not necessary for signal transmission, which continues after spiking has been blocked by the use of tetrodotoxin.

Bioelectrical Circuitry: Electrotonic Mechanisms in Neuronal Local Circuit Function   Bullock (1959) suggested that neuronal interaction may result from nonspike, graded electrotonic currents, and this hypothesis has received strong experimental support. In cell processes with high membrane resistance, the excitatory current can spread over neurites for relatively long distances with little attenuation (Shaw, 1972, this volume). Many arthropod motor neurons generate no spikes yet stimulate muscles over a centimeter away (Pearson, 1976, this volume). The bioelectrical language of neuronal local circuits is predominantly electrotonic; that is, intra- and interneuronal communication occurs by the passage into and out of cells of passive electrical currents, via the extracellular conducting milieu. These currents result from cellular activity and are graded and decrementing, unlike the all-or-nothing, self-regenerative spike action potentials. It has been suggested that electrotonic processing of information may play a significant role in brain function (Schmitt, Dev, and Smith, 1976), and the ISP explored in depth the biophysical and physiological basis of this hypothesis. Cable theory and its role in the computation of electrotonic effects was considered in detail by Julian Jack as a basis for discussion.

In compact neuronal tissue such as the retina where intercellular distances are small (measured in micrometers), electrotonic currents can serve instead of spike waves as the medium of fast information processing. Cortical columns and minicolumns are compact neuronal assemblies of this kind, but relevant bioelectrical data are not available for them. However, in view of the importance for higher brain function that Mountcastle attaches to neuronal interaction *within* minicolumns—perhaps more accurately within unitary functional assemblies—as well as between them and other brain tissue, and in view of the compactness of minicolumn structure, it seems plausible that information processing within the minicolumn is, at least in part, electrotonic. Minicolumns or other modular assemblies produced by D-D interaction of short-axon neurons have the property of both individual and parallel processing. Electrotonic interaction is to be expected between adjacent neuronal assemblies and also with more distant assemblies to form a "lateral" computation system, the output of

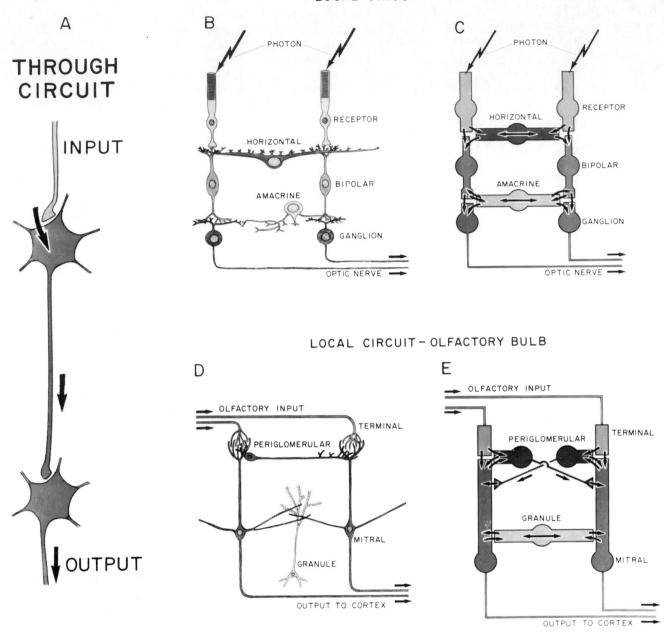

FIGURE 3 Comparison of through-projection Golgi Type I neurons (A) with neuronal local circuits of short-axon Golgi Type II neurons (B to E). B and C illustrate dendrodendritic synapses in the retina; these are shown in cellular arrays (B) and with respect to information transfer (C). D and E illustrate dendrodendritic synapses in the olfactory bulb, in cellular arrays (D) and with respect to information transfer (E). After Shepherd (1974).

which may not be the simple sum of the outputs of the individual assemblies (or minicolumns). Nonlinear interactions between local fields may be such that the resultant potential obeys other than algebraic summation rules (Schmitt, Dev, and Smith, 1976). Signaling and information processing in compact, particularly local circuit, tissue clearly are capable of

far more nuances and variability than in tissue activated by digital spike waves.

Decrementing, graded electrotonic potentials may be one or two orders of magnitude weaker than 50 to 100 mV spike trains. The question then arises whether such weak bioelectric vectors are capable of processing information in a system such as the brain.

Because this point is crucial for the entire theory of local circuit function in brain, it was considered in detail at the ISP. Technical limitations have made direct experimental evidence scarce, but three lines of indirect evidence strongly suggest that a positive answer may be given to the question.

First, that neuronal systems may be highly sensitive is shown by the fact that information processing by sensory transduction is in most cases at the limits of sensitivity: one photon for visual transduction, one or only a few tastant or olfactant molecules for chemical sensing, and near to K_T (Brownian movement) for auditory excitation. These exquisitely sensitive transductions are achieved each by its own molecular mechanism of amplification and transduction.

Visual transduction is the most thoroughly understood of the sensory transductions at the molecular level (see Figure 4). In the dark the receptor mem-

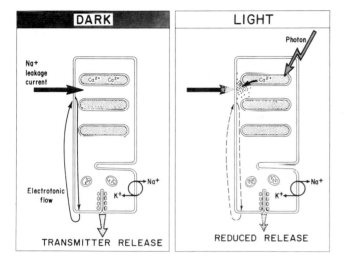

FIGURE 4 Proposed molecular mechanism of sensory transduction in the retina. Depolarization of receptor membrane in the dark, due to Na⁺ leakage, is modulated by calcium ions released from rhodopsin binding by absorption of a photon, altering flow of electrotonic current through the cell, thereby reducing transmitter released from ribbon terminal and hence the activity of other neurons in the retina.

brane is kept depolarized by a constant inflow of Na^+. Such ion leaks are apparently widely used by tissues to set the membrane at the most sensitive point in its sigmoidal curve of excitability. According to Hagins (this volume), absorption of an illuminating photon releases on the order of 10^2 Ca^{2+} ions from one rhodopsin molecule (out of 3×10^7 such molecules present in the outer limb of the retinal rod). Reduction of the Na^+ dark current by as little as 3% hyperpolarizes the receptor membrane slightly, thus

changing the passive electrotonic flow through the receptor cell and the medium and the rate of transmitter release at the ribbon synapse, leading eventually to the firing of spike impulses by the ganglion cells into the fibers of the optic nerve.

Two other more direct lines of evidence may be cited in support of the view that neurons may be sufficiently sensitive to be activated by electrotonic currents. The first concerns the amount of electrical energy required to liberate transmitter at the D-D synapses (which operate in a spikeless mode). Potentials of spike intensity at the synapse are not needed. Extremely small changes in presynaptic membrane potential may suffice (Bennett, 1968; Pearson and Fourtner, 1975; Llinás, this volume). Release of transmitter from vesicles does not require large transmembrane electrical gradients. Rather, release is due to the entrance into the terminal of Ca^{2+}; the amount of transmitter released is proportional to the calcium influx (Llinás and Heuser, 1977). In some synapses transmitter release is triggered by a relatively few millivolts, well within the range of electrotonic currents in local circuits.

A second direct line of evidence is the behavior of ion channels (e.g., for Na^+ and K^+) in the membrane of nerve axons. As a spike wave travels down an axon, sodium channels sense the approaching field and open the channel gates to Na^+ at the appropriate moment. This action is voltage-dependent. Presumably the field being sensed alters the conformation of the channel, thereby activiting the gating mechanism. According to Stevens (this volume), coupling of the electric field to the gating macromolecules is through the molecules' equivalent dipole moment, which varies for different conformations of the macromolecular gate. From a detailed and elegant study of the effect of electric fields on α-helix-coil transitions, Schwarz (this volume) points out that the field required to produce the transition (sensing) would be much smaller if the macromolecules or protein subunits interacted cooperatively (see also Schwarz and Seelig, 1968; Schwarz, 1978). He concludes that weak electric fields (such as might exist in electrotonic interactions in neuronal local circuits) would be effective, given a sufficient degree of cooperative interaction within or between channel macromolecules or their subunits. He suggests that such cooperative interaction might include cascade phenomena of the type discussed by Stadtman (this volume). Such enzyme cascades are an example at the chemical level of enormous signal amplification (see next section).

Dendritic membranes bearing no specialized organelles (synapses or gap junctions) are electrically passive, responding only with graded electrotonic activity (Bishop, 1956). Such electrotonic interaction may couple neighboring dendrites on the same or different neurons. In his pioneering work, Adey (1961) saw in such interactions a possible mechanism for the D-D processing of information by modulation of the electrical properties of dendritic membrane. Such a mechanism is likely to be very important in areas such as the cerebral cortex where extensive overlap of the dendritic arborizations of neighboring neurons occur (Adey, 1961, 1969; Adey, Walter, and Hendrix, 1961; Adey, Kado and Didio, 1962).

Another possible example of D-D interaction is provided by the parallelization of dendrites, perhaps induced by chemical specialization of the microenvironment (Scheibel and Scheibel, 1970; Fleischhauer and Detzer, 1975; Scheibel, this volume).

The evidence cited in this section strongly supports the view that electrotonic signals, although less intense than spike waves, suffice for information processing in neuronal local circuits. Admittedly we still are unable to measure electrical parameters simultaneously in many microscopic loci of cortical tissue, which is a prerequisite for laying the necessary biophysical basis. The reasoning must therefore be highly inferential at this time. However, new vistas on the physical basis of brain function open up if the sensitivity of neurons, particularly of their dendritic mechanisms, is so high as to intercept, transduce, and process electrical informational signaling deriving not only from members of local and neighboring assemblies, but also from distant cellular sources.

Such a view suggests that the cerebral cortex, like other nervous tissue rich in neuronal local circuitry, may constitute a system comparable to that discussed by Katchalsky, Rowland, and Blumenthal (1974) and by Haken (1977a,b), namely a system far from thermodynamic equilibrium in which dissipative dynamic interaction occurs with a high degree of cooperativity of the molecular and cellular components (see Schmitt, Schneider, and Crothers, 1975). The integrative and formative capabilities of such a system cannot be comprehended in terms of traditional connectionistic neurophysiological concepts but may well provide rich opportunities for creative investigation by the methods of biophysical chemistry.

CHEMICAL AND MOLECULAR CIRCUITRY Although we may not be accustomed to thinking of molecules as traveling in the brain in "circuits," this kind of chemical circuitry, which may be both local and extensive, is as fundamental to the operation of the brain as are structural and bioelectrical circuits. We shall consider circuits as circumscribed as those linking the interior of the cell with the external milieu and as extensive as the chemical traffic in the axon of a long motor neuron or the thin central-core regulatory axons that pass from the brain stem to all regions of the brain.

Intercellular space is a region where circuits of ions and metabolites flow incessantly. Nicholson (this volume) characterizes the brain as an electrically controlled chemical machine; he points out that alterations in the ionic milieu of the intercellular environment control the flow of electrotonic currents, hence of information, in those channels.

Intracellular communication, important for membrane-gene linkage, is mediated by the cytoskeleton (a rather inappropriate term because its role may not be exclusively mechanical). Energy for motility is transduced at the surface of the cytoskeleton, presumably through chemomechanical coupling between fibrous proteins (microtubules, myosin and actin filaments) by which substances are transported bidirectionally between the cell membrane and the genome (see Figure 5). The precise coupling mechanism that produces fast transport of substances through cells and neurites is still unknown, although several possibilities have been suggested (Schmitt, 1968; Schmitt and Samson, 1968; Ochs, 1972). Figure 5 illustrates the fibrous trabecular cytoskeletal differentiation of the ground substance, composed of tubulin, actin, and myosin, that mediates transport, as suggested by the high-voltage electron-microscope studies of Porter (this volume). The radial, intracellular orientation (i.e., normal to the plane of the cell membrane) has been studied by Weber (this volume), who observed the fibrous structures in cells treated with fluorescent antisera to actin, myosin, and actinin. Sëite and co-workers have shown that the fibrous arrays also penetrate into the substance of the nucleus presumably thereby approaching more closely to the genome (Sëite, Escaig, and Couineau, 1971; Sëite et al., 1977).

Energy mobilization through cyclic nucleotide-enzyme cascades and their coupling to excitable membranes This rapidly expanding field offers rich opportunities for research into psychopharmacology and neurobiochemistry. The lucid expositions by Rall and by Gilman in this volume emphasize the important role played by cyclic nucleotides throughout biosystems and particularly in metabolism, membrane permeability, transport, secretion, and the synthesis of specific proteins in the nervous system. Now being explored are reaction pathways extending from

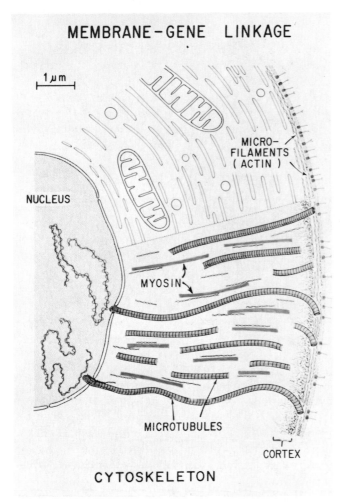

MEMBRANE–GENE LINKAGE

1 μm

NUCLEUS

MICRO-
FILAMENTS
(ACTIN)

MYOSIN

MICROTUBULES

CORTEX

CYTOSKELETON

FIGURE 5 Proposed mechanism of bidirectional information transfer between molecules in the region of the cell membrane and intranuclear genomic molecules by transport via a radially oriented cytoplasmic fibrous system consisting of microtubules, myosin, and microfilaments (actin).

membrane-borne receptors, after binding of the ligand (transmitter, modulator, hormone), through phosphorylating-enzyme-driven cascades, both in the cytosol and in the membrane, and leading eventually to the synthesis of specific membrane-bound proteins thought to mediate excitatory or inhibitory changes, slow polarization changes, and other regulatory mechanisms. At least one such membrane-bound protein, called "phospholamban," has been isolated from an excitable tissue, cardiac muscle, and has been chemically characterized (Katz, this volume). The cyclic nucleotide entrainment may also activate the genome to synthesize enduring (i.e., covalently linked) products that might play an important role in storage processes in brain cells. (For an excellent guide to the intricacies of cyclic nucleotide interactions see Daly, 1977.)

The sequential action of enzymes, as in the cyclic nucleotide entrainment from receptor to the deposition on the membrane of an electroactive phosphorylated protein, involves a cascade of directional, irreversible reactions with high kinetic amplification (about 100-fold at each enzymatically driven stage, according to Goldberg, 1975). Clearly, if it is shown that adenylate cyclase is activated not only by a receptor and chemical ligand but also by electrical signals via yet uncharacterized electroreceptors, a mechanism would be provided for the synthesis of enduring chemical substances within neurons through stimulation by weak electrotonic currents and fields.

Intraneuronal and interneuronal chemical circuitry via fast transport of metabolites and neuroactive substances In the decade since fast intraneuronal transport—an important outgrowth of Paul Weiss's discovery of "axoplasmic flow" (see Weiss and Hiscoe, 1948)—was characterized (Barondes, 1967), application of radioactive, immunochemical, and fluorescent labeling has demonstrated that intracellular transport is a vital process in living cells and is particularly important in neurons with elongate axonal and dendritic processes. Along these neurites macromolecules and particulates such as vesicles, lysosomes, and mitochondria are conveyed at a fairly uniform rate of ca 400 mm per day (5–7 μm per second). This presents a graphic illustration of *molecular circuitry*, that is, molecular traffic plying in both directions, anterograde and retrograde, within neurites and across synaptic junctions. The course of transport may lead from axonal terminals to the cell body and dendritic tips or in the reverse direction; or there may be local molecular transport circuits or loops, for example from an axonal terminal to the somatic center and back to a synaptic terminal (see Figure 6).

Direct microscopic observations of fast transport have been made in living nerve axons (Cooper and Smith, 1974; Smith and Koles, 1976; Forman, Padjen, and Siggins, 1977a,b; Hammond and Smith, 1977). In these studies particles and organelles were observed to move in a saltatory manner in both directions. The saltatory aspect of the direction-oriented movement of the vesicles puts constraints on possible theories of transport mechanisms.

Anterograde and retrograde transport convey trophic substances transsynaptically to and from innervated tissue. They also inform the soma of conditions such as injury at the axon periphery and elicit appropriate reparative (chromatolytic) action by the cell center. Retrograde transport has been demon-

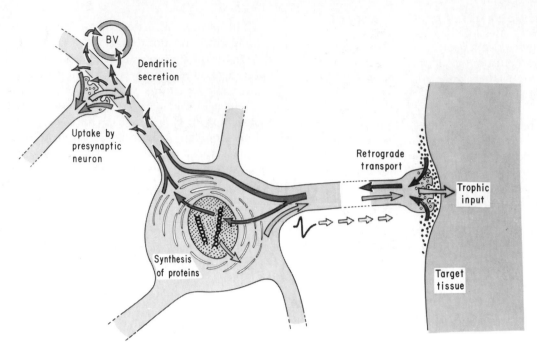

FIGURE 6 Bidirectional transport within neurites and transsynaptically between adjacent neurons and target cells. The effect of transported substances on gene expression and, by release from dendrites, upon the neuronal environment, including blood vessels (BV), is also indicated.

strated for an ever increasing list of substances including acetylcholine esterase, dyes, horseradish peroxidase, tetanus toxin, and sundry other proteins and viruses (herpes simplex, polio).

Labeled amino acids injected into the neuronal soma are incorporated into proteins that are transported to the tips of the largest dendritic trees in 15 to 30 minutes (Schubert and Kreutzberg, 1975). Certain solutes, such as adenosine, are released from dendrites into intercellular space and hence into blood vessels and may be absorbed by adjacent neurons and glia in which they aid in the biodynamic stimulation of metabolism. This constitutes a new idiom in neurobiology: the chemical integration of neurons in local areas through release of neuroactive substances from dendrites and their absorption into neighboring neurons and glia (Kreutzberg, this volume; Smith and Kreutzberg, 1976).

Retrograde transport of labeled precursors is being widely used to replace more tedious degeneration techniques for tracing neuronal circuits. These studies, together with immunochemical and Falck-Hillarp fluorescence techniques, have revealed neuronal circuits not previously mapped. This is thought by many neurophysiologists and neuroanatomists to be one of the greatest advances in neuroscience in recent years, and as techniques are further improved, neuronal circuitology will become a central theme of neuro-

science. It is hoped that the technique will also illuminate the structural logic underlying neuronal local circuits and neuronal assemblies such as columns and minicolumns.

Retrograde transport of nerve growth factor to the perikaryon is discussed by Thoenen (this volume) as a mechanism whereby effector target tissue, such as muscle, may influence the expression of genetic information within innervating neurons. It has also been shown by Schwab and Thoenen (1976, 1977) that tetanus toxin and its detoxified scission product may be transported retrogradely to neuronal cell centers and, very significantly from the therapeutic standpoint, that substances of therapeutic value such as antiviral agents may, by conjugation to a tetanus toxin fragment, be dispatched by fast transport to the cell center, where therapeutic results may be achieved that are possible by no other route of administration (Bizzini, Stoeckel, and Schwab, 1977). This constitutes an important application of advanced techniques of neurochemical circuitry.

Another local chemical circuit is the transfer of compounds of molecular weight up to about 1,000 daltons through electrotonic junctions. This process has been studied in crayfish lateral giant axons (Hermann et al., 1975) and in Retzius cells of the leech (Rieske, Schubert, and Kreutzberg, 1975).

Regulation of gene expression in the nervous system

Only a decade ago, little was known about the mechanisms of gene expression as it occurs specifically in neurons. In his excellent review of gene expression in the nervous system, Ebert (1968) could find little relevant data except in relation to differentiation of the nervous system during development. This situation has changed strikingly in the last few years. There is now a rapidly growing list of instances in which the molecular stimulus for gene expression is transmitted to the genome via dendrites or from innervated target tissue via transsynaptic and retrograde axonal transport. This subject, which is of central interest in neurobiology, was included in the biochemical circuit portion of this ISP because the vectors that evoke genetic expression in the neuronal genome can be identified and the route of transport is known; it is thus another example of a biochemical local circuit.

Transmitters delivered synaptically to a dendrite may have both an electrogenic effect (depolarization or hyperpolarization) on the target cell and also a metabolic effect, the latter being under certain conditions more significant than the former (Bloom, 1975). Thus an acetylcholine input to an adrenergic neuron may induce the synthesis of tyrosine hydroxylase, an enzyme necessary for the synthesis of norepinephrine, the transmitter utilized by the target cell (Axelrod, 1974).

The transsynaptic regulation of the synthesis of specific neuronal enzymes by electrical stimulation and by trophic interaction between neurons and target tissue is lucidly articulated by Thoenen (this volume), using the peripheral sympathetic nervous system as a model system. Nerve growth factor (NGF) proves to be a macromolecular mediator between effector cells and innervating neurons; retrograde axonal transport of NGF produces an effect on the synthesis of macromolecules which suggests that NGF may play a significant regulatory role.

Data are beginning to appear concerning the cellular mechanism by which transmitters influence enzyme synthesis. For example, L-dopa decreases protein synthesis by disaggregating polyribosomes in brain cells (Wurtman, this volume).

Hormones also stimulate gene expression in neurons, as indicated by the striking effects of sex hormones on both behavior and brain structure (Gorski, this volume).

From the evidence cited in this section, it is clear that the fast bidirectional transport of substances in neurites is not an experimental curiosity or epiphenomenon but rather a vital communication circuit by which the neuron is informed of the nature of its environment and can, to some extent, control its environment by release of appropriate substances. This communication system may mediate the neurohumoral signaling and regulation that are part of the integrative operations of the central nervous system.

Modulatory and transmitter action of locally released neuroactive substances: A model for local circuit chemical interaction That transmitters at chemical synapses might have functions other than electrogenic has been suggested succinctly by Bloom (1974, 1975). McMahon (1974) presented cogent evidence to support the view that, ontogenetically and phylogenetically, transmitters act as neural hormones prior to manifesting electrogenic functions.

An example of a modulatory transmitter is purinergic neuroactive material such as adenosine, which, in addition to altering the electrotonic length constant of neurites, profoundly influences metabolic reactions (Kreutzberg, this volume).

Another class of modulator substances is represented by the prostaglandins (Samuelsson, this volume). Yet another nonelectrogenic role of bona fide transmitters such as glycine, glutamic acid, and GABA is that of informing the cell center of conditions prevailing at the axon terminal by means of retrograde transport of signaling substances (Cuénod, this volume).

Figure 7 illustrates the fact that a modulatory transmitter (here norepinephrine) may be delivered to the neuron via a conventional synapse (in addition to inputs from conventional ionogenic transmitters, here illustrated by acetylcholine) or by diffusion after release from varicosities in the thin axons of adjacent central-core regulatory neurons.

The situation has been made more complicated and exciting by the discovery of a whole new family of "transmitters" in the form of neuroactive peptides, which appear to have endocrine or paracrine as well as neurotransmitter function. More than a dozen such neuropeptides are listed and characterized by Vale (this volume), and the list continues to grow. Another category of peptides constitutes the brain's major opioids, that is, "endogenous morphinelike substances"; these are discussed by Snyder (this volume). Whether these new neuroactive peptides qualify as transmitters under the conventional concept of the chemical synapse or whether their function warrants new functional categories will probably emerge from current research (Iversen, this volume).

One of the characteristics of the chemical synapse is that the transmitter released from the presynaptic terminal activates only the postsynaptic member of that particular synapse. This purpose is furthered by

MODULATION

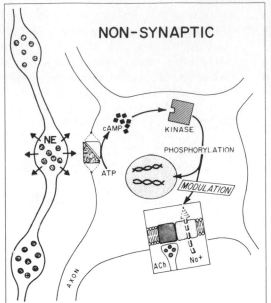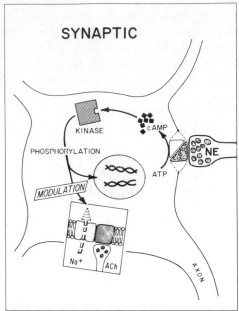

FIGURE 7 To illustrate the postulated modulatory action of a transmitter, here shown as norepinephrine (NE), which is introduced into the target cell via a conventional synapse (right) or by diffusion after hypothesized release from varicosity-borne vesicles in the thin axons of an adjacent central-core regulatory neuron (left). An electrogenic excitatory transmitter, acetylcholine (ACh), is shown as being introduced at a conventional synapse and is coupled to channel ionophores in the postsynaptic membrane. The hypothesized modulator transmitter, norepinephrine, is pictured as acting within membrane-borne receptors by entrainment in a cyclic nucleotide circuit that mediates the sometimes long-lasting modulatory effects.

the presence of hydrolytic enzymes that inactivate transmitter molecules left in the synaptic cleft, thus preventing their diffusion to other synapses, and by the active uptake of transmitter by the presynaptic terminal. This one-to-one relationship is not characteristic of neurons of the reticular formation that have central-core regulatory function.

Early findings in this very active field indicate that in systems such as the locus coeruleus (Bloom, 1974, 1975, 1976; Bloom, Hoffer, and Siggins, 1971; Moore and Bloom, 1978; Descarries, Beaudet, and Watkins, 1975; Beaudet and Descarries, 1976; Leger and Descarries, 1978) and the raphe nucleus (Chan-Palay, 1976, 1977), vesicle-containing varicosities stud the length of the frequently bifurcating 0.1-μm-thick C-fiber axons on their way to many parts of the brain. From the morphology it is believed by some that transmitters such as norepinephrine and serotonin, possibly acting as modulators, may be released from varicosities into intercellular space where, by diffusion, they bind to receptors on target neurons (see Figure 7, left side). Others (F. E. Bloom, for example) feel that such a process has yet to be proved by direct experimental evidence.

It has also been shown that transmitters can be released from dendrites, as was suggested by the work of Schubert and Kreutzberg (1975). Iversen (this volume) describes the evidence for this in the case of the release of dopamine from the dendrites of the substantia nigra; he uses nigral neurons as a model for the complex transmitter interactions that are known to exist in the neuropil of this brain region and that may be widespread in the CNS. Unlike the case of locus coeruleus and raphe axons, there appear to be no morphologically specialized synapses, varicosities, or even vesicles in the case of dendritic release in the substantia nigra. The transmitter is apparently stored in cisterns of the smooth endoplasmic reticulum; no exocytotic process is apparent.

The exciting conclusion that emerges from this new chapter of neuroscience is that the parenchyma over vast regions of the mammalian brain are "innervated" by very thin neurites emanating not from just one ("sympathetic"-type) class but from several classes of axons utilizing norepinephrine, serotonin, and (in some regions) oligopeptides as transmitters. Do all classes of "brain-innervating" neurons function side by side? And do yet other classes of neurons exist which release still undiscovered classes of neuroactive agents? Revolutionary new concepts of biochemical and physiological circuitry are being proposed on the basis of the newly discovered phenomena, concepts that must now be subjected to critical appraisal.

Paths to the future: The coming attack on higher brain function

This ISP was designed to present and evaluate new information about several areas of high priority in neuroscience. These include the functional anatomy of the brain, particularly the cerebral cortex; the properties of neuronal local circuits and of local integrative processes at several levels of complexity; the biophysics of information processing by graded electrotonic currents and fields; and new concepts of structural, bioelectric, and biochemical circuitry. It was hoped that on the basis of this information a realistic assessment might be made of the feasibility of constructing heuristic models of higher brain function at this time.

It became clear that the new information does indeed permit us to develop a new dynamic picture of brain functioning. It also clearly identifies an area that requires concentrated attack, namely the nature of the neuronal functional units or assemblies that are packed orthogonally in the cortex, the local circuitry within and between these functional units, and, very importantly, the connections between the functional units and subcortical structures. The difficulty is not due to sheer anatomical complexity alone but also to lack of recording techniques adequate to deal with the dynamics involved; a technical breakthrough comparable to the development of electronic techniques in the 1920s and of unit cell recording in the postwar period might permit the unraveling and defining of the dynamic circuitry involved. Here again the call goes out for a multidisciplinary attack; the challenge is as great as the one that unified the disparate areas of neurobiology into a unified discipline called neuroscience in the 1960s.

One of the ISP planners, Gerald Edelman, had for several years been considering basic problems of neurobiology from the viewpoint of selectional (as opposed to instructional) theory, which is the cornerstone of the theoretical edifice of modern immunology. A fairly elaborate, self-consistent theory began to crystallize in his mind during the spring months when the final program of the ISP was being hammered out. A basic assumption of Edelman's hypothesis was that the genetically determined func-

tional repertoire for the processing of memory, learning, perception, and consciousness (functionally analogous to but not homologous with the nucleotide codons of genetic theory) consists of cell assemblies that each contain 10^2 to 10^4 cells. This description agreed remarkably with that of the columnar units that Mountcastle, in his keynote lecture, characterized as the processing and the distributing units of the cerebral cortex. The similarity between Edelman's hypothetical repertoires and the cortical units depicted by Mountcastle, and the central role of neuronal local circuits in the functioning of cortical columns and minicolumns, suggested that a presentation of Edelman's hypothesis might be a fitting way to finish the ISP and, through the published proceedings of the ISP, to form a bridge to the next stage of neuroscience, the development of heuristic theories of higher brain function. (The papers by Edelman and Mountcastle have been published as a book entitled *The Mindful Brain,* Cambridge, MA: MIT Press, 1978.)

Edelman's hypothesis is rigidly selectionistic. The repertoires of cell assemblies are genetically determined, and incoming sensory signals play no instructional role in forming the basic anatomical connections that make up the primary and secondary repertoires.

In Edelman's scheme the intrinsic and extrinsic neuronal circuitry within the unitary neuronal local circuit assemblies and the circuitry connecting them to sensory, motor, and subcortical structures are also genetically and ontogenetically specified. The repertoire of neuronal groups, columns, or modules is present in large numbers (on the order of 600 million minicolumns comprising some 50 billion neurons), permitting matching of repertoire groups to sensory signals in a degenerate manner, that is, with more than one way by which the repertoire can recognize given input signals. The concept of degeneracy thus differs from redundancy, which characterizes identical structures.

Edelman sees "recognition" of unitary groups as being brought about by electrical, ultrastructural, and connectionistic action, and it is precise. Multiple signaling to primary repertoire groups leads to associative recognition and to the formation of a secondary repertoire of neuronal groups having a higher likelihood of response than the cell groups of the primary repertoire.

The concept of reentry is a critical one in the model. Because of the degenerate nature of the proposed selectional process, the absence of reentry would lead to a failure of continuity in the system as well as a failure to form coordinated abstract representations of external signals. In other words, reentry guarantees continuity in a distributed selectional system. Consciousness may be a kind of associative recollective updating by reentrant inputs that continually confirms or alters the theory of the self by parallel sensory or motor inputs and outputs.

One gauge of the heuristic value of a scientific theory, particularly one dealing with so complex a problem as that of higher brain function, is the number and clarity of the predictions suggested by the theory that can be used as a guide for future observations. Edelman has outlined some predictions and consequences suggested by his hypothesis; these include the following: The positions and interactions of single synapses are not determined by complementary interactions of surface protein molecules specific for each synapse, and no sizable precommitted molecular repertoire will probably be found to explain cell-cell interaction in neurodevelopment. Nor will a system having a substantial degree of plasticity be found to function as a pontifical neuron or single-neuron "decision unit." Neither molecules nor single neurons but groups of neurons, possibly of the kind now being identified as functional unit assemblies or modular units in the cerebral cortex, will prove to be the main units of selection in higher brain function. Such neuronal repertoire groups are multiply represented in a degenerate, isofunctionally overlapping manner. Neuronal local circuits and interconnecting axonal interconnections with extensive divergence facilitate the postulated degenerate relationship. However, multiple inputs from recognizer neurons are thought to converge on higher-level "recognizer-of-recognizer" neuronal groups; abstract cell-group codes are thus formed.

The notion of phased reentrant signaling on degenerate neuronal groups, the reentrance period being of the order of 0.1 second, agrees with many of the observational data obtained in studies of cognitive phenomena. Edelman suggests that correlations with such plasticity will probably be found in cortical, thalamocortical, and limbic-reticular signaling.

The degree to which these predictions are supported by future observations will provide a measure of the worth and usefulness of the hypothesis.

Our concepts of cortical organization and function have been revolutionized during the last two decades. On the basis of these new ideas and of the characterization of circuitry—structural, electrical, and chemical—considered in detail in the 1977 ISP and described in these proceedings, two general conclusions

seem justified. First, relevant data are at hand that warrant a broad attack on the problem of higher brain function utilizing all of the armamentarium of general neuroscience. Second, the most important target for concentrated attack is the structure and function of the cerebral cortex.

REFERENCES

ADEY, W. R., 1961. Brain mechanisms and the learning process. *Fed. Proc.* 20:617–627.

ADEY, W. R., 1969. Slow electrical phenomena in the central nervous system. *Neurosci. Res. Program Bull.* 7:75–180.

ADEY, W. R., R. T. KADO, and J. DIDIO, 1962. Impedance measurements in brain tissue of animals using microvolt signals. *Exp. Neurol.* 5:47–66.

ADEY, W. R., D. O. WALTER, and C. E. HENDRIX, 1961. Computer techniques in correlation and spectral analyses of cerebral slow waves during discriminative behavior. *Exp. Neurol.* 3:501–524.

AXELROD, J., 1974. Regulation of the neurotransmitter norepinephrine. In *The Neurosciences: Third Study Program*, F. O. Schmitt and F. G. Worden, eds. Cambridge, MA: MIT Press, pp. 863–876.

BARONDES, S. H., 1967. Axoplasmic transport. *Neurosci. Res. Program Bull.* 5:307–419.

BEAUDET, A., and L. DESCARRIES, 1976. Quantitative data on serotonin nerve terminals in adult rat neocortex. *Brain Res.* 111:301–309.

BENNETT, M. V. L., 1968. Similarities between chemically and electrically mediated transmission. In *Physiological and Biochemical Aspects of Nervous Integration*, F. P. Carlson, ed. Englewood Cliffs, N.J.: Prentice-Hall, pp. 73–128.

BENNETT, M. V. L., 1974. Flexibility and rigidity in electrotonically coupled systems. In *Synaptic Transmission and Neuronal Interactions*, M. V. L. Bennett, ed. New York: Raven Press, pp. 153–178.

BENNETT, M. V. L., and D. GOODENOUGH, 1978. Gap junctions. *Neurosci. Res. Program Bull.* 16:373–486.

BISHOP, G. H., 1956. Natural history of the nerve impulse. *Physiol. Rev.* 36:376–399.

BIZZINI, B., K. STOECKEL, and M. SCHWAB, 1977. An antigenic polypeptide fragment isolated from tetanus toxin: Chemical characterization, binding to gangliosides and retrograde axonal transport in various neuron systems. *J. Neurochem.* 28:529–542.

BLOOM, F. E., 1974. Dynamics of synaptic modulation: Perspectives for the future. In *The Neurosciences: Third Study Program*, F. O. Schmitt and F. G. Worden, eds. Cambridge, Mass.: MIT Press, pp. 989–999.

BLOOM, F. E., 1975. The role of cyclic nucleotides in central synaptic function. *Rev. Physiol. Biochem. Pharmacol.* 74:1–103.

BLOOM, F. E., 1976. Neuroanatomical network in relation to transmitter systems. *Proc. Neurological Symposium, Miami, Florida.*

BLOOM, F. E., B. J. HOFFER, and G. R. SIGGINS, 1971. Studies on norepinephrine containing afferents to Purkinje cells of rat cerebellum. I. Localization of the fibers and their synapses. *Brain Res.* 25:501–521.

BULLOCK, T. H., 1959. Neuron doctrine and electrophysiology. *Science* 129:997–1002.

CASPAR, D. L. D., D. A. GOODENOUGH, L. MAKOWSKI, and W. C. PHILLIPS, 1977. Gap junction structures. I. Correlated electron microscopy and x-ray diffraction. *J. Cell Biol.* 74:605–628.

CHAN-PALAY, V., 1976. Serotonin axons in the supra- and subependymal plexuses and in the leptomeninges; their roles in local alterations of cerebrospinal fluid and vasomotor activity. *Brain Res.* 102:103–130.

CHAN-PALAY, V., 1977. *Cerebellar Dentate Nucleus.* Berlin-Heidelberg-New York: Springer-Verlag.

COOPER, P. D., and R. S. SMITH, 1974. The movement of optically detectable organelles in myelinated axons of *Xenopus laevis. J. Physiol.* 242:77–97.

DALY, J., 1977. *Cyclic Nucleotides in the Nervous System.* New York: Plenum Press.

DESCARRIES, L., A. BEAUDET, and K. C. WATKINS, 1975. Serotonin nerve terminals in adult rat neocortex. *Brain Res.* 100:563–588.

EBERT, J. D., 1968. Gene expression. *Neurosci. Res. Program Bull.* 3:109–189.

FLEISCHHAUER, K., and K. DETZER, 1975. Dendritic bundling in the cerebral cortex. In *Physiology and Pathology of Dendrites* (Advances in Neurology, Vol. 12), G. W. Kreutzberg, ed. New York: Raven Press, pp. 71–77.

FORMAN, D. S., A. L. PADJEN, and G. R. SIGGINS, 1977a. Axonal transport of organelles visualized by light microscopy, cinemicrographic and computer analysis. *Brain Res.* 136:197–213.

FORMAN, D. S., A. L. PADJEN, and G. R. SIGGINS, 1977b. Effect of temperature on the rapid retrograde transport of microscopically visible intra-axonal organelles. *Brain Res.* 136:215–226.

GOLDBERG, N. D., 1975. Cyclic nucleotides and cell function. In *Cell Membranes,* G. Weissmann, and R. Claireborne, eds. New York: HP Publishing Co., pp. 185–201.

HAKEN, H., 1977a. *Synergetics: An Introduction.* Berlin-Heidelberg-New York: Springer-Verlag.

HAKEN, H., 1977b. *Synergetics: A Workshop.* Berlin-Heidelberg-New York: Springer-Verlag.

HAMMOND, G. R., and R. S. SMITH, 1977. Inhibition of the rapid movement of optically detectable axonal particles by colchicine and vinblastine. *Brain Res.* 128:227–242.

HERMANN, A., E. RIESKE, G. KREUTZBERG, and H. D. LUX, 1975. Transjunctional flux of radioactive precursors across electrotonic synapses between lateral giant axons of the crayfish. *Brain Res.* 95:125–131.

HUBEL, D. H., and T. N. WIESEL, 1977. *Ferrier Lecture:* Functional architecture of macaque monkey visual cortex. *Proc. R. Soc. B* 198:1–59.

JACOBSON, M., 1970. *Developmental Neurobiology.* New York: Holt, Rinehart and Winston.

JACOBSON, M., 1975. Development and evolution of type II neurons; conjectures and century after Golgi. In *Golgi Centennial Symposium: Perspectives in Neurobiology,* M. Santini, ed. New York: Raven Press, pp. 147–151.

KATCHALSKY, A. K., V. ROWLAND, and R. BLUMENTHAL, 1974. Dynamic patterns of brain cell assemblies. *Neurosci. Res. Program Bull.* 12:1–187.

KREUTZBERG, G. W., ed., 1975. *Physiology and Pathology of Dendrites* (Advances in Neurology, Vol. 12). New York: Raven Press.

KREUTZBERG, G. W., and P. SCHUBERT, 1975. The cellular dynamics of intraneuronal transport. In *The Use of Axonal Transport for Studies of Neuronal Connectivity.* W. M. Cowan and M. Cuénod, eds. Amsterdam-New York: Elsevier Scientific Publishing Company, pp. 83–112.

KREUTZBERG, G. W., P. SCHUBERT, and H. D. LUX, 1975. Neuroplasmic transport in axons and dendrites. In *Golgi Centennial Symposium: Perspectives in Neurobiology,* M. Santini, ed. New York: Raven Press, pp. 161–166.

KREUTZBERG, G. W., P. SCHUBERT, L. TÓTH, and E. RIESKE, 1973. Intradendritic transport to postsynaptic sites. *Brain Res.* 62:399–404.

LEGER, L., and L. DESCARRIES, 1978. Serotonin nerve terminals in the locus coeruleus of adult rat: A radioautographic study. *Brain Res.* (in press).

LLINÁS, R. R., and J. E. HEUSER, 1977. Depolarization-release coupling systems in neurons. *Neurosci. Res. Program Bull.* 15:557–687.

McMAHON, D., 1974. Chemical messengers in development: A hypothesis. *Science* 185:1012–1021.

MAKOWSKI, L., D. L. D. CASPAR, W. C. PHILLIPS, and D. A. GOODENOUGH, 1977. Gap junction structures. II. Analysis of the x-ray diffraction data. *J. Cell Biol.* 74:629–645.

MOORE, R. Y., and F. E. BLOOM, 1978. Central catecholamine neuron systems: Anatomy and physiology of the dopamine systems. *Ann. Rev. Neurosci.* 1:129–169.

OCHS, S., 1972. Fast axoplasmic transport of materials in mammalian nerve and its integrative role. *Ann. NY Acad. Sci.* 193:43–58.

OCHS, S., 1974. Trophic functions of the neuron. 3. Mechanisms of neurotrophic interactions. Systems of material transport in nerve fibers (axoplasmic transport) related to nerve function and trophic control. *Ann. NY Acad. Sci.* 228:202–223.

PEARSON, K. G., 1976. Nerve cells without action potentials. In *Simpler Networks and Behavior,* J. C. Fentress, ed. Sunderland, Mass.: Sinauer Associates, pp. 99–110.

PEARSON, K. G., and C. R. FOURTNER, 1975. Nonspiking interneurons in the walking system of the cockroach. *J. Neurophysiol.* 38:33–52.

PICKEL, V. M., M. SEGAL, and F. E. BLOOM, 1974. A radioautographic study of the efferent pathways of the nucleus locus coeruleus. *J. Comp. Neurol.* 155:15–42.

RAKIC, P., 1975. Local circuit neurons. *Neurosci. Res. Program Bull.* 13:291–446 (available as a separate hardcover book from MIT Press, Cambridge, MA).

RALL, W., 1970. Dendritic neuron theory and dendrodendritic synapses in a simple cortical system. In *The Neurosciences: Second Study Program,* F. O. Schmitt, Editor-in-Chief. New York: Rockefeller University Press, pp. 552–565.

RALL, W., and G. M. SHEPHERD, 1968. Theoretical reconstruction of field potentials and dendrodendritic synaptic interactions in olfactory bulb. *J. Neurophysiol.* 31:884–915.

RIESKE, E., P. SCHUBERT, and G. W. KREUTZBERG, 1975. Transfer of radioactive material between electrically coupled neurons of the leech central nervous system. *Brain Res.* 84:365–382.

ROCKEL, A. J., R. W. HIORNS, and T. P. S. POWELL, 1974. Numbers of neurons through full depth of neocortex. *Proc. Anat. Soc. Gr. Br. Ir.* 118:371.

SCHEIBEL, M. E., and A. B. SCHEIBEL, 1970. Organization of spinal motoneuron dendrites in bundles. *Exp. Neurol.* 28:106–112.

SCHMITT, F. O., 1968. Fibrous proteins, neuronal organelles. *Proc. Natl. Acad. Sci. USA* 60:38–47.

SCHMITT, F. O., P. DEV, and B. H. SMITH, 1976. Electrotonic processing of information by brain cells. *Science* 193:114–120.

SCHMITT, F. O., and F. E. SAMSON, 1968. Neuronal fibrous proteins. *Neurosci. Res. Program Bull.* 6:113–219.

SCHMITT, F. O., D. M. SCHNEIDER, and D. M. CROTHERS, eds., 1975. *Functional Linkage in Biomolecular Systems.* New York: Raven Press.

SCHUBERT, P., and G. W. KREUTZBERG, 1975. Dendritic and axonal transport of nucleoside derivatives in single motoneurons and release from dendrites. *Brain Res.* 90:319–323.

SCHWAB, M. E., and H. THOENEN, 1976. Electron microscopic evidence for a transsynaptic migration of tetanus toxin in spinal cord motoneurons: An autoradiographic and morphometric study. *Brain Res.* 105:213–227.

SCHWAB, M., and H. THOENEN, 1977. Selective transsynaptic migration of tetanus toxin after retrograde axonal transport in peripheral sympathetic nerves: A comparison with nerve growth factor. *Brain Res.* 122:459–474.

SCHWARZ, G., 1978. Chemical transition of biopolymers induced by an electrical field and their effects in dielectrics and birefringence. *Ann. NY Acad. Sci.* (in press).

SCHWARZ, G., and U. SCHRADER, 1975. The effects of cooperativity, finite change length, and field-induced changes of the conformational equilibrium on the electric birefringence of polypeptides in the range of the helix-coil transition. *Biopolymers* 14:1181–1195.

SCHWARZ., G., and J. SEELIG, 1968. Kinetic properties and electric field effect of the helix-coil transition of poly (γbenzyl L-glutamate) determined from dielectric relaxation measurements. *Biopolymers* 6:1263–1277.

SËITE, R., J. ESCAIG, and S. COUINEAU, 1971. Microfilaments et microtubules nucleaires et organisation ultrastructurale des batonnets intranucleaires des neurones sympathiques. *J. Ultrastruct. Res.* 37:449–478.

SËITE, R., J. LEONETTI, J. LUCIANI-VUILLET, and M. VIO, 1977. Cyclic AMP and ultrastructural organization of the nerve cell nucleus: Stimulation of nuclear microtubules and microfilaments assembly in sympathetic neurons. *Brain Res.* 124:41–51.

SHAW, S. R., 1972. Decremental conduction of the visual signal in barnacle lateral eye. *J. Physiol.* 220:145–175.

SHEPHERD, G. M., 1970. The olfactory bulb as a simple cortical system: Experimental analysis and functional implications. In *The Neurosciences: Second Study Program*, F. O. Schmitt, editor-in-chief. New York: Rockefeller University Press, pp. 539–551.

SHEPHERD, G. M., 1974. *The Synaptic Organization of the Brain.* New York: Oxford University Press.

SHEPHERD, G. M., 1978. Microcircuits in the nervous system. *Sci. Am.* 238:93–103.

SMITH, B. H., and G. W. KREUTZBERG, 1976. Neuron-target cell interactions. *Neurosci. Res. Program Bull.* 14:211–453.

SMITH, R. S., and Z. J. KOLES, 1976. Mean velocity of optically detected intraaxonal particles measured by a cross-correlation method. *Can. J. Physiol. Pharmacol.* 54:859–869.

SOTELO, C., 1975. Morphological correlates of electrotonic coupling between neurons in mammalian nervous system. In *Golgi Centennial Symposium: Perspectives in Neurobiology*, M. Santini, ed. New York: Raven Press, pp. 355–365.

WEISS, P., and H. B. HISCOE, 1948. Experiments on the mechanism of nerve growth. *J. Exp. Zool.* 107:315–395.

2 An Organizing Principle for Cerebral Function: The Unit Module and the Distributed System

VERNON B. MOUNTCASTLE

Introduction

THERE CAN BE little doubt of the dominating influence of the Darwinian revolution of the mid-nineteenth century upon concepts of the structure and function of the nervous system. The ideas of Spencer and Jackson and Sherrington and the many who followed them were rooted in the evolutionary theory that the brain develops in phylogeny by the successive addition of more cephalad parts. On this theory each new addition or enlargement was accompanied by the elaboration of more complex behavior and, at the same time, imposed a regulation upon more caudal and primitive parts and the presumably more primitive behavior they control. Dissolution of this hierarchy is thought to be revealed by disease or lesions of the brain in humans and by lesions or truncation of the neuraxis in experimental animals. The importance of these ideas can scarcely be exaggerated; for nearly a century they dominated the theory and practice of brain research, and experiments based on them yielded much of our present knowledge of the nervous system. They retained vigor and influence into the 1950s and still form a base for further advance in many fields of neuroscience.

Developments of recent decades require new formulations that include but transcend the hierarchical principle of brain organization. Prominent among them is the concept that the brain is a complex of widely and reciprocally interconnected systems and that the dynamic interplay of neural activity within and between these systems is the very essence of brain function. The large entities of advanced brains and their gross and microscopic inter- and intrasystem connections have developed in phylogeny in accord, it is thought, with evolutionary principles. They are determined genetically, but at the level of ultrastructure and of molecular events they are to some extent modifiable by postnatal experience. These entities are so widely, reciprocally, divergently, and convergently (but specifically) interconnected, and the ongoing activity within the systems they compose is so pervasive and continuous, that—particularly as regards the cerebral hemispheres—the hierarchical principle expressed by such antonyms as higher–lower or newer–older loses some of its heuristic value.

I present below a set of ideas that in sum compose an organizing principle or paradigm for cerebral function. It builds upon knowledge gained from experiments based upon evolutionary theory and its hierarchical principle, and it also includes the concept of the brain as a dynamic information-processing machine. More subtle and complex aspects of behavior are generally thought of as initiated and controlled by "higher" levels of the neuraxis: particularly perceiving, remembering, thinking, calculating, formulating plans for current and future action, and consciousness itself. I regard them as depending upon—that is, as the internally experienced and sometimes externally observable behavioral events produced by—the ensemble actions of large populations of neurons of the forebrain, organized into complex interacting systems. No external influences incompatible with the presently known laws of thermodynamics are imagined to exist. The principle is thus exactly consonant with that of Psychoneural Identity and exactly opposed to that of Cartesian

VERNON B. MOUNTCASTLE   Department of Physiology, The Johns Hopkins University School of Medicine, Baltimore, MD 21205

Dualism, whether in its original or its more recent formulations.

The general idea is as follows. The large entities of the brain we know as areas (or nuclei) of the neocortex, the limbic lobe, basal ganglia, dorsal thalamus, and so forth, are themselves composed of replicated *local neural circuits,* modules which vary in cell number, intrinsic connections, and processing mode from one large entity to another but are basically similar within any given entity (Szentágothai and Arbib, 1974; Szentágothai, 1975). Each module is a local neural circuit that processes information from its input to its output and in that processing imposes transforms determined by the general properties of the entity and its extrinsic connections. Modules are grouped into entities such as nuclei or cortical areas by a common or dominating extrinsic connection, by the need to replicate a function over a topographic representation, or by some other factor. The set of modules composing an entity may itself be fractionated into subsets by different linkages to similarly segregated subsets in other large entities. Closely linked and multiply interconnected subsets of modules in different and often widely separated entities thus form precisely connected but distributed systems. The preservation of neighborhood relations between the interconnected subsets of topographically organized entities results in nested distributed systems. *Such a distributed system is conceived to serve a distributed function.* A single module of an entity may be a member of several (but not many) such systems. Only in the limiting case might all the modules of an entity have identical connections.

I wish to explore these ideas, particularly as regards the neocortex, and the general proposition that the processing function of neocortical modules is qualitatively similar in all neocortical regions. Put shortly, there is nothing intrinsically motor about the motor cortex, nor sensory about the sensory cortex. Thus the elucidation of the mode of operation of the local modular circuit anywhere in the neocortex will be of great generalizing significance. This idea is unrelated to the equipotentiality concept of Lashley (1949).

I shall start with a brief résumé of what is known of the phylogenetic and ontogenetic development of the neocortex and its cytoarchitecture, facts which I believe are consonant with the general hypothesis.

Phylogenetic development of the neocortex

The avalanching enlargement of the neocortex is a major aspect of mammalian evolution and, in its degree, distinguishes primates from other mammals and man from other primates. A major goal of comparative neurology is to reconstruct the evolutionary development of man's brain by measuring both the endocranial casts of fossils and the brains of living primates and their putative insectivore ancestors (Jerison, 1973). Brain measurements in living primates are valuable for such a reconstruction largely by retrospective inference, for a salient feature of primate evolution is its parallel and radiating nature (Washburn and Harding, 1970; Hodos, 1970). For example, the living primates readily available for neurological research in significant numbers, the new and the old world monkeys, diverged from the line leading to man (and from each other) more than 30 million years ago. However, detailed measurements of the total brain and of the relative sizes of different brain parts in insectivores, prosimians, and simians do provide an ordinal ranking of species in terms of brain development, and the degree of brain development provides the best available correlation with the evolutionary level of achievement. Moreover, the careful measurements of Stephan and his colleagues (Stephan, 1967, 1969, 1972; Stephan and Andy, 1964, 1969; Stephan, Bauchot, and Andy, 1970) in more than sixty species have revealed that, of all cerebral parts, it is the absolute and relative development of the neocortex that correlates best with evolutionary achievement.

The living basal insectivores are thought to have evolved very little from their ancestors, from which man's line also arose. Stephan has used this idea to establish an index of the evolutionary development of a brain structure as the ratio of its observed volume to that expected in a basal insectivore of the same body weight. The progression index for neocortex is 156 for man, 60 for chimpanzee, and 40 for Cercopithecidae. Some unusual ratios occasionally occur when such an allometric method is used; for example, the high rank of miopithecus is thought to be due to secondary body dwarfing, while the low rank of the gorilla may be due to body gigantism. These aberrations disappear when the volume of the neocortex is related to the area of the foramen magnum (Radinsky, 1967) or to the volume of the medulla (Sacher, 1970). The degree of differential development of the neocortex in man is emphasized by the progression indices for different brain parts: neocortex, 156; striatum, 17; hippocampus, 4; cerebellum, 5; dorsal thalamus, 5; basal olfactory structures and olfactory bulb, 1 or less.

The progressive development of neocortex in primates is not uniform over its entire extent. For example, although the striate area is strongly progressive in prosimians, it is much less so in simians and especially in man, where it is reduced relative to overall neocortex. The striate area is not well defined in insectivores, and for this reason Stephan (1969) used the lepilemur as a base against which to measure the progression of this region, for this prosimian possesses the smallest clearly defined striate area. On this basis, the progression index for the striate area in man is less than one-fourth that of the neocortex as a whole. If the relative development of other sensory cortical areas is similar, one may infer that the progression index for the eulaminate homotypical cortex is even higher than the figure of 156 given for the total neocortex in man.

The enlargement of the neocortex in primates has been accomplished by a great expansion of its surface area, without striking changes in vertical organization. Indeed, Powell and his colleagues have shown that the number of neurons in a vertical line across the thickness of the cortex—that is, in a 30μm $\times$ 25μm cylinder—is remarkably constant at about 110 (Rockel, Hiorns, and Powell, 1974). The counts are virtually identical for the five areas studied in five species: the motor, somatic sensory, and frontal, parietal, and temporal homotypical cortices in the mouse, cat, rat, macaque monkey, and man. There is somewhat more than a doubling of the count in the striate cortex of most primates, for which no ready explanation is available.

Although with the one exception noted the number of cells in a small area of neocortex is invariant, the packing density does differ. The thickness of the cortex, the height of that small cylinder, varies by a factor of about three in different mammals, and there are some differences in thickness from one area to another in the same brain. It seems very likely that these differences are due to variations in the development of dendritic trees and synaptic neuropil (Bok, 1959). On the basis of electron-microscopic evidence, the ratio of the two main classes of neurons, the pyramidal and stellate cells, remains at about 2 to 1 in such diverse cytoarchitectural and functional areas as the motor, somatic sensory, and visual areas in the macaque (Sloper, 1973; Tömböl, 1974) and in the rat and cat (Gatter, Winfield, and Powell, 1977). A number of subtypes of these two major classes of cells have been described, but the appearance of new subtypes does not appear to be correlated with the evolutionary trend of neocortex, and it is unlikely that at any particular stage of mammalian evolution wholly new cell types have appeared that are unique to one brain as compared with other presumably more primitive or simpler ones.

Ontogenetic development of the neocortex

The ontogenetic development of the primate neocortex has been clarified by the work of a number of investigators using the radioactive labeling of dividing cells (for review, see Sidman, 1970) and, in the present context, particularly by the studies of Rakic in the monkey (Rakic, 1971, 1972, 1974, 1975, 1978; Sidman and Rakic, 1973). All of the cells destined for the neocortex of the macaque monkey arise from the ventricular and subventricular zones of the neural tube during the two-month period between the 45th and the 102nd day of the 165-day gestational period. Those cells destined for successively more superficial laminae arise in a regularly ordered temporal sequence: the neocortex is constructed from "inside to outside." Cells arising early, mainly from the ventricular zone, may move over their short migratory trajectories of 200 to 300 μm by extension of a process and nuclear translocation. Cells arising later apparently migrate over distances of up to 10 mm; they are guided to their final positions by moving along the surfaces of radially oriented glial cells which extend across the entire wall of the neural tube. The result is that the cortical cells are arranged in radially oriented cords or columns extending across the cortex, and it is has been suggested that the cells of such a column constitute a single clonal derivative (Meller and Tetzlaff, 1975). The special glial cells have been studied in detail by Rakic (1971, 1972) and by Schmechel and Rakic (1973). They can be identified in the monkey by the 70th day of gestation, after neuronal migration begins. They begin to decrease in number by the 120th day, two weeks after migration is complete, and thereafter show transitional forms.

From the data provided by these studies of neocortical development and an examination of a series of fetal brains (Powell and Mountcastle, 1977), it can be said that the cytoarchitectural differences characteristic of the neocortex of the newborn and the adult primate have not appeared at the time in fetal development when all the cortical cells have reached their final positions. Clear cytoarchitectural features can be recognized by E-108, a week after the generation of the last cortical cells, at the time when the fibers from the lateral geniculate nucleus are just reaching the cortex (Rakic, 1977). Area 17 has then become almost as distinct and sharply delimited as it is in the adult brain. Its boundaries lie along the banks of a calcarine sulcus whose depth has increased remarkably during the preceding 10 days. There is less marked but suggestive architectonic differentiation in other parts of the neocortex of the monkey at this stage on E-108. One example is seen between areas 3 and 4 in the walls of an incipient central sulcus. It thus appears that the intrinsic morphological differentiation of the neocortex begins immediately after the stage at which the cortical cells have reached their final position. Examination of fetal material has confirmed the finding of Rakic that at this stage of development the cells of the cortex are clearly arranged in columns.

Are cytoarchitectural differences causally related to differences in the function of different cortical areas?

Even brief inspection of serial sections reveals that there are differences in intrinsic structure between different regions of the cerebral cortex, particularly in the neocortex. The development of the field of cytoarchitectonics began with Meynert and is associated with the names of Campbell, Brodmann, Elliott Smith, von Economo, and the Vogts. Their efforts and the work of many who followed them resulted in detailed parcellations and hence maps of the cerebral cortex in a number of mammals, including man, based upon variations in the numbers and packing densities of cells of different types and sizes in homologous layers of different cortical regions. In some cases other criteria were used, such as the degree and temporal sequence of myelination of intrinsic or extrinsic nerve fibers. When pushed to the extreme by those sophisticated in its use, even minute parcellations of the cerebral cortex were thought to be valid. Some cytoarchitectonicists and neurologists of that era took the position that these morphologically identified regions were to be regarded as quasi-independent cerebral "organs," each functioning independently of its neighbors; this point of view has not been argued seriously for half a century. A period of sharp controversy followed the early years of cytoarchitectural study; the reaction against detailed parcellation was so great that some regarded all but the most obvious differences between cortical areas as subjective impressions (Lashley and Clark, 1946; Bonin and Bailey, 1947).

These old controversies now seem to be settled. There is general agreement that structural differences do exist between major regions of neocortex and that these differences can be defined objectively. They are a regular feature of the neocortex of any given species, and the areas so specified can be homologized over a series of mammals. Equally certain is the fact that cytoarchitecturally different cortical regions subserve different functions, where the term "function" takes its ordinary and usual sense (for example, the control of movement or the primary processing of a sensory input). That at least is the conclusion one must draw from nearly a century of study of the effects produced by electrical stimulation of the neocortex and of the behavioral changes that follow lesions confined to one or another of the major cytoarchitectural fields within it. This conclusion has been greatly strengthened by recent neuroanatomical studies, especially those in which new methods for defining connectivity have been used (important contributions have been made by Nauta, Powell, Jones, Kuypers, Akert, and others). One can now conclude that each neocortical area that has a distinctive cytoarchitecture and a distinctive "function" also possesses a unique set of extrinsic connections, that is, its own pattern of thalamic, corticocortical, interhemispheric, and long descending connections. Thus a major question concerning the neocortex is this: *To what degree are the three variables of cytoarchitecture, extrinsic connections, and "function" causally related?* It should be added that little is known of a possible fourth variable: differences in intrinsic microconnectivity in different cortical areas.

The discovery of the spontaneous electrical activity of the cerebral cortex led to the question of whether cortical areas defined cytoarchitecturally display differences in the pattern of electrical activity recorded on the cortical surface or from an overlying spot on the scalp. It was discovered that the electroencephalograms of very large regions such as the frontal, parietal, and occipital lobes are indeed quite different, but no characteristic differences have been found between records from areas, within those larger regions, which are clearly and sometimes strikingly different in structural organization. Until the present, at least, study of the spontaneous slow-wave activity of the neocortex has revealed little of its intrinsic functional organization.

A successful combination of descriptive cytoarchitecture and experimental analysis was first made in a series of studies by Rose and Woolsey. They found, for example, that the areas of the limbic cortex of the cat and rabbit upon which the three anterior nuclei of the dorsal thalamus project are clearly separated from one another by cytoarchitectural criteria and that each area thus defined receives the total projection of one nucleus and no other, with a narrow zone of transition between areas (Rose and Woolsey, 1948a). A similar coincidence was found between the orbitofrontal cortex of the cat defined by its intrinsic structure and the cortical projection zone of the mediodorsal nucleus of the thalamus (Rose and Woolsey,

1948b). These same investigators added a third and independent method for defining the extent of a cortical field in their study of the auditory cortex of the cat (Rose, 1949; Rose and Woolsey, 1949). Here the three methods of definition—cytoarchitecture, the cortical zone of projection of the medial geniculate nucleus of the dorsal thalamus, and the area of cortex activated by electrical stimulation of the spiral osseous lamina of the cochlea—produced virtually coincident definitions of the auditory cortex. This led to the general conclusion that a cortical area may be defined both by its intrinsic structure and as the zone of projection of a specific thalamic nucleus. This generality has since been confirmed in a large number of studies in many species, including primates (Jones and Burton, 1976; Jones and Wise, 1977). The results of more recent electrophysiological studies using single-unit analysis have strengthened this idea considerably, for it has been shown that both the static and the dynamic functional properties of cortical neurons can be correlated with the cytoarchitectural area in which they are located. This has been established in lightly anesthetized, unanesthetized but immobilized, and waking, behaving monkeys, in the somatic sensory (Powell and Mountcastle, 1959; Mountcastle and Powell, 1959a,b; Carli, LaMotte, and Mountcastle, 1971a,b; Mountcastle et al., 1969), the visual (Hubel and Wiesel, 1968, 1970, 1974a,b; Poggio et al., 1975; Poggio, Doty, and Talbot, 1977; Poggio and Fischer, 1977), the motor (Evarts, 1964, 1974), and the association areas (Duffy and Birchfiel, 1972; Lynch et al., 1973a,b; Sakata et al., 1973; Hyvärinen and Poranen, 1974; Mountcastle et al., 1975; Lynch et al., 1977).

In summary, I conclude that cytoarchitectural differences between areas of neocortex reflect differences in their patterns of extrinsic connections. These patterns are in no way accidental. They are detailed and precise for each area; indeed, they define it. The traditional or usual "functions" of different areas also reflect these differences in extrinsic connections; they provide no evidence whatsoever for differences in *intrinsic* structure or function. This suggests that neocortex is everywhere functionally much more uniform than hitherto supposed and that its avalanching enlargement in mammals and particularly in primates has been accomplished by replication of a basic neural module, without the appearance of wholly new neuron types or of qualitatively different modes of intrinsic organization. Cytoarchitectural differences may therefore reflect the selection or grouping together of sets of modules in particular areas by certain sets of input-output connections. In the primary motor and sensory cortices this selection is made by a single strongly dominant connection, and cytoarchitectural identification of heterotypical areas is clear and striking. Areas of the homotypical eulaminate cortex (95% of man's neocortex) are defined by more evenly balanced sets of extrinsic connections, and here cytoarchitectural differences, while clear, are less striking. Thus a major problem for understanding the function of the neocortex and therefore of the cerebrum is to unravel the intrinsic structural and functional organization of the neocortical module.

That module is, I propose, what has come to be called the *cortical column*.

The columnar organization of the cerebral cortex

It was von Economo, I believe, who first used the word "column" to describe the vertical alignment of neurons in rows extending across all the cellular layers of the cortex. So far as I know, von Economo made no statement concerning the functional organization of the cortex, and it was Lorente de Nó who first suggested a vertical model of cortical operation, an idea to which he was led from his own Golgi studies of intracortical connectivity. The idea of the columnar organization of the cortex has developed as a functional concept on the basis of a discovery made in physiological experiments, namely that the basic unit of operation in the neocortex is a vertically arrayed group of cells heavily interconnected along that vertical axis, sparsely so horizontally. This unit is envisaged to function in the operations of processing and distribution. I emphasize again [for my earlier statements see Mountcastle (1957) and Powell and Mountcastle (1959)] that on this theory the cortex is, nevertheless, not regarded as a collection of isolated units cemented together in a mosaic, as some authors infer (Towe, 1975; Creutzfeldt, 1976). In the sections below I give some of the physiological evidence for this hypothesis and then call attention to some of the many important new discoveries concerning the intrinsic structure and connectivity of the neocortex that lend strong support to the columnar hypothesis. First, however, I shall list a number of general principles that will be illustrated in what follows:

1. The cortical column is an input-output processing device. The number of other regions transmitting to and receiving from a traditionally defined cortical area may vary from about 10 to 30. The sample of that total entertained by any given subset of the modules of an area is much smaller and varies among subsets, with overlap.

2. The columnar arrangement allows the mapping of several variables simultaneously in a two-dimensional matrix, with a preservation of topology.

3. Specific connections are maintained between ordered sets of columns in different cortical areas and between sets of cortical columns and modules of subcortical structures. Thus topological relations may be preserved during transit through and between such areas, with or without topographic (geographic) mapping.

4. The identification parameters for columns and ordered sets of columns may vary within a given cortical region, as defined traditionally, and may differ strikingly between cortical regions.

5. The columnar functional model allows for a partially shifted overlap across a topographical representation that is compatible with a dynamic isolation of the active elements of a column by a form of lateral, pericolumnar, inhibition.

6. Divergent intracolumnar pathways to different outputs allow selective processing ("feature extraction") of certain input signal parameters for particular output destinations.

EVIDENCE FROM STUDY OF THE SOMATIC SENSORY CORTEX Study of the first somatic sensory area of anesthetized cats produced evidence that the basic functional unit of the neocortex is a vertically oriented column (or cylinder, or slab) of cells which extends across all the cellular layers. Such a column is capable of input-output functions of considerable complexity, independently of the horizontal spread of activity within the gray matter (Mountcastle, 1957). This hypothesis was confirmed and extended in studies of the homologous cortical area in anesthetized monkeys (Powell and Mountcastle, 1959). The identification parameters for columns in the somatic sensory cortex are the static properties of the neurons: the location of their receptive fields in the two dimensions of the body surface; the nature of the driving stimuli adequate to excite them, called the property of "modality"; and the rate of adaptation to a steady stimulus, a property determined at the level of the sensory receptor and thus one component of modality. These variables are set congruently by the segregated transsynaptic projection to the cerebral cortex of activity in small sets of first-order sensory fibers having common or closely overlapping receptive fields and a common sensory transducer capacity. They are mapped onto the X and Y dimensions of the postcentral somatic cortex, providing an example of an important general property of columnar organization:

it allows the mapping of a number of variables within the two dimensions of the cerebral cortex, with a preservation of topology.

Columnar organization for place and modality has now been observed in each of the topographical and cytoarchitectural divisions of the somatic sensory cortex, under a variety of experimental conditions and in several species: (1) in somatic area I of unanesthetized, neuromuscularly blocked squirrel and macaque monkeys (Werner and Whitsel, 1968; Mountcastle et al., 1969; Whitsel, Dryer, and Ropollo, 1971; Dryer et al., 1975); (2) in somatic I of waking, behaving macaque monkeys (Carli, LaMotte, and Mountcastle, 1971a,b); (3) in somatic area II in anesthetized cats (Carreras and Andersson, 1963) and unanesthetized, neuromusuclarly blocked macaque monkeys (Whitsel, Petrucelli, and Werner, 1969); and (4) in anesthetized neonatal (Armstrong-James, 1975) and adult rats (Welker, 1971).

Werner, Whitsel, and their colleagues have made a major contribution to understanding the mapping of the body upon the somatic sensory cortex, and their results bear directly upon the nature of the columnar organization of this region (for review, see Werner and Whitsel, 1973). Each segment or small portion of a segment is mapped on the cortical surface into a long, narrow, sometimes sinuous strip extending anteroposteriorly across all of the cytoarchitectural areas (3a, 3b, 1, and 2) of the postcentral somatic cortex. These strips are arranged in such a way that movement along a particular mediolateral path on the cortex specifies movement along a continuous path on the body surface, formed by the sequential combination of movements across the individual dermatomes. Movement anteroposteriorly along any one of the dermatomal representations traces a path along the dermatome on the body surface. It has been known for a long time that the parameter of modality is also mapped differentially within this spatial representation. This mapping process generates an image of the body in cortical space that is topological in the sense that it preserves the connectivity of the body along specific paths without regard to the exact metric of the body itself. Orderly relations are maintained between ordered sets of elements in the space of the body and other ordered sets of elements in the representational space of the cortex, over afferent pathways some of which are divergent and recombinant.

The differential gradient for modality in the anteroposterior direction of a strip varies somewhat from one topographic region to another (for example, foot, leg, hand, arm, face) (Whitsel and Dryer, 1976), but in all regions there is a high probability that the columns of area 3a are specified by deep afferents including muscle afferents; those of area 3b by slowly adapting cutaneous afferents; those of area 1 by quickly adapting cutaneous afferents (Paul, Merzenich, and Goodman, 1972); and those of area 2 by deep afferents from joints, with some mixing in regions of transition. Further evidence is needed to clarify this general arrangement, for a major uncertainty remains: Are cortical columns of the somatic sensory cortex specified for place only in the mediolateral direction, or is there also a defining parameter in the anteroposterior direction along the narrow dermatomal representation?

Only preliminary studies have been made of the dynamics of neuronal processing in the columns of the somatic sensory cortex. There is evidence that activity in one column leads to inhibition of neurons in adjacent columns, whether of the same or of different modality specification (Mountcastle and Powell, 1959a,b). The mechanism of this inhibition is unknown. It is generated intracortically, perhaps via the putatively inhibitory interneuron described by Marin-Padilla (1970; see also Jones, 1975b). The terminals of these cells are distributed in thin, anteroposteriorly oriented, extended vertical discs. Such a distribution of inhibition is what would be required to isolate an active column or slab from its neighbors. It is likely that the inhibition imposed transsynaptically via the recurrent axon collaterals of the projection neurons of layers V and VI (Stephanis and Jasper, 1964) also plays a role in creating a pericolumnar inhibition.

Some neurons of the somatic sensory cortex are differentially sensitive to the direction of a stimulus moving across their peripheral receptive fields. This feature of the central representation of peripheral events first appears after two or more stages of intracortical processing, for Whitsel, Ropollo, and Werner (1972) discovered that cells displaying this dynamic property are preferentially located in layer III of the sensory cortex, with a smaller number in layer V. Directional selectivity appears to be a much more common property of cutaneous neurons of area 5 (Sakata et al., 1973; Mountcastle et al., 1975), to which many of the layer III pyramidal cells of the sensory cortex project. Although the evidence is so far only preliminary, these observations suggest that within a cutaneously specified column of the sensory cortex, there is preferential processing and integration, within a given channel leading to a particular output, of the neuronal events signaling stimulus attributes that are further elaborated in the projection target of that output channel.

Woolsey and Van der Loos (1970) discovered in the somatic sensory cortex of the mouse a special anatomical arrangement that suggests a morphological basis for columnar organization in this area of this species. Each sinus hair of the contralateral face, and especially each of the mystacial vibrissae, is represented in a column of cells which, in layer IV, is clearly segregated into a "barrel" some 200–300 μm in diameter. The cell density in the wall of the barrel is 1.6 times that in its "hollow" center (Pasternak and Woolsey, 1975). Welker (1971) has shown by a single-neuron analysis that all the cells of a barrel, and the column of cells above and below it, are activated by movement of but a single contralateral vibrissa. Barrels are present also in the somatic sensory cortex of the mouse and of the Australian brush-tailed opossum, but they have not been found in any other of the large number of species examined (Feldman and Peters, 1974; Woolsey, Welker, and Schwartz, 1975).

In summary, the body form is mapped onto the postcentral somatic cortex of the primate with a preservation of topological order. Each small portion of the segmental innervation is projected to a long, sometimes sinuous, anteroposteriorly directed strip of cortex; strips vary in both A-P length and M-L width. Any single locus on the cortex is thus specified in its X and Y dimensions by the parameters of place. In addition, each column is further specified by the static parameter of modality. Thus the primary somatic sensory cortex illustrates several of the general characteristics of columnar organization:

1. Each local column is specified by the static parameters of place and modality, and rows of columns (or slabs) with the same dermatomal specification and those with the same modality specification are arranged more or less orthogonally to one another. There is preliminary evidence that other, more dynamic, variables are also mapped within this same two-dimensional matrix.

2. Its sets of columns are specifically linked to ordered sets of columns in other areas (see below).

3. This particular cortical area is dominated by its specific thalamocortical input, to such an extent that those regions in which sensory processing is thought to be most precise—the hand, foot, and face—are isolated from some corticocortical and callosal inputs.

4. The columnar organization is compatible with partially shifted overlap in the representation of the body form.

EVIDENCE FROM STUDY OF THE VISUAL CORTEX It is in the visual cortex that we possess the most information and the strongest evidence for columnar organization, thanks largely to the elegant studies of Hubel and Wiesel, which they have recently summarized (1977). The mapping of visual space upon the striate cortex is determined by the distribution of geniculocortical fibers, while the segregation parameters for the columnar mapping of a number of variables are formed during the initial stages of intracortical processing. I wish to emphasize this point, for *the columnar processing units of the cortex appear to be specified both by their afferent inputs and by the nature of the intracortical processing of that input.* Hubel and Wiesel have shown by a combination of electrophysiological and a number of independent experimental anatomical methods that the columns of area 17 "form vertically disposed alternating left-eye and right-eye slabs, which in horizontal sections form alternating stripes about 400 μm thick, with occasional bifurcations and blind endings." Much narrower columns whose cells are selectively tuned to the orientation of short line segments are stacked in a direction more or less orthogonal to that of the ocular dominance stripes, so that each member of a local couplet of ocular dominance columns contains a complete 180° sequence of the slim orientation columns (or slabs). For any given neuron, the right-left dominance is determined by the afferent input, but the degree of that dominance and the property of orientation are determined by intracortical processes. Such a cross-matched combination of the binocular and orientation sets occupies an area of about 800 μm × 800 μm. I define such a set as a macrocolumn; it is a superimposed couplet of the ocular dominance and orientation hypercolumns defined by Hubel and Wiesel. Thus the visual cortex presents an example par excellence of how a number of variables can be mapped or represented in a two-dimensional matrix, by virtue of columnar organization. The two dimensions of the representation of space, the visual field, are mapped congruently with the variables of ocular dominance and orientation and undoubtedly still others as well (see below).

The compatibility of the principles of columnar organization and of partially shifted overlap is as clearly demonstrated in the visual as in the somatic sensory cortex. Here the aggregate receptive field of each macrocolumn overlaps by about one-half that of the adjacent sets, and the linear relation between magnification factor and receptive field size means that this overlap factor is invariant across the entire cortical representation of the visual field. Thus any oriented line segment presented in the visual field will be mapped maximally into a set of macrocolumns whose position is determined by the spatial location and linear extent of the stimulus. Within that selected set of macrocolumns, the locus of maximal activity will be determined by orientation. The partially shifted overlap of the representation of visual space determines that the row of maximally activated macrocolumns will be flanked on either side by sets less vigorously active, a lateral spread sharply limited by inhibition.

It is important to emphasize, as Hubel and Wiesel have done, the isolation of the processing function of the striate cortex. This area as a whole is the least interconnected of cortical regions. It sends and receives callosal fibers only along the representation of the vertical meridian and appears to receive no ipsilateral corticocortical connections. No U-fibers link any part of area 17 with any other part of that area, the tangential spread of the large majority of the intragrisial fibers is limited to about 1–2 mm (Fisken, Garey, and Powell, 1973), and there are good reasons to suppose that the principal function of the intragrisial fibers is the creation of lateral walls of inhibition that contribute to the dynamic isolation of an active column from its neighbors. Thus, while intracortical processing within area 17 is an essential step leading to visual perception, it is probably correct to say that visual perception does not "occur" there, but rather within a series of complex distributed systems in each of which a locus in area 17 is an integral part. For the most complex aspects of vision, a primate possessing only area 17 among all visual and visual associative cortical areas would probably be perceptually blind.

Studies of the dynamic activity of visual cortical neurons suggest that within any given macrocolumn, processing for different stimulus attributes proceeds along parallel channels. The general rule seems to be that the attributes selected in a given pathway leading to an output channel are those further elaborated in the target area of the channel: the processing and distribution functions of a cortical column are then combined. This principle is shown, for example, by the recent findings of Poggio and his colleagues, who have studied the dynamic processing of neural activity in the foveal visual cortex of waking monkeys trained to fixate steadily on a target even when a variety of other visual stimuli are presented (Poggio, Doty, and Talbot, 1977; Poggio and Fisher, 1977). Poggio has measured the spatial-frequency tuning properties of striate neurons, their sensitivity to moving gratings, and certain aspects of binocular interaction including disparity sensitivity. As regards spatial-frequency sensitivity, the majority of cells of the deep layers of the cortex have the properties of "movement analyzers," appropriate for the brain stem oculomotor control system upon which many neurons of the infragranular layers project. In contrast, neurons of the supragranular layers appear to function as "form analyzers," to a certain degree independently of movement. The output trajectory from these layers is largely to areas 18 and 19, where it is likely that further processing leads eventually to the perception of spatial structure. Thus different sets of output neurons possess common static properties of locus of receptive field, ocularity, and orientation, but the channels leading to them accentuate and elaborate different dynamic properties of the input signals.

It has been known for some time that many neurons of the cat's visual areas (Barlow, Blakemore, and Pettigrew, 1967; Nikara, Bishop, and Pettigrew, 1968; Pettigrew, Nikara and Bishop, 1968) and in area 18 of the monkey cortex (Hubel and Wiesel, 1970) display receptive field disparity. It has been suggested that these neurons may therefore play a role in the central neural mechanisms in stereopsis. Poggio and Fisher (1977) have recently identified neurons with such receptive field disparities in area 17 of the waking, behaving monkey. They observed depth-tuned excitatory and inhibitory neurons that, in addition to playing a candidate role in the neural mechanisms for stereopsis, may serve to maintain visual fixation. These tuned neurons were found throughout the cortical layers, but in greatest proportion in the lower layers that project subcortically. By contrast, other neurons sensitive to a larger range of disparities either in front of ("near neurons") or behind ("far neurons") the plane of fixation are more plentiful in the supragranular layers. Cells of these layers (II and III) are known to project to other cortical regions, mainly 18 and 19, where it is believed the neural mechanisms for stereoscopic vision are further elaborated. These neurons may also contribute to the cortical control of oculomotor vergence leading to fusion.

This general idea has received further support from the combined electrophysiological and anatomical studies of Zeki, who has explored a set of projection zones of area 17 in areas 18 and 19 and in the cortex of the posterior bank of the superior temporal sulcus in the monkey. In each of these zones he has observed a further elaboration of the processing of a particular stimulus attribute (Zeki, 1974, 1975, 1977).

In summary, the striate visual cortex illustrates several of the general properties of columnar organization:

1. Several variables are mapped within its two-dimensional matrix.

2. Its macrocolumns function as input-output processing devices such that parallel processing within each allows the selection of certain dynamic stimulus attributes for elaboration along restricted channels leading to particular outputs (commonly those attributes are accentuated in the processing mechanisms of the target regions).

3. Its sets of columns are specifically linked to ordered sets of columns in other cortical areas and in modules of subcortical structures upon which it projects.

4. The visual cortex of the monkey is dominated by its geniculostriate projection and thus resembles the hand and foot areas of the somatic sensory cortex in the degree of input isolation.

5. The columnar organization of the visual cortex is compatible with the principle of partially shifted overlap in the representation of the visual fields in neural space.

EVIDENCE FROM STUDY OF THE AUDITORY CORTEX It has been known for a long time that the cochlear partition, and thus the frequency of stimulating sounds, is represented in the "primary" auditory cortex A-1 in an orderly fashion, a body of knowledge due in large part to the extensive series of evoked-potential experiments carried out by Woolsey and his colleagues (for review, see Woolsey, 1960). Similar methods have been used to identify the auditory cortex of the human brain on the superior surface of the temporal lobe in an area corresponding to the transverse temporal gyri (Celesia, 1976). The koniocortex of this region is the most markedly columniated of any heterotypical cortex; its radial arrangement of cells is obvious in sections cut normal to the cortical surface. Indeed, Sousa-Pinta (1973) has described in the cat's A-1 vertical cylinders of cells in the middle layers with diameters of 50–60 μm and with cell-poor centers. Studies of the physiological properties of single neurons of A-1 have revealed that cells encountered as a microelectrode passes down normal to the cortical surface are tuned to a nearly identical frequency and that their tuning curves have sharp roll-offs in both directions, due at least in part to lateral inhibition (Parker, 1965; Abeles and Goldstein, 1970; Merzenich and Brugge, 1973; Merzenich, Knight, and Roth, 1975; Imig and Adrian, 1977). A similar columnar organization for best frequency has been established for the anterior auditory area as well (Knight, 1977). The overlap of the tuning curves of neurons in adjacent isofrequency strips is sufficient to account for the partially shifted overlap of frequency representation observed in surface-mapping experiments.

It was Tunturi who first suggested that other properties of auditory signals might be mapped along each isofrequency contour or strip of the cortex, in a direction orthogonal to that of the change in frequency (Tunturi, 1952; Tunturi and Dudman, 1958). This has now been shown to be the case in the cat by the important new study of Imig and Adrian (1977), and in the monkey by the initial studies of Brugge and Merzenich (1973). In the high-frequency region of the cat's A-1, aural dominance and binaural interaction are the properties that vary along the long dimension of an isofrequency band. Neurons located along the perpendicular axis of the cortex, within such a band, display similar properties of frequency sensitivity and binaural interaction. Slanting penetrations within an isofrequency band often pass from a zone in which neurons exhibit one kind of binaural interaction to one in which they exhibit another.

Binaural stimulation may produce a suppression of response, as compared with the response to monaural stimulation, and in all such cases the contralateral ear is dominant. On the other hand, binaural stimulation may produce summation, and in this case either ear may dominate. The suppression and summation columns are arranged in continuous bands placed more or less orthogonally to the isofrequency contours. Within each summation set there is a further columniation for which the identification parameter is ear dominance. It is well known that the interaural intensity difference provides the cue for localization in space of high-frequency sounds (that is, sounds above about 3,000 Hz).

Studies of the auditory cortex of the monkey are much less advanced than those in the cat, but it is already clear that the representation of frequency in A-1 of the monkey is also in terms of isofrequency contours or bands located at right angles to the line of representation of the cochlear partition. These isofrequency bands extend throughout the cellular layers of the cortex, in accord with columnar organization (Brugge and Merzenich, 1973). One observation made by these investigators is of great interest in the present context. They observed in the bands for frequencies of 2,500 Hz and below that neurons in columns were most sensitive to the interaural delay. It is this property of interaural stimulus delay that accounts for the capacity to locate sound of low frequency in surrounding space.

Suga (1977) has discovered in the auditory cortex of the mustache bat an example of columnar organization that illustrates the advantage conferred by the freedom to map a number of variables in two dimensions. This animal emits orientation sounds with a long constant-frequency (CF) component followed by a short frequency-modulated (FM) component. The CF component is used for target detection and measurement of target velocity, with Doppler-shifted compensation. The FM component is used for localization and ranging of the target. The most intense part of the CF is the second harmonic at about 61kHz, which sweeps down to 51kHz during the last few msec of the signal. About 30% of the primary auditory cortex is devoted to columns that are closely specified for the CF component in the second harmonic of the orientation sounds and its Doppler-shifted echoes. Columns are specified along radial and concentric axes for the two identification parameters of frequency and amplitude, and this representation occupies a disproportionately large share of the auditory cortex.

In summary, the primary auditory cortex is organized in a columnar manner, and although the evidence is still incomplete, the identification parameters in the X and Y dimensions suggest that two intersecting bands of columns map sound frequency against the neural transforms of those stimulus attributes necessary for localizing sounds in space. These are the interaural intensity differences for high frequencies and interaural time differences for low frequencies (below 2,500 Hz). More evidence will be needed to establish this general model with certainty, and undoubtedly other dynamic parameters are also mapped along the axis of the isofrequency bands of columns, but the general similarity to the arrangements in the visual and somatic sensory cortices is obvious.

EVIDENCE FROM STUDY OF THE PRECENTRAL MOTOR CORTEX The precentral motor cortex was until recently the most intensively studied but least understood of the heterotypical areas of the neocortex. Significant advances in understanding the functional organization of this region and its role in the control of movement have been made in the last decade by the application of new methods. Notable among these are the recording of the electrical signs of the activity of single neurons in the motor cortex of waking monkeys trained to emit repetitively a defined movement (Evarts, 1975), intracortical stimulation and recording through a penetrating microelectrode (Asanuma, 1973, 1975), and several new methods for tracing projections to and from such a cortical region. I call attention to only a small part of the large literature that has resulted, in particular that dealing with the functional organization of the precentral motor cortex.

Asanuma and his colleagues have used the method of intracortical microstimulation to produce convincing evidence that those loci within the cortex at which stimulation with weak currents (4 μa) produces small movements of a distal joint, often executed by a single muscle, are arrayed in vertical columns of 0.5–1.0 mm in diameter, which match the radial cell columns so characteristic of this area (Asanuma and Rosen, 1972a,b). They were also able by recording through the stimulating microelectrode to define the afferent input to the motor cortical cells in the immediate vicinity. These cells were commonly activated by stimulation of receptors in deep tissues in and about the joint moved by the local intracortical stimulation. Only those columns in which stimulation produced movement of the fingers contained neurons with cutaneous receptive fields. These commonly lay on the glabrous skin of the hand in such locations as to be activated by the movement evoked by local stimulation. The input-output loop thus composed is thought to play a role in tactually guided movement of the hand and fingers and in instinctive grasping. These observations have been confirmed in principle by a number of investigators (Doetsch and Gardner, 1972; Lenon and Porter, 1976). Others have emphasized the more distributed nature of the "colonies" of pyramidal tract neurons related to a particular muscle (Phillips, 1969; Anderssen et al., 1975). A significant finding by Jankowska, Padel, and Tanaka (1975a,b) was that although the excited loci for a given muscle were more widely distributed than suggested by the observations of Asanuma, they were discontinuous. Thus one working hypothesis concerning the functional organization of the motor cortex is that radial columns of neurons processing input to output directed at a single motoneuron pool are clustered together, with an overlap where the thinning edge of a cluster meets the edges of clusters of columns related to other muscles. According to this idea there is complete compatibility between the columnar organization of the motor cortex and the partially shifted overlap emphasized by Phillips (1969) and others. One might suppose that the motor cortical patterns controlling movement result from the dynamic combination into continually forming and dissolving sets of active columns related to one, two, or many muscles involved in a particular phase of ongoing movement. The organizing commands for the composition of these *movement sets* are envisaged to arise elsewhere rather than in the precentral motor cortex per se. Thus the old and oft-repeated question, "Does the motor cortex think in terms of movements or muscles?" appears redundant. The motor cortex is an intermediate level in the true Jacksonian sense: it does not "think," and both movements and muscles are "represented" within it, though each in a different way.

Asanuma and Rosen (1973) have elucidated still further the columnar organization in the motor cortex by using two penetrating microelectrodes, one for stimulation and the other for recording. Stimulation in the upper layers was found to elicit excitation locally and in the lower layers as well, in a column slightly less than 1 mm in diameter; that same stimulation produced a pericolumnar zone of inhibition. Stimulation in the deeper layers produced local excitation, and the same pericolumnar inhibition, perhaps identical in mechanism to that described by Stephanis and Jasper (1964) as being caused by impulses in the recurrent axon collaterals of the cells of origin of pyramidal tract fibers. Surprisingly, no excitation of neurons in the supragranular layers was produced by stimulation in the deep layers.

In summary, the motor cortex is organized into cell columns about 1 mm in diameter, but the shape and geometry of the columns or strips is unknown. The groups of columns related to particular segmental interneuron and motoneuron pools appear in clusters, with overlap at their edges with adjacent clusters devoted to other muscles. The mapping parameter in the X and Y dimensions appears to be location in the pattern of the body musculature. One might predict that other, more dynamic aspects of the pattern of neuronal activity are mapped into these same X and Y dimensions, perhaps by a further columniation within the larger columns so far defined only in topographic terms. A dynamic pericolumnar inhibition appears to be exerted both by intragrisially projecting axons and by the action of recurrent collaterals of projection neurons of the infragranular layers.

EVIDENCE FROM STUDY OF THE PARIETAL HOMOTYPI-CAL CORTEX   The homotypical cortex of the parietal lobe of the monkey exhibits the vertical cording of neurons and the functional characteristics of columnar organization (Mountcastle et al., 1975; Lynch et al., 1977). These regions differ remarkably from the heterotypical areas considered hitherto, for they are neither dominated by a single afferent input, as are the primary sensory areas, nor linked unconditionally to peripheral effectors, as is the motor cortex. The specifying parameters for columnar sets in the homotypical parietal cortex must be sought in experiments in which electrophysiological observations can be made in animals trained to emit a series of behavioral acts—acts chosen because evidence obtained on other grounds suggests their relevance to the region under study. The columnar sets of areas 5 and 7, when studied in this way, all appear to have one common specifying characteristic: their cells are active in relation to the animal's action upon and within his immediately surrounding environment and also to the spatial relations between his body and its parts, the gravitational field, and that environment (Mountcastle, 1975, 1976, 1977). Within area 7 there are different sets of columns whose cells are active during (1) projection of the arm toward an object of interest; (2) manipulation of an object; (3) fixation of gaze and thus of visual attention; (4) visually evoked but not spontaneous saccadic movement of the eyes; (5) slow pursuit tracking movement of the eyes; as well as (6) a large group of neurons that are truly visual in nature, but whose properties are quite different from those of neurons of the striate cortex. The columnar segregation of these groups of cells with quite different properties is shown by the facts that (1) microelectrode penetrations normal to the cortical surface and along the vertically arranged cell columns have a high probability of encountering cells of only one class, and (2) penetrations that pass in directions slanting across the cell columns traverse blocks of tissue within which cells are all of one type or another rather than intermingled. So far little is known about the exact size or shape of the columns in the parietal cortex or about the dynamics of neuronal processing within them.

It is my proposition that each of these classes of columnar sets of the parietal cortex is related by specific extrinsic connections to similarly segregated sets of modules in other cortical regions and in subcortical nuclei as well, and that these closely interconnected modular sets of different large brain entities form precisely connected, distributed systems, serving distributed functions.

A CENTRAL CORE SYSTEM PROJECTING TO THE NEO-CORTEX, WITHOUT COLUMNAR ORGANIZATION   The general concept of columnar organization does not preclude the possibility that other systems may engage the cortex in different ways, particularly those involved in general regulatory functions rather than detailed information processing. One example is the noradrenergic system that arises in the locus coeruleus and projects to very widely distributed portions of the central nervous system, including the entire neocortex (for review, see Moore and Bloom, 1977). This direct neocortical projection system has been demonstrated in a number of species, including primates. The locus coeruleus emits two identifiable ascending tracts that reach the neocortex directly. They pass upward through the subthalamus; the medial component reaches the neocortex via the cingulum bundle, the lateral via the external capsule. The special aspect of this system is that from the two local points of entry, fibers pass tangentially to reach every cortical region and every cortical layer. Molliver and his colleagues (1977) have used an immunohistochemical method to trace this system in detail, and in their montage reconstructions the neocortex is seen to be interlaced in all directions by a web of fine noradrenergic fibers at 30–40 μm intervals. Each layer except IV contains radial, tangential, or oblique axons arranged in such a manner that any individual noradrenergic axon may influence adjacent cortical columns over very long distances. It appears that any single cell of the locus coeruleus may project very widely upon the brain, including large areas of the neocortex, and sustain an immense and divergent axonal field. The exact mode of termination of these fibers is still uncertain and may include both traditional synaptic terminations and transmitter release sites *en passage*, but it is obvious that the system has the capacity to influence directly every cell in the neocortex.

The functional significance of this system is equally uncertain. One may conjecture from its distribution that it exerts a controlling or regulating influence upon the neocortex and that this might occur by direct synaptic engagement, by release of synaptic transmitter agents "at a distance," by both of these means, or by regulation of blood flow and vascular permeability (Raichle et al., 1975). The role this system is known to play in sleep mechanisms may be only the most obvious of these controls. Whatever the nature of its influence upon the cortex—which may even include its maturation—there is no sign of "columnar organization" in the way it engages the neocortex.

Intrinsic organization of the neocortex

An understanding of the functional organization of the neocortical module requires a flow diagram of the structural linkages between its inputs and its outputs. It is not yet possible to construct such a diagram, though recent studies have provided many of the facts it will require, as regards both intrinsic and extrinsic connectivity. Szentágothai has summarized this growing body of information in a series of successively more complete models which have been of considerable heuristic value (Szentágothai, 1973, 1975, 1976; see also Garey, 1976, and Colonnier, 1966, 1968).

The general plan is as follows. Afferent fibers that reach the neocortex come from three major sources: from specifically related nuclei of the dorsal thalamus; from other cortical areas of the same hemisphere; and via the corpus callosum from usually homologous but sometimes heterologous areas of the contralateral hemisphere. Less dense and more diffusely distributed innervations arise in the generalized thalamic nuclei, the basilar forebrain regions, and certain monaminergic nuclei of the brain stem. The terminals of extrinsic afferents to the cortex are always of the excitatory type (asymmetrical profiles with round vesicles) (Garey and Powell, 1971; Jones and Powell, 1970), but they make up a relatively small portion of all excitatory terminals in the cortex: estimates vary from 5% to 20%. The major classes of corticofugal axons are ipsilateral corticocortical, commissural corticocortical, corticothalamic, and a large class whose targets include, in different combinations for different areas, the basal ganglia, mesencephalon, pons, medulla, and spinal cord. Afferent systems of different origin engage different but overlapping laminar targets within the cortex. The densest concentration of terminals of specific thalamocortical fibers is in layers IV and III-B (Jones and Powell, 1970; Hubel and Wiesel, 1972; Sloper, 1973; Jones, 1975a; Winfield and Powell, 1976; Jones and Burton, 1976). Those of the generalized thalamocortical system and those of brain stem origin terminate in all layers, but especially in layer I. Ipsilateral corticocortical and commissural fibers terminate predominantly in the supragranular layers, most densely in layers III and IV (see, for example, Jones, Burton, and Porter, 1975; Goldman and Nauta, 1977).

There are only rare exceptions to the general rules that all the pyramidal cells of the cortex emit extrinsically directed axons, that all extrinsic axons arising in the cortex come from pyramidal cells, and that all extrinsic axons are excitatory in synaptic action. The pyramidal cells of origin of different efferent systems are precisely segregated by layer. The cell bodies of corticothalamic fibers are located in layer VI (Lund et al., 1975; Gilbert and Kelly, 1975; Jones and Wise, 1977); those of the corticocortical systems in layer III (Shoumura, 1974; Shoumura, Ando, and Kato, 1975; Lund et al., 1975; Jones, Burton, and Porter, 1975; Jones and Wise, 1977; Glickstein and Whitteridge, 1976); and those of other descending systems to the basal ganglia, brain stem, and spinal cord in layer V (Berrevoets and Kuypers, 1975; Humphrey and Rietz, 1976; Jones et al., 1977; Jones and Wise, 1977).

There is evidence that some (unknown) proportion of the excitatory terminals of extrinsic afferents end monosynaptically upon the spiny processes of pyramidal cells, thus providing a monosynaptic "throughput" pathway. However, it is likely that the large majority of extrinsic afferents end upon the local interneurons of the cortex, the heterogeneous class of stellate cells. These interneurons vary in location, size, sign of synaptic action, extent and type of dendritic field, and axonal ramification. They have been classified in a number of ways (Lund, 1973; Jones, 1975b). It is likely that the spiny stellate cell of layers IV and III-B is a major target of the specific thalamocortical fibers. This cell is excitatory in synaptic action, and its terminals make powerful cascading synapses upon the spines of the apical dendrites of pyramidal cells (LeVay, 1973; Lund, 1973; Lund and Boothe, 1975; Jones, 1975a). Other interneurons are also excitatory and receive direct extrinsic input; together they must provide a system of echeloned pathways in both series and parallel configuration from input to output, undoubtedly encased by powerful feedback and feedforward loops as well. The pattern of distribution of the excitatory stellate interneurons in the neocortex is one of very dense and powerful synaptic connectivity to the output cells in the vertical direction across the cortical layers and rapidly thinning connectivity in the horizontal direction. One particular type of inhibitory interneuron, the large basket cell of layers III, IV, and V, emits an axonal distribution field arranged in a narrow, elongated vertical disc within which the individual axonal terminals clasp in basketlike arrangements the cell bodies of the pyramidal cells within that field (Marin-Padilla, 1969, 1970). This class of cells is likely to exert a strong synaptic pericolumnar inhibition. Other, smaller inhibitory basket cells are thought to isolate smaller cylinders of space within the larger column. The total number of inhibitory terminals (symmetrical profiles with flattened or multiform vesicles) in the cortex is small compared with the number of excitatory ones, but they are strategically placed upon the somata and proximal dendrites of pyramidal cells, so that their suppressive effects per synaptic event can be very powerful.

Almost all extrinsic axons emit recurrent collaterals that branch repeatedly in a spherelike domain up to 3 mm in diameter about the cell of origin, penetrating all the cellular layers from the place of recurrence, usually in layer VI. The exact terminations of the branches of these recurrent axons are not clear, but undoubtedly some emit axonal terminals to the spiny processes of the dendrites of adjacent pyramidal cells and are thus excitatory to them. However, it is likely that the large majority of the terminal branches of these axonal collaterals terminate upon inhibitory interneurons. This is suggested by the fact that the transsynaptic action of an antidromic impulse in an extrinsic axon, upon neighboring pyramidal cells, is a small and transient depolarization followed by a very large and prolonged hyperpolarization. The net result is a powerful inhibition (Stephanis and Jasper, 1964). The distribution pattern of the recurrent axonal collateral system suggests that intense activity in any small group of output cells will exert a powerful pericolumnar inhibition. Thus the cortical column is established by virtue of anatomical connections—its specific afferent input and its vertically oriented intrinsic connectivity—but also in a dynamic manner by a strong pericolumnar inhibition exerted by the large basket cell interneurons and the pyramidal cell axonal collaterals. It is this dynamic isolation which makes the concept of columnar organization compatible with that of partially shifted overlap.

It should be emphasized that the complexities of the neuronal processing mechanisms in the neocortex are not limited by classical synaptic connectivity. Recent studies have shown that in many places in the nervous system, including the neocortex, dendrites may themselves be presynaptic to other dendrites, or even to axon terminals. These elements are frequently arranged in "triads," which appear to be local processing units that may by their integrated outputs affect events in the neuronal elements of larger circuits (Schmitt, Dev, and Smith, 1976). Finally, a number of what are regarded as general regulatory systems engage the cortex in all its layers. It is presently surmised that these systems play a level-setting role, but it is possible that they exert a more focused and differential action upon cortical neuronal excitability.

Extrinsic connectivity of the neocortex

A major advance of the last two decades has been the discovery of a much more detailed and specific connectivity between brain parts than had hitherto been supposed. New methods for light microscopy, particularly the reduced silver methods for staining degenerating axon terminals, led to a series of important discoveries by a number of investigators. More recently, advantage has been taken of the axoplasmic transport of identifiable molecules to trace connections in both anterograde and retrograde directions. The labeling of transmitter agents or their synthesizing enzymes for fluorescent or immunofluorescent microscopy has made it possible to trace even the finest axons to their terminations.

The mass of information now available concerning neocortical connectivity cannot be summarized briefly, but certain general principles begin to emerge. Each neocortical region receives (is defined by) a projection from a dorsal thalamic nucleus and projects back to that nucleus in closely ordered registry. All neocortical regions receive, in addition, afferent inflows from a number of generalized regulating systems: from the basilar forebrain regions, from the generalized nuclei of the dorsal thalamus, and from certain monaminergic nuclei of the brain stem. Generally, homologous neocortical areas of the two hemispheres are reciprocally linked via the great commissures of the forebrain, but there are two known exceptions: the striate cortex (except for the region in which the vertical meridian is represented) and certain parts of the somatic sensory cortex have no commissural connections at all. Uncommonly, a cortical region is linked to heterologous as well as to homologous contralateral areas. Within a single hemisphere there is a step-by-step outward progression of corticocortical connections from primary sensory areas onto successively adjacent areas of the homotypical cortex of the parietal, occipital, and temporal lobes, and each of the successive "higher-order" convergent regions is reciprocally linked with more anterior areas of the frontal lobe. Those receiving the most highly convergent projections are linked via two-way connections with areas of the limbic lobe. There are, however, many exceptions to this general scheme, and many possible connections remain to be explored.

On the output side, the neocortex as a whole projects upon almost every other major entity of the nervous system: the basal ganglia, dorsal thalamus, mesencephalon, brain stem, and spinal cord, but the number and the patterns of their efferent projections differ greatly from one region to another. Many of them form massive reentrant systems, for example, the reciprocal systems linking dorsal thalamus and neocortex, or the large reentrant components converging upon the motor cortex from the basal ganglia and cerebellum, or the descending projections linked to brain stem relay nuclei of the auditory and somatic systems. These systems have many points of entry and exit. They should not be regarded as closed, reverberating circuits.

The number of extrinsic connections identified for single cytoarchitectural areas of the neocortex is much larger than had once been thought. Even the striate cortex, the least interconnected of those neocortical regions that have been studied intensively, is linked by fiber systems to and from at least 10 separate structures. Area 7 of the parietal lobe entertains 17 such connections, and area 3b of the postcentral somatic sensory cortex has connections with no fewer than 29 different targets/sources! Is it possible that each modular unit of a cytoarchitecturally defined area makes all the connections that have been identified for that area? Discoveries of the last two years suggest that this is not the case. Grant, Landgren, and Silvenius (1975) found that small lesions made in area 3a of the cat neocortex produce antegrade degeneration of terminals in restricted zones of areas 2, 3b, and 4. These zones are arranged in a columnar manner, each column is about 1 mm in diameter, and the columns are interspersed with zones of the same cytoarchitectural area free of any degeneration. Shanks, Rockel, and Powell (1975) and Jones, Burton, and Porter (1975) discovered independently that the terminals of commissural fibers linking the somatic sensory areas of the monkey are arranged in columns that cluster in mediolateral bands or groups at the transitional zones between the several cytoarchitectural areas of the postcentral gyrus, separated by columnar zones free of any terminals. Moreover, the cells of origin of these commissural fibers, which lie in layer III-B, were found to be clustered in groups, as if located in some columns but not in others. The columns that send and receive commissural fibers appear to be the same. Corticocortical fibers reaching the postcentral from the precentral gyrus also terminate in isolated clusters, but whether those columns sending and receiving ipsilateral association fibers are identical with those sending and receiving commissural fibers is not known. Shanks, Pearson, and Powell (1977) also found that the intrinsic fiber connections of the monkey's postcentral gyrus ter-

minate in bands or clusters that appear to be coincident with those linking the two postcentral gyri via the corpus callosum. Kunzle (1976) showed a similar alternating arrangement of vertically oriented zones that did and did not send and receive the commissural fibers linking areas 4 and 6 with homologous areas of the contralateral hemisphere.

Goldman and Nauta (1976a, 1977) found that both commissural and ipsilateral association fibers arising in the frontal granular cortex terminate within their diverse cortical targets in vertically oriented columns, 200–500 μm wide, which alternate in regular sequence with zones of comparable width that are free of such terminals. In a nearly reciprocal experiment, Jacobsen and Trojanowski (1977) found that the cells of origin of the commissural fibers arising in the frontal granular cortex of the monkey are located in clusters, alternating with zones free of such cells, a finding consonant with a vertical mode of organization. Goldman and Nauta (1976b) also made the important observation that the segregation of the zones of distribution of cortical efferents is not confined to cortical targets, for the terminals of axons projecting from the frontal granular cortex to the caudate nucleus, in the monkey, are segregated into clusters separated by zones free of such terminals. This finding has been confirmed by Jones et al. (1977).

These new experimental findings suggest that columniation of the intracortical terminal distributions of afferent fibers and of the cells that emit them is a common feature of neocortical organization, just as is the pattern of termination of thalamocortical afferents (Hubel and Wiesel, 1972). Moreover, it appears likely that the total set of columns composing a cytoarchitectural area is fractionated into subsets, each of which sends and receives a particular fraction of the total set of connections of the area. It is not likely that any one subset of columns has no extrinsic connections at all or that any other set entertains them all. A further specification of subset connections is obviously a major objective of present anatomical research.

General statements

THE MODULAR CONSTRUCTION OF THE NERVOUS SYSTEM   The general proposition is that the large entities of the nervous system which we know as the dorsal horn, reticular formation, dorsal thalmus, basal ganglia, neocortex, and so forth, are themselves composed of local circuits. These circuits form modules which vary from place to place in cell number, structural organization, or mode of neuronal processing, but which are at the first level of analysis similar within any single large entity. Modules are grouped into entities by virtue of a dominant extrinsic connection, the need to replicate a common function over a topographic field, or certain intermodular interactions. All the elements in the set of modules composing an entity may not be linked to all of its extrinsic connections; thus the total set of modules composing an entity is fractionated into subsets by different linkages to similarly segregated subsets in other large entities. These specific connections may preserve neighborhood relations in the topographic sense and in any case preserve topologic order. The closely linked subsets of several different large entities thus form precisely connected, distributed systems; these distributed systems are conceived as serving distributed functions.

THE COLUMNAR ORGANIZATION OF THE NEOCORTEX: THE BASIC UNIT   The basic unit of operation in the neocortex is a vertically arranged group of cells heavily interconnected in the vertical axis running across the cortical layers and sparsely connected horizontally. This idea originated as a prediction made from anatomical studies of intracortical cellular arrangements and received its strongest support from the results of electrophysiological studies of the primary sensory areas of the neocortex. More recently, additional evidence supporting this hypothesis has come from a large number of studies of both intrinsic and extrinsic cortical connectivity, particularly from those in which new methods have been used to identify the cells of origin and the locus of termination of connecting axons.

I define the basic modular unit of the neocortex as a minicolumn. It is a vertically oriented cord of cells formed by the migration of neurons from the germinal epithelium of the neural tube along the radial glial cells to their destined locations in the cortex, as described by Rakic. If this minicolumn is comparable in size to the cortical cylinders in which Rockel, Hiorns, and Powell (1974) made neuronal counts, it contains about 110 cells. This figure is almost invariant between different neocortical areas and different species of mammals, except for the striate cortex of primates, where it is 260. Such a cord of cells occupies a gently curving, nearly vertical cylinder of cortical space with a diameter of about 30 μm. Some uncertainty still exists in several major parameters of the human brain. Average reported values are: volume, 1,350 ml; surface area of neocortex, 3,000 cm² (range, 1,800–4,000 cm²); volume of neocortex,

750 ml (range, 500–1,000 ml). The average thickness is generally agreed to be about 2,500 μm, though it varies considerably from one cortical area to another. If the average figures are used for calculation, the human brain contains about 400 million minicolumns and more than 44 billion neurons. The true figures may be even higher.

THE LARGE PROCESSING UNIT OF THE NEOCORTEX: MANY-VARIABLE MAPPING IN A PACKAGE OF MINICOLUMNS   Studies of the primary sensory and motor cortices and of two areas of the homotypical cortex of the parietal lobe have revealed that it is possible to identify within the neocortex a much larger processing unit than the minicolumn. The diameters or widths of this larger unit have been given as 500 μm to 1,000 μm for different areas. Moreover, it is clear that this larger processing unit may vary in its cross-sectional form, being round, or oval, or slablike in shape. Given the dimensions of the larger processing unit of the visual cortex, the macrocolumn as I have defined it, one can estimate that the human neocortex contains about 1 million of these larger processing units, each packaging several hundred minicolumns. The calculations have a high degree of uncertainty and are given to indicate order of magnitude only.

The larger processing unit has been defined in terms of both the static and dynamic properties of its neurons. For the visual cortex, place on the visual cortex is of course in the first instance defined by place in the visual field. The larger processing unit is defined by ocularity and by orientation. The latter property results from intracortical processing and is specified by afferent input only in the topographical sense. In the somatic sensory cortex place on the body surface and modality type are the initial defining parameters, but it is still uncertain whether two dimensions are needed for the designation of place; if so, modality would then become a third defining parameter, mapped congruently. For the auditory cortex, sound frequency and those aspects of binaural interaction that define the location of a sound in space are the defining parameters. Further, it appears that within the domain of these larger processing units, other variables, particularly those of a dynamic nature, can be mapped onto the X and Y dimensions of the cortex, with no disturbance of topological relations. I propose that this "submapping" is ordered in terms of sets of minicolumns, and in the limit in terms of single ones. On this hypothesis the minicolumn is regarded as the irreducibly small processing unit of the neocortex. It may be, for example, that the minicolumn is the mapping unit for the parameter of orientation specificity within each ocular-dominant half of the couplet composing the macrocolumn of the striate cortex. A similar example is suggested by the mediolateral mapping for aural dominance and the various forms of binaural interaction observed along the isofrequency bands of the auditory cortex.

The property of many-variable representation is a salient feature of an organization in terms of vertical units and one of its important characteristics in terms of cortical function. A series of trade-offs must exist between the degree of fine-grainedness of a topographic representation and the number of variables mapped to it. In the somatic sensory or visual cortex, for example, the specificity required for the representation of place may limit markedly the number of variables simultaneously mapped to the regions. In those homotypical areas of neocortex where topography is much less precise or indeed absent altogether, a large number of variables can be mapped through a given area with preservation of ordered relations between sets on the source side, those within the area, and those in target structures. That is, a number of distributed systems can be mapped through a given area of cortex, thus allowing an integration of their activities (their functions) with properties of that area determined by some other input to it.

A cortical column is a complex processing and distributing unit that links a number of inputs to several outputs. The cells of origin of different output pathways appear to be sharply segregated by cortical layer. Although the intracolumnar channels making these links must certainly overlap and interact, there is evidence that the nature of neuronal processing may differ in different channels. Poggio and his colleagues have given examples of this phenomenon from their work on the visual cortex in waking monkeys. They found that the dynamic properties of spatial-frequency tuning, movement sensitivity, and fine and gross stereopsis are differentially emphasized in the different output channels. It appears likely that other pathways from input to output may be very short, even monosynaptic. Such "throughputs" emphasize the distribution function of a cortical column, as if certain aspects of input signals were being quickly routed to output targets for further processing.

An important property of the intracortical processing mechanisms is what I have termed *pericolumnar inhibition*. It is a powerful mechanism for the functional isolation of active columns from their neighbors, one that brings the concept of columnar organization into conformity with that of partially shifted overlap. The latter is the general principle that as a stimulus of restricted size is shifted in small steps across a receptor sheet, it brings to action a series of shifted but overlapping populations of cortical elements. Pericolumnar inhibition will tend to limit very sharply the lateral spread of activity around the columnar sets most strongly activated by such a local stimulus. This principle undoubtedly holds also for areas of the cortex other than sensory.

FUNCTIONAL PROPERTIES OF DISTRIBUTED SYSTEMS
It is well known from classical neuroanatomy that many of the large entities of the brain are interconnected by extrinsic pathways into complex systems, including massive reentrant circuits. Three sets of recent discoveries, described above, have put the systematic organization of the brain in a new light. The first is that many of the major structures of the brain are constructed by replication of identical multicellular units. These modules are local neural circuits of hundreds or thousands of cells linked together by a complex intramodular connectivity. The modules of any one entity are more or less similar throughout, but those of different entities may differ strikingly. The modular unit of the neocortex is the vertically organized group of cells I have described earlier. These basic units are single translaminar cords of neurons, the minicolumns, which in some areas are packaged into larger processing units whose size and form appear to differ from one place to another. Nevertheless, the qualitative nature of the processing function of the neocortex is thought to be similar in different areas, though that intrinsic processing apparatus may be subject to modification as a result of past history, particularly during critical periods in ontogenetic development.

The second important factor leading to a change in concepts concerning brain function is the accumulation of a vast amount of information concerning the extrinsic connectivity between large entities of the brain. These links are now known to be far more numerous, selective, and specific than previously supposed. The third fact of importance is the discovery that each one of the modules of a large entity does not entertain all the connections known for the entity. Thus the total set of modules of a large entity is fractionated into subsets, each linked by a particular pattern of connections to similarly segregated subsets in other large entities. The linked sets of modules of the several entities are defined as a distributed system. It is obvious that the total number of distributed systems within the brain is much larger than had once been thought, and perhaps by several orders of magnitude. Thus major entities are parts of many distributed systems, contributing to each a property determined for the entity by those connections common to all of its modular subsets and by the particular quality of their intrinsic processing. Even a single module of such an entity may be a member of several (though not many) distributed systems.

Distributed systems are thus composed of large numbers of modular elements linked together in echeloned parallel and serial arrangements. Information flow through such a system may follow a number of different pathways, and the dominance of one path or another is a dynamic and changing property of the system. Such a system has many entries and exits and has access to outflow systems of the brain at many levels. A distributed system displays a redundancy of potential loci of command, and the command function may from time to time reside in different loci of the system, in particular in that part possessing the most urgent and necessary information.

An important feature of such distributed systems, particularly those central to primary sensory and motor systems, is that the complex function controlled or executed by the system is not localized in any one of its parts. The function is a property of the dynamic activity within the system: it resides in the system as such. Part functions, or simple aspects of system function, may be executed by local operations in restricted parts of such a system. This may explain why local lesions of a distributed system scarcely ever destroy system function completely, but degrade it to an extent determined by lesion size and the critical role of the locus destroyed for system function. The remarkable capacity for improvement of function after partial brain lesions is viewed as evidence for the adaptive capacity of such distributed systems to achieve a behavioral goal, albeit slowly and with error, with the remaining neural apparatus.

Finally, distributed systems are by definition and observation both reentrant systems and linkages to inflow and outflow channels of the nervous system. This suggests that the large numbers of processing modules in the neocortex are accessible to both internally generated and externally induced neural activity. Phasic cycling of internally generated activity, accessing first primary sensory but then successively more general and abstract processing units of the homotypical cortex, should allow a continual updating of the perceptual image of self and self-in-the-world as well as a matching function between that perceptual image and impinging external events. This internal readout of internally stored information, and its match with the neural replication of the external continuum, is thought to provide an objective mechanism for conscious awareness. That mechanism is not beyond the reach of scientific enquiry.

REFERENCES

ABELES, M., and M. H. GOLDSTEIN, JR., 1970. Functional architecture in cat primary auditory cortex: Columnar organization and organization according to depth. *J. Neurophysiol.* 33:172–187.

ANDERSSEN, P., P. J. HAGAN, C. G. PHILLIPS, and T. P. S. POWELL, 1975. Mapping by microstimulation of overlapping projections from area 4 to motor units of the baboon's hand. *Proc. R. Soc. Lond.* B188:31–88.

ARMSTRONG-JAMES, M., 1975. The functional status and columnar organization of single cells responding to cutaneous stimulation in neonatal rat somatosensory cortex S-I. *J. Physiol.* 246:501–538.

ASANUMA, H., 1973. Cerebral cortical control of movement. *Physiologist* 16:143–166.

ASANUMA, H., 1975. Recent developments in the study of the columnar arrangement of neurons in the motor cortex. *Physiol. Rev.* 55:143–156.

ASANUMA, H., and I. ROSEN, 1972a. Functional role of afferent input to the monkey motor cortex. *Brain Res.* 40:3–5.

ASANUMA, H., and I. ROSEN, 1972b. Topographical organization of cortical efferent zones projecting to distal forelimb muscles in the monkey. *Exp. Brain Res.* 14:243–256.

ASAUNMA, H., and I. ROSEN, 1973. Spread of mono- and polysynaptic connections within cat's motor cortex. *Exp. Brain Res.* 16:507–520.

BARLOW, H. B., C. BLAKEMORE, AND J. D. PETTIGREW, 1967. The neural mechanisms of binocular depth discrimination. *J. Physiol.* 193:327–342.

BERREVOETS, C. E., and H. G. J. M. KUYPERS, 1975. Pericruciate cortical neurons projecting to brain stem reticular formation, dorsal column nuclei, and spinal cord in cat. *Neurosci. Letters* 1:257–262.

BOK, S. T., 1959. *Histonomy of the Cerebral Cortex*. Princeton: Van Nostrand-Reinhold.

BONIN, B. VON, and P. BAILEY, 1947. *The Neocortex of Macaca Mulatta*. Urbana: University of Illinois Press.

BRUGGE, J. F., and M. M. MERZENICH, 1973. Responses of neurons in auditory cortex of the macaque monkey to monaural and binaural stimulation. *J. Neurophysiol.* 36:1138–1158.

CARLI, G., R. H. LaMOTTE, and V. B. MOUNTCASTLE, 1971a. A comparison of sensory behavior and the activity of postcentral cortical neurons, observed simultaneously, elicited by oscillating mechanical stimuli delivered to the contralateral hand in monkeys. *Proc. 25th Int. Cong. Physiol.*

CARLI, G., R. H. LaMOTTE, and V. B. MOUNTCASTLE, 1971b. A simultaneous study of somatic sensory behavior and the activity of somatic sensory cortical neurons. *Fed. Proc.* 30:664.

CARRERAS, M., and S. A. ANDERSSON, 1963. Functional properties of neurons of the anterior ectosylvian gyrus of the cat. *J. Neurophysiol.* 26:100–126.

CELESIA, G. G., 1976. Organization of auditory cortical areas in man. *Brain* 99:403–414.

COLONNIER, M., 1966. The structural design of the neocortex. In *Brain and Conscious Experience*, J. C. Eccles, ed. New York: Springer-Verlag, pp. 1–23.

COLONNIER, M., 1968. Synaptic patterns on different cell types and the different laminae of the cat visual cortex. An electron-microscope study. *Brain Res.* 9:268–287.

CREUTZFELDT, O., 1976. The brain as a functional entity. *Prog. Brain Res.* 45:451–462.

DOETSCH, G. S., and E. B. GARDNER, 1972. Relationship between afferent input and motor output in sensorimotor cortex of the monkey. *Exp. Neurol.* 35:78–97.

DRYER, D. A., P. R. LOE, C. B. METZ, and B. L. WHITSEL, 1975. Representation of head and face in postcentral gyrus of the macaque. *J. Neurophysiol.* 38:714–733.

DUFFY, F. H., and J. L. BURCHFIEL, 1971. Somatosensory system: Organizational hierarchy from single units in monkey area 5. *Science* 172:273–275.

EVARTS, E. V., 1964. Temporal patterns of discharge of pyramidal tract neurons during sleep and waking in the monkey. *J. Neurophysiol.* 27:152–171.

EVARTS, E. V., 1974. Precentral and postcentral cortical activity in association with visually triggered movements. *J. Neurophysiol.* 37:373–381.

EVARTS, E. V., 1975. The Third Stevenson Lecture. Changing concepts of central control of movement. *Can. J. Physiol. Pharmacol.* 53:191–201.

FELDMAN, M. L., and A. PETERS, 1974. A study of barrels and pyramidal dendritic clusters in the cerebral cortex. *Brain Res.* 77:55–76.

FISKEN, R. A., L. J. GAREY, and T. P. S. POWELL, 1973. Patterns of degeneration after intrinsic lesions of the visual cortex (area 17) of the monkey. *Brain Res.* 51:208–213.

GAREY, L. J., 1976. Synaptic organization of afferent fibres and intrinsic circuits in the neocortex. In *Handbook of EEG Clin. Neurophysiol.*, Vol. 2, Pt. A, Sect. IV. A. Remond, ed. Amsterdam: Elsevier, pp. 57–85.

GAREY, L. J., and T. P. S. POWELL, 1971. An experimental study of the termination of the lateral geniculo-cortical pathways in the cat and the monkey. *Proc. R. Soc. Lond.* B179:41–63.

GATTER, K. C., D. A. WINFIELD, and T. P. S. POWELL, 1977. The neurons of the cortex of areas 4 and 17 in the cat and rat. In preparation.

GILBERT, C. D., and J. P. KELLY, 1975. The projections of cells in different layers of the cat's visual cortex. *J. Comp. Neurol.* 163:81–106.

GLICKSTEIN, M., and D. WHITTERIDGE, 1976. Degeneration of layer III pyramidal cells in area 18 following destruction of callosal input. *Brain Res.* 104:148–151.

GOLDMAN, P., and W. J. H. NAUTA, 1976a. Autoradiographic demonstration of cortico-cortical columns in the motor, frontal association, and limbic cortex of the developing rhesus monkey. *Neurosci. Abstr.*, p. 136.

GOLDMAN, P., and W. J. H. NAUTA, 1976b. An intricately patterned prefrontocaudate projection in the rhesus monkey. *J. Comp. Neurol.* 171:369–385.

GOLDMAN, P. S., and W. J. H. NAUTA, 1977. Columnar distribution of cortico-cortical fibers in the frontal association, limbic, and motor cortex of the developing rhesus monkey. *Brain Res.* 122:393–413.

GRANT, G., S. LANDGREN, and H. SILVENIUS, 1975. Columnar distribution of U-fibres from the postcruciate cerebral projection area of the cat's group I muscle afferents. *Exp. Brain Res.* 24:57–74.

HODOS, W., 1970. Evolutionary interpretation of neural and behavioral studies of living vertebrates. In *The Neurosciences: Second Study Program*, F. O. Schmitt, ed. New York: Rockefeller University Press.

HUBEL, D. H. and T. N. WIESEL, Receptive fields and functional architecture of monkey striate cortex. *J. Physiol.* 195:215–243.

HUBEL, D. H., and T. N. WIESEL, 1970. Cells sensitive to binocular depth in area 18 of the macaque monkey cortex. *Nature* (Lond.) 225:41–72.

HUBEL, D. H., and T. N. WIESEL, 1972. Laminar and columnar distribution of geniculo-cortical fibers in the macaque monkey. *J. Comp. Neurol.* 146:421–450.

HUBEL, D. H., and T. N. WIESEL, 1974a. Sequence, regularity and geometry of orientation columns in the monkey striate cortex. *J. Comp. Neurol.* 158:267–294.

HUBEL, D. H., and T. N. WIESEL, 1974b. Uniformity of monkey striate cortex: A parallel relationship between field size, scatter, and magnification factor. *J. Comp. Neurol.* 158:295–305.

HUBEL, D. H., and T. N. WIESEL, 1977. Functional architecture of macaque monkey cortex. *Proc. R. Soc. Lond.* B198:1–59.

HUMPHREY, D. R., and R. R. RIETZ, 1976. Cells of origin of corticorubral projections from the arm area of primate motor cortex and their synaptic actions in the red nucleus. *Brain Res.* 110:162–169.

HYVÄRINEN, J., and A. PORANEN, 1974. Function of the parietal associative area 7 as revealed from cellular discharges in alert monkeys. *Brain* 97:673–692.

IMIG, T. J., and H. O. ADRIAN, 1977. Binaural columns in the primary (AI) of cat auditory cortex. *Brain Res.* (in press).

JACOBSEN, S., and J. Q. TROJANOWSKI, 1977. Prefrontal granular cortex of the rhesus monkey. II. Interhemispheric cortical afferents. *Brain Res.* 132:235–246.

JANKOWSKA, E., Y. PADEL, and R. TANAKA, 1975a. The mode of activation of pyramidal tract cells by intracortical stimuli. *J. Physiol.* 249:617–636.

JANKOWSKA., E., Y. PADEL, and R. TANAKA, 1975b. Projections of pyramidal tract cells to alpha-motoneurons innervating hind-limb muscles in monkey. *J. Physiol.* 249:636–667.

JERISON, H. J., 1973. *Evaluation of the Brain and Intelligence.* New York: Academic Press.

JONES, E. G., 1975a. Lamination and differential distribution of thalamic afferents within the sensory motor cortex of the squirrel monkey. *J. Comp. Neurol.* 160:167–204.

JONES, E. G., 1975b. Varieties and distribution of non-pyramidal cells in the somatic sensory cortex of the squirrel monkey. *J. Comp. Neurol.* 160:205–267.

JONES, E. G., and H. BURTON, 1976. Areal differences in the laminar distribution of thalamic afferents in cortical fields of the insular, parietal and temporal regions of primates. *J. Comp. Neurol.* 168:197–247.

JONES, E. G., H. BURTON, and R. PORTER, 1975. Commissural and cortico-cortical "columns" in the somatic sensory cortex of primates. *Science* 190: 572–574.

JONES, E. G., J. D. COULTER, H. BURTON, and R. PORTER,

1977. Cells of origin and terminal distribution of corticostriatal fibers arising in the sensory motor cortex of monkeys. *J. Comp. Neurol.* 173:53–80.

JONES, E. G., and T. P. S. POWELL, 1970. An electron microscopic study of the laminar pattern and mode of termination of afferent fibre pathways in the somatic sensory cortex of the cat. *Phil. Trans. R. Soc. Lond.* B257: 1–11.

JONES, E. G., and S. P. WISE, 1977. Size, laminar and columnar distribution of efferent cells in the sensory-motor cortex of primates. *J. Comp. Neurol.* 175:391–438.

KNIGHT, P. L., 1977. Representation of the cochlea within the anterior auditory field (AAF) of the cat. *Brain Res.* 130:447–467.

KUNZLE, H., 1976. Alternating afferent zones of high and low axon terminal density within the macaque motor cortex. *Brain Res.* 106:365–370.

LASHLEY, K. S., 1949. Persistent problems in the evolution of mind. *Quart. Rev. Biol.* 24:28–42.

LASHLEY, K. S., and G. CLARK, 1946. The cytoarchitecture of the cerebral cortex of Ateles: A critical examination of cytoarchitectonic studies. *J. Comp. Neurol.* 85:223–305.

LENON, R. N., and R. PORTER, 1976. Afferent input to movement-related precentral neurones in conscious monkeys. *Proc. R. Soc. Lond.* B194:313–339.

LeVAY, S., 1973. Synaptic patterns in the visual cortex of the cat and monkey. Electron microscopy of Golgi preparations. *J. Comp. Neurol.* 150:53–86.

LORENTE DE NÓ, R., 1938. Cerebral cortex: Architecture, intracortical connections, motor projections. In *Physiology of the Nervous System*, J. F. Fulton, ed. New York: Oxford University Press, pp. 291–339.

LUND, J. S., 1973. Organization of neurons in the visual cortex area 17 of the monkey (*Macaca mulatta*). *J. Comp. Neurol.* 147:455–496.

LUND, J. S., and R. G. BOOTHE, 1975. Interlaminar connections and pyramidal neuron organization in the visual cortex, area 17, of the macaque monkey. *J. Comp. Neurol.* 159:305–334.

LUND, J. S., R. D. LUND, A. E. HENDRICKSON, A. H. BUNT, and A. F. FUCHS, 1975. The origin of efferent pathways from the primary visual cortex, area 17, of the macaque monkey as shown by retrograde transport of horseradish peroxidase. *J. Comp. Neurol.* 164:287–304.

LYNCH, J. C., C. ACUNA, H. SAKATA, A. GEORGOPOULOS, and V. B. MOUNTCASTLE, 1973a. The parietal association area and immediate extrapersonal space. *Proc. Soc. Neurosci.*

LYNCH, J. C., H. SAKATA, A. GEORGOPOULOS, and V. B. MOUNTCASTLE, 1973b. Parietal association cortex neurons active during hand and eye tracking of objects in immediate extrapersonal space. *Physiologist* 16:384.

LYNCH, J. C., V. B. MOUNTCASTLE, W. H. TALBOT, and T. C. T. YIN, 1977. Parietal lobe mechanisms of directed visual attention. *J. Neurophysiol.* 40:362–389.

MARIN-PADILLA, M., 1969. Origin of the pericellular baskets of the pyramidal cells of the human motor cortex: A Golgi study. *Brain Res.* 14:633–646.

MARIN-PADILLA, M., 1970. Prenatal and early postnatal ontogenesis of the human motor cortex: A Golgi study. II. The basket-pyramidal system. *Brain Res.* 23:185–191.

MELLER, K., and W. TETZLAFF, 1975. Neuronal migration during the early development of the cerebral cortex: A scanning electron microscopic study. *Cell Tissue Res.* 163:313–325.

MERZENICH, M. M., and J. F. BRUGGE, 1973. Representation of the cochlear partition on the superior temporal plane of the macaque monkey. *Brain Res.* 50:275–296.

MERZENICH, M. M., P. L. KNIGHT, and G. L. ROTH, 1975. Representation of cochlea within primary auditory cortex in the cat. *J. Neurophysiol.* 38:231–249.

MOLLIVER, M. E., R. GRZANNA, J. H. MORISON, and J. T. COYLE, 1977. Immunohistochemical characterization of noradrenergic innervation in the rat neocortex: A regional and laminar analysis. *Neurosci. Abstr.*

MOORE, R. Y., and F. E. BLOOM, 1977. Central catecholamine neuron systems: Anatomy and physiology. *Annu. Rev. Neurosci.* (in press).

MOUNTCASTLE, V. B., 1957. Modality and topographic properties of single neurons of cat's somatic sensory cortex. *J. Neurophysiol.* 20:408–434.

MOUNTCASTLE, V. B., 1975. The view from within: Pathways to the study of perception. *Johns Hopkins Med. J.* 136:109–131.

MOUNTCASTLE, V. B., 1976. The world around us: Neural command functions for selective attention. The F. O. Schmitt Lecture for 1975. *Neurosci. Res. Program Bull.* 14 (Suppl. 1).

MOUNTCASTLE, V. B., 1977. Brain mechanisms for directed attention. The Sherrington Memorial Lecture. *Proc. R. Soc. Med.* (in press).

MOUNTCASTLE, V. B., J. C. LYNCH, A. GEORGOPOULOS, H. SAKATA, and A. ACUNA, 1975. Posterior parietal association cortex of the monkey: Command functions for operations within extrapersonal space. *J. Neurophysiol.* 38:871–908.

MOUNTCASTLE, V. B., and T. P. S. POWELL, 1959a. Central nervous mechanisms subserving position sense and kinesthesis. *Bull. Johns Hopkins Hosp.* 105:173–200.

MOUNTCASTLE, V. B., and T. P. S. POWELL, 1959b. Neural mechanisms subserving cutaneous sensibility, with special reference to the role of afferent inhibition in sensory perception and discrimination. *Bull. Johns Hopkins Hosp.* 105:201–232.

MOUNTCASTLE, V. B., W. H. TALBOT, H. SAKATA, and J. HYVÄRINEN, 1969. Cortical neuronal mechanisms studied in unanesthetized monkeys. Neuronal periodicity and frequency discrimination. *J. Neurophysiol.* 32:454–484.

NIKARA, T., P. O. BISHOP, and J. C. PETTIGREW, 1968. Analysis of retinal correspondence by studying receptive fields of binocular single units in cat striate cortex. *Exp. Brain Res.* 6:353–372.

PARKER, D. E., 1965. Vertical organization of the auditory cortex of the cat. *J. Audit. Res.* 2:99–124.

PASTERNAK, J. R., and T. A. WOOLSEY, 1975. The number, size, and spatial distribution of neurons in lamina IV of the mouse SMI neocortex. *J. Comp. Neurol.* 160:291–306.

PAUL, R. L., M. MERZENICH, and H. GOODMAN, 1972. Representation of slowly and rapidly adapting cutaneous mechanoreceptors of the hand in Brodmann's areas 3 and 1 of *Macaca mulatta*. *Brain Res.* 36:229–249.

PETTIGREW, J. D., T. NIKARA, and P. O. BISHOP, 1968. Binocular interaction on single units in cat striate cortex: Simultaneous stimulation by single moving slit with receptive fields in correspondence. *Exp. Brain Res.* 6:391–410.

PHILLIPS, C. C., 1969. Motor apparatus of the baboon's hand. *Proc. R. Soc. Lond.* B173:141–174.

POGGIO, G. F., F. H. BAKER, R. J. W. MANSFIELD, A. SILLITO, and P. GRIGG, 1975. Spatial and chromatic properties of neurons subserving foveal and parafoveal vision in rhesus monkey. *Brain Res.* 100:25–59.

POGGIO, G. F., R. W. DOTY, JR., and W. H. TALBOT, 1977. Foveal striate cortex of the behaving monkey. Single neuron responses to square-wave gratings during fixation of gaze. *J. Neurophysiol.* 40:1369–1391.

POGGIO, G. F., and B. FISHER, 1977. Binocular interaction and depth sensitivity of striate and prestriate cortical neurons of the behaving rhesus monkey. *J. Neurophysiol.* 40:1392–1405.

POWELL, T. P. S., and V. B. MOUNTCASTLE, 1959. Some aspects of the functional organization of the cortex of the postcentral gyrus of the monkey: A correlation of findings obtained in a single unit analysis with cytoarchitecture. *Bull. Johns Hopkins Hosp.* 105:133–162.

POWELL, T. P. S., and V. B. MOUNTCASTLE, 1977. Unpublished observations of a series of fetal monkey brains kindly supplied by D. Bodian.

RADINSKY, L. B., 1967. Relative brain size: A new measure. *Science* 155:836–837.

RAICHLE, M. E., B. K. HARTMAN, J. O. EICHLING, and L. G. SHARPE, 1975. Central adrenergic regulation of cerebral blood flow and vascular permeability. *Proc. Natl. Acad. Sci. USA* 72:3726–3730.

RAKIC, P., 1971. Guidance of neurons migrating to the fetal monkey neocortex. *Brain Res.* 33:471–476.

RAKIC, P., 1972. Mode of cell migration to the superficial layers of fetal monkey neocortex. *J. Comp. Neurol.* 145:61–84.

RAKIC, P., 1974. Neurons in rhesus monkey visual cortex: Systematic relation between time of origin and eventual disposition. *Science* 183:425–427.

RAKIC, P., 1975. Timing of major ontogenetic events in the visual cortex of the rhesus monkey. In *Brain Mechanisms in Mental Retardation*, J. Buchwald and M. Brazier, eds. New York: Academic Press.

RAKIC, P., 1977. Prenatal development of the visual system in rhesus monkey. *Philos. Trans. R. Soc. Lond.* B278:245–260.

RAKIC, P., 1978. Neuronal migration and contact guidance in the primate telencephalon. *Postgrad. Med. J.* (in press).

ROCKEL, A. J., R. W. HIORNS, and T. P. S. POWELL, 1974. Numbers of neurons through full depth of neocortex. *Proc. Anat. Soc. Gr. Br. Ire.* 118:371.

ROSE, J. E., 1949. The cellular structure of the auditory region of the cat. *J. Comp. Neurol.* 91:409–440.

ROSE, J. E., and C. N. WOOLSEY, 1948a. Structure and relations of limbic cortex and anterior thalamic nuclei in rabbit and cat. *J. Comp. Neurol.* 89: 279–348.

ROSE, J. E., and C. N. WOOLSEY, 1948b. The orbitofrontal cortex and its connections with the mediodorsal nucleus in rabbit, sheep and cat. *Assoc. Res. Nerv. Ment. Dis.* 27:210–232.

ROSE, J. E., and C. N. WOOLSEY, 1949. The relations of thalamic connections, cellular structure and evocable electrical activity in the auditory region of the cat. *J. Comp. Neurol.* 91:441–466.

SACHER, G. A., 1970. Allometric and factorial analysis of brain structure in insectivores and primates. In *The Primate Brain*, C. R. Noback and W. Montagna, eds. New York: Appleton-Century-Crofts, pp. 245–287.

SAKATA, H., Y. TAKAOKA, A. KAWARASAKI, and H. SHIBUTANI, 1973. Somatosensory properties of neurons in the superior parietal cortex (area 5) of the rhesus monkey. *Brain Res.* 64:85–102.

SCHMECHEL, D. E., and P. RAKIC, 1973. Evolution of fetal radial glial cells in rhesus monkey telencephalon. A Golgi study. *Anat. Rec.* 175:436.

SCHMITT, F. O., P. DEV., and B. H. SMITH, 1976. Electrotonic processing of information by brain cells. *Science* 193:114–120.

SHANKS, M. F., R. C. A. PEARSON, and T. P. S. POWELL, 1977. The intrinsic connections of the primary sensory cortex of the monkey. *Proc. R. Soc. Lond.* (in press).

SHANKS, M. F., A. J. ROCKEL, and T. P. S. POWELL, 1975. The commissural fibre connections of the primary somatic sensory cortex. *Brain Res.* 98:166–171.

SHOUMURA, K., 1974. An attempt to relate the origin and distribution of commissural fibres to the presence of large and medium pyramids in layer III in the cat's visual cortex. *Brain Res.* 67:13–25.

SHOUMURA, K., T. ANDO, and K. KATO, 1975. Structural organization of "callosal" OBg in human corpus callosum agenesis. *Brain Res.* 93:241–252.

SIDMAN, R. L., 1970. Autoradiographic methods and principles for study of the nervous system with thymidine-H^3. In *Contemporary Research Techniques in Neuroanatomy*, O. E. Ebbesson and W. J. H. Nauta, eds. New York: Springer-Verlag.

SIDMAN, R. L., and P. RAKIC, 1973. Neuronal migration, with special reference to developing human brain: A review. *Brain Res.* 62:1–35.

SLOPER, J. J., 1973. An electron microscope study of the termination of afferent connections to the primate motor cortex. *J. Neurocytol.* 2:361–368.

SOUSA-PINTA, A., 1973. The structure of the first auditory cortex (AI) in the cat. I. Light microscopic observations on its organization. *Arch. Ital. Biol.* 111:112–137.

STEPHAN, H., 1967. Quantitative Vergleiche zur phylogenetischen Entwicklung des Gehirns der Primaten mit Hilfe von Progressionindices. *Mitt. Max-Planck-Ges.* 2:63–86.

STEPHAN, H., 1969. Quantitative investigations on visual structures in primate brains. In *Proc. 2nd Int. Cong. Primat.* Vol. 3: *Neurology, Physiology, and Infectious Diseases*, H. O. Hofer, ed. Basel: Karger, pp. 34–42.

STEPHAN, H., 1972. Evolution of primate brains: A comparative anatomical investigation. In *The Functional and Evolutionary Biology of Primates*, T. Tuttle, ed. Chicago: Aldine-Atherton, pp. 155–174.

STEPHAN, H., and O. J. ANDY, 1964. Quantitative comparisons of brain structures from insectivores to primates. *Am. Zool.* 4:59–74.

STEPHAN, H., and O. J. ANDY, 1969. Quantitative comparative neuroanatomy of primates: An attempt at a phylogenetic interpretation. *Ann. NY Acad. Sci.* 167:370–387.

STEPHAN, H., R. BAUCHOT, and O. J. ANDY, 1970. Data on size of the brain of various brain parts in insectivores and primates. In *The Primate Brain*, C. R. Noback and W. Montagna, eds. New York: Appleton-Century-Crofts, pp. 289–297.

STEPHANIS, C., and H. JASPER, 1964. Recurrent collateral

inhibition in pyramidal tract neurons. *J. Neurophysiol.* 27:855–877.

SUGA, N., 1977. Amplitude spectrum representation in the Doppler-shifted CF processing area of the auditory cortex of the mustache bat. *Science* 196:64–67.

SZENTÁGOTHAI, J., 1973. Synaptology of the visual cortex. In *Visual Centers of the Brain (Handbook of Sensory Physiology*, Vol. VII/3), R. Jung, ed. Berlin-New York: Springer-Verlag.

SZENTÁGOTHAI, J., 1975. The "module-concept" in cerebral cortex architecture. *Brain Res.* 95:475–496.

SZENTÁGOTHAI, J., 1976. Basic circuitry of the neocortex. *Exp. Brain Res.* (Suppl. 1): 282–287.

SZENTÁGOTHAI, J., and M. A. ARBIB, 1974. Conceptual models of neural organization. *Neurosci. Res. Program Bull.* 12:307–510.

TÖMBÖL, T., 1974. An electron microscopic study of the neurons of the visual cortex. *J. Neurocytol.* 3:525–531.

TOWE, A. L., 1975. Notes on the hypothesis of columnar organization in somatosensory cortex. *Brain Behav. Evol.* 11:16–47.

TUNTURI, A. R., 1952. A difference in the representation of auditory signals for the left and right ears in the isofrequency contours of the right middle ectosylvian auditory cortex of the dog. *Am. J. Physiol.* 168:712–727.

TUNTURI, A. R., and J. A. DUDMAN, 1958. Model of storage space in the MES auditory cortex. *Am. J. Physiol.* 192:437–446.

WASHBURN, S. L., and R. S. HARDING, 1970. Evolution of primate behavior. In *The Neurosciences: Second Study Program*, F. O. Schmitt, ed. New York: Rockefeller University Press, pp. 39–47.

WELKER, C., 1971. Microelectrode delineation of fine grain somatotopic organization of SMI cerebral neocortex in albino rat. *Brain Res.* 26:259–275.

WERNER, G., and B. L. WHITSEL, 1968. Topology of the body representation in somatosensory I of primates. *J. Neurophysiol.* 31:856–869.

WERNER, G., and B. L. WHITSEL, 1973. The somatic sensory cortex: Functional organization. In *The Somatosensory System (Handbook of Sensory Physiology*, Vol. II), A. Iggo, ed. Berlin-New York: Springer-Verlag.

WHITSEL, B. L., and D. A. DREYER, 1976. Comparison of single unit data obtained from the different topographic subdivisions of the postcentral gyrus of the macaque: Implications for the organization of somatosensory projection pathways. *Exp. Brain Res.* (Suppl. 1): 415–420.

WHITSEL, B. L., D. A. DREYER, and J. R. ROPOLLO, 1971. Determinants of the body representation in the postcentral gyrus of macaques. *J. Neurophysiol.* 34:1018.

WHITSEL, B. L., L. M. PETRUCELLI, and G. WERNER, 1969. Symmetry and connectivity in the map of the body surface in somatosensory area II of primates. *J. Neurophysiol.* 32:170–183.

WHITSEL, B. L., J. R. ROPOLLO, and G. WERNER, 1972. Cortical information processing of stimulus motion on primate skin. *J. Neurophysiol.* 35:691–717.

WINFIELD, D. A., and T. P. S. POWELL, 1976. The termination of thalamo-cortical fibres in the visual cortex of the cat. *J. Neurocytol.* 5:269–281.

WOOLSEY, C. N., 1960. Organization of cortical auditory system. In *Neural Mechanism of the Auditory and Vestibular Systems*, G. L. Rasmussen and W. F. Windle, eds. Springfield, Ill.: Thomas.

WOOLSEY, T. A., and H. VAN DER LOOS, 1970. The structural organization of layer IV in the somatosensory region (SI) of mouse cerebral cortex. The description of a cortical field composed of discrete cytoarchitectural units. *Brain Res.* 17:205–242.

WOOLSEY, T. A., C. WELKER, and R. H. SCHWARTZ, 1975. Comparative anatomical studies of the SMI face cortex with special reference to the occurrence of 'barrels' in layer IV. *J. Comp. Neurol.* 164:79–94.

ZEKI, S., 1974. The mosaic organization of the visual cortex in the monkey. In *A Festschrift for Professor J. Z. Young*, R. Bellairs and E. G. Gray, eds. London: Oxford University Press, pp. 327–343.

ZEKI, S. M., 1975. The functional organization of projections from striate to prestriate visual cortex in the rhesus monkey. *Cold Spring Harbor Symp. Quant. Biol.* 40:591–600.

ZEKI, S. M., 1977. Colour coding in the superior temporal sulcus of rhesus monkey visual cortex. *Proc. R. Soc. Lond.* (in press).

3 Evolving Concepts of Local Integrative Operations in Neurons

THEODORE HOLMES BULLOCK

ABSTRACT This chapter—and much of this Study Program—puts emphasis on the integrative operations and local interactions between parts of neighboring neurons. An accelerating pace of new insights added to accumulated clues points to a further quiet revolution in concepts at this level. Due for refinement are the ideas of the neuron membrane as a mosaic, in particular the "locus concept," which recognized differences in properties between parts of dendrites causing inhibitory and parts causing excitatory synaptic responses of slower and of faster time course; parts responsible for pacemaking, for impulse initiation, and for conducting; and points of failure or filtering, including terminal arbors with various properties such as facilitation. Interactions vary not only with anatomical relations and types of transmitter but due to different slopes of input-output curves and to cooperative effects. The list of variables available to neurons and small arrays of neurons with which they can integrate signals and states is sizable and still growing. These are permuted with the still greater number of different anatomical relations between definable types of cells. Typically, the combination of arrangement and properties is a consistent characterization of a locus—at least to some microscopic level. Below that, probabilistic statements are necessary. This means that consistent specification is high down to a small microscopic level. It is proposed that similar processes and mechanisms operate to account for common neuronal operations and for higher nervous functions.

CONFRONTED WITH an interesting device we first ask, "What's the principle?" or "How does it work?" This essay—and much of this ISP—will be focused on the operating principles of nervous systems. Although these are first-order questions in understanding a device like the brain, they have lagged behind questions of componentry at the cellular, subcellular, and chemical levels. Progress has been faster on the nature of membranes, nerve impulses, and transmitters. But it is well that we give attention to the more integrative levels without waiting for an adequate understanding of all the basic mechanisms.

THEODORE HOLMES BULLOCK Department of Neurosciences, School of Medicine and Neurobiology Unit, Scripps Institution of Oceanography, University of California, San Diego, La Jolla, CA 92093

Gerald Edelman speaks for many of us when he states that the most challenging problem in neurobiology is the determination of the structural substrates and cellular mechanisms of higher brain functions (see chapter 68). He is emphasizing the same point: the study of how neural elements work together. This concern is not new, but our concepts of the integrative operations of such elements have evolved greatly in a few decades.

Let me define my scope. Whatever components are involved, the neural transactions they accomplish must eventually be understood in terms of encoding and decoding signals, weighting, combining and filtering information, generating patterns in space and time—in short, operations we call integrative. Integration occurs at many levels, from subcellular interactions to long pathways between large entities. The domain of our concern here is called, for convenience, "local." This may be defined in terms of dimensions within the range of micrometers to millimeters.

The quiet revolution in concepts of neuronal operations, from the purely all-or-none impulse-bearing neuron of McCulloch and Pitts (1943), can be traced to the first preparation for studying single synapses introduced by Prosser in 1935 in the abdominal ganglion of crayfish (see also Prosser, 1937). Wiersma in 1933, Pantin in 1935, and Katz in 1936 demonstrated facilitation in the neuromuscular junction of crustaceans and medusae. Excitatory synaptic potentials were found at crayfish neuromuscular junctions by Wiersma and van Harreveld (1935, 1938), together with several of their labile integrative properties, including direct suppression by inhibitory synapses. This inhibition also shows facilitation. Hodgkin discovered the subthreshold local response of axons in crab's legs in 1938; Lloyd showed direct central inhibition upon the spinal motor neurons in 1941. Eccles and his collaborators recorded the inhibitory postsynaptic potential in 1952 (Brock, Coombs, and Eccles, 1952). By 1949 the dendrite was widely recognized as an integrating, graded, receptive region, and the spike-initiating zone was recognized as another integrative locus. Presynaptic inhibition was already clearly demonstrated by Marmont and Wiersma in 1938, and called α-inhibition by Katz (1949), but it took off anew with the work of Dudel and Kuffler in 1961. Only later did the notion take root that axonal terminals commonly carry a decrementing impulse and are therefore labile and integrative. Later still, and more hesitantly, the idea became recognized that in many places decremental spread is normal, even starting with overshooting action potentials (Bryant, 1977, 1978).

In 1955 Hagiwara and I recorded the EPSP from the squid giant synapse, with intracellular microelectrodes close to the junction, and showed positively that the current from the presynaptic spike is far too small to transmit (Bullock and Hagiwara, 1955, 1957). This laid to rest the possibility of electrical transmission at such synapses, an alternative until then very much alive. About the same time Furshpan and Potter (1957, 1959) demonstrated that electrical transmission does exist at some synapses. In 1959 Watanabe and I reported perhaps the first case of a subthreshold potential in one neuron causing an excitatory effect on another (Watanabe and Bullock, 1959, 1960). This was in the cardiac ganglion of the lobster; the communication between the cells in question requires a slow potential, so that spikes are quite ineffective. The communication link is electrotonic, attenuating, and low-pass filtering, incapable of propagating a spike.

By 1959 there was a significant list of integrative neuronal variables capable of contributing to the determination of output. The list has steadily expanded and may be expected to continue to grow. Table I is a revised version of a list of ways neurons can differ one from another in respect to integrative parameters (Bullock, 1976). I give it here in a condensed format that often places more than two alternatives under one item.

TABLE I

Partial list of variables available to neurons and small arrays of neurons with which integration of signals and states may be accomplished, apart from anatomical arrangements

1. Electrotonic connections between parts of neurons and between neurons may have high or low series resistance and high or low shunt capacitance.

2. Local potentials as active subthreshold responses can have higher or lower steepness of their nonlinear, input-output functions.

3. Safety factor can be locally high or low.

4. Accommodation can be large or small, fast or slow.

5. Recovery through the functional refractory period can be fast or slow.

6. Afterpotentials can be large or small, long or short.

7. Iterativeness can be high or low, tonic or phasic; firing rate/depolarization function can be steep or shallow, limited by autoinhibition earlier or later.

8. Autorhythmicity can be present, absent, contingent, high, low, regular, patterned, bursty, or irregular.

9. Miniature, quantal potentials can be absent, few or many, larger or smaller.

10. Synaptic transmission can be chemical, electrical, or both, polarized or unpolarized.

11. Synaptic transmission can be excitatory or inhibitory, low-gain or high-gain.

12. Postsynaptic potentials can be short or long, monophasic or biphasic; decaying passively or in part actively.

13. Postsynaptic response can be both potential change and conductance change or mainly one of these.

14. Postsynaptic response can exert an influence back on the presynaptic ending, or not.

15. Postsynaptic response after the end of input can continue or rebound or decay rapidly.

16. Inhibition can occur with increased or decreased conductance.

17. Inhibition can occur with discrete IPSP or slowly rising and long-lasting potential.

18. Facilitation and antifacilitation, early, late or both in sequence, may occur at different stages in transmission, homo- or heterosynaptically.

19. Influence of transmitters can be at close, intermediate, or long range.

20. Modulation by hormones, CO_2, temperature, field potentials, and various agents can differ in direction and degree.

21. Chemical transmission can modulate the effectiveness of electrical transmission, and vice versa.

22. Synchrony of subthreshold potentials between neurons can be strong or weak or at chance level.

23. Plasticity as a result of environmental influence or history can be high or low.

Source: Modified from Bullock (1975).

Let us look at the kinds of variables there are. Electrotonic connections (item 1) between neurons, like those between parts of the same neuron, are not merely present or absent. They range from slightly to severely attenuating, and some are low-pass filters.

The safety factor (item 3) is the ratio of depolarization, at a given locus, due to the approaching impulse, to the spike threshold at that place. In ordinary spike-conducting axons, it is higher than four. If it drops below 1.0, the spike dies out. What has become clear is that the safety factor sometimes drops below 1.0 at branch points and near the axon terminal and probably at some other loci in various neurons. This may be the result of certain intervals between impulses and can set up a filter for certain frequencies.

Spikeless neurons are not peculiar to the retina. They were shown already in 1968 by Ripley, Bush, and Roberts in crab leg stretch receptors (see also Bush and Roberts, 1968). These are large, long-axon neurons and give only graded subthreshold potentials to adequate stimuli that cause reflex responses. Penetration of the axon and depolarization of this single neuron to a subthreshold degree cause the normal reflex, although the ganglion is 10 mm away. Many interneurons in insect central ganglia also normally function without impulses, as Pearson and Fourtner (1975) have shown (see also Pearson, this volume). This has been predicted for a long time, and it remains one of the important general questions: How widespread are such neurons? The closely related question has not been as much studied: May some neurons that *can* spike perform some of their function without spiking, in the sense of exerting an influence, whether specific or diffuse, upon other neurons? By a modest extrapolation from what we know, I predict the answer will be affirmative.

Accommodation (item 4) is little studied today and not understood. I speak of intracellularly measured threshold shifts. In the squid giant axon the classical sodium theory predicted an early accommodation, that is, a rise in threshold with subthreshold depolarization, as when slowly rising stimuli are applied, but the finding was a small, delayed rise. Accommodation is still an empirical property, and it is widely different among neurons and parts of neurons; it can be dominating in somata and virtually absent in axons.

Variable aftereffects (item 6), degrees of the tendency to give impulses repetitively to maintained stimuli (item 7, "tonic" vs. "phasic" response), spontaneity (item 8), and other related properties are consistent personality features of each type of neuron and within certain sets may be correlated (Kernell, 1965; Koike et al., 1970).

The degrees of freedom increase when we take one or more additional neurons into consideration, as in junctional transmission (items 10–19), and again when we look at second-order effects such as modulations of transmission (items 20–23).

I direct your special attention to some items that go beyond the familiar or classical synaptic properties. First, remember that postsynaptic potentials (PSPs) show a wide variation in size, in duration (item 12), in the prominence of facilitation or antifacilitation (item 18), and in the tendency after the end of a burst of input to rebound or otherwise (item 15). Some PSPs decay passively, but others have a pronounced active decrementing component; some are diphasic (item 12). Perhaps less familiar are the possibilities of feedback effects of the postsynaptic unit upon the presynaptic endings (item 14), or the possibility that postsynaptic response can be accompanied by a decrease in membrane conductance (item 16) instead of the classical increase, or that a brief burst of input can cause a postsynaptic potential shift that lasts for many thousands of milliseconds (item 17).

Some forms of presynaptic interaction have been "classical" for more than 15 years. But new forms have been discovered that may have quite different bases. Electrical synapses can alter the effectiveness of chemical synapses and vice versa (item 21). Electrical synapses can even reverse the sign of electrotonic coupling, so that hyperpolarization and depolarization of one cell cause depolarization and hyperpolarization of other cells (Spira, Spray, and Bennett, 1976).

Another degree of freedom that slowly gained acceptance in the peripheral nervous system, particularly in smooth muscle, now appears to be potentially widespread in the CNS. This is the normal action of transmitters at a distance, far above the dimensions in angstrom units of classical synaptic clefts, possibly up to a few microns or even more (item 19). This relatively nonspecific action at a distance grades into a heterogeneous array of modulatory effects of more or less specific substances and agents such as electric fields (item 20).

This list of variables has been compressed in several ways. For example, I have not listed the available candidate codes or forms of representing information in neuronal activity. Clearly there is not a single code of the brain, waiting to be broken, but many ways in which states and signals can be represented, in graded changes in neurons, in spike trains with several statistical parameters besides mean frequency, and in spatiotemporal configurations of both the graded and the spike activity in ensembles or sets of neurons and associated glia. The number of codes used by nervous systems at the various levels of the "local circuit" or parts of interacting neurons—including graded unit behavior, spiking unit behavior and ensemble behavior—simply cannot be stated today. A lower bound would have to be in the dozens; an upper limit depends on the scope of one's taxonomy.

It would certainly be an important task for the future to discover the forbidden or unlikely combinations and the more likely combinations—in short, to find rules and to reduce the available permutations. At the same time, it is an important task to look for further variables available to neurons. The list has been growing and will surely continue to grow.

The range and variety of neuronal variables available to single units and small arrays of units, with which they may integrate signals and states, subthreshold as well as impulse signals, are so formidable that it is really beyond our ordinary human grasp to hold in mind at one time so many possibilities and permutations of them without imposing some simplification on the list. This is all the more staggering when we add the vast complexities available in anatomical arrangement and in arrays of larger and larger number, variety, and connectivity. The nervous system has large numbers of cell types; some three dozen distinct kinds of neurons have been defined in the insect optic ganglia; more than forty kinds in the human cerebral cortex.

Most of the distinguishing criteria used so far concern the branching of processes and the opportunities for connections with particular other cell types and on particular parts of the neuron. Comparative studies of nerve cells and their processes have revealed a long list of definable types of junctions (Bullock and Horridge, 1965; Bullock, Orkand, and Grinnell, 1977). To list just a few as samples, we have, at low magnification, climbing fiber contacts, mossy fiber claw contacts, basket endings, calyces, nests, shrubs, pannicles, and clubs; at high magnification (EM), we have Gray's types 1 and 2, serial axo-axonal, reciprocal dendrodendritic, ribbon, gap, spine, glomerular, and other types. Neuropil is the finest-textured tissue, with endings of processes—afferent, efferent, and mixed—undiluted by cell bodies. A few years ago we thought the neuropil was an unorganized chaos. The advances of modern anatomy—among the fastest-moving fields of neuroscience—are steadily reducing this chaos to order. We can now foresee the enunciation of rules and better and better descriptions of the synaptic complexes where not two but many neurons (pre- and postsynaptic) come together, and of the microcircuitry of neuropil in laminated regions and even in seemingly randomly arrayed regions. Progress in understanding in these respects is one-way—toward more and more definition, specification, and consistent order—and no end is in sight. Thus the list of available integrative mechanisms is lengthened substantially, since the functional variables of Table I can permute with the mi-croarchitectonic variables. Again I would emphasize that we must hope and look for rules, forbidden and favored combinations, at the same time that we expect still more possibilities, parameters, and complexities to be encountered.

It has been said as a first approximation to considerations of higher-level models that all nervous systems, low and high, obey the same principles of signal transmission, so that higher species and higher brain functions must depend solely on organization. Here I would underline that only for a few of the classical synaptic properties can we say that the principles are general. There is a great deal of room for at least quantitative differences, and especially for combinatorial differences, for unfamiliar principles, and for limitations upon the full range of the variable, among medusae, worms, slugs, insects, fish, and other creatures. Higher functions might well depend not only upon organization among millions of neurons but also upon parameter sets at the level of unit neurons and local circuits, as in the example of repetitive firing parameters within a defined neuron pool.

The degrees of freedom have increased—and show no sign of a plateau of discovery. The clues have accumulated that radical changes are likely in our classical picture of how nervous systems work. The "quiet revolution" noted in 1959 is continuing and accelerating.

For my own heuristic it is not yet enough to boil down all the presently known neuronal integrative parameters into a list of 23 items (Table I). It helps me, at any rate, to continue the distillation while broadening the scope beyond the single neuron, and I think it may serve through several years of the accelerating revolution to recognize three broad issues that embrace much of this list.

How far does the locus concept go? It will be of prime importance in the understanding of local interactions to learn how mosaic the membrane is. How many kinds of membrane are there? How do they differ and what influence do they have on each other? How small are the patches and how discrete? How fixed or how plastic are the properties or the boundaries? I shall not attempt any answers to these questions. They form a bridge for my purposes between the list of integrative parameters, suggestive of differentiated membrane properties, apparently without order or system, and the next issue, suggestive of considerable order and system.

How far does specification go? That is, how far does the concept of a specified or identifiable element go? Does it apply not only to the neuromere (telencephalon, diencephalon, mesencephalon, etc.), the lobe, the nucleus, the addressable subdivision of a nucleus, but also to the circuit, the glomerulus, the neuron, the dendrite—of the first, second, third, or higher order of branching—and to the synaptic contact? Does identifiability of neuronal specification apply only to giant neurons, motor neurons in species with very few of them, and exceptional interneurons in invertebrates with small numbers of cells?

I shall venture an opinion on this issue. It seems likely to me that we are far from seeing the end of the list of identifiable neurons, that the list will extend into the vertebrates well beyond the Mauthners, Müllers, and electromotor command cells of fishes. I believe that highly specified neurons, not quite individually identifiable but identifiable within an ambiguity of 2 or 3 or 10 or 20 neurons, will be found to be very common indeed, even at cortical levels.

Subcellularly, I believe the evolving concept as it stands today indicates that even in identifiable cells, among separate individuals, only a few of the lowest-order processes are rather constant (for example, first- and second-order dendrites), whereas the higher-order branches and the synaptic contacts as discrete anatomical elements are not identifiable. Nevertheless, based on physiology, a rather high degree of specification must obtain for the array of contacts that makes up the functional synapse. We can think of this in terms of an analogy. Trees of a given species have a characteristic silhouette, although no two are alike in detail. Other species, such as particular types (analogous to cell types) of birds and insects, make contact with them in characteristic ways and places. Both are far from random, although probabilistic statements are the most convenient descriptions.

This issue and this set of tentative answers leads me right into the next, and last, issue. How far can a knowledge of local circuits take us in understanding larger sets of cells and higher functions? This issue is a far cry from reciprocal synapses and spikeless neurons. Still, the ISP table of contents reflects the keen concern of many people, organizers and authors, for shedding light on behavior. A range of references culminates in Edelman's theory of higher brain function. We may show the bridge between these levels by raising a few key questions that represent the evolving conceptual issues. Are local circuits to be regarded as intermediate-level components in a hierarchical system of circuits? Or are they trivial and irrelevant to understanding higher functions, compared to the properties of very large numbers of elements, accessible to us only by studying the intact mass or the whole brain? Do the local circuits accomplish significant signal processing, filtering, mixing or evaluating, recognizing, deciding or formulating of output? Are they very sloppy and only useful probabilistically? Are gross field potentials merely epiphenomena?

Such questions call for a good deal of extrapolation from the firmer facts of lower levels. It is not only interest in the behavior of intact organisms that emboldens some of us to step out on such shaky ground. It is as well the need of neuroscience for synthesis, for heuristic propositions, for hard effort at the conceptual level. And it is in the expectation of breakthroughs, of further revolutions, especially those that span the gap between approaches and between levels of organization.

I shall not undertake to go very far toward an answer to these questions. But I think it may help to enunciate a few propositions bearing on them. An analogy may make these clearer—an extension of an old one developed in the last ISP (Bullock, 1974).

The nervous system may be thought of as similar in some ways to a complex social organization such as that of universities. Admitting severe limitations and dangers, let us see where it takes us to liken people, the units of the organization, to cells of the nervous system. All the units can do some things, such as receive inputs, integrate them, and formulate outputs—hear, remember, and speak. There are many local circuits—the relations between adjacent individuals in an office, a classroom, or on a committee. The larger connectivities—sources of input and destinations of output—determine the role of the local interactions in the department, the school, and the university.

Now, one suggestion from such a comparison, and I do not think it is rejectable out of hand, is that similar processes, interactions, and functional units operate at all levels—whether they be minimally specified masses as in the football stadium, or slightly organized groups as in the fraternities and faculties, or more specified committees, or even individuals, from janitor of the south wing to chairman of the neuroscience department. This does not exclude emergent phenomena in larger groups, but it says we can go a long way using only the phenomena seen in the "local circuit."

Another suggestion is that the system will work quite well after serious ablations, indeed with less perturbation when the chairman is sick than the janitor. There are plenty of individuals—nonredundant but capable—ready to assume the functions of anyone whose activities are needed. Still another conclusion that I believe fits both systems is that recognition, decision, and formulation of output can be accomplished either by the crowd, the faculty, the committee, or the individual. There is not one mechanism for these functions; all the candidate mechanisms are actually used. The personality is the aggregate of these operations, with more dependence on some than on others. Persistent effects of the environment and of its own activity, memory, and modifiability exist at many levels.

The main lesson of this far-fetched analogy is that I believe we should not discard as implausible any of the roles so far proposed for the single cell, or the local circuit, or the larger, well-specified mass in accomplishments even at higher levels of function.

In a climate where some are saying, "You have to get down to the single cell before meaningful analyses of mechanism can begin and you really need to know the connections of your cells," and others are saying, "Single-unit study is never going to explain much at higher levels," this sounds a bit too eclectic. I take this position not because I want to be friendly to everyone, or because I regard the alternatives as more or less equivalent. Far from it.

I believe our ignorance is so profound that we cannot dismiss either extreme ("units do everything" or "masses do everything"). But the two propositions are quite asymmetrical; we *know* that neuronal units can do things up to a considerable level of complexity, and we have no reason to place an upper limit on their responsibility or the complexity of the functional roles of single units *and* well-defined sets of units. We *believe* that ensembles or arrays of large numbers—"statistical configurations" in Roy John's term (1972)—can account for higher percepts, but we cannot prove or even test such an idea in a way that excludes the preceding alternative. The latter notion is plausible but less testable; the former is repugnant to many people, but on hard evidence it is merely limited by the question, How far does it in fact go in explaining behavior?

I have carefully couched the contrast in terms of extremes. Some may wish to avoid the more unpleasant aspects of the confrontation of views by espousing an intermediate or mixed position. Higher percepts, recognitions, and decisions may be assigned to moderately large, rather well-specified spatiotemporal patterns in constellations of cells, with adequate redundancy. In terms of plausibility, this notion is perhaps nearly maximal among a random assortment of physiologists today. I myself believe it—but only as one of the available, and probably actual, mechanisms used by nature. However, the democratic method of evaluating scientific plausibility has little weight or prognostic value (except in obtaining grants!). This apparently intermediate or safer view is not without its caveats. But this is not the place to develop this theme further. Only one corollary requires mention.

A fundamental consideration for the choice of models is how noisy—in the sense of sloppy—the neurons and local circuits are thought to be. The evolving concept, as I see it, points to a wide range of instances, showing that the brain cannot be called a noisy processor in this sense.

There are good cases to show that nature can, when she wishes, make neuronal units with extremely small percentages of unreliability or unexplained variation. I *know* that; I *believe* there are cases where unreliability is high. At least the unexplained variability is high. My experience as a comparative neurobiologist is that each of the candidate results is found, and I do not care to argue which is typical. Instead I would argue that the assumption that unexplained variation is unreliability or slop is unwarranted. We know that the brain changes its state from moment to moment. We know that jitter is often advantageous and may therefore have been selected for. We know that lots of averaging takes place—as when converging inputs bring independent spike trains or slow potential sources together. None of this is good evidence for unreliability. It would be much more heuristic to call unexplained variation in response just that instead of "noise," because it is then more likely to get studied and explained. I do not deny noise; of course there is noise. But how much of the unexplained fluctuation is noise, that is, how much is meaningless for the system? I do not deny redundant cells that reduce noise by averaging; certainly this is one of the operating principles of nervous systems, but how much of the brain of higher mammals is redundant in this sense? To be provocative I shall propose very much less than is often implied.

My assignment was to sketch evolving concepts, directions, and emphases as background for the meatier, factual chapters to follow. They may well argue quite the opposite on some points, or reverse a direction, and I shall cheer them on, for of such disputes are new revolutions made.

REFERENCES

BROCK, L. G., J. S. COOMBS, and J. C. ECCLES, 1952. The recording of potentials from motoneurones with an intracellular electrode. *J. Physiol.* 117:431–460.
BRYANT, H. L., 1977. Differential sensitivity of *Aplysia* axons to pharmacological and ionic manipulation. *Neurosci. Abs.* 3:173.

BRYANT, H. L., 1978. Graded action potentials and decremental conduction in *Aplysia* neurons. In preparation.

BULLOCK, T. H., 1959. The neuron doctrine and electrophysiology. *Science* 129: 997–1002.

BULLOCK, T. H., 1974. Comparisons between vertebrates and invertebrates in nervous organization. In *The Neurosciences: Third Study Program*, F. O. Schmitt and F. G. Worden, eds. Cambridge, Mass.: MIT Press, pp. 343–346.

BULLOCK, T. H., 1976. In search of principles in neural integration: Are there rules in the combination of elements in neural circuits? In *Simpler Networks: An Approach to Patterned Behavior and Its Foundations*, J. Fentress, ed. Sunderland, Conn.: Sinauer Assoc., pp. 52–60.

BULLOCK, T. H., and S. HAGIWARA, 1955. Further study of the giant synapse in the stellate ganglion of squid. *Biol. Bull.* 109:341–342.

BULLOCK, T. H., and S. HAGIWARA, 1957. Intracellular recording from the giant synapse of the squid. *J. Gen. Physiol.* 40:565–577.

BULLOCK, T. H., and G. A. HORRIDGE, 1965. *Structure and Function in the Nervous Systems of Invertebrates*. San Francisco: W. H. Freeman.

BULLOCK, T. H., R. ORKAND, and A. D. GRINNELL, 1977. *Introduction to Nervous Systems*. San Francisco: W. H. Freeman.

BUSH, B. M. H., and A. ROBERTS, 1968. Resistance reflexes from a crab muscle receptor without impulses. *Nature* 218:1172–1173.

DUDEL, J., and S. W. KUFFLER, 1961. Presynaptic inhibition at the crayfish neuromuscular junction. *J. Physiol.* 155:530–542.

FURSHPAN, E. J., and D. D. POTTER, 1957. Mechanism of nerve impulse transmission at a crayfish synapse. *Nature* (London) 180:342–343.

FURSHPAN, E. J., and D. D. POTTER, 1959. Transmission at the giant motor synapses of the crayfish. *J. Physiol.* 145:289–325.

HODGKIN, A. L., 1938. The subthreshold potentials in a crustacean nerve fiber. *Proc. R. Soc. Lond.* B126:87–121.

JOHN, E. R., 1972. Switchboard versus statistical theories of learning and memory. *Science* 177:850–864.

KATZ, B., 1936. Neuromuscular transmission in crabs. *J. Physiol.* 87:199–221.

KATZ, B., 1949. Neuromuscular transmission in invertebrates. *Biol. Rev.* 24:1–20.

KERNELL, D., 1965. The adaptation and the relation between discharge frequency and current strength of cat lumbosacral motoneurones stimulated by long-lasting injected currents. *Acta Physiol. Scand.* 65:65–73.

KOIKE, H., N. MANO, Y. OKADA, and T. OSHIMA, 1970. Repetitive impulses generated in fast and slow pyramidal tract cells by intracellularly applied current steps. *Exp. Brain Res.* 11:263–281.

LLOYD, D. P. C., 1941. A direct central inhibitory action of dromically conducted impulses. *J. Neurophysiol.* 4:184–190.

MARMONT, G., and C. A. G. WIERSMA, 1938. On the mechanism of inhibition and excitation of crayfish muscle. *J. Physiol.* 93:173–193.

McCULLOCH, W. S., and W. PITTS, 1943. A logical calculus of the ideas immanent in nervous activity. *Bull. Math. Biophys.* 5:115–133.

PANTIN, C. F. A., 1935. The nerve net of the Actinozoa. I. Facilitation. *J. Exp. Biol.* 12:119–138.

PEARSON, K. G., and C. R. FOURTNER, 1975. Nonspiking interneurons in the walking system of the cockroach. *J. Neurophysiol.* 38:33–52.

PROSSER, C. L., 1935. A preparation for the study of single synaptic junctions. *Am. J. Physiol.* 113:108.

PROSSER, C. L., 1937. Synaptic transmission in the sixth abdominal ganglion of the crayfish. *Biol. Bull. Woods Hole* 73:346.

RIPLEY, S. H., B. M. H. BUSH, and A. ROBERTS, 1968. Crab muscle receptor which responds without impulses. *Nature* 218:1170–1171.

SPIRA, M. E., D. C. SPRAY, and M. V. L. BENNETT, 1976. Electrotonic coupling: Effective sign reversal by inhibitory neuron. *Science* 194:1065–1067.

WATANABE, A., and T. H. BULLOCK, 1959. Modulation of activity by one neuron by subthreshold slow potentials in another. *Fed. Proc.* 18:167.

WATANABE, A., and T. H. BULLOCK, 1960. Modulation of activity of one neuron by subthreshold slow potentials in another in lobster cardiac ganglion. *J. Gen. Physiol.* 43:1031–1045.

WIERSMA, C. A. G., 1933. Vergleichende Untersuchungen über das periphere Nerven-Muskelsystem von Crustaceen. *Z. Vergl. Physiol.* 19:349–385.

WIERSMA, C. A. G., and A. van HARREVELD, 1935. On the nerve-muscle system of the hermit crab (*Eupagurus bernhardus*). 3. The action currents of the muscles of the claw in contraction and inhibition. *Arch. Néerl. Physiol.* 20:89–102.

WIERSMA, C. A. G., and A. van HARREVELD, 1938. The influence of the frequency of stimulation on the slow and the fast contraction in crustacean muscle. *Physiol. Zoöl.* 11:75–81.

4 Chemical Integrative Processes in the Central Nervous System

FLOYD E. BLOOM

ABSTRACT The chemical vocabulary of interneuronal communication resides in at least three specifiable variables: the transmitter molecules that neurons secrete, the temporal and spatial domains over which interconnected cells can regulate each other, and the resultant intracellular conditions imposed by these signals on their targets. The intracellular conditions imposed by the actions of transmitters on their target cells may provide the basis for a logic of intercellular operations which organizes individual neurons into responsive ensembles in order to produce phenomena recognizable as behavior. The ever-lengthening list of neuron-produced chemical signals allows ample possibilities for integrating time, space, and modality for rapid processing of biological information. The long-elusive principles of intercellular communication in the nervous system may take form through better comprehension of these chemical processes.

Introduction

A MAJOR THRUST for this Intensive Study Program is the search for new conceptual principles to explain how neurons interact to perform functional operations on the plane of psychological phenomena such as memory or learning. These higher-order operations remain abstractions, despite their intuitive reality, because we lack an understanding of how the operations are achieved in biological terms: which cells, doing what, over what domain, etc. In his chapter, Bullock examined the evolving concepts of local integrative operations from the perspective of a comparative electrophysiologist and has presented a tabulation of functional variables on which different anatomically defined neuronal units can achieve integrative actions. About a quarter of this listing refers to the general events of chemical interneuronal communication independent of the specific chemical agents involved. In this essay, I wish to address the issue of chemical integrative mechanisms more fully and to consider the several dimensions of neuronal specification from which I believe the integrative logic

FLOYD E. BLOOM Arthur Vining Davis Center for Behavioral Neurobiology, The Salk Institute, La Jolla, CA 92037

of neuron-neuron interaction may eventually be derived. In this highlighting of chemical processes capable of generating integrative actions, the issue of spiking versus "nonspiking" neurons—another major thrust of this program (see Shepherd, 1977, and the papers by Shepherd and by Dowling in this volume)—remains unengaged.

A brief historical survey of chemical transmitter ontology may provide some basis for my reasoning. When the list of putative neurotransmitter chemicals was relatively short, many members of the neuroscientific community shared the tacit belief that transmitter molecules were functionally equivalent elements differing only by virtue of whether the action they produced at their receptors was excitation or inhibition. Given that generalization, the transmitter for a given circuit did not really require identification provided the qualitative sign for the operation between the connected cells could be defined as either excitation or inhibition. With the logic operations restricted to excitation and inhibition, theoretical constructs of neuronal ensembles to explain information processing appeared to involve circuitry only. Such logic systems are trinary (excite, inhibit, or nothing) and allow for addition and subtraction in biologic units that can be weighted according to the distance from the cell soma and axon hillock at which that synapse excites or inhibits (Rose, 1977; Kent, 1978). If we view the neuron as a highly complex logic gate to do the functions we describe in other computational devices as AND, NAND, OR, and NOR, the chemically independent neuron takes on the properties of a living transistor or integrated circuit. For the purpose of academic debate, I can tolerate this view as a tool to understand the program of brain operations. However, such a view fails to encompass many highly developed biochemical properties of the nerve cell. Moreover, while this view might generate transistorized integrated-circuit devices that could process information like a brain, the problem we seek to solve here is how the brain itself processes information.

As more and more brain circuits became defined, and as new principles of intercellular anatomical organization such as the local circuit neuron were recognized, these details were readily incorporated into the circuitry-oriented schema. Identification of the transmitters involved remained an interesting aspect of the circuitry analysis, but nonetheless one that was superficial to the system's operation.

However, with the recognition of nonconforming synaptic operations in which membrane potential changes occurred over epochs of seconds unaccompanied by expected increases in membrane conductance (Weight, 1974), the monolithic view of synapse logic had to be reexamined (Bloom, 1975). Furthermore, neurochemically defined brain circuits producing these novel synaptic operations (Siggins, Hoffer, and Bloom, 1969; Hoffer et al., 1972, 1973; Bloom, 1975) also exhibited anatomic properties that did not conform to either the hierarchical or local circuit principles of neuroanatomy (Lindvall and Björklund, 1974; Moore and Bloom, 1978). Currently, synaptic pharmacology is besieged by an onslaught of new transmitterlike chemicals being discovered at rates far faster than the sites and mechanisms of operation for these substances can be determined. These newly recognized substances—mainly peptides (Barker and Smith, 1977; Nicoll, 1976; Vale, this volume)—pose an important challenge for the emerging logic of recognized synaptic operations: Are these substances acting in ways generally analogous to amino acids and small amines or do they represent one or more additional classes of chemical operations by which nerve cells communicate? Although data to settle this important conceptual issue are still lacking, I shall attempt here to develop a rational basis by which such communicative events can be evaluated and compared.

Domains of synaptic operations

The operations of all neurons can be charted on two domains, space and time, for comparative analysis. The spatial domain of a neuron refers to the target-cell areas to which it sends information and to all the neurons from which it receives information. Similarly, the temporal domain refers to the time courses of the neuron's effects on its targets and of its responses to its inputs.

Local circuit elements represent a special interest of this ISP. Here the operational unit may be spatially a synaptic triad or a restricted patch of dendrite, and the nonspiking local fields are found to be generated and abolished quickly. Thus, local circuits are located

at the far left of the domain graph (Figure 1). Currently available data indicate that amino acid–mediated interneuronal excitations and inhibitions operate over slightly longer times and greater spaces than the local circuits. The monoaminergic neurons operate over much larger spatial domains and even more prolonged temporal epochs (Aghajanian and Wang, 1978; Siggins, 1978). The dopamine-containing cell systems alone cover an extremely wide range, from the ultrashort systems of the retina (Dowling, Ehinger, and Hedden, 1975) and olfactory bulbs (Hökfelt et al., 1975) to the longer, more highly arborized mesocortical systems (Moore and Bloom, 1978). Within the spatial domain, the serotoninergic systems seem to be as divergent and extensive as the noradrenergic systems, but they are perhaps somewhat more succinct in the temporal display of their synaptic actions (compare Wang and Aghajanian, 1977; Hoffer et al., 1973; Segal and Bloom, 1974b). Cholinergic systems may also cover a broad spatial domain, but neither their circuitry nor their synaptic time spans of action within the CNS are as yet specifiable.

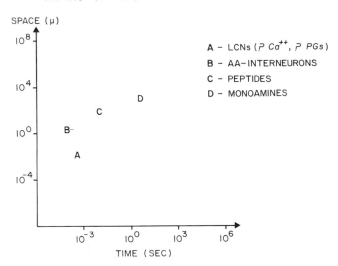

DOMAINS OF NEURONAL OPERATIONS

A – LCNs ($P\ Ca^{++}$, $P\ PGs$)
B – AA–INTERNEURONS
C – PEPTIDES
D – MONOAMINES

FIGURE 1   Four families of chemically coded neuronal elements are graphed onto two domains: space of efferent innervation and time. LCN: local circuit neuron. PG: prostaglandin. AA: amino acid.

Those neurons that can be determined to contain biologically active peptides on the basis of immunohistochemical observations (Hökfelt et al., 1977) do not fit as readily into this two-dimensional map as they might if such neurons all represented functionally equivalent units of a single coherent operational class: some presumptive peptidergic cells are small interneurons, such as the enkephalin- and neurotensin-containing cells (Snyder, this volume), while others cover significantly broader spatial domains, such as those cells in the CNS and peripheral nervous system, which are immunoreactive to antibodies against somatostatin, substance P, β-endorphin, or luteinizing hormone releasing factor (Vale, this volume). Unfortunately, we are as yet unable to specify for any of these peptidergic systems the duration of the synaptic actions they may mediate. Data from studies applying the peptides exogenously to test systems suggest that their durations of action under these conditions may be longer than the effects of simple amino acids (Nicoll, 1976; Renaud, 1977; Barker and Smith, 1977).

Although the spatial and temporal domains considered so far are those over which the chemically coded class of neurons send their efferent signals, strictly speaking—and perhaps of more importance to chemical and cellular concepts of integration—the spatial and temporal domains of the systems afferent to each element must also eventually be considered.

Other domains

Neuronal systems differ from each other in more ways than can be expressed simply in terms of the spatial and temporal domains over which they operate. At least one additional domain can be approached in this analysis, and that domain I will term for the present "energy." This third domain of neuronal operation defines the functional properties, that is, the mechanisms and consequences, of the synaptic operations of a given neuron. No one has yet calculated the dimensions of the energy shifts associated with a specifiable synaptic action (and indeed "energy" per se may not even be the correct quality in which to quantitate this domain). However, I use this term to distinguish transmitters that produce passive membrane responses (i.e., that permit responses to preexisting electrochemical gradients) from transmitters that produce active responses on the membrane and other segments of the target cell (e.g., the activation or inactivation of an enzyme or an ion-exchange carrier process). Along this energy dimension we can obtain further separation between the passive response operations mediated by simple amino acids and some amines (e.g., nicotinic cholinergic actions; see Weight, 1974) and those mediated by β-noradrenergic and dopaminergic actions (Bloom, 1975) in which one consequence is the activation of adenylate cyclase (Rall, this volume; Gilman,

this volume). While some peptide hormones act on their peripheral targets through activation of adenylate cyclase, there is as yet no compelling evidence to ascribe this sort of "energy" transduction in mammals to centrally active peptides (see Nathanson, 1977).

When only spiking neurons were considered to be pertinent components of integrative information-processing operations, all functionally important changes had to be related to shifts in firing rates or patterns. But given our present awareness that neurons can interact synaptically through small graded membrane potential changes without spikes, an extensive array of chemically derived responses become germane to information processing: local ion concentrations can be altered by sequestration or pumping, metabolic pools can be modified, enzymes and organelles needed for transmitter synthesis and storage can be called for, and longer-duration events such as genome expression or structural modification can be envisioned. As Bullock remarked in his chapter, the degrees of freedom available for synaptic operations are so numerous that one cannot keep them all in mind at one time. Yet very few of the myriad possible mechanisms for synaptic operation have been demonstrated to perform any integrative operation in any experimentally defined system.

Before dealing with one case in which such evidence is relatively strong, we should acknowledge briefly three chemical agents, of undoubted importance in integrative intercellular and intracellular events, whose sources and receptors cannot be well specified: Ca^{++} (Kretsinger, this volume), prostaglandins (Samuelsson, this volume), and adenosine (Kreutzberg, this volume; Rall, this volume). The last two certainly bear close scrutiny as local modulators of function because of their apparent rapid synthesis, release, and subsequent metabolism, but the nature of the events controlling their synthesis and release and the relation of these controlling events to underlying neuronal activity remain to be determined. One factor common to all of these regulators is the control of cyclic nucleotide concentrations within certain intracellular compartments. Although the properties of adenosine release and response have been held by some to suggest that this substance could be regarded as a local modulator released with other transmitters (Burnstock, 1975), it is possible that purines and pyrimidines may provide wholly separate controls on membrane properties (Siggins et al., 1977). As described more fully in the chapters in this volume by Rall, by Samuelsson, and by Berridge, the highly intricate interactions between cyclic nucleotides, Ca^{++}, adenosine, and prostaglandins, and the protein substrates through which these substances in turn express their actions, represent a microcosm of cross-integrating and self-regulating chemical systems that rivals any other known set of partially coupled chemical reactions. As powerful as these chemical levers may be for the regulation of all modes of neuronal activity—structural, chemical, and electrical—we as yet lack a framework that would allow us to monitor these substances within their compartments and to transform these metaphorical concepts of chemical intrigue into a program of cellular logic.

The three-dimensional domain map in Figure 2 attempts to provide an integrated comparison of the different properties now ascribable to those neural systems to which specific chemical mediators can be assigned. In order to lend greater substance to a chemically defined system with apparent integrative capacities, I offer the example of the central noradrenergic systems studied in our laboratory. Other chapters in this volume (Berridge; Levitan) as well as the recent literature (Libet, Kobayashi, and Tanaka, 1975; Brunelli, Castellucci, and Kandel, 1976; Kandel, 1976; Schulman and Weight, 1976) offer other biologic examples by which the nuances and unsolved problems of similar chemical integrative processes are becoming illuminated.

Central noradrenergic integrative actions: Paradigm or peculiarity?

The following arguments are based on studies of the central noradrenergic neurons of the nucleus locus coeruleus, and the data may well be applicable only for these neurons. Nevertheless, the central experimental logic of the approach being taken does seem to speak to the general question of how to relate the operations of chemically coded neurons to events on the behavioral level. This approach may eventually assist in transforming our concept-bound views of behavioral phenomena into more accurate descriptions of what neurons do under specific environmental conditions.

In my view, such a pursuit begins from the point at which the chemical nature of the biologically active material is established. Subsequent work can then be distilled into three major phases: (1) Where are the neurons that contain this material, which may be termed "source neurons," located, and on what other cells in the brain (target cells) do these source neurons produce effects? (2) What are the effects of this material on the target cells? (3) Under what conditions are these circuits called into action by the demands

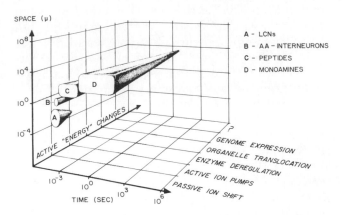

FIGURE 2 The same four families of neuronal elements as in Figure 1 theoretically related on a hypothetical third domain of functional control termed "energy." Possible control steps modulated by this energy domain are indicated from the molecular viewpoint ranging from events at the cell surface to events within the nucleus.

of the brain? A host of experimental problems require solutions between phases 2 and 3, such as characterizing the ionic basis of a specific neuron-neuron connection and determining its molecular mechanisms and pharmacological characteristics. All those problems have recently been reviewed for the central noradrenergic system (Bloom, 1977a), so we shall here consider the larger question of what principles of functional organization emerge when we consider this neuron system in three simultaneous contexts: neuroanatomy, time of operation, and mode of effect.

Space, time, and energy operations

The noradrenergic projection systems fit the descriptions of neither classical hierarchical or throughput systems (Schmitt, Dev, and Smith, 1976) nor the local neuron principles of organization (Rakic, 1975). Rather, noradrenergic projections follow highly divergent trajectories in which a few norepinephrine-containing neurons reach out to target cells in many distant regions of the brain bearing no obvious direct functional relationship to each other. This divergent anatomy strongly suggests that some still different principles of organization must be sought. Such principles may also underlie the organization of the widely separated targets of the serotonin-containing neurons of the raphe nuclei (Aghajanian and Wang, 1978) and the dopamine-containing neurons of the substantia nigra, ventral tegmentum, and dorsal hypothalamus (Moore and Bloom, 1978). Some perspective on the extent of the physiologic studies may be gained by considering that there are five major efferent systems from the nucleus locus coeruleus, which is the major source of central noradrenergic fibers: the central tegmental tract, the dorsal tegmental bundle, the dorsal periventricular system, the coeruleocerebellar fibers, which ascend through the superior cerebellar peduncle, and the descending fibers to medulla and spinal cord (Moore and Bloom, 1978).

One property that characterizes all of these major noradrenergic systems is their high degree of collateral arborization: each locus coeruleus neuron contributes terminal varicosities to a very large number of target cells in more than one region of the nervous system. I feel it important to note that although locus coeruleus fibers do innervate wide regions of the brain, the innervation patterns of the axons are neither random nor all-pervasive; within laminated cortical structures (Levitt and Moore, 1978) and within designated thalamic and hypothalamic nuclei (Lindvall et al., 1974), noradrenergic fibers show characteristic branching patterns and organized innervation densities (Lindvall and Björklund, 1974). In cerebral, cerebellar, and hippocampal cortices a major portion of the input seems to be directed toward the throughput output cells as targets (Bloom, 1977a). However, much more consideration needs to be devoted to the issue of how "the" target cells for an anatomically defined, cytochemically identified system are signified at the electron-microscopic level (see Moore and Bloom, 1978; Koda, Schulman, and Bloom, 1978) and to the related issue of the functional determination of transmitter release and response sites.

Within the group of noradrenergic projections that have been tested physiologically, operations on the time domain indicate that the effects have long latencies (80 msec or more) and long durations (300–600 msec or more), depending on the distance of the target cells from the locus coeruleus, the frequency with which the locus coeruleus is activated, and the contexts of the experiments (especially the presence or absence of anesthesia; see Segal, 1977). Here, an important area for further exploration is also worth noting. If the "effects" of the pathway are to be judged on the basis of changes in target-cell firing patterns or transmembrane properties, the source cells must be experimentally stimulated sufficiently to determine the quality and quantity of the effect. However, the locus coeruleus appears to exert a potent intranuclear feedback inhibition (Aghajanian, Cederbaum, and Wang, 1977), which would tend to dampen the physiologic occurrence of the types of

entrained higher-frequency stimuli that have been examined (Siggins, Hoffer, Oliver, and Bloom, 1971; Hoffer et al., 1973; Segal and Bloom, 1974b, 1976a,b; Segal 1977); these stimuli may therefore have been highly unphysiological.

On the third domain, the effects of the coeruleocerebellar and coeruleohippocampal projections and the iontophoretic simulations of the effects of coeruleocortical projections (Stone and Taylor, 1977) all adhere closely to the interpretation that the action of neurally released noradrenaline is mediated by β-adrenergic receptors coupled to adenylate cyclase; hence they are in accordance with the "second-messenger" scheme of Sutherland (see Bloom, 1975, and the papers by Rall and by Berridge in this volume). The effects as judged by firing rates and transmembrane effects are overtly inhibitory, with hyperpolarizations accompanied by increased membrane resistance (Siggins, Hoffer, Oliver, and Bloom, 1971; Siggins, Oliver, Hoffer, and Bloom, 1971; Hoffer et al., 1973). However, when examined with regard to other aspects of target-cell functioning in different experimental contexts (Foote, Freedman, and Oliver, 1975; Segal and Bloom, 1976a,b; Freedman et al., 1977; Segal, 1977), the effects of the locus coeruleus appear to fit better the designation of "biasing" or "enabling" (Hore, Meyer-Lohman, and Brooks, 1977) than they do simple "inhibition." The biasing or enabling function means only that in the epoch over which noradrenergic receptors are active, certain chemical messages received through other receptors can be enhanced or weighted (Bloom, 1975). Such enabling effects can be regarded as predictable outcomes of the observed changes in membrane properties (Weight, 1974).

Elsewhere I have suggested that the combination of electrophysiologic and biochemical changes produced in target cells by the noradrenergic fibers should be considered together as a holistic set of responsive changes and speculated that the observed electrophysiologic events may be mere epiphenomena of the biochemical actions (Bloom, 1975). For example, hyperpolarizing changes in transmembrane potential accompany the responses of many nonneural cells to hormones and neurotransmitters that activate cyclic nucleotide synthesis (Bloom, 1975). In the heart, catecholamines not only increase the force and frequency of cardiac contractions, but also activate lipolysis and glycogenolysis that provides the cardiac muscle with increased substrates for energy metabolism. Taken as a whole, the electrophysiologic shifts in the properties of the target-cell membrane and the concomitant shifts in intracellular metabolism could provide a cell state specific for an altered mode of information processing.

Documentation of that view will require better knowledge of when noradrenergic circuits are naturally called into action and of the purposes of those actions in the biologic functions of the target cells. Based on what is documentable now, however, this system would appear ideally suited to integrate across both time and space and to shift the metabolic "gears" of the cells to which that message is transmitted.

If the correlations between noradrenergic firing and sleep cycles indicate one purposeful aspect of the functioning circuitry of the noradrenergic system (see Chu and Bloom, 1974; Hobson, McCarley, and Wyzinski, 1975), the properties just defined might serve to explain the changes in synaptic efficacy or "gating" observed in awake animals with sleep (Winson and Abzug, 1977), circadian rhythms (Barnes et al., 1977), or attention (Burton, Rolls, and Mora, 1976; Sekuler and Ball, 1977). However, lest we relax in the misconceived notion that such correlations might explain the function of the locus coeruleus, we should realize that neither sleep nor attention is yet an explainable process. In fact, our comprehension of sleeping or attending may eventually be better served through recognition of the purposeful operation of the locus coeruleus than vice versa. Perhaps that recognition will provide more precise cellular meanings to the possibility that noradrenergic systems are important in psychological abstractions such as learning (Crow and Wendlandt, 1976; Stein, 1975; Hall, Bloom, and Olds, 1977) or extinction (Mason and Iversen, 1977).

Finally, let us assume, at least temporarily, that many classes of chemically coupled transductive systems exist to express the effects of transmitter receptors, and that these couplings can be ion- or substrate-specific, can be dependent or independent variables of energy production or Ca^{++} translocations, and can operate actively or passively over a wide range of transmitter-specific time periods. Where in this array of conceivable actions do we place the growing list of systems apparently mediated by peptides (Phillips et al., 1977; Kosterlitz et al., 1977), some of which may coexist within cells previously thought to be monoaminergic (Hökfelt et al., 1977)? Is there, in fact, any reason to assume that peptides secreted by neurons function differently than amino acid or monoamine transmitters? Are there still other "energy"-type operations to be described which, when understood, will encompass the roles played by these substances across their own unique temporal and spatial domains, and also explain the coexistence in brain, gut, and endocrine tissues of the same chemical signaling devices?

Concluding comments

Can an overall logic function of catecholamine-mediated messages in the CNS be derived from generalizations of the role suggested for catecholamines within the pacemaking cells of the heart (Pollack, 1977)? If we returned to the schematic circuit diagram view of the brain, identified cells whose basal activity exhibits properties of a biologic oscillator like the Purkinje cell and some other premotor reticular neurons (see Wiesenfeld, Halpern, and Tapper, 1977), would we find a good correlation with noradrenergic inputs? Does the holistic response of cardiac Purkinje fibers to sympathetic nerve impulses suggest that the central noradrenergic systems operate to enable or disenable target oscillator cells to execute preprogrammed subroutines in response to external information? Although tantalizing to me, such generalizations still require that the purposeful principle for which the operation occurs be formulated in a way that links molecular events to cellular events and cellular events to behaving ensembles of cells (see Nadel and O'Keefe, 1974). I will conclude by stating my own view that chemical identification of a transmitter substance is only one functional property of a neuronal signal; complete functional understanding also requires consideration of the spatial domain, temporal contexts, and operational logic of the signal. Together, these aspects of chemical integrative function define the principles by which nerve cells communicate, process information from the external and internal worlds, and integrate that information into the operation of the whole organism. We eagerly await that revelation of principles.

REFERENCES

AGHAJANIAN, G. K., J. M. CEDARBAUM, and R. Y. WANG, 1977. Evidence for norepinephrine-mediated collateral inhibition of locus coeruleus neurons. *Brain Res.* 136:570–577.

AGHAJANIAN, G. K., and R. Y. WANG, 1978. Physiology and pharmacology of central serotonergic neurons. In *Psychopharmacology: A Generation of Progress*, M. A. Lipton, A. diMascio, and K. Killam, eds. New York: Raven Press, pp. 171–182.

BARKER, J. L., and T. G. SMITH, JR., 1977. Peptides as neurohormones. *Neurosci. Symp.* 2:340–373.

BLOOM, F. E., 1973. Dynamic synaptic communication: Finding the vocabulary. *Brain Res.* 62:299–305.

BLOOM, F. E., 1974a. To spritz or not to spritz: The doubtful value of aimless iontophoresis. *Life Sci.* 14:1819–1834.

BLOOM, F. E., 1974b. Dynamics of synaptic modulation: Perspectives for the future. In *The Neurosciences: Third*

Study Program, F. O. Schmitt, ed. Cambridge, MA: MIT Press, pp. 989–999.

BLOOM, F. E., 1975. The role of cyclic nucleotides in central synaptic function. *Rev. Physiol. Biochem. Pharmacol.* 74:1–103.

BLOOM, F. E., 1976. The role of cyclic nucleotides in central synaptic function. In *Proceedings of the Satellite Symposium "New First and Second Messengers in Nervous Tissues,"* E. Costa, E. Giacobini, and R. Paoletti, eds. New York: Raven Press.

BLOOM, F. E., 1977a. Central noradrenergic systems: Physiology and pharmacology. In *Proceedings of the American College of Neuropsychopharmacology*, M. A. Lipton, A. diMascio, and K. F. Killam, eds. New York: Raven Press.

BLOOM, F. E., 1977b. Peptide transmitters: Clues to the chemical cryptogram of interneuronal communication? *BioSystems* 8:179–183.

BRUNELLI, M., V. F. CASTELLUCCI, and E. R. KANDEL, 1976. Synaptic facilitation and behavioral sensitization in *Aplysia*: Possible roles of serotonin and cyclic AMP. *Science* 194:1178–1181.

BUCHSBAUM, M. S., G. C. DAVIS, and W. E. BUNNEY, JR., 1977. Naloxone alters pain perception and somatosensory evoked potentials in normal subjects. *Nature* 270:620–622.

BURNSTOCK, G., 1975. Purinergic transmission. In *Handbook of Psychopharmacology*, L. L. Iversen, S. D. Iversen, and S. H. Snyder, eds. New York: Plenum Press, vol. 5, pp. 131–194.

BURTON, M. J., F. T. ROLLS, and F. MORA, 1976. Effects of hunger on the responses of neurons in the lateral hypothalamus to the sight and taste of food. *Exp. Neurol.* 51:668–677.

CASTELLUCCI, V., and E. R. KANDEL, 1976. Pre-synaptic facilitation as a mechanism for behavioral sensitization in *Aplysia*. *Science* 194:1176–1178.

CHU, N.-S., and F. E. BLOOM, 1974. Activity patterns of catecholamine-containing pontine neurons in the dorsolateral tegmentum of unrestrained cats. *J. Neurobiol.* 5:527–544.

CROW, T. J., and S. WENDLANDT, 1976. Impaired acquisition of a passive avoidance response after lesions induced in the locus coeruleus by 6-OH-dopamine. *Nature* 259:42–44.

DALY, J., 1975. Role of cyclic nucleotides in the nervous system. In *Handbook of Psychopharmacology*, L. L. Iversen, S. D. Iversen, and S. H. Snyder, eds. New York: Plenum Press, vol. 5, pp. 47–130.

DALY, J., 1977. *Cyclic Nucleotides in the Nervous System*. New York: Plenum Press.

DOWLING, J. E., B. EHINGER, and W. L. HEDDEN, 1975. The interplexiform cell: A new type of retinal neuron. *Invest. Ophthalmol.* 15:916–926.

FOOTE, S., R. FREEDMAN, and A. P. OLIVER, 1975. Effects of putative neurotransmitters on neuronal activity in monkey auditory cortex. *Brain Res.* 86:229–242.

FREEDMAN, R., B. J. HOFFER, D. J. WOODWARD, and D. PURO, 1977. Interaction of norepinephrine with cerebellar activity evoked by mossy and climbing fibers. *Exp. Neurol.* 55:269–288.

GAHWILER, B. H., 1976. Inhibitory action of noradrenaline and cyclic AMP in explants of rat cerebellum. *Nature* 259:483–484.

GARCIA, J., W. G. HANKINS, and K. W. RUSINIAK, 1974. Behavioral regulation of the milieu interne in man and rat. *Science* 185:824–832.

GUYENET, P. G. and G. K. AGHAJANIAN, 1977. Excitation of neurons in the nucleus locus coeruleus by Substance P and related peptides. *Brain Res.* 136:178–184.

HALL, R. D., F. E. BLOOM, and J. OLDS. 1977. Neuronal and neurochemical substrates of reinforcement. *Neurosci. Res. Program Bull.* 15:136–314.

HOBSON, J. A., R. W. McCARLEY, and P. W. WYZINSKI, 1975. Sleep cycle oscillation: Reciprocal discharge by two brain stem neuronal groups. *Science* 189:55–58.

HOFFER, B. J., G. R. SIGGINS, A. P. OLIVER, and F. E. BLOOM, 1972. Cyclic adenosine monophosphate mediated adrenergic synapses to cerebellar Purkinje cells. *Adv. Cyclic Nucleotide Res.* 1:411–423.

HOFFER, B. J., G. R. SIGGINS, and F. E. BLOOM, 1969. Prostaglandins and E antagonize norepinephrine effects on cerebellar Purkinje cells: Microelectrophoretic study. *Science* 166:1418–1420.

HOFFER, B. J., G. R. SIGGINS, and F. E. BLOOM, 1971. Studies on norepinephrine-containing afferents to Purkinje cells of rat cerebellum. II. Sensitivity of Purkinje cells to norepinephrine and related substances administered by microiontophoresis. *Brain Res.* 25:523–534.

HOFFER, B. J., G. R. SIGGINS, D. J. WOODWARD, and F. E. BLOOM, 1971. Spontaneous discharge of Purkinje neurons after destruction of Catecholamine-containing afferents by 6-hydroxydopamine. *Brain Res.* 30:425–430.

HOFFER, B. J., G. R. SIGGINS, A. P. OLIVER, and F. E. BLOOM, 1973. Activation of the pathway from locus coeruleus to rat cerebellar Purkinje neurons: Pharmacological evidence of noradrenergic central inhibition. *J. Pharmacol. Exp. Ther.* 184:553–569.

HÖKFELT, T., R. ELDE, O. JOHANSSON, A. LJUNGDAHL, M. SCHUTZBERG, K. FUXE, ET AL., 1977. The distribution of peptide-containing neurons in the nervous system. In *Psychopharmacology—A Generation of Progress*, A. diMascio, M. Lipton, and K. Killam eds. New York: Raven Press, pp. 39–66.

HORE, J., J. MEYER-LOHMANN, and V. B. BROOKS, 1977. Basal ganglia cooling disables learned arm movements of monkeys in the absence of visual guidance. *Science* 195:584–586.

KANDEL, E. R., 1976. *Cellular Basis of Behavior*. San Francisco: W. H. Freeman.

KENT, E. W., 1978. The brains of men and machines. *BYTE* 3:11–22, 96–106.

KODA, L. Y., J. A. SCHULMAN, and F. E. BLOOM, 1978. Ultrastructural identification of noradrenergic terminals in rat hippocampus: Unilateral destruction of the locus coeruleus with 6-hydroxydopamine. *Brain Res.* 145:140–146.

KOSTERLITZ, H. W., J. HUGHES, J. A. H. LORD, and A. A. WATERFIELD, 1977. Enkephalins, endorphins, and opiate receptors. *Neurosci. Symp.* 2:291–307.

LEVITT, P., and R. Y. MOORE, 1978. The adrenergic innervation of the neocortex of the rat. *Brain Res.* 139:219–232.

LIBET, B., H. KOBAYASHI, and T. TANAKA, 1975. Synaptic coupling into the production and storage of a neuronal memory trace. *Nature* 258:155–157.

LINDVALL, O., and A. BJÖRKLUND, 1974. The organization

of the ascending catecholamine neuron systems in the rat brain as revealed by the glyoxylic acid fluorescence method. *Acta Physiol. Scand. Suppl.* 412:1–88.

LINDVALL, O., A. BJÖRKLUND, A. NOBIN, and U. STENEVI, 1974. The adrenergic innervation of the rat thalamus as revealed by the glyoxylic acid fluorescence method. *J. Comp. Neurol.* 154:317–348.

MASON, S. T., and S. D. IVERSEN, 1977. An investigation of the role of cortical and cerebellar noradrenaline in associative motor learning in the rat. *Brain Res.* 134:513–527.

MOORE, R. Y., and F. E. BLOOM, 1978. Central catecholamine neuron systems: Anatomy and physiology of the dopamine systems. *Ann. Rev. Neurosci.* 1:129–169.

NADEL, L., and J. O'KEEFE, 1974. The hippocampus in pieces and patches: An essay on modes of explanation in physiological psychology. In *Essays on the Nervous System*, R. Bellairs and E. G. Gray, eds. Oxford: Clarendon Press, pp. 368–390.

NATHANSON, J., 1977. Cyclic nucleotides and nervous system function. *Physiol. Rev.* 57:157–256.

NICOLL, R. A., 1976. Peptide neurotransmitters. *Neurosci. Symp.* 1:99–122.

PHILLIPS, M. I., D. FELIX, W. E. HOFFMAN, and A. GANTEN, 1977. Angiotensin-sensitive sites in the brain ventricular system. *Neorosci. Symp.* 2:308–339.

POLLACK, G. H., 1977. Cardiac pacemaking: An obligatory role of catecholamines? *Science* 196:731–737.

RAKIC, P., 1975. Local circuit neurons. *Neurosci. Res. Program Bull.* 13:293–446.

RENAUD, L., 1977. Influence of medial pre-optic anterior hypothalamic area stimulation on the excitability of mediobasal hypothalamic neurones in the rat. *J. Physiol.* 264:541–564.

ROSE, D., 1977. On the arithmetical operation performed by inhibitory synapses onto the neuronal soma. *Exp. Brain Res.* 28:221–223.

SCHMITT, F. O., P. DEV, and B. H. SMITH, 1976. Electrotonic processing of information by brain cells. *Science* 193:114–120.

SCHULMAN, J. A., and F. F. WEIGHT, 1976. Synaptic transmission: Long lasting potentiation by a postsynaptic mechanism. *Science* 194:1437–1439.

SEGAL, M., 1977. Changes of interhemispheric hippocampal response during conditioning in the awake rat. *Exp. Brain Res.* 29:553–565.

SEGAL, M., and F. E. BLOOM, 1974a. The action of norepinephrine in the rat hippocampus. I. Iontophoretic studies. *Brain Res.* 72:79–97.

SEGAL, M., and F. E. BLOOM, 1974b. The action of norepinephrine in the rat hippocampus. II. Activation of the input pathway. *Brain Res.* 72:99–114.

SEGAL, M., and F. E. BLOOM, 1976a. The action of norepinephrine in the rat hippocampus. III. Hippocampal cellular responses to locus coeruleus stimulation in the awake rat. *Brain Res.* 107:499–511.

SEGAL, M., and F. E. BLOOM, 1976b. The action of norepinephrine in the rat hippocampus. IV. The effects of locus coeruleus stimulation on evoked hippocampal unit activity. *Brain Res.* 107:513–525.

SEKULER, R., and K. BALL, 1977. Mental set alters visibility of moving targets. *Science* 198:60–62.

SHEPHERD, G. M., 1977. Central processing of olfactory signals. In *Chemical Signals in Vertebrates*, D. Muller-Schwarze and M. M. Mozell, eds. New York: Plenum Publishing Co., pp. 489–497.

SIGGINS, G. R., 1978. Electrophysiological role of dopamine in striatum: Excitatory or inhibitory. In *Psychopharmacology—A Generation of Progress*. M. A. Lipton, A. diMascio, and K. Killam, eds. New York: Raven Press, pp. 143–158.

SIGGINS, G. R., D. L. GRUOL, A. L. PADJEN, and D. S. FORMAN, 1977. Purine and pyrimidine mononucleotides depolarise neurones of explanted amphibian sympathetic ganglia. *Nature* 270:263–264.

SIGGINS, G. R., B. J. HOFFER, and F. E. BLOOM, 1969. Cyclic 3'5' adenosine monophosphate: Possible mediator for the response of cerebellar Purkinje cells to microelectrophoresis of norepinephrine. *Science* 165:1018–1020.

SIGGINS, G. R., B. J. HOFFER, and F. E. BLOOM, 1971. Studies on norepinephrine-containing afferents to Purkinje cells of rat cerebellum. III. Evidence for mediation of norepinephrine effects by cyclic 3'5'-adenosine monophosphate. *Brain Res.* 25:535–553.

SIGGINS, G. R., B. J. HOFFER, A. P. OLIVER, and F. E. BLOOM, 1971. Activation of a central noradrenergic projection to cerebellum. *Nature* 233:481–483.

SIGGINS, G. R., A. P. OLIVER, B. J. HOFFER, and F. E. BLOOM, 1971. Cyclic adenosine monophosphate and norepinephrine: Effects on transmembrane properties of cerebellar Purkinje cells. *Science* 171:192.

STEIN, L., 1975. Norepinephrine reward pathways: Role in self-stimulation, memory consolidation, and schizophrenia. *Nebr. Symp. Motiv.* 22:113–159.

STONE, T. W., and D. A. TAYLOR, 1977. Microiontophoretic studies of the effects of cyclic nucleotides on excitability of neurone in the rat cerebral cortex. *J. Physiol.* 266:523–543.

WANG, R. Y., and G. K. AGHAJANIAN, 1977. Inhibition of neurons in the amygdala by dorsal raphe stimulation: Mediation through a direct serotonergic pathway. *Brain Res.* 120:85–102.

WEIGHT, F. F., 1974. Physiological mechanisms of synaptic modulation. In *The Neurosciences: Third Study Program*, F. O. Schmitt, ed. Cambridge, MA: MIT Press, pp. 929–942.

WIESENFELD, Z., B. P. HALPERN, and D. N. TAPPER, 1977. Licking behavior: Evidence of hypoglossal oscillator. *Science* 196:1122–1124.

WINSON, J., and C. ABZUG, 1977. Gating of neuronal transmission in the hippocampus: Efficiency of transmission varies with behavioral state. *Science* 196:1223–1225.

5 Selection and Control in Neurogenesis

W. M. COWAN

ABSTRACT   In this paper some of the factors involved in the developmental control of neuronal number, location, morphology, and connectivity are reviewed. The principal determinants of neuronal number are (1) the controlled proliferation of a population of precursor cells in one of the proliferative zones in the CNS or PNS, for a defined period of time, and (2) the subsequent elimination (at the time connections are being established) of a significant portion of the initial population generated. The final location and precise orientation of neurons are determined by their early migration along predetermined pathways and their selective aggregation and alignment with respect to their neighbors in the anlage of the nuclear group, cortical lamina, or peripheral ganglion in which they finally reside. The morphology of a neuron is largely determined by the pattern of its dendritic tree, which, in turn, is shaped by both genetic and epigenetic factors. Included among the latter are certain mechanical factors and the influence of specific afferents. The connections formed by a neuron, or group of neurons, are controlled by three factors: (1) the positional information which the cells acquire early in their development; (2) the expression of this information in axonal outgrowth; and (3) the identification of an appropriate terminal locus and the establishment of synaptic connections upon the appropriate parts of selected target cells within this terminal field. From the vast body of information bearing on these three issues, several generalizations have been drawn which appear to be relevant both for the formation of connections during normal development and for induced neuronal "plasticity."

Since the full-grown forest turns out to be impenetrable and indefinable, why not revert to the study of the young wood, in the nursery stages as we might say. . . . [If] the brain and other adult organs . . . are too complex to permit scrutinizing their structural plan . . . why not apply [the available methods] systematically to lower vertebrates and to the early stages of ontogenetic development, in which the nervous system should present a simple and, so to speak, diagrammatic organization.

S. Ramón y Cajal (1937)

W. M. COWAN   Department of Anatomy and Neurobiology, Washington University School of Medicine, St. Louis, MO 63110

Introduction

THE FORMATION of any neural center in the vertebrate nervous system[1]—be it a nuclear group or a cortical layer in the central nervous system (CNS) or a sensory or autonomic ganglion in the peripheral nervous system (PNS)—involves a number of related, but formally distinguishable, events. These include:

1. The proliferation of an appropriate number of neurons and glial cells from a definable precursor population in one of the four major proliferative zones: the *neuroepithelium* lining the ventricular system of the neural tube, the adjoining *subventricular zone*, the *neural crest*, and certain of the *ectodermal placodes*.

2. The migration of the cells from the proliferative zone in which they are generated to their definitive location. In the CNS this migration is usually of post-mitotic neurons. Migrating glial cells and the neuronal elements of the neural crest and ectodermal placodes usually retain their capacity for division and undergo further proliferation when they reach their final destination.

3. The selective aggregation of cells of like kind. In most neuronal systems this process also involves the precise orientation or alignment of the principal neurons in the population.

4. Cytodifferentiation, which involves both process formation and the commitment of the cells to a specific mode of conduction and a particular form of synaptic transmission.

5. The establishment of a specific set of afferent and efferent connections.

6. The selective death of a certain proportion of the neurons initially generated.

[1] Although there are many similarities in the pattern of neurogenesis in vertebrates and invertebrates, the differences between them are sufficiently striking that no general account can be given that adequately covers both. For reviews of the development of the invertebrate nervous system, reference should be made to the monographs edited by Young (1973) and by Fentress (1976).

7. The functional validation of certain of the connections that have been formed and the elimination of others.

Since each of these phases of neural development has been the subject of intensive study and since many have been reviewed at length elsewhere (see, for example, Hughes, 1968; Gaze, 1970; Jacobson, 1970b; Hunt and Jacobson, 1974; Hunt, 1975; and the articles by Angevine, Prestige, Sidman, and Jacobson in the second ISP book, 1970), in what follows a synoptic view will be presented of the selectional and control mechanisms that appear to be operative at each successive stage in neurogenesis. In particular, attention will be focused on four critical issues: (1) the control of neuron number, which includes a consideration of the factors involved in the regulation of cell proliferation in the nervous system, and the phenomenon of "naturally occurring cell death"; (2) the control of neuronal position, which includes both neuronal migration and selective cell aggregation; (3) the control of neuronal form and especially the interplay of genetic and environmental influences on dendritic growth and development; and (4) the control of neuronal connectivity, in which an attempt will be made to draw, from the vast body of experimental evidence bearing on this topic, a number of generalizations concerning normal and aberrant axonal growth and synapse formation.

The control of cell number

Among the many remarkable features about the development of the nervous system, one of the most remarkable is that it so consistently leads to the formation of neural centers which, from animal to animal within any given species, are strikingly constant not only in terms of their location and general form, but also in terms of the numbers of neurons they contain. In those systems for which precise quantitative data are available, the total numbers of nerve cells may vary by as little as 5% in a population of several hundred or even several thousand (see, for example, Fry and Cowan, 1972; Rogers and Cowan, 1973; Clarke and Cowan, 1976). This constancy implies that during the assembly of each neuronal population, a number of rather precise mechanisms must be involved in the regulation of cell number. And the fact that certain neuronal populations have been found to be more or less completely restored after the destruction of a sizable portion of their precursor pools suggests that the maintenance of appropriate

cell numbers is one of the major objectives of early neurogenesis. Most of the controlling factors still remain obscure, but as the result of the work of the past decade, it has become clear that in many, if not all, neuronal populations, the establishment of cell number is a two-stage process. Following the generation of an initial population of neurons from the relevant precursor pool, there is a secondary adjustment of the size of the population to match the functional needs of the system. That is to say, the controlled production of neurons is followed by a rigorous selection procedure. Since the known factors involved in the regulation of the two stages appear to be different, it is convenient to treat them separately even though they are clearly directed toward the same end result.

CELL PROLIFERATION   As there are significant differences in the pattern of cell proliferation in the CNS and PNS, and as the former has been rather more intensively studied, it will be dealt with first and at somewhat greater length. But it is evident that in both parts of the nervous system the size of the initial population of neurons generated is a function of three related factors: the size of the available precursor pool, the duration of the cell cycle, and the period over which cell proliferation is continued.

At present we have no reliable data about the size of any specific precursor pool, although estimates have been attempted for some neuronal populations by calculating back from the size of the established population and making some reasonable estimates about the duration of the cell cycle and the period of active cell proliferation as judged by ^{3}H-thymidine autoradiography. But at best these estimates are within a factor of perhaps two or four, and until techniques become available for selectively following the fate of individual precursor cells in the ventricular or subventricular zones of the neural tube, or in the various neural crest or placodal derivatives, it will be impossible to be more precise. This is not simply an academic issue: it is intimately related to the important issue of the determination of cell lineages in the nervous system, and to the problem of what determines the relative number of cells of different types in most complex neuronal populations. In all but the simplest peripheral ganglia and certain unusual central neuronal populations, there must be some rather delicately balanced relationship between the numbers of neurons of various classes within the population, and in particular between the numbers of cells with locally ramifying axons and the numbers of projection neurons.

On the other hand, by applying techniques which have now become commonplace in cell biology for determining the duration of the entire cell cycle or each of its major phases, it has been possible to measure these parameters in a number of neuronal populations, and several generalizations about the neuronal cell cycle can now be drawn with some confidence. First, it is evident that the duration of the cell cycle in most neuronal precursor pools is not significantly different from that in other somatic tissues. At early stages, when proliferation is at its peak, the total cell cycle has usually been found to be of the order of 8–12 hours. The phase of DNA synthesis (the so-called S phase) lasts approximately 5 or 6 hours; this is followed by the postsynthetic or second gap (G_2) phase lasting about 1–2 hours, and the mitotic (M) phase, which takes about 30–60 minutes. Following cytokinesis there is another gap period (the G_1 phase), which is initially quite short (usually less than 1 hour). Second, the total cell cycle tends to become increasingly prolonged as development proceeds, with most of the lengthening being due to an increase in the G_1 phase (Kauffman, 1968). This is of particular importance in those proliferative regions, such as the subventricular zone, in which cell proliferation is maintained long after it has ceased in the neuroepithelium lining the ventricular surface of the neural tube, and in which many of the smaller nerve cells (or microneurons) are generated. One important exception to this generalization may be the external granular zone of the cerebellum, in which most of the short-axon cells of the cerebellar cortex are generated. Here the cell cycle appears to be fairly long throughout the entire period of neurogenesis and shows little change over the three or four week period in which the stellate and granule cells are being formed (Fujita, Shimada, and Nakamura, 1966). Third, it is now evident that in some cases where the final numbers of cells are abnormally low (as in certain of the mouse neurological mutants, and after various types of experimental manipulation during embryonic life), the determining factor appears to be an unusual lengthening of the entire cell cycle, in which all phases may be involved (Wilson, 1974a,b). Whether other environmental factors (such as serious maternal malnutrition) act in the same way remains to be determined, but it is evident that a relatively minor alteration in the cell cycle, at a critical stage in development, could have major consequences for the size of many neuronal populations if it is not paralleled by a compensatory increase in the period of cell proliferation.

The duration of the proliferative period has been determined for a large number of neuronal populations,[2] using the technique of ^{3}H-thymidine autoradiography. As the principles underlying this method are well known and have been well reviewed elsewhere (Sidman, 1970), it is only necessary to emphasize that whereas the precursor cells in each of the several proliferative zones continue to divide for varying periods of time (and while so doing are able to incorporate the exogenously administered label into their DNA), there is a critical point in the life of each neuron when it abruptly ceases DNA synthesis.[3] By administering the label at different times, or for a suitably lengthy period of time, it is possible to define not only the time at which various subpopulations of neurons become postmitotic, but also the duration of the proliferative period of the population as a whole.

Unfortunately, although it is relatively easy to define the duration of the proliferative period and the "birthdate" of any given population of neurons, we do not know why the various populations are generated (i.e., become postmitotic) at particular times or why some populations cease dividing relatively early whereas others, often in the same proliferative zone, continue DNA synthesis for several days or even weeks. Hinds (1968) has suggested from his studies of cell proliferation in the mammalian olfactory bulb that one critical factor may be the overall extent of the neuroepithelium in which the proliferation occurs. According to this view the relatively small population of mitral cells is generated early, when the neuroepithelial lining of the olfactory ventricle is relatively small, whereas the enormous population of local circuit neurons (including the periglomerular cells and the granule cells) is generated over a much longer time period, when there has been

[2] The period of glial proliferation is more difficult to determine. Most types of glial cells, and the various peripheral supporting cells, seem to retain their capacity for DNA synthesis throughout the life of the organism and can readily be stimulated to divide by a variety of noxious agents, and especially by injury or death of the neighboring neurons (Sjöstrand, 1971; Watson, 1972).

[3] Earlier claims that certain large neurons in the vertebrate CNS, such as the cerebellar Purkinje cells, the larger pyramidal cells of the cerebral cortex and hippocampus, and most spinal motoneurons, are tetraploid, having undergone a further round of DNA synthesis without cytokinesis after leaving their respective proliferative zones (Lapham, 1968; Lapham et al., 1971), have not been substantiated (Fujita, 1974).

a corresponding expansion of the neuroepithelium. A somewhat similar view has been put forward by Smart (1972a,b) to account for differences in the sizes of various neuronal populations in the spinal cord and diencephalon. It is certainly true that in most neuronal populations the larger neurons (and these are usually the cells with distantly projecting axons) are generated earlier than the smaller, local circuit, neurons in the same region. For example, the ganglion cells of the retina are generated before the various retinal interneurons or the receptor cells (Sidman, 1961); the Purkinje and deep nuclear cells of the cerebellum are formed long before the various cortical interneurons and the enormous populations of granule cells (Miale and Sidman, 1961; Fujita, 1967); the hippocampal pyramidal cells are formed over a period of just 3 or 4 days whereas the associated granule cells in the dentate gyrus are generated later and over a period of some weeks (Angevine, 1965; Schlessinger, Cowan, and Gottlieb, 1975). There are, however, important exceptions to this generalization, of which one of the most striking is the finding that most of the short-axon (stellate) cells in layer IV of the mammalian cerebral cortex are generated before the larger pyramidal cells in the overlying layer III (Rakic, 1974).

This type of observation raises the intriguing question of what regulates the *relative numbers* of different classes of neurons in the various neuronal populations in the CNS. Although it has yet to be established that there is a precise relationship between, say, the number of local interneurons and the number of principal or projection cells in any neural center, it is generally believed that this is the case. The actual ratios seem to vary enormously from a minimum of just a few to one, to the many hundreds of cerebellar granule cells that exist for each Purkinje neuron, but it is likely that some delicately balanced control mechanism regulates the relative numbers of neurons of each type. At present it is difficult to see how such a regulatory mechanism may operate, but it is perhaps worth recalling that there is a good deal of evidence to suggest that probably all the cells in the neuroepithelium are coupled through low-resistance gap junctions (Sheridan, 1968) and that it is not until cells withdraw from the proliferative cycle that they lose this type of close relationship with their neighbors (Dixon and Cronly-Dillon, 1972).

Perhaps the most significant generalization that can be drawn from the published studies using ³H-thymidine autoradiography is that in every region of the nervous system, the various classes of neurons are always generated in distinctive sequences, and that often the population as a whole displays distinctive gradients in the time of origin of each subpopulation of cells. For example, in the neocortex (and this is especially clear in primates, in which the proliferative period is relatively long) the deepest-lying cells (the pyramidal and fusiform cells in layer VI) are generated first, and the more superficial cellular laminae (layers V through I) are sequentially added in a characteristic "inside-out" sequence (Rakic, 1974).[4] Exactly the reverse sequence is found in the retina, in which the first cells to be generated (the ganglion cells) come to lie farthest from the proliferative zone, while the last cells to be formed are the receptors, which remain along the surface of the original optic ventricle. While the retina has a simple "outside-in" sequence of cell generation (Sidman, 1961), the avian optic tectum displays a considerably more complex pattern: the earliest tectal neurons to be formed occupy the deepest layers; the next group to become postmitotic are those which form the most superficial group of laminae; lastly, the neurons which comprise the intermediate cell layers are generated (LaVail and Cowan, 1971). These contrasting patterns make it evident that no simple generalization as to the sequence of cell generation is possible.

In most regions of the CNS (and this is particularly true of those in which the period of cell genesis is fairly prolonged) it is usually possible to identify morphogenetic gradients in the sequence of cell proliferation—a phenomenon Hamburger (1948) has referred to as the "patterning of mitotic activity in space and time." Again a few examples will serve to make the point. In the retina of most vertebrates the earliest-formed neurons appear near the upper end of the choroid fissure, and as development proceeds, new cells are progressively added to this initial population in a series of more or less concentric rings (Straznicky and Gaze, 1971; Kahn, 1973). In the optic tectum, the major site of projection of retinal ganglion cell axons in submammals, the pattern is quite different; the initial focus of proliferation is near the rostrolateral pole, and it then spreads in a curvilinear manner toward the caudomedial end of the tectum (Cowan, Martin, and Wenger, 1968; Straznicky and Gaze, 1972). In most other regions the gradients are

[4] The terms "inside-out" and "outside-in" are used with respect to the proliferative layer in which the cells are generated. In the case of the cerebral cortex this is the neuroepithelial lining of the lateral ventricles; in the retina and optic tectum it is the ventricular surface of the original optic vesicle and the tectal ventricles, respectively.

more linear and generally proceed in a rostral-to-caudal direction. Thus in the spinal cord any given neuronal group (say, the motoneurons of the anterior horn) tends to be generated earlier at cervical levels than in the lumbosacral region (Hamburger, 1948; Nornes and Das, 1974), and a similar pattern holds for the greater part of the brain stem. Interestingly, in the thalamus this sequence is reversed: in general, neurons in the more posterior thalamic cell groups are generated earlier than those in the anterior nuclei (Angevine, 1970). One final generalization that seems justifiable on the basis of the available evidence is that in those parts of the CNS in which alar and basal plate regions are identifiable, proliferation in the basal region generally precedes that in the alar plate (Hamburger, 1948), and a comparable ventral-to-dorsal gradient is fairly common even in the forebrain (Schlessinger, Cowan, and Gottlieb, 1975; Smart and Smart, 1977).

At present we have no idea what establishes and controls these gradients of cell proliferation. Attempts have been made to see if they can be reversed by various forms of experimental manipulation such as dorsoventral rotation of the spinal cord. Most of these have either resulted in no change in the proliferative pattern (perhaps because, for technical reasons, they were carried out at too late a stage), but some preliminary observations suggest that the normal rostral-to-caudal progression of cell proliferation in the avian optic tectum may be reversible if the entire midbrain is excised and rotated 180° around its long axis (Cowan, 1971). Further work along these lines is clearly needed to determine whether each major region of the neuraxis has its own polarizing focus (Chung and Cooke, 1975) or whether there are extrinsic morphogenetic gradients acting more generally throughout the body, comparable to those which seem to control the positional cues that determine the axial polarity of the limbs, ear, and retina (Harrison, 1921, 1936; Stone, 1960; Hunt and Jacobson, 1974; Hunt, 1975).

One finding that seems to be generally true is that the highly ordered neuronal patterns of proliferation seen in most regions of the CNS are not determined by extrinsic signals from the major sources of afferents to these regions, or from the principal target regions to which they send their axons. Thus early removal of the optic cup has no effect on the rostrocaudal gradient of cell proliferation in the chick tectum, on the sequence in which its various layers are generated, or on the total number of neurons formed (Cowan, Martin, and Wenger, 1968; Kelly and Cowan, 1972). In frogs the same procedure has been shown to cause a slight, but statistically significant, reduction in the number of mitoses in the contralateral tectum (Kollros, 1953), but this occurs only after the period of neurogenesis and is almost certainly due to a reduction in the number of glial cells produced (Currie and Cowan, 1974). A comparable influence of afferent deprivation upon gliogenesis has been reported in the mammalian superior colliculus following postnatal enucleation of the contralateral eye (De Long and Sidman, 1962). Similarly, early limb bud removal or removal of all sensory inputs has been shown to have no effect upon the initial generation of motoneurons in the chick spinal cord (Hamburger, 1958; Hamburger, Wenger, and Oppenheim, 1966). And the same is true of the removal of the projection field of the nucleus of origin of centrifugal fibers to the avian retina (Cowan and Wenger, 1968).

That the generation of neurons in distinct, and invariable, sequences is a feature of certain complex neuronal populations has been recently demonstrated in a striking way in the avian optic tectum (Finger, Rogers, and Cowan, 1976). If the greater part of the alar plate at mesencephalic levels is removed on one side in early chick embryos (around 40 hours of incubation), the defect is promptly closed over by a regenerative proliferation of the adjacent neuroepithelium. This newly established neuroepithelium proceeds over the next 10 or 12 days to generate an essentially normal tectum, which will subsequently receive a retinotopically organized input from the contralateral eye. But what is of particular interest in the present context is that each of the several cellular layers that comprise the tectum can be shown (by the appropriate ^{3}H-thymidine autoradiographic experiments) to be generated in exactly the same sequence as on the control (normal) side—even though the whole process is delayed by about 36 hours. In addition to establishing that the orderly, sequential production of neurons is rigidly controlled, these experiments indicate that the regenerated neuroepithelium must contain a full complement of the precursors of all the various cell types that comprise the tectum, and that these cells must acquire the position-determining properties that control the later formation of the retinotectal projection totally independently of the regions from which the regenerated neuroepithelium is derived.

It is interesting that in the best experimental cases the regenerated tectum can achieve about 70–80% of its normal volume; since the density of cells in the various layers appears to be normal, the total number of cells generated must be of the same order of magnitude. This again implies that there must be a finely tuned control mechanism regulating the number of divisions each precursor cell can pass through and the precise sequence in which mitosis in the different precursor populations is terminated. However, if a similar operation is performed at a later period in tectal development, this control mechanism seems to break down, and a tumorlike overgrowth of tectal tissue may result. In such cases the total amount of tectal tissue formed may be substantially greater than that found in normal animals, but in many parts of the overgrown tissue mass there may be regions with a relatively normal cytoarchitectonic appearance (Källén, 1965). It is perhaps dangerous to draw conclusions from what is obviously a pathological development, but the appearance of normally laminated zones in an otherwise exuberant overgrowth of tissue suggests that the factors which control the sequential cessation of DNA synthesis in different populations of precursor cells in any one small sector of the proliferative zone may be quite different from those which control the overall level of proliferation in the tectum.

A similar regenerative proliferation has been found in the mammalian cerebellum. Following X-irradiation at a relatively early stage in the development of the external granular layer, the number of dividing cells in this zone may be severely depleted; but within a few days the precursor pool appears to be completely restored, and the final population of cortical interneurons and granule cells may be virtually normal (Altman, Anderson, and Wright, 1969). Controlled irradiation at successively later stages has a progressively severe effect on the genesis of specific classes of cells, so that it has been possible to eliminate essentially all the basket cells, or all the stellate cells, while leaving the granule cell population largely unaffected, or alternatively, with irradiation at later stages, to eliminate most of the granule cells while leaving the interneurons in the molecular layer intact (Altman and Anderson, 1975). Two obvious conclusions can be drawn from these experiments: first, there must be a critical stage in the genesis of each of the successive populations of cells derived from the external granular layer when, if the cells are irradiated, they are no longer capable of regeneration; and second, each of the various cell lines must be generated from its own precursor pool and the development of each line must proceed along its own time course. As a corollary, it follows that there must

be within the proliferative pool, as a whole, mechanisms that precisely determine the number of precursors of each cell type and the number of cell divisions each must pass through in order to generate an appropriate final number of neurons of each class. Superficially, at least, the process closely resembles wound healing in other organs and tissues, and it is not improbable that the same type of control mechanism is at work.

Most of the available evidence indicates that the control of cell proliferation in the CNS is regulated by local, or intrinsic, factors operating within the neuroepithelium itself, and as yet there is no convincing evidence that such external factors as circulating hormonal levels or malnutrition significantly affect the numbers of neurons generated. Most claims for such effects have not adequately distinguished between the numbers of neurons and glia generated (the estimates of cell number being usually based on total DNA content or crude estimates of total cell number), and few have distinguished between neuron production and neuron survival. However, there is evidence that cell proliferation in the PNS may be under some form of extrinsic control, although the mechanisms for this remain to be determined.

The first convincing demonstration of a peripheral influence of this kind came from the now classic study of Hamburger and Levi-Montalcini (1949) on the development of spinal ganglia in the chick. They observed that if a limb bud was extirpated, or if a supernumerary limb was added at an early stage, there could be a slight but statistically significant decrease or increase, respectively, in the numbers of mitoses in the related ganglia. They were also able to show that in the presence of an implanted mouse sarcoma, there could be an enormous proliferation of neurons and glia in both the adjacent and more distant autonomic ganglia. This latter observation, which led to the discovery of the celebrated nerve growth factor (NGF), clearly established that proliferation in both major components of the PNS can be influenced by extrinsic factors. And although it remains to be shown that NGF or any other agent *normally* plays a role in the control of proliferation in the PNS (as opposed to its undisputed role in the later maintenance of differentiated sympathetic neurons), it is clear that the CNS and PNS are significantly different in this respect. Just why this should be is not clear. It may be related to the fact that in the PNS proliferation is essentially a postmigratory event—in the sense that relatively small numbers of precursor cells migrate to the terminal loci and most proliferation then occurs in situ, whereas in the CNS cell migration nearly always follows the cessation of DNA synthesis.[5]

Before leaving the subject of cell proliferation in the nervous system, it is worth pointing out that the control of glial proliferation is clearly influenced by a number of extrinsic factors, of which the most interesting are perhaps those related to the state of the adjoining neurons and their processes. Reference has already been made to the marked reduction in gliogenesis that occurs if a significant portion of the afferents to a neural center are removed at an early stage (De Long and Sidman, 1962; Currie and Cowan, 1974). Equally marked is the increase in glial production in any region in which there is a significant degeneration of the constituent neurons or of axons passing through or terminating in the region. It is not yet clear what the appropriate mitogenic stimulus is in these cases. Since it can occur even if the related neurons do not actually degenerate but merely show some form of chromatolytic reaction to axotomy, it is not necessarily evoked by some neuronal breakdown product. It is tempting to suggest that there is a continuous two-way interaction between neurons and their supporting glia and that any alteration or disturbance in this interaction serves as stimulus to DNA synthesis in the glial elements. Recent in vitro studies of peripheral supporting cells, which have shown quite clearly that the addition of neurons or neuronal processes to a quiescent population of Schwann cells can act as a powerful mitogenic stimulus, may throw light on this important problem (Wood and Bunge, 1975).

NATURALLY OCCURRING NEURONAL DEATH In a number of neural centers it has been shown that the initial population of neurons generated exceeds, by a significant proportion, the number that finally survive to maturity. In these systems a phase of "spontaneous" or "naturally occurring" cell death serves as the final regulatory mechanism in determining the size of the definitive neuronal population. At present the number of systems in which this phenomenon has been adequately documented is rather limited.

[5] It is true that in the CNS some precursor cells leave the primitive neuroepithelium and set up secondary proliferative zones such as the subventricular layer or the external granular layer of the cerebellum, but even in these cases proliferation precedes the migration of the neurons to their definitive loci. Only in the dentate gyrus of the hippocampal formation has in situ neuronal proliferation been observed.

For obvious reasons studies of this phenomenon have been confined to neuronal populations consisting of only several hundred, or at the most a few thousand, neurons. In the absence of automated mechanisms for accurately counting neurons (as opposed to all the cells in any given area), only the most indirect attempts have been made to determine whether or not a comparable degree of cell death occurs in large, neuronal populations such as the cerebral cortex, and if so, whether it affects all classes of neurons including both local circuit neurons and projection cells. Where the numbers of cells are relatively small, it has been possible to estimate the size of the neuronal population at successive stages in development by serial cell counts. In other cases, where many thousands of neurons are involved, one approach has been to estimate the relative numbers of neurons that are labeled following a single injection of ^{3}H-thymidine in animals sacrificed within 24 or 48 hours after the administration of the isotope and in littermates that are allowed to survive to maturity. This approach is fraught with technical difficulties, and although in the one case in which it has been applied—the dentate gyrus of the rat (Schlessinger, Cowan, and Gottlieb, 1975)—it has given results compatible with the notion that this population of cells may undergo a significant degree of neuronal death during development, the data are by no means unequivocal. On the other hand, in every case in which it has been possible to follow the numbers of cells serially, it has been found that between 40% and 75% of the neurons that are initially generated die shortly after assembling to form the anlage of the relevant neural center.

Although it was more than seventy years ago that the first report of degenerating neurons in the developing nervous system appeared (Collin, 1906), it was not until the publication of Hamburger and Levi-Montalcini's (1949) study of the development of the spinal ganglia in the chick that the magnitude and potential significance of this apparently spontaneous death of neurons was recognized. And it was not until quite recently that its importance as a regulatory mechanism in the control of neuronal number came to be appreciated. As this topic was considered from a somewhat different point of view by Prestige (1970) at an earlier ISP and has recently been reviewed at length elsewhere (Cowan, 1973), it will suffice here to summarize some of the main features of the naturally occurring cell death and to indicate the critical role it may play in regulating neuronal number in the CNS.

The four aspects of this phenomenon that are of

particular interest are (1) its magnitude, (2) its timing, (3) the factors responsible for it, and (4) its distribution. Regarding the magnitude of the cell loss, it should be emphasized that we are not here dealing with the fortuitous death of an occasional neuron in a population of several thousand, as may be suspected from the relative infrequency with which frankly degenerating neurons are encountered in routine sections of the CNS. As has been pointed out, in those systems for which accurate data are available, the cell loss has been found to range from 40% (in the lateral motor columns of the chick spinal cord—Hamburger, 1975) to 75% (in the mesencephalic nucleus of the trigeminal nerve in the chick—Rogers and Cowan, 1973). Thus, in these systems cell death represents a major developmental event, and since there is no further reduction in the neuronal population, the naturally occurring neuronal degeneration serves as the final determinant of cell number.

This degeneration does not occur randomly throughout the entire period of development; it is generally limited to just a few days over a period that can now be predicted with some certainty for several systems. For example, in the mesencephalic nucleus of the trigeminal nerve in the chick, the cell death occurs over a period of about 96 hours during which the population is reduced from about 4,500 to its final number of 1,100. The sudden death of such a significant portion of the cells suggests that it is probably related to some critical event in normal neurogenesis. Earlier suggestions that only a fraction of the initial population of neurons actually sends processes to the periphery, or that cell death preferentially affects the last neurons in the population to be generated, have recently been ruled out. Thus, in the nucleus of origin of centrifugal fibers to the avian retina (the so-called isthmo-optic nucleus) and in the chick spinal cord, it is clear, from experiments with retrograde labeling with the enzyme marker horseradish peroxidase, that prior to the onset of the naturally occurring cell death essentially all of the cells extend axons to their respective targets (Clarke and Cowan, 1976; Oppenheim and Chu-Wang, 1977). And in the case of the isthmo-optic nucleus, in which there is a clear gradient in the time of origin of the neurons, the cell death has been found to be uniformly distributed across the entire population and not confined to the region containing the later-generated neurons (Clarke, Rogers, and Cowan, 1976).

Several lines of evidence suggest that the critical factors responsible for this naturally occurring cell death are to be found in the region in which the relevant processes terminate. The most significant of these (in addition to the finding that the processes actually reach their target field) is that any alteration in the size of the peripheral innervation field can significantly alter the magnitude of the cell death. This has generally been demonstrated by either total or partial extirpations of the projection field, which lead to a proportional accentuation of the cell death, the additional neuronal degeneration occurring over the same period as the naturally occurring cell loss (see Cowan, 1973, for a detailed review of this evidence). The most critical analysis, involving an artificial increase in the size of the periphery, has only recently been successfully carried out. By transplanting supernumerary limb buds close to the normal hindlimbs in a series of chicks, Hollyday and Hamburger (1976) have been able to reduce significantly the degree of naturally occurring cell loss in the lateral motor columns of the related spinal cord segments. This observation is of special interest because it suggests that the neurons that normally die are not genetically misspecified or for some other reason incapable of survival, and that it is the magnitude of some peripheral factor that determines the ultimate size of the neuronal population.

The simplest hypothesis is that the relevant factor is either the number of available synaptic sites (or sensory receptors in the case of sensory ganglion cells) or the amount of an essential "trophic agent." (These two views may, in fact, reflect two aspects of the same mechanism if, as seems eminently possible, the postulated trophic agent is available only at synaptic or receptor sites.) According to this view the number of processes generated normally exceeds the number of innervation sites (or the amount of trophic material available), and the various processes must compete among themselves for the available innervation sites (or for the particular trophic agent). As yet no alternative hypothesis has been found that satisfies all the available evidence; in particular, the finding that a proportion of the cells that might normally be expected to degenerate can be "rescued" by peripheral enlargement would seem to rule out the notion that the naturally occurring cell death is programmed in a manner comparable to that found in other tissues (see Saunders and Fallon, 1966) and in the nervous systems of certain invertebrates.

A still unresolved issue of considerable importance is whether the phenomenon of spontaneous cell death is limited to certain neural centers and particular types of neuron. As mentioned earlier, the phenomenon has been most intensively studied in small populations of neurons, and especially those with peripherally projecting processes. It would be of the greatest interest if it could be shown that a similar degree of cell death occurs in such regions as the cerebral cortex and if it also involves neurons with locally ramifying axons.

The control of neuronal position

The position a neuron occupies in the mature nervous system is determined by at least two developmental processes: (1) its migration from the proliferative zone in which it is generated; and (2) a complex of factors that we may collectively refer to as "selective neuronal aggregation." Although the two processes are closely related, it is convenient to deal with them separately. And again, since both have been the subject of a number of intensive studies in recent years (for reviews see Sidman and Rakic, 1973, 1974; Marchase, Vosbeck, and Roth, 1976), it will only be possible to consider some of the more important recent findings, and those which may have rather wide implications for the assembly of neuronal populations.

NEURONAL MIGRATION With the exception of certain granule cells of the dentate gyrus that are generated in situ (Angevine, 1965; Schlessinger, Cowan, and Gottlieb, 1975), all neurons in the vertebrate nervous system undergo at least one phase of migration before reaching their definitive location. The mechanism that triggers the onset of migration is not yet known, but it appears to be closely associated (at least in time) with the withdrawal of the cells from the mitotic cycle. As we have seen, at or close to the time of the final mitosis, neurons seem to acquire an address, in the sense that in any given region the neurons that become postmitotic at the same time come to occupy closely related positions in the mature brain or spinal cord. This has now been demonstrated for several neural systems and has in fact been one of the most significant contributions of ^{3}H-thymidine autoradiography (Sidman, 1970). Unfortunately it is not at all clear what the nature of the addressing mechanism may be, or how it is expressed during the migratory process. In many (but certainly not all) systems the migrating neurons seem to be closely applied to the surfaces of radially oriented glial processes which extend across the entire thickness of the wall of the early neural tube or its derivatives (Cajal, 1960; Rakic, 1975). Sidman and Rakic (1973, 1974) are of the opinion that this relationship is not simply a topographic one, and they have suggested that the radial glial processes actually serve to guide migrating neurons to their destinations, presumably through some as yet unknown cuing mechanism encoded on the opposed cell surfaces. In support of this view they cite their observation that in the *weaver* mutant mouse (in which the cerebellar granule cells fail to migrate across the molecular layer from their site of origin in the external granular zone) there is an early breakdown of the radial processes of the Bergmann glia (Rakic and Sidman, 1973). Although this observation has been questioned (Sotelo and Changeux, 1974), it is strongly suggestive, and the general hypothesis remains an attractive one. If it should be substantiated for the radial migration of neurons (and the initial migration of most neurons *is* radial), it would seem that many of the locus-determining properties commonly assigned to neurons should more correctly be thought of as involving an interactive association between neurons and the neighboring glia, and it would be of the greatest interest to determine what components on glial cell surfaces promote neuronal migration for a period of time and then at an appropriate point cause it to stop abruptly. At the same time it is clear that this hypothesis cannot account for all neuronal migrations, and in particular it fails to explain the migrations of many types of neurons that are clearly orthogonal to the radial orientation of the early glial processes. Unless there are as yet unrecognized glial cell surfaces or other types of preformed surfaces involved in such migrations, some alternative hypothesis is needed. It is also evident that in many instances the critical event is not the physical displacement of the entire cell but rather a progressive translocation of the neuronal nucleus within a growing process. The apparent migration of cerebellar granule cells is of this kind, and there is recent evidence to suggest that this may be true also of certain neurons in the avian optic tectum (Domesick and Morest, 1977). However, it seems unlikely that most classes of nonradially migrating neurons generate long-lasting processes of the type Domesick and Morest have described, and in these instances the entire cell must progressively move through the rather loosely structured neuropil of the developing nervous system.

Considering the problems involved, it is perhaps not surprising that in normal development some neurons become misdirected during their migratory period and end up in ectopic positions. Cajal (1960) seems to have been the first to recognize the existence of such ectopic cells in the spinal cords of early chick embryos, and he suggested that since such cells could not be found in mature animals, they were probably eliminated during the later stages of development. Direct evidence in support of this notion has come from the study of comparable ectopic neurons associated with the development of the isthmo-optic nucleus in normal chicks (Clarke and Cowan, 1976). In this system approximately 3% of the neurons migrate to ectopic positions ventral and lateral to the anlage of the nucleus; but despite their abnormal location, the axons of these ectopic cells successfully gain access to the isthmo-optic tract and through it reach the contralateral retina (from which they can be retrogradely labeled by intraocular injections of horseradish peroxidase). About 90% of these cells fail to survive the period of naturally occurring cell death in the rest of the isthmo-optic nucleus, apparently because they fail to receive a normal afferent input (Cowan and Clarke, 1976). It is not known how widespread this type of transient error of migration may be, since in most systems it is difficult, if not impossible, to identify specific classes of neurons at early developmental stages. However, it is evident that not all ectopically located neurons are eliminated during development. In fact a variety of neuronal ectopias have been described in the neuropathological literature, and some, such as those associated with cerebral lissencephaly, are strikingly constant in appearance and location (see Rakic, 1975, for review). It will be of considerable interest to determine why some ectopic neurons are selectively eliminated during development whereas others persist throughout the life of the animal. But it is worth noting in this context that the finding that the axons of certain ectopic neurons can successfully "find their way" to their appropriate target regions clearly implies that the factors responsible for the *directed migration* of neurons are formally distinguishable from those involved in the *directed outgrowth* of neuronal processes.

One important question that remains to be addressed is whether the process of migration is "instructive" (in the sense that it affects the ultimate phenotype of the migrating cells) or whether, from this point of view, it is essentially "neutral." At present there is no evidence bearing on this point in the CNS, but in the autonomic nervous system, which is more amenable to experimental analysis, there is a good deal of evidence to suggest that migration may be instructive. According to Cohen (1972) and Norr (1973), the "character" of the cells that come to form the pre- and paravertebral sympathetic ganglia is largely determined by an inductive effect exerted by the somitic mesoderm through which they normally migrate, and the capacity of the somitic mesoderm to exert this influence is predetermined by its earlier association with the adjoining neural tube. It is intriguing to speculate that similar inductive effects

may shape the morphology and function of central neurons, but it is difficult to anticipate how this will be experimentally analyzed.

Selective Neuronal Aggregation   On completing their primary migration, young neurons of related type specifically aggregate together to form the anlage of the future neural center or cortical lamina. In many, and perhaps all, systems this process involves both the coming together of functionally related neurons or neurons of like kind and also their specific alignment. Both processes are difficult to analyze in vivo, although few features of the mature nervous system are more characteristic than its precise parcellation into distinct nuclear groups or cortical laminae, and in many regions one of the most striking features is the distinctive orientation of the principal cell type. Fortunately, the analysis of certain genetic mutants and the development of in vitro methods for the analysis of neuronal reaggregation have begun to throw light on the factors that may be involved in both the aggregation and the alignment processes.

Among the neurological mutants, the so-called reeler mouse has been the subject of greatest interest from this point of view. In homozygous animals most (but, significantly, not all) cortical structures show a profound disruption of normal cell distribution. At first glance the appearance of these cortical areas seems totally chaotic when compared to that of normal animals; but on closer examination it is evident that the distorted architectural pattern is rather consistent from region to region, so that in some regions (such as the hippocampal formation) one can readily recognize systematic cytoarchitectonic disturbances (Caviness and Rakic, 1978). It has recently become clear from developmental studies that each class of cortical neurons is generated at the same time as its counterpart in normal animals, and in the appropriate sequence. Their abnormal distribution thus appears to be due to erroneous addressing or, to be more precise, to a failure of the cells to migrate to the appropriate region and there to aggregate in a normal manner. That the failure to aggregate selectively is probably the critical factor has been elegantly demonstrated by comparing the reaggregation patterns of dissociated cells from the cerebral cortex and hippocampus of normal and reeler animals (De Long, 1970; De Long and Sidman, 1970). Under appropriate conditions normal cortical neurons not only aggregate into distinct clumps but also show distinct evidence of lamination, indicating that the reaggregating neurons have appropriately realigned themselves with respect to their neighbors. No such lamination is seen in dissociated cortical cells from reeler mice that are allowed to reaggregate under the same conditions. Whether this is because they specifically lack the necessary surface components involved in cell–cell orientation, or because the relevant components are incorrectly distributed on the surfaces of the cells, remains to be determined. It is interesting that although the orientation and distribution of the cells in the cerebral cortex of the reeler mouse are quite abnormal, each class of cells seems to be capable of receiving and making a normal set of connections, and in the visual cortex at least, their functional properties and the topographic ordering of their afferent input seem quite normal (Dräger, 1976).

The second approach to this problem, which is proving to be singularly successful, derives from an early experimental finding of Holtfreter (1939) that chemically or mechanically dissociated embryonic cells that are allowed to reaggregate invariably sort themselves out according to type and can go on to form histotypic tissue aggregates following this sorting-out process. This approach has been extensively used by Moscona and his colleagues (see Moscona, 1974, for review) to identify neural-specific and brain-region-specific ligands that may be implicated in the reaggregation process. Others, notably Roth and his colleagues (Roth and Marchase, 1976; Barbera, 1975), have seen in the selectivity of this reaggregation a possible molecular approach to the problem of neuronal connectivity, and their early finding that isolated cells from the dorsal and ventral parts of the retina showed some degree of preferential affinity for the related ventral and dorsal halves of the optic tectum gave support to this view. At present this prospect seems less promising, but the work that it has stimulated may yet prove to be of considerable interest for our understanding of how nuclear groups and cortical laminae are formed. Since much of this work has been extensively reviewed in a recent monograph and in an admirable review (Barondes, 1976; Marchase, Vosbeck, and Roth, 1976) and is considered elsewhere in this volume by Rutishauser, only two observations need be made here.

One of the most intriguing findings is that cells dissociated from each of several tissues display a changing pattern of adhesive affinities. Thus the reaggregation of dissociated retinal cells from 8-day chick embryos is substantially inhibited by the presence of membrane fragments of cells of the same age; on the other hand, membranes from 7- or 9-day-old retinas have much less of an effect on the reaggregation of 8-day cells (Gottlieb, Merrell, and Glaser, 1974). Similar data are available for the reag-

gregation of cells from the optic tectum. Although it is not yet clear to what extent such temporal specifications are involved in the selective sorting out of tissue components during normal neurogenesis, it is tempting to suggest that some such mechanism may account for the characteristic laminar distribution of cells generated at different times in such structures as the cerebral cortex, retina, and optic tectum.

The second interesting finding is that there may also be *spatial* gradients of adhesive affinity during development, which may well be related to the characteristic gradients found during cell proliferation. We have already alluded to the preferential affinity of dorsal and ventral chick retinal cells for the ventral and dorsal parts of the optic tectum. In fact there is a very clear dorsal-to-ventral gradient in this pattern (although, interestingly, there is no evidence for a comparable rostral-to-caudal gradient), and more recent work suggests that there may be an overall rostral-to-caudal gradient operating over several regions of the neuraxis (Gottlieb and Arington, 1978).

The recent isolation of a "cell adhesion molecule" (see Rutishauser, this volume) suggests that this issue may be one of the first to be analyzed in molecular terms, but it is perhaps worth pointing out that selective aggregation is only one facet in the complex formation of neural centers. It will remain to be shown whether there are other molecular species with selective distributions over the surfaces of cells that could account for the precise orientation of the principal neurons, or whether, following aggregation, the critical surface determinants become selectively redistributed on the cells (perhaps in a manner analogous to capping), so that the same molecular species can serve both to bring the cells together and to impose upon them a characteristic polarity.

The control of neuronal form

Although some neurons begin to generate distinctive processes while still migrating toward their final location (Domesick and Morest, 1977), most only begin to generate a dendritic tree after aggregating with their neighbors. In this section we shall consider some of the factors which appear to be involved in determining the characteristic morphology of certain classes of neurons and which by inference may also be implicated in most other neuronal systems. It may seem invidious to focus on the factors controlling neuronal morphology, when clearly other aspects of the neuronal phenotype are at least as interesting and, from a functional point of view, possibly more important. The primary justification for this narrow view is that, at present, the analysis of neuronal morphology is a more manageable problem, and consequently rather more is known about it than about most other aspects of neuronal differentiation. That this situation may soon change is presaged by the exciting recent work on the control of transmitter synthesis in sympathetic neurons (see Patterson, this volume).

That each class of neurons has a distinctive and readily identifiable morphology has been recognized since the introduction of the Golgi method more than a century ago. What has not been evident, and indeed still remains unresolved for most neurons, is the extent to which their characteristic morphology is genetically determined as opposed to being shaped by purely local, or more general, environmental factors. Since the characteristic appearances of most neurons is determined in large part by the number, form, and distribution of their dendritic processes, this problem actually resolves itself into a series of questions concerning the control of process formation in general and of dendrogenesis in particular.

That there is a large genetic component in the determination of cell form is evident from several considerations. First, there is the obvious fact that certain classes of cells, such as the Purkinje cells of the cerebellum or the pyramidal cells of the cerebral cortex, are immediately recognizable from animal to animal within any given species, and often in quite widely separated species. However, as we shall see, this type of subjective "image identification" usually fails to take into account the considerable quantitative variability that may exist even between adjacent cells of the same phenotype. The second line of evidence has come from the careful study of physiologically identified neurons that have been filled with an appropriate dye or marker substance and then carefully reconstructed in three dimensions. Several studies of this kind have been carried out in the last decade (Macagno, Lopresti, and Levinthal, 1973; Pitman, Tweedle, and Cohen, 1973; Altman and Tyrer, 1977), and the general conclusion emerging from this work is that in isogenic organisms most types of identified neurons are remarkably constant in their morphology (at least as far as the primary and secondary dendritic branching patterns are concerned) and in the initial course taken by their axons; it is only in the fine terminal branches that significant variability is found. Third, there is now some evidence that certain types of neurons, when grown in vitro in complete isolation from other neurons, may develop a dendritic morphology which is sufficiently similar to that of their in vivo counterparts that there can be

no mistaking their original source (Banker and Cowan, 1977). Of course, the overall morphology of the dendritic arbor in vitro is two- rather than three-dimensional (since only processes that are in contact with the substratum can be extended).

At the same time it is equally clear that the final form of most neurons is largely shaped by epigenetic factors, both local and general. To date the latter have been much less intensively studied, and at present it is only possible to state that in certain forms of hormonal imbalance (e.g., experimental cretinism) dendritic growth is often quite stunted, and the frequency of dendritic branching is usually reduced (Eayrs, 1960, 1964). Similarly, generally malnourished animals, or animals reared in what are described as "deprived environments," are said to show defective dendritic growth and branching patterns (see, for example, Rosenzweig, Bennett, and Diamond, 1972; Greenough, 1976). While many of the reported changes require more careful evaluation with more quantitative methods, there seems to be little reason to question the general conclusion of this type of study, namely, that there is a considerable degree of developmental plasticity in many regions of the brain (and especially the cerebral cortex) and that one of the most readily modifiable components of the immature nervous system is its dendritic organization.

The effects of local environmental factors on neural morphology lend themselves more readily to experimental analysis, and it is now clear that local mechanical factors and connectional patterns play a major role in shaping the dendritic morphology of individual neurons. One of the best-documented examples of the former is the variable appearance of the stellate cells of the cerebellar cortex that are generated at different times. According to Rakic (1972), the earliest cells of this type to be generated from the external granular layer, the so-called basket cells, occupy the deepest zone within the molecular layer and have predominantly ascending dendrites. Later-formed cells in the midportion of the molecular layer have a characteristic stellate distribution of dendrites. The last-formed cells do not begin to generate dendrites until appreciably later and have only a restricted number of horizontally oriented dendrites. From what is known of the development of the molecular layer, it seems reasonable to conclude that the presence of the surrounding parallel fibers imposes major restraints on the growth and elaboration of the stellate cell dendrites.

A simpler type of mechanical effect has been found to affect the form of what have been termed "star pyramids" in the depths of the central sulcus of the monkey cerebral cortex (Jones, 1975). The general thinning associated with sulcus formation seems to alter significantly the growth and elaboration of the "apical" dendritic system of these cells, so that they appear essentially stellate in form. At the same time it is possible that the horizontal "splaying out" of the dendrites of these cells may also be due to the influence of the incoming thalamocortical afferents, and undoubtedly the most significant single influence in shaping the dendritic form of most neurons is the presence and arrangement of their afferents. A variety of experimental studies bear witness to this. These range from substantial but selective afferent deprivations to gross misalignment of afferents that normally have a high degree of spatial orientation. Depriving immature neurons of their major afferent input almost invariably leads to the rapid atrophy or death of the deprived cells (Cowan, 1970). More restricted deprivations may result in the failure of the denervated segment to grow normally, or in the loss of some specific dendritic feature, such as the characteristic dendritic spines. One of the most striking examples of the first effect is the localized failure of growth and collateral branching in the segment of the lateral dendrites of Mauthner cells that normally receives vestibular inputs, following early removal of the otocyst in axolotls (Kimmel, Schabtach, and Kimmel, 1977). Similarly, there are several reports of selective spine loss following various types of deafferentation, including the removal of specific thalamocortical fibers after sensory deprivation (Globus and Scheibel, 1967; Valverde, 1967). It has even been claimed that spines may reappear as a denervated zone becomes reinnervated (Parnavelas et al., 1974). These influences on dendritic spines are of particular interest since in other situations de novo spine formation appears to occur in severely denervated neurons, and such newly formed spines may survive indefinitely without becoming innervated (Herndon, 1968; Seil and Herndon, 1970; Herndon, Margolis, and Kilham, 1971). A remarkable realignment of dendritic processes is found in the cerebellar cortex after almost any type of experimental interference with parallel fiber development; invariably the distortion of the parallel fibers results in a gross disruption of the normal planar array of the Purkinje cell dendrites (Altman, 1973), and similar disturbances in Purkinje cell dendritic growth are seen in a number of genetic mutants in which there is either a malpositioning of the Purkinje cells themselves or a disorganization of their parallel fiber input (Caviness and Rakic, 1978).

Considering their pattern of growth, it is perhaps not surprising that dendrites should show considerable plasticity. As Cajal (1909) first pointed out, most young neurons bristle with many small "spinelike" appendages and enter a phase of exuberant dendritic growth when afferent fibers start arriving. Many of these early formed dendrites are subsequently retracted and disappear, so that the definitive form of the dendritic tree appears to be sculpted out of the initial more or less chaotic forest of processes. This sculpting process is readily observed in vitro; isolated neurons can be seen to generate and retract dendrites continuously, so that it is usually impossible to predict whether any given process will survive or not (Banker and Cowan, 1977).

The actual mechanism of dendritic growth appears to be similar to that of axons. Distinct dendritic growth cones have been observed in vitro and reconstructed from electron micrographs of sectioned neural tissues (Hinds and Hinds, 1972; Skoff and Hamburger, 1974). And the fact that even in adult animals the ends of dendrites may retain the appearance of growth cones (Sotelo and Palay, 1968) suggests that their potential for dendritic growth may persist throughout life, although presumably it is normally held under rather severe restraints. It is also evident from in vitro studies that most dendritic branching occurs at growth cones, and Hollingworth and Berry (1975) have suggested that normally much of this branching is stimulated by the formation of transient contacts with other neuronal processes. From a detailed network analysis of dendritic branching patterns in the cerebral and cerebellar cortices, they have concluded that the direction of dendritic growth, the order of branching, and the lengths of individual dendritic segments are all determined by local interactions between neighboring axons and dendritic growth cones. According to this view, the relatively high degree of trichotomous branching found in Purkinje cells is associated with a large number of such interactions, whereas their relative infrequency in the cerebral cortex could account for the long unbranched dendritic segments seen in cortical pyramidal neurons.

The control of neuronal connectivity

Of all the problems in developmental neurobiology, none is more intriguing or more important than the elucidation of the factors responsible for the establishment of specific patterns of connections between related neurons. Our understanding of this issue has advanced considerably in the past two decades, due largely to the imaginative studies of Sperry, of Gaze and his colleagues, and of Hunt and Jacobson on the development of the retinotectal projection, especially in the amphibian brain. Indeed, we now know more about the formation of this system than about almost any other. This is not to say that all the problems involved in its development have been resolved; in fact, several controversial issues continue to generate rather more heat than light. And perhaps because of the advances that have been made in our understanding of this system, the important question of whether or not other connectional patterns develop in the same way is often overlooked. In particular, it is a matter of the greatest importance to determine whether or not the "rules" governing axonal connectivity in systems such as this, with distantly projecting axons, also apply to the more numerous short-axon systems and to local neuron circuitry in general.

It is clear from several considerations that there are important developmental differences between projection neurons and cells with short axons, but it is not at all evident that these differences extend to the rules governing the types of connectional patterns that the two classes of cells can establish. For example, it seems misleading to suggest that because most locally projecting neurons do not display the same type of topographically organized connectional patterns that are formed by many distantly projecting neurons, they are in some way "less specific" or "under less rigid genetic control." In fact, one of the most impressive features of the known connections of these cells is that under normal circumstances they are remarkably constant, at least as to type. Among the best-known cells of this general class are the various interneurons and the innumerable granule cells in the cerebellar cortex. All the available evidence indicates that as long as the cortex is intact, each of these classes of cells forms a limited number of connections of readily definable morphological type (Palay and Chan-Palay, 1974). What is less clear is whether the *number* of connections formed by these cells is constant, within reasonable limits, or whether there is considerable variation from cell to cell. Technically this is a rather difficult point to establish. In some systems, such as the dentate gyrus, the distribution of connections to the relatively short-axon granule cells appears to be determined, in part at least, by a temporal competition between afferents of different types (Gottlieb and Cowan, 1972), and the impression one has is that such connections may show considerable variability in the numbers of synapses they form, although the type of synapse and the

zones in which they terminate are rather rigidly determined.

At present it would appear that the only significant difference between the connectivities of projection and of local circuit neurons is to be found in their topographic distribution: whereas most projection neurons seem to have some form of point-to-point (or, more correctly, an orderly "small region" to "small region") type of projection, the connections of many short-axon neurons seem to be more in the form of a lattice. This type of distribution should not be construed as evidence for a lack of specificity; in fact, from the point of view of the localized distribution of their axon terminals upon discrete segments of their target neurons, the connections formed by these cells are at least as specific as any formed by distantly projecting neurons. The reason for dealing with the point at such length is that the following series of generalizations concerning the formation of connections is based on studies of long-axon systems such as the retinotectal projection; it remains to be determined whether they apply with equal validity to the development of short axonal connections.

The first generalization that should be made is that topographic patterns of connectivity appear to be established (or rather to become irreversibly fixed) at about the time the first neurons in the population become postmitotic.[6] The mechanism whereby the first (and later) generated neurons in the population acquire such positional information, and how it becomes expressed in the directed outgrowth of their axons and in the selection of appropriate terminal loci, remains to be established. In the case of ganglion cells in the amphibian retina, the available evidence suggests that from an early stage the proliferating population has some type of position-determining information that is coordinate with the major axes of the body and can become irreversibly fixed if the isolated eye is allowed to develop beyond a critical stage (Hunt and Jacobson, 1972). However, until this critical stage, which seems to be closely related in time, if not causally, to the withdrawal of the first ganglion cells from the mitotic cycle (Jacobson, 1968), the intrinsic positional information within the cells

[6] Strictly this refers to the time when the neuronal population as a whole becomes axially polarized, in the sense of acquiring a coordinate set of position-dependent properties that serve to mark not only the positions of the cells in three dimensions (x, y, and z) but also the topographic distribution of their axons, again in the x, y, and z dimensions.

can be effectively overridden by certain position-determining cues operating throughout the body. This conclusion is based on a number of experiments involving eye rotations and the transplantation of eyes at different stages to various parts of the body and for varying periods of time, followed by mapping of the retinotectal projection after retransplantation of the eyes back to the orbit (Hunt and Jacobson, 1972; Hunt, 1975). Collectively these experiments indicate that as long as the integrity of the system is maintained, the ganglion cells behave as if they were rigidly "specified" in the sense that their axons distribute themselves within the optic tectum according to a fixed set of position-determining properties set by the position of the eye in relation to the primary axes of the body, at the time the retina passed through its critical period. It is important to emphasize that this is true only if the system retains its structural integrity. But if this is interfered with (for example, by bisecting the eye or by ablating a significant portion of the tectum), the system may be capable of adapting to the altered situation, presumably by some mechanism akin to embryonic regulation (Yoon, 1971; Hunt, 1975; Hunt and Berman, 1975).

There is some evidence to suggest that the later-generated cells can acquire positional information independently, and in the same manner as the first-formed cells, but since the experiments on which this is based involve disrupting the normal pattern of retinal development, it is possible that under normal circumstances the information is sequentially propagated throughout the population as each group of ganglion cells is generated (Hunt, 1975). Furthermore, the disappearance of gap junctions that occurs at this time may be implicated in this process (Dixon and Cronly-Dillon, 1972). But whatever the process, it is clear that the acquisition by any neuronal population of a fixed set of locus specificities is a sine qua non for the later formation of a set of connections with a precisely ordered distribution. And if, as seems likely, some of the other determining parameters of neuronal connectivity, such as the selection of an appropriate class of target cells and the predisposition to form synapses of a certain type upon a specific part of the target cells (the soma, proximal dendrites, etc.), are also established at this time, it is appropriate to describe this phase in the developmental history of the population as the critical period for its "specification."

The second generalization that appears to be justified by the available evidence is that connectionally related groups of neurons are independently speci-fied in the sense in which this term has just been used. The strongest evidence for this view derives from experiments in which the regenerated retinotectal projection upon a 180° rotated segment of the tectum has been mapped (Yoon, 1973; Levine and Jacobson, 1974). In these cases the regenerated fibers always grow back to the same portion of the rotated tectal segment that they formerly innervated. While certain other experiments may permit alternative explanations, these experiments with partial tectal rotations seem to point rather unequivocally to the persistence of some form of positional marker(s) on the neurons of the rotated tectal segment. Strictly this conclusion applies only to the situation in which axons regenerate back to their former terminal loci, and it could be argued that the displaced tectal neurons had previously acquired their positional markers from their earlier relationship with the retinal ganglion cell axons. However, there is some evidence that if the entire midbrain (including the optic tectum) is rotated at an appropriate stage in development (before the ingrowth of retinal fibers), the ensuing retinotectal projection may be similarly inverted (Crelin, 1952; Chung and Cook, 1975).

As yet the results of this type of experiment are not as clear-cut as one might wish; but if further studies of this kind clearly establish the independent specification of both the "projecting" and the "target" neurons,[7] it would provide strong evidence in support of Sperry's chemoaffinity hypothesis. According to this hypothesis (which was first put forward to account for the orderly regrowth of retinal fibers following interruption of the optic nerve, with or without rotation of the eye), at some point during development each retinal cell—or, more probably, each small population of ganglion cells—acquires a specific cytochemical label which is expressed on the growing tips of the axon(s), and it is through this label that the appropriate terminal region and the specific target neurons are identified, probably through a matching process involving similar, or complementary, labels on the surfaces of the target cells (Sperry, 1963). At present the evidence for this hypothesis is almost entirely indirect, but its general soundness may be judged from the fact that it has survived a number of fairly rigorous tests and re-

[7] It is worth pointing out in this context that within the central nervous system most neurons can be thought of as being both a source of a projection and also a target for the axons of other cells. This consideration by itself would seem to argue for the independent specification of each major class of neurons.

mains the most generally acceptable hypothesis, whereas most alternative explanations have fallen by the wayside.

A third generalization that can be made is that whereas the course taken by a group of axons may vary considerably, the pattern of connections they establish is fairly invariant. In other words, the route taken by nerve fibers is generally less critical than the destination to which they are addressed. The most striking evidence for this again comes from experimental studies of the retinotectal projection in lower vertebrates and is of two kinds. First, Gaze (1959) and Hibbard (1967) reported cases in which, after interruption of the optic nerve, the regenerating retinal fibers became associated with the oculomotor nerve; despite this highly aberrant course, the fibers were able to reach the optic tectum and were apparently able to innervate it appropriately. Second, Arora and Sperry (1962) were able to misdirect the retinal fibers by deliberately crossing the two divisions of the optic tract in goldfish. In these cases, although the fibers entered the tectum through an incorrect route, they successfully grew across the surface of the tectum and seemed to innervate the correct tectal region. The obvious implication of this type of experiment is that in some sense the axons "know" where they are to terminate, and they continue to grow until they "identify" an appropriate terminal locus. By emphasizing the ability of axons to "home in" on their target, we do not wish to imply that axonal pathfinding is a trivial problem or that the course the axons follow is unimportant. In fact, there is now a considerable body of evidence to show that during normal development the course selected by most groups of axons is rather carefully controlled and that even in genetic mutants in which aberrant axonal growth occurs (for example, in the visual pathways of most albino mammals), the abnormality is rather predictable from animal to animal (Guillery, 1974).

A fourth generalization that appears to be valid is that in most systems the final precise pattern of established connections is fashioned out of an earlier, less well-defined pattern. In the primate visual system, for example, Rakic (1977) has found that when retinal afferents first reach the dorsal lateral geniculate nucleus (around the 10th week of gestation), there is no indication of the precise laminar segregation of the fibers from the two eyes that characterizes the mature form. This pattern only becomes apparent 5 or 6 weeks later, and it is not until 3 or 4 weeks before birth that it begins to approach its mature form. The same appears to be true of the gen-

iculocortical projection insofar as this can be determined from an analysis of the distribution of transsynaptically transported label following the intraocular injection of tritium-labeled protein or glycoprotein precursors at different stages in development. Up to the 13th or 15th week of gestation, there is little or no indication of distinct eye dominance columns in layer IV of the visual cortex, in which the majority of the geniculocortical axons terminate. By the 18th or 19th week of gestation, alternating bands or stripes begin to appear in this layer, but they are by no means sharply defined (Rakic, 1977). And it is not until the first weeks after birth that the characteristic eye dominance pattern seen in mature animals becomes evident (Hubel, Wiesel, and LeVay, 1977). Furthermore, this pattern seems to result from the progressive withdrawal of axon terminals from an initial region of overlap between the relayed inputs from the two eyes; this is suggested by the finding that after monocular deprivation the "columns" associated with the nondeprived eye appear to be significantly expanded, at the expense of the adjoining columns related to the deprived eye (Hubel, Wiesel, and LeVay, 1977).

These and other observations suggest a further generalization, namely that there is usually a period of excessive axonal branching, and "hyperinnervation," followed by a phase during which different groups of terminals compete with each other for some as yet unidentified entity; the terminals that are unsuccessful in this competition are generally withdrawn, although the parent cell (and presumably the main part of the axon) persists. The most convincing evidence for a "hyperinnervation" of this kind comes from studies of the early innervation of muscle fibers, which in the mature animals normally receive only a single axon terminal. In many such cases there is an initial period (around the time of birth) during which the fibers may receive several independent inputs, but during the first two weeks after birth the number of inputs is progressively reduced until finally only one terminal persists (Redfern, 1970; Bennett and Pettigrew, 1974). However, there is also evidence for a similar type of hyperinnervation in certain neurons, the best-documented of which is perhaps the multiple innervation of immature cerebellar Purkinje cells by climbing fibers (Larramendi, 1969); here again, this early phase in which the cells receive inputs from a number of climbing fibers is followed by a period in which there is a selective elimination of all but one of the initial inputs. At present we do not know what factor(s) determine that some terminals will survive while others of the same general type will be eliminated. And if the selective elimination of some terminals is a result of their failure in some competitive process, we have no idea as yet what is being competed for. Changeux and Danchin (1976) have put forward an attractive model to account for some of the known developmental phenomena, based on what we might term the "functional validation" of synaptic contacts. According to this hypothesis, target cells are only capable of maintaining a limited number of any specific type of input, and appropriate patterns of activity in certain of these inputs give them a selective advantage over the other terminals of the same type.

At the same time a carefully regulated trophic relationship between target cells and their afferent inputs seems necessary to account for the large body of experimental evidence on the effects of deafferentation or the removal of neuronal projection fields on the survival of many classes of neurons. Since this subject has been extensively reviewed elsewhere (Hughes, 1968; Cowan and Wenger, 1968; Kelly and Cowan, 1972; Clarke and Cowan, 1976), it will suffice to mention here that, as a general rule, if a developing neuron is to survive, not only must it be able to make an appropriate number of connections of the correct type, it must also receive an adequate afferent input from other neurons.

One final generalization worth making is that although normally there must be some delicately programmed mechanism to ensure the formation of morphologically and functionally appropriate connections, growing axons appear to be under considerable pressure to form synapses; when deprived of their appropriate targets, their terminals may therefore occupy just about any unoccupied synaptic sites. This appears to be the basis of much of the "plasticity" seen during early development and perhaps also in adult animals subjected to various types of experimental manipulation. As Schneider and Jhaveri (1974) have pointed out, plasticity of this type can manifest itself in various forms. In some cases axons simply follow an aberrant course but nevertheless establish the correct connections. In others the aberrantly routed axons establish wholly inappropriate patterns of connections or innervate regions they would not normally invade. In still other cases the axons exhibit a "pruning" effect in that, when deprived of one of their projection fields, they often show an unusually rich innervation of another region. Or there may be some degree of "axonal sprouting" confined to the principal projection field, leading, in time, to the occupation of whatever vacated synaptic sites are present. A more detailed consideration of this important topic is clearly beyond the scope of this paper, but it is worth pointing out that the various forms of plasticity may reflect not only a certain pressure within axons to form a given number of synapses, but also a certain hierarchy of preferences. For example, in the dentate gyrus of the hippocampal formation, axons seem to sprout more readily within the territory of other afferent fiber systems with which they seem to share a common cytochemical specificity than into a vacated zone occupied by fibers with a quite different specificity (Lynch and Cotman, 1975). And in this connection it should be mentioned that at least some types of "plasticity" may simply be the persistence into adult life of an earlier pattern of connectivity that would normally have been eliminated. It remains to be shown to what extent this phenomenon can be experimentally controlled, and perhaps even directed, along adaptive lines.

ACKNOWLEDGMENT   The author's work is supported by research grants EY-01225 and NS-10943 from the National Institutes of Health.

REFERENCES

ALTMAN, J., 1973. Experimental reorganization of the cerebral cortex. IV. Parallel fiber re-orientation following regeneration of the external germinal layer. *J. Comp. Neurol.* 149:191–192.

ALTMAN, J., and W. J. ANDERSON, 1975. Experimental reorganization of the cerebellar cortex. I. Morphological effects of elimination of all microneurons with prolonged X-irradiation started at birth. *J. Comp. Neurol.* 146:355–406.

ALTMAN, J., W. J. ANDERSON, and K. A. WRIGHT, 1969. Early effects of X-irradiation of the cerebellum in infant rats: Decimation and reconstitution of the external granular layer. *Exp. Neurol.* 24:196–216.

ALTMAN, J. S., and N. M. TYRER, 1977. The locust wing hinge stretch receptors. II. Variation, alternative pathways and "mistakes" in the central arborizations. *J. Comp. Neurol.* 172:431–440.

ANGEVINE, J. B., 1965. The time of neuron origin in the hippocampal region. An autoradiographic study in the mouse. *Exp. Neurol. Suppl.* 2:1–70.

ANGEVINE, J. B., 1970. Critical cellular events in the shaping of neural centers. In *The Neurosciences: Second Study Program*, F. O. Schmitt, ed. New York: Rockefeller University Press, pp. 62–72.

ARORA, H. L., and R. W. SPERRY, 1962. Optic nerve regeneration after surgical cross-union of medial and lateral optic tracts. *Am. Zool.* 2:389.

BANKER, G. A., and W. M. COWAN, 1977. Rat hippocampal neurons in dispersed cell culture. *Brain Res.* 126:397–425.

BARBERA, A. J., 1975. Adhesive recognition between developing retinal cells and the optic tecta of the chick embryo. *Dev. Biol.* 46:167.

BARONDES, S. H., ed., 1976. *Neuronal Recognition*. New York: Plenum Press.

BENNETT, M. R., and A. G. PETTIGREW, 1974. The formation of synapses in striated muscle during development. *J. Physiol.* 241:515–545.

CAJAL, S. RAMÓN Y, 1909. *Histologie du Système Nerveux de l'Homme et des Vertébrés*, Vol. I. Paris: Malone. (Reprinted by Consejo Superior de Investigaciones Cientificas, Madrid, 1955.)

CAJAL, S. RAMÓN Y, 1937. *Recollections of My Life*, E. Horne Craigie, trans. Cambridge, MA: MIT Press.

CAJAL, S. RAMÓN Y, 1960. *Studies on Vertebrate Neurogenesis* L. Guth, trans. Springfield, IL: Thomas.

CAVINESS, V. S., and P. RAKIC, 1978. Mechanisms of cortical development: A view from mutations in mice. *Ann. Rev. Neurosci.* 1:297–326.

CHANGEUX, J.-P., and A. DANCHIN, 1976. Selective stabilization of developing synapses as a mechanism for the specification of neuronal networks. *Nature* 264:705–712.

CHUNG, S. H., and J. COOK, 1975. Polarity of structure and of ordered nerve connections in the developing amphibian brain. *Nature* 258:126–132.

CLARKE, P. G. H., and W. M. COWAN, 1976. The development of the isthmo-optic tract in the chick with special reference to the occurrence and correction of developmental errors in the location and connections of isthmo-optic neurons. *J. Comp. Neurol.* 167:143–164.

CLARKE, P. G. H., L. A. ROGERS, and W. M. COWAN, 1976. The time of origin and the patterns of survival of neurons in the isthmo-optic nucleus of the chick. *J. Comp. Neurol.* 167:125–142.

COHEN, A. M., 1972. Factors directing the expression of sympathetic nerve tracts in cells of neural crest origin. *J. Exp. Zool.* 179:167–182.

COLLIN, R., 1906. Récherches cytologiques sur le developpement de la cellule nerveuse. *Le Névraxe* 8:185–309.

COWAN, W. M., 1970. Anterograde and retrograde transneuronal degeneration in the central and peripheral nervous system. In *Contemporary Research Methods in Neuroanatomy*, W. J. H. Nauta and S. O. E. Ebbesson, eds. New York: Springer-Verlag, pp. 217–249.

COWAN, W. M., 1971. Studies on the development of the avian visual system. In *Cellular Aspects of Neural Growth and Differentiation*, D. S. Pease, ed. Berkeley: University of California Press, pp. 177–222.

COWAN, W. M., 1973. Neuronal death as a regulative mechanism in the control of cell number in the nervous system. In *Development and Aging in the Nervous System*, M. Rockstein, ed. New York: Academic Press, pp. 19–41.

COWAN, W. M., and P. G. H. CLARKE, 1976. The development of the isthmo-optic nucleus. *Brain Behav. Evol.* 13:345–375.

COWAN, W. M., A. H. MARTIN, and E. WENGER, 1968. Mitotic patterns in the optic tectum of the chick during normal development and after early removal of the optic vesicle. *J. Exp. Zool.* 169:71–92.

COWAN, W. M., and E. WENGER, 1967. Cell loss in the trochlear nucleus of the chick during normal development and after radical extirpation of the optic vesicle. *J. Exp. Zool.* 164:267–279.

COWAN, W. M., and E. WENGER, 1968. The development of the nucleus of origin of centrifugal fibers to the retina in the chick. *J. Comp. Neurol.* 133:207–240.

CRELIN, E. S., 1952. Excision and rotation of the developing Amblystoma optic tectum and subsequent visual recovery. *J. Exp. Zool.* 120:547–577.

CURRIE, J., and W. M. COWAN, 1974. Some observations on the early development of the optic tectum in the frog (*Rana pipiens*), with special reference to the effects of early eye removal on mitotic activity in the larval tectum. *J. Comp. Neurol.* 156:123–142.

DE LONG, G. R., 1970. Histogenesis of fetal mouse isocortex and hippocampus in reaggregating cell cultures. *Dev. Biol.* 22:562–575.

DE LONG, G. R., and R. L. SIDMAN, 1962. Effects of early eye removal at birth on histogenesis of the mouse superior colliculus: An autoradiographic analysis with tritiated thymidine. *J. Comp. Neurol.* 118:205–224.

DE LONG, G. R., and R. L. SIDMAN, 1970. Alignment defect of reaggregating cells in cultures of developing brains of reeler mutant mice. *Dev. Biol.* 22:584–599.

DIXON, J. S., and J. R. CRONLY-DILLON, 1972. The fine structure of the developing retina in *Xenopus laevis*. *J. Embryol. Exp. Morphol.* 28:659–666.

DOMESICK, V. B., and D. K. MOREST, 1977. Migration and differentiation of ganglion cells in the optic tectum of the chick embryo. *Neuroscience* 2:459–475.

DRÄGER, U. C., 1976. Reeler mutant mice: Physiology in primary visual cortex. In *Afferent and Intrinsic Organization of Laminated Structures in the Brain*, O. Creutzfeldt, ed. *Exp. Brain Res.* Suppl. 1:274–276.

EAYRS, J. T., 1960. Influence of the thyroid on the central nervous system. *Br. Med. Bull.* 16:122–126.

EAYRS, J. T., 1964. Endocrine influence on cerebral development. *Arch. Biol.* 75:529–565.

FENTRESS, J. C., ed., 1976. *Simple Networks and Behavior*. Sunderland, MA: Sinauer Assoc.

FINGER, T. E., L. A. ROGERS, and W. M. COWAN, 1976. Regulation in the retino-tectal system of early chick embryos. *Neurosci. Abstr.* 2:212.

FRY, F. J., and W. M. COWAN, 1972. A study of retrograde cell degeneration in the lateral mammillary nucleus of the cat, with special reference to the role of axonal branching in the preservation of the cell. *J. Comp. Neurol.* 144:1–24.

FUJITA, S., 1967. Quantitative analysis of cell proliferation and differentiation in the cortex of the postnatal mouse cerebellum. *J. Cell. Biol.* 32:277–287.

FUJITA, S., 1974. DNA constance in neurons of the human cerebellum and spinal cord as revealed by Feulgen cytophotometry and cytofluorometry. *J. Comp. Neurol.* 155:195–202.

FUJITA, S., M. SHIMADA, and T. NAKAMURA, 1966. ^{3}H-thymidine autoradiographic studies on the cell proliferation and differentiation in the external and internal granular layers of the mouse cerebellum. *J. Comp. Neurol.* 128:191–208.

GAZE, R. M., 1959. Regeneration of the optic nerve in *Xenopus laevis*. *J. Exp. Physiol.* 44:290–308.

GAZE, R. M., 1970. *The Formation of Nerve Connections*. New York: Academic Press.

GLOBUS, A., and A. B. SCHEIBEL, 1967. The effects of visual deprivation on cortical neurons: A Golgi study. *Exp. Neurol.* 19:331–345.

GOTTLIEB, D. I., and C. ARINGTON, 1978. Patterns of cell–cell adhesive specificity in the developing chick central nervous system. *Dev. Biol.* (in press).

GOTTLIEB, D. I., and W. M. COWAN, 1972. Evidence for a temporal factor in the occupation of available synaptic sites during the development of the dentate gyrus. *Brain Res.* 41:452–456.

GOTTLIEB, D. I., R. MERRELL, and L. GLASER, 1974. Temporal changes in embryonal cell surface recognition. *Proc. Natl. Acad. Sci. USA* 71:1800–1802.

GREENOUGH, W. T., 1976. Enduring brain effects of differential experience and training. In *Neural Mechanisms of Learning and Memory*, M. R. Rosenzweig and E. L. Bennett, eds. Cambridge, MA: MIT Press, pp. 255–278.

GUILLERY, R. W., 1974. Visual pathways in albinos. *Sci. Am.* 230:44–54.

HAMBURGER, V., 1948. The mitotic patterns in the spinal cord of the chick embryo and their relation to histogenetic processes. *J. Comp. Neurol.* 88:221–284.

HAMBURGER, V., 1958. Regression versus peripheral control of differentiation in motor hypoplasia. *Am. J. Anat.* 102:365–410.

HAMBURGER, V., 1975. Cell death in the development of the lateral motor column of the chick embryo. *J. Comp. Neurol.* 160:535–546.

HAMBURGER, V., and R. LEVI-MONTALCINI, 1949. Proliferation, differentiation and degeneration in the spinal ganglia of the chick embryo under normal and experimental conditions. *J. Exp. Zool.* 111:457–501.

HAMBURGER, V., E. WENGER, and R. OPPENHEIM, 1966. Motility in the chick embryo in the absence of sensory input. *J. Exp. Zool.* 162:133–160.

HARRISON, R. G., 1921. On relations of symmetry in transplanted limbs. *J. Exp. Zool.* 32:1–136.

HARRISON, R. G., 1936. Relations of symmetry in the developing ear of *Amblystoma punctatum*. *Proc. Natl. Acad. Sci. USA* 22:238–247.

HERNDON, R. M., 1968. Thiopen induced granule cell necrosis in the rat cerebellum. An electron microscopic study. *Exp. Brain Res.* 6:49–68.

HERNDON, R. M., G. MARGOLIS, and L. KILHAM, 1971. The synaptic organization of the malformed cerebellum induced by perinatal infection with the feline panleukopenia virus (PLV). II. The Purkinje cell and its afferents. *J. Neuropathol. Exp. Neurol.* 30:557–570.

HIBBARD, E., 1967. Visual recovery following regeneration of the optic nerve through the oculomotor nerve root in *Xenopus*. *Exp. Neurol.* 19:350–356.

HINDS, J. W., 1968. Autoradiographic study of histogenesis in the mouse olfactory bulb. I. Time of origin of neurons and neuroglia. *J. Comp. Neurol.* 134:287–304.

HINDS, J. W., and P. L. HINDS, 1972. Reconstruction of dendritic growth cones in neonatal mouse olfactory bulb. *J. Neurocytol.* 1:169–187.

HOLLINGWORTH, T., and M. BERRY, 1975. Network analysis of dendritic fields of pyramidal cells in the neocortex and Purkinje cells in the cerebellum of the rat. *Phil. Trans. R. Soc. Lond.* B270:227–262.

HOLLYDAY, M., and V. HAMBURGER, 1976. Reduction of the naturally occurring motor neuron loss by enlargement of the periphery. *J. Comp. Neurol.* 170:311–320.

HOLTFRETER, J., 1939. Gewebeaffinität, ein Mittel der embryonalen Formbildung. *Arch. Exp. Zellforsch.* 23:169–209.

HUBEL, D. H., T. N. WIESEL, and S. LEVAY, 1977. Plasticity of ocular dominance columns in monkey striate cortex. *Phil. Trans. R. Soc. Lond.* B278:377–409.

HUGHES, A. F. W., 1968. *Aspects of Neural Ontogeny*. New York: Academic Press.

HUNT, R. K., 1975. Developmental programming for retinotectal patterns. In *Cell Patterning* (Ciba Foundation Symposium 29), pp. 131–150.

HUNT, R. K., and N. BERMAN, 1975. Patterning of neuronal locus specificities in retinal ganglion cells after partial extirpation of the embryonic eye. *J. Comp. Neurol.* 162:43–70.

HUNT, R. K., and M. JACOBSON, 1972. Development and stability of positional information in retinal ganglion cells of *Xenopus*. *Proc. Natl. Acad. Sci. USA* 69:780–783.

HUNT, R. K., and M. JACOBSON, 1974. Neuronal specificity revisited. *Curr. Top. Dev. Biol.* 8:203–259.

JACOBSON, M., 1968. Cessation of DNA synthesis in retinal ganglion cells correlated with the time of specification of their central connections. *Dev. Biol.* 17:219–232.

JACOBSON, M., 1970a. Development, specification, and diversification of neuronal connections. In *The Neurosciences: Second Study Program*, F. O. Schmitt, ed. New York: Rockefeller University Press, pp. 116–129.

JACOBSON, M., 1970b. *Developmental Neurobiology*. New York: Holt, Rinehart and Winston.

JONES, E. G., 1975. Varieties and distribution of non-pyramidal cells in the somatic sensory cortex of the squirrel monkey. *J. Comp. Neurol.* 160:205–268.

KAHN, A. J., 1973. Ganglion cell formation in the chick neural retina. *Brain Res.* 63:285–290.

KÄLLÉN, B., 1965. Degeneration and regeneration in the vertebrate central nervous system during embryogenesis. *Prog. Brain Res.* 14:77–96.

KAUFFMAN, S. L., 1968. Lengthening of the generation cycle during embryonic differentiation of the mouse neural tube. *Exp. Cell Res.* 49:420–424.

KELLY, J. P., and W. M. COWAN, 1972. Studies on the development of the chick optic tectum. III. Effects of early eye removal. *Brain Res.* 42:263–288.

KIMMEL, C. B., E. SCHABTACH, and R. J. KIMMEL, 1977. Developmental interactions in the growth and branching of the lateral dendrite of Mauthner's cell (*Amblystoma mexicanum*). *Dev. Biol.* 55:244–259.

KOLLROS, J. J., 1953. The development of the optic lobes in the frog. II. The effects of unilateral enucleation in embryonic stages. *J. Exp. Zool.* 123:153–187.

LAPHAM, L. W., 1968. Tetraploid DNA content of Purkinje neurons of human cerebellar cortex. *Science* 159:310–312.

LAPHAM, L. W., D. J. WOODWARD, R. D. LENTZ, B. J. HOFFER, and C. J. HERMAN, 1971. Postnatal development of tetraploid DNA content in the Purkinje neuron of the rat: An aspect of cerebellar differentiation. In *Cellular Aspects of Neural Growth and Differentiation*, D. Pease, ed. Los Angeles: University of California Press, pp. 61–71.

LARRAMENDI, L. M. H., 1969. Analysis of synaptogenesis in the cerebellum of the mouse. In *Neurobiology of Cerebellar Evolution and Development*, R. Llinás, ed. Chicago: American Medical Association, pp. 803–843.

LAVAIL, J. H., and W. M. COWAN, 1971. The development of the chick optic tectum. II. Autoradiographic studies. *Brain Res.* 28:421–441.

LEVINE, R., and M. JACOBSON, 1974. Deployment of optic nerve fibers is determined by positional markers in the frog's tectum. *Exp. Neurol.* 43:527–528.

LYNCH, G., and C. W. COTMAN, 1975. The hippocampus as a model for studying anatomical plasticity in the adult brain. In *The Hippocampus. I. Structure and Development*, R. L. Isaacson and R. H. Pribram, eds. New York: Plenum Press, pp. 123–154.

MACAGNO, E. R., V. LOPRESTI, and C. LEVINTHAL, 1973. Structure and development of neuronal connections in isogenic organisms: Variation and similarities in the optic system of *Daphnia magna*. *Proc. Natl. Acad. Sci. USA* 70: 57–61.

MARCHASE, R. B., K. VOSBECK, and S. ROTH, 1976. Intercellular adhesive specificity. *Biochem. Biophys. Acta* 457:385–416.

MIALE, I. L., and R. L. SIDMAN, 1961. An autoradiographic analysis of histogenesis in the mouse cerebellum. *Exp. Neurol.* 4:277–296.

MOSCONA, A. A., ed., 1974. *The Cell Surface in Development*. New York: Wiley.

NORNES, H. O., and G. D. DAS, 1974. Temporal pattern of neurogenesis in spinal cord of rat. I. An autoradiographic study—time and sites of origin and migration and settling patterns of neuroblasts. *Brain Res.* 73:121–138.

NORR, S. C., 1973. *In vitro* analysis of sympathetic neuron differentiation from chick neural crest cells. *Dev. Biol.* 34:16–38.

OPPENHEIM, R. W., and I. W. CHU-WANG, 1977. Spontaneous cell death of spinal motoneurons following peripheral innervation in the chick embryo. *Brain Res.* 125:154–160.

PALAY, S. L., and V. CHAN-PALAY, 1974. *Cerebellar Cortex: Cytology and Organization*. New York: Springer-Verlag.

PARNAVELAS, J. B., G. LYNCH, N. BRECHA, C. W. COTMAN, and A. GLOBUS, 1974. Spine loss and regrowth in hippocampus following deafferentation. *Nature* 248:71–73.

PITMAN, R. M., C. D. TWEEDLE, and M. J. COHEN, 1973. The form of nerve cells. In *Intracellular Staining in Neurobiology*, S. B. Kater and C. Nicholson, eds. New York: Springer-Verlag, pp. 83–97.

PRESTIGE, M. C., 1970. Differentiation, degeneration, and the role of the periphery: Quantitative considerations. In *The Neurosciences: Second Study Program*, F. O. Schmitt, ed. New York: Rockefeller University Press, pp. 73–82.

RAKIC, P., 1972. Extrinsic cytological determinants of basket and stellate cell dendritic pattern in the cerebellar molecular layer. *J. Comp. Neurol.* 146:335–354.

RAKIC, P., 1974. Neurons in rhesus monkey visual cortex: Systematic relation between time of origin and eventual disposition. *Science* 183:425–427.

RAKIC, P., 1975. Cell migration and neuronal ectopias in the brain. *Birth Defects* 11:95–127.

RAKIC, P., 1977. Prenatal development of the visual system in rhesus monkey. *Phil. Trans. R. Soc. Lond.* B278:245–260.

RAKIC, P., and R. L. SIDMAN, 1973. Sequence of developmental abnormalities leading to granule cell deficit in cerebellar cortex of weaver mutant mice. *J. Comp. Neurol.* 152:103–132.

REDFERN, P. A., 1970. Neuromuscular transmission in newborn rats. *J. Physiol.* 209:701–709.

ROGERS, L. A., and W. M. COWAN, 1973. The development of the mesencephalic nucleus of the trigeminal nerve in the chick. *J. Comp. Neurol.* 147:291–320.

ROSENZWEIG, M. R., E. L. BENNETT, and M. C. DIAMOND, 1972. Brain changes in response to experience. *Sci. Am.* 226:22–29.

ROTH, S., and R. B. MARCHASE, 1976. An *in vitro* assay for retino-tectal specificity. In *Neuronal Recognition*, S. H. Barondes, ed. New York: Plenum Press, pp. 227–248.

SAUNDERS, J. W., and J. F. FALLON, 1966. Cell death in morphogenesis. In *Major Problems in Developmental Biology*, M. Locke, ed. New York: Academic Press.

SCHLESSINGER, A. R., W. M. COWAN, and D. I. GOTTLIEB, 1975. An autoradiographic study of the time of origin and the pattern of granule cell migration in the dentate gyrus of the rat. *J. Comp. Neurol.* 159:149–176.

SCHNEIDER, G. E., and JHAVERI, S. R., 1974. Neuroanatomical correlates of spared or altered function after brain lesions in the newborn hamster. In *Plasticity and Recovery of Function in the Central Nervous System*, D. G. Stein, J. J. Rosen, and N. Butters, eds. New York: Academic Press, pp. 65–109.

SEIL, F. J., and R. M. HERNDON, 1970. Cerebellar granule cells *in vitro*. *J. Cell Biol.* 45:212–220.

SHERIDAN, J. D., 1968. Electrophysiological evidence for low-resistance intercellular junctions in the early chick embryo. *J. Cell. Biol.* 37:650–659.

SIDMAN, R. L., 1961. Histogenesis of the mouse retina studied with tritiated thymidine. In *The Structure of the Eye*, G. K. Smelser, ed. New York: Academic Press, pp. 487–505.

SIDMAN, R. L., 1970. Cell proliferation, migration, and interaction in the developing mammalian central nervous system. In *The Neurosciences: Second Study Program*, F. O. Schmitt, ed. New York: Rockefeller University Press, pp. 100–107.

SIDMAN, R. L., 1970. Autoradiographic methods and principles for study of the nervous system with thymidine-H^3. In *Contemporary Research Techniques of Neuroanatomy*, S. O. L. Ebbesson and W. J. Nauta, eds. New York: Springer-Verlag, pp. 252–274.

SIDMAN, R. L., and P. RAKIC, 1973. Neuronal migration, with special reference to developing human brain: A review. *Brain Res.* 62:1–35.

SIDMAN, R. L., and P. RAKIC, 1974. Neuronal migrations in human brain development. In *Pre- and Post-Natal Development of the Human Brain*. (*Mod. Probl. Paediatr.* 13). Basel: Karger.

SJÖSTRAND, J., 1971. Neuroglial proliferation in the hypoglossal nucleus after nerve injury. *Exp. Neurol.* 30:178–189.

SKOFF, R. P., and V. HAMBURGER, 1974. Fine structure of dendritic and axonal growth cones in embryonic chick spinal cord. *J. Comp. Neurol.* 153:107–148.

SMART, I. H. M., 1972a. Proliferative characteristics of the ependymal layer during the early development of the spinal cord in the mouse. *J. Anat.* 111:365.

SMART, I. H. M., 1972b. Proliferative characteristics of the ependymal layer during the early development of the mouse diencephalon, as revealed by recording the number, location and plane of cleavage of mitotic figures. *J. Anat.* 113:109–129.

SMART, I. H. M., and M. SMART, 1977. The location of

nuclei of different labelling intensities in autoradiographs of the anterior forebrain of postnatal mice injected with [³H]-thymidine on the eleventh and twelfth days of conception. *J. Anat.* 123:515–525.

SOTELO, C., and J.-P. CHANGEUX, 1974. Bergmann fibers and granular cell migration in the cerebellum of homozygous weaver mutant mouse. *Brain Res.* 77:484–491.

SOTELO, C., and S. L. PALAY, 1968. The fine structure of the lateral vestibular nucleus in the rat. I. Neurons and neuroglial cells. *J. Cell Biol.* 36:151–179.

SPERRY, R. W., 1963. Chemoaffinity in the orderly growth of nerve fiber patterns and connections. *Proc. Natl. Acad. Sci. USA* 50:703–710.

STONE, L. S., 1960. Polarization of the retina and development of vision. *J. Exp. Zool.* 145:85–93.

STRAZNICKY, K., and R. M. GAZE, 1971. The growth of the retina in *Xenopus laevis*: An autoradiographic study. *J. Embryol. Exp. Morphol.* 26:67–79.

STRAZNICKY, K., and R. M. GAZE, 1972. The development of the tectum in *Xenopus laevis*: An autoradiographic study. *J. Embryol. Exp. Morphol.* 28:87–115.

VALVERDE, F., 1967. Apical dendritic spines of the visual cortex and light deprivation in the mouse. *Exp. Brain Res.* 3:337–352.

WATSON, W. E., 1972. Some quantitative observations upon the responses of neuroglial cells which follow axotomy of adjacent neurons. *J. Physiol.* 225:415–435.

WILSON, B. D., 1974a. Proliferation in the neural tube of the splotch (*Sp*) mutant mouse. *J. Comp. Neurol.* 154:249–256.

WILSON, B. D., 1974b. The cell cycle of ventricular cells in the overgrown optic tectum. *Brain Res.* 69:41–48.

WOOD, P. M., and R. P. BUNGE, 1975. Evidence that sensory axons are mitogenic for Schwann cells. *Nature* 256:662–664.

YOON, M. G., 1971. Reorganization of retinotectal projection following surgical operations on optic tectum of goldfish. *Exp. Neurol.* 33:395–411.

YOON, M. G., 1973. Retention of the original topographic polarity by the 180° rotated tectal reimplant in young adult goldfish. *J. Physiol.* 233:575–588.

YOUNG, D., ed., 1973. *Developmental Neurobiology of Arthropods*. Cambridge, Eng.: Cambridge University Press.

6 Functional Characterization of Neural Interactions through an Analysis of Behavior

W. REICHARDT

Introduction

Complex systems such as the central nervous system—or even parts of it—possess an enormous number of components. A determination of the detailed function of any individual component is rather hopeless at present, but fortunately this is not needed if one is interested in features on a macroscopic scale such as the behavior of an organism in its environment. The goal of such an investigation is therefore to select relevant parameters and to neglect all unnecessary information.

We have explored how optical information is processed by the fly's visual system. (For detailed information, see the review articles by Reichardt and Poggio, 1976, and Poggio and Reichardt, 1976.) The objective is to unravel the logical organization of the system and its underlying functional and computational principles. The approach is at a highly integrative level. There are three levels of analyzing and "understanding" complex systems. At the first, strictly "phenomenological" level, one investigates the overall function, the input-output behavior of the system, and its logical organization. At the second level, the functional principles of the subsystems are the object of the analysis. At the third level, one studies individual components and detailed circuitry.

From a reductionist point of view, one can reduce a complex behavior to fundamental laws at the cellular or even the molecular level. However, this does not imply the validity of the converse, the constructionist approach. The behavior of a complex system, composed of many components, cannot be easily understood in terms of a simple extrapolation of the properties of its components, because new properties

appear and their understanding requires an independent approach that is as fundamental in its nature as any other.

In this paper, a phenomenological theory of the fly's visual orientation behavior is outlined on the basis of experimental evidence. The theory describes and predicts, at the first level, a rather complex behavior in terms of some simple computations performed by nervous interactions on the visual input. At the second level, the functional properties of the interactions underlying the computations are described. We maintain that these two levels of analysis cannot simply follow from single-cell recordings or from histology. They are bound to be a prerequisite to any full understanding at the circuitry level. The ultimate goal of our research, however, is to relate function to structure, and there is no doubt that the neurophysiological and histological approaches are the basic tools at the third, the cellular, level.

A phenomenological approach to flight orientation behavior

The flight behavior of houseflies demonstrates an elaborate visual control system. Flies perceive motion relative to the environment and thereby stabilize their flight course; they locate and fly toward objects; they are able to track moving targets and to chase other flies; they discriminate or prefer some specific visual patterns; and they can in some cases separate a texture into "object" or "figure" and "ground."

EXPERIMENTAL PROCEDURES In free flight, an insect possesses six dynamic degrees of freedom: three of translatory and three of rotatory motion. The investigations undertaken so far have been confined to either one degree of rotation (the rotatory motion of a horizontally flying fly around its vertical axis: Reichardt, 1973) or one degree of translation (the ver-

W. REICHARDT Max-Planck-Institut für biologische Kybernetik, 74 Tübingen, Federal Republic of Germany

tical motion of a horizontally flying fly: Wehrhahn, 1974; Wehrhahn and Reichardt, 1975). Measurements were carried out by means of highly sensitive, fast mechanoelectric servotransducers, which sense either the flight torque or the lift force generated by the wings of a test fly.

When a contrasted optical environment is moved or intensity flickered in front of a fixed flying test fly, one is operating under so-called open loop conditions; when the transducer signal is used to control the position and speed of the environment by simulating the flight dynamics, the conditions are called closed-loop.

We shall confine ourselves mainly to the behavior of the fly around its vertical axis (rotatory degree of freedom). Many of the results, as well as their theoretical interpretations, have also been verified in one of the translatory degrees of freedom: the vertical motion of a fly in horizontal flight. Most of the experiments were carried out with female houseflies *Musca domestica* (head rigidly fixed to the thorax), though some of the results reported here refer to the fruitfly *Drosophila melanogaster,* and a few to the beetle *Chlorophanus viridis.*

DYNAMICS OF FLIGHT   Results from measurements on fixed flying flies, using fast torque-compensation techniques (Reichardt and Wenking, 1969; Reichardt, 1973), and comparison of these results with the behavior of freely flying flies (Land and Collett, 1974) have led to the conclusion that the aerodynamics of flight for rotation of a fly around its vertical axis can be described by a second-order ordinary differential equation.

We introduce an angular coordinate system describing the position of the fly on the horizontal plane. Here α_f designates the instantaneous direction of flight, and α_p the instantaneous angular position of an object. The angle $\psi = \alpha_p - \alpha_f$, called the error angle, represents the angular position of the object with respect to the coordinate system of the fly. When the head is fixed to the thorax, ψ also represents the location of the image of the object on the retina of the fly at a particular instant. The free-flight dynamics of rotation is well approximated by

$$\theta \ddot{\alpha}_f(t) + k \dot{\alpha}_f(t) = F(t), \qquad (1)$$

where $\theta = 1.5 \times 10^{-3}$ g cm^2 is the measured moment of inertia around the vertical axis of the fly (*Musca domestica*) and $k \approx 0.18$ g cm^2 sec^{-1} represents an aerodynamic friction constant. (Overdots indicate time derivatives.) Since $\theta/k \approx 8 \times 10^{-3}$ sec, the angular speed is always essentially proportional to the

instantaneous torque $F(t)$, which depends on the error-angle function $\psi(t)$. Equation 1 can be rewritten in terms of the error angle as

$$\theta \ddot{\psi}(t) + k \dot{\psi}(t) - \theta \ddot{\alpha}_p(t) - k \dot{\alpha}_p(t) = F[\psi(t), t] \quad (2A)$$

or

$$\theta \ddot{\psi}(t) + k \dot{\psi}(t) = -F[\psi(t), t] + S(t), \qquad (2B)$$

with

$$S(t) = \theta \ddot{\alpha}_p(t) + k \dot{\alpha}_p(t). \qquad (2C)$$

When $\alpha_p(t) \equiv 0$ (that is, the object does not move with respect to the environment), $S(t) \equiv 0$ and $\psi(t) \equiv -\alpha_f(t)$. Equation 2B describes the free-flight situation in the coordinate system of the fly. A method to simulate the free-flight conditions represented by equation 2B has been described in detail elsewhere (Reichardt, 1973). Although the orientation behavior of the fly can also be studied with other methods, most of the experiments described in this paper have been performed with the compensation method or modifications thereof (Virsik, 1974; Virsik and Reichardt, 1974, 1976). The characteristic variable directly observed in these experiments is the error angle $\psi(t)$.

A similar experimental setup was used to investigate the height-orientation behavior of flies (Wehrhahn, 1974; Wehrhahn and Reichardt, 1973, 1975). Corresponding to equation 2B, an ordinary differential equation in the vertical coordinate z (height) or angle ϑ relates the lift of the fly to its vertical displacement.

SPONTANEOUS BEHAVIOR   A fly flies in all directions α_f with equal probability in a no-contrast homogeneously illuminated environment. When these conditions are simulated in our experimental setup, the fly's torque turns out to be a stationary, zero-mean, stochastic signal $N(t)$ with a Gaussian density distribution and an exponential autocorrelation

$$C_{N,N}(\tau) = A \, e^{-\gamma|\tau|}. \qquad (3)$$

Under the assumption of a Gaussian distribution, the process $N(t)$ is completely and quantitatively characterized by its autocorrelation. Without visual contrast stimuli, the fly spontaneously "searches around," apparently in a random (but correlated) manner. Interestingly, a black object that does not move relative to the fly's retina does not affect the torque signal of the fly. Thus stabilized retinal images of this kind do not influence the orientation behavior of the fly.

VISUALLY INDUCED BEHAVIOR   Visually induced behavior is observed whenever a contrasted "panorama" moves relative to the fly's retina. The most elementary type of orientation behavior can be elicited when the cylindrical panorama used in the experiments contains a dark object in front of a white, illuminated background. Under closed-loop conditions, the fly's instantaneous torque determines an angular displacement of the object relative to the retina according to equation 2. In the equivalent free-flight situation, flies orient themselves toward the black object when they are either standing ($\alpha_p(t) = S(t) \equiv 0$) or moving ($\dot{\alpha}_p(t) \neq 0$; $S(t) \neq 0$), relative to the room coordinate system. In the first case, this orientation behavior will be called "fixation," in the second "tracking." In both cases, a random relative motion between the object and the fly's retina occurs continuously, apparently due to the continuous presence of the random torque process $N(t)$. The histograms of Figure 1 show the fraction of time the fly gazes at any part of the panorama that carries a black vertical stripe. The histograms show clearly that during stationary fixation the fly's "gaze" is directed in the mean toward the object ($\overline{\psi(t)} = 0$). The fixation of the stripe takes place irrespective of the initial position of the object on the fly's retina.

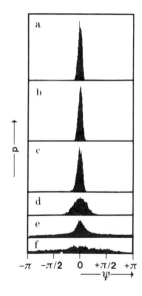

FIGURE 1 Stationary (asymptotic) fixation of a 5° wide, vertically oriented black stripe. The histograms show the fraction of time the fly fixated any part of the panorama—that is, the fraction of time associated with any value of the error angle ψ. The parameter is the average brightness of the panorama, ranging from 1.75×10^3 cd/m² (a) to 1.21×10^{-2} cd/m² (f) (lamp type: fluorescent ring bulbs, Philips TLE 40W/34 de Luxe). Decreasing light intensity degrades fixation until the ψ-distribution is in (f) almost flat. The light intensity used in most of the experiments described in this paper is that of part a. From Reichardt (1973).

THE PHENOMENOLOGICAL EQUATION   The observations described so far suggest that the fly's torque underlying the orientation behavior consists of two main components: a stationary, Gaussian random process $N(t)$, essentially independent of visual input; and a visually induced response $R[\psi(t), t]$, regarded as a functional of $\psi(t)$. The simplest assumption consistent with the experimental results is that $N(t)$ and $R[\psi(t), t]$ add in the nervous system; this assumption has been critically tested in the neighborhood of the fixation equilibrium and found to be valid (Poggio and Reichardt, 1973a). Consequently the fly's torque can be written as

$$F[\psi(t), t] = N(t) + R[\psi(t), t]. \qquad (4)$$

We shall now consider the term $R[\psi(t), t]$. Three points must be emphasized. First, the visually induced response does not depend on the visual motor loop being open or closed. It depends only on the history of the error angle $\psi(t)$ up to the instant t. Second, the response of the fly is time-invariant, under the experimental conditions, implying that R does not explicitly depend on t. Third, the value of $R[\psi(t)]$ at t is much more dependent on changes of ψ in the near past than to changes in the distant past. Under these conditions, one expects that if $\psi(t)$ does not change too quickly, the functional $R[\psi(t)]$ should be given in good approximation by a function R of the value of ψ and its first derivatives at t. In the case of the fly, R depends mainly on $\psi(t)$ and $\dot{\psi}(t)$ and can be written as

$$R[\psi(t), \dot{\psi}(t)] = T[\psi(t), \dot{\psi}(t)] + \rho[\psi(t), \dot{\psi}(t)], \qquad (5)$$

where T represents its even (symmetric) and ρ its odd (antisymmetric) part in $\dot{\psi}(t)$. It has been shown experimentally that equation 5 can be approximated by a linear expression in $\dot{\psi}(t)$ of the form

$$R = D[\psi(t)] + r[\psi(t)]\dot{\psi}(t) \qquad (6A)$$

or

$$R = \frac{\delta}{\delta\psi}U[\psi(t)] + r[\psi(t)]\dot{\psi}(t), \qquad (6B)$$

where U is the "potential" associated with D (Reichardt, 1973; Poggio and Reichardt, 1973a; Reichardt and Poggio, 1975; Virsik and Reichardt, 1976).

It should be mentioned that the description of R is based on a "quasi-stationary" phenomenological approximation. This simplification is the basic reason why equation (6) is valid only for $\overline{\dot{\psi}^2} > 0$.

The fact that the validity of equation 6 has been verified experimentally under a variety of conditions is of some significance. Even the dead time between visual input and a very small motor response can be neglected in most of the cases considered here. Land and Collett (1974) derived from their data a delay of less than 30 msec; Buchner and Reichardt (1978) determined the delay to a fast motion of a black stripe in female and male *Musca,* and at high brightness this turned out to be on the order of 20 msec (see Figure 2). (Srinivasan and Bernard, 1977, have reported delay values for the *Musca* "pursuit" system which differ by a factor of 5 between females and males. Our data do not confirm their experimental results.) Thus equation 2B can be rewritten as

$$\theta\ddot{\psi}(t) + k\dot{\psi}(t) = N(t) - D[\psi(t)] - r[\psi(t)]\dot{\psi}(t) + S(t). \quad (7)$$

The functions $D(\psi)$ and $r(\psi)$ depend on other parameters. In the case of a narrow vertical black stripe (5° wide, 90° long), the functions denoted $D^*(\psi)$ and $r^*(\psi)$, have been measured by different methods. Figure 3 shows the $D^*(\psi)$ and $r^*(\psi)$ associated with a black vertical segment: the instantaneous open-loop response $R(\psi)$ to the object rotating at small constant

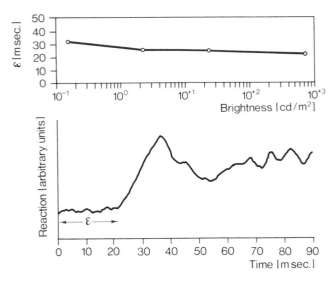

FIGURE 2   The delay ϵ of the torque response to a fast horizontal motion (0.5 msec per degree) of a vertical black stripe between the angular positions $\psi = 0°$ and $\psi = \pm30°$. The upper diagram shows how the delay decreases with increasing brightness of the panorama cylinder. Each point is an average from twenty female *Muscae*. The average standard error of the means amounts to ±0.7 msec. The lower diagram shows the time course of the reaction of an individual fly to a moving stripe. The motion of the stripe begins at time zero. The response of the fly was measured by a fast torque compensator whose transfer characteristic has no delay. The shape of the response curve indirectly reflects the reaction of the fly as it is convoluted with the (delay-free) pulse response of the compensator. Experiments with male *Muscae* carried out under the same conditions have led to the same results.

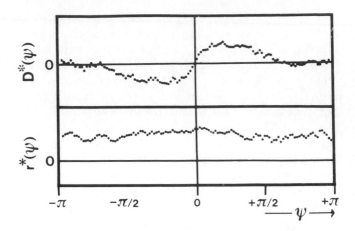

FIGURE 3   The functions $D^*(\psi)$, and $r^*(\psi)$, in relative units, associated with the response of the fly to a narrow vertical black stripe (5° wide, 22.5° long). The stripe segment was rotated with a constant angular speed (8°/sec), and the measured (open-loop) torque was decomposed into a direction-insensitive component $D^*(\psi)$ and into a direction-sensitive component $r^*(\psi)\dot{\psi}$. The stripe segment was presented to the lower parts (below the equator) of the compound eyes. Whereas $r^*(\psi)$ remains essentially unchanged, $D^*(\psi)$ is significantly smaller when the upper parts of the compound eyes are stimulated. The figure represents the average of five experiments, each lasting about 6 min. From Poggio and Reichardt (1976).

speed around the fly was measured for each ψ. Under the assumption that equation 6 holds, the two components $r^*(\psi)\dot{\psi}$ and $D^*(\psi)$ were identified through their respective symmetry properties in ψ. Both $D^*(\psi)$ and the associated potential $U^*(\psi)$ are shown in Figure 4a. The importance of these two functions derives from the fact that any small contrasted object will elicit a similar response, apart from scaling factors. It will be shown later that the $D(\psi)$ and $r(\psi)$ associated with an arbitrary pattern can be well approximated from the functions shown in Figure 4a. An important question concerns the "vertical" parameterization of D and r when small objects are used. The experimental tests suggest that the $r(\psi)$ term is homogeneously present all over the two eyes, whereas the term $D(\psi)$ is essentially present only in the lower part of the eyes, below the equator (Reichardt, 1973).

The visual control system of the fly consists of two basic operations: one transduces position (angular error) into torque through the term $D(\psi)$; the other converts velocity into torque through the term $r\dot{\psi}$.

An equation similar to equation 7 can be derived in an essentially equivalent way for the height-orientation behavior. The position term $L^*(\vartheta)$ is plotted in Figure 4b.

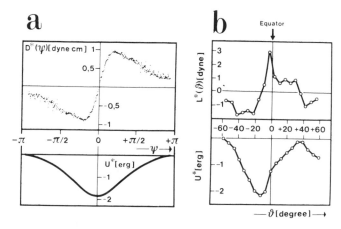

FIGURE 4 (a) The (direction-insensitive) torque response component $D^*(\psi)$ induced by a vertical black stripe (5° wide, $-45° \leq \psi \leq 45°$) and the associated "potential" (lower diagram). Average from measurements on 111 flies. The function $D^*(\psi)$ represents the mean attractiveness of the stripe for each ψ. To avoid a "stabilized retinal image," to which the fly would not respond, the stripe was randomly oscillated by the fly around each ψ position with small amplitude (partial closed-loop conditions; see Reichardt, 1973). The attractiveness profile $D^*(\psi)$ does not significantly depend on the motion spectrum of the stripe as long as the contrast changes at the level of the receptors are between 0.5 and 15 Hz. Redrawn from Reichardt (1973).

(b) The (direction-insensitive) response component $L^*(\vartheta)$ induced by a horizontally oriented black stripe moved in the vertical (z) direction (upper diagram) and its corresponding potential (lower diagram), according to $L^*(\vartheta) = \delta U^*(\vartheta)/\delta\vartheta$. Average from measurements on seven flies. Here ϑ is the vertical angle between the equator (the optical symmetry line between upper and lower half of the eye) and the angular position of the stripe. Redrawn from Wehrhahn and Reichardt (1975).

A LINEAR APPROACH TO SINGLE-OBJECT FIXATION

In the angular range $-30° \leq \psi \leq 30°$, equation 7 takes the linear form

$$\theta\ddot{\psi} + k\dot{\psi} + r^*\dot{\psi} + \beta\psi = N(t) + S(t) \qquad (8)$$

with

$$C_{N,N}(\tau) = A\, e^{-\gamma|\tau|},$$

where the coefficient β represents the slope of the $D^*(\psi)$ characteristics around $\psi = 0$ (see Figure 4a). For $S(t) = 0$, equation 8 is a linear stochastic equation in the error angle $\psi(t)$. Since $N(t)$ is a Gaussian random process, $\psi(t)$ must also be a Gaussian random process. The stationary solution is therefore simply given by the asymptotic probability distribution

$$p(\psi) = \sqrt{\frac{1}{2\pi\sigma^2}}\, \exp(-\psi^2/2\sigma^2). \qquad (9A)$$

The standard deviation σ can be obtained as

$$\sigma^2 = \frac{A}{\beta(k + r^*)}\, \frac{k + r^* + \gamma\theta}{\beta + (k + r^*)\gamma + \gamma^2\theta}. \qquad (9B)$$

The dependence on the fluctuation power A in this equation is not surprising. The parameter β plays the main role: whereas an increase in either β or r^* leads to a "better" stationary fixation (smaller σ), $\beta > 0$ is a necessary and sufficient condition for fixation. In terms of standard feedback language, the fly is equivalent to a position and velocity servomechanism: fixation cannot take place without position-sensitive information processing. However, speed-sensitive feedback can "improve" stationary fixation. The linear equation 8 quantitatively predicts the stationary distribution of the process $\psi(t)$ for normal θ/k couplings. An important point is that dynamic solutions in the expected value $\langle\psi(t)\rangle$, given by equation 8, agree with experimental results. A good example is provided by the chasing behavior of *Fannia* (Land and Collett, 1974), for which a linear equation of the type of equation 8 holds at least in the larger range $-100° < \psi < +100°$.

TRACKING AN OBJECT MOVING WITH CONSTANT ANGULAR VELOCITY

Orientation and tracking behavior of the fly can be precisely predicted by the phenomenological theory in a number of the experiments performed so far. The analysis of the case considered here can be derived from equation 8, with the term $S(t)$ taking the form $k\dot{\alpha}_p$, where $k\dot{\alpha}_p$ designates the constant angular speed of the object (black stripe). The conditions for stationary tracking are $\langle\ddot{\psi}\rangle = 0$, $\langle\dot{\psi}\rangle = 0$, which imply that the expected value of the error angle ψ is

$$\langle\psi_{tr}\rangle = \frac{k}{\beta}\, \dot{\alpha}_p. \qquad (10)$$

The fly lags behind the object by an average angle $\langle\psi_{tr}\rangle$, which is proportional to the speed of the object. For a black vertical stripe, the maximum speed $\dot{\alpha}_p$ for which tracking can occur is observed to be around 300°/sec, corresponding to a maximum lag of about 20°. For higher speeds, the target is lost more and more often, until no tracking takes place. The predictions have been fully confirmed by stationary tracking experiments (Virsik, 1974; Virsik and Reichardt, 1974).

If the object is embedded in a contrasted random dot pattern and rigidly connected to it, the description remains essentially the same. The only difference is that the parameters r and β are here different since they depend on the contrast of the background texture that "masks" the object. For equal object and background contrasts, $\beta = 0$: the object is not detected by the fly against the background. However, if "incoherent" relative motion takes place between object and background texture, the "masking" inhibition is destroyed and the parameter β, which is a measure of the "attractiveness" of the object, takes a value characteristic of the no-texture situation. The relevant point is that at this phenomenological level, it is possible to describe tracking of an object moving at constant speed in front of a contrasted texture. If one solves equation 8 for these conditions, one arrives at an angular lag of

$$\langle \psi_{\text{tr}} \rangle = \frac{k}{\beta} \left(1 + \frac{r_2}{k} \right) \dot{\alpha}_{\text{p}}, \tag{11}$$

where r_2 is associated with the direction-sensitive optomotor response elicited by the random dot background pattern (Virsik and Reichardt, 1974). The fly and the object would move under free-flight conditions with an average angular velocity $\dot{\alpha}_{\text{p}}$ with respect to the background pattern. Thus $\langle \psi_{\text{tr}} \rangle$ and $\dot{\alpha}_{\text{p}}$ are proportional to one another as in equation 10, but with a larger proportionality factor.

An interesting sidelight to this is that if the coupling of the fly to the background is artificially inverted, so that the background texture rotates in the same direction as the object but with twice its average speed, equation 11 becomes

$$\langle \psi_{\text{tr}} \rangle = \frac{k}{\beta} \left(1 - \frac{r_2}{k} \right) \dot{\alpha}_{\text{p}}. \tag{12}$$

Equation 12 predicts that the tracking angle decreases and eventually changes its sign when $r_2/k > 1$. In this case, the angular lag during tracking becomes an angular lead. Equations 10 through 12 have been tested in a series of experiments (Virsik, 1974; Virsik and Reichardt, 1976) and found to be in agreement with the theoretical predictions. Figure 5 illustrates the case in which the texture contrast amounts to $m = 55\%$.

A NONLINEAR THEORY OF PATTERN-INDUCED FLIGHT ORIENTATION The stationary solution of equation 7 was confined to the regions near the equilibrium states where a linear approximation holds. In general, $D(\psi)$ and correspondingly $U(\psi)$ are nonlinear functions associated with the surrounding pattern. A general solution of equation 7 for arbitrary $D(\psi)$ or $U(\psi)$ is therefore needed.

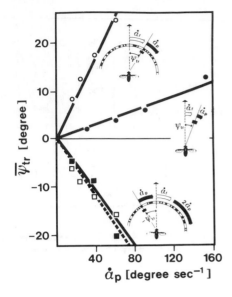

FIGURE 5 Tracking of a black (100% contrast) vertical stripe moving with constant angular speed $\dot{\alpha}_{\text{p}}$ in front of a background (360° around the fly). The fly tracks the stripe with an angular velocity $\dot{\alpha}_{\text{f}} = \dot{\alpha}_{\text{p}}$ and a mean angular lag $\langle \psi_{\text{tr}} \rangle$, shown in the figure as a function of object velocity $\dot{\alpha}_{\text{p}}$. The mean values plotted here were obtained from one fly.

Filled circles: Tracking of the stripe in front of a white background; see equation (10). Open circles: Tracking of the stripe in front of a random dot texture (360° angular extension) with an average contrast $m = 55\%$; see equation (11). Filled squares: Tracking of the stripe in front of the same random texture background but with reversed coupling of the fly to the background; see equation (12). Open squares: Predicted from the first two sets of data by equations (10)–(12). The full lines are regression lines (the dotted line corresponds to the open squares). Redrawn from Virsik and Reichardt (1976).

Equations of the type

$$\theta \ddot{\psi} + [k + r(\psi)] \dot{\psi} + \frac{\partial U(\psi)}{\partial \psi} = N(t) + S(t) \tag{13}$$

with

$$U(\psi) = U(\psi + 2\pi n), \qquad n = 0, 1, 2, \ldots,$$

where $N(t)$ is a noise process, are known as Langevin equations. The statistics of $\psi(t)$ can be given by the Fokker-Planck method, which associates with equation 13 a partial differential equation in the instantaneous probability density of ψ. Derivation of the solutions has been treated in detail by Poggio and Reichardt (1973a) and by Reichardt and Poggio (1975).

To simplify the treatment, one can make the assumption that θ is negligible, since its value (in the fly *Musca*) is very small. Moreover, it is assumed that the friction parameter associated with a given pattern is a constant, independent of ψ: $r(\psi) = r_0$. The "fixation" case, corresponding to $S(t) \equiv 0$, will be considered first. If the random process $N(t) = W(t)$ is Gaussian and "white," $\psi(t)$ is a Markov process defined by

$$\dot{\psi} + \frac{1}{k + r_0} \frac{\partial U(\psi)}{\partial \psi} = \frac{W(t)}{k + r_0}, \tag{14}$$

where $W(t)$ represents white noise with a spectral density c. In the more realistic case, $N(t)$ is a "colored" Gaussian process with an e-type first-order autocorrelation, and equation 14, written in the phase space, takes the form

$$\dot{\psi} + \frac{1}{k + r_0} \frac{\partial U(\psi)}{\partial \psi} = \frac{N(t)}{k + r_0}, \tag{15}$$

$$\dot{N} + \gamma N = W(t),$$

where $W(t)$ is a Gaussian white noise process with spectral density $A\gamma$.

While a Fokker-Planck equation can be derived for both equations 14 and 15, its stationary solution, rather simple in the white noise case, becomes difficult in the realistic case of equation 15. The white noise equation 14 will be considered first since the associated analytic solutions are illustrative.

The Fokker-Planck equation in the transition probability distribution function $p(\psi;t)$ associated with equation 14 is

$$\frac{\partial}{\partial t} p(\psi;t) = \frac{\partial}{\partial \psi} \left[\frac{1}{k + r_0} \frac{\partial U(\psi)}{\partial \psi} p(\psi;t) \right]$$

$$+ \frac{c}{(k + r_0)^2} \frac{\partial^2}{\partial \psi^2} p(\psi;t). \tag{16}$$

Its stationary solution (for $t \to \infty$) can be derived from equation 16 and the appropriate boundary conditions as

$$p(\psi) = C \exp\left[-U(\psi)(k+r_0)/c\right]. \tag{17}$$

Equation 17 relates an arbitrary nonlinear (cyclic) potential $U(\psi)$, associated with a given pattern, to the stationary error-angle distribution $p(\psi)$. Consequently, once the position and movement response associated with a pattern are known, the spontaneous orientation behavior of the fly is characterized in its stationary state by the stationary solution of the Fokker-Planck equation.

The mapping defined by equation 17 describes a one-to-one correspondence between a potential profile and $p(\psi)$. A large value of c (the spectral density of the fluctuation process) maps the entire potential with equal weight. Small values of c, however, result in a mapping of practically only the minima of $U(\psi)$ into $p(\psi)$. Thus the nonlinear cooperative superposition of simple, local computations determines a nontrivial pattern orientation behavior and underlies an elementary "classification" of patterns according to their order parameters. Numbers and positions of the minima can be considered as order parameters distinguishing different classes of patterns. As will be shown in the next section, the potentials of two or more objects show "symmetry breakings" with respect to the potential minima. These considerations, valid under the white noise hypothesis, apply in essence to equation 15 as well. Since equation 15 and the associated Fokker-Planck equation do not satisfy the condition of detailed balance (Graham and Haken, 1971), no general method is available to obtain the stationary distribution. An approximate solution (Reichardt and Poggio, 1975) nevertheless fully illustrates the role played by the colored spectrum. It shows that $p(\psi)$ may contain two maxima, even if $U(\psi)$ has only one minimum. Due to the nonwhite spectrum of the fluctuations, an "early" symmetry breaking in the peaks of the probability distribution can take place without a corresponding symmetry breaking in the potential minima. The effect illustrates the importance of the nature of the fluctuations, when not thermal, in determining the phase transition behavior of a system.

So far fixation of a stationary pattern ($S(t) = 0$) has been considered. The tracking case ($S(t) \neq 0$) is, in general, a more difficult problem. However, if $S(t)$ is a random process, it might be possible to solve the stochastic equation 13 by means of the Fokker-Planck method (Poggio and Reichardt, 1973a). In particular, if $S(t)$ is a white Gaussian process relative to which $N(t)$ can be neglected, the stationary distribution equation 17 gives the solution, with c now representing the spectral density of $S(t)$.

It has been pointed out already that another important tracking situation occurs when the target moves at constant angular speed $\dot{\alpha}_p$. In this case (for $\theta = 0$),

$$S(t) = k\dot{\alpha}_p(t), \qquad \dot{\alpha}_p = \text{const.} \tag{18}$$

Defining a new (noncyclic) potential (see Figure 6a) by

$$\tilde{U}(\psi) = k\dot{\alpha}_p\psi - U(\psi), \tag{19}$$

the associated Fokker-Planck equation has the solu-

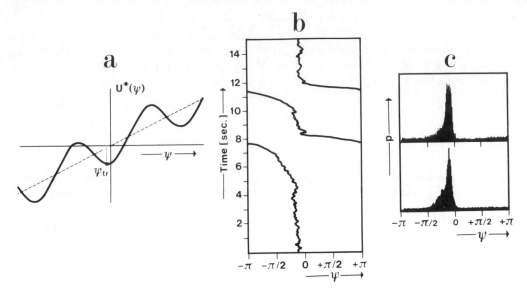

FIGURE 6 (a) Tracking of a target moving at constant angular speed $\dot{\alpha}_p(t)$ is formally equivalent to the motion of a particle in a wavy inclined surface. In the absence of fluctuations (the spontaneous torque process $N(t)$), the representative point comes to rest at the bottom of one of the wells. Tracking is impossible if there are no "bottoms" because of the excessive slope of the plane (the target's speed is too high). The fluctuation process dislodges the representative point now and then. Its average effect is to cause sliding of the point down the plane. Sliding occurs more rapidly the greater the slope (speed of the target), the shallower the wells (attractiveness of the target), and the stronger the random excitations ($N(t)$).

(b) A typical trajectory of the error angle $\psi(t)$, modulus 2π, during tracking of a black vertical stripe moving at fast, constant angular speed $\dot{\alpha}_p$. The fly lags more and more behind the target, suddenly makes what appears as a sort of nystagmus (a fast turn against the direction of the target motion), locks again on the target, and fixates for a while. Equation (20) and part a clearly explain this behavior, which has been also observed in walking *Tenebrio molitor* (Varjú, 1975) and in *Syritta pipiens* hovering in a rotating drum (Collett and Land, 1975).

The same fact is obvious in the histograms shown in part c. The upper histograms have been obtained through a digital simulation of equation (13) with $S(t) = k\dot{\alpha}_p$, $\dot{\alpha}_p = $ const., and the standard values for the parameters used throughout the paper. The lower histogram represents the result of a corresponding experiment. The fact that the peak of the distributions is shifted with respect to $\psi = 0$ means that the fly tracks the stripe with a certain mean angular lag ψ_{tr}. From Reichardt and Poggio (1975).

tion, under the hypothesis of a white fluctuation process $N(t)$,

$$p(\psi) \propto \exp\left[\frac{k+r}{c}\tilde{U}(\psi)\right]$$

$$\times \int_{\psi-2\pi}^{\psi} \exp\left[-\frac{k+r}{c}\tilde{U}(\psi')\right]d\psi'. \quad (20)$$

Equation 20 can be interpreted as the probability distribution of a Brownian particle in the noncyclic potential $\tilde{U}(\psi)$, shown in Figure 6a. A necessary condition for the tracking of a stripe is $k\dot{\alpha}_p < \max_\psi D^*(\psi)$. The average error angle $\langle\psi_{tr}\rangle$, which depends on the speed of the target, on r^*, and on $D^*(\psi)$, implies that the fly tracks the stripe with a certain lag (see Figure 6a, b). Figure 6c shows an experimental and a theoretical histogram for the probability distribution of the error angle ψ_{tr}, when a stripe is lost repeatedly.

The height-orientation behavior can be also described with the same mathematical method.

AN ENVIRONMENT OF HIGHER COMPLEXITY Equation 17 also describes the orientation behavior of the fly toward more complex patterns, if the associated $r(\psi)$ and $D(\psi)$ are known. Figure 7 shows the $D(\psi)$ and $U(\psi)$ profiles corresponding to two stripe patterns, for different angular separations $\Delta\psi$ of two identical stripes. The parameter r (small compared to k; see Reichardt and Poggio, 1975) is obtained under the assumption that the contributions from the two stripes are simply additive. With these parameter values, equation 17 gives the stationary probability distribution of error angle ψ with respect to the zero of the pattern (the center line between the two stripes). However, an analytic solution of the equation, taking into account the nonwhite spectral properties of $N(t)$, is difficult. An approximate solution, illustrating the qualitative effects of the nonwhite spectral density, has been derived by Reichardt and Poggio, (1975). Figure 8 shows a digital simulation of equation 13 and the corresponding experimental histograms in-

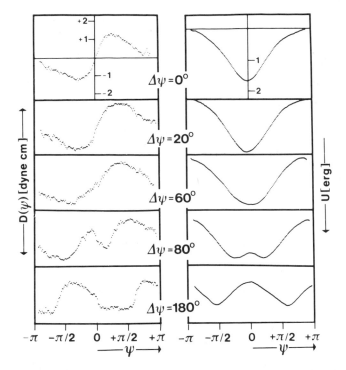

FIGURE 7 The attractiveness functions $D(\psi)$ associated with one- and two-stripe patterns: the parameter $\Delta\psi$ is the angular separation between the black vertical stripes (5° wide). $\Delta\psi = 0$ indicates that the direction of flight coincides with the symmetry line of the pattern, which was oscillated (maximum amplitude ±5°) around each ψ position. The mean torque was recorded under open-loop conditions. The $D(\psi)$ profiles shown in the left figure are averages of 6–15 individuals and agree well with corresponding measurements performed under the conditions of Figure 4a. The potentials $U(\psi)$ (right figure) are derived from $D(\psi)$ according to equation (6B). Redrawn from Reichardt and Poggio (1975).

dicating the amount of time the fly oriented toward any part of the patterns. The agreement is satisfactory, since no best fitting is involved in the determination of the parameters (for instance, those characterizing $N(t)$). Moreover, the measurement technique introduces some smoothing of the $D(\psi)$ profile, which especially affects the theoretical prediction for those patterns in which the two minima of the potential just build up ($\Delta\psi \approx 60°$). It is interesting to observe that the two maxima in the theoretical fixation histogram for $\Delta\psi = 60°$ arise from *one* potential minimum because of the nonwhite spectral composition of $N(t)$. Thus a two-maxima fixation distribution is observed even when the associated potential distribution contains only one minimum, an effect which may be called an "early phase transition." From the point of view of the associated stationary orientation behavior, it is clear that the first three patterns

of Figure 8 are essentially equivalent and in this sense belong to the same class.

Functional specification of the neural interactions

The phenomenological theory characterizes the basic logical organization of the behavior we are studying at the level of the responsible neural interactions. However, it does not allow us to specify these interactions because the variables ψ and $\dot{\psi}$ are only indirectly related to the organization of the receptor inputs and to the interaction processes in the central nervous system. Therefore one needs a description at a deeper level by which receptor organization and neural computations can be conceptually taken into account.

MOVEMENT AND POSITION COMPUTATIONS The phenomenological theory described above deals with the fixation and tracking behavior of flies. The central dogma of the theory is that closed-loop orientation behavior can be derived from the results of open-loop experiments. This means that we need only consider open-loop experiments, in which the visual stimulus is well defined and the motor output is measured.

Consider the following experimental example. If a periodic grating is moved to the right or to the left in front of a fly, an average optomotor response, designated $\vec{R}$ or $\overleftarrow{R}$, can then be measured. This response may or may not be selectively sensitive to directed movement. In fact, one can always distinguish in the average optomotor response a direction-sensitive component, which changes sign under the operation of inverting the direction of motion of the stimulus, and a direction-insensitive component, which is invariant under the same operation (Poggio and Reichardt, 1973b; Poggio, 1974, 1975; Buchner, 1974; Pick, 1974b; Geiger and Poggio, 1975). These two components can be associated with the terms $r\dot{\psi}$ and $D(\psi)$, respectively, in the phenomenological equation. An important consequence is that the two components can be identified with the movement and the position-dependent computations.

The decomposition of the averaged optomotor response of a network into two components is always possible for any given stimulus (see Geiger and Poggio, 1975). A system that is truly direction-sensitive does not give any mean response to a flickered stimulus; a system that is direction-insensitive (for instance, when no lateral interactions exist between the inputs) may give the same mean output for flicker as

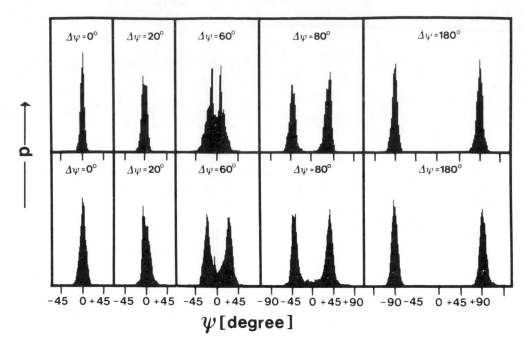

FIGURE 8 Distributions of ψ during stationary fixation of one- and two-stripe patterns (lower figure). The parameter is $\Delta\psi$ as in Figure 7. The duration of the experiments, from individual flies, was either 3 min (for $\Delta\psi = 0°$ and $\Delta\psi = 20°$) or 2×3 min. The upper figure shows corresponding histograms obtained from digital simulation of equation (13) (with $S(t) = 0$). The $D(\psi)$ functions shown in Figure 7 have been used in the simulations; the other parameters have the standard values used throughout this paper. The value of θ/k was 8×10^{-3} both in the experiments and in the simulations. The simulated time is also equivalent (although the normalization in the two cases is only approximate). Redrawn from Reichardt and Poggio (1975).

for constant motion of a periodic grating, independently of its direction of motion. A distinction of the two computations in the optomotor response is conceptually much more difficult if transient inputs and outputs are considered. Therefore our attention will be restricted to experiments in which average responses have been measured. In this way a clear characterization of the underlying interactions is possible.

Consider now two experimental paradigms. In the first experiment, a periodic grating (sinusoidal contrast) is moved at constant speed in one and then in the opposite direction, in front of two adjacent photoreceptors. This experiment has been performed by Kirschfeld (1972) through optical stimulation of specific pairs of photoreceptors in one ommatidium. The light stimuli that form the inputs to the two receptors are sinusoidally modulated with the same frequency, the same amplitude, and a phase shift whose sign reflects the direction of movement. The experimental result shows that the fly responds with a strong direction-sensitive average optomotor response, which changes sign if the direction of motion is reversed. It is clear that a necessary condition for the evaluation

of directed movement is a system with at least two inputs. Furthermore, the overall interaction between the two input signals must be nonlinear, since the average output of a linear system depends on the mean values of the inputs and not on their phase relationship.

In the second experiment, a narrow, vertical stripe is brightness flickered in front of one eye of the fly at the position ψ_0. Again, the light stimuli onto the receptors near ψ_0 are sinusoidally modulated in time, with an identical frequency and phase. A similar stimulus is generated by a stripe oscillating around ψ_0 with a small amplitude. Both types of stimulations elicit an average tendency to turn toward the stimulus (Reichardt, 1973; Pick, 1974a). The response is essentially direction-insensitive, by definition. In addition, the response is position-dependent, corresponding to the term $D(\psi)$ in the phenomenological equation. Again, no linear system can perform this computation. The reason is that in the time average of the response, no significant reaction is found for a stabilized retinal image. Receptor input modulation is necessary to elicit a direction-insensitive response.

Hence the operation on the inputs cannot be linear, since the average output of a linear system is independent of the input modulation.

From these considerations it follows that spatially distributed nonlinear functional interactions between channels following the receptor outputs are essential for the computations of position and movement information in the fly's visual system.

AN INTERACTION APPROACH   In this section we shall outline a conceptual framework which appears appropriate for describing a large class of nonlinear systems with interacting inputs.

A nonlinear system with many inputs and outputs can be represented by a "function" whose domain and range are sets of functions of time (inputs and outputs, respectively). Such a function is usually called an "operator." Alternatively, we can consider the dependence of the response, at a particular time *t,* on the previous input. This constitutes a relation between an ordinary function (the input) and a number (the output at *t*), conventionally called a "functional." Time-invariant systems, which are the main focus of interest, can be represented by functionals.

Interaction formalism and graphs   We shall restrict ourselves here to a Volterra-like integral representation. We consider a time-invariant system with *n* "receptors" indexed by $1, \ldots, n$ and one output; an integral polynomial representation, if it exists, is given by

$$y(t) = g_0 + \sum_{i=1}^{n} g_i * x_i + \sum_{i_1, i_2}^{n} g_{i_1 i_2} *^2 x_{i_1} x_{i_2} + \ldots \quad (21)$$

$$+ \sum_{i_1, \ldots, i_N}^{N} g_{i_1 \ldots i_N} *^N x_{i_1} \ldots x_{i_N},$$

where $*^\ell$ is defined by

$$g_{i_1 \ldots i_\ell} *^\ell x_{i_1} \ldots x_{i_\ell} = \int_{-\infty}^{+\infty} \ldots \int_{-\infty}^{+\infty} g_{i_1 \ldots i_\ell}(\tau_1, \ldots, \tau_\ell)$$

$$\times x_{i_1}(t - \tau_1) \ldots x_{i_\ell}(t - \tau_\ell) d\tau_1 \ldots d\tau_\ell. \quad (22)$$

Equation 22 can be considered a straightforward generalization of the well-known convolution integral. The input functions $x_i(t)$ are real-valued functions of time, each indexed by the associated receptor. In the following, one can assume that $x_i(t)$ is represented by a Fourier polynomial. The kernels $g_0, g_i, g_{i_1 i_2}, \ldots$ are of the Volterra type: $g(\tau) = 0$ if $\tau < 0$. Kernels with identical indices, g_{ii}, are called self-kernels, otherwise cross-kernels. The Fourier transform of a kernel is given by

$$G_{i_1 \ldots i_\ell}(\omega_1, \ldots, \omega_\ell) = \int_{-\infty}^{+\infty} \ldots \int_{-\infty}^{+\infty} d\tau_1 \ldots d\tau_\ell$$

$$\times g_{i_1 \ldots i_\ell}(\tau_1, \ldots, \tau_\ell) \exp\left[-j(\omega_1 \tau_1 + \ldots + \omega_\ell \tau_\ell)\right], \quad (23)$$

where $j = \sqrt{(-1)}$. The ℓ-linear mapping equation 22 is said to be of ℓth degree, and the associated kernel $g_{i_1 \ldots i_\ell}(\tau_1, \ldots, \tau_\ell)$ will be referred to as a ℓth-order kernel. For instance, $g_{i_1 i_2 i_3}(\tau_1, \tau_2, \tau_3)$ is of third order. The alternative notation $g_{2;1}^{(3)}$ may be introduced: $g_{m_1; m_2; \ldots; m_k}^{(N)}$ indicates that there are k separate inputs and the kernel is of order m_i in the ith: its total order is $m_1 + m_2 + \ldots + m_k = N$.

The representation equation 21 is equivalent to a conceptual decomposition of the network into a sum of interactions of different orders.

Properties of symmetry or structure can be symbolized in a graphical representation. As an example, consider the second-order interaction $g_{i_1 i_2}(\tau_1, \tau_2)$. In Figure 9, the interaction is shown decomposed into the eigenfunctions of the operator "input inversion." If the input functions $x_i(t)$ are generated by a motion of a pattern, invariance properties of the interactions can be connected to invariance properties of the network output with respect to operations on the pattern. For instance, for symmetric patterns moving at constant speed, the direction-sensitive component of the output of the second-order interaction of Figure 9 is due to g^a; the direction-insensitive component is due to g^s.

In summary, the "canonical" decomposition of a network in a series of multilinear functionals (or their associated graphs) reduces complicated systems to the sum of simpler subsystems. The important point is the possibility of associating functional and computational properties with interactions of a given order and type.

Multi-input systems   In this section, we shall consider a one-dimensional array of receptors. The system receiving inputs from these receptors is assumed to have the Nth-order approximate representation shown in equation 21. The input functions are $x_i(t) = I_i(t) - I_0$, where I_0 is the light intensity value around which the representation (21) is valid and $I_i(t)$ is the effective light intensity stimulating receptor i. Receptor i has the spatial coordinate ψ_i and the angular sensitivity $\rho_i(\psi) = \rho_0(\psi - \psi_i)$. The input functions $x_i(t)$ can be obtained from the actual stimulus, a space- and time-dependent light intensity distribu-

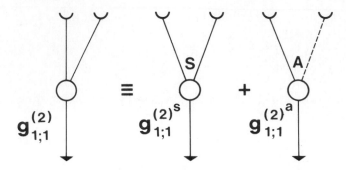

FIGURE 9 A two-input, second-order interaction can be always decomposed into symmetric (s) and antisymmetric (a) second-order, two-input interactions. By antisymmetry (symmetry) is meant that a permutation of the input functions does (not) change the sign of the time-dependent output. Correspondingly, the associated kernel can be decomposed in a symmetric (g^s) and an antisymmetric (g^a) component associated with the graphs of the figure, with

$$g_{1;1}^{(2)s}(\tau_1,\tau_2) = \tfrac{1}{2}[g_{1;1}^{(2)}(\tau_1,\tau_2) + g_{1;1}^{(2)}(\tau_2,\tau_1)],$$

$$g_{1;1}^{(2)a}(\tau_1, \tau_2) = \tfrac{1}{2}[g_{1;1}^{(2)}(\tau_1, \tau_2) - g_{1;1}^{(2)}(\tau_2, \tau_1)].$$

Thus the interaction is decomposed into the eigenfunctions of the operator "input inversion." The input signals x_1 and x_2 may be generated by motion of a pattern. If inversion of direction of motion simply exchanges the inputs x_1 and x_2, the direction-sensitive and direction-insensitive components of the optomotor response are given by

$$y_{ds} = \tfrac{1}{2}(\vec{y} - \overleftarrow{y}) = g_{1;1}^{(2)a} *^2 x_1 x_2,$$

$$y_{di} = \tfrac{1}{2}(\vec{y} + \overleftarrow{y}) = g_{1;1}^{(2)s} *^2 x_1 x_2.$$

From Poggio and Reichardt (1976).

tion determined by the transmission function of the pattern, by its motion, by the possibly time-dependent illumination, and by $\rho_i(\psi)$. General formulas provide, for various stimulus configurations, the coefficients b_{ij} which characterize the Fourier series of $x_i(t)$ in the basic frequency ω^*:

$$x_i(t) = \sum_k b_{ik} e^{jk\omega^* t}, \tag{24}$$

where $j = \sqrt{(-1)}$ (Geiger and Poggio, 1975). An application of equation 21 or its Fourier transform yields, for instance, the average output of the network, given by

$$\bar{y} = g_0 + \sum_i^n G_i(0)b_{i,0} + \sum_{i,k}^n \sum_q G_{ik}(q\omega^*, -q\omega^*)\, b_{i,q}b_{k,-q}$$

$$+ \sum_{ikh}^n \sum_{pq} G_{ikh}(q\omega^*, p\omega^*, (-p-q)\omega^*)$$

$$\times\, b_{i,q}b_{k,p}b_{k,-p-q} + \ldots . \tag{25}$$

We consider two special cases:
1. Sinusoidal grating with spatial wavelength λ

moving at constant speed w. The basic frequency ω^*, called the contrast frequency, is here

$$\omega^* = \omega = \frac{2\pi}{\lambda}\, w, \tag{26}$$

and the average output for motion in one direction in front of equally spaced receptors ($\psi_i - \psi_{i-1} = \Delta\phi$) is (for the right eye)

$$\vec{y} = \bar{y}_{ds} + \bar{y}_{di}, \qquad \overleftarrow{y} = \bar{y}_{ds} - \bar{y}_{di},$$

$$\bar{y}_{ds} = \sum_{n=1}^{N^*} h_n^*(\omega_0) \sin n\, \frac{2\pi\Delta\phi}{\lambda},$$

$$\bar{y}_{di} = \sum_{n=1}^{N^*} k_n^*(\omega) \cos n\, \frac{2\pi\Delta\phi}{\lambda} + k_0^*(\omega), \tag{27}$$

where $\bar{y}_{ds}$ and $\bar{y}_{di}$ are the direction-sensitive and direction-insensitive components of the average output. N^* depends both on the degree of nonlinearity of the network and on the maximum distance of interacting receptors. The "reduced" kernels $h_n^*(\omega)$ and $k_n^*(\omega)$ are derived, for $n \geq 1$, from antisymmetric and symmetric components of the cross-kernels G, respectively; the self-kernels generate, together with cross-kernels of order >1, the term $k_0^*(\omega)$. They depend not only on ω but also on I_0 and on the effective contrast. In $\bar{y}_{ds}$ the first zero crossing occurs for $\lambda \geq 2\Delta\phi$. Thus the response is "right" (has the same sign as the direction of movement) for $\lambda \geq 2\Delta\phi$, in agreement with Shannon's sampling theorem. Interestingly, the limit $\lambda = 2\Delta\phi$ is obtained if only second-order interactions are present (Poggio and Reichardt, 1973b; Buchner, 1974).

2. Two input networks with sinusoidal inputs. If

$$x_1(t) = L_1 \sin(\omega t), \tag{28}$$

$$x_2(t) = L_1 \sin(\omega t + \delta),$$

then

$$\bar{y} = \sum_{n=0}^{N/2} k_{2n}(\omega) \cos n\delta + \sum_{n=0}^{N/2} h_{2n}(\omega) \sin n\delta, \tag{29}$$

where N represents the maximum even degree of nonlinearity of the network. Under the condition $k_n(\omega) \neq 0$, the dependency of the average output on δ uniquely characterizes N and thus the order of nonlinearity of the system.

DIRECTION-SENSITIVE OPTOMOTOR RESPONSE AND ASSOCIATED INTERACTIONS The average direction-sensitive response corresponds to the "classical" optomotor reaction studied in insects for a long time (Hassenstein, 1951; Varjú, 1959; Götz, 1964; Reichardt, 1969, 1970). In these investigations, the optomotor response was time-averaged and "antisymmetrized." This resulted in the quantity

$$\bar{y}_{ds} = \frac{\overrightarrow{y} - \overleftarrow{y}}{2}, \qquad (30)$$

which has been defined as the direction-sensitive component of the optomotor response.

Two major questions should be discussed. The first concerns the topology of these interactions, and the second their functional properties. Characterization of the interacting topology has been attempted by two different methods: selective stimulation of single receptors (Kirschfeld, 1972; Kirschfeld and Lutz, 1974; Franceschini, 1975) and stimulation of restricted arrays of receptors by sinusoidal gratings with specific wavelengths and orientations (Buchner, 1974, 1976). The results are summarized in Figure 10. The emerging web of interactions between receptors of the system R_1-R_6 and receptors of the system R_7-R_8 is rather complex and highly specific. The overall picture is not yet complete. A still open problem concerns the exact role played by the two receptor systems R_1-R_6 and R_7-R_8 in the movement and position computations in *Musca* and *Drosophila* (Wehrhahn, 1976, 1977; Heisenberg and Buchner, 1977). In the following, we identify with the term "receptor" each receptor or group of receptors that share the same visual field. The topology of these interactions is not the major concern of this paper (see Kirschfeld, this volume). Important for the second question is the demonstration by Kirschfeld (1972) that two single photoreceptors in the fly's eye can elicit an average direction-sensitive response. From older investigations, we know that the direction-sensitive optomotor response often depends, at low input modulations, on the square of the contrast of a moving grating (Fermi and Reichardt, 1963; McCann and

a   b

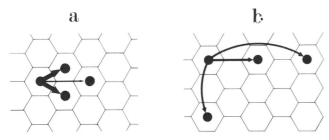

FIGURE 10 Topology of the direction-sensitive interactions underlying movement computation. (a) "Elementary movement detectors" (with relative weights) associated with each visual element in the visual system of *Drosophila* (Buchner, 1974, 1976). (b) Elementary interactions, determined in *Musca* for the R_1-R_6 system by Kirschfeld (1972), using the method of single-receptor stimulation, are mapped onto the mosaic of visual elements. From Buchner (1976).

MacGinitie, 1965; Eckert, 1973; Götz, 1964, 1965; Hengstenberg and Götz, 1967; Buchner, 1974, 1976). In terms of the canonical decomposition, these two results would imply that "essential" interactions involved in the direction-sensitive movement computation are second-order nonlinear and receive their information from two inputs (*p*-order 2). The associated kernel must be antisymmetric. Thus the corresponding graph, basic to the movement computation, can be recognized as the antisymmetric one of Figure 9.

Antisymmetric second-order interactions represent a minimal model for movement computation. Interestingly, they are also optimal in terms of the "resolution limit." It is well known that the resolving power and the acuity of the compound eye are determined, respectively, by the angular separation and by the angular sensitivity distribution of individual receptors (Götz, 1964; Reichardt, 1969). For one dimension they coincide with $\Delta\phi$ and $\rho_0(\psi)$. The general equation 27 shows, in agreement with the Shannon sampling theorem, that a periodic array of equidistant receptors can resolve uniquely the direction of movement of a periodic grating only if $\lambda \geq 2\Delta\phi$. The "resolution limit" $\lambda = 2\Delta\phi$ is already obtained by second-order interactions between neighboring receptors. In this case, equation 27 gives

$$\bar{y}_{ds} = h_1^*(\omega)\sin\frac{2\pi\Delta\phi}{\lambda}. \qquad (31)$$

Nonlinearities of higher order may introduce "artificial" sampling intervals greater than the ones physically present in the system: as wide-angle interactions, they can only (but not necessarily) deteriorate the resolution limit set by the sampling theorem (Thorson, 1966; Poggio and Reichardt, 1973b; Buchner, 1974).

Second-order antisymmetric interactions also have a number of other characteristic properties susceptible to experimental testing (Poggio and Reichardt, 1973b; Buchner, 1974; Geiger and Poggio, 1975). In the following, we shall briefly consider some of the results.

1. Experimental tests of equation 27 and comparison with independent data on the topology of the interactions are consistent with second-order nonlinearities. Equation 27 cannot, however, directly distinguish between multiple spacings and nonlinearities of higher order than the second. The difficulty can be circumvented through a two-input stimulation. In this case, equation 29 can be applied. The experimental data (Pick, 1974a, 1976), shown in Figure 11, clearly imply $N = 2$ for the direction-sensitive com-

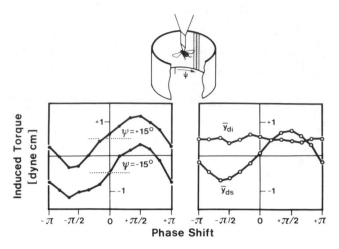

FIGURE 11   The mean torque response of a test fly elicited by two 2.7° wide, vertically oriented filament lamps whose intensities are sinusoidally modulated and phase-shifted with respect to one another. The phase lag is defined as positive if the luminance modulation of the right lamp follows that of the left lamp. The background luminance amounted to 60 cd/m². The degree of the light modulation of the two lamps was 40%. Left diagram: the upper (lower) curve represents the mean torque induced by the two lamps located in the mean position $\psi = +15°$ ($\psi = -15°$). Right diagram: half-sum ($\bar{y}_{ds}$) and half-difference ($\bar{y}_{di}$) of the reaction curves drawn in the left diagram. Redrawn from Pick (1974a).

ponent $\bar{y}_{ds}$; that is, they imply second-order interactions.

2. The mean of the direction-sensitive optomotor response shows the property of "phase invariance." Inspection of equation 25 shows that different temporal Fourier components in the input functions never interfere in the mean output for interactions up to second order. As a consequence of this "superposition property," the mean response does not depend upon the relative phases of the spatial Fourier components of an arbitrary pattern moved at constant speed in front of the photoreceptors. The property of "phase invariance" leads to the striking experimental result that two quite different patterns elicit an identical mean optomotor response $\bar{y}_{ds}$ (Varjú and Reichardt, 1967; Götz, 1972; Zimmermann, 1973). In general, for higher-order nonlinearities, phase invariance and superposition do not hold.

3. A third property can be conjectured on the basis of the essential homogeneity and the restricted spatial range of second-order interactions: the interactions between the different channels should have the same frequency dependence. This means that the coefficients in equation 27 should satisfy

$$h_n^*(\omega) = \alpha_n h^*(\omega) \quad \text{for all } n, \tag{32}$$

leading to the following property of the mean response:

$$\bar{y}_{ds}(\omega,\lambda) = T(\omega) \, I(\lambda), \tag{33}$$

where the function $T(\omega)$ must approach zero in the limit of either $\omega \to 0$ or $\omega \to \infty$ (Götz, 1975). The data plotted in Figure 12 show that this is indeed the case. The response depends upon the frequency $\omega/2\pi = w/\lambda$ rather than upon the angular velocity w (Götz, 1972; Eckert, 1973). Equation 33 again shows the essential simplicity of the interactive structure underlying movement computation.

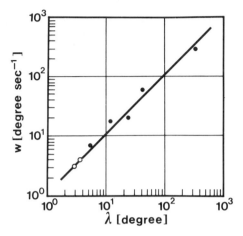

FIGURE 12   Relation between angular wavelength λ of a moving periodic grating and its most efficient angular velocity w. The maximum reactions, either positive (●) or reversed (○), are determined by the contrast frequency ω and not by the velocity w. From Eckert (1973).

Psychophysical, behavioral, and electrophysiological data have suggested a few specific models of selective motion detection (Barlow and Levick, 1965; Thorson, 1964, 1966; Foster, 1971; Grüsser and Grüsser-Cornehls, 1973; van Doorn and Koenderink, 1976). Clearly the formalism discussed here is not a "model" of movement detection. Its aim is to illustrate how such a theory may be developed. One of the first models of movement detection was proposed by Hassenstein and Reichardt (1956) and outlined in more detail by Reichardt (1957, 1961) and Hassenstein (1958, 1959). The scheme, which depends upon evaluating the cross-correlation between signals from two neuro-ommatidia, can account for the antisymmetric mean optomotor response of the beetle *Chlorophanus*; it has also led to predictions that have been experimentally verified in other insects (Reichardt and Varjú, 1959; Varjú and Reichardt, 1967; Reichardt, 1969; Kunze, 1961). Other versions of the original *Chlorophanus* model have been proposed in different contexts (Thorson, 1966; Foster, 1971; Kirschfeld, 1972); they are in fact correlation models, characterized by the time-averaged output

$$\bar{y}_{ds} = \int \tilde{W}(\omega)\, X_1(\omega)\, X_2(-\omega)d\omega, \qquad (34)$$

where $\tilde{W}(\omega)$ is an odd, imaginary function, reflecting the overall filter properties of the network, and $X_1(\omega)$ and $X_2(\omega)$ are the Fourier transforms of time-dependent inputs. The generality of the correlation model can be easily interpreted in terms of the formalism discussed here. Equations 21 and 25 show that all n-input systems that admit a Volterra-like expansion lead to contributions of the type of equation 34, if nonlinearities of order higher than the second are negligible. Consequently the class of correlation models is the most general representation of second-order interactions if the mean direction-sensitive output is considered.

Other models of motion detection have focused on understanding the physiological circuitry rather than the functional properties of the direction-sensitive response. A well-known example is the scheme proposed by Barlow and Levick (1965) to account for the activity of directionally selective units in the rabbit's retina. The model of Barlow and Levick is not inconsistent with the functional structure derived in this section. However, the data so far available (see also Michael, 1968; Montero and Brugge, 1969) do not seem to allow a functional characterization of the underlying interactions similar to the one described in this paper. Some analogies may also be expected in the responsible neural circuitry. Some support for this conjecture comes from recordings of Marmarelis and McCann (1973) from movement-sensitive, direction-selective neurons in *Musca* and *Phaenicia*. Their recordings show that, at the level of these neurons, cross-interactions of second order are present and higher-order interactions are negligible.

DIRECTION-INSENSITIVE RESPONSES AND ASSOCIATED INTERACTIONS As has been pointed out before, the computation of position that results in the function $D(\psi)$ is the basis of visual orientation and tracking behavior in flies. In the open-loop experiments, the direction-insensitive component of the optomotor response corresponds to the transduction of the position information into a mean torque response. The underlying interactive structure is not yet completely understood; the information available so far is mainly limited to the horizontal, ψ-dependent organization. As for the movement computation, we shall use the canonical decomposition equation 21 to classify the

interactions underlying the direction-insensitive optomotor response by means of input-output experiments.

Direct, nonlateral interactive computations As a first restriction on the possible graphs, it can be easily shown that only symmetric interactions (kernels) can provide the direction-insensitive optomotor responses considered here. Experiments with flickering light or small-angle oscillations with narrow stripes suggest that the simplest possibility of this type, a sequence of self-interactions (self-kernels) parameterized by their two-dimensional location, may actually be realized in the fly's eye. The $D(\psi)$ response shown in Figure 4a can be also elicited by flickering a narrow, dark stripe against a steady, bright background, in different ψ positions, as Pick (1974a) has shown, correcting an earlier hypothesis (Reichardt, 1973). The degree of these interactions is still an unsolved problem, but it must be higher than one.

The graphs shown in Figure 13 are of degree 2, but there is no conclusive experimental reason for this. The existence of operations of degree higher than one is supported by a series of closed-loop experiments (Reichardt, 1973, and unpublished data). Fixation of a vertical stripe was measured for various stripe contrasts. The dependence of $D(\psi)$ on contrast turns out to be roughly quadratic at low contrast values. Moreover, $D(\psi)$ is invariant under contrast inversion in a pattern if the contrast values involved are not too high. Since linearization with small input modulations does not occur, essential self-interactions (self-kernels) of degree higher than one are required. From a computational point of view, however, nonlinear self-kernels ($N > 1$; p-order 1) are all essentially similar. Very small horizontal oscillations ($\ll \Delta\phi$) of a very narrow vertical stripe also elicit a significant

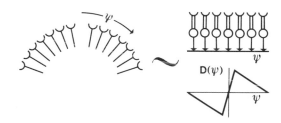

FIGURE 13 Schematic representation of the spatially distributed organization responsible for the extraction of position information in the case of a narrow object (6° to 10°). There is no experimental evidence requiring the nonlinear self-interactions to be only second-order (as they are drawn here for simplicity); however, the p-order is 1. The lateral interactions that affect the attractiveness of broader patterns (6° to 10°) are not drawn here. From Poggio and Reichardt (1976).

rage response, again suggesting that the computation does not require interactions between neighboring receptors on the horizontal coordinate ψ. Support for this conjecture is given by the experiment shown in Figure 11. The mean direction-insensitive, position-dependent component of the response ($\bar{y}_{di}$) turns out to be a constant, independent of the phase of the two light inputs. Accordingly, equation 29 would imply

$$k_0 > 0, \qquad k_{2n}(\omega) = 0 \quad (n > 0). \qquad (35)$$

Thus, in the restricted angular range ($<10°$), lateral interactions between input channels would not exist. This conclusion, however, must be accepted with caution. Due to the two-dimensional geometry of the eye, a number of alternative possibilities are conceivable. For instance, "vertical" interactions would also be consistent with the experimental results. However, Pick (1977) has given some experimental evidence that "vertical" interactions of the type discussed here do not exist. Other, special cases of nonlinear lateral interactions would also be phase-independent under the conditions of Figure 11 (see Pick, 1974b). Self-interactions (self-kernels) are the simplest candidates, and they are in agreement with all data so far available. We therefore conjecture that nonlinear operations on the single photoreceptor channels, associated with self-kernels, provide, in this angular range, the position-dependent computation. The resulting interactive structure, shown in Figure 13, is simple and computationally trivial (p-order 1). However, the ψ-parameterization of the self-kernels implied by the shape of the function $D(\psi)$ yields a nontrivial, closed-loop behavior. It is clear that the dependence of the self-kernels on ψ is the critical carrier of position information.

It is quite obvious that such a simple computational structure, which leads to the superposition rule, cannot by itself give a highly selective, pattern-dependent response. Only nonlinear interactions between channels can provide a mechanism for nontrivial pattern selectivity. Only through nonlinear lateral interactions can a composed pattern become a new, independent configuration (Poggio, 1974). In fact, many recent experimental data suggest that, in addition to the self-interactions, nonlinear inhibitory interactions also take place on a broader angular range. In this range, they are the cause of the quantitative failure of the superposition rule.

Lateral, nonlinear, inhibitory interactions The first hint that inhibitory interactions affect the position computation came from the experiments with two vertical stripes. The attractiveness of a pattern composed of two vertical stripes turned out to be less than the sum of their individual attractivenesses.

In a similar way, the attractiveness (corresponding to $\bar{y}_{di}$) of a flickered vertical stripe (Figure 14) does not increase proportionally to its width and even decreases when its lateral dimensions exceed about 10° or five ommatidia columns. (Similar measurements carried out by Pick, 1974b, led to the same result, except that his data suggest 6° and consequently three ommatidia columns.) Thus the emerging organization seems to include self-interactions and surrounding lateral interactions, on an angular range larger than about 10° (or 6°) certainly less than about 80°. Figure 14 also shows how the time-averaged response of the fly depends upon a stimulus consisting of a black stripe oscillated sinusoidally with different amplitudes A and the same frequency as the flicker signal. Under these experimental conditions, mainly the self-interactions are stimulated. Consequently the reaction measured builds up approximately linearly with an increase in the oscillation amplitude A, whereas the response to a flickering bar decreases when the lateral interactions come into play.

In addition to the data reported here, experiments with periodic luminance gratings also show the presence of lateral interactions. Interestingly, Geiger and

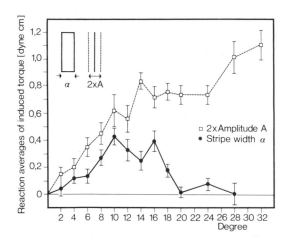

FIGURE 14 Mean open-loop attractiveness responses from test flies to a stationary, flickered vertical stripe as a function of its width α and to a black stripe oscillated sinusoidally with an amplitude A (2.5 Hz frequency). The data refer to a mean object position $\psi = \pm 30°$. The average brightness of the flickered stripe amounted to 468 cd/m², the brightness of the background to 64 cd/m². Modulation degree was $m = 88\%$. The stripe was oscillated with a background illumination of 700 cd/m². Each point in both measurements is the mean of 30 measurements with 15 individual flies. Each measurement lasted 2 min. The vertical bars denote standard errors of the mean.

Poggio (1975) determined that the direction-sensitive component is confined to the lower half of the compound eye. This result clearly supports the theoretical argument that the interactions underlying the orientation behavior also underlie the direction-insensitive response. Furthermore, both cross-kernels and self-kernels seem to be present only in the lower half of the compound eye.

An important question for understanding the position computation concerns the order of the lateral interactions and, possibly, their spatial organization. The first answer to this problem was again provided by two-input experiments (Pick, 1974b). Two adjacent vertical dark stripes, 4.5° broad, were sinusoidally flickered at $\psi = 20°$ on the fly's right eye, with various phase shifts. The results (Figure 15) require, in terms of equation 29, interactions of degree 2 or higher ($k_4 \neq 0$). The geometry and the number of interacting photoreceptors are not as yet clear. At least two receptors, and perhaps more, are required; the p-order is thus at least 2, possibly 4. In Figure 16, some of the simplest alternatives are presented. A few other schemes are, however, experimentally indistinguishable at this stage of analysis. For instance, interactions in the vertical direction (ϑ)

may well be present and may in fact control the position-dependent "attractiveness" of objects with different vertical extensions. It is quite possible that a set of fourth- and/or higher-order inhibitory interactions with various topologies is actually present in the visual system of the fly. The simple organization shown in Figure 16a envisages excitatory second-order self-kernels surrounded by lateral inhibitory fourth-order interactions with various spacings. Other interactive structures are also consistent with the data. It is especially important to stress that some recurrent inhibitory interactions may have a "forward" Volterra representation with infinitely many graphs, the first ones corresponding to the graphs of parts a or b of Figure 16. An example of such a recurrent inhibitory interaction is given in Figure 16d, together with its "forward" Volterra representation. In such a case, the problem of the range and sign of interactions would take on a new aspect.

Object-ground and figure-ground discrimination When a small black object is embedded in a "noisy" background texture, it may be quite difficult or even impossible to distinguish the object from the background. However, small relative motions between object and background allow an easy detection. Does the orientation behavior of flies indicate a similar process? That this is indeed the case was shown by Virsik (1974) and by Virsik and Reichardt (1976). Under natural (closed-loop) conditions, flies can fixate and track small objects in front of a random texture, if the object moves relative to the background (Figure 5). Open-loop experiments demonstrate the same effect, in agreement with the main thesis of the phenomenological theory, which maintains that closed-loop behavior can be directly predicted from open-loop responses.

It is quite clear that computations which allow us to apply the superposition rule cannot account for this effect. As we shall discuss later, however, it is possible to prove formally, using equation 21, that the simplest graphs capable of this computation have order 4 and two receptor inputs (p-order 2) (see Figure 16).

To find out whether this computation can be accounted for (in flies) by the "minimal" fourth-order graphs of Figure 16, a series of open-loop experiments has been performed (Heimburger, Poggio, and Reichardt, 1976; Poggio and Reichardt, 1978). The inset of Figure 17 shows the basic experimental design. A black vertical stripe is sinusoidally oscillated around a fixed position in front of one eye. A complex noiselike background can also be oscillated with preset amplitude A, frequency ω^*, and phase ϕ. The

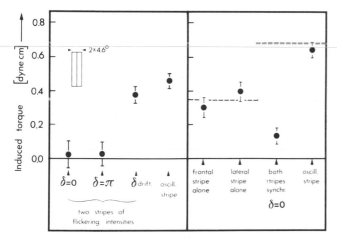

FIGURE 15   Mean torque attractiveness to different stimuli of sinusoidally flickering and oscillating stripes. Mean angular position of the stimulus $\psi = \pm 20°$. The data are from 6 (left) and 8 (right) female *Musca* (4–10 days old), respectively. The flicker and oscillation frequency amounted to 3 Hz, the amplitude of the oscillation to $A = 4.6°$. No attractiveness is observed toward the two stripes flickering simultaneously ($\delta = \pi$). However, flickering of the two stripes with two slightly different frequencies (3 Hz and 3.25 Hz) elicits a mean attraction (δ drift) that is of the same order as the response elicited by the oscillating stripe. The attractiveness of an oscillating stripe is almost the sum of the attractivenesses of the single flickering stripes. Redrawn from Pick (1974b).

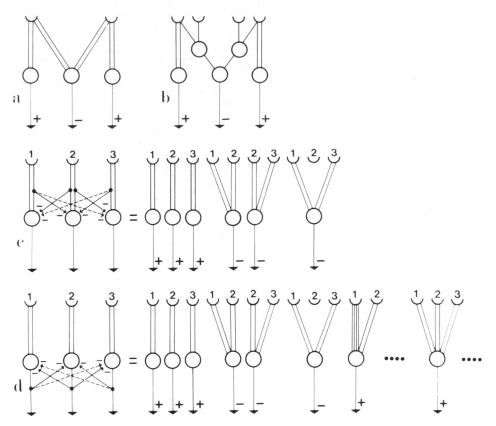

FIGURE 16 Four interactive organizations that could underlie the figure-ground discrimination effect in the fly. Parts a and b show two lateral inhibitory interaction schemes, containing second-order self-graphs and fourth-order cross-graphs, with p-orders 2 (a) and 4 (b). In part c, a forward inhibitory network is decomposed in its polynomial graph representation (see equation (21)). Self-kernels and fourth-order inhibitory cross-kernels (with p-order 2) occur. (d) Recurrent inhibitory network and its equivalent polynomial representation (when it exists). In addition to the graphs of part c, an infinite number of other graphs appear, both excitatory and inhibitory, of increasing order (and p-order!). In particular, the (excitatory) graph at the extreme right provides disinhibition effects, expected from the recurrent structure of the network at the left (compare with part c). Interestingly, the p-order of the network of part d is "infinite" (that is, equal to the total number of receptors). It can be shown that in all experimental situations described in this paper, only the first four graphs of part d play a significant role. They underlie the "object-ground" effect shown in Figures 17, 18, and 19 (see equation (36)) and the orientation responses shown in Figure 15. From Poggio and Reichardt (1976).

average "attractiveness" of the object (given in terms of the average fly's torque) is measured in units of the standard response to the stripe oscillating in front of the stationary background texture. For equal frequencies of oscillation (the amplitude is 0.5° for the background, 1° for the stripe), Figure 17 shows that the "detection" of the stripe is reduced when the phase is either $\phi = 0$ (in phase, the two movements are "coherent") or $\phi = \pi$ (antiphase, the two movements are in phase apposition). The attractiveness of the object reaches its maximum for $\phi = \pi/2$ and is also strong when foreground and background oscillate with different frequencies. An opaque white screen interposed between the stripe and the background, as shown in the inset of Figure 17, does not

have any influence on the effect. This indicates the existence of lateral (nonlinear) interactions between receptors stimulated by the object and receptors stimulated by the background. A more complete version of the experiment reported in Figure 17 is shown in Figure 18. Again, equal frequencies of oscillation were used; however, the amplitudes for the background and for the stripe were equal and amounted to $\pm 1°$. As can be read from the phase dependence of the average response, plotted in Figure 18, the object is not detected for phases $\phi = 0$ and $\phi = \pi$, whereas the attractiveness of the object reaches its maximum for about $\phi = \pi/2$ and $\phi = 3\pi/2$. It can be shown that for small oscillation amplitudes (such as the ones used in the experiments plotted in Figures

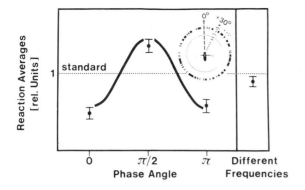

FIGURE 17 Average (direction-insensitive) torque response of 10 flies to sinusoidally oscillating "object" and "ground" patterns, under open-loop conditions. The object consists of a black vertical stripe, 3° wide, positioned in the lower part of the panorama oscillated around the mean positions $\psi = \pm 30°$. The ground pattern consists of a random dot texture (Julesz, 1975), which can be moved independently from the foreground. A white stationary screen (12° wide) is mounted between the stripe and the background pattern. In all experiments represented in the figure, the oscillation amplitude of the stripe was $\pm 1°$ (at 2.5 Hz frequency) and $\pm 0.5°$ for the random texture (when oscillating). The standard response measures the attractiveness of the stripe when oscillated alone, while the random texture was stationary. When object and ground are both oscillated with the same frequency, the average attraction toward the stripe depends on the relative phase, as shown in the left side of the figure. When object and ground are oscillated with different frequencies (2.5 and 1.8 Hz, respectively) the average attraction is about "standard." Each point is the mean of 10 individual measurements. Each individual measurement lasted 2 min. The vertical bars denote standard errors of the mean. The continuous line is given by (hand) fitting the experimental data with equation (36), where k_0 is determined by the "standard" response ($k_0 = 1$) and k_4 is the free parameter. From Poggio and Reichardt (1976).

17 and 18), the light signals onto the receptors are periodic functions of time, containing mainly the first harmonic of the oscillation frequency. Thus, at least for a qualitative discussion, we may neglect higher harmonics. Under this assumption, fourth-order interactions of the kind shown in Figure 16 fully account for the mean response of Figures 17 and 18, which is, in fact, rather well fitted by the typical fourth-order response:

$$\bar{y}_{\text{di}} = k_0 + k_4 \cos 2\phi \qquad (36)$$

with $k_0 > 0$, $k_4 < 0$ in general, and $|k_0| = |k_4|$ for equal amplitudes of background and stripe oscillations. Here ϕ represents the phase difference between the sinusoidal motions of the two patterns. Detailed calculations show that the various graphs of Figure 16 are indeed consistent with all experimental results

(Poggio and Reichardt, 1978). (Even the sixth-order graphs arising from the recurrent interactions of Figure 16d would give terms of the type of equation 36 with $k_6 > 0$ under our experimental conditions.) Moreover, the simplest (in terms of equation 21) interactive network that can discriminate relative motion of object and ground is the fourth-order one of Figure 16a.

Let us now consider the main steps of the argument:

1. Self-interactions (self-kernels) provide the "excitatory" attraction toward the stripe. What is additionally needed is a mean inhibitory influence, effective for coherent oscillations of the two patterns and ineffective for coherent motion. The lowest-level interactions that should be considered have degree 2; the next higher ones have degree 4. It will be shown that degree 2 cannot provide the required inhibition.

2. The only second-order graph we need consider is a graph with symmetry properties and two inputs, one stimulated by the stripe, the other by the noise. The ensemble average of the mean outputs of such nets is zero because of the random nature of the texture and because of the spatial distribution of the stripe's first harmonic. Next, however, it can be shown that the fourth-order interactions of Figure 16a satisfy the above-specified requirements.

3. An oscillation of the stripe at frequency ω^* generates a periodic signal of double frequency at the output of the second-order self- (a) or cross- (b) interactions of Figure 16. Oscillation of the noise yields

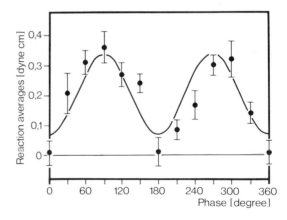

FIGURE 18 Experimental conditions as described in the legend and in the inset of Figure 17, except for the equal oscillation amplitudes of $\pm 1°$ for the stripe and the noise background. Each point represents the average from 10 flies. The average responses are given in absolute units. The vertical bars denote standard errors of the mean. The continuous line is the component $-k_4 \cos 2\phi$ in equation (36) derived from a Fourier analysis of the data plotted in the figure. From Poggio and Reichardt (1978).

a similar result. For simplicity, the case of the self-kernels is considered. The important point here is that the frequency and phase of the ensemble average of the quadratic operations (self-kernels) depend on the frequency and phase of the motion and not on the structure of the pattern if the oscillation amplitude is small. Due to the frequency doubling, phase differences ϕ between the oscillations of the stripe and the texture are mapped into a double phase difference at the input of the second-order cross-interaction. Thus the mean output of the latter interaction depends on 2ϕ (see equation 29). The additional assumption that this output is "inhibitory" ($k_4 < 0$) whereas the output of the self-kernels is "excitatory" ($k_0 > 0$, attraction toward the object) yields equation 36.

Different oscillation frequencies of object and ground lead to a zero mean contribution from the fourth-order inhibitions. The contributions of the self-kernels, elicited by the background, cancel, because (besides being homogeneously distributed on the two eyes) they are counteracted by those fourth-order inhibitory interactions whose inputs are all stimulated by the (in-phase) background texture. Consequently, only the "excitatory" contributions elicited by the stripe are left, as in the case of a stationary background.

Even in terms of the simplified analysis outlined here, it is obvious that an increasing background amplitude should increase the effect of the lateral inhibitions. Figure 19 shows that this is indeed the case. For $\phi = 0$ or $\phi = \pi$, the attractiveness reduces to zero for equal amplitudes of stripe and background. For increasing background amplitudes, the inhibition overrides the excitatory contributions of the self-kernels. The fly is then repelled by the stripe ("escape response"). In an equivalent way, for $\phi = \pi/2$, the inhibition turns into excitation and the stripe attractiveness increases. At large amplitudes, a number of factors reduce the effect. Higher harmonics now become significant and higher-order terms, possibly due to the recurrent structure of the inhibitions (Figure 16d), could play a larger role.

So far we have discussed the computational properties of the visual system which enable the fly to discriminate moving objects from noiselike textured grounds. More recently the experiments have been extended to figures consisting of noiselike contrasted vertical stripes (5° to 22° width) moved in front of a ground that carries the same noiselike texture (Poggio and Reichardt, 1978). Results from experiments with different phases and frequencies were in principle the same as the one reported in connection with

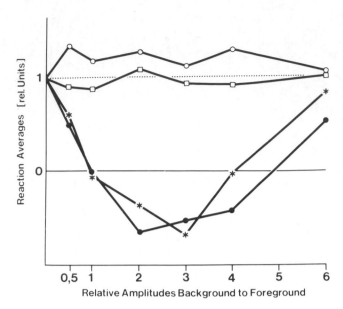

FIGURE 19 Experimental details as described in the legend of Figure 17, except for the various oscillation amplitudes of the ground with respect to the stripe's "unity" amplitude of ±1°. The relative phase relations between stripe and background are 0° (filled circles), 90° (open circles), or 180° (stars). Squares designate measurements with different frequencies (2.5 Hz for stripe and 1.8 Hz for random texture). The average standard error of the means is ±0.1 (relative units). From Poggio and Reichardt (1976).

the object-ground discrimination, suggesting that incoherent motion of the figure leads (as in the case of an object) to a separation of figure from ground. Under the functional condition of incoherency, the influence of the fourth-order inhibitory interactions is reduced to zero across the boundary of the figure, so that the nerve net responsible for the computations "breaks" into two parts, one part responding only to the figure, the other responding only to the ground. That is to say, the influence of the noise figure becomes context-free and therefore independent of the ground under the conditions of incoherent relative motion.

The next experimental step in the analysis of the figure-ground problem was the use of figures that did not consist of the same contrast texture as the ground. Figure 20 shows the outcome of such an experiment in which the figure was constructed from alternating noiselike and white stripes moved in different phase relations in front of a noiselike ground. The result shows that the fly is already attracted by the figure when figure and ground are moved in synchrony ($\phi = 0$). The attraction increases when the phase is set to either $\phi = \pi/2$ or $\phi = 3\pi/2$ and becomes slightly negative or zero for $\phi = \pi$. The im-

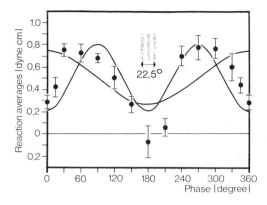

FIGURE 20 Average (direction-insensitive) torque response of 10 flies to sinusoidally oscillating "figure" and "ground" patterns, under open-loop conditions. The figure consists of five vertical stripes, each 4.5° wide (inset), positioned in the lower part of the panorama, oscillated with the center line around the mean positions $\psi = \pm 30°$. Three stripes carry a fine-grain random dot texture, whereas two stripes are white. They are organized in an alternating sequence (inset). The ground is a fine-grain random dot pattern that can be moved independently of the figure. In all experiments represented in this diagram, the oscillation amplitudes of the figure and the ground amounted to $\pm 3.5°$ (both at 2.5 Hz). The average response (given in absolute units) measures the attractiveness of the figure when figure and ground are oscillated with different relative phases. In contrast to the experiment reported in Figure 18, the flies are attracted by the figure at phase zero. The attraction increases for increasing phase angles and declines to about zero for 180° phase shift. Each point is the mean of 10 individual measurements. Each individual measurement lasted 2 min. The vertical bars denote standard errors of the mean. The two continuous lines represent the components $k_2 \cos \phi$ and $-k_4 \cos 2\phi$ in equation (37), derived from a Fourier analysis of the data points plotted in the diagram. From Poggio and Reichardt (1978).

portant new information gained by this experiment is that the dependence of the average reaction on the phase contains not only a periodic component with a periodicity of π, but also one, of about equal amplitude, with a periodicity of 2π, so that instead of equation 36, the response can be approximated by

$$\bar{y}_{\mathrm{di}} = k_0 + k_2 \cos\phi + k_4 \cos 2\phi \qquad (37)$$

with $k_0 > 0$, $k_2 > 0$, and $k_4 < 0$. One can show by arguments similar to the ones discussed in connection with the object-ground separation (Poggio and Reichardt, 1978) that the term $k_2 \cos \phi$ cannot be due to a second-order symmetric interaction. The only possible candidate we can see at present is a second-order symmetric cross-interaction between two second-order antisymmetric cross-interactions of the type g^a presented in Figure 9. The graphical representation of this interaction is given in Figure 21. It

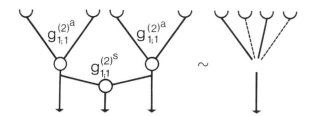

FIGURE 21 A graphical representation of the computational structure responsible for the 360° component in Figure 20. The results of two second-order antisymmetric cross-interactions are cross-correlated by a second-order symmetric cross-interaction which provides an excitatory contribution to the average response (left side of the diagram). This interaction type can be also represented by the $p = 4, N = 4$ graph plotted on the right side of the diagram.

should be mentioned that the contribution of this interaction to the response is excitatory. It provides a component of vectorial position information for the evaluation system, whereas the self-interactions make a scalar contribution.

Résumé

Experimental evidence and theoretical considerations lead to the conclusion that the visual orientation behavior of the fly can be quantitatively predicted from the corresponding open-loop reactions by a phenomenological theory. The part of the visual system responsible for these reactions operates like a parallel organized network with many receptors and building blocks, interacting in an essentially nonlinear way. Only four types of nonlinear functional interactions are required for the explanation of the behavioral responses. One of these interactions underlies the direction-sensitive optomotor response and is related to the speed-dependent term in the phenomenological equation. The other three interactions are responsible for the direction-insensitive response, which mediates the attractiveness of a pattern and appears in the phenomenological equation as a position-dependent term.

Antisymmetric second-order cross-interactions between pairs of receptors compose the part of the network responsible for the direction-sensitive response. The two-dimensional topology of these mechanisms has been only partially unraveled so far. These interactions are present in both the upper and lower parts of the compound eyes and seem to be rather homogeneously distributed.

Self-interactions compute the position-dependent response for narrow objects. They are weighted according to their two-dimensional location through gradients of their density and/or their synaptic properties. Self-interactions are consistent with the superposition property. That is to say, the attractiveness of a pattern, computed by self-interactions, would be the sum of the attractivenesses of its components. However, inhibitory and excitatory fourth-order symmetric cross-interactions also affect, at least on a certain angular range, the position-dependent response and therefore violate the superposition property. The topology of these types of interactions is not known in detail, except that the inhibitory cross-interactions are confined to the lower parts of the compound eyes. The interplay between the inhibitory fourth-order interaction and the excitatory self-interaction is responsible for the object and figure-ground separation, whereas the excitatory fourth-order interactions probably mediate the figure perception.

The complex visual orientation behavior rests on the cooperation of a few different types of elementary, but essentially nonlinear interactions which are mainly organized in parallel. One of the major questions remaining concerns the organization of the actual neural network underlying the interaction mechanisms. The electrophysiological and anatomic analysis should be much simplified by the behavioral analysis since only four different types of local circuit building blocks (or linear combinations of them) must be localized and unraveled in the mass of neurons in the visual system of the fly.

REFERENCES

BARLOW, H. B., and W. R. LEVICK, 1965. The mechanism of directionally sensitive units in rabbit's retina. *J. Physiol.* 178:477–504.

BUCHNER, E., 1974. Bewegungsperzeption in einem visuellen System mit gerastertem Eingang. Dissertation Eberhard Karls-Universität Tübingen.

BUCHNER, E., 1976. Elementary movement detectors in an insect visual system. *Biol. Cybernetics* 24:85–101.

BUCHNER, S., and W. REICHARDT, 1978. Delay time between light stimulation and motor response in the fly. In preparation.

COLLETT, T. S., and M. LAND, 1975. Visual control of flight behaviour in the hoverfly, *Syritta pipiens. J. Comp. Physiol.* 99:1–66.

ECKERT, H. E., 1973. Optomotorische Untersuchungen am visuellen System der Stubenfliege *Musca domestica. Kybernetik* 14:1–23.

FERMI, G., and W. REICHARDT, 1963. Optomotorische Reaktionen der Fliege *Musca domestica. Kybernetik* 2:15–28.

FOSTER, D. H., 1971. A model of the human visual system in its response to certain classes of moving stimuli. *Kybernetik* 8:69–84.

FRANCESCHINI, N., 1975. Sampling of the visual environment by the compound eye of the fly: Fundamentals and applications. In *Photoreceptor Optics*, A. W. Snyder and R. Menzel, eds. Berlin, Heidelberg, New York: Springer-Verlag.

GEIGER, G., and T. POGGIO, 1975. The orientation of flies towards visual patterns: On the search for the underlying functional interactions. *Biol. Cybernetics* 17:1–16.

GÖTZ, K. G., 1964. Optomotorische Untersuchungen des visuellen Systems einiger Augenmutanten der Fruchtfliege *Drosophila. Kybernetik* 2:77–92.

GÖTZ, K. G., 1965. Die optischen Übertragungseigenschaften der Komplexaugen von *Drosophila. Kybernetik* 2:215–221.

GÖTZ, K. G., 1972. Principles of optomotor reactions in insects. *Bibl. Ophthalmol.* 82:252–259.

GÖTZ, K. G., 1975. The optomotor equilibrium of the *Drosophila* navigation system. *J. Comp. Physiol.* 99:187–210.

GRAHAM, B., and H. HAKEN, 1971. Generalized thermodynamic potential for Markov systems in detailed balance. *Z. Phys.* 243:289.

GRÜSSER, O.-J., and U. GRÜSSER-CORNEHLS, 1973. Neuronal mechanisms of visual movement perception and some psychophysical and behavioral correlations. In *Handbook of Sensory Physiology* Vol. VII/3A, R. Jung, ed. Berlin, Heidelberg, New York: Springer-Verlag, pp. 333–429.

HASSENSTEIN, B., 1951. Ommatidienraster und afferente Bewegungsintegration (Versuche am Rüsselkäfer *Chlorophanus viridis). Z. Vergl. Physiol.* 33:301–326.

HASSENSTEIN, B., 1958. Über die Wahrnehmung der Bewegung von Figuren und unregelmässigen Helligkeitsmustern. *Z. Vergl. Physiol.* 40:556–592.

HASSENSTEIN, B., 1959. Optokinetische Wirksamkeit bewegter periodischer Muster. *Z. Naturforsch.* 14b:659–674.

HASSENSTEIN, B., and W. REICHARDT, 1956. Systemtheoretische Analyse der Zeit-, Reihenfolgen- und Vorzeichenauswertung bei der Bewegungsperzeption des Rüsselkäfers *Chlorophanus. Z. Naturforsch.* 11b:513–524.

HEIMBURGER, L., T. POGGIO, and W. REICHARDT, 1976. A special class of nonlinear interactions in the visual system of the fly. *Biol. Cybernetics* 21:103–105.

HEISENBERG, M., and E. BUCHNER, 1977. The role of retinula cell types in visual behavior of *Drosophila melanogaster. J. Comp. Physiol.* (in print).

HENGSTENBERG, R., and K. G. GÖTZ, 1967. Der Einfluss des Schirmpigmentgehalts auf die Helligkeits- und Kontrastwahrnehmung von *Drosophila*-Augenmutanten. *Kybernetik* 3:276–285.

JULESZ, B., 1975. Experiments in the visual perception of texture. *Sci. Am.* 232:34–43.

KIRSCHFELD, K., 1972. The visual system of *Musca*: Studies on optics, structure and function. In *Information Processing in the Visual System of Arthropods*, R. Wehner, ed. Berlin, Heidelberg, New York: Springer-Verlag, pp. 61–74.

KIRSCHFELD, K., and B. LUTZ, 1974. Lateral inhibition in the compound eye of the fly, *Musca. Z. Naturforsch.* 29c:95–97.

KUNZE, P.L, 1961. Untersuchung des Bewegungssehens fixiert fliegender Bienen. *Z. Vergl. Physiol.* 44:656–684.

LAND, M. F., and T. S. COLLETT, 1974. Chasing behaviour of houseflies (*Fannia canicularis*): A description and analysis. *J. Comp. Physiol.* 89:331–357.

MARMARELIS, P., and G. D. McCANN, 1973. Development and application of white-noise modeling techniques for studies of insect visual nervous system. *Kybernetik* 12:74–90.

McCANN, G. D., and G. F. MacGINITIE, 1965. Optomotor response studies of insect vision. *Proc. R. Soc. Lond.* B 163:369–401.

MICHAEL, C. R., 1968. Receptive fields of single optic nerve fibers in a mammal with an all-cone retina. II. Directionally sensitive units. *J. Neurophysiol.* 31:257–267.

MONTERO, V. M., and J. F. BRUGGE, 1969. Direction of movement as a significant stimulus parameter for some lateral geniculate cells in the rat. *Vision Res.* 9:71–88.

PICK, B., 1974a. Visual flicker induces orientation behavior in the fly *Musca*. *Z. Naturforsch.* 29c:310–312.

PICK, B., 1974b. Das stationäre Orientierungsverhalten der Fliege *Musca*. Dissertation Eberhard-Karls-Universität Tübingen.

PICK, B., 1976. Orientation behaviour of the fly implies visual pattern discrimination. *Biol. Cybernetics* 23:171–180.

PICK, B., 1977. Visuelles Orientierungsverhalten von Fliegen: Eine nichtlineare Systemanalyse. In *Kybernetik 1977*, E. Butenandt and G. Hauske, eds. München, Wien: R. Oldenbourg Verlag. In print.

POGGIO, T., 1974. Processing of visual information in flies: From a phenomenological model towards the nervous mechanisms. In *Atti della prima riunione Scientifica* (Camogli, 1973). Soc. Ital. Biofis. Pura e Applicata, pp. 217–225.

POGGIO, T., 1975. Processing of visual information in insects: Outline of a theoretical characterization. In *Biokybernetik*, Band V, H. Drischel and P. Dettmar, eds. Jena: VEB Gustav Fischer Verlag, pp. 235–243.

POGGIO, T., and W. REICHARDT, 1973a. Considerations on models of movement detection. *Kybernetik* 13:223–227.

POGGIO, T., and W. REICHARDT, 1973b. A theory of the pattern induced flight orientation of the fly *Musca domestica*. *Kybernetik* 12:185–203.

POGGIO, T., and W. REICHARDT, 1976. Visual control of orientation behaviour in the fly. Part II. Towards the underlying neural interactions. *Quart. Rev. Biophys.* 9:377–438.

POGGIO, T., and W. REICHARDT, 1978. In preparation.

REICHARDT, W., 1957. Autokorrelations-Auswertung als Funktionsprinzip des Zentralnervensystems. *Z. Naturforsch.* 12b:448–457.

REICHARDT, W., 1961. Autocorrelation; a principle for the evaluation of sensory information by the central nervous system. In *Sensory Communication*, W. A. Rosenblith, ed. Cambridge, Mass.: MIT Press, pp. 303–318.

REICHARDT, W., 1969. Movement perception in insects. In *Processing of Optical Data by Organisms and Machines*, W. Reichardt, ed. London, New York: Academic Press, pp. 465–493.

REICHARDT, W., 1970. The insect eye as a model for analysis of uptake, transduction, and processing of optical data in the nervous system. In *The Neurosciences: Second Study Program*, F. O. Schmitt, ed. New York: Rockefeller University Press, pp. 494–511.

REICHARDT, W., 1973. Musterinduzierte Flugorientierung. Verhaltens-Versuche an der Fliege *Musca domestica*. *Naturwissenschaften* 60:122–138.

REICHARDT, W., and T. POGGIO, 1975. A theory of pattern induced flight orientation of the fly *Musca domestica*: II. *Biol. Cybernetics* 18:69–80.

REICHARDT, W., and T. POGGIO, 1976. Visual control of orientation behaviour in the fly. Part I. A quantitative analysis. *Quart. Rev. Biophys.* 9:311–375.

REICHARDT, W., and D. VARJÚ, 1959. Übertragungseigenschaften im Auswertesystem für das Bewegungssehen. *Z. Naturforsch.* 14b:674–689.

REICHARDT, W., and H. WENKING, 1969. Optical detection and fixation of objects by fixed flying flies. *Naturwissenschaften* 56:424–425.

SRINIVASAN, M. V., and G. D. BERNARD, 1977. The pursuit response of the housefly and its interaction with the optomotor response. *J. Comp. Physiol.* 115:101–117.

THORSON, J., 1964. Dynamics of motion perception in the desert locust. *Science*, N.Y. 145:69–71.

THORSON, J., 1966. Small signal analysis of a visual reflex in the locust: I, II. *Kybernetik* 3:41–66.

VAN DOORN, A. J., and J. J. KOENDERINK, 1976. A directionally sensitive network. *Biol. Cybernetics* 21:161–170.

VARJÚ, D., 1959. Optomotorische Reaktionen auf die Bewegung periodischer Helligkeitsmuster. *Z. Naturforsch.* 14b:724–735.

VARJÚ, D., and W. REICHARDT, 1967. Übertragungseigenschaften im Auswertesystem für das Bewegungssehen II. *Z. Naturforsch.* 22b:1343–1351.

VIRSIK, R., 1974. Verhaltens-Studie der visuellen Detektion und Fixierung bewegter Objekte durch die Fliege *Musca domestica*. Dissertation Eberhard-Karls-Universität Tübingen.

VIRSIK, R., and W. REICHARDT, 1974. Tracking of moving objects by the fly *Musca domestica*. *Naturwissenschaften* 61:132–133.

VIRSIK, R., and W. REICHARDT, 1976. Detection and tracking of moving objects by the fly *Musca domestica*. *Biol. Cybernetics* 23:83–98.

WEHRHAHN, C., 1974. Verhaltensstudie zur musterorientierten Höhenorientierung der Fliege *Musca domestica*. Dissertation Eberhard-Karls-Universität Tübingen.

WEHRHAHN, C., 1976. Evidence for the role of retinal receptors R 7/8 in the orientation behaviour of the fly. *Biol. Cybernetics* 21:213–220.

WEHRHAHN, C., 1977. Experimental evidence for the role of receptors R 1–6 and R 7–8 in the optomotor and orientation response of *Musca*. In preparation.

WEHRHAHN, C., and W. REICHARDT, 1973. Visual orientation of the *Musca domestica* toward a horizontal stripe. *Naturwissenschaften* 60:122.

WEHRHAHN, C., and W. REICHARDT, 1975. Visually induced height orientation of the fly *Musca domestica*. *Biol. Cybernetics* 20:37–50.

ZIMMERMANN, G., 1973. Der Einfluss stehender und bewegter Musteranteile auf die optomotorische Reaktion der Fliege *Drosophila*. Dissertation Eberhard-Karls-Universität Tübingen.

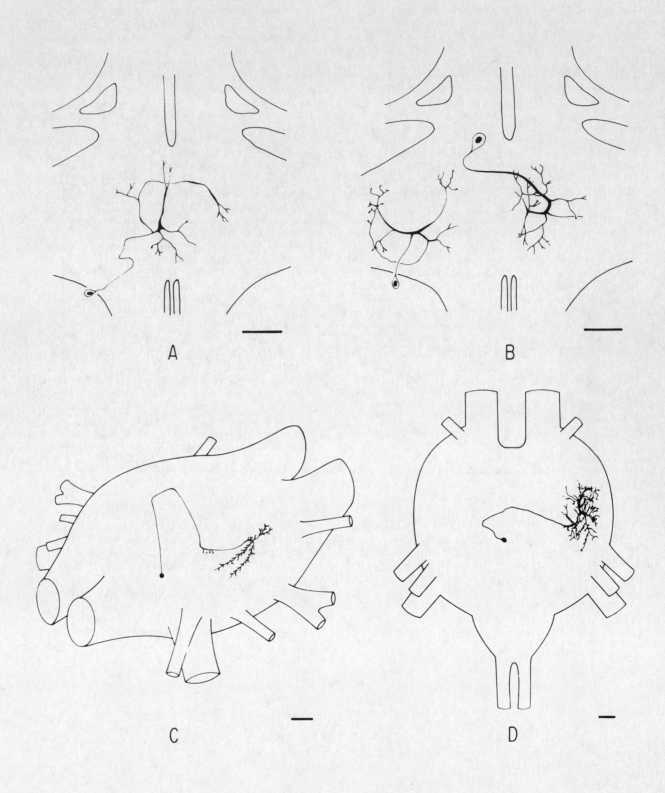

A

B

C

D

INTRODUCTION TO
LOCAL CIRCUITS

*Local neurons in the thoracic ganglia of dragonfly
larva (A, B), cockroach (C), and locust (D). The
calibration bars represent 100 μm. (A and B are
redrawn from a paper by A. Zawarzin, C from a paper
by K. G. Pearson and C. R. Fourtner, and D from a
paper by M. Burrows and M. V. F. Siegler. For
detailed credits see Pearson, this volume.)*

Introduction

GORDON M. SHEPHERD

THIS SECTION will introduce and analyze several types of local circuits. The aim is to illustrate the range of methods that can be brought to bear, the research strategies that have been developed, the kinds of information that have been generated, and the insights to be gained into the nature of nervous organization.

What is meant by the term *local circuit*? Not surprisingly, this question generated a good deal of discussion among the participants at the ISP; perhaps also not surprisingly, there was no clear consensus on a definition. For our purposes in this section, it is sufficient to recognize that the nervous system is composed of different regions, each with a characteristic histological structure. Local circuits are then defined as the connections and pathways that are wholly contained within the bounds of a given region. In most cases this simple definition will be quite adequate. The trouble comes when we must deal with extended structures, such as the cerebral cortex, that have basic structures that are subject to many local variations. This defiance of convenient categories is, of course, part of the innate cussedness of neuronal matter. One can, however, adopt a practical approach in such cases by focusing on the most local level and asking to what extent the circuits and properties contained therein are common to or different from those of surrounding regions.

Another point worth noting is the possible confusion between "local circuits" and "local neurons." Local, or intrinsic, neurons are cells with processes contained entirely within a given region; they can thus take part only in local circuits. However, a distinction between local and nonlocal, or projection, neurons is artificial with respect to local organization, for in many regions the projection neurons also participate in local circuits through their dendritic as well as their axonal synaptic connections. A similar point may be made with respect to spiking and nonspiking neurons: projection neurons generate impulses in their axons, but they may also have presynaptic dendrites that function by graded synaptic potentials in a manner similar to that of anaxonal cells and nonspiking interneurons. In other words, spiking neurons may also have nonspiking, local, outputs. The fact that parts of a neuron may function as independent units in relation to local circuits will be discussed further in the papers in this section.

The section opens with a consideration of the processes at work during the development of local circuits. Pasko Rakic reviews the historical background of ideas about the interplay between genetically determined structures and their modification by experience, and brings them into focus in the context of neuronal connections and properties at the local circuit level. He then illustrates how these questions are being studied in two different systems. The first involves analysis of the development and modification of synaptic connections onto Purkinje cells in the cerebellum as they are affected by single gene mutations. The second involves the mechanisms for the development of the pathways and connections that mediate binocular vision in primates. In both cases he shows with great clarity how incoming terminals of axons from other regions enter into the local circuits of their target regions and how these connections are progressively remodeled during normal development.

My own paper analyzes the organization of the olfactory bulb. Because of its accessibility and the relatively simple arrangement of its neuronal elements, the olfactory bulb is advantageous for the application of a number of experimental techniques. Information processing in this structure is carried out largely through dendritic synaptic circuits by an interplay of impulse and graded activity, and this has provided useful examples of some of the distinguishing characteristics of local circuits. The importance of correlating results from a variety of experimental approaches, including theoretical models that realistically incorporate the essential properties of the local systems, is emphasized. These results, and the discovery of similar types of local circuits in other nervous regions, have necessitated revision and extension of many of the classical notions about the principles underlying nervous organization. Some of the directions for developing new concepts are discussed.

In the third and final paper in this section, Keir Pearson extends the analysis of local circuits to the nervous systems of invertebrates. It may not seem quite right to phrase it this way, since it was the study of invertebrates that provided the earliest and clearest evidence about many basic properties of synapses and types of neuronal circuits. The discovery of nonspiking neurons and the identification of synaptic connections within the neuropil of invertebrate ganglia have been more recent developments. Pearson reviews his own work and that of others that has begun to establish these key aspects of local organization in several types of systems and several different species. He points to the striking similarities in local organization and local properties that have been found in vertebrates and invertebrates and discusses how they may provide insights into some of the basic functional units common to all neural tissue.

7

Genetic and Epigenetic Determinants of Local Neuronal Circuits in the Mammalian Central Nervous System

PASKO RAKIC

ABSTRACT Studies of normal and experimentally perturbed development of neuronal circuitry in the mammalian cerebellar cortex and visual system reveal a complex interplay between intrinsic (genetic) and extrinsic (epigenetic) factors that determine the pattern of adult synaptoarchitecture. The first part of this essay concerns temporal sequences, redistribution, and selective elimination of synaptic terminals upon Purkinje cells in primate and rodent cerebellum and the effect of specific cerebellar neuron deleting mutations or of aberrant neuron positions on the pattern of synaptic circuitry. The second part describes the genesis of connections subserving binocular vision in primates and the consequences of prenatal and postnatal perturbation on their normal development and/or maintenance by unilateral eye enucleation or sensory deprivation. These studies provide evidence that a balance between genetic and epigenetic factors is essential for normal development and maintenance of local synaptic circuits although the mechanisms underlying this interplay are not understood.

THE STRUCTURAL and functional organization of the mammalian brain is the end product of a complex interplay between genetic endowment and individual experience. It has proven very difficult, however, to distinguish between the effect of genes and the impact of the environment on the development of any part of the central nervous system and, even more so, on the evolution of specific patterns of behavior. This is to be expected, since the mammalian CNS is composed of billions of cells, immensely varied in shape and size, all interconnected in a complex, almost hopelessly intricate synaptic network. It is therefore not surprising that the functional potential of such a network is at present elusive and refractory to precise analysis. However, recent reviews of trends in neuroscience research indicate that answers to basic questions about mechanisms governing development

PASKO RAKIC Section of Neuroanatomy, Yale University School of Medicine, New Haven, CT 06510

of brain and behavior will eventually be obtained by analysis of local neuronal circuits[1] at the synaptic level (Jacobson, 1970; Sidman, 1973; Stent, 1973; Barlow, 1975; Changeux and Danchin, 1976; Goldman, 1976; Rakic, 1974b, 1976a,c; Schmitt, Dev, and Smith, 1976; Caviness and Rakic, 1978). The general premise of contemporary approaches is that local synaptic circuits are continuously changing in response to a fluctuating environment and that these changes can occur only within genetically determined limits.

Revival of an old concept

The hypothesis that a changing pattern of connectivity between nerve processes is the biological basis of adaptive behavior is not a new one. In the field of brain research, however, the old usually does not date back more than 100 years. Although naturalists in the mid-19th century set the stage for the revolutionary idea that neuronal links serve as a biological basis of brain activity (Sechenov, 1863), it was not until the discovery of the metallic-impregnation method by Camillo Golgi in 1873 that it became possible to vis-

---

[1] At the recent Work Session on "Local Circuit Neurons" at the Neuroscience Research Program, the term *local neural circuit* was defined very generally as any portion of the neuron (or neurons) that under given conditions functions as an independent integrative unit. Although local circuit neurons (short-axon cells) are principal components of local circuits clearly terminals of afferent neurons, as well as somas and dendrites of efferent cells, are also integral parts. Thus local circuits may have a wide range of morphological and functional boundaries: they might be simply multisynaptic local units (Shepherd, 1972) or indepent dendritic arborizations involving only a part of the dendritic tree (Ralston, 1971; Shepherd, 1972), or they may involve one or many local circuit neurons. In each case, the function of the local circuit is to process information at the local level rather than to propagate it out of a given structure. (For more details see Rakic, 1976c.)

ualize the axonal and dendritic ramifications and cell bodies of neurons in the CNS (Golgi, 1885). Even then, however, the functional significance of cell processes was not fully appreciated. Golgi, for example, deleted spines from illustrations of dendritic shafts as artifacts. Even as late as the occasion of his Nobel Prize address in 1906, he assigned to the dendrites a mainly nutritive or metabolic supportive role. Ramón y Cajal, who shared the Nobel award with Golgi, held a different view. Already in 1890 he had suggested that axonal terminals and dendritic arborizations were functionally significant and, remarkably, that these structures of the neuron could be modified by life experience (Ramón y Cajal, 1890). In his autobiography (Ramón y Cajal, 1937, p. 459), he states: "Adaptation and professional dexterity, or rather the perfecting of function by exercise (physical education, speech, writing, piano-playing, mastery in fencing, and other activities) were explained by either a progressive thickening of the nervous pathways (suggestion made by Tanzi and Lugaro) . . . or the formation of new cell processes (non-congenital growth of new dendrites and extension and branching of axone collaterals) capable of improving the suitability and the extension of the contacts, and even of making entirely new connections between neurons primitively independent."

In the more than half century since Ramón y Cajal's inspiring remarks, neurobiologists have been painfully aware of the difficulties involved in the analysis of minute connections in the brain. Only in recent years—a period, perhaps appropriately designated by Bodian (1972) as "a revolutionary decade"—have new facts emerged that urge us to address ourselves again to the structure, function, and modifiability of local circuits. To some, it may appear that any generalizations are still premature; they may justifiably argue that we should wait until new findings are accumulated and confirmed. On the other hand, such a self-defeating attitude may be contrasted with Ramón y Cajal's bold statement at Clark University that short-axon cells play a critical role in the development of human intelligence (Ramón y Cajal, 1899). At the time the remark was nothing more than speculation, and he knew that this was a matter to be determined by quantitative scientific analysis in the future, rather than one to be left to personal opinion and imagination: "It is a rule of wisdom, and of my scientific prudence as well, not to theorize before completing the observation of facts. But who is so master of himself as to be able to wait calmly in the midst of darkness until the break of dawn? Who can tarry prudently until the epoch of

the perfection of truth (unhappily as yet very far off) shall come?"

Indeed many neuroscientists did not wait for improvements in technology to continue pursuing this attractive idea. The concept of the modifiability of synaptic connection is the essence of various theories of learning and memory (e.g., Pavlov, 1927; Hebb, 1949; Young, 1964). Numerous hypotheses evolved to explain the mechanisms of synaptic development and modifiability implicit in these theories (e.g., Keating, 1968; Gaze and Keating, 1972; Jacobson, 1970; Stent, 1973; Changeux and Danchin, 1976; Prestige and Willshaw, 1975; Malesburg and Willshaw, 1976). However, the central question remains unanswered: Are regional physiological processes in local neuronal circuits capable of producing measurable structural changes in the shape of cell processes or in focal areas of the cell membrane? If so, the actual output of the neuron depends in the broadest sense on previous experience.

Recently it has become possible to adduce new and pertinent evidence in support of these ideas. Technical advances in morphological and physiological methodology have made possible the analysis of synaptic mechanisms at a new level of resolution. Moreover, the advances in methods have been accompanied by a revision of prevailing concepts of both the static nature of neuronal structure and also the scientific strategies necessary for unraveling this structure. These refinements in technique and concepts have made research on the structure and function of the central nervous system among the most exciting and promising endeavors in contemporary biology. It should be underscored that analysis of the complex mammalian brain has contributed as much to these developments as studies of simpler organisms.

It is not my intention to review comprehensively the great variety of conditions under which neuronal structure and connectivity can be modified. Instead, I shall limit my discussion to two current approaches to the analysis of genetic and epigenetic contributions to the development of the nervous system in which I have had some degree of personal involvement: (1) Analysis of the formation and modification of synaptic connections of Purkinje cells in the cerebellar cortex induced by single gene mutations; and (2) Studies of the mechanisms involved in the genesis of connections subserving binocular vision in primates.

These examples were selected because they illustrate the principle that progressive remodeling of local circuits occurs during normal development and because they reveal the degree to which a sequence of interdependent cellular events can be modified.

The apparent difference in the nature of biological information revealed by the analysis of these two neuronal systems probably stems more from the research techniques that can be applied to each than from any inherent biological differences between them. Thus the first example is based largely on ultrastructural evidence and demonstrates how synapses develop and how their pattern of development can be changed by a single gene mutation. The second example shows, by the method of axonal transport, how the distribution of axon terminals can be altered by experimental manipulation of the nervous system, either directly by extirpations of relevant components or indirectly by manipulation of the sensory environment. Together, the two examples illustrate that in the CNS cellular developmental events do not occur in isolation; rather, the pattern of synaptic connectivity in an individual brain at any given time is an end product of complicated interdependencies between genetic endowment and external environment. The nature of these interrelationships has only begun to emerge.

Development of synaptic input to Purkinje cells in normal and mutant cerebellum

The differentiation of the synaptology of cerebellar Purkinje cells furnishes an excellent example of the remodeling of synaptic connections during development. The remarkable succession of cellular events that occurs during histogenesis of cerebellar cortex has been the subject of frequent studies since Ramón y Cajal (1890, 1911) first described these basic morphogenetic events. The use of autoradiography and electron microscopy in recent years has added many new details, as well as some important concepts (for reviews see Rakic, 1974b, 1976a; Sidman and Rakic, 1973; Sidman, 1973; Sotelo, 1975; Caviness and Rakic, 1978; and many others). This essay will therefore consider only selected aspects of Purkinje-cell differentiation. The findings discussed will illustrate dynamic changes in synaptic relations during development and the extent to which mutation at a single genetic locus can alter the normal chain of cellular events during Purkinje-cell morphogenesis.

In all species examined so far, Purkinje cells are generated well in advance of the birth of most other neuronal classes in the cerebellum (Ramón y Cajal, 1911; Miale and Sidman, 1961; Rakic, 1971, 1974b; Das and Nornes, 1972; Altman, 1973; Zecevic and Rakic, 1976). Soon after their final division, the Purkinje cells assume a bipolar form and migrate from the ventricular zone toward the external cerebellar surface below the embryonic marginal zone; there their fusiform somas form an irregular cellular band several rows thick. In the course of subsequent differentiation, Purkinje cells in all species examined pass through three stages described originally by Ramón y Cajal (1911); fusiform, multipolar-stellate form, and the stage of orientation and flattening of the dendritic tree. The protracted development and large size of the Purkinje cell's dendritic tree in primates allows convenient visualization of these stages and an analysis of their temporal interrelationships. (Figure 1 shows Purkinje cells at various ages in the rhesus monkey; for comparable stages in man see Zecevic and Rakic, 1976.)

The morphogenesis of Purkinje cells in the rhesus monkey begins around the fortieth embryonic day (E40), when they are generated, and continues until the ninetieth postnatal day (P90), when they have reached their mature shape (Rakic, 1971, 1974b). The entire process involves an enormous increase in cell surface area (see Figure 1). As the dendrites of the cells grow, they become studded with numerous spines. The cell surface membrane forms a variety of types of synaptic contacts with at least eight classes of axons (Palay and Chan-Palay, 1974). The Purkinje-cell dendrites normally grow exclusively within a bed of parallel fibers—the granule-cell axons—from which they receive their major synaptic input. The interdependencies of these two classes of neuronal processes during development have been described in detail (e.g., see Figure 15 in Rakic, 1973) and will not be discussed here. Instead, I shall emphasize the changing pattern of the climbing-fiber Purkinje-cell synaptic relationship during development and the aberration of this synaptic arrangement associated with abnormalities in the Purkinje-cell dendritic arbor.

REDISTRIBUTION OF CLIMBING-FIBER SYNAPTIC INPUT

Studies of normal development In the rhesus monkey during the second half of gestation, the young Purkinje cell bristles with perisomatic spines (Figure 1B,C and 2); these were first described in rodents by Ramón y Cajal (1890) from observations using the Golgi method and later confirmed by electron microscopy in a variety of species (Larramendi, 1969; Mugnaini, 1969; Kornguth and Scott, 1972; Zecevic and Rakic, 1976). At this stage the major afferent input is from climbing fibers, but both the spines and their contacts with climbing fibers appear to be transient. In the course of Purkinje-cell differentiation, climbing-fiber terminals become transferred from the cell soma to the dendritic trunk, where they form synapses with

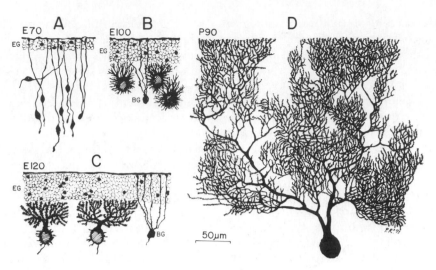

FIGURE 1 Composite drawing of Purkinje cell impregnated according to the Golgi method in macaque cerebellar cortex at various embryonic (E) and postnatal (P) ages. All sections were made transverse to the folium. Purkinje cells are from the anterior lobe in the sections close to the midline. Except for the external granular layer (EG) and occasional Bergmann glia (BG), other cellular elements are omitted, and all cells are drawn at the same magnification. In rhesus monkey, all Purkinje cells are generated and enter the cerebellar cortex during the first quarter of the 165-day gestation period (Rakic, unpublished data). (A) At the 70th embryonic day (E70) most cells are still in the bipolar stage of development. (B) Between E80 and E100, some cells are in the multipolar stage; that is, they have considerably enlarged in volume and surface area, somatic spines project in all directions, and apical dendrites become more apparent (although they are still not oriented in a single plane). (C) By E120, the Purkinje-cell dendritic tree has been flattened and oriented in the plane perpendicular to the folium. (D) By P90, the cell has attained the adult configuration, which is characterized by a smooth-surfaced soma and an elaborate espaliered dendritic tree studded with spines.

different types of spines; at the same time the Purkinje-cell soma becomes smooth (Figure 1) and receives an input from basket-cell axons (Figure 2).

It is worth emphasizing that the temporary climbing-fiber synapses upon the Purkinje-cell body are of the asymmetrical type (Figure 2B) and are presumably excitatory, as in mature cortex (Eccles, Ito, and Szentágothai, 1967). The function of such a powerful and dense complex of synaptic junctions on the body of the immature Purkinje cells in the middle of gestation is a complete mystery. One reasonable assumption is that they play an important role in the morphogenesis of the Purkinje cells (Ramón y Cajal, 1911; Kornguth and Scott, 1972). Following selective removal of climbing fibers by chemical destruction of the inferior olive (Sotelo et al., 1975) or after cutting of the cerebellar peduncle (Sotelo and Arsenio-Nunes, 1976), there appears to be an increase in the density of Purkinje-cell dendritic spines and a change in the geometry of their dendritic arborization. In normal development, climbing-fiber synapses appear to be exchanged on the cell surface with basket-cell axon terminals. The latter are of the symmetrical type (Figure 2C) and are presumably inhibitory in the mature cerebellar cortex. Initially, therefore, only

climbing-fiber terminals are present on the cell perikaryon, then both climbing and basket-cell axon terminals are intermixed (this stage occurs around E100 in the monkey fetus and is depicted in Figure 2); finally, only basket-cell terminals remain on the cell body. The process of synaptic remodeling is concurrent with the disappearance of perisomatic spines (Figure 2). The mechanism by which the remodeling of synaptic input upon the Purkinje-cell surface occurs is unknown (Larramendi, 1969). Despite several attempts, it has not been possible to determine with certainty whether already-established synaptic junctions are broken down and new ones formed on the dendritic spines or whether the entire area of the cell membrane, together with its synaptic attachment, is passively transferred from the body to the dendritic trunk as new membrane surface is generated at the level of the cell body. The latter hypothesis derives from Ramón y Cajal's (1911) assumption that the perisomatic spines are subsumed into the membrane of the Purkinje cell during the course of normal development.

There are several other somewhat different examples of temporary synaptic junctions in the developing mammalian central nervous system. Thus syn-

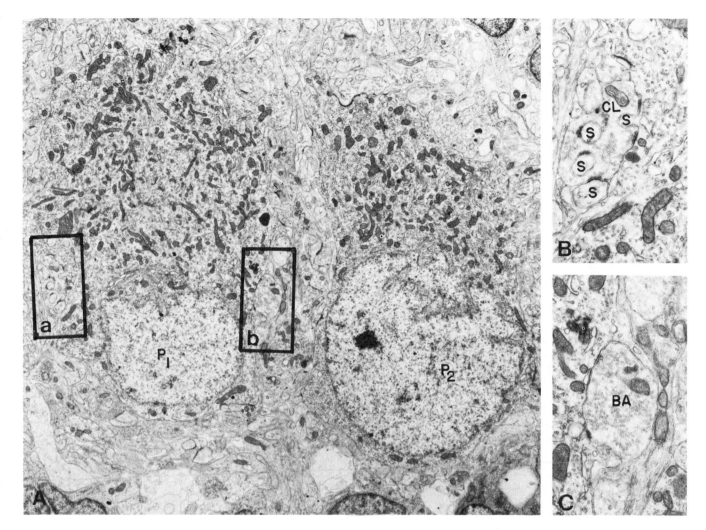

FIGURE 2 (A) Low-magnification electron micrograph of two Purkinje cells (P_1 and P_2) in the cerebellar cortex of the rhesus monkey fetus at E105. The two cells are slightly older than those illustrated in Figure 1B (E100); they are still in the multipolar phase of differentiation, however, and their bodies contain numerous perisomatic spines. This embryonic age was selected for illustration because at this stage synaptic input on the Purkinje-cell soma is in transition; it still receives a certain number of climbing-fiber synaptic terminals on the somatic spines (rectangle a), while newly formed basket-cell axons have begun to invade the smooth cell surface (rectangle b). (B, C) Higher magnification electron micrographs of synaptic terminals shown within rectangles a and b show that climbing-fiber terminals are asymmetrical (excitatory), whereas basket-cell synapses are symmetrical (inhibitory). Eventually, all climbing-fiber synapses will move to the spines in the dendritic shafts, and only basket-cell terminals will remain on the cell soma. *Abbreviations*: BA, basket-cell axon terminal; CL, climbing-fiber terminal; S, perisomatic spines.

apses form transiently on filopodia of growing dendrites of spinal neurons, then become repositioned as the cell processes grow and differentiate (Skoff and Hamburger, 1974). In this case, however, it appears that a portion of the filopodial membrane may be incorporated into the distal part of the dendritic trunk, so that synaptic sites may actually not change position.

The mechanism behind the translocation of synapses on developing neurons will remain in the sphere of speculation until a suitable marker for the distribution and turnover of specific synaptic sites of neuronal membrane becomes available. In this respect, analysis of synaptic remodeling in the peripheral nervous system is somewhat more advanced and has already furnished some important information (e.g., see Purves, 1977). Studies using iontophoretic mapping techniques in cultured tissues show that locations of acetylcholine receptor sites on developing neuromuscular junctions in the chick change in the absence of neural contact. These results suggest that the redistribution of synaptic sites may be under the genetic control of the postsynaptic cell (Fischbach et al., 1976). It is not certain that the same mechanisms will prove to be valid for the CNS. The development of postsynaptic membrane specializations on Purkinje-cell dendritic spines in the absence of their presynaptic partners, the granule-cell axons, is observed in mutants as well as under various experimental conditions (Altman and Anderson, 1973; Hirano and Dembitzer, 1973; Rakic and Sidman, 1973; Sotelo, 1975). The inner surface of these membrane specializations is by freeze-fracture criteria identical to the normal postsynaptic thickenings (Hanna, Hirano, and Pappas, 1975; Landis and Reese, 1977). These findings suggest that the development of postsynaptic sites may proceed independently in at least some synaptic relations of the central neurons (Rakic, 1976a). However, until more is known, competition between climbing-fiber axon terminals and basket-cell axon terminals for the available sites on the Purkinje-cell surface cannot be ruled out as an alternative hypothesis. Whatever the mechanism may be, the climbing-fiber/Purkinje-cell synapse is perhaps the most clearly documented example of redistribution of specific synaptic inputs on different compartments of the same neuron in the course of normal differentiation in the central nervous system.

Genetically perturbed synaptic development   Mutations at a single genetic locus can affect the completion of the translocation of the climbing-fiber input on Purkinje cells. Among several cerebellar mouse mutants, three—reeler, weaver, and staggerer—modify the arrangement, morphology, or connectivity of Purkinje cells (see Figure 3). Although the primary targets of these mutations are unknown, all three exhibit a cerebellar malformation associated with death and/or malposition of one or more classes of neurons (Sidman, 1968; Rakic and Sidman, 1973; Rakic, 1976a; Sotelo, 1975; Caviness and Rakic, 1978; Landis and Sidman, 1978). Systematic changes in Purkinje-cell morphology and synaptology occur in relation to the absence, alteration, or malposition of interrelated cells that are affected by the mutant gene. Essentially similar effects can be obtained when granule cells are depleted by a variety of teratologic agents (Altman and Anderson, 1973; Llinás, Hillman, and Precht, 1973; Herndon and Oster-Granite, 1975). Collectively these studies indicate that the initiation and growth of Purkinje-cell primary and secondary dendrites, as well as the development of their dendritic spines, may be uninfluenced by parallel-fiber input; the orientation and volume of the dendritic arbor and development of tertiary branchlets do, however,

depend on the presence of parallel fibers. The abnormality of Purkinje-cell morphology is therefore a secondary phenomenon explained in terms of cell interactions with parallel fibers (Rakic and Sidman, 1973; Rakic, 1974b). In staggerer, however, it is thought that gene action may affect the Purkinje cells more directly, and granule-cell death is considered to be a consequence of the failure of these cells to establish synaptic contact with Purkinje cells (Sotelo and Changeux, 1974; Herrup and Mullen, 1976; Mullen, 1977; Landis and Sidman, 1978). The consequences of these abnormalities for the organization of local synaptic circuits can be analyzed by electron microscopy, since most synaptic elements that impinge upon Purkinje cells can be distinguished by their ultrastructural characteristics (e.g., Mugnaini, 1972; Palay and Chan-Palay, 1974). One might well expect the resulting synaptic mismatching to have a profound effect on behavior, so it is not surprising that these neurological mutants were first identified because of behavioral abnormalities (Falconer, 1951; Lane, 1964).

In all three neurological mutants illustrated in Figure 3—reeler (Mariani et al., 1977), staggerer (Sotelo, 1975; Landis and Sidman, 1968), and weaver (Rakic and Sidman, 1973; Sotelo, 1975; Rakic, 1976a)—the immature pattern of synaptic arrangement may persist in mature Purkinje cells in the form of perisomatic spines and aberrant climbing-fiber connections with cell bodies. In another mutant mouse, "nervous," the Purkinje-cell dendritic arbor is smaller than normal, and many climbing-fiber terminals remain on the Purkinje-cell body for an abnormally long period (Landis, 1973). The persistence of perisomatic spines in all these mutants may be related to the decreased size of the Purkinje-cell soma and dendritic arbor (Figure 3) when the growth of the Purkinje cell is stunted by failure to establish contact with a normal complement of parallel fibers (Caviness and Rakic, 1978).

Recently, application of the Golgi method to various neuropathological conditions associated with several genetic abnormalities in man (Purpura, Hirano, and French, 1976; Williams et al., 1978) has demonstrated structural changes that resemble the arrested structural differentiation described in mutant mice. The polydendritic Purkinje-cell somas in Menkes's disease are of particular interest. In this inherited condition, somatic spines normally present in man until about the thirty-fifth week of gestation (Zecevic and Rakic, 1976) fail to resorb; instead they differentiate into spine-bearing dendritic protoplasmic extensions. Aberrant growth of spine-bearing

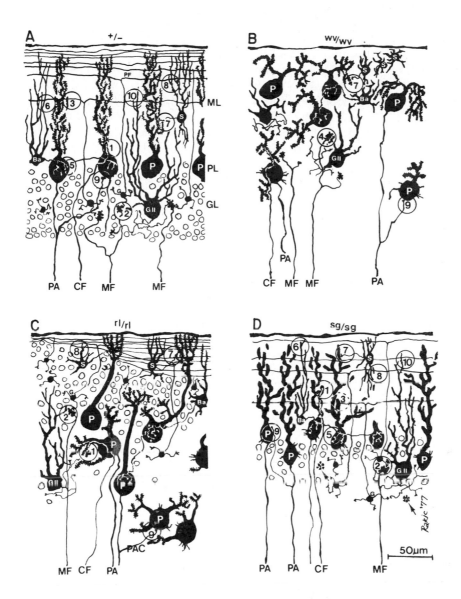

FIGURE 3 Composite semischematic drawing of the neuronal arrangement and synaptic circuitry of the normal (A), homozygous weaver (B), reeler (C), and staggerer (D) cerebellum (based on Rakic, 1976a and D. Landis, personal communication). The neuronal silhouettes are drawn from Golgi preparations, and the positions of unimpregnated granule cells are outlined. All sections are longitudinal to the folium and drawn at approximately the same magnification. (A) Normal cerebellum of a three-week-old mouse (C57BL/6J +/+). (B) Cerebellar cortex of a three-week-old homozygous weaver mouse (C57BL/6J −wv/wv) in a parasagittal plane where granule cells are absent. (C) Midsagittal outline of the three-week-old reeler mouse (C57BL/6J rl/rl). The area represented in the drawing is an area of transition between relatively well-organized cortex, in which the molecular layer contains properly oriented parallel fibers (right side), and an abnormal segment of cortex, with numerous granule cells situated close to the pia above the Purkinje cells (left side). (D) Cerebellar cortex of 2½-week-old staggerer mouse (C57BL/6Ra). Many granule cells are still present at this age, although many are in the process of degeneration (arrows). Note the presence of all classes of synapses except the class between parallel-fiber and Purkinje-cell dendritic spines (broken circle marked by number 3). *Abbreviations*: Ba, basket cell; CF, climbing fiber; G, granule cell; GII, Golgi type II cell; MF, mossy fiber; P, Purkinje cell; PA, Purkinje-cell axon; PF, parallel fiber; S, stellate cell. The major classes of synapses, all identified ultrastructurally, are encircled and numbered: 1, climbing fiber to Purkinje-cell dendrite; 2, mossy fiber to granule-cell dendrite; 3, granule-cell axon (parallel fiber) to Purkinje-cell dendrite; 4, mossy fiber to Golgi type II cell dendrite; 5, basket-cell axon to Purkinje-cell soma; 6, parallel fiber to basket-cell dendrite; 7, stellate-cell axon to Purkinje-cell dendrite; 8, parallel fiber to stellate-cell dendrite; 9, Purkinje-cell axon collateral to Purkinje-cell soma; 10, parallel fiber to Golgi type II cell dendrite. (Slightly modified from Caviness and Rakic, 1978.)

cytoplasmic expansions and synaptic contacts has also been reported in an inherited lysosomal storage disease in man (Purpura and Suzuki, 1976). This general type of mismatch, in which specific axons establish synaptic contact with an inappropriate site on the surface of the target neuron, is also encountered on improperly oriented pyramidal cells in the cerebral cortex in the reeler mouse (Caviness and Rakic, 1978) and may be the most common aberration of synaptic circuits, although until recently it usually went undetected.

ELIMINATION OF CLIMBING-FIBER SYNAPTIC INPUTS

Studies of normal development   The development of the climbing-fiber input to the Purkinje cell also provides an illustration of another type of synaptic rearrangement during development, one which involves an absolute reduction rather than an apparent change in the position of already-established synaptic contacts. Here again, the primary observation was made by Cajal. As his drawings vividly illustrate (Figures 74 and 75 in Ramón y Cajal, 1911), Purkinje cells in the course of their development receive multiple inputs from several climbing fibers. As the Purkinje cell differentiates, some of these axons are gradually eliminated until only a single climbing fiber remains spread along the main dendritic trunk of each Purkinje cell. The regression from multiple to single innervation in the course of normal development has been recently confirmed by unit recordings (Crepel, Mariani, and Delhaye-Bouchard, 1976). This mode of synaptic elimination may not be an isolated example confined to cerebellar Purkinje cells. Another well-documented example of synaptic elimination comes from the study of peripheral junctions in rat. Both anatomical and physiological evidence indicate that during the embryonic development of the neuromuscular junction, striated muscle cells receive inputs from several motoneurons. All but one disappear in the course of maturation (Hughes, 1964; Redfern, 1970; Bennett and Pettigrew, 1974; Brown, Jansen, and van Essen, 1976).

Arrested development in mutants   Elimination of climbing-fiber synapses can be arrested by genetic mutations, as documented by physiological studies in the weaver (Crepel and Mariani, 1976) and reeler (Mariani et al., 1977) mutant mice. Purkinje cells in the agranular weaver cerebellum and those situated in aberrant positions in reeler cerebellum usually retain a multiple climbing-fiber innervation, as if the embryonic synaptic arrangement were preserved. Also, when granule cells in the cerebella of rats are depleted by low level X-ray irradiation, individual

Purkinje cells may receive multiple climbing-fiber innervation (Woodward, Hoffer, and Altman, 1974). Whatever the mechanism of gene action or X-ray effect (and as shown by Sotelo, 1977, it may be quite complex), the end product is an altered number of synapses of a given class upon a single cell.

COMMENT   The findings described should not, of course, be taken as support for the extreme, and by now generally discredited, postulate that neuronal connections are at first randomly distributed and that the adult synaptic pattern is achieved simply by functional reinforcement. (After all, climbing fibers that grow selectively to the developing cerebellar cortex do not form synaptic junctions with other neuronal elements, even when they are in direct proximity (Rakic, 1976a)). On the other hand, the concept that the exact details of cell-to-cell connections are strictly specified (Sperry, 1963) may not be completely sufficient. This will become even more obvious when we discuss the genesis of visual connections in primates. A somewhat more moderate view is that connections are genetically specified between classes of cells and that the "fine tuning" of synaptic pattern is achieved, at least in part, by functional validation (to use the term favored by Jacobson, 1970), functional interaction (Keating, 1968), or selective stabilization (Changeux and Danchin, 1976) of developing synapses.

Although the analysis of alterations in Purkinje-cell connectivity described above provides no evidence that the functional activity of presynaptic input has any effect on shaping the pattern of synaptic connections, this may be due in part to present technology, which allows only visualization of an anatomical picture of changes encountered as a consequence of aberrant cellular relationships. These studies are therefore mainly useful for illustrating that synaptic junctions are indeed in constant flux during development and that the final pattern must depend to a large extent directly or indirectly on genetic information. The possible effect of the external environment on the formation of synapses is not presently detectable at the cellular level in this system. Sensory systems, as described below, have proven more favorable for the analysis of environmental impact on neural networks.

Genesis of visual connections

Evidence for interactions between the developing brain and the external environment, which may be critical for establishing normal synaptic connections, has recently been obtained from a series of studies on the postnatal development of the primate visual system (Baker, Grigg, and von Noorden, 1974; Hubel and Wiesel, 1977; Hubel, Wiesel, and LeVay, 1977). At these relatively late developmental stages, most neurons in the primate neocortex have assumed their final locations, and the principal long-tract projections in the telencephalon are largely established (Goldman and Nauta, 1976, 1977a,b; Rakic, 1976b, 1977a; Hubel, Wiesel, and LeVay, 1977). The neuropil, however, is still gaining new axonal and dendritic branches and synapses as well as glial processes, and glial cells are also increasing in number (Rakic, 1975). In this section I shall describe some recent work on the development of synaptic circuitry subserving binocular vision in the monkey.

The primate visual system is an excellent model for study of the development of central connections. Input from the two eyes in this species is separated in the dorsal lateral geniculate nucleus (LGd) as well as in the primary visual cortex (Figure 4). Thus, in the LGd, three laminae (1, 4, and 6) receive direct inputs only from the contralateral eye, and the remaining three (2, 3, and 5) from the ipsilateral eye (Minkowski, 1920; Brouwer and Zeeman, 1926; Polyak, 1957; Matthews, Cowan, and Powell, 1960). The organization of the afferents subserving two eyes in the primary visual cortex can be examined by injecting one eye with radioactive amino acids and sugars and allowing the radioactively labeled metabolites to be transported first to the LGd and then, by means of transneuronal transport (Grafstein, 1971), to the cortex, where it can be visualized autoradiographically. As shown by Wiesel, Hubel, and Lam (1974), radioactivity transported transneuronally to the monkey's primary visual cortex (area 17 of Brodmann, 1905), is distributed within cortical layer 4 in sublayers 4A and 4C in a system of stripes approximately 350 μm wide. These alternate with unlabeled stripes of the same width corresponding to regions of layer 4 that receive input from the uninjected eye (Figure 4, enlarged square of area 17). These stripes correspond to the system of ocular dominance columns as physiologically defined (Hubel and Wiesel, 1968, 1977; LeVay, Hubel, and Wiesel, 1975).

It is becoming accepted that the great majority of geniculocortical afferents terminate on local circuit neurons (stellate cells) situated in layer 4 (Figure 5). The short axons of these cells may either ascend or descend to synapse directly or indirectly, through additional (one or more) local circuit neurons, upon dendrites of efferent pyramidal cells situated in other cortical layers (Valverde, 1971; Lund, 1973, 1976; Lund and Boothe, 1975). The efferent cells situated

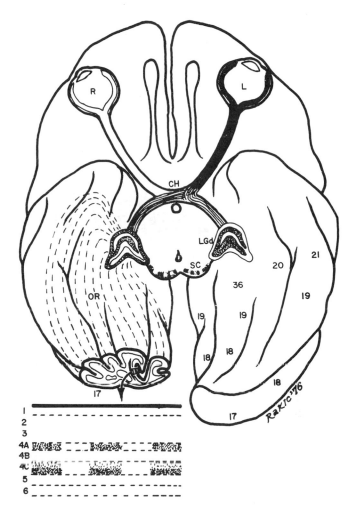

FIGURE 4 Semischematic illustration of the connections underlying binocular vision in the rhesus monkey. On the brain viewed from below, the dorsal lateral geniculate body (LGd) and superior colliculus (SC) are slightly enlarged to render the details of binocular representation legible. For the same reason, a small region of area 17 in the depth of the calcarine fissure (curved arrow) is enlarged at lower left. The axons originating from retinal ganglion cells of each eye partially cross at the optic chiasm (CH) and are distributed in the three appropriate laminae of the LGd and to the appropriate territories representing each eye in the SC. Principal neurons of the LGd project to the primary visual cortex (area 17) through the optic radiation (OR) and mostly terminate in sublayers 4A and 4C in the form of alternating columns that receive input from one or the other eye. (From Rakic, 1977a.)

at different strata of the cortex have unique targets of projection: the small- and medium-sized pyramids of layer 2 and 3 give rise to corticocortical projections, whereas large cells situated in layers 5 and 6 project to the superior colliculus (SC), pulvinar, and LGd (Figure 5; Lund et al., 1975). Thus visual information received by local neuronal circuitry within the pri-

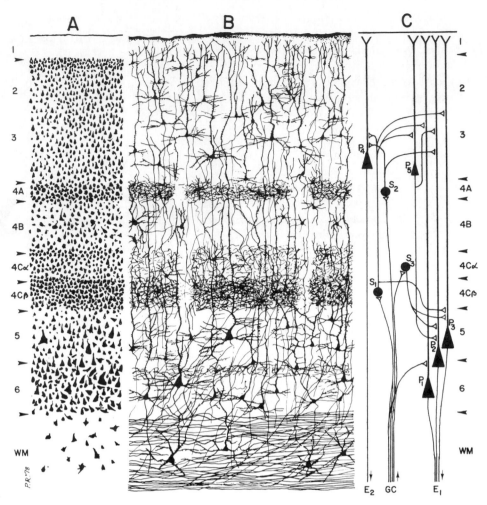

FIGURE 5 Diagram of the laminar and columnar organization of neuronal circuits in the primary visual cortex of the rhesus monkey. Our understanding of synaptic connectivity in this structure is both less detailed and less certain than that of the cerebellar cortex (compare Figure 3). The simplified scheme integrates observations derived by several techniques. On the left (A) the cytoarchitectonic appearance of the visual cortex (area 17) in Nissl stain displays horizontal-cell stratification designated according to Lund's (1975) modification of Brodmann's (1905) original scheme. The middle diagram (B) is a composite drawing of neurons impregnated by the Golgi method and superimposed afferent axonal plexuses in sublayers 4A and 4C stained by a modification of Liesegang's reduced silver method (LeVay, Hubel, and Wiesel, 1975). As verified by the autoradiographic method, these afferents form stripes or columns 350–400 μm wide, only two of which (one complete column flanked by two half-columns) are illustrated. At the right (C) is a grossly simplified diagram of the organization of local neuronal circuits in the primary visual cortex of rhesus monkey based on recent studies by Valverde (1971), Lund, (1973, 1976), Lund et al. (1975), and Lund and Boothe (1975). It appears that only a small number of geniculocortical (GC) axons synapse directly on efferent pyramidal cells (P_1); the largest number presumably terminate on local circuit neurons (stellate cells) situated in sublayers 4A and 4C. The stellate cells of sublayers $4C\beta$ (S_1) and 4A (S_2) project predominantly to layer 3, where they synapse either directly upon dendrites of efferent pyramidal cells (P_{1-4}) or indirectly through another local circuit neuron (small pyramidal cells, P_5). The majority of stellate cells of sublayer 4C (S_3) probably contact efferent pyramids within layer 5. The large pyramids of layers 5 and 6 (P_{1-3}) form a cortical efferent pathway (E_1) that projects mostly to subcortical structures (superior colliculus, pulvinar, and lateral geniculate nucleus, respectively), whereas the small- and medium-sized pyramids of layer 2 and 3 (P_4) form an efferent system (E_2) that projects to other cortical areas.

mary visual cortex is transferred to secondary visual centers for further processing. Although anatomical and physiological details of this connectivity are far from fully understood, it is obvious that geniculate terminals in the cortex are an integral part of local neuronal circuits within each ocular dominance column and that any alteration in their distribution would have profound effects on the processing of information received from each eye. The advantage of the autoradiographic method is that by injecting one eye, regions of the LGd and the visual cortex occupied by afferents serving each eye can be precisely determined in each specimen. (Hereafter such regions will be termed *ocular dominance domains*.)

NORMAL DEVELOPMENT OF OCULAR DOMINANCE DOMAINS   Recently the pattern of distribution of retinogeniculate, retinotectal and geniculocortical connections following unilateral eye injection of a mixture of ^{3}H-proline and ^{3}H-fucose has been examined in monkey fetuses exteriorized by hysterotomy (Rakic, 1976b, 1977a). After the injection, the fetuses were returned to the uterus. Either 20 hours or 14 days later, they were removed by a second caesarian section, and their brains were processed for autoradiography.

In a fetus injected with radioactive tracers at embryonic day 64 (E64) and killed at E78 and in a fetus injected at E67 and killed 20 hours later, radioactivity was transported orthogradely and distributed uniformly throughout the full extent of the LGd on both sides, without the segregation into laminae characteristic of this nucleus in the adult monkey (Rakic, 1976b) (Figure 6A, B). It is important to underscore the fact that at this fetal age all neurons of the LGd have been generated and are already situated within the nucleus, although the nucleus has still not attained its mature configuration, characteristic laminar pattern, and adult position within the diencephalon (Rakic, 1977b). In a fetus injected at E77 and killed at E91 (E77–E91), the separation of the axons and/or axon terminals that originate from one or the other eye is discernible at the caudal pole of the LGd as irregularly shaped areas of lower and higher silver grain densities (Figure 6C). The laminae also first appear between E90 and E95 at the caudal pole of the monkey LGd (Hendrickson and Rakic, 1977), which receives input from the central retina. In an E110–E124 specimen, the projections from the two eyes are segregated in the form of a somewhat irregular six-layered pattern throughout the entire LGd; prospective laminae 2, 3, and 5 are labeled on the side ipsilateral to the injected eye, and 1, 4, and 5 are labeled on the contralateral side (Figure 6D). The distribution of grains over the territory of appropriate laminae assumes the typical adult pattern in the E130–E144 specimen (Figure 6E). Thus, since gestation lasts 165 days in the rhesus monkey, the segregation of afferents from the two eyes into monocular domains at the thalamic level is completed at least three weeks before birth (Rakic, 1976b, 1977a)

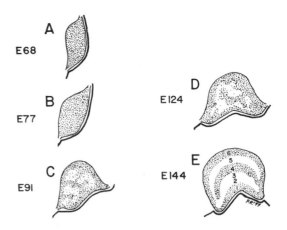

FIGURE 6   Schematic representation of the distribution of radioactive tracers over the lateral geniculate body (LGd) following injections of radioactive tracers (^{3}H-proline and ^{3}H-fucose mixture) into the contralateral eye in five monkey fetuses of various prenatal ages temporarily exteriorized by hysterotomy. After injection, each fetus was replaced in the uterus and sacrificed 20 hours (A) or 14 days (B–E) later by caesarian section at the embryonic (E) days indicated at the right side of each LGd. The position and shape of the LGd is outlined as it appears in coronal sections of the diencephalon aligned identically in relation to the midline in each monkey. Although all neurons of the LGd are generated before E45 (Rakic, 1977b), the nucleus changes considerably in size and shape during development and rotates from a lateral to ventral position in the thalamus. Note that between E68 and E78 radioactivity is distributed uniformly over the entire nucleus; the segregation of the input from the two eyes occurs mainly between E91 and E124 and is completed before E144. (For details see Rakic, 1976b, 1977a.)

Radioactive label was transported transneuronally to the LGd neurons and their axons in the same fetuses (Rakic, 1976b). The optic radiation is distinct in the occipital lobes of the fetus killed at E78, 14 days after unilateral eye injection. However, geniculocortical fibers do not enter the cortical plate at this age, but instead accumulate below the developing cortex (Rakic, 1977a). ^{3}H-thymidine autoradiographic analysis shows that at this fetal age in the monkey, only a small fraction of neurons destined for layer 4 of the visual cortex have been generated in the ventricular zone (Rakic, 1974a); and of the neurons that have already undergone their last divisions, many have not yet reached their final position in the cortex (Rakic, 1975). In the slightly older, E77–E91 specimen, some geniculocortical axons do invade the territory of the prospective primary visual cortex and become uniformly distributed within layer 4; again, however, there is no evidence of preferential segregation into the ocular dominance columns of sublayers 4A and 4C. After all visual cortical neurons have been generated (Rakic, 1974a) and have attained their final positions (Rakic, 1975), the number of visual afferents entering the cortex increases further so that somewhere between E110 and E124, sublayers 4A and 4C become delineated; at the same time, the territories corresponding to ocular dominance columns are not yet discernible (Figure 7A).

In the fetus injected a few weeks later at E130 and killed at E144, the segregation of input vertically into sublayers 4A and 4C becomes more visible; the horizontal segregation of the axons carrying input from the two eyes into incipient ocular dominance columns also begins to emerge (Figure 7B). The subtle fluctuation in density of grains is difficult to discern upon inspection, but grain counts and measurements (Figure 8) clearly demonstrate alternating territories 250–300 μm wide that contain slightly higher and lower grain densities (Rakic, 1976b). Thus the combined width of an ipsilateral and contralateral ocular dominance column, as determined by the distance between two peaks of grain concentrations (Figure 8) is about 20–25% smaller than in the mature monkey, indicating that there is a substantial increase in the cortical surface area between E144 and maturity (Rakic, 1977a). The process of segregation of the geniculocortical afferents into ocular dominance columns continues in the immediate postnatal period; by about three weeks of age (Hubel, Wiesel, and LeVay, 1977), the adult pattern is attained (Figure

7C). A recent study indicates that the process of segregation of the geniculocortical projection proceeds similarly in the visual cortex of the cat, except that corresponding stages occur later with respect to birth (LeVay, Stryker, and Shatz, 1978). A similar analysis of the formation of retinogeniculate projections during postnatal development in the golden hamster shows a pattern of initial overlap, although the timing and sequence of development are somewhat different (So, Schneider, and Frost, 1978).

It appears then that the genesis of visual connections subserving binocular vision passes through two broad phases. In the first phase, axons derived from each eye invade their target structures, and their endings are distributed in an overlapping manner. In the second phase, the axon terminals derived from the two eyes become segregated from each other into separate territories concerned predominantly with one eye or the other (Rakic, 1976b). Moreover, the biphasic mode of genesis of central neuronal connections seems not to be confined to the visual system. Thus, in the pyriform cortex, olfactory and association input initially overlap before being separated into different strata of the molecular layer (Price, Moxley, and Schwab, 1976). In neither the visual system nor the olfactory cortex is it yet clear whether the overlapping endings of axons of different origin initially contact and/or synapse on the very same class of neurons before they are redistributed to different

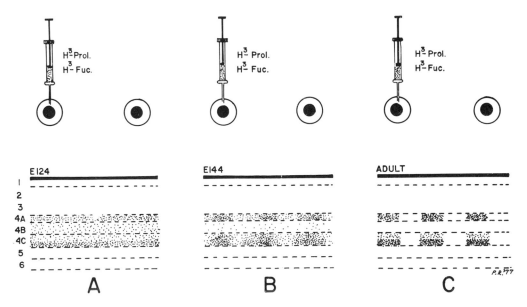

FIGURE 7 Schematic representation of the development of ocular dominance columns in layer 4 of the primary visual cortex of the rhesus monkey of various ages (E124, E144, adult), as visualized in autoradiograms following transneuronal transport of radioactive tracers (³H-fucose and ³H-proline) injected into one eye 14 days before sacrifice. Cortical layers indicated by numerals 1–6 are delineated according to Brodmann's (1905) classification. (Based on data from Rakic, 1976b, 1977a.)

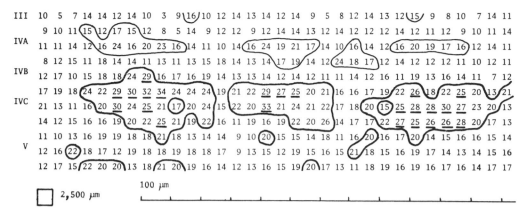

FIGURE 8 Results of grain counts over a 0.8 mm² area of layers 3, 4, 4B, 4C, and 5 of the primary visual cortex in monkey fetuses injected at E130 and killed at E144. The autoradiogram is photographed in dark-field illumination and its negative projected by a Prado (Leitz GMBH) apparatus onto grid paper in which each square corresponds to a 2,500 μm² area of the cortex. Grains were counted in 352 unit areas along a 1.6 mm length of the calcarine cortex. Areas with 15 grains or more per 2,500 μm² in sublayer 4A are outlined by a thin line. Areas with 20 grains or more per 2,500 μm² in sublayer 4C are outlined by a thick line. Areas with 25 grains or more are underscored

by a short, thick line. The distance between the two regions of highest grain counts that correspond to the pair of ocular dominance columns is approximately 500 μm. Note that the width of areas with higher grain counts is not half of the double column. Presumably territories of terminals from the uninjected eye still considerably overlap the territories of the injected eye, and only a narrow, approximately 100–150 μm wide zone of highest and lowest grain counts may be considered to correspond to areas that receive projections derived predominantly from one eye. (From Rakic, 1976b.)

classes or whether they remain uncommitted and unattached until a specific signal emerges from the appropriate differentiated target neurons.

ALTERED DEVELOPMENT OF OCULAR DOMINANCE

Manipulation of development by unilateral eye enucleation Considerable rearrangement of the terminations of axons in the visual system can be demonstrated in the mature monkey when one eye is enucleated by intrauterine surgery at critical periods of fetal life (Rakic, 1977c). In a monkey in which one eye was enucleated at E64, radioactive tracers injected in the remaining eye before sacrifice at the third postnatal month were distributed uniformly over the entire LGd in both hemispheres (Figure 8a). Preliminary analysis shows that the number and position of neurons in the two LGds are not substantially affected by such early unilateral eye removal, even though the characteristic laminae fail to develop (Rakic, 1977c, 1978). ³H-thymidine autoradiographic analysis of the distribution of labeled neurons within the LGd at various short intervals following exposure to this nucleotide indicates that during the rotation and shifting of this nucleus in the course of thalamic development, the positions of LGd cells relative to each other generally do not change (Rakic, 1977b). Neurons situated in presumptive layers 1 and 6 at the ventral and dorsal peripheries of the nucleus,

which normally receive input from the contralateral (enucleated) eye, now come in contact with axons originating from the ipsilateral (remaining) eye. The projections from the remaining eye therefore occupy twice as large a territory within the mature LGd as they would occupy under normal circumstances. This large domain is not necessarily achieved through expansion of the fibers from the remaining eye into new territories. Rather, since projections from the two eyes initially overlap in the LGd of fetal monkeys (Rakic, 1977a), terminals from the remaining eye may simply fail to *retract* in the absence of competition from the contralateral eye (compare Figures 6 and 9).

Light-microscopic autoradiography displays only the density of projections from the remaining eye; it does not provide any clues as to whether or not axon terminals from the remaining eye actually form synaptic contacts with all LGd neurons. Theoretically synapses could be established exclusively with the set of neurons that are originally "committed" to the remaining eye—that is, those in presumptive layers 2, 3, and 4. Axons may be intermixed with neurons "committed" to the contralateral eye in layers 1, 4, and 6 without making synaptic junctions. To resolve this problem, the LGd was examined electron-microscopically. A uniform distribution of synaptic profiles throughout the entire LGd, including the extreme periphery of the nucleus, was found (Figure 9). Synapses between retinal afferents and LGd neurons can be recognized by their multiple contacts with large dendritic profiles and by their loosely packed, round synaptic vesicles and large, pale mitochondria with wide intercristal spaces (Guillery and Collonier, 1970; LeVay, 1971). Since neurons in layers 1 and 6 of the LGd normally receive synapses exclusively from the contralateral (removed) eye, the retinal synapses encountered in this territory must belong to the remaining, ipsilateral eye. Thus not only are axons that originate from the remaining eye present in the territory normally occupied by the enucleated eye, they also seem to be able to establish ultrastructurally defined synaptic junctions with neurons they do not normally contact in the adult (Rakic, 1977c).

When the visual cortex of the monkey was unilat-

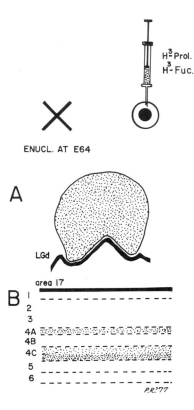

FIGURE 9 Schematic representation of the distribution of radioactive tracers in the LGd and primary visual cortex of a two-month-old monkey 14 days after injection of a mixture of ³H-proline and ³H-fucose into one eye. In this animal, the other eye had been removed on E64. The fetus was then returned to the uterus and delivered near term. Under these circumstances, orthogradely transported radioactive label is distributed uniformly over the entire LGd, and transneuronally transported label forms a uniform band over sublayers 4A and 4C without a trace of alternating ocular dominance columns. (Based on data from Rakic, 1977c, 1979.)

erally enucleated at E64, the distribution of transneuronally transported radioactive label in sublayers 4A and 4C was continuous and uniform (Figure 8B). Since retinal terminals from the remaining eye cover the entire volume of the LGd (Figure 9), all LGd neurons are exposed to equal amounts of radioactive label; thus a continuous line of silver grains can be expected in the cortex, whether or not there is any change in the genetically prescribed pathway from retina to cortex. This poses a major problem in the interpretation of the autoradiographic results in the cortex obtained from the enucleation experiment. If two separate sets of LGd neurons genetically predetermined to subserve one or the other eye still exist, the transneuronal transport method is inadequate to determine the size of their respective terminal projections in the cortex. However, it may be significant that the geniculate input to the cortex has been sorted out "vertically," as indicated by the denser radioactivity over sublayers 4A and 4C, which suggests that competition between afferents serving the two eyes is not essential for the completion of the process of laminar differentiation. This rearrangement of afferent input to the LGd and cortex must have a significant effect on the organization of local neuronal circuits in these structures. Indeed, in the mouse, there is some evidence that the pattern of dendritic arborization of local circuit neurons in the visual cortex of the mouse changes after eye enucleation (Valverde, 1968).

Manipulation of development of ocular dominance columns by eye deprivation A series of studies has shown that balanced binocular visual input is particularly critical for normal development during the early postnatal period in both cat and monkey (Hubel and Wiesel, 1965; Hubel and Wiesel, 1970; Baker, Grigg, and von Noorden, 1974; Hubel, Wiesel, and LeVay, 1977). Thus early simultaneous stimulation from corresponding points in the visual fields of the two eyes is necessary if cortical cells are to retain the capacity for binocular responsiveness (Hubel, Wiesel, and LeVay, 1977). This pattern, however, can be dramatically changed if one eye is occluded at birth by suture of the eyelid (Figure 10). Four independent experimental methods—physiological recording, transneuronal autoradiography, Nauta anterograde fiber degeneration, and reduced silver stain for normal fibers—have convincingly demonstrated that the ocular dominance columns belonging to the deprived eye are considerably reduced in width, while those of the nondeprived eye are broadened (Hubel, Wiesel, and LeVay, 1977).

Failure to attain the normal pattern of ocular dom-

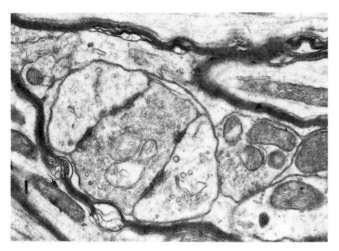

FIGURE 10 A retinal axon terminal making typical multiple synaptic junctions with two dendrites in the left LGd nucleus of a monkey in which the contralateral eye was enucleated at E64. This retinal terminal is located at the periphery of the LGd in a presumptive area of layer 6, which normally receives input exclusively from the contralateral eye. Since this eye is not present, this synapse most likely originates from the ipsilateral eye. This may be the first ultrastructural evidence for synaptic plasticity in the developing visual system. For details see text and Rakic (1977a, 1979).

inance columns as a consequence of abnormal visual experience (Hubel, Wiesel, and LeVay, 1977) can be viewed with reference to the mode of normal development of visual connections (Rakic, 1976b, 1977a). For example, the widths of the ocular dominance stripes subserving the functional eye in a monkey that was monocularly deprived from the neonatal period (Figure 11B) are similar to the widths of stripes subserving each eye at the time around birth (Figure 7B). Since the two sets of stripes overlap in the prenatal period, the comparison of the relative width of the ocular dominance stripes in the two sets of experiments raises the possibility that terminals subserving the functional eye fail to retract—that is, they simply retain the territory they had occupied at the time monocular deprivation began—while terminals from the deprived eye regress. Although LGd neurons subserving the functional eye need not have invaded new territory or expanded as such, the possibility that they form a larger number of synapses in the cortex is not ruled out. Thus, as in prenatal unilateral eye enucleation (Rakic, 1977c), the effect of monocular deprivation on the ocular dominance domains in primates can be explained by the hypothesis of synaptic competition for space on the postsynaptic cell (Guillery, 1972; Hubel, Wiesel, and LeVay, 1977). Therefore, these changes most likely represent arrest of normal development and regression of nonfunc-

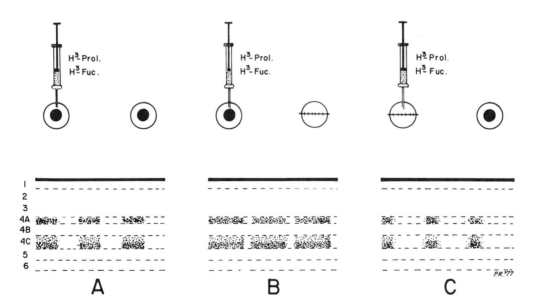

FIGURE 11 Schematic representation of the distribution of transneuronally transported radioactive label over layer 4 in the primary visual cortex in three monkeys 3–4 weeks after unilateral injections of ³H-proline and ³H-fucose. (A) Ocular dominance columns in the normal mature monkey. (B) Ocular dominance columns in the monkey with unilateral eyelid suture during the neonatal period followed by injection into the functional eye several months later. (C) Ocular dominance columns in the monkey with unilateral eye suture during the neonatal period injected into the deprived eye several months later. (Based on data from Hubel, Wiesel, and LeVay, 1977.)

tional circuits, rather than active rearrangement of central connections.

Developmental considerations may also help to explain why monocular deprivation in the monkey in the neonatal period does not affect the size of the territory occupied by input from each eye in the LGd. To explain the relative stability of the distribution of retinal terminals in the LGd in deprivation experiments, one must consider that in the LGd the separation of input from the two eyes is completed prenatally, whereas in the cortex it continues after birth (Rakic, 1976b). It appears, then, that a given structure may be particularly susceptible to changes only during a restricted developmental period. This critical period for LGd in primates occurs prenatally, as shown by the finding that eye enucleation performed before birth can dramatically affect the organization of ocular dominance domains (Rakic, 1977c). After birth, already-segregated retinal terminals are less susceptible to changes in visual input.

Conclusions and future perspectives

A general lesson to be drawn from the studies of the visual system and of the cerebellum described in this chapter is that once a critical phase in the development of neuronal circuitry is completed, whether it be normal or aberrant, a series of subsequent steps is set in motion. A normal or mutant gene, a circumscribed lesion in a distant but related brain structure, or an abnormal sensory input may exert a limited direct effect, which in turn provides the setting for subsequent cellular events and for the emergence of further new neuronal relationships, the net outcome of which is a unique brain with its individual behavioral capabilities.

The examples reviewed indicate that the interplay between genetic and epigenetic factors is essential for normal development and maintenance of local synaptic circuits. At present, the mechanisms underlying this balance are not fully understood. It is unlikely, however, that a breakthrough will come from a single discovery or from single sets of experiments, as occurred in the field of molecular biology more than two decades ago. The biological system and the questions asked are so different as to require different research strategies. One approach consists of the reconstruction of synaptic relationships among neurons and, particularly, the gathering of quantitative data on minute changes in the synaptic pattern under different experimental conditions. This is a formidable task, but it may be one of the most exciting and most promising challenges of neuroscience research.

REFERENCES

ALTMAN, J., and W. J. ANDERSON, 1973. Experimental reorganization of the cerebellar cortex. II. Effects of elimination of most microneurons with prolonged X-irradiation started at four days. *J. Comp. Neurol.* 149:123–152.

BAKER, F. H., P. GRIGG, and G. K. VON NOORDEN, 1974. Effects of visual deprivation and strabismus on the response of neurons in the visual cortex of the monkey, including studies on the striate and prestriate cortex in the normal animal. *Brain Res.* 66:185–208.

BARLOW, H. B., 1975. Visual experience and cortical development. *Nature* 258:199–204.

BENNETT, M. R., and A. G. PETTIGREW, 1974. The formation of synapses in striated muscle during development. *J. Physiol.* 241:515–545.

BODIAN, D., 1972. Neuron junctions: A revolutionary decade. *Anat. Rec.* 174:73–82.

BRODMANN, K., 1905. Beitrage zur histologischen Lokalization der Grosshirnrinde Dritte Mitteilung: Die Rinderfelder der niederen Affen. *J. Psychol. Neurol. (Leipzig)* 9:177–226.

BROUWER, B., and W. P. C. ZEEMAN, 1926. The projection of the retina in the primary optic neuron in monkeys. *Brain* 49:11–35.

BROWN, M. C., J. K. S. JANSEN, and D. VAN ESSEN, 1976. Polyneuronal innervation of skeletal muscle in new-born rats and its elimination during maturation. *J. Physiol.* 261:387–422.

CAVINESS, V. S., JR., and P. RAKIC, 1978. Mechanisms of cortical development: A view from mutations in mice. *Annu. Rev. Neurosci.* 1:297–326.

CHANGEUX, J.-P., and A. DANCHIN, 1976. Selective stabilization of developing synapses as mechanism for the specification of neuronal networks. *Nature* 264:705–712.

CREPEL, F., and J. MARIANI, 1976. Multiple innervation of Purkinje cells by climbing fibers in the cerebellum of the weaver mutant mouse. *J. Neurobiol.* 7:579–582.

CREPEL, J., J. MARIANI, and N. DELHAYE-BOUCHARD, 1976. Evidence for a multiple innervation of Purkinje cells by climbing fibers in the immature rat cerebellum. *J. Neurobiol.* 7:567–578.

DAS, G. D., and H. O. NORNES, 1972. Neurogenesis of the cerebellum of the rat: An autoradiographic study. *Z. Anat. Entwicklungsgesch.* 138:155–165.

ECCLES, J. C., M. ITO, and J. SZENTÁGOTHAI, 1967. *The Cerebellum as a Neuronal Machine.* Berlin, Heidelberg, New York: Springer-Verlag.

FALCONER, D. S., 1951. Two new mutants "trembler" and "reeler," with neurological actions in the house mouse (*Mus musculus*). *J. Genet.* 50:192–201.

FISCHBACH, G. D., D. K. BERG, S. A. COHN, and E. FRANK, 1976. Enrichment of nerve-muscle synapses in spinal cord-muscle cultures and identification of relative peaks of ACh sensitivity at sites of transmitter release. *Cold Spring Harbor Symp. Quant. Biol.* 30:347–357.

GAZE, R. M., and M. J. KEATING, 1972. The visual system and "neuronal specificity." *Nature* 237:375–378.

GOLDMAN, P. S., 1976. Maturation of mammalian nervous system and the ontogeny of behavior. In *Advances in the Study of Behavior*, vol. 7, J. S. Rosenblatt, R. A. Hinde, E. Shaw, and C. Beer, eds. New York: Academic Press, pp. 1–90.

GOLDMAN, P. S., and W. J. H. NAUTA, 1976. Autoradiographic demonstration of a projection from prefrontal association cortex to the superior colliculus in the rhesus monkey. *Brain Res.* 116:145–149.

GOLDMAN, P. S., and W. J. H. NAUTA, 1977a. An intricately patterned prefronto-caudate projection in the rhesus monkey. *J. Comp. Neurol.* 171:369–386.

GOLDMAN, P. S., and W. J. H. NAUTA, 1977b. Columnar organization of association and motor cortex: Autoradiographic evidence for cortico-cortical and commissural columns in the frontal lobe of the newborn rhesus monkey. *Brain Res.* 122:369–385.

GOLGI, C., 1885. Sulla fina anatomia degli organi centrali del sistema nervoso. In *Opera omnia.* Milan: Hoepli, 1903, pp. 397–536.

GRAFSTEIN, B., 1971. Transneuronal transfer of radioactivity in the central nervous system. *Science* 172:177–179.

GUILLERY, R. W., 1972. Binocular competition in the control of geniculate cell growth. *J. Comp. Neurol.* 144:117–130.

GUILLERY, R. W., and M. COLONNIER, 1970. Synaptic patterns in the dorsal lateral geniculate nucleus of the monkey. *Z. Zellforsch.* 103:90–108.

HANNA, R. B., A. HIRANO, and G. D. PAPPAS, 1975. Membrane specializations of dendrite spines and glia in the weaver mouse cerebellum: A freeze fracture study. *J. Cell Biol.* 68:403–410.

HEBB, D. O., 1949. *The Organization of Behavior.* New York: Wiley.

HENDRICKSON, A., and P. RAKIC, 1977. Histogenesis and synaptogenesis in the dorsal lateral geniculate nucleus (LGd) of the fetal monkey brain. *Anat. Rec.* 187:602 (abstract).

HERNDON, R. M., and M. OSTER-GRANITE, 1975. Effect of granule cell destruction on development and maintenance of the Purkinje cell dendrite. *Adv. Neurol.* 12:361–371.

HERRUP, K., and R. J. MULLEN, 1976. Intrinsic Purkinje cell abnormalities in staggerer mutant mice revealed by analysis of a staggerer-normal chimera. *Neurosci. Abst.* 2:101.

HIRANO, A., and H. DEMBITZER, 1973. Cerebellar alteration in the weaver mouse. *J. Cell Biol.* 56:478–486.

HUBEL, D. H., and T. N. WIESEL, 1965. Binocular interaction in striate cortex of kittens reared with artificial squint. *J. Neurophysiol.* 28:1041–1059.

HUBEL, D. H., and T. N. WIESEL, 1968. Receptive fields and functional architecture of monkey striate cortex. *J. Physiol.* 195:215–243.

HUBEL, D. H., and T. N. WIESEL, 1970. The period of susceptibility to the physiological effects of unilateral eye closure in kittens. *J. Physiol.* 206:419–436.

HUBEL, D. H., and T. N. WIESEL, 1977. Functional architecture of macaque monkey visual cortex. *Proc. R. Soc. Lond.* B198:1–59.

HUBEL, D. H., T. N. WIESEL, and S. LEVAY, 1977. Plasticity of ocular dominance columns in monkey striate cortex. *Philos. Trans. R. Soc. Lond.* B278:377–409.

HUGHES, A., 1964. Further experiments on innervation and function of grafted supranumary limbs in the embryo of *Eleutorodactylus martinicensis. J. Embryol. Exp. Morphol.* 12:229–245.

JACOBSON, M., 1970. The development, specification, and diversification of neuronal connections. In *Neurosciences: Second Study Program*, F. O. Schmitt, ed. New York: Rockefeller Univ. Press, pp. 116–129.

KEATING, M. J., 1968. Functional interaction in the development of specific nerve connections. *J. Physiol.* 198:75–77.

KORNGUTH, S. E., and G. SCOTT, 1972. The role of climbing fibers in the formation of Purkinje cell dendrites. *J. Comp. Neurol.* 146:61–82.

LANDIS, D. M. D., and T. S. REESE, 1977. Structure of the Purkinje cell membrane in staggerer and weaver mutant mouse. *J. Comp. Neurol.* 171:247–260.

LANDIS, D. M. D., and R. L. SIDMAN, 1978. Electron microscopic analysis of post-natal histogenesis in the cerebellar cortex of staggerer mutant mice. *J. Comp. Neurol.* (in press).

LANDIS, S., 1973. Ultrastructural changes in the mitochondria of cerebellar Purkinje cells of nervous mutant mice. *J. Cell Biol.* 57:782–797.

LANE, P., 1964. In *Mouse News Letter* 30:32.

LARRAMENDI, L. M. H., 1969. Analysis of synaptogenesis in the cerebellum of the mouse. In *Neurobiology of Cerebellar Evolution and Development*, R. Llinás, ed. Chicago: AMA Education and Research Fdn., pp. 803–843.

LEVAY, S., 1971. On the neurons and synapses of the lateral geniculate nucleus of the monkey and the effects of eye enucleation. *Z. Zellforsch.* 113:396–419.

LEVAY, S., D. H. HUBEL, and T. N. WIESEL, 1975. The pattern of ocular dominance columns in macaque visual cortex revealed by a reduced silver stain. *J. Comp. Neurol.* 159:559–576.

LEVAY, S., M. P. STRYKER, and C. J. SHATZ, 1978. Ocular dominance columns and their development in layer IV of the cat's visual cortex: A quantitative study. *J. Comp. Neurol.* 179:223–244.

LLINÁS, R., D. E. HILLMAN, and W. PRECHT, 1973. Neuronal circuit reorganization in mammalian agranular cerebellar cortex. *J. Neurobiol.* 1:60 04.

LUND, J. S., 1973. Organization of neurons in the visual cortex, area 17, of the monkey (*Macaca mulatta*). *J. Comp. Neurol.* 147:455–496.

LUND, J. S., 1976. Laminar organization of the primary visual cortex, area 17, of Macaque monkey. *Exp. Brain Res. Suppl.* 1:288–291.

LUND, J. S. and BOOTHE, R. G., 1975. Interlaminar connections and pyramidal neuron organization in the visual cortex, area 17, of the macaque monkey. *J. Comp. Neurol.* 159:305–334.

LUND, J. S., R. D. LUND, A. E. HENDRICKSON, A. H. BUNT, and F. FUCHS, 1975. The origin of efferent pathways from the primary visual cortex, area 17, of the macaque monkey as shown by retrograde transport of horseradish peroxidase. *J. Comp. Neurol.* 164:287–304.

MALESBURG, C. V. D., and D. J. WILLSHAW, 1976. A mechanism for producing continuous neural mappings: Ocularity dominance stripes and ordered retino-tectal projections. *Exp. Brain Res.* Suppl. 1:463–469.

MARIANI, J., F. CREPEL, K. MIKOSHIBA, J.-P. CHANGEUX, and C. SOTELO, 1977. Anatomical, physiological and biochemical studies of the cerebellum from reeler mutant mouse. *Philos. Trans. R. Soc. Lond.* B281:1–28.

MATTHEWS, M. R., W. M. COWAN, and T. P. S. POWELL, 1960. Transneuronal degeneration in the lateral geniculate nucleus of the macaque monkey. *J. Anat.* 94:145–169.

MIALE, I. L., and R. L. SIDMAN, 1961. An autoradiographic

analysis of histogenesis in the mouse cerebellum. *Exp. Neurol.* 4:277–296.

MINKOWSKI, M., 1920. Über den Verlauf, die Endigung und die zentrale Reprasentation von gekreuzten und ungekreuzten Schnervenfasern bei eingen Säugetieren und beim Menschen. *Schweiz. Arch. Neurol. Neurochir. Psychiatr.* 6:201–252; 7:268–302.

MUGNAINI, E., 1969. Ultrastructural studies on the cerebellar histogenesis. II. Maturation of the nerve cell populations and establishment of synaptic connections in the cerebellar cortex of the chick. In *Neurobiology of Cerebellar Evolution and Development*, R. Llinás, ed. Chicago: AMA Education and Research Fdn., pp. 749–782.

MUGNAINI, E., 1972. The histology and cytology of the cerebellar cortex. In *The Comparative Anatomy and Histology of the Cerebellum*, vol. 3: *The Human Cerebellum, Cerebellar Connections, and Cerebellar Cortex*, O. Larsell and J. Jansen, eds. Minneapolis: Univ. Minnesota Press, pp. 201–264.

MULLEN, R. J., 1977. Genetic dissection of the CNS with mutant-normal mouse and rat chimeras. *Neurosci. Symp.* 2:47–65 (abstract).

PALAY, S. L, and V. CHAN-PALAY, 1974. *Cerebellar Cortex: Cytology and Organization.* Berlin, Heidelberg, New York: Springer-Verlag.

PAVLOV, I. P., 1927. *Conditional Reflexes*, 6 vols. London: Oxford Univ. Press.

POLYAK, S. L., 1957. *The Vertebrate Visual System.* Chicago: Univ. Chicago Press.

PRESTIGE, M. C., and D. J. WILLSHAW, 1975. On the role of competition in the formation of patterned neuronal connexions. *Proc. R. Soc. Lond.* B190:77–98.

PRICE, J. L., G. F. MOXLEY, and J. I. SCHWOB, 1976. Development and plasticity of complementary afferent fiber systems to the olfactory cortex. *Exp. Brain Res. Suppl.* 1:148–154.

PURPURA, D. P., A. HIRANO, and J. H. FRENCH, 1976. Poly-dendritic Purkinje cells in X-chromosome linked copper malabsorption: A Golgi study. *Brain Res.* 117:125–129.

PURPURA, D. P., and K. SUZUKI, 1976. Distortion of neuronal geometry and formation of aberrant synapses in neuronal storage disease. *Brain Res.* 116:1–21.

PURVES, D., 1977. The formation and maintenance of synaptic connections. In *Function and Formation of Neural Systems.* Dahlen Workshop (in press).

RAKIC, P., 1971. Neuron-glia relationship during granule cell migration in developing cerebellar cortex. I. Golgi and electronmicroscopic study in *Macacus rhesus. J. Comp. Neurol.* 141:283–312.

RAKIC, P., 1973. Kinetics of proliferation and latency between final division and onset of differentiation of the cerebellar stellate and basket neurons. *J. Comp. Neurol.* 147:523–546.

RAKIC, P., 1974a. Neurons in rhesus monkey visual cortex: Systematic relation between time of origin and eventual disposition. *Science* 183:425–427.

RAKIC, P., 1974b. Intrinsic and extrinsic factors influencing the shape of neurons and their assembly into neuronal circuits. In *Frontiers in Neurology and Neuroscience Research*, P. Seeman and G. M. Brown, eds. Toronto: Univ. Toronto Press, pp. 112–132.

RAKIC, P., 1975. Timing of major ontogenetic events in the

visual cortex of the rhesus monkey. In *Brain Mechanisms in Mental Retardation.* N. A. Buchwald and M. Brazier, eds. New York: Academic Press, pp. 3–40.

RAKIC, P., 1976a. Synaptic specificity in the cerebellar cortex: Study of anomalous circuits induced by single gene mutation in mice. *Cold Spring Harbor Symp. Quant. Biol.* 40:333–346.

RAKIC, P., 1976b. Prenatal genesis of connections subserving ocular dominance in the rhesus monkey. *Nature* 261:467–471.

RAKIC, P., 1976c. *Local Circuit Neurons.* Cambridge, MA: MIT Press.

RAKIC, P., 1977a. Prenatal development of the visual system in the rhesus monkey. *Philos. Trans. R. Soc. Lond.* B278:245–260.

RAKIC, P., 1977b. Genesis of the dorsal lateral geniculate nucleus in the rhesus monkey: Site and time of origin, kinetics of proliferation, routes of migration and pattern of distribution of neurons. *J. Comp. Neurol.* 176:23–52.

RAKIC, P., 1977c. Effects of prenatal unilateral eye enucleation on the formation of layers and retinal connections in the dorsal lateral geniculate nucleus (LGd) of the rhesus monkey. *Neurosci. Abstr.* 3:573.

RAKIC, P., 1979. Structural alterations and rearrangement of connections in the dorsal lateral geniculate body of the rhesus monkey following prenatal enucleation of one eye. In preparation.

RAKIC, P., and R. L. SIDMAN, 1973. Organization of cerebellar cortex secondary to deficit of granule cells in weaver mutant mice. *J. Comp. Neurol.* 152:133–162.

RALSTON, J. J., III, 1971. Evidence for presynaptic dendrites and a proposal for their mechanism of action. *Nature* 230:585–587.

RAMÓN Y CAJAL, S., 1889. Conexión general de los elementos nerviosos. In *La Medicina Practica.* Madrid.

RAMÓN Y CAJAL, S., 1890. A propos de certain éléments bipolaires du cervelat avec quelques détails nouveaux sur l'evolution des fibres cerebelluses. *J. Int. Anat. Physiol.* (Paris) 7:1–22.

RAMÓN Y CAJAL, S., 1899. Comparative study of the sensory areas of the human brain. In *Clark University, 1889–1899: Decennial Celebration.* Worcester, MA: Clark Univ.

RAMÓN Y CAJAL, S., 1911. *Histologie du système nerveux de l'homme et des vertébrés.* Paris: Maloine. Reprinted by Consejo Superior de Investigaciones Cientificas, Madrid, 1955. vol. 2.

RAMÓN Y CAJAL, S., 1937. *Recollections of My Life.* Cambridge, MA: MIT Press.

REDFERN, P. A., 1970. Neuromuscular transmission in newborn rats. *J. Physiol.* 209:701–709.

SCHMITT, F. O., P. DEV, and B. H. SMITH, 1976. Electrotonic processing of information by brain cells. *Science* 193:114–120.

SECHENOV, I. M., 1863. *Reflexes of the Brain.* Cambridge, MA: MIT Press (1965, reissue).

SHEPHERD, G. M., 1972. The neuron doctrine: A revision of functional concepts. *Yale J. Biol. Med.* 45:584–599.

SIDMAN, R. L., 1968. Development of interneuronal connections in brain of mutant mice. In *Physiological and Biochemical Aspects of Nervous Integration*, F. D. Carlson, ed. Englewood Cliffs, NJ: Prentice-Hall, pp. 163–193.

SIDMAN, R. L., 1973. Cell-cell recognition in the developing central nervous system. In *Neurosciences: Third Study Program*, F. O. Schmitt and F. G. Worden, eds. Cambridge, MA: MIT Press, pp. 743–758.

SIDMAN, R. L., and P. RAKIC, 1973. Neuronal migration, with special reference to developing human brain: A review. *Brain Res.* 62:1–35.

SKOFF, R. P., and V. HAMBURGER, 1974. Fine structure of dendritic and axonal growth cones in embryonic chick spinal cord. *J. Comp. Neurol.* 153:107–148.

SO, K., G. E. SCHNEIDER, and D. O. FROST, 1978. Postnatal development of retinal projections to the lateral geniculate body in Syrian hamsters. *Brain Res.* 142:575–583.

SOTELO, C., 1975. Dendritic abnormalities of Purkinje cells in cerebellum of neurological mutant mice (weaver and staggerer). *Adv. Neurol.* 12:335–351.

SOTELO, C., 1977. Formation of presynaptic dendrites in the rat cerebellum following neonatal X-irradiation. *Neuroscience* 2:275–283.

SOTELO, C., and M. L. ARSENIO-NUNES, 1976. Development of Purkinje cells in the absence of climbing fibers. *Brain Res.* 111:389–395.

SOTELO, C., and J.-P. CHANGEUX, 1974. Transynaptic degeneration "en cascade" in the cerebellar cortex of staggerer mutant mice. *Brain Res.* 67:519–526.

SOTELO, C., D. E. HILLMAN, A. J. ZAMORA, and R. LLINÁS, 1975. Climbing fiber deafferentation: Its action on Purkinje cell dendritic spines. *Brain Res.* 98:574–581.

SPERRY, R. W., 1963. Chemoaffinity in the orderly growth of nerve fiber patterns and connections. *Proc. Natl. Acad. Sci. USA* 50:703–710.

STENT, G. S., 1973. A physiological mechanism for Hebb's postulate of learning. *Proc. Natl. Acad. Sci. USA.* 70:997–1001.

VALVERDE, F., 1968. Structural changes in the area striata of the mouse after enucleation. *Exp. Brain Res.* 5:274–292.

VALVERDE, F., 1971. Short axon neuronal subsystems in the visual cortex of the monkey. *Int. J. Neurosci.* 1:181–197.

WIESEL, T. N., D. H. HUBEL, and D. M. K. LAM, 1974. Autoradiographic demonstration of ocular-dominance columns in the monkey striate cortex by means of transneuronal transport. *Brain Res.* 79:273–279.

WILLIAMS, R. S., P. C. MARSHALL, I. T. LATT, and V. S. CAVINESS, JR., 1978. The cellular pathology of Menkes' steely hair syndrome. *Neurology* 28:575–583.

WOODWARD, D. J., B. J. HOFFER, and J. ALTMAN, 1974. Physiological and pharmacological properties of Purkinje cells in rat cerebellum degranulated by postnatal X-irradiation. *J. Neurobiol.* 5:283–304.

YOUNG, J. Z., 1964. *A Model of the Brain.* London: Oxford Univ. Press.

ZECEVIC, N., and P. RAKIC, 1976. Differentiation of Purkinje cells and their relationship to other components of developing cerebellar cortex in man. *J. Comp. Neurol.* 167:27–48.

8 Functional Analysis of Local Circuits in the Olfactory Bulb

GORDON M. SHEPHERD

ABSTRACT An understanding of the functional organization of any region of the nervous system depends on the experimental methods used and the accessibility of the region and its constituent elements to the application of these methods. Any one method may provide essential clues or evidence about the functions of the region, but it can never be sufficient; for evidence gains creditability only through support from other independent methods, and its significance can only be judged within the fabric of all the information available about that region. Coherent concepts therefore require the correlation of results from as many approaches as possible. It is well to recognize this principle as a guide to experimental analysis and a means of qualifying the interpretation of results, particularly during a period when neuroscientific methods are multiplying rapidly in number and variety.

In this paper I shall outline briefly how such a multidisciplinary approach has evolved in the study of synaptic circuits in the vertebrate olfactory bulb. While describing this work I shall attempt to draw attention to some general considerations relevant to the analysis of local circuits and to some implications of local circuit organization for our understanding of the basic units for information processing in the nervous system.

Anatomical methods

GOLGI STUDIES have shown that there are three main neuronal types in the olfactory bulb (see Figure 1). The main output neuron is the *mitral cell*, the cell bodies of which are arranged in a thin layer. A subtype, the *tufted cell*, is scattered through the external plexiform and glomerular layers. There are two main types of intrinsic neuron: the *periglomerular cell* is confined to the glomerular layer, where the olfactory axons terminate; the *granule cell* has its cell body located in the deep, granule layer and has central and peripheral dendrites, the latter ramifying extensively in the external plexiform layer. The granule layer also contains scattered short-axon cells.

The termination of olfactory axons among mitral-,

tufted-, and periglomerular-cell dendrites implies synaptic connections onto those dendrites (Ramón y Cajal, 1911), and electron-microscopic (EM) studies have confirmed these axodendritic synapses (see insert, Figure 1). It has also been shown that the mitral- and periglomerular-cell dendrites are interconnected by numerous dendrodendritic synapses (Pinching and Powell, 1971). And there is evidence in some mammalian species that the axons may terminate on mitral-cell but not on periglomerular-cell dendrites (White, 1972, 1973). None of these details could have been deduced from the Golgi material itself; the Golgi method can indicate in what layer synapses are likely to occur, but the electron microscope is necessary to identify the synapses.

The intermingling of mitral secondary dendrites and granule-cell dendrites in the external plexiform layer similarly implies a connection between the two (Ramón y Cajal, 1911). Again the electron microscope has shown that the predominant connection is in the form of reciprocal synapses located side-by-side with opposite morphological polarities (Hirata, 1964; Andres, 1965; Rall et al., 1965; Reese and Shepherd, 1972). A modest proportion of the dendrodendritic synapses in the glomeruli have this arrangement, and nearly all the mitral and granule synapses are of this type.

EM studies of the bulb are greatly aided by the ease with which cell processes can be recognized. It has been found that mitral-to-granule synapses are characterized by spheroidal vesicles and asymmetric membrane thickenings, whereas granule-to-mitral synapses are characterized by flattened vesicles and symmetric membrane thickenings (Price and Powell, 1970). This correlates with the excitatory and inhibitory actions, respectively, of these synapses suggested by physiological studies (see below). A similar correlation has been suggested for synapses in other parts of the nervous system (Uchizono, 1966), and the evidence in the olfactory bulb is among the clearest for this morphophysiological correlation. Freeze-fracture

GORDON M. SHEPHERD Department of Physiology, Yale University School of Medicine, New Haven, CT 06510

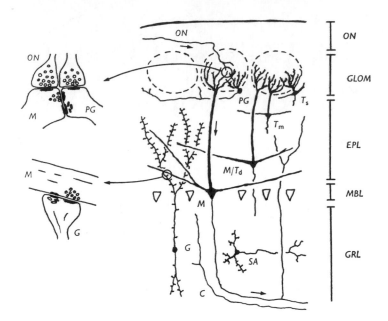

FIGURE 1 Schematic diagram summarizing neuronal elements and synaptic connections in the rabbit olfactory bulb. Insets at left show main types of synaptic connections in the glomeruli (above) and external plexiform layer (below). *Abbreviations*, for this and following figures: ON, olfactory nerves; PG, periglomerular short-axon cell; T$_s$, superficial tufted cell; T$_m$, middle tufted cell; M/T$_d$, displaced mitral or deep tufted cell; M, mitral cell; G, granule cell; SA, short-axon cell of deep layer; C, centrifugal fibers. Histological layers shown at right: GLOM, glomerular layer; EPL, external plexiform layer; MBL, mitral body layer; GRL, granule layer. (From Getchell and Shepherd, 1975a.)

studies (Landis, Reese, and Raviola, 1974) showed that the mitral-to-granule synapse is characterized by accumulations of intramembranous particles on the postsynaptic side. This correlation with a presumed excitatory synapse is similar to the findings in the cerebellum (Landis and Reese, 1974). In both regions, particle accumulations are absent at presumed inhibitory synapses (e.g., granule-to-mitral in the bulb).

From these and other studies in the olfactory bulb it appears that individual synapses have a morphology similar to that of simple contacts seen in other regions of the nervous system. Thus the same basic type of junction can serve synaptic transmission from an axon to a dendrite or between two dendrites. Another important point is that dendrodendritic synapses are not specific for a given neuronal type or neuronal process. In the bulb, the long-axon (mitral) cell, the short-axon (periglomerular) cell, and the anaxonal (granule) cell all take part in dendrodendritic connections in which their processes occupy presynaptic as well as postsynaptic positions. This may be taken as evidence that functional circuits are organized in terms of patterns of synaptic connections rather than in terms of the particular geometry of the neuronal processes involved.

Physiological methods

By virtue of its distinct neuronal types and separation into layers, the olfactory bulb is a favorable site for electrophysiological analysis. The afferent and efferent pathways can be separately stimulated, and mitral cells can be identified by antidromic volleys in the lateral olfactory tract. Numerous extracellular single-unit studies (reviewed in Shepherd, 1972a) have verified that mitral cells undergo a period of suppression after antidromic impulse invasion. Intracellular recordings have shown this period to be correlated with a long-lasting hyperpolarization of the mitral-cell membrane that has the properties of an inhibitory postsynaptic potential (IPSP). Typical recordings are shown in Figure 2A, B.

The interval between impulse invasion and the onset of the IPSP is dependent on the strength of the volley and has a minimum duration of approximately 2 msec, which is sufficient for two synaptic delays. The evidence suggests that the granule cell acts as an interneuron in this pathway, in analogy with the Renshaw pathway for inhibition in the spinal cord. However, in contrast with Renshaw cells, in which inhibitory action is ascribed to high-frequency, long-lasting impulse discharges, impulse activity in the granule-

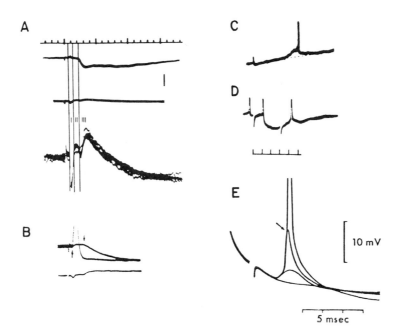

FIGURE 2   Intracellular recordings from mitral cells. (A, B) Responses to LOT volley. (A) Upper trace shows long-lasting IPSP, middle trace the field potential, lower trace the field potential at higher gain with time components 1–3. Time scale in 2 msec divisions; voltage calibration 10 mV (upper traces), 2mV (lower traces). (Modified from Shepherd, 1970.) (B) Response straddling threshold for axon of this cell, with field potential trace shown below. Arrows show onset of spike and onset of inhibition. (From Nicoll, 1969.) (C, D, E) Responses to ON volley. (C) Spike response arising from EPSP. (From Yamamoto, Yamamoto, and Iwama, 1963.) (D) Succession of spontaneous impulse, first ON shock artifact, spike response followed by IPSP; second ON shock artifact, spike response arising from small EPSP. Time in 5 msec divisions. (From Getchell and Shepherd, 1975). (E) Response during hyperpolarization of cell membrane by applied current, showing EPSP, fast prepotential, and full spike. (From Mori and Takagi, 1975.)

cell layer is rare, and discharges are brief. Long-lasting synaptic inhibition is, in fact, common in neurons of the brain. The possibility that such inhibition might be mediated wholly or in large part without concurrent impulse activity was recognized early in the bulb (Phillips, Powell, and Shepherd, 1963; Shepherd, 1963).

Orthodromic volleys in the olfactory nerves also set up a sequence of impulse generation followed by inhibition in mitral cells. In some cases the impulse can be seen to arise from a depolarizing EPSP (Figure 2C); in other cases it arises more abruptly from the baseline (Figure 2D). Note in Figure 2D that in the response to the second volley, a small EPSP is revealed. This is consistent with the idea that hyperpolarization following the first volley moves the membrane potential away from the equilibrium potential for the EPSP and toward that for the IPSP. It appears that depolarization due to electrode entry into this cell is a complication in the activity recorded. This complication requires continual assessment in intracellular recordings, particularly the smaller neurons of the CNS.

In Figure 2E, the cell has been hyperpolarized by injected current, and a fast prepotential is revealed. Similar potentials have been seen in several other sites; for example, in chromatolytic motoneurons (Eccles, Libet, and Young, 1958), hippocampal pyramidal cells (Spencer and Kandel, 1961), and Purkinje cells (Llinás and Nicholson, 1971). In analogy with those cells, Mori and Takagi (1977) have suggested that the fast prepotential in the mitral cell represents "booster" activity in the distal part of the primary dendrite. EM studies have shown that this part of the dendrite is surrounded by glial membranes; in the monkey these appear as a thin myelin sheath (Pinching, 1971). The latter finding shows that myelination is not an exclusive property of axons; whether it is associated with active or passive properties in the mitral dendrite has not yet been established.

Physiological identification of mitral cells by antidromic criteria and by correlation with evoked potentials can be carried out relatively easily. Identification by means of intracellular dyes has not yet been reported, although in vertebrates, intracellular staining has been effective in identifying cells in several central regions (retina, spinal cord, cerebellum, cortex). However, for both recording and staining, the largest cells and processes have offered the best targets. Small cells and small processes present a severe challenge in the vertebrate nervous system and also in invertebrate neuropil. Information at this level is essential for analysis of local circuits, but assessment of the effects of electrode penetration on physiological properties will be of critical importance.

Evidence for the properties of periglomerular short-axon cells will be discussed after consideration of computer simulation studies of mitral and granule cells.

Theoretical models

Neurophysiologists traditionally have been hesitant to apply theoretical methods to the interpretation of experimental data relating to neuronal organization. This reluctance derives in part from a healthy skepticism that the theoretical assumptions can adequately incorporate the complexities of the regions and systems under study. The methods of Rall for describing the electrotonic properties of dendritic trees have shown that theory can in fact be applied to neurons

to provide the essential basis for interpreting experimental results (Rall, 1977; see also Jack, this volume). Rall has emphasized the need for an ongoing interplay between experiments on the living system and experiments on realistic models of that system.

In the olfactory bulb we first attempted to reconstruct intracellular and extracellular potentials with computational models of the mitral- and grade-cell populations, as they are activated by an antidromic volley in the lateral olfactory tract (Rall et al., 1966; Rall and Shepherd, 1968). This work has been reviewed before (Shepherd, 1972a); Figure 3 displays representative computations of antidromic impulse spread in the mitral cells and synaptic excitation of the granule cells. The computations in the mitral-cell model explored the effects on impulse propagation of the geometrical hurdle from axon to cell body to dendritic equivalent cylinder. Goldstein and Rall (1974) subsequently analyzed this interesting theoretical problem in detail, and computer simulations of the effects of similar changes in nerve-process diameters on impulse propagation have now been carried out for several types of neuron (see the chapters by Parnas and by Pellionisz, this volume). Our computations also explored the alternatives of active versus passive dendritic properties, and we concluded

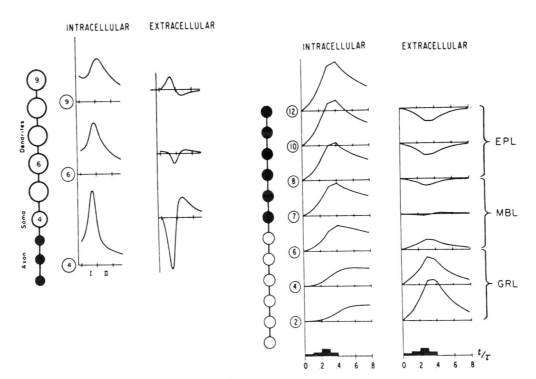

FIGURE 3 Computed intracellular and extracellular potentials generated by mitral-cell (left) and granule-cell (right) compartmental models in response to a LOT volley. Filled compartments indicate sites of active impulse generation (left) and EPSP (right); open compartments have only passive electrical properties. (From Rall and Shepherd, 1968.)

that active properties might be present in some of the mitral-cell dendrites but could be ruled out to any significant extent in granule-cell dendritic branches if the computed extracellular transients were to agree with the recorded field potentials.

The extracellular transients were computed on the basis of a potential divider model for describing the relation of the recording electrodes to primary and secondary extracellular current flows. Subsequent studies showed that partial activation of the bulb produces potentials in active and inactive regions as predicted by the model (Shepherd and Haberly, 1970). Recently the theoretical basis for the potential divider model has been described by Klee and Rall (1977) (See Figure 4.)

The sequence of activity in the computer simula-

tions, together with reasonable assumptions about the laminar locus and timing relative to the mitral-cell IPSP, led to the postulate of mitral-to-granule excitation followed by granule-to-mitral inhibition through the dendrites of these two cell types. The reciprocal synapses in the external plexiform layer, as described above, provide a morphological basis for this pathway (Rall et al., 1965; Rall and Shepherd, 1968).

The computations using the potential divider model were for the case of synchronous activation of large populations of mitral and granule cells. Recently Robert Brayton and I focused on the situation at the other extreme—the minimum parts of individual mitral and granule dendritic trees involved in mediating self-inhibition and lateral inhibition

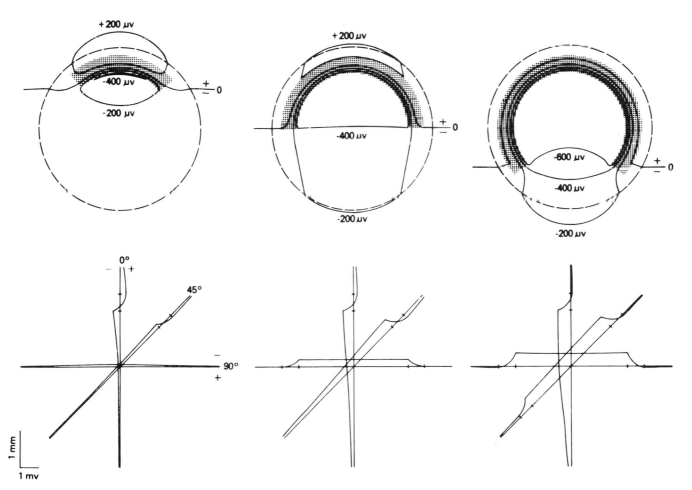

FIGURE 4 Computed field potentials generated by populations of synchronously active cells of differing cortical extents. Extents of active populations are indicated by shaded areas. Activity consists of depolarization of 10 mV in cell somata, which are arranged along the inner border with dendrites extending radially outward. Isopotential contours are indicated in upper diagrams, and depth profiles through the entire region (dashed sphere) are shown below. Resistivity within the region is 250 Ω-cm, outside is 2,500 Ω-cm. Note superficial positivity and deep negativity for recording tracks through active zones, in agreement with experiments on olfactory bulb. (From Klee and Rall, 1977.)

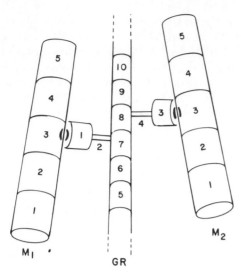

FIGURE 5 Compartmental model of dendrodendritic synaptic circuit, comprised of two mitral secondary dendrites (M$_1$ and M$_2$) and a branch of a granule-cell dendrite (GR) with two spines. Reciprocal synapses connect the spines to the mitral cells. The mitral dendrites are 4 μm in diameter; each compartment is 100 μm in length, with specific membrane resistance of 2,000 Ω-cm^2 and specific cytoplasmic resistance of 80 Ω-cm. For the granule-cell dendrite, the corresponding values are 4,000 Ω-cm^2 and 80 Ω-cm; compartments 5–10 are 1 μm in diameter and 50 μm in length; the spine necks (2 and 4) are 0.2 μm in diameter and 3 μm in length; the spine heads (1 and 3) are 1 μm in diameter and 3 μm in length.

through the reciprocal synapses. Figure 5 shows these parts, which consist of secondary dendrites of two mitral cells and a part of a granule dendrite with two spines connecting to the two mitral dendrites. The model is in compartmental form. An action potential is generated in the first compartment of mitral cell M$_1$, simulating antidromic invasion. The subsequent events are passive impulse spread into the M$_1$ dendrite, activation of the excitatory synapse from compartment 3 to the spine head of the granule dendrite, and activation of the inhibitory synapse back onto the mitral dendrite, producing self-inhibition of the mitral cell. This sequence is illustrated in Figure 6. During this same period, the EPSP in the first spine head spreads electrotonically through the granule-cell tree and into the second spine head. The depolarization activates the inhibitory synapse of the second spine head onto the second mitral dendrite, producing lateral inhibition of the second mitral cell.

The computer simulation thus reproduces the basic properties of the responses recorded from the mitral cells (cf. Figure 2) by the postulated dendrodendritic pathway. A key point is that the pathway involves only certain parts of the dendritic trees of the neu-

rons involved. These parts define the functional unit (Shepherd, 1972b, 1977) for self-inhibition and lateral inhibition under these conditions. The functional unit is in fact a dendritic synaptic network with this specific morphological locus and these specific physiological properties. Two levels of local circuits are included in this unit: the reciprocal synapse and the dendritic circuits in which they are embedded. We will return to the question of levels of organization in the discussion section.

Previous attempts to model neuronal networks have generally treated the nerve cell as a single node or integrating locus and described the network as being built up by axonal connections between the nodal points. The present approach begins with Rall's recognition of the extended dendritic nature of the neuronal integrative surface and builds the relevant functional network within that context. This, of course, requires specific estimates of dendritic and synaptic properties. The present results represent a first step toward analyzing the dynamic relations between synaptic inputs and outputs in individual parts of dendrodendritic networks.

Short-axon cells

The granule cell is unusual among local interneurons in that it combines a large population with a parallel orientation of extended dendritic trees. These factors were, in fact, necessary morphological preconditions for modeling the field potentials described above.

The other interneuron in the olfactory bulb—the periglomerular (PG), short-axon cell—operates under very different conditions. PG cells are confined within a narrow layer; their dendritic trees are short and have different orientations as they enter and ramify within the glomeruli. Thus field-potential analysis has limited value in unraveling the functional properties of these cells; unfortunately the same limitation applies to many other kinds of short-axon cells in other parts of the nervous system. Fortunately, in the case of the periglomerular cell, there are counterbalancing advantages.

Single unit recordings have provided some understanding of PG cell properties (Shepherd, 1963, 1971; Getchell and Shepherd, 1975b). PG cells characteristically respond to a strong volley in the olfactory nerves with a brief burst of impulses. The impulse frequency tends to increase with increasing volley strength, although the amount of increase varies in different cells. The results indicate that in the rabbit the PG cells, like the mitral cells, are excited monosynaptically by the olfactory-nerve terminals in

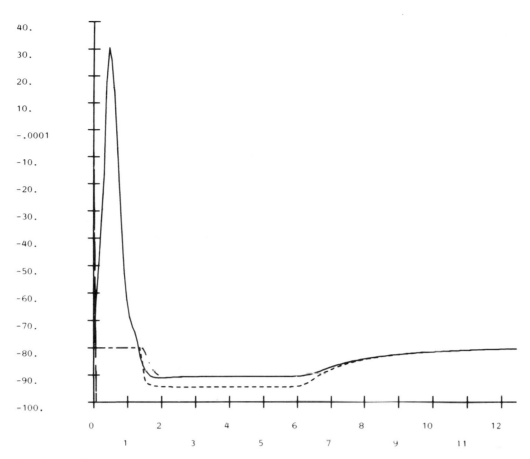

FIGURE 6 Computed activity in the dendrodendritic circuit of Figure 5, elicited by an impulse generated in compartment 1 of M_1. The impulse recorded from M_1 is shown as a solid line; it spreads electrotonically through compartments 2–5, activating the reciprocal synapse connecting mitral compartment 3 to granule spine head 1, which feeds back self-inhibition onto mitral compartment 3 (note the hyperpolarizing IPSP in M_1 dendrite in the aftermath of the impulse). The depolarization set up in granule-cell spine head 1 spreads into the granule dendrite and into the second spine 3 (see Figure 5), activating the inhibitory part of the reciprocal synapse onto compartment 3 of the M_2 dendrite. This mediates lateral inhibition onto the M_2 dendrite, as seen in the hyperpolarizing IPSP in compartment 3 (dashed line) and compartment 1 (dashed-dotted line). Note the similarity of these traces to the experimental recordings in Figure 2B.

the glomeruli. Following this excitatory period, there is characteristically a period during which the response to a second volley is suppressed or shortened in duration. This period may last for several hundred milliseconds. A similar period occurs in mitral cells, where, of course, the IPSP due mainly to granule-cell inhibition occurs (see Figure 2). The suppression of PG cells at longer testing intervals can be shown to be independent of the olfactory-nerve recovery cycle, leaving us to assess the effects of PG-cell impulse activity.

To do this we studied PG-cell units at threshold for single-spike initiation by weak ON volleys. In some cells the test response was facilitated in terms of threshold and/or latency; this response characteristically began early and could last up to 30 msec. In some cases the test response was suppressed. In Figure 7, for example, there is early blockage due to absolute refractoriness, a relative refractory recovery phase, and, finally, blockage at 15 msec intervals and beyond. Although electrophysiologists often use strong volleys to elicit clear-cut response patterns, the use of very weak ones, as in these studies, may be more productive of evidence about synaptic connections and the properties of small intrinsic neurons.

Mitral cells undergo similar periods of facilitation and suppression following an ON volley (Getchell and Shepherd, 1975a); this raises the interesting question of the relation between the PG-cell and mitral-cell responses. The Renshaw-cell model (Eccles, Fatt, and Koketsu, 1955) requires the IPSP mediated by an interneuron to be coincident with an impulse

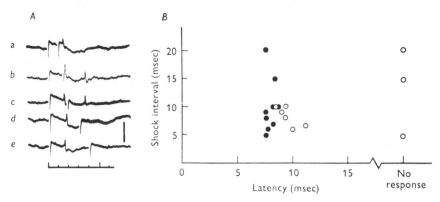

FIGURE 7 Extracellular unit responses in glomerular layer to paired ON volleys. (A) Responses shown at increasing shock intervals; note suppression of test response at shortest (a) and longest (d, e) intervals. Time in 5 msec divisions. (B) Plots of data; filled circles indicate spike responses to conditioning volleys, open circles to testing volleys. (From Getchell and Shepherd, 1975b.)

discharge in the interneuron; but how can the PG cell be an inhibitory interneuron for the mitral cell when it appears to be inhibited itself? The answer lies in a consideration of the dendrodendritic arrangements in the glomeruli. As shown in Figure 8, beginning on the left, the simplest types of synaptic pathways identified in EM studies are the monosynaptic olfactory-nerve connections onto mitral-cell and PG-cell dendrites and the disynaptic pathways through dendrodendritic synapses. PG cells also have reciprocal synapses onto mitral cells. A circuit thus exists whereby the PG-cell dendrite can inhibit the mitral-cell dendrite and, by so doing, block further excitatory input to itself; that is, it presynaptically inhibits itself from responding to further olfactory-nerve input. This mechanism provides a tentative explanation for the physiological results described above and indicates that dendrodendritic pathways can provide for a relationship between impulse firing

and the inhibitory action of a short-axon cell that is different from that of the Renshaw-cell model.

This example also underscores the caution one must exercise in basing interpretations of synaptic interactions on extracellular spike data. Studies of spike discharge patterns in other parts of the nervous system may warrant reinvestigation on this account, particularly in regions where dendrodendritic synapses are known to exist or are suspected. In many such regions, "impulse flow" may give only a limited indication of the actual information flow through the synaptic circuits. This consideration appears to be important in developing strategies for studying the functional properties of local neuronal circuits.

Natural stimulation

Thus far we have considered methods of analysis that involve brief, artificial activation of local circuits from volleys produced by electrical shocks. The next step is to use natural stimulation. For this purpose we need synchronous activation by a stimulus defined in time course and in spatial locus. The ability to control stimuli in this way has been fundamental to the analysis of neuronal properties and mechanisms in the visual (Kuffler, 1953), auditory (Galambos and Davis, 1943), and somatosensory (Mountcastle, 1957) systems, to name only the best-known examples. In these systems it has been relatively easy to generate well-defined step pulses, ramps, and sinusoidal stimuli. In the olfactory system, however, we are dealing with stimuli—volatile gases—that are very difficult to work with. In fact, when we began our experiments several years ago there were no methods for delivering and monitoring the stimuli equivalent to those used for other sensory systems.

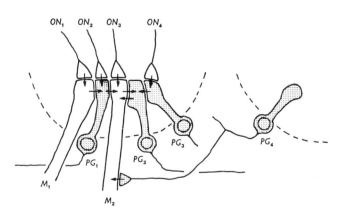

FIGURE 8 Schematic diagram summarizing evidence from EM and electrophysiological studies for synaptic circuits in the glomerular layer of the olfactory bulb. (From Getchell and Shepherd, 1975b.)

The instrumentation we have developed (Kauer and Shepherd, 1975a,b) consists of a system of concentric nozzles that deliver step pulses of odor to the exposed olfactory receptor sheet of a salamander. The step pulses have a relatively abrupt onset, a steady plateau phase, and an abrupt termination. The duration and concentration of the stimulus can be independently varied. For monitoring the stimulus a low percent CO_2 is introduced into the odor carrier stream; this is measured by a CO_2 analyzer with a small inlet port positioned over the olfactory receptor sheet at the site of stimulation.

Typical results obtained with these methods are shown in Figure 9. These are recordings of extracellular spike activity in a mitral cell. The stimulus is the odor of amyl acetate, delivered in step pulses lasting 4 sec, as shown by the lower traces. At the lowest concentration (d), just over threshold for this unit, there is a prolonged impulse discharge. At a higher concentration (c), the discharge has a higher frequency, shorter onset latency, and briefer duration, and it is followed by a period of suppression. These changes become more pronounced at higher concentrations (b, a). Note that at the highest concentration (a), the response consists of only two spikes separated by a brief interval and followed by complete suppression for the remainder of the pulse.

We found that there are three main types of activity correlated with pulse stimuli: initially excitatory, initially suppressive, and no change (unaffected). These categories were originally described by Kauer (1974), and our results confirm them and show the precise relation between the timing of the response and the stimulus. As in the earlier study, cells are not specific for particular odors; among the battery of odors used, a given cell may show all three response categories.

With regard to synaptic circuits, the results have some interesting implications. The prolonged discharge at threshold suggests a prolonged impulse input through the receptor axons and correspondingly prolonged excitatory synaptic drive in the glomeruli, but with minimal inhibitory synaptic actions. As odor concentration increases, it appears that the receptor impulse activity increases pari passu, causing earlier and more intense excitatory synaptic drive to the mitral cells, but it also activates circuits that provide for suppression, which cuts off the impulse response; suppression then continues for the duration of stimulation. It is tempting to correlate this suppression with synaptic inhibition through the dendrodendritic pathways as described above. Our present work is directed to obtaining further evidence for the properties of this inhibition and attempting to identify the contributions at the external plexiform and glomerular levels.

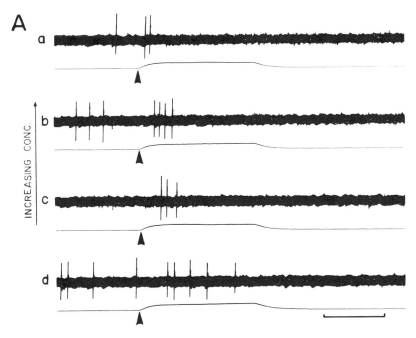

FIGURE 9 Extracellular unit responses in salamander olfactory bulb to odor pulse stimuli delivered to the olfactory mucosa. Lower traces are pulse monitors, with onsets indicated by arrows. Successive trials at increasing concentration as shown; test odor was amyl acetate. Time, 4 msec. (From Kauer and Shepherd, 1977.)

These results demonstrate that odor stimuli can be controlled and monitored in a manner equivalent to that in other sensory systems. This control greatly facilitates the analysis of response properties of neurons and synaptic circuits under conditions of natural stimulation; and in some cases findings can be directly compared with results from electrical stimulation. For example, the prolonged discharge at threshold, with little evidence of inhibition, correlates well with the finding that the mitral-cell response to a test volley in the olfactory nerves shows little evidence of suppression when the shocks are very weak. With odor stimulation at higher concentrations, the excitatory-suppressive sequence in some mitral cells is very clear, which correlates with the excitatory-inhibitory sequence in the mitral-cell response to strong olfactory-nerve volleys. We need close correlations of this type, using both electrophysiological and natural modes of stimulation, in the analysis of local circuits. Our results indicate that they are possible in the olfactory bulb; they show further that the functional properties of local circuits are not rigidly set but may change dramatically in relation to submodality of stimulus and levels of activation.

Metabolic mapping

One traditionally thinks of functional analysis of the nervous system in terms of electrophysiological methods; but other approaches are possible for detecting changes in activity of cells. One of the most promising is the use of 2-deoxyglucose (2DG), as introduced by Sokoloff and his colleagues (Kennedy et al., 1975; Plum, Gjedde, and Sampson, 1976). This glucose analog is taken up by nervous tissue and phosphorylated by the same mechanisms as glucose, but it cannot be further metabolized. Thus, when radioactively labeled with ^{14}C and introduced in tracer amounts, 2DG can be used to give autoradiograms revealing regions in which nerve cells have changed their activity and hence their glucose requirements. Early results have shown local regions of activity-related 2DG uptake in relation to sciatic-nerve stimulation, ocular ablations, and focally induced epilepsy (Kennedy et al., 1975; Collins et al., 1976). These results have been consistent with evidence from previous studies using electrophysiological methods, but they have gone further in providing maps of the simultaneous activity changes throughout the nervous system.

Our interest in this method was based on the rationale that it was particularly sensitive to activity changes in neuropil, that is, in synaptic terminals and local synaptic circuits. It was therefore well suited for determining whether or not spatial patterns of activity are present in olfactory bulb neuropil during odor stimulation. The possibility of such patterns had been suggested (Mozell, 1971; Moulton, 1976), but the electrophysiological evidence was fragmentary and unsatisfactory.

Our experiments involve injecting rats with a pulse of ^{14}C-2DG and placing them in a closed glass chamber with a controlled olfactory environment for 45 minutes (Sharp, Kauer, and Shepherd, 1975, 1977). The brains are then rapidly removed and frozen, the bulbs are sectioned, and X-ray autoradiograms are prepared according to the Sokoloff method.

In control rats breathing room air, there is a broad band of relatively high activity in the autoradiograms of the olfactory bulb, extending from the glomerular layer to the granule layer. Individual layers can be discerned in favorable sections, and the glomerular and mitral-cell layers typically have high levels of resting activity. A characteristic finding is the presence of scattered very small dense foci, and careful correlation with the histology shows that these are located over groups of glomeruli. It appears that these foci are in some way related to olfactory input under conditions of minimal stimulation of olfactory receptors by odors in the ambient room air.

Under conditions of odor stimulation, larger areas of increased activity are characteristically found in the olfactory bulb. Figure 10 shows a typical result for the case of stimulation with the odor of amyl acetate. A broad band of increased activity is found in the anterolateral aspect of the bulb, and another similar band is found in the posteromedial aspect. Histological correlations show that these bands have peak density in the glomerular layer and spread into adjacent olfactory-nerve and external plexiform layers. This general pattern of activity is found in different animals subjected to this odor, suggesting that the pattern may represent a spatial distribution of activity important for transmission of this olfactory input. Furthermore, preliminary evidence indicates that patterns may be different for different odors and may thus reveal an essential aspect of the mechanisms of discrimination between odors. The results in the rat olfactory bulb have been confirmed and extended in studies of the olfactory bulb of the tree shrew (Skeen, 1977).

Synaptic transmitters

I shall conclude this review of experimental methods by considering briefly the identification of transmitter

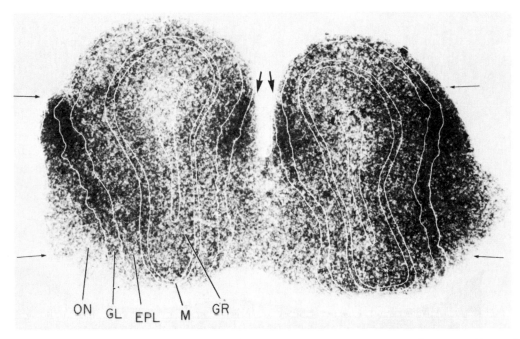

ON GL EPL M GR

FIGURE 10 Autoradiograph of frontal sections of olfactory bulbs of a rat exposed to strong odor of amyl acetate. The outlines of the histological layers of the olfactory bulb, as determined from the subsequently stained sections, are shown superimposed on the autoradiographs. Small arrows indicate extent of lateral active regions; large arrows indicate medial active regions. Scale bar is 500 μm. (From Sharp, Kauer, and Shepherd, 1977.)

substances. Only in very recent years have adequate techniques become available so that one can begin to approach this problem with confidence in the central nervous system. A number of later chapters in this volume testify to the range of methods now available.

In the olfactory bulb the best case for a specific transmitter substance can be made for the granule-to-mitral dendrodendritic synapse. Microiontophoretic studies, combined with single unit recordings, have provided evidence that GABA is the transmitter substance at this synapse (McLennan, 1971; Nicoll, 1971). Iontophoresis of GABA produces suppression of mitral-cell activity, mimicking the suppression following LOT volleys. Iontophoresis of bicuculline, a known blocker of GABA, blocks the LOT-induced inhibition of mitral cells. More recently it has been shown that radioactively labeled GABA is taken up by granule cells. (Halász, Ljungdahl, and Hökfelt, 1978). Moreover, an immunocytochemical study has provided evidence for the localization of the GABA-synthesizing enzyme GAD in granule cells (Ribak et al., 1977). High GAD activity has been reported in the external plexiform layer and presumably reflects GABA synthesis in granule-cell dendrites and spines in that layer (Graham, 1973).

With regard to the other half of the reciprocal synapse in the external plexiform layer, microiontophoretic studies have shown that mitral cells are also suppressed by amino acids such as aspartate and D-L homocysteate (McLennan, 1971; Nicoll, 1971). At first this seemed paradoxical, since these substances have excitatory actions at many other central synapses. The explanation appears to be that they may exert their excitatory action on the granule cells, thereby mimicking the excitatory dendrodendritic synaptic actions of the mitral-to-granule half of the reciprocal synapse. The excited granule cells then inhibit the mitral cells reciprocally, so that the observed effect is mitral-cell inhibition. This interpretation awaits further testing, but it serves as an important caution for the interpretation of microiontophoretic studies in other parts of the nervous system. It is clear that one cannot assume that the substance iontophoresed acts directly on the cell recorded from. Any synaptic terminal or local circuit element that carries receptors, specific or nonspecific, for that substance may be activated by it and transmit the ultimate effect on the cell recorded from by its own local action or that of the circuits of which it is a part.

In the glomerular layer there has long been evidence for catecholamine uptake and synthesis (Lichtensteiger, 1965). Recently Halász et al. (1977) have shown with immunocytochemical methods that periglomerular-cell bodies are positive for dopamine (DA)-synthesizing enzymes. The reaction extends

LOCAL CIRCUITS IN THE OLFACTORY BULB   139

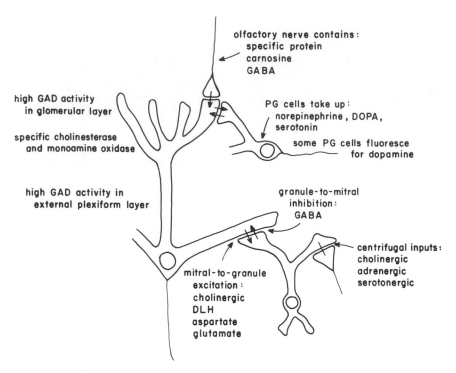

olfactory nerve contains:
specific protein
carnosine
GABA

high GAD activity
in glomerular layer

specific cholinesterase
and monoamine oxidase

PG cells take up:
norepinephrine, DOPA,
serotonin

some PG cells fluoresce
for dopamine

high GAD activity in
external plexiform layer

granule-to-mitral
inhibition:
GABA

centrifugal inputs:
cholinergic
adrenergic
serotonergic

mitral-to-granule
excitation:
cholinergic
DLH
aspartate
glutamate

FIGURE 11 Summary of evidence for neurotransmitter substances in the olfactory bulb. For details see text. (Modified from Shepherd, 1977.)

into the dendrites, suggesting that DA may function as the transmitter at dendrodendritic as well as axodendritic synapses of the PG cells. However, only a part of the population of cells around the glomeruli contain these enzymes. This fact provides a most interesting hypothesis—that the periglomerular-cell population may consist of metabolically distinct subpopulations that use different transmitter substances and, therefore, could have different synaptic actions. This hypothesis suggests a biochemical fractionation of an anatomically defined and otherwise homogeneous cell type. A new complexity is thus introduced into the functional significance of cell types in the nervous system—a complexity that is obviously relevant to the organization of the local circuits within a given region. Similar observations have been made in the amacrine-cell population in the retina (see Miller, this volume). In the olfactory bulb further work is needed to determine the subtypes of PG cells that subserve the inhibitory actions attributed to PG cells by the electrophysiological studies. The PG cell appears to be the first short-axon cell type in the CNS in which DA has been identified as a possible neurotransmitter. Some tufted cells also appear to synthesize DA (Halász et al., 1977). Recently a second subpopulation of PG cells, which synthesize GABA, has been identified (Ribak et al., 1977).

The biochemical constituents of the olfactory nerves have been studied intensively in recent years. A protein has been described that is unique to these nerves and the receptor cells from which they arise (Margolis, 1974). A dipeptide, carnosine, has also been found in these cells and axons; it is present in higher concentration there than in any other region of the nervous system (Margolis, 1974; Neidle and Kandera, 1974). Its function and possible relation to chemical transmission by the nerve terminals in the glomeruli is intriguing but as yet unknown.

The other main extrinsic fiber systems to the olfactory bulb are the efferent pathways from the CNS. The bulb is one of the regions that receives terminals from the adrenergic and serotoninergic fibers arising in the brain stem (Halász, Ljungdahl, and Hökfelt, 1978). These terminals are found on granule-cell spines, where they are strategically located for producing inhibition of the mitral cells or biasing the mitral- and granule-cell interactions. Some connections to the periglomerular regions are also known.

From this brief review it can be seen that there is evidence regarding possible neurotransmitters for most of the main neuronal types and extrinsic fiber systems in the olfactory bulb. In this respect progress is equivalent to that in regions such as retina or cerebellum. A special significance of the olfactory bulb for these studies may rest in the evidence for neurotransmitters at dendrodendritic synapses. The optic tectum is another central region where considerable progress has been made, including evidence for possible transmitters at dendrodendritic synapses (see Cuénod, this volume). Other regions, such as the basal ganglia, have also been studied intensively, and there is tentative evidence for important synaptic interaction between dendrites in some of these regions. Progress in neurochemical studies will be closely dependent on knowledge of the organization of the local circuits within the regions under study.

Discussion

The experiments that have been reviewed illustrate the proposition set out in the introduction to this section—that a correlation of results from different methodologies is essential in the effort to understand the nature of nervous organization. In addition, general comment may be made on two further aspects, one practical and the other theoretical.

On the practical side, it is worth remembering that physiological study of the olfactory bulb was initially based on traditional methods of electrophysiological analysis suitable for motoneurons and other large impulse-generating projection neurons in the nervous system. Electron-microscopic study of synaptic connections was also begun at a time when only the types of synapses made by projection neurons with long axons had been recognized. These approaches by themselves have been successful in the olfactory bulb up to a point; but one of the lessons emerging most clearly from this work is that our methods and the tactics of applying them must be reevaluated and modified for the task of analyzing local synaptic circuits and local synaptic properties. Evidence of the presence of output synapses on dendrites and their activation by local graded potentials is the most urgent need. I pointed out earlier that "impulse flow" as monitored by extracellular unit recordings can no longer be relied upon as an accurate reflection of "synaptic flow"—that is, of the activity mediated by local synaptic circuits. Even with intracellular recordings, the compartmentalization of dendritic trees severely restricts the utility of a soma recording site in monitoring or testing the input-output relations mediated by circuits into and out of distant dendritic compartments. The development of improved recording techniques and isolated preparations are important steps toward obtaining stable recordings from intrinsic neurons and dendrites; even so, the effects of electrode impalement on local properties

and the electrotonic constraints on the sampling of activity will have to be rigorously assessed. With regard to neurochemical aspects, it is likely that the simple picture of brief synaptic potentials mediated by punctate synaptic junctions will be much embellished as more is learned about the variety of morphophysiological relations at different junctions and the variety of longer-term effects a terminal may exert through substances acting on neighboring terminals as well as on itself. Considerations such as these indicate that the practical problems facing experimental analysis of local circuits are considerable; but they also leave little doubt that it is here that the basic mechanisms of neuronal organization are to be found.

On the theoretical side, a key problem is to develop a conceptual framework for the new types of organization that have come into view through the work on local circuits. In the olfactory bulb, some clues have been provided by the organization of synaptic circuits in relation to the dendrites of the principal and intrinsic neuronal populations. I have discussed this elsewhere on several occasions (Shepherd, 1972b, 1974, 1975, 1977, 1978). Here it will suffice to say that, beginning with the single synapse as the basic unit, several levels of organization of increasing extent and complexity can be identified in terms of synaptic clusters, dendritic branching compartments, whole dendritic trees, the whole neuron, and multineuronal chains and loops. This view of the olfactory bulb emerges rather naturally from simple structural considerations. Present analysis of functional operations is being carried out within this context, as illustrated by the model of the reciprocal synapse and the dendritic branch compartments of the mitral and granule cells, as in Figure 5.

There is evidence that similar types of synaptic circuits and functional properties are found in a number of other regions. We thus face two key questions. First, can logical hierarchies of levels of organization be identified in all regions? Second, can the levels in any given region be systematically correlated in a meaningful way with those in other regions? Against these propositions it has been argued that every neuron is unique and that the information processed in each is different in kind from that of any other region. However, the evidence seems to be increasing that, behind the welter of detail, there may indeed be some relatively limited and common principles of organization along the lines indicated above, that apply, to a greater or lesser extent, to all types of nervous organization. Both points of view were expressed in the formal and informal discussions at this Study Program and represent at least a preliminary attack on this important issue.

Although these matters are speculative, they touch on a requirement of any field for a consensus on the basic units of organization. We have traditionally thought of the basic structural unit as the neuron and its basic functional property as the impulse. But at the level of local circuits, these units lose their force and generality: input-output operations may be carried out through restricted parts of whole neurons, and local synaptic transmission and integration may take place in the absence of impulse activity. Impulse activity of course underlies the excitability that has always been regarded as the hallmark of nervous tissue; yet not only do some nerve cells function without this activity, there are a number of nonnervous types of cells, in both animals and plants, that also exhibit this property (see Mueller, this volume).

It thus appears that the study of local synaptic circuits in the olfactory bulb, retina, and other regions requires a reassessment of our traditional beliefs about the essential nature of nervous organization. The case for retaining traditional tenets in the face of the new evidence has been argued eloquently by Peters, Palay, and Webster (1976). The problem, in fact, is not to discard these tenets, but rather to incorporate them into a new framework. I have suggested elsewhere (Shepherd, 1972b, 1977) that this can be developed around the functional operations carried out at the different levels of organization. In this view, neuronal units are replaced by functional units, and the traditional neuron doctrine is incorporated into a set of functional principles that begins with the single synapse as the simplest unit and builds in complexity through the successive levels of organization. At each level the synaptic circuits comprise the basic units for information processing, the processing being carried out by the ensemble of units at that level of complexity. Since the functional operations are largely defined by synaptic properties and circuits, it is possible that the organizing principles we seek will be eventually subsumed under the heading of a synaptic doctrine. If this can serve as a means to orient the search for common principles that account for the diversity of nervous-system structures and functions, it will have some heuristic value.

REFERENCES

Andres, K. H., 1965. Der Feinbau des Bulbus Olfactorius der Ratte unter besonderer Berücksichtigung der Synaptischen Verbindungen. *Z. Zellforsch.* 65:530–561.

Collins, R. C., C. Kennedy, L. Sokoloff, and F. Plum, 1976. Metabolic anatomy of focal seizures. *Arch. Neurol.* 33:536–542.

Eccles, J. C., P. Fatt, and K. Koketsu, 1955. Cholinergic and inhibitory synapses in a pathway from motor-axon collaterals to motoneurones. *J. Physiol.* 216:524–562.

Eccles, J. C., B. Libet, and R. R. Young, 1958. The behavior of chromatolyzed motoneurons studied by intracellular recording. *J. Physiol.* 143:11–40.

Galambos, R., and H. Davis, 1943. The response of single auditory-nerve fibers to acoustic stimulation. *J. Neurophysiol.* 6:424–437.

Getchell, T. V., and G. M. Shepherd, 1975a. Synaptic actions on mitral and tufted cells elicited by olfactory nerve volleys in the rabbit. *J. Physiol.* 251:497–522.

Getchell, T. V., and G. M. Shepherd, 1975b. Short-axon cells in the olfactory bulb: Dendrodendritic synaptic interactions. *J. Physiol.* 251:523–548.

Goldstein, S. S., and W. Rall, 1974. Changes of action potential shape and velocity for changing core conductor geometry. *Biophys. J.* 14:731–757.

Graham, L. T., 1973. Distribution of glutamic acid decarboxylase activity and GABA content in the olfactory bulb. *Life Sci.* 12:443–447.

Halász, N., A. Ljungdahl, T. Hökfelt, O. Johansson, M. Goldstein, D. Park, and P. Biberfeld, 1977. Transmitter histochemistry of the rat olfactory bulb. I. Immunohistochemical localization of monoamine synthesizing enzymes: Support for intrabulbar, periglomerular dopamine neurons. *Brain Res.* 126:455–474.

Halász, N., A. Ljungdahl, and T. Hökfelt, 1978. Transmitter histochemistry of the rat olfactory bulb. II. Fluorescence histochemical, autoradiographic and electron microscopic localization of monoamines. *Brain Res.* (in press).

Halász, N., A. Ljungdahl, and T. Hökfelt, 1978. Transmitter histochemistry of the olfactory bulb. III. Autoradiographic localization of ^{3}H-GABA, glycine and leucine. *Brain Res.* (in press).

Hirata, Y., 1964. Some observations on the fine structure of the synapses in the olfactory bulb of the mouse, with particular reference to the atypical synaptic configuration. *Arch. Histol. Jap.* 24:293–302.

Kauer, J. S., 1974. Response patterns of amphibian olfactory bulb neurones to odour stimulation. *J. Physiol.* 243:695–715.

Kauer, J. S., and G. M. Shepherd, 1975a. Olfactory stimulation with controlled and monitored step pulses of odor. *Brain Res.* 85:108–113.

Kauer, J. S., and G. M. Shepherd, 1975b. Concentration-specific responses of salamander olfactory bulb units. *J. Physiol.* 252:49–50.

Kennedy, C., M. H. Des Rosiers, J. W. Jehle, M. Reivich, F. R. Sharp, and L. Sokoloff, 1975. Mapping of functional neural pathways by autoradiographic survey of local metabolic rate with (^{14}C) deoxyglucose. *Science* 187:850–853.

Klee, M., and W. Rall, 1977. Computed potentials of cortically arranged populations of neurons. *J. Neurophysiol.* 40:647–666.

Kuffler, S. W., 1953. Discharge patterns and functional organization of mammalian retina. *J. Neurophysiol.* 16:37–68.

Landis, D. M. D., and T. S. Reese, 1974. Differences in

membrane structure between excitatory and inhibitory synapses in the cerebellar cortex. *J. Comp. Neurol.* 155:93–126.

LANDIS, D. M. D., T. S. REESE, and E. RAVIOLA, 1974. Differences in membrane structure between excitatory and inhibitory components of the reciprocal synapse in the olfactory bulb. *J. Comp. Neurol.* 155:67–92.

LICHTENSTEIGER, W., 1965. Uptake of norepinephrine in periglomerular cells of the olfactory bulb in the mouse. *Nature* 210:955–956.

LLINÁS, R., and C. NICHOLSON, 1971. Electrophysiological properties of dendrites and somata in alligator Purkinje cells. *J. Neurophysiol.* 34:532–551.

McLENNAN, H., 1971. The pharmacology of inhibition of mitral cells in the olfactory bulb. *Brain Res.* 29:177–184.

MARGOLIS, F. L., 1974. Carnosine in the primary olfactory pathway. *Science* 184:909–911.

MARGOLIS, F. L., and J. F. TARNOFF, 1973. Site of biosynthesis of the mouse brain olfactory bulb protein. *J. Biol. Chem.* 248:451–455.

MORI, K., and S. F. TAKAGI, 1975. Spike generation in the mitral cell dendrite of the rabbit olfactory bulb. *Brain Res.* 100:685–689.

MOULTON, D. G., 1976. Spatial patterning of responses to odors in the peripheral olfactory system. *Physiol. Rev.* 56:578–593.

MOUNTCASTLE, V. B., 1957. Modality and topographic properties of single neurons of cat's somatic sensory cortex. *J. Neurophysiol.* 20:408–434.

MOZELL, M. M., 1971. Spatial and temporal patterning. In *Handbook of Physiology*, vol. 4, *Chemical Senses 1: Olfaction*, L. M. Beidler, ed. Berlin: Springer, pp. 205–215.

NEIDLE, A., and J. KANDERA, 1974. Carnosine—An olfactory bulb peptide. *Brain Res.* 80:359–364.

NICOLL, R. A., 1971. Pharmacological evidence for GABA as the transmitter in granule-cell inhibition in the olfactory bulb. *Brain Res.* 35:137–149.

PETERS, A., S. L. PALAY, and H. DE F. WEBSTER, 1976. *The Fine Structure of the Nervous System.* Philadelphia: Saunders.

PHILLIPS, C. G., T. P. S. POWELL, and G. M. SHEPHERD, 1963. Responses of mitral cells to stimulation of the lateral olfactory tract on the rabbit. *J. Physiol.* 168:65–88.

PINCHING, A. J., 1971. Myelinated dendritic segments in the monkey olfactory bulb. *Brain Res.* 29:133–138.

PINCHING, A. J., and T. P. S. POWELL. 1971b. The neuropil of the glomeruli of the olfactory bulb. *J. Cell Sci.* 9:347–377.

PLUM, F., A. GJEDDE, and F. E. SAMSON, 1976. Neuroanatomical functional mapping by the radioactive 2-deoxy-D-glucose method. *NRP Bulletin* 14:457–518.

PRICE, J. L. and T. P. S. POWELL, 1970. The synaptology of the granule cells of the olfactory bulb. *J. Cell Sci.* 7:125–155.

RALL, W., 1977. Core conductor theory and cable properties of neurons. In *Handbook of Physiology*, section 1, volume 1, E. R. Kandel, ed. Baltimore: Williams & Wilkins, pp. 39–97.

RALL, W., and G. M. SHEPHERD, 1968. Theoretical reconstruction of field potentials and dendrodendritic synaptic interactions in olfactory bulb. *J. Neurophysiol.* 31:884–915.

RALL, W., G. M. SHEPHERD, T. S. REESE, and M. W. BRIGHTMAN, 1965. Dendro dendritic synaptic pathway for inhibition in the olfactory bulb. *Exp. Neurol.* 14:44–56.

RAMÓN Y CAJAL, S., 1911. *Histologie du système nerveux de l'homme et des vertébrés.* Paris: Maloine.

REESE, T. S., and G. M. SHEPHERD. 1972. Dendro-dendritic synapses in the central nervous system. In *Structure and Function of Synapses*, G. D. Pappas and D. P. Purpura, eds. New York: Raven, pp. 121–136.

RIBAK, C. E., J. E. VAUGHN, K. SAITO, R. BARBER, and E. ROBERTS, 1977. Glutamate decarboxylase localization in the neurons of the olfactory bulb. *Brain Res.* 126:1–18.

SHARP, F. R., J. S. KAUER, and G. M. SHEPHERD, 1975. Local sites of activity-related glucose metabolism in rat olfactory bulb during odor stimulation. *Brain Res.* 98:596–600.

SHARP, F. R., J. S. KAUER, and G. M. SHEPHERD, 1977. Laminar analysis of 2-deoxyglucose uptake in olfactory bulb and olfactory cortex of rabbit and rat. *J. Neurophysiol.* 40:800–813.

SHEPHERD, G. M., 1963. Neuronal systems controlling mitral cell excitability. *J. Physiol.* 168:101–117.

SHEPHERD, G. M., 1970. The olfactory bulb as a simple cortical system: Experimental analysis and functional implications. In *The Neurosciences: Second Study Program*, F. O. Schmitt, ed. New York: Rockefeller Univ. Press, pp. 539–552.

SHEPHERD, G. M., 1971. Physiological evidence for dendro-dendritic synaptic interactions in the rabbit's olfactory glomerulus. *Brain Res.* 32:212–217.

SHEPHERD, G. M. 1972a. Synaptic organization of the mammalian olfactory bulb. *Physiol. Rev.* 52:864–917.

SHEPHERD, G. M., 1972b. The neuron doctrine: A revision of functional concepts. *Yale J. Biol. Med.* 45:584–599.

SHEPHERD, G. M., 1974. *The Synaptic Organization of the Brain.* New York: Oxford Univ. Press.

SHEPHERD, G. M., 1975. Models of local circuit neuron function in the olfactory bulb. In *Local Circuit Neurons*, P. Rakic, ed. Cambridge, MA: MIT Press, pp. 50–58.

SHEPHERD, G. M., 1977. The olfactory bulb: A simple system in the mammalian brain. In *Handbook of Physiology*, section 1, volume 1, E. R. Kandel, ed. Baltimore: Williams & Wilkins, pp. 945–968.

SHEPHERD, G. M., 1978. Microcircuits in the nervous system. *Sci. Am.* 238(2):92–103.

SHEPHERD, G. M., and L. B. HABERLY, 1970. Partial activation of olfactory bulb: Analysis of field potentials and topographic relation between bulb and lateral olfactory tract. *J. Neurophysiol.* 33:643–653.

SKEEN, L. C. 1977. Odor-induced patterns of deoxyglucose consumption in the olfactory bulb of the tree shrew, *Tupaia glis.* *Brain Res.* 124:147–153.

SPENCER, W. A., and E. R. KANDEL, 1961. Electrophysiology of hippocampal neurons. IV. Fast prepotentials. *J. Neurophysiol.* 24:272–285.

UCHIZONO, K., 1967. Synaptic organization of the Purkinje cells in the cerebellum of the cat. *Exp. Brain Res.* 4:97–113.

WHITE, E. L., 1972. Synaptic organization in the olfactory glomerulus of the mouse. *Brain Res.* 37:69–80.

WHITE, E. L., 1973. Synaptic organization of the mammalian olfactory glomerulus: New findings including an intraspecific variation. *Brain Res.* 60:299–313.

YAMAMOTO, C., T. YAMAMOTO, and K. IWAMA, 1963. The inhibitory system in the olfactory bulb studied by intracellular recording. *J. Neurophysiol.* 26:403–415.

9 Local Neurons and Local Interactions in the Nervous Systems of Invertebrates

K. G. PEARSON

ABSTRACT Local neurons are now known to be widespread throughout the nervous systems of invertebrates. Many of those in the thoracic ganglia of insects function without generating action potentials, so that the patterning of motor activity is to a large extent dependent on graded interactions between nonspiking neurons. Little is known about the functions and properties of other local neurons in invertebrates. Three recent findings indicate that interactions between neurons may sometimes be restricted to localized regions of the processes of invertebrate neurons: (1) the occurrence of reciprocal and serial arrangements of synapses; (2) the location of pre- and postsynaptic sites on the distal ends of secondary processes; and (3) the spatial separation of two or more arborizing regions of the processes of some nonspiking neurons. The different arborizing regions may be electrically isolated from each other and may therefore function independently.

Introduction

ALTHOUGH TREMENDOUS advances in our understanding of the nervous system have been made by studying neurons with long axons, it is now quite apparent that a full description of the integrative events within the nervous system requires a thorough knowledge of the properties and organization of the far more abundant short-axon and axonless neurons, referred to as *local neurons*. This point has been emphasized in a number of recent books and articles (Shepherd, 1974; Rakic, 1975; Gray, 1974; Schmitt, Dev, and Smith, 1976). In general we know little about the properties and function of these neurons. However, one important fact has emerged in recent years: the dendrites of many local neurons, as well as those of some long-axon neurons, can form synaptic connections with dendrites of other neurons. That is, dendrites of some neurons can be both presynaptic and postsynaptic elements and can thus give rise to serial and reciprocal arrangements of synapses between dendrites. Thus we can envisage local interactions involving feedback and/or feedforward loops as oc-

curring at three different levels: (1) interactions through reciprocal and serial synaptic junctions localized to discrete regions of single dendrites; (2) interactions through assemblies of these junctions localized to parts of the dendritic trees; and (3) interactions through local neurons restricted to a small region of the nervous system. Furthermore, it is obvious that many neurons cannot be regarded as single functional units, since different regions of the same neuron may have quite different functions (Nelson et al., 1975).

Shepherd (1972) has suggested that a functional unit be regarded as the anatomical structure serving a specific function. At the lowest level, a single synapse may be a functional unit, whereas at a higher level, specific arrangements of synapses may form a functional unit. For example, many reciprocal synapses found throughout the vertebrate nervous system provide localized inhibitory feedback to the input neuron. Increasingly complex functional units, in which simpler units may be embedded, can easily be envisaged (see Shepherd, this volume).

The concept of a hierarchical arrangement of functional units has been developed exclusively from anatomical and physiological studies on vertebrates (Shepherd, 1972, 1974). However, there is no reason why this concept should not be used when considering integrative processes in the nervous systems of invertebrates.

At present we know very little about local interactions between neurons in invertebrates. The widespread occurrence of local neurons throughout invertebrates, together with the finding of reciprocal and serial synaptic junctions in many regions of their nervous systems, clearly indicates that local interactions play a prominent part in the integration of neural events in these animals. However, there is not a single case in which we fully understand the function of any particular local neuron (or group of local neurons), and the function of none of the reciprocal and serial synaptic junctions so far described is known with certainty. With these caveats in mind, this chap-

K. G. PEARSON Department of Physiology, University of Alberta, Edmonton, Canada

ter will review what we do know about the occurrence, properties, and possible functions of local neurons and about the occurrence and possible functions of reciprocal and serial synapses in these animals.

Local neurons

The usual criterion for classifying a neuron as a local neuron is that all its processes are contained within an anatomically discrete region of the nervous system. However, this criterion is not always satisfactory, since some regions of the nervous system are not structurally well defined. Moreover, at one level certain regions can be considered as discrete, whereas at a finer level they are found to be composed of many distinct regions. For example, each thoracic ganglion in arthropods can be considered a discrete region of the nervous system; yet within each ganglion there are numerous localized regions of neuropil. Are we to classify as local neurons only those whose processes are contained wholly within one region of neuropil, or should all neurons contained entirely within the ganglion be referred to as local neurons? Obviously we could arbitrarily choose one or the other of these criteria. With our present rudimentary knowledge of axonless and short-axon neurons in invertebrates, however, such narrow definitions seem pointless. Thus the general definition given by Bullock (1977) is quite appropriate for the purposes of this article: *a local neuron is one without processes that spread to other neuropil masses, lobes, or other ganglia.*

OCCURRENCE AND STRUCTURE OF LOCAL NEURONS Table I lists the animals and regions within the nervous system in which local neurons have been described. It must be stressed that the table probably indicates only a very small fraction of the cases in which local neurons exist, reflecting the abysmal lack of neuroanatomical data in invertebrates. Perhaps most surprising is the fact that very little is known about the anatomy of some animals upon which an enormous amount of physiological work has been done. For example, there are only a few anatomical studies on the processes of neurons in *Aplysia* (Coggeshall, 1967; Thompson, Schwartz, and Kandel, 1976; Winlow and Kandel, 1976; Gillette and Pomeranz, 1975), and none of these has provided information about the occurrence of local neurons in this animal. This seems strange in light of the fact that large numbers of local neurons have been found in other gastropod molluscs such as the snail (see Bullock and Horridge, 1965, p. 1312). Neuroanatomical studies on the leech segmental ganglion have also failed to reveal the existence of local neurons, but the relatively small number of interganglionic fibers and the existence of local neurons in other annelids such as the earthworm suggest that local neurons are in fact contained within each ganglion (Bullock and Horridge, 1965, p. 688).

Despite our limited knowledge of invertebrate neuroanatomy, it is clear that there is an extraordinary variation in the number of local neurons from one region of the nervous system to another and from one animal to another. There are few, if any, local neurons in nemotodes, for example, whereas there may be as many as 10^8 in the octopus brain (Young, 1971). Some lobes of the octopus brain are composed almost entirely of local neurons; in the vertical lobe there are approximately 25 million local neurons and only 65,000 neurons with axons that leave the lobe. Densely packed masses of small local neurons are also found in certain brain regions of gastropod molluscs, arthropods, some polychaetes, and some nemertineans. These neurons have large, dense, chromatin-rich nuclei and are commonly known as globuli cells. The corpora pedunculata (mushroom bodies) in the insect brain consist almost entirely of globuli cells. The highest numbers of these cells occur in insects that display the most complex patterns of behavior—for example, bees and ants—and the lowest in those with a simple behavioral repertoire—for example, butterflies (Howse, 1974). Within a single order, however, there is not always a correlation between the size of the corpora pedunculata and behavioral complexity; for example, in termites there is a decrease in brain size and number of neurons as behavioral complexity increases (Howse, 1974). The occurrence of globuli cells in polychaete worms is also related to behavior; they are entirely absent from sedentary worms but occur in some, but not all, families of active worms.

It is tempting to suggest that, in general, the number of local neurons is related to the complexity of the behavioral repertoire. Certainly they exist in large numbers in the brains of cephalopod molluscs and social insects, two groups that have a rich behavioral repertoire; and they may be entirely absent from simpler animals such as nematodes, sedentary polychaetes, and many coelenterates that possess limited behavioral repertoires. However, because of the enormous diversity in the structure of the nervous system and the behavior of invertebrates, this general correlation has little heuristic value. This situation contrasts with that in vertebrates, where the progressive increase with phylogeny in the absolute and relative numbers of local neurons in the cortex and

TABLE I
Descriptions of local neurons in invertebrates

Phylum	Animal	Location	Reference
Coelenterates	Jellyfish	Marginal ganglion	Horridge, 1956
Platyhelminths	Flatworm	Brain/commissures	*Hanstrom, 1926 (547)
Nemertineans	Ribbonworm	Brain	*Burger, 1891 (584)
Annelids	Polychaete worm	Brain	*Hanstrom, 1927 (717)
		Segmental ganglia	Smith, 1957
	Earthworm	Brain	*Ogawa, 1939 (724)
		Ventral cord ganglia	*Ogawa, 1939 (686)
Arthropods			
Arachnids	Horseshoe crab	Corpora pedunculata	*Hanstrom, 1926 (1256)
	Spider	Ventral ganglia	*Hanstrom, 1919 (886)
Crustaceans	Crab	Brain/optic lobe	*Hanstrom, 1924 (833)
		Ventral cord	*Bethe, 1897 (859)
	Crayfish	Abdominal ganglia	*Retzius, 1890 (855)
Insects	Ant	Corpora pedunculata	Vowles, 1955
		Optic ganglia	Ribi, 1975b
	Bee	Corpora pedunculata	Vowles, 1955
		Optic ganglia	Ribi, 1975b
	Butterfly	Corpora pedunculata	L. Pearson, 1971
	Cockroach	Corpora pedunculata	Maynard, 1967
		Thoracic ganglion	Pearson and Fourtner, 1975
	Dragonfly	Optic ganglia	Arnett Kibel et al., 1977
		Thoracic ganglia	Zawarzin, 1924
		Abdominal ganglia	Zawarzin, 1924
	Fly	Optic ganglia	Strausfeld, 1970
	Locust	Thoracic ganglion	Burrows and Siegler, 1976
Molluscs	Clam	Visceral ganglion	*Freidenfelt, 1904 (1394)
	Snail	Brain	*Hanstrom, 1925 (1312)
	Octopus	Brain/optic lobe	Young, 1971
		Stellate ganglion	Gray, 1974
	Squid	Subesophageal lobes	Young, 1976
		Optic lobe	Young, 1974

* Cited in Bullock and Horridge (1965). The number in parentheses is the page number of the citation.

other brain regions (Ramón y Cajal, 1911) suggests that local neurons are critically involved in those behaviors which are most highly elaborated in humans (see Rakic, 1975, for a discussion of this point).

The structure of local neurons in invertebrates is quite varied (see Figures 1 and 2), although in general they have small somata (less than 20 μm) and fine, highly branched processes. The majority of invertebrate local neurons described so far lack axons and can therefore be classified as amacrine cells. By contrast, there are very few local neurons resembling the short-axon, Golgi type II neurons found in vertebrates. This is a striking difference between verte-

brates and invertebrates, for the majority of local neurons in vertebrates have short axons (Rakic, 1975). Globuli cells in the corpora pedunculata of polychaetes and insects have a long axonlike process (Figure 2A); in the cockroach this process appears to conduct action potentials away from the processes located near the soma (Maynard, 1967). In this respect globuli cells resemble vertebrate Golgi type II neurons. The resemblance is superficial, however, since the axonlike processes make numerous synaptic contacts along their length with the processes of other neurons (Schürmann, 1971). Thus these processes are doing more than simply relaying information

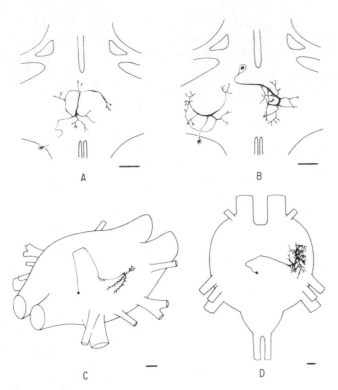

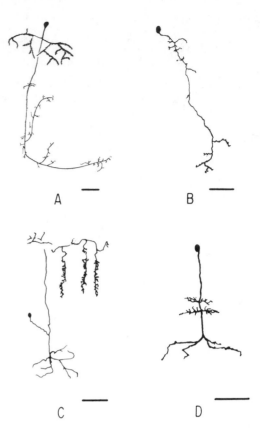

FIGURE 1 Local neurons in the thoracic ganglia of insects. (A, B) Dragonfly larva (redrawn from Zawarzin, 1924). (C) Cockroach (from Pearson and Fourtner, 1975). (D) Locust (from Burrows and Siegler, 1976). (Calibration = 100 μm.)

FIGURE 2 Examples of local neurons in the invertebrate brain. (A) Intrinsic neuron in the corpora pedunculata of a butterfly (redrawn from L. Pearson, 1971). (B) Microneuron in the pedal lobe of the squid (from Young, 1976). (C) Amacrine cell in the medulla of a bee (from Ribi, 1975a). (D) Amacrine cell in the optic lobe of the octopus (from Young, 1964). (Calibration = 50 μm.)

from one region to another. Another possible example of a short-axon local neuron in invertebrates has been described in the thoracic ganglia of dragonfly larvae (Figure 1A). Although this neuron has a long, unbranched process, it is not certain that it is an axon (Zawarzin, 1924); nor is there any evidence that this process conducts action potentials. So neither this neuron nor the neurons of the corpora pedunculata can be confidently classified as short-axon neurons; and since there are no other descriptions of short-axon local neurons in invertebrates, we must conclude that they are rare or nonexistent.

There are numerous examples of identified interneurons in the central nervous systems of invertebrates (Kandel, 1976; Bullock, 1977), and even the smallest may be identifiable (Goodman, 1976). However, only a few can be classified as local neurons. Three different local neurons in the thoracic ganglia of dragonfly larvae are shown in Figures 1A and 1B. There is only one of each of these neurons for each half-ganglion (Zawarzin, 1924). A single local neuron has been described in the cockroach metathoracic ganglion (Pearson and Fourtner, 1975); it may be responsible for controlling the flexion phase of leg movement during walking (Figure 1C). A homolo-

gous local neuron may exist in the locust (Figure 1D). Large local neurons have also been described in the abdominal ganglia of crayfish (Retzius, 1890, cited in Bullock and Horridge, 1965, p. 855), and by comparison with insects it is probable that each of these neurons is unique. Two classes of local neurons exist in the segmental ganglia of the polychaete worm *Neris* (Smith, 1957): one has processes running horizontally and the other vertically through the ganglion. The number of neurons in each class is small (30–40 vertical and 10–15 horizontal in each ganglion), and individual neurons are spatially separated. Thus it would be possible to identify each local neuron; since no physiological studies have yet been done on these neurons, we do not know whether each has a unique function.

The sheer number of local neurons in certain regions of the brains of cephalopod molluscs, in the corpora pedunculata of insects, and in the optic ganglia of molluscs and insects makes it exceedingly improbable that individual local neurons will be uniquely identifiable. Within the first optic ganglion (the lamina) of the fly visual system, however, there are specialized groups of processes termed *cartridges* (see Shaw, this volume). There is one cartridge per ommatidium, and a small number of processes from local neurons (amacrine cells) are associated with each cartridge. Thus, insofar as single ommatidia can be identified, we can consider the different local neurons associated with each cartridge to be identified.

An intriguing structural feature of some amacrine cells in the optic ganglia of insects and the optic lobes of cephalopod molluscs is the fact that they have more than one region in which arborization of the processes is prolific (Figures 2C and 2D; see Strausfeld, 1970, 1976). These regions are separated by a thin nonbranching process. What is the function of the connecting process? Does it transmit information from one branching region to another, somewhat like a conventional axon? Or does it have no real electrical function but simply connect two regions that function independently? If the latter is true, then each arborizing region would require its own output synapses as well as means of receiving inputs. Unfortunately the ultrastructure of these amacrine cells has not been analyzed sufficiently well to tell us whether each branching region is both pre- and postsynaptic to other neurons. Some support for this notion that different branches can function independently does come from observations in the fly that inputs to the outer layers of the second optic ganglion (the medulla) differ from those to the inner layers and that many single amacrine cells have separate branching regions in the inner and outer layers (Strausfeld, 1976). This feature appears analogous to the situation in the cat and rabbit retina, where one type of horizontal cell has two highly branched regions separated by a fine process and where the soma/dendritic region receives input mainly from the cones and the terminal region receives input mainly from the rods (Nelson et al., 1975). To date this horizontal cell is the only clear example we have of two regions of the same neuron functioning independently.

Besides the amacrine cells of the optic lobes of insects and cephalopod molluscs, two other examples of local neurons with spatially separated branching regions are known. Figure 1A shows one such neuron in the thoracic ganglion of the dragonfly larva. No electrophysiological or ultrastructural studies have been done on this neuron, so we have no evidence that the different regions function independently. Burrows (personal communication) has also found local neurons in the metathoracic ganglion of the locust that have two branching regions separated by approximately 500 μm. Again ultrastructural studies have not been done on this neuron, and it is not known whether each region receives inputs as well as having output connections. However, physiological studies suggest that the two regions could function independently. These neurons do not generate action potentials; thus the connecting process is not functioning like a conventional axon, propagating action potentials from one region to another. Moreover, the long length and small diameter of the process connecting the branching regions seems to preclude the possibility that electrical potentials electrotonically propagate from one branching region to another. It seems very likely, therefore, that the different branching regions are electrically isolated from each other and, therefore, function independently.

Electrical Properties of Local Neurons   The electrical properties of local neurons are, in general, very poorly understood. In fact the only intracellular recordings so far made from local neurons have come from neurons in the metathoracic ganglia of cockroaches and locusts (Pearson and Fourtner, 1975; Burrows and Siegler, 1976). These recordings have shown that the local neurons have the following properties: (1) a low resting potential, (2) a high level of synaptic activity, and (3) the absence of action potentials when depolarized. In sum, graded changes in membrane potential cause marked excitation or inhibition of identified motoneurons (Figure 3); and even large depolarizing currents do not generate action potentials in these local neurons.

It is extremely important to ask whether these neurons function without action potentials in an intact animal. The nonspiking behavior seen in electrophysiological experiments could be the normal behavior of these local neurons; or it could be an artifact caused by one or more of the following factors: (1) the site of recording is far from the site of spike generation; (2) penetration of the neuron damages the cell and causes the spike-generating mechanism to become refractory; and (3) changes in metabolism due to dissection cause refractoriness of the spike-generating mechanism. There are several reasons, however, for believing that none of these factors is responsible for the observed nonspiking behavior of local neurons in insect thoracic ganglia. First, intracellular recordings are made from the processes of the local neurons that are close to the processes of the motoneurons influenced by graded changes in membrane potential in the interneurons. Thus the recording site is presumably quite close to the sites of

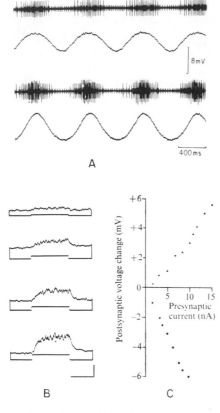

A

B   C

FIGURE 3   Effect of nonspiking interneurons on motoneurons in the thoracic ganglia of insects. (A) Sinusoidal depolarizations (bottom traces) of an interneuron in the cockroach metathoracic ganglion excites at least three motoneurons to the coxal levator muscles (top traces). Note that the motoneurons are excited without the generation of action potentials in the interneuron. (From Pearson and Fourtner, 1975.) (B) Depolarizing current pulses (bottom traces) in a nonspiking interneuron of the locust metathoracic ganglion causes subthreshold depolarizations in a fast motoneuron innervating the tergotrochanteral muscle. Note the increased amplitude of the synaptic activity in the motoneuron with the larger current pulses. (Calibration: voltage = 3.8 mV; current = 33nA.) (C) Plots showing a linear relationship between the magnitude of the current injected into nonspiking neurons and the change in membrane potential in the fast tergotrochanteral motoneuron of the locust (filled triangle = excitatory interneuron; filled circle = inhibitory interneuron). (B and C from Burrows and Siegler, 1976.)

transmitter release; yet no action potentials are observed. Second, although it is impossible to be certain that penetration of the local neurons does not cause refractoriness of the spike-generating mechanisn, this does seem unlikely, for no spikes are ever observed immediately after penetration. Furthermore, stable recordings lasting up to an hour can often be obtained in these interneurons (indicating little or no damage to the interneuron); and in none of these

recordings have spikes been observed. Finally, no consistent signs of extracellular spike activity are seen immediately prior to penetrating a nonspiking neuron. The possibility that changes in metabolism due to dissection cause nonspiking behavior is also unlikely because (1) in the cockroach the rhythmic leg movements and patterns of EMG from flexor and extensor muscles are similar in dissected and normal animals; and (2) in the locust and cockroach, certain leg reflexes are unchanged by dissection (Pearson, unpublished observations; Burrows, personal communication). Thus dissection does not significantly influence the generation of normal motor patterns and transmission in reflex pathways. Since interneurons are involved in the generation of these motor patterns (Pearson and Fourtner, 1975), it follows that spike activity in these interneurons is not required for the production of normal patterns of motor output. In summary, there is no reason to believe that those local neurons in insect thoracic ganglia that in electrophysiological experiments have been found incapable of producing action potentials, do produce action potentials under normal conditions. Of course, under some artificial conditions these neurons might be made to produce action potentials. Gerschenfeld (this volume) has shown that the normally nonspiking horizontal cells of the vertebrate retina can be induced to spike when strontium is added to the external medium. And Hengstenberg (1978) has found that light-induced depolarizations in one type of interneuron of the fly visual system will produce spikes *only* when the membrane is hyperpolarized by current injection (see also Kirschfeld, this volume). However, there are no data showing that spikes are normally generated by this neuron, and it is quite conceivable that it functions without action potentials.

The extent to which local interneurons in other regions of the insect nervous system, and in other invertebrates, function without action potentials is not known (for a review of nerve cells without action potentials see Pearson, 1976). Since the receptors and second-order neurons in the visual system of insects function without action potentials (Laughlin, 1973; Zettler and Järvilehto, 1973), it is quite likely that amacrine cells in the first optic ganglion, and possibly the second, do not generate spikes. However, at present there is no clear example of a nonspiking or even a spiking amacrine cell in the insect visual system. The local neurons of the corpora pedunculata of insects do generate action potentials (Maynard, 1967), but the occurrence of reciprocal and serial synaptic connections between the processes of these neurons suggests that graded interactions may occur.

There have been no physiological studies on the electrical properties of local neurons in animals other than insects.

Transmission from the nonspiking local neurons in the insect thoracic ganglion appears to be chemically mediated with graded changes in the presynaptic membrane potential modulating the continuous release of transmitter. Four results support this notion: (1) current injections or action potentials in the motoneurons have no effect on the membrane potential of local neurons; (2) brief presynaptic current pulses cause long-lasting postsynaptic potentials; (3) at some junctions a presynaptic depolarization gives a postsynaptic hyperpolarization (see Figure 3C); and (4) there is an increase in synaptic noise in motoneurons when they are depolarized by potential changes in local neurons (Figure 3B). Many local neurons in the cockroach and locust appear to release transmitter continuously while at rest, since changes in motoneuronal activity or postsynaptic potentials often occur in response to both depolarizing and hyperpolarizing currents (Pearson, unpublished observations; Burrows, personal communication). The relationship between the pre- and postsynaptic potentials (that is, the input-output relationship) has not yet been determined for any local neuron in insect thoracic ganglia. However, if the input-output relationship is similar to that at the squid giant synapse (see Llinás, this volume) or at synapses in the lamprey spinal cord (see Martin and Ringham, 1975), then the continuous release of transmitter at rest would require the resting membrane potential of the local neurons to be less than −50 mV. It follows that the low resting potentials of many nonspiking neurons indicate that they are continuously releasing transmitter.

FUNCTION OF LOCAL NEURONS In only a few cases do we have any idea of the function of local neurons in invertebrates. The large concentrations of such neurons in some brain regions of insects and cephalopod molluscs have led to speculation that they are intimately involved in controlling higher forms of behavior, particularly learning behavior (Howse, 1975; Young, 1964). Removal of brain regions containing large numbers of local neurons does in fact abolish previously learned behavior and adversely influence the acquisition of new memories (Young, 1964; Menzel, Erber, and Masuhr, 1974). There are no data to indicate how local neurons are involved in the formation and retention of memories.

Young (1964) has speculated that certain local neurons of the optic and vertical lobes of the octopus are inhibitory and that they function to suppress inappropriate commands. There are no anatomical, pharmacological, or physiological data to support this idea, but it is appealing nonetheless because of the considerable body of evidence that most local neurons in the mammalian nervous system are inhibitory (Gray, 1974; Rakic, 1976). Local neurons may also be involved in mediating reflex inhibitory influences in the thoracic ganglia of insects (Pearson, Wong, and Fourtner, 1976) and lateral inhibitory effects in the insect visual system (Strausfeld, 1976).

The only system in which we have clear information about the function of local neurons is the walking system of the cockroach (Pearson and Fourtner, 1975). Graded depolarizations of one local neuron (Figure 1C) excite flexor motoneurons that are normally active during the protraction phase of walking (Figure 3A). These flexor motoneurons innervate muscles acting at different joints. During rhythmic leg movements the membrane potential of the local neuron oscillates, with the depolarizing phases occurring in phase with the flexor bursts, and the application of short-duration current pulses can reset the rhythm. These and other data indicate that depolarizations in this local neuron are entirely responsible for eliciting flexor bursts during walking; they show, in addition, that the locomotor rhythm is generated in a network of nonspiking local neurons. Although the involvement of local neurons in the generation of other motor patterns in insects is not known, it must be considered very likely, since these neurons also exist in the thoracic ganglia of the locust (Burrows and Siegler, 1976). Moreover, preliminary calculations indicate that more than 70% of the neurons within each locust thoracic ganglion are local neurons (Pearson, 1977).

Local interactions

The discovery of dendrodendritic synapses in the central nervous system of vertebrates has been one of the major causes of the "quiet revolution" in neurobiology (Schmitt, Dev, and Smith, 1976); it has meant that for many neurons the dendrites, as well as the axon, are output elements. Thus the classical idea that all neurons are functionally polarized, with inputs terminating on the soma and dendrites and the output transmitted through an axon, is obviously incorrect. The close location of input and output sites on dendrites provides a means by which interactions can be restricted to small parts of the dendritic tree and may allow different dendritic regions to function independently. From a comparative viewpoint it is interesting to consider the extent to which the synaptic organization of invertebrate nervous systems is similar to that in vertebrates, and in particular whether local interactions also occur between parts of the processes of invertebrate neurons. Unfortunately we know very little about the synaptic organization of invertebrate nervous systems, and any comparison with vertebrates must be quite superficial. Nevertheless, there are some striking similarities and considerable anatomical evidence that local interactions between processes are common in invertebrates.

The structure of chemically transmitting synapses is basically similar in all animals. The presynaptic terminal contains numerous vesicles, which aggregate close to a densely staining inclusion near the presynaptic membrane. The vesicle diameter can vary between different junctions (from about 40 nm to 80 nm) but is relatively constant for any one type of junction. Usually there is thickening of the pre- and postsynaptic membranes, and the synaptic cleft is slightly wider than the adjacent intercellular gap. A notable exception is in the gastropod mollusc *Aplysia,* where specialization of the synaptic membranes is only rarely seen (Coggeshall, 1967). The appearance of the densely staining presynaptic inclusions can vary considerably between different junctions, but some of them are similar in vertebrates and invertebrates. For example, presynaptic ribbons and bars in visual receptors of crustaceans (Hamori and Horridge, 1966; Hafner, 1974) and thoracic neurons of the cockroach (Wood, Pfenninger, and Cohen, 1977) closely resemble the presynaptic ribbons in some vertebrate neurons (Dowling and Boycott, 1966; Hama, 1969; Bennett, 1971); and presynaptic dense projections commonly found in vertebrate synapses (Gray, 1974) are also seen in some invertebrate junctions (Wood, Pfenninger, and Cohen, 1977). At some synapses in insects the presynaptic bars and dense projections are capped with a flat platelike structure parallel to the presynaptic membrane (Schürmann, 1971; Burkhardt and Braitenberg, 1976). These types of inclusions have not been observed in vertebrates. In general it appears that there is greater diversity in the structure of the presynaptic inclusion in invertebrates than in vertebrates, but the functional significance of these inclusions is not known. An exciting possibility is that we may find a correlation between the occurrence of a certain type of inclusion and the functional properties of the synapse.

Apart from similarities in the structure of single synapses in vertebrates and invertebrates, there are also similarities in the structural organization of groups of synapses. Dyad junctions, in which a single terminal is presynaptic to two closely adjacent postsynaptic processes, are common in the arthropod visual system (Arnett-Kibel, Meinertzhagen, and Dowling, 1977; Hafner, 1974), the leech and cockroach ventral cord (Muller and McMahan, 1976; Wood, Pfenninger, and Cohen, 1977), and the lobster stomatogastric ganglion (King, 1976a); these junctions closely resemble dyad synapses in the inner plexiform layer of the vertebrate retina (Dowling and Boycott, 1966). They may be functionally similar to the triad arrangement of processes in glomeruli in the thalamus, olfactory bulb, and cerebellum (Rakic, 1976). Triad junctions in which a single terminal is presynaptic to three, immediately adjacent postsynaptic processes are also common in the visual systems of vertebrates and invertebrates (Dowling and Boycott, 1966; Arnett-Kibel, Meinertzhagen, and Dowling, 1977). Finally, the reciprocal and serial arrangements of synapses so common in many regions of the vertebrate nervous system have also been found in invertebrates (Table II; Figure 4).

The occurrences of reciprocal and serial synapses listed in Table II undoubtedly indicate only a very small fraction of the cases where such synapses exist in invertebrates. It is obvious that serial arrangements of synapses are widespread throughout annelids, arthropods, and molluscs. On the other hand, vertebratelike reciprocal synapses, in which two junctions are polarized in opposite directions and slightly separated from each other, have been found only in arthropods; all but two of the latter were located in the optic neuropil. The two exceptions are reciprocal synapses between processes of globuli cells in the corpora pedunculata of bees and crickets (Schürmann, 1974) and between motoneurons and an interneuron in the flight system of the fly *Drosophila* (King, 1977). A second type of reciprocal junction, in which there is a single junction with vesicles arranged symmetrically on both sides, is quite common in coelenterates (Horridge and MacKay, 1962; Westfall, 1970) but is not seen in vertebrates.

The function of none of the reciprocal and serial synapses described in the CNS of invertebrates is known with certainty. Some serial synapses may be the basis for presynaptic modulation of transmission—for example, in the giant fiber systems of the crayfish (Stirling, 1972) and cockroach (Castel et al., 1976) and the oculomotor system of the crab (Sandeman and Mendum, 1971). However, in none of these systems has such a function been demonstrated physiologically. Where presynaptic modulation has been demonstrated in invertebrates (Waziri, 1977; Kennedy, Calabrese, and Wine, 1974; Thompson and

TABLE II
Description of reciprocal (R) and serial (S) synapses in invertebrates

Phylum	Animal	Location	Type*	Reference
Coelenterates	Jellyfish	Marginal ganglia	*R	Horridge and MacKay, 1962
Annelids	Leech	Segmental ganglia	S	Muller and McMahan, 1976
Arthropods				
Arachnids	Horseshoe crab	Optic neuropil	R	Whitehead and Purple, 1970
	Spider	Optic neuropil	R	Trujillo-Cenoz, 1965
Crustaceans	Crab	Brain	S	Sandeman and Mendum, 1971
	Crayfish	Abdominal ganglia	S	Stirling, 1972
	Lobster	Optic neuropil	R, S	Hamori and Horridge, 1966
		Stomatogastric ganglion	S	King, 1976a,b
Insects	Bee	Corpora pedunculata	R, S	Schürmann, 1971
	Cockroach	Thoracic ganglia	S	Castel et al., 1976
	Cricket	Corpora pedunculata	R, S	Schürmann, 1974
	Dragonfly	Median ocellus	R, S	Dowling and Chappell, 1972
		Optic neuropil	R, S	Arnett-Kibel, Meinertzhagen, and Dowling, 1977
	Fly	Optic neuropil	R	Braitenberg and Debbage, 1974
			R, S	Strausfeld, 1976
		Thoracic ganglion	R	King, 1977
Molluscs	Octopus	Optic lobe	S	Gray, 1974
		Vertical lobe	S	Gray, 1970
		Stellate ganglion	S	Gray, 1974

* R = vesicles on both sides of a *single* junction

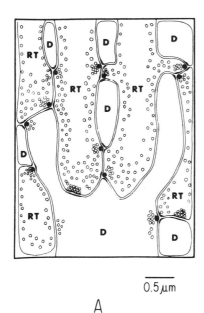

0.5 μm

A

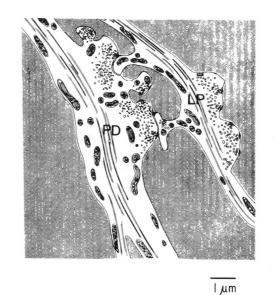

1 μm

B

FIGURE 4 Examples of reciprocal and serial synapses in invertebrates. (A) Reciprocal connections between the median ocellus receptor terminals (RT) of the dragonfly and between the receptor terminals and dendrites (D) of second-order neurons. (From Dowling and Chappell, 1972.)

(B) Serial arrangement of synapses in the lobster stomatogastric ganglion. The LP neuron receives synaptic contact from the PD neuron, and also makes synapses onto other neurons not shown on this drawing. (From Selverston et al., 1976.)

Stent, 1976), the structural organization of the neurons involved is not known. In the neuromuscular system of the crayfish, however, serial synapses in which an inhibitory axon forms axoaxonal synapses close to the terminals of an excitatory axon undoubtedly mediate presynaptic inhibition of excitatory input to the claw opener muscle (Jahromi and Atwood, 1974). Similarly, serial synapses are the basis of presynaptic inhibition in the mammalian spinal cord (Gray, 1974). Another function of serial synapses in mammals, which has not yet been suggested for serial synapses in invertebrates, may be to provide feedforward inhibition of relay neurons (Liebermann, 1973). Dowling and Chappell (1972) have speculated that delayed inhibitory feedback through reciprocal junctions in the dragonfly median ocellus system (Figure 4A) functions to enhance the transient *on* and *off* responses observed in the receptor cells. On the other hand, Schürmann (1974) has suggested that reciprocal synapses between the processes of neurons in the corpora pedunculata of bees and crickets function to positively couple these processes. The function of reciprocal synapses between flight motoneurons and an interneuron in *Drosophila* is obscure (King, 1977). By comparison there is now good evidence for at least two functions of reciprocal synapses in vertebrates: (1) to provide local inhibitory feedback onto relay neurons (Shepherd, 1974); and (2) to provide mutual inhibitory coupling between local neurons (Liebermann, 1973).

One of the extremely important functional implications of the occurrence of reciprocal and serial synapses is that they provide a means by which interactions between neurons can be restricted to small regions of one or a few processes of the interacting neurons. Although there is not yet a single example in invertebrates where this is known to occur, there are two reasons, in addition to the mere existence of reciprocal and serial synapses, why this must be considered very likely. First, many local neurons have two or more widely separated regions where their processes arborize, and the arborizing regions can be electrically isolated from the others and function independently. Second, recent ultrastructural studies on the leech segmental ganglion (Muller and McMahan, 1976) and on the lobster stomatogastric ganglion (King, 1976a,b) have shown that pre- and postsynaptic connections are made close to each other on the *distal* ends of the secondary processes and almost exclusively at specialized fingerlike swellings and varicosities on the secondary processes (Figure 5). The close location of pre- and postsynaptic sites within these specialized swellings suggests that interactions

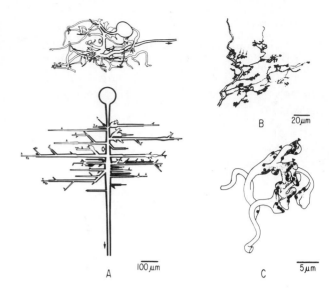

FIGURE 5 Diagrams showing the location of synapses on the distal ends of secondary processes of invertebrate neurons. (A) Anterior median neuron of the lobster stomatogastric ganglion. Top, reconstruction based on serial sections; bottom, the same neuron with all the processes diagrammatically straightened. The large, open arrows indicate the primary process. Presynaptic and postsynaptic contacts are represented by the filled triangles pointing away and toward the processes, respectively. Note that all the synapses are formed near the ends of the secondary processes and that pre- and postsynaptic sites are often located close to each other. Not all the synapses are indicated on this diagram. (From King, 1976b.) (B) Secondary branches of a pressure-sensitive sensory neuron in the leech ventral cord. The synaptic contacts are made on irregular swellings (arrows) near the ends of the secondary processes. (C) A swelling on a secondary process of a pressure cell, showing the sites of presynaptic (filled circles) and postsynaptic (filled triangles) contacts. Note the close location of the pre- and postsynaptic sites. (B and C from Muller and McMahan, 1976.)

at these sites could occur without exerting any influence on interactions at other synaptic sites. However, the likelihood that a specific type of interaction occurs at a single swelling is low, since this would require an enormous amount of structural specificity. It is more conceivable that an assembly of swellings could all function in a similar manner and thus act as a single complex functional unit. For some interactions in the stomatogastric ganglion, however, even this possibility is unlikely, since the sites of synaptic connection from one neuron to another are widely distributed over the processes of the postsynaptic neuron (King, 1976b). It is too early to know whether this latter finding applies to connections between other neurons in invertebrates. There are certainly two cases in which it does not: different processes of neurons in the corpora pedunculata and the second optic ganglion of insects are known to receive inputs from different sets of afferents (L. Pearson, 1971; Schürmann, 1974; Strausfeld, 1976). If, in general, we find that the different inputs to a neuron are spatially separated and that the various postsynaptic connections made to a neuron are also spatially separated, the probability of local interactions between processes will be high. To speculate further about the possibility of these local interactions is pointless. We urgently require ultrastructural analyses of many more systems and their correlation with intracellular recordings from different regions of the processes of identified neurons.

Conclusions

Local neurons are widely distributed throughout the nervous systems of invertebrates (Table I). Until now there have been only a few electrophysiological studies on these neurons, and we know very little about their properties. The only invertebrate local neurons studied in detail have been those in the thoracic ganglia of insects. So far all these neurons have been found not to generate action potentials. This observation, together with the obvious fact that local neurons do not need action potentials to communicate over the short distances covered by their processes, raises the possibility that the vast majority of local neurons function in a graded manner without generating spikes. Unfortunately it is going to be extremely difficult, if not impossible, to determine the electrophysiological properties of most local neurons, for their small size does not easily permit the use of intracellular recording and staining techniques. In the immediate future most of our ideas about the functioning of local neurons will probably be based on neuroanatomical data. It is hoped that similarities in synaptic organization between small local neurons and those neurons upon which electrophysiological studies are possible will give us further insight into their functional roles.

In invertebrates there is now considerable evidence that pre- and postsynaptic sites in many neurons are immediately adjacent to each other and thus form serial and reciprocal arrangements of synapses (Table II). The data suggest that a variety of functions could be carried out by the different processes of single neurons. In other words, many single neurons in invertebrates, as well as in vertebrates, may not be acting as functional units. Shepherd (1972) has proposed that a functional unit be regarded simply as the anatomical structure for a given function. If com

plex functional units can be recognized, then neuroanatomical studies may quickly give us important insight into the functioning of certain regions of the nervous system. What, then, are the chances that functional units will be recognized? From detailed ultrastructural studies on the vertebrate nervous system we now recognize certain repeating features of neuronal organization in different regions of the brain. For example, glomeruli involving the interactions of three neurons are widespread (Shepherd, 1974), and it is conceivable that they serve the same function in different regions of the brain. At a finer level, we find reciprocal synapses in which the ultrastructure of the vesicles and membranes suggests that many of them function to provide local inhibitory interactions. In invertebrates we are also seeing similarities in the synaptic organization in a variety of animals. For example, dyad junctions in which a single release site is presynaptic to two adjacent postsynaptic processes are common in the insect visual system, annelid ventral cord, and crustacean stomatogastric ganglion. Other common features include: the location of most synapses on the distal end of secondary processes; presynaptic sites restricted to swellings and varicosities; and postsynaptic sites on the ends of thin spikelike processes. Thus we are beginning to find identifiable structures involving processes of a number of different neurons in widespread regions of the nervous systems in vertebrates and invertebrates. Within the near future other multineuronal structures will probably be identified. If we can specify the function of these structures, it seems very likely that a wide variety of functional units will be identified. It is important to keep in mind, however, that the same function may be achieved by anatomically quite different structures.

The striking similarities between vertebrates and invertebrates in structures such as dyads and serial and reciprocal junctions, as well as in the ultrastructure of single synapses, is somewhat surprising, since presumably the two groups evolved from animals that had very rudimentary nervous systems. The common structures we see in the two groups, therefore, must be either very primitive or have arisen independently. The latter possibility suggests that efficient organization of neural tissue allows only a limited number of structural units. In any event, it is now clear that not only are the electrical properties of nerve cells and the characteristics of transmission at single synapses similar in invertebrates and vertebrates, but also, at a higher level, there are many similarities among integrative events involving interactions between neurons.

REFERENCES

ARNETT-KIBEL, C., I. A. MEINERTZHAGEN, and J. E. DOWLING, 1977. Cellular and synaptic organization in the lamina of the dragon-fly, *Sympetrum rubicundulumn. Proc. R. Soc. Lond.* B196:385–412.

BENNETT, M. V. L., 1971. Electroreception. In *Fish Physiology*, vol. 5, W. S. Hoar and D. J. Randall, eds. New York: Academic Press, pp. 493–574.

BRAITENBERG, V., and P. DEBBAGE, 1974. A regular set of reciprocal synapses in the visual system of the fly, *Musca domestica. J. Comp. Physiol.* 90:25–31.

BULLOCK, T. H., 1977. *Introduction to Nervous Systems.* San Francisco: W. H. Freeman.

BULLOCK, T. H., and G. A. HORRIDGE, 1965. *Structure and Function in the Nervous Systems of Invertebrates.* San Francisco: W. H. Freeman.

BURROWS, M., and M. V. S., SIEGLER, 1976. Transmission without spikes between locust interneurons and motoneurons. *Nature* 262:222–224.

BURKHARDT, W., and V. BRAITENBERG, 1976. Some peculiar synaptic complexes in the first visual ganglion of the fly, *Musca domestica. Cell Tiss. Res.* 173:287–308.

CASTEL, M., M. E. SPIRA, I. PARNAS, and Y. YAROM, 1976. Ultrastructure of region of a low safety factor in inhomogeneous giant axon of the cockroach. *J. Neurophysiol.* 39:900–908.

COGGESHALL, R. E., 1967. A light and electron microscopy study of the abdominal ganglion of *Aplysia californica. J. Neurophysiol.* 30:1263–1288.

DOWLING, J. E., and B. B. BOYCOTT, 1966. Organization of the primate retina: Electron microscopy. *Proc. R. Soc. Lond.* B166:80–111.

DOWLING, J. E., and R. L. CHAPPELL, 1972. Neural organization of the median ocellus of the dragonfly. II. Synaptic structure. *J. Gen. Physiol.* 60:121–165.

GILLETTE, R., and B. POMERANZ, 1975. Ultrastructural correlates of interneuronal function in the abdominal ganglion of *Aplysia californica. J. Neurobiol.* 6:463–474.

GOODMAN, C. S., 1976. Constancy and uniqueness in a large population of small interneurons. *Science* 193:502–504.

GRAY, E. G., 1970. The fine structure of the vertical lobe of the octopus brain. *Philos. Trans. R. Soc. Lond.* B258:379–395.

GRAY, E. G., 1974. Synaptic morphology with special reference to microneurons. In *Essays on the Nervous System*, R. Bellairs and E. G. Gray, eds. Oxford: Clarendon Press, pp. 155–178.

HAFNER, G. S, 1974. The ultrastructure of retinula cell endings in the compound eye of the crayfish. *J. Neurocytol.* 3:295–311.

HAMA, K., 1969. A study of the fine structure of the saccular macula of the goldfish. *Z. Zellforsch.* 94:155–171.

HAMORI, J., and G. A. HORRIDGE, 1966. The lobster optic lamina. II. Types of synapse. *J. Cell Sci.* 1:257–270.

HENGSTENBERG, R., 1978. Spike responses of "non-spiking" visual interneurons. *Nature* 270:338–340.

HORRIDGE, G. A., 1956. The nervous system of the ephyra larva of *Aurellia amita. Q. J. Microsc. Sci.* 97:59–74.

HORRIDGE, G. A., and B. MACKAY, 1962. Naked axons and symmetrical synapses in coelenterates. *Q. J. Microsc. Sci.* 103:531–541.

HOWSE, P. E., 1974. Design and function in the insect brain. In *Experimental Analysis of Insect Brain*, L. Barton Browne, ed. New York: Springer-Verlag, pp. 180–194.

HOWSE, P. E., 1975. Brain structure and behavior in insects. *Annu. Rev. Entomol.* 20:359–379.

JAHROMI, S. S., and H. L. ATWOOD, 1974. Three-dimensional ultrastructure of the crayfish neuromuscular apparatus. *J. Cell. Biol.* 63:599–613.

KANDEL, E. R., 1976. *Cellular Basis of Behavior.* San Francisco: W. H. Freeman.

KENNEDY, D., R. L. CALABRESE, and J. J. WINE, 1974. Presynaptic inhibition: Primary afferent depolarization in crayfish neurons. *Science* 186:451–454.

KING, D. G., 1976a. Organization of crustacean neuropil. I. Patterns of synaptic connections in lobster stomatogastric ganglion. *J. Neurocytol.* 5:207–237.

KING, D. G., 1976b. Organization of crustacean neuropil. II. Distribution of synaptic contacts on identified motor neurons in lobster stomatogastric ganglion. *J. Neurocytol.* 5:239–266.

KING, D. G., 1977. An interneuron in *Drosophila* synapses within a peripheral nerve onto the dorsal longitudinal muscle motor neurons. *Neurosci. Abst.* 3:180.

LAUGHLIN, S. B., 1973. Neural integration in the first optic neuropile of dragonflies. *J. Comp. Physiol.* 84:335–355.

LIEBERMANN, A. R., 1973. Neurons with presynaptic perikarya and presynaptic dendrites in the rat lateral geniculate nucleus. *Brain Res.* 59:35–59.

MARTIN, A. R., and G. L. RINGHAM, 1975. Synaptic transfer at a vertebrate central nervous system synapse. *J. Physiol.* 251:409–426.

MAYNARD, D. M., 1967. Organization of central ganglia. In *Invertebrate Nervous Systems*, C. A. G. Wiersma, ed. Chicago: Univ. Chicago Press, pp. 231–255.

MENZEL, R., J. ERBER, and T. MASUHR, 1974. Learning and memory in the honeybee. In *Experimental Analysis of Insect Behaviour*, L. Barton Browne, ed. New York: Springer-Verlag, pp. 195–217.

MULLER, K. J., and V. J. MCMAHAN, 1976. The shapes of sensory and motor neurones and distribution of their synapses in ganglia of the leech: A study using intracellular injection of horseradish peroxidase. *Proc. R. Soc. Lond.* B194:481–499.

NELSON, R., A. V. LÜTZOW, H. KOLB, and P. GOURAS, 1975. Horizontal cells in cat retina with independent dendritic systems. *Science* 189:137–139.

PEARSON, K. G., 1976. Nerve cells without action potentials. In *Simpler Networks and Behavior*, J. C. Fentress, ed. Sterling, MA: Sinauer Assoc., pp. 99–110.

PEARSON, K. G., 1977. Interneurons in the ventral nerve cord of insects. In *Identified Neurons and Behavior in Arthropods*, G. Hoyle and C. A. G. Wiersma, eds. New York: Plenum Press, pp. 329–338.

PEARSON, K. G., and C. R. FOURTNER, 1975. Non-spiking interneurons in the walking system of the cockroach. *J. Neurophysiol.* 38:33–52.

PEARSON, K. G., R. K. S. WONG, and C. R. FOURTNER, 1976. Connections between hair-plate afferents and motoneurons in the cockroach leg. *J. Exp. Biol.* 64:251–266.

PEARSON, L., 1971. The corpora pedunculata of *Sphinx ligustri* L. and other lepidoptera: An anatomical study. *Philos. Trans. R. Soc. Lond.* B259:477–516.

RAKIC, P., 1976. *Local Circuit Neurons.* Cambridge, MA: MIT Press.

Ramón y Cajal, S., 1911. *Histologie du système nerveux de l'homme et des vertébrés.* Paris: Maloine.

Ribi, W. A., 1975a. The neurons of the first optic ganglion of the bee, *Apis mellifera. Adv. Anat. Embryol. Cell. Biol.* 50:1–43.

Ribi, W. A., 1975b. Golgi studies of the first optic ganglion of the ant, *Cataglyphis bicolor. Cell Tiss. Res.* 160:207–217.

Sandeman, D. C., and C. M. Mendum, 1971. The fine structure of the central synaptic contacts on an identified crustacean motoneuron. *Z. Zellforsch. Anat.* 119:515–525.

Schmitt, F. O., P. Dev, and B. H. Smith, 1976. Electrotonic processing of information by brain cells. *Science* 193:114–120.

Schürmann, F. W., 1971. Synaptic contact of association fibers in the brain of the bee. *Brain Res.* 26:169–176.

Schürmann, F. W., 1974. Bemerkungen zur Funktion der Corpora pedunculata in Gehirn der Insekten aus morphologische Sicht. *Exp. Brain Res.* 19:406–432.

Selverston, A. I., D. F. Russel, J. P. Miller, and D. G. King, 1976. The stomatogastric nervous system: Structure and function of a small neural network. *Prog. Neurobiol.* 7:215–290.

Shepherd, G. M., 1972. The neuron doctrine: A revision of functional concepts. *Yale J. Biol. Med.* 45:584–599.

Shepherd, G. M., 1974. *The Synaptic Organization of the Brain.* New York: Oxford University Press.

Smith, J. E., 1957. The nervous anatomy of the body segments of nereid polychaetes. *Philos. Trans. R. Soc. Lond.* B240:135–196.

Stirling, C. A., 1972. The ultrastructure of giant fiber and serial synapses in crayfish. *Z. Zellforsch.* 131:31–45.

Strausfeld, N. J., 1970. Golgi studies on insects. II. The optic lobes of *Diptera. Philos. Trans. R. Soc. Lond.* B258:135–223.

Strausfeld, N. J., 1976. Mosaic organizations, layers and visual pathways in the insect brain. In *Neural Principles in Vision*, F. Zettler and R. Weiler, eds. Berlin: Springer-Verlag, pp. 245–279.

Thompson, E. B., J. H. Schwartz, and E. R. Kandel, 1976. A radioautographic analysis in the light and electron microscope of identified *Aplysia* neurons and their processes after intrasomatic injection of L-[³H] fucose. *Brain Res.* 112:251–281.

Thompson, W. J., and G. S. Stent, 1976. Neuronal control of heartbeat in the medicinal leech. III. Synaptic relations of the heart interneurons. *J. Comp. Physiol.* 111:309–333.

Trujillo-Cenoz, O., 1965. Some aspects of the structural organization of the arthropod eye. *Cold Spring Harbor Symp. Quant. Biol.* 30:371–382.

Vowles, D. M., 1955. The structure and connections of the corpora pedunculata in bees and ants. *Q. J. Microsc. Sci.* 96:239–255.

Waziri, R., 1977. Presynaptic electrical coupling in *Aplysia*: Effects on postsynaptic chemical transmission. *Science* 195:790–792.

Westfall, J. A., 1970. Ultrastructure of synapses in a primitive coelenterate. *J. Ultrastruct. Res.* 32:237.

Whitehead, R., and R. L. Purple, 1970. Synaptic organization in the neuropile of the lateral eye of *Limulus. Vision Res.* 10:129–133.

Winlow, W., and E. R. Kandel, 1976. The morphology of identified neurons in the abdominal ganglion of *Aplysia californica. Brain Res.* 112:221–250.

Wood, M. R., K. H. Pfenninger, and M. J. Cohen, 1977. Two types of presynaptic configurations in insect central synapses: an ultrastructural analysis. *Brain Res.* 130:25–45.

Young, J. Z., 1964. *A Model of the Brain.* Oxford: Clarendon Press.

Young, J. Z., 1971. *The Anatomy of the Nervous System of Octopus vulgaris.* Oxford: Clarendon Press.

Young, J. Z., 1974. The central nervous system of *Loligo.* I. The optic lobe. *Philos. Trans. R. Soc. Lond.* B267:263–302.

Young, J. Z., 1976. The nervous system of *Loligo.* II. Suboesophageal centres. *Philos. Trans. R. Soc. Lond.* B274:104–167.

Zawarzin, A., 1924. Zur Morphologie der Nervenzentren. Das Bauchmark der Insekten. Ein Beitrag zur vergleichenden Histologie (Histologische Studien über Insekten VI). *Z. Wiss. Zool.* 122:323–424.

Zettler, F., and M. Järvilehto, 1973. Active and passive axonal propagation of non-spike signals in the retina of *Calliphora. J. Comp. Physiol.* 85:89–104.

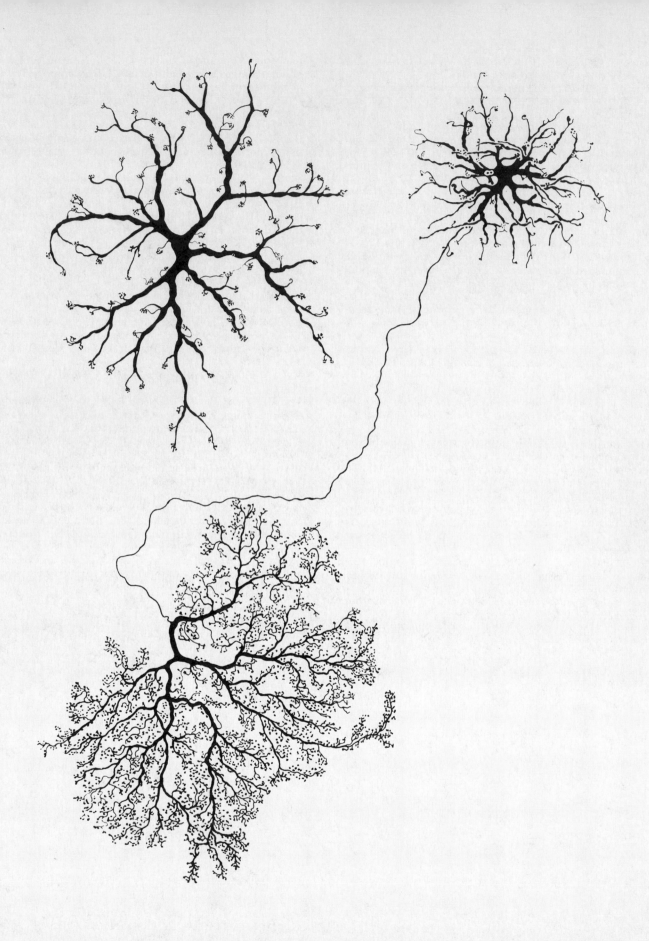

ELEMENTS OF
RETINAL FUNCTION

Golgi-impregnated horizontal cells viewed in flat mounts of the retina of the domestic cat. The A-type cell, top left, is axonless and has a dendritic spread of about 250 μm × 250 μm. The B-type cell is a short-axon cell; its dendritic spread is about 150 μm × 150 μm. Its axon is 0.5–1.0 μm in diameter, and the axon terminal system has a field about twice the size of the dendritic field of the parent cell. Both types of cells appear to function only with sustained, graded potentials. (From B. B. Boycott, Aspects of the comparative anatomy and physiology of the vertebrate retina. In Essays on the Nervous System: A Festschrift for Professor J. Z. Young, *R. Bellairs and E. G. Gray, eds. Oxford: Clarendon Press, 1974, pp. 223–257.)*

Introduction

JOHN E. DOWLING

OVER THE PAST THREE DECADES, significant progress has been made in our understanding of information processing in the vertebrate brain. At the same time, we have learned a good deal about the properties of the single neurons that occur throughout neural systems. These advances have come about largely because of the development and exploration of two very successful experimental approaches. First, by means of extracellular microelectrodes, the spike outputs of neurons in many parts of the brain have been recorded, thus giving us some understanding of the types of analyses occurring in many brain areas. Second, with intracellular probes, the biophysical and biochemical nature of neurons and their synaptic junctions has been uncovered, providing us with much information about how the single nerve cell is excited, carries signals along its processes, and passes information to other cells. There has been, however, relatively little progress in integrating the knowledge gained by these two approaches; we still know little about the details of the neural mechanisms underlying the data processing that occurs throughout much of the brain. This is primarily because of the complexity of much of the neural coding that takes place in the brain and the lack of information about, and inaccessibility of, the small, short-axon or intrinsic neurons involved in local circuit interactions that underlie a good deal of signal processing.

In the vertebrate retina, we have begun to understand the information processing occurring in the two synaptic or plexiform layers in terms of neuronal mechanisms. To be sure, many details remain to be uncovered; nonetheless, the types of processing occurring in the plexiform layers have been deduced, the cells involved in the synaptic interactions underlying the signal processing are known, and many of the individual synapses have even been identified and to some extent studied. So, for example, we can now say that in the outer plexiform layer of the retina a spatial analysis of the visual input is carried out by interactions between receptor, horizontal, and bipolar cells; and in the inner plexiform layer a temporal analysis is added through the interactions of bipolar, amacrine, and ganglion cells. Furthermore, it is the intrinsic, short-axon or axonless neurons—the horizontal and amacrine cells—that play a key role in the transformations occurring in the plexiform layers. The nature of the intrinsic neurons' activity is impressed on the output cells, mainly in an inhibitory way. That is, the sustained activity of horizontal and amacrine cells provides a tonic surround inhibition on bipolar cells and on *on* and *off* ganglion cells. On the other hand, the phasic activity of the so-called transient amacrine cells is clearly reflected in the responses of the *on-off* ganglion cells. Presumably, complex interactions of the transient amacrines among themselves and with the *on-off* ganglion-cell dendrites give rise to the more complex receptive field properties, such as movement and directional selectivity, of these ganglion cells.

Thus, the vertebrate retina is an ideal system in which to seek insights into the local circuit mechanisms underlying information processing. The retina is rich in local circuits and is amenable to detailed extracellular and intracellular recordings. The analysis of synaptic interactions mediated by local circuits has progressed well beyond similar efforts in other parts of the vertebrate brain. The contributions in this section attempt to explain retinal function in terms of neuronal and synaptic mechanisms. Following my overview of the anatomy, physiology, and pharmacology of the retina, William Hagins provides a discussion of the transductive processes occurring in the photoreceptor cell. Frank Werblin then analyzes the synaptic interactions occurring between the different cell types of the retina and discusses some of the functional implications of these interactions. Hersh Gerschenfeld next discusses the neurotrans-

mitters that may play a role in the outer plexiform layer of the retina and describes experiments that show how neuropharmacological drugs can be used to dissect synaptic circuits in this layer.

Robert Miller describes how altering the ionic environment of the retina by superfusion selectively affects certain of the retinal neurons. Such studies provide insights into the functional organization of the retina and information on the polarity of certain retinal synapses. Miller also analyzes the electrical properties of the axonless amacrine cells. Otto Grüsser describes the kinds of ganglion cells found in the cat retina and compares the frequency-transfer characteristics of intracellularly recorded horizontal-cell responses with those of ganglion-cell receptive fields. These studies show how the properties of distal neurons in the retina may be expressed in the properties of more centrally located neurons. Finally, Stephen Shaw and Kuno Kirschfeld contribute discussions of signal transmission and neuronal integration in invertebrate eyes. The invertebrate visual system offers certain advantages over the vertebrate in analyzing aspects of signal transmission, and there are both similarities and differences in the ways information processing is accomplished by invertebrate and vertebrate retinas.

The emphasis in this volume on the retina serves to underscore the fact that the vertebrate retina is a true part of the brain in every sense, even though it is displaced into the eye. In the past, research on the retina has too often been ignored by those working on brain mechanisms because it has been felt that the retina is special or unusual. For example, when it was first shown that some retinal neurons are axonless and that they can function without action potentials, it was not generally believed that such phenomena would also be found in the brain itself. Recent work, however, has indicated that retinal mechanisms are not unique, and my view is that they may well represent prototype mechanisms that are likely to be found generally in the vertebrate brain. A detailed description of the retina, such as the following papers begin to develop, may provide insights into how the rest of the brain functions in ways we cannot yet predict.

10 Information Processing by Local Circuits: The Vertebrate Retina as a Model System

JOHN E. DOWLING

ABSTRACT   The vertebrate retina is a part of the central nervous system well suited to studies of local circuit interactions. With the techniques of electron microscopy and intracellular recordings, it is possible to visualize synaptic contacts between retinal neurons and to monitor the electrical activity of individual cells. Such information, coupled with our knowledge of retinal organization derived from light-microscopic techniques, permits us to identify probable sites of interactions and synaptic pathways in the retina. This chapter reviews recent anatomical, physiological, and pharmacological studies and presents a scheme of the functional organization of the vertebrate retina.

The vertebrate retina is an ideal part of the brain in which to conduct a detailed analysis of local circuit interactions and mechanisms. It consists of a small number of neurons whose perikarya and processes are organized in discrete layers. The electrical activity of the individual cells can be recorded intracellularly and the retina naturally stimulated by patterns of light focused on the receptors. The output of the retina is readily monitored by recording optic-nerve discharges, so that the types of information processing occurring within the synaptic layers is known. Last, but not least, the retina is highly accessible, and it can be removed from the eye and readily maintained in an artificial environment. This paper will review the functional organization of the retina. Subsequent papers will provide more detailed experimental data concerning many of the points and ideas raised here.

Cellular organization

Figure 1 shows a light micrograph of the retina of the mudpuppy, *Necturus maculosus*. Because they have especially large cells, the mudpuppy and related am-

JOHN E. DOWLING   The Biological Laboratories, Harvard University, Cambridge, MA 02138

phibia have been extensively employed in recent retinal research (see, for example, Miller and Werblin, this volume). Like other vertebrate retinas, the mudpuppy retina viewed in longitudinal section displays three cellular and two plexiform layers. The most distal cellular layer, the outer nuclear layer, consists of the perikarya of the receptor cells. The inner nuclear layer contains the perikarya of the horizontal, bipolar, and amacrine cells, while the ganglion cell perikarya are found in the most proximal cellular layer, along the inner margin of the retina. In addition, there are prominent glial elements, the Müller cells, which extend vertically through the entire retina; their nuclei are usually situated in the inner nuclear layer. Thus, within the retina are five major types of neuronal elements and one principal type of glial cell.

Virtually all the synapses occurring in the retina are confined to the two plexiform layers, and in each of these synaptic layers the processes of 3 major cell types interact. The drawing in Figure 1, based on tissue processed by the Golgi method, illustrates schematically the form of the principal cell types in the mudpuppy retina. Cells with similar characteristics are found in all vertebrates (Ramón y Cajal, 1911; Polyak, 1941; Boycott and Dowling, 1969).

The receptor cells provide the input to the outer plexiform layer, where they interact synaptically with the dendrites of the bipolar cells and the processes of the horizontal cells. The bipolar cells are the output neurons for the outer plexiform layer; all visual information passes from outer to inner plexiform layer through them. The horizontal cells, on the other hand, have processes that extend widely in the outer plexiform layer, and their processes are, for the most part, confined to that layer.

The inner plexiform layer is organized in basically the same fashion. The bipolar cells provide the input to the layer; their terminals within the plexiform

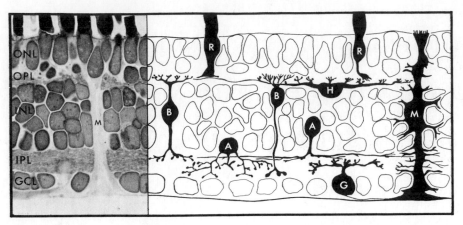

FIGURE 1 *Left*: Light micrograph of the mudpuppy retina showing the three nuclear layers, the two plexiform layers, and the prominent Müller (glial) cells (M). ONL: outer nuclear layer; OPL: outer plexiform layer; INL: inner nuclear layer; IPL: inner plexiform layer; GCL: ganglion cell layer (×235). (Modified from Miller and Dowling, 1970.)

Right: Principal cell types found in the vertebrate retina. Drawing is based on observations of cells in the mudpuppy retina impregnated by the Golgi method. R: receptors; H: horizontal cells; B: bipolar cells; A: amacrine cells; G: ganglion cells; M: Müller (glial cell). (Modified from Dowling, 1970.)

layer come into synaptic contact with the dendrites of the ganglion cells and the processes of the amacrine cells. The ganglion cells and their axons provide the output pathway for the inner plexiform layer and, indeed, for the entire retina; the processes of amacrine cells reside strictly within the inner plexiform layer.

The horizontal and amacrine cells are of particular interest. They have long been supposed to play key roles in the integration of information within the plexiform layers, and recent research clearly bears out this notion. Anatomically, many horizontal cells and probably all amacrine cells are without axons (see the frontispiece for this section). The processes of these axonless cells appear alike when viewed by light microscopy, and electron microscopy shows that they may be both pre- and postsynaptic (Figure 2) (Dowling and Boycott, 1966; Dowling, 1970). Elsewhere in the brain, similar axonless or short-axon cells (Golgi type II) have been observed and they also have processes that are both pre- and postsynaptic (see Ralston, this volume). Thus the retinal neurons may provide a model for short-axon or axonless brain cells.

Synaptic organization

Two prominent types of contacts believed to represent chemical synapses have been described by electron microscopy in vertebrate retinas and are found in both plexiform layers. The first, *ribbon synapses*, are characterized by an electron-dense ribbon or bar in the presynaptic cytoplasm (Figure 2a–d) (Sjöstrand, 1958; Missotten, 1965). The ribbon is typically sur-

rounded by a cluster of synaptic vesicles and is oriented at right angles to the presynaptic membrane. Multiple postsynaptic elements are usually found at ribbon synapses in the retina, and electron-dense material is often observed along the postsynaptic membranes, giving them a slightly thickened appearance (Figure 2b). Ribbon synapses are made by the receptor terminals in the outer plexiform layer (Figure 2a, c) and by the bipolar terminals in the inner plexiform layer (Figure 2b, d) (Missotten, 1965; Dowling and Boycott, 1966). Thus the input neurons to the two plexiform layers make synapses of this type.

The other type of synapse observed in retinas is similar to synaptic contacts observed throughout the vertebrate brain; they have therefore been termed *conventional synapses* (Figure 2b–e) (Kidd, 1962; Dowling and Boycott, 1966). They are characterized by a cluster of synaptic vesicles in the presynaptic terminal close to the presumed synaptic site. Only a single

FIGURE 2 Examples of synaptic contacts observed by electron microscopy in vertebrate retinas. (a) Ribbon synapses (arrows) of a cone receptor terminal in the rhesus monkey retina. Three processes penetrate into invaginations along the terminal base. The lateral processes within the invagination are from horizontal cells (H); the central elements are bipolar-cell dendrites (B) (×28,500). (b) A ribbon synapse of a bipolar terminal (B) (filled arrow) and a conventional synapse of an amacrine process (open arrow) in the inner plexiform layer of the chicken retina. There are usually two postsynaptic processes at ribbon synapses of bipolar terminals and one postsynaptic process at conventional synapses of amacrine cells. Note that the amacrine-cell process (A) is both a presynaptic and a postsynaptic element (×33,750). (c) Conventional synapse (open arrow)

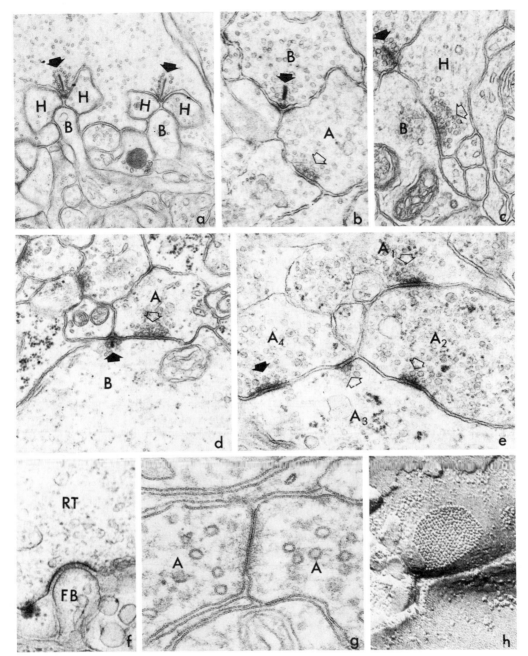

made by a horizontal-cell process (H) onto a bipolar-cell dendrite (B) in the mudpuppy retina. Note that this horizontal-cell process is itself postsynaptic at a ribbon synapse of a receptor terminal (filled arrow) (×33,750). (d) Reciprocal synaptic arrangement between a bipolar terminal (B) and amacrine-cell process (A) in the skate retina. The bipolar terminal contacts the amacrine process at a ribbon synapse (filled arrow); the amacrine makes a conventional synapse (open arrow) back onto the bipolar terminal (×30,000). (e) Serial (open arrows) and reciprocal (closed arrow) synaptic arrangements between four amacrine processes (A₁–A₄) in the frog retina. This micrograph illustrates clearly that amacrine processes may be presynaptic and postsynaptic along short portions of their length (×37,500). (f) Superficial or basal contact of a flat bipolar-cell dendrite

(FB) on the base of a receptor terminal in frog. Note that there is no synaptic ribbon or aggregation of synaptic vesicles associated with these junctions. However, some membranous specializations are seen along the junction along with filamentous material in the junctional cleft (×56,250). (g) An electrical (gap) junction in the inner plexiform layer of the rat retina between two amacrine-cell processes (A). Note that the extracellular space between the contacting processes is virtually obliterated at the junction (×75,000). (h) A gap junction in the inner plexiform layer of the rat retina demonstrated by the freeze-fracture method. The numerous, tightly packed particles, 80–100 Å in diameter, are characteristic of gap junctions seen in a variety of tissues (×75,000).

postsynaptic process is observed at these synapses; and on and between the pre- and postsynaptic membranes some electron-dense material is often observed. In the retina, conventional synapses are made principally by the axonless or short-axon cells, that is, the horizontal and amacrine cells (Dowling and Boycott, 1966; Dowling, 1970).

Since the processes of the horizontal and amacrine cells may be both pre- and postsynaptic, both serial and reciprocal synaptic arrangements are often observed (Kidd, 1962; Dowling, 1968). Figures 2b, 2c, and 2e illustrate serial synapses; that is, the amacrine- or horizontal-cell processes that receive a synapse make a synapse onto another element. Figures 2d and 2e illustrate reciprocal synapses; that is, the amacrine processes that receive a synapse, make a synapse back onto the processes that contact them.

Two other types of presumed synaptic contacts have also been observed in vertebrate retinas. The first, which is also believed to be chemical, is made exclusively by the receptor terminals; it has been termed a *superficial*, *basal*, or *flat contact* (Figure 2f) (Missotten, 1965; Dowling, 1968; Lasansky, 1969). In mammals basal contacts are made only by cones, but in other animals basal contacts are made by both rods and cones (Dowling, 1968, 1974). Basal contacts are found along the base of the terminal and are made with the dendrites of one subclass of bipolar cell, the flat bipolar (Missotten, 1965; Kolb, 1970). At these junctions some electron-dense material is seen on both membranes as well as within the synaptic cleft. However, no ribbon or cluster of synaptic vesicles is seen on either side of the contact. The evidence that these junctions are synaptic is twofold: first, the only contacts with receptors made by flat bipolars are these basal junctions (Kolb, 1970); second, freeze-fracture observations show that the intramembranous particle distribution at these junctions is similar to that seen at excitatory synapses elsewhere in the nervous system (Raviola and Gilula, 1975).

In addition, junctions that have the morphological characteristics of electrical (gap) junctions have been observed in many retinas (Figure 2g, h). Prominent gap junctions between horizontal cells or between their processes are commonly observed (Yamada and Ishikawa, 1965; Kolb, 1977). Gap junctions between photoreceptor cells have also been observed in a number of species (Raviola and Gilula, 1973; Witkovsky, Shakib, and Ripps, 1974; Fain, Gold, and Dowling, 1976). Presumed electrical junctions between amacrine cells have also been occasionally reported as well as some between bipolar terminals and amacrine-cell processes (Raviola and Raviola, 1967;

Kolb and Famigletti, 1974; Dowling, unpublished observations). As yet no systematic study of the occurrence of gap junctions in the retinas of various species has been made.

Figure 3 is a summary diagram showing typical synaptic pathways observed in many retinas. For simplicity, only the chemical synapses are illustrated. Although this drawing was originally prepared to illustrate synaptic contacts made in the frog retina, it is now clear that the synaptic pathways illustrated are rather general. Differences between species are quantitative rather than qualitative; that is, all the synaptic arrangements shown exist in virtually all retinas, although certain retinas have more of one kind of arrangement than another. Differences are especially evident in the inner plexiform layer.

In the outer plexiform layer (upper half of Figure 3), the receptor terminals make junctions with the processes of the horizontal cells and the dendrites of the bipolar cells. The flat bipolar cells are postsynaptic at basal junctions, and the invaginating bipolars at ribbon contacts (Kolb, 1970). We have already noted freeze-fracture evidence suggesting that the junction between the receptors and flat bipolars has characteristics of an excitatory synapse; these observations also suggest that the junction between the receptors and the invaginating bipolar cells resembles inhibitory synapses seen elsewhere in the brain (see also Stell, Ishida, and Lightfoot, 1977).

Horizontal cells also make contact with receptor terminals at the ribbon synapses. These contacts usually occur within invaginations of the receptor terminal, and often there is a precise arrangement of processes within the invagination (Stell, 1965; Missotten, 1965). Typically two horizontal-cell processes penetrate deeply into the invagination and come to lie on either side of the synaptic ribbon. The more superficially and centrally positioned processes in the invagination are usually the dendrites of the bipolar cells (Stell, 1965; Missotten, 1965; but see also Stell, 1976). What the significance of the invagination may be or what the precise arrangement of the processes within the invagination may mean is still obscure. One suggestion is that the invagination facilitates interactions between the horizontal process and the bipolar processes and/or receptor terminal (Dowling and Boycott, 1966).

In a number of species, synapses made by the horizontal cells have been identified (Dowling, Brown, and Major, 1966; Dowling, 1970). These synapses are of the conventional type and are made predominantly on bipolar dendrites (Figures 2c and 3). A horizontal-cell synapse feeding back onto a receptor

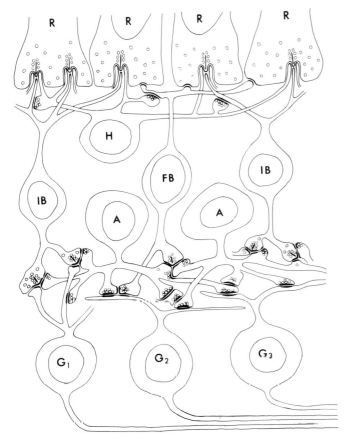

FIGURE 3 Summary diagram of the arrangements of synaptic contacts found in vertebrate retinas. In the outer plexiform layer, processes from invaginating bipolar (IB) and horizontal (H) cells penetrate into invaginations in the receptor terminals (RT) and terminate near the synaptic ribbons of the receptors. The processes of flat bipolar cells (FB) make superficial (basal) contacts on the bases of some receptor terminals. Horizontal cells make conventional synaptic contacts onto bipolar dendrites.

In the inner plexiform layer, bipolar terminals most commonly contact one ganglion-cell (G) dendrite and one amacrine-cell (A) process at the ribbon synapse (left side of drawing), or two amacrine-cell processes (right side of drawing). When the latter arrangement predominates in a retina, numerous conventional synapses between amacrine-cell processes (serial synapses) are observed. Amacrine-cell synapses in all retinas make synapses back onto bipolar terminals (reciprocal synapses). The input to ganglion cells may differ in terms of the proportion of bipolar and amacrine synapses. Ganglion cells may receive mainly bipolar input (G_1), an even mix of bipolar and amacrine input (G_2), or exclusively amacrine input (G_3). (Modified from Dowling, 1968.)

terminal has never been observed, even though physiological evidence for feedback onto certain receptor cells, especially cones, has been found (Baylor, Fuortes, and O'Bryan, 1971). So there remains some question of how horizontal cells interact with both bipolar cells and receptor terminals in many retinas (see the papers by Gerschenfeld and by Grüsser in this volume).

In summary, receptors make synapses with both horizontal and bipolar cells. Anatomy suggests that the flat bipolar cell may be excited by the receptor, whereas the invaginating bipolar cell is inhibited. Horizontal cells appear to interact with both bipolar dendrites and receptor terminals, but synapses mediating these interactions have not been firmly identified in many cases. Since horizontal cells spread their processes much further laterally in the outer plexiform layer than do bipolar cells, the cellular and synaptic organization of this layer suggests that bipolar cells are driven directly by nearby receptors and indirectly by distant receptors through horizontal cells (Figure 3).

The inner plexiform layer of the retina in all vertebrates is thicker than the outer plexiform layer; more synaptic contacts are seen per unit area, and a greater variety of junctions is observed. As already noted, differences between species are much more apparent in the inner plexiform layer (Dowling, 1968; Dubin, 1970). Bipolar-cell terminals contact amacrine-cell processes and ganglion-cell dendrites at ribbon synapses (Figures 2b, d, 3). In virtually all cases two postsynaptic elements are observed at the synapses. This arrangement has been termed a *dyad* (Dowling and Boycott, 1966). The postsynaptic elements at a dyad consist of a ganglion-cell dendrite and an amacrine-cell process, or two amacrine-cell processes, or, rarely, two ganglion-cell dendrites. Which of the pairings predominates is species-dependent.

In all retinas numerous conventional synapses made by amacrine-cell processes are observed in the inner plexiform layer. Amacrine-cell synapses are observed on ganglion-cell dendrites, on bipolar terminals, and on other amacrine-cell processes. As already noted, synapses involving amacrine-cell processes may be organized in a serial or reciprocal fashion. Such synaptic arrangements suggest the possibility of very local interactions between amacrine-cell processes and other elements within the inner plexiform layer.

Indications of alternate synaptic pathways in the inner plexiform layer have come from comparative studies of vertebrate retinas focusing on ganglion-cell physiology. For example, the receptive-field organization of many of the ganglion cells in the monkey and cat is simple in the sense that their fields can be satisfactorily mapped using static spots of light projected onto the retina (Kuffler, 1953; Hubel and

Wiesel, 1960). These receptive fields are organized into two concentric and antagonistic zones: stimulation of one zone excites or inhibits firing of the cell; stimulation of the other zone elicits the opposite response.

On the other hand, the receptive-field organization in animals such as the frog and pigeon is more complex; more than simple static spots of light are needed to map their receptive fields adequately (Maturana et al., 1960; Maturana and Frenk, 1963). Many receptive fields in these species respond best to spots, bars, or edges of light moving through the receptive field in a specific direction. Stimulated with static spots of light, such cells respond only with transient *on* and/or *off* bursts of impulses.

When the anatomies of the various species are compared, it is found that retinas with simpler receptive-field organizations (monkey and cat) have many dyad pairings of one amacrine-cell process and one ganglion-cell process, a relatively low number of amacrine synapses per unit area, and few serial synapses (Dowling, 1968; Dubin, 1970). On the other hand, retinas with more complex receptive-field organizations (frog and pigeon) have dyad pairings consisting mostly of two amacrine-cell processes, abundant amacrine synapses per unit area, and many serial synapses. Retinas with numerous examples of both types of receptive fields (e.g., rabbit, ground squirrel, and mudpuppy) show about equal numbers of amacrine-ganglion cell and amacrine-amacrine pairings at the dyads and intermediate numbers of amacrine synapses and serial synapses per unit area.

Comparative observations indicate that (1) in retinas where the simple type of receptive-field organization predominates, bipolar terminals make numerous direct contacts with ganglion-cell dendrites, whereas in retinas where the complex type of receptive-field organization predominates, relatively fewer direct bipolar-ganglion cell contacts occur; and (2) there are significantly more amacrine synapses and amacrine-amacrine interactions in retinas with complex receptive fields than in retinas with simpler receptive fields. The amacrine cells thus appear to mediate complex interactions—such as motion detection and directional selectivity—in the inner plexiform layer. A further implication of the above data is that in retinas with more complexly organized receptive fields, amacrine cells may be interposed between bipolar terminals and ganglion-cell dendrites. In such a pathway there may be a four-neuron chain through the retina: receptors to bipolars to amacrines to ganglion cells. Recent work on the ground squirrel retina showing that some ganglion cells do receive their input entirely from amacrine cells apparently confirms this notion (West and Dowling, 1972).

In the inner plexiform layer, therefore, different synaptic pathways to the ganglion cell are suggested. These ideas are summarized in the lower half of Figure 3. The left-hand side of the drawing represents a "simple" inner plexiform layer organization; the ganglion cell receives its input mainly via direct bipolar-ganglion cell junctions, and there are relatively few amacrine-cell junctions. The ganglion cell in the middle, on the other hand, receives a more equal input from the bipolar and amacrine cells, and there are more amacrine-cell contacts associated with this pathway. Finally, on the right side, a "complex" inner plexiform organization is pictured. Here the ganglion cell receives its input mainly or exclusively from amacrine-cell processes, which make many contacts among themselves and onto the ganglion-cell dendrites. The anatomy thus suggests that the physiological properties of a ganglion cell depend on the kind of input into that cell, that is, whether it is predominantly bipolar or amacrine. Evidence provided below and elsewhere in this volume (see the papers by Werblin and by Miller) indicates that in general this is the case.

Intracellular activity

In most animals, especially mammalian species, retinal neurons are relatively small. Thus intracellular recordings are difficult, and only in a few cold-blooded animals have such recordings been made from all of the retinal cells (Werblin and Dowling, 1969; Kaneko, 1970; Matsumoto and Naka, 1972; Naka and Ohtsuka, 1975). However, in a number of species, recordings from one or a few of the types of cells have been reported (Schwartz, 1974; Nelson et al., 1976). The results indicate that the response characteristics of retinal cells are quite similar across species and that a number of generalizations can be made. The discussion here will focus on recordings from the mudpuppy (Werblin and Dowling, 1969), but, where relevant, results from other species will also be discussed.

Figure 4 shows responses from each of the neuronal types in the mudpuppy elicited with a spot of light about 100 μm in diameter focused on the electrode with a centered annulus of 500 μm radius. These responses were assigned to their respective cell types after intracellular staining with Niagara Sky Blue, which permits identification of perikaryon shape and location within the retina (Werblin and Dowling, 1969). More recent intracellular staining in

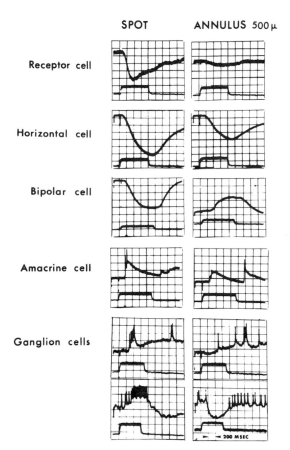

SPOT   ANNULUS 500μ

Receptor cell

Horizontal cell

Bipolar cell

Amacrine cell

Ganglion cells

200 MSEC

FIGURE 4 Intracellular recordings from neurons in the mudpuppy retina. Responses were elicited with a spot of light focused over the electrode (left column) or with an annulus (right column). (Modified from Werblin and Dowling, 1969.)

the retina has employed the dye Procion Yellow, which has the great advantage of diffusing throughout the cell into both dendritic and axonic processes (Kaneko, 1970; Matsumoto and Naka, 1972). Thus identification of retinal cell types after Procion Yellow staining is often unequivocal. These records represent typical examples of about 80% of the recordings made in mudpuppy; when this work was done, the cellular origin of the other 20% of recordings could not be firmly established (Werblin and Dowling, 1969). More recently, Müller (glial) cell potentials in the mudpuppy retina have been identified and characterized (Miller and Dowling, 1970). It also appears that there is a second type of amacrine-cell response in many species; it is more sustained than those shown in Figure 4 (Kaneko, 1971a; Matsumoto and Naka, 1972).

The more distal neurons—the receptors, horizontal cells, and bipolar cells—respond to retinal stimulation with sustained potentials that are graded with

intensity. Nerve impulses have never been associated with these responses. The neurons in the proximal retina—the amacrine cells and ganglion cells—respond with mostly depolarizing and transient potentials, on which are superimposed nerve impulses. The absence of impulses in the distal retina is of considerable interest and may be explained by the fact that these are neurons with relatively short processes that do not need to transmit information over long distances. Thus electrotonic spread of slow potentials is probably sufficient for information to reach the most distant extension of these cells.

The other finding of unusual interest is that these distal neurons respond mostly with hyperpolarizing potentials. In spike-generating neurons, hyperpolarization is usually associated with inhibition. Here, however, no impulses are fired by the cells, and presumably excitation can be signaled by hyperpolarization of the cells. That all vertebrate photoreceptors so far recorded hyperpolarize when excited by light seems compelling evidence that excitation can be signaled by hyperpolarizing potentials in the distal retina (Bortoff, 1964; Tomita, 1970; Toyoda, Nosaki, and Tomita, 1969; Baylor and Fuortes, 1970).

With spot and annular stimulation, it is possible to characterize the responses of each cell type and to describe its receptive-field organization. For example, receptors in mudpuppy give large responses to spot illumination, but only small responses when annuli are presented. Experiments using spot and annular stimuli together show only small differences when compared with spot stimulation alone. This suggests that receptors in mudpuppy are not substantially affected by surround illumination. The same appears to be true for rod receptors in toad (Brown and Pinto, 1974), but in turtle it has been shown that surround illumination can significantly depolarize cone receptors, apparently through feedback from horizontal cells (Baylor, Fuortes, and O'Bryan, 1971). Evidence for feedback from horizontal cells onto receptors also has been obtained in gecko retinas (Kleinschmidt and Dowling, 1973), in perch, and in goldfish (Figure 8c) (Burkhardt, 1977; Hedden and Dowling, 1978). The evidence so far suggests that feedback from horizontal cells is more obvious in cone receptors than in rods.

In turtle and marine toads, it has further been shown that adjacent receptors electrically interact, probably by gap junctions between receptors (Baylor, Fuortes, and O'Bryan, 1971; Schwartz, 1975; Fain, Gold, and Dowling, 1976). In turtle cones the summation area between receptors is only about 50 μm in diameter, but toad and turtle rods summate over an area about 200 μm in diameter. The functional significance of receptor coupling is not yet entirely clear, although recent work suggests that such coupling may serve to average the intrinsic noise of photoreceptors (Lamb and Simon, 1976; see also Shaw, this volume).

Horizontal cells in mudpuppy respond with large hyperpolarizing potentials over a retinal area several hundred microns in diameter. Thus both spot and annular stimulation evoke sizable potentials (Figure 4), and when spots and annuli are presented together, their effects summate. It has further been shown that horizontal cells are electrically coupled to one another, which serves to increase their receptive-field spread (Kaneko, 1971b; Dowling and Ripps, 1972; Naka, 1972). In mudpuppy, virtually all horizontal cells only hyperpolarize in response to light, regardless of stimulus intensity, wavelength, and configuration. In other species, particularly those with color discrimination, horizontal cells may both hyperpolarize and depolarize depending on the wavelength of the stimulus (Svaetichin and MacNichol, 1958; Tomita, 1963). Such horizontal cells have been termed C-type (chromaticity) cells; horizontal cells that only hyperpolarize are called L-type (luminosity) cells.

Two physiological types of bipolar cells have been found in the mudpuppy and in all other retinas in which bipolar responses have been recorded (Kaneko, 1970; Matsumoto and Naka, 1972; Schwartz, 1974). One type hyperpolarizes in a sustained fashion to central-spot illumination (Figure 4); the other depolarizes to spot illumination (Figure 8b). With either cell type, annular illumination antagonizes or reduces the sustained potential produced by the central spot. In mudpuppy, annular illumination does not drive the membrane potential back beyond the resting potential of the cell; so to see the effects of the surround illumination, central illumination must be present. In other species, annular stimulation alone may polarize the cell (Figure 8b; Kaneko, 1970; Matsumoto and Naka, 1972). In all species studied, however, an antagonistic center-surround receptive-field organization is observed at the bipolar-cell level, so that with appropriate stimulus conditions potentials of opposite polarity may be obtained from the bipolar cell (Figures 4 and 8b).

In mudpuppy, the predominant response of amacrine cells to retinal illumination is transient regardless of the stimulus configuration used. The amacrines are the first cell type along the visual pathway to respond primarily in a transient fashion, and they usually give on and off responses to illumination any-

where within their receptive fields. Some differences between amacrine-cell responses in the relative sizes of the on and off components are observed, and these differences usually depend on the geometry and position of stimulation used. For example, Figure 4 illustrates a cell with a large on response to central spot illumination; with annular illumination, the off response is enhanced and is comparable in size to the on response.

Superimposed on the transient depolarizing responses of the amacrine cells are nerve impulses. In mudpuppy, however, more than two spikes are seldom observed riding on the transient depolarization, regardless of intensity or configuration of the stimulus. It is therefore unclear whether the slow-potential part of the response or the spikes are most important for signal transmission by amacrine cells.

As noted earlier, sustained amacrine-cell responses have been observed in several species (Kaneko, 1971a; Toyoda, Hashimoto, and Ohtsu, 1973). Such cells may either hyperpolarize or depolarize to light, and the response polarity may depend on wavelength. Intracellular amacrine responses that show both transient and sustained components have also been observed in several species (Norton et al., 1970; Matsumoto and Naka, 1972; Toyoda, Hashimoto, and Ohtsu, 1973).

Two basic types of ganglion-cell responses are found in the mudpuppy retina. One ganglion-cell type strongly resembles the amacrine-cell response, giving transient responses at both the onset and cessation of stimulation (Figure 4). Differing amounts of on and off contributions may be evoked with different stimulus configurations, as with amacrine-cell responses. These ganglion-cell responses differ from the amacrine-cell responses in having numerous spikes riding on the transient depolarization, and in that the number of spikes fired appears closely related to the amount of depolarization. The second type of ganglion cell (lower records, Figure 4) has a receptive-field organization that closely resembles that of bipolar cells. With central illumination a sustained slow potential and a steady discharge of spikes are evoked. When some central illumination is maintained, large annular illumination hyperpolarizes the cell and inhibits firing in a sustained fashion. The cell shown in Figure 4 is an on-center cell. Off-center cells that hyperpolarize to central illumination and depolarize to annular illumination are also found in the mudpuppy retina (Figure 5).

Figure 5 is a summary diagram that suggests how some of the potentials and certain of the receptive-field properties of the mudpuppy neurons may be

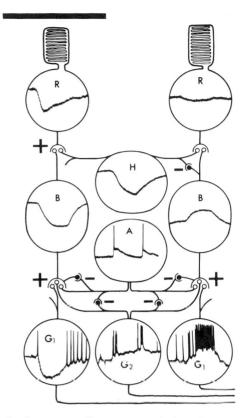

FIGURE 5 Summary diagram correlating the synaptic organization of the vertebrate retina with some of the intracellularly recorded responses from the mudpuppy retina. This figure attempts to show how the receptive-field organization of the hyperpolarizing bipolar cells, *off*-center ganglion cells, and *on-off* ganglion cells is established. The responses occurring in the various neurons upon illumination of the receptor are indicated on the left side (bar). The hyperpolarizing bipolar cells and *off*-center ganglion cells (G_1) respond to direct central illumination (left side) by hyperpolarizing; to indirect surround illumination (right side) by depolarizing. Note that the switch from hyperpolarizing to depolarizing potentials along the surround illumination pathway occurs at the horizontal-bipolar junction. The *on-off* ganglion cell (G_2) receives strong inhibitory input from amacrine cells; the figure suggests that these cells receive their excitatory input from bipolar cells. Inhibitory feedback synapses from amacrine cells onto the bipolar terminals are also indicated. R: receptors; H: horizontal cell; B: bipolar cells; A: amacrine cells; G: ganglion cells; + with open circles: excitatory synapses; − with filled circles: inhibitory synapses. (Modified from Dowling, 1970.)

produced by the synaptic interactions occurring in the retina. This drawing correlates a simplified wiring diagram of the retina (based on the connections suggested in Figure 3) with typical potentials recorded from the mudpuppy. The array of neurons in the scheme is activated by a flash of light presented to the receptor on the left (indicated by the bar above the receptor). As already noted, receptors in mud-

puppy respond relatively autonomously. Surround illumination does not significantly alter the receptor response. Thus a large receptor response is observed only in the illuminated receptor; the adjacent (non-illuminated) receptor shows only a small response, which may reflect some direct coupling between receptors (see Werblin, this volume).

The anatomy suggests that bipolar and horizontal cells are both activated by the receptors (Figures 2, 3). The scheme of Figure 5 suggests further that bipolar cells are polarized strongly in a graded, sustained fashion by direct contacts with receptors (Figure 5, left side) and that such bipolar-cell potentials are antagonized by horizontal-cell contacts (right side). Anatomical evidence suggests that such horizontal-bipolar interactions in mudpuppy could occur at horizontal-bipolar synapses (Figure 5), or perhaps within the receptor terminal invaginations, or in both locations (Dowling and Werblin, 1969).

Since horizontal cells usually have a greater lateral reach in the outer plexiform layer than do the bipolar cells, a center-surround receptive-field organization is observed in the bipolar-cell response. The central response appears to be mediated by the direct receptor-bipolar junctions and the antagonistic surround response by the receptor-horizontal-bipolar pathway. In the mudpuppy, the bipolar-receptive field center matches closely in area the dendritic spread of the bipolars, whereas the surround response approximates the lateral spread of the horizontal cells. The only other cell type in the mudpuppy retina spreading far enough laterally to account for the antagonistic surround in the bipolar-cell response is the amacrine cell, which also synaptically contacts the bipolar cells. Mudpuppy amacrine cells, however, respond transiently to retinal illumination at both *on* and *off*. The surround inhibition observed in the bipolar-cell response is, on the other hand, graded and sustained and has the approximate form of the horizontal-cell response.

Naka and his colleagues have provided impressive evidence in favor of the hypothesis that horizontal cells form the surrounds of the bipolar cells by injecting hyperpolarizing current into catfish and dogfish horizontal cells. They find that such currents mimic the effect of surround illumination in both bipolar and ganglion cells (Naka, 1972; Naka and Witkovsky, 1972). However, Gerschenfeld and his colleagues have recently provided evidence that some horizontal cells in turtle may not contribute to the surround responses of certain of the bipolar cells (see Gerschenfeld and Piccolino, this volume).

Amacrine cells respond transiently at both the onset and cessation of static illumination placed any-where in the receptive field. How the sustained responses of the distal retinal cells are converted to transient responses at the level of amacrine cells and certain of the ganglion cells (G₂) is not known, but the anatomy of the bipolar-amacrine synaptic complex provides the basis of a suggestion. That is, the reciprocal synapses of the amacrine-cell processes back onto the bipolar terminals just adjacent to the bipolar ribbon synapses could conceivably turn off the bipolar excitation locally, and a transient response in the amacrine and ganglion cells could result (see Miller, this volume).

The responses of the two types of ganglion-cell responses found in the mudpuppy retina appear to be closely related to the primary type of input to each type of cell. For example, the G_1 type of ganglion cell has a receptive-field organization quite similar to that of the bipolar cells. Central illumination hyperpolarizes the cell in a sustained fashion; surround illumination depolarizes the activity of the cell in a sustained fashion. This type of ganglion cell appears to receive most of its synaptic input directly from the bipolar terminals through excitatory synapses (see below and Miller, this volume).

The G_2 type of ganglion cell responds transiently to retinal illumination, much as amacrine cells do. This type of ganglion cell appears to receive a major part of its synaptic input from the amacrine cells. Indeed strong inhibitory (hyperpolarizing) input from the amacrine cells to these ganglion cells has been identified (Werblin, 1970; Miller, this volume). The origin of the excitatory (depolarizing) input to these cells is not so clear; it may come from bipolar cells (Miller, this volume) or perhaps from other amacrine cells (Werblin, this volume). Evidence has recently been provided that such *on-off* ganglion cells respond very well to motion, and many may show directionally selective responses (Norton et al., 1970; Werblin, 1970). This suggests, as does the anatomy, that the amacrine cells are the retinal neurons most responsible for mediating complex ganglion-cell activity such as motion and directional selectivity. Experiments demonstrating that bipolar and more distal neurons show no directional selectivity provide further evidence that amacrine cells must play such a role (Werblin, 1970).

How amacrine-cell interactions might account for directionally selective responses is yet to be determined (see Dowling, 1970; Miller, this volume). The amacrine responses being transient in nature and occurring at both the onset and cessation of illumi-nation, seem well suited for mediating the motion-sensitizing responses. For example, amacrine cells respond similarly to a bright spot on a light background or a dark spot on a light background, which is a feature of many motion-sensitive and directionally selective cells (Barlow and Levick, 1965; Michael, 1968).

In conclusion, the outer plexiform layer of the vertebrate retina appears to be concerned mainly with the static and spatial aspects of the illumination of the receptors. The neurons contributing processes to that layer respond primarily with sustained, graded potentials, and the neuronal interactions there accentuate contrast in the retinal image by forming an antagonistic center-surround organization at the level of the bipolar cells.

The inner plexiform layer, on the other hand, appears concerned with the more dynamic or temporal aspects of illumination on the receptors. Amacrine cells and transient ganglion cells accentuate the changes in retinal illumination and respond vigorously to moving stimuli. Interactions in the inner plexiform layer probably account for the motion- and direction-selective responses of certain ganglion cells.

Synaptic mechanisms

Once we have some understanding of the functional organization of the vertebrate retina, a number of questions arise concerning retinal synaptic mechanisms. For example, it is well established that neurons release neurotransmitters when depolarized (Katz and Miledi, 1967). However, when the retina is excited with light, most of the distal neurons hyperpolarize. How, then, do the retinal synapses work?

A clue to an answer came some years ago when intracellular horizontal-cell responses were first recorded and it was found that in the dark the resting potentials of horizontal cells are low (−25 to −40 mV) relative to other neurons (Svaetichin and MacNichol, 1958). In the light, on the other hand, the cells hyperpolarize to a level that is similar to the resting potential of most neurons (−60 to −80 mV). Thus horizontal cells appear to be maintained in a partially depolarized state in the dark, whereas light decreases the depolarization. On the basis of this and other evidence, it was proposed that photoreceptors continuously release a depolarizing transmitter in the dark and that light interrupts the flow of this transmitter (Trifonov and Byzov, 1965; Trifonov, 1968).

Subsequent studies on photoreceptors showed that in the dark there is a steady inward flow of Na^+ across the plasma membrane of the outer segment of the vertebrate photoreceptor; light decreases the Na^+ conductance of the outer segment, causing the cell to hyperpolarize (see Hagins, this volume). Thus photoreceptors also appear to be partially depolarized in the dark, a condition consistent with the notion of transmitter release from receptor synapses in darkness.

Figure 6 shows an experiment that tests this hypothesis directly. It is well known that high levels of extracellular Mg^{2+} and certain other divalent cations such as Co^{2+} and Mn^{2+} block neurotransmitter release from the presynaptic terminal at chemical synapses (Del Castillo and Katz, 1954; Takeuchi and Takeuchi, 1962; Katz and Miledi, 1967). If photoreceptors release transmitter in the dark, application of Mg^{2+} to the retina should block this release and cause horizontal cells to hyperpolarize, as they do in light. Figure 6 shows that this is indeed the case. Within a few minutes of the application of Mg^{2+} to skate retinas, horizontal cells hyperpolarized from -25 to -30 mV to -55 to -60 mV and light responses were lost.

These and similar results strongly support the notion that receptors release transmitter in darkness and that light decreases the flow. Can bipolar-cell activity also be explained on the basis of this hypothesis? As described earlier, there are two basic types of bipolar cells in vertebrate retinas—one that hyperpolarizes in response to central illumination of its receptive field and another that depolarizes.

The hyperpolarizing bipolar cells exhibit an increase in membrane resistance during light stimulation of the center of their receptive fields (Tomita, 1970; Nelson, 1973); thus generation of these responses could be similar to that of horizontal-cell potentials. The responses of depolarizing biopolar cells, on the other hand, provide a more difficult problem. The center response of these cells in the mudpuppy is accompanied by a decrease in membrane resistance (Nelson, 1973; Toyoda, 1973). If these bipolar cells also receive their central input directly from receptors, this implies that the effect of the receptor neurotransmitter is to decrease conductance of the cell. Thus in the light, when trans-

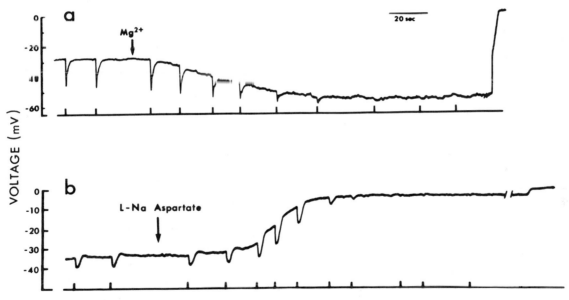

FIGURE 6 (a) An experiment showing the effects of magnesium on a skate horizontal cell. Ringer's containing magnesium was applied to the retina (arrows), and within 15–25 sec the cell began to hyperpolarize. Over the next few minutes the cell hyperpolarized to approximately -60 mV, and light-evoked activity was lost. At the end of the experiment the pipette was withdrawn from the cell (break in record). The rapid positive shift of potential of 55–60 mV confirmed the increase in membrane potential in the presence of high levels of magnesium. Test flash intensity and duration (0.2 sec) were kept constant throughout both experiments. The markers along the lower trace of each record indicate flash presentations. (Modified from Dowling and Ripps, 1973.) (b) The effects of L-aspartate on a skate horizontal cell. Ringer's containing L-Na aspartate was applied to the retina (arrow), and after 15–25 sec the cell began to depolarize. The light-evoked responses were initially larger than control potentials, but they diminished in amplitude and gradually disappeared. The cell was depolarized by aspartate to a membrane potential of -5 to -7 mV, confirmed by the withdrawal of the pipette from the cell (end of record). (Modified from Dowling and Ripps, 1972.)

mitter release is decreased, a conductance increase would be observed in the bipolar cell. Although it is an unconventional neurotransmitter action, recent experiments suggest that this does occur in neurons of the frog sympathetic ganglion (Weight, 1973). Elsewhere in this volume, Miller provides evidence that depolarizing bipolar cells are maintained in a hyperpolarized state in the dark, and that hyperpolarizing bipolars are maintained in a depolarized state—findings that also support these views.

If the above notions are correct, the synapse between the receptor and the hyperpolarizing bipolar cell can be viewed as an excitatory one, whereas the synapse between the receptor and depolarizing bipolar is analogous to an inhibitory junction. As noted earlier, the basal junctions made by the receptor onto the dendrites of the flat bipolars have certain morphological features consistent with those of excitatory synapses, whereas the junctions between receptors and invaginating bipolars appear more inhibitory in nature. These observations suggest that the flat bipolars in the retina are hyperpolarizing, whereas the invaginating bipolars are depolarizing (see also Famiglietti and Kolb, 1976; Stell, Ishida, and Lightfoot, 1977).

It may further be supposed that the retinal neurons that are maintained in a partially depolarized state in the dark—that is, horizontal and hyperpolarizing bipolar cells—themselves release transmitter in the dark. Their light effects are exerted, presumably, by withdrawal of their transmitter. As yet, however, little is known of the synaptic mechanisms of these cells (but see the papers by Miller and by Gerschenfeld in this volume).

Another question about retinal synaptic mechanisms concerns the amount of voltage change across the presynaptic membrane that is required to alter transmitter flow, thus allowing a signal to be detected postsynaptically. Distal retinal neurons respond to light with sustained, graded potentials whose amplitudes are only 20–30 mV at most. With dim illumination, the responses of the distal retinal neurons may be only one or a fraction of a millivolt. At other chemical synapses that have been studied, on the other hand, potential changes across the presynaptic membrane of more than 20–30 mV are required for any significant release of neurotransmitter (Takeuchi and Takeuchi, 1962; Katz and Miledi, 1967; Kusano, 1970; Llinás, this volume).

Some recent measurements on rod receptors stimulated with near-threshold lights have provided some insight on this question. It has long been known that rods respond to a single quantum of light and that the perception of light requires the absorption of one quantum by 5–10 rods in a field of 5,000 (Hecht, Shlaer, and Pirenne, 1942; Pirenne, 1962). When a field of toad rods is illuminated with a light providing on average only one quantum per receptor, a signal of about 1 mV is generated in each rod. However, when the light is dimmed to near-threshold levels— one quantum absorbed per 500 to 1,000 rods—all rods continue to see a signal because of the coupling between photoreceptors. The signal generated in any one rod, however, including those that capture a photon, is reduced significantly because of the coupling. Indeed, under these conditions the signals in all rods are so small that they cannot be detected with present techniques. A calculation indicates that a potential change of no more than 50–100 μV occurs in any rod at threshold levels of illumination (Fain, 1975; Fain, Gold, and Dowling, 1976). These results indicate, therefore, that exceedingly small presynaptic voltages must be capable of modulating the flow of synaptic transmitter at the receptor terminal. It may well be that synapses made by other retinal neurons that respond with graded potentials are also exceedingly sensitive to voltage changes. The papers by Llinás and by Shaw (this volume) discuss high-sensitivity synapses found elsewhere in the nervous system.

How the photoreceptor synapse manages this high degree of voltage sensitivity is not known. However, the fact that photoreceptor cells are maintained in a partially depolarized state in the dark provides the basis for a suggestion. Where studied, it has been shown that the relation between presynaptic voltage and transmitter release is an S-shaped function. Transmitter release begins when the terminal is depolarized by 10–30 mV and is maximal when the terminal is depolarized by 50 mV or more from rest (Katz and Miledi, 1967). If the photoreceptor has a similar voltage-release relationship, it would be well along this function in the dark because the rod is depolarized by at least 30–40 mV under these conditions (Hagins, this volume). Thus small, light-induced changes in the presynaptic voltage will significantly alter transmitter flow. One reason why receptors and other retinal neurons are maintained in a partially depolarized state in the dark may relate to these considerations.

Pharmacology; the interplexiform cell

Identifying the specific neurotransmitters employed at the various retinal synapses has proved to be a difficult task. The most compelling information presently available relates to the inner plexiform layer and the cells that contain and presumably use dopamine. Elsewhere in the retina our information is quite fragmentary (see Gerschenfeld, this volume).

In the outer plexiform layer it has been shown that the acidic amino acids, glutamate and aspartate, have effects on second-order cells that closely mimic the effects of the receptor transmitter; that is, horizontal and hyperpolarizing bioplar cells are depolarized by these agents (Figure 6), whereas the depolarizing bipolars are hyperpolarized (Dowling and Ripps, 1972; Cervetto and MacNichol, 1973; Murakami, Ohtsu, and Ohtsuka, 1972; Murakami, Ohtsuka, and Shimazaki, 1975). No other substances so far tested appear to have these specific effects, and it has been proposed on this basis that one of these amino acids may be the receptor transmitter. However, objections to this view have been raised (see, for example, Waloga and Pak, 1976), and other transmitter candidates are presently under examination (Gerschenfeld, this volume). The inhibitory neurotransmitter GABA has also been observed by histochemical methods to be present in the outer plexiform layer of certain species. In goldfish this agent has been localized to certain of the horizontal cells (Lam, 1975).

In the inner plexiform layer five neurotransmitters (acetylcholine, GABA, glycine, dopamine, and an indoleamine, perhaps serotonin) have been identified by histochemical and, in some cases, other methods (Graham, 1974; Neal, 1976; Voaden, 1976; Ehinger, 1976; Masland, 1976). All of these transmitters have been associated with amacrine cells, and it has been convincingly demonstrated that certain amacrine cells have the capability of accumulating one or another of these substances. It thus appears that there are pharmacologically distinct types of amacrine cells, perhaps as many as five, each containing and presumably employing a different neurotransmitter. It is likely that these pharmacological types of amacrine cells make specific and different connections within the inner plexiform layer and mediate different functions. Evidence supporting this view has come from studies of the dopaminergic amacrine cells of the rabbit retina (Dowling and Ehinger, 1978). These cells make synaptic contacts only with other amacrine cells, suggesting that they may play a modulating role in the retina.

As noted above, our best evidence relating a particular neurotransmitter to a specific cell type involves the dopamine-containing retinal cells. The principal reason for this is that cells containing dopamine and certain other catecholamines and indoleamines can be demonstrated by fluorescence microscopy, employing the Falck Hillarp method (Falck, 1962). Since the entire cell usually fluoresces with this method, the nature and type of cell containing the neurotransmitter can often be unequivocally identified.

It has been observed that in most retinas a small percentage (5–10%) of the amacrine cells show dopamine fluorescence (Ehinger, 1976). However, in two groups of animals, teleost fish and New World monkeys, such studies have revealed a sixth type of retinal neuron whose existence had not previously been generally recognized (Ehinger, Falck, and Laties, 1969). The perikarya of these neurons reside in the inner portion of the inner nuclear layer among the amacrines, and their processes extend widely in the inner plexiform layer, like many amacrines. They differ from amacrine cells in that they also extend processes to the outer plexiform layer, where they arborize extensively. Recent Golgi studies have shown that this type of neuron is present in a variety of species (Gallego, 1971; Boycott et al., 1975), so it appears that they are a general feature of vertebrate retinas. Curiously, only in teleost fish and New World monkeys do these cells show dopamine fluorescence; the transmitter employed by these cells in other animals is unknown. These neurons have been termed *interplexiform cells,* and their role in the retina is presently under active investigation.

Most of the information available on the interplexiform cell has come from two types of studies on the dopamine-containing cells of the goldfish retina. In the first, the synaptic organization of these cells was studied by injecting into goldfish eyes dopamine-analogs, which are taken up by the interplexiform cells and which selectively alter their fine structure (Dowling and Ehinger, 1975, 1978). In the second, the possible physiological role of the interplexiform cell has been investigated by applying dopamine to various retinal neurons while recording their activity intracellularly (Hedden and Dowling, 1978).

Figure 7 shows a summary diagram of the synapses made by the interplexiform cells in the goldfish. The input to the interplexiform cells is exclusively in the inner plexiform layer from amacrine cells. In the inner plexiform layer the interplexiform cells themselves make synapses on amacrine cells only. They never contact bipolar terminals or ganglion-cell dendrites. In the outer plexiform layer the interplexiform cells are exclusively presynaptic. They form abundant synapses on the externally positioned horizontal cells and some onto bipolar dendrites. They do not contact receptor terminals. The interplexiform cells thus appear to provide a centrifugal pathway for information flow in the retina from inner to outer plexiform layers. All of the input to these cells

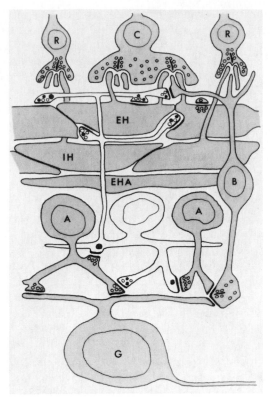

FIGURE 7   A schematic diagram of the synaptic connections of the interplexiform cells of the goldfish retina. The input to these neurons is in the inner plexiform layer from amacrine cells (A). The interplexiform-cell processes make synapses onto amacrine-cell processes in the inner plexiform layer, but they never contact the ganglion cells (G) or their dendrites. In the outer plexiform layer the processes of the interplexiform cells surround the external horizontal cells (EH). They make synapses on the external horizontal-cell perikarya and onto bipolar-cell dendrites. The interplexiform-cell processes have never been observed as postsynaptic elements in the outer plexiform layer at either rod (R) or cone (C) receptor terminals or at the occasional external horizontal synapse. Nor are synapses seen between interplexiform-cell processes and elements of the intermediate and internal horizontal-cell layers. IH: intermediate (rod) horizontal cell; EHA: external horizontal-cell axon processes; B: bipolar cell. (From Dowling, Ehinger, and Hedden, 1976.)

is in the inner plexiform layer, whereas their output is in both plexiform layers and is especially prominent in the outer plexiform layer. Recent studies on interplexiform cells in the cat and New World monkey indicate a similar synaptic organization: input in the inner plexiform layer and output in both plexiform layers (Kolb and West, 1977; Dowling and Ehinger, in preparation).

The effects of dopamine on the intracellular activity of the three major cell types contributing processes to the outer plexiform layer is shown in Figure 8. On

horizontal cells, applied dopamine causes a substantial depolarization and a decrease in the amplitude of light-evoked responses. On a depolarizing bipolar cell, dopamine slightly hyperpolarizes the cell, increases the amplitude of response to central spot illumination, and decreases the amplitude of response to annular illumination. On a cone photoreceptor, dopamine causes no change in resting membrane potential or in the maximum amplitude of the light-evoked response; it does, however, cause an alteration in the form of the receptor response, namely, a significant reduction in amplitude of the late depolarizing component.

These results can be interpreted in the following way. Dopamine depolarizes horizontal cells and depresses their responsiveness to light. This results in a decrease of lateral inhibition in the outer plexiform layer, expressed in the receptor response by an alteration in waveform and in the bipolar cell by a decrease in the response to annular illumination. In addition, dopamine appears to have a direct effect on bipolar cells, which results in a small change in dark-resting potential and an increase of responsiveness to central illumination.

It would appear, therefore, that one role of interplexiform cells is the regulation of the center-surround antagonism in the outer plexiform layer. The activation of these cells depresses lateral inhibitory effects mediated by horizontal cells and enhances bipolar-cell center responsiveness. There is less information on the role interplexiform cells may play in the inner plexiform layer. Dopamine appears to depolarize and desensitize the transient amacrine cells but not the sustained amacrine cells. It is thus conceivable that interplexiform cells could suppress lateral inhibitory effects mediated by transient amacrine cells in the inner plexiform layer.

Ganglion-cell receptive-field organization

Figure 9 puts together much of the currently available information on synaptic interactions in the retina and how the major types of ganglion-cell receptive fields may be formed. This diagram is derived from the work of a number of laboratories (see, for example, Werblin, this volume; Miller, this volume; Naka, 1976); and it focuses mainly on the physiological interactions that have been described. Synapses are indicated as excitatory (open circles) or inhibitory (closed circles). (Whether a synapse is excitatory or inhibitory is often not easy to decide in the retina. In this paper a synapse is referred to as excitatory if the postsynaptic response is of the same polarity as the

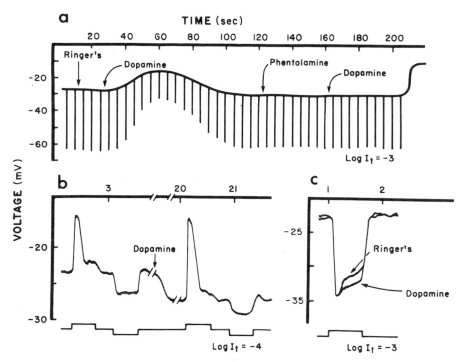

FIGURE 8 The effects of dopamine on the intracellularly recorded activity of neurons that contribute processes to the outer plexiform layer in goldfish. In all cases, atomized control and test solutions were applied to the isolated retina (arrows). (a) Dopamine depolarizes horizontal cells and decreases their light responsiveness. These effects of dopamine are completely blocked by phentolamine. (b) Dopamine hyperpolarizes bipolar cells that depolarize to spot illumination (raised abscissa) and that hyperpolarize to annular illumination (lowered abscissa). After dopamine application, bipolar responses to center illumination are enhanced, whereas responses to surround illumination are depressed. (c) Dopamine causes no change in the resting membrane potential of cones. It does, however, affect the waveform of the response. Cone responses were elicited with diffuse light flashes (raised abscissa). Log I_t: relative flash intensity. (Modified from Hedden and Dowling, 1978.)

response in the presynaptic elements. Conversely an inhibitory synapse is one where the postsynaptic response is of opposite polarity to the presynaptic potential or where the postsynaptic response is diminished as a result of synaptic action.) Known reciprocal interactions between two elements are indicated by an open triangle.

The first synaptic interaction in the retina occurs between the receptors. This is an electrical interaction, shown in Figure 9 as mediated by junctions between the receptor terminals. However, electrical junctions between receptors have also been observed at the level of the inner segments (Custer, 1973; Fain, Gold, and Dowling, 1976). Specificity of the coupling has been reported (Baylor and Hodgkin, 1973); that is, coupling between receptor types of the same class (rod and rod, or red cone and red cone) is strong; coupling between classes of receptor is very weak or not detectable (Schwartz, 1975; Fain, Gold, and Dowling, 1976). Also, rod-rod coupling is more extensive than cone-cone coupling. As noted above, the role of the electrical coupling between receptors is not entirely clear; it may function to reduce the intrinsic noise of the receptors (Lamb and Simon, 1976).

The receptors make chemical synapses with the bipolar and horizontal cells. The basal junctions made by the receptors onto the flat bipolar cells appear to be excitatory; these cells (HB) respond to central illumination with hyperpolarizing responses. On the other hand, the ribbon contacts between receptors and invaginating bipolars appear to be inhibitory; these cells (DB) respond to central illumination with depolarizing responses. Receptors also drive the horizontal cells at the ribbon synapses, and these junctions are excitatory; horizontal cells mainly hyperpolarize in response to illumination, like the receptors. With some receptors, primarily cones, horizontal cells interact with the receptor terminal reciprocally (open triangles). That is, the horizontal cells feed back onto the receptors depolarizing them (Figure 8c).

The horizontal cells (H) also appear to mediate the surround antagonism observed in bipolar cells (but

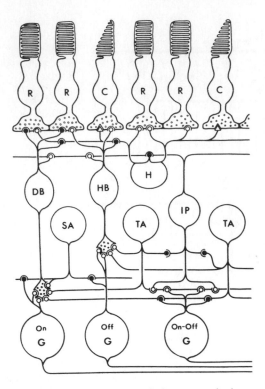

FIGURE 9 Summary scheme of the synaptic interactions that occur in the retina and that underlie the receptive-field properties of *on*, *off*, and *on-off* ganglion cells. Excitatory synapses are indicated by open circles, inhibitory junctions by filled circles, and reciprocal synapses by triangles.

see Gerschenfeld, this volume). This surround antagonism may in some cases be mediated presynaptically through the receptors, or by direct interactions with bipolar-cell dendrites. The final chemical synaptic interaction described in the outer plexiform layer involves the interplexiform cells (IP), about which we know little physiologically. In goldfish, however, the evidence suggests that these cells depress the light-evoked activity of the horizontal cells and enhance the responsiveness of the bipolar cells. Thus they appear to regulate lateral inhibitory effects mediated by horizontal cells and the strength of center-surround antagonism.

There are also electrical synapses observed in the outer plexiform and inner nuclear layers. These involve mainly the horizontal cells. In some species, such as fish (Figure 7), the junctions are between the cell perikarya; in other species the junctions are observed between cell processes. In all cases it appears that the electrical coupling between horizontal cells serves to increase the receptive field of these cells, allowing the effects of the cells to be seen over a much wider area.

In the inner plexiform layer the bipolar terminals appear to make primarily excitatory contacts with ganglion cells (Naka, 1976; Miller, this volume). Ganglion cells that make contacts with depolarizing bipolars are the *on*-center ganglion cells; those that make contacts with the hyperpolarizing bipolars are therefore the *off*-center ganglion cells. Naka (1976) and his colleagues have further shown that the sustained amacrines in the catfish retina interact with the *on*-center and *off*-center ganglion cells. The sustained amacrines provide a surround antagonism to the responses of these cells in the inner plexiform layer similar to the surround antagonism imparted by horizontal cells to bipolar-cell responses in the outer plexiform layer.

The *on-off* ganglion cells are more complicated. Clearly they receive substantial input from amacrine cells of the transient type (see the papers by Werblin and by Miller in this volume), and much of this input is inhibitory. Whether they receive their excitatory input from bipolars or amacrine cells is unclear (compare the papers by Werblin and by Miller). The diagram indicates that all of the input into these cells, both excitatory and inhibitory, is coming from amacrine cells; that some ganglion cells have only amacrine input has been shown anatomically. On the other hand, Figure 5 indicated an *on-off* ganglion cell receiving input from both bipolar and amacrine cells. Regardless of the case, it appears that the *on-off* ganglion cells receive substantial inhibitory input from the transient amacrine cells, which affects significantly the responses of these ganglion cells and is probably responsible for determining their complex properties. How these inhibitory circuits work—presumably the various pharmacological subtypes of amacrine cells are involved—is for future research to tell us.

The amacrine cells receive their input from the bipolar cells. Miller (this volume) has proposed that transient amacrine cells receive input from both the hyperpolarizing and the depolarizing bipolar cells; the opposite polarities of response of the two cell types, coupled with small latency differences, could explain the transient nature of these amacrine-cell responses. It might be supposed, therefore, that sustained amacrines receive their input from one or another of the types of bipolar cells, depending on whether the sustained amacrine is primarily hyperpolarizing or depolarizing. Reciprocal synapses between bipolar cells and amacrine cells have been described anatomically; but no physiological evidence for such an interaction has as yet been described. As noted above, the feedback synapses between bipolar and amacrine cells may enhance the transient responses of certain amacrine and ganglion cells.

The last synaptic interactions in the inner plexiform layer that will be considered are those of the interplexiform cells. Some indirect evidence indicates that the interplexiform cells are driven by transient amacrines, and because dopamine only affects transient amacrines in the goldfish retina, it may be that the interplexiform cells synapse only onto the transient amacrines (Hedden and Dowling, 1978). What role the interplexiform cell plays in the inner plexiform layer is unclear. By analogy to their role in the outer plexiform layer, these cells may modulate the inhibitory interactions mediated by the transient amacrine cells in the inner plexiform layer.

In summary, the responses of the output neurons of the two plexiform layers of the retina, the bipolar and ganglion cells, are shaped substantially by inhibitory interactions mediated by the intrinsic interneurons of the plexiform layers, the horizontal and amacrine cells. These inhibitory interneurons, in turn, appear to be under the influence of another class of neuron, the interplexiform cells, which may modulate the primary inhibitory interactions within the retina. Thus there may be two levels of control exerted within each plexiform layer on the responses of the output neurons.

Finally, it should be stressed that Figure 9, although complex, probably reflects only the simplest of interactions that occur within the retina. The ganglion-cell receptive-field organization observed in many species shows a remarkable diversity and complexity that we cannot yet explain. Directionally selective responses represent only one example that can be cited. How the retina processes color information is likewise understood only in a rudimentary way. Although we have come a long way in understanding this tiny piece of the brain, there is much left to explore.

ACKNOWLEDGMENTS Our research has been generously supported by the National Eye Institute, National Institutes of Health, under grants EY-00811 and EY-00822. Patricia A. Sheppard expertly prepared the figures, and Donna S. Hall assisted with the preparation of the manuscript.

REFERENCES

BARLOW, H. B., and W. R. LEVICK, 1965. The mechanism of directionally selective units in the rabbit's retina. *J. Physiol.* 178:477–504.

BAYLOR, D. A. and M. G. F. FUORTES, 1970. Electrical responses of single cones in the retina of the turtle. *J. Physiol.* 207:77–92.

BAYLOR, D. A., M. G. F. FUORTES, and P. M. O'BRYAN, 1971. Receptive fields of single cones in the retina of the turtle. *J. Physiol.* 214:265–294.

BAYLOR, D. A., and A. L. HODGKIN, 1973. Detection and resolution of visual stimuli by turtle photoreceptors. *J. Physiol.* 234:163–198.

BORTOFF, A., 1964. Localization of slow potential responses in the *Necturus* retina. *Vision Res.* 4:626–627.

BOYCOTT, B. B., and J. E. DOWLING, 1969. Organization of the primate retina: Light microscopy. *Philos. Trans. R. Soc. Lond.* B255:109–184.

BOYCOTT, B. B., J. E. DOWLING, S. K. FISHER, H. KOLB, and A. M. LATIES, 1975. Interplexiform cells of the mammalian retina and their comparison with catecholamine-containing retinal cells. *Proc. R. Soc. Lond.* B191:353–368.

BROWN, J. E., and L. H. PINTO, 1974. Ionic mechanisms for the photoreceptor potential of the retina of *Bufo marinus*. *J. Physiol.* 236:575–592.

BURKHARDT, D. A., 1977. Responses and receptive-field organization of cones in perch retinas. *J. Neurophysiol.* 40:53–62.

CERVETTO, L., and E. F. MacNICHOL, JR., 1972. Inactivation of horizontal cells in turtle retina by glutamate and aspartate. *Science* 178:767–768.

CUSTER, N. V., 1973. Structurally specialized contacts between the photoreceptors of the retina of the axolotl. *J. Comp. Neurol.* 151:35–56.

DEL CASTILLO, J., and B. KATZ, 1954. The effects of magnesium on the activity of motor nerve endings. *J. Physiol.* 124:553–559.

DOWLING, J. E., 1968. Synaptic organization of the frog retina: An electron microscopic analysis comparing the retinas of frogs and primates. *Proc. R. Soc. Lond.* B170:205–227.

DOWLING, J. E., 1970. Organization of vertebrate retinas. *Invest. Ophthalmol.* 9:655–680.

DOWLING, J. E., 1974. Synaptic arrangements in the vertebrate retina: The photoreceptor synapse. In *Synaptic Transmission and Neuronal Interaction*, M. V. L. Bennett, ed. New York: Raven Press, pp. 87–101.

DOWLING, J. E., and B. B. BOYCOTT, 1966. Organization of the primate retina: Electron microscopy. *Proc. R. Soc. Lond.* B166:80–111.

DOWLING, J. E., J. E. BROWN, and D. MAJOR, 1966. Synapses of horizontal cells in rabbit and cat retinas. *Science* 153:1639–1641.

DOWLING, J. E., and B. EHINGER, 1975. Synaptic organization of the interplexiform cells of the goldfish retina. *Science* 188:270–273.

DOWLING, J. E., and B. EHINGER, 1978. The interplexiform cell system I. Synapses of the dopaminergic neurons of the goldfish retina. *Proc. R. Soc. Lond.* B201:7–26.

DOWLING, J. E., and B. EHINGER, 1978. Synaptic organization of the dopaminergic neurons in the rabbit retina. *J. Comp. Neurol.* 180:203–220.

DOWLING, J. E., B. EHINGER, and W. HEDDEN, 1976. The interplexiform cell: A new type of retinal neuron. *Invest. Ophthalmol.* 15:916–926.

DOWLING, J. E., and H. RIPPS, 1971. S-Potentials in the skate retina: intracellular recordings during light and dark adaptation. *J. Gen. Physiol.* 58:163–189.

DOWLING, J. E., and H. RIPPS, 1973. Neurotransmission in the distal retina: The effect of magnesium on horizontal cell activity. *Nature* 242:101–103.

DOWLING, J. E., and F. S. WERBLIN, 1969. Organization of retina of the mudpuppy, *Necturus maculosus*. I. Synaptic structure. *J. Neurophysiol.* 32:315–338.

DUBIN, M., 1970. The inner plexiform layer of the vertebrate retina: A quantitative and comparative electron microscopic analysis. *J. Comp. Neurol.* 140:479–506.

EHINGER, B., 1976. Biogenic monoamines as transmitters in the retina. In *Transmitters in the Visual Process*, S. L. Bonting, ed. New York: Pergamon Press, pp. 145–163.

EHINGER, B., B. FALCK, and A. M. LATIES, 1969. Adrenergic neurons in teleost retina. *Z. Zellforsch* 97:285–297.

FAIN, G. L., 1975. Quantum sensitivity of rods in the toad retina. *Science* 187:838–841.

FAIN, G. L., G. H. GOLD, and J. E. DOWLING, 1976. Receptor coupling in the toad retina. *Cold Spring Harbor Symp. Quant. Biol.* 40:547–561.

FALCK, B., 1962. Observations on the possibilities of the cellular localization of monoamines by a fluorescence method. *Acta Physiol. Scand.* 56 (Suppl. 197):1–25.

FAMIGLIETTI, E. V., JR., and H. KOLB, 1976. Structural basis for ON- and OFF-center responses in retinal ganglion cells. *Science* 194:193–195.

GALLEGO, A., 1971. Horizontal and amacrine cells in the mammal's retina. *Vision Res. Suppl.* 3:33–50.

GRAHAM, L. T., JR., 1974. Comparative aspects of neurotransmitters in the retina. In *The Eye*, H. Davson and L. T. Graham, Jr., eds. New York: Academic Press, vol. 6, pp. 283–342.

HECHT, S., S. SHLAER, and M. H. PIRENNE, 1942. Energy, quanta, and vision. *J. Gen. Physiol.* 25:819–840.

HEDDEN, W. L., and J. E. DOWLING, 1978. The interplexiform cell system II. Effects of dopamine on goldfish retinal neurons. *Proc. R. Soc. Lond.* B201:27–55.

HUBEL, D. H., and T. N. WIESEL, 1960. Receptive fields of optic nerve fibers in the spider monkey. *J. Physiol.* 154:572–80.

KANEKO, A., 1970. Physiological and morphological identification of horizontal, bipolar, and amacrine cells in the goldfish retina. *J. Physiol.* 207:623–633.

KANEKO, A., 1971a. Physiological studies of single retinal cells and their morphological identification. *Vision Res. Suppl.* 3:17–26.

KANEKO, A., 1971b. Electrical connexions between horizontal cells in the dogfish retina. *J. Physiol.* 213:95–105.

KATZ, B., and R. MILEDI, 1967. A study of synaptic transmission in the absence of nerve impulses. *J. Physiol.* 192:407–436.

KIDD, M., 1962. Electron microscopy of the inner plexiform layer of the retina in the cat and the pigeon. *J. Anat.* 96:179–188.

KLEINSCHMIDT, J., and J. E. DOWLING, 1975. Intracellular recordings from gecko photoreceptors during light and dark adaptation. *J. Gen. Physiol.* 66:617–648.

KOLB, H., 1970. Organization of the outer plexiform layer of the primate retina: Electron microscopy of Golgi-impregnated cells. *Philos. Trans. R. Soc. Lond.* B258:261–283.

KOLB, H., 1977. The organization of the outer plexiform layer in the retina of the cat: Electron microscopic observations. *J. Neurocytol.* 6:131–153.

KOLB, H., and R. WEST, 1977. Synaptic connections of the interplexiform cell in the retina of the cat. *J. Neurocytol.* 6:155–170.

KUFFLER, S. W., 1953. Discharge patterns and functional organization of mammalian retina. *J. Neurophysiol.* 16:37–68.

KUSANO, K., 1970. Influence of ionic environment on the relationship between pre- and postsynaptic potentials. *J. Neurobiol.* 1:435–457.

LAM, D. M. K., 1975. Synaptic chemistry of identified cells in the vertebrate retina. *Cold Spring Harbor Symp. Quant. Biol.* 40:571–579.

LAMB, T. D., and E. J. SIMON, 1976. The relation between intercellular coupling and electrical noise in turtle photoreceptors. *J. Physiol.* 263:257–286.

LASANSKY, A., 1969. Basal junctions at synaptic endings of turtle visual cells. *J. Cell. Biol.* 40:577–581.

MASLAND, R. H., and C. J. LIVINGSTONE, 1976. Effect of stimulation with light on synthesis and release of acetylcholine by an isolated mammalian retina. *J. Neurophysiol.* 39:1210–1219.

MATSUMOTO, N., and K-I. NAKA, 1972. Identification of intracellular responses in the frog retina. *Brain Res.* 42:59–71.

MATURANA, H. R., and S. FRENK, 1963. Directional movement and horizontal edge detectors in the pigeon retina. *Science* 142:977–979.

MATURANA, H. R., J. Y. LETTVIN, W. S. MCCULLOCH, and W. H. PITTS, 1960. Anatomy and physiology of vision in the frog (*Rana pipiens*). *J. Gen. Physiol.* 43:129–175.

MICHAEL, C. R., 1965. Receptive fields of directionally selective units in the optic nerve of the ground squirrel. *Science* 152:1092–1094.

MILLER, R. F., and J. E. DOWLING, 1970. Intracellular responses of the Müller (glial) cells of the mudpuppy retina: Their relation to the b-wave of the electroretinogram. *J. Neurophysiol.* 33:323–341.

MISSOTTEN, L., 1965. *The Ultrastructure of the retina.* Brussels: Arscia Uitgaven N.V.

MURAKAMI, M., K. OHTSU, and T. OHTSUKA, 1972. Effects of chemicals on receptors and horizontal cells in the retina. *J. Physiol.* 227:899–913.

MURAKAMI, M., T. OHTSUKA, and H. SHIMAZAKI, 1975. Effects of aspartate and glutamate on the bipolar cells in the carp retina. *Vision Res.* 15:456–458.

NAKA, K-I., 1972. The horizontal cell. *Vision Res.* 12:573–588.

NAKA, K-I., 1976. Neuronal circuitry in the catfish retina. *Invest. Ophthalmol.* 15:926–934.

NAKA, K-I., and T. OHTSUKA, 1975. Morphological and functional identifications of catfish retinal neurons. II. Morphological identification. *J. Neurophysiol.* 38:72–91.

NAKA, K., and P. WITKOVSKY, 1972. Dogfish ganglion cell discharge resulting from extrinsic polarization of the horizontal cell. *J. Physiol.* 223:449–460.

NEAL, M. J., 1976. Acetylcholine as a retinal transmitter substance. In *Transmitters in the Visual Process*, S. L. Bonting, ed. New York: Pergamon Press, pp. 127–143.

NELSON, R., 1973. A comparison of electrical properties of neurons in *Necturus* retina. *J. Neurophysiol.* 36:519–535.

NELSON, R., H. KOLB, E. V. FAMIGLIETTI, JR., and P. GOURAS, 1976. Neural responses in the rod and cone systems of the cat retina: intracellular records and procion stains. *Invest. Ophthalmol.* 15:946–953.

NORTON, A. L., H. SPEKREIJSE, H. G. WAGNER, and M. L. WOLBARSHT, 1970. Responses to directional stimuli in retinal preganglionic units. *J. Physiol.* 206:93–107.

PIRENNE, M. H., 1962. Absolute thresholds and quantum

effects. In *The Eye*, H. Davson, ed. New York: Academic Press, vol. 2, pp. 123–140.

POLYAK, S. L., 1941. *The Retina.* Chicago: University of Chicago Press.

RAMÓN Y CAJAL, S., 1911. *The Structure of the Retina*, compiled and translated by S. A. Thorpe and M. Glickstein. Springfield, IL: Thomas (1972).

RAVIOLA, E., and N. B. GILULA, 1973. Gap junctions beteen photoreceptor cells in the vertebrate retina. *Proc. Natl. Acad. Sci. USA* 70:1677–1681.

RAVIOLA, E., and N. B. GILULA, 1975. Intramembrane organization of specialized contacts in the outer plexiform layer of the retina. *J. Cell Biol.* 65:192–222.

RAVIOLA, G., and E. RAVIOLA, 1967. Light and electron microscopic observations on the inner plexiform layer of the rabbit retina. *Am. J. Anat.* 120:403–426.

SCHWARTZ, E. A., 1974. Responses of bipolar cells in the retina of the turtle. *J. Physiol.* 236:211–224.

SCHWARTZ, E. A., 1975. Cones excite rods in the retina of the turtle. *J. Physiol.* 246:639–651.

SCHWARTZ, E. A., 1975. Rod-rod interaction in the retina of the turtle. *J. Physiol.* 246:617–638.

SJÖSTRAND, F. S., 1958. Ultrastructure of retinal rod synapses of the guinea pig eye as revealed by three-dimensional reconstructions from serial sections. *J. Ultrastruct. Res.* 2:122–170.

STELL, W. K., 1976. Functional polarization of horizontal cell dendrites in goldfish retina. *Invest. Ophthalmol.* 15:895–908.

STELL, W. K., 1965. Correlation of retinal cytoarchitecture and ultrastructure in Golgi preparations. *Anat. Rec.* 153:389–397.

STELL, W. K., A. T. ISHIDA, and D. O. LIGHTFOOT, 1977. Structural basis for on- and off-center responses in retinal bipolar cells. *Science* 198:1269–1271.

SVAETICHIN, G., and E. F. MacNICHOL, 1958. Retinal mechanisms for chromatic and achromatic vision. *Ann. NY Acad. Sci.* 72:385–404.

TAKEUCHI, A., and N. TAKEUCHI, 1962. Electrical changes in pre- and post-synaptic axons of the giant synapse of *Loligo. J. Gen. Physiol.* 45:1181–1193.

TOMITA, T., 1970. Electrical activity of vertebrate photoreceptors. *Quart. Rev. Biophys.* 3:179–222.

TOMITA, T., 1963. Electrical activity in the vertebrate retina. *J. Opt. Soc. Am.* 53:49–57.

TOYODA, J., H. HASHIMOTO, and K. OHTSU, 1973. Bipolaramacrine transmission in the carp retina. *Vision Res.* 13:295–307.

TOYODA, J., H. NOSAKI, and T. TOMITA, 1969. Light-induced resistance changes in single photoreceptors of *Necturus* and *Gekko. Vision Res.* 9:453–463.

TRIFONOV, Y. A., 1968. Study of synaptic transmission between the photoreceptor and the horizontal cell using electrical stimulation of the retina. *Biofizika* 13, 5:809–817.

TRIFONOV, Y. A., and A. L. BYZOV, 1965. The response of the cells generating S-potential on the current passed through the eye cup of the turtle. *Biofizika* 10:673–680.

VOADEN, M. J., 1976. Gamma-aminobutyric acid and glycine as retinal neurotransmitters. In *Transmitters in the Visual Process*, S. L. Bonting, ed. New York: Pergamon Press, pp. 107–125.

WALOGA, G., and W. L. PAK, 1976. Horizontal cell potentials: Dependence on external sodium ion concentration. *Science* 191:964.

WEIGHT, F. F., 1972. In *Synaptic Transmission and Neuronal Interaction*, M. V. L. Bennett, ed. (Soc. Gen. Physiologists Series, vol. 28) New York: Raven Press, pp. 141–152.

WERBLIN, F. S., 1970. Response of retinal cells to moving spots: Intracellular recording in *Necturus maculosus. J. Neurophysiol.* 33:342–351.

WERBLIN, F. S., and J. E. DOWLING, 1969. Organization of the retina of the mudpuppy, *Necturus maculosus.* II. Intracellular recording. *J. Neurophysiol.* 32:339–355.

WEST, R. W., and J. E. DOWLING, 1972. Synapses onto different morphological types of retinal ganglion cells. *Science* 178:510–512.

WITKOVSKY, P., M. SHAKIB, and H. RIPPS, 1974. Interreceptor junctions in the teleost retina. *Invest. Ophthalmol.* 13:996–1009.

YAMADA, E., and T. ISHIKAWA, 1965. The fine structure of the horizontal cells in some vertebrate retinae. *Cold Spring Harbor Symp. Quant. Biol.* 30:383–392.

11 Excitation in Vertebrate Photoreceptors

W. A. HAGINS

ABSTRACT Physical theory predicts that transmission of sensory signals along rod and cone cells of vertebrate retinas requires single-photon absorption in the outer segments to control the flow of tens of thousands of ions through the cell membranes. Experiments in rods of the rat retina directly confirm this prediction. The control mechanism by which photon absorptions influence the ionic permeability of the plasma membrane of rods and cones requires release, diffusion, and removal of an intracellular transmitter substance that conveys information from photolyzed photopigment molecules to control sites on the plasma membrane, where a continuous flow of Na$^+$ ions enters. The transmitter temporarily suppresses this Na$^+$ current, thus producing the first electrical event in visual excitation. Much evidence now indicates that the transmitter substance is free Ca^{++} ions. The transmitter cycle requires the expenditure of free energy other than that available in the photons. There is now evidence that this free energy may be derived from the light-sensitive hydrolysis of guanosine triphosphate. The biochemical machinery involved in visual excitation in rods and cones is complex.

VERTEBRATE ROD and cone cells, like the photoreceptors of invertebrates, are machines whose function is to convert photons into neural information. In this short essay, I shall consider some of the events that link the absorption of light with synaptic events in the visual system. The entire process of photoreception is complex, however, and some of its most important stages are still not well understood. So I shall give more emphasis to unsolved problems than to what seems well established at present.

Figure 1 shows a generalized drawing of a verte-

W. A. HAGINS   Laboratory of Chemical Physics, NIAMDD, National Institutes of Health, Bethesda, MD 20014

brate rod or cone. Photons are absorbed in photopigment molecules in the outer segment at the left, and the synapse at the right quickly responds. The latency of vision is so short that signal transmission along the visual cell cannot depend upon molecular diffusion of photoproducts released by light in the outer segment to span the length of the cell; small molecules diffuse much too slowly in liquids. Instead, when photons are absorbed, rods and cones behave as short electric cables, transmitting neural signals from end to end as displacements of their membrane potentials from some steady-state value. Signal transmission in rods and cones is both fast and very reliable. Single rods in the human retina count single photons (Hecht, Shlaer, and Pirenne, 1942), but they give false photon responses in darkness at a rate of less than once in 10 sec (Barlow, 1956). These two properties of vertebrate rods set bounds on the size of the electrical event that must occur in a rod outer segment when it responds to an absorbed photon (Hagins, 1965). If the total electrical capacitance of the rod membrane between outer segment and synapse is C, then the minimum electric charge flowing into C must be large enough to change the membrane potential by an amount that exceeds the spontaneous charge fluctuations due to thermal noise, conductance fluctuations, and the random charge displacements due to the action of ionic membrane pumps. If only the thermal membrane noise is taken into account, it has been shown that the minimum membrane charge Q that must be produced in a photon response is given by the inequality

$$Q > (2C\xi kT \ln 2)^{1/2}, \tag{1}$$

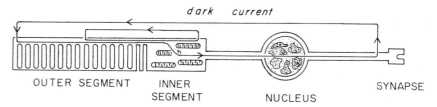

FIGURE 1   Schematic diagram of a generalized vertebrate retinal rod or cone, showing lines of flow of the dark current.

where k is Boltzmann's constant, T is the absolute temperature, and ξ is a parameter that depends on the quantum efficiency of photon detection by the rod and on its rate of spontaneous responses in darkness. For human rods ξ is of the order of 1. Solutions to relation 1 for photoreceptors of squid (representing most large invertebrate rhabdomeric cells) and of vertebrates are shown in Figure 2. The two lines were computed for cells with responsive quantum efficiencies α of 1 or 1/3 and for spontaneous thermal excitation rates of about 0.0001 and 0.01 per sec (the response time of a cell being about 0.1 sec).

It is clear from Figure 2 that many electronic charges must flow into the plasma membrane of the cell in a photon response. That is, the photoelectric conversion process in a receptor outer segment must have a large numerical current gain. This prediction was tested and confirmed in squid photoreceptors and is consistent with the behavior of vertebrate rods and cones as well. It has important biochemical implications; the excitatory machinery in a photoreceptor must provide either a way to convert the free energy of an absorbed photon into the motion of many charged particles through the plasma membrane, or there must be some way for the cell to use its own energy resources to sustain the photoelectric conversion process, even at an early stage in visual excitation. Direct measurements on responses of squid photoreceptors indicate that cellular metabolism must drive the photocurrent (Hagins, 1965). What about vertebrate rods and cones?

Electrical responses of rods and cones

The first intracellular recordings from vertebrate cones by Tomita (1965), Bortoff (1964), and Bortoff and Norton (1967) revealed that the cells had lower resting membrane potentials than most neurons and that light caused hyperpolarization to a level more typical of a cell with a high intracellular K^+ and a plasma membrane predominantly permeable to potassium ions. Toyoda, Nosaki, and Tomita (1969) then showed that the lumped membrane resistance of the cell increased during hyperpolarization and suggested that light might act by reducing the membrane conductance to some ion whose flow in darkness depolarized the membrane potential. Subsequent work (Sillman, Ito, and Tomita, 1969; Yoshikami and Hagins, 1973) indicated that the ion whose flux is suppressed by light is Na^+. Direct elemental analyses of frozen hydrated frog photoreceptors are consistent with this (Table I). In the outer segments, the potassium content of the cells is relatively low and the chloride content is high. If all the K^+ and Cl^- are free, the resting potential of the cells would be about -30 mV, a value similar to levels recorded with intracellular electrodes (Hagins, Robinson, and Yoshikami, 1975; Hagins and Yoshikami, 1975; Baylor and Fuortes, 1970; Brown and Pinto, 1974).

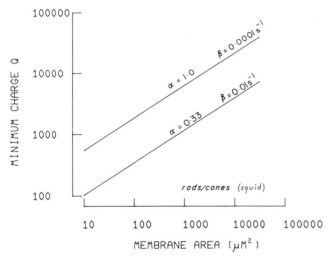

FIGURE 2 Minimum charge that must be produced in the membrane capacitance of a photoreceptor in response to absorption of a single photon plotted against total receptor-cell membrane area. The upper line is for a cell with a responsive quantum efficiency of 1 and a spontaneous dark excitation rate $\beta = 0.0001$/sec. The lower line is for a cell with $\alpha = 0.33$ and $\beta = 0.01$/sec. (From Hagins, 1965.)

TABLE I

Elemental composition of Rana pipiens *rod outer segments from electron microprobe analyses of flash-frozen and cleaved dark-adapted retinas*

	Concentration (mM/liter)		
Element	Perfusion fluid	Gross outer segment layer	Outer segment water
K	2.5	15 ± 4	37
Ca	0.1	2.5 ± 0.8	
Cl	125.0	62 ± 5	58
S	0.0	25 ± 5	
P	0.7	190 ± 20	
Na*	115.0		68

* Calculated by the difference between cationic content of the perfusion fluid and K content of outer segments. Direct Na determinations were of doubtful accuracy for technical reasons.

Source: Hagins and Yoshikami (1975).

The distribution of the depolarizing inward membrane current has been measured directly in rat rods by computing the divergence of the interstitial current in the receptor layer of the isolated rat retina with extracellular electrodes (Penn and Hagins, 1969; Hagins, Penn, and Yoshikami, 1970). In darkness there is a net inward current through the plasma membrane of the outer segment, while the remainder of the cell shows a balancing outward current. When light is absorbed in the outer segment, the current is reduced transiently over a spatial region within 10 μm of the point where photons are incident.

Two remarkable features of this "dark current" are its enormous size and sensitivity to light. In rat rods the current is at least 20 pA and perhaps 70 pA per cell (Hagins, Penn, and Yoshikami, 1970) and is sufficient to turn over all of the univalent cations in the cytoplasm about once a minute. This explains why ouabain abolishes both dark current and light response so quickly (Yoshikami and Hagins, 1973). It also gives a good reason why the vertebrate retina is so dependent upon a good supply of nutrients and oxygen; the production of ATP in quantities sufficient to expel the Na^+ carried in by the dark current requires that the Q_{O_2} of the rod layer be about 50 mm³/hr/mg dry wt, a level equaling that of the most active vertebrate cells. More remarkable still is the size of a photon response; a single absorbed photon produces a transient reduction of the dark current amounting to 3% at its peak. The entire area under a photon response amounts to the suppression of the flow of more than 2 million Na^+ ions, which greatly exceeds the minimum requirements demanded by relation (1). How is this accomplished?

Control of the dark current by light

Besides the sensitivity of the dark current to light, there are two other curious features of the light responses of rods. First, the time course of the transient suppression of the dark current bears no simple relation to the kinetics of the transformation of rhodopsin or any of its known intermediates during photolysis (Penn and Hagins, 1972; Hagins, 1972). Second, the rhodopsin-bearing membranous disks inside rod outer segments are not confluent with the plasma membrane. There is no doubt about this: electron micrographs show no continuity between the two structures (Cohen, 1968, 1972). The membrane capacitance of rod outer segments is that of a smooth cylindrical lipid bilayer (Penn and Hagins, 1972; Ruppel and Hagins, 1973), and the dye-staining behavior of rod outer segments in living retinas (Yoshikami, Robinson, and Hagins, 1974; Hagins, Robinson, and Yoshikami, 1975) clearly shows that whereas the infolded disks of cone outer segments are accessible to extracellular fluorescent dyes, those of rods are not.

Clearly some mechanism must exist in the outer segments of rods to transmit signals between rhodopsin molecules in the disks and sites on the plasma membrane where the dark current enters. A diffusible intracellular transmitter released by photochemical changes in a disk would be adequate for this, because distances are so short in an outer segment. Consider a quantity of a transmitter substance M whose diffusion coefficient in the cytoplasm of an outer segment is D. Let it be released at the center of a rod disk on the axis of an outer segment of radius R. If the plasma membrane is impermeable to M and its reabsorption is neglected, radial diffusion will relax the spatial inhomogeneity with a time course that ultimately becomes an exponential time function with a time constant t_r given by

$$t_r - R^2/\alpha_1^2 D, \qquad (2)$$

where α_1 is the first root of the Bessel function J_1 (Crank, 1956, eq. 5.56). For a frog rod outer segment with a radius of 3 μm and a transmitter with a diffusion coefficient of 3×10^{-6} cm²/sec, such as would apply for most small molecules in water, $t_r \approx 2$ msec. This time is well within the latency of light's effect on the dark current (Penn and Hagins, 1972).

A scheme that would incorporate an intracellular transmitter into excitation of both rods and cones is shown in Figure 3. Its essential features are:

1. M is postulated to be Ca^{++}, an ion known to act as an intracellular transmitter in other cells.

2. Since M is a normal constituent of the extracellular medium, cone disks could control M's flow into the cytoplasm.

3. Some concentration of M would be expected to be present in the cytoplasm even in darkness.

4. Any change that would affect the cytoplasmic level of M would affect the flow of the dark current.

There is now a good deal of evidence supporting the scheme of Figure 3. The size of the dark current of rat rods is increased when the extracellular activity of Ca^{++} is lowered and is reduced to zero when it is raised to about 20 mM. At 1 mM external Ca^{++}, the dark current is about 20% of its maximum size in low-Ca^{++} solutions (Yoshikami and Hagins, 1973). When the rods are treated with divalent ionophores, X-537A or A23187, the dark current becomes much

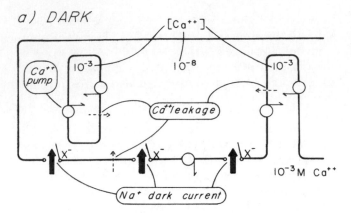

a) DARK

b) LIGHT

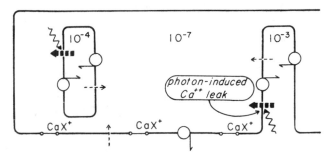

FIGURE 3 Schematic model of the hypothesis that Ca^{++} ions act as the internal transmitter of visual excitation in vertebrate rods and cones. Ca^{++} concentrations indicated are only approximate and are derived from studies of skeletal muscle. (From Hagins, 1972.)

more sensitive to externally supplied Ca^{++}; 10^{-5} M Ca^{++} will suppress both dark current and light responses of such cells (Hagins and Yoshikami, 1974). The effects of external Ca^{++} on the dark current are rapid and reversible. Removing the external Ca^{++} from the extracellular fluid with metal buffers such as ethylene glycol-*bis* (β-amino-ethyl ether)-N-N'-tetra-acetic acid (EGTA) causes rat rods to become desensitized to light by about tenfold, as if their internal store of transmitter were depleted. However, it is not possible to completely desensitize the cells under such conditions without additional treatment such as light adaptation. Lizard cones can, however, be completely desensitized by Ca^{++} deprivation (Yoshikami and Hagins, 1978). The greater effectiveness of EGTA in desensitizing cones is understandable, since their infolded disk membranes can lose Ca^{++} directly to the extracellular fluid.

While these results support the scheme of Figure 3 qualitatively, a more stringent test can be applied by studying the effects of intracellular Ca^{++} buffers on the light responses of rods.

Stoichiometry of transmitter release in rods

Theoretical considerations require that a rod response to a single absorbed photon cause release of many transmitter particles (Yoshikami and Hagins, 1973; Cone, 1973; Hagins and Yoshikami, 1975). For a 3% change in the dark current to be detectable against a background of continuously opening and closing Na$^+$ channels in the plasma membrane of a rod, the total number of channels, open and closed, must be more than 3,600. If 3% of those open are closed by a photon response, at least twenty transmitter particles must be bound. This also means that the specific conductance of an open Na$^+$ channel must be less than 1 pS, a prediction that has recently been confirmed experimentally (Schwartz, 1977; Lamb and Simon, 1977).

The quantity of M released in a photon response can be estimated experimentally if a known amount of a suitable buffer that binds M is introduced into the cytoplasm of the rod outer segments. The buffer must have an affinity for M that is high enough to compete with the sites on the plasma membrane where the dark current is admitted, but not so high that it is saturated with the transmitter in darkness. Figure 4 shows the principle of the experiment. Let A be the concentration of M released from the disks into the rod cytoplasm per absorbed photon, Q the number of photons absorbed from a stimulus flash, and E the steady-state concentration of M in the cytoplasm as free transmitter and as transmitter bound to "D" sites on the plasma membrane and to cytoplasmic buffers. Further, let K and R be the binding constants of the D sites and the cytoplasmic buffer, respectively, for M. Then if S is the fraction of "D" sites having Ms bound to them at some instant after a stimulus flash,

$$E + AQ = \frac{(1/K)S}{1-S} + DS + \frac{BRS}{K + (R-K)S}. \quad (3)$$

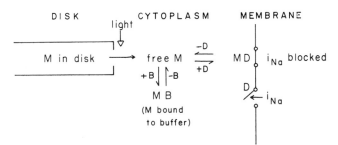

FIGURE 4 Diagram of the reactions of a diffusible transmitter substance M in a rod outer segment in the presence of a cytoplasmic buffer B that reversibly binds M in competition with the Na$^+$-gating D sites on the plasma membrane. A steady-state level of M is present in the dark.

This is the titration relation for two types of binding sites, D and B. The first term on the right represents the concentration of free M, while the second and third denote the concentrations of M bound to the D sites and the cytoplasmic buffer, respectively.

Experiments in which Equation 3 can be tested, using the relative size of the dark current of rat rods following a stimulus flash as a measure of S, are described in detail elsewhere (Hagins and Yoshikami, 1977). Metal buffers such as EGTA were introduced into live rat rods by incubating the retinas for 1–2 hr with suspensions of unilamellar phospholipid vesicles containing the buffer and a fluorescent dye, 6-carboxyfluorescein. The fluorescent dye was slowly transferred to the retinal cells as the vesicles apparently fused with their plasma membranes (Weinstein et al., 1977). From the amount of 6-carboxyfluorescein in the cells, it was inferred that cytoplasmic concentrations of EGTA of about 10 μM were achieved. Retinas so treated showed the predicted desensitizing effects to be expected if EGTA competed with the D sites for the transmitter. Figure 5 shows typical families of retinal responses from vesicle-treated retinas. 2 μsec flashes of wavelength 560 nm were used as stimuli. Flash energies in units of photons absorbed per rod per flash are marked on the curves. The curves show voltage differences between two extracellular pipette electrodes, one at the rod tips and the other 60 μm deep in the receptor layer. If the Na⁺ conductance of the plasma membrane is not too large, this voltage is a good measure of the size of the dark current and, after normalization, of S.

Rods treated with vesicles containing the proton buffer piperazine N,N'-bis (2-ethane sulfonic acid) (PIPES) gave responses shown in Figure 5a. The corresponding responses for rods treated with EGTA-containing vesicles appear in Figure 5b. The curves have been normalized to unit amplitude in the dark, but the full dark voltage difference between the electrodes was always 130–500 μV.

When the responses of the two retinas are compared, it is clear that EGTA reduces the sensitivity of the dark current to dim flashes but not to bright ones. This can be understood qualitatively if the EGTA competes with the D sites for M; but if enough M is released by a bright flash, the free buffer saturates and finally the D sites do too. The desensitization seen in these experiments is permanent, but it is much smaller than that reported by Brown and Pinto (1977), who injected metal buffers directly into rods with intracellular pipettes.

Equation 3 can be fit to families of responses to obtain estimates of the cytoplasmic levels E of transmitter in darkness and the quantity A released in light. If it is assumed that M is free Ca⁺⁺, and K is deduced from the free Ca⁺⁺ activity that suppresses the dark current in rods treated with the divalent ionophore X-537A, the computed solutions of Equation 3 that fit responses of a retina treated with EGTA-filled vesicles are as shown in Figure 6. The

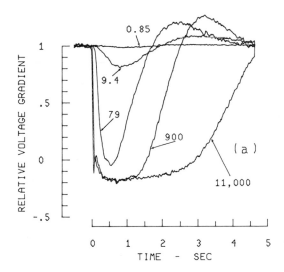
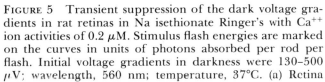
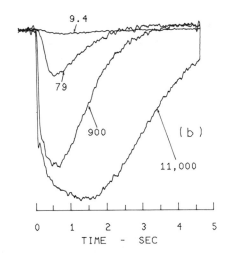

FIGURE 5 Transient suppression of the dark voltage gradients in rat retinas in Na isethionate Ringer's with Ca⁺⁺ ion activities of 0.2 μM. Stimulus flash energies are marked on the curves in units of photons absorbed per rod per flash. Initial voltage gradients in darkness were 130–500 μV; wavelength, 560 nm; temperature, 37°C. (a) Retina incubated for 1.5 hr in a suspension of unilamellar dioleoyl phosphatidyl choline vesicles containing 430 mM PIPES buffer. (b) Same but vesicles contained 450 mM EGTA. The EGTA-treated retina showed desensitization to weak light flashes. (From Hagins and Yoshikami, 1977.)

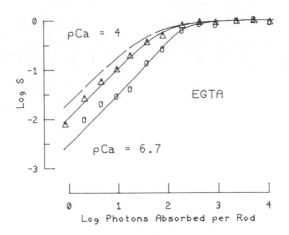

FIGURE 6 Amplitude versus flash energy curves for a retina like that of Figure 5b treated with EGTA-containing phospholipid vesicles. Δ: external Ca^{++} activity 100 μM. $\bigcirc$: external Ca^{++} activity of 0.2 μM. Solid lines are fits of equation (3) to the data, with A and E adjustable (*see* text). Dashed line: amplitude:flash energy relation for a rat retina without cytoplasmic buffer. The desensitizing effect of cytoplasmic EGTA is less at high external Ca^{++} than at low values because much of the EGTA is saturated with Ca^{++} at the higher value. (From Hagins and Yoshikami, 1977.)

data points are taken from responses in solutions whose free Ca^{++} activities were 100 μM (triangles) and 0.2 μM (circles). The dashed curve indicates the amplitude:flash energy relation to be expected in the absence of added cytoplasmic EGTA; the two solid lines are least-squares fits of Equation 3 to the data, with A and E adjustable. Table II shows the results obtained. Similar numbers were derived from curve-

TABLE II

Cytoplasmic levels of Ca^{++} and numbers of Ca^{++} ions added to outer segment cytoplasm per absorbed photon

	Free Ca^{++} activity in extracellular fluid	
	100 μM	0.2 μM
E (Cytoplasmic free Ca^{++} in dark)	1.2 ± 0.1 μM	0.44 ± 0.6 μM
A (Extra Ca^{++} ions in cytoplasm 0.4 sec after stimulus flash per absorbed photon)	880 ± 70	460 ± 85

Notes: (1) Derived from least-squares fits of solutions of equation 3 to amplitude: flash energy relations like that of Figure 6. Cytoplasmic levels of EGTA were 10–12 μM, and cytoplasmic pH was 6.8. (2) Ca^{++} affinity constant of "D" sites was estimated at about 10^6 from data of Yoshikami and Hagins (1974). (3) Indicated errors are uncertainties in parameters associated with scatter of the observations about the best-fitting solutions of equation 3.

Source: Hagins and Yoshikami (1977).

fits on data from retinas treated with two other divalent metal buffers, trans-1,2,cyclohexylenediamine N,N,N′,N′-tetra-acetic acid (CDTA) and ethylenediamine N-hydroxyethyl, N,N′,N′-triacetic acid (HDTA).

Three conclusions can be drawn from Table II. First the buffering effect of EGTA is consistent with the transmitter being Ca^{++}. A more detailed analysis by Hagins and Yoshikami (1977) suggests that only Ba^{++} has an affinity for EGTA in the range that might produce similar desensitizations. Second, the cytoplasmic free Ca^{++} in rat rods is quite comparable with that of other neurons and is relatively well stabilized against changes in external [Ca^{++}] below the level of 100 μM. Third, at least several hundred Ca^{++} ions appear in the cytoplasm of the outer segments for each photon absorbed by rhodopsin. Is this result consistent with what is known of the metabolism of Ca^{++} by isolated preparations of rod disks?

Calcium in rod outer segments

The outer segment layers of flash-frozen frog and rat retinas contain at least 2 mM of total Ca (Hagins and Yoshikami, 1975). Analyses of isolated outer segment suspensions yield figures ranging from 0.1 mM (Szuts and Cone, 1977) to 20 mM (Hendriks, Daemen, and Bonting, 1974). Even the lower figure would provide sufficient Ca^{++} to respond to flashes causing several thousand photon absorptions per rod outer segment.

Do rod disks release Ca^{++} when illuminated? The evidence on this point is not yet satisfactory. Several workers have reported small light-stimulated Ca^{++} losses from outer segment preparations (Hendriks, Daemen, and Bonting, 1974; Liebman, 1974), but Szuts and Cone (1977) have failed to find any such effect. When outer segment membrane preparations are sonicated in the presence of Ca^{++}, the resulting particles have been reported to lose varying amounts of the ion on illumination (Smith, Fager, and Litman, 1977; Hubbell, 1977; Kaupp and Junge, 1977); but effluxes as large as those predicted by the EGTA buffer experiments described above have not been seen. Direct measurements of Ca^{++} efflux from the receptor layer of live rat retinas have also shown no light effects, even though the technique used is sensitive enough to detect less than 1% of the total predicted flux (Yoshikami and Hagins, 1978). The presence of a Ca^{++}-impermeable plasma membrane might explain this result, but why are isolated rod disks apparently so inert? The answer may be that their metabolism is not maintained after isolation.

Thus we must consider the metabolic requirements of the transmitter cycle.

Calcium and metabolism in outer segments

The substantial numerical gain required by the Ca^{++} release would not seem to demand a contribution from the rod's sources of metabolic free energy, but in fact such a contribution is probably necessary. In principle, the degradation of a photon of green light containing 2.5 electron volts of energy to heat could be used to move 1,000 Ca^{++} ions from an infinite reservoir into the cytoplasm of an outer segment without violating the first law of thermodynamics. But there are few cellular mechanisms capable of subdividing a quantum of energy into such efficiently used small fractions. Instead, one high-energy phosphate ester bond is probably hydrolyzed to displace 1–3 Ca^{++} ions from a store in a light response or in recovery from one. What evidence is there for light-stimulated dissipation of phosphate bond energy in photoreception?

Ostwald and Heller (1972) and others have described ATPase activity in preparations of outer segments. More sensitive methods have revealed that adenosine triphosphate (ATP) released from isolated rod outer segments with intact plasma membranes is consumed at a higher rate when the rod fragments are subsequently illuminated (Hagins, Robinson, and Yoshikami, 1975; Robinson, Yoshikami, and Hagins, 1975; Carretta and Cavaggioni, 1976). This effect has been traced to the combined effect of guanosine 5′ triphosphate (GTP) hydrolysis by a GTPase that is activated by light within 0.2 sec coupled to transfer of the terminal phosphate of ATP to the light-created GDP (Robinson and Hagins, 1977). The light-activated GTPase has recently been confirmed (Wheeler, Matuo, and Bitensky, 1977; Wheeler and Bitensky, 1977), but its measured specific activity at low light levels is presently too small to furnish the numerical gain demanded by transmitter release.

There is a second energy-yielding reaction found in isolated fragments of rod outer segments: light-activated hydrolysis of cyclic nucleotide phosphates (Bitensky et al., 1975). It has a specific activity equal to that of the GTPase and is activated to the same degree by light exposure; 1 photon absorbed per 1,000 rhodopsin chromophores is sufficient to activate it fully. But its function is still unknown. The possible connection between guanosine 3′-5′ cyclic monophosphate (cGMP) metabolism and photoreception is subject to much speculation (Rasmussen and Goodman, 1977) and is currently being investi-

gated in live retinas with cGMP analogs and phosphodiesterase inhibitors (Lipton, Rasmussen, and Dowling, 1977).

Whatever biochemical machinery is finally discovered behind the excitatory responses of retinal rods and cones, it is likely to be much more complex than that suggested by the simple cartoon of Figure 3. There is a hint of how elaborate the final scheme must be in the very successful mathematical model proposed by Baylor, Hodgkin, and Lamb (1974) to describe the amplitudes and time courses of the electrical responses of turtle cones to light. It is shown in Figure 7. In essence it consists of a catenary sequence of first-order reactions, beginning with an intermediate produced by light and resulting in a transmitter substance Y (possibly Ca^{++}) appearing in the cytoplasm. Y is then removed by another first-order chain whose first step has a rate coefficient that is itself proportional to the concentration of the first decay product of Y. If the rate constants in the scheme are chosen carefully, the model reproduces cone responses quite accurately.

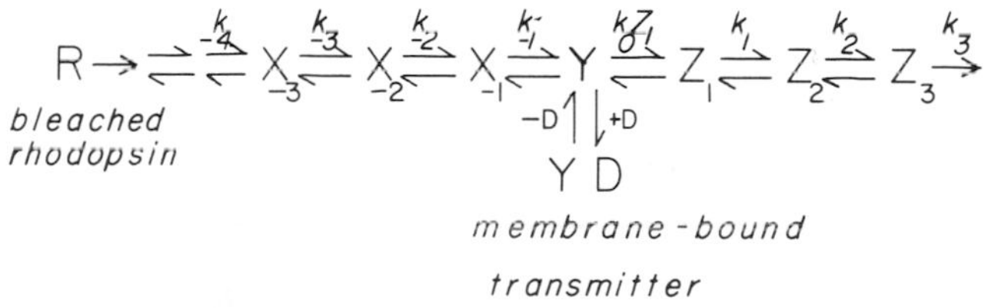

$$R \to \underset{k_{-4}}{\overset{k_4}{\rightleftharpoons}} X_{-3} \underset{k_{-3}}{\overset{k_3}{\rightleftharpoons}} X_{-2} \underset{k_{-2}}{\overset{k_2}{\rightleftharpoons}} X_{-1} \underset{k_{-1}}{\overset{k_1}{\rightleftharpoons}} Y \underset{-D}{\overset{+D}{\rightleftharpoons}} Z_1 \underset{}{\overset{k_1}{\rightleftharpoons}} Z_2 \overset{k_2}{\rightleftharpoons} Z_3 \overset{k_3}{\to}$$

bleached rhodopsin

YD

membrane-bound

transmitter

FIGURE 7 Kinetic scheme proposed by Baylor, Hodgkin, and Lamb (1974) to account for the electrical responses of turtle cones.

There are several features of the model that are difficult to explain. First, the catenary sequence of reactions invoked to produce the correct shape for low-intensity light responses (Penn and Hagins, 1972) requires at least four intermediates, none of which are identified products of photolysis of rhodopsin. Second, the rate constants of these reactions are reduced when the external Ca^{++} level is lowered (Yoshikami and Hagins, 1972; Bertrand, Fuortes, and Pochobradsky, 1977). Third, the model offers no simple explanation of the finding that Ca^{++} deprivation reversibly abolishes the light responses of lizard cones (Yoshikami and Hagins, 1978) but not that of rat rods (Yoshikami and Hagins, 1973). Nevertheless, the model provides a useful framework within which to draw a picture of visual excitation that blends electrophysiology and biochemistry. Future progress in the study of rod-and-cone excitation will surely depend heavily on biochemical methods.

REFERENCES

BARLOW, H. B., 1956. Retinal noise and absolute threshold. *J. Opt. Soc. Am.* 46:634–639.

BAYLOR, D., and M. G. F. FUORTES, 1970. Electrical responses of single cones in the retina of the turtle. *J. Physiol.* 207:77–92.

BAYLOR, D. A., A. L. HODGKIN, and T. LAMB, 1974. The electrical response of turtle cones to flashes and steps of light. *J. Physiol.* 242:685–728.

BERTRAND, D., M. G. F. FUORTES, and J. POCHOBRADSKY, 1977. Actions of EGTA and high calcium on the cones in the turtle retina. *J. Physiol.*, in press.

BITENSKY, M. W., N. MIKI, J. J. KEIRNS, M. KEIRNS, J. M. BARABAN, J. FREEMAN, M. A. WHEELER, J. LACY, and F. R. MARCUS, 1975. Activation of photoreceptors disk membrane phosphodiesterase by light and ATP. *Adv. Cyclic Nucleotide Res.* 5:213–255.

BORTOFF, A., and A. L. NORTON, 1965. Simultaneous recordings of photoreceptor potentials and the PIII component of the ERG. *Vision Res.* 5:527–533.

BROWN, J. E., and L. H. PINTO, 1974. Ionic mechanism for the photoreceptor potential of the retina of Bufo marinus. *J. Physiol.* 236:575–591.

BROWN, J. E., and L. H. PINTO, 1977. Effects of intracellularly injected EGTA on responses of toad rods. In *Vertebrate Photoreception*, H. B. Barlow and P. Fatt, eds. New York: Academic Press.

CARRETTA, A., and A. CAVAGGIONI, 1976. On the metabolism of rod outer segments. *J. Physiol.* 257:687–698.

COHEN, A. I., 1968. New evidence supporting the 1:00Kage to extracellular space of outer segment saccules of frog cones but not rods. *J. Cell Biol.* 37:424–444.

COHEN, A. I., 1970. Further studies on the question of the patency of saccules in outer segments of vertebrate photoreceptors. *Vision Res.* 10:445–453.

CONE, R. A., 1;73. The internal transmitter model for visual excitation: Some quantitative implications. In *Physiology and Biochemistry of Visual Pigments*, H. Langer, ed. New York: Springer-Verlag, pp. 275–282.

CRANK, J., 1956. *Mathematics of Diffusion*. London: Oxford University Press.

HAGINS, W. A., 1965. Electrical signs of information flow in photoreceptors. *Cold Spring Harbor Symp. Quant. Biol.* 30:403–418.

HAGINS, W. A., 1972. The visual process: Excitatory mechanisms in the primary receptor cells. *Annu. Rev. Biophys. Bioengr.* 1:131–158.

HAGINS, W. A., R. D. PENN, and S. YOSHIKAMI, 1970. Dark current and photocurrent in retinal rods. *Biophys. J.* 10:380–412.

HAGINS, W. A., W. E. ROBINSON, and S. YOSHIKAMI, 1975. Ionic aspects of excitation in rod outer segments. In *Energy Transformation in Biological Systems* (CIBA Found. Symp. 31), pp. 169–189.

HAGINS, W. A., and S. YOSHIKAMI, 1974. A Role for Ca^{++} in excitation of retinal rods and cones. *Exp. Eye Res.* 18:299–305.

HAGINS, W. A., and S. YOSHIKAMI, 1975. Ionic mechanism in excitation of photoreceptors. *Ann. NY Acad. Sci.* 264:314–325.

HAGINS, W. A., and S. YOSHIKAMI, 1977. Intracellular transmission of visual excitation in vertebrate photoreceptors: Electrical effects of chelating agents introduced into rods by vesicle fusion. In *Vertebrate Photoreception*, H. B. Barlow and P. Fatt, eds. New York: Academic Press, pp. 97–139.

HECHT, S., S. SHLAER, and M. H. PIRENNE, 1942. Energy, quanta and vision. *J. Gen. Physiol.* 25:819–840.

HENDRIKS, TH., F. J. M. DAEMEN, and S. L. BONTING, 1974. Biochemical aspects of the visual process XXV. Light-induced calcium movements in isolated frog rod outer segments. *Biochem. Biophys. Acta* 345:468–473.

HUBBELL, W., 1977. Molecular anatomy and light-dependent processes in photoreceptor membranes. In *Vertebrate Photoreception*, H. B. Barlow and P. Fatt, eds. New York: Academic Press.

KAUPP, U., and W. JUNGE, 1977. Rapid calcium release by passively loaded retinal disks on photoexcitation. *FEBS Lett.* 81:229–232.

LAMB, T. D., and E. J. SIMON, 1977. Analysis of electrical noise in turtle cones. *J. Physiol.* 272:435–468.

LIEBMAN, P. A., 1974. Light-dependent Ca^{++} content of rod outer segment disk membranes. *Invest. Ophthalmol.* 13:700–702.

LIPTON, S., H. RASMUSSEN, and J. E. DOWLING, 1977. Adaptation of vertebrate photoreceptors. II. Similar effects of Ca^{++}, cyclic nucleotides and prostaglandins as intracellular messengers. *J. Gen. Physiol.* 70:771–791.

OSTWALD, T. J., and J. HELLER, 1972. Properties of a magnesium or calcium-dependent adenosine triphosphatase from frog photoreceptor outer segment disks and its inhibition by illumination. *Biochemistry* 11:4679–4686.

PENN, R. D., and W. A. HAGINS, 1969. Signal transmission in retinal rods and the origin of the electro retinographic a-wave. *Nature* 223:201–203.

PENN, R. D., and W. A. HAGINS, 1972. Kinetics of the photocurrent of retinal rods. *Biophys. J.* 12:1073–1094.

RASMUSSEN, H., and D. B. P. GOODMAN, 1977. Relationships between calcium and cyclic nucleotides in cell activation. *Physiol. Rev.* 57:421–509.

ROBINSON, W. E., and W. A. HAGINS, 1977. A light-activated GTPase in retinal rod outer segments. *Biophys. J.* 17:196a.

ROBINSON, W. E., S. YOSHIKAMI, and W. A. HAGINS, 1975. ATP in retinal rods. *Biophys. J.* 15:168a.

RUEPPEL, H., and W. A. HAGINS, 1973. Spatial origin of the fast photovoltage in retinal rods. In *Physiology and Biochemistry of Visual Pigments*, H. Langer, ed. New York: Springer-Verlag, pp. 257–261.

SCHWARTZ, E. A., 1977. Voltage noise observed in rods of the turtle retina. *J. Physiol.* 272:217–246.

SILLMAN, A. J., H. ITO, and T. TOMITA, 1969. Studies on the mass receptor potential of isolated frog retina. II. On the basis of the ionic mechanism. *Vision Res.* 9:1443–1451.

SMITH, H. G., R. S. FAGER, and B. J. LITMAN, 1977. Light-activated calcium release from sonicated bovine retinal rod outer segment disks. *Biochemistry* 16:1399–1405.

SZUTS, E., and R. A. CONE, 1977. Calcium content of frog rod outer segments and disks. *Biochem. Biophys. Acta* 468:194–208.

TOMITA, T., 1965. Electrophysiological study of the mechanism subserving color coding in the fish retina. *Cold Spring Harbor Symp. Quant. Biol.* 30:559–566.

TOYODA, J., H. NOSAKI, and T. TOMITA, 1969. Light-induced resistance changes in single photoreceptors of *Nec-*

turus and *Gecko. Vision Res.* 9:453–463.

WEINSTEIN, J. N., S. YOSHIKAMI, P. HENKART, R. BLUMEN-THAL, and W. A. HAGINS, 1977. Lipsome-cell interaction: Transfer and intracellular release of a trapped fluorescent marker. *Science* 195:489–491.

WHEELER, G. L., and M. W. BITENSKY, 1977. A light-activated GTPase in vertebrate photoreceptors: Regulation of light-activated cyclic GMP phosphodiesterase. *Proc. Natl. Acad. Sci. USA* 74:4238–4242.

WHEELER, G. L., Y. MATUO, and M. W. BITENSKY, 1977. Light-activated GTPase in vertebrate photoreceptors. *Nature* 269:822–824.

YOSHIKAMI, S., and W. A. HAGINS, 1973. Control of the dark current in vertebrate rods and cones. In *Biochemistry and Physiology of Visual Pigments*, H. Langer, ed. New York: Springer-Verlag, pp. 245–255.

YOSHIKAMI, S., and W. A. HAGINS, 1978. Calcium and excitation of vertebrate rods: Retinal efflux of Ca^{++} studied with dichlorophosphonazo III. *Ann. NY Acad. Sci.*, in press.

YOSHIKAMI, S., W. E. ROBINSON, and W. A. HAGINS, 1974. Topology of the outer segment membranes of retinal rods and cones revealed by a fluorescent probe. *Science* 185:1176–1179.

12 Integrative Pathways in Local Circuits between Slow-Potential Cells in the Retina

FRANK S. WERBLIN

ABSTRACT This chapter illustrates how visual sensitivity can be controlled by synaptic interactions at specific local circuits involving processes from slow-potential retinal neurons. The direct pathway from photoreceptors to bipolars to ganglion cells forms the receptive-field centers and is intersected by two separate systems of lateral interneurons. The topography and activity of the interneurons acting at local circuits form the properties of the antagonistic surrounds. Each lateral system responds best to a specific form of illumination, and each modulates the sensitivity at the receptive-field center.

Synaptic transmitter is released in the dark by the photoreceptors, and release is reduced with illumination. The receptor transmitter depolarizes the *off* bipolar and the horizontal cells by increasing conductance, but it hyperpolarizes the *on* bipolar cells by decreasing conductance. Steady illumination therefore hyperpolarizes the horizontal cells that act at local circuits to alter bipolar sensitivity, probably by feeding back and resetting the relation between illumination and response in the receptors via a sign-inverting synapse.

Ganglion-cell activity is organized through convergent inputs from the bipolar and amacrine cells. The *on* ganglion cells are excited by the *on* bipolars. This synapse is silent in the dark. The *off* ganglion cells are excited by the *off* bipolars. This synapse is active in the dark. All ganglion cells are inhibited by the amacrine-cell system. Thus changing illumination, which activates amacrine cells, modulates ganglion-cell sensitivity.

Introduction

ONE OF THE striking features of the organization of the retina is the clear distinction between centrally and laterally directed neural pathways. The signal is carried centrally by the chain of neurons consisting of photoreceptors and bipolar and ganglion cells. This chain intersects two distinct systems of lateral

FRANK S. WERBLIN Department of Electrical Engineering and Computer Science and the Electronics Research Laboratory, University of California, Berkeley, CA 94720

neurons, the horizontal and amacrine cells, at two different levels in the retina. It can be shown that each system of lateral interneurons forms a concentric antagonistic surround for the central pathways. Therefore, the functionally defined center and surround components of receptive fields in the retina may be related to anatomically defined systems of cell types. It follows that ganglion cells actually possess at least two overlapping antagonistic surround regions, each mediated by one of the lateral systems of interneurons.

Each of the systems of lateral interneurons can be activated by a specific form of visual stimulus, so that either or both of the lateral antagonistic pathways can be selectively driven under experimental control, this makes it possible to assess the role of each system of lateral interneurons in modifying the quality of the signal along the central pathway.

One of the functions of the lateral antagonistic pathways is the control of sensitivity along the central pathway. Each system of lateral interneurons has a specific and different effect upon sensitivity; the ways in which they modify visual sensitivity are described in the first part of this chapter.

The synaptic interactions that control visual function in the retina are of particular neurobiological interest because they involve communication of slow-potential neurons in local circuits. These cells are normally polarized to a steady potential near the mid-range of their response limits, and some steadily release synaptic transmitter at a high rate, which can be modulated by light-elicited activity. Synaptic function can be inferred by studying the electrical properties of these cells and the changes that take place when either central or lateral pathways are activated. Studies of synaptic function constitute the second part of the chapter.

We shall eventually be able to describe in detail the

neural basis for visual function in the retina. I attempt part of that process here by correlating the studies of visual function in terms of sensitivity control with those of synaptic activity in terms of electrical properties of the cells; the correlations are expressed in Table I at the end of the chapter. The process was begun at least a hundred years ago by Ernst Mach, who observed:

Since each point perceives itself, so to speak as above or below the average of its neighbors, there results a characteristic type of perception. Whatever is near the mean of the surroundings becomes effaced, whatever is above or below is disproportionately brought into prominence. One could say that the retina schematizes and caricatures. The teleological significance of the process is clear in itself. It is an analog of abstraction and of the formation of concepts. (Quoted in Ratliff, 1965)

Synaptic interactions controlling sensitivity

Dowling (this volume) has outlined the basic synaptic organization of the vertebrate retina, along with the characteristic forms of cellular activity measured at each retinal level (see also Werblin and Dowling, 1969). He showed that there exists a vertical or centrally directed pathway from photoreceptors to bipolar to ganglion cells, which is intersected at two levels—by lateral pathways formed by horizontal cells at the outer retina and by amacrine cells at the inner retina. Even a cursory examination of the anatomy suggests that the systems of neurons in the lateral pathways are appropriately situated to mediate lateral interactions and thereby to form the antagonistic surrounds for single units in the central pathway. It was shown how the horizontal cells, for example, seem to be involved in the formation of the concentric antagonistic surround for the bipolar cells. It will be shown below that the amacrine-cell system forms yet another kind of antagonistic surround for the ganglion cells (Werblin, 1972). Furthermore, an important role of each of the antagonistic surrounds will be characterized: they seem to control the intensity domain and response range for the cells in the central pathway as a function of the patterns of illumination falling in local surrounding retinal regions.

LATERAL PATHWAYS IN THE RETINA   Figure 1 outlines the retinal pathways and experimental arrangement used to define the role of lateral interactions for the horizontal and amacrine cells. It is abstracted from anatomical studies of Dowling and Werblin (1969), Lasansky (1973), Wong-Riley (1974), and others. Very simply, the central test spot is used to elicit

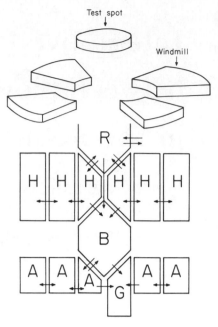

FIGURE 1   Synaptic organization of the retina. The central vertical pathway, leading from receptor (R) to bipolar (B) to ganglion cell (G), is intersected by two systems of lateral interneurons: the horizontal cells (H) and the amacrine cells (A). The arrows indicate the direction and presence of possible synaptic pathways. Each cell type receives synaptic input from at least two cell types. Lateral interneurons feed across to each other and may feed both forward and back to cells in the central pathway. Most of these synaptic pathways have been analyzed by deriving current-voltage relations for the dark and light states of activity (see text). Position of the test stimuli for eliciting center and surround illumination are shown above the synaptic diagram. The test spot for eliciting the center response was set to cover the center of the receptive center field for the cells in the central pathway, usually about 400 μm in diameter for tiger salamander and mudpuppy. The "windmill" pattern was truncated inside 400 μm to avoid stimulating the central pathway and extended to about 2,000 μm to encompass the receptive-field surround. The windmill activates the horizontal-cell system when stationary but activates both horizontal and amacrine cells when rotating. Under these conditions, the lateral pathways interact with the center pathway to modify activity elicited by the test spot.

activity in the central pathway (see Dowling for the forms of cellular activity), and the "windmill" vanes are used to selectively activate lateral antagonistic interactions mediated by either the horizontal-cell system or the amacrine-cell system as described below. Then the effect of activity in either lateral antagonistic system can be evaluated by measuring the changes in response properties of the cells along the central pathway elicited by the test spot.

The strategy for selectively activating the lateral

systems follows from the difference in the response properties of the horizontal and amacrine cells outlined earlier (see Dowling, this volume; Werblin, 1972). Horizontal cells respond tonically to the presence of illumination within their receptive fields, but amacrine cells respond only transiently to *changes* in illumination within their receptive fields. Therefore, when the windmill is stationary, the horizontal cells will be activated, but the amacrine cells will be silent. However, when the windmill begins to spin, a local population of amacrine cells beneath the edges of the moving vanes of the windmill will be brought into activity. The specific population of amacrine and horizontal cells always changes as the windmill spins, but the concentric organization of the stimuli ensures that the effects from all the vanes will converge at the center pathway; and the homogeneity of the retinal pathways ensures that the strength of the lateral signals converging at the center will be relatively constant during the rotation of the windmill.

LATERAL INTERACTIONS AT THE OUTER PLEXIFORM LAYER   The role of the horizontal cells alone can be studied using the stationary windmill. The results are shown in Figure 2. Bipolar cells (Figure 2A) respond with graded polarization to test flashes of the center spot of different intensities, but only over a limited domain of log-test intensities varying by less than 50 to 1. For any fixed surround condition, the bipolar response is not measurable at test intensities below this domain and is of maximal level for all test intensities above it (Werblin, 1974; Thibos and Werblin, 1978). The important point here is that the specific domain (of log intensities) over which the bipolar response is graded is not fixed, but depends upon the level of surround illumination. Figure 2A shows that the graded response range tends to shift bodily to the right along the log intensity axis as the surround intensity increases. Under optimal conditions, when the entire surround is illuminated, an increase in surround intensity of 1 log unit results in a shift to the right of the graded response curve by about 1 log unit. Also, the graded response curves are shifted so that the midpoint of the graded response curve falls very near the intensity of the surround.

The cells postsynaptic to the bipolars are also affected by lateral interactions at the outer retina, and Figure 2B shows that the graded response curves for the ganglion cells are similarly shifted to the right along the log intensity axis by increasing levels of surround illumination.

LATERAL INTERACTIONS AT THE INNER PLEXIFORM LAYER   The amacrine-cell system appears to be silent in the presence of the fixed windmill; but when the vanes begin to spin, the amacrine cells are strongly and steadily depolarized (Werblin, 1972). Under these conditions it has been shown that the ganglion cells are hyperpolarized but the bipolar cells are unaffected by the spin. The hyperpolarization affects the entire graded response range for the ganglion cells, as shown in Figure 2C. The primary effect of the spinning windmill is to decrease the level of response in the ganglion cells for all center test intensities. As a result, the threshold for ganglion-cell activity appears to be elevated, and the maximum response level is reduced. In the tiger salamander, all ganglion cells are affected by the spinning windmill, but the activity recorded from the change-sensitive ganglion cells is more strongly modified (see also Schwartz, 1973).

These studies suggest at least one clear role for each of the systems of lateral interneurons in the retina, the horizontal and amacrine cells. Each forms an antagonistic surround for cells in the center pathway, and activation of the antagonistic surround reduces the response of the cells in the center pathway over all of their graded response domain. The horizontal cells, responding tonically to the presence of illumination in the surround, act to tonically reset the relationship between response and log intensity by bodily shifting the S-shaped response curve to the right. The amacrine cells respond to change by acting to suppress the response, primarily of the change-sensitive ganglion cells, over their entire response domain (see Naka, 1977). These two systems operate in tandem, so that the effects initiated at the outer retina affect all proximal cells, whereas those initiated at the inner retina affect primarily the change-sensitive ganglion cells.

SIGNIFICANCE OF LATERAL INTERACTIONS   Studies of single cells at the visual cortex have consistently shown that the neural vocabulary of the visual system is concerned with information about the presence, movement, and orientation of boundaries within the visual field. The abstraction of this kind of information about boundaries begins at the retina, and the lateral interactions described above seem to be involved in the organization of this information.

It has been known for more than a decade that the response properties of retinal ganglion cells to many physiological stimuli remain relatively invariant with differing levels of ambient illumination (Maturana et

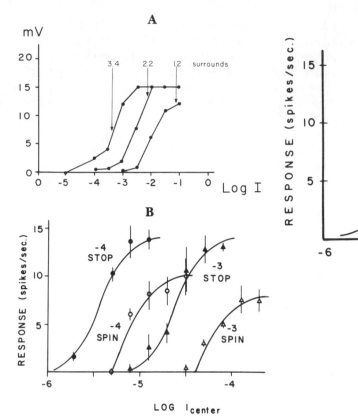

FIGURE 2 Shift in response domain for central-pathway cells as a function of conditions of surround illumination. (A) Intensity-response curves for a depolarizing bipolar cell measured with varying center test intensities at three levels of fixed-surround illumination. Numbers at arrows indicate surround intensity relative to the center test intensity plotted along the abscissa. The entire graded response domain

is increased by about 1 log unit for each log unit increase in surround intensity. (B) Similar experiment with fixed surround, but measured in an *on* ganglion cell of a mudpuppy. Again, the graded response curve for the cell is shifted to a brighter intensity domain by about 1 log unit for each log unit increase in surround intensity. (C) Effect of spinning and stationary windmill patterns on the graded response of an *on-off* ganglion cell. Increase in the intensity of the fixed surround by 1 log unit causes the graded response to shift from −5.5 to −4.5 log units along the abscissa, as in A and B. At each level, spinning of the windmill in the surround causes a compression of the center-elicited response as indicated by the downward shift in the curves marked "spin." This ganglion cell reflects lateral interactions at the outer plexiform layer (lateral shift) and interactions at the inner plexiform layer (downward shift) on the intensity-response relation.

al., 1963). This is due to a variety of retinal mechanisms responsible for *adaptation,* processes that adjust the response domain of the retina to correspond to the ambient light conditions. A major process of adaptation takes place in the photoreceptors themselves (Dowling, 1963; Normann and Werblin, 1974; Kleinschmidt and Dowling, 1975; Fain, 1976; Dowling and Ripps, 1972); but neural interactions proximal to the photoreceptors are also involved in optimizing signals as a function of local ambient conditions. The adjustment of the bipolar intensity-response domain shown in Figure 2 is an example of a neurally mediated form of sensitivity control. Another form of proximal control of sensitivity is described by Green et al. (1975).

The response domain for the bipolar cells is relatively narrow: the response grows from threshold to saturation within less than a fiftyfold range in test intensity. This is useful for boundary detection because a small change in intensity across a boundary

will be converted into a large potential change in the bipolar cells. Because the response curve spans a very narrow domain of log intensities, it must be carefully positioned along the intensity domain so that it spans just those intensities that include the boundary. Apparently the strategy for domain control at the outer plexiform layer is to position the graded response range of the bipolars at the intensity of the local surrounding regions. Horizontal cells compute a local average of surround intensities and, through the synaptic interactions described below, act to align the bipolar graded response with this local intensity average.

The significance of the lateral interactions at the inner plexiform layer is more difficult to interpret, probably because we do not have a good idea of the physiological stimuli to which this neural system is tuned. Change is introduced by the spinning windmill in these experiments for convenience, but a variety of other stimuli that generate changing patterns work equally as well to activate amacrine-cell and suppress ganglion-cell activity (Copenhagen, 1975; Werblin and Copenhagen, 1974). Figure 2B shows that the range of response in the change-sensitive cells is compressed when the level of change or movement in the local surround is high. As a result, the levels of response generating the neural image, represented by the activity of the mosaic of change-sensitive ganglion cells, are compressed by change in light or pattern in the local surround. The compression of the overall range of response to change is analogous to a reduction in the contrast of the neural image.

The above discussion provides a brief introduction to some of the forms of processing related to the neural control of sensitivity taking place in the retina. It is of interest now to determine how functions such as local intensity averaging, domain shifting, and range control expressed above in terms of *visual processing*—are performed through specific *neuronal interactions* at local circuits in the retina.

Analysis of the electrical properties of synaptic interactions in the retina

There are numerous approaches to understanding the details of synaptic activity in the retina. Most involve modifying the normal electrical or chemical conditions of the neurons and making inferences about synaptic mechanisms based upon precedents derived from other preparations and how modifications affect cellular activity. The papers in this volume by Miller and by Gerschenfeld deal with changes in retinal activity due to altered ionic or pharmacological environments. In this section I summarize work in which the synaptic inputs to each retinal neuron were studied by measuring the changes in the characteristics of the light response as the membranes of the postsynaptic cells were polarized to different potential levels by extrinsic currents.

The method of membrane polarization is useful for determining the magnitude and direction of conductance changes associated with synaptic inputs and for measuring the approximate equilibrium potentials for the ionic species whose permeability channels are modified by the action of impinging synaptic transmitter. It works best when a neuron receives a single synaptic input and when the subsynaptic membrane is not too distant from the recording site. Under these conditions the current-voltage curves derived for the membrane in the active and nonactive states provide sufficient information. In the retina

the conditions are less than ideal: each cell type receives at least two synaptic inputs, which tend to overlap in time (see Figure 1), and the recordings are usually taken by penetrating the cell body, which is a significant electrotonic distance from the subsynaptic membrane at the dendrites. Despite these limitations, the patterns of activity measured in the cells reveal important information about the synaptic inputs and serve to establish some constraints on the possible modes of synaptic communication between retinal cells.

ELECTRICAL COUPLING BETWEEN RODS   As an example of the strategy involved in interpreting the current-voltage relations for a cell that receives two simultaneous synaptic inputs, we take the tiger salamander rod. Hagins (this volume) suggests that the rod response is generated by a decrease in sodium conductance at the outer segment. If we could measure the current-voltage relations for the rod in the dark and in the light, we should find a consistently higher resistance for the light condition. The current-voltage curves derived for light and dark should reveal, at their intersection, a "reversal potential" for the light response that is close to the equilibrium potential for sodium.

When these measurements are actually made in the rod, the current-voltage curves appear to be parallel: there is no evidence for a conductance change associated with the light response, as shown in Figure 3A. This apparent violation of the rules is in fact expected because the light-elicited conductance changes at the outer segment are obscured by a second synaptic input to the rods, namely, the electrotonically coupled input from neighboring rods (Werblin, 1975; Copenhagen and Owen, 1976; Schwartz, 1976; Fain, Gold, and Dowling, 1976). As a result of this second input, the mosaic of inner segments in the retina can be considered as one broad cell, encompassing many rod inner segments. The light-elicited inputs to this "cell" are distributed over a region much greater than the area of the impaled rod alone; such a distributed input tends to lack any clear sign of conductance change measured at a single site, even though each outer segment in the mosaic probably polarizes as a result of a conductance change. This can be explained by considering that most of the input to a single rod comes through electrical rather than chemical synaptic input, or that the polarization of a single rod by extrinsic current has little effect on the potential of the neighboring cells, which supply most of the light-elicited current to the impaled rod (Lamb, 1976, Lamb and Simon, 1976). Therefore the input

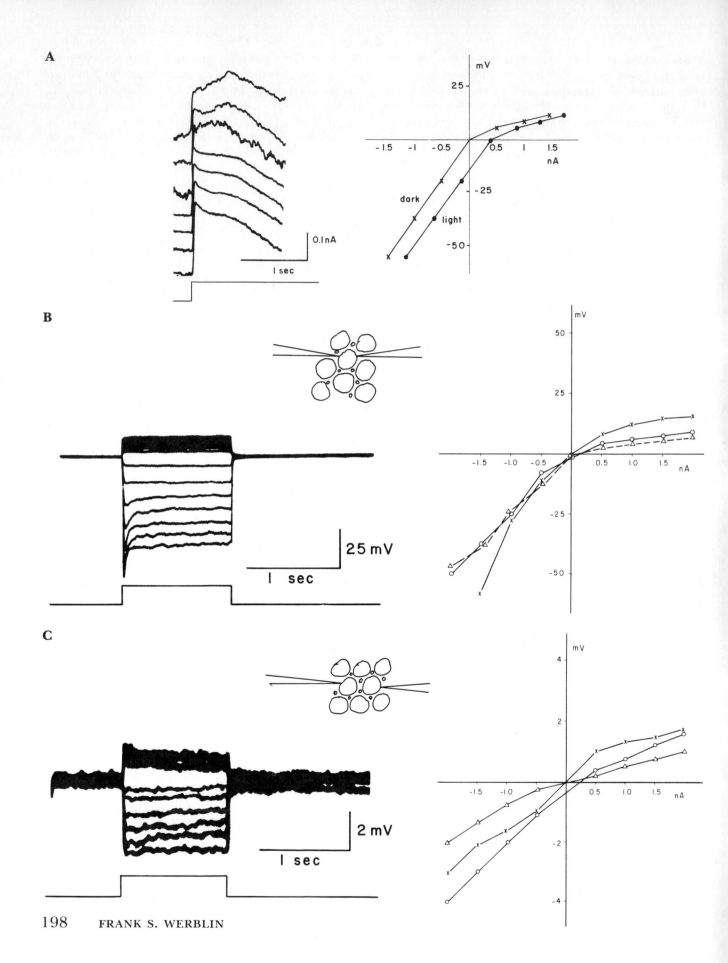

FRANK S. WERBLIN

from neighbors is relatively constant at all potential levels in the impaled rod.

The electrical coupling can be shown more directly by passing current through one rod while recording the potential change generated in a neighbor. Figures 3B and 3C show that the potential in the neighbor is only about 20% of that generated at each current level in the rod receiving the extrinsic current. This measure is consistent for rod pairs in the tiger salamander; and if it is assumed that the rods are coupled to each other in a square array, it means that the activity in any one rod is affected by about eighty of its neighbors (see Werblin, 1978). Direct measurements of the receptive field of the individual rods in the tiger salamander indicate a diameter of about 8–10 rods, verifying that each individual rod is coupled to about eighty neighbors. These measurements also indicate that less than half of the response in any one rod is generated by its own outer segment (see also Fain, 1975), which helps to explain why the current-voltage curves in Figure 5 show no resistance change due to light and do not converge.

The study of the electrical properties of the rod response outlined above indicates how one synaptic input can obscure the electrical measurements of an-other when both occur simultaneously. Since Hagins (this volume) has given more information about the rod response, we can use the apparently paradoxical finding of no conductance associated with the rod response to help characterize the other synaptic input, namely, the electrotonic coupling between the rods themselves. Similar problems arise in the following studies on the electrical properties of the response of more proximal retinal cells, which also receive simultaneous inputs from at least two sources.

COUPLING BETWEEN HORIZONTAL CELLS   The strategy developed above for the study of the rods will also be useful in studying the horizontal cells, for they too seem to receive two synaptic inputs. One input, from the photoreceptors, appears to be due to a chemically mediated conductance change; the other, from neighboring horizontal cells, seems to be associated with no conductance change and may not be chemical (Marshall and Werblin, 1978).

In the tiger salamander under normal conditions there is a distribution in the diameter of the receptive fields of the horizontal cells. About 25% have very narrow fields, about 0.5 mm in diameter, corresponding roughly to the diameter of the processes of a single horizontal cell (Lasansky, 1973). The remaining units have much broader receptive fields.

The horizontal cells with narrow receptive fields appear to be driven by a simple excitatory synapse. The heavier current-voltage curves in Figure 4A indicate that the membrane conductance in the dark is greater by about 20% than that in the light. The dashed curve along the steeper heavy curve shows the electrical state of the membrane in the presence of Co++, which blocks the release of transmitter from the photoreceptors. The coincidence of the electrical state of the membrane in the presence of light and Co++ suggests that the photoreceptor transmitter is liberated at its highest rate in the dark, is reduced to insignificant levels by bright lights (Trifonov, 1968; Dowling and Ripps, 1973; Cervetto and Piccolino, 1974; Kaneko and Shimazaki, 1975), and acts to depolarize the horizontal cells by increasing conductance (Marshall and Werblin, 1978). The light and dark curves converge at about +50 mV, a rough measure for the null potential for the response. This is probably an overestimate of the null potential, since the subsynaptic membrane is located at some considerable electrotonic distance from the recording site at the cell soma.

The horizontal cells with broad receptive fields probably receive an additional synaptic input from neighboring horizontal cells, since the spread of proc-

---

FIGURE 3   Current-voltage relations for a rod, derived under voltage clamp. (A) *Left*: Response current measured at seven different potential levels, indicated by the points on curves at right in response to full-field test flash eliciting half-maximal response. The response currents are of almost equal magnitude at each potential level from −90 mV to −25 mV, indicating no clearly measurable conductance change associated with the light response. *Right*: Current-voltage curves for dark and light derived from the responses. The curves are roughly parallel over the entire potential range for which the measurements were made. The dark level of about −35 mV is at the origin. Axes on the graph are inverted (current along the abscissa) for comparison with most of the other curves in the paper. (B) Coupling between rods. *Left*: Current-voltage curves derived from penetration of single rod with two separate electrodes in isolated retina under visual control, using modulation-contrast optics. The rod membrane is rectifying, having input resistance of about 10 MΩ for depolarizing currents and about 50 MΩ for hyperpolarizing currents. (C) Current voltage curves derived by passing current into one rod and recording potential changes in a neighbor under visual control. The current-voltage curves are of the same form as in A and B, but decreased in magnitude by a factor of about five. Typical attenuation in neighbors varied from five to ten. The relation between potential between the two rods is roughly linear between −90 and −10 mV and is unaffected by Co++, suggesting that coupling is mediated by electrotonic conduction. This is consistent with the result in Figure 3A, suggesting distributed inputs to rods (see text).

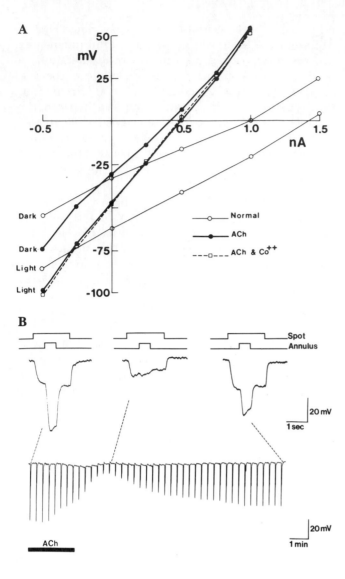

FIGURE 4 Current-voltage curves for horizontal cells, showing also the effect of ACh application. (A) Dark curves show typical results for narrow-field horizontal cells receiving input primarily from photoreceptors. The curves converge at a measured null potential near +50 mV. The dashed curve, indicating the state of the membrane with Co^{++} (without endogenous transmitter), is close to the curve for bright light, suggesting that light turns off transmitter and that transmitter depolarizes by exciting horizontal cells, thereby increasing conductance to ions that depolarize the membrane. Most horizontal-cell current-voltage curves resemble the lighter curves in the figure, showing an extrapolated null potential near +200 mV. In the presence of ACh, these curves become similar to the heavy curves. (B) ACh also decreases the size of the receptive field of the horizontal cells. The figure shows that the response to the annulus is abolished, while the response to the center test spot is reduced by only about 25% in the presence of ACh. Upper figures are time-expanded records taken from the total time record shown below.

esses for any one cell is much narrower than its measured receptive field. These cells seem to receive an additional synaptic input, which is not associated with a conductance change, as shown by the lighter curves in Figure 4A. The almost parallel trajectory for these curves, with extrapolated intersection near +200 mV, precludes a simple conductance-mediated response. The argument for a second input, associated with no conductance change, is strengthened by the following finding, which we hit upon quite by accident.

In trying to evaluate the effect of putative transmitter substances on the response of the horizontal cell, we used acetylcholine (ACh), since it had been reported to be synthesized by the cones in turtle (Lam, 1972). Instead of depolarizing the horizontal cells by increasing conductance, a property of the endogenous transmitter (see Figure 4A), ACh caused a decrease in conductance. Surprisingly, ACh also seemed to uncouple the horizontal cells. The broad-field cells (shown by light lines in Figure 4) reverted to narrow-field cells (shown by heavy lines). The receptive field was reduced from 2.0 mm to about 0.5 mm (see Figure 4B), and the curves' intersection was reduced from over 200 mV to about 50 mV. Most important, in cases where we were able to make the measurement, the *absolute* change in conductance between dark and light remained roughly the same before and after ACh, indicating that the increased surround response, mediated through the coupling and eliminated in the presence of ACh, was not associated with an additional conductance change.

These studies suggest that the receptor-to-horizontal synapse is chemically mediated but that the horizontal-to-horizontal coupling may be electrotonic because it is associated with no conductance change. However, this argument is only tentative because a distributed chemically mediated synaptic input, initiated in the periphery of the horizontal-cell receptive field, might not be measurable by these techniques, just as the distributed conductance change in rods was not measured. Also, there is no precedent for ACh interrupting an electrical synapse. The studies establish the excitatory nature of the receptor-to-horizontal synapse and lead to speculation about the nature of coupling between horizontal cells. Further studies of the effects of cholinergic agents on the response properties of the horizontal cells are needed, and some of these are discussed by Gerschenfeld (this volume).

SYNAPTIC INPUTS TO BIPOLAR CELLS As indicated in Figure 1, there are possibly two synaptic inputs to the bipolar cells; they are driven directly, probably chemically, by the photoreceptors. In addition, anatomical studies (Dowling and Werblin, 1969; Lasansky, 1973) show conventional chemical synaptic morphology, indicating a pathway from horizontal cells directly to bipolar dendrites and somata. There is also physiological evidence for a feedback pathway from horizontal cells to the cones of turtle (Baylor, Fuortes, and O'Bryan, 1971) and perchpike (Burkhardt, 1976); but no unequivocal evidence for this pathway has been revealed in anatomical studies.

The second, lateral input to bipolars or photoreceptors from the horizontal cells is of particular interest, for it is the pathway that mediates the surround antagonism that resets bipolar sensitivity, as described earlier in this paper. An argument has been made that the sensitivity control, by which the intensity domain for the graded bipolar response is reset by lateral antagonism due to surround illumination, might be mediated via a feedback pathway (Werblin, 1978b; Thibos and Werblin, 1978). It is therefore of special interest to determine the synaptic mechanisms responsible for surround antagonism in the bipolar cells.

The current-voltage curves for the two kinds of bipolar cells, the depolarizing or *on* type and the hyperpolarizing or *off* type, are shown in Figure 5 for response to center alone and to center plus antagonistic surround. All current-voltage curves appear to pivot around a potential near +50 mV, suggesting that channels permeable to ions with equilibrium potentials positive with respect to the dark level are modulated by both synaptic inputs to the bipolars. The antagonistic surround causes a diminution of the center response by reducing the associated conductance change. In a sense, the antagonistic surround appears to reverse the effect of center illumination on both the potential and conductance change of the bipolar cells.

The simplest explanation for these effects is that the antagonistic surround feeds back to the photoreceptors and reverses the light-elicited potential change at the receptor terminals. This is probably true for the cone pathway, where illumination at the periphery has been shown to depolarize the cones (Baylor, Fuortes, and O'Bryan, 1971), but no such effect has ever been measured in the rod system. There is also the possibility, based on anatomical observations, that horizontal cells feed forward to the bipolars; and if this pathway is operating, the forms of conductance change associated with each input to the bipolar cells require some special explanation. Since we showed earlier that the photoreceptor

transmitter is released at the highest rate in the dark, it is convenient here to use darkness as the stimulus so that we can refer to the effect of the transmitter itself. Although the measurement has not yet been made, we assume here that the horizontal cells also liberate a chemical transmitter and that it is released at the highest rate in the dark when the horizontal cells are most depolarized. Under dark conditions, the *off* bipolar (Figure 5A) would be depolarized by the photoreceptor transmitter but hyperpolarized by direct input from the horizontal-cell transmitter. Conversely, the depolarizing bipolar cells (Figure 6B) would be hyperpolarized by photoreceptor transmitter but depolarized by a horizontal-cell transmitter. All conductance changes involve ions with an equilibrium potential positive with respect to the dark level in these cells, since the null potential for all effects is at about +50 mV in Figure 5 for both cell types. Therefore, the photoreceptor transmitter must increase conductance in the *off* bipolar but decrease conductance in the *on* bipolar. Conversely the horizontal cell transmitter must increase conductance in the *on* bipolar but decrease conductance in the *off* bipolar.

The notion of a transmitter-elicited conductance decrease is unusual but not unprecedented (see Gerschenfeld, 1973, and this volume). Moreover, although the ionic channels involved here cannot be ascertained from these experiments, some of the work of Miller (this volume; Miller and Dacheux, 1976; Waloga and Pak, 1976) suggests that chloride ions are involved in the depolarization of *on* bipolars and sodium in the depolarization of *off* bipolars.

The results for the bipolar cells, and above for the horizontal cells, can provide the beginning of an explanation of visual phenomena in terms of synaptic mechanisms. The broad antagonistic surround for the bipolar-cell receptive field is formed through (possibly electrotonic) coupling between horizontal cells, as discussed above. Horizontal cells seem to form chemical synapses, which are fed either back or forward according to the constraints indicated above and which antagonize the response mediated by the direct receptor-to-bipolar chemical synapse. The resetting of the graded bipolar response characteristic along the log intensity domain, as a function of average surround illumination (Figure 2A), can be best explained in terms of a feedback synapse that reduces the light-elicited hyperpolarization at the receptor terminal, thereby requiring a greater receptor polarization (brighter test flash) to maintain the same bipolar response (for details see Werblin, 1978b; Thibos and Werblin, 1978).

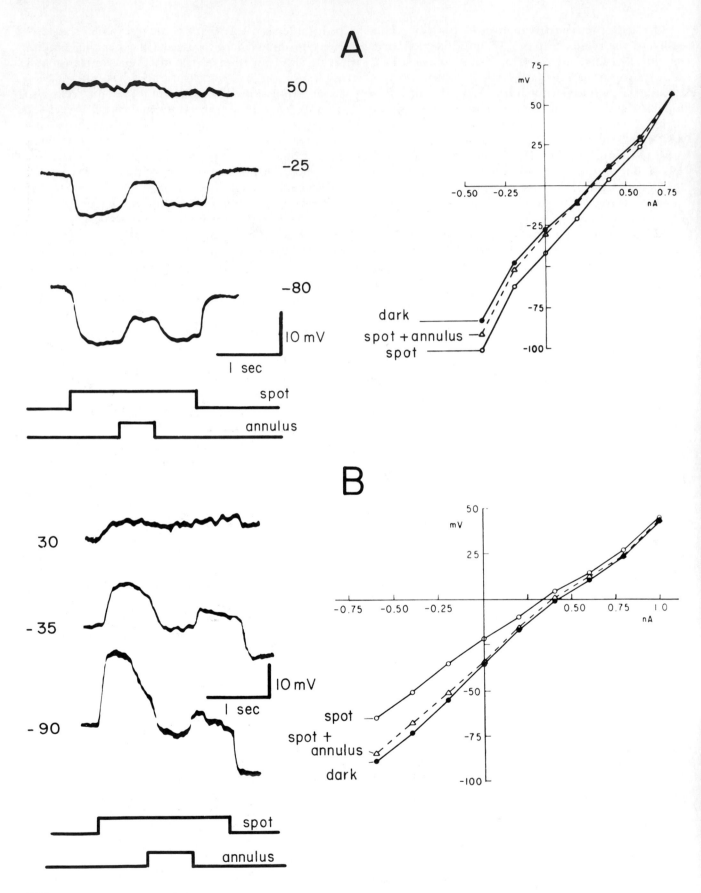

50

−25

−80

10 mV

1 sec

spot

annulus

A

mV
75

50

25

−0.50 −0.25   0.50 0.75

nA

−25

−75

−100

dark

spot + annulus

spot

30

−35

−90

10 mV

1 sec

spot

annulus

B

mV
50

25

−0.75 −0.50 −0.25   0.50 0.75 1.0

nA

−50

−75

−100

spot

spot +
annulus

dark

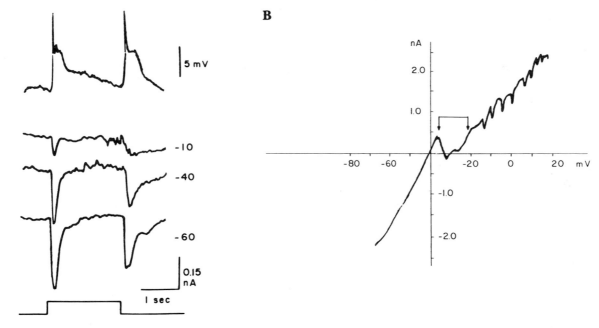

A

5 mV

−10

−40

−60

0.15 nA

1 sec

B

nA

2.0

1.0

−80   −60   −20   0   20   mV

−1.0

−2.0

FIGURE 6 Electrical properties of the amacrine-cell response. (A) Top trace shows typical response. Lower traces show synaptic currents measured under voltage clamp to eliminate spiking. All inputs are transient and excitatory with null potential near 0 mV. There is no evidence for the sustained bipolar input, and no sign of an inhibitory component. (B) Current-voltage curve under voltage clamp during a ramp depolarization. A large negative-resistance region is encountered about 4 mV positive to the dark level (at origin), which boosts the voltage response by about 20 mV (arrows). At more depolarized levels there is a series of smaller repetitive spikes, presumably at the amacrine-cell dendrites, which are capable of propagating depolarizations initiated at the soma.

INITIATION OF TRANSIENT ACTIVITY IN THE RETINA: THE AMACRINE-CELL RESPONSE The transition from purely slow-potential activity to more classical spike-like phenomena seems to take place proximal to the bipolar terminal (for anatomy see Wong-Riley, 1974). The first suggestion of transient activity is found in the amacrine cells, which respond with a brief depolarization and a few spikes at the onset and termination of a step of illumination, as shown in Figure 6A. Amacrine cells also receive at least two kinds of synaptic input: they are driven by the bipolars and by neighboring amacrine cells.

In an effort to evaluate the postsynaptic potentials (PSPs) associated with the amacrine-cell response, the amacrine cell was voltage-clamped as shown in Figure 6A (Werblin, 1977). This eliminated the voltage-dependent spiking activity and revealed the currents associated with the synaptic inputs. In all cases the PSPs associated with the light response were reduced and became nulled at membrane depolarizations near 0 mV. All PSPs were purely transient, so the bipolar input, which might have shown some sustained component, was obscured—perhaps by a much stronger lateral transient input from neighboring amacrine cells. There was never any indication of an outward-going current component at any membrane potential level, which suggests that all inputs to the amacrine cells are excitatory. The synapse from bipolar to amacrine cells may be phasic and cannot maintain a sustained level of activity (for another explanation see Miller, this volume).

Small transient PSPs in the amacrine cell are boosted to large spikelike potentials with rapid leading edge by a regenerative mechanism that is probably located at the amacrine-cell soma. Figure 6B shows a current-voltage curve for an amacrine cell derived under voltage clamp. There is a large negative-resistance region, which appears when the amacrine cell is depolarized by just a few millivolts. The negative-resistance zone indicates that a small PSP will be boosted to more than 20 mV in a spikelike

FIGURE 5 Current-voltage curves for the bipolar cells for center and center-plus-annulus illumination. (A) Hyperpolarizing or *off* bipolar cell responses all pivot around a null potential near +50 mV. Center illumination causes a conductance decrease, but addition of the surround to the center flash reverses this effect, increasing conductance and depolarizing the cell. (B) Depolarizing or *on* bipolar cell. Center illumination causes a conductance increase, but addition of the surround causes a hyperpolarization and concomitant decrease in conductance. (See text for an explanation of the effects of transmitter on the membrane.)

manner. With further depolarization of the amacrine-cell membrane, a series of smaller spikes appears, suggesting another regenerative site, probably at the amacrine-cell processes (Werblin, 1977). Both spike systems are blocked by tetrodotoxin (TTX) (see Miller, this volume; Miller and Dacheux, 1976d), so they probably involve sodium activation. Receptive fields for the amacrine cells are generally quite large in the mudpuppy, spanning more than 400 μm (Thibos and Werblin, 1978b); they are sometimes smaller in the tiger salamander (Wunk and Werblin, 1978). As shown below, inhibitory PSPs (IPSPs) with response and receptive-field properties similar to those of the amacrine cells seem to form a broad, transient, change-sensitive antagonistic surround for all the ganglion cells in the tiger salamander. This antagonistic surround compresses the ganglion-cell response, as shown in Figure 2C.

FORMATION OF THE GANGLION-CELL RECEPTIVE FIELDS: SYNAPTIC INPUTS   The studies outlined above help to define the forms of activity associated with each of the cell types—*on* and *off* bipolar cells and amacrine cells—that can make synaptic input to the ganglion cells. These activity profiles are shown in Figure 7 for both center and surround illumination. The *on* and *off* bipolar responses are nearly mirror images of each other and show primarily sustained phases of opposite polarity for center and surround illumination. The transient overshoot in the responses is due to some residual delayed antagonism from the horizontal-cell system interacting with the center response, even when "pure" center and surround stimuli are used. This occurs either because of scatter inherent in the stimuli or because the antagonistic surround extends through the center of the receptive field for the bipolar cells (Wunk and Werblin, 1978).

In addition to sustained inputs from bipolars, the anatomy also suggests that amacrine cells can make either direct or indirect (through feedback to the bipolars) contact with the ganglion cells. The amacrine cells have broad, homogeneous receptive fields, as indicated by the fact that the response remains roughly the same for both spot and annular stimulation. Finally, a narrow-field transient form of activity is included in the figure. We have no clear cell type with which to associate this form of response (amacrine cells usually show a much broader receptive field); but there appears to be a narrow-field transient input to the ganglion cells, as shown below, so this form of activity is included in the vocabulary list of forms of synaptic input available to the ganglion cells of tiger salamander. This narrow-field response may represent the resultant antagonistic interaction of two populations of broad-field transient

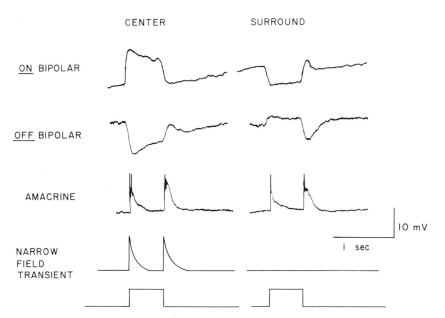

FIGURE 7   Vocabulary of inputs to the ganglion cells. Center and surround responses of the *on* and *off* bipolars, as well as amacrine cells, are shown. In addition, there appears to be a narrow-field transient input to the ganglion cells of uncertain origin. It is shown separately here, and no attempt is made to identify the cell or interacting populations of cells that generate the narrow field. Individual PSPs, isolated from the ganglion cells in subsequent figures, will consist of these four components.

cells, the activity of cells not recorded from, or the interaction of inputs from bipolar cells (see Miller, this volume).

Figure 8 shows the forms of response found in the ganglion cells of the tiger salamander. There are four basic ganglion-cell response types: (1) a sustained center *on* response with no surround activity; (2) a sustained center *off* response, with surround activity of opposite polarity; (3) a transient *on-off* response with relatively narrow receptive field; and (4) a "hybrid" response with transient *on-off* activity in response to center illumination but sustained activity in response to surround illumination. These four ganglion-cell types appear to be formed through combinations of synaptic input from the four precursor waveforms shown in Figure 7. It is possible to dissect the responses to reveal separate synaptic components by polarizing the membrane to the null potential of one component, thereby unveiling the waveform(s) of the other component(s). The synaptic inputs tend to overlap in time, so some of the problems previously

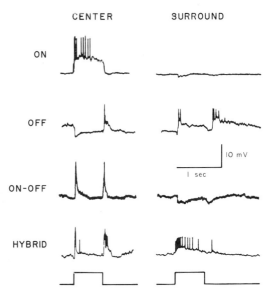

FIGURE 8 Ganglion-cell types in the tiger salamander. There are four basic types of response measured in the retina: (1) *on*-center units, which depolarize tonically to center illumination but show no sustained surround response; (2) *off*-center units, which hyperpolarize tonically to center and depolarize tonically to surround illumination; (3) *on-off* units, which depolarize transiently at center *on* and *off* but show little depolarization for surround illumination; and finally (4) hybrid units, which respond transiently to center illumination at *on* and *off* but tonically to surround illumination. All units show some sign of transient inhibition, seen most clearly at *on* and *off* of surround illumination. The synaptic components of these responses, composed of the forms of activity of the presynaptic cells shown in Figure 7, are outlined in Figure 9.

encountered, in which one input is obscured by another, are also present here.

Figure 9A shows sample responses of an *on* ganglion cell at different levels of membrane polarization, determined by the level of extrinsic current. At all potential levels the center response is almost purely depolarizing and sustained, but the surround response is transient and tends to reverse near -60 mV. These records are taken from just one of many ganglion cells, and in this particular case the transient surround component is not very large.

The current-voltage curve for the membrane in the dark and the response versus potential curves for the sustained and transient components of the response are shown in Figure 9A. The sustained response seems to result from an excitatory PSP (EPSP) that nulls near $+70$ mV and is therefore the result of an excitatory synaptic input. The transient component appears to reverse polarity near -60 mV, a few millivolts negative with respect to the dark level for this cell, and is therefore an IPSP. The fact that there is no sustained inhibitory potential associated with the surround response in the *on* ganglion cell but always a surround response in the bipolars (see Figure 7) suggests (1) that the sustained inhibition is not fed forward to the ganglion cell and (2) that the ganglion cell is probably not driven tonically by a bipolar cell in the dark.

The observations above, coupled with the work of Naka (1977) and Miller and Dacheux (1976), which suggest that the *on* ganglion cells are driven directly by the *on* bipolars, indicate that the *on* bipolars drive the *on* ganglion cells through an excitatory synapse. The synapse is silent in the dark but brought into activity when the bipolar cell is somewhat depolarized. This pathway is therefore not appropriate for signaling small changes near threshold because there is some "dead space" between the initial polarization of the bipolar and the initiation of activity in the ganglion cell. Also, since there is no direct tonic inhibition to this ganglion cell, all tonic sensitivity control, at least in this cell type, is probably mediated at the outer plexiform layer.

Figure 9B shows the responses for an *off* ganglion cell to center and surround illumination at different potential levels. Again, there appear to be at least two inputs to this ganglion cell. A transient PSP that reverses at about -50 mV is best seen at the initial onset of the center response, although it can be also followed to a lesser degree at the onset and offset of all response components. In addition, there is a sustained hyperpolarization in response to the center flash, and a sustained depolarization in response to

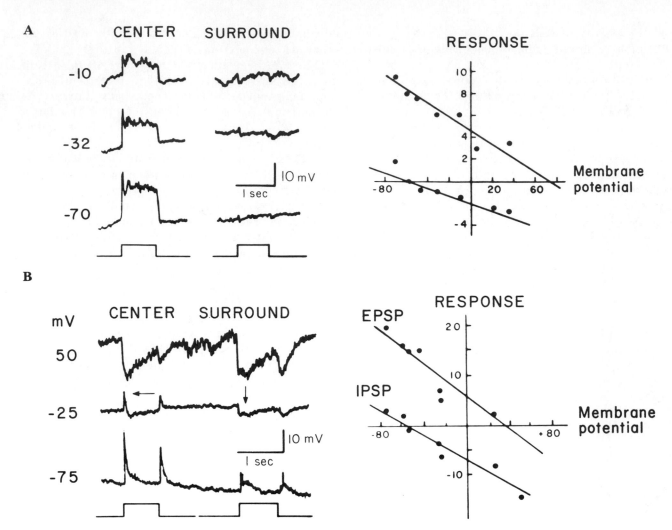

FIGURE 9 Response versus potential for the four kinds of ganglion cell, revealing the PSPs corresponding to the four kinds of synaptic input shown in Figure 8. (A) *On*-center cell at three different sample potential levels, showing that the center-elicited sustained EPSP diminishes as the membrane is depolarized. A small transient IPSP is also measured in the response to surround illumination, increasing with depolarization. *Right*: Response versus potential curves measured for the cell in A reveal an EPSP with null potential near +70 mV and an IPSP with reversal potential near −60 mV. There is no sign of a sustained hyperpolarization at any potential, suggesting that there is no sustained antagonism fed forward to the ganglion synapse from the cell and that the *on* bipolar that drives this ganglion cell (see text) does not drive the ganglion cell in the dark. (B) Responses in an *off* ganglion cell at four potential levels reveal a sustained IPSP to center illumination and a sustained EPSP to surround illumination, mimicking the response of the *off* bipolar cell. Some hint of a transient IPSP, reversing near −55 mV, is evident at the onset of the center flash.

the surround flash, both of which decrease together with membrane depolarization and become too small to measure near +40 mV.

Since the sustained components of the response to center and surround illumination resemble the response of the *off* bipolar cell, and since Naka (1977) and Miller and Dacheux (1976) have shown that *off* bipolar cells seem to drive the *off* ganglion cells, it is reasonable to conclude from these results that the *off* bipolar cell provides a sustained excitatory input to the *off* ganglion cell. Unlike the excitatory input in

the *on* bipolar–*on* ganglion synapse, which appears to be silent in the dark, the *off* system seems to be tonically active in the dark. The evidence supporting this notion is that, although the synapse is shown to be excitatory, there is a clear hyperpolarization of the ganglion cell when the bipolar cell hyperpolarizes during the center test flash. The response versus potential curves in Figure 9B suggest that the null potential for this excitatory synapse is near +40 mV.

The transient PSP reverses polarity near −50 mV, and is an IPSP, since the resting membrane potential

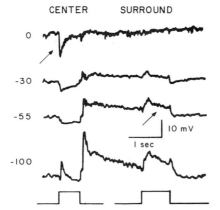

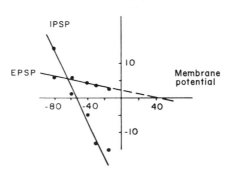

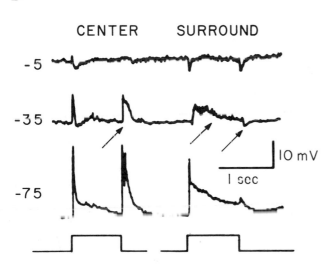

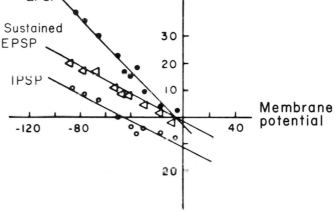

Right: Response versus intensity curves for the EPSP and IPSP in the *off*-center ganglion cell. Results suggest that the *off*-center ganglion cell is tonically driven by the *off* bipolar cell in the dark (see text). (C) Responses for an *on-off* ganglion cell at three representative potential levels. An EPSP with narrow receptive field, driven only by center illumination, reverses sign between −25 and +50 mV. A broad-field transient IPSP seen best at *on* and *off* of the surround, reverses sign between −75 and −25 mV. *Right*: Response versus potential curves for the EPSP and IPSP of the *on-off*

ganglion cell. (D) Responses at three representative potentials for a hybrid ganglion cell. Response consists of a narrow-field transient EPSP, seen best at center *on* and *off*, reversing near 0 mV, a sustained EPSP seen during surround illumination, also reversing near 0 mV, and finally a transient IPSP seen best at the offset of surround illumination that reverses near −50 mV. *Right*: Response versus potential curves for the three components of the hybrid ganglion-cell response.

for these ganglion cells is normally more positive than −50 mV. The transient IPSP has the response and receptive-field properties of the amacrine cell (Figure 7).

The response of an *on-off* ganglion cell at three representative potential levels is shown in Figure 9C. This response consists of transient EPSPs and IPSPs that overlap in time and are difficult to sort out. However, it is apparent that the EPSP at the onset and termination of the center flash reverses between −25 and +50 mV, whereas the IPSP at the onset and

termination of the surround flash reverses at a much more negative potential, between −75 and −25 mV. The response versus potential curves for this cell are shown in Figure 9C. In these and other records it seems that the total response is composed of inputs from a narrow-field EPSP elicited only by center illumination (see Figure 7) and a broad-field IPSP, probably of amacrine-cell origin, elicited by both center and surround flashes but visible primarily with surround illumination.

Finally, the responses for the hybrid cell are shown

at four representative potential levels in Figure 9D. This is the most complex response of all and can be decomposed into at least three components. A sustained EPSP is seen best during the surround flash and has an apparent reversal near 0 mV. A transient EPSP, seen best at the onset and termination of the center flash, also reverses near 0 mV. Finally, as with all the other ganglion cells in the tiger salamander, there is a transient IPSP that is seen most clearly at the termination of the surround flash, which reverses near −50 mV. The response versus potential curves for these three response components are shown in Figure 9D.

The hybrid ganglion cell seems to have the two inputs of the *off* ganglion cell: a sustained excitatory input from the *off* bipolar and a transient broad-field inhibitory input from the amacrine-cell system. But in addition, this cell type has a narrow-field transient input like the excitatory input in the *on-off* cell.

The full complement of inputs to the tiger salamander ganglion cells is summarized in Figure 10. *On* bipolars excite *on* ganglion cells, *off* bipolars excite *off* ganglion cells and hybrid cells. A narrow-field transient system excites the *on-off* and hybrid ganglion cells. All ganglion cells are inhibited by a broad-field transient system, which is probably formed by the amacrine cells.

SYNAPTIC MECHANISMS THAT MEDIATE VISUAL FUNCTION   The first part of this chapter summarized the roles of specific retinal layers in mediating visual function: lateral interactions mediated by horizontal cells at the outer plexiform layer seem to control the response domain of the bipolars; lateral interactions involving amacrine cells at the inner plexiform layer are responsible for the compression of the response of change-sensitive ganglion cells as a function of the level of change in the local visual field. The second part has summarized the electrical properties of specific synaptic inputs to each cell type. It has been shown that lateral interactions at the outer plexiform layer are most easily explained in terms of a feedback synapse from horizontal cells to bipolars but that lateral interactions at the inner plexiform layer involve at least one feedforward synapse from amacrine to ganglion cells. These two areas of study can be correlated and allow us to begin to describe visual function in terms of specific synaptic mechanisms. Table I summarizes the specific synaptic mechanism proposed here for mediating each visual function.

The table expresses, in rudimentary form, some of the neural mechanisms that control visual function. Further development of this kind of table should be

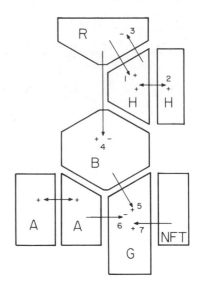

FIGURE 10   Summary diagram showing synaptic pathways that mediate concentric antagonism, thereby controlling sensitivity in the retina. Each pathway, its postsynaptic properties, and its role in control of sensitivity is outlined. (1) Excitatory synapse from photoreceptors to horizontal cells (Figure 4A). Transmitter from photoreceptors depolarizes the horizontal cell by increasing conductance to ions with equilibrium potential more positive than the dark level. (2) Coupling between horizontal cells. This coupling (Figure 4), which is probably electrical, creates broad receptive fields for the horizontal cells. The horizontal-cell system forms a broad antagonistic surround for bipolar and subsequent cells in the visual pathway. (3) Feedback pathway from horizontal cells to the photoreceptors. The synaptic mechanism here is uncertain. Feedback acts to antagonize the light response and reset the relation between illumination and membrane potential or release of transmitter, thereby controlling sensitivity (Figure 2). The current-voltage curves for the bipolars suggest that the feedback pathway is primarily responsible for surround antagonism at the outer plexiform layer (Figure 5). (4) Synapse from photoreceptors to the bipolar cells. Transmitter excites the *off* bipolars by increasing conductance but inhibits the *on* bipolars by decreasing conductance—both to ions with an equilibrium potential positive with respect to the dark level. In both cases this pathway is antagonized by synaptic feedback from the horizontal cells to the photoreceptors (Figure 5). (5) Excitatory pathway from the bipolars to the sustained ganglion cells of like phase: *on* bipolars excite the *on* ganglion cells; *off* bipolars excite the *off* ganglion cells. The *off* bipolar also makes excitatory synaptic input to the hybrid ganglion cell (Figure 9). (6) Inhibitory synaptic input to the ganglion cells. This pathway exists in all ganglion-cell types in the tiger salamander retina. It is mediated by a conductance increase to ions with an equilibrium potential slightly negative with respect to the dark membrane potential (Figure 9). This is the pathway that compresses the ganglion-cell response in the presence of movement in the surround (Figure 2). (7) Narrow-field transient input. This input forms the center of the receptive field for the hybrid and the *on-off* ganglion cells. It is of uncertain origin.

TABLE I
Neural mechanisms of visual function

Visual Function	Synaptic Mechanism
Spatial averaging of local intensities to form local antagonistic surround signal.	Coupling between horizontal cells, possibly electrical, extends the receptive field of individual cells (Werblin, 1974; Thibos and Werblin, 1978; Marshall and Werblin, 1978).
Formation of sustained concentric receptive fields.	Broadly coupled horizontal cells feed back or forward with sign-inverting synapse to form antagonistic surround; narrow dendritic field of bipolars, driven by photoreceptors, forms center.
Formation of *on* and *off* systems.	Postsynaptic membrane of the bipolar cells have different responses to the photoreceptor transmitter: it causes a conductance increase in *off* bipolars but a conductance decrease in *on* bipolars (Figure 5; Miller and Dacheux, 1976; Murakami, Ohtsuka, and Shimazaki, 1975).
Response domain reset to different log intensities by the antagonistic surround.	A feedback synapse from horizontal cells to receptors resets the relation between the potential at the receptor terminal and light (Werblin, 1978b).
Initiation of transient activity.	Postsynaptic to the bipolar cells; may involve phasic synapses from bipolars to amacrines (Werblin, 1977; Werblin and Wunk, 1978).
Amplification of transient activity at the inner plexiform layer.	Regenerative depolarization at the soma of the amacrine cells (Werblin, 1977).
Formation of broad, change-sensitive antagonistic surround for ganglion cells.	Coupling between amacrine cells, probably chemical, and propagation of activity by dendritic spikes along amacrine-cell processes (Werblin, 1977; Thibos and Werblin, 1978; Miller and Dacheux, 1976).
Change-sensitive antagonistic surround in ganglion cells.	Chemically coupled amacrine cells form broad antagonistic field.
Compression of response range in change-sensitive ganglion cells.	Feedforward chemical synaptic input from amacrine cells to ganglion cells, generating an IPSP, and probably shunting the membrane (Werblin and Copenhagen, 1974; Werblin, 1977; Thibos and Werblin, 1978).

most exciting, the retina being a neural subsystem for which we can define behavior and in which we have access to detailed analysis of cellular activity. At present it appears that processing of the visual message by local circuits in the retina is performed by classical synaptic mechanisms involving either the release of transmitters or electrotonic coupling. The identity of the transmitters remains unknown (but see Dowling, this volume). I have suggested that these transmitters affect the postsynaptic membranes of most cells by modulating conductance. (Some of the inputs to bipolars may decrease conductance.) The ionic channels affected by the transmitters are also unknown, but it should be possible to determine their identity with available techniques.

Spatial averaging functions, such as those at the level of the rods and the horizontal cells, seem to be mediated by electrotonic coupling. This is clear for the rods of lower vertebrates, although such coupling is not found in mammalian retinas. Coupling between horizontal cells appears to be electrical (see Figure 4), but measurements will have to be improved to understand why this "electrical" coupling should be interrupted by ACh.

Neural control of retinal sensitivity, as expressed by the effect of the steady antagonistic surround on the graded response of the bipolar cells (see Figure 2A), is an intriguing problem. How can conventional neural interactions, probably involving transmitter-mediated conductance changes, cause a shift in the levels of illumination to which the retina is sensitive? I have elsewhere offered a possible explanation (Werblin, 1978b). Briefly, the feedback synapse from horizontal cells to receptors may reset the relation between receptor potential (and therefore tonic level of transmitter release) and stimulus intensity. This resets the range of intensities over which the postsynaptic cells can respond to the photoreceptor transmitter.

On and *off* systems in the retina seem to be established at the level of the postsynaptic membrane of the bipolars receiving transmitter from the photoreceptors (Miller and Dacheux, 1976; Murakami, Ohtsuka, and Shimazaki, 1975; Figure 5). These systems seem to remain segregated by specific connectivity from *on* bipolars to *on* ganglion cells and from *off* bipolars to *off* ganglion cells (Miller and Dacheux, 1976; Naka, 1977; Figures 9 and 10).

The *on-off* systems in the retina are still not clearly understood. They probably involve input from both the *on* and *off* bipolars, but the ways in which these signals combine is not known. Transient activity is initiated at the input to the amacrine cells (Figure 6) and amplified by regenerative sodium channels at the cell soma (Werblin, 1977; Miller and Dacheux, 1976, 1977). But is there also a direct, narrow-field, transient pathway from the bipolars to the ganglion cells (Figure 9)? My own studies have suggested that two broad-field amacrine systems can interact antagonistically to generate a narrow-field transient system (Werblin, 1977); but Miller (this volume) suggests that the narrow-field transient can be formed from bipolar inputs alone.

Compression of the ganglion-cell response in the presence of broad-field change in the surround (Figure 2C) is probably mediated by a direct inhibitory input from the amacrine cells. All ganglion cells in the tiger salamander receive a broad-field transient IPSP with reversal potential near the dark level (Figures 9 and 10). Therefore the "contrast control" referred to with reference to Figure 2C may simply be mediated by an IPSP at the ganglion cells and an associated conductance increase.

ACKNOWLEDGMENT   The research reported was sponsored by the National Eye Institute Grant EY 00561; the Miller Foundation, University of California, Berkeley; and the John Simon Guggenheim Foundation and Fight for Sight. Some of the studies presented in this paper are part of doctoral dissertations presented at Berkeley by Larry Marshall, Larry Thibos, Dan Wunk, and Josef Skrzypec.

REFERENCES

BAYLOR, D. A., M.G.F. FUORTES, and P. M. O'BRYAN, 1971. Receptive fields of cones in the retina of the turtle. *J. Physiol.* 214:265–294.

BROWN, J. E., and L. PINTO, 1974. Ionic mechanism for the photoreceptor potential of the retina of *Bufo marinus*. *J. Physiol.* 236:575–591.

BURKHARDT, D. A., 1977. Responses and receptive-field organization of cones in perch retina. *J. Neurophysiol.* 40:53–62.

CALVIN, W. H., 1969. Dendritic synapses and reversal potential: Theoretical implications of the view from the soma. *Exp. Neurology* 24:248–254.

CERVETTO, L., and M. PICCOLINO, 1974. Synaptic transmission between photoreceptors and horizontal cells in the turtle retina. *Science* 183:417–419.

CHAN, R. Y., and K. I. NAKA, 1976. The amacrine cell. *Vision Res.* 16:1119–1129.

COPENHAGEN, D. R., 1975. Time course of threshold elevation in on-off ganglion cells of *Necturus* retina: Effects of lateral interactions. *Vision Res.* 15:573–581.

COPENHAGEN, D. R., and W. G. OWEN, 1976. Functional characteristics of lateral interactions between rods in the retina of the snapping turtle. *J. Physiol.* 259:251–282.

DOWLING, J. E., 1963. Neural and photochemical mechanisms of visual adaptation in the rat. *J. Gen. Physiol.* 46:1287–1301.

DOWLING, J. E., and H. RIPPS, 1972. Adaptation in skate photoreceptors. *J. Gen. Physiol.* 60:698–719.

DOWLING, J. E., and H. RIPPS, 1973. Effect of magnesium on horizontal cell activity in the skate retina. *Nature* 242:101–103.

DOWLING, J. E., and F. S. WERBLIN, 1969. Organization of retina of the mudpuppy, *Necturus maculosus*, I. Synaptic structure. *J. Neurophysiol.* 32:315–338.

FAIN, G. L., 1976. Sensitivity of toad rods: Dependence on wave-length and background illumination. *J. Physiol.* 261:71–102.

FAIN, G. L., G. H. GOLD, and J. E. DOWLING, 1976. Receptor coupling in the toad retina. *Cold Spring Harbor Symp. Quant. Biol.* 40:547–561.

GERSCHENFELD, H. M., 1973. Chemical transmission in invertebrate central nervous system and neuromuscular junction. *Physiol. Rev.* 53:1–119.

GREEN, D. G., J. E. DOWLING, I. M. SIEGEL, and H. RIPPS, 1975. Retinal mechanisms of visual adaptation in the skate. *J. Gen. Physiol.* 65:483–502.

KANEKO, A., 1970. Physiological and morphological identification of horizontal, bipolar, and amacrine cells in goldfish retina. *J. Physiol.* 207:623–633.

KANEKO, A., 1973. Receptive field organization of bipolar and amacrine cells in the goldfish retina. *J. Physiol.* 235:133–153.

KANEKO, A., and H. HASHIMOTO, 1969. Electrophysiological study of single neurons in the inner nuclear layer of the carp retina. *Vision Res.* 9:37–55.

KANEKO, A., and H. SHIMAZAKI, 1975. Effects of external ions on the synaptic transmission from photoreceptors to horizontal cells in the carp retina. *J. Physiol.* 252:509–522.

KLEINSCHMIDT, J., and J. E. DOWLING, 1975. Intracellular

recordings from gecko photoreceptors during light and dark adaption. *J. Gen. Physiol.* 66:617–648.

LAM, D.M.K., 1972. Biosynthesis of acetylcholine in turtle photoreceptors. *Proc. Natl. Acad. Sci. USA* 69:1987–1991.

LAMB, T. D., 1976. Spatial properties of horizontal cells in the turtle retina. *J. Physiol.* 263:239–256.

LAMB, T. D., and E. J. SIMON, 1976. The relation between intercellular coupling and electrical noise in turtle photoreceptors. *J. Physiol.* 263:257–286.

LASANSKY, A., 1973. Organization of the outer synaptic layer in the retina of the larval tiger salamander. *Philos. Trans. R. Soc. Lond. (Biol. Sci.)* 265:471–489.

LASANSKY, A., and P. L. MARCHIAFAVA, 1974. Light induced resistance changes in retinal rods and cones of the tiger salamander. *J. Physiol.* 236:171–191.

MARSHALL, L. M., and F. S. WERBLIN, 1978. Synaptic transmission to the horizontal cells in the retina of the tiger salamander. *J. Physiol.* 279:321–346.

MATSUMOTO, N., and K. I. NAKA, 1972. Identification of intracellular responses in the frog retina. *Brain Res.* 42:59–71.

MATURANA, H. R., J. Y. LETTVIN, W. H. PITTS, and W. S. McCULLOCH, 1960. Physiology and anatomy of vision in the frog. *J. Gen. Physiol.* 43:129–175.

MILLER, R. F., and R. F. DACHEUX, 1976a. Synaptic organization and ionic basis of on and off channels in mudpuppy retina. I. Intracellular analysis of chloride sensitive electrogenic properties of receptors, horizontal cells, bipolar cells, and amacrine cells. *J. Gen. Physiol.* 67:639–659.

MILLER, R. F., and R. F. DACHEUX, 1976b. Synaptic organization and ionic basis of on and off channels in mudpuppy retina. II. Chloride-dependent ganglion cell mechanisms. *J. Gen. Physiol.* 67:661–678.

MILLER, R. F., and R. F. DACHEUX, 1976c. Synaptic organization and ionic basis of on and off channels in mudpuppy retina. III. A model of ganglion cell receptive field organization based upon chloride-free experiments. *J. Gen. Physiol.* 67:679–690.

MILLER, R. F., and R. F. DACHEUX, 1976d. Dendritic spikes in mudpuppy amacrine cells: Identification and TTX sensitivity. *Brain Res.* 104:157–162.

MURAKAMI, M., T. OHTSUKA, and H. SHIMAZAKI, 1975. Effects of aspartate and glutamate on the bipolar cells in the carp retina. *Vision Res.* 15:456–458.

NAKA, K. I., 1976. Neuronal circuitry in the catfish retina. *Invest. Ophthalmol.* 15:926–935.

NAKA, K. I., 1977. Functional organization of catfish retina. *J. Neurophysiol.* 40:26–43.

NORMANN, R., and F. S. WERBLIN, 1974. Control of retinal sensitivity: I. Light and dark adaptation of vertebrate rods and cones. *J. Gen. Physiol.* 63:37–61.

RATLIFF, F., 1965. *Mach Bands: Quantitative Studies on Neural Networks in the Retina.* San Francisco: Holden Day.

SCHWARTZ, E. A., 1973. Organization of on-off cells in the retina of the turtle. *J. Physiol.* 230:1–14.

SCHWARTZ, E. A., 1976. Electrical properties of the rod syncytium in the retina of the turtle. *J. Physiol.* 257:379–406.

THIBOS, L. N., and F. S. WERBLIN, 1978. The response properties of the steady antagonistic surround in the mudpuppy retina. *J. Physiol.* 278:79–99.

THIBOS, L. N., and F. S. WERBLIN, 1978. The properties of surround antagonism elicited by spinning windmill patterns in the mudpuppy retina. *J. Physiol.* 278:101–116.

TRIFONOV, Y. A., 1968. Study of synaptic transmission between photoreceptors and horizontal cells by means of electrical stimulation of the retina. *Biofizika.* 13:809–817.

WALOGA, G., and W. L. PAK, 1976. Horizontal cell potentials: Dependence on external sodium ion concentration. *Science* 191:964–966.

WEAKLY, J.N.C., 1973. The action of cobalt ions on neuromuscular transmission in the frog. *J. Physiol.* 234:597–612.

WERBLIN, F. S., 1970. Response of retinal cells to moving spots: Intracellular recording in *Necturus maculosus. J. Neurophysiol.* 33:342–350.

WERBLIN, F. S., 1971. Adaptation in a vertebrate retina: Intracellular recording in *Necturus. J. Neurophysiol.* 34:228–241.

WERBLIN, F. S., 1972. Lateral interactions at inner plexiform layer of a vertebrate retina: Antagonistic response to change. *Science* 175:1008–1010.

WERBLIN, F. S., 1974. Control of retinal sensitivity. II. Lateral interactions at the outer plexiform layer. *J. Gen. Physiol.* 63:62–87.

WERBLIN, F. S., 1975a. Regenerative hyperpolarization in rods. *J. Physiol.* 224:53–81.

WERBLIN, F. S., 1975b. Anomalous rectification in horizontal cells. *J. Physiol.* 244:639–657.

WERBLIN, F. S., 1977. Regenerative amacrine cell activity and formation of on-off ganglion cell response. *J. Physiol.* 264:767–786.

WERBLIN, F. S., 1978a. Transmission along and between rods. *J. Physiol.* 280:449–470.

WERBLIN, F. S., 1978b. Synaptic mechanisms mediating bipolar response in the retina of the tiger salamander. *International Symposium on Phototransduction,* H. B. Barlow and P. Fatt, eds. London: Academic Press.

WERBLIN, F. S., and D. COPENHAGEN, 1974. Control of retinal sensitivity. III. Lateral interactions at the inner plexiform layer. *J. Gen. Physiol.* 63:88–110.

WERBLIN, F. S., and J. E. DOWLING, 1969. Organization of the retina of mudpuppy, *Necturus maculosus.* II. Intracellular recording. *J. Neurophysiol.* 32:339–355.

WONG-RILEY, M.T.T., 1974. Synaptic organization of the inner plexiform layer in the retina of the tiger salamander. *J. Neurocytol.* 3:1–33.

WUNK, D. F., and F. S. WERBLIN, 1978. Synaptic inputs to ganglion cells in the tiger salamander retina. In preparation.

13 Pharmacology of the Connections of Cones and L-Horizontal Cells in the Vertebrate Retina

H. M. GERSCHENFELD and M. PICCOLINO

ABSTRACT   Glutamate and acetylcholine (ACh) agonists are good mimics of some of the postsynaptic effects of the unknown cone synaptic transmitter in the turtle retina. Although transmission from cones to L-horizontal cells is sensitive to both nicotinic and muscarinic ACh agonists, only the muscarinic antagonists preferentially block transmission at the postsynaptic level. Thus glutamate and atropine, which block the L-horizontal cell responses to light by different mechanisms, can be used to analyze pharmacologically the interneuronal role of L-horizontal cells in the outer plexiform layer.

Peripheral light stimulation evokes in the cone a depolarizing potential that can be converted into a Ca^{2+} spike by current injection and Sr^{2+}-containing media. Both atropine and glutamate block the depolarizing potential and the Ca^{2+} spike in the cones, thus confirming that they result from a negative feedback effect of the L-horizontal cells. However, atropine block of the L-horizontal cells enhances rather than blocks the depolarizing responses evoked in hyperpolarizing bipolar cells by light stimulation at the periphery of their receptor field. This suggests that in the turtle retina the antagonism between the responses of the hyperpolarizing bipolar cells to stimulation of the center and the surround of their receptor fields is not totally due to an effect of the L-horizontal cells.

FEW PROBLEMS in neurobiology are as difficult as that of establishing beyond doubt that a substance is a transmitter at a specific synapse. This has proven to be the case in the vertebrate retina as well, so that if one consults recent reviews (Graham, 1974; Bonting, 1976), one will be amazed both by the complexity of the existing experimental data and by the absence of positive transmitter identification at the cellular level (with probably one exception: see Dowling, this volume). Table I lists some of the substances that have been proposed as transmitter candidates for various retinal cells in a number of studies using different

H. M. GERSCHENFELD and M. PICCOLINO Laboratoire de Neurobiologie, École Normale Supérieure, 75005 Paris, France; Laboratorio di Neurofisiologia del C.N.R., 56100 Pisa, Italy

TABLE I
Transmitter candidates in retinal cells

Cell	Proposed Transmitter Candidates
Photoreceptors	Acetylcholine
	Glutamate
	Aspartate
	Glycine
	Taurine
Horizontal cells	GABA
Bipolar cells	Acetylcholine
	Glutamate
Amacrine cells	Dopamine
	Acetylcholine
	GABA
	Glycine
	Taurine
Interplexiform cells	Dopamine (fish, New World monkeys)
	Others
Ganglion cells	Glutamate

approaches on different vertebrate retinas. The multiplicity of transmitter candidates listed for some of the cells may reflect the existence of different populations of the same cell type, each reacting to a different transmitter. At present, however, it seems more likely that the multiplicity of candidates results from insufficient analysis.

The synaptic transmitter released by the cones is still unknown; nor is it known if all the cones of the same retina use the same transmitter. It is possible, however, to clearly define the physiological requirements of this synaptic transmitter.

Requirements for the synaptic transmitter of retinal cones

Most well-known synapses are *phasic*; that is, in their resting conditions they release transmitter in small quantal packets, and only when the physiological signal, the action potential, depolarizes the presynaptic ending and induces a Ca^{2+} influx is the transmitter massively released (see Llinás, this volume).

As first postulated by Trifonov (1968), the cone synapses are *tonic* synapses. Unlike the phasic synapses, they continuously release transmitter in the dark; and the physiological signal, the cone hyperpolarization evoked by light, interrupts a continuous Ca^{2+} influx at the nerve terminal and causes either depression or suppression of transmitter release. When the ionic content of the extracellular medium is manipulated, either by totally removing Ca^{2+} ions or by adding divalent cations (Mg^{2+}, Co^{2+}) that block the Ca^{2+} membrane permeability, the effects mimic well those of light stimulation on the second-order neurons (Dowling and Ripps, 1973; Cervetto and Piccolino, 1974; Kaneko and Shimazaki, 1975a,b; Dacheux and Miller, 1976; see also Miller, this volume).

When the transmitter release from cone synapses is suppressed, either by light stimulation or by manipulating the divalent ion content of the extracellular medium, the three main types of postsynaptic cells respond in different ways (see Werblin, this volume). The L-horizontal cells become hyperpolarized (Tomita, 1965; Werblin and Dowling, 1969; Kaneko, 1970; Nelson, 1973), and this hyperpolarization involves a *decrease* in membrane conductance (Toyoda, Nosaki, and Tomita, 1969; Nelson, 1973; Trifonov, Byzov, and Chailahian, 1974). The two types of bipolar cells show two different responses to either light stimulation at the center of their receptor field (see Dowling, this volume) or to the blockage of Ca^{2+} permeability (see Miller, this volume). Hyperpolarizing bipolar cells are hyperpolarized by both light stimulation of the center of their receptor field (Werblin and Dowling, 1969; Kaneko, 1973; Toyoda, 1973; Schwartz, 1974) and by adding Co^{2+} ions to the

extracellular medium (Kaneko and Shimazaki, 1975b; Dacheux and Miller, 1976). As in the L-horizontal cells, the hyperpolarizing responses are accompanied by a *decrease* in membrane conductance (Toyoda, 1973; Nelson, 1973; Werblin, this volume). On the contrary, depolarizing bipolar cells are depolarized by both central light spots (Werblin and Dowling, 1969; Toyoda, 1973; Nelson, 1973; Schwartz, 1974; Richter and Simon, 1975) and by blocking transmission with Co^{2+} ions (Kaneko and Shimazaki, 1975b; Dacheux and Miller, 1976). The light depolarization of the depolarizing bipolars involves an *increase* in membrane conductance (Toyoda, 1973; Nelson, 1973; see also Werblin, this volume). The result of this experimental evidence is, therefore, that the cone transmitter must (1) depolarize the L-horizontal cells by *increasing* their membrane conductance; (2) depolarize the hyperpolarizing bipolar cells by *increasing* their membrane conductance; and (3) hyperpolarize the depolarizing bipolar cells by *decreasing* their membrane conductance (Table II).

Some questions immediately arise from such a complex set of postsynaptic requirements. The retina is part of the vertebrate central nervous system, in which excitation and inhibition are thought to be mediated by different neurons (see Eccles, 1969; Krnjević, 1974). Does the cone then constitute an exception to this organization pattern? On the other hand, is it possible for a single cell releasing one transmitter to perform such opposite actions? Or does the cone release more than one transmitter?

There are reports that some neurons can release two different transmitters (see Hanley et al., 1974; Brownstein et al., 1974). Although this appears quite likely for neurons during short periods of their differentiation (see Patterson, this volume), the evidence for neurons of adult animals is much less compelling.

In contrast, invertebrate central nervous systems,

TABLE II

Properties of the cone transmitter

Post Cell	Effect on Cell	Effect on Membrane Conductance	Effect of Release Suppression (light or Co^{2+} ions)
L-horizontal cell	Depolarization	Increase	Hyperpolarization, Decrease of membrane conductance
Hyperpolarizing bipolar cell	Depolarization	Increase	Hyperpolarization, Decrease of membrane conductance
Depolarizing bipolar cell	Hyperpolarization	Decrease	Depolarization, Increase of membrane conductance

especially the molluscan nervous systems that have been intensely investigated in this respect, offer many examples of single neurons that, by releasing a single identified transmitter, can produce multiple and sometimes opposite actions on different postsynaptic neurons. Such an organizational pattern has been demonstrated for neurons using acetylcholine (Kandel et al., 1967; Kehoe, 1972), serotonin (Gerschenfeld and Paupardin-Tritsch, 1974a,b), dopamine (Berry and Cottrell, 1975), and histamine (Weinreich, 1977). The multiplicity of actions of each of these transmitters on the different postsynaptic neurons involves the activation of different receptors, each of them associated with a specific ionic channel (see Gerschenfeld, 1973, 1977).

Of the multireceptor systems that have been described in molluscan CNS, the one that appears most germane to the cone synapses is the serotoninergic system. Serotonin (5-hydroxytryptamine, 5-HT) is very probably *not* the transmitter of the cones; but its postsynaptic effects bear a marked resemblance to those expected from the cone transmitter. 5-HT applied to molluscan neurons can produce different effects by either increasing or decreasing the membrane conductance to different ions. Thus it depolarizes different neurons by increasing their Na^+ conductance or by decreasing their K^+ conductance and/or hyperpolarizes other neurons either by increasing their conductance to K^+ or Cl^- ions or by decreasing their Na^+ conductance. Each of these actions is mediated through the activation of a different 5-HT receptor (Gerschenfeld and Paupardin-Tritsch, 1974a). Moreover, 5-HT released as a transmitter from an identified cerebral neuron in *Aplysia californica* was shown to evoke in different postsynaptic neurons at least three of the effects described above: excitation associated with a Na^+ conductance increase, inhibition associated with a K^+ conductance increase, and a second type of inhibition involving a decrease in Na^+ conductance (Gerschenfeld and Paupardin-Tritsch, 1974b).

On the basis of such a model, it is plausible that one substance liberated from the cones can be sufficient to depolarize both the L-horizontal and the hyperpolarizing bipolar cells by increasing their Na^+ conductance and to hyperpolarize the depolarizing bipolar cells by decreasing their Na^+ conductance.

Pharmacological attempts to identify the cone synaptic transmitter

Of the photoreceptor transmitter candidates listed in Table I, we have reliable pharmacological informa-

tion at the cellular level for only glutamate and acetylcholine (ACh). L-glutamic acid, which is very likely a transmitter at many excitatory neuromuscular junctions of arthropods (see Kravitz et al., 1970; Takeuchi, 1977), is ubiquitously distributed in the cells of vertebrate retinas (see Graham, 1974). This is not surprising since glutamic acid is involved in other metabolic functions; but it is possible that a specific synaptic pool of glutamate exists.

Cervetto and MacNichol (1972) observed that application of high concentrations (50–100 mM) of glutamate to the turtle retina in an eyecup preparation results in a depolarization of the L-horizontal cells and in the blocking of their light responses. Under the same conditions, cone responses were slightly affected; this was confirmed by Murakami, Ohtsu, and Ohtsuka (1972) in the carp retina. More recently Kaneko and Shimazaki (1975a,b, 1976) showed in isolated perfused carp retinas that glutamate can depolarize the L-horizontal cells at lower concentrations. Moreover, glutamate mimics closely the expected effects of the cone transmitter on the other postsynaptic cells (Murakami, Ohtsuka, and Shimazaki, 1975; Kaneko and Shimazaki, 1975b, 1976).

Figure 1A shows a recording from a L-horizontal cell of the carp stimulated at short intervals with light flashes. When glutamate (5 mM) is applied to the preparation, the L-horizontal cells are depolarized, and its light responses gradually diminish and are almost completely blocked. This effect is reversible, and the cell rapidly recovers its initial potential level. The effect does not appear to result from a presynaptic effect of glutamate, for when the cone transmitter release is blocked by a high Mg^{2+} medium, the light responses are blocked but the glutamate action persists (Figure 1B). Glutamate ions appear to have the same depolarizing effect on the hyperpolarizing bipolar cells (Kaneko and Shimazaki, 1976).

The effect of glutamate on the depolarizing bipolar cells is different. Figure 1C corresponds to an intracellular recording from such a depolarizing bipolar, which shows opposite responses to stimulation at the center (depolarizations) and the periphery (hyperpolarizations) of its receptor field. Application of glutamate to the preparation causes a hyperpolarization of the cell and a complete and rapid block of both types of light response. These recover after the glutamate is washed out. The washout is accompanied by a peculiar off-depolarization.

All these effects of glutamate are obtained with rather high concentrations (1–5 mM). It is possible that diffusion barriers and uptake mechanisms inside

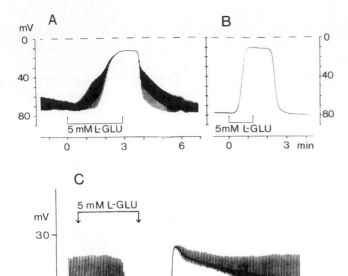

FIGURE 1 Effect of L-glutamate (5 mM) on second-order cells of isolated-perfused carp retina. (A) When applied to a retina bathed in a normal saline solution, glutamate depolarizes an L-horizontal cell and blocks its light responses. (B) Glutamate is applied to the same cell in a high Mg^{2+} medium, which prior to the drug application hyperpolarizes and blocks the light responses. Even in this case, glutamate continues to depolarize the L-horizontal cell. (C) Effect of glutamate on a depolarizing bipolar cell, which responds by depolarizations to white light spot stimuli (700 μm diameter) and by hyperpolarizations to white light annuli (900 μm inner diameter, 10 mm outer diameter). The two types of light stimuli are presented alternately. The application of glutamate hyperpolarizes the cell, and its washout is accompanied by an off-depolarization (Kaneko and Shimazaki, 1976).

the retina interfere with achieving an effective concentration at the receptor sites.

Glutamate appears to fulfill the requirements for a cone transmitter candidate, at least in terms of its effects on membrane potential. No data are available on its effects on the membrane conductance of postsynaptic cells, and unfortunately the absence of known specific antagonists of glutamate constitutes an impediment to further investigations.

Another substance that has been proposed as a possible transmitter for the cones is acetylcholine. Early biochemical studies of the retina detected the presence of ACh, and later extensive analyses showed that its concentration in retina varies between 5.7 nM/g wet wt in the pig to 33 nM/g wet wt in the

chicken. Cone retinas appear to be richer in ACh. The enzymatic systems related to the synthesis and inactivation of ACh have also been extensively analyzed in many vertebrate retinas. All the data have been recently reviewed by Graham (1974).

However, it is worth mentioning that, some years ago, Lam (1972) reported that isolated cones of turtle retina incubated in the presence of labeled precursors of ACh were able to synthesize ACh. These results were criticized by Lam (1975) himself on the grounds that he did not observe the enrichment in the concentration of acetylcholine transferase that might be expected if this enzyme were preferentially concentrated in the photoreceptors. Recent results on a possible transmitter role for ACh at the turtle outer plexiform layer appear contradictory. On the one hand, Yazulla and Schmidt (1976) report that binding sites for ^{125}I-labeled α-bungarotoxin can be detected by histoautoradiography in the retina of the turtle (as well in the goldfish) and that an important part of these binding sites are located at the outer plexiform layer. On the other hand, Baughman, Bader, and Schwartz (1976) have shown that uptake of labeled choline, known to be an important step in ACh metabolism in synapses, is almost exclusively localized in cell structures at the inner synaptic regions and that little or no uptake is observed in the distal retina. Contradictory data have also been reported concerning the effects of ACh on L-horizontal cells. Murakami, Ohtsu, and Ohtsuka (1972) observed no effect when ACh aerosol was sprayed on the vitreal surface of the carp retina. Kaneko and Shimazaki (1976) observed that when 10^{-5} M ACh perfused to an isolated carp retina, it depolarizes the L-horizontal cells and markedly diminishes their light responses. These authors report that high concentrations of Mg^{2+} ions in the extracellular medium cause a block of such ACh effects; they interpret this by suggesting that ACh depolarizes the cone endings, which would increase the release of the natural transmitter.

In an attempt to reevaluate these data, we recently studied the effects of ACh agonists and antagonists on the L-horizontal cells of the turtle retina (Gerschenfeld and Piccolino, 1977, and unpublished data). The principal results of this study are summarized in Table III.

In the perfused turtle eyecup preparation, with the drug applied from the vitreal side, application of ACh (up to 5 mM) has no effect, either on the cones or on the L-horizontal cells. This might be due to active hydrolysis of ACh at the proximal layers of the retina, which are very rich in acetylcholinesterase (see Graham, 1974) or some other uncontrolled factor.

TABLE III
Effect of cholinergic drugs on the L-horizontal cells

Class	Compound	Effect on L-Horizontal Cells	
		Depolarization	Hyperpolarization plus block
General agonists	ACh	−	−
	Carbachol	±	−
Nicotinic agonists	Nicotine	+++	−
	Decamethonium	−	−
Nicotinic antagonists	Tubocurarine	−	−
	Gallamine	−	−
	β-Erytroidin	−	−
	Hexamethonium	−	−
	TEA	−	−
Muscarinic agonists	Pilocarpine	+++	−
	Arecoline	+	++
	Methacolin	−	−
Muscarinic antagonists	Atropine	−	+++
	Scopolamine	−	++
	Probanthine	−	++
Inhibitors of ACh esterase	Eserine	++	+++
	Neostigmine	+	+++
	Edrophonium	+	++

Carbachol (5 mM), an ACh agonist that is not hydrolyzed by acetylcholinesterase, causes a depolarization of L-horizontal cells in some experiments and markedly reduces their responses. However, these effects are capricious and cannot be observed in all retinas. Several other ACh agonists, such as 1–5 mM nicotine and 1–5 mM pilocarpine (a muscarinic agonist), always cause L-horizontal cell depolarization and a reduction of the light responses. This is illustrated in Figure 2 for pilocarpine. The effects of both agonists are reversible. Another nicotinic agonist, decamethonium, does not produce any effect on L-horizontal cells. Among the other muscarinic agonists we tried, 1–5 mM arecoline causes a slight depolarization of L-horizontal cells, always followed by what appears to be an antagonistic effect (see below), whereas acetyl-β-methylcholine (metacholin), at the same concentrations shows no effect.

Application of three inhibitors of acetylcholinesterase—eserine, neostigmine, and edrophonium (at concentrations of 1–5 mM)—show similar and rather complex actions on L-horizontal cells and do not block the cone responses. Figure 3 illustrates an experiment using eserine. Application of this inhibitor causes first a depolarization and then a decrease of

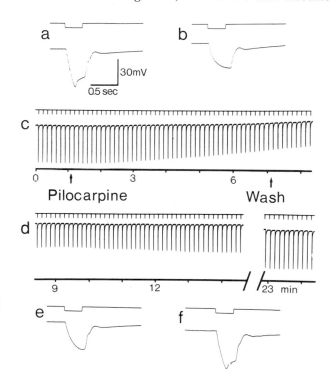

FIGURE 2   Effect of pilocarpine on an L-horizontal cell of turtle retina. Pilocarpine (1 mM) depolarizes the cell and decreases the amplitude of the light responses (c, d). The responses in a, b, e, and f are high-speed recordings obtained before applying pilocarpine (a), just before washing-out the drug (b), and during the washout (e, f). The traces above each recording give the timing of the light stimuli (spot of white light of 3,600 μm diameter). The voltage calibration is valid for both the low- and the high-speed recordings.

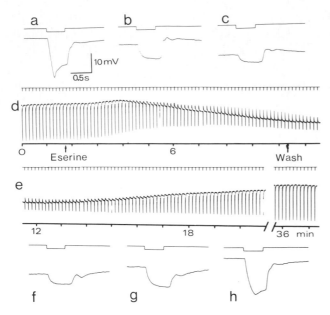

FIGURE 3   Effect of eserine on an L-horizontal cell of the turtle retina. The stimulus parameters are the same as in Figure 2. In d and e, application of eserine (5 mM) causes a depolarization of the L-horizontal cell, followed by a hyperpolarization and a block of the light responses. Note the depolarizing shift of the light potential and the off-depolarization that develops under the drug action. The high-speed recordings a–c and f–h are from the same experiment: a is a control response; b and c were obtained during the eserine application; and f–h correspond to different stages of the response recovery after washing-out of the drug.

the light responses of an L-horizontal cell, followed by a hyperpolarization and progressive blocking of the light responses. Moreover, these light responses develop an off-depolarization, and the light potential gradually shifts to more depolarized levels. This behavior can be interpreted as caused by a mixture of a primary potentiating effect and a secondary antagonist effect, since it is known that anticholinesterase drugs can also act as ACh antagonists.

The most interesting results of these experiments come from those with the ACh antagonists. First, none of the nicotinic antagonists assayed (see Table III) showed any blocking action on the L-horizontal cells. Even methyl-β-erythroidin (5 mM), which is known to be highly diffusible in vertebrate CNS, is totally ineffective. In contrast, three muscarinic antagonists (atropine, scopolamine, and probanthine) have similar blocking actions on the L-horizontal cells. Figure 4 is from an experiment demonstrating the effect of atropine sulfate (5 mM) on an L-horizontal cell. Atropine application causes a hyperpolarization of the L-horizontal cell and a gradual decrease

of the amplitude of the light responses (Figure 4c,d). After twenty minutes of atropine application, responses to light are almost completely blocked and show an off-depolarization. The action of atropine can be reversed only after prolonged washing. Atropine also exerts some depressing action on the cones (Figure 4a,b); it slightly hyperpolarizes them and causes some reduction of their light responses (at most, to three-fourths or two-thirds of the original amplitude). This decrease is much smaller than the blocking of the L-horizontal cell responses (which are reduced to one-twelfth or less). Moreover, and most important, the action of atropine on the L-horizontal cells cannot be accounted for by its effects on the cones, for prolonged atropine application does not much affect the responses of the hyperpolarizing bipolar cells to light stimulation at the center of their receptor field—that is, to the activation of the direct connection between cones and bipolar cells (Figure 5). If transmitter release from the cones were impaired by atropine, the hyperpolarizing bipolar cells should also become hyperpolarized and their light responses should be blocked. It is therefore evident that atropine blocks synapses between cones and L-horizontal cells by acting mainly on the L-horizontal cells.

It is difficult, at present, to unequivocally relate these observations on the effects of ACh agonists and antagonists on both the dark and light potentials of the L-horizontal cells to a possible transmitter role for ACh at the cone synapses. More complete information on the effect of these drugs on both types of bipolar cells and, more precisely, on the membrane conductance of postsynaptic cells is necessary. Furthermore, as in the case of glutamate, the effective concentrations of the ACh agonists and antagonists used are very high, and we do not know whether such high concentrations are necessary because of the existence of diffusion barriers or because the effects observed are nonspecific and only appear at such concentrations.

However, it is of interest that if ACh is the cone transmitter, the hyperpolarizing bipolar cells must be endowed with ACh receptors different from the muscarinic receptors.

Pharmacological analysis of local circuits in the outer plexiform layer

Even if future work eliminates glutamate and/or ACh from consideration as the cone transmitter, the experiments described in the previous section demonstrate (1) that glutamate blocks, by depolarization, the

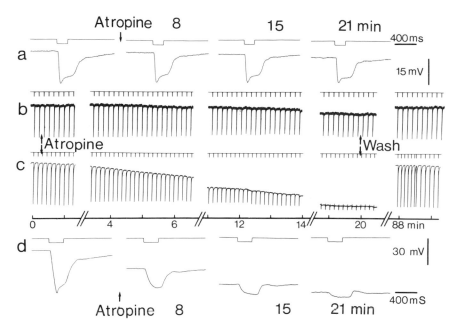

FIGURE 4   Effect of atropine on the turtle retina. Atropine sulfate (5 mM) is applied both on a cone (a, b) and on an L-horizontal cell (c, d). Both cells were stimulated with white light of the same intensity, the cone with a spot of 155 μm diameter and the L-horizontal cell with a larger spot (3,600 μm). Atropine application hyperpolarizes the L-horizontal cell and almost completely blocks its light responses (c), whereas it slightly hyperpolarizes the cone (b). The responses recover only after very prolonged washing. In a and d, the responses of the cone and the L-horizontal cell were recorded at high speed. (From Gerschenfeld and Piccolino, 1977.)

responses of the L-horizontal cells and (2) that muscarinic antagonists block, by hyperpolarization, the light responses of L-horizontal cells by acting preferentially at the postsynaptic level. Therefore, these drugs may constitute interesting pharmacological tools with which to analyze the possible interactions of L-horizontal cells and other cellular elements of the distal retina. Two of these interactions will be analyzed here: (1) the feedback action of L-horizontal cells on the cones, and (2) their feedforward action on the hyperpolarizing bipolar cells.

L-HORIZONTAL-CELL FEEDBACK ON THE CONES   In the last few years it has become increasingly evident that the responses of the photoreceptor to light depend not only on the impinging photons but also on the illumination of nearby areas of the retina. Over short distances, photoreceptors interact electrotonically among themselves through a series of gap junctions (Baylor, Fuortes, and O'Bryan, 1971; Raviola and Gilula, 1973; Baylor and Hodgkin, 1973; Schwartz, 1975; Fain, 1975; Fain, Gold, and Dowling, 1975; Copenhagen and Owen, 1976). These lateral interactions are reported to be additive for distances up to 300 μm for rods and up to 120 μm for cones. In cones, extending the area of illumination further adds a depolarizing wave to the hyperpolarizing responses to light; this is the depolarizing feedback potential (Baylor, Fuortes, and O'Bryan, 1971). This negative feedback effect onto the cones shows a large receptive field, and it is graded with regard to both the light intensity and the area of peripheral stimu-

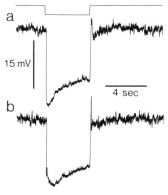

FIGURE 5   Atropine application on a hyperpolarizing bipolar cell of the turtle retina. (a) Control response of a hyperpolarizing bipolar cell to stimulation at the center of its receptor field with a white light spot (600 μm diameter). Note the membrane noise decrease during hyperpolarization. (b) Response to the same light stimulus of the same cell obtained after 25 min of atropine application. The response is slightly decreased in amplitude, but no alteration in membrane noise is observed. (From Gerschenfeld and Piccolino, 1977.)

lation (O'Bryan, 1973). This suggests that the depolarizing feedback potential is mediated by the L-horizontal cells (which are also electrically coupled to one another). In experiments in the turtle in which cones and L-horizontal cells were simultaneously impaled, the cone depolarized when hyperpolarizing current was injected into the L-horizontal cell; this strongly suggests that the cone feedback potential originates from an L-horizontal cell hyperpolarization (Baylor, Fuortes, and O'Bryan, 1971). Measurements of the input resistance of the cone during the feedback depolarization show that it is associated with an alteration of the membrane conductance that appears to consist of two separate components with different time courses; the slower of these, which may outlast the light stimulus, is an *increase* in membrane conductance (O'Bryan, 1973).

Figure 6a–c shows how a depolarizing feedback potential is elicited in a turtle cone responding with a typical 15 mV amplitude hyperpolarization to central spot stimulation (Figure 6a). The same cone responds with a fast, large hyperpolarization when stimulated with a very bright light annulus alone; the hyperpolarization is due to light scattering to the

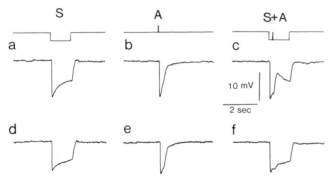

FIGURE 6 Atropine effect on the feedback depolarizing potential of a turtle cone. The top row of traces shows the timing and the duration of the light stimuli. (a–c) Control recordings of the cone responses. In a, the cone responds with a hyperpolarization to a centered spot of white light (diameter 250 μm). In b, the cone is stimulated with an annulus (430 μm inner diameter, 3,600 μm outer diameter, 2 log units brighter than central spot). This stimulation causes a fast hyperpolarization, mainly due to light scattering from the center. The recording in c shows a feedback depolarizing potential that appears when the annulus is presented during the center stimulation, 180 msec after its onset. The recordings d–f were obtained from the same cone, using the same stimulation parameters, during application of atropine sulfate (5 mM). Notice in f that the depolarizing feedback potential has been blocked and that the flashing of the annulus, in the same temporal relation with the center stimulation, evokes only a small hyperpolarization due to light scattering. (From Piccolino and Gerschenfeld, 1977a.)

center of the cone receptor field (Figure 6b). When the background spot illumination and the light annulus are combined with appropriate timing (Figure 6c), the time course of the control hyperpolarization is markedly altered by the development of a depolarizing wave—the depolarizing feedback potential.

Under some experimental conditions, when the retina is stimulated with large spots of dim monochromatic light, the depolarizing feedback potential develops into a 20 mV spike (Fuortes, Schwartz, and Simon, 1973); furthermore, O'Bryan (1973) demonstrated that the depolarizing feedback potential can be converted into a spikelike signal by injecting outward current into the cone.

We recently analyzed such spikes in the retina of the turtle *Pseudemys scripta* (Piccolino and Gerschenfeld, 1977b, 1978). When the feedback depolarizing potentials are converted to spikes by injecting outward current into the cone, the resulting spikes are resistant to tetrodotoxin (TTX) in concentrations up to 10^{-6} mM, which suggests that they do not involve the activation of a regenerative Na^+ conductance. As in many other cells (see Hagiwara, 1974), these spikes may be due to a Ca^{2+} conductance change. Unfortunately, it is not possible to alter the extracellular Ca^{2+} concentration to study the feedback potential, since one or two chemical synapses may be involved in the generation of the feedback potential and increases in the Ca^{2+} outer concentration hyperpolarize the vertebrate photoreceptors and depress their light responses (Brown and Pinto, 1974). Nevertheless, it has recently been shown that Sr^{2+} ions permeate the photoreceptor membrane through the Ca^{2+} channels (Fain, Quandt, and Gerschenfeld, 1977), and they are able to replace Ca^{2+} ions in the maintenance of cone-to-L-horizontal cell transmission without affecting the cone light responses (Piccolino, 1976). Therefore, the effect on the feedback potential of media containing different Sr^{2+} concentrations was studied.

Figure 7a is an intracellular recording from a turtle cone, which responds with a 22 mV hyperpolarization to a centered light spot and with a fast hyperpolarization (due again to light scattering to the center) to a bright annulus. When the annular flash is presented during the center background stimulation, a small feedback depolarization is evoked which, at the low recording speed, remains hidden in the noise. Figure 7b is a recording from the same cone at faster speed; it does not show any response when stimulated only with an annulus of dim green light (550 nm). Figures 7a' and 7b' show the responses of the same cone to the same series of stimuli while bathing the retina in

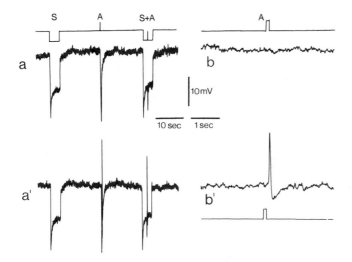

FIGURE 7 Effect of Sr²⁺ ions on the feedback depolarizing potential. (a, a') Control recordings from a turtle cone. In a, the cone is stimulated first with a step of central light (spot S, 250 μm diameter), then with a peripheral light flash (annulus A, 150 μm inner diameter, 3,600 μm external diameter), and finally with an appropriate combination of both stimuli (S + A). The depolarizing feedback potential is practically obscured by the noise. In a', a dim monochromatic annulus (550 nm, delivering 5 × 10⁴ photons/μm²/sec) is flashed on the retina without any apparent cone response. (b, b') Responses of the same cone to a similar series of stimuli as in a and a' during perfusion of the retina with a saline solution containing 6 mM SrCl₂. In b, a spike appears in response to peripheral stimulation and to proper combination of center and peripheral stimulation. In b', a spike, uncontaminated by any parasite hyperpolarization, can be evoked at the dark potential level by stimulation of the periphery in a Sr²⁺-containing Ringer's (see text).

a medium containing 6 mM SrCl₂. The responses to the central light spot remains unchanged, but now the bright annular flash, whether presented during central background light stimulation or not, evokes a spike (Figure 7a'). Moreover, in Figure 7b', at the dark potential level, the green annular stimulus now evokes a spike of more than 20 mV in amplitude and 150 msec in duration, showing an undershoot (see also Figure 8). In other experiments using higher concentrations of SrCl₂, the spikes reach amplitudes of 30–40 mV and durations up to 300 msec. Addition to the extracellular medium of Ba²⁺ ions, which are known to permeate Co²⁺ channels and to block K⁺ channels in other preparations (see Hagiwara, 1974), also converts the depolarizing feedback potential into a spike. In experiments using Ca²⁺ ions, which impair the cone-to-L-horizontal cell transmission only slightly when Sr²⁺ ions are present in the medium, the spikes are rapidly blocked. The same is observed with low concentrations (0.5 mM) of the Ca²⁺-channel

blocker, isoverapramil (D600). All these data strongly support the idea that the feedback spikes are due to a regenerative increase in Ca²⁺ conductance.

To confirm that the depolarizing feedback potential and the feedback spikes result from the activation of a connection from the L-horizontal cells to the cones, we used drugs that have been shown to decrease or block the L-horizontal-cell light responses, either by depolarizing or hyperpolarizing them. In the experiment shown in Figure 6, atropine was used for this purpose. The control responses of the cone in parts a–c have already been described to illustrate the depolarizing feedback potential. If we compare these recordings to those of parts d and e, it is evident that atropine application (5 mM) results in a complete disappearance of the depolarizing feedback potential. Such blocking of the feedback can also be observed when the depolarizing potential is converted into a spike by using current injection or a Sr²⁺-containing media.

Another pharmacological experiment that confirms the origin of the feedback effects from the horizontal cell is shown in Figure 8. The upper row

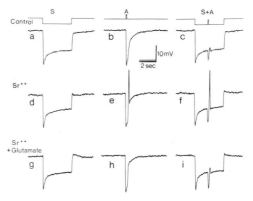

FIGURE 8 Effect of glutamate on the feedback spike of a turtle cone. (a–c) Control recordings from a turtle cone. In a, the cone responds by a hyperpolarization to a step of central light (spot S, 155 μm diameter). In b, stimulation of the cone with a peripheral bright light (annulus A, 150 μm inner diameter, 3,600 μm outer diameter, 2 log units brighter than the central spot) causes a "parasite" hyperpolarization. In c, proper combination of both stimuli (S + A) evokes a small depolarizing feedback potential, which appears contaminated by a previous parasite hyperpolarization. (d–f) Responses to the same stimulus in the presence of 6 mM Sr²⁺ in the medium: both the stimulation with the annulus (e) and the combination of both stimuli (f) evoke the discharge of a spike. (g–i) Glutamate (50 mM) application, in the presence of 6 mM Sr²⁺, completely blocks the feedback spike. In i, a feedback depolarizing potential can still be observed, but the application of glutamate for few more minutes causes a complete disappearance of the feedback potential (see text).

of recordings (a–c) correspond, respectively, to the responses of a turtle cone to a bright light spot, a short bright annulus, and a bright annulus flashed during presentation of the background spot. The depolarizing feedback potential in Figure 8c is small and appears to be preceded by a "parasite" hyperpolarization. In recordings d–f the same stimuli were applied with 6 mM $SrCl_2$ in the medium; spikes now developed when the cone was stimulated with the annular flash (e and f). Application to the preparation of a high concentration of glutamate (50 mM), which depolarizes the L-horizontal cells and depresses their light responses, blocks the feedback spikes (h and i). Figure 8i, in which a depolarizing potential can still be observed, was recorded shortly before the complete blocking of all feedback effects.

The pharmacological experiments of Figures 6 and 8 confirm that the depolarizing potentials and/or the spikes evoked in turtle cones by stimulating the periphery of their receptor field with light result from a negative feedback effect from the L-horizontal cells. What, then, is the synaptic mechanism associated with such feedback effects?

The exact mechanism controlling the connection between L-horizontal cells and cones is still unknown; but the measurement of a conductance change during the feedback potential (O'Bryan, 1973) supports the idea of a chemical synapse from the L-horizontal cell to the cone. The ultrastructural data, however, do not favor this hypothesis. No vesicles have been observed in the horizontal processes invaginated within the cone pedicle in the lower vertebrate retinas (see, e.g., Dowling and Werblin, 1969; Lasansky, 1971; Schaeffer and Raviola, 1975; Stell, 1976). Schaeffer and Raviola (1975) observed some membrane clusters of particles in the E-face of the cone synaptic ridge of freeze-etched turtle retinas, which would suggest a postsynaptic specialization of the cone terminal. Stell (1976) reports that in goldfish, horizontal-cell processes present membrane specializations and undercoatings *away* from the region facing the cone; he suggests that these specialized zones may form the site where the feedback action takes place. Alternatively, Raviola (1976) has pointed out that synaptic vesicles are not observed in the horizontal-cell processes because the probability of catching the vesicle during exocytosis at the time of fixation is very low. Since L-horizontal cells, like cones, are hyperpolarized by light stimulation, if a feedback chemical synapse exists, it is very likely to function tonically—that is, by continuous release of transmitter in the dark. In that case, the problem will be the identification of the conductance change evoked in the cone by the L-horizontal-cell transmitter.

From the measurements of O'Bryan (1973), it is known that the second component associated with the feedback potential is an increase in membrane conductance. But from O'Bryan's data, as well as from unpublished experiments in which we injected small constant-current pulses across the cone membrane, it is very difficult to evaluate the first component. As Byzov and Cervetto (1977) recently reported, short depolarizing pulses passed across the cone membrane during large light spot stimuli produce larger electrotonic potentials than hyperpolarizing pulses of the same current intensity. We also observed this phenomenon; moreover, when we increased the amplitude of the depolarizing current pulses during a light annulus stimulation, the electrotonic potentials gave rise to regenerative spikelike responses. Moreover, it is evident that the feedback effect from the L-horizontal cells can involve an overt increase in Ca^{2+} conductance, as revealed by the experiments in Sr^{2+}-containing media (Piccolino and Gerschenfeld, 1977b) and also in normal medium (Fuortes and Simon, 1973; O'Bryan, 1973). The threshold of activation of this Ca^{2+} conductance has not yet been defined with precision.

These data point to several alternative explanations of the synaptic mechanism, if indeed it is chemically mediated. (1) The continuously liberated transmitter of the L-horizontal cells causes a decrease of the Na^+ conductance in the dark; its suppression by peripheral light stimulation increases the Na^+ conductance of the cone ending, depolarizes it, and brings the membrane to the threshold of activation of the Ca^{2+} conductance. (2) In the dark, the L-horizontal-cell transmitter controls the Ca^{2+} conductance of the cone. The suppression of this transmitter action by light causes an increase of Ca^{2+} conductance, which becomes regenerative. One possible mechanism by which the transmitter of the L-horizontal cells could control the Ca^{2+} conductance is by maintaining in the dark an increased K^+ conductance of the cone endings. When peripheral light stimulation suppresses the transmitter release, it decreases the K^+ conductance of the cone membrane, thus removing an important shunt; the Ca^{2+} conductance increases and becomes regenerative.

Of these possible synaptic mechanisms, the last is the most likely, for it appears to be the only one capable of operating at both the dark and the light potential levels of the cone (Figure 7). Moreover, it has been demonstrated that a regenerative Ca^{2+} conductance can be activated by suppressing a membrane ionic shunt (see Hagiwara, 1974), which is the case in the nerve terminals of the squid giant synapse (Katz and Miledi, 1969). Another example from the retina also illustrates this possibility: the partial suppression of K^+ permeability in toad rods by tetraethylammonium ions depolarizes the rods and produces Ca^{2+} spikes. Unlike the feedback spikes of turtle cones, the rod spikes are activated by either central or peripheral stimuli and are insensitive to dicarboxylic amino acids and muscarinic blockers (Fain, Quandt, and Gerschenfeld, 1977; Piccolino and Gerschenfeld, 1977b).

It has not yet been possible to obtain crucial evidence favoring any of these mechanisms. Moreover, given the lack of ultrastructural evidence in favor of a chemical connection from the L-horizontal cells to the cones, an alternative, electrical mechanism can be imagined. Since the L-horizontal-cell processes are deeply invaginated in the cone endings, it is possible that a field effect, such as that operating between the Mauthner cell and the surrounding small cells in fish medulla (Furukawa and Furshpan, 1963; Korn and Faber, 1975; Korn, this volume), could be responsible for the feedback effect. According to this model, if the electrical resistance of the extracellular space between the cone and the L-horizontal-cell processes is very high, a hyperpolarization of the numerous invaginated cell processes of the L-horizontal cells could cause a depolarization of the cones, which on reaching threshold could activate a regenerative Ca^{2+} conductance. This hypothesis has not been tested.

L-HORIZONTAL-CELL FEEDFORWARD EFFECTS   No special consideration will be given in this article to the role of L-horizontal cells in the generation of the opposite color-coded responses of the C-type horizontal cells. Different mechanisms have been proposed to explain these responses (see Fuortes and Simon, 1974; Stell, 1976). All of the explanations involve the intervention of the L-horizontal cells, which pharmacological experiments appear to confirm (Piccolino and Gerschenfeld, 1977a).

The most important of the proposed feedforward actions of L-horizontal cells is their involvement in the production of the center-surround antagonism of the receptor field of bipolar cells (Werblin and Dowling, 1969; Naka, 1972; Kaneko, 1973; Richter and Simon, 1975). All of these authors agree that the responses of both types of bipolar cells to small spots presented in the center of their receptor field involve activation of a direct connection between photorecep-

tors and bipolar cells, whereas the antagonistic responses elicited by light stimulation of the periphery of the receptor field involve activation of a polysynaptic pathway in which L-horizontal cells play a fundamental role.

This hypothesis was recently tested in the retina of the turtle *Pseudemys* by studying the effect of blocking the L-horizontal cell with atropine on the center-surround antagonism of the hyperpolarizing bipolar-cell receptor field (Piccolino and Gerschenfeld, 1977a). Figure 9 shows one of the twelve hyperpolarizing

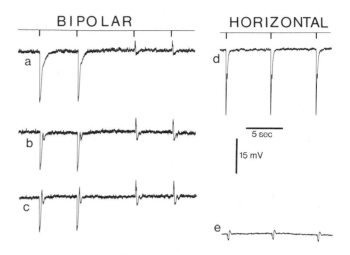

FIGURE 9   Effect of atropine on the center-surround antagonism of the receptor field of hyperpolarizing bipolar cells. At left (a–c), recordings from an hyperpolarizing bipolar cell; at right (d–e), recordings from two different horizontal cells. The top traces on both sides mark the timing of the light stimulations. At left, the first two stimuli in each row were centered light spots (diameter 380 μm), and the two following stimuli were white light annuli (500 μm inner diameter, 3,600 μm outer diameter, 2 log units less intense than the central spot). (a) Control recordings of the bipolar-cell response to the spot and annulus. (b) After 10 minutes of atropine application, the central responses are slightly diminished and show off-hyperpolarizations, whereas the responses to the periphery become increased in amplitude. (c) After 20 minutes of atropinization, the center responses are not much changed, except for the increasing complexity of the off responses, while the amplitude of the responses to the annulus have further increased. (d) Recording from an L-horizontal cell impaled just before penetrating the bipolar cell at left, showing a hyperpolarizing response to large white light spots (diameter 3,600 μm, similar brightness to the central spot in a). The recording in e is from another L-horizontal cell penetrated at the end of the experiment, just after removing the pipette from the bipolar cell at left, while the preparation was still bathed in atropine. Notice the block of L-horizontal cell responses after more than 25 minutes of atropine application. (From Piccolino and Gerschenfeld, 1977a.)

bipolars studied for this purpose. All of these cells were recognized by the following criteria (Schwartz, 1974; Richter and Simon, 1975; Simon, Lamb, and Hodgkin, 1975): (a) their high sensitivity to light; (b) the center-surround antagonism of their receptor field; (c) the typical off-depolarization after prolonged light stimuli; and (d) the attenuation of membrane noise during the hyperpolarizing response to light stimulation of the center of their receptor field (see also Figure 5). The hyperpolarizing bipolar cell of Figure 9 responded with a 20 mV depolarization to a white light central spot and gave a few mV depolarization to stimulation with a light annulus concentric with the central spot (Figure 9a). Application of atropine (5 mM) to the retina causes, after a short time, a small reduction of the center response (parallel to the cone response decrease described earlier) and a small increase in the depolarizing response (Figure 9B). After 20–25 min of atropine application, the center hyperpolarizing responses show unchanged amplitude and a still-unexplained, complex off-response. At the same time, it can be observed that depolarizing responses to the periphery are not blocked; on the contrary, their amplitude is increased.

In the same preparation, many L-horizontal cells were impaled before (Figure 9d) and after (Figure 9e) 20–25 min of atropine application; atropine hyperpolarized and almost blocked all the L-horizontal cell responses. In d and e, the light parameters used to evoke the L-horizontal cell responses were similar to those used to stimulate the center of the receptor field in a–c. It was found that atropine blocks the L-horizontal-cell responses to dim light equally as well as those to brighter stimuli; that is, the blocking effect of atropine does not depend on the intensity of light stimulus.

These results show that blocking the cone–to–L-horizontal-cell synapses accentuates rather than blocks the response of the hyperpolarizing bipolar cell to peripheral light stimulation. Therefore they do not support the hypothesis that the center-surround antagonism of hyperpolarizing bipolars depends exclusively on L-horizontal cells. It is possible, however, that, since under atropine the L-horizontal cell potential is moved to a very hyperpolarized level, any further small hyperpolarization evoked by light annuli could induce a depolarizing response in hyperpolarizing bipolar cells. Further experiments are needed to clarify this problem.

Concluding remarks

Although we do not know the synaptic transmitter released by the cones, its main properties can be predicted from our present knowledge of the physiological properties of the cone synapses. It is probable that, in contrast to the vertebrate CNS, in which opposite synaptic actions are mediated by separate sets of neurons using different transmitters, retinal cones resemble certain multiaction cells of the molluscan CNS which, by releasing a single transmitter, can elicit multiple and opposite synaptic actions involving both increases and decreases of the postsynaptic membrane conductance.

Microelectrophysiological analysis of the action of some cone transmitter candidates reveals that glutamate produces effects on the L-horizontal and bipolar cells similar to those expected of the cone transmitter. ACh agonists also mimic the effects of the transmitter on L-horizontal cells. A systematic analysis of the action of agonists and antagonists of ACh shows that, in spite of the sensitivity of the L-horizontal cells to both nicotinic and muscarinic agonists, only the muscarinic antagonists, such as atropine (in high concentrations, as in the case of glutamate and the cholinergic agonists), effectively block the light responses by acting preferentially at the postsynaptic level.

Although these data are insufficient to prove the involvement of either glutamate or ACh (and, therefore, the muscarinic ACh receptors) in the synaptic transmission from the cone to the L-horizontal cell, these agonists and blockers can be used to analyze pharmacologically the function of L-horizontal cells in the local circuits at the outer plexiform layer of the retina.

The feedback action of L-horizontal cells on the cones has been analyzed. The depolarizing feedback potential evoked in the cones by peripheral light stimulation can be converted under some conditions (current injection or addition of Sr^{2+} ions to the medium) into a spike, which involves the activation of a regenerative Ca^{2+} conductance. However, the nature of the L-horizontal connection to the cone remains to be clarified. Atropine, which blocks the L-horizontal-cell light response by hyperpolarization, and glutamate, which blocks the same responses by depolarization, both suppress the depolarizing feedback potential and the Ca^{2+} spike evoked in the cones by peripheral illumination, thus confirming their origin from a response of the L-horizontal cells.

The blocking by atropine of the L-horizontal cells

of turtle retina accentuates the antagonism between the responses of the hyperpolarizing bipolar cells to stimulation of the center and the periphery of their receptor field.

More research is necessary to identify the cone transmitter and to unravel the local circuits in the lower vertebrate retinas. A combination of microphysiological methods with pharmacological analysis appears a promising way to investigate these problems.

ACKNOWLEDGMENTS The authors are indebted to Dr. R. T. Kado for suggesting the possibility of an electrical mechanism to explain the negative feedback potential in the cones. They thank Mr. B. Lacaisse for technical assistance and Dr. Eve Marder for reviewing the manuscript. The work of the authors was supported by grants of the Centre National de la Recherche Scientifique, Délégation Générale à la Recherche Scientifique, and Institut National de la Santé et de la Recherche Médicale, France.

REFERENCES

BAUGHMAN, R. W., C. R. BADER, and E. A. SCHWARTZ, 1976. Autoradiographic localization of cholinergic cells in retina. Neurosci. Abstr. 2:1102.

BAYLOR, D. A., M.G.F. FUORTES, and P. M. O'BRYAN, 1971. Receptive fields of cones in the retina of the turtle. J. Physiol. 214:265–294.

BAYLOR, D. A., and A. L. HODGKIN, 1973. Detection and resolution of visual stimuli by turtle photoreceptors. J. Physiol. 234:163–108.

BERRY, M. S., and G. A. COTTRELL, 1975. Excitatory, inhibitory and biphasic synaptic potentials mediated by an identified giant dopamine neuron. J. Physiol. 244:589–612.

BONTING, S. L., ed., 1976. Transmitters in the Visual Process. Oxford: Pergamon Press.

BROWN, J. E., and L. H. PINTO, 1974. Ionic mechanism for the photoreceptor potential of the retina of Bufo marinus. J. Physiol. 236:575–591.

BROWNSTEIN, M. J., J. M. SAAVEDRA, J. AXELROD, G. H. ZEMAN, and D. O. CARPENTER, 1974. Coexistence of several putative neurotransmitters in single identified neurons of Aplysia. Proc. Natl. Acad. Sci. USA 71:4662–4665.

BYZOV, A. L., and L. CERVETTO, 1977. Effects of applied currents on turtle cones in darkness and during the photoresponse. J. Physiol. 265:85–102.

CERVETTO, L., and E. F. MacNICHOL, 1972. Inactivation of horizontal cells in turtle retina by glutamate and aspartate. Science 178:767–768.

CERVETTO, L., and M. PICCOLINO, 1974. Synaptic transmission between photoreceptors and horizontal cells in the turtle retina. Science 183:417–419.

COPENHAGEN, D. R., and W. G. OWEN, 1976. Functional characteristics of lateral interactions between rods in the retina of the snapping turtle. J. Physiol. 259:251–282.

DACHEUX, R. F., and R. F. MILLER, 1976. Photoreceptor-bipolar cell transmission in the perfused retina eyecup of the mudpuppy. Science 191:963–964.

DOWLING, J. E., and J. H. RIPPS, 1973. Effect of magnesium on horizontal cell activity in the skate retina. Nature 242:101–103.

DOWLING, J. E., and F. S. WERBLIN, 1969. Organization of the retina of the mudpuppy Necturus maculosus. II. Synaptic structure. J. Neurophysiol. 32:315–338.

ECCLES, J. C., 1969. The Inhibitory Pathways of the Nervous System. Springfield, IL: Thomas.

FAIN, G. L., 1975. Quantum sensitivity of rods in the toad retina. Science 187:838–841.

FAIN, G. L., G. H. GOLD, and J. E. DOWLING, 1975. Receptor coupling in the toad retina. Cold Spring Harbor Symp. Quant. Biol. 40:547–561.

FAIN, G. L., F. N. QUANDT, and H. M. GERSCHENFELD, 1977. Calcium-dependent regenerative responses in rods. Nature (in press).

FUORTES, M.G.F., E. A. SCHWARTZ, and E. J. SIMON, 1973. Colour-dependence of cone responses in the turtle retinas. J. Physiol. 234:199–216.

FUORTES, M.G.F., and E. J. SIMON, 1974. Interactions leading to horizontal cell responses in turtle retina. J. Physiol. 240:177–198.

FURUKAWA, T., and E. J. FURSHPAN, 1963. Two inhibitory mechanisms in the Mauthner neurons of goldfish. J. Neurophysiol. 26:140–176.

GERSCHENFELD, H. M., 1973. Chemical transmission in invertebrate central nervous systems and neuromuscular junctions. Physiol. Rev. 53:1–119.

GERSCHENFELD, H. M., 1977. Multiple receptor activation by single transmitters. In Synapses, G. A. Cottrell and P. N. R. Usherwood, eds. Glasgow: Blackie & Son, pp. 157–176.

GERSCHENFELD, H. M., and D. PAUPARDIN-TRITSCH, 1974a. Ionic mechanisms and receptor properties underlying the responses of molluscan neurons to 5-hydroxytryptamine. J. Physiol. 243:427–456.

GERSCHENFELD, H. M., and D. PAUPARDIN-TRITSCH, 1974b. On the transmitter role of 5-hydroxytryptamine at excitatory and inhibitory monosynaptic junctions. J. Physiol. 243:457–481.

GERSCHENFELD, H. M., and M. PICCOLINO, 1977. Muscarinic antagonists block cone to horizontal cell transmission in turtle retina. Nature 268:257–259.

GRAHAM, L. T., 1974. Comparative aspects of neurotransmitters in the retina. In The Eye, H. Davson and L. T. Graham, eds. New York: Academic Press, vol. 6, pp. 283–342.

HAGIWARA, S., 1974. Ca-dependent action potential. In Membranes—A Series of Advances, G. Eisenman, ed. New York and Basel: Marcel Dekker, pp. 359–381.

HANLEY, M. R., G. A. COTTRELL, P. C. EMSON, and F. FONNUM, 1974. Enzymatic synthesis of acetylcholine by a serotonin-containing neuron from Helix. Nature (Lond.) 251:631–633.

KANDEL, E. R., W. T. FRAZIER, R. WAZIRI, and R. E. COGGESHALL, 1967. Direct and common connections among identified neurons of Aplysia. J. Neurophysiol. 39:1352–1376.

KANEKO, A., 1970. Physiological and morphological identification of horizontal, bipolar and amacrine cells in the goldfish retina. J. Physiol. 207:623–633.

KANEKO, A., 1973. Receptive field organization of bipolar

and amacrine cells in the goldfish retina. *J. Physiol.* 235:133–154.

KANEKO, A., and H. SHIMAZAKI, 1975a. Effects of external ions on the synaptic transmission from photoreceptors to horizontal cells in the carp retina. *J. Physiol.* 252:509–522.

KANEKO, A., and H. SHIMAZAKI, 1975b. Synaptic transmission from photoreceptors to bipolar and horizontal cells in the carp retina. *Cold Spring Harbor Symp. Quant. Biol.* 40:537–546.

KANEKO, A., and H. SHIMAZAKI, 1976. Synaptic transmission from receptor to the second-order neurons in the carp retina. In *Neural Principles of Vision*, F. Zettler and R. Weiler, eds. Berlin and Heidelberg: Springer-Verlag, pp. 143–157.

KATZ, B., and R. MILEDI, 1969. Tetrodotoxin-resistant electric activity in presynaptic terminals. *J. Physiol.* 203:459–487.

KEHOE, J. S., 1972. The physiological role of three acetylcholine receptors in synaptic transmission. *J. Physiol.* 225:115–146.

KORN, H., and D. S. FABER, 1975. An electrically mediated inhibition in goldfish medulla. *J. Neurophysiol.* 38:452–471.

KRAVITZ, E. A., C. R. SLATER, K. TAKAHASHI, M. D. BOWNDS, and R. GROSSFELD, 1970. Excitatory transmission in invertebrates-glutamate as a potential neuromuscular transmitter compound. In *Excitatory Synaptic Mechanisms*, P. Andersen and J. K. S. Jansen, eds. Oslo: Universitetsforlaget, pp. 84–93.

KRNJEVIĆ, K., 1974. Chemical nature of synaptic transmission in vertebrates. *Physiol. Rev.* 54:418–540.

LAM, D. M. K., 1972. Biosynthesis of acetylcholine in turtle photoreceptors. *Proc. Natl. Acad. Sci. USA* 68:2777–2781.

LAM, D. M. K., 1975. Synaptic chemistry of identified cells in the vertebrate retina. *Cold Spring Harbor Symp. Quant. Biol.* 40:571–579.

LASANSKY, A., 1971. Synaptic organization of cone cells in turtle retina. *Philos. Trans. R. Soc. Lond.* B262:365–381.

MURAKAMI, M., K. OHTSU, and T. OHTSUKA, 1972. Effects of chemicals on receptors and horizontal cells in the retina. *J. Physiol.* 227:899–913.

MURAKAMI, M., T. OHTSUKA, and H. SHIMAZAKI, 1975. Effects of aspartate and glutamate on the bipolar cells in the carp retina. *Vision Res.* 15:456–458.

NAKA, K. I., 1972. The horizontal cells. *Vision Res.* 4:573–588.

NELSON, R., 1973. A comparison of electrical properties of neurons in *Necturus* retina. *J. Neurophysiol.* 36:519–535.

O'BRYAN, P. M., 1973. Properties of the depolarizing synaptic potential evoked by peripheral illumination in cones of the turtle retina. *J. Physiol.* 235:207–223.

PICCOLINO, M., 1976. Strontium-calcium substitution in synaptic transmission in turtle retina. *Nature* 261:554–555.

PICCOLINO, M., and H. M. GERSCHENFELD, 1977a. Lateral interactions in the outer plexiform layer of turtle retinas after atropine block of horizontal cells. *Nature* 268:259–261.

PICCOLINO, M., and H. M. GERSCHENFELD, 1977b. Calcium spikes evoked in turtle cones by peripheral light stimulation. *Neurosci. Abstr.* (in press).

PICCOLINO, M., and H. M. GERSCHENFELD, 1978. Activation of a regenerative calcium conductance in turtle cones by peripheral stimulation. *Proc. R. Soc. Lond.* B201:309–315.

RAVIOLA, E., 1976. Intercellular junctions in the outer plexiform layer of the retina. *Invest. Ophthalmol.* 11:881–895.

RAVIOLA, E., and N. B. GILULA, 1973. Gap junctions between photoreceptor cells in the vertebrate retina. *Proc. Natl. Acad. Sci. USA* 65:192.

RICHTER, A., and E. J. SIMON, 1975. Properties of centre hyperpolarizing, red sensitive bipolar cells in the turtle retina. *J. Physiol.* 248:317–334.

SCHAEFFER, S. F., and E. RAVIOLA, 1975. Ultrastructural analysis of functional changes in the synaptic endings of turtle cone cells. *Cold Spring Harbor Symp. Quant. Biol.* 40:521–528.

SCHWARTZ, E. A., 1974. Responses of bipolar cells in the retina of the turtle. *J. Physiol.* 236:211–224.

SCHWARTZ, E. A., 1975. Rod-rod interaction in the retina of the turtle. *J. Physiol.* 246:617–638.

SIMON, E. J., T. D. LAMB, and A. L. HODGKIN, 1975. Spontaneous voltage fluctuations in retinal cones and bipolar cells. *Nature* 256:661–662.

TAKEUCHI, A., 1977. Excitatory and inhibitory transmitter actions at the crayfish neuromuscular junction. In *Motor Innervation of Muscle*, S. Thesleff, ed. New York: Raven Press, pp. 231–261.

TOYODA, J. I., 1973. Membrane resistance changes underlying the bipolar cell response in the carp retina. *Vision Res.* 13:283–294.

TOYODA, J., H. NOSAKI, and T. TOMITA, 1969. Light induced resistance changes in single photoreceptors of *Necturus* and *Gekko*. *Vision Res.* 13:283–294.

TOMITA, T., 1965. Electrophysiological study of the mechanisms subserving color coding in the fish retina. *Cold Spring Harbor Symp. Quant. Biol.* 30:559–566.

TRIFONOV, Y. A., 1968. Study of synaptic transmission between photoreceptors and horizontal cells by means of electrical stimulation of the retina (in Russian). *Biofizika* 13:809–817.

TRIFONOV, Y. A., A. L. BYZOV, and L. M. CHAILAHIAN, 1974. Electrical properties of subsynaptic and non-synaptic membranes of horizontal cells in fish retina. *Vision Res.* 14:229–241.

WEINREICH, D., 1977. Synaptic responses mediated by identified histamine-containing neurons. *Nature* 268:854–856.

WERBLIN, F. S., and J. E. DOWLING, 1969. Organization of the retina of the mudpuppy *Necturus maculosus*. II. Intracellular recording. *J. Neurophysiology* 32:339–355.

YAZULLA, S., and J. SCHMIDT, 1976. Radioautographic localization of ^{125}I-α-bungarotoxin binding sites in the retinas of goldfish and turtle. *Vision Res.* 16:878–880.

14 The Neuronal Basis of Ganglion-Cell Receptive-Field Organization and the Physiology of Amacrine Cells

ROBERT F. MILLER

ABSTRACT The neuronal pathways that underlie the receptive fields of *on*, *off*, and *on-off* ganglion cells have been examined by intracellular recording techniques in perfused retina-eyecup preparations of rabbit and mudpuppy. Replacement of external chloride ions restricts light-evoked excitation to off responses of *off* and *on-off* ganglion cells. Intracellular recordings of chloride-free effects permit the identity of preganglion cell types associated with *on* and *off* pathways.

Amacrine cells form an inhibitory input to ganglion cells, and it appears that separate amacrine-cell units interact with *on*, *off*, and *on-off* ganglion cells. Amacrine cells generate dendritic and somatic spike activity in addition to large-amplitude EPSPs. Studies of spike thresholds suggest that the amacrine cells may function in one of two different states. When stimuli are below somatic spike threshold, dendrites may function independently from one another through dendrodendritic synapses. A synaptic booster role is proposed for the dendritic spikes. When stimuli reach somatic spike threshold, the dendritic operations may be much more uniform as the somatic spikes invade the dendritic tree.

Ganglion-cell receptive-field organization

THE FIRST electrophysiological studies of ganglion-cell receptive-field properties in the vertebrate retina (Hartline, 1938) demonstrated three classes of neurons (*on*, *off*, *on-off*), based on the discharge pattern evoked by focal illumination. Later work showed that some ganglion cells had center-surround organization (Kuffler, 1952; Barlow, 1953), whereas others seemed to respond best to complex forms and moving targets (Lettvin et al., 1959; Barlow, Hill, and Levick, 1964). Despite the rich variety of ganglion-cell types that have been discovered among vertebrates, Hartline's classification remains a useful way of describing a very elemental feature of ganglion-cell organization. Superimposed on the *on*, *off*, and

ROBERT F. MILLER Department of Ophthalmology, Washington University School of Medicine, St. Louis, MO 63110

on-off classification, one finds cells of differing complexity. Thus, an *on* cell could be an *on*-center cell or an *on*-motion-selective unit described in rabbit.

The mechanism by which ganglion cells are encoded for responding to the onset and termination of a light stimulus was unknown until intracellular recordings from preganglion-cell neurons were first described (Werblin and Dowling, 1969; Kaneko, 1970). These studies described both hyperpolarizing (HPBC) and depolarizing (DPBC) bipolar cells and seemed to provide an explanation for the way in which *on* and *off* channels might be organized. The technique of single-cell intracellular recording falls short of providing a detailed explanation of the pathways or synaptic polarities of cell interactions. Are bipolar cells inhibitory or excitatory? How are the DPBCs and HPBCs encoded? What role do amacrine cells play in integrating receptive-field properties? During the past few years, I have approached these problems by using an isolated, perfused retina-eyecup preparation of mudpuppy and rabbit. Ion-substitution experiments and pharmacological studies have provided insight into the fundamental pathways, synaptic polarities, and amacrine-cell function that underlie the organization of *on*, *off*, and *on-off* channels.

The organization of the vertebrate retina is uniquely altered when external chloride ions are replaced by a suitably large anion in the perfused retina-eyecup preparations of the rabbit and mudpuppy. The chloride-free (C-F) changes in retinal organization are best appreciated by an examination of ganglion-cell impulse activity using extracellular recording techniques (Figure 1). The recordings were obtained from the rabbit retina, but identical changes were also observed in mudpuppy ganglion cells (Miller and Dacheux, 1973, 1974, 1976b). Both small spot (240 μm) and full-field light stimulation were employed to study receptive-field properties of *on*

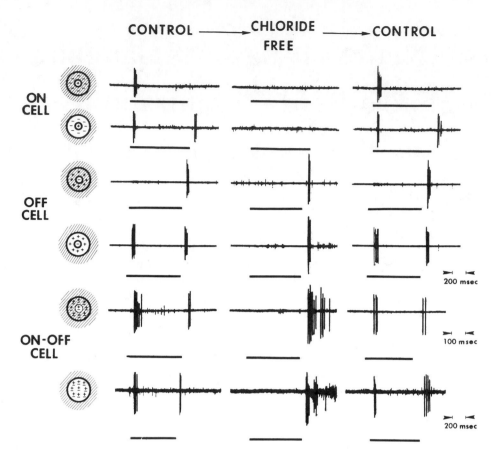

FIGURE 1 C-F effects on an *on*-center cell (upper two horizontal rows), an *off*-center cell (middle two horizontal rows), and an *on-off* cell (lower two horizontal rows). The left-hand drawing indicates by the absence of shading whether small or large spot stimulus was used. The left-hand vertical column shows discharge patterns observed in a control environment, the middle column shows responses in a C-F environment after steady-state conditions were observed, and the right-hand column shows discharge patterns after a return to normal medium. All responses are photographic reproductions of impulse activity displayed on a storage oscilloscope. The 200 msec calibration applies to all traces except second lowest horizontal row. Negative down. White light energy was constant for all stimuli at 1.6×10^{-6} W/cm². (From Miller and Dacheux, 1975.)

center (upper two horizontal rows), *off*-center (middle two horizontal rows), and *on-off* ganglion cells (lower two horizontal rows). The recordings illustrate responses obtained in normal perfusate (left vertical column), about 3 min after introducing a C-F Ringer's (middle vertical column) and following a return to the control environment (right vertical column). The diagrams on the left illustrate, by the absence of shading, whether small-spot or diffuse-light stimulation was employed. In a control medium, focal-light stimulation evoked a transient *on* or *off* burst in *on*-center and *off*-center ganglion cells, respectively (first and third responses). Diffuse-light stimulation evokes both *on* and *off* responses, which demonstrate the center-surround antagonistic organization of these cells. In contrast, both focal- and diffuse-light stimulation evoke *on* and *off* responses

in *on-off* cells, showing that these neurons do not have a center-surround antagonistic organization, but give *on-off* responses throughout a large region of their receptive field. These cells usually show an inhibitory or silent surround. In a C-F medium, ganglion-cell discharge is restricted to *off* activity of *off*-center and *on-off* ganglion cells. *On*-center cells are insensitive to light stimulation under these conditions and cannot be excited by either focal or diffuse stimulation. The *off*-center cell loses excitation through the surround pathway, but the *off*-center excitation persists. The on component of *on-off* cells is abolished, but the off discharge remains.

The loss of on activity under C-F conditions suggested that this altered ionic environment separated *on* and *off* channels and encouraged further exploration with the objective of evaluating chloride-sen-

228   ROBERT F. MILLER

sitive cellular responses and identifying the pathways that mediate *on, off,* and *on-off* activity. Further analysis required intracellular recording experiments for which the mudpuppy was selected because of the large size of the retinal neurons and also because the major cell types had been identified by Werblin and Dowling (1969). In these experiments intracellular recordings were maintained during a perfusion sequence of control–chloride-free–return to control (Miller and Dacheux, 1976a,b,c). In this way alterations in responses could be attributed to the C-F environment and not to extraneous causes. A summary of these experiments is presented in Figure 2. Responses obtained in control Ringer's are illustrated on the left, and those observed in a C-F Ringer's are shown on the right. The configuration of the light stimulus (large spot, small spot, annulus) is illustrated below the responses. Not surprisingly, receptors (R) are relatively insensitive to chloride replacement (Miller and Dacheux, 1973; Winkler, 1973; Cervetto and Piccolino, 1974; Brown and Pinto, 1974). Both light-evoked responses and input resistance are minimally affected by this procedure. On the other hand, horizontal-cell (HC) responses, which hyperpolarize to light stimulation, are abolished in a C-F medium. The loss of light-evoked activity in these neurons is associated with a large (30–40 mV) hyperpolarization and is commonly accompanied by an increase in input resistance.

The two types of bipolar cells are differentially affected by a C-F environment. The left portion of Figure 1 illustrates some of the organizational features of DPBCs and HPBCs. Annular-light stimulation evokes a transient hyperpolarization at *on* and a transient depolarization at *off.* Focal-light stimulation evokes a relatively sustained hyperpolarization. If an annulus is superimposed on continuous focal illumination, a depolarization results. These stimuli and their combination demonstrate the center-surround organization of these cells, with center stimulation giving rise to a hyperpolarization and surround activation opposing the center response with a depolarizing influence. Under C-F conditions, the antagonistic surround of HPBCs is abolished, but the center response persists. Both annulus and focal-light stimulation evoke sustained hyperpolarizations, and the annulus superimposed on continuous focal illumination also evokes hyperpolarization. Apparently all stimuli evoke center responses.

The DPBC becomes insensitive to light stimulation under C-F conditions. These cells are organized in a mirror image of the HPBC, with center stimulation evoking depolarization and annular stimulation, su-

perimposed on continuous focal illumination, giving rise to a hyperpolarization. These cells become insensitive to both center and surround stimulation under C-F conditions. However, unlike the horizontal cells, DPBCs are not markedly hyperpolarized by C-F medium; the membrane potential is minimally affected, and light-evoked responses gradually diminish and finally disappear.

The loss of center-surround antagonism in the HPBC is compatible with the loss of HC activity and the suggestion of Werblin and Dowling (1969) that this neuron mediates the surround response. However, recent observations by Gerschenfeld (this volume) have raised doubts that the HC is the exclusive surround pathway in the turtle.

The amacrine cells are the most distal neurons in the retina that show evidence of impulse activity. The only type of amacrine cell identified in the mudpuppy is an *on-off* type, which responds to both the onset and offset of a light stimulus with transient depolarizations associated with spikes. In a C-F medium, the *on* response is abolished, leaving an *off* response preceded by a small sustained hyperpolarization. The lower traces of Figure 1 show examples of intracellular recordings from ganglion cells in control and C-F Ringer's. In a C-F environment, only *off* activity is observed, and *off* responses are usually preceded by a relatively sustained hyperpolarization during the light stimulus. In summary, a C-F environment simplifies the organization of the retina and reduces the pathway from receptors to neurons of the inner retina to a nonconcentrically organized HPBC. The HPBC must, therefore, subserve the ganglion-cell discharge that persists under C-F conditions. By elimination, the DPBC must underlie the pathway for the chloride-sensitive *on* excitation, and the horizontal cells may be principally responsible for center-surround organization of the bipolar cells. These experiments suggest a model for the organization of ganglion cells as well as the polarities of intervening synaptic interactions.

In order to understand more fully the polarities of synaptic connections in the vertebrate retina, it is helpful to consider the nature of synaptic interactions between photoreceptors and postreceptor neurons. Trifonov and Byzov (1965) first suggested that photoreceptors release a transmitter in the depolarized dark state and that the light-evoked hyperpolarization is associated with a decrease in transmitter release. Later studies supported this hypothesis by showing that horizontal cells are hyperpolarized by externally applied synaptic blocking agents (Dowling and Ripps, 1973; Cervetto and Piccolino, 1974; Da-

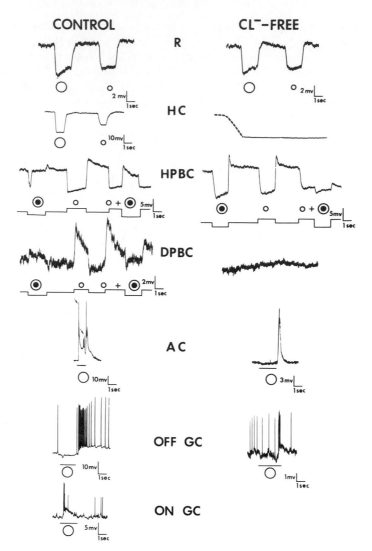

FIGURE 2 Summary diagram of chloride-sensitive and chloride-insensitive retinal neurons. The left-hand column shows responses observed in control Ringer's; the right-hand column shows responses obtained in a C-F medium. Receptors (R) are relatively unaffected by the C-F environment. Horizontal cells (HC) become insensitive to light stimulation in a C-F medium as the cell is hyperpolarized. Hyperpolarizing bipolar cells (HPBC) show antagonistic center-surround organization in control, but the surround mechanism is abolished in C-F medium, leaving only center-mediated hyperpolarization. Depolarizing bipolar cells (DPBC) show antagonistic center-surround organization in control but lose both center and surround responses in a C-F medium. Amacrine cells (AC) show *on* and *off* somatic spikes (first arrow), followed by smaller dendritic spikes (second arrow) in control Ringer's. Some amacrine cells show light-evoked hyperpolarization in C-F medium, accompanied by loss of on depolarization. *On* and *off* ganglion cells are evident in the control environment. *Off* impulse activity shown in the *on* cell represents spontaneous activity resulting from cell penetration. Only *off* cells are observed in a C-F medium. Note that the *off* cell in C-F shows light-evoked hyperpolarization preceding *off* discharge. (From Miller and Dacheux, 1976a.)

cheux and Miller, 1976), suggesting that a dark-released transmitter maintained them in a depolarized state. Figure 3 demonstrates that this concept is applicable to all postreceptor neurons. In these experiments intracellular recordings were maintained from receptors, HCs, DPBCs, and HPBCs in the perfused retina-eyecup preparation of the mudpuppy. Externally applied cobalt was used to block synaptic transmission. A brief exposure to cobalt had little effect on receptors but had rapid, reversible effects on postreceptor neurons. HCs and HPBCs were hyperpolarized by cobalt application, but DPBCs were depolarized. In other words, the action of light and transmitter block produce equivalent changes in membrane polarization, and such experiments strongly support the view that a transmitter released

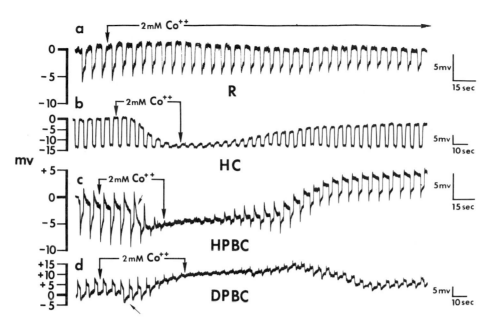

FIGURE 3 Effects of 2 mM cobalt on intracellularly recorded responses obtained from a receptor (R), a horizontal cell (HC), a hyperpolarizing bipolar cell (HPBC), and a depolarizing bipolar cell (DPBC). A diffuse, intermittent light stimulus (irradiance 8.25×10^{-6} W/cm²) was used in all studies. Each trace is an uninterrupted display of the effects on the light response and membrane potential of changing the perfusate from a normal Ringer's solution to a Ringer's solution with 2 mM Co^{2+} added. The duration of Co^{2+} exposure is indicated. A 3 min exposure had relatively little effect on receptors (some reduction in ampli- tude is observed). However, very brief (1 min or less) exposures abolished the light-evoked activity of the postreceptor neurons. In the horizontal cell (b) and the HPBC (c) Co^{2+} application is associated with hyperpolarization. However, Co^{2+} perfusion results in a depolarization of the DPBC (d). In both bipolar cells, the initial effect of Co^{2+} is an enhancement of transient on and off responses. Recovery of response amplitude in bipolar cells was incomplete after return to the initial perfusate, probably because of some deterioration of the cell. Positivity is indicated by an upward deflection. (From Dacheux and Miller, 1976.)

by receptors in the dark depolarizes HCs and HPBCs but hyperpolarizes DPBCs. When the above observations are combined with the C-F data, it becomes possible to describe the pathways and polarities of synaptic interactions which underlie ganglion-cell receptive-field organization.

Figure 4 presents a model of the retina based on the above experiments. Chloride-sensitive cells are hashmarked and include the HC and the DPBC. *On*-center cells are connected to the DPBC, as the activity of both cell types is abolished in a C-F medium. Furthermore, the DPBC releases an excitatory transmitter during light stimulation since *on* cells are depolarized by a conductance increase that gives rise to impulse activity (personal observation).

Off-center cells are connected to the HPBC since both cells remain light-responsive in a C-F environment. In addition, the loss of surround excitation in *off*-center cells corresponds to the loss of surround organization of the HPBC, which probably reflects the absence of HC activity.

On-off ganglion cells are connected to both DPBCs and HPBCs, since *on* activity is abolished but *off* activity persists under C-F conditions. This arrangement helps explain the similar latency of *on* and *off* discharge observed in *on-off* ganglion-cell recordings since an identical number of neuronal elements mediate *on* and *off* responses. On the other hand, the *on* or surround discharge of an *off*-center cell, evoked by diffuse-light stimulation or selective surround stimulation, has a much longer latency than the *off* discharge, since an additional neuron (HC) is involved in this pathway. It is possible, however, that amacrine cells contribute to surround excitation.

As the model of Figure 4 illustrates, amacrine cells, like *on-off* ganglion cells, receive input from both DPBCs and HPBCs. Under C-F conditions, the amacrine-cell response consists of an off EPSP preceded by a sustained hyperpolarizing response. Evidence has been presented elsewhere indicating that the absence of the *on* responses is not due to a chloride-dependent mechanism of EPSP generation, but reflects an absence of synaptic input from the DPBC (Miller and Dacheux, 1976a). Amacrine cells inhibit *on-off* ganglion cells by activation of a chloride-dependent IPSP. That *on-off* amacrine cells are inhibi-

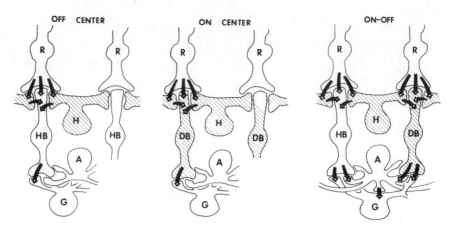

FIGURE 4   A model of receptive-field organizaton and synaptic polarities for *on*-center, *off*-center, and *on-off* ganglion cells. Chloride-sensitive cells are shaded and include depolarizing bipolars and horizontal cells. The synaptic polarities indicate the action of the cell when it is in a relatively depolarized state. Cells that release a transmitter in the dark include receptors, horizontal cells, and hyperpolarizing bipolar cells. Cells that release a transmitter in response to light stimulation include the depolarizing bipolars and *on-off* amacrine cells. (From Miller and Dacheux, 1976c.)

tory to *on-off* ganglion cells is not in agreement with the original suggestion of Werblin and Dowling (1969). These workers proposed that such amacrine cells were excitatory to *on-off* ganglion cells. The evidence in favor of an inhibitory relationship has been summarized by Miller and Dacheux (1976b). More recently, I have obtained simultaneous recordings from amacrine cells and nearby *on-off* ganglion cells. Depolarizing current injection into the amacrine cells does not evoke excitation, but rather inhibits the excitatory response to light. Additional properties of amacrine-cell inhibition are discussed below.

The receptor-postreceptor polarities in Figure 4 indicate the action of the transmitter in the dark, which depolarizes HCs and HPBCs and hyperpolarizes DPBCs. These polarities also indicate whether the synapse inverts the sign of the response, with + indicating a noninverting synapse and − indicating a sign reversal. The horizontal-bipolar connections are indicated as opposite to those of the receptor-bipolar action, indicating the antagonist influence of this contact. In turtle (Baylor, Fuortes, and O'Bryan, 1971) and Gecko (Pinto and Pak, 1974), horizontal cells feed back into cones to produce transient-sustained components of the cone response. In mudpuppy, there is evidence that HC processes contact bipolar cells (Dowling and Werblin, 1969), and the action of HCs is drawn at this point. HC action could not account for surround activity of bipolar cells solely through a cone-feedback system, since the HC responses themselves would show evidence of it. In any case it is assumed that the HCs, like the receptors, release a transmitter in the depolarized dark state. Thus, at this junction, receptor transmitter and HC influences are driving the bipolar cell in opposite directions.

Bipolar cells communicate through excitatory transmitters

According to the model of Figure 4, *off*-center ganglion cells receive input from HPBCs. Intracellular recordings of *off* cells demonstrate that these neurons are hyperpolarized by light stimulation (Wiesel, 1959; Werblin and Dowling, 1969; Kaneko, 1970). A hyperpolarizing response can result from inhibition or disfacilitation (a reduction in EPSP). Figure 5 presents evidence in favor of the disfacilitation mechanism and suggests that HPBCs release an excitatory transmitter at maximal rate in the depolarized dark state. The top row of recordings in Figure 5 were obtained from an *off* ganglion cell in the perfused mudpuppy retina eyecup. The light stimulus was followed by a brief current pulse (−0.1 nA) applied to a bridge circuit. Perfusion with a 2 mM cobalt solution resulted in hyperpolarization of the cell as the response to light was diminished. The hyperpolarizing action of cobalt was associated with an increase in input resistance, as indicated by the increased negative pulse amplitude. This is the expected result if the HPBC releases an excitatory transmitter in the dark which depolarizes the *off*-center ganglion cell by a conductance increase. The lower-left recording shows the change in input resistance of an *off* cell before and during light stimulation. A light-evoked increased negative deflection during application of a negative current pulse demonstrates that the hyperpolarizing response is associated with a decrease in conductance and further supports the disfacilitatory nature of the response. The right-hand portion of Figure 5 shows that when light-evoked activity in *off* cells is completely abolished during cobalt application (same cell as upper row), depolarizing current injection gives rise to impulse activity, indicating that the loss of light-evoked responsiveness is not due to deterioration of the intracellular recording. Similar experiments have been carried out in *on-off* ganglion cells and *on-off* amacrine cells. These neurons also show significant hyperpolarization and an increase in input resistance during cobalt application, an observation that further supports the idea that the HPBC communicates with all postreceptor neurons by releasing an excitatory transmitter at maximal rate in the depolarized dark state. Similar experiments in some *on* cells, however, show neither a hyperpolarization nor a change in input resistance during cobalt

application, suggesting that in the dark-adapted state, depolarizing bipolars release very little transmitter and require light-evoked depolarization in order to excite postsynaptic neurons. The depolarization of *on* ganglion cells is associated with a large conductance increase; thus DPBCs release an excitatory transmitter at maximal rate during light stimulation.

Ganglion-cell mechanisms

Figure 6 illustrates intracellular recordings obtained from the three major types of ganglion cells. The *on-off* cells respond with an EPSP-IPSP sequence at the onset and termination of a light stimulus. An annulus can effectively isolate the IPSP response, indicating that the pathways for IPSPs and EPSPs have different spatial properties. The IPSPs have been extensively studied by Miller and Dacheux (1976b) and are generated by an increased chloride conductance, with the chloride equilibrium potential maintained below

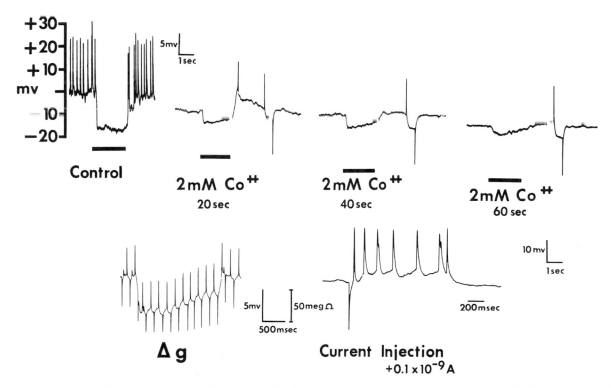

FIGURE 5   Top traces illustrate an intracellular recording obtained from an *off* ganglion cell. Following the introduction of 2 mM Co²⁺, the cell was hyperpolarized as the light-evoked response declined. The traces are vertically displaced according to the potential values on the left-hand margin. A brief negative current pulse (0.1 nA) was presented to the microelectrode, and a bridge device was used to evaluate changes in input resistance. The increased negative deflection indicates that the action of Co²⁺ was associated with an increase in input resistance. The lower left-

hand trace was obtained from an *off* cell while intermittent negative current pulses were applied. Light-evoked hyperpolarization is associated with increased resistance, suggesting a disfacilitatory mechansim. The lower right-hand recording was obtained from the same cell as that shown in the upper traces and illustrates that after Co²⁺ completely blocked light-evoked activity, depolarizing-current injection elicited spike activity, indicating that the absence of light responsiveness was not caused by deterioration of the recording.

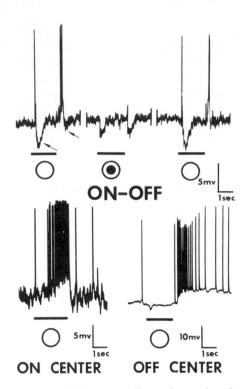

ON-OFF

ON CENTER   OFF CENTER

FIGURE 6 Intracellular recordings from the three ganglion-cell types. Upper traces show the response of an *on-off* ganglion cell to a diffuse-light stimulus (left recording) followed by an annulus (O.D., 2 mM; I.D., 600 μm) (middle response) and then a second diffuse-light stimulus (right trace). The diffuse-light stimulus evoked *on* and *off* impulse activity, followed by *on* and *off* hyperpolarizing transient responses (arrows). The annulus evoked *on* and *off* hyperpolarizations, with a small *off* EPSP but no impulse activity. Lower traces show *on*-center and *off*-center cells in response to a diffuse-light stimulus that did not evoke surround excitation. Note that *on* and *off* hyperpolarizations are not observed in *on*-center and *off*-center cells. All traces are photographic reproductions of response recorded on a penwriter, which caused some attenuation of impulse activity. Stimulus irradiance equal for all stimuli: 3.7×10^{-7} W/cm². (From Miller and Dacheux, 1976c.)

the resting membrane potential, as demonstrated by intracellular measurements of chloride activity using chloride-selective electrodes (Miller and Dacheux, 1975). Evidence previously described indicates that the IPSPs are generated by amacrine cells; thus the difference in EPSP and IPSP latency, in response to diffuse-light stimulation, can be ascribed to the additional neuron interposed in the inhibitory pathway. As Figure 6 demonstrates, *on* and *off* IPSPs are not observed in either *on*-center or *off*-center ganglion cells, suggesting that these neurons do not receive input from *on-off* amacrine cells; these types of ganglion cells may receive input from other types of amacrine cells. In the catfish, Naka (1976) has dem-

onstrated that sustained amacrines are inhibitory to *on*-center and *off*-center ganglion cells. It seems likely that the three major ganglion cell types are each related to a different amacrine-cell type with similar organizational features. Thus there is little doubt that a major function of amacrine cells is to provide an inhibitory input to ganglion cells. This does not eliminate the possibility that some amacrine cells form an excitatory pathway to a small class of ganglion cells, but such a pathway has not been physiologically identified.

In summary, *on* and *off* channels are first separated in the outer retina and are subserved by DPBCs and HPBCs, respectively. In the inner retina, the properties of ganglion cells and amacrine cells are determined by the type(s) of bipolar cells with which they connect. Synaptic input from DPBCs or HPBCs forms the basis for *on*-center and *off*-center ganglion cells, respectively, whereas *on-off* ganglion cells receive input from both types of bipolars. All bipolar-cell inputs are excitatory, with the DPBC releasing a transmitter at maximal rate during light stimulation and the HPBC releasing a transmitter at maximal rate in the dark. In addition, *on-off* amacrine cells receive input from both types of bipolars and in turn generate chloride-dependent IPSPs in *on-off* ganglion cells. *On*-center and *off*-center cells appear to have inhibitory amacrine cells that are independent of the *on-off* cell system.

The model of the *on-off* ganglion cell illustrated in Figure 4 differs from that presented by Dowling (see his Figure 9, this volume). Dowling suggests that excitation and inhibition are mediated by amacrine-cell input. Attempts to demonstrate excitatory amacrine input to the *on-off* ganglion cell have not succeeded; only an inhibitory relationship has been shown (but see Werblin, this volume). Furthermore, Miller and Dacheux (1976c) have demonstrated with simultaneous amacrine-cell and *on-off* ganglion-cell recording that these two cell types are coactivated and that the period of large-amplitude EPSP in the amacrine cell is associated in time with inhibition of the *on-off* ganglion cell. These results favor the concept that the *on-off* amacrine and ganglion cells receive direct excitatory input from bipolar cells.

The physiology of amacrine cells

The amacrine cells constitute a unique class of neurons, which lack axons and have dendrites that form postsynaptic and presynaptic relationships. These neurons receive input from bipolars and other amacrines and form feedback synapses onto bipolar-cell terminals and feedforward synapses onto ganglion cells and other amacrines. Although classical morphologists considered the amacrine cell to be axonless, physiological experiments suggest that the synaptic processes of amacrine cells possess both axonal and dendritic properties; that is, amacrine cell processes generate both postsynaptic potentials and tetrodotoxin (TTX)-sensitive spikes (Miller and Dacheux, 1976d). Golgi stains of amacrine cells (Figure 7) indicate that these neurons do not form a homogeneous class of neurons, and physiological experiments also suggest that different amacrine types may exist (Toyoda, 1973; Naka, 1975).

In the mudpuppy retina the *on-off* amacrine cell is the only type of amacrine identified by intracellular staining techniques (Werblin and Dowling, 1969). Evidence from C-F studies indicates that these neurons receive input from both DPBCs and HPBCs. Since these bipolar cells are nearly mirror images of one another, why don't signals from the two bipolars simply cancel one another to produce little if any response in the postsynaptic neurons? The answer to this apparent predicament probably resides in the relationship between membrane potential and transmitter release, assuming that the major basis of post–bipolar cell communication is chemically mediated transmitter action. In the squid giant synapse, Katz and Miledi (1966) demonstrated that a threshold for transmitter release exists and that suprathreshold depolarizations increase the number of vesicles released until a saturation level is reached. More recent experiments into this problem (Llinás, 1976, and this volume) suggest that there is no threshold for the calcium current necessary for transmitter release, but that a nonlinear relationship exists, so that small depolarizations near the resting membrane potential are not as effective as small depolarizations superimposed on a more depolarized state. The relationship between pre- and postsynaptic potential is sigmoidal. In our experiments, recordings from cells that receive input from DPBCs suggest that these neurons release a transmitter maximally during light, but that transmitter release is minimal in the dark-adapted state. Thus, in these neurons, some threshold level for significant transmitter release may exist. It is also possible that a threshold for transmitter release exists for HPBCs and that the maximum hyperpolarization evoked by light reaches a potential at which no or very little transmitter is released. The evidence for the latter view comes from observations of cells receiving input from HPBCs. Light stimulation that evokes prominent transient and sustained responses in HPBCs causes very little evidence of the transient response detected in *off* ganglion cell recordings (Figure 5). Figure 8 applies this concept to illustrate how DPBCs and HPBCs may interact to form *on-off* responses in amacrine cells. In the upper trace the response of a DPBC is illustrated, with the dashed line representing the membrane potential above which transmitter is released. The middle trace shows the response of an HPBC, and the dashed line marks the membrane potential below which transmitter release is terminated. Thus at light *on*, the amacrine cell, illustrated in the bottom trace, receives an excitatory input from the DPBC and a disfacilitatory influence from the HPBC. The subtraction of the two responses (*a − b*) gives a net depolarization. At the termination of the light stimulus, the amacrine cell receives disfacilitation from the DPBC and excitation from the HPBC, and the net result (*c − d*) gives a depolarizing *off* response. Notice that this type of interaction gives transient *on* and *off* responses and does not depend on any feedback from amacrines to bipolars. Nevertheless, amacrine-to-bipolar feedback

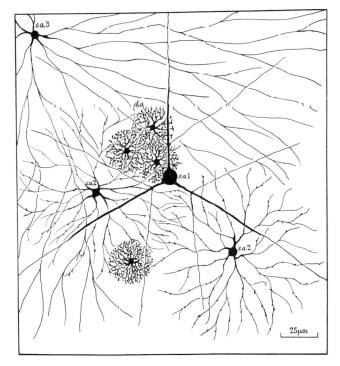

FIGURE 7 Diagram of amacrine cells viewed flatmount from Golgi material of monkey central retina. In this view, there is considerable variability in dendritic expansion. In addition, diffuse amacrine cells (d.a.) terminate extensively in all sublamina of the inner plexiform layer, but the dendrites of stratified amacrines (s.a.) terminate in a single sublamina. Three different types of stratified amacrines are indicated, based mainly on the shape of dendritic expansion as viewed from flatmount preparation. (From Boycott and Dowling, 1969.)

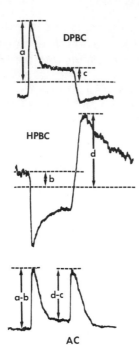

FIGURE 8 This diagram illustrates how depolarizing (DPBC) and hyperpolarizing (HPBC) bipolars might synaptically activate an amacrine cell (AC) to give phasic *on* and *off* depolarizations. The DPBC releases an excitatory transmitter during the light stimulus, while the HPBC decreases its rate of transmitter release during light-evoked hyperpolarization. In the DPBC recording, the bottom dashed line indicates the membrane potential that must be exceeded for transmitter release. At light *on*, the excitation into the AC is a reflection of *a*. The HPBC releases an excitatory transmitter in the dark, and the bottom dashed line in this recording indicates the membrane potential below which transmitter release terminates or is significantly reduced. Thus the onset of a light stimulus evokes DPBC excitation *a* minus the disfacilitation *b* from the HPBC. This gives net excitation as illustrated in the AC. At the termination of the light stimulus, the AC receives a disfacilitation *c* from the DPBC and an excitatory input *d* from the HPBC, giving a net excitation *d − c*. This type of interaction is capable of explaining the transient *on* and *off* responses without additional synaptic mechanisms. However, feedback synapses from amacrines to bipolars and between amacrines could contribute to waveform shaping of the phasic response.

has been demonstrated anatomically, and such a synaptic mechanism could contribute to the transient nature of the response. In fact, we have demonstrated that the application of picrotoxin or bicuculline markedly slows the decaying phase of *on* and *off* responses in amacrine cells; and it is possible that this reflects a loss of a GABA-mediated feedback onto bipolar-cell terminals or interactions between amacrine cells. We have presented evidence elsewhere that about half of the *on-off* amacrine cells release

GABA, while the other half are glycinergic (Miller, Dacheux, and Frumkes, 1977).

Figure 9 illustrates an intracellular recording from an *on-off* amacrine cell in the mudpuppy retina. In part a, a diffuse-light stimulus evokes *on* and *off* EPSPs associated with impulse activity. Both large- and small-amplitude spikes are apparent, but during the light stimulus only a continuous train of small spikes is observed. Trace b illustrates, at a faster time base, details of the on response. The first detectable response consists of a relatively slow rising EPSP (1), followed by a much sharper response (2), which after a notch in the recording (3) is followed by a large-amplitude spike. The remainder of the response con-

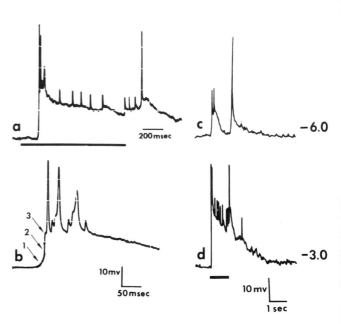

FIGURE 9 (a) Intracellularly recorded amacrine-cell response evoked by diffuse-light stimulation (duration indicated by dark bar). Slow potential consists of early transient and later sustained components. Impulses consist of two early large-amplitude spikes followed by a low-frequency train of small spikes. Termination of the light stimulus evoked a large-amplitude spike associated with a slow potential. (b) The early response components of an amacrine cell. The initial light-evoked response consists of a slow-rising EPSP component (arrow 1), followed by a fast pre-potential (arrow 2), followed by a large-amplitude spike (arrow 3). The remaining response consists of two large spikes of decreasing amplitude, each associated with an FPP, with small spikes interposed. (c) A moderately low-level light stimulus evoked an *on* EPSP with two dendritic spikes; at the termination of the light stimulus, a larger EPSP resulted in a somatic spike. (d) An increase in stimulus intensity (+6.0 and −3.0 indicate log reductions of stimulus intensity, with 0 value equal to 4.6 nW/cm²) evoked somatic spikes and a train of dendritic spikes. Thus dendritic spikes have a lower light-evoked threshold than somatic spikes. (Modified from Miller and Dacheux, 1976d.)

236   ROBERT F. MILLER

sists of small and large spikes, with each of the large spikes preceded by a fast rising response. Consistent with the terminology of Spencer and Kandel (1961), we have termed the fast-rising responses fast prepotentials (FPPs). The FPPs and small spikes probably represent equivalent responses and result from dendritic-spike (DS) activity that decays passively into the soma, the probable site of recording. The large amplitude spikes are probably generated by the soma. In the type of recording illustrated in Figure 9, large spikes of up to 100 mV have been observed, but dendritic spikes rarely exceed 10 mV (Miller and Dacheux, 1976d). That these two spikes have different loci of origin can be demonstrated by two different techniques. In part c, stimulus intensity was reduced; at light onset, an EPSP was evoked, which gave rise to two DSs. At the termination of the light stimulus, the EPSP was larger and gave rise to a single somatic spike (SS) preceded by a DS. The lowest threshold response of amacrine cells consists of EPSPs followed by DSs. The SSs are the highest threshold responses of amacrine cells. In part d, an increase in stimulus intensity of 3 log units more than that of c evoked a large EPSP with SSs and sustained DSs apparent.

Further evidence that DSs and SSs are generated at different loci in amacrine cells has been obtained from studies of spike threshold using depolarizing current injection. The results of these studies strongly suggest that in some fortuitous recordings the microelectrode impaled an amacrine-cell dendrite; under these conditions, we believe some evidence of amacrine-to-bipolar feedback activity may be present. Figure 10 shows a soma recording. In these recordings the SS is large and the DSs are commonly less than 10 mV. The middle trace, left-hand section, demonstrates that a small depolarizing current injection evoked a single SS. Note that near the peak of the SS, a notch is apparent, suggesting that the SS invaded the dendritic tree and evoked a single DS. This phenomenon is never observed in response to light stimulation, probably because the SS invades the dendrites during the refractory period of the DS. The upper right-hand recording shows this phenomenon more clearly. In the lower left-hand recording, a series of depolarizing-current injections are superimposed. The lowest trace in the series shows a single SS in response to a maintained depolarization of about 500 msec. The uppermost trace shows the spike activity that resulted from 0.1 nA of current injection. Note that a single SS is followed by a train of DSs. Thus, in the somatic recordings, the SS has a lower threshold than the DS. Furthermore, the SS shows

rapid accommodation, whereas the DS mechanism is less rapidly accommodated. When recorded from the soma, the DSs are not strictly uniform in amplitude. In general, the first DS that appears as an FPP is larger than DSs that occur later in the response. The decreased amplitude in later DSs could result from multiple DS generation loci, which begin to passively invade the soma at different electrotonic distances. We wondered, therefore, whether the EPSP itself might be composed of DSs that are too small in amplitude to be readily resolved as spike activity. Both SSs and DSs are TTX-sensitive, suggesting that these spikes are sodium-dependent (Miller and Dacheux, 1976d). The lower two right-hand traces show an amacrine-cell response in control Ringer's and the same cell observed a few minutes after perfusion with TTX. Impulse activity was abolished under these conditions but the *on* and *off* EPSPs are not affected. Thus severely attenuated DSs do not appear to make a contribution to the EPSP of amacrine cells.

If the small-amplitude impulses are indeed generated by the dendrites of amacrine cells, it should be possible to detect them with extracellular recording techniques. Extracellular spike activity has been observed at a retinal level just beyond (20–30 μm), the depth at which somatic-type (positive-negative) ganglion-cell spikes are commonly encountered (Miller and Dacheux, 1976d). These spikes are always purely negative in waveform and have properties similar to DSs observed intracellularly. Low-level light stimulation usually evokes *on* and *off* bursts, but higher-intensity light stimulation commonly results in a sustained low-frequency level of activity. Somatic spikes, however, have not been clearly identified by extracellular recording techniques. Werblin (1977) has also suggested that amacrine cells generate somatic and dendritic spikes.

In a few intracellular recordings from amacrine cells, studies of response properties and DS threshold suggest that the recordings are coming from dendrites (Miller, in preparation). Such recordings are difficult to maintain and are commonly observed immediately following an intracellular recording from a ganglion cell. On a few occasions, a presumed intradendritic recording was obtained, after which a somatic recording was observed on further penetration. The main criterion that separates these recordings from somatic recordings is the observation that DSs show a lower threshold to depolarizing-current injection than SSs. Furthermore, DSs are much larger, while SSs are smaller, than those recorded in the soma. These responses also show large fluctuations in the recording and strongly suggest that in a

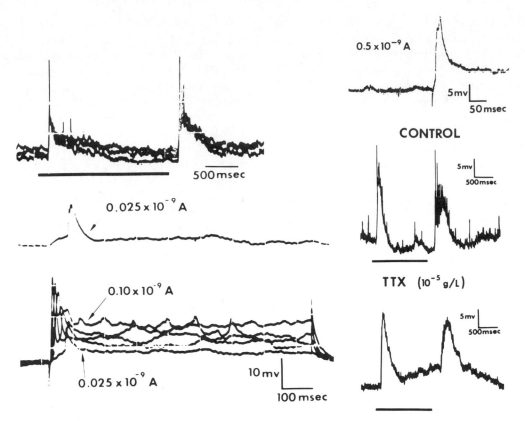

FIGURE 10   Upper left-hand trace illustrates superimposed light-evoked amacrine-cell responses, showing large- and small-amplitude spikes. Middle trace, left, illustrates a single large-amplitude spike evoked by a depolarizing-current injection. The large-amplitude spike has a notch near the peak, suggesting that a somatic spike gave rise to a dendritic spike. Note that only a single somatic spike is generated, even though the depolarizing-current injection lasted for about 500 msec. The lower left-hand traces are superimposed amacrine-cell responses evoked by different levels of depolarizing-current injection. The topmost trace was elic-ited by a 0.1 nA current injection and shows a single somatic spike followed by a train of smaller spikes (same cell as upper left traces). Thus this type of recording shows so-matic spikes have a lower threshold than dendritic spikes. The upper right-hand trace illustrates another recording at a faster time scale. Depolarizing-current injection evoked a single large spike with a notch near the peak. The middle and lower right-hand traces show an amacrine-cell response before and after TTX application. TTX blocked large and small spikes, but *on* and *off* EPSPs are relatively unaffected. (Modified from Miller and Dacheux, 1976d.)

single dendrite, DSs are generated by EPSPs that have a duration of about 100 msec. Depolarizing-current injection into these neurons reveals large fluctuations in the baseline recording, with groups of dendritic spikes followed by transient hyperpolariz-ing responses. I have suggested that this type of fluc-tuation may represent the activation of dendroden-dritic synaptic activity. Large baseline fluctuations are much less evident when depolarizing-current injec-tion studies are carried out in somatic recordings. These observations suggest that DSs may serve as a powerful booster to the synaptic actions of amacrine-cell dendrites. Since the DS amplitude is larger than the EPSP amplitude, a group of DSs could markedly enhance the probability of vesicular release at sites of synaptic interaction along a dendrite.

We propose that one function of dendritic spikes is to provide a synaptic amplification for the network operations of amacrines. Since it is not presently known where on the dendrites such spikes are generated, one immediate question raised by this hypothesis is whether dendritic spikes are generated sufficiently close to sites of transmitter re-lease to perform, from either active or passive prop-agation, the proposed function. Figure 11 (lower three traces) shows a light-evoked IPSP recorded from an *on-off* ganglion cell; only the *on* response is shown. Notice that in addition to a smooth IPSP, FHPs are also evident. Hyperpolarizing the cell in-verts the smooth IPSP as well as the fast responses (lowest trace). Figure 11 (upper three traces) shows another example of FHPs. This type of recording shows a much smaller, smooth IPSP, with large-am-plitude FHPs. It is possible that such recordings are

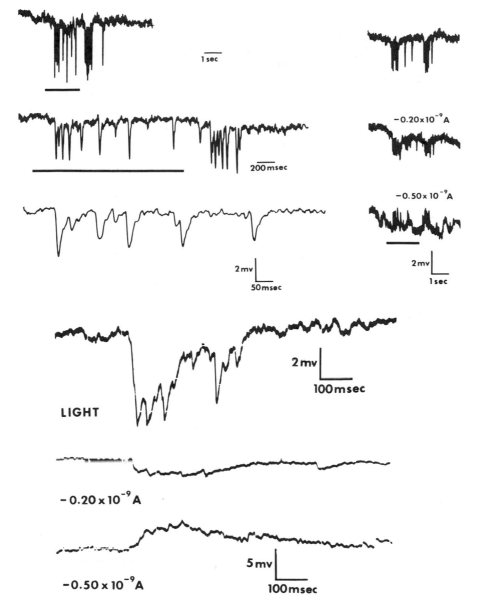

FIGURE 11 The upper three traces on the left show, at different time scales, an intracellular recording that shows prominent, large-amplitude, fast hyperpolarizing potentials (FHPs). The dark bar indicates the duration of the light stimulus, and the third trace shows only the *on* response. The third trace demonstrates that the FHPs are of variable amplitude and show temporal summation properties similar to other synaptic potentials. The FHPs demonstrate light-evoked properties similar to dendritic spikes of amacrine cells; intermediate- and high-intensity flashes evoke sustained activity, in addition to *on* and *off* bursts.

On the right, FHPs are inverted to depolarizing responses with negative-current injection demonstrating the IPSP nature of the responses. The lower three traces illustrate an intracellular recording, which shows a relatively large, smooth IPSP (only the *on* response is illustrated) and smaller FHPs compared to the upper responses. Unlike the upper responses, these recordings usually show some evidence of impulse activity on initial penetration. The lower two traces show (at a reduced gain) that reversal of the smooth IPSP also inverts the FHPs.

intradendritic from *on-off* ganglion cells. Impulse activity is never observed in these recordings, whereas spikes are usually observed in the type illustrated in the lower three traces of Figure 11. The third trace shows the FHPs with an expanded time scale. FHPs are typically about 20 msec in duration and show temporal summation properties. The upper right-hand section of Figure 11 shows that the FHPs recorded under these conditions can be inverted to depolarizing responses by negative current injection, demonstrating the true IPSP nature of the response. The FHPs have functional properties similar to DSs. Low-intensity stimuli evoke brief *on* and *off* bursts of responses, whereas more intense stimuli often evoke a train of FHPs such as that illustrated in Figure 11. The evidence presented in this figure suggests that DS generation effects transmitter release from amacrine-cell dendrites and supports a synaptic-booster role for DS function. The fact that two different spike-generation sites exist in amacrine cells and that such spikes show different threshold properties in response to light stimulation suggests that amacrine cells may operate in one of two functional states.

Figure 12 presents a model illustrating these two different amacrine-cell states. The upper portion illustrates the type of activity that is possible under stimulus conditions below SS threshold. The dark regions represent areas of active spike generation, and the hashed regions areas of passive spike decay into the soma. Spike-generation sites have been drawn near synaptic processes only to illustrate, as previous results have demonstrated, that DSs partic-

ipate in synaptic operations of amacrine cells. Since amacrine-cell inhibition is dendritic, stimuli that are below SS threshold may permit local dendritic operations in isolation from other dendritic activity. In other words, under these conditions the amacrine cell is parcellated into a number of functional subsets, each performing local synaptic operations in relation to other dendrites or dendritic regions. It is possible that DSs will propagate, either actively or passively, and result in a relatively uniform response within a single dendrite. However, the impedance load of the soma and other dendrites would probably attenuate such spikes and would make them less effective in other dendritic branches. When stimuli are sufficiently intense so that SSs are generated, these spikes invade the dendritic tree (lower illustration) and provide a more uniform synaptic operation. Even though the propagation of SSs into the dendrites is probably passive, there may be very little attenuation of spike amplitude at the distal ends of the dendrites, and this is illustrated by the relatively constant spaces between the hatched marks. The fact that very few (1-5) SSs

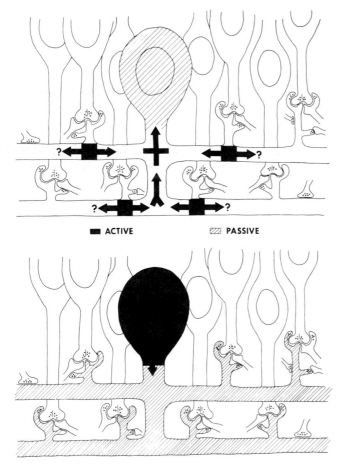

■ ACTIVE   ▨ PASSIVE

FIGURE 12 A two-state functional model of the *on-off* amacrine cell. The upper diagram represents the condition in which stimuli are below somatic-spike threshold. The dark regions indicate areas of active spike initiation, and the hatched areas represent passive propagation. Unmarked areas could represent regions of either active or passive propagation. According to the model, each dendrite is capable of relatively independent operations with minimal influences on other dendrites, through dendrodendritic operations. Dendritic spikes, through passive or active spread, are restricted largely to a single dendrite, since they do not actively invade the soma and would probably be markedly attenuated in other dendrites. The proposed function of dendritic spikes is to increase the probability of transmitter release and thereby serve as a synaptic boosting or amplifying device, providing a powerful nonlinear enhancement to the inhibitory operations of amacrine-cell dendrites with respect to bipolar-cell terminals, ganglion-cell dendrites, and neighboring amacrine cells.

When stimuli are large enough to reach somatic-spike threshold, the soma actively generates spikes, which invade the dendrites. The dendritic invasion is passive because it usually occurs during the refractory period of dendritic spikes. The density of the hatched lines roughly indicates the amount of electrotonic decay in the dendrites. Because the somatic spike is a large current source, it seems reasonable that the somatic-spike invasion of the dendrites is accomplished with very little electrotonic attenuation, but this suggestion is tentative and must await a more quantitative understanding of amacrine-cell membrane properties. The two-state model implies independent dendritic operations until somatic spikes are generated; during this time dendritic operations are more uniform and are dictated by dendritic invasion of the somatic spike.

are generated in response to diffuse-light stimulation does not mean that other forms of stimuli, such as moving targets, could not evoke a higher frequency of SSs and make this state of amacrine-cell function more tonic in its operation. In other words, we might consider the SSs to provide a kind of safety device, assisting the dendrites at times when the excitatory input is great and thereby contributing to dendritic operations by feeding onto bipolar-cell terminals and increasing the inhibition fed to ganglion-cell dendrites. It remains for future research, using additional forms of light stimulation and quantitative analysis of the electroanatomy of amacrine cells, to evaluate further the significance of the two-state functional model of the amacrine cell.

The significance of dendritic inhibition in retinal information processing

The morphology of amacrine cells indicates that these neurons provide synaptic contacts to bipolar-cell terminals and the dendrites of other amacrine and ganglion cells. Very few somatic contacts onto ganglion cells have been reported. As Llinás and Nicholson (1971) have pointed out, the existence of dendritic inhibition permits functional amputation of dendrites or regions of dendrites so that local operations in one area are relatively independent of those in other dendrites or other dendritic regions. In the rabbit retina, a large number of *on-off* ganglion cells are motion-selective (Barlow, Hill, and Levick, 1964)—a spot or bar moving in one direction (preferred) evokes ganglion-cell discharge, whereas movement in the opposite (null) direction produces no response.

Figure 13 shows an intracellular recording from an *on-off* ganglion cell from a rabbit (Dacheux, 1977). The upper trace shows the response to a diffuse-light stimulus, which evokes *on* and *off* EPSP-IPSP sequences identical to the response characteristics of *on-off* ganglion cells of mudpuppy. The lower trace shows the response of the cell evoked by a 100 μm slit moved first in the preferred direction. This stimulus evoked an EPSP; but note that the EPSP is not smooth but consists of positive and negative components interacting to produce net excitation. If the slit is moved in the opposite, null direction, an IPSP results; but here too the IPSP shows fluctuation during movement. These findings therefore indicate that amacrine-cell inhibition to the ganglion cell probably provides a major synaptic component of the motion-selective mechanism. Furthermore, even in the pre-

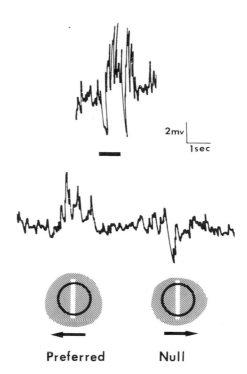

Preferred   **Null**

FIGURE 13 Intracellular recording obtained from an *on-off* motion-selective ganglion cell in the perfused rabbit retina. The upper trace shows prominent *on* and *off* IPSPs evoked by diffuse-light stimulation. Impulse activity was initially present but soon lost due to injury-induced depolarization. The lower response shows the PSP evoked by a moving slit in the preferred and null directions. In the preferred direction the net effect is excitation, but in the null direction net inhibition is present. This observation suggests that amacrine-to-ganglion inhibition plays an important role in the motion-selective synaptic mechanism.

ferred direction, there is some evidence of inhibitory influences, although these seem to be outweighed by the excitatory input.

Barlow and Levick (1965) have studied motion-selective cells in the rabbit and have demonstrated that the receptive field can be divided into multiple subsets, with each portion encoding a preferred-null synaptic operation that has little effect on the operation of nearby regions. They suggested that the horizontal cells were the interneurons mediating motion selectivity, but more recent anatomical (Dowling, 1970) and physiological (Werblin, 1970) studies favor the amacrine cell as the critical neuron in motion-selective coding. The functional subdivisions of the motion-selective mechanism give precisely the behavior anticipated from considerations of dendritic inhibition.

A model of this type of arrangement is illustrated in Figure 14. The left-hand section shows a flatmount

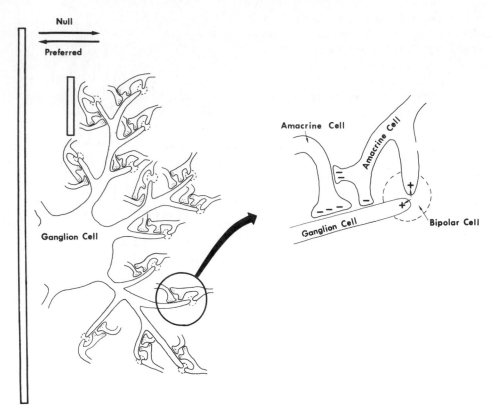

FIGURE 14 A model of the synaptic mechanism underlying motion selectivity, which takes into account that (1) the motion-selective mechanism is largely amacrine-to-ganglion inhibition; and (2) dendritic inhibition is the basis of amacrine-ganglion interaction. The left-hand diagram is a flat-mount view of a ganglion cell. Dashed circles represent bipolar-cell input contacting ganglion and amacrine dendrites. An expanded view of the proposed synaptic connections is illustrated on the right. Movement in the preferred direction evokes net excitation due to amacrine-to-amacrine inhibitory connections. In the null direction, net inhibition results because amacrine inhibitory input precedes the excitatory bipolar-cell input. The coding network is repeated throughout the dendritic expansion of the ganglion cell, so that motion selectivity is encoded to small as well as large stimuli. Furthermore, dendritic inhibition may permit functional amputation, so that activity in one dendrite has very little influence on other dendrites. This may explain why null movement in one part of the receptive field may not inhibit preferred movement in a more remote region, since the inhibitory operation would be localized.

view of a ganglion cell. The dotted circles represent bipolar-cell input, which contacts both amacrine and ganglion cells. The amacrine-cell processes in turn contact ganglion-cell dendrites and the dendrites of other amacrines. The details of a single dendritic region are represented on the right-hand section. In this example, movement in the null direction results in arrival of inhibitory amacrine input, which outweighs the excitatory influences received from the bipolar. In the preferred direction, the amacrine-to-amacrine contact reduces the inhibitory input to the ganglion cell so that the excitatory bipolar-cell input is relatively greater. In this arrangement, stimulation with a moving bar covering the entire receptive field will evoke net excitation and impulse discharge in the preferred direction and net inhibition in the null direction. Furthermore, a much smaller stimulus will produce the same type of response. In addition, movement in the null direction in one dendritic region will evoke inhibitory influences that are localized and will not effect activity in other dendrites; this has been demonstrated by the experiments of Barlow and Levick (1965) and has been more thoroughly studied by Wyatt and Daw (1976). Note that the model in Figure 14 also gives inhibitory responses for movement in the preferred direction, a result that is consistent with the type of response presented in Figure 13. The existence of dendritic inhibition through functional isolation of dendrites, or even dendritic regions, may provide an explanation for some of the organizational features of complex receptive fields; that is, subtle operations of this type may help in reducing the number of neurons required for complex synaptic operations.

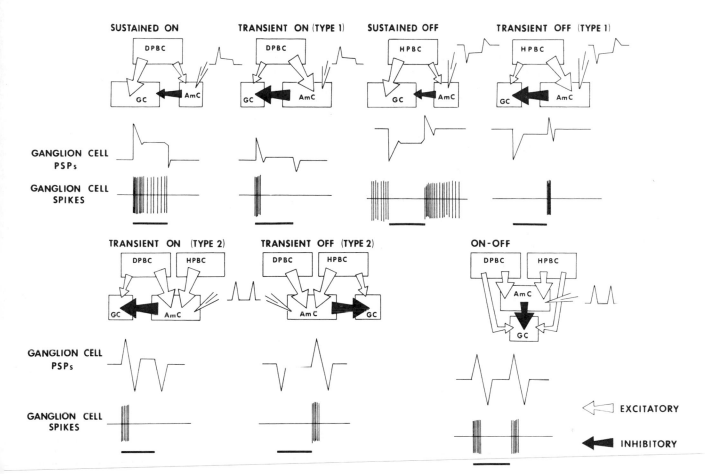

FIGURE 15 The synaptic current divider model based on intracellular recordings and electron-microscopic analysis (Dowling, 1968; Dubin, 1970). The diagrammatic responses demonstrate ganglion-cell PSPs based on experimental observations of mudpuppy and rabbit. The lower trace in each section illustrates the expected impulse activity from each cell type. The size of the block represents relative synaptic input into ganglion or amacrine cells. Clear arrows indicate inhibition, dark arrows excitation. In the top row it is assumed that *on* cells interact with a sustained (depolarizing) amacrine cell, and *off* cells interact with a sustained (hyperpolarizing) amacrine; the *on-off* cells interact with *on-off* amacrines.

In simple retinas, sustained cells (*on* and *off*) result from a relatively large input to ganglion cells and a small input to amacrines. This leads to a small amacrine-ganglion inhibition, and the light-evoked response characteristics more closely reflect the organizational mechanisms of the outer retina. Transient ganglion cells result when a relatively large synaptic input enters the amacrine cells; this provides a much stronger amacrine-ganglion inhibition and gives only transient excitation. In the *transient off* cells, the enhanced inhibition is expressed as a tonic inhibition in the dark from an *off*-type amacrine that abolishes spontaneous activity. A second type of *transient on* cell (type II) appears to receive excitation from the DPBC but inhibition from the *on-off* amacrine system. A much less common, but similar, arrangement appears to underlie type II *transient off* cells. The *on-off* ganglion-cell system receives input from DPBCs and HPBCs and inhibition from the *on-off* system.

Species differences in the organization of the vertebrate retina

From a variety of physiological studies it has become apparent that receptive-field properties of ganglion cells differ widely among species (Kuffler, 1952; Lettvin et al., 1959; Barlow, Hill, and Levick, 1964), with somewhat simpler center-surround cells predominating in mammals with binocular vision and more complex cells predominating in monocular mammals and lower vertebrates. Dowling (1968) and Dubin (1970), on the basis of electron-microscopic studies, have suggested that increasing ganglion-cell complexity is associated with enhanced input into amacrine cells and larger numbers of amacrine synapses. I would like to advance a physiological interpretation of these observations. We can consider that the post-bipolar synapses represent a synaptic current divider. In complex retinas with a large input into amacrine cells, the synaptic input current is unevenly divided and excitatory input into amacrine cells outweighs that received by ganglion cells. This is particularly evident in the *on-off* system of the mudpuppy, where the EPSPs of *on-off* amacrine cells are up to 45 mV in amplitude; as far as I know, they represent the largest EPSPs reported in the central nervous system. In contrast, the EPSPs of *on-off* ganglion cells are smaller and rarely exceed 10 mV. Assuming that the input resistances of the two cell types are similar, these observations clearly suggest that the synaptic current from bipolars has been weighted toward amacrine cells. This weighting will, in turn, enhance the inhibition from amacrines to ganglion cells. Thus complex retinas are characterized by large amacrine responses, which provide an enhanced inhibitory function. A greater number of amacrine synapses is probably a major factor too. Recent pharmacological experiments in the rabbit retina have demonstrated that complex receptive-field properties of ganglion cells can be simplified, some by strychnine, some by picrotoxin (Wyatt and Daw, 1976; Caldwell, 1977). We have recently presented evidence that the *on-off* amacrine cells consist of two populations, one releasing GABA and the second releasing glycine (Miller, Dacheux, and Frumkes, 1977). Thus the pharmacological experiments in the rabbit suggest that complex receptive fields are largely determined by inhibitory responses from amacrine cells. According to the synaptic current divider concept, the more current fed into amacrine cells, the more powerful the inhibition and the more precise and selective the stimulus configuration must be in order to evoke excitation. This concept can account for a large variation in ganglion-cell types. Based on extensive intracellular recording experiments in mudpuppy and rabbit (Dacheux, 1977), Figure 15 illustrates different ganglion-cell types and the properties that depend on amacrine-cell inhibition. The size of the block and arrow represents relative input into the ganglion cell and amacrine cell, with dark arrows for inhibition and light arrows for excitation. A *sustained on* cell is represented by a large bipolar-to-ganglion input and relatively little input into a sustained (depolarizing) amacrine cell. A *transient on* cell of type I has a much stronger bipolar-to-amacrine input and hence a strong amacrine-ganglion inhibition, which makes the excitation phasic. Similar differences between *sustained off* and *transient off* can be attributed to interaction between HPBCs and *off* (hyperpolarizing) amacrines. The *on*-center and *off*-center cells in Figure 15 all show transient characteristics. A second type of *transient on* appears to receive excitation primarily from the DPBP but a strong inhibition from the *on-off* amacrine system. Another arrangement is the type II *transient off*, which receives excitation from HPBPs and inhibition from *on-off* amacrines. The most common arrangement for *on-off* ganglion cells is that shown in the *on-off* system, which receives excitation from DPBCs and HPBCs and inhibition from *on-off* amacrines. In essence, ganglion cells that receive very little amacrine inhibition will more clearly show the influence of integration in the outer retina, whereas cells with strong amacrine inhibition will show more complex properties, and their complexity may reveal the subtlety of dendritic inhibition.

The findings presented in this paper do not eliminate the possibility that a small class of amacrine cells are excitatory to ganglion cells, as suggested by Dowling (1968) and Werblin and Dowling (1969) (see Dowling, Figure 9, this volume). In the ground squirrel, a small group of ganglion cells appear to receive input exclusively from amacrine cells (West and Dowling, 1974). In the cat, Kolb (1974) has provided evidence that rod bipolars feed into ganglion cells through an amacrine cell. It is therefore possible that some amacrine cells are excitatory to ganglion cells, although physiological evidence favoring this view has not been presented.

ACKNOWLEDGMENT   I wish to thank Ramon Dacheux, whose research skills have contributed greatly to much of this work. The research reported here has been supported by grant EY-00844 from the National Eye Institute, National Institutes of Health.

REFERENCES

BARLOW, H. B., 1953. Summation and inhibition in the frog's retina. *J. Physiol.* 119:69–88.

BARLOW, H. B., R. M. HILL, and W. R. LEVICK, 1964. Retinal ganglion cells responding selectively to direction and speed of image motion in the rabbit. *J. Physiol.* 173:377–407.

BARLOW, H. B., and W. R. LEVICK, 1965. The mechanism of directionally selective units in rabbit's retina. *J. Physiol.* 178:477–504.

BAYLOR, D. A., M.G.F. FUORTES, and P. M. O'BRYAN, 1971. Receptive fields of cones in retina of the turtle. *J. Physiol.* 214:256–294.

BOYCOTT, B. B. and J. E. DOWLING, 1969. Organization of the primate retina: light microscopy. *Philos. Trans. R. Soc. Lond.* B255:109–184.

BROWN, J. E., and L. H. PINTO, 1974. Ionic mechanism for the photoreceptor potential of the retina of *Bufo marinus*. *J. Physiol.* 236:575–592.

BURKHARDT, D. A., 1970. Proximal negative response of frog retina. *J. Neurophysiol.* 33:405–420.

CALDWELL, J. H., 1977. Ganglion cell receptive fields and synaptic organization in the rabbit retina. Ph.D. dissertation, Washington University, St. Louis, MO.

CERVETTO, L., and M. PICCOLINO, 1974. Synaptic transmission between photoreceptors and horizontal cells in the turtle retina. *Science* 183:417–418.

DACHEUX, R., 1977. A physiological study of the ontological formation of synaptic interactions in the rabbit retina. Ph.D. dissertation, State University of New York at Buffalo.

DACHEUX, R. F., and R. F. MILLER, 1976. Photoreceptor-bipolar cell transmission in the perfused retina eyecup of the mudpuppy. *Science* 191:963–964.

DOWLING, J. E., 1968. Synaptic organization of the frog retina: An electron microscopic analysis comparing the retinas of frogs and primates. *Proc. R. Soc. Lond.* B170:205–228.

DOWLING, J. E., 1970. Organization of vertebrate retinas. *Invest. Ophthalmol.* 9:655–680.

DOWLING, J. E., and H. RIPPS, 1973. Effects of magnesium on horizontal cell activity in the skate retina. *Nature* 242:101–103.

DOWLING, J. E., and F. S. WERBLIN, 1969. Organization of retina of the mudpuppy, *Necturus maculosus*. I. Synaptic structure. *J. Neurophysiol.* 32:315–338.

DUBIN, M. W., 1970. The inner plexiform layer of the vertebrate retina: A quantitative and comparative electron microscopic analysis. *J. Comp. Neurol.* 140:479–505.

HARTLINE, H. K., 1938. The response of single optic-nerve fibers of the vertebrate eye to illumination of the retina. *Am. J. Physiol.* 121:400–415.

KANEKO, A., 1970. Physiological and morphological identification of horizontal, bipolar and amacrine cells in goldfish retina. *J. Physiol.* 207:623–633.

KATZ, B., and R. MILEDI, 1966. Input-output relation of a single synapse. *Nature* 212:1242–1245.

KOLB, H., and E. V. FAMIGLIETTI, 1974. Rod and cone pathways in the inner plexiform layer of cat retina. *Science* 186:47–49.

KUFFLER, S. W., 1952. Neurons in the retina: Organization, inhibition and excitation problems. *Cold Spring Harbor Symp. Quant. Biol.* 17:281–292.

LETTVIN, J. Y., H. R. MATURANA, W. S. MCCULLOCH, and W. H. PITTS, 1959. What the frog's eye tells the frog's brain. *Proc. Inst. Radio Engrs.* 47:1940–1951.

LLINÁS, R. R., 1976. Calcium and transmitter release in squid synapse. In *Approaches to the Cell Biology of Neurons* (Society for Neuroscience Symposia VII), W. M. Cowan and J. A. Frerendelli, eds. Bethesda, MD: Society for Neuroscience.

LLINÁS, R., and C. NICHOLSON, 1971. Electro-physiological properties of dendrites and soma in alligator Purkinje cells. *J. Neurophysiol.* 34:532–551.

MILLER, R. F., and R. F. DACHEUX, 1973. Information processing in the retina: Importance of chloride ions. *Science* 181:266–268.

MILLER, R. F., and R. F. DACHEUX, 1975a. Chloride-sensitive receptive field mechanisms in the isolated retina-eyecup of the rabbit. *Brain Res.* 90:329–334.

MILLER, R. F., and R. F. DACHEUX, 1975b. Intracellular chloride activity in retinal neurons. ARVO Meeting, Sarasota, FL.

MILLER, R. F., and R. F. DACHEUX, 1976a. Synaptic organization and ionic basis of on and off channels in mudpuppy retina. I. Intracellular analysis of chloride-sensi-

tive electrogenic properties of receptors, horizontal cells, bipolar cells and amacrine cells. *J. Gen. Physiol.* 67:639–659.

MILLER, R. F., and R. F. DACHEUX, 1976b. Synaptic organization and ionic basis of on and off channels in mudpuppy retina. II. Chloride-dependent ganglion cell mechanisms. *J. Gen. Physiol.* 67:661–678.

MILLER, R. F., and R. F. DACHEUX, 1976c. Synaptic organization and ionic basis of on and off channels in mudpuppy retina. III. A model of ganglion cell receptive field organization based on chloride-free experiments. *J. Gen. Physiol.* 67:679–690.

MILLER, R. F., and R. F. DACHEUX, 1976d. Dendritic and somatic spikes in mudpuppy amacrine cells: Identification and TTX sensitivity. *Brain Res.* 104:157–162.

MILLER, R. F., R. F. DACHEUX, and T. FRUMKES, 1977. Amacrine cells in *Necturus* retina: Evidence for independent GABA and glycine releasing neurons. *Science* 198:748.

NAKA, K. I., 1976a. Neuronal circuitry in the catfish retina. *Invest. Ophthalmol.* 15:926–935.

NAKA, K. I., and N.R.G. CARRAWAY, 1975. Morphological and functional identifications of catfish retinal neurons. I. Classical morphology. *J. Neurophysiol.* 38:53–71.

PINTO, L. H., and W. L. PAK, 1974. Light-induced changes in photoreceptor membrane resistance and potentials in gecko retinas. II. Preparations with active lateral interactions. *J. Gen. Physiol.* 64:49–69.

SPENCER, W. A., and E. R. KANDEL, 1961. Electrophysiology of hippocampol neurons. IV. Fast prepotentials. *J. Neurophysiol.* 24:272–285.

TOYODA, J. E., H. HASHIMOTO, and K. OHTSU, 1973. Bipolar amacrine transmission in the carp retina. *Vision Res.* 13:295–307.

TRIFONOV, Y. A., and A. L. BYZOV, 1965. The response of the cells generating S-potential on the current passed through the eyecup of the turtle. *Biofizika* 10:673–680.

WERBLIN, F. S., 1970. Response of retinal cells to moving spots: Intracellular recording in *Necturus maculosus*. *J. Neurophysiol.* 33:342–350.

WERBLIN, F. S., 1977. Regenerative amacrine cell depolarization and formation of on-off ganglion cell responses. *J. Physiol.* 264:767–785.

WERBLIN, F. S., and J. E. DOWLING, 1969. Organization of the retina of the mudpuppy, *Necturus maculosus*. II. Intracellular recording. *J. Neurophysiol.* 34:228–241.

WEST, R. W., and J. E. DOWLING, 1972. Synapses onto different morphological types of retinal ganglion cells. *Science* 178:510–512.

WIESEL, T. N., 1959. Recording inhibition and excitation in the cat's retinal ganglion cells with intracellular electrodes. *Nature* 183:264–265.

WINKLER, B. S., 1973. Dependence of fast components of the electroretinogram of the isolated rat retina on the ionic environment. *Vision Res.* 13:457–463.

WYATT, H. J., and N. W. DAW, 1976. Specific effects of neurotransmitter antagonists on ganglion cells in rabbit retina. *Science* 191:204–205.

WYATT, H. J., and N. W. DAW, 1975. Directionally sensitive ganglion cells in the rabbit retina: Specificity for stimulus direction, size and speed. *J. Neurophysiol.* 38:613–626.

15 Cat Ganglion-Cell Receptive Fields and the Role of Horizontal Cells in Their Generation

O.-J. GRÜSSER

ABSTRACT In ganglion cells of the light-adapted cat retina, the spatial summation of excitatory processes elicited from the receptive-field (RF) center, or of inhibitory processes elicited from the RF periphery, revealed frequency-dependent nonlinear properties. The interaction of RF center processes and RF periphery, however, was linear within a wide range. The same was true for the interaction of inhibitory with excitatory processes elicited from the RF center. The experimental data indicated the existence of at least two types of lateral inhibition in the cat retina: lateral inhibition 1 (shunting type), probably located at the horizontal-cell level, and lateral inhibition 2 (subtractive type), located at the amacrine-cell level.

Intracellular recordings from horizontal cells of the light-adapted eye in situ revealed three different classes of H-units. The frequency-transfer characteristics of these three classes differed, but most H-units reached a maximum response in a frequency range of 1–3 Hz. Discrete Fourier analysis of the nonlinear H-unit responses and the frequency-transfer properties indicate that H_n-units are rod-dominated, H_m-units have a mixed rod-cone response, and the response of H_w-units is dominated by two or three different cones. The possible mechanisms for horizontal-cell influence on the signal transmission between receptors and bipolar cells are discussed.

Introduction

The neuronal network of the retina contains neurons (horizontal, bipolar, and amacrine cells) that transmit signals by slow electrotonic conduction of the membrane potential changes along dendrites and axons (Figure 1). It also contains the ganglion cells, in which the cell soma membrane potential is transformed into a sequence of conducted "all-or-nothing" action potentials, as "classical" neurons ought to do (Eccles, 1964). This sequence of action potentials constitutes the output signal of the retina; it is transmitted through the ganglion-cell axons to the visual centers of the brain. In its two synaptic layers (outer and inner plexiform layer) the synaptic terminals of retinal neurons form numerous structures with reciprocal synaptic complexes (see Dowling, Figure 3, this volume). Thus the retina is a useful neuronal network for testing old and new ideas about dendrodendritic interaction, the modulator function of dendrites, signal transmission by electrotonic conduction, and the function of synapses in local circuits (Jung, 1953; Schmitt, Dev, and Smith, 1976).

In his introductory lecture Dowling (this volume) stated that the synaptic organization of retinal neurons is fairly similar across species. Species differences in the retinal synaptic pathways are believed to be quantitative rather than qualitative. Therefore intracellular work carried out in some nonmammalian "model" retinas (e.g., *Necturus*: Dowling and Werblin, 1969; Werblin and Dowling, 1969; *tiger salamander*: Werblin, 1978; *turtle*: Gerschenfeld, 1978; *fish*: Svaetichin, 1953; Svaetichin et al., 1965, 1971; Laufer et al., 1971; Kaneko, 1970, 1971a,b, 1973; Kaneko and Shimazaki, 1975; Naka, 1972, 1977; Naka and Rushton, 1966, 1967, 1968; Naka and Nye, 1971; Marmarelis and Naka, 1973a–c; Naka and Ohtsuka, 1975; Naka and Carraway, 1975; Naka, Marmarelis, and Chan, 1975) can be used as a guide in the interpretation of findings in the mammalian retina. In the light of phylogenetic development, this is not necessarily expected. The early mammals, developing about 200 million years ago from diurnal reptiles, adapted to nocturnal ecological niches inaccessible to the poikilotherm reptiles. Thus the mesozoic mammalian visual system developed a strong rod dominance, and a "secondary" cone system appeared only much later as the mammals became, with the extinction of the ruling reptiles, in part diurnal (Walls, 1967; Jerison, 1973). Simultaneously, the neocortical visual centers developed, and a strong retinothalamocortical projection appeared. In lower vertebrates

O.-J. GRÜSSER Physiologisches Institut, Freie Universität Berlin, Berlin 33, Federal Republic of Germany

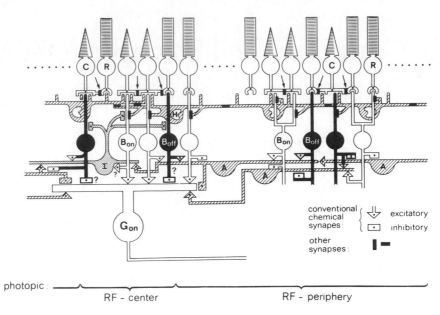

photopic :

RF - center ⏜ RF - periphery

FIGURE 1 Schematic diagram of the network forming the receptive field of an *on*-center ganglion cell in the light-adapted cat retina. Receptors (C = cones, R = rods), A-type horizontal cells (H), bipolar cells (B; *off* bipolar cells are black), amacrines (A), interplexiform cells (I), *on*-center ganglion cell (G). Conventional chemical synapses of excitatory and inhibitory type are marked by different symbols. Nonconventional synapses are marked by black bars. Whether *off* bipolar cells have direct contacts with *on*-center ganglion cells is an open question.

the main neuronal specialization seems to have occurred at the ganglion-cell level, while in higher mammals part of this specialization seems to have shifted to the cortical level (Hubel and Wiesel, 1968, 1970; Zeki, 1977a,b). The high degree of specialization of many nonmammalian vertebrate retinas during phylogenesis imposes some restrictions on the comparison of ganglion-cell function in nonmammalian amd mammalian vertebrates. In the frog retina, for example, Ramón y Cajal (1894) described eleven morphological classes of ganglion cells (excluding Dogiel cells). To date, ten different classes of retinal ganglion cells can be distinguished by neurophysiological techniques in *Rana esculenta*. These retinal ganglion cells exhibit considerable specialization with respect to the effective stimulus parameters: moving visual stimuli of a certain size, velocity, and black-white or chromatic contrast are necessary for effective neuronal activation. The simple center-surround model of cat retinal ganglion-cell receptive fields is therefore not applicable (Maturana et al., 1960; Grüsser and Grüsser-Cornehls, 1976; Grüsser-Cornehls and Saunders, 1978). In addition, the majority of lower vertebrate ganglion cells send their axons to the optic tectum and the pretectal visual nuclei, while in higher mammals the bulk of retinal ganglion cells studied to date connect the retina with the thalamic visual-relay nuclei.

The neurons of the cat retina

The domestic cat has a retina well adapted to both nocturnal and diurnal functions, although a major portion of cat behavior is nocturnal. I shall summarize here the main specializations of the cat retina.

Rods and cones. In the area centralis, the region of highest visual acuity, about 16,500 cones and 280,000 rods are found per mm². In the region about 15° outside of the area centralis, the corresponding values are about 6,000 cones and 450,000 rods/mm² (Steinberg, Reid, and Lacy, 1973). Nearly all recordings that will be mentioned were made from retinal neurons with receptive fields within 15° of the area centralis. There is good physiological evidence that the cat retina contains one class of rods (maximum chromatic sensitivity at about 502 nm) and three classes of cones with maximum sensitivities of about 470, 556, and 600 nm (Granit, 1947, 1950; Donner, 1950; Donner and Willmer, 1950; Daw and Pearlman, 1969, 1970; Andrews and Hammond, 1970a,b; Saunders, 1973, 1977). For the cat retina, physiological and anatomical evidence has shown that cones have a direct rod input (Raviola and Gilula, 1973; Nelson, 1977; Kolb, 1977).

Horizontal cells. Two types of horizontal cells are distinguished by morphological criteria: one type has a dominant cone input to its dendrites and a separate rod input to an axonal "terminal arborization" (Cajal-type H-cell: see Ramón y Cajal, 1894; B-horizontal cell of Fisher and Boycott, 1974; Kolb, 1974; Nelson et al., 1975). The second, axonless Gallego-type H-cell seems to form a syncytium with other axonless H-cells and receives a direct input only from cones (Gallego, 1965, 1971; A-cell of Fisher and Boycott, 1974). Gallego (personal communication, 1977) has recently found another type of short-axon H-cell in the monkey retina. One can therefore conjecture that further morphological studies of the cat retina might also lead to a morphological subdivision of the Cajal-type H-cells. Physiologically, all horizontal cells studied so far are of the hyperpolarizing L-type; that is, no antagonistic response with respect to chromatic stimuli has been found (Grüsser, 1957; Steinberg, 1969a–c; Niemeyer, 1973; Niemeyer and Gouras, 1973; Nelson et al., 1975; Nelson, 1977).

Bipolar cells. Three major bipolar cell types have been described in the cat retina (Boycott and Kolb, 1973). Rod bipolars make connections only with rods. The invaginating cone bipolars contact 4–10 cones and form the central dendrites of the synaptic triads. The flat cone bipolars make basal contacts with the pedicles of 8–14 cones. According to Kolb (1974), the rod bipolar cells make synaptic contacts only with amacrine-cell processes, while the cone bipolar cells form synaptic ribbon-type contacts with ganglion and amacrine dendrites. The synaptic terminals of flat cone bipolar cells are found in the outer part of the inner plexiform layer and those of the invaginating cone bipolar cells in the inner part of the outer plexiform layer. Based on morphological criteria, Famiglietti and Kolb (1976) believe that the invaginating cone bipolars are the *on*-center bipolar cells (they are depolarized as the RF center is illuminated) and the flat bipolar cells are the *off*-center bipolar cells (see Dowling, this volume). Correspondingly, they assume that ganglion cells with their dendritic branchings mainly in the outer part of the inner plexiform layer are *off*-center ganglion cells and that ganglion cells with their main dendrites within the inner part of the inner plexiform layer are *on*-center ganglion cells.

As yet, intracellular recordings from bipolar cells of the cat retina have been reported only from the perfused eye (Niemeyer, 1975; Nelson, 1977). Given these data we presume that in the light-adapted cat retina the *on* bipolars are depolarized by illumination of the RF center and hyperpolarized by illumination of the RF periphery, while the *off* bipolars exhibit the reversed responses (RF center hyperpolarization and RF periphery depolarization).

Amacrines. These axonless cells receive their input from bipolar-cell terminals (ribbon synapses) as well as from other amacrine cells. They form conventional chemical synapses on ganglion-cell dendrites and on the dendrites of other amacrines. Thus amacrines form the second layer of lateral signal conduction in the retina. We obtained a few intracellular recordings from amacrine cells of the cat retina: all responded with a phasic *on* and *off* depolarization that was partly superimposed by a few low-amplitude action potentials. No tonic *on* or *off* amacrine cells like those found by Naka in the fish retina have been recorded so far in the cat retina. Nevertheless, I would assume that tonic *on* amacrines and *off* amacrines also exist there.

Interplexiform cells. The morphology of these cells and of their synaptic contacts has been studied by Kolb (1977). She is of the opinion that all conventional synapses in the outer plexiform layer are formed by interplexiform-cell dendritic terminals, but other research workers (Boycott, personal communication, 1977) question this conclusion.

Ganglion cells. Three different techniques were applied to classify cat retinal ganglion cells: morphological criteria, analysis of the RF organization as revealed by visual stimuli of different properties, and measurement of the axonal conduction velocity, calculated from the latency of single-axon responses to electrical stimuli of the optic nerve or optic chiasm. The main properties of the three large ganglion-cell categories found in the cat retina are listed in Table I.

The morphological criteria were cell size (perikarya), size and complexity of dendritic arborization (Stone, 1975; Boycott and Wässle, 1974; Levick, 1975; Wässle, Levick, and Cleland, 1975; Rowe and Stone, 1976). There is good evidence that the three morphological classes (α, β, γ) correspond to three functional classes of ganglion cells called Y-, X-, and W-cells (Enroth-Cugell and Robson, 1966; Levick, 1975; Stone and Hoffmann, 1972; Hoffmann, 1973). Y-, X-, and W-cells in turn correlate with latency class I, II, and III neurons. The W-cells are not a homogeneous group; color-coded neurons, direction-selective neurons, movement-sensitive neurons, uniformity detectors, and others are grouped into this class.

As shown in Table I, the three different neuronal classes project only in part to the same regions of the central visual system. As the present report deals only with Y- and X-cells, I shall restrict the following description to these two categories of retinal ganglion cells. Both have a concentric receptive-field organization: half of the neurons of each class have *on*-center receptive fields, and the other half have *off*-center receptive fields.

TABLE I
Classes of retinal ganglion cells (domestic cat)

Classification Criteria	Neuron Classes			References
Morphology	α	β	γ	Boycott and Wässle, 1974; Stone, 1965; Wässle, Levick, and Cleland, 1975; Leicester and Stone, 1967; Hughes, 1975; Cleland, Levick, and Wässle, 1975
Dendritic field diameter	180–1000 μm	25–300 μm	180–500 μm	
Perikarya size	22–38 μm	12–22 μm	8–18 μm	
Frequency	3.5%	45%	50%	
Axon diameter	6–13 μm	2–5 μm	0.5–2 μm	Donovan, 1967; Hughes and Wässle, 1976; Stone and Holländer, 1971
Central projection sites				
LGN layer A, A$_1$	+	+	∅	Hoffmann, Stone, and Sherman, 1972; Eysel and Grüsser, 1975; Kelly and Gilbert, 1975
LGN C-layer	+	∅	+	
Colliculi superiores	+		+	
Electrical Stimulation of Optic Nerve or Chiasm	class I	class II	class III	Bishop, Jeremy, and Lance, 1953; Grüsser-Cornehls, and Grüsser, 1960; Bishop, Clare, and Landau, 1969; Fukuda and Stone, 1974; Kirk et al., 1975; Stone and Freeman, 1971; Eysel and Grüsser, 1974, 1975; Cleland et al., 1975; Eysel, 1976
Latency[a]	0.33–0.60 msec	0.65–1.2 msec	>1.2 msec	
OT-evoked potential wave	t_1	t_2	post t_2	
Conduction speed of the axon	30–55 m/sec	15–27 m/sec	<15 m/sec	
Visual Stimuli	Y	X	W	Granit, 1947, 1950; Kuffler, 1952, 1953; Wiesel, 1960; Rodieck, 1965; Enroth-Cugell and Robson, 1966; Stone and Fabian, 1966; Grüsser, 1971; Enroth-Cugell and Pinto, 1972; Cleland, Levick, and Sanderson, 1973; Stone and Fukuda, 1974; Cleland and Levick, 1974; Enroth-Cugell, Lennie, and Shapley, 1975; Saito and Fukuda, 1975; Freund, Hennerici, and Rabenschlag, 1977
	on-center/ *off*-center	*on*-center/ *off*-center	mainly *on-off*	
RF center diameter	0.3°–3.0°	0.1°–1.5°	1°–4°	
RF organization	center-surround; concentric	concentric; center-surround	concentric or specialized; in part movement-sensitive	
Response to 30 sec of *on* and *off* stimulation of RF center (photopic adaptation)	transient	sustained	transient *on/off*	Cleland, Dubin, and Levick, 1971; Saito, Shimahara, and Fukada, 1970, 1971; Ikeda and Wright, 1972; Cleland and Levick, 1974; Sato, Yamamoto, Nakahama, 1976
McIlwain's periphery effect	+	?	?	McIlwain, 1964, 1966
Receptor Connections	cones domi- nant / rods and cones	rods and cones / rods only	rods and cones	Donner, 1950; Granit, 1950; Donner and Willmer, 1950; Barlow, Fitzhugh, and Kuffler, 1957; Andrews and Hammond, 1970; Daw and Pearlman, 1970; Rodieck and Rushton, 1976; Saunders, 1977

Visual Stimuli	Y		X		W	
Flicker-fusion frequency (maximum, large-field stimuli, 400 cd/m²)	80 Hz	60–70 Hz	45–55 Hz	25–28 Hz	?	Enroth, 1952; Dodt and Enroth, 1953; Grüsser, 1956; Grüsser and Reidemeister, 1959; Ogawa, Bishop, and Levick, 1966; Fukuda et al., 1966
Response enhancement by border contrast	+	+	+	∅	?	Baumgartner and Hakas, 1962; Grüsser, 1977; Grüsser and Grüsser-Cornehls, 1977
Response to moving slit of light (1° × 10°)						Hamasaki et al., 1973; Grüsser and Grüsser-Cornehls, 1973
20°/sec	+	+	+	+	+	
200°/sec	+	+				
Change of RF organization with dark-adaptation scotopic stimuli	no response	+	+	∅	?	Barlow, Fitzhugh, and Kuffler, 1957; Domberg, 1968; Sakmann and Creutzfeldt, 1969; Jakiela and Enroth-Cugell, 1976
Rhythmic discharge pattern to large-field short flashes	++	+	+	∅	?	Grüsser and Grützner, 1958; Grüsser and Grüsser-Cornehls, 1962; Steinberg, 1966, 1967; Büttner, Grüsser, and Schwanz, 1975

a Values for 18 mm distance between stimulation and recording site.

On-center neurons in the light-adapted retina respond to a small spot of light projected to the RF center with an *on* activation and with a transient *off* inhibition as the light spot is turned off (Figure 2). A light stimulus projected to the RF periphery leads to an *on* inhibition of the maintained activity and to a transient *off* activation as the RF periphery stimulus is turned off (Kuffler, 1952, 1953). The receptive-field organization of the *off*-center neurons (X- or Y-ganglion cells) exhibits the reversed response type: *on* inhibition and *off* excitation from the RF center and *on* excitation and *off* inhibition from the RF periphery. An outer surround of the RF periphery has again a reversed function and is responsible for the disinhibition visible when the inhibitory effect of the RF periphery is measured (Ikeda and Wright, 1972).

The concentric RFs are usually conceptualized as circular in shape, but most of them are elliptical. There is a tendency for the preferred orientation of the major RF axis to be along the horizontal meridian (Hammond, 1974). Y-cells recorded from the same region of the retina as X-cells always have larger RF centers, but the average size of the RF centers of both X- and Y-ganglion cells increases with the distance of the RF from the area centralis (Hammond, 1975).

When one records with conventional tungsten microelectrodes (Hubel, 1957) from the optic tract, one has an approximately equal probability of recording latency-class I neurons (Y) or latency-class II neurons (X), although only 3.5% of retinal ganglion cells are Y-type and about 45% are X-type (Wässle, Levick, and Cleland, 1975; Wässle and Peichl, personal communication, 1977). This bias of recording probability is due to the size of Y-cell axons, which constitute the myelinated fibers with the largest diameter in the fiber-diameter spectrum of cat optic nerve (Donovan, 1967; Hughes and Wässle, 1976).

The majority of Y- and X-cells have a mixed rod-cone input. Some Y-cells, however, are cone-dominated, while some X-cells in the light-adapted state have only a rod input, a corresponding chromatic sensitivity curve with the maximum sensitivity at 502 nm, and a low flicker fusion frequency (Table I). The other main functional differences in Y- and X-cells are presented in the table. Enroth-Cugell and Robson (1966), who introduced the X/Y classification, used a sinusoidal spatial grating with a period about twice the RF center diameter. This pattern was presented in two ways: stationary at different positions within the RF, or moving. For all X-cells a null position was found at which the appearance and disappearance of the grating against a homogeneous field of the same average luminance did not lead to any response. In contrast, such a null position could not be established

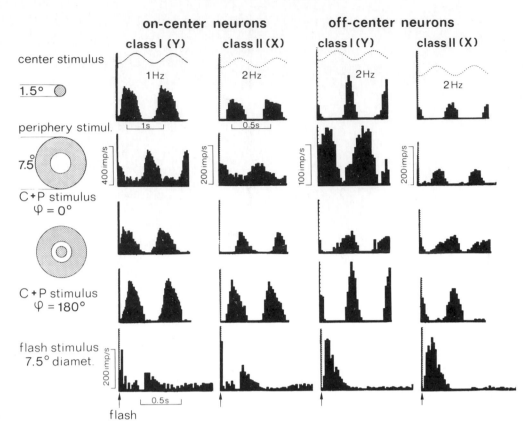

FIGURE 2   PST histograms (average of 10 responses) of latency class I *on*-center neuron, class II *on*-center neuron, class I *off*-center neuron and class II *off*-center neuron (ganglion-cell response) to sinusoidal light stimulation of the RF center, the RF periphery, and both together (syn-chronous or alternating stimuli) in the light-adapted cat retina (background luminance = 2 cd/m², L_0 = 120 cd/m², m = 0.7). The lower row shows responses of the same neurons to 10 msec light flashes (arrows).

in Y-cells. This finding indicates that in X-cells, the excitatory and inhibitory processes elicited from the RF center or the RF periphery, respectively, might compensate each other, whereas this is not the case in Y-cells. This finding was also taken as an indication that the interaction between RF center and RF periphery processes (center-surround interaction) is linear in X-cells. This topic will be discussed in more detail below.

With some experience, the classification Y/X is fairly unequivocal. The same is true for the correlation between Y/class I and X/class II. We performed double-blind tests (one experimenter measured the response latency to optic chiasm electrical stimuli and the other determined the RF properties) and found more than 95% agreement (Eysel, Grüsser, and Hoffmann, unpublished observations, 1976). A similarly high coincidence exists between physiological properties and the morphological classifications listed in

Table I, as Cleland, Levick, and Wässle (1974) demonstrated in their careful study.

Pathways of spatial interaction within the receptive field of ganglion cells

Different pathways, that is, different types of interaction between the cells of the retina, are involved in the RF center and RF periphery mechanisms of retinal ganglion cells mentioned in the preceding and following sections. Before I present the results of black-box experiments in which we tried to measure these interactions quantitatively, I shall first describe some possible mechanisms that might be responsible for the functional organization of ganglion-cell receptive fields in cat. This will be done for an *on*-center ganglion cell, but the same mechanisms also apply for *off*-center ganglion-cell receptive fields (reverse excitation with inhibition and vice versa).

Direct excitation is the activation of an *on*-center ganglion cell elicited by light stimulation of the RF center. The presumed pathway is: receptors located within the RF center (hyperpolarization by light) → *on* bipolar cells of the RF center (depolarization by light) → ganglion-cell membrane (depolarization and generation of action potentials, Figure 1).

Direct inhibition of an *on*-center ganglion cell is the *off* inhibition elicited by a decrease in the luminance of an RF center stimulus. Its pathway is: receptors located within the RF center (decrease in hyperpolarization at light *off*) → *off* bipolar cells of the RF center (depolarization at light *off*) → *on*-center ganglion cells (postsynaptic hyperpolarization and reduction in impulse activity). Intracellular recordings of *on*-center ganglion cells revealed that light *off* in the RF center leads to a sustained hyperpolarization of the resting membrane potential (Wiesel, 1965; Foerster, Grüsser, and van de Grind, unpublished observations, 1971; van de Grind, Grüsser, and Lunkenheimer, 1973). If *off*-center bipolar cells do not contact ganglion-cell dendrites directly (see Dowling, this volume; Miller, this volume), a narrow-receptive-field amacrine must be assumed to be intercalated between *off* bipolars and *on*-center ganglion cells.

Lateral excitation is the *off* activation appearing when a spot or ring of light projected to the RF periphery of an *on*-center ganglion cell is turned off (Figure 2). The pathway is: receptors of the whole RF → *off* bipolar cells (depolarization at light *off*) → sustained *off* amacrines (depolarization) → ganglion cell (postsynaptic depolarization and increase in impulse activity).

Lateral inhibition 1 is the inhibitory interaction between horizontal cells and *on*-center or *off*-center bipolar cells. A possible pathway is: receptors (hyperpolarization at light *on*) → horizontal cells (hyperpolarization at light *on*) → bipolar cells (shunting inhibition of receptor-bipolar interaction). As Dowling mentioned in his paper, a possible feedback detour must also be considered: receptors → horizontal cells → receptors → bipolar cells. Possible receptor-receptor interactions are included.

Lateral inhibition 2 is the inhibition of *on*-center ganglion-cell activity caused by illumination of the RF periphery. For this mechanism we assume activation of the following pathway: receptors of the whole RF (hyperpolarization) → *on* bipolar cells of the whole RF (depolarization) → sustained *on* amacrines (depolarization) → *on*-center ganglion cells (postsynaptic inhibition by hyperpolarization, Figure 2).

Lateral disinhibition is the inhibition of lateral inhibition 2, which can be demonstrated in a three-stimulus experiment. A spot of light is projected to the

RF center of an *on*-center neuron. If a ring of light is simultaneously projected to the RF periphery, the center activation is reduced (Figure 2). If a second ring is then projected to the outer RF periphery, the neuronal activation again increases. The simplest explanation is that the outer ring activates receptors and horizontal cells, which in turn inhibit the *on*-center bipolar cells (lateral inhibition 1) activated by the inner ring and transmitting the signals of lateral inhibition 2. The outer ring does not inhibit the direct excitation elicited from the RF center because the distance between the outer ring and the RF center is too great (see Ikeda and Wright, 1972).

A quantitative study of the spatial summation within the ganglion-cell receptive field

In this section I shall discuss some quantitative properties of the mechanisms proposed in the preceding section and will describe results of black-box experiments, that is, data from measurements at the output level of the retina. The stimulus patterns were chosen to enable a quantitative estimation of the different inhibitory and excitatory mechanisms acting within the retinal network. The present report will be restricted to findings in *on*-center ganglion cells of the light-adapted retina, although excitatory and inhibitory mechanisms found for the receptive field of *off*-center ganglion cells reveal the same properties.

I shall discuss both linear and nonlinear modes of interaction within the RF. In addition to the nonlinear lateral inhibitory mechanisms described below, two other nonlinearities are easily recognizable in the PST histograms of Figure 2. The half-wave rectification with a negative cutoff, appearing particularly in the center responses, is caused by the threshold mechanisms of impulse generation. The nonsinusoidal distortion of the positive half-wave is probably due to a similar deformation at the receptor level (Cleland and Enroth-Cugell, 1966; Rackensperger and Grüsser, 1966). Despite these overall nonlinear response properties, it is the interaction of nonlinear and linear components of the intraretinal signal processing that gives rise to the functional organization of the ganglion-cell RF.

SUMMATION OF DIRECT EXCITATION   Direct excitation is seen in the increased neuronal discharge rate as the RF center is stimulated. When photopic sinusoidal light stimuli with a modulation depth greater than 0.4 were applied, the time course of the neuronal response as expressed by the PST histograms revealed considerable nonlinearities (Figures 2, 3).

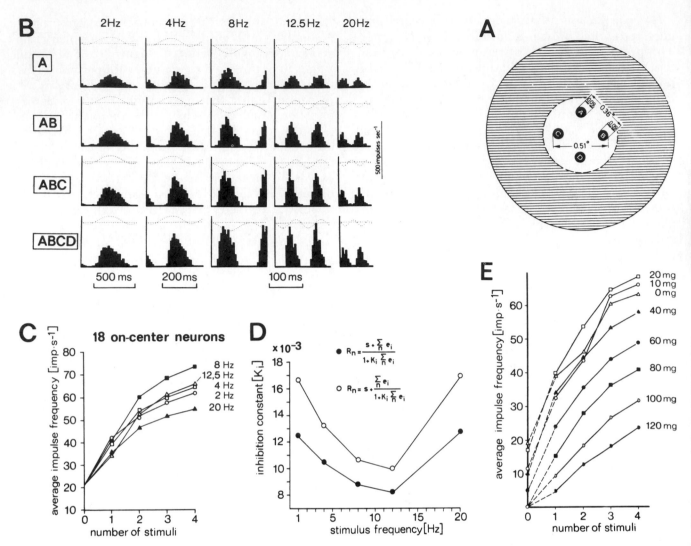

FIGURE 3 Spatial summation within the RF center of retinal *on*-center ganglion cells. (A) Schematic drawing of the stimulus pattern. The four light spots (A, B, C, D) were projected into equally sensitive parts of the RF center. (B) PST histograms of a Y-type *on*-center neuron. Average responses to 1–4 light spots projected to the RF center. Responses to 20 sine-wave stimuli were averaged. $L_0 = 22$ cd/m², $m = 0.9$. (C) Quantitative analysis of spatial summation of excitation within the RF center. The average impulse rate of 18 *on*-center neurons is plotted as a function of the number of stimuli. Stimulus parameters as in B. (D) Dependence of the inhibition constant k_i of Equation (1) on the stimulus frequency; k_i was computed from the curves of Figure 2C (minimal chi-square sum technique). (E) Spatial summation in the RF center of an *on*-center neuron at different levels of Na-pentobarbital anesthesia. The overall amount of barbiturate injected intravenously is marked on each curve. Weight of animal (encéphale isolé preparation) = 2.0 kg. Overall recording time of the neuron is about 2 hours. The neuronal activation decreased with barbiturate doses above 15 mg/kg. (From Grüsser, Schaible, and Vierkant-Glathe, 1970.)

Either the average impulse rate $\bar{R}$ or the maximal rate R_{max} was chosen to represent the level of neuronal excitation; the two were closely correlated. Both rates increased as the frequency of the photopic stimuli was increased above 0.5 Hz, then in most neurons reached a maximum between 8 and 15 Hz and decreased again with a further increase in the stimulus frequency up to the critical flicker-fusion frequency (Grüsser, 1956; Grüsser and Creutzfeldt, 1957; Grüs-ser and Reidemeister, 1958; cf. van de Grind, Grüsser, and Lunkenheimer, 1973). The increase in the neuronal response at medium stimulus frequencies was more pronounced in Y-cells than in X-cells.

To measure the spatial summation of direct excitation within the RF center, one to four spots of light (Figure 3A) were projected into the RF center. Each spot elicited approximately the same neuronal response (synchronous sinusoidal light stimuli: 0.5–25

Hz; $m = 0.9$; average stimulus luminance, $L_0 = 17$–38 cd/m²; background illumination, about 0.3–0.5 cd/m²). The response to all possible combinations of the four spots of light was measured. Examples of the PST histograms obtained in such experiments are shown in Figure 3D. The average spatial summation curves (Figure 3C) are well described by the following nonlinear equation:

$$\bar{R}_n = S + \frac{k_0 \sum\limits_n e_i}{1 + k_i \sum\limits_n e_i}, \qquad (1)$$

where $\bar{R}_n$ represents the average impulse rate (impulses/sec) elicited by n spots of light applied simultaneously, S the spontaneous activity obtained at the background luminance, and e_i the increase above the spontaneous activity elicited by the ith spot of light ($e_1 = e_2 = e_3 = e_4$). The inhibition constant k_i was a function of the stimulus frequency and decreased above 1–2 Hz, reaching a minimum between 10 and 15 Hz (Figure 3D)—that is, within a frequency range at which neuronal activation was at its maximum. k_i also decreased with the distance between the spots of light (Büttner and Grüsser, 1968; Grüsser, Schaible, and Vierkant-Glathe, 1970). In addition, the nonlinearity of spatial summation expressed by equation 1 depended on the level of anesthesia (Figure 3E).

We assume that lateral inhibition 1 is responsible for the nonlinear spatial summation of excitation and has the following properties:

1. Location distal to the ganglion-cell dendrites.
2. Attenuation above 1–3 Hz.
3. Flicker fusion reached at a frequency around 18–20 Hz (photopic stimuli).
4. Efficiency reduced by pentobarbital anesthesia.
5. Effect of lateral inhibition 1 better described by an equation applying shunting inhibition (Varjú, 1965; Furman, 1965) than by a model of linear subtractive inhibition.

It is conjectured that horizontal cells mediate lateral inhibition 1.

SPATIAL SUMMATION WITHIN THE RF PERIPHERY   If horizontal cells are responsible for lateral inhibition 1, one can predict that similar nonlinearities should appear when the spatial summation within the RF periphery is investigated because the signal transmission between receptors and bipolar cells will be influenced by lateral inhibition 1, independent of the relative location of the interacting neurons within the RF of an individual ganglion cell (Figure 1). To measure the spatial summing properties of the RF periphery, sectors of a light ring were projected there, the sector width being the experimental variable (Figure 4A). The neuronal activation (*off* activation in *on*-center neurons) was measured with PST histograms ($\bar{R}$, R_{max}, Figure 2), and again equation 1 was found to be valid.

According to the model in Figure 1, horizontal cells mediating lateral inhibition 1 should affect not only the excitatory processes elicited from the RF center, but also the lateral inhibition elicited by stimulation of the RF periphery (lateral inhibition 2). In order to study the summing properties of lateral inhibition 2, we had to apply a technique to measure inhibition quantitatively. To this end, we measured the responses of retinal ganglion cells to either stimulation of the RF center alone ($\bar{R}_c$) or a combined synchronous stimulation of RF center and periphery, whereby the area of the light stimuli projected to the RF periphery, A_p, and the sine-wave frequency were varied (Figure 4A,B). The overall effect of lateral inhibition 2 (I_2) was then expressed as the difference between the responses to the center stimulus $\bar{R}_c$ and to the combined stimulation of center and periphery $\bar{R}_{c+p}$. For stimulus frequencies below 10 Hz, the following relationship held (Figure 4B):

$$I_2 = \bar{R}_c - \bar{R}_{c+p} = \frac{\alpha A_p}{1 + k_i A_p} \text{ (impulses/sec)}. \qquad (2)$$

The structure of equation 2 is identical to that of equation 1 and suggests that the lateral inhibition 2 elicited by light stimulation of the RF periphery is indeed controlled by another lateral inhibitory mechanism acting distal to the ganglion-cell and amacrine-cell layers. The inhibition constant k_i of equation 2, like k_i of equation 1, decreased as the sine-wave frequency rose above 2 Hz. The constant α also decreased when the frequency exceeded 2 Hz. Thus the higher the stimulus frequency, the more linear the spatial summation of lateral inhibition 2, but the smaller its overall efficiency as expressed by the constant α. The relative efficiency of lateral inhibition 2 was, as a rule, stronger in class I (Y)-cells than in class II (X)-cells. In most of the *on*-center neurons and many *off*-center neurons (X- and Y-cells), however, neuronal activation caused by a photopic flicker stimulus greater than 10 Hz and covering the entire RF was stronger than the response obtained when a stimulus of the same frequency was restricted to the RF center only. This indicates that the lateral excitation is attenuated much less at a higher stimulus frequency than lateral inhibition 2.

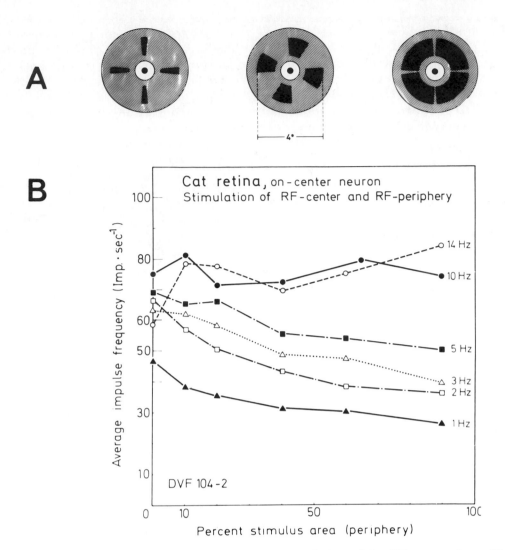

FIGURE 4 Summation of inhibition within the RF periphery. (A) Stimulus pattern: light ring sectors of different overall areas were projected to the RF periphery, and a spot of light to the RF center. (B) Spatial summation of RF periphery inhibition in an *on*-center neuron. Stimuli as in part A; the abscissa shows the percentage of stimulus area. For stimulus frequencies below 10 Hz, the neuronal activation elicited by the combined stimulation of the RF center and RF periphery was smaller than the responses obtained by stimulation of the RF center alone. The spatial summation of this inhibitory effect was a nonlinear function of the stimulus area. The average inhibitory effect decreased as the stimulus frequency increased. Above 10 Hz, the facilitatory RF periphery effect was stronger than the inhibitory effects. Photopic adaptation: $L_0 = 10$ cd/m², $m = 0.9$. (Grüsser and Lütgert, 1972; from van de Grind, Grüsser and Lunkenheimer, 1973.)

SUMMATION OF DIRECT EXCITATION AND DIRECT INHIBITION WITHIN THE RF CENTER The results described above led to questions of whether the low-frequency attenuation of lateral inhibition 1 is a general property of retinal inhibitory mechanisms and whether the spatial summing properties of the RF are generally of the nonlinear type. To answer these questions, two further series of experiments were performed.

In the first series of experiments, the superposition of *direct excitation* (i.e., *on* excitation in *on*-center neu-

rons) and *direct inhibition* (*off* inhibition in *on*-center neurons) was studied. Two spots of light were projected to equally sensitive parts of the RF center (Figure 5A), and the phase angle φ between the two sinusoidally modulated light stimuli (0.5–30 Hz, $m = 0.95$) was varied between 0 and 360°. Figure 5B exhibits recordings from such an experiment and Figure 5C demonstrates the neuronal activity $\bar{R}_{AB}$ to be a function of φ:

$$\bar{R}_{AB} = 4bA^* \cos\frac{\varphi}{2} + S, \qquad (3)$$

256   O.-J. GRÜSSER

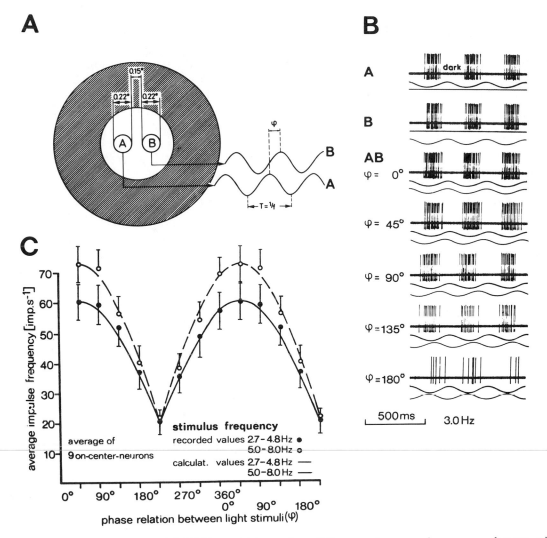

FIGURE 5 Summation of excitation and inhibition within the RF center of an *on*-center ganglion cell. (A) Stimulus pattern: two spots of light were projected onto equally sensitive parts of the RF center. The temporal frequency and the phase angle φ of the two sine-wave light stimuli were variable. (B) Responses of an *on*-center ganglion cell to the stimulus pattern of part A. The neuronal responses to each of the two stimuli and to combined stimulation with five different phase angles φ are shown; stimulus frequency = 3.0 Hz. $L_0 = 36$ cd/m², $m = 0.95$. (C) Average neuronal impulse rate ($\bar{R}$, ordinate) of nine *on*-center neurons stimulated with stimulus pattern of part A at two different frequency ranges and different phase angles. Stimulus parameters as in part B. (From Büttner, Büttner, and Grüsser, 1971.)

where b is a constant and A^* is the amplitude of the neuronal response elicited by each of the two light spots alone ($A_1^* = A_2^*$). Büttner, Büttner, and Grüsser (1971) showed that this equation results if a linear summation between direct excitation and direct inhibition occurs at the ganglion-cell membrane. The assumption is made that *on*-center bipolar cells and *off*-center bipolar cells act as separate channels, one leading to postsynaptic excitation, the other to postsynaptic inhibition at the ganglion-cell membrane. Intracellular recordings (Wiesel, 1959; Foerster, van de Grind, and Grüsser, unpublished observations, 1971) indeed indicate that *on*-center ganglion cells are depolarized by increasing and hyperpolarized by decreasing the stimulus luminance within the RF center (see also van de Grind, Grüsser, and Lunkenheimer, 1973).

Equation 3 is the solution of

$$\bar{R}_{AB} (\varphi) = bA^* \int_{\varphi/2}^{\pi+\varphi/2} [\sin \alpha + \sin (\alpha - \varphi)]d\alpha, \quad (4)$$

where $\alpha = \omega t$, which expresses the linear summing properties of the ganglion-cell membrane. To avoid misunderstanding, it should be noted that this linear summation of direct excitation and direct inhibition is located distal to the half-wave rectification and does not imply that the retinal network acts linearly in its overall performance. The boundaries of the integration take into consideration the fact that the ganglion cells act as half-wave rectifiers, which necessarily limits the analysis of impulse data to the excitation level suprathreshold for the impulse generation.

DYNAMIC INTERACTION BETWEEN RF CENTER AND RF PERIPHERY MECHANISMS   A second mode for studying the summation of excitation and inhibition at the ganglion-cell membrane was provided by applying the stimulus patterns shown in Figure 4A. The RF center stimulus C and the RF periphery stimulus P were modulated with the same frequency, but the phase angle φ between the two stimuli was varied in steps of 20° or 40° between 0° and 360° (Figure 6A, X-neuron). Figure 6B demonstrates the dependence of the neuronal activation $\bar{R}_{c+p}$ on the phase angle φ for selected stimulus frequencies:

$$\bar{R}_{c+p}(\varphi) = (\bar{R}_c + \bar{R}_p)\,[a + b\,\sin(\varphi/2 + \lambda)], \quad (5)$$

where $\lambda, a \leq 1$, and $b \leq 1$ are constants and $\bar{R}_c$ and $\bar{R}_p$ are the average impulse rates obtained when the RF center and periphery, respectively, are stimulated alone. One can write this as

$$R_{c+p}(\varphi) = (R^*_{min} + R^*_{max})\,\sin(\varphi/2 + \lambda), \quad (6)$$

where R^*_{min} and R^*_{max} are the minimal and maximal values obtained at a given frequency when φ was varied between 0° and 360°.

Depending on the phase angle φ, in this type of experiment the direct excitatory and inhibitory processes elicited by light stimuli in the RF center are superimposed on the lateral excitatory and lateral inhibitory processes elicited by the ring of light projected to the RF periphery. Because equations 5 and 6, like 3, are solutions of a linear model, linear spatial summing properties (of the ganglion-cell membrane) might again be assumed for the interaction of RF center and RF periphery mechanisms. The same statement is applicable to data from experiments in which either the center or the periphery stimulus was kept constant and the other was sinusoidally modulated at 1–3 Hz (Buettner, 1973; Buettner-Mönninghoff, 1976). Enroth-Cugell and Robson (1966) and Enroth-Cugell and Pinto (1970) reached the same conclusion by analyzing data from other types of experiments.

OSCILLATORY RESPONSES OF GANGLION CELLS   In the experiments described above, steady-state sine-wave stimuli were applied. This type of stimulation is not suitable for discovering nonlinear interactions in the neuronal network elicited by the simultaneous appearance of different nonharmonic frequency components (either in the stimulus or in the response). A useful stimulus for overcoming this restriction is the application of very short light flashes, which have a flat frequency spectrum within a wide frequency range. A small spot of light illuminating the RF center of an *on*-center ganglion cell for up to 20 msec elicited an activation lasting 30–120 msec, followed by an inhibitory period of 50–200 msec. Thereafter the neuronal impulse rate returned to the spontaneous level. As the diameter of the flash stimulus increased, the neuronal response exhibited alternating periods of excitation and inhibition (Figure 2) lasting up to 2 sec. In most Y-neurons the oscillatory response pattern was more pronounced than in X-neurons. The flash responses of *off*-center neurons began with the primary inhibitory period followed by a single excitatory period (as in Figure 2) or 2–4 excitatory periods interrupted by short discharge pauses. In the frequency range characteristic of sequential activation and inhibition of retinal ganglion cells (3–12 Hz), neither receptors nor horizontal cells exhibited oscillatory responses to flash stimuli. Hence inhibitory and excitatory mechanisms originating proximal to these structures induce the oscillatory response. Neurons contributing to an internal retinal feedback loop are, of course, candidates for the structures responsible for such a low-frequency oscillation of the retinal network. Perhaps the interplexiform neurons are responsible for the intraretinal feedback mechanisms.

The nonlinear spatial summing properties of some of the RF mechanisms also became apparent in these experiments. We found a very limited range in which the Bunsen law and the Ricco law were valid (Grüsser and Grützner, 1958; Grüsser and Kapp, 1958; Grüsser and Grüsser-Cornehls, 1962; Büttner, Grüsser, and Schwanz, 1975).

THE FREQUENCY PROPERTIES OF EXCITATORY AND INHIBITORY MECHANISMS   Direct and lateral excitation, direct inhibition, and the two types of lateral inhibition differ not only with respect to their relative efficiency and the different parts of the RF in which they occur, but also with respect to their temporal frequency properties. Direct excitation and direct inhibition had a response maximum of 8–15 Hz in the light-adapted retina. Lateral excitation reached a response maximum in a similar range, while lateral

on-center-neuron

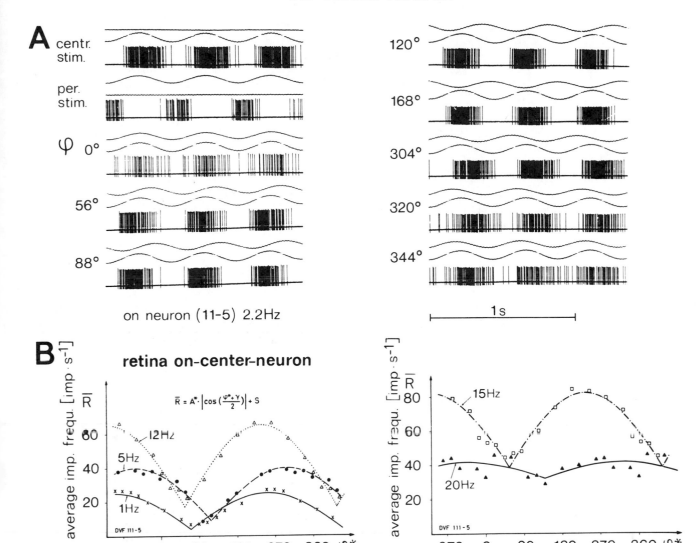

FIGURE 6 Measurement of the dynamic interaction between RF center and RF periphery responses of *on*-center ganglion cells. An RF center light stimulus and an RF periphery stimulus (ring of light) were modulated at the same sine-wave frequency *f* but at different phase angles φ. (A) Recording examples from an X-type *on*-center neuron. Responses to the central stimulus alone (*on* activation) and to the periphery stimulus alone (*off* activation). The neuronal response pattern depended on the φ, which was varied between 0 and 360° (Grüsser and Rackensperger, unpublished observations, 1967; from Grüsser, 1971). (B) Relationship between φ and the average impulse frequency of an *on*-center neuron. The curves were computed from the experimental data according to Equation (6) (minimal chi-square method). Average stimulus luminance $L_0 = 60$ cd/m², $m = 0.9$. (Grüsser, Lütgert, and Rackensperger, unpublished observations, 1970; from van de Grind, Grüsser, and Lunkenheimer, 1973.)

inhibition 2 reached a maximum around 4–8 Hz in most neurons. In contrast, lateral inhibition 1 had its maximum between 1 and 3 Hz. We were tempted to presume that the "distal" lateral inhibition 1 is mediated by the horizontal-cell layer, whereas the faster

"proximal" lateral inhibition 2, like the lateral excitation, is due to a signal processing in amacrines in which the feedback effects through the interplexiform cells and the feedforward effects through conventional amacrines are lumped together. These con clusions derived from black-box experiments can be tested by direct intracellular recordings from neurons located distal to the ganglion-cell layer. So far we have gathered enough intracellular data only from horizontal cells. They will be described in the following section.

Neurophysiology of horizontal cells

The first intracellular recordings from cat retinal horizontal cells were obtained about twenty years ago (Motokawa et al., 1957; Grüsser, 1957, 1958, 1960, 1961; Grüsser and Kapp, 1958; Brown and Wiesel, 1959). Due to the depth measurements of the microelectrode tip, I initially believed the source of the intracellular slow potentials to be synaptic structures of receptors or the inner segments of cones. The work of Steinberg and Schmidt (1970) and of Nelson et al. (1975, 1976), however, provided convincing evidence that the large RF hyperpolarizing potentials recorded in the outer plexiform layer originate in the horizontal cells. We therefore call these potentials *H-potentials*.

THREE DISTINCT TYPES OF HORIZONTAL-CELL RESPONSES   When the bandwidth of the responses to white, photopic flicker stimuli is used as the criterion, our data indicate the existence of at least three types of H-cell responses in the cat retina. To date we have not applied chromatic flicker stimuli, but all H-potentials tested so far with square-wave monochromatic light stimuli have revealed hyperpolarizing responses (Grüsser, 1957; Nelson et al., 1975). The H-cell responses to large ($15° \times 15°$), high modulation ($m = 0.6–0.9$), photopic ($L_0 = 140–200$ cd/m²), sine-wave light stimuli could be grouped unequivocally into three distinct classes on the basis of the critical flicker frequency (CFF): H_n-units had a CFF of 25–40 Hz; H_m-units, 55–70 Hz; and H_w-units, 95–110 Hz. These three classes, H-potentials also had easily distinguishable responses to photopic square-wave stimuli (Figure 7). All of the H-potentials had the following properties:

1. They were all recorded near the margin between the inner nuclear and outer plexiform layer (depth estimated according to Brown and Wiesel, 1959).

2. H-potentials never discharged action potentials.

3. A stable membrane potential of -25 to -50 mV was found (background luminance level ≈ 0.1 cd/m²).

4. A well-defined receptive field exhibiting nonlinear spatial summing properties over areas of at least 4° existed.

5. Independent of stimulus size, shape, intensity, or position within the RF, H-units always responded to illumination with a hyperpolarization of their membrane potential; that is, we did not find an antagonistic depolarizing surround.

6. The increase in hyperpolarization by a luminance increase was considerably faster than the hyperpolarization decrease by an equal luminance decrease. This led to waveform distortions in the sine-wave response, which is characteristic of a system that is nonlinear in the time domain.

THE DYNAMIC RESPONSE OF H-UNITS H_n-units had no oscillatory potentials in their responses to square-wave stimuli (Figure 7). Because of the low CFF, we assume that this class of H-units has a predominant rod input (see also Steinberg, 1969a–c; Niemeyer and Gouras, 1973; Niemeyer, 1975). The photopic H_n-unit responses were at maximum at frequencies up to 2 Hz and attenuated slowly with a slope of about -3 dB/octave up to a "corner" frequency of about 15 Hz. Above this frequency, a maximum attenuation of about -18 dB/octave was found (Figure 9C). The phase relationship between the sine-wave responses and the stimuli is described by the following equation for the phase angle ψ (in degrees):

$$\psi = \Delta t \, 2\pi f. \qquad (7)$$

This is a constant-delay phase relation; Δt was between 40 and 50 msec.

The responses of an H_m-unit to sinusoidally flickering light are illustrated in Figure 8. At low stimulus frequencies (<5 Hz), nonlinear components appeared: the hyperpolarizing phase of the sine-wave response lasted longer than the depolarizing phase, and the hyperpolarization increased faster than it decreased.

The amplitude and phase-response characteristics (Bode plots) of an H_m-unit are shown in Figures 9A and 9B. At photopic stimulus conditions, H_m-units reached a response maximum between 1 and 4 Hz, above which the amplitude of the sine-wave responses was attenuated at -3 dB/octave. All H_m-unit Bode plots obtained with photopic flicker stimuli of a sufficient size exhibited a second maximum at frequencies between 30 and 45 Hz. This second resonance frequency corresponded to the oscillatory potentials seen in the square-wave response (Figure 7F). Above the second maximum, the attenuation of H_m-unit responses reached values up to 36 dB/octave. For the phase angle ψ between stimulus and response, equation 7 was again valid with a constant delay Δt of 25–30 msec (Figure 9B). When the stimulus lumi-

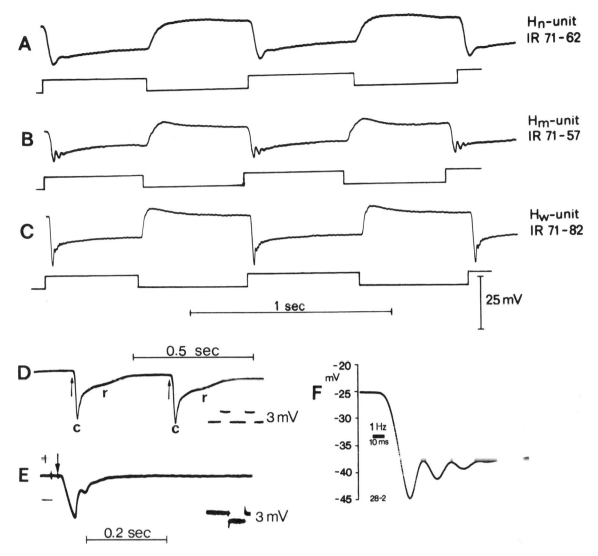

FIGURE 7   Response of three different types of H-units in the light-adapted cat retina. (A–C) Square-wave modulation, $15° \times 15°$ stimulus area. H_n-unit: $L_0 = 200$ cd/m², $m = 0.9$. H_m-unit: $L_0 = 190$ cd/m², $m = 0.72$. H_w-unit: $L_0 = 190$ cd/m², $m = 0.8$. (D) Responses of an H_m-unit to a short (1 msec) light flash. The presumed cone response is marked "c," the presumed rod response "r." (E) Flash response of an H-unit lacking the rod response. (F) Average responses of an H_m-unit to 10 square-wave 1/sec photopic light stimuli. Note the oscillatory potentials. (A–C from Foerster, van de Grind, and Grüsser, 1977a; D from Grüsser, 1961; E from Grüsser and Kapp, 1958; F from Grehn and Stange, unpublished observations, 1976.)

nance was shifted from the photopic to the mesopic range, or when small spots of light were projected to the RF center (e.g., Figure 9A, stimulus diameter 1.5°), the amplitude-frequency response characteristics of H_m-units became similar to those found in H_n-units. One can conclude from these findings that H_m-units received signals from at least two classes of receptors: one was brought to flicker fusion between 20 and 28 Hz (rods), and the other, a cone, reached a response maximum at 30–40 Hz and a flicker fusion frequency of 55–70 Hz.

H_w-units were only recorded at or near the center of the area centralis. Figure 10A shows some of the square-wave responses recorded from one H_w-unit; the amplitude response characteristics are shown in Figure 9D. The latter exhibits two response peaks obtained in a frequency range in which only cones can be assumed to have a flicker response. The lower frequency peak was at 40–45 Hz, the higher at 90–95 Hz. With a fast-frequency sweep, these peaks are easily visible (Figure 10B). When the average intensity L_0 of the sine-wave flicker stimuli was reduced to

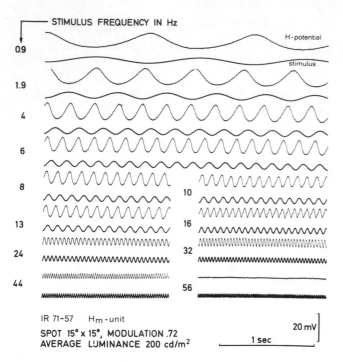

IR 71-57   Hₘ-unit

SPOT 15° x 15°, MODULATION .72
AVERAGE LUMINANCE 200 cd/m²

20 mV

1 sec

FIGURE 8 H_m-unit response to a sinusoidal flicker stimulus. Stimulus parameters as indicated. The upper tracing of each pair is the H_m-potential, the lower tracing is the signal from a photocell monitoring the light stimulus. Note the distortion of the H_m-potential in the low-frequency range. Hyperpolarization is recorded in the downward direction. (From Foerster, van de Grind, and Grüsser, 1977b.)

mesopic stimulus levels and several minutes were allowed for adaptation to this new level, the Bode plots reached a maximum near 2 Hz and again had many similarities with the response characteristics of H_n-units.

As for H_m-units, their upper frequency response maximum (90–95 Hz) corresponded to the frequency of the fast oscillatory potentials seen in the response to photopic square-wave stimuli (Figure 7C).

RECEPTIVE FIELDS AND THE EFFECT OF STIMULUS AREA   All H_n-units had their maximum sensitivity in the RF center. From this point the responses decreased approximately symmetrically, with an exponential function toward the RF periphery (see Nelson, 1977). At low stimulus frequencies (< 2 Hz), the average RF size of H_n-units was consistently larger than that of H_m-units. To compare RF sizes obtained at different stimulus frequencies, we defined a parameter d^* (degrees), the diameter of the round light stimulus (centered to the RF) for which half of the maximum response was obtained. d^* was about 1.4° for H_m-units and 2.2° for H_n-units at 2 Hz. In both H_m- and H_n-units, d^* increased with increasing stim-

ulus frequency. This implies that the spatial and temporal nonlinearities of H-responses influenced each other.

In all H-units, the d^*-values and the sizes of the receptive fields were much larger than the dendritic or axonic spread of single H-cells. Therefore, one has to assume that signals were transmitted within the H-cell syncytium, in accordance with the morphological findings that gap junctions exist between the Cajal-type H-cells in the cat retina (Sobrino and Gallego, 1970).

A nonlinear area-response function is expected from the exponential spatial-sensitivity function (Naka and Rushton, 1967; Werblin, 1970). A test was performed to determine whether linear or nonlinear spatial summation is valid for H-cells. We computed the expected area-response function of the H-cells—assuming linear summing properties to be valid—by applying a linear convolution between the exponential spatial-weighting function and the stimulus area. The area-response relation of H_n-units corresponded well to the computed function, whereas the data obtained in H_m-units deviated significantly from the computed functions. Hence, for H_m-units one has to assume, in addition to the exponential spatial-sensitivity function, a nonlinear spatial summation of the membrane potential changes (for details see Foerster et al., 1977).

HARMONIC ANALYSIS   The intensity functions of all types of horizontal responses formed S-shaped curves when plotted on a semilogarithmic coordinate system. The nonlinear compression of the H-cell responses is well described by a hyperbolic function first applied to vision physiology by Ewald Hering more than a hundred years ago (see also Naka and Rushton, 1966):

$$R = \frac{-k_0 L_0}{1 + k_i L_0}, \qquad (8)$$

where R is the membrane potential change (in mV) and L_0 is the stimulus intensity. The constants k_0 and k_i were different for H_n- and H_m-units and decreased in both types of H-units as the stimulus frequency increased above 2–3 Hz. As Figure 8 demonstrates, the H_m-unit response to low-frequency sine-wave stimuli had a nonsinusoidal shape; that is, nonlinear components appeared. Moreover, the hyperpolarizing phase of the sine-wave response lasted longer than the depolarizing phase, and the hyperpolarization increased faster than it decreased. Similar nonlinearities were obtained in H_n- and H_w-units at low stimulus frequencies. The nonlinear temporal asym-

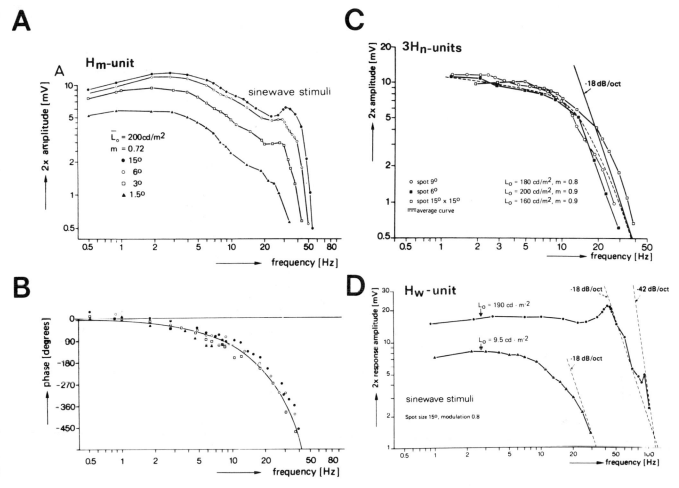

FIGURE 9 Frequency-transfer properties of H-units. (A) Bode plot of an H_m-unit stimulated by sine-wave flicker stimuli of different areas (as indicated). (B) Phase relationship of the responses of the same H_m-unit. The line was computed according to Equation (7). (C) Bode plots of three H_n-units. (D) Bode plots of an H_w-unit with two different L_0 values (as indicated). (From Foerster, van de Grind, and Grüsser, 1977a,b.)

metry can be expressed by a modification of equation 8:

$$R(t) = \frac{-k_0 L(t)}{1 + k_i L(t - \tau)}, \qquad (9)$$

with the delay τ. For sine-wave stimuli this becomes

$$R(t) = \frac{-k_0 L_0 \sin 2\pi f}{1 + k_i L_0 \sin (2\pi f - \tau)}. \qquad (9a)$$

A discrete Fourier analysis performed at an experimental uncertainty level below 3% was used to analyze the nonlinear components in detail. We computed the distortion coefficients

$$d_i = C_i / C_1, \qquad i \geq 2, \qquad (10)$$

where C_i is the constant of the ith harmonic of the

Fourier equation

$$F(x) = C_0 + C_1 \sin (x + \psi_1) + C_2 \sin (2x + \psi_2) \\ + \ldots + C_n \sin (nx + \psi_n), \qquad (11)$$

where C_i and ψ_i represent the amplitude and phase of the ith harmonic component. The significant higher harmonics were lumped together in a *harmonic distortion factor* h:

$$h = \sqrt{\sum_{i=2}^{n} d_i^2}. \qquad (12)$$

The influence of area and frequency on harmonic distortion was quantified by the values of d^* and h. Figure 11 demonstrates that the stimulus frequency has a much stronger effect on the nonlinearity of H-potentials than either area or luminance. Increasing the frequency from 1 Hz to 8 Hz led to a decrease in

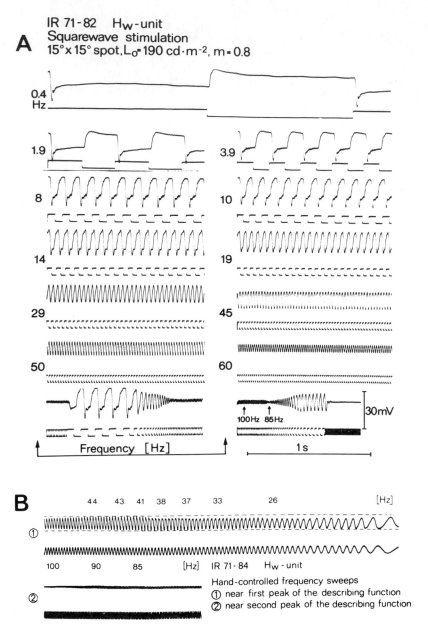

A

IR 71-82 H_W-unit
Squarewave stimulation
$15° × 15°$ spot, $L_0 = 190$ cd·m^{-2}, m = 0.8

0.4 Hz

1.9   3.9

8   10

14   19

29   45

50   60

↑ ↑
100Hz 85Hz

30mV

Frequency [Hz]   1s

B

44 43 41 38 37 33   26   [Hz]

①

100   90   85   [Hz]   IR 71-84 H_W-unit

②

Hand-controlled frequency sweeps
① near first peak of the describing function
② near second peak of the describing function

FIGURE 10   Flicker responses of cone-dominated H_w-units. (A) H_w-unit response to square-wave flicker stimuli. Note the high-frequency oscillatory response at light *on*. Square-wave stimulus frequencies as indicated. The bottom row shows responses to rapid changes in stimulus frequency. A resonance is visible at about 95 Hz. (From Foerster, van de Grind, and Grüsser, 1977a.) (B) Responses of H_w-unit to a fast-frequency sweep (sine-wave flicker stimuli) in the frequency range of the two peaks of the describing function (peak 1: 43 Hz; peak 2: 95 Hz). (From Foerster, van de Grind, and Grüsser, unpublished observations, 1971.)

the distortion factor h from 24% to 10% (Figure 11A), whereas the response amplitude within this range changed by no more than 20% (Figure 9A). This contrasts with the influence of stimulus area A on the distortion factor and on the amplitude. A hundred-fold decrease in A led to decrease in h from 24% to 17% (Figure 11B), but to a reduction of approximately 50% in the amplitude (Figure 9B). Thus the

harmonic distortion was not simply proportional to the H-potential amplitude and was, therefore, not due to a simple "saturation" effect.

INTERPRETATION OF H-UNIT RESPONSES   The rod-cone ratio is 17:1 in the cat retina centralis and about 100:1 in the retinal periphery (Holländer and Stone, 1972; Steinberg, Reid, and Lacy, 1973). Besides dif-

264   O.-J. GRÜSSER

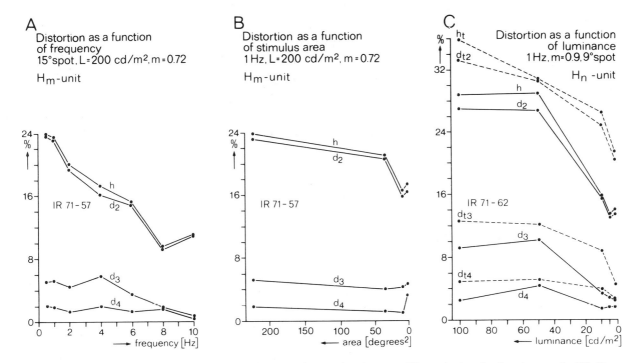

A

Distortion as a function
of frequency
15° spot, L=200 cd/m², m=0.72

H_m-unit

B

Distortion as a function
of stimulus area
1 Hz, L=200 cd/m², m=0.72

H_m-unit

C

Distortion as a function
of luminance
1 Hz, m=0.9, 9° spot

H_n-unit

FIGURE 11 Harmonic distortion factor h and the contribution of the second (d_2), third (d_3), and fourth (d_4) harmonics are plotted as a function of stimulus frequency (A), stimulus area (B), and stimulus luminance L_0 (C). Responses from H_m-unit (A, B) and an H_n-unit (C). (From Foerster, van de Grind, and Grüsser, 1977b.)

ferent spectral sensitivities, rod and cone responses differ in the maximum CFF. Under optimal stimulus conditions, rods are believed to reach flicker fusion in a frequency range ≤25 Hz (Schatternikoff, 1902; von Kries, 1903), whereas cones can obtain values of up to 110 Hz (see van de Grind et al., 1973). This high-frequency CFF for at least one type of cone is corroborated by our present findings in H_w-cells. "Red," "green," and "blue" cones are believed to have different frequency-response characteristics; that is, they reach their response maximum and their CFF at different flicker frequencies. Again this fits in well with the multipeak H_w-unit Bode plots, if one assumes that H_w-units receive more than one cone input. Under these conditions, a fairly clear-cut interpretation of the experimental data in H-units is possible:

1. All H-units recorded receive a mixed rod-cone input. The cone component in H_n-units, however, is very small. H_n-unit responses are rod-dominated. H-units that have a rod spectral sensitivity curve have been described by Steinberg (1969a), Niemeyer (1975) and Nelson et al. (1975, 1976) and have been attributed to the axon terminals of the Cajal-type H-cells.

2. H_m-units receive a mixed rod-cone input in which one of the two receptor types dominates, depending on the stimulus intensity and frequency. Therefore, H_m-units should have a mixed rod-cone spectral sensitivity curve. The green cone, which is dominant for the cat retina (maximum sensitivity at 556 nm: Granit, 1950), is proposed as a probable candidate. This cone type also dominates ganglion-cell responses in the light-adapted cat retina (Daw and Pearlman, 1969, 1970; Andrews and Hammond, 1970a,b; Hammond and James, 1971). Steinberg (1969b,c), Niemeyer and Gouras (1973), Niemeyer (1975), and Nelson (1977) described H-unit responses with a mixed rod-green cone input.

3. H_w-units have an input from *more* than two types of receptors: rods plus two or three types of cones. For the two H_w-units recorded for a sufficient length of time, only the upper-frequency maximum of the Bode plots was at similar frequencies; the lower one differed significantly. This indicates that only one type of cone input was identical for both H_w-units, and the other differed. We therefore postulate the existence of three different cones in the cat retina (somewhat surprising considering that cats have such poor color vision). Saunders (1973, 1977), however, has recently described chromatic response properties of cat retinal ganglion cells and lateral-geniculate-body neurons that can be explained only if one assumes the existence of three different types of cones.

4. The A-horizontal cells form a syncytium. Hence the effective receptive field of a single H-unit, and also the area from which the receptor-bipolar synapses are modifiable, are considerably larger than would be expected on the basis of the dendritic trees of individual H-cells.

5. The upper-frequency responses of H-cells reflect nothing other than the response limits of the fastest receptors acting as inputs to the horizontal cells. There is no experimental evidence that the horizontal-cell membrane by itself acts as a low-pass filter effective in the frequency range up to 100 Hz. In recent experiments (Grüsser, Lindau, and Schreiter, unpublished observations, 1977), we found that *on*-center and *off*-center ganglion cells respond to sine-wave electrical polarization of the retina up to frequencies between 150 and 180 Hz. These findings indicate that the excitatory retinal structures proximal to the receptor layers, especially the ganglion cells, probably do not constitute the frequency-limiting parts for normal retinal signal transmission.

6. H-units, especially of the most often encountered H_m-type, reach a response maximum between 1 and 3 Hz. This is also true of the maximum found for lateral inhibition 1. This correspondence supports the view that horizontal cells mediate lateral inhibition 1. One possible objection stems from the rather low flicker-fusion frequency of lateral inhibition 1, in the range of about 20 Hz (photopic stimulus conditions). This may, however, express the upper frequency limit of the shunting inhibitory mechanisms between the horizontal cells and the receptor-bipolar synaptic complex discussed in the next section.

7. Comparing the responses of H_n-, H_m-, and H_w-units at different luminance levels, it seems probable that the H-unit response maximum reached between 1 and 3 Hz is due to a corresponding maximum of the rod input. Rods respond more slowly and contribute a larger value to Δt in equation 7. The longer delay and lower frequency-response characteristics of the rod component of H_m-units appearing in the flash responses after the initial fast hyperpolarization also support this view. This late rod response, however, is not found in all H-units (Figure 7D,E).

How do horizontal cells interact with the signal transmission between receptors and bipolar cells?

In the preceding sections, data were presented from which one can deduce that horizontal cells form a network that regulates the signal flow between receptors and bipolar cells. Due to the relatively isomorphic structure of the retina, this lateral interaction affects not only the signals elicited from the receptors located in the RF center of a ganglion cell, but also the signals elicited from the RF periphery and mediated predominantly through the amacrines to the ganglion-cell membrane.

One can conceive of different modes by which horizontal cells might interact with the signal transmission between receptors and bipolar cells:

1. The first possibility to be considered is the feedback mechanism from the horizontal cells to the receptor membrane (see Dowling, this volume). This mechanism, like the receptor-receptor contacts, would increase the effective receptive field of a single photoreceptor beyond the area of its outer segment.

2. The second possibility is the synaptic interaction between conventional chemical synapses or nonconventional synapses formed by horizontal-cell dendrites on bipolar-cell dendrites outside the triad structure (Figure 12). According to Fisher and Boycott (1974), such conventional synapses are formed by A-horizontal cells, whereas the efferent synaptic connections of B-horizontal cells have not yet been uncovered. In a recent study, however, Kolb (1977) concluded from her electron-microscopic data that all chemical synapses found at bipolar-cell dendrites in the outer plexiform layer are endings from interplexiform cells and that A-horizontal cells form nonconventional synapses with the membrane of bipolar-cell dendrites.

3. There are several other alternatives by which horizontal cells, without using conventional synaptic contacts, might still modify signal transmission between receptors and bipolar cells. A few years ago,

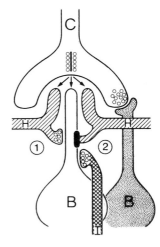

FIGURE 12 Scheme of the possible connections between A-type horizontal cells (H) and bipolar cells (B). 1: Fisher-Boycott-type. 2 = Kolb-type. C = cone. I = interplexiform cell.

266   O.-J. GRÜSSER

Svaetichin et al. (1965, 1971) proposed a chemical interaction between the transmitter released from the receptor terminals and an inactivating enzyme released by horizontal-cell dendrites (see also Rodieck, 1973). This interaction is supposed to take place within the synaptic cleft. Svaetichin et al. presumed that the enzyme counteracting the transmitter is released according to the level of polarization of the bipolar-cell dendrites.

4. Another possibility is interaction by "competition" for the transmitter released at a very restricted part of the presynaptic photoreceptor membrane in the region of the ribbon structure. If the transmitter is an electrically charged molecule, it does not move by free diffusion across the synaptic cleft alone; its movement and distribution also depend on the voltage gradient across the synaptic cleft. This gradient depends in turn on the current flowing through the outer and inner segments of the photoreceptors, as well as on the membrane potential and the current flowing through the bipolar-cell and horizontal-cell dendrites within the receptor pedicles. The fraction of the transmitter molecules discharged per unit of time which reach either the bipolar-cell dendrite or the horizontal-cell dendrite would therefore depend on the relative membrane potentials of the two structures. Thus the horizontal-cell membrane potential can control the relative number of transmitter molecules reaching the molecular receptors in the bipolar-cell membrane without a direct contact to this membrane. I like to call this interaction "control of synaptic efficacy by competition for the same transmitter."

5. Another mechanism falling into the same class of neuronal interaction is conceivable if one assumes that the transmitter turnover in the postsynaptic membrane depends on the activity level of the receptor molecule in the subsynaptic membrane. The data presented by Schwartz (this volume) indicate that the electrical potential across the cell membrane might influence the configuration of large molecules. If this is also true for receptor molecules in horizontal-cell and bipolar-cell dendritic membranes, and if a change in molecular configuration changes the speed of transmitter/receptor interaction, a further mechanism would be added by which horizontal cells could influence the interaction between receptors and bipolar cells. The concentration gradient between the site of transmitter release and the sites of transmitter action then becomes dependent on the speed of transmitter/receptor interaction at the postsynaptic membranes competing for the same transmitter.

Indirect interactions between horizontal cells and bipolar cells by competition for the same transmitter would certainly constitute a rather unorthodox way for neighboring neurons to interact. I think, however, that this interpretation has the advantage of making meaningful the extremely restricted location of vesicles at a ribbon-type synapse and the highly focalized transmitter release from the presynaptic membrane.

What do horizontal cells contribute to ganglion-cell receptive-field organization?

I have described above experimental data indicating the existence of at least two types of lateral inhibitory mechanisms interacting with the signal flow between receptors and ganglion cells and contributing to the functional organization of the ganglion-cell receptive field. When one compares the frequency properties of the lateral shunting inhibition 1 and the lateral subtractive inhibition 2 with the frequency-transfer properties of horizontal cells in the light-adapted retina, one finds that the class of horizontal cells most frequently encountered in our experiments (H_m-units) has a response maximum in a frequency range 1–3 Hz, which corresponds to the maximum of lateral inhibition 1. This coincidence of frequency properties does not exist, however, for the higher-frequency portion (>20 Hz). Therefore, if our conjecture that H_m-units transmit lateral inhibition 1 is correct, we have to assume that a low-pass filter with a frequency cutoff around 20 Hz limits the interaction between horizontal cells and the signal flow between receptors and bipolar cells. It is conceivable that such a low-pass filter is present for the nonconventional forms of synaptic interaction between horizontal cells and bipolar cells discussed in the preceding section.

The idea of a *shunting inhibition* mediated by horizontal cells is expressed by the following equation, in which B is the depolarization of *on* bipolar cells (in mV), r_i the receptor potential of one of the n receptors feeding directly into the bipolar cell considered, and h_j is the membrane potential of one of m horizontal cells connected with the bipolar cell:

$$B = \frac{-k_r \sum_n r_i}{1 + k_h \sum_m h_j};$$ \hfill (13)

k_r and k_h would be differently dependent on the flicker frequency; k_h is attenuated at a lower flicker frequency than k_r, thus making the functional organization of the bipolar cell dependent on flicker frequency. Because B is an input signal to the ganglion cell, the horizontal cells not only control this input, but modify it in relation to the temporal stimulus frequency.

Horizontal cells might also functionally connect receptors with each other, although no direct physiological evidence is found in the cat retina for such a feedback function. Nevertheless, horizontal cells should be kept in mind as possibly responsible for receptor-receptor interactions, including the suppression of cone signals in the dark-adapted retina.

Finally, horizontal cells might form an adaptation pool integrating the average retinal illumination level over a region far beyond the diameter of a ganglion-cell RF and making signal flow between receptors and bipolars dependent on the average retinal illumination. Such a function is consistent with equation 13 if k_r, k_h and h_j are not zero at frequencies near 0 Hz. This condition is fulfilled at least by h_j, because the horizontal-cell light-induced hyperpolarizing potential is still visible two minutes after the light stimulus is turned on.

ACKNOWLEDGMENT This work was supported by grants from the Deutsche Forschungsgemeinschaft (Gr 161). The skillful technical assistance of M. Klingbeil, J. Dames, and K. Krawczynski and the accurate typing of J. Axhausen are gratefully acknowledged. Part of the experiments were supported by a twinning grant from the European Training Program in Brain and Behavior (1975, 1976) to the working groups of the author in Berlin and to W. A. van de Grind in Amsterdam. Much of the experimental data described in the section on the neurophysiology of horizontal cells was obtained in collaboration with M. Foerster and W. A. van de Grind.

REFERENCES

ANDREWS, D. P., and P. HAMMOND, 1970a. Mesopic increment threshold spectral sensitivity of single optic tract fibres in the cat: Cone-rod interaction. *J. Physiol.* 209:65–81.

ANDREWS, D. P., and P. HAMMOND, 1970b. Suprathreshold spectral properties of single optic tract fibres in cat, under mesopic adaptation: Cone-rod interaction. *J. Physiol.* 209:83–103.

BARLOW, H. B., R. FITZHUGH, and S. W. KUFFLER, 1957. Change of organization in the receptive fields of the cat's retina during dark adaptation. *J. Physiol.* 137:338–354.

BAUMGARTNER, G., and P. HAKAS, 1962. Die Neurophysiologie des simultanen Helligkeitskontrastes. Reziproke Reaktionen antagonistischer Neuronengruppen des visuellen Systems. *Pflügers Arch.* 274:489–510.

BAYLOR, D. A., M. G. F. FUORTES, and P. M. O'BRYAN, 1971. Receptive fields of cones in the retina of the turtle. *J. Physiol.* 214:265–294.

BISHOP, G. H., M. H. CLARE, and W. U. LANDAU, 1969. Further analysis of fiber groups in the optic tract of the cat. *Exp. Neurol.* 24:386–399.

BISHOP, P. O., D. JEREMY, and J. W. LANCE, 1953. The optic nerve: Properties of a central tract. *J. Physiol.* 121:415–432.

BOYCOTT, B. B., J. E. DOWLING, S. K. FISCHER, H. KOLB, and A. M. LATIES, 1975. Interplexiform cells of the mammalian retina and their comparison with catecholamine-containing retinal cells. *Proc. R. Soc. Lond.* B191:353–368.

BOYCOTT, B. B., and H. KOLB, 1973. The connections between the bipolar cells and photoreceptors in the retina of the domestic cat. *J. Comp. Neurol.* 148:92–114.

BOYCOTT, B. B., and H. WÄSSLE, 1974. The morphological types of ganglion cells of the domestic cat's retina. *J. Physiol.* 240:397–419.

BROWN, K. T., and M. MURAKAMI, 1968. Rapid effects of light and dark adaptation upon the receptive field organization of S-potentials and late receptor potentials. *Vision Res.* 8:1145–1171.

BROWN, K. T., and T. N. WIESEL, 1959. Intraretinal recording with micropipette electrodes in the intact cat eye. *J. Physiol.* 149:537–562.

BUETTNER, U. W., 1973. Quantitative Untersuchungen zur Wechselwirkung zwischen Zentrum und Peripherie des rezeptiven Feldes retinaler Ganglienzellen der Katze. Phasische Reizung im Zentrum des rezeptiven Feldes bei konstanter Belichtung der Peripherie. Doctoral dissertation, Freie Universität Berlin.

BUETTNER-MÖNNINGHOFF, E., 1976. Quantitative Untersuchungen zur Wechselwirkung zwischen Zentrum und Peripherie des rezeptiven Feldes retinaler Ganglienzellen der Katze. Phasische Reizung in der Peripherie des rezeptiven Feldes bei konstanter Belichtung des Zentrums. Doctoral dissertation, Freie Universität Berlin.

BÜTTNER, CH., U. BÜTTNER, U. EYSEL, O.-J. GRÜSSER, H.-U. LUNKENHEIMER, and D. SCHAIBLE, 1971. Spatial summation in the receptive fields of cat's retinal ganglion cells. I. Summation within the RF-center. In *Proceedings of the First European Biophysics Congress,* E. Broda, A. Locker, and H. Springer-Lederer, eds. Vienna: Verlag der Wiener Medizinischen Akademie, pp. 257–261.

BÜTTNER, CH., U. BÜTTNER, and O.-J. GRÜSSER, 1971. Interaction of excitation and direct inhibition in the receptive field center of retinal neurons. *Eur. J. Physiol.* 322:1–21.

BÜTTNER, U., and O.-J. GRÜSSER, 1968. Quantitative Untersuchungen der räumlichen Erregungssummation im rezeptiven Feld retinaler Neurone der Katze. I. Reizung mit zwei synchronen Lichtpunkten. *Kybernetik* 4:81–94.

BÜTTNER, U., O.-J. GRÜSSER, and E. SCHWANZ, 1975. The effect of area and intensity on the response of cat retinal ganglion cells to brief light flashes. *Exp. Brain Res.* 23:259–278.

CLELAND, B. G., M. W. DUBIN, and W. R. LEVICK, 1971. Sustained and transient neurones in the cat's retina and lateral geniculate nucleus. *J. Physiol.* 217:473–496.

CLELAND, B., and CH. ENROTH-CUGELL, 1966. Cat retinal ganglion cell responses to changing light intensities: Sinusoidal modulation in the time domain. *Acta Physiol. Scand.* 68:365–381.

CLELAND, B. G., C. ENROTH-CUGELL, 1970. Quantitative aspects of gain and latency in the cat retina. *J. Physiol.* 206:73–91.

CLELAND, B. G., and W. R. LEVICK, 1974a. Brisk and sluggish concentrically organized ganglion cells in the cat's retina. *J. Physiol.* 240:421–456.

CLELAND, B. G., and W. R. LEVICK, 1974b. Properties of rarely encountered types of ganglion cells in the cat's retina and an overall classification. *J. Physiol.* 240:457–492.

CLELAND, B. G., W. R. LEVICK, and K. J. SANDERSON, 1973. Properties of sustained and transient ganglion cells in the cat retina. *J. Physiol.* 228:649–680.

CLELAND, B. G., W. R. LEVICK, and H. WÄSSLE, 1975. Physiological identification of a morphological class of cat retinal ganglion cells. *J. Physiol.* 248:151–171.

CLELAND, B. G., R. MORSTYN, H. G. WAGNER, and W. R. LEVICK, 1975. Long-latency retinal input to lateral geniculate neurones of the cat. *Brain Res.* 91:306–310.

DAW, N. W., and A. L. PEARLMAN, 1969. Cat colour vision: One cone process or several? *J. Physiol.* 201:745–764.

DAW, N. W., and A. L. PEARLMAN, 1970. Cat colour vision: Evidence for more than one cone process. *J. Physiol.* 211:125–137.

DODT, E., and C. ENROTH, 1954. Retinal flicker response in cat. *Acta Physiol. Scand.* 30:375–390.

DOMBERG, H., 1972. Die Veränderungen der Größe des rezeptiven Feldzentrums retinaler on-Zentrum-Neurone der Katze bei verschiedener Lichtadaptation. Doctoral dissertation, Freie Universität Berlin.

DONNER, K. O., 1950. The spike frequencies of mammalian retinal elements as a function of wave-length of light. *Acta Physiol. Scand.* 21:7–59.

DONNER, K. O., and E. N. WILLMER, 1950. An analysis of the response from single visual-purple-dependent elements, in the retina of the cat. *J. Physiol.* 111:160–173.

DONOVAN, A., 1967. The nerve fibre composition of the cat optic nerve. *J. Anat.* 101:1–11.

DOWLING, J. E., and F. S. WERBLIN, 1969. Organization of retina of the mudpuppy, Necturus maculosus. I. Synaptic structure. *J. Neurophysiol.* 32:315–338.

ECCLES, J. C., 1964. *The Physiology of Synapses.* Berlin-Göttingen-Heidelberg-New York: Springer-Verlag.

ENROTH, CH., 1952. The mechanism of flicker and fusion studied on single retinal elements in the dark-adapted eye of the cat. *Acta Physiol. Scand.* 27 (Suppl., 100): 1–67.

ENROTH-CUGELL, CH., and P. LENNIE, 1975. The control of retinal ganglion cell discharge by receptive field surrounds. *J. Physiol.* 247:551–578.

ENROTH-CUGELL, CH., P. LENNIE, and R. M. SHAPLEY, 1975. Surround contribution to light adaptation in cat retinal ganglion cells. *J. Physiol.* 247:579–588.

ENROTH-CUGELL, CH., and L. PINTO, 1970. Algebraic summation of centre and surround inputs to retinal ganglion cells of the cat. *Nature* 226:458–459.

ENROTH-CUGELL, CH., and L. H. PINTO, 1972. Properties of the surround response mechanism of cat retinal ganglion cells and centre-surround interaction. *J. Physiol.* 220:403–439.

ENROTH-CUGELL, CH., and L. H. PINTO, 1972. Pure central responses from off-centre cells and pure surround responses from on-centre cells. *J. Physiol.* 220:441–461.

ENROTH-CUGELL, CH., and J. G. ROBSON, 1966. The contrast sensitivity of retinal ganglion cells of the cat. *J. Physiol.* 187:517–552.

EYSEL, U. TH., 1976. Quantitative studies of intracellular postsynaptic potentials in the lateral geniculate nucleus of the cat with respect to optic tract stimulus response latencies. *Exp. Brain Res.* 25:469–486.

EYSEL, U. TH., and O.-J. GRÜSSER, 1974. Simultaneous recording of pre- and postsynaptic potentials during degeneration of optic tract fiber input to the cat lateral geniculate nucleus. *Brain Res.* 81:552–557.

EYSEL, U. TH., and O.-J. GRÜSSER, 1975. Intracellular postsynaptic potentials of cat lateral geniculate cells and the effects of degeneration of the optic tract terminals. *Brain Res.* 98:441–455.

FAIN, G. L., G. H. GOLD, and J. E. DOWLING, 1975. Receptor coupling in the toad retina. *Cold Spring Harbor Symp. Quant. Biol.* 40:547–561.

FAMIGLIETTI, E. V., and H. KOLB, 1975. A bistratified amacrine cell and synaptic circuitry in the inner plexiform layer of the retina. *Brain Res.* 84:293–300.

FAMIGLIETTI, E. V., and H. KOLB, 1976. Structural basis for on- and off-center responses in retinal ganglion cells. *Science* 194:193–195.

FISHER, S. K., and B. B. BOYCOTT, 1974. Synaptic connections made by horizontal cells within the outer plexiform layer of the cat and the rabbit. *Proc. R. Soc. Lond.* B186:317–331.

FOERSTER, M. H., W. A. VAN DE GRIND, and O.-J. GRÜSSER, 1977a. Frequency transfer properties of three distinct types of cat horizontal cells. *Exp. Brain Res.* 30:347–366.

FOERSTER, M. H., W. A. VAN DE GRIND, and O.-J. GRÜSSER, 1977b. The response of cat horizontal cells to flicker stimuli of different area, intensity and frequency. *Exp. Brain Res.* 30:367–385.

FREUND, H.-J., and G. GRÜNEWALD, 1969. Räumliche Summation und Hemmungsvorgänge im rezeptiven Feldzentrum von Retina-Neuronen der Katze. *Exp. Brain Res.* 8:37–52.

FREUND, H.-J., M. HENNERICI, and U. RABENSCHLAG, 1977. Reversal of surround-into-centre-type responses of cat retinal ganglion cells by local darkening of the receptive field centre. *Vision Res.* 17:487–494.

FUKUDA, Y., 1971. Receptive field organization of cat optic nerve fibers with special reference to conduction velocity. *Vision Res.* 11:209–226.

FUKUDA, Y., and J. STONE, 1974. Retinal distribution and central projections of Y-, X-, and W-cells of the cat's retina. *J. Neurophysiol.* 37:749–772.

FUKUDA, Y., K. MOTOKAWA, A. C. NORTON, and K. TASAKI, 1966. Functional significance of conduction velocity in the transfer of flicker information in the optic nerve of the cat. *J. Neurophysiol.* 29:698–714.

FURMAN, G. G., 1965. Comparison of models for subtractive and shunting lateral inhibition in receptor-neuron fields. *Kybernetik* 2:257–274.

GALLEGO, A., 1965. Connexions transversales au niveau des couches plexiformes de la rétine. *Actualités Neurophysiologiques*, 6e ser., M. Monnier, ed. Paris: Masson, pp. 5–27.

GALLEGO, A., 1964–1965. Connexions transversales au niveau des couches plexiformes de la rétine. *Ann. Inst. Farm. Exp.* 13/14:181–204.

GALLEGO, A., 1971. Horizontal and amacrine cells in the mammal's retina. *Vision Res.* (Suppl.) 3:33–50.

GRANIT, R., 1943. The spectral properties of the visual receptors of the cat. *Acta Physiol. Scand.* 3:219–229.

GRANIT, R., 1947. *Sensory Mechanisms of the Retina.* London: Oxford University Press.

GRANIT, R., 1948. Neural organization of the retinal elements, as revealed by polarization. *J. Neurophysiol.* 11:239–251.

GRANIT, R., 1950. The organization of the vertebrate retinal elements. *Ergeb. Physiol.* 46:31–70.

GRIND, W. A. VAN DE, O.-J. GRÜSSER, and H. U. LUNKENHEIMER, 1973. Temporal transfer properties of the afferent visual system. Psychophysical, neurophysiological and theoretical investigations. *Handbook of Sensory Physiology,* VII/3, R. Jung, ed. Berlin-Heidelberg-New York: Springer-Verlag, chapter 7.

GRÜSSER, O.-J., 1956. Reaktionen einzelner corticaler und retinaler Neurone der Katze auf Flimmerlicht und ihre Beziehungen zur subjektiven Sinnesphysiologie. Doctoral dissertation, Freiburg i.Br.

GRÜSSER, O.-J., 1957. Rezeptorpotentiale einzelner retinaler Zapfen der Katze. *Naturwissenschaften* 44:522.

GRÜSSER, O.-J., 1958. Rezeptorpotentiale einzelner retinaler Zapfen der Katze. *Pflügers Arch.* 268:47.

GRÜSSER, O.-J., 1960. Rezeptorabhängige Potentiale der Katzenretina und ihre Reaktionen auf Flimmerlicht. *Pflügers Arch.* 271:511–525.

GRÜSSER, O.-J., 1961. Rezeptorabhängige R-Potentiale der Katzenretina. In *Neurophysiologie und Psychophysik des visuellen Systems.* R. Jung und H. Kornhuber, eds. Berlin: Springer-Verlag, pp. 56–61.

GRÜSSER, O.-J., 1971. A quantitative analysis of spatial summation of excitation and inhibition within the receptive field of retinal ganglion cells of cats. *Vision Res.* (Suppl.) 3:103–127.

GRÜSSER, O.-J., 1977. Subcortical and cortical mechanisms of visual contrast: Behavioural, electrophysiological, and developmental aspects. In *Spatial Contrast,* H. Spekreijse and L. H. van der Tweel, eds. Amsterdam: North-Holland, pp. 96–99.

GRÜSSER, O.-J., and O. CREUTZFELDT, 1957. Eine neurophysiologische Grundlage des Brücke-Bartley-Effektes: Maxima der Impulsfrequenz retinaler und corticaler Neurone bei Flimmerlicht mittlerer Frequenzen. *Pflügers Arch.* 263:668–681.

GRÜSSER, O.-J., and U. GRÜSSER-CORNEHLS, 1962. Periodische Aktivierungsphasen visueller Neurone nach kurzen Lichtreizen verschiedener Dauer. *Pflügers Arch.* 275:292–311.

GRÜSSER, O.-J., and U. GRÜSSER-CORNEHLS, 1973. Neuronal mechanisms of visual movement perception and some psychophysical and behavioral correlations. In *Handbook of Sensory Physiology,* VII/3A, R. Jung, ed. Berlin-Heidelberg-New York: Springer-Verlag, pp. 334–428.

GRÜSSER, O.-J., and U. GRÜSSER-CORNEHLS, 1976. Neurophysiology of the anuran visual system. In *Frog Neurobiology: A Handbook,* R. Llinás and W. Precht, eds. Berlin-Heidelberg-New York: Springer-Verlag, pp. 297–385.

GRÜSSER, O.-J., and A. GRÜTZNER, 1958. Neurophysiologische Grundlagen der periodischen Nachbildphasen nach kurzen Lichtblitzen. *Graefes Arch. Ophthalmol.* 160:65–93.

GRÜSSER, O.-J., and H. KAPP, 1958. Reaktionen retinaler Neurone nach Lichtblitzen. II. Doppelblitze mit wechselndem Blitzintervall. *Pflügers Arch.* 266:111–129.

GRÜSSER, O.-J., H.-U. LUNKENHEIMER, M. LÜTGERT, W. RACKENSPERGER, and W. WUTTKE, 1971. Spatial summation in the receptive fields of cat's retinal ganglion cells. II. Summation within the RF-periphery. In *Proceedings of the First European Biophysics Congress,* E. Broda, A. Locker, and H. Springer-Lederer, eds. Vienna: Verlag der Wiener Medizinischen Akademie, pp. 263–266.

GRÜSSER, O.-J., and C. REIDEMEISTER, 1959. Flimmerlichtuntersuchungen an der Katzenretina. II. Off-Neurone und Besprechung der Ergebnisse. *Z. Biol.* 111:254–270.

GRÜSSER, O.-J., D. SCHAIBLE, and J. VIERKANT-GLATHE, 1970. A quantitative analysis of the spatial summation of excitation within the receptive field centers of retinal neurons. *Pflügers Arch.* 319:101–121.

GRÜSSER, O.-J., U. GRÜSSER-CORNEHLS, and D. STANGE, 1977. Simultaneous contrast experiments in cat retinal ganglion cells. *Eur. J. Physiol.* 368:R.42.

GRÜSSER-CORNEHLS, U., and O.-J. GRÜSSER, 1960. Mikroelektrodenuntersuchungen am Geniculatum laterale der Katze: Nervenzell-und Axonentladungen nach elektrischer Opticusreizung. *Pflügers Arch.* 271:50–63.

GRÜSSER-CORNEHLS, U., and R. McD. SAUNDERS, 1978. The chromatic responses of frog retinal neurons to stationary and moving stimuli. Submitted.

HAMASAKI, D. I., R. CAMPBELL, J. ZENGEL, and L. R. HAZELTON, 1973. Response of cat retinal ganglion cells to moving stimuli. *Vision Res.* 13:1421–1432.

HAMMOND, P., 1974. Cat retinal ganglion cells: Size and shape of receptive field centres. *J. Physiol.* 242:99–118.

HAMMOND, P., 1975. Receptive field mechanisms of sustained and transient retinal ganglion cells in the cat. *Exp. Brain Res.* 23:113–128.

HAMMOND, P., and C. R. JAMES, 1971. The Purkinje shift in cat: Extend of the mesopic range. *J. Physiol.* 216:99–109.

HERING, E., 1874. Zur Lehre vom Lichtsinne. V. Grundzüge einer Theorie des Lichtsinnes. *Sitzungsber. Kais. Akad. Wiss. Wien* (Math.-Nat. Classe, Abth. III) 69:179–217.

HOFFMANN, K. P., J. STONE, and S. M. SHERMAN, 1972. Relay of receptive field properties in dorsal lateral geniculate nucleus of the cat. *J. Neurophysiol.* 35:518–531.

HOLLÄNDER, H., and J. STONE, 1972. Rod pedicle density in the cat's retina. *Brain Res.* 42:497–502.

HUBEL, D. H., 1957. A tungsten microelectrode for recording from single units. *Science* 125:549–550.

HUBEL, D. H., and T. N. WIESEL, 1968. Receptive fields and functional architecture of monkey striate cortex. *J. Physiol.* 195:215–243.

HUBEL, D. H., and T. N. WIESEL, 1972. Laminar and columnar distribution of geniculo-cortical fibers in the macaque monkey. *J. Comp. Neurol.* 146:421–450.

HUGHES, A., 1975. A quantitative analysis of the cat retinal ganglion cell topography. *J. Comp. Neurol.* 163:107–128.

HUGHES, A., and H. WÄSSLE, 1976. The cat optic nerve: Fibre total count and diameter spectrum. *J. Comp. Neurol.* 169:171–184.

IKEDA, H., and M. J. WRIGHT, 1972. The outer disinhibitory surround of the retinal ganglion cell receptive field. *J. Physiol.* 226:511–544.

IKEDA, H., and M. J. WRIGHT, 1972. Receptive field organization of "sustained" and "transient" retinal ganglion cells which subserve different functional roles. *J. Physiol.* 227:769–800.

JAKIELA, H. G., and C. ENROTH-CUGELL, 1976. Adaptation

and dynamics in x-cells and y-cells of the cat retina. *Exp. Brain Res.* 24:335–342.

JERISON, H. J., 1973. Evolution of the brain and intelligence. New York: Academic Press, p. 482.

JUNG, R., 1953. Allgemeine Neurophysiologie. In *Handbuch der Inneren Medizin*, V/1, pp. 1–181.

KANEKO, A., 1970. Physiological and morphological identification of horizontal, bipolar, and amacrine cells in goldfish. *J. Physiol.* 207:623–633.

KANEKO, A., 1971a. Physiological studies of single cells and their morphological identification. *Vision Res.* (Suppl.) 3:17–26.

KANEKO, A., 1971b. Electrical connexions between horizontal cells in the dogfish retina. *J. Physiol.* 213:95–105.

KANEKO, A., 1973. Receptive field organization of bipolar and amacrine cells in the goldfish retina. *J. Physiol.* 235:133–153.

KANEKO, A., and H. SHIMAZAKI, 1975. Effects of external ions on the synaptic transmission from photoreceptors to horizontal cells in the carp retina. *J. Physiol.* 252:509–522.

KELLY, J. P., and CH. D. GILBERT, 1975. The projections of different morphological types of ganglion cells in the cat retina. *J. Comp. Neurol.* 163:65–80.

KIRK, D. L., B. G. CLELAND, H. WÄSSLE, and W. R. LEVICK, 1975. Axonal conduction latencies of cat retinal ganglion cells in central and peripheral retina. *Exp. Brain Res.* 23:85–90.

KOLB, H., 1974. The connections between horizontal cells and photoreceptors in the retina of the cat: electron microscopy of Golgi preparations. *J. Comp. Neurol.* 155:1–14.

KOLB, H., 1977. The organization of the outer plexiform layer in the retina of the cat: electron microscopic observations. *J. Neurocytol.* 6:131–153.

KOLB, H., and R. W. WEST, 1977. Synaptic connections of the interplexiform cell in the retina of the cat. *J. Neurocytol.* 6:155–170.

KRIES, J. VON, 1903. Über die Wahrnehmung des Flimmerns durch normale und durch total farbblinde Personen. *Z. Sinnesphysiol.* 32:113–117.

KUFFLER, ST. W., 1952. Neurons in the retina: Organization, inhibition and excitation problems. *Cold Spring Harbor Symp. Quant. Biol.* 17:281–292.

KUFFLER, S. W., 1953. Discharge patterns and functional organisation of mammalian retina. *J. Neurophysiol.* 16:37–68.

LASANSKY, A., 1972. Cell junctions at the outer synaptic layer of the retina. *Invest. Ophthalmol.* 11:265–275.

LAUFFER, M., E. E. MILLÁN, and H. VANEGAS, 1971. Spectral sensitivity of L-type S-potentials in a teleost retina. *Vision Res. Suppl.* 3:77–86.

LEICESTER, J., and J. STONE, 1967. Ganglion, amacrine and horizontal cells of the cat's retina. *Vision Res.* 7:695–705.

LEVICK, W. R., 1975. Form and function of cat retinal ganglion cells. *Nature* 254:659–662.

LEVICK, W. R., and B. G. CLELAND, 1974. Receptive fields of cat retinal ganglion cells having slowly conducting axons. *Brain Res.* 74:156–160.

LÜTGERT, M., 1976. Die Interaktion von Zentrum und Peripherie des rezeptiven Feldes. Frequenzeigenschaften und räumliche Summation der ON-Hemmung innerhalb der rezeptiven Feldperipherie bei retinalen ON-Zentrum

Ganglienzellen der Katze. Medical dissertation, Freie Universität Berlin.

MAFFEI, L., 1968. Inhibitory and facilitatory spatial interactions in retinal receptive fields. *Vision Res.* 8:1187–1194.

MAFFEI, L., 1968. Spatial and temporal averages in retinal channels. *J. Neurophysiol.* 31:283–287.

MARMARELIS, P. Z., and K. I. NAKA, 1973a. Nonlinear analysis and synthesis of receptive-field responses in the catfish retina. I. Horizontal cell–ganglion cell chain. *J. Neurophysiol.* 36:605–618.

MARMARELIS, P. Z., and K. I. NAKA, 1973b. Nonlinear analysis and synthesis of receptive-field responses in the catfish retina. II. One-input white-noise analysis. *J. Neurophysiol.* 36:619–647.

MARMARELIS, P. Z., and K. I. NAKA, 1973c. Nonlinear analysis and synthesis of receptive-field responses in the catfish retina. III. Two-input white-noise analysis. *J. Neurophysiol.* 36:634–648.

MATURANA, H. R., J. Y. LETTVIN, W. S. McCULLOCH, and W. H. PITTS, 1960. Anatomy and physiology of vision in the frog (*Rana pipiens*). *J. Gen. Physiol.* 43:129–175.

McILWAIN, J. T., 1964. Receptive fields of optic tract axons and lateral geniculate cells: Peripheral extent and barbiturate sensitivity. *J. Neurophysiol.* 27:1154–1173.

McILWAIN, J. T., 1966. Some evidence concerning the physiological basis of the periphery effect in the cat's retina. *Exp. Brain Res.* 1:265–271.

MOTOKAWA, K. T., T. OIKAWA, and K. TASAKI, 1957. Receptor potential of vertebrate retina. *J. Neurophysiol.* 20:186–199.

NAKA, K.-I., 1972. The horizontal cells. *Vision Res.* 12:573–588.

NAKA, K.-I., 1977. Functional organization of catfish retina. *J. Neurophysiol.* 40:26–43.

NAKA, K.-I., and N. R. G. CARRAWAY, 1975. Morphological and functional identifications of catfish retinal neurons. I. Classical morphology. *J. Neurophysiol.* 38:53–90.

NAKA, K.-I., P. Z. MARMARELIS, and R. Y. CHAN, 1975. Morphological and functional identifications of catfish retinal neurons. III. Functional identification. *J. Neurophysiol.* 38:92–131.

NAKA, K.-I., and P. W. NYE, 1971. Role of horizontal cells in organization of the catfish retinal receptive field. *J. Neurophysiol.* 34:785–801.

NAKA, K.-I., and T. OHTSUKA, 1975. Morphological and functional identifications of catfish retinal neurons. II. Morphological identification. *J. Neurophysiol.* 38:72–91.

NAKA, K.-I., and W. A. H. RUSHTON, 1966. S-potentials from luminosity units in the retina of fish (Cyprinidae). *J. Physiol.* 185:587–599.

NAKA, K.-I., and W. A. H. RUSHTON, 1967. The generation and spread of S-potentials in fish (Cyprinidae). *J. Physiol.* 192:437–461.

NAKA, K.-I., and W. A. H. RUSHTON, 1968. S-potential and dark adaptation in fish. *J. Physiol.* 194:259–269.

NELSON, R., 1977. Cat cones have rod input: A comparison of the response properties of cones and horizontal cell bodies in the retina of the cat. *J. Comp. Neurol.* 172:109–136.

NELSON, R., H. KOLB, E. V. FAMIGLIETTI, and P. GOURAS, 1976. Neural responses in the rod and cone systems of the cat retina: Intra-cellular records and procion stains. *Invest. Ophthalmol.* 15:946–953.

NELSON, R., A. VON LÜTZOW, H. KOLB, and P. GOURAS, 1975. Horizontal cells in cat retina with independent dendritic systems. *Science* 189:137–139.

NIEMEYER, G., 1973. Intracellular recording from the isolated perfused mammalian eye. *Vision Res.* 13:1613–1618.

NIEMEYER, G., 1975. The function of the retina in the perfused eye. *Doc. Ophthalmol.* 39:53–116.

NIEMEYER, G., and P. GOURAS, 1973. Rod and cone signals in S-potentials of the isolated perfused cat eye. *Vision Res.* 13:1603–1612.

OGAWA, T., P. O. BISHOP, and W. R. LEVICK, 1966. Temporal characteristics of responses to photic stimulation by single ganglion cells in the unopened eye of the cat. *J. Neurophysiol.* 29:1–30.

RACKENSPERGER, W., and O.-J. GRÜSSER, 1966. Sinuslichtreizung der rezeptiven Felder einzelner Retinaneurone. *Experientia* 22:192.

RAMÓN Y CAJAL, S., 1894. *Die Retina der Wirbelthiere*, translated by A. Graeff. Wiesbaden: Bergmann.

RAVIOLA, E., and N. B. GILULA, 1973. Gap junctions between photoreceptor cells in the vertebrate retina. *Proc. Natl. Acad. Sci. USA* 70:1677–1681.

REIDEMEISTER, C., and O.-J. GRÜSSER, 1959. Flimmerlichtuntersuchungen an der Katzenretina. I. On-Neurone und On-Off-Neurone. *Z. Biol.* 111:241–253.

RODIECK, R. W., 1965. Quantitative analysis of cat retinal ganglion cell response to visual stimuli. *Vision Res.* 5:583–601.

RODIECK, R. W., 1973. *The Vertebrate Retina: Principles of Structure and Function.* San Francisco: W. H. Freeman.

RODIECK, R. W., and W. A. H. RUSHTON, 1976. Isolation of rod and cone contributions to cat ganglion cells by a method of light exchange. *J. Physiol.* 254:759–773.

RODIECK, R. W., and W. A. H. RUSHTON, 1976. Cancellation of rod signals by cones, and cone signals by rods in the cat retina. *J. Physiol.* 254:775–785.

ROWE, M. H., and J. STONE, 1976. Properties of ganglion cells in the visual streak of the cat's retina. *J. Comp. Neurol.* 169:99–126.

SAITO, H.-A., and Y. FUKUDA, 1973. Repetitive firing of the cat's retinal ganglion cell. *Vision Res.* 13:263–270.

SAITO, H.-A., T. SHIMAHARA, and Y. FUKUDA, 1970. Four types of responses to light and dark spot stimuli in the cat optic nerve. *Tohoku J. Exp. Med.* 102:127–133.

SAITO, H.-A., T. SHIMAHARA, and Y. FUKUDA, 1971. Phasic and tonic responses in the cat optic nerve fibers: Stimulus-response relations. *Tohoku J. Exp. Med.* 104:313–323.

SAKMANN, B., and O.-D. CREUTZFELDT, 1969. Scotopic and mesopic light adaptation in the cat's retina. *Pflügers Arch.* 313:168–185.

SAKMANN, B., O.-D. CREUTZFELDT, and H. SCHEICH, 1969. An experimental comparison between the ganglion cell receptive field and the receptive field of the adaptation pool in the cat retina. *Pflügers Arch.* 307:133–137.

SATO, T., M. YAMAMOTO, and H. NAKAHAMA, 1976. Variability of inter-spike intervals of cat's on-center optic tract fibres activated by steady light spot: A comparative study on X- and Y-fibres. *Exp. Brain Res.* 24:285–293.

SAUNDERS, R. McD., 1973. Colour vision in the cat by microelectrode studies at the optic tract level. *Eur. J. Physiol.* 343:R91.

SAUNDERS, R. McD., 1977. The spectral responsiveness and the temporal frequency response (TFR) of cat optic tract and lateral geniculate neurons: sinusoidal stimulation studies. *Vision Res.* 17:285–292.

SCHATTERNIKOFF, M., 1902. Über den Einfluß der Adaptation auf die Erscheinung des Flimmerns. *Z. Sinnesphysiol.* 29:241–263.

SCHMITT, F. O., P. DEV., and B. H. SMITH, 1976. Electrotonic processing of information by brain cells. *Science* 193:114–120.

SCHWARTZ, E. A., 1975a. Rod-rod interaction in the retina of the turtle. *J. Physiol.* 246:617–638.

SCHWARTZ, E. A., 1975b. Cones excite rods in the retina of the turtle. *J. Physiol.* 246:639–651.

SOBRINO, J. A., and A. GALLEGO, 1970. Celulas amacrinas de la capa plexiform externa de la retina. *Actas Soc. Esp. Cien. Fisiol.* 12:373–375.

SPEKREIJSE, H., and A. L. NORTON, 1970. The dynamic characteristics of color-coded S-potentials. *J. Gen. Physiol.* 56:1–15.

STEINBERG, R. H., 1966. Oscillatory activity in the optic tract of cat and light adaptation. *J. Neurophysiol.* 29:139–156.

STEINBERG, R. H., 1969a. Rod and cone contributions to S-potentials from the cat retina. *Vision Res.* 9:1319–1329.

STEINBERG, R. H., 1969b. Rod-cone interaction in S-potentials from the cat retina. *Vision Res.* 9:1331–1344.

STEINBERG, R. H., 1969c. The rod after-effect in S-potentials from the cat retina. *Vision Res.* 9:1345–1355.

STEINBERG, R. H., M. REID, and P. L. LACY, 1973. The distribution of rods and cones in the retina of the cat (*Felix domesticus*). *J. Comp. Neurol.* 148:229–248.

STEINBERG, R. H., and R. SCHMIDT, 1971. The evidence that horizontal cells generate S-potentials in the cat retina. *Vision Res.* 11:1029–1031.

STONE, J., 1965. A quantitative analysis of the distribution of ganglion cells in the cat's retina. *J. Comp. Neurol.* 124:337–352.

STONE, J., and M. FABIAN, 1966. Specialized receptive fields of the cat's retina. *Science* 152:1277–1279.

STONE, J., and R. B. FREEMAN, JR., 1971. Conduction velocity groups in the cat's optic nerve classified according to their retinal origin. *Exp. Brain Res.* 13:489–497.

STONE, J., and Y. FUKUDA, 1974. The naso-temporal division of the cat's retina re-examined in terms of Y-, X- and W-cells. *J. Comp. Neurol.* 155:377–394.

STONE, J., and Y. FUKUDA, 1974. Properties of cat retinal ganglion cells: A comparison of W-cells with X- and Y-cells. *J. Neurophysiol.* 37:722–748.

STONE, J., and H. HOLLÄNDER, 1971. Optic nerve axon diameters measured in the cat retina: Some functional considerations. *Exp. Brain Res.* 13:498–503.

SVAETICHIN, G., 1956. The cone function related to the activity of retinal neurons. *Acta Physiol. Scand.* 39 (Suppl. 134): 67–92.

SVAETICHIN, G., K. NEGISHI, B. DRUJAN, and C. MURIEL, 1971. S-potentials and retinal automatic control systems. In *Proceedings of the First European Biophysics Congress,* E. Broda, A. Locker, and H. Springer-Lederer, eds. Vienna: Verlag der Wiener Medizinischen Akademie, vol. 5, pp. 77–88.

SVAETICHIN, G., K. NEGISHI, R. FATEHCHAND, B. D. DRUJAN, and A. S. DE TESTA, 1965. Nervous function based on interactions between neuronal and non-neuronal elements. *Prog. Brain Res.* 15:243–266.

VARJÚ, D., 1965. Über nichtlineare Analogschaltungen zur Simulierung biologischer Adaptationsvorgänge. *Prog. Brain Res.* 17:74–101.

WÄSSLE, H., W. R. LEVICK, and B. G. CLELAND, 1975. The distribution of the alpha type of ganglion cells in the cat's retina. *J. Comp. Neurol.* 159:419–438.

WALLS, G. L., 1967. *The Vertebrate Eye and Its Adaptive Radiation.* New York: Hafner.

WERBLIN, F. S., 1970. Response of retinal cells to moving spots: Intracellular recording in Necturus maculosus. *J. Neurophysiol.* 33:342–350.

WERBLIN, F. S., and J. E. DOWLING, 1969. Organization of the retina of the mudpuppy, *Necturus maculosus.* II. Intracellular recording. *J. Neurophysiol.* 32:339–355.

WIESEL, T. N., 1959. Recording inhibition and excitation in the cat's retinal ganglion cells with intracellular electrodes. *Nature* 183:264–265.

WIESEL, T. N., 1960. Receptive fields of ganglion cells in the cat's retina. *J. Physiol.* 153:583–594.

ZEKI, S. M., 1977. Simultaneous anatomical demonstration of the representation of the vertical and horizontal meridians in areas V2 and V3 of rhesus monkey visual cortex. *Proc. R. Soc. Lond.* B195:517–523.

ZEKI, S. M., 1977. Colour coding in the superior temporal sulcus of rhesus monkey visual cortex. *Proc. R. Soc. Lond.* B197:195–223.

16 Signal Transmission by Graded Slow Potentials in the Arthropod Peripheral Visual System

STEPHEN R. SHAW

ABSTRACT After a summary account of the compound eye's functional construction, the generation and spread of slow-potential visual signals in the first two layers of the arthropod eye is discussed. Single photon captures by receptors are sufficient to evoke behavioral responses from an insect, and the millivolt-sized potentials that these elicit are followed from photoreceptors through second-order monopolar cells. It is argued that both cell types transmit slow potentials along their axons decrementally and communicate through a high-sensitivity synapse. Electrical coupling between photoreceptors, passive cable conduction, and input convergence onto the monopolars all probably function as a reliable noise reduction, signal-averaging amplifier system. Synaptic amplification of the input signal improves the output sensitivity of the monopolar cell, analogous to vertebrate retina mechanisms, but it also contracts the cell's dynamic range. At the synaptic level, evidence for range-switching has been found in response to changes in ambient light conditions. The large electrical fields generated across the blood-brain barrier of the eye are discussed as a probable part of this autoranging mechanism and as an explanation of the lateral inhibitory interactions reported at the monopolar cell level.

Introduction

THE COMPOUND EYES are the main visual organs of arthropods, usually supplemented in insects by three smaller ocelli. Judged from unit recording, visual processing is the main function of the nerve neuropils behind the eyes, although tactile and auditory modalities have input to visual cells even in the two outermost layers, which in insects are called the lamina and medulla (Horridge et al., 1965; Northrop and Gugnion, 1970).

The layout of the insect optic lobe itself can be compared, with a little rearrangement, to the retina proper of the vertebrates (see Figure 1). Some other,

physiological, similarities have emerged between the two within the last few years. For example, both the receptors and the second-order monopolar cells in insects and crustaceans transmit information by way of graded slow potentials, without nerve impulses to the following cells, as it is supposed that vertebrate rods, cones, and bipolar cells do. This idea seemed rather unconventional when it was first voiced seriously for insect photoreceptors in the early 1960s (Burkhardt, 1962), before the first premonitions of the even stranger and then much-smaller hyperpolarizing signals from vertebrate cones (Bortoff, 1964; Tomita, 1965). More recently there has been a proliferation of examples in both camps, and, backed by cell identification, minority opinion has solidified into currently accepted truth.

A major objective of this study program is to draw on several areas of nerve research to assess the significance of such changed beliefs on signal transmission. Are such systems widespread, or are they the exception to the rule? Is there anything special about the systems that use them, or can their cable and synaptic properties be fitted easily within the framework of existing neurophysiological concepts? In pursuit of this question, the present review is restricted narrowly to summarizing the properties of graded-potential visual systems in the eyes and ocelli of arthropods, mainly insects. (For a more general introduction to insect vision, see Goldsmith and Bernard, 1974.) The origins, sizes, interactions, and significance of the small potentials resulting from photoexcitation in the receptors are discussed and followed into the second-order cells. Discussion is limited mainly to these first two nervous layers of arthropod eye, and to the cell species about which most is known: the larger photoreceptors with short axons and the secondary monopolar cells (LMCs) of the lamina synaptic neuropil, which corresponds to the vertebrate outer plexiform layer. Other cell types

STEPHEN R. SHAW Department of Neurobiology, Research School of Biological Sciences, Australian National University, Canberra, A.C.T. 2601, Australia

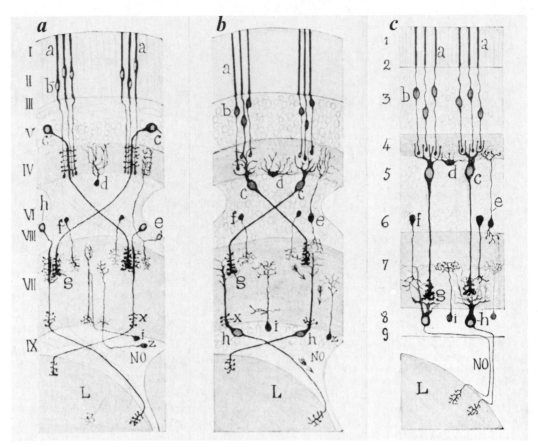

FIGURE 1 (a) insect compound eye organization seen in Golgi-stained material, compared with (c) the vertebrate retina after Ramón y Cajal and Sánchez (1915). In (b) the authors redrew the insect optic lobe with some of the neuronal cell bodies displaced into the positions occupied by corresponding cells in the vertebrate, thus revealing the anatomical similarities of the two systems. In the insect, the layers I–III correspond to the photoreceptor somata; IV to the lamina; VII to the medulla; and L to the lobula complex. (b, photoreceptors; c, lamina monopolar cells.)

are known anatomically in this complex (see, e.g., Strausfeld and Campos-Ortega, 1977), and some of them must give rise to the unidentified extracellular recordings of impulse discharges recorded (Northrop and Guignon, 1970; Arnett, 1972; Mimura, 1974). While conventional impulse traffic must be the province of some cells (whether afferent, efferent, or intrinsic is unknown), the major output from the lamina synapse is believed to be the slow potentials of the LMCs.

Work on *Limulus* lateral eye has dominated invertebrate vision until recently, but since it has been extensively reviewed (Hartline and Ratliff, 1972; Fuortes and O'Bryan, 1972), it will not be emphasized here. Dominated in the adult by a 10 cm optic nerve, the receptor groups appear to signal only by conventional nerve impulse trains to largely unknown postsynaptic centers; to what use the information is put is so far unknown, for want of demonstrable laboratory behavior (Campenhausen, 1967). Some insects behave better, and it is to them we briefly turn.

Behavioral relevance of slow potential phenomena

The relevance of studying small potentials from single visual cells may be shown by a few excerpts from the behavioral literature. Since Ramón y Cajal, it has not been difficult to defend the dignity of the individual cell, but the recidivists of recent vertebrate photoreceptor research suggest that each cell there shares potentials with most others. Arthropod photoreceptors are at least somewhat more selective, as will be shown here by electrical coupling evidence and a few behavioral examples.

Kirschfeld and Lutz (1974) have shown that it is possible to detect behavioral (turning) responses from insects using phased stimulation of just two individual photoreceptors in neighboring ommatidia and to inhibit this behavior selectively by stimulating other single receptors nearby. The outcome is similar with the structurally much simpler ocelli of barnacles. These can contain as few as three photoreceptors, and darkening of one ocellus is sufficient to promote reflex withdrawal of the legs (Gwilliam, 1963; Shaw, 1972).

A second lesson also comes from the turning response of house flies, again from Tübingen, exposed to moving patterns. Flies can see and turn to follow these patterns even in very dim light (Reichardt, 1966), and when the calibrations take account of the now more accurately known narrow receptive fields and spectral sensitivity, it is found that this behavior occurs even when single receptors are catching less than one photon per second.

It is therefore appropriate to inquire about the nature of the response of a single photoreceptor, especially at these photon-scarce levels, since it is obviously adequate to promote behavior: the receptor signals are indeed "seen" and are not just subthreshold epiphenomena. But to set the scene, I will first briefly describe the relevant optics and anatomy.

Functional anatomy and optics of insect eyes

RECEPTOR LAYER The photoreceptor or retinular cells are bunched together in groups rather like elongate orange segments; eight or nine usually make up an *ommatidium*, each with its own separate lenslet (Figure 2). In most insects the inner borders of each photoreceptor send out parallel, tubular microvilli about 700 Å in diameter; these meet to form a closely packed, central rod or *rhabdom* only 1–3 μm in diameter but very long—over 1 mm in dragonflies. In flies the microvilli from separate cells never touch; they remain grouped about 1 μm apart, as separate *rhabdomeres* (Kirschfeld, this volume). In most insects there are two or three smaller retinular cells with few rhabdomeric microvilli; tiered retinas with some rhabdoms overlying others are also common.

Each ommatidium is separated from its neighbor groups by a sheath of glial cells, between which, in the locust, lies the main body of extracellular space (ECS) of the eye: electron-dense tracers indicate, however, that a small ECS reservoir lies at the base of the rhabdom microvilli and even between microvilli, and this reservoir is in free and rapid communication with the rest (Figure 3; Perrelet and Baumann, 1969; Shaw, 1977b, 1978). The glial cells probably regulate the ionic and osmotic environment of the receptors.

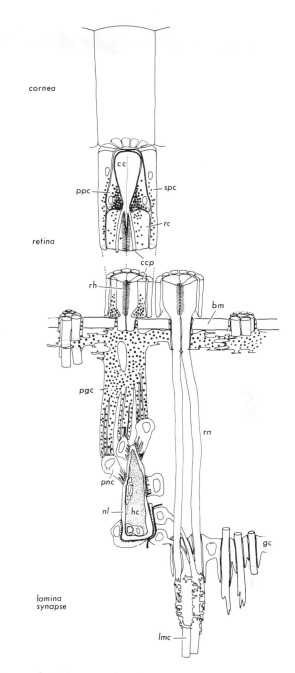

FIGURE 2 Diagram showing the main cell types in the retina of the locust. *Abbreviations*: bm, basement membrane; ccp, cone-cell processes; gc, glial cell; hc, haemocoel channels; lmc, lamina monopolar cell axon; nl, neural lamella; pgc, pigmented glial cell; pnc, perineurial cell; ppc, principal pigment (glial) cell; ra, receptor axon; rc, photoreceptor-cell soma, eight making up each ommatidium; rh, rhabdom; spc, secondary pigment cell.

Light focused near the end of the rhabdom or individual rhabdomere by each lenslet is expected to remain trapped within the structure by internal reflection, since the higher refractive index of the rhab-

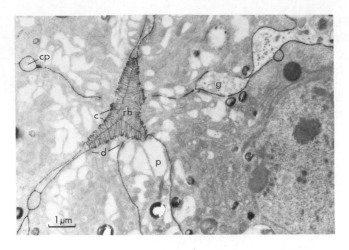

FIGURE 3 Cross section through a grasshopper ommatidium after the eye has been exposed to a Ringer's containing the extracellular marker ruthenium red. Tracer shows up black in the clefts between the six large and two smaller photoreceptors. It passes through the desmosomal ring (d) encircling the central rhabdom (rh), and penetrates to some extent between microvilli and particularly into cisternae (c) at their bases. (p, intracellular palisade vacuole; cp, cone-cell process; g, glial cell.) Fixed formaldehyde/gluteraldehyde and osmium, but not counterstained. (After Shaw, 1978.)

dom, relative to the surrounding cytoplasm, creates an optical waveguide. These effects have been observed elegantly and directly by reversing the illumination path (Kirschfeld and Franceschini, 1968). Consequently, the receptive field (RF) of each receptor is set mainly by the cross section of its rhabdom and the optical diffraction pattern from its lens, predicting a roughly Gaussian acceptance function. In several insects this RF has been measured directly, usually by recording from individual photoreceptors. Values of 1°–3° at half-width sensitivity are usual in diurnal insects, and there is a similar angular spacing between neighboring ommatidia. In diurnal insects, very little light scatters between lenslets (Shaw, 1969a; Scholes, 1969), probably due to dense but physiologically inert screening pigments around the lens focal plane. Other species (moths, beetles, some crustaceans, etc.), particularly nocturnal ones or those inhabiting dim environments, enlarge the effective aperture to catch every last photon, each cell absorbing through many lenslets with no intervening pigment screen (Shaw, 1969a; Kunze, 1969, 1972; Walcott, 1974). The RF is then much broader, so that visual acuity suffers. The optimum trade-off strategy between high acuity and maximum photon capture has been quantified by Snyder, Stavenga, and Laughlin (1977) for different sorts of eyes and conditions.

To concentrate the light into a tiny central rod would make sense only if the visual pigment were also confined there, and this now seems certain. Microspectrophotometry (Langer and Thorell, 1966; Goldsmith, 1975) shows that a photoisomerizable pigment resides within the rhabdom with a respectably high extinction coefficient—a "rhodopsin," although this familiar name conceals some unfamiliar properties, such as ultraviolet sensitivity and stable photoproducts (Kirschfeld, this volume). In addition, freeze-fracture studies now show that the rhabdom membrane contains particles thought to represent individual or aggregate molecules of this photopigment (Fernandez and Nickel, 1976; Boschek and Hamdorf, 1976).

In summary, optics and receptor anatomy show that light is optically concentrated onto the rhabdom membranes, wherein lies the photopigment. This region has access to the nearby ECS, which contains the store of ions drawn on during generation of the receptor potential.

ANATOMICAL ORGANIZATION OF THE RECEPTOR AXON AND THE LAMINA SYNAPSE REGION The acellular basement membrane conveniently marks the end of the rhabdomeres and the start of the receptor axons (Figure 2). Below this level in the locust (Shaw, 1978) the extracellular space is reduced, and a different set of glial cells surrounds and separates each axon. These glial cells are themselves linked together by numerous septate and gap junctions. ECS tracers lanthanum and ruthenium red can get through the individual outermost junctions, but, presumably because of cumulative effects, they penetrate no further than 30 μm below the basement membrane. The extracellular space thus appears to be at least partially closed off to small tracers around the axons (Shaw, 1977b, 1978), and diffusion of ECS radiotracers through this region is very slow (Shaw, 1977a). These findings parallel electrical measurements described later, which indicate a barrier of increased extracellular resistance extending about 200 μm along the axons down to the lamina synapse. This has physiological consequences for interaction between cells and is believed to be part of the blood-brain barrier already known at the insect nerve cord. A row of blood channels in fact runs between the axons within the barrier in most of the sixteen insect orders examined (Shaw, in preparation).

The lamina synaptic zone is itself about 100 μm deep and sees the termination at one elongated site of six axons (Trujillo-Cenóz, 1972; Strausfeld, 1976) to form a synaptic complex—the neurommatidium or optic cartridge. These six come from the larger photoreceptors and form repeating synaptic complexes with the secondary monopolar cells (LMCs), often as dyads or triads with presynaptic dense bars and vesicles (Trujillo-Cenóz, 1965; for recent work see Armett-Kibel, Meinertzhagen, and Dowling, 1977). The LMCs project together to the second synaptic neuropil (medulla) to end in topographical register, in flies at least, with the long visual fibers of the two small photoreceptors, which are supposed to bypass the first synapse (Campos-Ortega and Strausfeld, 1972). In dragonflies, however, at least one of the long fibers appears to synapse en route through the lamina. Feedback synapses are also seen from one monopolar back onto particular receptors in dragonfly and from presumed efferent fibers from the medulla in the fly; tangential fibers are also known. Figure 4 suggests the complexity of wiring currently envisaged for the most thoroughly studied synaptic cartridge, that of the fly. Even there the picture is not complete; recently small junctions have been found to connect intracartridge receptor terminals (Chi and Carlson, 1976). The most recent synopsis of the interconnections is by Strausfeld and Campos-Ortega (1977). It is well to remember that such a complex edifice rests entirely upon the assumption that the tiny presynaptic densities, where seen, are truly synapses made flesh and not just local factories or other nondescripts. No one, of course, has seriously challenged this idea; it gives the only fine structural lead there is, and certainly provides a wealth of suggestive detail as yet not matched by the physiologist, whose realm we have at last reached.

Electrical responses of the photoreceptors in compound eyes

THE CELL SOMA RESPONSE In most species examined, the photoreceptors respond, as a pulse of light is increased in intensity, with a corresponding, graded-amplitude, delayed wave of membrane depolarization (Figure 5). At higher intensities, the response develops an initial peak, which increases up to a maximum of about 40–60 mV depolarization in bright lights. In some of the larger photoreceptors, where coarse electrodes allow the baseline potential to be measured properly, resting potentials of 30–50 mV are found, and the peak response overshoots zero by about 20 mV. The response is caused by a graded membrane-conductance increase to Na^+ ions (Millechia and Mauro, 1969; Brown et al., 1970; Fulpius and Baumann, 1969), and the cutback from the initial peak is associated with a rise in intracellular

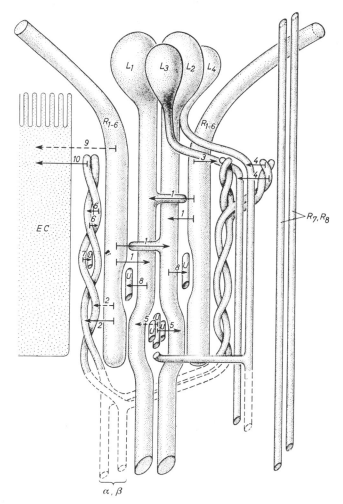

FIGURE 4 The clearest summary diagram available to illustrate the complex interrelationship within a single synaptic complex, or optic cartridge, in the fly lamina. The numbers refer to possible synaptic interactions between the various elements. Photoreceptors, R1–R6; monopolars, L1–L4; centrifugal elements, u; and epithelial glial cells, EC. Since 1970, other elements have been described and the interrelations clarified further. (From Boschek, 1970; see also Campos-Ortega and Strausfeld, 1974.)

free Ca^{++} (Brown and Blinks, 1974), plus probably a delayed increase in K^+ conductance (Hanani and Shaw, 1977).

The dynamic range of the transient response to light is about 4–5 log units, depending on the limits specified. On a semilog plot, the transient (but not the later plateau phase) follows a growth-curve type of function (see Figure 9), first identified by Naka and Rushton (1966) in the vertebrate eye by the hyperbolic relationship

$$\frac{V_I}{V_{max}} = \frac{I}{I + I_{max/2}} = \frac{1 + \tanh(\ln J^{1/2})}{2},$$

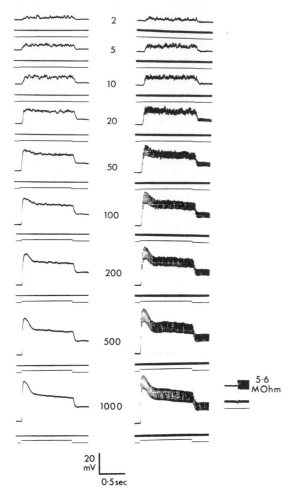

FIGURE 5 Intracellular responses from a single locust photoreceptor to light flashes of increasing intensity (relative values in the center) from a small source aligned along the visual axis. *Left*: The response is graded in amplitude and develops an initial transient with brighter flashes. At low intensity, the response is composed of small fluctuations, which represent single photon captures and which appear to summate in the larger responses. *Right*: The cell resting impedance drops considerably during illumination, as monitored by a bridge circuit passing a 60 Hz sine wave. Studies on other arthropods indicate that this drop mainly reflects an increase in sodium permeability of the photoreceptor surface membrane.

where V_{max} and V_I are the voltage at saturation and at some intensity I, $I_{max/2}$ is the scaling constant, and $J = I/I_{max/2}$. The interest in this nonlinear formalism is that the voltage-intensity relation produced is exactly what is predicted for a fixed-membrane potassium conductance, in parallel with a sodium conductance that varies linearly with light intensity during the initial peak. If each photon capture by each photopigment molecule activates one or some fixed number of sodium conductance sites, the initial

response would be predicted quite well (Shaw, 1968a). As expected by this view, the quantized response at low intensity is demonstrably linear, and Lisman and Brown (1975) have shown that the superposed photocurrent produced in voltage clamp is also linear over a wide range in *Limulus*. These details are given to bolster a point more relevant to the present concern of information transmission by the receptors: that by transducing light into membrane voltage in this way, the photoreceptors are necessarily burdened with an output function covering a large range of light intensity (10^4, between 1% limits) but concomitantly with rather poor sensitivity in terms of millivolts per intensity unit. The range of environmental contrast available for perception at any one time of day is much smaller than this (~100:1 on the ground) and is in any case limited, as in the vertebrate eye, by entoptic scatter (perhaps to less than 10^3–10^2:1; Shaw, 1969a). It would be advantageous to have some means to magnify the meter needle—to examine just a part of the receptor range but with higher sensitivity—and this appears to be one "improvement" performed by the first synaptic relay.

In passing we may mention one further limitation of the receptors in all the species studied: the inability to signal well at high frequency, where output modulation falls off rapidly. This may be important to fast-flying and turning insects such as dragonflies and flies in detecting low-contrast modulations in the environment. The amplitude part of the frequency-response function of the receptor cells is flat only up to quite low values (10–20 Hz in barnacle: Shaw, 1972; about 40 Hz in fly: French and Järvilehto, 1978a), after which it drops off steeply. The transmission characteristic resembles that of a multistage low-pass filter with about eleven stages (*Limulus*: Fuortes and Hodgkin, 1964) or five stages (fly: French and Järvilehto, 1978b). There is no convincing insight as to what the physical embodiment of these stages might be, although chemical reactions have been suggested (Borsellino and Fuortes, 1968). Whatever the stages represent, the number of them decreases during light adaptation (Fuortes and Hodgkin, 1964).

THE QUANTAL RESPONSE TO LIGHT At low intensity the photoresponse is irregular, and in very dim lights it finally breaks down into individual discrete potentials (*Limulus*: Yeandle, 1958; locust: Scholes, 1964; fly: Kirschfeld, 1966; cockroach: Laughlin, 1975), the frequency of which is linear with light intensity, although in some species the individual "bumps" are difficult to resolve. These were seized upon immediately as possible direct registrations of photon captures, and while this seems ever more likely in *Limulus*, the argument continues (e.g., Kaplan and Barlow, 1976; Weiss and Yeandle, 1975). In fact, the evidence seems most compelling in the locust eye, which will be summarized next.

Scholes (1964, 1965) compiled frequency-of-response counts of bumps to dim flashes. These clearly fit the statistics expected for a one-event, random process (Poisson parameter $m = 1$) and exclude a process in which the coincidence of two or more events is required ($m = 2, 3, \ldots$). However, the presence of noise can degrade the $m = 2, 3, \ldots$ curves to look like the $m = 1$ curve (Kaplan and Barlow, 1976), and the presence of spontaneous "dark bumps" in *Limulus* weakens the force of such evidence for that animal. In locust, however, dark bumps are rare (Scholes, 1964): Lillywhite (1977) finds an entirely negligible frequency of less than 1 per 5 min when stray light is cut to a minimum. By selection, Scholes also minimized the fluctuation in cell threshold that occurs with time and so minimized this source of distortion. Scholes's evidence that we are dealing with a one-event process in locust therefore remains very strong. That this individual event is really a single photon capture and not something else, however, was seriously undermined by Scholes's calibrations, which showed an extremely poor (0.1%) quantum capture efficiency (QCE); because his stimulator could not be properly aligned with the narrow receptive fields, however, this result is not really surprising, as he was aware. I reexamined this casually for a few cells and came up with a best QCE per cell of about 8% (Shaw, 1968b). Since six large cells under each facet dominate absorption, the QCE per facet must be about six times larger than this. Lillywhite (1977) has recently measured this properly and quantitatively, using axial monochromatic light; for dark-adapted cells he finds a QCE per facet of about 60% ($\pm$ 20% S.D.). If the quantum efficiency of the actual photopigment is about 0.66, as in vertebrates (Dartnall, 1968), we can conclude that practically every last (axial, best-wavelength) photon entering a facet lens ends up producing one bump. There is one last loophole: that capture could be less efficient than this, with one photon generating several bumps, n. If n is fixed, at a number as small as two, this alternative is easily dismissed by repeated trials near threshold; these show neither alternations of misses with pairs (or triplets, etc.) nor a predominance of short intervals in a long sequence of bumps (Lillywhite, 1977). Likewise, Scholes (1965) found no serial correlation between interbump intervals. There perhaps remains the more subtle possibility raised by Weiss and Yeandle (1975) that n is on

average only a little greater than unity, is not fixed, but is instead a probabilistic function. They point out that this generates an expected statistical distribution of bumps different from the simple $m = 1$ case; but it can be distinguished from it only if QCE is large ($\geq 10\%$), which, in locust, it fortunately is. Lillywhite has tested this by examining the distribution of interbump intervals and decisively rejects the probabilistic model in favor of 1 photon $\rightarrow$ 1 bump. The interesting deterministic corollary would seem to be that in locust, the effect of a photon must cease following its bump. This might be expected if one photon opened one membrane conductance channel, but this seems unlikely (see below). One alternative—a multichannel response activated by multiple transmitter molecules (Cone, 1973)—would require the extra constraint that these molecules must all arrive and act during one bump and not linger on unattached for later activation.

Each bump must stem from light absorbed where the photopigment is, in the rhabdom membrane. The photocurrent in invertebrates and vertebrates originates close to the site of photon absorption, although, because of optical limitations, this cannot be refined better than, at most, a few microns (Hagins and Jennings, 1959; Hagins, Zonana, and Adams, 1962; Baumann, 1966; Fein and Charlton, 1975). Only in the fortuitously favorable receptors of the leech is it possible to show that the photocurrent passes through or very close to the rhabdomeric microvilli and not through the main cell surface (Lasansky and Fuortes, 1969). The conductance changes underlying single bumps have never been properly measured except in *Limulus*; Walther (1966) quotes 0.2–1 nS for leech, and a few rough measurements of my own gave values as high as 5 nS in locust. Although considerably smaller than those for *Limulus* (*ca.* 300 nS: Cone, 1973), such values are still 10^2–10^3 larger than the most recent estimates, from noise analysis, of the conductance of single sodium-selective channels in a variety of excitable membranes (2–10 pS: Neher and Stevens, 1977). Since there is evidence that the photoreceptor membrane in some invertebrates becomes sodium-selective during light activation (Millechia and Mauro, 1969; Fulpius and Baumann, 1969), this suggests by analogy that several hundred channels must be activated to produce one bump. How such a multiple event is linked to the conformational change in only one rhodopsin molecule is not known: the multiplication seems likely to involve either intermediate transmitter molecules (Cone, 1973), local electrical regeneration (Bass and Moore, 1970), or some cooperative interaction between excited and unexcited molecules. The experiments of Martinez and Srebro (1976) seem to rule out regenerativeness.

Lastly, it may be asked what is the smallest of these small potential changes known to transmit information in arthropod eyes? This appears to be about 300 μV for barnacle photoreceptor cell bodies, decreasing to under 100 μV in the terminals (Shaw, 1972). Extrapolating the careful measurements of Scholes and Reichardt (1969) down to light levels where behavior is only just detectable (Fermi and Reichardt, 1963; Reichardt, Braidenberg, and Weidel, 1968) produces even lower values (40 μV soma, probably 20 μV in the terminals). However, we already know that this extrapolation procedure is invalid: the response at low intensity fragments into intensity-independent bumps. Some of the quantum response estimates in vertebrate eye are based on a similar extrapolation from high-intensity averages and give similarly small values. At the other extreme, what are presumed to be single photon bumps of 10 mV amplitude have been recorded from photoreceptors of a nocturnal spider (Blest and Laughlin, personal communication) and in deeply dark-adapted *Limulus*, where they are larger still and apparently regenerative (Dowling, 1968). Like the optical specializations discussed earlier, these seem obvious adaptations for the extremely low light levels of nocturnal life. There is no information on the minimum amplitude modulation necessary to effect behavior in normal diurnal conditions.

In summary, single bumps probably originate in or close to the rhabdomeric microvilli, probably as multichannel conductance changes, and in one insect at least they are direct registrations of single photon captures. These millivolt-sized events form the photoreceptor output during the low-light behavioral events we have described and are therefore worth following further. Model studies suggest that the light response at all intensity levels may be no more than the nonlinear superposition of these unitary events, with a slightly faster time course at high intensities (Dodge, Knight, and Toyoda, 1968).

ELECTRICAL COUPLING BETWEEN PHOTORECEPTORS
Comprehensive measurements on the *Limulus* lateral eye established that the photoreceptors and the eccentric cell in one ommatidium (but not in neighboring ommatidia) are strongly coupled, through rectifying electrical junctions (Smith and Baumann, 1969). A similar degree of coupling was observed within drone bee ommatidia; weaker coupling in locust (Shaw, 1969b) and within an ommatidium seemed to involve all the cells penetrated. In crayfish

ommatidia, Muller (1973) cites very strong coupling, but only between cells with microvilli similarly aligned, that is, microvilli that touch end-on or lie side-by-side. In flies the rhabdomeres are separate, and it is unlikely that the cells in one ommatidium are coupled strongly, if at all (Scholes, 1969; see below). This, and the absence of any specialized contacts (except desmosomes) between receptor somas or between axons, suggests that coupling must be by way of microvillar end or side contact, but special junctions at the tips could not be found by Fernandez and Nickel (1976). Ribi (1978) has recently found particles lying between microvilli, in a wasp. The alternative of coupling caused by a high-shunt resistance between microvilli makes it difficult to explain the high degree and selectivity of coupling demonstrated in some species; in addition, the intervilli spaces seem partially open to tracers (Perrelet and Baumann, 1969; Shaw, 1978). Coupling between the same pair of large photoreceptors in different specimens of a barnacle gave enormously variable results (Shaw, 1972), so that the origin of the coupling variability in the earlier results in arthropods is uncertain. My guess is that the lower values reflect cell damage and that coupling in vivo is even stronger than was estimated on average.

In *Limulus*, single bumps clearly spread effectively among the dozen or so ommatidial cells, so that the result in each receptor and the output eccentric cell is an average of the ensemble's catch. The same is true for local spikes in the drone bee ommatidium (Shaw, 1969b), although here each cell has a separate functional axon. The effect of coupling is obviously to decrease the unit size but to increase the smoothness of the output response, especially when coupled with the low-pass action of the intercell junctions (Smith and Baumann, 1969): in effect, it is a low-pass filter and averager. Recently, Lillywhite (personal communication) has demonstrated the spread of bumps within locust ommatidia; as with the electrical coupling, the effects appear weaker than in *Limulus*.

Signal propagation in photoreceptor axons

ABSENCE OF REGENERATIVE IMPULSES In recordings from both the visual cell bodies and the axons of many species of insects and crustaceans, no impulses have been reported, although a single small potential is frequently found on the rising edge of the receptor waveform and probably indicates a failed local response. An exception is the drone bee retinular cell, in which this response sometimes becomes a full-blown spike. Baumann (1968), however, found that the spike is much reduced compared to the receptor potential when recorded from the axon. Chappell and Dowling (1972) recorded a similar spike in dragonfly ocellar receptors; when this was eliminated with tetrodotoxin, leaving just the slow potential, synaptic transmission from the axon was not detectably impaired. This suggests that single spikes, where present, are functionally redundant. Nevertheless, they provide a useful reply to the criticism, once heard quite frequently, that spikes are absent in recordings because the cells have been damaged by the electrode penetration. In the bee the spikes can be easily seen in extracellular records in which no damage could have taken place (Figure 6). Thus, if they are generally present in other species, they should also be observable extracellularly; they are not, however.

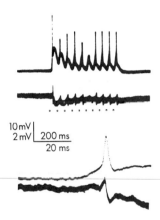

10 mV | 200 ms
2 mV | 20 ms

FIGURE 6 Intracellular (upper traces) and simultaneous extracellular (lower traces) recordings from a drone bee photoreceptor. Each light flash (dots) produces a receptor potential with a single local spike on its rising phase, although this may fail at high repetition rates. When the intracellular spike occurs, it can be clearly detected as a diphasic response by the nearby extracellular electrode. The lower frame is on an expanded time scale. (After Shaw, 1969b.)

DECREMENTAL CONDUCTION   Recordings from the photoreceptor axons in several species show similar characteristic differences from the photoreceptor somata. The receptor potential appears basically to be little different from that of the soma, although it is somewhat smaller and the initial transient is disproportionately reduced (Järvilehto and Zettler, 1970; Baumann, 1968; Ioannides and Walcott, 1971; Shaw, 1972; Ozawa et al., 1976). This would be expected for passive propagation down a leaky cable in which the length constant is longer than the axon and the time constant more rapidly attenuates the higher frequencies in the visual signal. Even in the very long axons

of barnacles, which scaled up would have the dimensions of a long garden hose, the specific membrane resistance required to give the attenuation observed is not unprecedentedly high (10^5 Ω-cm^2: Shaw, 1972). In the barnacle no evidence was obtained of regenerative potentials, and potentials resulting from extrinsic polarization duplicated the action of light on postsynaptic cells.

Steady-state attenuations by a factor of two or three seem usual in most of the reported recordings, although this has not been examined systematically. At least in the locust, the attenuation must be reduced and the axon length constant increased by the much larger extracellular resistance around the axons (Shaw, 1975; Shaw, in preparation).

Decremental conduction can introduce a significant time delay into signal conduction because the potential change propagates quite slowly, with an effective velocity of $v = 2\lambda/\tau$ in an infinite axon (Hodgkin and Rushton, 1946; see Jack, this volume). A delay averaging 24 msec was recorded in the very long barnacle axons (Shaw, 1972), and about 2 msec in paired comparisons in the fly eye (Scholes, 1969). Conduction is thus very slow; in the fly eye, for example, it is roughly a factor of ten slower than expected from a regenerative, unmyelinated fiber of similar size (Rushton, 1951).

The electrical recordings of Scholes (1969), identified later as coming from the axon terminals of fly photoreceptors (Järvilehto and Zettler, 1970), clearly show selective strong excitatory coupling between the six axon terminals that converge onto one lamina cartridge, presumably mediated electrically by the junctions recently found there by Chi and Carlson (1976). Attenuation in individual axons in the fly appears to be larger than in other eyes (at least sixfold: Scholes, 1969); but with normal optical stimulation that illuminates all the cells, it is offset by the (presumed) electrical coupling. This is another way of saying that the relatively large attenuations at individual terminals recorded by Scholes must largely reflect the loading of each by five others when only one is active; if coupling were absent, attenuation would be much less. By appropriate masking techniques, Scholes (personal communication) has also detected coupling back in the cell soma. It has been suggested that this coupling functions, as in the cell bodies of other species, as a signal averager and low-pass filter to improve the signal/noise (S/N) ratio in the terminals by a factor of almost six (Shaw, 1972; Gemperlein and Smola, 1972). The actual improvement depends on the effective bandwidth of the voltage noise. This would account for the smoother appearance and absence of photon bumps in axon terminals in the fly, even in records that are definitely intracellular (e.g., Järvilehto and Zettler, 1970). On the other hand, intracellular responses from the lamina from what are almost certainly receptor terminals—in dragonfly (Laughlin, 1974a) and in locust (Shaw, unpublished)—do show distinguishable fluctuations. Laughlin argues strongly against such universal coupling in dragonfly axons, which would degrade the distinct color sensitivities of the receptors in one ommatidium, contrary to his findings. In the fly, all the converging axons, R_{1-6}, are believed to be of one spectral type, green-sensitive, and their differing polarized light sensitivities *are* obliterated at convergence (Scholes, 1969).

The actual noise present has not been measured in any photoreceptor terminal. Laughlin's (1976) measurements of response variability in the dragonfly cell soma show the S/N ratio improving as $\sqrt{I}$, as would be expected if the only noise contributor were due to the irregular, random arrival of photons. Considering the optimal optical eye design, Snyder, Stavenga, and Laughlin (1977) show theoretically that this source of variability will never become negligible even at high intensities, contrary to popular belief. Recently, Lillywhite and Laughlin (1978) have directly measured the overall response variance at low intensity in insect photoreceptors and have separated from this the component due to photon shot noise. It turns out that this last source contributes only half the total variance, the rest being what they call transducer noise, the amplitude of which also follows $\sqrt{I}$ over the range examined. The important corollary is that adherence to a square-root law can no longer be considered as unambiguous evidence that thresholds in a visual system are limited by photon-capture variability alone, but could conceal a large contribution from intrinsic noise sources in the system.

The electrical coupling between receptor somas, that between axons where it exists, and passive decrement down a capacitive cable must to some extent all act to partially smooth out high-frequency fluctuations in the response and in the background noise if this is at all significant. If the effective signal lies in a lower frequency band than the overall noise (Hagins, Penn, and Yoshikami, 1970), the S/N ratio will improve accordingly. It is difficult to see how these several forms of smoothing could work in a regenerative system, where the coupling coefficients would have to be very weak so as not to exceed spike threshold and so saturate the averaging process. The penalties paid by a slow-potential system are some worsening of frequency response, a reduction in response

amplitude, and the introduction of a small cable delay (1–2 msec). It is shown below that the first two drawbacks are remedied by the properties of the first synapse. The third is a misconception, since synaptic transmission from the insect photoreceptor becomes effective very early in the rising phase of the receptor potential, whereas a spike train would be (and is, in *Limulus* eye) triggered at much higher and therefore delayed depolarizations; for the short insect axon cable, slow-potential conduction combined with no apparent synaptic threshold is in effect a *faster* process than regenerative transmission by several milliseconds, and the gap widens at low intensity.

Postsynaptic responses: the lamina monopolar cells (LMCs) and ocellar L-cells

SYNAPTIC TRANSMISSION   Recordings described from the lamina region in locust (Shaw, 1968b), fly (Järvilehto and Zettler, 1971), and dragonfly (Laughlin, 1973) appear to come mostly from the large monopolars (Figure 8). Similar recordings may be obtained from the large second-order L-cells below the dragonfly ocellus (Chappell and Dowling, 1972) and locust ocellus (Patterson and Goodman, 1974; Wilson, 1978). The responses of all these cells appear basically similar: light produces graded hyperpolarization but no action potentials, even when recordings are taken several hundred microns down the axon (Zettler and Järvilehto, 1971, 1973). At low intensities, particularly in dark-adapted LMCs and L-cells of the locust (Shaw, 1968b; Wilson, 1978), the response is seen to comprise unitary hyperpolarizations up to 10 mV in amplitude, which fuse at higher intensities (Figure 11). Since the LMC response is initially much bigger and of opposite polarity to the corresponding photoreceptor response, it is agreed by all authors that the intervening synapse is chemically mediated, possibly with acetylcholine as transmitter (Chappell and Klingman, 1974). The synaptic latency is not exactly known because of the circular problem that the exact amplitude-transfer function is not known; but Ozawa et al. (1976), in a similar situation in barnacle eye, found an irreducible, minimum latency of about 5 msec. In locust, if an amplitude criterion of 1 mV in the receptors is chosen arbitrarily, the latency so determined remains constant over a wide intensity range at 3–4 msec (Figure 7), of which about 2 msec must represent the cable delay measured by Scholes (1969). The amplitude criterion of 1 mV must be approximately correct, since much larger values produce a negative latency, with LMCs leading. Measuring from the first appearance of the potentials,

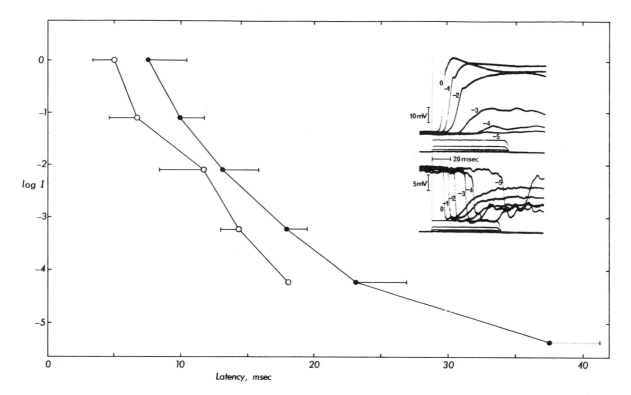

Figure 7 Measurement of conduction plus synaptic delay between photoreceptors and second-order cells in locust eye, over a range of light intensities (I), made to a criterion of 1 mV and half-height in the respective cell types. Each point is the average ±1 S.D. of 5–9 cells. Individual responses are shown in the inset. (From data in Shaw, 1968a,b.)

Järvilehto and Zettler (1971) obtained a synaptic delay of 1 msec. This establishes that potentials of about 1 mV, and probably less, do promote synaptic transmission, as Shaw (1972) demonstrated directly in barnacle.

The necessary corollary is that isolated photoreceptor bumps, which in a dark-adapted locust can exceed this size, must produce a direct postsynaptic equivalent. Thus the unitary hyperpolarizing bumps in locust LMCs are almost certainly the postsynaptic response to presynaptic receptor bumps (Shaw, 1968). In fly and dragonfly, where these unitary events are not as easily distinguishable, the presynaptic receptor bumps are similarly less distinct. A further interesting corollary follows: if there is any input convergence onto LMCs, as is suggested above by the anatomy and by Scholes (1969) for the fly, this should show up as a higher effective QCE for the unitary hyperpolarizations; and for the most sensitive cells, I found a factor of roughly six (Shaw, 1968a,b). Different amplitude classes of hyperpolarizing events (Shaw, 1968a,b) would on this interpretation directly indicate input convergence from different presynaptic sources.

The response recorded near the synapse, at both low and high intensities, can be altered by polarization through the microelectrode, and reversed in polarity, as should be expected for a postsynaptic conductance increase mechanism (Shaw, 1968a,b; Laughlin, 1974c; Wilson, 1978), perhaps to K^+ (Zimmerman, 1977). The complicated effects reported in the axons by Zettler and Järvilehto (1973) are perhaps to be reconciled by Wilson's (1978) demonstration that the rectification properties are different for synaptic and for axon membrane.

The LMC and L-cell response at high intensity appears to result from the summation of individual conductance changes, but exhibits a much more pronounced transient behavior than the receptors (Figure 8). The maximum voltage excursion in the LMCs in the best recordings is 40–50 mV, close to that of receptors (Laughlin, 1973). The operational voltage amplification across the synapse varies with intensity and, in the absence of latency data, has been estimated by Laughlin—by relating the *peaks* of the pre- and postsynaptic events—to be as high as fourteen over the middle operating range. Since the postsynaptic response is driven by potentials even smaller

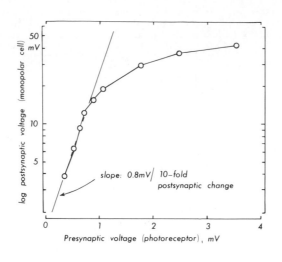

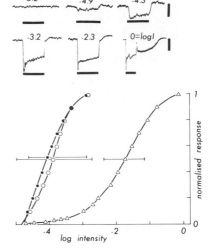

FIGURE 8 *Right*: Responses from a dragonfly lamina monopolar neuron to flashes of light of increasing relative brightness. Vertical bars: 20 mV; horizontal bars: stimulus duration (0.5 sec). The lower curves show the normalized response amplitude vs. log intensity functions averaged from the photoreceptor initial transient (triangle) and the much steeper curves from the initial transient (white dot) and plateau response (black dot) of monopolar cells. (After Laughlin, 1973.) *Left*: The log postsynaptic transient response plotted against the presynaptic transient voltage taken from the curves at the right. The relationship has a very steep initial slope, about 0.8 mV/decade.

than the presynaptic peak, the *synaptic* gain will be somewhat larger still.

In terms of the voltage necessary for transmitter release, the synapse is effectively much more sensitive than the motor-system synapse of the squid stellate ganglion, at which only presynaptic potentials exceeding 10–30 mV produce measurable postsynaptic output (Katz and Miledi, 1967; Llinás, this volume). This in part reflects the low input conductance resulting from the small size of the lamina postsynaptic neurons, which scales up the synaptic characteristic. For comparative purposes, this scaling effect and that due to the convergence of several photoreceptors can be eliminated by plotting the postsynaptic response semilogarithmically (Figure 8); this shows a maximum slope of about 0.8 mV presynaptic per tenfold postsynaptic change. Since this method of plotting Laughlin's (1973) results again takes no account of synaptic latency, the actual slope must be steeper still (<0.8 mV/decade). This value is comparable to that found at the electroreceptor synapse of a fish by Bennett (1968: about 0.8 mV/decade, assuming linear proportionality between impulse frequency and generator potential amplitude) and Obara (1976: 1–2 mV/decade, from extracellular measurements, which must underestimate the slope). These characteristics appear to set these sensory synapses apart from the squid giant, where the slope at best is no more than 8 mV/decade.

Since the amplitude range of LMCs does not ex-

ceed that of receptors, large amplifications must contract the dynamic range to less than 2 log units (Laughlin, 1973), so that the ceiling is reached sooner. This contrasts with 4–5 log units for receptors (Figure 9). Thus while the sensitivity in mV/intensity unit is greatly improved, the dynamic range is contracted, to span the approximate contrast range in the earthly environment at one particular intensity level. This parallels closely the transformations occurring between receptors and some ganglion-cell types in vertebrates (Werblin, 1974; Werblin and Copenhagen, 1974) but requires in both cases some additional mechanism for shifting the operating range to cope with the very large changes in mean ambient light level encountered in daily life.

The work on locust suggests a major cause of amplification to be synaptic—the unit hyperpolarization is much larger than its presynaptic precursor. Secondly, the convergence of up to six inputs onto some monopolars, and even more for the wide-field cells of Mimura (1976), either directly or through presynaptic interaction (as in the fly) will increase the frequency and (with superposition) the amplitude of the LMC response. A third source of amplification may stem from multiple synapses between receptors and LMC spines (Laughlin, 1973). This is supposed not only to amplify the signal but also to improve the S/N ratio in proportion to the square root of the number of spine synapses; since this is $\sqrt{40} \approx 6$, it is a powerful effect. Taken at face value this could be mis-

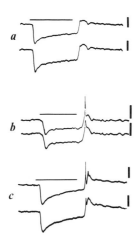

FIGURE 9 Simultaneous intracellular recordings from two points separated along the axon of a large second-order cell in three separate experiments on the locust ocellus. In each case, the lower record shows the response near the ocellar synapse to a 200 msec light flash (horizontal bars); the upper record shows the response some distance downstream. (a) In most recordings, a small decrement in the hyperpolarizing response is evident in the direction away from the synapse. (b, c) Light *off* in some cases triggers an impulse downstream in the cell, which can then be seen to decrement sharply back in the reverse direction. (Vertical bars: 10 mV.) (Courtesy of Martin Wilson; see Wilson, 1978a,b.)

leading, for although it is certainly expected that the same voltage in a larger synapse would be more effective—because more transmitter packets would be available for release—this is not related to the number of synaptic subdivisions per se, but only to the overall size of the transmitter store. Whether the LMC synapse itself is large in the sense that the immediately available store is large—comparable say to the amphibian neuromuscular junction—has not been quantitatively evaluated; therefore, the relative contribution of size to synaptic amplification and S/N improvement cannot yet be assessed. It seems a reasonable proposition at this stage.

NOISE IN POSTSYNAPTIC CELLS   Most LMCs and L-cells show several millivolts of low-frequency background noise, which Laughlin estimated to be equivalent to a 400 μV mean signal in the receptors, larger than that usually recorded from them. This postsynaptic fluctuation may represent random background release of transmitter at the synapse, and in locust its amplitude increases accordingly if the cell is depolarized by applied current, contrary to what would be predicted for a depolarizing synapse upon the LMC (cf. Zimmerman, 1977). This source of variability in LMCs is relatively modest, and, especially at low in-

tensity, the response variability in LMCs probably reflects mainly the fluctuation in photon catch and variation in bump amplitude in the receptors, plus possibly the size of the transmitter packet.

ADDITIONAL S/N IMPROVEMENT AT THE SYNAPSE   In addition to the presynaptic mechanisms treated earlier, it seems necessary that the postsynaptic convergence of as many as six receptor axons must reduce variability due to the independent photon captures in the six. The additional effect of synaptic size is uncertain (see above). Another possible and powerful mechanism, which Hagins, Penn, and Yoshikami (1970) were forced to postulate for vertebrate rods (to reduce the calculated noise below the estimated signal), would be to filter the presynaptic response through a low-pass transmitter-release process with extremely sharp high-frequency rolloff above 2 Hz. This possibility may now be dismissed at least in the fly, where the amplitude gain across the synapse actually increases modestly but continuously with frequency, between 1 Hz and 100 Hz (French and Järvilehto, 1978b). Thus the frequency characteristics of the synapse compensate somewhat for antecedent factors that degrade high-frequency performance: the intrinsic properties of the transducer process, the electrical couplings, and passive cable propagation (of which the first is certainly the most important).

SIGNAL CONDUCTION IN LMCs AND OCELLAR L-CELLS   Some investigators (Shaw, 1968b; Laughlin, 1975a) have concluded provisionally that signal transmission along the LMC axons may be passive, since spikes are usually absent and the axons little different dimensionally from those of the receptors (roughly 0.7 mm in length by 2 μm in diameter), which do transmit decrementally. The illumination response is clearly graded with intensity, and it is difficult to reconcile preservation of this gradation with any active signaling mechanism. Finally, hyperpolarizing regenerative mechanisms are not too common in the nervous system, although they are not unknown (Werblin, 1975). Zettler and Järvilehto (1971, 1973), however, examining the LMC waveform at different points along the axon, concluded instead that there was active propagation.

Zettler and Järvilehto's primary observations were (1) that there was no detectable decrement in signal amplitude out along the axon and (2) no detectable propagation delay either. Since some delay would be expected for either passive or active cable propagation, its apparent absence does not speak against either; it means only that the delay was too small to be observed reliably. A small amount of decrement (perhaps 20%) could be concealed within the (surprisingly small) scatter of their measurements, which are thus compatible with passive conduction, but with a relatively large length constant (λ). But Zettler and Järvilehto reject this conclusion because the measured input resistance of their cells is very low, indicating a small λ. If this in turn were caused by damage, the light response should also have been reduced in proportion at the recording site, which it was not. Laughlin (1974c) reports much higher values of LMC input resistance in dragonfly, although these cells have wider axons.

New evidence that may reconcile this controversy comes from Wilson's (1978) data on ocellar L-cells; they indicate a low membrane resistance for the synaptic region itself but a much higher value for the axon membrane. Because λ for the axon is consequently large, input resistance measured even well away from the synaptic membrane is still dominated by the high conductance of the latter, and so appears paradoxically low. This high conductance where the response is actively generated would, of course, not impair the passive propagation of the signal away from this site. If these results apply also to the LMCs of the fly, the existing data are thus equally compatible with decremental conduction in the LMC axon, with a large λ. If the specific membrane resistance were 20,000 Ω-cm^2 (λ = 1.6 mm), the steady-state decrement over 500 μm would be less than 10%, smaller than the measurement scatter of Zettler and Järvilehto (Wilson, personal communication).

In the case of L-cells, Wilson (1978) was able to penetrate the axon simultaneously at two points and found a small but significant decrement, going away from the synapse. This might be thought to be merely the result of greater damage at the site downstream, but the measurements have a nice inbuilt control. Light *off* triggers a depolarizing response, often surmounted by a small spike, from some deeper part of the cell, and this decrements in the reverse direction, toward the synapse (Figure 9). It is not yet certain whether the spike originates in the same cell or across an electrical junction or whether it is functionally important. Some results of mine (MS in preparation) provide some support for passive conduction in LMC axons in locust. One-dimensional measurements of extracellular resistance show this to be fairly constant below the lamina, so that radial voltage-difference measurements between two electrodes indicate local radial currents directly. The records show that these local currents from the LMCs can be separated from those of receptors over some distance and that the

currents decline with distance from the synapse. The monotonic decline of the ERG gradient always observed below the lamina is the extracellular indication of this decrement in the LMC signal (Figure 1 of Shaw, 1975).

In conclusion, the sum of evidence now seems to favor passive conduction of LMC and L-cell signals and to oppose some form of regenerative signaling. If correct, this would happily reconcile the problem of the incompatibility of graded transmission of information with the regenerative signaling system proposed by Zettler and Järvilehto.

Temporal and spatial integration of slow potentials in LMCs; electrical field interactions

Interpretation of much of the published work requires some knowledge of the unusual electrical recording situation in the insect eye, which will be summarized first. It is condensed from a manuscript in preparation (but see also Shaw, 1975, 1977a, 1978).

LOCAL ELECTRICAL FIELDS AND THEIR ORIGINS   Surprisingly large voltages, up to 40 mV (Mote, 1970), are set up in the extracellular space (ECS) of insect eyes, especially if wide-field flashes of light falling on many cells are used. Most investigators have used intracellular-type electrodes, the tip locations of which are therefore often ambiguous and sometimes intracellular; but very large voltages can also be recorded with extracellular pipettes with 30 μm tips (Leutscher-Hazelhoff and Kuiper, 1964; Shaw, 1968b, 1975). Measurements of extracellular conductivity based on techniques used by Hagins, Penn, and Yoshikami (1970) on intact locusts reveal a consistently large ECS conductivity change around the receptor axons, occasionally as much as 90:1. Extracellular resistance is highest around the axons, down to 10-fold to 100-fold less near the cell bodies, and intermediate in the lamina and below. Interpretation of the measurements is complicated by extensive cellular penetration by the DC measuring currents, which are almost 90% intracellular halfway along the receptors, and by a series of large blood channels that run between the axons (Figure 2). These channels shunt much of the current around, instead of through, the tissue and also effectively locate a remotely placed indifferent electrode between the retina and lamina, where the channels intersect. An important outcome is that the photocurrent follows a path on the return leg of which it must, by the same set of rules, largely penetrate cells and travel intracellularly (Figure 10). It is the small fraction of pho-

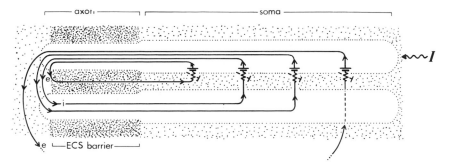

FIGURE 10 Electrical-field inhibitory interaction between insect photoreceptors, based on the scheme of Shaw (1975) and illustrated for two receptors only. The extracellular space around the receptor axons (heavy stippling) has an elevated resistance, forming part of the blood-eye barrier. Receptor current from a cell activated by light (I) exits from the axon terminal but returns intracellularly, mostly through neighboring, nonactivated cells (i), partly because the extracellular return pathway (e) is blocked by the barrier. The neighboring terminals will be hyperpolarized and transmitter release from them suppressed.

tocurrent still remaining in the high-resistance ECS that creates large voltage gradients in the region around the receptor axons. If the receptors in the region recorded are all evenly illuminated, the tangential voltage gradients disappear and the net photocurrent from each receptor is confined to flow along its own local portion of the ECS. Three independent estimates put this compartment at only 3% of tissue volume in the outer retina (Shaw, 1976, 1977a, 1978), giving an intracellular:extracellular resistance ratio of about 1:9. Across the barrier between retina and lamina, this ratio becomes 1:100 or more. It is therefore not surprising that with wide-field illumination, voltages approaching that of the transmembrane receptor potential itself can be recorded across the ECS; this is the major resistance in the circuit with simultaneous activation of all the cells. Consequently, the maximum voltage drop across the receptor presynaptic membrane during such illumination must be reduced from perhaps 25 mV (axonal attenuation factor of two) to just a few millivolts. If the illumination is made selectively stronger on some cells, depolarization of the terminals of their neighbors is not just reduced or abolished, but reversed (Figure 10; Shaw, 1975).

Because of synaptic amplification and the early saturation of the LMC waveform, the voltage change in the ECS at the synapse lags behind that across the LMC membrane. Since transmitter release from visual receptors appears to be voltage-dependent, as elsewhere (Shaw, 1972; Ozawa et al., 1976), altogether the synaptic zone has built into it the means by which, in principle, (1) general activation of many cells can lead to a reduction in the whole ensemble's synaptic output, through buildup of antagonistic fields around the terminals; (2) individual cells or classes of cell with relatively weak outputs can be suppressed completely by more active units; and (3) time-dependent suppression can be effected. A final outcome is that intracellular recording sites in the retina and lamina, no matter how professionally penetrated, are isolated from the usual remote placement of the indifferent electrode by a large series extracellular resistance, across which large photovoltages develop and add inexorably to the recorded response. Since this has not hitherto been fully understood, most of the published work has not been corrected for the distortion it can introduce.

LATERAL INHIBITION IN LMCs   Zettler and Järvilehto (1970) and Zettler and Autrum (1975) discovered that the angular fields of view of the fly LMCs were narrower than for either receptor somata or terminals, suggesting a lateral inhibitory system at synaptic level. Some caution is needed here, since such an effect would be expected anyway from a series extracellular potential of a millivolt or two with a wider receptive field (and smaller opposite effect in the retina). Such fields are present at this level in the fly (Mote, 1970), although possibly so delayed as to little affect the result. Avoiding this problem by calibrating at each angle, Laughlin (1974b) also finds the same effect, as do I in preliminary attempts in locust. In the fly no anatomical or dye-marked processes have turned up connecting either receptor axons or the larger LMCs from different stations, and measurements from a few locust LMCs using single-facet stimulation have so far revealed no direct interaction either (Figure 11).

A possible explanation is the lateral suppression via lamina electrical fields mentioned above, as suggested from different measurements by Laughlin (1974a)

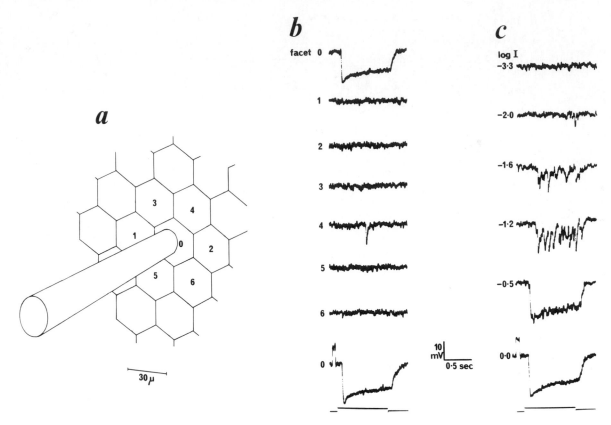

FIGURE 11   The projection of photoreceptors onto second-order cells in locust eye. When light is piped into single facets of the eye (*a*), responses can only be detected when stimulation is delivered through one particular lens, indicating that one ommatidium only drives the second-order cell (*b*). The intensity calibration in (*c*) indicates that activation through each surrounding facet was probably less than 1% of that through facet 0 in this case. No postsynaptic inhibitory interactions have been detected so far in the small sample of cells examined.

and Shaw (1975). An important qualification is that exactly the reverse would occur (facilitation) if the field potential peaked *peripheral* to the synapse, but fortunately, at least in locust, the two coincide exactly (Shaw, in preparation).

Strausfeld and Campos-Ortega (1977) instead implicate laterally spreading amacrine cells as possible inhibitory intermediaries, through conventional synapses. Local potassium accumulation from the terminals in the lamina might also be involved in axial pre- and postsynaptic facilitation, with the same end result. The relative importance of these or other mechanisms remains to be demonstrated, as does the potency of field-potential suppression upon the terminals.

The use of depolarizing signals by the receptors but hyperpolarizing ones by the follower cells may be viewed here as a specialization that enhances the field-potential amplitude and effectiveness. During illumination the LMC synapse behaves as an active source and the receptor terminal as a passive source of current, facing the extracellular space. The local extracellular fields therefore add together to form the large, positive compound potential recorded extracellularly at the synapse. Had the receptors and LMCs used the *same* polarity signals within the same structure, the resulting source and sink would oppose and partly cancel each other.

TRANSIENT RESPONSE AND LIGHT ADAPTATION IN LMCs   Especially at high intensities, during light adaptation and with wide-field stimuli, the transient appearance of the LMC response is undoubtedly a partial distortion caused by the delayed rise of the ECS potential, series recorded. However, single-facet stimulation, which reduces the fields to about 1 mV, still indicates large residual transient behavior (Laughlin, personal communication; see also Figure 11). Laughlin (1974a, 1975a) suggested that this effect may be controlled by the lamina ECS potential. While this would be much smaller than its supposed effect, a synapse that amplifies transmembrane voltage differences in the forward direction must do the same in reverse, so there is no conflict here. Recent preliminary pharmacological results indicate that local, reciprocal feedback synapses between photoreceptors and L-cells may be prominent in controlling the transient behavior at the ocellar first synapse (Chappell and Klingman, 1974; Chappell and Kuhar, 1976). Again, more work is needed to determine the contributions of each mechanism. They probably account for the rate-sensitive behavior of the first photoreceptor synapse observed with ramp stimuli by Järvilehto (personal communication) and Ozawa et al. (1976).

Related to the transient behavior is the functionally important role of range-setting in light adaptation, explored by Laughlin (1975b). The very contracted range of LMC output needs to be steered along the log I axis to cope with changes in ambient intensity, and this is what Laughlin found. At high intensities this is partly caused by receptor range-shifting, but it occurs over a wide lower range where the receptor curve itself remains unmoved. The result is that the LMCs obey much better than the receptors the desirable Weber-Fechner relation (equal output change for equal incremental stimuli, whatever the absolute level) shown by many visual systems (Figure 12). It is probable that the feedback process responsible for response transience, whether electrical or chemical, is a main agent in this range-setting, adaptive behavior. It seems likely that the same mechanism is responsible for both the spatial and the temporal suppression outlined above, but direct experiments in this area remain to be done.

Slow potentials in higher-order cells

The higher ganglia have mostly been examined by extracellular recording techniques, which have selected out only the impulse-firing cells. Exceptions are some wide-field, motion-sensitive neurons of the lobula complex, which have been penetrated and stained intracellularly. Some of these also carry impulses, but two types of cell have been suggested to function using only slow potentials (Hausen, 1976). However, the status of this result is at present controversial (see Kirschfeld, this volume).

Independent processing by separate arms of the same cell

This intriguing possibility is raised elsewhere in this volume. Pearson (this volume) points out that some thin neurons in the optic lobe (such as type h of

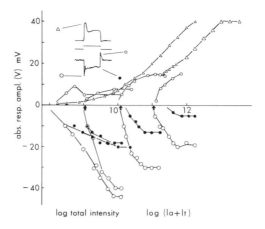

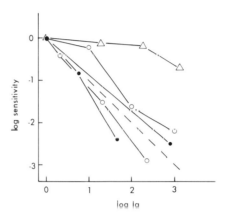

FIGURE 12 *Top*: The effect of light adaptation on the response-intensity curves of photoreceptors and second-order cells in dragonfly eye. As the eye is adapted to brighter backgrounds, the second-order cell response is readily densitized, as its curve translates to the right (from white to black dots), although the receptor curve shows little change, except at the brightest adapting backgrounds. This indicates that some extra mechanism is involved in scaling down the second-order signal at synaptic level to cope with increased ambient illumination. *Bottom*: The second-order cells obey the Weber-Fechner scaling law quite well (dashed line), but the receptors (triangles) do not. (After Laughlin, 1975b.)

Figure 1) have several arborizations at widely separate depths. This, of course, could have exactly the opposite significance—it could couple these sites rather than isolate them. Which actually occurs depends on cell geometry and local length constant (Graubard and Calvin, this volume). A small degree of isolation, with increased local weighting, might even be possible between the individual synaptic apparatuses on neighboring monopolar cell spines; this is unlikely to be anything like absolute, with realistic membrane parameters. The calculations for this case have been made by Jack, Noble, and Tsien (1975, pp.

220ff.). It seems more likely that the stalks described are merely an economical means of connecting one axon to several others in a closely packed system.

One example from the insect visual system in which functional isolation between parts of a cell does exist was mentioned earlier in connection with the ocellar L-cells. Wilson (1978) found very little decrement of the slow potential in these cells orthodromically toward the brain; but he found a very marked loss in amplitude of the deeper spike that this triggers and that spreads back centrifugally up the cell. The spike cannot usually be recorded at all at the synapse itself. This indicates failure of antidromic spike invasion well before the synapse, and isolation probably results both from the shorter axon length constant for the high-frequency components of the spike and from shunting by the higher resting conductance in the region of synaptic arborization. It is not yet known whether the spike forms an active signaling mechanism in these cells or whether it is merely redundant, as suggested earlier for some insect photoreceptors. It appears that at least the distal part of the cell acts as a passive, decremental conductor.

Final perspective

A good case can now be made that the first two types of neuron in the compound eye transmit signals decrementally, as small graded potentials which derive from single photon absorptions. This article has focused on the known details of the interactions and synaptic specializations associated with these small potentials. Signal processing in both photoreceptors and monopolar cells is qualitatively similar to that believed to occur in the counterpart cells in the vertebrate eye. Here also, the rods, cones, horizontal cells, and bipolars conduct small decremental signals; some of the receptors are also electrically intercoupled, and center-surround inhibitory systems are believed to operate as ranging and sharpening devices at bipolar level (see Werblin, this volume). The detailed operations of the two systems are sometimes different. Thus the conductance and transmitter-release systems in vertebrate receptors are activated in darkness—the reverse of the insect eye—and lateral interactions involve the horizontal-cell networks, as opposed to the large extracellular field effects implicated, at least in part, in insects.

At higher levels, a large gulf appears between our current understanding of visual processing in arthropods and in vertebrates. Although light-microscopic studies have advanced our knowledge of the anatomy of the deeper optic lobe, the physiology lags far behind. Indeed, so far, little has been done to relate the physiology to identified cell types, and the research is conducted at a rather primitive phenomenological level. Until this imbalance is corrected, it will not be possible to make more meaningful comparisons with the visual organization of vertebrates.

ACKNOWLEDGMENTS I hope that the frequency of reference to their recent work bears some evidence of my indebtedness to several colleagues and visitors in neurobiology at the Australian National University. My particular thanks to Drs. S. B. Laughlin, M. Wilson, A. S. French, and P. Lillywhite for fruitful discussions.

REFERENCES

ARMETT-KIBEL, C., I. A. MEINERTZHAGEN, and J. E. DOWLING, 1977. Cellular and synaptic organisation in the lamina of the dragonfly Sympetrum rubicundulum. Proc. R. Soc. Lond. B196,385–413.

ARNETT, D. W., 1972. Spatial and temporal integration properties of units in the first optic ganglion of dipterans. J. Neurophysiol. 35:429–444.

BASS, L., and W. J. MOORE, 1970. An electrochemical model for depolarisation of a retinula cell of Limulus by a single photon. Biophys. J. 10:1–19.

BAUMANN, F., 1966. Stimulation lumineuse de différents secteurs d'une céllule retinienne de L'Abeille. J. Physiol. (Paris) 58:458.

BAUMANN, F., 1968. Slow and spike potentials recorded from retinula cells of the honey bee drone in response to light. J. Gen. Physiol. 52:855–875.

BENNETT, M. V. L., 1968. Similarities between chemically and electrically mediated transmission. In Physiological and Biochemical Aspects of Nervous Integration, F. D. Carlson, ed. Englewood Cliffs, NJ: Prentice-Hall, pp. 73–128.

BORSELLINO, A., and M.G.F. FUORTES, 1968. Responses to single photons in visual cells of Limulus. J. Physiol. 196:507–539.

BORTOFF, A., 1964. Localisation of slow potentials in the Necturus retina. Vision Res. 4:627–635.

BOSCHEK, C. B., 1970. On the structure and synaptic organisation of the first optic ganglion in the fly. Z. Naturforsch. 25b:560.

BOSCHEK, C. and B., and K. HAMDORF, 1976. Rhodopsin particles in the photoreceptor membrane of an insect. Z. Naturforsch. 31c:763.

BROWN, H. M., S. HAGIWARA, H. KOIKE, and R. W. MEECH, 1970. Membrane properties of a barnacle photoreceptor examined by the voltage-clamp technique. J. Physiol. 208:385–413.

BROWN, J. E., and J. R. BLINKS, 1974. Changes in intracellular free calcium concentration during illumination of invertebrate photoreceptors. J. Gen. Physiol. 64:643–665.

BURKHARDT, D., 1962. Spectral sensitivity and other response characteristics of single visual cells in the arthropod eye. Symp. Soc. Exp. Biol. 16:86–109.

CAMPENHAUSEN, C. VON, 1967. The ability of Limulus to see visual patterns. J. Exp. Biol. 46:557–570.

CAMPOS-ORTEGA, J. A., and N. J. STRAUSFELD, 1972. The columnar organisation of the second synaptic region of the visual system of *Musca domestica*(L.) *Z. Zellforsch. Mikrosc. Anat.* 124:561–585.

CHAPPELL, R. L., and J. E. DOWLING, 1972. Neural organisation of the median ocellus of the dragonfly. I. Intracellular electrical activity. *J. Gen. Physiol.* 60:121–147.

CHAPPELL, R. L., and A. D. KLINGMAN, 1974. Synaptic feedback in the retina: A model from pharmacology of the dragonfly ocellus. *Proc. Int. Union. Physiol. Sci.* (New Delhi), 11.

CHAPPELL, R. L., and M. J. KUHAR, 1976. Evidence for acetylcholine in dragonfly retina. *Assoc. Res. Vis. Ophthalmol. Mtg., Sarasota*, p. 17.

CHI, C., and S. D. CARLSON, 1976. Close apposition of photoreceptor axons in the housefly. *J. Insect Physiol.* 22:1153–1157.

CONE, R. A., 1973. The internal transmitter model for visual excitation: Some quantitative implications. In *Biochemistry and Physiology of Visual Pigments*, H. Langer ed. Berlin: Springer-Verlag, pp. 275–282.

DARTNALL, H. J. A., 1968. The photosensitivities of visual pigments in the presence of hydroxylamine. *Vision Res.* 8:339–358.

DODGE, F. A., B. W. KNIGHT, and J. TOYODA, 1968. Voltage noise in *Limulus* visual cells. *Science* 160:88–90.

DOWLING, J. E., 1968. Discrete potentials in the dark-adapted eye of the crab *Limulus*. *Nature* 217:28–31.

FEIN, A., and J. S. CHARLTON, 1975. Local membrane current in *Limulus* photoreceptors. *Nature* 258:250–252.

FERMI, G., and W. REICHARDT, 1963. Optomotorische Reaktionen der Fliege *Musca domestica*. *Kybernetik* 2:15–28.

FERNANDEZ, H. R., and E. E. NICKEL, 1976. Ultrastructural and molecular characteristics of crayfish photoreceptor membranes. *J. Cell Biol.* 69:721–732.

FRENCH, A. S., and M. JÄRVILEHTO, 1978a. The dynamic behaviour of photoreceptor cells in the fly in response to random (white noise) stimulation at a range of temperatures. *J. Physiol.* 273:311–322.

FRENCH, A. S., and M. JÄRVILEHTO, 1978b. The transmission of information by first and second-order neurons in the fly visual system. *J. Comp. Physiol.* 126:87–96.

FULPIUS, B., and F. BAUMANN, 1969. Effects of sodium, potassium and calcium ions on slow and spike potentials in single photoreceptor cells. *J. Gen. Physiol.* 53:541–561.

FUORTES, M.G.F., and A. L. HODGKIN, 1964. Changes in time scale and sensitivity in the ommatidia of Limulus. *J. Physiol.* 172:239–263.

FUORTES, M.G.F., and P. M. O'BRYAN, 1972. In *Handbook of Sensory Physiology* VII/2, M. G. F. Fuortes, ed. Berlin: Springer-Verlag, pp. 279–338.

GEMPERLEIN, R., and U. SMOLA, 1972. Ubertragungseigenschaften der Sehzelle der Schmeissfliege *Calliphora erythrocephala*. 3. Verbesserung des Signal-Storungs-Verhaltnisses durch präsynaptische Summation in der Lamina ganglionaris. *J. Comp. Physiol.* 79:393–409.

GOLDSMITH, T. H., 1975. The polarisation sensitivity—dichroic absorption paradox in arthropod photoreceptors. In *Photoreceptor Optics*, A. W. Snyder and R. Menzel, eds. Berlin: Springer-Verlag, pp. 392–409.

GOLDSMITH, T. H., and G. D. BERNARD, 1974. The visual system of insects. In *The Physiology of Insecta* (2nd ed.), M.

Rockstein, ed. New York: Academic Press, vol. 2, pp. 165–272.

GWILLIAM, G. F., 1963. The mechanism of the shadow reflex in Cirripedia. I. Electrical activity in the supraoesophageal ganglia and ocellar nerve. *Biol. Bull. Woods Hole* 125:470–485.

HAGINS, W. A., and W. H. JENNINGS, 1959. Radiationless migration of electronic excitation in retinal rods. *Disc. Faraday Soc.* 27:180–190.

HAGINS, W. A., R. D. PENN, and S. YOSHIKAMI, 1970. Dark current and photocurrent in retinal rods. *Biophys. J.* 10:380–412.

HAGINS, W. A., H. V. ZONANA, and R. G. ADAMS, 1962. Local membrane current in the outer segments of squid photoreceptors. *Nature* 194:844–846.

HANANI, M., and C. SHAW, 1977. A potassium contribution to the response of the barnacle photoreceptor. *J. Physiol.* 270:151–163.

HARTLINE, H. K., and F. RATLIFF, 1972. *Handbook of Sensory Physiology* VII/2, M. G. F. Fuortes, ed. Berlin: Springer-Verlag, pp. 381–447.

HAUSEN, K., 1976. Functional characterisation and anatomical identification of motion sensitive neurons in the lobula plate of the blowfly, *Calliphora erythrocephala*. *Z. Naturforsch.* 31c:629–633.

HODGKIN, A. L., and W. A. H. RUSHTON, 1946. The electrical constants of a crustacean nerve fibre. *Proc. R. Soc. Lond.* B133:444–479.

HORRIDGE, G. A., J. A. SCHOLES, S. R. SHAW, and J. TUNSTALL, 1965. Recordings from neurones in the locust brain and optic lobe. In *The Physiology of the Insect Central Nervous System*, J. E. Treherne and J. W. L. Beament, eds. New York: Academic Press, pp. 165–202.

IOANNIDES, A. C., and B. WALCOTT, 1971. Graded illumination potentials from retinula cell axons in the bug *Lethocerus*. *Z. Vergl. Physiol.* 71:315–325.

JACK, J. J. B., D. NOBLE, and R. W. TSIEN, 1975. *Electric Current Flow in Excitable Cells*. Oxford: Clarendon Press.

JÄRVILEHTO, M., and F. ZETTLER, 1970. Micro-localisation of lamina-located visual cell activities in the compound eye of the blowfly *Calliphora*. *Z. Vergl. Physiol.* 69:134–138.

JÄRVILEHTO, M., and F. ZETTLER, 1971. Localised intracellular potentials from pre- and postsynaptic components in the external plexiform layer of an insect retina. *Z. Vergl. Physiol.* 75:422–440.

KAPLAN, E., and R. B. BARLOW, 1976. Energy, quanta and *Limulus*. *Vision Res.* 16:745–751.

KATZ, B., and R. MILEDI, 1967. A study of synaptic transmission in the absence of nerve impulses. *J. Physiol.* 192:407–436.

KIRSCHFELD, K., 1966. Discrete and graded receptor potentials in the compound eye of the fly *Musca*. In *The Functional Organisation of the Compound Eye*, C. G. Bernhard, ed. Oxford: Pergamon Press, pp. 291–307.

KIRSCHFELD, K., and N. FRANCESCHINI, 1968. Optische Eigenschaften der Ommatidien im Komplexauge von *Musca*. *Kybernetik* 5:47–52.

KIRSCHFELD, K., and B. LUTZ, 1974. Lateral inhibition in the compound eye of the fly *Musca*. *Z. Naturforsch.* 29c:95–97.

KUNZE, P., 1969. Eye glow in the moth and superposition theory. *Nature* 223:1172–1174.

KUNZE, P., 1972. Comparative studies of arthropod superposition eyes. *Z. Vergl. Physiol.* 76:347–357.

LANGER, H., and B. THORELL, 1966. Microspectrophotometry of single rhabdomeres in the insect eye. *Exp. Cell Res.* 41:673–676.

LASANSKY, A., and M. G. F. FUORTES, 1969. The site of origin of electrical responses in visual cells of the leech, *Hirudo medicinalis. J. Cell Biol.* 42:241–252.

LAUGHLIN, S. B., 1973. Neural integration in the first optic neuropile of dragonflies. I. Signal amplification in dark-adapted second-order neurons. *J. Comp. Physiol.* 84:335–355.

LAUGHLIN, S. B., 1974a. Neural integration in the first optic neuropile of dragonflies. II. Receptor signal interactions in the lamina. *J. Comp. Physiol.* 92:357–375.

LAUGHLIN, S. B., 1974b. Neural integration in the first optic neuropile of dragonflies. III. The transfer of angular information. *J. Comp. Physiol.* 92:377–396.

LAUGHLIN, S. B., 1974c. Resistance changes associated with the response of the insect monopolar neurons. *Z. Naturforsch.* 29c:449–450.

LAUGHLIN, S. B., 1975a. The function of the lamina ganglionaris. In *The Compound Eye and Vision of Insects,* G. A. Horridge, ed. Oxford: Oxford University Press, pp. 341–358.

LAUGHLIN, S. B., 1975b. Receptor and interneuron light-adaptation in the dragonfly visual system. *Z. Naturforsch.* 30c:306–308.

LAUGHLIN, S. B., 1976. The sensitivities of dragonfly photoreceptors and the voltage gain of transduction. *J. Comp. Physiol.* 111:221–247.

LEUTSCHER-HAZELHOFF, J. T., and J. W. KUIPER, 1964. Responses of the blowfly (*Calliphora erythrocephala*) to light flashes and to sinusoidally modulated light. *Doc. Ophthalmol.* 18:275–283.

LILLYWHITE, P. G., 1977. Single photon signals and transduction in an insect eye. *J. Comp. Physiol.* 122:189–200.

LILLYWHITE, P. G., and S. B. LAUGHLIN, 1978. A neglected source of intrinsic noise in photoreceptors. *Proc. Austral. Physiol. Pharmacol. Soc.* 9:49P.

LISMAN, J. E., and J. E. BROWN, 1975. Light-induced changes of sensitivity in *Limulus* ventral photoreceptors. *J. Gen. Physiol.* 66:473–488.

MARTINEZ, J. M., and R. SREBRO, 1976. Calcium and the control of discrete wave latency in the ventral photoreceptor of *Limulus. J. Physiol.* 261:535–562.

MILLECHIA, R., and A. MAURO, 1969. The ventral photoreceptor cells of *Limulus. J. Gen. Physiol.* 54:310–330, 331–351.

MIMURA, K., 1974. Analysis of visual information in lamina neurones of the fly. *J. Comp. Physiol.* 88:335–372.

MIMURA, K., 1976. Some spatial properties in the first optic ganglion of the fly. *J. Comp. Physiol.* 105:65–82.

MOTE, M. I., 1970. Focal recording of responses evoked by light in the lamina ganglionaris of the fly *Sarcophaga bullata. J. Exp. Zool.* 175:149–158.

MULLER, K. J., 1973. Photoreceptors in the crayfish compound eye: Electrical interaction between cells as related to polarised-light sensitivity. *J. Physiol.* 232:573–595.

NAKA, K. I., and W. A. H. RUSHTON, 1966. S-potentials from colour units in the retina of fish (Cyprinidae). *J. Physiol.* 185:536–555.

NEHER, E., and C. F. STEVENS, 1977. Conductance fluctuations and ionic pores in membranes. *Ann. Rev. Biophys. Bioeng.* 6:345–381.

NORTHROP, R. B., and E. F. GUIGNON, 1970. Information processing in the optic lobes of the lubber grasshopper. *J. Insect Physiol.* 16:691–714.

OBARA, S., 1976. Mechanism of electroreception in ampullae of Lorenzini of the marine catfish *Plotosus.* In *Electrobiology of Nerve and Muscle,* J. P. Reuben, D. P. Purpura, M. V. L. Bennett, and E. R. Kandel, eds. New York: Raven Press, pp. 129–147.

OZAWA, S., S. HAGIWARA, K. NICOLAYSEN, and A. E. STUART, 1976. Signal transmission from photoreceptors to ganglion cells in the visual system of the giant barnacle. *Cold Spring Harbor Symp. Quant. Biol.* 40:563–570.

PATTERSON, J. A., and L. J. GOODMAN, 1974. Intracellular responses of receptor cells and second-order cells in the ocelli of the desert locust *Schistocerca gregaria. J. Comp. Physiol.* 95:237–250.

PERRELET, A., and F. BAUMANN, 1969. Evidence for extracellular space in the rhabdom of the honeybee drone eye. *J. Cell Biol.* 40:825–830.

RAMÓN Y CAJAL, S. R., and D. SÁNCHEZ, 1915. Contribución al conocimiento de los centros nerviosos de los insectos. *Trab. Lab. Invest. Biol. Univ. Madrid* 13:1–164. (English translation by M. E. Power and B. L. Trustcott available at Yale University Library.)

REICHARDT, W. E., 1966. Detection of single quanta by the compound eye of the fly *Musca.* In *The Functional Organisation of the Compound Eye,* C. G. Bernhard, ed. Oxford: Pergamon Press, pp. 267–289.

REICHARDT, W., V. BRAITENBERG, and G. WEIDEL, 1968. Auslösung von Elementarprozessen durch einzelne Lichtquanten im Fliegenauge. *Kybernetik* 5:148–170.

RIBI, W. A., 1978. A unique and phylogenetically primitive hymenopteran compound eye: The retina of the digger wasp *Sphex cognatus,* Smith (Hymenoptera, Sphecidae). *Zool. Jb. Anat., Jena* (in press).

RUSHTON, W. A. H., 1951. A theory of the effects of fibre size in the medullated nerve. *J. Physiol.* 115:101–122.

SCHOLES, J. H., 1964. Discrete subthreshold potentials from the dimly lit insect eye. *Nature* 202:572–573.

SCHOLES, J. H., 1965. Discontinuity of the excitation process in locust visual cells. *Cold Spring Harbor Symp. Quant. Biol.* 30:517–527.

SCHOLES, J. H., 1969. The electrical responses of the retinal receptors and the lamina in the visual system of the fly *Musca. Kybernetik* 6:149–162.

SCHOLES, J. H., and W. REICHARDT, 1969. The quantal content of optomotor stimuli and the electrical responses of receptors in the compound eye of the fly *Musca. Kybernetik,* 6:74–80.

SHAW, S. R., 1968a. Polarised light detection and receptor interaction in the arthropod eye. Ph.D. dissertation, University of St. Andrews, Scotland.

SHAW, S. R., 1968b. Organisation of the locust retina. *Symp. Zool. Soc. Lond.* 23:135–163.

SHAW, S. R., 1969a. Optics of arthropod compound eye. *Science* 165:88–90.

SHAW, S. R., 1969b. Interreceptor coupling in ommatidia of drone honeybee and locust compound eyes. *Vision Res.* 9:999–1029.

SHAW, S. R., 1972. Decremental conduction of the visual signal in barnacle lateral eye. *J. Physiol.* 220:145–175.

SHAW, S. R., 1975. Retinal resistance barriers and electrical lateral inhibition. *Nature* 255:480–483.

SHAW, S. R., 1976. Neural effects of extracellular fields in insect eyes. *Assoc. Res. Vis. Opthalmol., Sarasota Mtg.* p. 17.

SHAW, S. R., 1977a. Restricted diffusion and extracellular space in the insect retina. *J. Comp. Physiol.* 113:257–282.

SHAW, S. R., 1977b. Blood-brain barrier and extracellular space in the insect eye. *Proc. Austral. Physiol. Pharmacol. Soc.* 8:90P.

SHAW, S. R., 1978. The extracellular space and blood-eye barrier in an insect retina: An ultrastructural study. *Cell Tiss. Res.* 188:35–61.

SMITH, T. G., and F. BAUMANN, 1969. The functional organisation within the ommatidia of the lateral eye of *Limulus. Prog. Brain Res.* 31:313–340.

SNYDER, A. W., D. G. STAVENGA, and S. B. LAUGHLIN, 1977. Spatial information capacity of compound eyes. *J. Comp. Physiol.* 116:183–207.

STRAUSFELD, N. J., 1976. *Atlas of an Insect Brain.* Berlin: Springer-Verlag.

STRAUSFELD, N. J., and J. A. CAMPOS-ORTEGA, 1977. Vision in insects: Pathways possibly underlying neural adaptation and lateral inhibition. *Science* 195:894–897.

TOMITA, T., 1965. Electrophysiological study of the mechanisms subserving color coding in the fish retina. *Cold Spring Harbor Symp. Quant. Biol.* 30:559–566.

TRUJILLO-CENÓZ, O., 1965. Some aspects of the structural organisation of the intermediate retina of dipterans. *J. Ultrastruct. Res.* 13:1–33.

TRUJILLO-CENÓZ, O., 1972. In *Handbook of Sensory Physiology* VII/2, M. G. F. Fuortes, ed. Berlin: Springer-Verlag, 5–62.

WALCOTT, B., 1971. Unit studies on light adaptation in the retina of the crayfish, *Cherax destructor. J. Comp. Physiol.* 94:207–218.

WALTHER, J. B., 1966. Single cell responses from the primitive eyes of an annelid. In *The Functional Organisation of the Compound Eye,* C. G. Bernhard, ed. Oxford: Pergamon Press, pp. 329–336.

WEISS, G. H., and S. YEANDLE, 1975. Distribution of response times in visual sense cells after weak stimuli. *J. Theor. Biol.* 55:519–528.

WERBLIN, F. S., 1974. Control of retinal sensitivity. II. Lateral interactions at the outer plexiform layer. *J. Gen. Physiol.* 63:62–87.

WERBLIN, F. S., 1975. Regenerative hyperpolarisation in rods. *J. Physiol.* 244:53–81.

WERBLIN, F. S., and D. R. COPENHAGEN, 1974. Control of retinal sensitivity. III. Lateral interactions at the inner plexiform layer. *J. Gen. Physiol.* 63:88–110.

WILSON, M., 1978a. The functional organisation of locust ocelli. *J. Comp. Physiol.* 124:297–316.

WILSON, M., 1978b. Generation of graded potential signals in the second order cells of locust ocellus. *J. Comp. Physiol.* 124:317–331.

YEANDLE, S., 1958. Electrophysiology of the visual system—Discussion. *Am. J. Ophthalmol.* 46:82–87.

ZETTLER, F., and H. AUTRUM, 1975. Chromatic properties of lateral inhibition in the eye of a fly. *J. Comp. Physiol.* 97:181–188.

ZETTLER, F., and M. JÄRVILEHTO, 1971. Decrement-free conduction of graded potentials along the axon of a monopolar neuron. *Z. Vergl. Physiol.* 75:402–421.

ZETTLER, F., and M. JÄRVILEHTO, 1972. Lateral inhibition in an insect eye. *Z. Vergl. Physiol.* 76:233–244.

ZETTLER, F., and M. JÄRVILEHTO, 1973. Active and passive axonal propagation of nonspike signals in the retina of Calliphora. *J. Comp. Physiol.* 85:89–104.

ZIMMERMAN, R. P., 1977. Pharmacology of the second-order neuron of the compound eye of the fly. *Invest. Ophthalmol.* (Suppl., April 1977), p. 25.

17 The Visual System of the Fly: Physiological Optics and Functional Anatomy as Related to Behavior

K. KIRSCHFELD

ABSTRACT The thermally quasi-stable metarhodopsin in insect photoreceptors is photoreisomerizable back into rhodopsin. It is shown in the specialized dorsal compound eye of Simuliid flies that matching of the absorption properties of the screening pigments to the absorption properties of the rhodopsin-metarhodopsin system enables receptors to maintain a high rhodopsin concentration even in bright illumination. Behaviorally relevant consequences are illustrated.

There are small groups of anatomically defined neurons in the dipteran visual system that are highly specialized in function and reminiscent of "grandmother neurons." A group may be as small as two neurons, one in each side of the brain; they may detect, for example, a rotation of the animal's optical environment. Strategies are discussed that allow us to relate their activities to such specific behavior responses as optomotor turning response or landing response.

Introduction

COMPOUND EYES and lens eyes are thought to be adapted to different functions. This view was put forward by Exner (1891), based mainly on the fact that compound eyes usually have a relatively low angular resolution compared, for example, to the human eye. It can be shown, however, that the low resolution of compound eyes is caused by their small size rather than by the principles of their construction. In other words, at the level of the output of the photoreceptors there is no obvious difference between the two kinds of eyes (Kirschfeld, 1976).

Nevertheless the number of points resolved by a fly's eye is considerably less (6,000 ommatidia in *Musca*: Braitenberg, 1967) than that of a human eye (4×10^5: Steinbuch, 1965), and we may ask whether we may expect higher functions such as pattern recognition to be performed at all by a visual system limited in information capacity.

To illustrate the situation Figure 1 shows the same photograph represented by 4×10^5, 11,200, 6,000, and 1,400 points, corresponding to the number of points resolved by the human eye and by the ommatidia in the compound eyes of several species of Diptera. It is obvious that a fly like *Musca*, with its 6,000 ommatidia, has sufficient input elements within its eyes to transmit quite a detailed image. In fact it may be four times better than the image shown, as the optical resolution of individual facet lenses is better than would be expected on the basis of the divergence angles of the ommatidia (Kirschfeld, 1976).

The figures illustrate only the number of points transmitted by the eyes of man and flies. They do not incorporate the anisotropic distribution of the resolved points in the visual field of man, which decays rapidly with distance from the fovea. It also does not illustrate the fact that the number of points transmitted by the two compound eyes of *Musca* are distributed over almost the whole solid angle of 360 degrees, whereas the angle of the human eye is very limited. The figure merely indicates the amount of information the visual system of *Musca* has to deal with. To get an idea of what a housefly might actually "see," we might ask at what distance an individual human face would be recognized by *Musca* with respect to the number of points scanned by its compound eyes. As has been shown by Harmon (1971), a lower limit of recognizability is reached if the separation of the points scanned from a human face is approximately 2 cm. A fly with a divergence angle $\Delta\varphi$ between neighboring ommatidia of $2°$ reaches this resolution at a distance of 60 cm. If we introduce the optical resolution of individual facet lenses, the critical distance increases further to 2.4 m.

These general considerations show that, as regards the capacity of dipteran eyes to acquire information,

K. KIRSCHFELD Max-Planck-Institut für Biologische Kybernetik, Spemannstrasse 38, 7400 Tübingen, Federal Republic of Germany

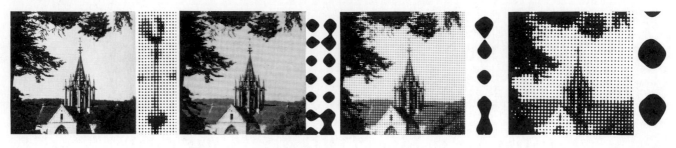

FIGURE 1 The same photograph reproduced with different numbers of points to illustrate the information capacity of the visual systems of man (4×10^5 points), *Calliphora* (1.12×10^4 points), *Musca* (6×10^3 points), and *Drosophila* (7×10^2 points). At the right of each photograph is an enlarged detail.

there is no a priori reason why visual performances of vertebrates should not also be realized in the visual system of the fly. We should also consider that—in addition to their well-known capabilities in such areas as movement detection, color vision, and pattern recognition—flies might also be able to analyze polarized light, since photoreceptors with microvillar fine structure are, in principle, capable of this (Moody and Parriss, 1961).

After a brief description of the anatomy of the dipteran visual system, I shall discuss the functional properties of the compound eye and the individual neurons of the three optic neuropils, insofar as they can be defined anatomically and have known relationships to animal behavior.

Outline of the structure of the dipteran visual system

The eye of the housefly is composed of approximately 3,000 ommatidia. The corneal lens of each ommatidium projects an image of the optical environment onto the distal endings of the seven rhabdomeres. Whereas six rhabdomeres (labeled 1 to 6), extend over the whole length of the ommatidia and belong to one receptor cell each (Figure 2, ommatidia C–E), rhabdomere 7 is formed by two receptor cells (7 and 8), which are arranged in tandem, one below the other (Figure 2, ommatidium G). Receptors 1–6 have the same spectral sensitivity, with one maximum at 360 nm and a second close to 500 nm (Burkhardt, 1962; for the most recent data see Horridge and Mimura, 1975). According to experiments with *Drosophila* mutants (Harris, Stark, and Walker, 1976), receptor 7 is probably an ultraviolet (UV) receptor and receptor 8 probably a receptor with maximal sensitivity in the UV and blue spectral range. The situation must be more complicated, however, since there are two kinds of receptor 7 available in each eye, differing in regard to the existence of a pho-

tostable pigment (Kirschfeld and Franceschini, 1977). This difference may explain the controversy in the literature over the spectral and polarization sensitivities of these receptors (Eckert, Bishop, and Dvorak, 1976; Järvilehto and Moring, 1976; Smola and Meffert, 1976). The ocelli of *Calliphora* have broad-band sensitivity from 340 nm to 450 nm (Kirschfeld and Lutz, 1977).

Since the rhabdomeres are unfused (in contrast to the rhabdomeres of the bee, for example) and act as separate lightguides, their optical axes diverge (Figure 2, ommatidium I). The optical axes of rhabdomeres in different ommatidia are aligned in a rather peculiar way: optical axes of seven rhabdomeres of seven different ommatidia are basically parallel, each "looking" toward the same point in the environment (Figure 2, ommatidia C–E are three of them in the section plane; see Kirschfeld, 1967). Careful investigation has shown that they actually are not exactly parallel but deviate from parallel by 0.4°. This means that their alignment is optimized with respect to optical crosstalk and absolute sensitivity (Pick, 1977).

Receptor axons of receptors 1–6 terminate in the first optic neuropil (the lamina), those of receptors 7 and 8 in the second optic neuropil (the medulla). Signals are carried further to the third optic neuropil, which is subdivided into the lobula and the lobula plate. The first two optic neuropils are composed of many equivalent subunits, called *cartridges* in the lamina and *columns* in the medulla, which are the same in number as the ommatidia and hence represent so-called retinotopic projections, each subunit corresponding to one ommatidium. The third optic neuropil is also composed of a matrix of columns, but there is only one lobular column for every six medullar columns and thus for their respective ommatidia (Braitenberg, 1970; Campos-Ortega and Straussfeld, 1972a,b; Trujillo-Cenóz, 1972; Straussfeld, 1976b).

Within all three optic neuropils there are, besides the periodic elements, subperiodic neurons that allow

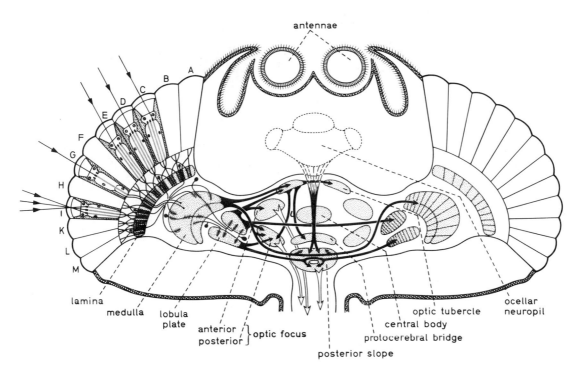

FIGURE 2   Schematic representation of the visual system of the fly. In several ommatidia (C–E, G, I) cornea lens, crystalline cone, and receptor cells have been drawn. Black arrows indicate projections from optic neuropils to higher-order centers of the midbrain. Open arrows: output projections to the thoracic ganglia. (Modified from Kirschfeld, 1973; Hausen, 1976b; Straussfeld, 1976a.)

for tangential connections between the retinotopic elements and/or for convergence of signals from many of the retinotopic elements onto one or a few subperiodic neurons.

Signals from the medulla and the lobuli, so far as is currently known, are conveyed to the following neuropils located in the midbrain: anterior optic tubercle, anterior and posterior optic focus, and posterior slope. From the last three neuropils direct connections are mediated to the thoracic neuropil and possibly to motoneurons (Figure 2; for review see Straussfeld, 1976a).

Since the number of fibers arriving at the optic centers of the midbrain is obviously considerably smaller than the number of ommatidia, all small-field interactions and abstraction processes will take place in the first three optic neuropils.

Visual pigments of invertebrates and their significance for vision

A light quantum absorbed by a visual pigment molecule isomerizes the chromophore retinal from the 11-cis to the all-trans form. Subsequent "dark" reactions lead to a number of intermediates. In contrast to vertebrate visual pigments, in many invertebrates,

including insects, metarhodopsin is quasi-thermostable: that is, it does not hydrolyze into opsin and all-trans retinal (Hamdorf, Schwemer, and Gogala, 1971; Stavenga, Zantema, and Kuiper, 1973; Hamdorf and Schwemer, 1975; for review see Goldsmith, 1972). Reisomerization is due basically to light absorbed by the metarhodopsin (Figure 3). The equi-

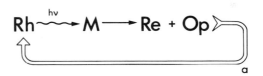

FIGURE 3   (a) Scheme of photochemical reaction in vertebrate photoreceptor cells. Rhodopsin (Rh) absorbs a light quantum and—through several intermediate steps—is transformed into metarhodopsin (M), which decomposes into retinene (Re) and opsin (Op). Resynthesis of rhodopsin is metabolically mediated (large arrow). (b) In insects rhodopsin, by absorbing a light quantum, is isomerized into metarhodopsin, which, also by absorbing a light quantum, is photoreisomerized into rhodopsin.

librium is determined primarily by the ratio between the absorption coefficients of the two pigments. There is also a slow metabolic regeneration that takes place in several insect photoreceptors (Stavenga, 1975b).

This difference between vertebrate and invertebrate visual pigments is of considerable functional significance for the two kinds of visual systems. With increasing light intensity in insect photoreceptors, the concentration of rhodopsin does not decrease, as it does in the vertebrates, because photoisomerization and photoreisomerization increase to the same degree with intensity (see, e.g., Hamdorf and Schwemer, 1975). Hence dark adaptation is not a time-consuming process as far as visual pigments are concerned. On the other hand, adjustment of the sensitivity of the receptors to different light intensity levels (light adaptation) cannot make use of changing rhodopsin concentrations with varying absorption probabilities of light, but must be based on different mechanisms.

To illustrate how this ability of the invertebrate visual pigment to be photoreisomerized, coupled with some elementary physical principles, affects the design and function of compound eyes, I shall describe the structure and function of a highly specialized dipteran compound eye: the compound eye of simuliid males. Specialized, rather than "all-around" sense organs sometimes offer a better chance of assessing function since the latter can be more easily recognized.

THE SPECIALIZED EYES OF SIMULIID FLIES Male simuliid flies have subdivided compound eyes. The dorsal eye differs in several characteristic features from the ventral eye and also from the (nonsubdivided) female eye (Figure 4).

1. The corneal facets are considerably larger in diameter in the dorsal eye (diameter 25–40 μm) than in the ventral one (diameter 10–15 μm).

2. In the dorsal eye, the retinular cells and their rhabdomeres are extremely elongated (length approximately 300 μm), so that they penetrate the basement membrane and extend into the ventral region of the head (Figure 5).

3. The screening pigment in the dorsal eye is translucent for light of longer wavelengths. It is light brown in color, whereas the ventral eye has dense, dark, red-brown screening pigments.

The specializations noted in the first two points are easily interpreted functionally. Since the resolution of insect corneal lenses is basically diffraction-limited (Kirschfeld and Franceschini, 1968; Franceschini and

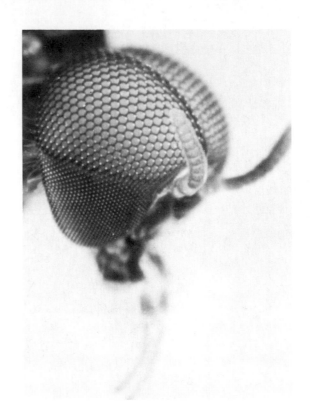

FIGURE 4 Head of male simuliid fly (*Wilhelmia equina*). The exceptionally large facets of the dorsal eye are easily recognizable. (From K. Kirschfeld and P. Wenk, in preparation.)

Kirschfeld, 1971) and since the number of quanta absorbed in a rhabdomere increases with its length, according to Lambert-Beers absorption law, the combination of large facet lenses and elongated rhabdomeres in the dorsal eye of male *Simulium* allows for high angular resolution and high absolute sensitivity (light quanta absorbed per second).

The translucent screening pigments can only be understood functionally on the basis of the thermally stable metarhodopsin. Spectrophotometry shows that the screening pigment is not translucent at all wavelengths, but that it acts like a color filter that absorbs strongly in the short-wavelength part of the spectrum (380 to 520 nm) and weakly or not at all at wavelengths longer than 550 nm. This suggests that the rhodopsin of the visual cells absorbs in the blue spectral range where screening is optimal, whereas the metarhodopsin absorbs at longer wavelengths, in the range where the screening pigment is translucent. A primary consequence of this is that the angular resolution of the receptors is high since within their spectral sensitivity range (rhodopsin absorption), optical isolation between ommatidia is high. Second,

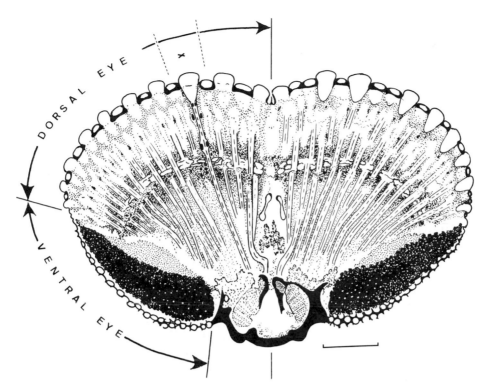

FIGURE 5 Frontal section through the head of a simuliid male (*Wilhelmia equina*). The ommatidia pentrate the basal membrane and extend into the ventral part of the head, as can be seen at an idealized ommatidium (x). (From K. Kirschfeld and P. Wenk, in preparation.)

screening is low in the absorption range of metarhodopsin. This means that reisomerization employs not only light from the small area at which a receptor is looking, but light entering the eye from all directions. This light, however, because of the screening pigments, is changed in spectral composition in such a way that the equilibrium between rhodopsin and metarhodopsin is shifted to rhodopsin; therefore a high probability for the absorption of blue quanta by rhodopsin is maintained. This kind of interpretation of colored screening pigments was first given by Stavenga, Zantema, and Kuiper (1973) for the red and yellow screening pigments of *Calliphora*. Such a selective screening filter mechanism, of course, limits the spectral band that can be used for vision; it seems most favorable for an eye that does not mediate wideband color vision. And this is, as we shall see, not necessary for the simuliid dorsal eye.

The adaptations that have been mentioned are adequate for one purpose: the detection of small, rapidly moving objects against the sky. The behavioral analysis showed that the females cross above the swarm of males and are pursued by them for mating. Detecting a rapidly moving female (size approximately 1 mm × 3 mm) over some distance might be

a difficult task for a small insect eye, since the modulation of light flux within the rhabdomere would be rather small, and therefore quantum fluctuations of light would become a limiting factor for detectability. By means of dummy experiments in which a small lead ball similar in size to a female is moved above swarming males, it can be shown that at noon males stop chasing the dummy if it is more than approximately 50 cm (angular subtense about 0.2°) away (Kirschfeld and Wenk, 1976). A calculation shows that quantum noise in these conditions is small compared with the signal induced within the receptors. The situation is different at dawn, however. Then light quantum fluctuations are closer to the size of the signal; consequently the dummies are no longer followed even if they are as close as 10 cm above the swarm.

The rhabdomeres of the dorsal eye are five to six times longer than those of the ventral eye. This increases the number of absorbed quanta by a factor of about four, if a reasonable absorption coefficient of $0.01/\mu m$ (Kirschfeld, 1969) for the absorption maximum is taken into account. This means that the threshold for detectability of females is reached 1–2 hr later in the evening, as estimated on the basis of luminance decay with time. This, in turn, increases the probability of mating and explains the high selection pressure for elongated rhabdomeres.

We may ask why rhodopsin absorption in dorsal eyes occurs in the short-wavelength spectral range and metarhodopsin absorption at longer wavelengths, whereas in principle the opposite may also occur (for review see Hamdorf and Schwemer, 1975). This seems to be advantageous for several reasons. First, natural light has a quantum emission maximum at blue wavelengths. Second, resolution of insect cornea lenses is diffraction-limited, hence in the short-wavelength part of the spectrum, optical resolution will be higher, and the signals within the receptors induced by females larger, than when rhodopsin is absorbing at longer wavelengths.

Functional properties of anatomically identified neurons

THE LAMINA Although the structure of the dipteran lamina is known in considerable detail, down to the synaptic interconnections (for review see Straussfeld and Campos-Ortega, 1977), only little is known of the functional properties of individual neurons.

The pattern of retinula-cell axon projection between retina and lamina exhibits a conspicuous interweaving of fibers. This results from the fact that receptor axons of different ommatidia, namely those of receptors 1–6, looking at the same point in space, converge to the same cartridge, where they are synaptically connected to second-order neurons (Trujillo-Cenóz and Melamed, 1966; Braitenberg, 1967). Within the cartridges the signals of these receptors (all carrying essentially the same information) are summated (superimposed), thus yielding a system with increased absolute sensitivity (Kirschfeld, 1967; Scholes, 1969). The dipteran eye, according to the terminology of Exner (1891), is an *apposition eye*. To distinguish the type of eye realized in *Musca* from apposition eyes with fused rhabdoms and without the special kind of retina-lamina projection, the former is called a *neural superposition eye* (Kirschfeld, 1967, 1972b, 1973; Stavenga, 1975c).

Axons of receptors 7 and 8 bypass the lamina without synaptic contact and terminate in the medulla. Their signals do not contribute to the neural superposition but deliver the input to a second visual subsystem. This second system—besides such differences as the spectral sensitivity of its receptors—has a lower absolute sensitivity. This is due primarily to the fact that it does not share the neural superposition; in addition, the rhabdomeres of receptors 7 and 8 are shorter than those of 1–6 and hence cannot absorb as many quanta. It has been shown, however, that the potential amplitude in receptor 8 is comparable to that of receptors 1–6 at equivalent stimulus intensities (Zettler and Järvilehto, 1972). This is not a contradiction of the statement that receptors 1–6 have higher sensitivity, since sensitivity in functional terms is defined adequately only as signal-to-noise ratio and not as absolute receptor potential amplitude for a given rate of incidence of light quanta. It is obvious from the recordings, however, that at equivalent stimulus intensities and receptor potential amplitudes, the noise level in receptor 8 is considerably higher than in receptors 1–6; that is, they have a higher gain (a higher receptor potential amplitude per absorbed quantum) but a lower sensitivity according to the definition formulated above. The higher gain seems to be an adaptation to the need of receptors 7 and 8 to transmit their signals directly over a larger distance to the medulla, whereas receptors 1–6 have only to transmit signals over a short distance to the lamina. Since the presynaptically superimposed (Scholes, 1969) signals of six receptors should not exceed the dynamic range of the axonal membrane (some 60 mV), the contribution of the individual receptor has to be reduced by a factor of approximately six.

The fact that receptors 1–6 in the dipteran compound eye have the highest absolute sensitivity does not necessarily mean that they mediate all visually induced performance at very low light intensities. For example, diurnal rhythms in *Drosophila* are synchronized by extraocular receptors that have not yet been anatomically determined. The absolute threshold of this synchronization is similar to that of the ommatidial photoreceptors (Truman, 1976). Nevertheless, the absolute sensitivity of the extraocular receptors,

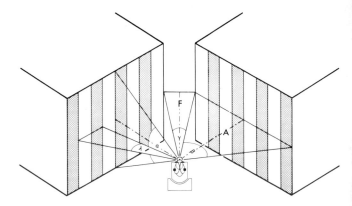

FIGURE 6 Experimental setup for stimulation of the visual system of a fly by means of moving stripe patterns. (From Hausen, 1976b.)

in terms of signal-to-noise ratio, may be considerably lower than those of the ommatidial receptors, since diurnal synchronization needs only very low temporal resolution.

Besides the six receptor input axons, there are eight more retinotopic neurons contributing to each cartridge, as well as three well-known subperiodic elements with their synaptic interconnections. Electrophysiological responses of identified cells, however, have only been recorded from two centripetal second-order neurons of the lamina, the so-called L_1 and L_2 neurons. These neurons show hyperpolarizing, maintained graded potentials in response to illumination and represent the summated activity of all six receptor inputs (Autrum, Zettler, and Järvilehto, 1970; Järvilehto and Zettler, 1971; Zettler and Weiler, 1976). Their hyperpolarizing activity is inhibited (depolarized) if receptors of neighboring ommatidia are illuminated. This inhibitory effect is mediated by light from 340 to 600 nm; hence it seems probable that it is caused by receptors 1–6 (Zettler and Autrum, 1975; Zettler and Weiler, 1976). Since the sum of activity of receptors 7 and 8 also covers this spectral range, the inhibition could result from a summated effect of these receptors. An unsolved question is whether this inhibition is mediated by neural interconnections—and, if so, by which neu-

rons—or whether it is possibly due to "field effects" within the lamina such as have been shown for epithelial receptors in insects (Thurm, 1973) and suggested for visual neuropils as well (Laughlin, 1974a,b; Shaw, 1975).

THE MEDULLA   Some sixty different types of neurons in the medulla have been described, and each retinotopic column consists of at least thirty-four of these types. Only a few synaptic connectivities have been described (Campos-Ortega and Straussfeld, 1972a,b). Intracellular recordings, combined with dye-marking techniques, have only just begun (DeVoe and Ockleford, 1976).

THE LOBULI   A whole set of giant lobula-plate neurons has been investigated electrophysiologically and identified anatomically by means of dye injections (Dvorak, Bishop, and Eckert, 1975; Hausen, 1976a,b). Figure 6 shows a typical setup for this kind of experiment, and Figure 7 shows the lobula-plate neurons that have been identified (Hausen, 1976b). All neurons described are movement-sensitive. Cells labeled "H" respond maximally to movement in the horizontal direction; cells labeled "V" to movement in the vertical direction.

The neurons may be classified into two types: those

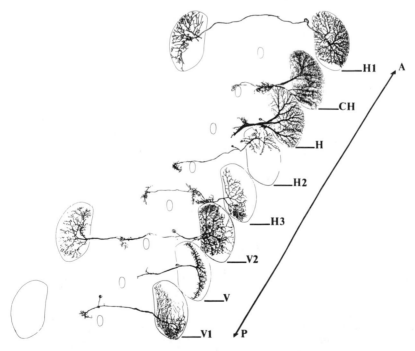

FIGURE 7   Diagram of some lobula-plate neurons of *Calliphora* that have been investigated electrophysiologically and defined anatomically. Neurons responding to horizontal movement (H1, CH, H, H2, and H3) are localized in the front of the plate; those responding to vertical movement (V2, V, and V1) are arranged in the central and caudal part of the lobula plate. (From Hausen, 1976b.)

generating classical spikes and those responding with graded potentials to visual stimulation. All neurons with axons extending into the contralateral part of the brain ("heterolateral" neurons) exhibit spikes; graded potentials were recorded from neurons with axons restricted to one half of the brain ("homolateral" neurons).

The large lobula-plate neurons obviously get input from small, periodic lobula-plate and/or medulla neurons. Their activity is further modulated by interactions among themselves. In Figure 8 a double recording of an H2 cell (extracellular) and a CH cell (intracellular) shows that each spike in H2 elicits an EPSP in CH. There are, in addition to these EPSPs of known origin, still others, larger in size, that are obviously triggered by a third element. The synaptic delay from the presynaptic spike to the EPSPs is 0.72 msec.

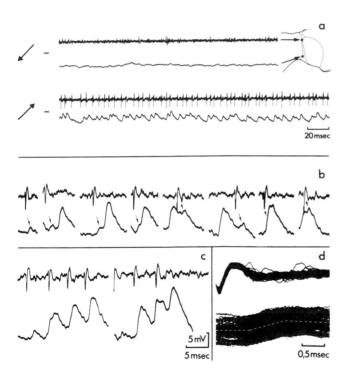

FIGURE 8 Double recording of an H1 cell (extracellular) and a CH cell (intracellular). Recording sites (in the right optic lobe) are indicated on the inset, upper right. (a) The two upper tracks (from H1) show responses to motion of a pattern in the left visual field from front to back (progressive); the two lower tracks (from CH) from back to front (regressive). Regressive movement induces spikes in the H1 cell and EPSPs without spikes in the CH cell. (b, c) Details of recording with higher time resolution. H1 spikes induce EPSPs in the CH cell (arrows). A second kind of EPSP with high amplitude occurs independently of the H1 spikes. (d) Superposition of approximately 200 H1 spikes and CH EPSPs. Latency approximately 0.72 msec. (From Hausen, 1976b.)

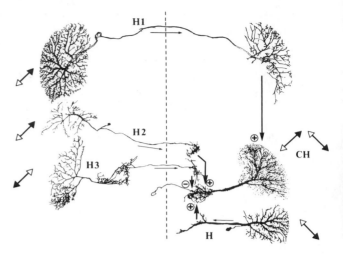

FIGURE 9 Input elements of the CH cell. CH cells are excited by H1 and H2 cells of the contralateral optic lobe (sensitive to regressive movement; black arrows indicate excitation, open arrows inhibition). Anatomical and physiological data indicate that there is also an excitatory input to the CH cell from the ipsilateral H cell (sensitive to progressive movement). The contralateral H3 cell (sensitive to progressive movement) possibly mediates an inhibitory input to the CH cell. The whole pattern of interconnections makes the CH cell sensitive to rotary movement. (From Hausen, 1976b.)

Figure 9 summarizes the interactions that have been demonstrated directly by double recording or that are suggested by the properties of the cells and their anatomical relationships. It can be seen that, by inhibitory and excitatory interactions, cells with new properties can be created. The CH cell is excited by contralateral "regressive" (back-to-front) movement through H1 and H2; it is inhibited by contralateral progressive (front-to-back) movement through H3 and excited by progressive ipsilateral movement through H. Thus the CH neuron is stimulated maximally if the optical environment is rotated relative to the animal.

Besides the neurons with connections restricted to the lobula complex, at least one neuron that has been repeatedly recorded interconnects the lobula plate with the heterolateral medulla (Figure 10). It generates spikes and is sensitive to upward movement in the frontal ventral eye region (Figure 11).

Recently the nonspiking properties of some of the lobula-plate neurons have been critically investigated in more detail. Actually nonspiking neurons in insects are known not only in the lobula plate of the fly but also in the nervous systems of other invertebrates, for example, the cockroach (Pearson and Fuortner, 1975) and locust ventral cord (Burrows and Siegler, 1976). These neurons have some properties in com-

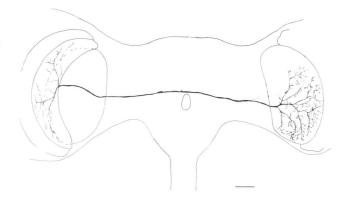

FIGURE 10 Histologically defined neuron of *Calliphora* that interconnects the lobula plate with the contralateral medulla. Calibration: 0.1 mm. (Courtesy of R. Hengstenberg.)

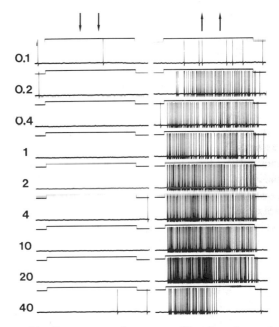

FIGURE 11 Responses of a neuron like that shown in Figure 10 to movement of a stripe pattern downwards (left side) or upwards (right side). The parameter indicated at the left is contrast frequency w/λ (Hz). It is shown that upward movement with a contrast frequency of 10–20 Hz is the maximally efficient stimulus. (Courtesy of R. Hengstenberg.)

mon that can be formulated as follows (see Pearson and Fuortner, 1975):

1. They do not produce detectable spike activity.

2. Their resting potential is low (-30 mV to -50 mV) compared to the normal resting potential in spiking cells (> -50 mV).

3. The most characteristic feature of these neurons is a high level of "synaptic" noise. It is only rarely possible, however, to observe complete individual

IPSPs and EPSPs. The noise is completely different from that recorded in spiking cells.

Hengstenberg's (1977) investigation of the nonspiking giants in the lobula plate has shown that the nonspiking giants of the dipteran lobula plate with the characteristics listed above can be transformed into spiking neurons by hyperpolarizing them with current injections (Figure 12). With increasing hyperpolarization first the noise level increases; then clearly detectable spikes appear, which sometimes do not reach full amplitude. Finally, classically shaped spikes are generated, which "ride" on slow-potential waves. With a further increase of hyperpolarization the frequency of spikes again drops to zero.

Obviously these "nonspiking" neurons have electrically excitable membranes; but under the usual recording conditions, the membrane is in a permanent refractory state and is therefore unable to generate spikes. The relatively large noise that is typical of the nonspiking neurons is explained by the fact that in the depolarized state of the refractory membrane there is a range in which even small changes in current lead to considerable changes in the ampli-

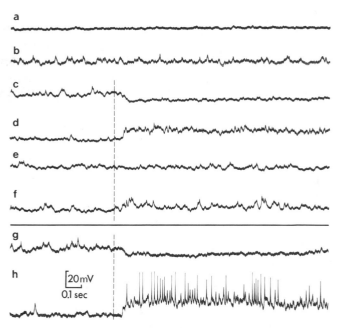

FIGURE 12 Intracellular responses of the neuron labeled V in Figure 7 in darkness (a), with constant illumination (b), and responding to movements of a stripe pattern (c–h). The pattern is illuminated throughout and starts moving at the broken line. Upward (c), downward (d), clockwise (e), and counterclockwise (f) movements elicit no significant response. No spikes can be seen in a–f. With steady hyperpolarization, by injecting -2.4 nA, upward movement (g) hyperpolarizes the cell, downward movement (h) depolarizes it and also elicits spikes. (From Hengstenberg, 1977.)

tude and frequency of the "mini" spikes. Noise will be maximal in the membrane potential range just before ordinary spikes occur—that is, just before the membrane regains full regenerating properties.

In the depolarized situation, there must be a considerable potassium outflow from the neuron, since the potassium channels will be open in this situation. This current must be compensated for by inward flow of other positive ions, presumably sodium. To prevent complete loss of electrochemical gradients, considerable pump activity would have to be maintained permanently.

The findings indicate that in these lobula-plate neurons the depolarization to refractoriness, together with a graded type of information processing, might be a result of preparation and/or recording procedures. In intact animals these neurons are expected to generate spikes. To test whether they do, it will be necessary to improve recording conditions.

The contribution of individually characterized neurons to behavioral responses

At present there is no possibility of tracking signals from the receptor, neuron by neuron, to the effector in the visual system of the fly, for too many neurons contribute to visually induced responses and many of them are neither anatomically defined nor electrophysiologically specified. However, indirect approaches may overcome the "tables of properties of neurons" and help us gain some understanding of the relevance of neuronal function for behavioral responses.

The main approach is to determine, by means of input-output analysis, the functional organization that leads to a particular kind of behavior and to specify the underlying computational principles. As Reichardt (this volume) has shown, this can be done not only for the system as a whole but also for subsystems that can be precisely defined in their topology. If such subsystems for different behaviors differ in their basic properties, analysis of their analogies will provide a means of relating neurons of known function to behavioral responses.

A first step is to try to specify the kinds of photoreceptors that contribute to a given response. Since spectral sensitivities of photoreceptors in the ommatidia, as well as in the ocelli of the fly, are fairly well known, the action spectrum measured for a behavioral response, possibly combined with selective adaptation, can provide a guide for this sort of analysis.

It has been shown that the optomotor turning response—at least at low intensity levels—exhibits the same spectral sensitivity as receptors 1–6. Hence these receptors can be considered the input elements to this kind of behavior (Eckert, 1971). This approach, however, is not always directly conclusive. Possible contributions of the ocelli cannot be easily discriminated from interactions between ommatidial receptors, as for example in the phototaxis (Schümperli, 1973; Stark, Ivanyshyn, and Hu, 1976). Moreover, changes in the spectral properties of a given type of receptor—caused perhaps by pigment migration within the photoreceptors (Kirschfeld and Franceschini, 1969; Stavenga, Zantema, and Kuiper, 1973)—might obscure the results.

The analysis of mutants has considerably increased our knowledge of the properties of photoreceptor cells and their contribution to behavioral responses (Harris, Stak, and Walker, 1976; Heisenberg and Buchner, 1977). Experiments with *Drosophila* mutants lacking special kinds of photoreceptors show that the function of receptors 1–6 is sufficient to explain optomotor turning responses, pattern-induced fixation, and visually controlled landing responses.

A second question concerns the minimal number of receptors necessary for the performance of certain behavioral responses. It can be shown, by experiment or by theoretical analysis, that one receptor is sufficient to trigger the pattern-induced fixation response (Poggio and Reichardt, 1973a,b; 1976; Pick, 1974). Two are necessary and sufficient to induce directionally sensitive turning responses (Hassenstein and Reichardt, 1953; Reichardt and Varjü, 1959; Kirschfeld, 1972b; Reichardt and Poggio, 1976), and three to determine the direction of the electric vector of linearly polarized light (Kirschfeld, 1972a,c; Wehner, 1976). For these three tasks, one receptor is, in theory, also sufficient if temporal scanning methods are applied.

To which kind of behavior, we may finally ask, do the lobula-plate giant neurons contribute? Since these neurons are sensitive to the direction of movement, the following behavioral responses must be considered: the optomotor turning response, the lift response, and the landing response.

The strength of movement-sensitive responses in insects depends on the angular velocity w of a pattern, or, more precisely, on the ratio of angular velocity w to pattern spatial wavelength λ, if the pattern is a grating (Kunze, 1961; Götz, 1964; Eckert, 1973). Figure 13 shows this dependence of the optomotor turning response (Reichardt, 1965) and the mean spike frequency of a Lobula H1 neuron of flies on contrast frequency. It is obvious that both functions have similar characteristics, especially as far as the maximum

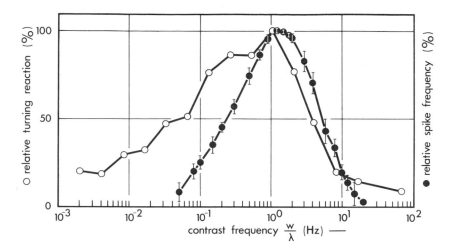

FIGURE 13 Open circles: Optomotor turning response of the fly (*Musca*) as a function of the contrast frequency. (From Reichardt, 1965.) Filled circles: Relative spike frequency of fly (*Phaenicia*) cells labeled H1 in Figure 7 to stripe patterns with various contrast frequencies. (From H. Eckert, in preparation.)

($w/\lambda \approx 2$ Hz) is concerned. Landing response, by contrast, has a maximum response close to 10 Hz—that is, at considerably higher frequencies (Hengstenberg, unpublished data). Therefore, the H1 lobula giant neuron probably is part of the optomotor turning response system. The difference between the two curves in Figure 13 may be due to species differences, differences in the stimulus conditions, or the fact that more than one kind of neuron contributes to the behavioral response.

As Figure 11 shows, one more type of identified lobula-plate/medulla neuron, sensitive to upward movement, in fact shows a maximal spike frequency at w/λ frequencies higher ($w/\lambda \approx 10$–20 Hz) than are characteristic for the lift response, which is also in-

duced by upward moving patterns (~3 Hz: Wehrhahn, unpublished data). It fits, however, with the landing response, insofar as the maximum of w/λ and the direction of movement are concerned.

One might argue that "rapid"-movement detectors, maximally responding to pattern frequencies $w/\lambda >$ 10 Hz, might also serve the lift or optomotor turning responses just by adding a low-pass filter with a cutoff of 2–3 Hz before the motor output. This would not work, however, because the frequency characteristic of a movement detector is determined by the filters at the *input* channels (Figure 14). A filter at the output cannot affect w/λ since the mean value of the signal at the output after the nonlinear interaction represents the mean of the turning reaction. This

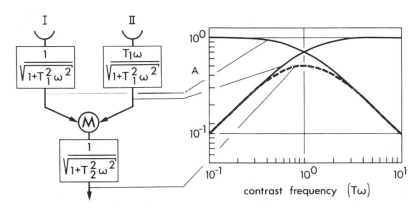

FIGURE 14 *Left*: An elementary movement detector that allows the basic functions of detecting speed and direction. It consists of two input elements (I, II), one with a low-pass filter and one with a high-pass filter (each with time constant T_1) at the input channels. The nonlinear interaction is represented by the multiplier M. Mean response is in-dicated at the output of a second low-pass filter (time constant T_2). *Right*: Frequency response curves at the output of the three linear filters at the left. Amplitude frequency response functions are indicated within the symbols for the linear filters.

mean value, however, is no longer affected by low-pass filtering. Hence movement detectors with different w/λ characteristics must be neurally represented separately from the input channels. This example shows that it is possible, on the basis of quantitative data from behavioral analysis, to draw conclusions about structural details of the neural substrate.

Conclusion

The fly visual system provides a suitable neural system for the study of the reception and processing of information in nerve networks.

The visual system of the housefly is composed of a considerable number of neurons—approximately 5×10^5. This has several consequences. On the one hand, our knowledge of the anatomical substrate is still quite limited. Considerable effort will be needed to work out the principles on which the medulla, lobula, and possibly higher centers are organized at the cellular and synaptic level. Further, the large number of neurons in a brain of limited size implies that many of them must be rather small and—in contrast to many of the giant neurons—not yet routinely accessible to present-day electrophysiological methods. It is hoped that other kinds of approaches, for example, activity-dependent staining methods, might be applied to bridge this gap. On the other hand, the large number of neurons enables flies to perform quite complex kinds of behavior, such as movement perception or pattern discrimination, that might even be relevant to our understanding of human psychophysics. It is because of these higher functions that analysis of the visual system of the fly is justified, even though there are several disadvantages in electrophysiological accessibility compared with such simpler systems as the *Limulus* lateral eye, the *Hermissenda* nervous system, or *Aplysia* ganglia.

Many kinds of fly behavior seem quite stereotyped and not subject to modification by learning processes. Thus flies are not as useful as bees, for example, for the study of learning or the analysis of memory. But this behavioral rigidity does have the advantage of being highly reproducible, which provides a basis for quantitative analysis. Several kinds of behavior can be separated from each other by means of an input-output analysis of the underlying computational principles. On the basis of such detailed functional knowledge, it may be possible to determine the behavioral responses to which specific neural elements contribute. This should be possible even if the properties of all the interneurons are not known.

ACKNOWLEDGMENTS It is a pleasure to acknowledge the valuable comments and discussion of Drs. K. Hausen, R. Hengstenberg, and B. Pick. I also thank E. Freiberg, L. Heimburger, M. Heusel, and B. Lutz for preparing the figures and Dr. R. M. Cook for reading the English manuscript.

REFERENCES

AUTRUM, H., F. ZETTLER, and M. JÄRVILEHTO, 1970. Postsynaptic potentials from a single monopolar neuron of the ganglion Opticum I of the blowfly *Calliphora. Z. Vergl. Physiol.* 70:414–424.

BARLOW, B. R., JR., and E. KAPLAN, 1977. Properties of visual cells in the lateral eye of *Limulus* in situ. *J. Gen. Physiol.* 69:203–220.

BRAITENBERG, V., 1967. Patterns of projection in the visual system of the fly. I. Retina-lamina projections. *Exp. Brain Res.* 3:271–298.

BRAITENBERG, V., 1970. Ordnung und Orientierung der Elemente im Sehsystem der Fliege. *Kybernetik* 7:235–242.

BURKHARDT, D., 1962. Spectral sensitivity and other response characteristics of single visual cells in the Arthropod eye. *Symp. Soc. Exp. Biol.* 16:86–109.

BURROWS, M., and M. V. S. SIEGLER, 1976. Transmission without spikes between locust interneurones and motoneurones. *Nature* 262:222–224.

CAMPOS-ORTEGA, J. A., and N. J. STRAUSSFELD, 1972a. Columns and layers in the second synaptic region of the fly's visual system: The case for two superimposed neuronal architectures. In *Information Processing in the Visual System of Arthropods,* R. Wehner, ed. Berlin-Heidelberg-New York: Springer-Verlag, pp. 31–36.

CAMPOS-ORTEGA, J. A., and N. J. STRAUSSFELD, 1972b. The columnar organization of the second synaptic region of the visual system of *Musca domestica L.* I. Receptor terminals in the medulla. *Z. Zellforsch.* 124:561–585.

DeVoe, R. D., and E. M. OCKLEFORD, 1976. Intracellular responses from cells of the medulla of the fly *Calliphora erythrocephala. Biol. Cybernetics* 23:13–24.

DVORAK, D. R., L. G. BISHOP, and H. E. ECKERT, 1975. Intracellular recording and staining of directionally selective motion detecting neurons in fly optic lobe. *Vision Res.* 15:451–453.

ECKERT, H., 1971. Die spektrale Empfindlichkeit des Komplexauges von *Musca. Kybernetik* 9:145–156.

ECKERT, H., 1973. Optomotorische Untersuchungen am visuellen System der Stubenfliege *Musca domestica L. Kybernetik* 14:1–23.

ECKERT, H., L. G. BISHOP, and D. R. DVORAK, 1976. Spectral sensitivities of identified receptor cells in the blowfly *Calliphora. Naturwissenschaften* 63(1):47.

EXNER, S., 1891. *Die Physiologie der facettierten Augen von Krebsen und Insekten.* Leipzig-Wien: Franz Deuticke.

FERMI, G., and W. REICHARDT, 1963. Optomotorische Reaktionen der Fliege *Musca domestica.* Abhängigkeit der Reaktion von der Wellenlänge, der Geschwindigkeit, dem Kontrast und der mittleren Leuchtdichte bewegter periodischer Muster. *Kybernetik* 2:15–28.

FRANCESCHINI, N., and K. KIRSCHFELD, 1971. Etude optique

in vivo des éléments photorécepteurs dans l'oeil composé de *Drosophila. Kybernetik* 8:1–13.

GOLDSMITH, T. H., 1972. The natural history of invertebrate visual pigments. In *Handbook of Sensory Physiology*, VII/1, H. J. A. Dartnall, ed. Berlin-Heidelberg-New York: Springer-Verlag, pp. 685–719.

GÖTZ, K. G., 1964. Optomotorische Untersuchung des visuellen Systems einiger Augenmutanten der Fruchtfliege *Drosophila. Kybernetik* 2:77–92.

HAMDORF, K., and J. SCHWEMER, 1975. Photoregeneration and the adaptation process in insect photoreceptors. In *Photoreceptor Optics*, A. W. Snyder and R. Menzel, eds. Berlin-Heidelberg-New York: Springer-Verlag, pp. 263–289.

HAMDORF, K., J. SCHWEMER, and M. GOGALA, 1971. Insect visual pigment sensitive to ultraviolet light. *Nature* 231:458–459.

HARMON, L. D., 1971. Some aspects of recognition of human faces. In *Pattern Recognition in Biological and Technical Systems* (Proceedings of the Fourth Congress of the Deutsche Gesellschaft für Kybernetik), O.-J. Grüsser and R. Klinke, eds. Berlin: Springer-Verlag, pp. 196–219.

HARRIS, W. A., W. S. STARK, and J. A. WALKER, 1976. Genetic dissection of the photoreceptor system in the compound eye of *Drosophila melanogaster. J. Physiol.* 256:415–439.

HASSENSTEIN, B., and W. REICHARDT, 1953. Der Schluss von Reiz-Reaktions-Funktionen auf System-Strukturen. *Z. Naturforsch.* 8b(9).

HAUSEN, K., 1976a. Functional characterization and anatomical identification of motion sensitive neurons in the lobula plate of the blowfly *Calliphora erythrocephala. Z. Naturforsch.* 31c:629–633.

HAUSEN, K., 1976b. Struktur, Funktion und Konnektivität bewegungsempfindlicher Interneurone im dritten optischen Neuropil der Schmeißfliege *Calliphora erythrocephala.* Ph.D. dissertation, Eberhard-Karls-Universität, Tübingen.

HEISENBERG, M., and E. BUCHNER, 1977. The role of retinula cell types in visual behaviour of *Drosophila melanogaster. J. Comp. Physiol.* 117:127–162.

HENGSTENBERG, R., 1977. Spike responses of "nonspiking" visual interneurons. *Nature* 270:338–340.

HORRIDGE, G. A., and K. MIMURA, 1975. Fly photoreceptors. I. Physical separation of two visual pigments in *Calliphora* retinula cells 1–6. *Proc. R. Soc. Lond.* B190:211–224.

JÄRVILEHTO, M., and J. MORING, 1976. Spectral and polarization sensitivity of identified retinal cells of the fly. In *Neural Principles in Vision*, E. Zettler and R. Weiler, eds. Berlin: Springer-Verlag, pp. 214–226.

JÄRVILEHTO, M., and F. ZETTLER, 1971. Localized intracellular potentials from pre- and postsynaptic components in the external plexiform layer of an insect retina. *Z. Vergl. Physiol.* 75:422–440.

KIRSCHFELD, K., 1967. Die Projektion der optischen Umwelt auf das Raster der Rhabdomere im Komplexauge von *Musca. Exp. Brain Res.* 3:248–270.

KIRSCHFELD, K., 1969. Absorption properties of photopigments in single rods, cones and rhabdomeres. In *Rendiconti S.I.F.*, vol. 43. W. Reichardt, ed. New York: Academic Press, pp. 116–136.

KIRSCHFELD, K., 1972a. Die notwendige Anzahl von Rezeptoren zur Bestimmung der Richtung des elektrischen Vektors linear polarisierten Lichtes. *Z. Naturforsch.* 27b:578–579.

KIRSCHFELD, K., 1972b. The visual system of *Musca*: Studies on optics, structure and function. In *Information Processing in the Visual Systems of Arthropods*, R. Wehner, ed. Berlin-Heidelberg-New York: Springer-Verlag, pp. 61–74.

KIRSCHFELD, K., 1972c. Vision of polarised light. In *Symposia Proceedings of the Fourth International Biophysics Congress, Moscow*, pp. 289–296.

KIRSCHFELD, K., 1973. Das neurale Superpositionsauge. In *Fortschritte der Zoologie*, M. Lindauer, ed. Stuttgart: Gustav Fischer, Band 21: Heft 2/3, pp. 229–257.

KIRSCHFELD, K., 1976. The resolution of lens and compound eyes. In *Neural Principles in Vision*, F. Zettler and R. Weiler, eds. Berlin-Heidelberg-New York: Springer-Verlag, pp. 354–370.

KIRSCHFELD, K., and N. FRANCESCHINI, 1968. Optische Eigenschaften der Ommatidien in Komplexauge von *Musca. Kybernetik* 5:47–52.

KIRSCHFELD, K., and N. FRANCESCHINI, 1969. Ein Mechanismus zur Steurung des Lichtflusses in den Rhabdomeren des Komplexauges von *Musca. Kybernetik* 6:13–22.

KIRSCHFELD, K., and N. FRANCESCHINI, 1977. Photostable pigments within the membrane of photoreceptors and their possible role. *Biophys. Struct. Mechanism.* 3:191–194.

KIRSCHFELD, K., and B. LUTZ, 1977. The spectral sensitivity of the ocelli of *Calliphora* (Diptera). *Z. Naturforsch.* 32c:439–441.

KIRSCHFELD, K., and P. WENK, 1976. The dorsal compound eye of simuliid flies: An eye specialized for the detection of small, rapidly moving objects, *Z. Naturforsch.* 31c:764–765.

KUNZE, P., 1961. Untersuchung des Bewegungssehens fixiert fliegender Bienen. *Z. Vergl. Physiol.* 44:656–684.

LAUGHLIN, S. B., 1974a. Neural integration in the first optic neuropile of dragonflies. II. Receptor signal interactions in the lamina. *J. Comp. Physiol.* 92:357–375.

LAUGHLIN, S. B., 1974b. Neural integration in the first optic neuropile of dragonflies. III. The transfer of angular information. *J. Comp. Physiol.* 92:377–396.

MOODY, M. F., and J. R. PARRISS, 1961. The discrimination of polarized light by octopus: A behavioural and morphological study. *Z. Vergl. Physiol.* 44:268–291.

PEARSON, K. G., and C. R. FUORTNER, 1975. Nonspiking interneurons in walking system of the cockroach. *J. Neurophysiol.* 38:33–52.

PICK, B., 1974. Visual flicker induces orientation behaviour in the fly *Musca. Z. Naturforsch.* 29c:310–312.

PICK, B., 1977. Specific misalignments of rhabdomere visual axes in the neural superposition eye of dipteran flies. *Biol. Cyb.* 26:215–224.

POGGIO, T., and W. REICHARDT, 1973a. Considerations on models of movement detection. *Kybernetik* 13:223–227.

POGGIO, T., and W. REICHARDT, 1973b. A theory of the pattern induced flight orientation of the fly *Musca domestica. Kybernetik* 12:185–203.

POGGIO, T., and W. REICHARDT, 1976. Visual control of orientation behaviour in the fly. Part II. Towards the underlying neural interactions. *Q. Rev. Biophys.* 9(3):377–438.

REICHARDT, W. E., 1966. Detection of single quanta by the

compound eye of the fly *Musca*. In *The Functional Organization of the Compound Eye*, C. G. Bernhard, ed. Oxford: Pergamon Press, pp. 267–289.

REICHARDT, W., and T. POGGIO, 1976. Visual control of orientation behaviour in the fly. I. A quantitative analysis. *Q. Rev. Biophys.* 9(3):311–375.

REICHARDT, W., and D. VARJÚ, 1959. Übertragungseigenschaften im Auswertesystem für das Bewegungssehen (Folgerungen aus Experimenten an dem Rüsselkäfer Chlorophanus viridis). *Z. Naturforsch.* 14b:674–689.

SCHOLES, J., 1969. The electrical responses of the retinal receptors and the lamina in the visual system of the fly *Musca*. *Kybernetik* 6:149–162.

SCHÜMPERLI, R. A., 1973. Evidence for colour vision in *Drosophila melanogaster* through spontaneous phototactic choice behaviour. *J. Comp. Physiol.* 86:77–94.

SHAW, S. R., 1975. Retinal resistance barriers and electrical lateral inhibition. *Nature* 255:480–483.

SMOLA, U., and P. MEFFERT, 1976. Die spektrale Empfindlichkeit der zentralen Sehzellen im Auge der Schmeißfliege *Calliphora erythrocephala*. In *Verhandlungen der Deutschen Zoologischen Gesellschaft*, vol. 69, W. Rathmeyer, ed. pp. 282.

STARK, W. S., A. M. IVANYSHYN, and K. G. HU, 1976. Spectral sensitivities and photopigments in adaptation of fly visual receptors. *Naturwissenschaften* 63:513–518.

STAVENGA, D. G., 1975a. Optical qualities of the fly eye: An approach from the side of geometrical, physical and waveguide optics. In *Photoreceptor Optics*, A. W. Synder and R. Menzel, eds. Berlin: Springer-Verlag, pp. 126–144.

STAVENGA, D. G., 1975b. Dark regeneration of invertebrate visual pigments. In *Photoreceptor Optics*, A. W. Snyder and R. Menzel, eds. Berlin: Springer-Verlag, pp. 290–295.

STAVENGA, D. G., 1975c. The neural superposition eye and its optical demands. *J. Comp. Physiol.* 102:297–304.

STAVENGA, D. G., A. ZANTEMA, and J. W. KUIPER, 1973. Rhodopsin processes and the function of the pupil mechanism in flies. In *Biochemistry and Physiology of Visual Pigments*, H. Langer, ed. Berlin: Springer-Verlag, pp. 175–180.

STEINBUCH, K., 1965. *Automat und Mensch*. Berlin: Springer-Verlag.

STRAUSSFELD, N. J., 1976a. *Atlas of an Insect Brain*. Berlin-Heidelberg-New York: Springer-Verlag.

STRAUSSFELD, N. J., 1976b. Mosaic organizations, layers, and visual pathways in the insect brain. In *Neural Principles in Vision*, F. Zettler and R. Weiler, eds. Berlin: Springer-Verlag, pp. 245–279.

STRAUSSFELD, N. J., and J. A. CAMPOS-ORTEGA, 1977. Vision in insect: Pathways possibly underlying neural adaptation and lateral inhibition. *Science* 195:894–897.

THURM, U., 1973. Basics of the generation of receptor potentials in epidermal mechanoreceptors of insects. In *Abhandlungen der Rheinisch-Westfälischen Akademie der Wissenschaften*, Band 53 (Symposium Mechanoreception), pp. 355–385.

TRUJILLO-CENÓZ, O., 1972. The structural organization of the compound eye in insects. In *Handbook of Sensory Physiology VII/2*, M. G. F. Fuortes, ed., Berlin-Heidelberg-New York: Springer-Verlag, pp. 5–62.

TRUJILLO-CENÓZ, O., and J. MELAMED, 1966. Compound eye of dipterans: Anatomical basis for integration—an electron microscope study. *J. Ultrastruct. Res.* 16:395–398.

TRUMAN, J. W., 1976. Extraretinal photoreception in insects. *Photochem. Photobiol.* 23:215–225.

WEHNER, R., 1976. Polarized-light navigation by insects. *Sci. Am.* 235(1):106–115.

ZETTLER, F., and H. AUTRUM, 1975. Chromatic properties of lateral inhibition in the eye of a fly. *J. Comp. Physiol.* 97:181–188.

ZETTLER, F., and M. JÄRVILEHTO, 1972. Intraaxonal visual responses from visual cells and second-order neurons of an insect retina. In *Information Processing in the Visual Systems of Arthropods*, R. Wehner, ed. Berlin-Heidelberg-New York: Springer-Verlag, pp. 217–222.

ZETTLER, F., and R. WEILER, 1976. Neuronal processing in the first optic neuropile of the compound eye of the fly. In *Neural Principles in Vision*, F. Zettler and R. Weiler, eds. Berlin-Heidelberg-New York: Springer-Verlag, pp. 227–237.

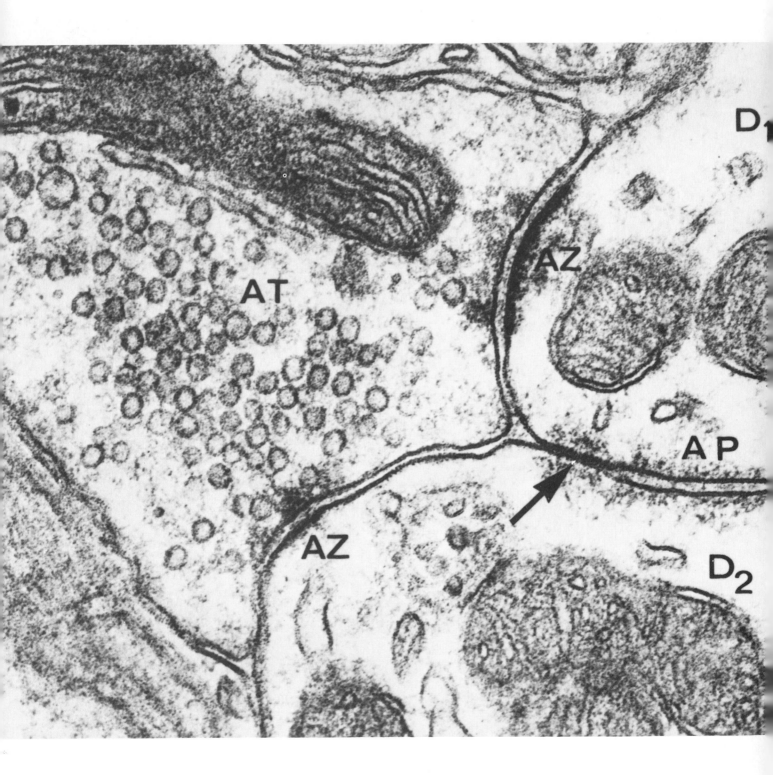

SPIKELESS

AND

ELECTROTONIC

INFORMATION

PROCESSING

An electron micrograph of an inferior-olive glomerulus of the cat. A peripheral axon (AT) establishes a chemical synapse or active zone (AZ) on each of two adjacent dendritic profiles (D$_1$, D$_2$). The membrane interface between the two apposing dendritic processes bears a gap junction (arrow) and an attachment plaque (AP). (Micrograph provided by C. Sotelo.)

Introduction

GORDON M. SHEPHERD

THIS SECTION picks up the main themes of local organization and follows them into other parts of the nervous system. We shall be particularly concerned with the level of the individual synapse and synaptic terminal, with chemical and electrical types of synapses, and with the graded electrical potentials that appear to constitute the controlling signals for transmission and integration in many local circuits.

Katherine Graubard and William Calvin describe recent experiments analyzing dendrodendritic synapses. In lobster neurons there is now anatomical evidence for input and output synapses intermingled on dendritic processes in the neuropil. Graubard and Calvin examine some of the input-output properties of these neurons and relate them to the geometry and electrotonic properties of the dendritic branches. The manner of spread of potentials is characterized, and comparisons are made with neurons in *Aplysia* and with motoneurons and superior colliculus neurons in the vertebrate nervous system. A modeling approach is used, building on the work of Rall and the principles discussed in this volume by Julian Jack. The results support the idea that there is a degree of autonomy in local computational operations within the dendritic branches of these neurons.

Henri Korn and D. S. Faber take up the subject of electrical interactions between nerve cells and differentiate two main types. One is caused by field effects in which currents generated by one neuron directly alter the excitability of a neighboring neuron without specialized junctions between the two. The other results from the spread of current through specific low-resistance junctions (gap junctions or electrical or electrotonic synapses) connecting two neurons. On the basis of their experiments in the Mauthner cell, Korn and Faber show how field effects can produce either excitation or inhibition, depending on the specific morphological constraints on current flows in and around particular neuronal branches and terminals. Transmission through electrical synapses is described for fish oculomotor neurons and for the lateral vestibular neurons of fish and rat. Electrical and chemical synapses may function independently or together, as in mixed synapses; the relation between the two, and their significance for local circuit organization in the vertebrate nervous system, are discussed.

Norton Gilula devotes further attention to electrotonic junctions. He summarizes the fine structure of gap junctions as revealed by the electron microscope, primarily for nonnervous tissue. There is now evidence about the steps involved in the formation of these junctions during development, their significance for cell differentiation, their protein and lipid composition and rates of turnover, and their stability in the face of various experimental procedures. The junctional channels not only provide high-conductance pathways for electric current flow but also accommodate and possibly regulate the intercellular movement of a variety of ions and molecules of low molecular weight. Gilula discusses recent studies of gap junctions in culture populations with paricular regard to the specificity of cell-to-cell communication and the transmission of hormonal stimulation.

18 Presynaptic Dendrites: Implications of Spikeless Synaptic Transmission and Dendritic Geometry

KATHERINE GRAUBARD and WILLIAM H. CALVIN

ABSTRACT   Two recent developments have modified our traditional concept of the neuron: output synapses have been discovered intermixed with input synapses and synaptic transmission has been shown to grade with presynaptic voltage. In a number of invertebrate spikeless and spiking neurons, synaptic transmission lasts for the duration of the presynaptic depolarization. There is a threshold presynaptic voltage, but it is sometimes below the spike threshold, or even below the resting potential. Above the release threshold, the postsynaptic potential (PSP) grades over a wide range of presynaptic voltages. The steady-state cable equation can be used to predict how PSPs spread within a complex dendritic geometry. Input synapses located on long, thin processes develop large PSPs, although these PSPs attenuate markedly before reaching central structures. Whereas a proximal dendrodendritic output synapse would see proximal and distal input synapses as approximately equal, a distal output synapse would see many-fold differences in the relative PSP sizes. Thus regional computations could take place in distal dendritic trees; a given neuron could compute many different functions of its inputs. Models are made of *Aplysia* and lobster neurons, of a cat spinal motoneuron, and of a neuron in the rat superior colliculus.

Introduction

DOES THE NEURON function as a unit, or are some processes allowed a measure of regional autonomy? In the classic view of the neuron, synaptic input and output sites are strictly segregated, with all inputs onto the dendrites and soma and all output from the far ends of the axon. Synaptic inputs affect outputs only through the intermediary spike mechanism, and thus all output synapses receive the same message, generated by the summation of postsynaptic potentials (PSPs) at the spike trigger zone. The discovery of presynaptic inhibition (Frank, 1959) and its ana-

tomical correlate of axoaxonic synapses (Gray, 1962) modified this simple description of nerve cells but did not seriously challenge the basic concepts of the neuron as the computational unit of the nervous system. The finding of dendrodendritic synapses (Rall et al., 1966), however, has raised a question: Can local PSP inputs evoke transmitter release from nearby output synapses without the need for spikes? If true, this creates the possibility of dendrites functioning in a semiautonomous fashion, with each dendrite capable of sending a message based largely on its local inputs and with the spike trigger zone computing still another function, perhaps more broadly representative of all inputs to the cell.

Since neurons with intermixed input and output synapses are common in both vertebrate and invertebrate nervous systems, the need to understand dendrodendritic synapses is vital. This paper will discuss two questions that are basic to such an understanding. (1) What are the input-output properties of spikeless synaptic transmission? (2) How do PSPs spread within complex dendritic geometries? Answers to these questions, together with considerations discussed elsewhere (Calvin and Graubard, this volume), should help us to assess which neurons with presynaptic dendrites are likely candidates for regional computation.

Input-output properties of synapses

To understand how synaptic outputs from dendrites could function, it is necessary to know what amplitude of depolarization will just evoke transmitter release, how that release will grade with depolarizations larger than this threshold, and whether that release is transient or sustained when a depolarization is maintained for many seconds.

The best studies of individual synaptic regions come from the squid giant synapse; a detailed analysis

KATHERINE GRAUBARD and WILLIAM H. CALVIN   Departments of Zoology and Neurological Surgery, University of Washington, Seattle, WA 98195

of that synapse by Llinás may be found elsewhere in this volume. Earlier studies of that synapse (e.g., Hagiwara and Tasaki, 1958; Katz and Miledi, 1966) and of the lamprey giant synapse (Martin and Ringham, 1975) showed that a substantial depolarization is required to reach the threshold for synaptic release and that there is a steep input-output curve above this threshold. Recent studies of squid by Charlton and Atwood (1977) show a low threshold when long-lasting depolarizations are used. Such synaptic properties as high thresholds and steep input-output relations seem well adapted to operation via spikes but poorly adapted for grading release; indeed, no input synapses (e.g., axoaxonics) seem to occur within electrical proximity of these giant output synapses. The giant synapses seem to be specialized for fail-safe transmission of spikes through a multineuronal escape-behavior pathway, not for integrative purposes.

There are systems with neurons lacking spikes (Ripley, Bush, and Roberts, 1968; Werblin and Dowling, 1968; Mendelson, 1971; Zettler and Järvilehto, 1971; Paul, 1972; Shaw, 1972; Maynard and Walton, 1975; Pearson and Fourtner, 1975; Burrows and Siegler, 1976). However, synaptic input-output curves for these systems have so far been calculated only by indirect means (Maynard and Walton, 1975; Burrows and Siegler, 1976).

One system that might provide a useful model for cells with dendrodendritic synapses is the lobster stomatogastric ganglion. It contains many spiking and nonpsiking neurons that make inhibitory synaptic connections and have a cell structure that appears to favor PSP-modulated release (Figure 1D). Recently, Graubard (1978a) and Graubard, Raper, and Hartline (1977) studied graded synaptic transmission between some of these neurons.

LOBSTER STOMATOGASTRIC NEURONS   The stomatogastric ganglion of *Panulirus interruptus* consists of the

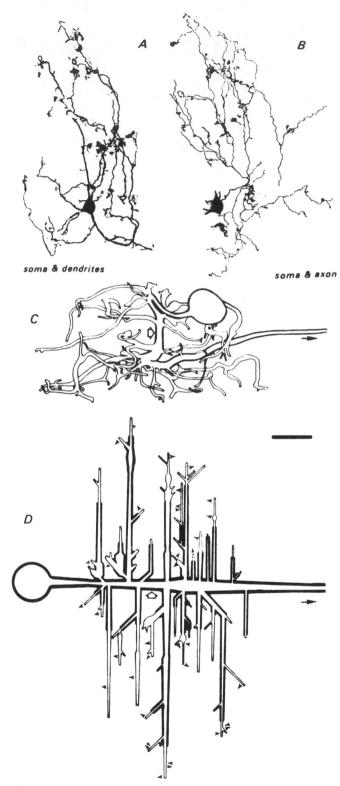

soma & dendrites

soma & axon

FIGURE 1 Neurons with intermingled input and output synapses. (A, B) Golgi type II neuron in lateral geniculate nucleus of cat is an intrinsic neuron with outputs onto the principal neurons projecting to visual cortex, both via its axon terminals (B) but also via dendrodendritic synapses from its dendritic tree (A). Invertebrate neurons also have intermixed input and output synapses. (C) The AM neuron of lobster stomatogastric ganglion has extensive secondary and tertiary processes ending in the neuropil, in addition to the axon exiting from the ganglion. (D) The neuron in part C straightened out into a stick figure; the small arrowheads of opposite direction show input and output synapses located on short tertiary processes. The heavy outlining indicates the extent of glial covering and, thus, regions where neither input nor output synapses can be found.

Bar: 50 μm for A and B, 100 μm for C and D. (A and B from Famiglietti and Peters, 1972, reprinted by permission of the *Journal of Comparative Neurology*; C and D from King, 1976, reprinted by permission of the *Journal of Neurocytology*.)

cell bodies and neuropilar processes of about thirty neurons, most of which are motor neurons to the striated muscle of the gut. The physiological interconnections between these neurons have been described in detail (Selverston et al., 1976). Neuron structure has been demonstrated by King (1976) using the method of serial section reconstruction; Figure 1C, D shows the branching pattern of one such neuron. Input and output synapses occur near each other on fine processes within the neuropil; they are thus at some distance from both the soma and the spike-initiating region. The soma and the larger-diameter processes appear to be sites prohibited for synaptic interconnection, as they are entirely ensheathed in glia (King, 1976; heavy lines in Figure 1D). Since there are many sites of interconnection between a given pair of neurons, the PSP recorded intrasomatically is a composite of contributions from a multitude of sites on a number of different processes.

While such a system is complex, it has some advantages over the giant synapses. It is possible to examine both spiking and nonspiking presynaptic neurons (Maynard, 1972; Maynard and Walton, 1975). There are a large number of monosynaptic inhibitory connections from which to choose. Such synapses are not obligatory and occur in a location where they will be exposed to the voltage fluctuations caused by both local synaptic inputs and attenuated PSPs from distant input synapses. Additionally, some of the presynaptic neurons are bursting pacemaker neurons with endogenous voltage swings of considerable amplitude; such voltage oscillations might also drive

graded transmitter release (Graubard, Raper, and Hartline, 1977).

POSTSYNAPTIC WAVEFORMS FOR PRESYNAPTIC VOLTAGE STEPS   Transneuronal input-output properties were measured by depolarizing the presynaptic cell with steps of current injected into the soma while recording the voltage change produced in both the pre- and postsynaptic cell bodies (Figure 2). Tetrodotoxin (TTX) blocks spikes in this system; its use allowed input-output properties to be studied without interference by spikes or spontaneous PSP input in either the pre- or the postsynaptic cell. For a long presynaptic depolarizing current step above the threshold for transmitter release, one typically obtains pre- and postsynaptic responses like those shown in Figure 2A. This example is for a spiking presynaptic neuron in which the spikes have been blocked by 2×10^{-7}M TTX; the waveform is identical for spiking neurons in TTX (Graubard, Raper, and Hartline, 1977) and for nonspiking neurons with or without TTX (Graubard, 1978a). This typical postsynaptic waveform consists of a synaptic delay followed by a hyperpolarization to a peak of inhibition and then a decay to a maintained plateau. In most neuron pairs, the plateau hyperpolarization is maintained for the duration of the presynaptic depolarization. These peak-plateau postsynaptic responses have been shown to have the characteristics of typical chemical synapses; both peak and plateau have the same reversal potential. They have been successfully demonstrated between all tested neuronal pairs having a large, spike-evoked, monosynap-

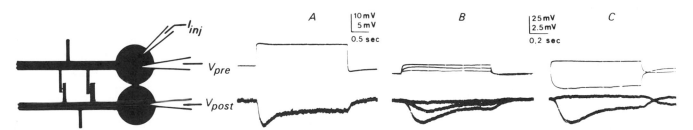

FIGURE 2   Spikeless synaptic transmission. At left is a diagram of stimulation and recording conditions. Electrodes are intrasomatic, but chemical synapses are distributed on secondary neurites in the neuropil. Records are shown of spiking neurons with spikes blocked with 2×10^{-7}M TTX. A long presynaptic current pulse (not shown) produces a steplike presynaptic voltage change, as shown in the upper traces of A, B, and C. (A) Depolarization of presynaptic neuron produces a hyperpolarizing response in the postsynaptic neuron. The response has a synaptic delay, a peak response, and a plateau level of hyperpolarization that lasts

for the duration of presynaptic depolarization. (B) Grading the presynaptic voltage causes a grading of both peak and plateau components of postsynaptic response. (C) A hyperpolarization of some presynaptic cells causes a depolarization in the postsynaptic cell, indicating that the presynaptic neuron continuously releases transmitter while at rest, thus inhibiting the postsynaptic cell continuously. Presynaptic cells are PD cells; postsynaptic neurons are PY cells. B, C share common calibration; B, C, and Figure 3B are from the same preparation. (Data from Graubard, Raper, and Hartline, 1977.)

tic IPSP and from spikeless presynaptic neurons as well.

The size of the peak response depends on the past history of the synaptic activity (Graubard, 1978a); it decreases to the plateau size if there has been massive release in seconds prior to the presynaptic depolarization. Peak-plateau shaped responses occur at the squid giant synapse but have not been found in studies of nonspiking neurons of the locust (Burrows and Siegler, 1976); there is also no evidence for a peak-plateau response at motor endplate when the rate of miniature endplate potentials is studied as a function of presynaptic depolarizing current (Quastel, 1974).

TRANSNEURONAL INPUT-OUTPUT CURVES A transneuronal input-output curve, similar to the synaptic input-output curves obtained for the giant synapses (Katz and Miledi, 1966; Martin and Ringham, 1975), can be constructed by applying a series of current steps to the presynaptic neuron soma (Figure 2B). The current causes a steplike change in the intrasomatic voltage of the presynaptic neuron (for spiking neurons this procedure is performed in 2×10^{-7}M TTX). The amplitude of both peak and plateau components of the postsynaptic response can then be plotted as a function of the presynaptic voltage (Figure 3). There is a presynaptic voltage threshold for obtaining any detectable postsynaptic response. Beyond that threshold, the postsynaptic peak and plateau responses both grow with increases in presynaptic voltage.

The position of the release threshold relative to the resting potential is of paramount importance for the functional interpretation of such curves. If the threshold were high, release from output synapses in fine processes might only occur when spikes retrogradely invaded the processes from the spike trigger zone (usually thought to reside on the main axon).

In Figure 3A the release threshold is about 18 mV depolarized from the presynaptic neuron's resting potential. Thus only individual PSPs of substantial size (as seen at the output synapses, not the soma) could cause release. Smaller PSPs could not cause release unless background levels of other inputs biased the resting potential upwards.

Some presynaptic neurons, however, have resting potentials much closer to the release threshold. In Figure 2C a neuron pair demonstrates the typical peak-plateau hyperpolarizing waveform to presynaptic depolarization. If the presynaptic neuron is hyperpolarized, the postsynaptic response is not absent, as might be predicted. Instead, a small depolarization is observed. The input-output curve (Figure 3B) still

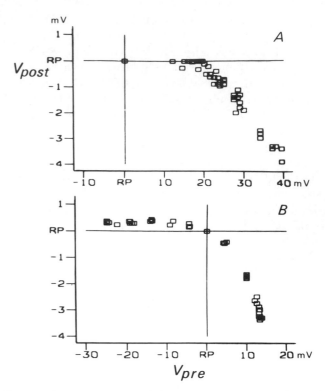

FIGURE 3 Transneuronal input-output curves derived from experiments like that of Figure 2. *Abscissa*: Amplitude of presynaptic soma voltage produced by a current step. *Ordinate*: Peak response in postsynaptic neuron. (A) Nonspiking presynaptic neuron EX1 and spiking postsynaptic neuron GM (data from Graubard, 1978a). (B) Spiking neurons PD and PY; data from the experiment used for Figure 2B, C (Graubard, Raper, and Hartline, 1977). For both cell pairs, increasing depolarization of the presynaptic neuron above the release threshold causes increasing hyperpolarization of the postsynaptic neuron. In A, however, the release threshold is about 18 mV depolarized from the presynaptic cell's resting potential (RP), while in B, the release threshold is about 5 mV below the resting potential.

has the usual shape, but the release threshold is more negative than the cell's resting potential. Thus the presynaptic neuron is continuously releasing transmitter at its resting level, and any small fluctuation in presynaptic membrane potential causes an inverted fluctuation in the postsynaptic membrane potential. The resting potential of the postsynaptic neuron therefore includes a bias of −0.5 mV from this particular presynaptic neuron's resting release; the contribution from the postsynaptic cell's other inputs is unknown. Both neurons of this pair are spiking neurons recorded in TTX. These results suggest that graded release might be important for this cell pair even in the absence of TTX when the presynaptic cell is free to fire.

Figure 4 shows a different cell pair that has an

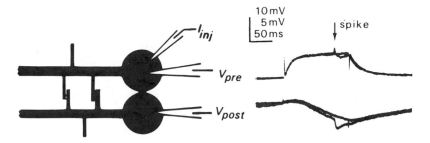

FIGURE 4 Augmentation of graded release by a presynaptic spike. Long current pulse in the presynaptic LP neuron straddles the threshold for causing a spike. Spike-evoked IPSP is small in comparison to graded release. Such spikeless release is probably important in the function of many spiking neurons within this ganglion. (Data from Graubard, Raper, and Hartline, 1977.)

input-output curve similar to that of Figure 3B. There is no TTX in the bathing medium, and just enough current is injected into the presynaptic soma to straddle the condition for eliciting a presynaptic spike. Two superimposed sweeps are shown, demonstrating the hyperpolarizing response of the postsynaptic neuron with and without the increment caused by the spike (the spike is greatly attenuated in the somatic recording). The spike causes a standard transient IPSP to be superimposed on the hyperpolarizing waveform of the graded response; note that the graded response is larger than the spike-evoked contribution. Thus graded release can be at least as significant as spike-evoked communication between neurons. Some of these presynaptic neurons exhibit endogenous pacemaker oscillations, which can produce significant postsynaptic effects even when subthreshold for spike production (Graubard, Raper, and Hartline, 1977).

PROPERTIES OF SPIKELESS SYNAPTIC TRANSMISSION Such studies, and the studies of giant synapses and of spikeless neurons that preceded them (see the papers by Llinás and by Pearson in this volume), allow several important conclusions to be drawn regarding graded synaptic transmission. (1) It can occur from either spiking or nonspiking presynaptic neurons. (2) It can be long-lasting, with the postsynaptic plateau response maintained for the duration of the presynaptic depolarization. (3) The presynaptic release threshold can be well above the resting potential in some cases but below the presynaptic resting potential in other cases. (4) Postsynaptic response grades with presynaptic voltage and can be sensitive to small presynaptic voltage fluctuations. (5) The peak component may be absent or large and, in the lobster neurons described, quite depressed by a recent history of synaptic release.

These transneuronal input-output properties are

presumably the result of many individual synapses located on numerous pre- and postsynaptic processes acting together to form the composite response. Simply because the composite exhibits a threshold and grades with presynaptic depolarization does not imply that the individual synapses have such properties. Just as the distribution of thresholds in a motoneuron pool contributes to grading muscle tensions, so might the individual synapses have distributed properties not detectable by the transneuronal input-output method.

If the presynaptic release threshold were so high that only spikes could cross it, the output synapse could be interpreted in terms similar to those used for axoaxonic synapses and presynaptic inhibition (as Ralston, 1971, pointed out in his discussion of presynaptic dendrites in thalamus). If the threshold were low relative to the sizes of local PSPs, incoming PSPs might continuously modulate release. This might permit some measure of regional autonomy for each dendritic branch, in contrast to the picture of dendritic output synapses being driven synchronously by a spike from an axonal trigger zone. Much depends upon the PSPs within the dendritic tree: How big are they at the input synapse? How do they decrement as they spread passively throughout the dendritic tree? The influence of cell shape and membrane resistivity on PSP spread is the subject of the second portion of this paper.

Influence of dendritic geometry on synaptic potentials

Vertebrate and invertebrate neurons come in an enormous variety of sizes and shapes. Membrane resistivity can vary by a factor of a thousand between neurons. There is a large variation in dendritic geometry, even when one considers only neurons that make serial synapses. Can we derive general principles about how the members of this varied group function? In particular, for neurons with intermixed input and output sites, do the shape of the cell and the location of the input and output synapses say anything about how that cell operates?

It would be convenient if we could resolve this question by directly recording PSPs at a number of different sites around the cell. Technically, however, this is an unrealistic approach for most neurons, so we must resort to calculations based on measurements of neuron geometry and estimates of the resistivity of the cytoplasm and membrane. We will use cable theory calculations to make educated guesses about what such experiments might reveal.

The steady-state cable equation can be easily applied to neurons with complex branching patterns (Rall, 1959; Graubard, 1973; Jack, Noble, and Tsien, 1975). The soma of the neuron is transformed into an isopotential sphere and the dendritic geometry into a series of finite or infinite cable segments. With such a system, it is easy to calculate how voltage (or current) spreads within a cell. Synaptic inputs are also considered in the steady state, as an approximately quantal (0.1 nanomho) synaptic conductance change and a 60 mV driving potential. Thus the PSPs we will describe resemble the long-lasting responses of the stomatogastric neurons in Figure 2. Spike-evoked PSPs are transients; the peak of such PSPs will be attenuated even more than the results from our steady-state calculations. The area under such a transient PSP, however, is directly comparable to our steady-state results (Jack, Noble, and Tsien, 1975). Other non-steady-state effects, such as those caused by varying membrane resistivities or by the historic effects of synaptic transmission, will not be discussed in this paper.

In order to cover a wide range of neuron shapes and membrane resistivities, we will consider four different neurons. Our first example from *Aplysia* represents one extreme: the cell has a branching pattern in which very small processes branch from very large ones (Figure 5A); the neuron's membrane resistivity is so high that little current leaks across the cell membrane within the neuropil (the length constant is large). Thus the cell demonstrates, almost purely, the effect of branching pattern. The second neuron, from the stomatogastric ganglion, has a more typical membrane resistivity and branching pattern. The third cell, a cat spinal motoneuron, has become the classic neuron to which other cells are compared. The fourth cell, a horizontal cell from the rat superior colliculus, presents another extreme: a cell with long, thin, relatively unbranched dendrites. Of these four

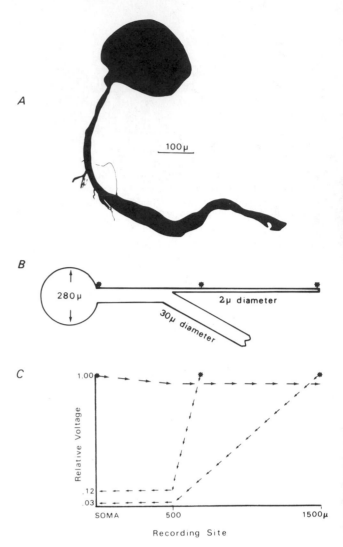

FIGURE 5 *Aplysia* L12–L13 neuron voltage attenuation. (A) Drawing of a Procion dye injection (after Graubard, 1973); only a few of the thin secondary branches are shown. (B) Schematic drawing of cell, showing (not to scale) the 280 μm soma, the 30 μm main axon, and a 2 μm diameter secondary process beginning 500 μm from the soma. The secondary process terminates 1,000 μm from the branch point. The figure is arranged so that the processes from soma to distal tip fall on a straight line to facilitate plotting the voltage gradient. (C) Simulated movement of a recording electrode along the neuron (Rinzel and Rall, 1973). Ordinate is voltage relative to applied voltage at a given point (stars). Graph of voltage spread calculated from steady-state cable equations (R_m = 550,000 Ω-cm², R_i = 90 Ω-cm; membrane infolding taken into account as in Graubard, 1975). A voltage applied to the soma (star) falls to 95% of its original value by the 500 μm branching, but little additional attenuation occurs distally along the 2 μm $\times$ 1,000 μm secondary process (large arrows). A voltage applied at the distal tip (star) falls to 3% of its original value before reaching the branch point (small arrows). Voltages applied more proximally along the secondary process attenuate less.

neurons, all but the motoneuron probably make serial synapses, much like the dendrodendritic synapses of the Golgi type II cell shown in Figure 1A, B. Consideration of these neurons has led to some surprising conclusions:

1. Input synapse location may make only a minor difference in somatic PSP size; there is often little disadvantage in placing an input synapse on the distal dendrites rather than on the soma.

2. PSPs within the dendritic tree can be large, especially in distal dendrites; moving an input synapse from soma to distal tip could greatly increase the PSP size in the distal tip. Thus input synaptic location would be very important to a distally located output synapse, even if it were unimportant to a centrally located spike trigger zone.

ANALYSIS OF AN APLYSIA NEURON   The L12–L13 neuron of *Aplysia* abdominal ganglion (Figure 5A) is hardly a typical neuron, but an analysis of it is particularly instructive as preparation for understanding the effects of branching patterns, as distinct from those of length constant, on voltage transmission within neurons. Initially the cell was studied (Graubard, 1973, 1975) because of its long, large axon: the sphere-plus-cable shape allows intrasomatic current injection and voltage measurements to be interpreted with the aid of the Rall (1960) method. The membrane and axoplasmic resistivities were estimated; these values, together with the cell geometry, allow calculations to be made of the voltage profiles within the neuron that result from various locations of an input synapse.

Synapses on *Aplysia* neurons are almost never associated with the cell soma and are relatively infrequent on the large-diameter processes. Synapses are commonly found between small processes in the neuropil; input and output synapses can be near each other on the same fine process (a serial synapse) (Graubard, 1973, 1978b). Thus, in some respects, these neurons may have a structure analogous to the Golgi type II cell of Figure 1A, B, with both axonal and dendritic output synapses.

Voltages do attenuate within cablelike structures because of the imperfect insulation provided by the surface membrane. As it happens, the *Aplysia* neuron has an exceptionally high membrane resistivity ($R_m \approx 550,000$ Ω-cm², although infolding of surface membrane in the soma and large-diameter processes may make the effective R_m as much as a factor of ten lower); this resistivity greatly reduces the effect current leakage has on voltage profiles. For example, the length constant of the 30-μm-diameter axon (Figure

5A) is in the range 5–15 mm; only about 1 mm of this axon is within the ganglion, so it is within about 10% of being isopotential within the ganglion.

Voltages spread very well from the soma or axon out to the tips of the small-diameter processes (Figure 5C). This property makes it possible to measure the reversal potential of a PSP with little error, providing the membrane resistivity remains constant over the surface of the cell (Graubard, 1975). However, there is asymmetry in the transmission of voltage. Voltages are sharply attenuated as they spread from the tips of the small-diameter processes toward the axon and soma. This attenuation results from the branching pattern of the cell and not from the length constant of the small-diameter process. To understand the mechanism, one must consider the effects of the loading of the fine process by the large-diameter axon.

LOADING OF CABLE SEGMENTS   Along an infinite cable, it is quite simple to compute voltage decrements: voltages decrement exponentially with distance in the steady state; the length constant is the distance at which the voltage falls to 37% of its original value.

A fine cylindrical process 2 μm in diameter and 1,000 μm long will be considered initially. If this 2 μm process were infinitely long, voltage would fall about 17% over 1,000 μm (Figure 6). It is not infinite, however, so its 5.6 mm length constant is of little use as an index of the attenuation to be expected. Looking outwards from the main axon, one effectively sees a 1,000 μm segment of cable with a sealed end. The voltage will decrement only 1.6% in this case, not 17%. Conversely, if one is looking down this 1,000 μm cable from its distal end, one sees it terminated by a 30 μm axon. This termination "loads" the cable segments so that the original voltage will fall to 3% of its original value (Figure 6), showing that the voltage attenuation is very asymmetrical because the terminations are asymmetrical. Thus the PSP generated at a distal site will lose most of its original size by the time it reaches the main axon, even if the main axon itself spreads it into the soma with little further decrement. By itself, this might suggest that, as seen from the soma or the spike-initiating region on the axon, distal synapses will be weak whereas somatic synapses will be much more effective.

THE LOCAL PSP SIZE COMPENSATES FOR ATTENUATION   The large attenuation of the PSP from the distal synapse would seem to contradict our earlier conclusion that the location of the input synapse often makes relatively little difference in the deter-

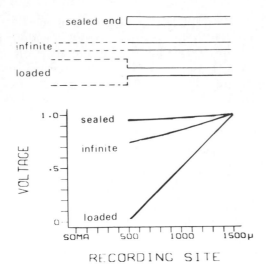

FIGURE 6 Attenuation as a function of terminating load. Graph follows the convention of Figure 5C. Secondary process of 2 μm × 1,000 μm exhibits very different voltage attenuations, depending on its termination. Were the cylinder to extend infinitely, the exponential fall of the voltage applied at the distal tip would reach the 83% level by 1,000 μm. Were the termination a sealed end, it would only fall to the 98% level (illustrating why voltages spreading distally toward a sealed end decrement so little; see Figure 5C, large arrows). However, centripetal spread of voltages along the secondary process is strongly affected by the 30 μm main axon, which terminates the process centrally; this loading results in a nearly linear fall of the voltage to the 3% level. Thus length constant per se gives little indication of the severity of voltage attenuation.

mination of somatic PSP size. But what determines the size of the PSP at the site of the synapse (the "local PSP")? The size of the PSP at the synaptic site (V_{psp}) is a function of the synaptic conductance (g_{psp}) and driving potential (E_{psp}) and of the input conductance of the cell computed for that specific location (g_{in}):

$$V_{psp} = \frac{g_{psp} E_{psp}}{g_{psp} + g_{in}} .$$

The input conductance of the cell, g_{in}, is not constant; it varies as a function of the location where it is measured. It will be small at the tip of a thin process and it will get larger when measured nearer the axon or the soma. For example, if the input conductance were 10 times the synaptic conductance change, then the local steady-state PSP would be 9% of the synaptic battery—e.g., 5.4 mV for a 60 mV battery. This is approximately the situation for distal synapses on very thin, long neurites; when the input conductance is 1,000 times the synaptic conductance, as can happen at central sites such as a 30 μm axon or on the

soma, then the local PSP would be 0.1% of the battery—e.g., 60 μV for a 60 mV battery. Sixty microvolts is about the size of the "quantal PSPs" observed intrasomatically in *Aplysia* neurons (Castellucci and Kandel, 1974).

Thus, while distal sites are associated with severe attenuation, they are also associated with large local PSP sizes. This compensation is not complete, but the size of the PSP measured in the soma is often only 10–20% lower for a distally originating PSP than for a somatically originating one.

PSP SIZE PROFILES Figure 7 shows the calculated version of a hypothetical experiment in which the recording microelectrode is moved from the distal tip, past the input synaptic site, down onto the main axon and into the soma. As in Figure 5B, C, we have rearranged the cell's geometry so that the soma, the first 500 μm of the large axon, and the 1,000 μm of the thin neurite are stretched out in a line. This allows a simple plot to be made of PSP size as a function of the position of the recording site.

For an input synapse on the distal tip (point 3 in Figure 7), the local PSP size is large. The PSP falls

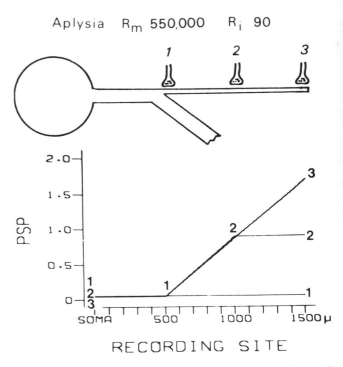

FIGURE 7 Profile of PSP amplitude and attenuation with distance for three different input synapse locations along a secondary process. *Ordinate*: Steady-state PSP (in mV) resulting from 0.1 nanomho conductance and 60 mV driving potential. *Abscissa*: Location of simulated recording electrode.

almost linearly until it reaches the junction with the large axon, where it is 3% of its original size of 1.7 mV. For the 500 μm between the junction and the soma, the voltage loss is very small. For an input synapse located halfway out the secondary process (point 2 in Figure 7), the local size of the PSP is 900 μV; it too falls almost linearly as the large axon is approached. What is notable is that this 900 μV PSP spreads distally to the tip with very little decrement, as one might expect from Figure 5C. An input synapse at the junction of the primary and secondary processes produces a 48 μV PSP locally; this voltage also spreads distally virtually unattenuated.

Thus the voltage as measured at the distal tip would be strongly influenced by the location of the synaptic inputs, even though the somatic voltages are not. Figure 8 explicitly plots the size of the PSP measured in the soma as a function of synaptic location, not only for the three sites shown in Figure 7 but for all points. The maximum differences between somatic and distal input sites are less than 10% for this example. Figure 8 also shows the voltage measured at the distal tip as a function of synaptic location. The voltage grows from 46 μV to 1,700 μV, a 37-fold increase and quite in contrast to the 10% effect of synaptic location on the somatic PSP. If the thin neurite is 4 μm in diameter, the input conductances are larger and the local PSPs smaller; thus the distal PSP increases by only 10-fold.

LONG THIN DENDRITES AND SYNAPTIC EFFICACY The longer and thinner the neurites on which the input synapses are located, the larger the distal-tip voltages can become. Utilizing long, thin neurites for locating input synapses does not appreciably affect the sizes of somatic or axonal PSPs (provided that the electrotonic length of the process is short and synaptic conductance is much less than the input conductance of the cell at that location).

The bar histograms in Figure 9 summarize the steady-state PSP sizes for four input synaptic locations, as seen at four different measuring locations within the neuron. Measured at the soma, all four inputs appear nearly the same size (exact sizes can be found in Figure 8); such equipotentiality is also the case at the axonal recording site (approximately where the spike trigger zone might be located). A dendrodendritic output synapse at the tip of the proximal neurite would naturally see input 1 as very large. It is considerably larger than input 2, located 200 μm out the 1,000 μm neurite. Inputs 3 and 4 are approximately the same size at this distal tip as they are in the soma and at the axonal recording sites.

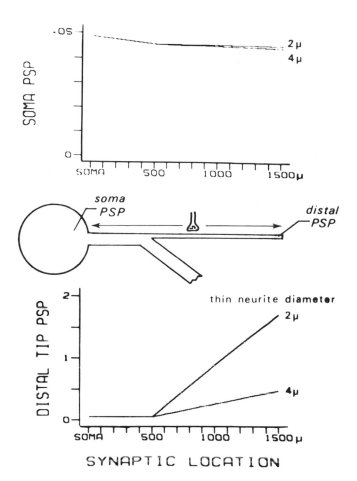

FIGURE 8 Effect of moving the input synapse site on the size of the PSP measured at the soma or distal tip. Calculations for 2 μm and 4 μm secondary process diameters. *Abscissa*: Location of input synapse (not recording site as in Figure 7). *Top*: PSP size in the soma changes little as the input synapse is moved; secondary process diameter makes little difference within the observed anatomical range. *Bottom*: PSP size at the distal tip is markedly dependent on input synapse location because the local PSP depends on the input conductance of the cell seen from the synaptic site. An increase in secondary process diameter increases input conductance and thus reduces distal-tip PSP size. Distal-tip PSP varies over 37-fold range for 2 μm diameter secondary process, over 10-fold for 4 μm diameter process.

Thus an output synapse at the distal tip will see nearly all inputs as about equal to one another, except for input synapses on its parent neurite; those inputs will grade dramatically with location. Similarly the distal tip of the other thin neurite will weigh its local inputs more strongly and see inputs on other neurites as small and equal.

Thus, in theory, this cell has the property that each neurite is able to compute a picture of the input information somewhat different from that of any other neurite and different from that of an axonal

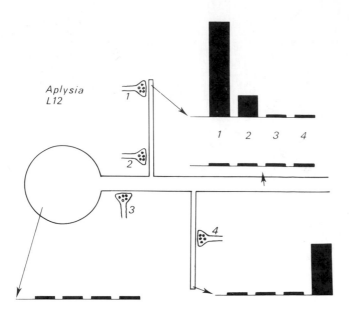

FIGURE 9 *Aplysia* summary schematic, showing the PSPs from four input synaptic locations (represented in bar histogram form) measured at the soma, on the axon distally, and at the distal tips of two different secondary processes. Measured in the soma and main axon, all input sites are within 10% of their mean. An output synapse at a distal tip, however, would be much more strongly affected by inputs along the same secondary process than by inputs elsewhere.

trigger zone. Should the output synapse be located on the proximal end of the long neurite, this would not be true; regional autonomy requires isolation by a long thin neurite (Figure 8). Midway out a long, thin neurite, an output synapse would weigh all distal synapses strongly but relatively equally (as may be inferred from Figure 7); PSP strengths will fall as the input locations move proximally along the neurite. One could design a variety of circuits in this manner, all using the single neuron; it remains to be seen whether any *Aplysia* neurons actually make use of this potential for simultaneously computing many different functions of their inputs. There are indications (e.g., Waziri, 1976) that they do.

More typical cell geometries and resistivities

Although the synaptic location properties noted thus far have been a result of geometric aspects of the L12–L13 *Aplysia* neuron, the so-called cable properties, which are markedly dependent on the membrane leakage of currents, have affected voltage attenuations in only very minor ways. This neuron is extreme in at least two ways: (1) a very high R_m, which minimizes leakage; and (2) large differences in diameter between the thin neurites and the more central processes (e.g., diameter changes at the junctions from 2 μm to 30 μm), which exaggerate geometric effects.

This extreme case is educational because it enables one to identify the geometric, as opposed to the cable, factors that control the PSP size and interactions. Yet we were most curious to see how PSPs would behave in neurons that did not share these extreme membrane and geometric properties.

THE LOBSTER   As noted in Figure 1D, neurons in the lobster stomatogastric ganglion have input and output synapses intermixed on fine processes of the nerve cell. Although they are like *Aplysia* neurons in this respect, their geometry and their membrane resistivities are much less extreme.

We have not modeled all of the processes shown in Figure 1D, but the 10 μm axon, 7 μm × 200 μm secondary processes, and 2 μm × 100 μm tertiary processes (Figure 10) exhibit characteristic properties not especially sensitive to inaccuracies in the central loading that might result from our incomplete model. More extensive electrical reconstructions have been done by Glasser (1977; see also Selverston et al., 1976); our Figure 10 cell diagram is greatly simplified but will serve to illustrate a few basic points in comparison to the *Aplysia* results in Figure 9. Figure 10 summarizes our calculations based on an R_m of 3,600 Ω-cm² and an R_i of 90 Ω-cm; this yields an intrasomatic input resistance of 3.2 MΩ.

These 2–7–10–15 μm diameter changes at junctions are more typical of most "standard" neurons than 2-to-30 diameter jumps. Also more typical is the R_m, which falls into the range estimated for cat spinal motoneurons (see Barrett and Crill, 1974). A model for this lobster neuron thus eliminates the two extreme features of the *Aplysia* neuron.

There are significant membrane leakage losses that affect the PSP profiles in Figure 10; the geometric factors, however, still provide the major features. A recording site near input synapse 1 at the distal end of the dendrite receives a potent effect from the local synapse, less potent effects from other inputs on the same secondary process, and much smaller inputs from elsewhere in the cell. Recording in the soma, the four inputs are not all equal, as they were in the *Aplysia* example: inputs 1 and 2, from the more proximal secondary branch, are somewhat stronger than those from the more distal secondary branch. Just the opposite relative weighting is seen at a distal recording site on the axon, approximately where the spike trigger may reside. This situation occurs be-

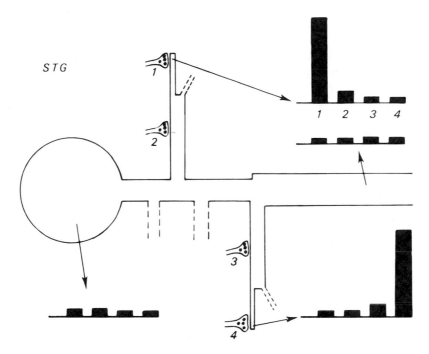

STG

FIGURE 10 Lobster neuron summary schematic, showing the PSPs from four input synaptic locations (represented in bar histogram form). Inputs are at 100 μm along a 7 μm × 200 μm secondary process (points 2 and 3) and at the tip of a 2 μm × 100 μm tertiary process (points 1 and 4); the secondary processes are 100 μm and 200 μm from the soma along a 10 μm diameter axon that enlarges to 15 μm distally. Unlike the *Aplysia* example (Figure 9), membrane leakage of current significantly decrements PSPs along the main axon so that the branch point location is important (compare soma and axon bar histograms). Input synapse location along secondary-tertiary process produces less than 30% difference in central PSP size, but a 7-fold difference in distal PSP size.

cause of the membrane leakage losses along the 10 μm main axon. Unlike the *Aplysia* example, the 1 mm length constant estimated for the stomatogastric axon is not appreciably longer than the distance the axon traverses within the neuropil. This means that the position where the secondary processes branch from the main axon may have some influence on relative PSP sizes, but there is still little influence of actual synaptic location along the secondary process itself. The length of the tertiary processes, and their takeoff point along the secondary process, have little significance for central PSP sizes.

Thus the old notion that proximal synapses are potent and distal synapses are relatively ineffective (Chang, 1952; Eccles, 1957) does not hold for this lobster neuron, but leakage losses do create some effects. However, it is the leakage along the primary axon rather than in the finer processes that is important. Thus the axon within the neuropil, near the spike trigger zone, will exhibit a different weighting of input PSPs than would be recorded in the cell soma. The propensity of invertebrate nervous systems for locating the cell body on a synapse-free side process, rather than at the center of the funneling of

dendrites into the axon as in mammalian CNS neurons, creates problems of technical interpretation for PSP sizes and spike thresholds. As we shall see, however, the electrical reconstruction of a cat spinal motoneuron is otherwise little different from our lobster case in its implications for synaptic location.

THE SPINAL MOTONEURON We have created a traditional model neuron (see Rall, 1962) in which the 3/2 power of the branch diameter is conserved looking peripherally at branchings, with an electrotonic length of the equivalent cylinder of 1.0, a membrane resistivity of about 3,100 Ω-cm², and a soma diameter of 80 μm. With nine such dendrites, this results in an intrasomatic input resistance of 1.1 MΩ and a dendritic dominance of 14, quite consistent with a large cat spinal motoneuron and probably with many other large CNS neurons. Our goal here is not to model particular motoneurons accurately (see Barrett and Crill, 1974) but to provide a comparison of our previous examples with a class of the larger neurons in the central nervous system.

As in the lobster case and unlike the *Aplysia* example, retrograde voltage spreading out the dendrites exhibits some loss. The synaptic reversal potential of a PSP from a distal-tip input would be overestimated by 50% using intrasomatic current injection and voltage measurement (Calvin, 1969). Again, central loading brings down the PSP size as the measurement point approaches the soma; unlike the *Aplysia* and lobster cases, the soma here has another eight identical dendrites leaving it, which contribute the central loading on our model branch. A plot of soma PSP size as a function of synaptic location (in a manner analogous to the *Aplysia* plot in Figure 8) shows that a distal synapse is 36% "less effective" than a somatic input. A major culprit is the leaky membrane, aided by the side branches, which provide significant diversion paths. Looking at the distal-tip PSP as a function of input synaptic location, one sees again the enormous range (35-fold) that characterized the *Aplysia* example. Cat spinal motoneurons have not, however, been reported to possess dendrodendritic output synapses (see Conradi, 1976). To the extent that CNS neurons with dendrodendritic synapses have branching patterns that conserve the 3/2 power of branch diameters, this result indicates that distal dendrodendritic output synapses can achieve significant local computation.

THE SUPERIOR COLLICULUS HORIZONTAL CELL   Neurons, such as those illustrated in Figure 11, that have long, thin dendrites and a small soma will, in many cases, not fit the descriptive model we have just given for neurons with significant central loading on the dendritic processes. This is perhaps best shown by examining another extreme case: the horizontal cells

of superior colliculus. They are located in the superficial layer where dendrodendritic synapses are common (Lund, 1969; Sterling, 1971); indeed, Sterling (1971) has hypothesized a role for inhibitory dendrodendritic synapses and graded synaptic release in the receptive-field organization of this layer. While it is not known whether the horizontal cells are spiking or nonspiking, they have both dendrodendritic synapses (Langer and Lund, 1974; Cuénod, this volume) and a respectable axon. This cell is thus particularly suitable for an analysis of the implications of spikeless transmission and dendritic geometry for regional computation within neurons.

We have modeled the entire dendritic tree shown in Figure 11. Unlike our previous examples in which values of R_m were chosen to satisfactorily predict the typical values of intrasomatic input resistance obtained experimentally, there are no intracellular recordings from these horizontal cells from which to obtain input resistances. We have therefore explored R_m values that generally bracket the values obtained in other CNS neurons (1,000–4,000 Ω-cm^2), although increasing R_m even to 20,000 Ω-cm^2 does not appreciably affect our conclusions. Figure 11 is based on $R_m = 3,600$ Ω-cm^2 and $R_i = 90$ Ω-cm.

Figure 11 shows four different locations for an input synapse. The bar histogram beneath each site shows the relative strength of the PSP recorded at that site from each of the four inputs; this is the weighting that a dendrodendritic output site would perceive.

Because the dendrites are long and thin (diameter usually less than 1–2 μm), there is considerable mem-

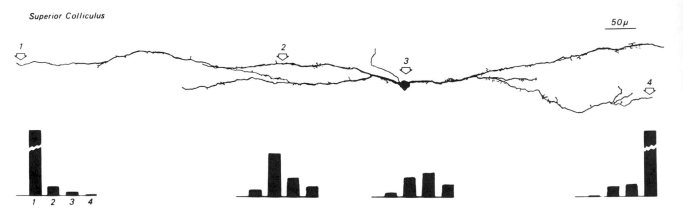

Superior Colliculus

50μ

FIGURE 11   Horizontal cell from rat superior colliculus. Neuron spans about 1,000 μm, but diameters are seldom larger than 1–2 μm. Four input synapse locations (numbered arrows) are shown; bar histograms beneath each arrow show relative strengths of all four input synapses measured at that site. Broken bars indicate the local PSP is actually 3–5 times larger than shown. Besides the local PSPs

becoming large at the distal tips of long processes (as in Figures 9 and 10), the primary feature of these PSP profiles is the large loss due to membrane current leakage along the long, thin processes; central loading and branching do not play important roles here. A dendrodendritic output synapse would perceive input synapse strengths very differently, depending on its location.

brane leakage affecting the voltage profiles. This can be appreciated by looking at input 3 (on the soma), comparing the heights of the third bar in each of the four histograms. The somatic input falls to 53% of its original height before reaching the right distal tip (site 4) and falls to 16% of its original height before reaching the left distal tip (site 1). Local inputs at the distal tip are very large in size because of the low input conductance at those sites; the broken bars in histograms 1 and 4 are actually 5 and 3 times higher than shown. Synaptic efficacy at the soma also varies considerably (bar histogram beneath site 3), in contrast to earlier examples where the soma did not see much variation in the synaptic efficacy with input location.

If there were a dozen output synapses scattered along the dendritic tree, a dozen different sets of weightings of the input array would be computed, all within this one neuron. These 1,000-μm-wide horizontal cells project their dendritic trees a substantial distance across the topographic representation of the visual space mapped onto the superior colliculus (Langer and Lund, 1974); thus each output synapse should weigh the light patterns in the visual field differently. Such a horizontal cell with a dozen output synapses distributed along its dendritic tree could do the job that might otherwise require a dozen different neurons with smaller dendritic trees scattered throughout the colliculus.

This conclusion, of course, depends on the assumptions made in the model and on the dendrodendritic synapses having input-output properties similar to those presented earlier. We do not know the role of spikes in such neurons; the weighting of inputs seen at the soma is presumably that seen by an initial-segment spike trigger zone. If spikes retrogradely invaded the dendritic tree, the output from a dendrodendritic synapse would also be occasionally augmented by a spike (in a manner in Figure 4) with an input weighting corresponding to that of the soma rather than the local weighting.

Discussion

The compensation for attenuation provided by increases of local PSP size with isolation suggests that dendritic spines may not affect central PSP sizes by simple, passive cable properties; thus changes in the neck of the dendritic spine would not produce a significant modulation of central PSP sizes. Of course, if the synaptic conductance change were so large that the local PSP always approached the synaptic reversal potential, then the compensation capability would be

lost and spine necks could modulate central PSP sizes (see Rall and Rinzel, 1971). To the extent that the transient and steady-state components of PSPs behave differently in passive spread and local PSP size, then the implications of dendritic geometry will vary. Our conclusions address only the implications of sustained PSPs (such as those shown in Figure 2) in which synaptic conductances are small relative to input conductances.

In this paper, we have attempted only a consideration of passive and synaptic properties. The intraneuronal cascade of processes connecting the input synapses with the output synapses is simplified in spikeless transmission, and one may examine the steady-state passive properties for the implications of dendritic geometry. In our companion paper (Calvin and Graubard, this volume), we try to place the passive and synaptic properties in the perspective of subexcitable phenomena (local resistance changes, rebounds), nonpropagated local responses and dendritic spikes, repetitive firing from an initial-segment trigger zone, intermittent conduction, and presynaptic inhibition/facilitation.

Using four exemplary neuron shapes, we have gone from one extreme (membrane leakage is unimportant, branching determines everything) to another (branching is minor, but leakage is quite significant). In all cases, distal-tip output synapses could see their local inputs as far more important than other input synapses. This potential for regional computation is markedly augmented by locating output synapses far out on long, thin dendrites, thus isolating them from larger central structures. Such isolation has the effect of keeping input conductances low at distal tips, thus allowing local PSPs to become many times larger than PSPs spreading retrogradely to the distal tip from inputs elsewhere.

Coming back to our original question—How do dendrites function when they contain output synapses as well as input synapses?—we can make the following statement: Unless the release threshold is unusually high, it is likely that dendrodendritic synapses will operate even without spikes because of the large size of local PSPs in the distal dendritic tree. Unless the membrane resistivity is so high that it forces the dendritic tree toward isopotentiality, it is likely that different output synapses from the same neuron will integrate input synaptic activity differently. Thus it seems hard to escape the conclusion that regional computation exists.

Many neurons with dendrodendritic synapses will still, by PSP summation at the initial segment, produce a spike train that activates the distant output synapses on the end of the axon. As the spike retrogradely invades the dendritic tree (Calvin, 1978), dendrodendritic output synapses will be similarly activated, although such release may be conditioned by local inputs in the manner suggested for presynaptic inhibition at axoaxonic synapses. A proximal dendrodendritic synapse would see about the same weighting of input synapses as an initial-segment trigger zone, but it might have a threshold for graded release that is lower than the spike threshold. As dendrodendritic synapses are located more distally, weighting of input synapses will change to favor local inputs. Output synapses isolated from more proximal structures by long, thin dendrites would have the greatest opportunity for regional computation, simply because local PSPs would be very large. Thus neurons with *distal* dendrodendritic synapses are the cells most likely to produce semiautonomous regional computation.

ACKNOWLEDGMENTS The spikeless synaptic transmission experiments were done at the University of California, San Diego, with support from NIH grant NS 13138 and the Sloan Foundation. Daniel K. Hartline and Jonathan A. Raper collaborated on the data presented in Figures 2, 3B, and 4. KG is the recipient of a postdoctoral fellowship NS 05060 from NIH. The dendritic geometry work in Seattle was supported by NIH grants NS 09677 and NS 04053. We thank Thomas Langer and David King for the loan of their original cell drawings and Susan M. Johnston for assistance in the calculations.

REFERENCES

BARRETT, J. N., 1975. Motoneuron dendrites: Role in synaptic integration. *Fed. Proc.* 34:1398–1407.

BARRETT, J. N., and W. E. CRILL, 1974. Specific membrane properties of cat motoneurones. *J. Physiol.* 239:301–324.

BURROWS, M., and M. V. S. SIEGLER, 1976. Transmission without spikes between locust interneurones and motoneurones. *Nature* 262:222–224.

CALVIN, W. H., 1969. Dendritic synapses and reversal potentials: Theoretical implications of the view from the soma. *Exp. Neurol.* 24:248–264.

CALVIN, W. H., 1978. Re-excitation in normal and abnormal repetitive firing of CNS neurons. In *Abnormal Neuronal Discharges*, N. Chalazonitis and M. Boisson, eds. New York: Raven Press.

CASTELLUCCI, V. F., and E. R. KANDEL, 1974. A quantal analysis of the synaptic depression underlying habituation of the gill-withdrawal reflex in *Aplysia. Proc. Natl. Acad. Sci. USA* 71:5004–5008.

CHANG, H. T., 1952. Cortical and spinal neurons. Cortical neurons with particular reference to the apical dendrites. *Cold Spring Harbor Symp. Quant. Biol.* 17:189–202.

CHARLTON, M. P., and H. L. ATWOOD, 1977. Slow release of transmitter at the squid giant synapse. *Neurosci. Lett.* 5:165–169.

CONRADI, S., 1976. Functional anatomy of the anterior horn motor neuron. In *The Peripheral Nerve*, D. N. Landon, ed. London: Chapman and Hall, pp. 279–329.

ECCLES, J. C., 1957. *The Physiology of Nerve Cells.* Baltimore: The Johns Hopkins Press.

FAMIGLIETTI, E. V., and A. PETERS, 1972. The synaptic glomerulus and the intrinsic neuron in the dorsal lateral geniculate nucleus of the cat. *J. Comp. Neurol.* 144:285–334.

GLASSER, S. M. W., 1977. Computer reconstruction and passive modeling of identified nerve cells in the lobster stomatogastric ganglion. Ph.D. dissertation, Department of Physics, University of California, San Diego.

GRAUBARD, K., 1973. Morphological and electrotonic properties of identified neurons of the mollusc, *Aplysia californica.* Ph.D. dissertation, University of Washington, Seattle.

GRAUBARD, K., 1975. Voltage attenuation within *Aplysia* neurons: The effect of branching pattern. *Brain Res.* 88:325–332.

GRAUBARD, K., 1978a. Synaptic transmission without action potentials: Input-output properties of a nonspiking presynaptic neuron. *J. Neurophysiol.* 41:1014–1025.

GRAUBARD, K., 1978b. Serial synapses in *Aplysia. J. Neurobiol.* 9:325–328.

GRAUBARD, K., J. A. RAPER, and D. K. HARTLINE, 1977. Non-spiking synaptic transmission between spiking neurons. *Neurosci. Abstr.* 3.

GRAY, E. G., 1962. A morphological basis for presynaptic inhibition? *Nature* 193:82–83.

HAGIWARA, S., and I. TASAKI, 1958. A study of the mechanism of impulse transmission across the giant synapse of the squid. *J. Physiol.* 143:114–137.

JACK, J. J. B., D. NOBLE, and R. W. TSIEN, 1975. *Electrical Current Flow in Excitable Cells.* London: Oxford University Press.

KATZ, B., and R. MILEDI, 1966. Input-output relation of a single synapse. *Nature* 212:1242–1245.

KING, D. G., 1976. Organization of crustacean neuropil. II. Distribution of synaptic contacts on identified motor neurones in lobster stomatogastric ganglion. *J. Neurocytol.* 5:239–266.

LANGER, T. P., and R. D. LUND, 1974. The upper layers of the superior colliculus of the rat: A Golgi study. *J. Comp. Neurol.* 158:405–436.

LUND, R. D., 1969. Synaptic patterns of the superficial layers of the superior colliculus of the rat. *J. Comp. Neurol.* 135:179–208.

MARTIN, A. R., and G. L. RINGHAM, 1975. Synaptic transfer at a vertebrate central nervous system synapse. *J. Physiol.* 251:409–426.

MAYNARD, D. M., 1972. Simpler networks. *Ann. NY Acad. Sci.* 193:59–72.

MAYNARD, D. M., and K. D. WALTON, 1975. Effects of maintained depolarization of presynaptic neurons on inhibitory transmission in lobster neuropil. *J. Comp. Physiol.* 97:215–243.

MENDELSON, M., 1971. Oscillator neurones in crustacean ganglia. *Science* 171:1170–1173.

PAUL, D. H., 1972. Decremental conduction over "giant" afferent processes in an arthropod. *Science* 176:680–682.

PEARSON, K. G., and C. R. FOURTNER, 1975. Nonspiking interneurons in walking system of the cockroach. *J. Neurophysiol.* 38:33–52.

QUASTEL, D. M. J., 1974. Excitation-secretion coupling at the mammalian neuromuscular junction. In *Synaptic Transmission and Neuronal Interaction* (Society of General Physiologists Series, vol. 28), M. V. L. Bennett, ed. New York: Raven Press.

RALL, W., 1959. Branching dendritic trees and motoneuron membrane resistivity. *Exp. Neurol.* 1:491–527.

RALL, W., 1960. Membrane potential transients and membrane time constant of motoneurons. *Exp. Neurol.* 2:503–532.

RALL, W., 1962. Electrophysiology of a dendritic neuron model. *Biophys. J.* 2:145–167.

RALL, W., and J. RINZEL, 1971. Dendritic spines and synaptic potency explored theoretically. *Int. Cong. Physiol. Sci. Proc.* 9:1384.

RALL, W., and J. RINZEL, 1973. Branch input resistance and steady attenuation for input to one branch of a dendritic neuron model. *Biophys. J.* 13:648–688.

RALL, W., G. M. SHEPHERD, T. S. REESE, and M. W. BRIGHTMAN, 1966. Dendrodendritic synaptic pathway for inhibition in the olfactory bulb. *Exp. Neurol.* 14:44–56.

RALSTON, H. J., III, 1971. Evidence for presynaptic dendrites and a proposal for their mechanism of action. *Nature* 230:585–587.

RIPLEY, S. H., B. M. H. BUSH, and A. ROBERTS, 1968. Crab muscle receptor which responds without impulses. *Nature* 218:1170–1171.

SELVERSTON, A. I., D. F. RUSSELL, J. P. MILLER and D. G. KING, 1976. The stomatogastric nervous system: Structure and function of a small neural network. *Prog. Neurobiol.* 7:215–290.

SHAW, S. R., 1972. Decremental conduction of the visual signal in barnacle lateral eye. *J. Physiol.* 220:145–175.

STERLING, P., 1971. Receptive fields and synaptic organization of the superficial gray layer of the cat superior colliculus. *Vision Res. Suppl.* 3:309–328.

WAZIRI, R., 1976. Modulation of chemical postsynaptic efficacy by electrical presynaptic transmission in *Aplysia*. *Neurosci. Abstr.* 2:1441.

WERBLIN, F. S., and J. E. DOWLING, 1969. Organization of the retina of the mudpuppy, *Necturus maculosus*. II. Intracellular recording. *J. Neurophysiol.* 32:339–355.

ZETTLER, F., and M. JÄRVILEHTO, M., 1971. Decrement-free conduction of graded potentials along the axon of a monopolar neuron. *Z. Vergl. Physiol.* 75:401–421.

19 Electrical Interactions between Vertebrate Neurons: Field Effects and Electrotonic Coupling

H. KORN and D. S. FABER

ABSTRACT   The excitability of one neuron can be directly altered by extracellular currents generated by adjacent cells. Such field effects, which do not require specialized junctions, are dependent on the orientation and electrical properties of the neurons involved as well as the properties of their surrounding medium. An example is the electrical inhibition of fish medullary neurons by an action potential in the adjacent Mauthner cell. This inhibition results from transmembrane channeling of the Mauthner-cell action currents in the affected neurons due to the high extracellular resistance around these cells. (In this network the same identified neurons mediate both electrical and chemical inhibitions of the Mauthner cell.) For electrically mediated transmission (and electrotonic coupling), currents generated in a cell spread into adjacent neurons through low-resistance pathways or gap junctions, where the intercellular space is narrowed. The functional characteristics of electrotonic transmission can be demonstrated in such effector systems as fish oculomotor neurons and in the lateral vestibular neurons of fish and rat. The occurrence of electrotonic coupling in mammals is also emphasized and reviewed. Electrically and chemically mediated transmission are not mutually exclusive; both can be observed at the same axon terminal (thus yielding a "mixed synapse") or in adjacent synaptic loci. These recent findings and also a possible modulation of electrotonic transmission by chemically induced conductance changes are discussed in this paper.

THE CONCEPT of electrical interactions between neurons is already implicit in the classical reticular network theory of the central nervous system. Hypothetical models for both electrical excitation and inhibition were developed in the 1940s (Eccles, 1946; Brooks and Eccles, 1947) but were then generally neglected with the advent of intracellular recordings and the first evidence obtained for chemically me-

H. KORN and D. S. FABER   Laboratoire de Physiologie, C.H.U. Pitié-Salpétrière, 75634 Paris Cedex 13, France; Department of Physiology, State University of New York at Buffalo and Research Institute on Alcoholism, Buffalo, NY 14203

diated synaptic transmission. The concepts remained tenable, however, and there has recently been a renaissance of interest in electrical transmission. Electrotonic coupling, mediated through gap junctions, has become firmly established physiologically in the last twenty years and is now known to operate not only in invertebrates and lower vertebrates but also in higher vertebrates, including mammals. On the other hand, field effects do not require specialized junctions; in this case the extracellular currents generated by one neuron directly alter the excitability of adjacent ones. They have been described only for a few vertebrate systems, and we are just beginning to appreciate their underlying mechanisms.

Electrical interactions mediated by extracellular currents: Field effects

The term *field effects* refers to the situation in which the extracellular currents generated by one neuron alter the excitability of another by being channeled across the plasma membrane of the latter; they involve specific cells and have been shown to be critically dependent on the orientation and electrical properties of the cells as well as on the properties of the extracellular medium. A functional contribution to neuronal communication and network behavior can also be attributed to field effects, at least in instances in which they have been well analyzed. Theoretically they could result in excitation and/or inhibition of the postsynaptic neuron. So far, however, only monophasic actions have been described for the vertebrate central nervous system.

The reported effects can be separated into two different categories based on possible distinctions between pre- and postsynaptic neurons. (1) Instances in which fields generated by synchronous activation of a homogeneous population of neurons enhance the synchronization of those neurons; for example, the

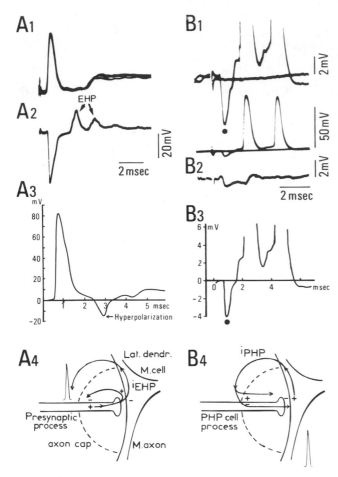

FIGURE 1   Generation of electrical inhibition in goldfish medullary networks involving the Mauthner cell. (A_1–A_4) Hyperpolarization of the M-cell during the EHP. (A_1, A_2) Intra- and extracellular recordings, respectively, of the M-cell antidromic action potential and the subsequent EHP evoked by stimuli applied to the spinal cord. (A_3) To determine the actual change in membrane potential, A_2 was subtracted algebraically from A_1. At the peak of the EHP, this M-cell was hyperpolarized by 15 mV. Note that the antidromic spike in A_1 was followed by an IPSP, the polarity of which was inverted by intracellular Cl⁻ injections. (A_4) Conceptual model of EHP generation. A failure of active impulse propagation in the presynaptic process sets up the extracellular current flow (iEHP) and is responsible for the EHP. (A_1–A_3 are modified from Furukawa and Furshpan, 1963.) (B_1–B_4) Evidence that the M-cell action current produces a passive hyperpolarizing potential (PHP) in adjacent medullary neurons. (B_1, B_2) Intra- and extracellular recordings, respectively, from a medullary neuron in which antidromic invasion of the M-cell (spinal stimulation) evoked an all-or-none PHP followed by a PSP and two spikes. (B_3) In order to determine the net membrane hyperpolarization during the PHP, B_2 was subtracted from B_1. The black dot indicates a PHP in this and the following two figures. Upper and lower traces in B_1 are high-gain AC and low-gain DC recordings, respectively. (B_4) Model for PHP generation. The M-cell antidromic action potential is only actively propagated to the level of the axon hillock,

field-generated depolarizations of cat and frog spinal motoneurons associated with their antidromic invasion (Nelson, 1966; Magherini, Precht, and Schwindt, 1976). Theoretically, however, such synchronous activity could, in some structures, result in an inhibition of a second population of neurons (Rall and Shepherd, 1968). (2) Instances in which impulse activity in a presynaptic neuron produces, without synaptic delay, either monophasic excitation (Werman and Carlen, 1976) or inhibition (Furukawa and Furshpan, 1963; Faber and Korn, 1973; Korn and Faber, 1975a) of the postsynaptic cell(s).

The two examples of electrically mediated inhibitions to be described below concern the goldfish Mauthner cell (M-cell) and fall into the second category. In this section we shall focus on M-cell properties since their analysis has led to the most complete understanding of the mechanisms underlying the generation of field effects. It should be pointed out that M-cells do not require specialized junctions and provide a basis for actions of a purely inhibitory nature, in contrast to electrotonic coupling by way of gap junctions. Furthermore, our recent work on this system has demonstrated that interneurons mediating electrical inhibition have a dual postsynaptic action, with their terminal depolarization also evoking the release of an inhibitory chemical neurotransmitter (Korn and Faber, 1976). This finding suggests that under appropriate conditions other inhibitory interneurons might also mediate an early phase of electrical inhibition.

ELECTRICAL INHIBITION OF THE M-CELL   Furukawa and Furshpan (1963) first demonstrated that an early inhibition of the M-cell can be evoked by its antidromic or orthodromic activation; this inhibition is correlated with a positive extrinsic hyperpolarizing potential (EHP), which can be recorded extracellularly (see Figure 1A_2) in the axon cap—that is, in the vicinity of the cell's axon hillock. This positive potential is not observed during intracellular recording from the neuron itself (A_1); but when the true transmembrane potential change (i.e., the difference between the intra- and extracellularly recorded potentials) is calculated, one finds a 15–20 mV membrane hyperpolarization (A_3). Such observations suggest

and the extracellular local current (iPHP) that is associated with the spike flows back toward this active region from the distal electrically inexcitable soma and dendrites. Some of this return current enters PHP cells, which have processes parallel with the lines of current flow. This inward current produces the PHP. (From Korn and Faber, 1975a.)

that the M-cell is not the EHP generator and that the source for hyperpolarization is outside this neuron. These authors further demonstrated that the EHP is functionally inhibitory and can be mimicked by an anode located in the vicinity of the M-cell's axon hillock. They therefore linked the EHP to an external anodal source and postulated that it was the consequence of a failure in impulse conduction in fibers invading the axon cap surrounding the M-cell's axon hillock; the inactive terminals of these fibers would serve as passive current sources for the more distal sinks (A₄). Some of this extracellular current is drawn into the M-cell at the region of the axon hillock, inhibiting this membrane area and exciting the neuron at more distal points as it leaves the cell. This experiment illustrates a basic property of field-effect interactions: an external current source that hyperpolarizes one region of the postsynaptic neuron should depolarize another more remote area as it leaves it. Therefore, the functional nature of the field effect depends on the relative orientation of the neurons involved; in the present case, the inward current is inhibitory because it hyperpolarizes the axon hillock, which is the site of impulse initiation (Furshpan and Furukawa, 1962), and the outward current depolarizes the distant, electrically inexcitable soma and dendrites.

ELECTRICAL INHIBITION MEDIATED BY THE M-CELL

The second example of electrical inhibition was discovered more recently (Faber and Korn, 1973; Korn and Faber, 1975a) and has served as the foundation for our present understanding of the generation of field effects. Furshpan and Furukawa (1962) reported that the M-cell action currents generate an extracellular negative field (Figure 1A₂), which can be as large as 35 mV in magnitude at its focus in the axon cap but falls off steeply from that point. We subsequently observed that this extracellular current produces a passive hyperpolarizing potential (PHP) in some neighboring medullary neurons (Figure 1B₁, B₃). PHPs are intracellularly recorded hyperpolarizations (B₁) that are larger than the corresponding extracellular field potentials (B₂) monitored in the immediate vicinity of the neurons being investigated. The conclusion that the PHP is passively generated has been reviewed in detail elsewhere (Korn and Faber, 1975a,b); briefly, it is based on evidence that the PHP has the same latency, threshold, time course, and all-or-none character as the M-cell antidromic spike. Furthermore, as is generally the case with electrically mediated postsynaptic responses, it is not associated with a change in membrane conductance,

and its amplitude and time course are independent of membrane potential (Figure 2A). However, it does exhibit the same dependence on membrane conductance as do electrotonically mediated coupling

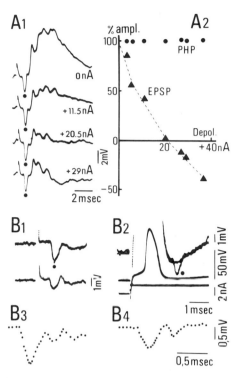

FIGURE 2 (A₁, A₂) PHP independence of membrane potential. (A₁) Intracellular recordings from a PHP-exhibiting neuron using a double-barreled microelectrode—one for potential measurements and one for current injections. A spinal stimulus produced a PHP followed by an EPSP. Steady depolarizing currents sufficient to cause a polarity reversal of the EPSP left the PHP unaffected. The current amplitude is indicated on each record. (A₂) Graph of the PHP and EPSP amplitudes versus current magnitude. *Ordinate*: EPSP and PHP amplitudes in percentages of their control values in the absence of membrane polarization. *Abscissa*: depolarizing (Depol) current magnitude, nA (circles: PHP amplitude; triangles: EPSP amplitude). (From Faber and Korn, 1973.) (B₁–B₄) Reduction of the PHP during the increased membrane conductance associated with the spike after hyperpolarization. (B₁) *Upper trace*: PHP produced by a threshold spinal-cord stimulation. *Lower trace*: Corresponding extracellular field potential. (B₂) Adequate timing of a direct stimulation of the cell sufficient to evoke a spike and the spinal-stimulus result in a reduced PHP during the spike after hyperpolarization (superimposed sweeps with and without a spinal stimulus). *Upper and middle traces*: Recordings at high AC and low DC gains, respectively. *Lower trace*: Depolarizing current pulse used to evoke the direct spike. (B₃, B₄) Net PHPs calculated by a subtraction process for the control and increased conductance conditions, respectively. The PHP was reduced by 45%, and membrane resistance was decreased by 1.2 MΩ (not shown) during the afterhyperpolarization. (Modified from Korn and Faber, 1975b.)

potentials being reduced in amplitude during conductance increases (Figure 2B).

GENERATION OF FIELD EFFECTS Our conclusion for the mechanism of PHP generation is that it is the result of an intercellular channeling across the cell's membrane of the M-cell action current flowing back to the axon hillock, with the inward transmembrane current producing the passive membrane hyperpolarization (Figure 1B$_4$). Clearly this model is analogous to that postulated for electrical inhibition of the M-cell, and its experimental confirmation has demonstrated that the two field effects are actually consequences of a common network. Specifically we have shown that: (1) the PHP can be mimicked with an external cathode situated in the axon cap, whereas cathodal current pulses applied outside this region do not produce such transmembrane hyperpolarizations; (2) axons of the PHP-exhibiting neurons (as determined by intracellular injections of Procion Yellow dye) project into the axon cap; and (3) although the input resistance and estimated specific membrane resistance of these neurons are not unusually low, the extracellular resistivity of the axon cap appears to be at least 2.5 times that of the surrounding tissue (Korn and Faber, 1975a). These results demonstrate that processes of the PHP cells lie parallel with the lines of the M-cell action current flowing back to the axon cap and serve as a return path for some of that current. In this context, then, the PHP and the EHP would both depend on the high extracellular resistivity of the axon cap, which favors the intercellular channeling of the "presynaptic" action currents.

The evidence that PHP-exhibiting neurons send their processes into the axon cap (i.e., into this region of high extracellular resistance surrounding the axon hillock of the M-cell) further suggested that action potentials in the former could generate electrical inhibition (i.e., an EHP) in the latter. This postulate, which requires that the "presynaptic impulses" not actively invade the cell's terminals, was confirmed by simultaneous intracellular recordings from the PHP-exhibiting neurons and the M-cell (Figure 3A); action potentials in the PHP-exhibiting neurons produce unitary EHPs in the axon cap of about 0.2–1.0 mV magnitude (Figure 3B$_1$). That is, the common electrical network coupling the M-cell and the PHP-exhibiting neurons results in a reciprocal electrical inhibition between these two elements.

As mentioned earlier, the functional sign of a field effect is determined by the relative orientation of the neurons involved. Both the EHP and the PHP are inhibitory because the inward hyperpolarizing current flow is at or near the site of spike initiation, whereas electrically inexcitable membrane regions are depolarized by the passive outward current flow. Similarly, Rall and Shepherd (1968) have postulated that in the olfactory bulb, extracellular currents generated by synaptic activation of granule cells substantially hyperpolarize mitral-cell bodies and depolarize their terminals. On the other hand, under appropriate conditions field-effect excitation could be expected of axodendritic or axosomatic synapses, with excitation occurring at the spike-generating initial segment of the postsynaptic neuron. Of interest here is the recent suggestion that the rising phase of the Ia EPSP in cat spinal motoneurons is a field-effect excitation (Werman and Carlen, 1976). This hypothesis is based on the observation that the early phase is much less sensitive to shifts in membrane potential than are either the decaying phase of the Ia EPSP or other EPSPs generated at more distal dendritic sites. Although the mechanism underlying this presumed electrical excitation has not yet been elucidated, it appears quite compatible with the model developed here.

ELECTRICAL AND CHEMICAL INHIBITION OF THE M-CELL MEDIATED BY PHP-INHIBITING NEURONS The electrical inhibition of the M-cell following its activation is only the first component of the recurrent inhibition of that cell; it is followed by a powerful chemically mediated IPSP (Figure 1A$_1$). The PHP-exhibiting neurons belong to the recurrent collateral network of the M-cell, and we have recently tested and proven the hypothesis that they mediate the chemical component of the inhibition as well (Korn and Faber, 1976), as originally suggested by Furukawa and Furshpan (1963). In our experiments, response to direct stimulation of the identified PHP neurons were recorded successively in the axon cap and in the M-cell (Figure 3A, B$_1$, B$_2$). Since the recurrent IPSP in the M-cell is not normally associated with a significant potential change, the probability of detecting unitary IPSPs was increased by intracellular Cl$^-$ injections, which converted them into depolarizing responses. Under these conditions direct stimulation of the presynaptic interneurons produced typical monophasic unitary EHPs in the axon cap (Figure 3B$_1$) and monosynaptic unitary IPSPs in the postsynaptic M-cell (B$_2$). These evoked IPSPs were Cl$^-$-dependent and were associated with a conductance increase that lasted for the duration of the IPSP (10–20 msec). Although these experiments have provided a unique opportunity to study the properties of an inhibitory chemical synapse in the vertebrate central

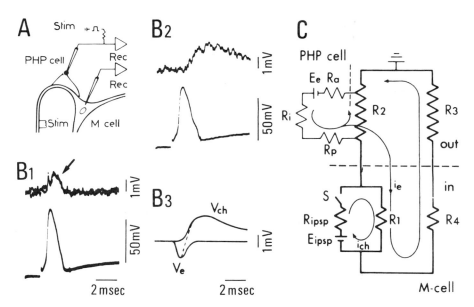

FIGURE 3 Unitary electrically and chemically mediated postsynaptic potentials produced by a single PHP neuron. (A) Diagram of the experimental setup for simultaneous recording and stimulation of a PHP neuron and the Mauthner cell. (B_1, B_2) Comparison of the potentials evoked outside and inside the M-cell (upper traces) by a directly evoked presynaptic spike (lower traces). (B_1) A unitary positive EHP (arrow) was recorded in the axon cap (two superimposed traces). (B_2) The cap electrode was advanced into the M-cell, and recordings were made after intracellular injection of Cl$^-$; the presynaptic spike produced a monosynaptic depolarizing IPSP in the M-cell. (B_3) Superposition of the potential changes recorded in the upper traces of B_1 and B_2. The electrical component, V_e, has been inverted with respect to the observed extracellular recording, since external positivity represents a hyperpolarization of the M-cell; the chemical IPSP (V_{ch}) is left in the depolarizing direction because of the difficulty of assessing the magnitude of the true hyperpolarization brought about prior to Cl$^-$ injection. The net transmembrane potential change is thus biphasic, with the electrically mediated component being curtailed by the rising phase of the chemical one (dashed line). (C) Model for the generation of the two inhibitory components. The lower half of the diagram represents the M-cell, with R_1 being the passive membrane resistance of the soma and axon hillock and R_4 that of the distal dendrites. The equivalent network for the PHP cell is to the left of the vertical dashed line, with E_e and R_a being, respectively, the driving electromotive force and resistance of the active spike-generating membrane, R_i the internal resistance, and R_p the passive resistance of the noninvaded terminal processes of the cell; i_e symbolizes the portion of the action current that flows inward across the M-cell's axon hillock and somatic membranes, thereby producing the electrical inhibition. The current i_e returns to the active site through R_4 and the distal extracellular resistance R_3. The remainder of the action current flows back through the high extracellular resistance of the axon cap, R_2. In addition, the release of transmitter by the PHP cell, which depends on terminal depolarization, produces an inhibitory Cl$^-$-dependent current, i_{ch}, in the M-cell; the analog for this additional chemical inhibitory process is represented by the network parallel with R_1. (E_{ipsp}, driving force for i_{ch}; R_{ipsp}, resistance of the activated inhibitory channels; S, switch illustrating the opening of these channels.) (Modified from Korn and Faber, 1976.)

nervous system, their relevance to this paper lies in the unequivocal demonstration that one neuron can mediate both inhibitions. The consequence of such a mixed synaptic action is that by incorporating the advantages of the two components (B_3), it has a rapid onset that is synchronous with the arrival of the presynaptic terminal depolarization (electrical component) and a prolonged duration (chemical component).

The model for one neuron generating both electrical and chemical inhibitions is shown in Figure 3C. The requirements, or assumptions, underlying this model are quite modest and can be summarized as follows:

1. The failure of the presynaptic spike to actively invade the terminal processes is necessary for this monophasic inhibitory field effect.

2. The chemically mediated component either depends on the remaining passively conducted terminal depolarization being above threshold for the inhibitory transmitter release (Katz and Miledi, 1967) or is a result of impulses in other terminals of the same neurons. (For details see Triller and Faber, 1978.)

3. The terminal presynaptic processes should lie, at least in part, in a region of increased extracellular resistance in order to have a significant intercellular channeling of the inhibitory electrical current.

In addition, the PHP neurons, which bring about

both electrical and chemical inhibitions, otherwise appear functionally similar to interneurons mediating typical postsynaptic chemical inhibition in the vertebrate central nervous system. Thus it can be speculated that other, similar interneurons might also mediate an electrical phase of inhibition in circumstances compatible with the three conditions described above. Along this line it should be pointed out that some of these morphological requirements are indeed satisfied by interneurons of the vertebrate cerebellar cortex (Sotelo and Llinás, 1972).

FUNCTIONS OF ELECTRICAL INHIBITION   Electrically mediated inhibition might serve two functions: (1) synchronization and/or (2) inhibition of the postsynaptic cells. First, since unitary EHPs are quite small, the maximal EHP recorded in the axon cap must involve the synchronous activity of a sizable number of neurons. The PHP contributes significantly to this synchronization: it resets the activity of the inhibitory interneurons and increases the probability that they will be excited by the collaterals. This concept has been supported by observations that in some of the neurons the PHP is followed by a depolarizing pickup of the EHP, so that the PHP-EHP sequence aids in the recruitment of the less excitable cells, which otherwise would not be brought to the firing level by the collateral input alone (Korn and Faber, 1975b). This synchronizing system, which guarantees maximal short-latency inhibition of the M-cell, could not operate so quickly with a longer-latency chemically mediated transmission alone. The second alternative, that of a functional inhibition not related to a rebound synchronization, would appear more relevant for PHP neurons not involved in collateral inhibition of the M-cell, such as some of the vestibular neurons (Korn and Faber, 1975a). For example, electrical inhibition of the M-cell, although brief, is often large enough to prevent a suitably timed antidromic or orthodromic impulse from invading the axon hillock of this neuron (Furukawa and Furshpan, 1963). Similarly, excitation of the vestibular neurons by an eighth nerve input, which at the same time triggers an M-cell spike, could conceivably degrade the startle reflex through an antagonistic vestibulospinal pathway. Therefore, it might be expected that the M-cell exerts an inhibitory control over these neurons without delay—that is, electrically.

Electrical transmission and coupling

The reality of electrotonic transmission and coupling is now well established, although as recently as the mid-1960s it was still questioned by a number of authors. When the first results of early intracellular investigations were published, this mode of synaptic transmission was considered by many to be exceptional and restricted to primitive forms of phylogeny (for the early history of this concept see Eccles, 1964). However, more recent electrophysiological data have demonstrated the presence of electrotonic coupling between neurons, not only in the invertebrate but in the vertebrate phyla as well, including mammals (Bennett, 1972; Korn and Bennett, 1972; Llinás, 1975). Furthermore, in most instances electrical transmission was found to take place by way of morphologically distinct junctions of the zonula occludens variety (Farquhar and Palade, 1963) where the membrane of the coupled cells come together, thus narrowing the extracellular space to about 20–40 Å. This type of junction was first considered to constitute low-resistivity pathways between nerve cells (Robertson, 1963; Bennett et al., 1963; Pappas and Bennett, 1966). It now appears that although proofs of a strict correlation between electrophysiological and histological data are still missing in a few cases (see Bennett et al., 1967b), the structural correlate for electrotonic coupling belongs to the class of the so-called gap junctions (Robertson, 1963; Payton, Bennett, and Pappas, 1969; Revel and Karnovsky, 1967; Asada and Bennett, 1971; Pappas, Asada, and Bennett, 1971). These junctions have been found in numerous neuronal structures, including several regions of the CNS, where they can form axosomatic, axoaxonic, or somasomatic close appositions between neurons (see Sotelo, 1975, 1977; Sotelo and Korn, 1978).

In this paper we shall survey some recent findings concerning the electrophysiology of electrotonic transmission in the vertebrates. Newly identified coupled nuclei (especially in mammals) will be emphasized; some of the possibilities that remain, such as that of dual chemical and electrotonic transmission at the same synapse, will be discussed, and the synaptic control of electrotonic coupling will be described. Other major topics, such as the role of intercellular transport through gap junctions during growth and embryonic development (Furshpan and Potter, 1968; Bennett, 1973a) and gap junctions as pathways for metabolic interactions between neurons (see Bennett, 1973b; Simpson, Rose, and Loewenstein, 1977), will not be reviewed. Nor shall we analyze the mode of operation of electrical synapses and the respective advantages of or similarities between the electrical and chemical modes of synaptic transmission, topics that have been extensively described in a series of exhaustive reports by Bennett (1966,

1972, 1974). We will make, whenever possible, a distinction between the generalized concept of electrotonic coupling between neurons and the more specific situation of electrotonic transmission, which includes the implication of identifiable pre- and postsynaptic neuronal elements.

ELECTROPHYSIOLOGICAL CRITERIA FOR THE PRESENCE OF ELECTROTONIC TRANSMISSION AND COUPLING IN THE VERTEBRATE CNS   The most convincing demonstration of electrotonic coupling requires simultaneous recording from and intracellular stimulation of adjacent cells: polarization in one cell (usually by injecting transmembrane current pulses) must result in an appreciable polarization of the adjacent cell— that is, more polarization than would be obtained from positioning the electrodes extracellularly. However, since recording simultaneously from two cells in deep central structures is often not feasible technically, less direct criteria are generally used in the CNS.

Electrical transmission from a presynaptic fiber to a postsynaptic neuron can be suspected when the interval between the presynaptic volley (or spike) and the onset of the resulting postsynaptic potential is shorter than a chemical synaptic delay. For electrotonic coupling in a nucleus, intracellular recordings are obtained from single cells, while polarization of the adjacent neurons is produced by their antidromic activation. The principle underlying this method (Bennett et al., 1964; Bennett, 1966) is as follows: Where neurons are coupled, an impulse will not propagate actively to neighboring neurons if the coupling ratio is low; the action currents set up by this impulse will, however, produce a small depolarization in the nearby cells. Consequently, if the threshold of the axon of the impaled neuron is high relative to that of a significant proportion of the neurons in the nucleus, antidromic stimulation of graded intensities will produce graded subthreshold depolarizations in that cell. The latency of the antidromic depolarizations may be slightly longer than that of the antidromic spike in the impaled cell because of slowing during electrotonic spread (Bennett, 1966), but the delay between the two should be consistently shorter than a chemical synaptic delay in order to exclude depolarizations evoked by chemical synapses through afferent fibers or recurrent collaterals.

Although their evidence may be considered somewhat indirect, graded antidromic depolarizations leave little doubt of the reality of coupling between cells (provided it is demonstrated that they are not EPSPs). They have been recorded in many different kinds of neurons in experiments where electrical transmission has been demonstrated more directly and confirmed by ultrastructural data as well (Bennett, Nakajima, and Pappas, 1967; Bennett et al., 1967a; Korn and Bennett, 1972, 1975). Their presence in association with close membrane apposition has therefore been considered as sufficient physiological proof of coupling in other systems (Bennett et al., 1964; Bennett and Pappas, 1965; Pappas and Bennett, 1966; Bennett et al., 1967b). Techniques using antidromic stimulations were also used in studies of coupling in the mammalian brain (see below). Although these depolarizations have been named differently by different authors, they shall be referred to as *graded antidromic depolarizations* in this paper.

It is also important to demonstrate that graded antidromic depolarizations in a neuron are not dependent on events associated with antidromic activation of the neuron's own axon (such as M-spikes). For this purpose a collision technique can be used: neurons that exhibit graded depolarizations are directly activated by a pulse applied through the bridge circuit, and this activation is followed by an antidromic stimulus. Under these conditions the directly evoked spike prevents the antidromic one from reaching the recording site during a period equal to the sum of the conduction time of this spike down the axon, the refractory period following spike propagation, and the conduction time of the antidromic action potential; graded depolarizations observed during this period of axonal block are necessarily brought about by invasion of neurons other than the impaled one.

Finally, one should be able to demonstrate the absence of a membrane-potential dependence or of an equilibrium potential for the graded depolarizations. However, due mainly to geometrical factors (Rall et al., 1967), the lack of a reversal potential for graded depolarizations is often difficult to establish and is of limited value in distinguishing an electrotonically transmitted potential from a chemical PSP.

ELECTROTONIC SYNAPTIC TRANSMISSION IN VERTEBRATES   In comparison with chemically mediated transmission, electrotonic transmission, since it does not involve a significant synaptic delay, can result in a shorter-latency postsynaptic excitation. Consequently it may mediate rapid reflexes in the escape systems of both vertebrates (Auerbach and Bennett, 1969; Furshpan, 1964) and invertebrates (Watanabe and Grundfest, 1961). In recent years a large body of evidence has been generated for electrotonic transmission from primary afferent vestibular fibers to vestibular neurons in species ranging from lower vertebrates such as the toadfish *Opsanus tau* (Korn, Sotelo, and Bennett, 1977), frog (Precht et al., 1974), and the lizard *Lacerta viridis* (Richter, Precht, and Ozawa, 1975) to pigeons (Wilson and Wylie, 1970) and even a mammal, the rat (Wylie, 1973). In each case, the short latency of the earliest component of the complex EPSP recorded in vestibular neurons following afferent stimulation provided the evidence for an electrotonic spread of the presynaptic impulses.

Results from experiments on the toadfish lateral vestibular nucleus (LVN) are shown in Figure 4A. Part A_1 illustrates the experimental setup used for all the species mentioned above. Part A_2 gives an example of the EPSPs induced by stimulation of the ipsilateral vestibular nerve; they were recorded from a cell identified as a vestibulospinal neuron by its antidromic activation from the spinal cord (not shown). The PSPs A_2 and A_4 appeared at the same stimulus strengths as the positive-negative wave of the extracellularly recorded presynaptic volley A_5. These EPSPs had an amplitude of 7–8 mV and a latency of about 0.35 msec. A comparison between this intracellular response and the corresponding extracellular field potential indicates that most of this latency was in conduction time of the primary afferent-nerve volley (A_4 and A_5). The vertical dotted line drawn from the positive peak (P-wave) of the extracellular field potential, which signals the time of arrival of the presynaptic volley, indicates that the synaptic delay was close to zero for this neuron. The delay was determined by this method for 34 neurons, and the histogram A_6 shows that it ranged from 0 to 0.21 msec ($m = 0.08$ msec; S.D. = 0.06). Therefore, in all cells it was too fast for chemical mediation at this temperature (Hubbard and Schmidt, 1963; Katz and Miledi, 1965; Bennett, Nakajima, and Pappas, 1967) and so was brought about by electrical transmission between primary afferents and vestibular neurons. This finding is consistent with the fact that in the toadfish LVN neurons are coupled (see below) and also with the presence of gap junctions at the synaptic terminals on the cell bodies and dendrites of the LVN neurons (Korn, Sotelo, and Bennett, 1977). Since the only axon terminals to establish gap junctions with the LVN neurons are the large boutons with rounded vesicles and a few club endings it follows that these terminals belong to primary vestibular fibers and that they mediate the electrical component of the vestibular EPSP.

Short-latency depolarizations (or EDPs: early depolarizing potentials) were also recorded in vestibular neurons of the frog following ipsilateral vestibular nerve stimulations. Figure 4B shows a sample of these PSPs; the stimulus intensity for evoking them (B_1) was close to the threshold for the field potential in the vestibular nucleus; when the stimulus strength was slightly increased, action potentials were generated by a PSP of increased amplitude (B_2). Because of their latency, and also because similar EDPs can be obtained by spinal stimulation, it can be inferred that these potentials are generated by electrotonic transmission between primary afferents and vestibular neurons and/or by means of electrotonic coupling between secondary neurons and vestibular efferents projecting into the labyrinth. Early and similar monosynaptic EPSPs were recorded from vestibular neurons in the lizard (Figure 4C).

The first demonstration of electrical transmission in a mammal was obtained in the rat by Wylie (1973). In 18 vestibular cells, the synaptic delay of the vestibular-evoked EPSPs, measured from the peak of the P-wave to the onset of the initial component, was 0.25 msec or, if evaluated from the mean latency from the onset of response of afferent fibers, 0.13 msec; these values are less than the minimal ones reported for a chemical synaptic delay in this species. Such PSPs were found to be insensitive to the displacement of membrane potential in either the hyperpolarizing or depolarizing directions. As we shall see, these results are in good agreement with the fact that the giant cells of the rat lateral vestibular nucleus are electrotonically coupled (Korn, Crepel, and Sotelo, 1972; Korn, Sotelo, and Crepel, 1973) and the fact that large terminals synapsing on the perikaryon and on the main dendritic trunk of these neurons bear gap junctions (Sotelo and Palay, 1967, 1970). Gap junctions between large synaptic boutons (probably emerging from primary vestibular fibers) and vestibular neurons have also been observed in the lamprey vestibular nuclei (Stefanelli and Caravita, 1970), in the goldfish tangential nucleus (Hinojosa and Robertson, 1967), in the LVN of the rat (Sotelo and Palay, 1970), and in the rat descending vestibular nucleus (Sotelo, 1975). Thus, from a comparative point of view, the mode of transmission from primary afferent fibers to postsynaptic LVN neurons is rather homogeneous, at least up to cat, in which electrical transmission and coupling of LVN neurons are missing (for references see Korn, Sotelo, and Crepel, 1973). Although the significance of electrical transmission in the vestibular system is still unclear, it appears to produce a reduction in the latency of escape and balancing responses. It would be interesting to determine whether mammalian species

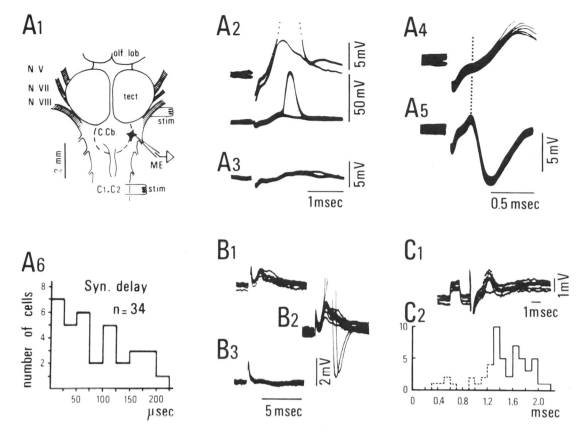

FIGURE 4 Electrical EPSPs induced in lateral vestibular neurons by ipsilateral vestibular nerve stimulations. (A₁–A₆) Experiments performed on the toadfish *Opsanus tau*. (A₁) Diagram of stimulating and recording electrodes. (*Abbreviations*: C.Cb, corpus cerebellum; ME, recording microelectrode; N.V., N.VII, N.VIII: trigeminal, facial, and vestibular nerves, respectively; olf. lob, olfactory lobe; stim, stimulating electrodes; tect., optic tectum.) The dark area indicates the LVN. (A₂–A₆) Evidence for electrically mediated synaptic transmission. Intracellular recordings obtained from an LVN neuron. (A₂, upper and lower traces) Intracellular potentials recorded at high and low gain, respectively. The ipsilateral vestibular nerve was stimulated at strengths straddling threshold for spike generation in the recorded cell. The stimulus set up a short-latency EPSP, which could be large enough to generate a full sized action potential (two superimposed traces, one with and one without a spike.) (A₃) Extracellular potential evoked just outside the cell by the same stimuli. (A₄–A₅) Superimposed traces recorded at high gain and at a faster sweep speed. The ipsilateral vestibular nerve was activated at a strength just below threshold for spike generation. (A₄) Short-latency EPSP intracellularly recorded. (A₅) Corresponding extra-

cellular field potential monitored outside the cell. The records in A₄ and A₅ are aligned with respect to the stimulus artifacts; a vertical dotted line drawn from the positive peak of the extracellular field potential allows evaluation of the relative timing between the presynaptic volley and the onset of the EPSP (synaptic delay). (A₆) Histogram showing the distribution of the EPSP synaptic delay in 34 lateral vestibular neurons. (Modified from Korn, Sotelo, and Bennett, 1977.) (B₁–B₂) Intracellular recordings from a frog vestibular neuron. (B₁) Short-latency electrical PSP alone. (B₂) As the stimulus intensity was increased, the PSP reached the firing level and full action potentials were generated. (B₃) Extracellular potential produced outside the cell by the same stimulus as for C₂. (Modified from Precht et al., 1974.) (C₁, C₂) Electrical EPSPs in lateral vestibular neurons of the lizard, *Lacerta viridis*. (C₁) All-or-none, short-latency depolarization evoked with a low-intensity stimulus applied to the ipsilateral vestibular nerve. (C₂) Histogram showing the frequency distribution of the early depolarization (dashed line) and of later, presumably chemical EPSPs (solid line). (Modified from Richter, Precht, and Ozawa, 1975.)

more closely related to rodents than the cat also use electrical transmission at the synapses between the vestibular nerve and neurons of the vestibular nuclei.

ELECTROTONIC COUPLING IN VERTEBRATES   The toadfish LVN has produced not only an example of

electrical transmission from primary afferents but also a remarkable case of electrotonic coupling between neurons (Korn, Sotelo, and Bennett, 1977). The responses of an LVN neuron to spinal stimulations of increasing strength are shown in Figure 5. In this cell, graded antidromic depolarizations up to

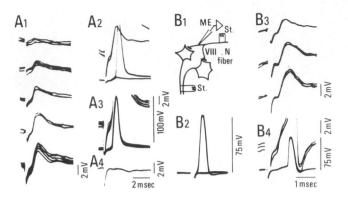

FIGURE 5 Electrotonic coupling of lateral vestibular neurons in the toadfish *Opsanus tau*. (A$_1$–A$_4$) Recordings from a lateral vestibular neuron; the spinal cord was stimulated at increasing intensities from A$_1$ to A$_3$. (A$_1$) High-gain recording. Top to bottom: as the stimulus strength was increased, a graded depolarization increased to an amplitude of about 5 mV. (A$_2$–A$_3$) Upper and lower traces are at high and low gain, respectively. A 5.5 mV depolarization reached the firing level of the penetrated cell and was adequate to generate a spike (two superimposed sweeps, one with and one without a spike.) (A$_3$) A stronger spinal stimulus evoked an antidromic action potential (several superimposed sweeps). (A$_4$) Extracellular field potential produced outside this neuron by the same stimulus as in A$_3$. (B$_1$–B$_4$) Evidence for electrotonic spread of graded antidromic depolarizations from postsynaptic neurons to prejunctional fibers. (B$_1$) The experimental setup. (*Abbreviations*: ME, recording microelectrode; St, stimulating electrodes; VIII N fiber, primary vestibular afferent axon.) (B$_2$–B$_4$) Intracellular recordings from a presynaptic fiber. (B$_2$) Identification of the impaled neuron as a prejunctional fiber (low-gain recording); stimuli just threshold for excitation of the unit were applied to the vestibular nerve. When the orthodromic spike failed, there was no underlying PSP observed that would have initiated the impulse (superimposed sweeps at constant stimulus strength where a spike did or did not occur.) (B$_3$) High-gain recordings; stimuli adequate to evoke antidromic graded depolarizations in postsynaptic neurons were applied to the spinal cord. Short-latency depolarizations, presumably due to spread from the postsynaptic cells, were also recorded in the presynaptic fiber; their amplitude reached a peak of about 5.4 mV as the stimulus strength was progressively increased (from top to bottom). (B$_4$) Stronger spinal stimulation evoked a depolarization large enough to generate a spike in the impaled presynaptic fiber. Upper and lower traces are at high AC and low DC gain, respectively. (Modified from Korn, Sotelo, and Bennett, 1977.)

5 mV were observed (A$_1$) with stimuli below threshold for the antidromic spike; with a stronger stimulus, they increased in size and became adequate to excite the cell (A$_2$). These important findings indicate that coupling between LVN neurons is close enough that a cell can be excited by activity spread from its neighbors when enough of them are active. Finally, the antidromic spike itself was evoked as the intensity of

the spinal stimulus was increased (A$_3$). Several properties that distinguish the graded antidromic depolarizations from EPSPs could be demonstrated. First, in all cases the antidromic spike preceded the depolarizations by a delay that was too short for chemical transmission by recurrent collaterals (for 29 neurons the computed delay of the antidromic depolarizations was about 0.09 msec longer than that of the antidromic spikes). Second, the interval between the positive peak of the extracellular field potential generated by the fastest elements of the incoming volley and the onset of graded antidromic depolarizations was about 0.13 msec—too short for chemical transmission by afferent fibers. Third, comparison of extracellular with intracellular potentials showed that the graded antidromic depolarizations started during or after the early part of the negative field potential (compare A$_2$ with A$_4$)—that is, during or after the antidromic invasion of cell bodies adjacent to the investigated cells. Finally, the time courses of the graded antidromic depolarizations were comparable to those of the electrically mediated component of the vestibular evoked PSPs.

Spread of postsynaptic neuronal activity to presynaptic fibers could also be demonstrated in this material. Axons identified as primary afferent vestibular fibers were impaled, and graded depolarizations that could become large enough to set up presynaptic spikes were recorded following graded stimulation of the spinal cord (Figure 5B). The short latency and the all-or-none character of the action potential (see B$_2$) confirmed that in this case recordings were from a primary vestibular axon. Spinal stimulations of increasing intensity evoked depolarizations that had a short latency (about 0.45 msec) and increased to an amplitude of 5.4 mV as the stimulus strength was increased (B$_3$); as the stimulus strength was further increased, the depolarizations became larger and induced action potentials (B$_4$). The mean latency of the graded depolarizations recorded in presynaptic fibers was 0.51 msec (S.D. = 0.18; $n = 15$) and that of the antidromic spikes in the vestibular neurons was 0.37 msec (S.D. = 0.16; $n = 29$). The 0.14 msec difference, which is the time for spread of activity from the LVN neurons to the recording site, is too short for chemical transmission. It follows that the prejunctional potentials were brought about by direct electrotonic spread of antidromic impulses from LVN neurons to eighth-nerve fibers.

Lateral vestibular neurons are not directly connected: gap junctions occur exclusively between fibers and somata (or dendrites) of postsynaptic cells and are not found between dendrites or somata themselves. The implication is that cells are coupled by way of afferent fibers, which give rise to the large boutons with rounded vesicles, and the less numerous club endings, both of which synapse on these neurons with gap junctions. Physiological results such as those shown in Figure 5B demonstrate that the fibers each end on many neurons and that they can provide the required coupling pathway. Electrotonic spread between cells by way of presynaptic fibers has been demonstrated in other morphologically similar situations on the basis of physiological data (Bennett et al., 1964; Bennett and Pappas, 1965; Bennett, 1966; Pappas and Bennett, 1966; Bennett et al., 1967b; Kriebel et al., 1969; Korn, Sotelo, and Crepel, 1973). Morphological data from different fish nuclei have also confirmed that a single axon terminal can establish gap junctions on two adjacent neurons (Meszler, Pappas, and Bennett, 1972; Pappas, Waxman, and Bennett, 1975; Sotelo, Rethelyi, and Szabo, 1975; references in Korn, Sotelo, and Bennett, 1977).

Evidence that in the toadfish LVN postsynaptic impulses causing graded potentials in prejunctional axon can initiate presynaptic spikes (see Figure 5B$_4$) must be emphasized. Comparable observations have been made in some gymnotids (Bennett et al., 1967), in the frog (Precht et al., 1974), and in the electric catfish *Malapterurus* (Bennett, Nakajima, and Pappas, 1967). These results led to an interesting concept: antidromic impulses in presynaptic terminals presumably propagate to the vestibular receptors and leave them refractory; thus invasion of these terminals may provide negative feedback by preventing their reexcitation at short intervals following a synchronous discharge of an adequate number of postsynaptic cells.

In a number of nuclei where highly synchronous firing controls specialized systems, including sonic muscles and electric organs, the synchronization is mediated by electrotonic junctions that provide positive feedback between neighboring neurons; for this reason they have been termed *synchronizing synapses* (for reviews, see Bennett, 1972, 1974). A study of the neural control of rapid eye movements in fish (Korn and Bennett, 1971, 1972, 1975) was undertaken to determine whether the same organizational principle applies to more ordinary effector systems. Previous work had shown that the somata of puffer fish oculomotor neurons innervating the same muscle are electrotonically coupled and that impulses can arise at different sites in the neurons (Kriebel et al., 1969). It was then suggested that, when the cell bodies are depolarized by EPSPs (following ophthalmic-nerve stimulation), the weak coupling between cells might

exert a significant synchronizing influence, leading to synchronous muscle activity and rapid eye retraction, whereas slow, graded compensatory movements might arise from impulse activity originating in the dendrites, where the coupling is negligible. Impulses would not spread between cells because of the weakness of the coupling between cell bodies and the absence of any EPSPs in them. Thus it became interesting to determine whether coupling was involved in synchronization of fish oculomotor neurons during such rapid eye movements as occur in the fast phase of vestibular nystagmus.

Figure 6A shows the experimental setup. As in mammals, horizontal nystagmus can be produced by touching the ampulla of the horizontal semicircular canal of the puffer fish (Figure 6B). There are slow deviations of both eyes away from the stimulated side, followed by rapid returns to that side. The nystagmus generally outlasts the stimulus, but the frequency slows late in the response. As frequency decreases, the duration of the fast phase remains about the same and the slow phase lengthens. In addition, trains of electrical stimuli (200–300 per second) applied to the nerve of either horizontal semicircular canal evoke a vestibular nystagmus in fish. Intracellular recordings from medial rectus motoneurons indicate that, during the fast phase of a nystagmus evoked by contralateral nerve stimulation, impulses arise from large PSPs (Figure 6C$_1$) generated at or near the cell body. During the slow phase (induced by ipsilateral stimulation), impulses arose abruptly from the base line (C$_2$) and were generated in the dendrites. Intracellular recordings in curarized fish confirmed these conclusions; for example, stimulation of the nerve from the contralateral horizontal canal (which induces the fast phase) evoked spikes that arose from large PSPs (D$_1$) and were blocked relatively easily by hyperpolarizing currents (D$_2$). Stimulation of the nerve from the ipsilateral horizontal canal evoked spikes that arose abruptly from the baseline (D$_3$) and were much more difficult to block by hyperpolarizing currents; little if any underlying PSP was observed when these impulses were delayed or blocked (D$_4$).

To establish the synchronizing role of coupling between cell bodies, antidromic stimuli were paired with stimuli to the nerve from the contralateral horizontal semicircular canal. The former evoked graded antidromic depolarizations (Figure 7A), indicating coupling with neighboring cells (because the coupling is weak, these depolarizations never reached the threshold of the penetrated neuron). The neighboring cells evoked somatic PSPs (Figure 7B). As expected, subthreshold PSPs induced by weak stimulations (B$_2$)

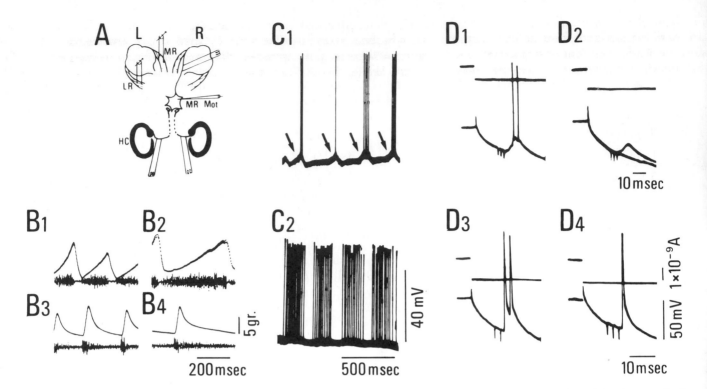

FIGURE 6 Evidence that impulses recorded in medial rectus motoneurons of the Puffer fish *Spheroides maculatus* arise at a distance from the cell body (presumably in dendrites) during the slow phase of the vestibular nystagmus, while impulses arise from large PSPs generated in or near the cell body during the fast phase. (A) Diagram of stimulating and recording electrodes. (*Abbreviations*: HC, horizontal semicircular canal; L, left side; LR, lateral rectus muscle; MR, medial rectus muscle; MR Mot, medial rectus motoneurons.) (B_1–B_4) Isometric responses (upper trace) and EMG recording (lower trace) from the right medial rectus. (B_1, B_2) Slow-phase responses recorded at the beginning (B_1) and near the end (B_2) of a nystagmus evoked by mechanical stimulation of the ampulla of the right horizontal semicircular canal. (B_3, B_4) Fast-phase responses at the beginning (B_3) and near the end (B_4) of the mechanical stimulation of the ampulla of the left horizontal semicircular canal. As the frequency during nystagmus decreases, there is a lengthening of the slow phase, while the duration of the fast phase remains constant. (C_1, C_2) Intracellular recordings from medial rectus motoneuron of an uncurarized fish during a vestibular nystagmus. The nystagmus was evoked by short trains of pulses (250 Hz; 0.1 msec; 2V) applied to the nerve of the horizontal semicircular canal of either side prior to the recording. (C_1) A stimulation of the nerve from the left horizontal semicircular canal evoked periodic bursts of spikes that appear to rise from EPSPs (arrows). (C_2) The same stimulation was applied to the nerve from the right semicircular canal; there were long-lasting bursts of spikes, which arose abruptly from the baseline. (D_1–D_4) Different impulse-initiating sites in a single neuron. Intracellularly recorded responses were evoked by trains of three stimuli to the nerve from contralateral (D_1, D_2) and ipsilateral (D_3, D_4) horizontal semicircular canals. *Upper traces*: Hyperpolarizing current. Spikes evoked by contralateral stimulation were blocked by relatively small hyperpolarizing currents and were initiated by large EPSPs. Spikes evoked by ipsilateral stimulation were more difficult to block; delay and block of early responses in D_4 did not reveal EPSPs. The third stimulus artifact in D_2 is superimposed on the falling phase of the first spike. Most of the gradual negative-going potential change during the current pulses is due to bridge imbalance arising from changing electrode properties. (C_1–C_2 and D_1–D_4 are from two different motoneurons; figure modified from Korn and Bennett, 1975.)

could summate with the graded antidromic depolarizations to fire the cell (B_3). A similar but less precise synchronization is illustrated in Figure $7C_1$; here the penetrated cell, unlike that in B_3, was made to fire a long time after the antidromic depolarization. In another mode of synchronization (C_2), an impulse can be advanced by an earlier graded depolarization; here there is improvement in synchronization instead of a recruitment of unexcited cells. Experiments similar to those just described indicate that there is no significant coupling between dendrites; antidromic graded depolarizations did not summate with a dendritic input to fire otherwise unexcited cells or to generate more spikes in the ones that were already excited (Figure 7D), although it could be demonstrated that antidromic impulses do propagate out the dendrites to the impulse-initiating sites (Korn and Bennett, 1972, 1975). Figure 7E summarizes these

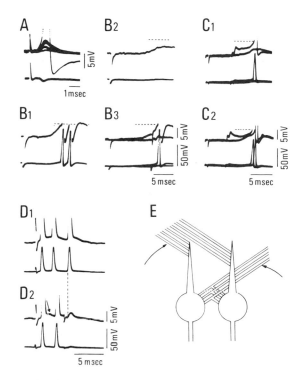

FIGURE 7 Synchronization mediated by electrotonic coupling between somata of oculomotor neurons in the puffer fish *Spheroides maculatus*: interaction of somatic EPSPs with graded antidromic depolarizations. (A) *Upper trace*: Graded depolarizations produced in a medial rectus motoneuron by graded antidromic stimulation (five superimposed traces). As the stimulus strength was increased, an increasing depolarization was recorded; it reached a maximum amplitude of about 4 mV before the axon of the impaled cell was excited. *Lower trace*: Potential later recorded just outside the cell with an antidromic stimulus near threshold for the cell. (B₁–B₃) Recording from another motoneuron; higher gain on upper trace. (B₁) A relatively strong stimulus to the contralateral horizontal semicircular canal evoked two spikes preceded by a large, slowly rising PSP. The firing level of the cell for somatic input is indicated by the dashed line. (B₂) A weaker vestibular stimulus evoked only a subthreshold PSP. (B₃) Two superimposed sweeps, one with an antidromic stimulus just subthreshold for the impaled cell, one with the antidromic stimulus preceded by vestibular stimulation as in B₂. The antidromic stimulus evoked a depolarization that summated with the vestibular PSP to excite the cell at the firing level for somatic inputs (dashed line) (C₁, C₂) Recording from a different motoneuron, higher gain on upper trace. (C₁) Two superimposed sweeps, one with a weak vestibular stimulus that evoked only a PSP and one with this vestibular stimulus followed by an antidromic stimulus. The antidromic stimulus evoked a depolarization that summated with the PSP to reach the firing level (dashed line). (C₂) As in C₁, but with vestibular stimulation adequate to excite the cell. Summation of inputs advanced firing of the cell by causing it to reach firing level sooner. The firing level and the spike amplitude decreased slightly between C₁ and C₂, presumably due to injury. (D₁, D₂) Lack of coupling between dendrites as indicated by failure of dendritic inputs to facilitate spread of antidromic

results; the absence of significant coupling between dendrites allows the cells to fire independently when excited by dendritic inputs (left arrow), thus allowing mediation of slow, graded eye movements. The coupling of cell bodies through afferent terminals provides a synchronizing influence that facilitates mediation of rapid eye movements, such as the fast phase of the vestibular nystagmus, when cells are excited by somatic inputs (right arrow). It should be pointed out that this model is not relevant for mammals because there is no evidence of electrotonic coupling of oculomotor neurons in the cat, although certain puzzling results might indicate a yet-unclear kind of interaction between abducens neurons (Gogan et al., 1974; for discussion see Korn and Bennett, 1975). However, electrical transmission provides an effective way of interconnecting cells, and as discussed elsewhere (Korn and Bennett, 1972), it is possible to anticipate that electrotonic coupling will be found in the command cells that are presynaptic to oculomotor neurons and that initiate the signals for the fast phase of the nystagmus.

ELECTROTONIC COUPLING IN THE MAMMALIAN CNS

In recent years, EM studies have shown that a large number of areas in the mammalian CNS exhibit gap junctions, including the mesencephalic trigeminal nucleus of both the mouse (Hinrichsen and Larramendi, 1968) and the rat (Imamoto and Shimizu, 1970; Sotelo, 1975), the lateral and inferior vestibular nuclei of the rat (Sotelo and Palay, 1967, 1970; Sotelo,

impulses between cells. (D₁) Three abruptly rising dendritic spikes were evoked by stimulation of the nerve to the ipsilateral horizontal semicircular canal. (D₂) The stimulus intensity was reduced slightly, and two (instead of three) dendritic spikes were recorded. An antidromic stimulus was given just prior to the time of occurrence of the third spike in D₁ (vertical dashed line); the stimulus was subthreshold for the penetrated cell but excited many adjacent cells, as indicated by the large graded antidromic depolarization. This antidromic activity failed to excite the impaled cell. The recording at high gain (upper trace) shows a small depolarization (arrow) that could represent a dendritic PSP as well as electrotonic spread of impulses from somata of adjacent neurons. (Modified from Korn and Bennett, 1972.) (E) Diagram of somatic and dendritic inputs to medial rectus oculomotor neurons. The dendritic inputs (left arrow) are activated by stimulation of the ipsilateral eighth nerve. There is no coupling, and movements are smoothly graded in amplitude. The somatic inputs (right arrow) are activated by stimulation of contralateral eighth nerve. There is weak coupling between the cell bodies (by way of the presynaptic fibers) and, therefore, some increase in synchronization of firing during the fast phase of the vestibular nystagmus. (Modified from Korn and Bennett, 1975.)

1975), the cochlear nucleus of the rat (Sotelo, Gentschev, and Zamora, 1976), and the inferior olivary complex of the cat (Sotelo, Llinás, and Baker, 1974), the opossum (King, Martin, and Bowman, 1975), the monkey (Sotelo, 1975), and the rat (Sotelo, unpublished). Gap junctions have been also encountered in the cerebellum of the cat (Sotelo and Llinás, 1972) and of mutant mice (Sotelo, unpublished), in cat olfactory bulb (Pinching and Powell, 1971), in primate neocortex (Sloper, 1972), and in the inner and outer layers of primate retina (Dowling and Boycott, 1966). Freeze-fractured electrical synapses have been studied in the olfactory bulb of the rabbit (Landis, Reese, and Raviola, 1974; for review see Sotelo and Korn, 1978). It follows that, far from being an exception, electrotonic junctions are now frequently found in the mammalian brain. Three examples of neuronal electrotonic coupling in mammals have been confirmed by electrophysiological evidence; in all of them gap junctions are present in the structures investigated.

Mesencephalic nucleus of the fifth nerve in the rat Baker and Llinás (1971) gave the first electrophysiological demonstration of electrotonic coupling in the mammalian brain: it was based on the presence of short-latency depolarizations (SLDs) in about 10% of the impaled cells of the rat mesencephalic nucleus following peripheral masseteric-nerve stimulation (see Figure 8A, B). Although similar in principle to the graded antidromic potentials, SLDs cannot be so named, for the nucleus is sensory. When measured from the incoming volley, their latency appears to be too short for chemically evoked potentials (Figure 8C); some of them were graded, and on some occasions the larger depolarizations directly generated full spikes (as in Figure 8D, E). Collision experiments conclusively demonstrated that the graded depolarizations were independent of events in their own axons and were brought about by invasion of neighboring cells (Figure 8F). This procedure allowed the uncovering of graded depolarizations in neurons with low threshold for somatopetal invasion.

Lateral vestibular nucleus of the rat The second example is the Deiters nucleus of the rat (Korn, Crepel, and Sotelo, 1972; Korn, Sotelo, and Crepel, 1973). In this structure 69% of the neurons exhibited graded antidromic depolarizations following spinal-cord stimulations of graded intensities (two examples are shown in Figure 9A, B). As the stimulus strength was increased, the amplitude of the intracellularly recorded depolarizations increased (in A_1 the stimulus strength, expressed as a percentage of the threshold T for antidromic invasion of the impaled neurons,

is indicated at the right of each record); finally, an antidromic spike was generated. Demonstration that the graded depolarizations were not M-spikes required collision experiments: a stimulating pulse was applied through the recording microelectrode prior to the stimulation of the spinal cord; under these conditions the control antidromic spike (Figure $9C_1$) was blocked and the antidromic depolarization was uncovered (C_2–C_3). Despite the block, their graded nature could still be demonstrated by varying the intensity of the spinal stimulus. The time interval between the foot of the antidromic spike and the onset of the graded depolarizations was measured systematically: the histogram of Figure 9D indicates that in all cases it ranged between 0 and 150 μsec, which is shorter than any chemical synaptic delay and rules out chemically mediated PSPs from recurrent collaterals. An alternative explanation of the origin of the graded depolarizations would be EPSPs induced by rapidly conducting afferents from the spinal cord. This possibility was eliminated for the following reasons:

1. Their latencies (as measured from the onset of the incoming volley) were often shorter than any synaptic delay ever observed at a chemical synapse.

2. No significantly larger (i.e., faster) fibers than those of the presumptive vestibulospinal tract were observed in the spinal cord.

3. As indicated by lesion experiments, afferent fibers from the spinal cord terminate exclusively in the dorsal part of the nucleus, and no degeneration was observed in the ventral part of this structure, even though graded depolarizations were recorded in neurons located at all depths in the nucleus.

On the other hand, longer-latency inhibitory postsynaptic potentials (Figure 9E) and EPSPs (Figure 9F), which are presumably chemically mediated, could be evoked in the impaled neurons by strong spinal stimuli. The importance of this finding to the synaptic control of electrotonic coupling in these cells will be discussed in the last section of this paper.

These results are in good agreement with the fact that large terminals synapsing on the perikaryon and the main dendrites of the giant lateral vestibular neurons bear both "active zones" and gap junctions (Figure 10). However, these neurons are not directly connected; gap junctions occur exclusively between presynaptic fibers and postsynaptic cells. Thus coupling is mediated by way of presynaptic fibers (as shown in the insert of Figure 10).

Inferior olive in the cat Recently electrotonic coupling was demonstrated indirectly by the presence of finely graded antidromic depolarizations evoked by

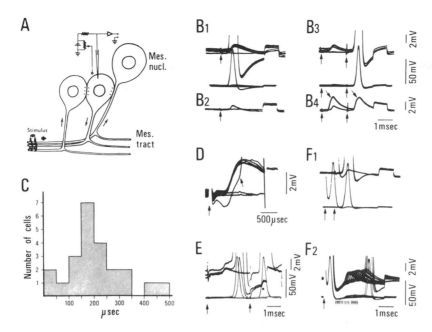

FIGURE 8 Electrotonic coupling between mesencephalic neurons in the rat. (A) The experimental setup; three cells and the projections of their axons are shown. The neurons were electrically activated from the trigeminal nerve (stimulus) or directly through the recording microelectrode by means of a bridge circuit. Somatosomatic (left) and axosomatic (right) arrangements of gap junctions are indicated by arrowheads. Upgoing arrows at the axon of lateral cells indicate somatopetal conduction of action potentials; the downgoing arrow in the central cell indicates somatofugal conduction. (B₁–B₄) Intracellular recordings from a mesencephalic neuron. (B₁) The stimulation (arrow) activated the cell. When the stimulus failed to generate a full spike, a small all-or-none depolarization was observed; it occurred at a slightly longer latency. (B₂) The stimulus intensity was reduced in order to demonstrate the all-or-none character of the short-latency depolarization. (B₃, B₄) Double trigeminal stimulation. The first stimulus was subthreshold and the second was suprathreshold for invasion of the impaled neuron. (B₃) The first stimulus evoked an all-or-none short-latency depolarization. (B₄) As the cell was hyperpolarized by 20 mV through the recording microelectrode, the full action potential following the second stimulus was blocked, and only an M-spike could be observed. Note that following the first stimulus, a failure of the M-spike shows a short-latency depolarization, which could also be observed as a

slight indentation at the peak of the M-spike (downgoing arrows). (C) Latency distribution of short-latency depolarizations recorded from 23 mesencephalic neurons; their mean value was found to be 180 μsec. Parts D, E, and F are from three different neurons. (D) A subthreshold stimulus evoked an all-or-none depolarization, which in one case (arrow) initiated a full spike. (E) Double trigeminal nerve stimulation; the second stimulus was suprathreshold. When action potentials were initiated by the short-latency depolarization (first stimulus), the full spike was blocked by collision, but not the underlying short-latency potential (dot). (F₁, F₂) Collision experiments. A direct activation of the impaled neuron (first arrow) preceded the nerve stimulus. (F₁) The directly evoked spike produced a block of the somatopetal invasions but did not block the depolarization. The second sweep was taken without the first stimulus to show the latency of the depolarization with respect to that of the full spike. (F₂) Blockage of orthodromic invasion by the directly evoked spike. Note that the depolarization did not block or show refractoriness as the trigeminal stimuli were moved closer in time to the direct activation (arrows). In parts B₁, B₃, E, F₁, and F₂, the upper and lower traces were taken at high and low DC gain, respectively; B₂, B₄, and D are high-gain recordings. (Modified from Baker and Llinás, 1971.)

cerebellar white-matter stimulations (Llinás, Baker, and Sotelo, 1974; Figure 11A, B). These depolarizations were insensitive to membrane polarization (Figure 11C) and did not collide with either antidromic or direct stimulations at short intervals (Figure 11D). Most important was the finding that in a number of olivary neurons the graded depolarizations evoked by white-matter stimulations were followed by hyperpolarizations that could be inverted by Cl⁻ injections and appear to be IPSPs. These IPSPs

were graded, and their latency decreased as stimulus strength was increased (Figure 11E). Although there is at present no evidence of interneurons in the inferior olive itself, some of the reticular cells in the periphery of this nucleus may be candidates for evoking this recurrent inhibitory action. The functional meaning of this inhibition, which could modify the internal organization of the inferior olive coupling, will be discussed with respect to the strategic location of the gap junctions below.

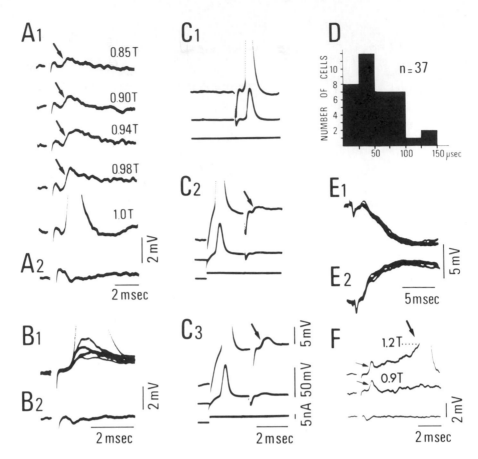

FIGURE 9 Electrotonic coupling between lateral vestibular neurons in the rat. (A, B) Evidence for electrotonic coupling obtained by antidromic stimulations (high-gain recordings). (A_1) Top to bottom are successive traces obtained with increasing spinal stimuli. As the stimulus strength was increased from 0.85 to 0.98 T, a graded depolarization increased to a peak amplitude of about 1.5 mV; a 1.0 T stimulus evoked an antidromic spike. (B_1) Recording from another neuron. Five successive sweeps have been superimposed; graded antidromic depolarizations up to 2.2 mV were evoked by stimuli of increasing strengths, the largest of which induced an antidromic spike. (A_2, B_2) Extracellular field potentials generated by near-threshold stimuli outside the cells recorded in A_1 and B_1, respectively. (C_1–C_3) Persistence of the graded antidromic depolarizations during collision experiments. In all three records a stimulus was applied to the spinal cord; it evoked an antidromic spike alone in C_1. (C_2, C_3) A depolarizing pulse was applied through the recording microelectrode prior to the spinal stimulus; it evoked a direct spike, which blocked the antidromic action potential and uncovered a graded antidromic depolarization (downgoing arrow); as the strength of the antidromic stimulation was progressively increased, the size of the graded antidromic depolarization increased in am-plitude up to 3.2 mV despite the block in the axon of the impaled cell. *Upper and middle traces*: Simultaneous recordings at high and low gain, respectively. *Lower traces*: Depolarizing current. (D) Histogram of the distribution of the graded antidromic depolarizations' delayed onset relative to the foot of the antidromic spike in 37 intracellularly recorded neurons. Mean time interval was found to be 55 μsec. (E_1, E_2, and F) Synaptic inputs to lateral vestibular neurons. (E_1) IPSPs produced by stimulation of the spinal cord. (E_2). Same potential as in E_1 but reversed after intracellular injection of Cl^- through the recording microelectrode (several superimposed sweeps in E_1 and E_2). (F) EPSPs evoked by spinal stimulations. *Upper trace*: The spinal cord was stimulated at a strength above threshold (1.2 T) for antidromic activation of the impaled neuron; failure of antidromic invasion uncovered a graded antidromic depolarization (thin arrow), which was followed by a short-latency EPSP (thicker arrow); this PSP reached the firing level (dotted horizontal line) and set up a spike. *Middle trace*: A 0.9 T stimulus induced a graded antidromic depolarization (arrow) and a small delayed EPSP. *Lower trace*: Extracellular field potential recorded outside the neuron. (Modified from Korn, Sotelo, and Crepel, 1973.)

The functional meaning of electrotonic coupling in mammals is still obscure. However, its occurrence in the olivary system strongly suggests that, as in other nuclei, it might generate synchronous neuronal fir-ing. For example, Llinás (1975) has proposed that in the inferior olive, coupling might be essential for synchrony of cerebellar nuclear neurons and their corresponding Purkinje cells; indeed, synchronous

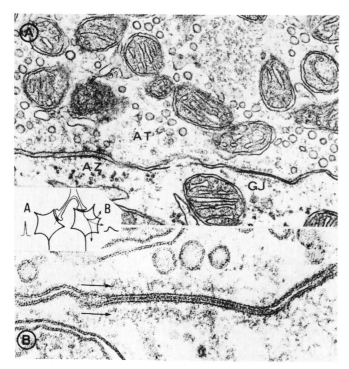

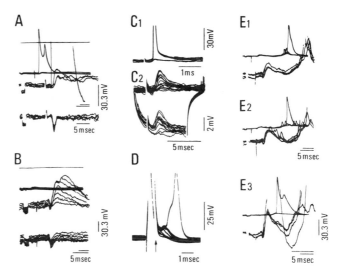

FIGURE 10   Gap junctions in the lateral vestibular nucleus of the rat. (A) Electron micrograph of a large-axon terminal (AT) synapsing on the perikaryon of a giant cell (× 50,000). Two types of junctional complexes are present at this synaptic interface. At the left there is an active zone (AZ), with its associated dense projections and synaptic vesicles; at the right the apposed plasma membranes converge to form a typical gap junction (GJ), which represents the morphological correlate of electrotonic transmission. The association of these two complexes constitutes a morphological "mixed synapse." (B) High magnification of the gap junction (× 122,000). There is a seven-layered structure, and dense bands (arrow) undercoat the junction on each side. *Insert*: Diagram indicating the direction of current flow between LVN neurons that are electrotonically coupled by way of presynaptic fibers. A prefiber, which branches and synapses through gap junctions (dark areas), is shown with two postsynaptic cells, A and B. The action currents set up by a spike in A flow through the terminals of this axon to B, where a depolarizing potential is generated. (Modified from Korn, Sotelo, and Crepel, 1973.)

FIGURE 11   Electrotonic coupling between neurons in the inferior olive of the cat. (A, B) Demonstration of electrotonic coupling. (A) Intracellular recording from an inferior-olive neuron. White-matter stimulations at intensities straddling threshold level evoked short-latency, graded antidromic depolarizations when the stimulus intensity was subthreshold for antidromic invasion of the cell. (B) Graded antidromic depolarizations evoked in another cell by stimulations applied in the cerebellar white matter. In both A and B, the upper trace indicates the extracellular reference potential, and the upper and lower middle traces are high- and low-gain recordings, respectively; the lower trace is the corresponding extracellular potential evoked just outside each cell. (C_1, C_2) Lack of effect of membrane hyperpolarization on the graded antidromic potential. (C_1) Control antidromic identification of an inferior-olive neuron (low-gain recording). (C_2) Graded antidromic depolarization (upper traces) evoked in the same cell were not significantly changed in amplitude and time course when this cell was hyperpolarized through the recording microelectrode (lower traces). (D) Collision experiment. Graded antidromic stimulations were delivered (arrow) following direct activation of an impaled cell. The direct spike blocked the antidromic action potentials (not illustrated here) but did not block the graded antidromic depolarizations, the largest of which reached the firing level and set up a full spike. (E_1–E_3) Demonstration of short-latency, graded antidromic depolarization and IPSPs in the same inferior-olive cells. *Upper trace*: High-gain AC recording. *Lower trace*: Low-gain DC recording. (E_1) An antidromic (cerebellar white matter) stimulation evoked an antidromic depolarizing potential, which was followed by a large depolarization (reversed IPSP). (E_2, E_3) As the intensity of the stimulus was increased, both potentials increased in amplitude and with strong stimuli. (E_3) Action potentials were occasionally evoked by the short-latency, antidromic depolarizations. (Several traces are superimposed in the records of this figure; modified from Llinás, Baker, and Sotelo, 1974.)

activations have been observed by Bell and Grimm (1969) at the level of cerebellar Purkinje cells in the cat. It has also been postulated (Llinás, Baker, and Sotelo, 1974) that when near-simultaneous activation of inferior-olive cells is generated through electrotonic coupling during rhythmic activity induced by harmiline, the inferior olive nucleus behaves as a 10 Hz oscillator (Llinás and Volkind, 1973).

POSSIBILITY OF A DUAL MODE OF SYNAPTIC TRANSMISSION   In the vertebrate CNS, axosomatic and axodendritic synapses with gap junctions also exhibit some of the morphological features of chemical synapses such as presynaptic vesicles and postsynaptic densities (Pappas and Bennett, 1966, Bennett et al.,

1967a; Pfenninger and Rovainen, 1974; Cantino and Mugnaini, 1975; Sotelo, 1975; Bennett, Sandri, and Akert, 1978). In fact, from fish to rodents, all synapses between primary vestibular fibers and postsynaptic neurons studied with the electron microscope (Robertson, Bodenheimer, and Stage, 1963; Hinojosa, 1973; Nakajima, 1974; see also Sotelo and Palay, 1970; Korn, Sotelo, and Bennett, 1977) exhibit both the active zones characteristic of chemical synapses and gap junctions, although an increasing proportion of the surface is occupied by the active zones as we go from fish to rats (Sotelo, 1977). Thus these synapses can be considered as morphologically "mixed" (Sotelo and Palay, 1970). These and other findings have raised the possibility of dual electrical and chemical mediation of synaptic transmission.

The physiological evidence for mixed synapses has not always been conclusive. In the electromotor systems and the toadfish sonic-muscle system, transmission at morphologically mixed synapses was described as purely electrical (Pappas and Bennett, 1966; Bennett et al., 1967). In other systems, it is not clear that dual mediation involves the same terminals. For example, following ipsilateral vestibular nerve stimulations, complex EPSPs can be recorded in the goldfish Mauthner cell (Figure 12A). Their first component appears to be electrically mediated (Furshpan, 1964), but the latency and properties of the second one are similar to those of chemically mediated synaptic PSPs (Labeyrie and Korn, 1975; see also the review by Diamond, 1971), since the second peak of the vestibular-evoked EPSP disappeared during high-rate repetitive stimulations (A_1) or when the extracellular Mg^{++} concentration was increased (A_2–A_3).

In the vestibular nuclei of the toadfish the situation was also found to be quite complicated (Korn, Sotelo, and Bennett, 1977). The vestibular-evoked EPSP exhibited two distinct components (Figure 12B). The first of these was shown to be transmitted electrically. The second, indicated by arrowheads on part B_1, generally appeared at vestibular-nerve stimulations of higher intensities than were required to evoke the first peak; this potential had a longer latency (about 1.6 msec in A_1 and A_2), a rather slow time to peak, and a prolonged decay time. Further evidence that it is due to chemical transmission comes from the fact that this peak was preceded by a small positivity (arrows in B_1 and B_2), presumably representing intracellular pickup of the presynaptic volley. The interval between the summit of this presynaptic component and the onset of the resulting PSP was compatible with a monosynaptic chemical delay from slow fibers. Moreover, this second component was reduced in

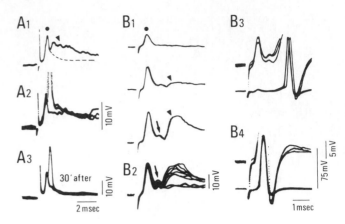

FIGURE 12 Composite EPSPs evoked by stimulation of the ipsilateral vestibular nerve. (A_1–A_3) Effects of extracellular high-magnesium content on the composite EPSP recorded from the lateral dendrite of the goldfish Mauthner cell. (A_1) Control diphasic PSP induced by a stimulus that was below threshold to fire the cell; the early electrotonic component and a subsequent prolonged peak (presumably chemical) are indicated by a black dot and an arrowhead, respectively. The falling phase of the electrotonic component elicited singly during repetitive stimulation at 50 Hz is reproduced by a dashed line. (A_2) As the stimulus strength was increased, the early electrotonic peak of the PSP reached the firing level of the neuron, and a spike was generated. (A_3) 30 min after intraventricular injection of Mg^{++} ions, the second component of the vestibular-evoked EPSP disappeared, while the first one remained unaffected and could still generate a spike. Note that the gain was reduced by half in A_3. (B_1–B_4) Intracellular recordings obtained from an LVN neuron in the toadfish Opsanus tau as the strength of the stimulus applied to the nerve was progressively increased. (B_1) Subthreshold EPSPs. The stimulus first evoked a short-latency EPSP alone (black circle), followed, with stronger stimulation, by a second, longer-lasting depolarization (arrowheads). The second PSP was preceded by a small response, less than 1 mV in amplitude (arrow in the bottom trace), which may be the corresponding postsynaptic volley recorded internally. (B_2) As the frequency of the stimulation at the strongest value used in B_1 was increased to 50 Hz, the late PSP decreased in amplitude and finally disappeared, while the first PSP and the presumed presynaptic volley (arrow) remained unchanged. (B_3, B_4) With stronger stimulus intensities, spikes were generated by the second PSP (B_3) and finally by the first one (B_4) (upper and lower traces at high and low gain, respectively). (Modified from Korn, Sotelo, and Bennett, 1977.)

amplitude and finally abolished when the repetition of the stimulation was increased to 50 per second (B_2); in contrast, the presumed presynaptic component of the intracellularly recorded potential remained unchanged. That the electrical component can be evoked alone by weak stimulations (B_1, upper trace) indicates that the afferent fibers transmit electrically with essentially no chemical component. Higher-threshold fibers may conceivably exhibit both electrical and chemical transmission, but present data cannot distinguish between this possibility and that of two separate populations of fibers each transmitting exclusively in one mode. In the lateral dendrite of the Mauthner cell in goldfish, weak eighth-nerve stimulation can also produce a short-latency, and therefore electrical, EPSP with no significant later, and therefore chemical, component; in some cases, however, no separation of the two components can be obtained.

At other synapses, both chemical and electrical modes of transmission clearly occur at the same ending, as in the chick ciliary ganglion (Martin and Pilar, 1963) and in the leech (Nicholls and Purves, 1970); but in this latter example, the morphological basis is nuclear. In spinal motoneurons of the teleost *Sternachus*, gap junctions and vesicle attachment sites defined by freeze etching can be present at the same terminal (Bennett, Sandri, and Akert, 1978).

The most convincing evidence for dual transmission has been obtained at an identified synapse of the spinal cord of the sea lamprey (Rovainen, 1974; Ringham, 1975; Martin and Ringham, 1975). Figure 13A illustrates the pre- and postsynaptic elements of this synapse between a Müller axon and a lateral interneuron. Two microelectrodes, one for passing current and the other for voltage recordings, were placed in the presynaptic axon, and another electrode for recording the potentials produced by coupling and by transmitter release was placed in the postsynaptic cell. EPSPs were produced in the lateral cells by intracellular stimulation of the Müller axon (Figure 13B, upper trace); they were composite, with a small first component, which remained constant in latency and amplitude during repetitive stimulation, and a larger second component (1–10 mV), which had an additional delay of about 2 msec and fluctuated or decreased in amplitude during repetitive stimulation. Both of them always followed presynaptic action potentials one-to-one at constant latencies up to frequencies of at least 50 per second in normal bathing fluid. With closely spaced electrodes, the latency of the first component was less than 1 msec, and electrical coupling could be demonstrated between cell and axon (Figure 13C); thus the first component was electrical. In bathing fluid containing 4 mM Mg, the second component declined and disappeared (Figure 13B, lower trace), indicating that it was induced by chemical transmission. Interneurons intercalated between the Müller axon and the lateral cell might still have mediated this second peak; however, after poisoning the spinal cord with tetrodotoxin, short depolarizing current pulses in the Müller axon near the lateral cell still elicited the second component of the EPSP (D_1–D_3). Furthermore, the plot of EPSP amplitude against axonal depolarization was the same for the decreasing action potential after tetrodotoxin was added as it was for the artificial depolarization with current (D_4). Thus the release of transmitter can be accounted for by the depolarization of the presynaptic axon. Depolarizing the axon with prolonged pulses (50 msec) resulted in an increase of the postsynaptic response because of a summation of the electrical coupling potential with the chemical EPSP. Electrotonic coupling could be seen with depolarizing (E_1) and hyperpolarizing pulses; when the presynaptic depolarization was increased, EPSPs appeared on top of the coupling potentials (E_2–E_3). The synaptic transfer curve for this experiment is shown in E_4. The postsynaptic responses in the hyperpolarizing region and the responses in the early part of the depolarizing region were due to electrical coupling. At about 35–40 mV depolarization, the EPSP appeared; it reached its maximum amplitude at about 80 mV peak depolarization. Above this level, the response continued to increase at a rate consistent with that expected for the electrical coupling potential alone (dashed line). When the coupling potential amplitudes are plotted against steady-state depolarization (crosses on the graph in Figure 13E_4), it can also be seen that this electrical synapse is highly rectifying.

Thus several lines of evidence indicate that the composite EPSP produced by Müller axons in lateral cells is monosynaptic for both electrical and chemical components. It is likely that a similar dual transmission is operant at many if not most of the identified morphologically mixed synapses.

SYNAPTIC CONTROL OF ELECTROTONIC COUPLING Some experimental ways by which reversible changes in coupling resistance can be obtained have been reported (Asada and Bennett, 1971; Rose and Loewenstein, 1971; Socolar and Politoff, 1971), but an original and more natural mechanism by which cells are uncoupled has been observed by Spira and Bennett (1972). Although it was first described in an invertebrate, it is worth considering in detail, for it is obviously of general significance for most systems in which neurons are coupled.

Two neurons, the G- and M-cells of the buccal ganglion of the mollusc *Navanax* are electrotonically coupled (Levitan, Tauc, and Segundo, 1970) and can be simultaneously impaled. Spira and Bennett (1972) observed a decrease in the degree of coupling either spontaneously or following brief trains of stimuli applied to the pharyngeal nerve; this phenomenon,

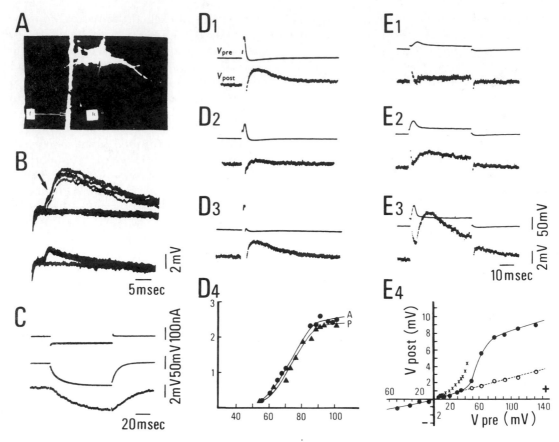

FIGURE 13 Evidence for dual electrical and chemical transmissions at a single synapse in the lamprey spinal cord. (A) Photomicrograph of a presynaptic Müller fiber (f) and an adjacent postsynaptic lateral cell (lc), which have been injected with Procion Yellow. During the experiments, simultaneous intracellular recordings were obtained from similar cells. (Modified from Ringham, 1975.) (B) Composite EPSP in a lateral cell evoked from a bulbar axon. *Upper trace*: A single spike (not illustrated) directly evoked through the recording presynaptic axon induced an all-or-none composite postsynaptic EPSP with a small first peak followed by a larger second component (arrow). *Lower trace*: Effects of Ca^{++}-free fluid. After switching to 0 Ca^{++}, 4 mM Mg fluid, the second component disappeared, while the first remained unaffected in amplitude. (From Rovainen, 1974.) (C) Evidence for electrotonic transmission. A prolonged hyperpolarizing current pulse (upper trace) injected in the presynaptic fiber (middle trace) also produced a hyperpolarizing potential (lower trace) in the postsynaptic cell. (From Ringham, 1975.) (D_1–D_4) Evidence for chemical transmission. Intracellular recordings from the presynaptic axon (upper traces) and from the postsynaptic cell (lower traces). (D_1) A synaptic potential was produced in the neuron by a directly evoked spike in the presynaptic fiber. (D_2, D_3) Recordings obtained after addition of 0.2 μg/ml tetrodotoxin in the bathing solution. (D_2) As the presynaptic spike was reduced in amplitude, the EPSP was also reduced. (D_3) An artifical depolarizing pulse 2 msec in duration injected in the presynaptic fiber after the tetrodotoxin block produced a postsynaptic EPSP similar to those pro-

duced in D_1 by the action potential. (D_4) Synaptic transfer curves from the experiment illustrated in D_1–D_3. *Abcissa*: Amplitude of presynaptic depolarization. *Ordinate*: EPSP amplitude. Curve A was obtained with progressively reduced action potentials during development of the tetrodotoxin block, curve P with depolarizing pulses after a completed block. (E_1–E_3) Responses to prolonged presynaptic depolarizing pulses in textrodotoxin experiment, showing electrotonic coupling between presynaptic axon and postsynaptic cell (E_1) and EPSPs evoked by a stronger depolarizing current (E_2). As the intensity of the presynaptic current was increased, large EPSPs were superimposed on coupling potentials (E_3). *Upper traces*: Low-gain recording in presynaptic fiber (note delayed rectification). *Lower traces*: High-gain recording in postsynaptic cell. (E_4) Synaptic transfer curve for the experiment illustrated in E_1–E_3, with 50 msec presynaptic hyperpolarizing and depolarizing pulses. For points indicated by open circles and black circles the abcissa represents the peak of the presynaptic depolarization. Black circles represent the total amplitude of the postsynaptic response, open circles the contribution of the electrotonic coupling potential. The difference between the two curves indicates the amplitude of the chemical EPSP. The curve with crosses shows the coupling-potential amplitude replotted with the abcissa representing now steady-state presynaptic depolarizations; these points and those in the hyperpolarizing quadrant represent the synaptic transfer curve for the electrotonic coupling potential. (Modified from Martin and Ringham, 1975.)

which is associated with increased synaptic activity, can be attributed to a decrease in input resistance of the coupled cells caused by activation of chemical afferent synapses (Figure 14). Electrotonic coupling is obvious in A_1, B_1, C_1, and D_1; the records show that the coupling coefficient for spread of maintained hyperpolarizations and small depolarizations was greater from the G-cell to the M-cell than in the opposite direction. When long-lasting excitatory pulses were applied (as in C_1 and D_1), the spread of maintained depolarizations was underlying that of the spikes. Strong depolarization of the G-cell could generally excite the M-cell (C_1). If both cells were depolarized to the point of spiking, there was a considerable synchronization of their impulse activity, and synchronized spontaneous activity was occasion-

ally observed. When a short train of impulses was applied to the ipsilateral pharyngeal nerve, the spread of potential between cells was strongly reduced (A_1', B_1', C_1', and D_1'). The coupling coefficients for maintained depolarization and hyperpolarization decreased drastically. During decoupling, a strong depolarization of the G-cell failed to excite the M-cell (C_1'). Decoupling was associated with a decrease in the input resistance of both cells, which fell to about half their resting values (A_1' and B_1').

Spira and Bennett (1972) demonstrated that this decrease was due to persistent synaptic bombardment mediated by afferent inhibitory fibers; decoupling lasting at least 5 sec was not uncommon. The functional implications of such a variable coupling are great: motor neurons are thus able to fire synchron-

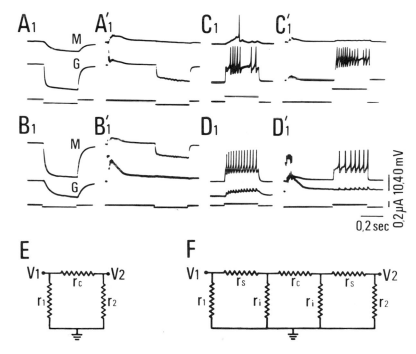

FIGURE 14 Synaptic control of electrotonic coupling. (A) Coupling and decoupling of G- and M-cells in *Navanax*. *Upper traces*: Recording from M-cell. *Middle traces*: Recording from G-cell (note the higher gain in B_1, B_1', D_1, and D_1'). *Lower traces*: Polarizing current applied in the G-cell for the upper records, and in the M-cell for the lower records. A train of stimuli that decoupled cells was applied to the large ipsilateral pharyngeal nerve at the beginning of each of the sweeps labeled by a primed letter. (A_1–D_1) Evidence for electrotonic coupling between the G- and M-cells. (A_1, B_1) Spread of hyperpolarization. (C_1, D_1) Spread of depolarization: spikes in the polarized neuron produced small, slowed depolarizing potentials in the unpolarized cell, which were superimposed on a slow depolarization (the irregularity of firing in C_1 was due to activation of an inhibitory interneuron). (A_1', B_1') Electrotonic spread of hyperpolarization was eliminated by decoupling stimuli, and

the input resistance was reduced by about half. (C_1', D_1') Spread of depolarization was also reduced by decoupling stimuli; reduction in spread of maintained depolarization was greater than that of spikes. Note that stimulation in the G-cell (C_1') could no longer excite the M-cell, although the M-cell could still be excited by stimuli applied to its own soma (D_1'). (From Spira and Bennett, 1972.) (E) Simplest equivalent circuit of two electrotonically coupled cells. Each of them and the coupling pathway are represented by a single resistor, r_1, r_2, and r_c, respectively. (Modified from Bennett, 1966.) (F) Equivalent circuit for synaptic decoupling. r_1 and r_2: cell resistances; r_s: series resistances of collaterals that are presumed to mediate coupling of the cells; r_c: junctional resistance; r_i: resistance of inhibitory synapses localized at the site of coupling. (From Bennett, 1974.)

ously during the rapid movement required for prey capture and asynchronously during the slow movement of peristalsis. To confirm this Spira and Bennett also showed that uncoupling can be evoked by physiological stimuli such as inflation of the pharynx.

Initially Spira and Bennett postulated that the decoupling was ascribable to a decrease in the nonjunctional resistance, as indicated by the simple equivalent circuit of Figure 14E; in this diagram the two coupled cells are represented as single resistances r_1 and r_2, and the junctional resistance as r_c. The coupling coefficient, when current is applied in cell 1, is given by

$$\frac{V_1}{V_2} = \frac{r_2}{r_c + r_2},$$

where V_1 and V_2 are the resulting potentials in the two cells. Thus, if only the input resistance of cell 2 decreases, the coefficient in the direction from cell 1 to cell 2 also decreases. However, the decrease in input resistance was found insufficient to explain the change observed in these experiments. Thus Bennett (1974) postulated that inhibitory synapses are distributed along the coupling pathway according to the model shown in Figure 14F; this situation could lead to a reduction of electrotonic coupling with less change in input resistance than required by the first model: if r_1 goes to zero, the coupling pathway between cells is shunted, and the cells will be decoupled.

On the other hand, a synaptically induced decrease in membrane conductance can lead to an increased electrotonic coupling, as observed in the abdominal ganglion of *Aplysia* by Carew and Kandel (1976). The motor neurons labeled L14A, B, and C, which mediate the *Aplysia* inking response provoked by brief noxious stimuli, were simultaneously impaled with microelectrodes (Figure 15A₁). When a single current pulse was applied to one, the responses of all three cells indicated that they were coupled electrotonically (Figure 15A₂). A single brief electrical stimulus to the connectives (i.e., to nerve traces that carry input from the head ganglia) produces in all three cells a complex EPSP with a fast initial peak followed by a slower component (indicated respectively by a dot and an arrow in Figure 15B). Several lines of evidence demonstrate that the fast EPSP results from an increase in ionic conductance and that the slow component results from a conductance decrease. For example, membrane depolarization reduced the amplitude of the fast EPSP and increased the amplitude of the slow one, whereas hyperpolarization had opposite effects. Carew and Kandel further investigated the modulating effect of these two types of PSPs on electrotonic transmission by injecting hyperpolarizing

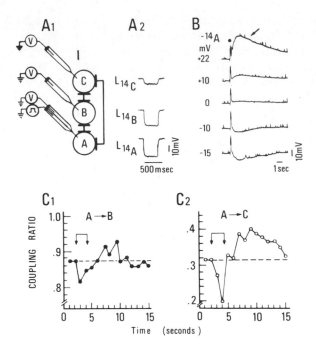

FIGURE 15 Evidence that increased-conductance EPSPs reduce electrotonic coupling, whereas decreased-conductance EPSPs increase electrotonic coupling between motor neurons in *Aplysia californica*. (A₁, A₂) Demonstration that cells are coupled. (A₁) The experimental setup. Simultaneous recordings were made from three cells labeled L14A, B, and C. (A₂) Membrane potential changes were recorded in all three cells when a hyperpolarizing current pulse was injected in cell L14A. (B) Effects of membrane potentials on fast and slow EPSPs. Stimulation of the connectives by a single (1.5 msec) electrical pulse produced a composite EPSP, with a fast and a slow phase (indicated in the upper trace by a dot and an arrow, respectively); numbers at the left indicate displacement of the membrane potential from resting level (0 mV). Note that depolarization reduced the amplitude of the fast EPSP and increased the slow EPSP; hyperpolarization increased the fast EPSP and reduced and inverted the slow one. This result is consistent with the interpretation that the fast EPSP results from an increase in ionic conductance and the slow EPSP results from a decrease in ionic conductance. (C₁, C₂) Evolution of coupling during fast and slow EPSPs. Coupling was monitored with hyperpolarizing pulses, 400 msec in duration. Repetitive connective stimulation (six per second for two seconds, indicated by arrows) produced a complex fast EPSP during the train and a slow EPSP following the train. (C₁) Coupling between L14A and B. (C₂) Coupling between L14A and C. The decrease in coupling during the fast EPSP and the increase during the slow EPSP were proportionately greater for the weakly coupled pair, L14A and C. (Modified from Carew and Kandel, 1976.)

constant-current pulses into one motor cell, while simultaneously recording from the others. The coupling ratio between the cells decreased during the fast EPSP, showing that cells were uncoupled by the excitatory increased conductance (Figure 15C₁, C₂).

During the slow EPSP, however, the coupling ratio between cells increased; presumably the junctional resistance did not change, and coupling was enhanced because the slow EPSP increased the input resistance of the postsynaptic cells. Inking evoked by a noxious stimulus is predominantly triggered by the fast EPSP; however, since the slow EPSP provides a second means of activating the inking system when the fast one fails to do so, an increase in coupling between cells might ensure that this reflex will occur.

Although synaptic uncoupling has not yet been demonstrated in the vertebrate CNS, it is probably operative there. In this respect, the morphology of the inferior olivary complex in cat reproduces all the strategic locations of synapses suggested by Bennett (1974; see Figure 14F). As shown by Sotelo, Llinás, and Baker (1974), coupling in this structure appears to be restricted to the rather specialized inferior-olive glomerulus. A correlation of Golgi and electron-microscopic studies has revealed that the central core of each glomerulus is composed of intermingled dendritic processes arising from different inferior-olive neurons. Gap junctions occur mainly between the dendritic profiles that form the central region of the glomeruli. Importantly, the peripheral zone of each glomerulus is covered by numerous axon terminals, which are in synaptic contact with the central dendritic profiles. These structural features, illustrated in Figure 16A, give morphological support for the occurrence of coupling between inferior cells (see the first diagram in Figure 16B). In addition, the location of electrotonic coupling may allow a "functional amputation" (Llinás, Baker, and Sotelo, 1974; Llinás, 1975) of the electrotonic interactions by the shunting effects of the surrounding chemical synapses on the core glomerular elements. This postulate is summarized by the second model in Figure 16B. Thus inhibitory inputs (e.g., those mediating the IPSPs of Figure 11E$_1$–E$_3$) could serve as a switching system to regulate the degree of coupling between cells; it has been suggested that such an inhibitory control of coupling occurs in a number of other vertebrate nuclei where dendrodendritic electrotonic synapses have been found recently (see Bennett, 1974). Finally, we would like to suggest that, although conclusive data are still missing, variable coupling might also be possible at functionally mixed synapses during repetitive firing of the presynaptic fibers.

Summary and conclusions

Electrical interactions between neurons are now well established as a legitimate mode of neuronal com-

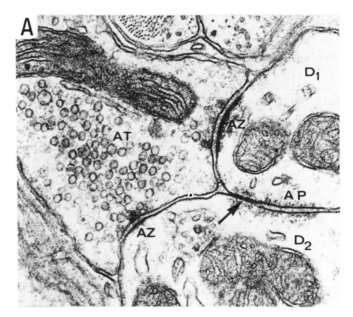

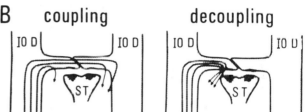

FIGURE 16 (A) Electron micrograph of an inferior-olive glomerulus of the cat ($\times$ 55,000). A peripheral axon (AT) establishes a chemical synapse or active zone (AZ) on each of two adjacent dendritic profiles (D$_1$, D$_2$). The membrane interface between the two apposing dendritic processes bears a gap junction (arrow) and an attachment plaque (AP). (Courtesy of C. Sotelo, unpublished figure.) (B) Hypothetical model for decoupling of cells belonging to an inferior-olive glomerulus. *Left:* Inferior-olive dendrites (IOD) are coupled through a gap junction. *Right:* When the presynaptic terminal (ST) is active and releases transmitter, the membrane resistance of the postsynaptic dendrites drops because of the increase in synaptic conductance. Current flows through the shunted membrane rather than through the gap junctions, and cells are thereby decoupled. (From Llinás, 1975.)

munication and information processing. Clear-cut mechanisms have been ascribed to the generation of both field effects and electrotonic coupling, and these fast forms of synaptic transmission appear to play significant functional roles in mediating escape reactions and in neuronal synchronization. It is hoped that future experimentation will not be restricted to assessing the relative importance of electrical and chemical transmission in the vertebrate CNS, but will deal instead with the potential power and flexibility of neuronal networks that combine the two. In this paper we have reviewed some of the recent advances that highlight this potential. Both field effects and electrotonic coupling, for example, can be but the first component of a mixed synaptic action combining the speed of electrical transmission with the more prolonged character of chemically mediated synaptic transmission. In the case of field-effect inhibitions, this concerted action can be extremely effective in preventing repetitive firing of a postsynaptic neuron, as has been described for the Mauthner-cell system; and with electrical excitation it can increase the relative synchrony and speed of neuronal postsynaptic responses. Furthermore, the interaction of electrical and chemical mechanisms provides a basis for modulating synaptic effectiveness: the former can be either enhanced or depressed by the latter, depending on the nature of the ionic conductance change involved. Consequently, the degree of coupling and synchrony between neurons depends not only on the properties of the junctional resistance and the pre- and postsynaptic neurons, but also on activity in other input neurons. Although synaptic control of coupling and decoupling has been best described in two invertebrate systems, the morphological substrate for a similar control does exist in the vertebrate CNS, and we expect that it will be demonstrated there as well.

REFERENCES

ASADA, Y., and M. V. L. BENNETT, 1971. Experimental alterations of coupling resistance at an electrotonic synapse. *J. Cell Biol.* 49:159-172.

AUERBACH, A. A., and M. V. L. BENNETT, 1969. A rectifying electrotonic synapse in the central nervous system of a vertebrate. *J. Gen. Physiol.* 53:211-237.

BAKER, R., and R. LLINÁS, 1971. Electrotonic coupling between neurons in the rat mesencephalic nucleus. *J. Physiol.* 212:45-63.

BELL, C. C., and R. J. GRIMM, 1969. Discharge properties of cerebellar Purkinje cells recorded with single and double microelectrodes. *J. Neurophysiol.* 32:1044-1055.

BENNETT, M. V. L., 1966. Physiology of electrotonic junctions. *Ann. NY Acad. Sci.* 137:509-539.

BENNETT, M. V. L., 1972. A comparison of electrically and chemically mediated transmission. In *Structure and Function of Synapses*, G. D. Pappas and D. P. Purpura, eds. New York: Raven Press, pp. 221-256.

BENNETT, M. V. L., 1973a. Function of electrotonic junctions in embryonic and adult tissues. *Fed. Proc. Am. Soc. Exp. Biol.* 32:65-75.

BENNETT, M. V. L., 1973b. Permeability and structure of electrotonic junctions and intercellular movements of tracers. In *Intracellular Staining in Neurobiology*, S. B. Katel and C. Nicholson, eds. Berlin: Springer-Verlag, pp. 115-134.

BENNETT, M. V. L., 1974. Flexibility and rigidity in electrotonically coupled systems. In *Synaptic Transmission and Neuronal Interactions*, M. V. L. Bennett, ed. New York: Raven Press, pp. 153-177.

BENNETT, M. V. L., E. ALJURE, Y. NAKAJIMA, and G. D. PAPPAS, 1963. Electrotonic junctions between teleost spinal neurons: Electrophysiology and ultrastructure. *Science* 141:262-264.

BENNETT, M. V. L., M. GIMENEZ, Y. NAKAJIMA, and G. D. PAPPAS, 1964. Spinal and medullary nuclei controlling electric organ in the eel, *Electrophorus. Biol. Bull. Marine Biol. Lab. Woods Hole* 127:362.

BENNETT, M. V. L., Y. NAKAJIMA, and G. D. PAPPAS, 1967. Physiology and ultrastructure of electrotonic junctions. III. Giant electromotor neurons of *Malapterurus electricus. J. Neurophysiol.* 30:180-208.

BENNETT, M. V. L., and G. D. PAPPAS, 1965. Neurophysiology and ultrastructure of a synchronously firing nucleus in toadfish *Opsanus. Fed. Proc.* 24:462.

BENNETT, M. V. L.,, G. D. PAPPAS, E. ALJURE, and Y. NAKAJIMA, 1967a. Physiology and ultrastructure of electrotonic junctions. II. Spinal and medullary electromotor nuclei in mormyrid fish. *J. Neurophysiol.* 30:180-208.

BENNETT, M. V. L., G. D. PAPPAS, M. GIMENEZ, and Y. NAKAJIMA, 1967b. Physiology and ultrastructure of electrotonic junctions. IV. Medullary electromotor nuclei in gymnotid fish. *J. Neurophysiol.* 30:236-300.

BENNETT, M. V. L., C. SANDRI, and K. AKERT, 1978. Neuronal gap junctions and morphologically mixed synapses in the spinal cord of the teleost *Sternachus Albifrons* (gymnotodei). *Brain Res.* 143:43-60.

BROOKS, C., and J. C. ECCLES, 1947. An electrical hypothesis of central inhibition. *Nature* 159:760-764.

CANTINO, D. and E. MUGNAINI, 1975. The structural basis for electrotonic coupling in the avian ciliary ganglion. A study with thin sectioning and freeze-fracturing. *J. Neurocytol.* 4:505-536.

CAREW, T. J. and E. KANDEL, 1976. Two functional effects of decreased conductance EPSPs: Synaptic augmentation and increased electrotonic coupling. *Science* 192:150-152.

DIAMOND, J., 1971. The Mauthner cell. In *Fish Physiology*, W. S. Hoar and D. J. Randall, eds. New York: Academic Press, vol. 5, pp. 265-346.

DOWLING, J. E., and B. B. BOYCOTT, 1966. Neural connections of the retina: Fine structure of the inner plexiform layer. *Cold Spring Harbor Symp. Quant. Biol.* 30:393-402.

ECCLES, J. C., 1946. An electrical hypothesis of synaptic and neuro-muscular transmission. *Ann. NY Acad. Sci.* 47:429-455.

ECCLES, J. D., 1964. *The Physiology of Synapses*. Berlin: Springer-Verlag.

FABER, D. S., and H. KORN, 1973. A neuronal inhibition mediated electrically. *Science* 179:577-578.

FARQUHAR, M. G., and G. E. PALADE, 1963. Junctional complexes in various epithelia. *J. Cell Biol.* 17:375-412.

FURSHPAN, E. J., 1964. Electrical transmission at an excitatory synapse in a vertebrate brain. *Science* 144:878-880.

FURSHPAN, E. J., and T. FURUKAWA, 1962. Intracellular and extracellular responses of the several regions of the Mauthner cell of the goldfish. *J. Neurophysiol.* 25:732-771.

FURSHPAN, E. F., and D. D. POTTER, 1968. Low resistance junctions between cells in embryos and tissue culture. *Curr. Top. Dev. Biol.* 3:95-127.

FURUKAWA, T., and E. J. FURSHPAN, 1963. Two inhibitory

mechanisms in the Mauthner neurons of goldfish. *J. Neurophysiol.* 24:140–176.

GOGAN, P., J. P. GUERITAUD, G. HORSCHOLLE-BOSSAVIT, and S. TYC-DUMONT, 1974. Electrotonic coupling between motoneurons in the abducens nucleus of the cat. *Exp. Brain Res.* 21:139–154.

HINOJOSA, R., 1973. Synaptic ultrastructure in the tangential nucleus of the goldfish (*Carassius auratus*). *Am. J. Anat.* 137:159–199.

HINOJOSA, R., and J. D. ROBERTSON, 1967. Ultrastructure of the spoon type synaptic endings in the nucleus vestibularis tangentialis of the chick. *J. Cell Biol.* 34:421–430.

HINRICHSEN, C. F., and L. M. LARRAMENDI, 1968. Synapses and cluster formation of the mouse mesencephalic fifth nucleus. *Brain Res.* 7:296–299.

HUBBARD, J. J., and R. F. SCHMIDT, 1963. An electrophysiological investigation of mammalian motor nerve terminals. *J. Physiol.* 166:145–167.

IMAMOTO, K., and N. SHIMIZU, 1970. Fine structure of the mesencephalic nucleus of the trigeminal nerve in the rat. *Arch. Histol. Jap.* 32:51–67.

KATZ, B., and R. MILEDI, 1965. The measurements of synaptic delay and the time course of acetylcholine release at the neuromuscular junction. *Proc. R. Soc. Lond.* B161:483–495.

KATZ, B., and R. MILEDI, 1967. A study of synaptic transmission in the absence of nerve impulses. *J. Physiol.* 192:407–436.

KING, J. S., G. F. MARTIN, and M. H. BOWMAN, 1975. The direct spinal area of the inferior olivary nucleus: An electron microscopic study. *Exp. Brain Res.* 22:13–24.

KORN, H., and M. V. L. BENNETT, 1971. Dendritic and somatic impulse initiation in fish oculomotor neurons during vestibular nystagmus. *Brain Res.* 27:169–175.

KORN, H., and M. V. L. BENNETT, 1972. Electrotonic coupling between teleost oculomotor neurons: Restriction to somatic regions and relation to function of somatic and dendritic sites of impulse initiation. *Brain Res.* 38:433–439.

KORN, H., and M. V. L. BENNETT, 1975. Vestibular nystagmus and teleost oculomotor neurons: Functions of electrotonic coupling and dendritic impulse initiation. *J. Neurophysiol.* 38:430–451.

KORN, H., F. CREPEL, and C. SOTELO, 1972. Couplage électrotonique entre les neurones géants du noyau vestibulaire chez le rat. *C. R. Acad. Sci. Paris D* 274:1365–1368.

KORN, H., and D. S. FABER, 1975a. An electrically mediated inhibition in goldfish medulla. *J. Neurophysiol.* 38:452–471.

KORN, H., and D. S. FABER, 1975b. Mechanisms and functions of electrically mediated inhibition in the vertebrate central nervous system. In *Sensory Physiology and Behavior*, R. Galun, P. Hillman, I. Parnas, and R. Werman, eds. New York: Plenum Press, pp. 289–305.

KORN, H., and D. S. FABER, 1976. Vertebrate central nervous system: Same neurons mediate both electrical and chemical inhibitions. *Science* 194:1166–1169.

KORN, H., C. SOTELO, and M. V. L. BENNETT, 1977. The lateral vestibular nucleus of the toadfish *Opsanus tau*: Ultrastructural and electrophysiological observations with special reference to electrotonic transmission. *Neuroscience* 2:851–884.

KORN, H., C. SOTELO, and F. CREPEL, 1973. Electrotonic coupling between neurons in the rat lateral vestibular nucleus. *Exp. Brain Res.* 16:255–275.

KORN, H., C. SOTELO, N. KOTCHABHAKDI, and M. V. L. BENNETT, 1974. Fish lateral vestibular neurons: Electrotonic transmission from primary vestibular afferents, electrotonic coupling between vestibulo spinal neurons and identification of efferent cells to the labyrinth. *Biol. Bull.* 147:486–487.

KORN, H., A. TRILLER, and D. S. FABER, 1978. Structural correlates of recurrent collateral interneurons producing both electrical and chemical inhibitions of the Mauthner cell. *Proc. R. Soc. Lond.* B202:533–538.

KRIEBEL, M. E., M. V. L. BENNETT, S. G. WAXMAN, and G. D. PAPPAS, 1969. Oculomotor neurons in fish: Electrotonic coupling and multiple sites of impulse initiation *Science* 166:520–524.

LABEYRIE, E., and H. KORN, 1975. Depolarisations paroxystiques induites par le cardiazol au niveau de la cellule de Mauthner: Effets comparés de cette substance et de l'EGTA sur les modes de transmission électrique et chimique de l'excitation afférente. *J. Physiol.* (Paris) 71:336–337A.

LANDIS, D. M., T. S. REESE, and E. RAVIOLA, 1974. Differences in membrane structure between excitatory and inhibitory components of the reciprocal synapse in the olfactory bulb. *J. Comp. Neurol.* 155:67–91.

LEVITAN, H., L. TAUC, and J. P. SEGUNDO, 1970. Electrical transmission among neurons in the buccal ganglion of a mollusc, *Navanax inermis*. *J. Gen. Physiol.* 55:484–496.

LLINÁS, R., 1975. Electrical synaptic transmission in the mammalian central nervous system. In *Golgi Centennial Symposium Proceedings*, M. Santini, ed. New York: Raven Press, pp. 379–386.

LLINÁS, R., R. BAKER, and C. SOTELO, 1974. Electrotonic coupling between neurons in cat inferior olive. *J. Neurophysiol.* 37:560–571.

LLINÁS, R., and R. A. VOLKIND, 1973. The olivo-cerebellar system: Functional properties as revealed by harmaline induced tremor. *Exp. Brain Res.* 18:69–87.

MAGHERINI, P. C., W. PRECHT, and P. C. SCHWINDT, 1976. Evidence for electrotonic coupling between frog motoneurons in the in situ spinal cord. *J. Neurophysiol.* 39:474–483.

MARTIN, A. R., and G. PILAR, 1963. Dual mode of synaptic transmission in the avian ciliary ganglion. *J. Physiol.* 168:443–463.

MARTIN, A. R., and G. L. RINGHAM, 1975. Synaptic transfer at a vertebrate central nervous system synapse. *J. Physiol.* 251:409–426.

MESZLER, R. M., G. D. PAPPAS, and M. V. L. BENNETT, 1972. Morphological demonstration of electrotonic coupling of neurons by way of presynaptic fibers. *Brain Res.* 36:412–415.

NAKAJIMA, Y., 1974. Fine structure of the synaptic endings on the Mauthner cell of the goldfish. *J. Comp. Neurol.* 156:379–402.

NELSON, P. G., 1966. Interaction between spinal motoneurons of the cat. *J. Neurophysiol.* 29:275–287.

NICHOLLS, J. G., and D. PURVES, 1970. Monosynaptic chemical and electrical connexions between sensory and motor cells in the central nervous system of the leech. *J. Physiol.* 209:647–667.

PAPPAS, G. D., Y. ASADA, and M. V. L. BENNETT, 1971. Morphological correlates of increased coupling resistance at an electrotonic synapse. *J. Cell Biol.* 49:173–188.

PAPPAS, G. D., and M. V. L. BENNETT, 1966. Specialized junctions involved in electrical transmission between neurons *Ann. NY Acad. Sci.* 137:495–508.

PAPPAS, G. D., S. G. WAXMAN, and M. V. L. BENNETT, 1975. Morphology of spinal electromotor neurons and presynaptic coupling in the gymnotid *Sternarchus albifrons. J. Neurocytol.* 4:469–478.

PAYTON, B. W., M. V. L. BENNETT, and G. D. PAPPAS, 1969. Permeability and structures of junctional membranes at an electrotonic synapse. *Science* 166:1641–1643.

PFENNINGER, K. H., and C. M. ROVAINEN, 1974. Stimulation- and calcium-dependence of vesicle attachment sites in the presynaptic membrane: A freeze-cleave study on the lamprey spinal cord. *Brain Res.* 72:1–23.

PINCHING, A. J., and T. P. POWELL, 1971. Ultrastructural features of transneuronal cell degeneration in the olfactory system. *J. Cell Sci.* 8:253–287.

PRECHT, W., A. RICHTER, S. OZAWA, and S. SCHIMAZU, 1974. Intracellular study of frog's vestibular neurons in relation to the labyrinth and spinal cord. *Exp. Brain Res.* 19:377–393.

RALL, W., and G. M. SHEPHERD, 1968. Theoretical reconstruction of field potentials and dendrodendritic synaptic interactions in olfactory bulb. *J. Neurophysiol.* 31:884–915.

RALL, W., R. E. BURKE, T. G. SMITH, P. G. NELSON, and K. FRANK, 1967. Dendritic location of synapses and possible mechanisms for the monosynaptic EPSP in motoneurons. *J. Neurophysiol.* 30:1169–1193.

REVEL, J. P., and M. J. KARNOVSKY, 1967. Hexagonal array of subunits in intracellular junctions of the mouse heart and liver. *J. Cell Biol.* 33:C7–C12.

RICHTER, A., W. PRECHT, and S. OZAWA, 1975. Responses of neurons of lizard's, *Lacerta viridis*, vestibular nuclei to electrical stimulation of the ipsi- and contralateral VIIIth nerves. *Pflügers Arch.* 355:85–94.

RINGHAM, G. L., 1975. Localization and electrical characteristics of a giant synapse in the spinal cord of the Lamprey. *J. Physiol.* 251:395–407.

ROBERTSON, J. D., 1963. The occurrence of a subunit pattern in the unit membrane of club endings in Mauthner cell synapses in goldfish brains. *J. Cell Biol.* 19:201–221.

ROBERTSON, J. D., T. S. BODENHEIMER, and D. E. STAGE, 1963. The ultrastructure of Mauthner cell synapses and nodes in goldfish brains. *J. Cell Biol.* 19:159–199.

ROSE, B., and W. R. LOEWENSTEIN, 1971. Junctional membrane permeability: Depression by substitution of Li for extracellular Na, and by lack of Ca and Mg; restoration by cell repolarization. *J. Membrane Biol.* 5:20–50.

ROVAINEN, C. M., 1974. Synaptic interactions of reticulospinal neurons and nerve cells in the spinal cord of the sea lamprey. *J. Comp. Neurol.* 154:207–224.

SIMPSON, I., B. ROSE, and W. R. LOEWENSTEIN, 1977. Size limit of molecules permeating the junctional membrane channels. *Science* 195:294–296.

SLOPER, J. J., 1972. Dendro-dendritic synapses in the primate motor cortex. *Brain Res.* 34:186–192.

SOCOLAR, S. J., and A. L. POLITOFF, 1971. Uncoupling cell junctions in a glandular epithelium by depolarizing current. *Science* 172:492–494.

SOTELO, C., 1975. Morphological correlates of electrotonic coupling between neurons in mammalian nervous system. In *Golgi Centennial Symposium Proceedings*, M. Santini, ed. New York: Raven Press, pp. 355–365.

SOTELO, C., 1977. Morphological basis for electrical communications between neurons in the central nervous system of vertebrates. In *Neuron Concept Today*, J. Szentágothai, H. Hamori, and E. Vizi, eds. Budapest: Akadémiai Kiadó, pp. 17–26.

SOTELO, C., and H. KORN, 1978. Morphological correlates of electrical and other interactions through low-resistance pathways between neurons of the vertebrate central nervous system. *Int. Rev. Cytol.* 55:67–107.

SOTELO, C., T. GENTSCHEV, and A. J. ZAMORA, 1976. Gap junctions in retinal cochlear nucleus of the rat: A possible new example of electrotonic junctions in the mammalian CNS. *Neuroscience* 1:5–7.

SOTELO, C., and R. LLINÁS, 1972. Specialized membrane junctions between neurons in the vertebrate cerebellar cortex. *J. Cell Biol.* 53:271–289.

SOTELO, C., R. LLINÁS, and R. BAKER, 1.74. Structural study of inferior olivary nucleus of the cat: Morphological correlates of electrotonic coupling. *J. Neurophysiol.* 37:541–559.

SOTELO, C., and S. L. PALAY, 1967. Synapses avec des contacts étroits (tight junctions) dans le noyau vestibulaire latéral du rat. *J. Microscopie* 6:86a.

SOTELO, C., and S. L. PALAY, 1970. The fine structure of the lateral vestibular nucleus in the rat. II. Synaptic organization. *Brain Res.* 18:93–115.

SOTELO, C., M. RETHELYI, and T. SZABO, 1975. Morphological correlates of electrotonic coupling in the magnocellular mesencephalic nucleus of the weakly electric fish *Gymnotus carapo. J. Neurocytol.* 4:587–607.

SPIRA, M. E., and M. V. L. BENNETT, 1972. Synaptic control of electrotonic coupling between neurons. *Brain Res.* 37:294–300.

STEFANELLI, A., and S. CARAVITA, 1970. Ultrastructural features of the synaptic complex of the vestibular nuclei of *Lampetra planeri* (Bloch). *Z. Zellforsch.* 108:282–296.

WATANABE, A., and H. GRUNDFEST, 1961. Impulse propagation at the septal and commisural junctions of crayfish lateral giant axon. *J. Gen. Physiol.* 45:267–308.

WERMAN, R., and P. L. CARLEN, 1976. Unusual behavior of the Ia EPSP in cat spinal motoneurons. *Brain Res.* 112:395–401.

WILSON, V. J., and R. M. WYLIE, 1970. A short latency labyrinthine input to the vestibular nuclei in the pigeon. *Science* 168:124–127.

WYLIE, R. M., 1973. Evidence of electrotonic transmission in the vestibular nuclei of the rat. *Brain Res.* 50:179–183.

20 Electrotonic Junctions

NORTON B. GILULA

ABSTRACT Electrotonic junctions have been identified as low-resistance pathways between cells in most of the animal phyla. These electrical-coupling pathways exist in excitable as well as nonexcitable tissues. They are capable of allowing an exchange of diffusable molecules, such as inorganic ions and low-molecular-weight metabolites, between cells. The permeability of these junctions may be regulated by intracellular changes in pH or in calcium concentrations. A structural pathway for this cell-to-cell communication appears to be located within the membrane specialization referred to as a gap junction or nexus. This structure is comprised of a polygonal lattice of 8–9 nm particles containing a 2 nm dot that is presumably the site of a hydrophilic channel for the electrotonic coupling property.

ELECTROTONIC JUNCTIONS have now been characterized in a wide variety of tissues, both excitable and nonexcitable. In fact, much of the contemporary information about these junctions has been generated from studies on nonnervous tissues. In excitable tissues, it has been recognized for almost twenty years that electrotonic junctions provide the basis for electrical or low-resistance synapses. These synapses permit the electrotonic spread of current from cell to cell, providing a mechanism for rapidly synchronizing certain neuronal and muscle-cell systems. Unfortunately, the role of electrotonic junctions in nonnervous tissues has been much more difficult to determine.

In this presentation I shall review the cell biology of electrotonic junctions, with particular emphasis on the structural, biochemical, and biological properties of these junctions in nonneuronal systems.

Structure and distribution of junctions

Electrotonic junctions were first described ultrastructurally in the late 1950s (for reviews, see McNutt and Weinstein, 1973; Gilula, 1974a; Staehelin, 1974). The first description of an electrotonic junction in the nervous system was made in 1963 by Robertson. These junctions were described between Mauthner fibers in the goldfish brain, and Robertson called

NORTON B. GILULA   The Rockefeller University, New York, NY 10021

them *synaptic discs*. Before then, Dewey and Barr (1962) had detected these junctions in smooth and cardiac muscle, and they used the term *nexus* to describe them. In 1967 Revel and Karnovsky used an extracellular tracing substance, lanthanum hydroxide, to define the thin-section characteristics of the electrotonic junction as it is resolved today. They described these junctions in mammalian myocardium and liver as septilaminar structures comprised of two closely apposed membranes of adjacent cells, with the two membranes separated by a 2–4 nm space or "gap" (Figure 1). This characteristic appearance led to use of the term *gap junction* to describe the electron-microscopic appearance of electrotonic junctions. Cur-

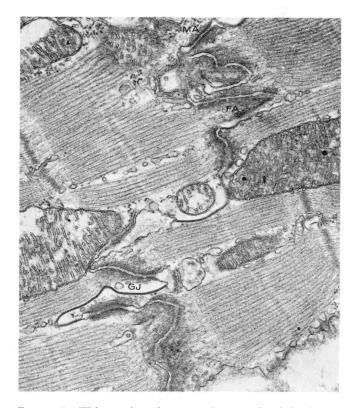

FIGURE 1 Thin-section electron micrograph of the intercalated disc components of the mouse myocardium. The intercalated disc contains a gap junction (GJ) for electrotonic coupling, a fascia adhaerens (FA) for insertion of the myofilaments, and a desmosome or macula adhaerens (MA) for cell-cell adhesion. (× 51,000.)

rently the terms *gap junction* and *nexus* are used synonymously to describe this structure. In *en face* views of the lanthanum-impregnated gap junction, the gap region contains a polygonal lattice of subunits 8–9 nm in diameter with a 9 nm center-to-center spacing. The central region of the subunits frequently contains a 1.5–2 nm electron-dense dot.

In freeze-fracture replicas at the site of gap junctional contact, the internal membrane fracture faces are characterized by a polygonal arrangement of intramembrane particles that are homogeneous in size (~ 8.5 nm in diameter) on the inner membrane half (fracture face P), and a complementary arrangement of pits or depressions on the outer membrane half (fracture face E) (Figure 2). Gap junctions in a variety of different organisms have now been examined, and it has been demonstrated that these structural features are common in organisms from almost all phyla, with the exception of arthropods. In arthropod organisms, the intramembrane particles are heterogeneous in size and they are located on the outer membrane half (fracture face E).

Gap junctions are widely distributed in animal organisms as plaquelike contacts between cells. The plaques can exist in a variety of pleiomorphic forms,

and the particle packing within a plaque can also vary considerably (Larsen, 1977). Contemporary cytological technology permits an unambiguous identification of gap junctions that exist as sites of close contact between cells, where the intervening extracellular space can be penetrated by lanthanum (or some other similar material), and where two or more intramembrane particles (homogeneous in size) are aggregated at the specific site of contact (Raviola and Gilula, 1973). It is currently impossible to identify a gap-junctional particle existing as a single, isolated element in a freeze-fracture face. In mammalian organisms, gap junctions have been detected between cells from all four basic tissues, and they are ubiquitous cell-membrane elements in most culture systems as well. Thus far, gap-junctional structures have not been identified between lymphoid cells, erythroid cells, mature skeletal-muscle fibers (mammalian), and many neurons in both the central and peripheral nervous system. In addition, gap junctions are formed between homologous cells, as well as between heterologous cells in vivo and in culture (Hyde et al., 1969; Johnson, Herman, and Preus, 1973; Epstein and Gilula, 1977).

Experimental manipulation of junctions

Gap junctions are adhesive elements that are strikingly insensitive to a variety of perturbing treatments. The structure is not detectably altered by treatment with proteases, divalent-cation chelators, a variety of nonionic and anionic detergents, urea, and other substances. However, the junctional gap can be affected by treatment with phospholipase C or extraction with acetone (Goodenough and Revel, 1971).

In most systems, the junctions can be considered as static elements that have a slow turnover rate, and their incidence can, at least in one system, be influenced (increased) by hormonal stimulation (Merk, Botticelli, and Albright, 1972).

During cell dissociation procedures that employ treatments with proteases, divalent-cation chelators, physical pipetting, and similar techniques, the junctions are retained as intact complexes that remain on the surface of the dissociated cells (Muir, 1967; Berry and Friend, 1969; Amsterdam and Jamieson, 1974). For example, when two cells joined by a single gap junction are dissociated by means of these procedures, one cell will retain the entire junctional complex, while the other will have no junctional element (Gilula, 1977). In actuality, a lesion or tear is present in one cell as a result of the removal of the entire

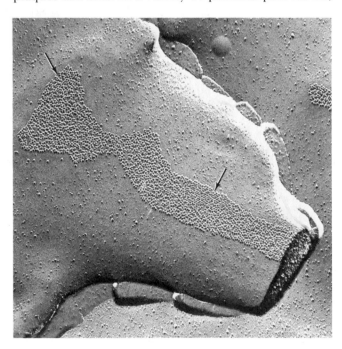

FIGURE 2 Freeze-fracture electron micrograph of a gap-junctional membrane (fracture face P) between rat ovarian granulosa cells. The gap junction is comprised of a lattice of homogeneous intramembrane particles that can vary in packing; for example, both loose packing and tight packing (arrows) are present in this plaque. (× 58,000.)

junctional complex. This lesion dramatically illustrates the physical adhesive property of the gap junction.

There is one experimental treatment capable of separating or splitting the gap-junctional complex. This approach involves the perfusion of intact tissue, such as the myocardium or liver, with hypertonic sucrose solutions. After a short perfusion time, the two junctional membranes are separated, but the particle lattices are maintained in the separated membranes (Goodenough and Gilula, 1974). The separation occurs in the gap region, and the process can be rapidly reversed by simply replacing the hypertonic sucrose with a buffered salt solution. This procedure affects gap junctions and tight junctions but not desmosomes; therefore it was initially utilized to demonstrate the electrotonic role of gap junctions in mammalian myocardium (Barr, Dewey, and Berger, 1965; Dreifuss, Girardier, and Forssman, 1966).

Junctional formation and turnover

The formation of gap junctions has recently been described as a sequence of structural events detected in several different biological systems (Revel, Yip, and Chang, 1973; Johnson et al., 1974; Decker and Friend, 1974; Benedetti, Dunia, and Bloemendal, 1974; Albertini and Anderson, 1974; Decker, 1976). The events, as visualized with freeze-fracturing, can be summarized as follows: (1) the appearance of formation plaques; (2) the appearance of large "precursor" particles with a reduction of the intercellular space; (3) the appearance of smaller "junctional" particles in polygonal arrangements; and (4) the enlargement of junctions. At present there is no information about the biochemical events related to the structural formation process. Attempts to perturb the formation process by inhibiting protein synthesis have failed in at least one system (Epstein, Sheridan, and Johnson, 1977). However, there has been a report indicating that protein synthesis may be required for junctional formation in a system that is under hormonal control (Decker, 1976).

Indirect information generated from a study on mammalian liver plasma membranes indicates that a subcellular fraction containing gap junctions has a slow turnover rate (Gurd and Evans, 1973). Morphologically, gap junctions can be detected as internalized structures in the cytoplasm. These are currently referred to as annular gap junctions or annular nexuses (Merk, Albright, and Botticelli, 1973; Albertini and Anderson, 1974; Albertini, Fawcett, and Olds, 1975). The annular structures are frequently associated with phagolysosomal vacuoles, where they are apparently degraded beyond recognition (Gilula, 1977). These structures are observed frequently in a variety of tissues, particularly those under hormonal control, and may reflect a viable mechanism for the turnover and degradation of gap junctional elements.

Physiological properties of electrotonic junctions

The physiological properties of electrotonic junctions have been extensively characterized in excitable tissues, most notably the arthropod nervous system, the vertebrate nervous system, and the mammalian myocardium (for reviews see Loewenstein, 1966; Furshpan and Potter, 1968; Bennett, 1977). In excitable tissues the major function for these junctions or electrical synapses is the rapid electrotonic spread of an action potential from one cell to the next without a significant time delay. This property permits the myocardium to function as a syncytium, even though the tissue is comprised of individual cells. The major contemporary features of electrotonic junctions in the nervous system have been discussed by Korn (this volume). I shall therefore use this section to review the physiological information that has been obtained from studies on nonexcitable tissues.

The electrotonic spread of current has been detected in a wide variety of interacting cell populations. The determinations are made directly by passing a current pulse between intracellular microelectrodes positioned in adjacent cells that are in physical contact. When current is readily transferred between the two cells with little voltage attenuation, it is concluded that a specialized intercellular low-resistance pathway is present. In most cellular systems examined, current moves equally well in both directions. Paradoxically, rectification was observed in the initial physiological study of an electrotonic synapse (Furshpan and Potter, 1969). Cells joined by a low-resistance junction or electrotonic synapse are referred to as being electrically or ionically coupled. In a variety of nonexcitable tissues, this property has been termed intercellular communication (Loewenstein, 1966). From the microelectrode determinations, it is possible to predict the existence of a specialized region of intercellular contact where membrane resistance is significantly different ($10-100$ Ω-cm^2 instead of 10^6-10^8 Ω-cm^2). In addition, channels of finite dimensions should be present to accommodate the movement of current, in the form of ions (presumably Na$^+$, K$^+$, Cl$^-$), from cell to cell. Based on the hydrated ionic radii of such ions, these channels should have diameters around 1.5 nm. Fluorescent molecules of higher molecular weight, such as sodium fluorescein (330 daltons), can also move between cells that are ionically coupled. A recent study has demonstrated that the dipteran salivary-gland epithelial cells can transfer molecules up to 1,200 daltons; molecules above that size fail to move from cell to cell (Simpson, Rose, and Loewenstein, 1977). Thus it appears that the junctional channels resemble molecular sieves possessing a selective permeability based on molecular weight and that the movement of molecules from cell to cell simply occurs at a rate of passive diffusion in cytoplasm.

Contact-dependent movement of metabolically significant molecules has also been described. This phenomenon was originally termed *metabolic cooperation* between cells (Subak-Sharpe, Bürk, and Pitts, 1969). During metabolic cooperation or metabolic coupling, cells are able to exchange a variety of low-molecular-weight metabolites. Currently the list of communicated metabolites includes nucleotides, sugars, amino acids, and vitamin intermediates (Rieske, Schubert, and Kreutzberg, 1975; Pitts and Simms, 1977; Pitts, 1977).

In 1972 a study was designed to determine whether there was a relationship between the two reported contact-dependent phenomena—ionic coupling and metabolic coupling—and if so, what was the specific junctional structure associated with communication between cells (Gilula, Reeves, and Steinbach, 1972). The observations from this study clearly demonstrated that ionic and metabolic coupling can occur simultaneously between cells and that a specific junctional structure, the gap junction, can be detected between communicating cells. Utilizing a cell type lacking in gap junctions, it was also possible to demonstrate that cells are not coupled when the gap junction is absent. The same conclusion was reported in a similar series of studies (Azarnia, Michalke, and Loewenstein, 1972; Azarnia, Larsen, and Loewenstein, 1974). At present it can be concluded that the gap junction most likely provides a structural pathway for electrotonic coupling between cells, but this may not be the only pathway for low-resistance coupling.

Regulation of junctional permeability

So far it has not been possible to demonstrate a localized junctional regulation of permeability between cells. However, several recent studies have provided substantial evidence that intracellular calcium concentrations can have a significant effect on both physiological and structural properties of electrotonic junctions.

Most of the information about calcium and junctional permeability has been generated by Loewenstein and his colleagues (see Loewenstein, 1966). Their observations suggested that the intracellular content of calcium is important for regulating permeability; hence, an abnormal elevation or depression in the level of calcium leads to an uncoupling. The most direct confirmation of this hypothesis came from an elegant experiment by Rose and Loewenstein (1975) using the dipteran salivary-gland cells. They demonstrated that uncoupling occurs as a result of an elevation in the intracellular calcium concentration in the vicinity of the presumptive junctional interaction. Although uncoupling is directly related to elevated calcium levels, there is no indication that the uncoupling achieved by this process can be readily reversed. Recent structural observations also suggest that the gap-junctional particle lattices are detectably altered (closer packing of the particles) in the uncoupled state (Peracchia and Dulhunty, 1976; Peracchia, 1977). In fact, this structural alteration is reported to occur by addition of calcium to isolated gap junctions in vitro (Peracchia, 1978).

Although most of the calcium studies have been performed on arthropod tissues, there are recent indications that a similar mechanism may be operative in mammalian systems as well (Oliveira-Castro and Barcinski, 1974; De Mello, 1975). In general, it has been difficult to translate the calcium information into nonarthropod coupled systems (for discussion see Gilula and Epstein, 1976). This may be related to the fact that arthropods have a unique gap-junctional structure (Gilula, 1974a).

A biologically attractive mechanism for regulating permeability has recently been reported in a study on amphibian embryos by Turin and Warner (1977). They reported that changes in intracellular pH (from 7.4 to 6.7) caused an uncoupling of the embryonic cells; more importantly, the pH-induced uncoupling is rapidly reversible.

Communication specificity

Electrotonic junctions have been observed between homologous, as well as heterologous, cells in vivo and in culture (Hyde et al., 1969; Michalke and Loewenstein, 1971; Johnson, Herman, and Preus, 1973; Raviola and Gilula, 1973; Pitts, 1977). In general, the gap-junctional structures described in vivo are strikingly similar, except for those in arthropod tissues

(Gilula, 1974a). In vertebrate cell-culture populations, it has been demonstrated that cells from different organs, different tissues, and different organisms (from a variety of vertebrate phyla) can communicate with each other (heterologous cell interactions) providing they are communication-competent in homologous cell cultures (Epstein and Gilula, 1977). Communication between heterologous vertebrate cells in culture appears to occur readily if the cells (1) can physically contact each other and (2) are communication-competent. There is no apparent specificity for this interaction.

A communication specificity has, however, been detected in arthropod culture systems; communication-competent arthropod cells fail to communicate with communication-competent cell cultures of vertebrate cells (Epstein and Gilula, 1977). This specificity may be related to the different gap-junctional structures expressed by the two cell types (arthropod versus vertebrate). Furthermore, only cells from arthropod organisms within the *same* order can communicate with each other. This specificity may be a reflection of the unique gap-junctional structure and significant evolutionary diversification of the organisms within the phylum.

Isolation and biochemical characterization of gap junctions

Gap junctions have been isolated as enriched subcellular fractions, primarily from rat and mouse liver (Benedetti and Emmelot, 1968; Goodenough and Stoeckenius, 1972; Evans and Gurd, 1972; Gilula, 1974b; Dunia et al., 1974; Duguid and Revel, 1975; Ehrhart and Chaveau, 1977; Culvenor and Evans, 1977). No endogenous activity or binding properties have been detected in the isolated fraction, so the purity of the fractions must be determined by ultrastructural criteria (Figures 3A and 3B). The most convenient assay for determining an enrichment is negative staining (Figure 3C), which provides a detailed image of the characteristic junctional lattice of 8–9 nm particles. This lattice is virtually identical to the ones exposed in lanthanum-impregnated thin sections and freeze-fracture replicas. A small, 1.5–2.0 nm, electron-dense dot occupies the central region of the 8–8.5 nm particles; this stainable region has been interpreted in thin sections and freeze-fracturing to represent the hydrophilic channel for cell-to-cell communication (Payton, Bennett, and Pappas, 1969; McNutt and Weinstein, 1970).

Protein and lipid are both present in the isolated gap-junction fractions, but no carbohydrate has been

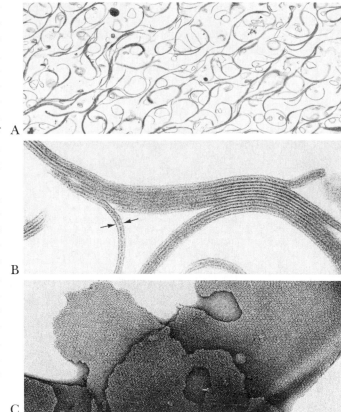

FIGURE 3 (A) Thin-section micrograph of an enriched subcellular fraction of gap junctions from rat liver. (× 16,000.) (B) Higher magnification image of the isolated junctions in Figure 3. Note that the isolated junctions still maintain their structural integrity (arrows), and the structures can often aggregate to produce a myelinlike image. (× 140,000.) (C) Negative stain appearance of isolated rat-liver gap junctions. The isolated structures are comprised of a lattice of particles that contain a central electron-dense dot. This dot may represent the location of the polar channel for electrotonic coupling. (× 103,000.)

reported. In most of the reports on isolated gap junctions from liver, the junctional polypeptides have been affected by a proteolytic treatment used to reduce collagen contamination. Thus far it appears that a 25,000–26,000 dalton polypeptide can be detected, together with other less-prominent polypeptides. Junctions have been isolated in another tissue, bovine lens fibers, and a 34,000 dalton polypeptide is the prominent component in this fraction (Dunia et al., 1974).

A recent combined electron-microscopic and X-ray diffraction analysis of an isolated gap-junction fraction from mouse liver (Caspar et al., 1977; Makowski et al., 1977) determined that the lattice constant of the junctional particles (termed *connexons*) varies from about 8 nm to 9 nm. There is significant short-range disorder in the lattice, and the long-range order is quite regular. The interpretation of the X-ray diffraction data is that the gap-junctional membranes are comprised of a hexagonal lattice of connexon units that are intercalated in a lipid bilayer. The connexons are protein structures (presumably a hexameric arrangement of a polypeptide) that form an axial channel with a maximum diameter of about 2 nm. This channel would be a reasonable location for the hydrophilic pathway required for cell-to-cell communication.

Electrotonic junctions in differentiating systems

The idea that gap-junctional communication plays a regulatory role in differentiating systems became very attractive when cell-to-cell communication was documented in a variety of embryonic tissues. Nevertheless, it has been very difficult to demonstrate a direct or indirect involvement of gap-junctional communication in any differentiation process. In fact, it is clear from a study on the differentiation of insect epidermis that junctional communication can exist across apparent differentiation boundaries (Warner and Lawrence, 1973; Lawrence and Green, 1975). In the past few years, however, there have been several encouraging studies that may provide us with an opportunity to assess the role of gap junctions in differentiation.

Blackshaw and Warner (1976) found that the myotome cells in the segmented regions of amphibian somite formation are coupled; the cells in the segmenting somite are poorly coupled to the cells in the segmented region, and the mesodermal cells in the unsegmented region are completely uncoupled from the cells in the segmented region. These data have been interpreted as indicating that the coupling pattern potentially reflects the number of cells that have completed their morphogenetic movements. In these embryos, coupling is reestablished between cells of adjacent somites after segmentation is completed. Thus, during the differentiation process, communication initially present is lost, and is then reestablished after the morphogenetic movements have ceased.

Another example of uncoupling during differentiation has been reported between the oocyte and the cumulus oophorus (granulosa) cells in the mammalian ovarian follicle (Epstein, Beers, and Gilula, 1976). Communication is present between the granulosa cells and the oocyte in immature follicles. During follicular development, however, the communication gradually decreases as the time of ovulation approaches. After ovulation, communication is no longer detectable. It is possible that this pattern of communication between the cumulus and oocyte is closely related to the pattern of oocyte maturation that occurs during the same stages of development.

In avian muscle differentiation, communication has been documented between myoblasts prior to fusion (Kalderon, Epstein, and Gilula, 1977). This communication is not qualitatively altered by experimentally inhibiting the fusion process. Therefore, communication is not a sufficient event by itself to promote the formation of a multinucleated muscle fiber. These studies have recently been extended to the process of innervation; gap-junctional interactions compatible with the previous detection of electrotonic junctions (Fischbach, 1972) have been detected between neurons and muscle fibers during the synaptogenesis process (Kalderon and Gilula, unpublished observations). Communication may therefore provide an important mechanism for transmitting signals from cell to cell that can regulate the differentiation process during myogenesis and neuromuscular junction formation.

A co-culture approach for studying cell communication

We have recently utilized co-cultures of mouse neonatal ventricular myocardial cells and rat ovarian granulosa cells to examine a potential role of gap-junctional communication in the transmission of hormonal stimulation (Lawrence, Beers, and Gilula, 1977). The myocardial cells can be stimulated with the catecholamine norepinephrine to increase their beat frequency and alter the amplitude and duration of their action potentials. The granulosa cells can be stimulated with the hormone FSH to produce plasminogen activator. In both instances, the hormonal stimulations are cAMP-dependent. In co-cultures, communication is readily established between the two cell types. After treatment of the co-cultures with FSH, the myocardial cells respond as if they were directly stimulated by norepinephrine. Conversely, in co-cultures the granulosa cells respond to norepinephrine treatment as if they were stimulated by FSH. Thus the co-culture approach has demonstrated that hormonal stimulation can be transmitted between heterologous communicating cells. Moreover, the communicator or cytoplasmic signal for this response may be cAMP.

Conclusion

Information about electrotonic junctions has expanded significantly in the past five years due to important advances in structural, physiological, and biochemical approaches. Much of the novel information has been derived from junctions outside of the nervous system. In the next few years, the probes being developed with isolated junctions should provide us with an exciting opportunity to focus on the junctional elements in the nervous system as well.

ACKNOWLEDGMENTS The work in the author's laboratory has been supported by the Irma T. Hirschl Trust, USPHS Grant HL-16507, and NIH Career Development Award HL-00110.

REFERENCES

ALBERTINI, D. F., and E. ANDERSON, 1974. The appearance and structure of intercellular connections during the ontogeny of the rabbit ovarian follicle with particular reference to gap junctions. *J. Cell Biol.* 63:234–250.

ALBERTINI, D. F., D. W. FAWCETT, and P. J. OLDS, 1975. Morphological variations in gap junctions of ovarian granulosa cells. *Tiss. Cell* 7:38–405.

AMSTERDAM, A., and J. D. JAMIESON, 1974. Studies on dispersed pancreatic exocrine cells. I. Dissociation technique and morphologic characteristics of separated cells. *J. Cell Biol.* 63:1037–1056.

AZARNIA, R., W. MICHALKE, and W. R. LOEWENSTEIN, 1972. Intercellular communication and tissue growth. VI. Failure of exchange of endogenous molecules between cancer cells with defective junctions and noncancerous cells. *J. Membr. Biol.* 10:247–258.

AZARNIA, R., W. J. LARSEN, and W. R. LOEWENSTEIN, 1974. The membrane junctions in communicating and noncommunicating cells, their hybrids and segregants. *Proc. Natl. Acad. Sci. USA* 71:880–884.

BARR, L., M. M. DEWEY, and W. BERGER, 1965. Propagation of action potentials and the structure of the nexus in cardiac muscle. *J. Gen. Physiol.* 48:797–823.

BENEDETTI, E. L., and P. EMMELOT, 1968. Hexagonal array of subunits in tight junctions separated from isolated rat liver plasma membranes. *J. Cell Biol.* 38:15–24.

BENEDETTI, E. L., I. DUNIA, and H. BLOEMENDAL, 1974. Development of junctions during differentiation of lens fiber. *Proc. Natl. Acad. Sci. USA* 71:5073–5077.

BENNETT, M. V. L., 1977. Electrical transmission: A functional analysis and comparison to chemical transmission. In *Handbook of Physiology*, I/1, E. R. Kandel, ed. Baltimore: Williams & Wilkins, pp. 357–416.

BERRY, M. N., and D. S. FRIEND, 1969. High yield preparation of isolated rat liver parenchymal cells: A biochemical and fine structure study. *J. Cell Biol.* 43:506–520.

BLACKSHAW, S. E., and A. E. WARNER, 1976. Low resistance junctions between mesoderm cells during development of trunk muscles. *J. Physiol.* 255:209–230.

CASPAR, D. L. D., D. A. GOODENOUGH, L. MAKOWSKI, and W. C. PHILLIPS, 1977. Gap junction structures. I. Correlated electron microscopy and X-ray diffraction. *J. Cell Biol.* 74:605–628.

CULVENOR, J. G., and W. H. EVANS, 1977. Preparation of hepatic gap (communicating) junctions. *Biochem. J.* 168:475–481.

DECKER, R. S., 1976. Hormonal regulation of gap junction differentiation. *J. Cell Biol.* 69:669–685.

DECKER, R. S., and D. S. FRIEND, 1974. Assembly of gap junctions during amphibian neurulation. *J. Cell Biol.* 62:32–47.

DE MELLO, W. C., 1975. Effect of intracellular injection of calcium and strontium on cell communication in heart. *J. Physiol.* 250:231–245.

DEWEY, M. M., and L. BARR, 1962. Intercellular connection between smooth muscle cells: The nexus. *Science* 137:670–672.

DREIFUSS, J. J., L. GIRARDIER, and W. G. FORSSMAN, 1966. Etude de la propagation de l'excitation dans le ventricule de rat du moyen de solutions hypertoniques. *Pflügers Arch.* 292:13–33.

DUGUID, J. R., and J. P. REVEL, 1975. The protein components of the gap junction. *Cold Spring Harbor Symp. Quant. Biol.* 60:45–47.

DUNIA, I., K. SEN, E. L. BENEDETTI, A. ZWEERS, and H. BLOEMENDAL, 1974. Isolation and protein pattern of eye lens fiber junctions. *FEBS Lett.* 45:139–144.

EHRHART, J.-C., and J. CHAVEAU, 1977. The protein component of mouse hepatocyte gap junctions. *FEBS Lett.* 78:295–299.

EPSTEIN, M. L., and N. B. GILULA, 1977. A study of communication specificity between cells in culture. *J. Cell Biol.* 75:769–787.

EPSTEIN, M. L., W. H. BEERS, and N. B. GILULA, 1976. Cell communication between the rat cumulus oophorus and the oocyte. *J. Cell Biol.* 70:302a.

EPSTEIN, M. L., J. D. SHERIDAN, and R. G. JOHNSON, 1977. Formation of low resistance junctions *in vitro* in the absence of protein synthesis and ATP production. *Exp. Cell Res.* 104:25–30.

EVANS, W. H., and J. W. GURD, 1972. Preparation and properties of nexuses and lipid-enriched vesicles from mouse liver plasma membranes. *Biochem. J.* 128:691–700.

FISCHBACH, G. D., 1972. Synapse formation between dissociated nerve and muscle cells in low density cell cultures. *Dev. Biol.* 28:407–429.

FURSHPAN, E. J., and D. D. POTTER, 1959. Transmission at giant motor synapses of the crayfish. *J. Physiol.* 143:289–325.

FURSHPAN, E. J., and D. D. POTTER, 1968. Low-resistance junctions between cells in embryos and tissue culture. *Curr. Top. Dev. Biol.* 3:95–127.

GILULA, N. B., 1974a. Junctions between cells. In *Cell Communication*, R. P. Cox, ed. New York: Wiley, pp. 1–29.

GILULA, N. B., 1974b. Isolation of rat liver gap junctions and characterization of the polypeptides. *J. Cell Biol.* 63:111a.

GILULA, N. B., 1977. Gap junctions and cell communication. In *International Cell Biology* (1976–1977), B. R. Brinkley and K. R. Porter, eds. New York: Rockefeller Univ. Press, pp. 61–69.

GILULA, N. B., and M. L. EPSTEIN, 1976. Cell-to-cell communication, gap junctions and calcium. *Soc. Exp. Biol. Symp.* 30:257–272.

Gilula, N. B., O. R. Reeves, and A. Steinbach, 1972. Metabolic coupling, ionic coupling and cell contacts. *Nature* 235:262–265.

Goodenough, D. A., and J. P. Revel, 1971. The permeability of isolated and *in situ* mouse hepatic gap junctions studied with enzymatic tracers. *J. Cell Biol.* 50:81–91.

Goodenough, D. A., and W. Stoeckenius, 1972. The isolation of mouse hepatocyte gap junctions. Preliminary chemical characterization and X-ray diffraction. *J. Cell Biol.* 61:575–590.

Goodenough, D. A., and N. B. Gilula, 1974. The splitting of hepatocyte gap junctions and zonulae occludentes with hypertonic disaccharides. *J. Cell Biol.* 61:575–590.

Gurd, J. W., and W. H. Evans, 1973. Relative rates of degradation of mouse liver surface membrane proteins. *Eur. J. Biochem.* 36:273–279.

Hyde, A., B. Blondel, A. Matter, J. P. Cheneval, B. Filloux, and L. Girardier, 1969. Homo- and heterocellular junctions in cell cultures: An electrophysiological and morphological study. *Prog. Brain Res.* 31:283–311.

Johnson, R. G., W. S. Herman, and D. M. Preus, 1973. Homocellular and heterocellular gap junctions in Limulus: A thin-section and freeze-fracture study. *J. Ultrastruct. Res.* 43:298–312.

Johnson, R. G., M. Hammer, J. Sheridan, and J. P. Revel, 1974. Gap junction formation between reaggregated Novikoff hepatoma cells. *Proc. Natl. Acad. Sci. USA* 71:4536–4540.

Kalderon, N., M. L. Epstein, and N. B. Gilula, 1977. Cell-to-cell communication and myogenesis. *J. Cell Biol.* 75:788–806.

Larsen, W. J., 1977. Structural diversity of gap junctions. A review. *Tiss. Cell* 9:373–394.

Lawrence, P. A., and S. M. Green, 1975. The anatomy of a compartment border: The intersegmental boundary in *Oncopeltus*. *J. Cell Biol.* 65:373–382.

Lawrence, T. S., W. H. Beers, and N. B. Gilula, 1977. Hormonal stimulation and cell communication in co-cultures. *J. Cell Biol.* 75:63a.

Loewenstein, W. R., 1966. Permeability of membrane junctions. *Ann. NY Acad. Sci.* 137:441–472.

Makowski, L., D. L. D. Caspar, W. C. Phillips, and D. A. Goodenough, 1977. Gap junction structures. II. Analysis of the X-ray diffraction data. *J. Cell Biol.* 74:629–645.

McNutt, N. S., and R. S. Weinstein, 1970. The ultrastructure of the nexus: A correlated thin-section and freeze-cleave study. *J. Cell Biol.* 47:666–687.

McNutt, N. S., and R. S. Weinstein, 1973. Membrane ultrastructure at mammalian intercellular junctions. *Prog. Biophys. Mol. Biol.* 26:45–101.

Merk, F. B., C. R. Botticelli, and J. T. Albright, 1972. An intercellular response to estrogen by granulosa cells in the rat ovary: An electron microscope study. *Endocrinology* 90:992–1007.

Merk, F. B., J. T. Albright, and C. R. Botticelli, 1973. The fine structure of granulosa cell nexuses in rat ovarian follicles. *Anat. Rec.* 175:107–125.

Michalke, W., and W. R. Loewenstein, 1971. Communication between cells of different types. *Nature* 232:121–122.

Muir, A. R., 1967. The effect of divalent cations on the ultrastructure of the perfused rat heart. *J. Anat.* 101:239–262.

Oliveira-Castro, G. M., and M. A. Barcinski, 1974. Calcium-induced uncoupling in communicating lymphocytes. *Biochim. Biophys. Acta* 352:338–343.

Payton, B. W., M. V. L. Bennett, and G. D. Pappas, 1969. Permeability and structure of junctional membranes at an electrotonic synapse. *Science* 166:1641–1643.

Peracchia, C., 1977. Gap junctions: Structural changes after uncoupling procedures. *J. Cell Biol.* 72:628–641.

Peracchia, C., 1978. Calcium effects on gap junction structure and cell coupling. *Nature* 271:669–671.

Peracchia, C., and A. F. Dulhunty, 1976. Low-resistance junctions in crayfish: Structural changes with functional uncoupling. *J. Cell Biol.* 70:419–439.

Pitts, J. D., 1977. Direct communication between animal cells. In *International Cell Biology* (1976–1977), B. R. Brinkley and K. R. Porter, eds. New York: Rockefeller Univ. Press, pp. 43–49.

Pitts, J. D., and J. W. Simms, 1977. Permeability of junctions between animal cells: Intercellular transfer of nucleotides but not macromolecules. *Exp. Cell Res.* 104:153–163.

Raviola, E., and N. B. Gilula, 1973. Gap junctions between photoreceptor cells in the vertebrate retina. *Proc. Natl. Acad. Sci. USA* 70:1677–1681.

Revel, J. P., and M. J. Karnovsky, 1967. Hexagonal array of subunits in intercellular junctions of the mouse heart and liver. *J. Cell Biol.* 33:C7–C12.

Revel, J. P., P. Yip, and L. L. Chang, 1973. Cell junctions in the early chick embryo: A freeze etch study. *Dev. Biol.* 35:302–317.

Rieske, E., P. Schubert, and G. W. Kreutzberg, 1975. Transfer of radioactive material between electrically coupled neurons of the leech central nervous system. *Brain Res.* 84:365–382.

Robertson, J. D., 1963. The occurrence of a subunit pattern in the unit membranes of club endings in Mauthner cell synapses in goldfish brains. *J. Cell Biol.* 19:201–221.

Rose, B., and W. R. Loewenstein, 1975. Permeability of cell junction depends on local cytoplasmic calcium activity. *Nature* 254:250–252.

Simpson, I., B. Rose, and W. R. Loewenstein, 1977. Size limit of molecules permeating the junctional membrane channels. *Science* 195:294–296.

Staehelin, L. A., 1974. Structure and function of intercellular junctions. *Int. Rev. Cytol.* 39:191–283.

Subak-Sharpe, J. H,. R. R. Bürk, and J. D. Pitts, 1969. Metabolic cooperation between biochemically marked mammalian cells in tissue culture. *J. Cell Sci.* 4:353–367.

Turin, L., and A. Warner, 1977. Carbon dioxide reversibly abolishes ionic communication between cells of early amphibian embryo. *Nature* 270:56–57.

Warner, A. E., and P. A. Lawrence, 1973. Electrical coupling across developmental boundaries in insect epidermis. *Nature* 245:47–48.

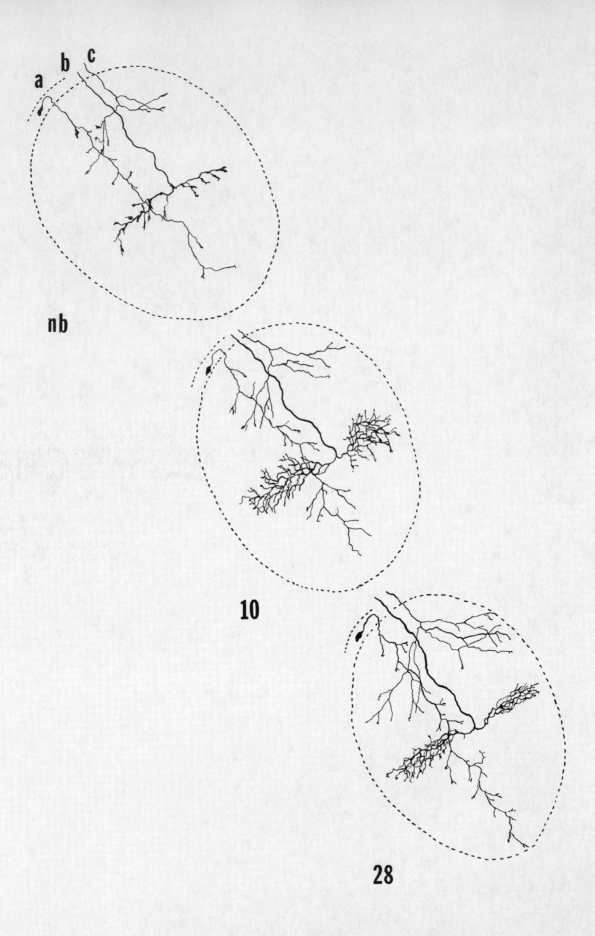

STRUCTURAL ASPECTS OF LOCAL CIRCUITS

*Development and maturation of terminal axonal
neuropil generated by three descending thalamopetal
afferent systems in the newborn (nb), 10-, and 28-day-
old rat. Fiber* a *comes from the nucleus reticularis
thalami and fibers* b *and* c *from cerebral cortex. All
three are present in rudimentary fashion at birth.
Slightly schematicized drawings based on Golgi
preparations. (From M. E. Scheibel, T. L. Davies, and
A. B. Scheibel, Ontogenetic development of
somatosensory thalamus. I. Morphogenesis.*
Experimental Neurology *51:392–406, 1976.)*

Introduction

GORDON M. SHEPHERD

OUR PRESENT IDEAS about the importance of dendrites and axon collaterals for the organization of local circuits rely heavily on anatomical work carried out over the past decade. This section is devoted to a consideration of some of this work.

From the point of view of morphology, the characterization of a synapse requires identification of the pre- and postsynaptic profiles of the terminals involved. A synapse oriented from an axon terminal to a dendrite is termed *axodendritic*. For many years it was assumed that the presynaptic element of a synapse is always an axon terminal, but the identification of dendrodendritic synapses negated this generalization. At this point the term *presynaptic dendrite* came into use. The term is in fact somewhat redundant—after all, one does not refer to "presynaptic axons"—but it has obvious practical use in labeling dendritic profiles containing output synapses when they are observed in morphological studies.

The thalamus of the mammalian brain is one region in which presynaptic dendrites are prevalent and constitute an important element in the local synaptic circuits. The early anatomical work on these regions was important in showing that dendrodendritic synapses are not confined to the olfactory bulb and retina but are also present in the telencephalon, in structures that appeared relatively late in evolution and are related to the growth of the cerebral cortex.

H. J. Ralston was one of the pioneers in this work. In his chapter he reviews the essential steps involved in characterizing synaptic terminals in central neuropil and tracing them back to their dendritic or axonal branches and cells of origin. Ralston has inferred that graded synaptic release, which had been suggested for the olfactory granule cell, and for which there is evidence at several different types of synapses, also occurs at the presynaptic dendrites of thalamic neurons; here the sites of output synapses on distal dendritic processes and spines suggest semi-independent functional units. This idea is applied to other types of neurons in the papers by Shepherd, Pearson, Graubard, and Calvin elsewhere in this volume. Ralston describes the possible significance of this type of organization for the functional operations carried out by the thalamic neurons.

A generalization that has emerged from recent anatomical investigations is that the neuropil is not diffusely arranged with respect to neuronal elements and synaptic pathways. Instead, the dominant theme appears to be specific types and patterns of synaptic connections, compartmentalization of neuronal parts, and clustering of neuronal subpopulations. Arnold Scheibel discusses how the idea of structural and functional units, or modules, arose in his work. He focuses on the ramifications of axons and groupings of dendrites into bundles as two structural configurations with significance for input-output relations. He describes these forms of organization in several central systems—spinal cord, thalamus, olfactory bulb, and cerebral cortex—and places them in an evolutionary and behavioral context.

The clearest information on local circuits has come from regions that are organized in especially simple and stereotyped ways. At the opposite end of the spectrum stands the cerebral cortex. Although we have learned much about the neuronal elements of the cortex and about some basic properties of cortical functioning, the identification of specific synaptic circuits is still at a very early stage of development. The problems come from the great expanse of the cortex, the many local variations within it, and the intermingling of so many different types of inputs, outputs, and synaptic pathways.

Some basic strategies for approaching the problems of the cortex at a structural level are discussed by John Szentágothai. The essential steps that he describes include the identification of neuronal and synaptic types and the characterization of sequences of neuronal connections mediating excitation and local circuits mediating inhibition. He emphasizes the importance of modularization, as exemplified by the cortical columns, and outlines the ways in which this structural organization may provide the substrate for the input-output operations of the cortex.

21 Neuronal Circuitry of the Ventrobasal Thalamus: The Role of Presynaptic Dendrites

H. J. RALSTON III

ABSTRACT Within thalamic relay nuclei of rat, cat, and monkey, there are structures that contain synaptic vesicles, receive synaptic input from primary-afferent axons to the nucleus, and frequently exhibit characteristics of dendrites. Designated presynaptic dendrites by several authors, they synapse upon conventional dendrites or other presynaptic dendrites. Frequently they form a triadic relationship in which the primary-afferent axon is presynaptic to both a thalamocortical relay (TCR) cell dendrite and a presynaptic dendrite; the latter in turn synapses upon the same TCR-cell dendrite. It is thus apparent that presynaptic dendrites must somehow interact with both the primary-afferent axon and dendrites of thalamic neurons to modify the character of primary-afferent input upon thalamic neurons. The physiological character of this synaptic interaction mediated by presynaptic dendrites is as yet unknown. It is most likely that presynaptic dendrites release transmitter because of local depolarization resulting from primary-afferent or other synaptic input; they may therefore act as independent synaptic units and be relatively unaffected by the activities of other dendritic branches of the parent neuron.

DURING THE past decade there has been a gradual recognition by many investigators that neurons may communicate with one another by graded release of synaptic transmitters and that these transmitters may be released from nonaxonal regions of nerve cells. Neuroscientists studying invertebrate neurons, such as those of insects, have long recognized that substantial numbers of the intrinsic neurons of ganglia do not conduct propagated action potentials but appear to release transmitter from their distal branches following local depolarization (see Pearson, this volume). In the invertebrate it is often possible to directly visualize, and inject with dyes, particular neurons under study; one may thus characterize the morphology of the cells that had been characterized physiologically. Such direct correlations of structure

H. J. RALSTON III   Department of Anatomy, University of California, San Francisco, CA 94143

and function are much more difficult in most regions of the vertebrate central nervous system. Although there is now ample evidence that many cell bodies and dendrites of various types of vertebrate neurons contain synaptic vesicles and are thus likely to be release sites of synaptic transmitter, there is little direct evidence linking particular neurons viewed by light and electron microscopy with proven synaptic transmitter release from somatic or dendritic sites. This chapter deals with the available evidence about the structure and function of vertebrate neurons postulated to have presynaptic dendrites.

Presynaptic dendrites in vertebrate CNS

There are two regions of the vertebrate CNS in which investigators have demonstrated that neurons may interact by local depolarization leading to dendritic transmitter release: the retina and the olfactory bulb. Horizontal cells of the retina do not appear to have propagated axon potentials associated with transmitter release (see Dowling, 1976, for a recent review). Retinal amacrine neurons do not have axons, although individual dendritic processes may spike; but it appears that individual dendritic branches may act independently of other regions of the neuron (see Miller, this volume). In the olfactory bulb, the projection neuron (the mitral cell) has action potentials generated in the initial segment of the axon; these also invade the cell body and dendritic tree, resulting in local transmitter release from mitral dendrites onto adjacent granule-cell dendritic branches. Local depolarization of the granule-cell process results, and transmitter is consequently released back upon the mitral-cell dendrite (Rall et al., 1966). A similar spike-initiated process occurs when periglomerular-cell dendritic branches release transmitter upon mitral-cell dendrites, resulting in local mitral dendritic depolarization with transmitter release back upon periglomerular cells (Shepherd, 1971). It is evident that transmitter release in these two regions of the vertebrate nervous system may take place following the invasion of dendritic branches by action potentials arising in the region of the neuron cell body or by graded depolarizations of the dendritic branches as a result of local synaptic input. It is likely that one or both of these mechanisms is also operative in presynaptic dendrites within the brain and spinal cord, although there is as yet little direct evidence bearing on this issue.

In the retina and olfactory bulb, the light-microscopic morphology of neurons thought to have presynaptic dendrites can be compared with electron-microscopic profiles that are found to be both pre- and postsynaptic. Such a correlation is more difficult in thalamic nuclei that contain neurons having presynaptic dendrites or cell bodies. The idea that thalamic neurons might interact by means of presynaptic dendrites in a manner similar to that seen in the retina and olfactory bulb evolved gradually during the late 1960s. Several authors, including Szentágothai, Hamori, and Tombol (1966) and Colonnier and Guillery (1964), found that the retinal afferent axon in the lateral geniculate nucleus synapsed upon the dendritic branches of the geniculocortical relay cells and upon profiles with synaptic vesicles. The retinal afferent was invariably the *presynaptic* element in all the synapses, a finding that conflicted with the earlier model for presynaptic inhibition in the thalamus in which the primary-afferent axon was presumed to be *postsynaptic* to other axons (Andersen et al., 1964). It was stated that the synapses between the retinal afferent and the vesicle-filled profile were examples of axoaxonal contacts.

Jones and Powell (1969a) published an extensive study of the fine structure of several thalamic relay nuclei and again reported that the primary-afferent fiber was invariably presynaptic to other vesicle-filled profiles. They found that several of the latter profiles contained ribosomes or patches of rough endoplasmic reticulum (RER), organelles thought to occur primarily in dendrites and rarely, if ever, in axons. They considered whether the profiles with both synaptic vesicles and organelles usually found in dendrites might be dendrites with vesicles, but they finally concluded that it was more likely they were branches of initial segments of axons.

In the same year Ralston and Herman (1969) found several profiles in the cat ventrobasal thalamus with both the characteristics of dendrites and the presence of synaptic vesicles. They concluded that these structures were indeed presynaptic dendrites

and that they received input from primary-afferent fibers (the dorsal-column lemniscal axon) and in turn were presynaptic to thalamocortical-cell dendrites. Many reports followed in which it was shown that various thalamic relay nuclei contain cells with presynaptic dendrites: the medial geniculate nucleus of the cat (Morest, 1971); the lateral geniculate nucleus of the cat (Famiglietti, 1970; Famiglietti and Peters, 1972), rat (Lieberman and Webster, 1972, 1974; Lieberman, 1973), and monkey (Wong, 1970; Pasik et al., 1973); and the monkey ventrolateral nucleus (Harding, 1973a). Most authors pointed out that there is a consistent triadic relationship between the primary afferent, the presynaptic dendrite, and the presumed relay-cell dendrite in the thalamus. This triad is arranged so that the primary afferent is presynaptic to both the presynaptic dendrite and the relay-cell dendrite; the presynaptic dendrite in turn synapses upon the relay-cell dendrite. This arrangement provides a direct synaptic contact between the incoming primary afferent and the relay-cell dendrite and an indirect one in which the presynaptic dendrite is interposed between primary afferent and relay dendrite. It is presumed that the indirect synaptic arrangement somehow permits modification of the effect of the primary afferent upon the relay cell.

Evidence for the dendritic origin of presynaptic structures

The evidence that these synaptic structures are dendrites rather than axons is reasonably sound. In many cases the presynaptic profiles contain ribosomes or RER (Figure 2) or can be traced back to mainstem dendrites in serial sections (Ralston and Herman, 1969; Famiglietti and Peters, 1972). The presumed presynaptic dendrites have sometimes been traced back to parent cell bodies that also contain synaptic vesicles (Wong, 1970). To date no investigator has been able to demonstrate that the presumed presynaptic dendrites can be traced back to a structure having a myelin sheath. Frequently the presynaptic dendrites have a substantially greater diameter than any known axons in the thalamus. Often, however, it is not possible to find ribosomes or RER or other features of the presumed presynaptic dendrite that would provide a fairly certain identification of the profile as dendritic (Figure 1). Even extensive serial-section analysis may fail to trace the profile back to a stem dendrite or a neuronal cell body. Figures 3, 4, and 5 illustrate serial sections of a typical synaptic arrangement within cat lateral geniculate nucleus. The series is one of several by Dr. S. Rapisardi at the

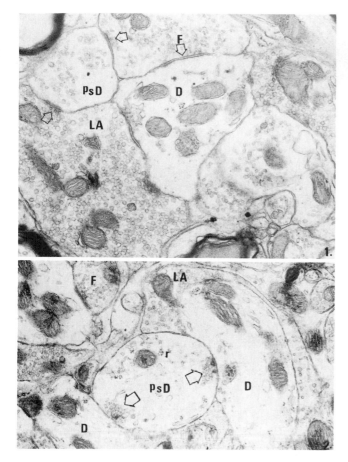

may find profiles containing synaptic vesicles that are both pre- and postsynaptic and that are in continuity with dendrites, whereas in other cases such proof of dendritic origin is difficult to obtain.

Cells of origin of presynaptic dendrites

What cell type in the thalamus might give rise to presynaptic dendrites? If one makes a large lesion in a region of the cortex to which a given thalamic nucleus projects, the thalamocortical neurons of the nucleus will degenerate, leaving behind only neurons that do not have a major projection to that cortical site. Using such techniques, it has been found that presynaptic dendrites are still present in various thalamic nuclei following death of the thalamocortical

FIGURES 1, 2 Cat ventrobasal thalamus. In Figure 1 a lemniscal afferent axon (LA) is presynaptic to both a conventional dendrite (D) and a presumed presynaptic dendrite (psD). The latter also receives a synapse from an axon containing flattened synaptic vesicles (F). In serial sections, the presynaptic dendrite formed synaptic contact with dendrite (D). In a series of 10 serial sections the psD profile was not found to contain ribosomes. (× 19,000.) In Figure 2 a presynaptic dendrite (psD) containing ribosomes (r) forms synapses upon conventional dendrites (D). In this section the edge of a lemniscal afferent axon (LA) appears at the top of the figure. Twelve sections away, the lemniscal axon synapses upon psD. (× 16,000.)

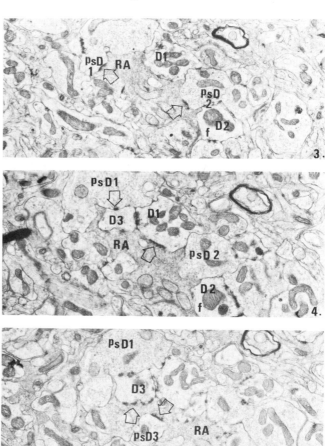

FIGURES 3, 4, 5 Serial sections from cat lateral geniculate nucleus (courtesy Dr. S. Rapisardi). These sections are numbers 78, 81, and 83 of a series over 120 consecutive sections long. The retinal afferent (RA) contacts both presynaptic dendrites psD1 and psD2. psD1 subsequently synapses upon D3, and psD2 contacts D1. The rapidly changing contour of individual profiles is evident even in this short series. Note that the ring of filaments present in D2 in Figures 3 and 4 disappears by Figure 5. (× 6,500.)

University of California, San Francisco, in which he analyzed synaptic arrangements in the lateral geniculate nucleus in more than a dozen cases of 60 to 200 consecutive serial sections. He frequently found presynaptic dendrites similar to those shown by other authors. However, in the analysis of presumed presynaptic dendrites that receive synaptic input from retinal afferents, he was unable to find evidence that presumed presynaptic dendritic profiles were in continuity with undoubted dendritic structures. On the other hand, the profiles were never shown to have any characteristics of axons. Thus, in some cases one

relay (TCR) cell; examples include the cat ventrobasal thalamus (Ralston, 1971), the cat lateral geniculate nucleus (Famiglietti and Peters, 1972), and the monkey lateral geniculate nucleus (Pasik et al., 1973). Therefore, at least some of the presynaptic dendrites arise from neurons that may be presumed to be intrinsic to the thalamus.

Several authors have attempted to compare the morphology of thalamic neurons seen with the Golgi method with the appearance of presynaptic dendrites under the electron microscope. From such an analysis, Morest (1971, 1975) has concluded that presynaptic dendrites arise from Golgi type II neurons—that is, neurons with processes confined to the particular thalamic nucleus. Similar conclusions have been reached by other authors comparing light- and electron-microscopic studies of thalamic neurons (Famiglietti and Peters, 1972; Scheibel, Davies, and Scheibel, 1972a,b; Lieberman, 1973; Lieberman and Webster, 1974). Famiglietti (1970) had suggested that TCR cells might also give rise to presynaptic dendrites. He based this suggestion on the beaded appearance of TCR-cell dendrites stained by the Golgi method and the similar beaded appearance of presynaptic dendrites under the electron microscope. In an analysis of similar material in the rat, Lieberman (1973) concluded that the evidence suggesting that TCR cells give rise to presynaptic dendrites was not strong.

It is very likely that intrinsic neurons (Golgi type II cells) of thalamic nuclei have presynaptic dendrites. Whether or not thalamocortical relay cells also give rise to presynaptic dendrites must be considered an open question for the moment. As yet there is no direct evidence associating a particular neuronal type with cells having presynaptic dendrites. Such evidence may be forthcoming when it becomes possible to inject single identified neurons intracellularly with a substance (such as horseradish peroxidase) that permits the cell to be analyzed by both light and electron microscopy. Recent advances in staining cells by the Golgi method, which enables their electron-microscopic analysis (Fairen, Peters, and Saldanha, 1977), should also permit a direct correlation between the light- and electron-microscopic appearance of cells.

Further evidence that presynaptic dendrites arise from cells within a particular nucleus of the thalamus is provided in Figures 6–9. A series of normal cats underwent microinjections (0.1–0.2 microliters) of tritiated leucine into the ventrobasal thalamus. The radioactive amino acid is taken up by the cell bodies of neurons and incorporated into protein, and the radioactive protein is subsequently transported along

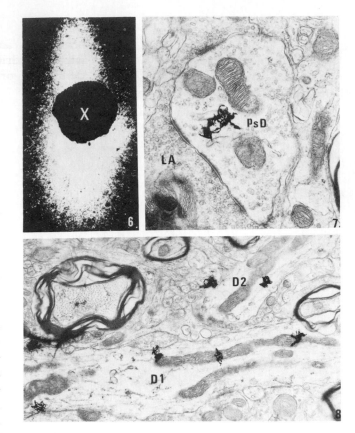

FIGURES 6, 7, 8 Autoradiographic studies of cat ventrobasal thalamus. Figure 6 is a dark-field micrograph showing the radioactive injection site indicated by the bright region, within the thalamus. The circle (X) is a core of tissue removed for electron microscopy. Figures 7 and 8 are electron micrographs of the tissue core in Figure 6. Figure 7 shows a lemniscal afferent (LA) synapsing upon a presynaptic dendrite (psD), which has an overlying cluster of silver grains as a result of being labeled with tritiated amino acid incorporated into protein. Figure 8 depicts conventional dendrites within the nucleus, with overlying silver grains. (Figure 6, × 17; Figure 7, × 21,000; Figure 8, × 11,000.)

dendritic and axonal branches. Axons of passage do not incorporate the amino acid into protein (Cowan et al., 1972). After surviving for 24–48 hours, the anesthetized animal is killed by intracardiac perfusion with a paraformaldehyde-glutaraldehyde mixture, and the tissue is processed for light- and electron-microscopic autoradiography. The radioactive cells and their processes are revealed by the presence of silver grains overlying sources of radioactivity, with the radioactive source estimated by the probability circle method of Bachmann and Salpeter (1965). There is a built-in control in the nucleus for nonspecific labeling since the lemniscal afferent is readily recognized. Because this terminal has its parent cell body in the dorsal-column nuclei, several centimeters

376   H. J. RALSTON III

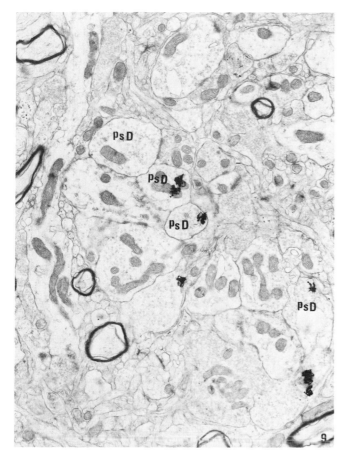

FIGURE 9 A typical synaptic zone in ventrobasal thalamus following injection of radioactive amino acid as shown in Figure 6. Several of the presynaptic dendrites may be seen to have overlying silver grains. Some of the silver grains lie on the edges of structures, and it is not possible to determine precisely the source of radioactivity. (× 10,500.)

distant, the lemniscal afferent should never appear any more radioactive than background levels.

An example of a single injection site into the ventroposterolateral (VPL) thalamus is shown in Figure 6 in a dark-field micrograph. The bright area is the region of radioactivity (8 weeks' exposure to Kodak NTB-2 emulsion). The circle in the center (X) is the core of tissue removed for electron-microscopic analysis (Ralston and Herman, 1969). Figure 7 reveals silver grains overlying a single presynaptic dendrite, which is in turn postsynaptic to a lemniscal axon (LA). There are in the nucleus radioactive dendrites that lack synaptic vesicles (Figure 8, D1, D2). It is not known whether these dendrites arise from TCR cells or from intrinsic neurons. Figure 9 shows a low-power view of a typical synaptic zone in the thalamus. Several of the presumed postsynaptic dendrites are

overlaid with silver grains; several others are not. Whether the latter structures had their cell bodies in a zone other than that injected, or whether they were radioactive but the radioactive emission (a beta particle) was not captured by the overlying photographic emulsion, is not known.

These autoradiographic studies support previous suggestions that presynaptic dendrites arise from cells with cell bodies within a particular thalamic relay nucleus. The present autoradiographic-examination technique, however, does not distinguish between radioactive labeling of intrinsic and projection cells. This issue is being approached in another study in which TCR cells are removed by retrograde degeneration and the surviving cells in the nucleus are labeled with tritiated amino acid.

Functions of presynaptic dendrites

The function of presynaptic dendrites within the mammalian CNS is as yet unknown. All authors examining the morphological features of these structures have found that presynaptic dendrites receive input from the primary-afferent fiber to the particular relay nucleus (lemniscal afferent to ventrobasal thalamus; retinal afferent to the lateral geniculate nucleus; brachium of the inferior colliculus to the medial geniculate nucleus). Cortical axons have also been found to project to presynaptic dendrites in many cases (e.g., Jones and Powell, 1969b; Harding, 1973b; Morest, 1975). On the other hand, Lieberman and Webster (1974) did not find cortical projections to presynaptic dendrites in rat lateral geniculate nucleus; the rat appears to be different from the cat and monkey in other respects, in that presynaptic dendrites were found to be uncommon in its ventrobasal thalamus (Spacek and Lieberman, 1974). Presynaptic dendrites may also receive input from axons with flattened vesicles from a source as yet unknown (Figure 1). In cat and monkey the presynaptic dendrites can be activated by either primary-afferent or cortical input and in turn synapse upon other dendrites in the nucleus or even upon one another. In 1971 it was suggested that presynaptic dendrites may release transmitter by one of two mechanisms: either synchronous release from many branches of the dendritic tree upon invasion by an action potential generated in the cell body or local depolarization as a result of direct synaptic input upon a particular dendritic branch containing synaptic vesicles (Ralston, 1971; Shepherd, 1971). In the latter case, each dendritic branch would act as an independent synaptic unit like those found by Graubard in her studies of lobster neurons (see Graubard and Calvin, this volume). She finds that graded synaptic transmitter release occurs in both spiking and nonspiking neurons and that voltages applied to distal neuronal processes attenuate markedly as they travel toward the parent cell body. Her work in invertebrate neurons supports the suggestion that vertebrate cells can have dendritic branches that release transmitter as a result of local depolarization and that each dendritic branch can undergo depolarization changes with little effect on other branches of the same neuron.

To date there are relatively few intracellular studies on thalamic neurons in mammals. Purpura (1972) reported a diphasic postsynaptic potential as a result of brief excitatory potentials (EPSPs) interrupted by inhibitory potentials (IPSPs). He found that the IPSP component of the diphasic potential is generated prior to the initiation of an impulse that can activate a recurrent inhibitory pathway. He suggested that dendrodendritic synapses activated by the primary-afferent fiber might mediate this inhibitory potential. It will take many more intracellular studies with thalamic neurons to work out the functional consequences of the dendrodendritic interactions demonstrated in morphological studies.

In summary, there is ample evidence that thalamic relay nuclei contain profiles resembling dendrites that contain synaptic vesicles and form contacts with other neuronal structures. These contacts meet the morphological criteria for chemical synaptic junctions. In many cases the synaptic-vesicle-containing profiles exhibit the morphological features of dendrites, or they can be traced back to stem dendrites or even to cell bodies. In other cases serial reconstructions have not been able to demonstrate that these profiles arise from dendrites. On the other hand, presumed presynaptic dendrites have never been shown to be branches of undoubted axons. The presynaptic dendrites receive input from the primary-afferent axon to the nucleus, frequently from cortical axons and axons with flattened vesicles. They may synapse upon other presynaptic dendrites or on dendrites without vesicles. Golgi-staining evidence suggests that in most cases the portions of the dendritic tree that give rise to the presynaptic dendrites are far removed from the parent cell body; therefore, the fine dendritic branches are not likely to be affected by events in other dendritic branches or even by spikes arising in the cell body. It is likely that the individual dendritic branches act as separate synaptic units independent of the other activities of the parent neuron. They probably release synaptic transmitter in a graded fashion as a result of local synaptic input.

They are ideally placed to change the character of the synaptic input mediated by primary-afferent axons, since the primary afferent typically synapses directly upon a relay-cell dendrite and at the same time upon a presynaptic dendrite, which then contacts the relay cell. This placement of the presynaptic dendrite in the primary-afferent path would allow it to modify the effects of the primary-afferent input upon thalamic neurons immediately after an impulse arrives at the primary-afferent synaptic terminal. The precise character of the functional interactions among the primary-afferent fiber, the presynaptic dendrite, and the thalamic neuron will be examined more thoroughly as techniques for intracellular recording in small central neurons improve. There is no doubt, however, that our concept of neuronal interactions must include a substantial place for dendrites capable of releasing transmitter, for it is now evident that such dendrites are present in many areas of vertebrate and invertebrate nervous systems.

ACKNOWLEDGMENTS Research reported in this paper is supported by grant NS-11614 from the U.S. Public Health Service. I am indebted to Diane Daly Ralston for carrying out the experimental procedures upon animals and for performing the autoradiography, to Helen Krawchuk for preparation of electron-microscopic materials, and to Peter V. Sharp for preparation of histological materials.

REFERENCES

ANDERSEN, P., C. McC. BROOKS, J. C. ECCLES, and T. A. SEARS, 1964. The ventrobasal nucleus of the thalamus: Potential fields, synaptic transmission and excitability of both presynaptic and post-synaptic components. *J. Physiol.* 174:348–369.

BACHMANN, L., and M. M. SALPETER, 1965. Autoradiography with the electron microscope: A quantitative evaluation. *Lab. Invest.* 14:1041–1053.

COLONNIER, M., and R. W. GUILLERY, 1964. Synaptic organization in the lateral geniculate nucleus of the monkey. *Z. Zellforsch.* 62:333–355.

COWAN, W. M., D. I. GOTTLIEB, A. E. HENDRICKSON, J. L. PRICE, and T. A. WOOSLEY, 1972. An autoradiographic demonstration of axonal connections in the central nervous system. *Brain Res.* 37:21–51.

DOWLING, J. E., 1976. Local circuit neurons in the vertebrate retina. In *Local Circuit Neurons*, P. Rakic, ed. Cambridge, MA: MIT Press, pp. 40–49.

FAIREN, A., A. PETERS, and J. SALDANHA, 1977. A new procedure for examining Golgi-impregnated neurons by light and electron microscopy. *J. Neurocytol.* 6:311–337.

FAMIGLIETTI, E. V., 1970. Dendro-dendritic synapses in the lateral geniculate nucleus of the cat. *Brain Res.* 20:181–192.

FAMIGLIETTI, E. V., JR, and A. PETERS, 1972. The synaptic glomerulus and the intrisic neuron in the dorsal lateral geniculate nucleus of the cat. *J. Comp. Neurol.* 144:285–334.

HARDING, B. N., 1973a. An ultrastructural study of the centre median and ventrolateral thalamic nuclei of the monkey. *Brain Res.* 54:335–340.

HARDING, B. N., 1973b. An ultrastructural study of the termination of afferent fibers within the ventrolateral and centre median nuclei of the monkey thalamus. *Brain Res.* 54:341–346.

JONES, E. G., and T. P. S. POWELL, 1969a. Electron microscopy of synaptic glomeruli in the thalamic relay nuclei of the cat. *Proc. R. Soc. Lond.* B172:153–171.

JONES, E. G., and T. P. S. POWELL, 1969b. An electron microscope study of the mode of termination of corticothalamic fibers within the sensory relay nuclei of the thalamus. *Proc. R. Soc. Lond.* B172:173–185.

LIEBERMAN, A. R., 1973. Neurons with presynaptic perikarya and presynaptic dendrites in the rat lateral geniculate nucleus. *Brain Res.* 59:35–59.

LIEBERMAN, A. R., and K. E. WEBSTER, 1972. Presynaptic dendrites and a distinctive class of synaptic vesicle in the rat dorsal lateral geniculate nucleus. *Brain Res.* 42:196–200.

LIEBERMAN, A. R., and K. E. WEBSTER, 1974. Aspects of the synaptic organization of intrisic neurons in the dorsal lateral geniculate nucleus. *J. Neurocytol.* 3:677–710.

MOREST, D. K., 1971. Dendrodendritic synapses of cells that have axons: The fine structure of the Golgi type II cell in the medical geniculate body of the cat. *Z. Anat. Entwichlungsgesch.* 133:216–246.

MOREST, D. K., 1975. Synaptic relationships of Golgi type II cells in the medical geniculate body of the cat. *J. Comp. Neurol.* 162:157–194.

PASIK, P., T. PASIK, J. HAMORI, and J. SZENTÁGOTHAI, 1973. Golgi Type II interneurons in the neuronal circuit of the monkey lateral geniculate nucleus. *Exp. Brain Res.* 17:18–34.

PURPURA, D. P., 1972. Synaptic mechanisms in coordination of activity in thalamic internuncial common paths. In *Corticothalamic Projections and Sensorimotor Activities*, T. Frigyesi, E. Rinvik, and M. D. Yahr, eds. New York: Raven Press, pp. 21–56.

RALL, W., G. SHEPHERD, T. S. REESE, and M. W. BRIGHTMAN, 1966. Dendrodendritic synaptic pathway for inhibition in the olfactory bulb. *Exp. Neurol.* 14:44–56.

RALSTON, H. J., III, 1969. The synaptic organization of lemniscal projections to the ventrobasal thalamus of the cat. *Brain Res.* 14:99–116.

RALSTON, H. J., III, 1971. Evidence for presynaptic dendrites and a proposal for their mechanism of action. *Nature* 230:585–587.

RALSTON, H. J., III, and M. M. HERMAN, 1969. The fine structure of neurons and synapses in the ventrobasal thalamus of the cat. *Brain Res.* 14:77–99.

SCHEIBEL, M. E., T. L. DAVIES, and A. B. SCHEIBEL, 1972a. An unusual axonless cell in the thalamus of the adult cat. *Exp. Neurol.* 36:512–518.

SCHEIBEL, M. E., T. L. DAVIES, and A. B. SCHEIBEL, 1972b. On dendrodendritic relations in the dorsal thalamus of the adult cat. *Exp. Neurol.* 36:519–529.

SHEPHERD, G. M., 1971. Physiological evidence for dendrodendritic interactions in the rabbit's olfactory glomerulus. *Brain Res.* 32:212–217.

SPACEK, J., and A. R. LIEBERMAN, 1974. Ultrastructure and three-dimensional organization of synaptic glomeruli in rat somatosensory thalamus. *J. Anat.* 117:487–516.

SZENTÁGOTHAI, J., J. HAMORI, and T. TOMBOL, 1966. Degeneration and electron microscope analysis of the synaptic glomeruli in the lateral geniculate body. *Exp. Brain Res.* 2:283–301.

WONG, M. T. T., 1970. Somato-dendritic and dendro-dendritic synapses in the squirrel monkey lateral geniculate nucleus. *Brain Res.* 20:135–139.

22 Development of Axonal and Dendritic Neuropil as a Function of Evolving Behavior

ARNOLD B. SCHEIBEL

ABSTRACT Neuropil comprises the great mass of neural membranes involved in the processing of information in the central nervous system. It is accordingly conceived as being made up largely of dendrites and axon terminals, but it should also include neurons and even neuroglia where they are directly involved in the transfer and modulation of signals. Neuropil evolves as behavior develops and its progressive evolution may be conceived as both the causative factor and the matrix most reactive to the evolving behavioral spectrum.

We will cite one example of axonal and three examples of dendritic evolutionary change that appear closely linked to functional development. Each case will exemplify, in its own way, the unique and idiosyncratic patterning of neuropil structure. The maturation of thalamopetal terminals, originating at both more caudal and more rostral stations in the ventrobasal complex, can be related to the maturation of thalamocortically based behavior. The differential development of dendrite bundles in cervical and lumbosacral areas of the anterior horn of cat spinal cord appear related to appearance of typical fore- and hind-limb activities. The precocious appearance of dendrite bundles in the olfactory bulb may correlate with the onset of nipple search, suckling activity, and nipple preference. Finally, the development and maturation of highly specific patterns of basilar (circumferential) dendrite systems of the giant pyramidal cells of Betz in feline and human motor cortex are putatively related to characteristic downstream motor activities, as is the later degeneration of these systems in the aged and senescent brain.

OUR PRESENT conceptions of the neuropil are based largely on the structural studies of Ramón y Cajal (1911) and the other great first-generation Golgi anatomists. In the twentieth century, Herrick (1948) and Beritoff (1943) were among the earliest to redirect attention to the intricacy and functional implications of this tissue matrix. The development of

electron-microscopic techniques by Fernández-Morán (1954), Palade (1953), Palay (1956), Pease (1955), Robertson (1953), and others in the 1950s provided deeper insights into the structural interrelations involved; but even today, we cannot improve on Herrick's conceptions of the growth, development, and functional significance of this tissue that provides the substrate warp and woof of all neural activities.

From the primordial diffuse neuropil, differentiation advanced in two diverse directions. One of these . . . led to the elaboration of the stable architectural framework of nuclei and tracts, the description of which comprises the larger part of current neuroanatomy. This is the heritable structure, which determines the basic patterns of those components of behavior which are common to all members of the species. The second derivative of the primordial neuropil is the apparatus of individually modifiable behavior, conditioning, learning and ultimately the highly specialized associational tissues of the cerebral cortex. In both phylogeny and ontogeny, differentiation of the first type precedes that of the second. Primitive animals and younger developmental stages exhibit more stable and predictable patterns of behavior; and the more labile patterns are acquired later. This . . . close-meshed web of finest axons, within which all cell bodies are imbedded . . . is everywhere present providing continuous activation (or potential activation) of every neuron, summation, reinforcement, or inhibition of whatever activities may be going on . . . and seems to be the basic apparatus of integration. (Herrick, 1948)

Over the years, our efforts have been directed toward dissection of specific neuropil patterns in an attempt to learn more about circuitry and organization as a function of the specific output. Beginning in the mid-1950s, we have sought constant features in circuit design that, through their repetition and high recognition factor, might qualify them as putative organizational building blocks or modules in much the same way that systems engineering attempts to modularize complex instrumentation or

ARNOLD B. SCHEIBEL Departments of Anatomy and Psychiatry, University of California, Los Angeles, and Brain Research Institute, UCLA Medical Center, Los Angeles, CA 90024

electronic devices. While many configurations have been suggested from work in our laboratory (Scheibel and Scheibel, 1958, 1966a,b, 1970a,b,c, 1971a,b,c; Globus and Scheibel, 1967) and in those of others (e.g., Szentágothai, 1967, 1971, 1972; Mannen, 1960), no model has yet been delimited that can demonstrably fill a least-common-denominator role, either functionally or anatomically. The basic problem lies not so much in circuit complexity—for many, such as those of the cerebellum, have been reasonably well worked-out—but rather in deciding how to establish the topographic limits of the module.

How basic should a basic element or module be? If metabolic viability is a sufficient criterion, then a single cerebellar Purkinje cell, with its dendritic domain, might be considered a module. But from the informational point of view, a single neuron with its dendritic domain is meaningless. Is it, then, the Purkinje cell with climbing-fiber input to its larger dendrite shafts and granule-cell/parallel-fiber input to its smaller branchlets? In the normal state in situ, Fox and Barnard (1957) have shown that 200,000–500,000 or more parallel fibers can form real or potential synaptic contacts with such a cell. What, then, constitutes the minimal number of contacts whose summated activity can make this type of connection functionally meaningful? And to have functional significance, of course, the granule-cell/parallel-fiber system must, in turn, be driven. We look to the input mossy-fiber system, which carries us, in terms of origin, as far as spinal cord and brain stem. To further compound the issue, there is compelling evidence that in many vertebrates, particularly birds and mammals (Ramón y Cajal, 1909–1911; Hillman, 1969), the Purkinje complex cannot function appropriately without the restraining influences of allied inhibitory circuitry, basket- and stellate-cell systems for feedforward control, and Golgi type II cell loops for feedback control. The inhibitory activities of these elements must, in turn, be controlled through recurrent collateral systems of the Purkinje neurons and of the climbing fibers for meaningful sculpting of the excitatory, inhibitory, and disinhibitory sequences. Our problems are compounded when we look to even more complex neuronal systems, such as those of spinal cord, brain stem, and cerebral cortex. It would appear that appropriate delineation of the irresolvable functional element or module in any portion of the CNS requires decisions combining the wisdom of Solomon and the optimism of Dickens's Mr. Micawber.

During the past few years, as an alternative to our search for the pontifical—and perhaps, mythical—module, we have sought structural configurations that appear to correlate functionally with output, achieving maximal forward expression as behavior matures, and perhaps regressing as the behavior deteriorates or disappears with age. Two structural complexes in particular appear to fulfill the requirements in varying degrees. One of these is the terminal plexus generated by an axon; the other is the dendrite bundle, found widely throughout the CNS and made up of shafts from a number of different neurons, often from mutually distant sites and with functionally distinct signatures.

The patterns generated by terminal-axon ramifications become more complex as the brain matures, indicating wider patterns of connectivity, more intensive synaptic patterns, or both. And yet, as we shall demonstrate, maturation may also bring an apparent decrement or paring down in plexus size and/or density, possibly as an expression of evolving roles—a more precise specification of the processing function this axon species plays during the adult life of the organism. Indeed, loss of elements—whether at the level of the individual synapse or the cell—seems to be a very significant part of the process of maturation of brain and behavior. Technical limitations of our methodology have so far prevented us from determining whether such axonal systems show more extensive regression with senescence.

The dendrite bundle has emerged as a structural entity of surprisingly wide distribution and quite accurately reflective of the state of maturation of output characteristics in the system. In one or two cases, it has been possible to study bundle systems from infancy, through the stage of maximal adult vigor, and into senescence. In such cases, the bundle again mirrors (or determines) the state of the output. For this reason, it is tempting to suggest cause-and-effect connections, and, in the case of the bundle, an hypothesis is presented linking bundle system to the central code responsible for the item of output behavior to which it appears temporally correlated.

Axon terminals

At the level of resolution provided by the light microscope, Golgi methods have revealed a number of axonal terminal systems showing well-documented age-related changes. A particularly effective paradigm is provided by the sensory "relay" nuclei of the thalamus. We shall use the somatosensory fields comprising ventroposterolateral and ventroposteromedial nuclei—the ventrobasal complex—as our model. The system is particularly useful since at least four discrete patterns are provided by the four major specific afferent systems, exclusive of inputs from nonspecific systems of the brain stem and intralaminar thalamus (Ramón y Cajal, 1909–1911; Scheibel and Scheibel, 1966a,b, 1970a,b). The convergence and maturation of these systems provide a complex and highly idiomatic neuropil structure that remains, nonetheless, dissectable, and for which there exists correlative neurophysiological data (Andersen, Eccles, and Sears, 1964; Davies et al., 1976; Mountcastle, Poggio, and Werner, 1963; Purpura, 1969; Schlag and Waszak, 1971; Steriade and Wyzinski, 1972; Waszak, 1974). Our Golgi material does not include examples of the earliest appearance of such fibers at their terminal sites, but late prenatal mouse and rat materials facilitate reconstruction of most aspects of their early development.

It should be noted that young rodent material is particularly useful for studying the development of axonal patterns, principally because of the small brain size. Favorably oriented and impregnated tissue sections of 150–200 μm may include 15–20% of the total thickness of newborn mouse ventrobasal complex and, frequently, the entire length of tissue specimen from cortex through upper brain stem. Under such conditions, it may be possible to describe the complete course and structure of a single fiber and its terminal neuropil. More fragmentary data from larger mammals, including cat and monkey, indicate that within limits, the rodent-derived material provides a reliable model of developing mammalian thalamus. Such larger animals as the cat are more useful in the description of cell types, dendrite patterns, and such complex dendrite formations as bundles. In particular, the ontogenesis of local circuit or short-axon cells is easier to follow in these forms. In fact, we have had some difficulty in recognizing such cells in the rodent and have, on occasion, raised the question of whether the mouse has significant representation of these small neurons (Scheibel and Scheibel, 1966).

Ascending lemniscal afferents are present in the late postnatal period (5–7 days before term), bearing small calyxes or exaggerated growth-cone-like structures (Figure 1, nb). Small pseudopod-like extensions rapidly lengthen in the perinatal period into a number of short-axon stalks that form primitive nests around the somata of developing thalamic neurons. These still-primitive, bushy terminals increase in complexity along with the postsynaptic dendritic domain in a manner reminiscent of the coeval growth of cerebellar climbing fibers and Purkinje-cell dendrites (Ramón y Cajal, 1909–1911). The full expression of this afferent sensory arbor in rat and mouse

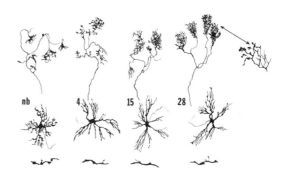

FIGURE 1 Development and maturation of components of the ventrobasal nucleus in the newborn (nb), 4-, 15-, and 28-day-old rat. The upper series of drawings illustrates development of the lemniscal afferent terminal, starting with calyxlike structures closely applied to the cell bodies of immature thalamocortical neurons. There is progressive division of the terminal filaments producing recognizable bushy arbors by day 15. Clusters of nodules later develop on these terminal branchlets (inset drawing, right); apparently it is those small terminal structures that participate in the formation of synaptic glomeruli. The middle and lower series outline the parallel maturation of the thalamocortical neuron and the development of dendritic spinelike extensions or excrescences. Drawings based on Golgi preparations. (From Scheibel, Davies, and Scheibel, 1976.)

seems to lag somewhat behind the pattern in the young kitten, where such arbors are already quite dense and nearer maturity at birth. The small terminal clusters of nodules, which are now known to characterize the individual terminal axon branches of each arbor (Szentágothai, 1963), and which undoubtedly take part in formation of thalamic glomeruli, do not appear in our preparations until 14–20 days after birth, and then only in rudimentary form (Figure 1, day 28).

In previous papers we have discussed a highly organized topographical arrangement of these terminal arbors (Scheibel and Scheibel, 1966), which produce a concentrically laminated onionskin motif spreading throughout the ventrobasal field from the ventrolateral hilar area. This apparent parcellation of the thalamic sensory-processing area by successive phalanxes of lemniscal terminals has been considered to be of significant substrate value in the development of the rather precise somatotopic organizational patterns that have been demonstrated here by physiological means (Mountcastle, 1961). It is interesting that study of routine cell stains of this nucleus (Nissl, Klüver, etc.) at this point reveals no bunching or clustering of thalamic neurons which would provide evidence of topographical or representational specificities. The arrival and distribution of the rostrally developing lemniscal afferents themselves may impose topographical specificity upon this thalamic-cell field. However, we have no evidence so far about the state of maturity of the thalamocortical projection itself, although we know it is present in rudimentary form in the immediately prenatal period. So we cannot yet decide whether the precise intrathalamic distribution of lemniscal afferents is the initial organizing influence or whether the thalamic-cell ensembles are already labeled for locus and mode specificities (Mountcastle, 1961) and selectively attract the appropriate terminal axons into their area.

Descending afferents have been described coming from cerebral cortex and nucleus reticularis thalami (Ramón y Cajal, 1909–1911; Minderhoud, 1971; Scheibel and Scheibel, 1966a,b; Scheibel, Scheibel, and Davies, 1972). At least two distinct fiber systems seem to be associated with corticothalamic elements, although their respective cortical origins have not yet been determined. Two major terminal patterns have been described (Ramón y Cajal, 1909–1911; Scheibel and Scheibel, 1966a): a system of large-caliber axons generating dense discoid terminal plexuses oriented perpendicular to the parent fiber (Figure 2, fiber *b*) and a somewhat finer fiber system terminating in diffuse, bifurcating fields, each of which covers an appreciable area of the thalamic sensory matrix (Figure 2, fiber *c*).

The discoid terminal plexus pattern is recognizable in the earliest stages (a few days before term); we have studied it because of the characteristic right-angled turn generated by the stem fiber. Secondary branching from this transverse preterminal is initially rudimentary (Figure 1, nb) but becomes increasingly complex, forming rather dense transverse plexuses by postnatal day 10 in the rat. Maturation of this

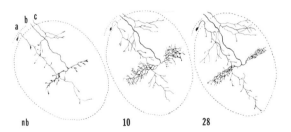

FIGURE 2 Development and maturation of terminal axonal neuropil generated by three descending thalamopetal afferent systems in the newborn (nb), 10-, and 28-day-old rat. Fiber *a* comes from the nucleus reticularis thalami and fibers *b* and *c* from cerebral cortex. All three are present in rudimentary fashion at birth. Note that the terminal elaborations of fiber *b* are somewhat more extensive at 10 days than at 28 days. Slightly schematicized drawings based on Golgi preparations. Rostral pole is at reader's upper left. (From Scheibel, Davies, and Scheibel, 1976.)

system is achieved at approximately postnatal day 28; and comparison with the earlier stage now indicates that there has occurred not only active growth through multiple-order rebranching, but also a dynamic process of reshaping. This reshaping appears to entail *selective loss* of many axonal branchlets to achieve the final morphological pattern. In Figure 1 note the obvious thinning of the transverse neuropil segment or disc between postnatal days 10 and 28.

The second fiber generates a diffuse bifurcating plexus covering appreciable amounts of the thalamic sensory matrix. In the young but mature mouse, a single terminal field appears to envelope as much as 25–35% of the area of the ventrobasal complex. We have not yet attempted quantitative studies of three-dimensional reconstructions of the nucleus, however. As maturation proceeds, the rather formless terminal system of each element gradually expands during the first two weeks of extrauterine life to form the characteristic conical field that appears to "stack" along the rostrocaudal axis of the nucleus with others of its kind.

The caudally directed axons of the nucleus reticularis thalami are identifiable at birth by thin, long, relatively straight projections and the occasional short collaterals that issue from each parent fiber throughout the thalamic ventral complex of nuclei (Figure 2, fiber *a*). Judging from the extent of these branches and the growth cones on their tips, it seems unlikely that they have established significant numbers of synaptic connections with the postsynaptic ensemble at this time. In the 12–15-day-old kitten and in the 7–10-day-old rat, these fibers seem more mature. They ordinarily terminate in small bouton clusters on the receptive postsynaptic neurons, which may be the thalamocortical projection cells (Figure 3). We have suggested that they bear a significant relationship to the genesis of thalamic slow waves (Scheibel, Davies, and Scheibel, 1973), and recent electrophysiological evidence appears to provide support for this notion (Yingling and Skinner, 1977).

The studies so far cited indicate a progressive growth and maturation in presynaptic elements during the first 2–4 weeks of postnatal life in small laboratory animals. In addition, there is evidence of structural shaping and a loss of portions of the axonal neuropil during maturation; this is particularly noticeable in the thinning of the terminal fields of one species of corticothalamic axons, which are progressively reshaped from transversely oriented bushes into much thinner—and denser—discoid plexuses. We infer that such changes decrease the pool of postsynaptic candidate elements for any one presynaptic

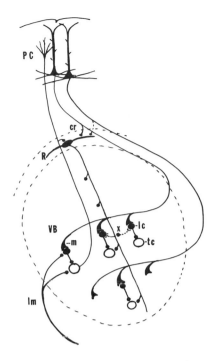

FIGURE 3 Simplified schematic drawing of some connections between the ventrobasal nucleus (VB) of the thalamus and pericruciate cortex (PC). Medial lemniscus fibers (lm) terminate on both thalamocortical (TC) and local circuit (lc) interneurons. Thalamocortical projection cells send axons through the nucleus reticularis thalami (R), giving off collaterals en route to cortex. Caudal projections of cortical pyramids, after sending collaterals (cr) to reticularis cells, terminate via their specialized mossy tuftlike terminals (m) on thalamic local circuit neurons. These synapse, in turn, with thalamocortical cells and may also be linked to each other by small axonless cells (x). Descending projections from nucleus reticularis cells establish contacts with linear arrays of thalamocortical neurons. (From Scheibel, Scheibel, and Davies, 1972.)

fiber and increase the effective density of synaptic interaction loci for those remaining within the pool.

Another interesting aspect to the sequence of maturation of thalamic neuropil has emerged from our studies. The entire roster of postsynaptic and intranuclear components mature somewhat later than the presynaptic components we have been describing. Dendrite systems of thalamic neurons, both projection and local circuit cells, and particularly the specialized structures on their surfaces such as dendritic excrescences, are among the last components to achieve full growth. As a matter of fact, an entire species of small neurons recently described in adult thalami—the axonless cell (Scheibel, Davies, and Scheibel, 1972)—has not been seen at all in tissue sampled during the first 4–5 weeks of postnatal life. From these observations we draw the tentative con-

clusion that structures imposing extranuclear control upon thalamic somatosensory operations become functional—or at least reach their fullest expression—earlier than intrinsic systems. This may provide the opportunity for thalamopetal influx from both "above" and "below" to help shape the final organizational pattern of thalamic neuropil. A number of physiological studies over the past decade have explored the effects of sensory input, or its deprivation, on the functional characteristics of receptive neuropil elements, especially in the visual system (Hubel and Wiesel, 1970; Blakemore, 1974). The results underline the need for afferent sensory barrage in later stages of maturation of the neuropil systems involved in information processing.

Dendrite bundles

Only in the last decade have we become aware that during maturation of the nervous system dendrites can arrange, or rearrange, themselves in very close associations called *bundles*. Because of the dramatic physiological implications of such structural associations, it seems remarkable that the phenomenon had not previously been noted in more detail. Ramón y Cajal (1909–1911) illustrates a bundle-like formation among the basilar shafts of large Meynert pyramids in the visual cortex of a 15-day-old child (see his Figure 388, p. 610, vol. 2). His textual description is appropriate, if brief: "Ces prolongements [the basilar dendrites] se ramifient en cours de route et forment ainsi des faisceaux presque horizontaux. En allant à la rencontre les uns des autres, ces faisceaux, venus de cellules plus ou moins distantes, s'enchevêtrent et constituent alors un *plexus dendritique* touffu d'expansions plus ou moins parallèles."

In 1953 Barron called attention to an earlier structural study by Laruelle (1937) of longitudinally sectioned rabbit spinal cord in which dendrites were described as "absolutely interwoven." At about the same time as our own first studies (Scheibel and Scheibel, 1970a), Marsh, Matlovsky, and Stromberg (1971) published a brief communication describing the apparent existence of dendrite bundles in Nissl preparations of spinal cord. Somewhat later, Fleischauer, Petsche, and Wittkowski (1972) described bundle formations among the apical dendrites of the neocortex, while Matthews, Willis, and Williams (1971) confirmed our initial Golgi-based spinal-cord study with the electron microscope. Thus there can be little doubt of the existence of the structural complex. However, its mode of development and functional significance raise provocative questions that may have significant implications for CNS function as a whole. We shall consider them in three loci: spinal cord, olfactory bulb, and motor cortex.

THE SPINAL CORD   Our initial observations were based on Golgi-stained, longitudinally sectioned (horizontal) slabs of lumbosacral spinal cord from perinatal kittens, adolescent (4–5-month) cats, adult cats, and one adult monkey. Although we found that there was already a general tendency for longitudinal arrangement of some motoneuronal dendrites in the very late fetal cord, there was little evidence of dendrite bundling until at least the end of the second week of postnatal life; nor was the bundle fully developed until the fourth month (Figure 4).

The organization of these bundles is of special interest. It has been well known since the studies of Romanes (1964) that ventral-horn motoneurons are

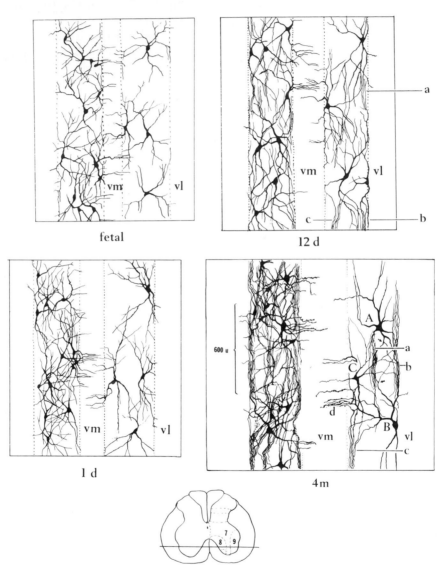

fetal

12 d

1 d

4 m

FIGURE 4   Drawings of horizontal sections through feline ventral horn showing developing of motoneuron dendrites and dendrite bundles. In fetal cord, dendrites are essentially radiative. At postnatal day 1, the beginnings of sagittal orientation are visible. At 12 days, sagittal orientation is well advanced, and bundle complexes are just beginning to form at a, b, and c. At four months, the motoneuron system is essentially mature, rostrocaudal orientation of dendrites is predominant, and dendrite bundles at a, b, and c are well developed and project along the cord for several hundred millimicrons. Neurons A, B, and C each contribute dendrites to several bundles. (Other abbreviations: vm, ventromedial white matter; vl, ventrolateral white matter; d, small bundle of commissural dendrites, which can sometimes be seen as early as the first postnatal day.) Inset diagram shows plane of section and location of relevant spinal laminae. Drawn from Golgi preparations (× 100). (From Scheibel and Scheibel, 1970c.)

386   ARNOLD B. SCHEIBEL

organized in longitudinal ensembles segregated by function—that is, according to the muscle innervated. Furthermore, there is some degree of higher-order segregation of the cell columns themselves, based on whether the muscle innervated is a morphological flexor or extensor and whether it is located proximally or distally along the extremity (Balthasar, 1952; Romanes, 1946).

Dendritic shafts of these highly segregated neurons mingle extensively in the bundles, which may continue in recognizable form for several millimeters along the longitudinal axis of the spinal cord. Mingling seems to occur with high frequency among dendrites of neurons innervating several flexor (or extensor) elements that can operate as agonists and, even more interestingly, among processes from neurons innervating muscles whose actions nominally antagonize one another across a joint. Thus the dendrite bundle seems to bring together dendrite shafts from cells of heterogeneous origins whose functions are complementarily related in one way or another. Equally interesting is the fact that we have seldom seen evidence of dendrite-bundle formation among elements from neurons innervating a proximal and a distal muscle.

Each bundle may contain as few as three or four dendrites, or as many as 15–25. The diameter of each bundle may vary from 10 μm to 75 μm and its constitution changes constantly as dendrite branches join the bundle, leave it, or play out. In addition, a certain proportion of motor neuron dendrites (~20%) and, apparently, a majority of interneuronal processes seen in horizontal sections, do not enter the dendrite bundles at all.

Within individual bundles, the intervals between pairs of facing dendritic membranes may be very small, often averaging less than one micron for distances of several hundred microns. In many cases, the extraneuronal space between two or more dendrite shafts cannot be resolved with the light microscope. Our electron microscopy confirms intervals limited, in the case of the olfactory bulb for instance, to tens of angstroms in some cases, without any sign of interposed structures (Scheibel and Scheibel, 1975a). Glial leaves and synaptic terminals may be interposed among elements of the bundle; but in our experience, these structures, especially the latter, tend to be concentrated on the external dendritic surface, while the intrafascicular surfaces bear fewer formed elements that could interfere with the "tightness of fit" of the bundled shafts.

In our analysis of the development of dendrite bundles in the lumbosacral cord of the kitten, it rapidly became clear that their initial appearance paralleled the development of weight-bearing and stepping-walking phenomena in the limbs (Scheibel and Scheibel, 1970c). For approximately the first two weeks of postnatal life, the kitten uses its legs like the flippers of an aquatic mammal, making swimming or rowing motions, primarily through the use of the most proximal muscle masses, while the body remains on the ground. At about day 12–15, most kittens attempt to bring their legs under them to raise the weight of the body off the ground and commence stepping-walking movements. These motor capacities improve rapidly during the ensuing 3–4 weeks, and by the third or fourth postnatal month the young cat has achieved maximal motor control, especially during the period of social play. This appears to be the period of maximal dendrite-bundle growth, and electromyographic analysis of activity in a nominal agonist-antagonist pair such as the gastrocnemius and anterior tibial shows maturation of reciprocal activities during this period (Figure 5).

The unusual commingling of dendrites from motor neurons supplying functionally antagonistic muscle pairs and the maturation of the bundle systems coeval with that of weight-bearing, stepping, walking functions led us to speculate on the possible relation of one to the other. Sherrington (1910) suggested that each element of limb movement in a chain reflex such as walking served as stimulus to the next and that the relevant excitation was initiated at deep receptors in the limbs. However, Brown (1914) demonstrated that alternating activity of flexors and extensors could be elicited following deafferentation, which led him to postulate an intrinsic mechanism in spinal cord capable of controlling the alternating activities in stepping. Liddell and Sherrington (1924) subsequently conceived of the stretch reflex as an adjustment mechanism modulating a motor rhythm of central origin, similar to that of Brown. A contemporary version of this centrally programmed motor rhythm has been advanced by Lundberg (1969), who favors the interplay of paired half-centers in the generation of alternating sequences of flexors and extensors. Our own conceptions increasingly attribute to the dendrite bundle itself a significant role in the information-processing capacity of the spinal cord, particularly as the repository for certain stereotypic central programs, such as those responsible for reciprocal activity of leg-muscle pairs in stepping, walking, and weight-bearing.

One test of this notion immediately suggested itself. Although the newborn kitten shows little evidence of patterned control over leg muscle activities, especially

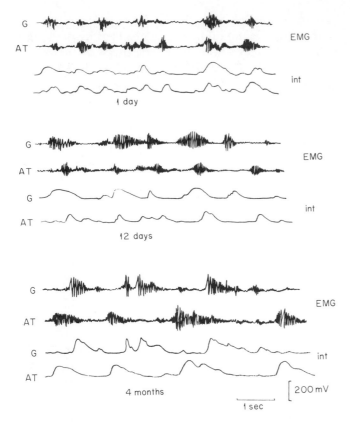

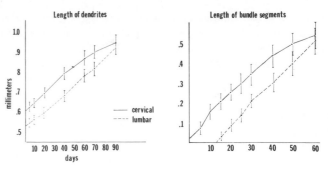

FIGURE 6 Graphs comparing the level of maturation of the dendrite systems in the ventral horns of cervical and lumbosacral cord during the first 2–3 months of life. *Left*: Development of average dendrite length during the first 90 days of life. At birth, the dendrites of the cervical region are approximately 15% longer than those of the lumbosacral region. By the end of the third month, the difference is no longer significant. *Right*: The development of motoneuron dendrite bundles, as evidenced by the length of bundle segments at various periods during the initial 60 days of life. At birth, bundle complexes averaging 30–40 millimicrons are seen in the cervical cord, but none are visible in lumbosacral cord until 12-14 days of age; the difference is no longer significant at about 50 days of age. The short vertical lines represent one standard deviation at each data point. (From Scheibel and Scheibel, 1971b.)

FIGURE 5 Electromyograms (EMG) from gastrocnemius (G) and anterior tibial (AT) muscles of kitten taken at 1 day, 12 days, and four months after birth. No reciprocal activity can be seen in the first series of traces; there is a suggestion of alternating sequences in the second series, and well-developed reciprocal patterning in the third series. The second pair of traces in each series is the integrate of the first pair. (From Scheibel and Scheibel, 1972.)

where weight-bearing and progression are involved, one item of peripheral, patterned motor activity appears available to it virtually at birth, or within the first day or two of postnatal life. This is the alternate treading motions of its two front legs used to help express milk from the maternal nipple. The obvious flexor-extensor sequencing necessitated in the production of this pattern suggested to us that if dendrite bundles were, in fact, involved in generating stereotyped sequential activities, dendrite-bundle complexes to support this precocious motor activity should be present in the cervical portion of the anterior horn considerably earlier than in the lumbosacral area.

Comparative study of the two zones in a number of kittens, ranging from immediately postnatal to several weeks of age, confirmed this notion. As indicated by Figure 6, at the time of birth dendrites of cervical motoneuron dendrites were on average 15% longer than those of the lumbosacral zone; the difference was no longer significant by the end of the third month. Of even greater interest, bundle groupings averaging 30–40 μm in length were seen at birth throughout the cervical anterior horn, whereas none were visible in the lumbosacral area until postnatal day 12–14. These differences ceased to be significant after postnatal day 50. At the time when the first evidence of lumbosacral bundle formations could be seen (end of the second postnatal week), cervical dendrite bundles already showed average lengths of 150–200 μm (Scheibel and Scheibel, 1971b). In this regard, it should be recalled that development in the prenatal organism advances in the rostrocaudal direction along the long axis of the body and from proximal to distal regions (Coghill, 1943; Windle and Griffin, 1931). Further evidence is found in the studies of Langworthy (1929), who described more precocious development rostrally in kittens, and by Fox, Irman, and Himwich (1967), who showed that myelinization is somewhat more advanced in the cervical region at birth.

The apparent temporal relationship between the appearance of dendrite bundles in an area and the development of a specific item of behavior characteristic of that area is suggestive, but at this point it was only inferential. More examples were clearly necessary if we were to further define the relationship we had sketched out. A number of bundle systems were subsequently described throughout the brain stem, diencephalon, and cortex; we shall cite two of these for their didactic value.

THE OLFACTORY BULB   The secondary dendrites of the mitral cells of the olfactory bulb provide another example of a dendrite-bundle system that is present at birth. The mitral cells themselves are essentially pyramids, as the olfactory bulb is basically displaced or emigrated telencephalon; as such, it provides a small, semidetached model of primitive cortex. Further, it provides a teloreceptive function which, unlike most others, is already apparently in operational condition at birth and may, in fact, be absolutely necessary if the newborn mammal is to institute nipple-searching activities and begin to suckle.

Our own interest in this system was stimulated by the dramatic difference in dendrite status between the olfactory mitral cells and the similarly derived pyramid cells of adjacent cerebral cortex. As Figure 7 indicates, although mitral elements of the newborn rat (A) are undeniably immature, their primary or apical shafts show moderate development and the secondary (basilar) dendrites are already long and densely intertwined in bundle formations very similar to those of the mature 100-day-old animal (B). In comparison, the typical cortical pyramid is just beginning to develop a basilar fringe, which will take at least two months to achieve full maturity. We have stressed the enormous length of these secondary mitral dendrites (Scheibel and Scheibel, 1975a) and their tendency toward directional polarization; they run round the olfactory bulb in the sagittal, but not in the coronal plane.

Figure 8 emphasizes the rather large number of secondary dendrite shafts generated by three typical mitral cells. Clearly, the dendrite plexus actually formed by shafts from all of the mitral cells in this tiny area alone (note the unstained somata in the layer of mitral cells, a) must be incomparably denser and more complex. The physical approximation achieved by many of these dendritic processes for appreciable portions of their trajectory is at least suggested by the electron micrograph in Figure 9. As in spinal-cord dendrite membranes, these membrane segments may parallel each other for appreciable distances (20–100 μm), with separation intervals of only 20–100 Å and without interposed structures or membranes, except for small amounts of a fine granular

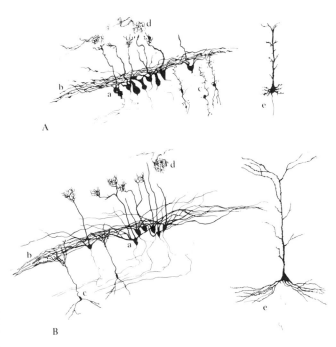

FIGURE 7   Contrast in appearance between olfactory bulb structure in newborn (A) and 100-day-old (B) rat. Note that the secondary (basilar, b) dendrites of mitral cells (a) are well developed at birth; those of neocortical pyramids (e) are in earliest stages of formation. Granule cells (c) are also present at birth but are only partially developed. Drawn from sections stained by rapid Golgi modification. Original magnification × 125. (From Scheibel and Scheibel, 1975a.)

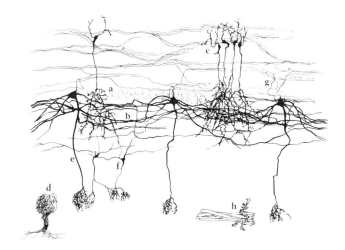

FIGURE 8   Components contributing to the synaptic organization of the olfactory bulb in adult rat. Note the complexity of the dendrite-bundle system (b) generated by only three neurons of the mitral-cell layer (a) and the apparent partition of this system by spiny dendrites of the granule cells (c). Enlargement at h shows detail of this interaction. (Other abbreviations: d, olfactory glomerulus; e, primary dendrite of mitral cell; f, small tufted cell; g, masses of centripetal axons of mitral cells.) Drawn from rapid Golgi preparation. Original magnification × 200. (From Scheibel and Scheibel, 1975a.)

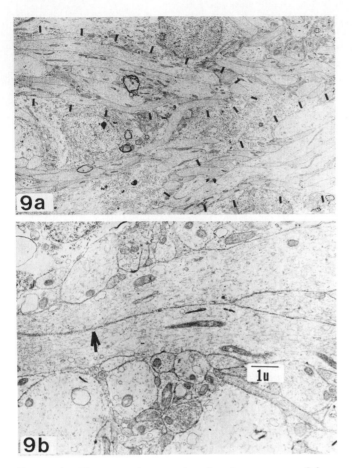

FIGURE 9 Electron micrographs of various aspects of dendrite-bundle structure in the external plexiform layer of the olfactory bulb. (a) Section cut almost parallel to parts of two dendrite bundles whose approximate outlines are delimited by the series of small perpendicular bars. Segments of dendrites can be seen entering or leaving the upper bundle. (b) Section cut almost longitudinally through part of a dendrite bundle, showing long stretches of close approximation between facing membranes of adjacent dendrites. These micrographs of nemestrine monkey bulb were obtained in collaboration with Dr. U. Tomiyasu. Original magnifications: a, × 1,800; b, × 8,400.

material. These enormous skeins of dendritic tissue are partitioned by the spine-rich dendrites of the deeper-lying granule-cell system, which, as Shepherd (1967) has shown, appear to provide a recurrent type of dendrodendritic inhibitory control. But we have also suggested (Scheibel and Scheibel, 1975a) that this synaptic system, whose effects may be generated along a patch of dendritic membrane several hundred to several thousand microns distant from the mitral-cell body, may generate consequences via local field gradients—both electrical and chemical— beyond that achieved through manipulation of mem-

brane thresholds by means of synaptic potentials alone.

We have provisionally related the initial output of the lumbosacral dendrite-bundle complexes to standing-stepping-walking operations and the more precocious cervical complexes to forepaw treading in the suckling neonate. Can we point to an output equally closely related to the dendrite-bundle systems of the olfactory bulb, which is far from any obvious motor outflow? Indeed, its central connections do seem to bypass those thalamocortical channels familiar to other input systems in which sensory data must be processed prior to the sculpting of a response. Most common laboratory mammals are blind at birth and essentially incapable of significant weight-bearing and walking activity. Yet almost immediately after birth, they unerringly seek out the maternal nipple and repeatedly return to it. Although somesthetic systems of the snout and face may be involved to some extent, we know that the thalamocortical systems into which they feed are very immature. Dendrites in the ventrobasal complex are in early stages of development (Scheibel, Davies, and Scheibel, 1976). In fact, microelectrode analysis of unit activity in various thalamic sites in kittens reveals little or no evidence of sensory responsiveness or spontaneous activity before the third to fifth day of life (Davies et al., 1976). Sensorimotor zones of the cerebral neocortex are equally immature and in the earliest stages of horizontal dendrite proliferation (Scheibel and Scheibel, 1971c).

We believe that rudimentary recognition codes for nipple-milk odors are already laid down at birth along the mitral secondary dendrite bundles and that these genetically induced trace systems are immediately reinforced with initiation of suckling. Progressive modulation and refinement of the code occurs as nipple preference develops in each neonate. This may also be the period when the surprisingly powerful centrifugal input from the contralateral olfactory nucleus (Lohman and Mentink, 1969; Powell, Cowan, and Raisman, 1965; Valverde, 1964) is of most use, enabling the blind neonate to compute the difference between his location and that of the target nipple.

These proposed recognition codes in mitral dendrite bundles serve as input governing approach or retreat behavior depending on odor cues. With most primary and secondary olfactory cortical systems still in an immature state, we believe that mitral output impinges directly upon old motor systems of the mesencephalic tegmentum via projections through mediodorsal thalamus, habenular nucleus, and the hypothalamus (MacLeod, 1971). These "sensorimotor" connections may operate reflexly in the same sense that frog retina and tectum automatically select appropriate output responses based on the computed size of an impinging visual stimulus (Lettvin et al., 1959). With subsequent growth of the suckling and maturation of visual and somesthetic systems, these archaic links between olfactory input and old motor systems are superseded, but they are never entirely lost. Maturation brings with it a wider repertoire of olfactory experience and full development of thalamocortical processing systems. However, the earlier-appearing connections through amygdala, basal forebrain, and hypothalamus undoubtedly continue to function as a significant part of the appetitive-response mechanism of the macrosmatic animal that can still operate without significant thalamocortical participation (Scheibel and Scheibel, 1975a).

GIANT PYRAMIDS OF THE MOTOR CORTEX The sequence of growth, maturation, and senescence of cortical pyramidal cells has provided a useful model, not only for relating the parallel development of structure to waxing function, but also for the equally correlatable waning of both during the period of senescence. Among the tens of millions of pyramids undoubtedly associated with cortical "motor output" functions, the giant pyramidal cells of Betz may be the test objects of choice, not only because of the ease with which they can be identified at all stages of their development and their vigorously stated anatomical configuration (Ramón y Cajal, 1909–1911; Scheibel and Scheibel, 1977), but also because of their very limited numbers (approximately 40,000 per hemisphere according to Lassek, 1954) and apparently selective vulnerability to the processes of aging and senescence (Scheibel, Tomiyasu, and Scheibel, 1977).

In previous studies we have described the maturation of cortical pyramids in detail (Scheibel and Scheibel, 1971c). The apical shafts are the earliest elements of the dendritic domain to appear (Figure 10) and are followed, usually in the perinatal period, by the development of horizontal elements, which include the terminal arches and oblique branches of the apical shaft and the basilar dendrite system. Complete maturity of the cortical pyramid is apparently reached when the basilar dendrite system achieves its fullest expression (Figure 11); and it is this system that first shows degenerative changes with the onset of senescence.

The giant pyramids of Betz are characterized by the enormous development of their basilar dendrite

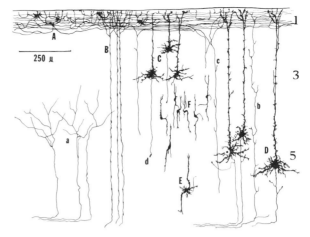

FIGURE 10 Simplified drawing of immature cortex (1-day-old kitten) showing the almost complete lack of horizontal dendrite systems and the well-developed horizontal axon system in layer 1. (A) Cajal-Retzius cells and horizontal fibers of layer 1. (B) Fibers from ependymal glial cells. (C) Developing third-layer pyramids. (D) Developing fifth-layer pyramids. (E) Immature bipolar spindle cell. (F) Fourth-layer granule cells at immature bipolar stage. Also shown, a, a specific thalamocortical afferent; b, a nonspecific afferent; c, an ascending collateral of unknown origin; d, a pyramidal-cell axon with growth cone. (From Scheibel and Scheibel, 1975b.)

skirt and by the dramatic bundle systems that these elements form with those of nearby Betz elements and also—particularly in subhuman primates and man—with those of pyramidal cells throughout the fifth and sixth cortical layers (Figure 12). In fact, the dendrodendritic relations into which these neurons enter are, with the possible exception of the very similar Meynert pyramids of visual area 17, apparently unique to the telencephalon.

In our study of Betz-cell systems in laboratory animals, we showed how the extraordinary length of the basilar dendrite systems (1–2 mm) enabled them to project well beyond the confines of the individual cortical cell column as presently understood (Asanuma and Rosen, 1972; Mountcastle, 1957). Despite some tendency toward clumping of these elements in the cat and apparently in man (Lassek, 1954), giant pyramidal cells are located at average intervals of 240 ± 54 μm in cat pericruciate cortex (Scheibel et al., 1974), thereby providing a considerable degree of overlap in the extension of these shafts. It is this overlap that enables the fifth layer of pericruciate cortex in the cat, and portions of the motor strip in man, to generate a veritable shelf of interlacing dendrite shafts approximately parallel to the pial surface and perpendicular to the apical shafts (Figure 12). Sections cut tangentially through cortex reveal

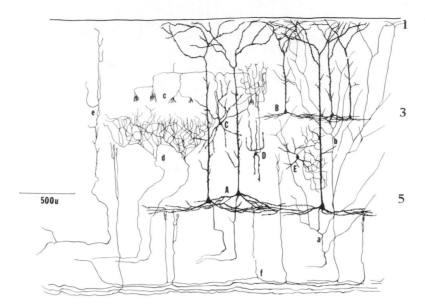

FIGURE 11 Simplified and somewhat schematicized drawing of mature cortex, showing full development of horizontal dendrite systems and loss of the horizontal fiber system in the first layer. (A) Basilar shaft systems of fifth-layer pyramids. (B) Basilar dendrites of third-layer pyramids. (C) Fourth-layer, stellate-cell-generating axon with basket-type terminals. (D) Lower fourth-layer stellate cell with ascending axon. (E) Lower fourth-layer stellate cell with very localized axon system. Also shown: a, a pyramidal axon with recurrent collaterals; b, the axon system of a third-layer pyramid; c, basket terminals of a stellate cell; d, specific thalamocortical afferents; e, nonspecific thalamocortical afferent; f, ascending collaterals from association fibers in subcortical white matter. No attempt has been made to present the full diversity of cell types and the complexity of the resulting neuropil. (From Scheibel and Scheibel, 1975b.)

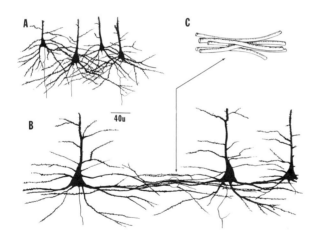

FIGURE 12 Details of dendritic organization in precruciate gyrus of the adult cat. (A) Medium-sized pyramids of layer 3 show the generally oblique course of most basilar dendrites. (B) Three giant pyramidal cells of Betz from the fifth layer, showing the horizontal trajectory of the long basilar dendrites and their organization in bundles. (C) An enlargement of the circled field in B, showing details of dendrite-bundle organization. Drawn from several Golgi sections through precruciate gyrus of the adult cat. A and B were drawn to the same scale. (From Scheibel et al., 1974.)

densely interlaced skeins of dendrites formed principally by the basilar shafts of giant pyramids radiating out from each parent cell body, entering and emerging from bundle systems for hundreds—and sometimes thousands—of microns along their courses. Visually, these generate a coarse net of ever-changing dendritic makeup, providing potential channels for communicative interaction that would seem, on intuitive grounds at least, to be enormous.

In human cortex, the Betz-cell systems are even more complex. The number of major basilar shafts emerging from each cell body is so extensive that they may cover the entire circumference of the cell body (Figure 13), and we have suggested the term *circumferential* as more appropriate than *basilar* in these cases (Scheibel and Scheibel, 1977). As with laboratory animals, these massive horizontal dendrite systems are not present in the newborn infant, but they begin to develop rapidly as the organism attempts to bear weight on its extremities and to initiate standing-walking-playing activities. Differential cell counts by Lassek (1954) show that 75% of human Betz cells are located in motor areas supplying the leg, 17.9% in the arm region, and only 6.6% in the

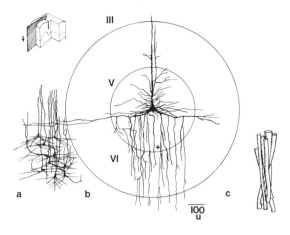

FIGURE 13 Drawing of one typical pattern generated by the circumferential dendrite domain of a human Betz cell. Here the most elaborate portion of the dendrite system, made up largely of secondary branches from the primary basilar components, descends through layer V into layer VI. The ensemble of fifth- and sixth-layer pyramids, shown at a, are actually located within the dendritic domain, b, centered on the +. Many of the apical dendrites of the pyramidal-cell ensemble appear to form bundle complexes, c, with the descending Betz-cell dendrites. Drawn from a Golgi section cut perpendicular to the surface. (From Scheibel and Scheibel, 1977.)

"head" area, despite the dedication of much more extensive cortical areas to head and arm than to leg. A positive correlation is thereby suggested between Betz elements and muscle mass or antigravity status, or both. The major responsibility for maintenance of antigravity tone in bipeds is, of course, localized to the lower extremities and back.

Antidromic studies indicate a division of pyramidal tract cells into two major groups on the basis of conduction velocity (Evarts, 1965; Takahashi, 1965; Oshima, 1969). A small group of rapidly conducting axons are phasically active during movement and precede EMG activity by 40–100 msec (Evarts, 1965, 1967). The great remaining mass of more slowly conducting pyramidal elements tends to be tonically active, with less dramatic changes in firing activity in either direction, no matter what the activity status at the level of motor output. The limited numbers of rapidly conducting elements are assumed to be the largest axons and are undoubtedly of Betz origin.

There is increasing evidence that the phasically programmed early output of Betz cells is selectively directed toward extensor inhibition and flexor enhancement (Lundberg and Voorhoeve, 1962) as an obligatory initial event in any patterned motor act superimposed on the background set of supportive,

antigravity tone. It seems probable that the rapid burst of early activity in the largest pyramidal-cell axons initiates partial lysis in supportive activities across weight-bearing joints immediately prior to the development of definitive motor patterns guided by the masses of surrounding pyramidal cells. The primary role of the Betz cell is, accordingly, conceived as preparative of the peripheral motor apparatus for the specific output program about to be implemented.

Seen from this perspective, the maturation of the great horizontal circumferential dendrite skirts and the development of bundles becomes a telencephalic prerequisite to acquisition of weight-bearing, stepping, and walking activities of the extremities and, in fact, any kind of motor activity that must be superimposed on a weight-bearing element. Studies of developing human infant cortex emphasize the dramatic growth of these horizontal systems between term and 24 months (Conel, 1939, 1959); and examination of appropriately impregnated sections document the rapid appearance and partial maturation of the dendrite-bundle systems in the periods between 18 and 24 months and between 36 and 48 months (Scheibel and Scheibel, unpublished data), when the child develops most of his initial locomotor skills. Our data are not complete, but we have reason to believe that horizontal dendrite systems and their bundle complexes continue to grow in length and complexity for the first 7–10 years of life and, under special instances of motor challenge, perhaps still longer.

It is also worth noting, in regard to the role of the horizontal dendritic complex, that in hooved animals, where the young must stand and follow the mother within a few hours of birth, the sensorimotor cortex appears to be remarkably mature at birth; it has completely formed horizontal and circumferential dendrite systems (Persson, 1973) and a moderately advanced horizontal dendrite-bundle system in layer V (Scheibel and Scheibel, unpublished data).

Study of the Betz cells has also provided us with the unique opportunity to follow the deterioration of an easily identifiable neuronal element whose limited total number is likely to make any appreciable loss functionally significant (Figure 14). This is further aided by the fact that the giant Betz pyramids appear especially vulnerable to aging processes (Scheibel, Tomiyasu, and Scheibel, 1977). As emphasized by Figure 15, our data from Golgi and ancillary methods indicate that by the eighth decade of life, 75% or more of all Betz cells are severely affected or de-

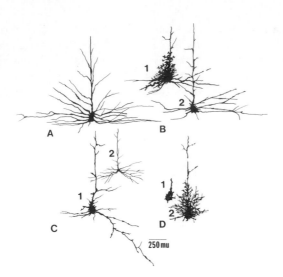

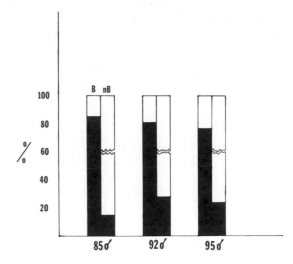

FIGURE 14 Drawings of progressive pathological changes in Betz cells in an 85-year-old man. (A) Early changes with irregular swelling of the cell body and dendrite shafts. (B1) Protoplasmic astrocyte surrounds swollen Betz cell, which has lost most of its circumferential dendrite system. (B2) Betz cell with moderately advanced changes, including loss of many circumferential dendrites (note stumps), dendritic swelling, etc. (C1) Cell with advanced changes showing large degenerating taproot dendrite. Almost all circumferential shafts are in late stages of destruction. (C2) Moderate-sized layer-V pyramid, which appears relatively intact. (D1) Adendritic Betz cell, showing final phase of deterioration. (D2) Betz cell completely ensheathed by transitional type of astrocyte. The dendrites appear in final stages of disruption. Based on Golgi variants drawn at original magnification of × 200. (From Scheibel, Tomiyasu, and Scheibel, 1977.)

FIGURE 15 Bar graph comparing the proportion of Betz (B) and non-Betz (nB) cell pathology, as seen in Golgi material in the motor strip area of three male patients aged 85, 92, and 95 years. In each case, the non-Betz bar is broken to indicate that the total number of cells in that category is much greater than the total number of Betz cells. Note that in each case 75% or more of the Betz elements show age-related changes, while less than 30% of the non-Betz cells are similarly affected.

stroyed, while less than 30% of the great surrounding pool of pyramidal cells appear affected. Since the former initially numbered only 40,000 or less per hemisphere and the latter are present in the tens of millions (Lassek, 1954), it is clear that losses suffered by the Betz-cell pool are statistically highly significant.

Just as the horizontal dendrite systems of pyramidal cells are the last to develop (Figure 10), so also are they the first to suffer in the aging process (Scheibel et al., 1975). This is particularly true in the case of Betz cells, where the dissolution of the great fifth-layer dendrite bundles with shortening and eventual disappearance of the circumferential shafts is an inevitable precursor to death of the entire Betz cell. Assuming that the dendrite bundle, as suggested above, serves as repository for certain types of central programs (Scheibel and Scheibel, 1973), selective attrition of this system should clearly affect the output sequences for which it has borne responsibility.

We have recently suggested that an important sequella to age-related Betz-cell pathology is an increas-

ing inability to relax antigravity tone across weight-bearing joints prior to patterned motor activity (Scheibel, Tomiyasu, and Scheibel, 1977). This may contribute to the well-known joint stiffness of the lower extremities and hips and the slowdown in motor performance and agility that is characteristic of the aged. In addition, the low-grade but persistent leg pains of which so many elderly persons complain may result in part from the unrelieved extensor tone that must increasingly be fought in all motor acts involving these members as Betz-cell function is lost. It has been usual in the past to attribute these developing infirmities to degenerative joint changes and to low-grade pathology in the basal ganglia. We believe that progressive deterioration and loss of the major dendrite bundles of the fifth layer of motor cortex, culminating in total loss of the parent Betz cells, frequently exceeding 75% by the eighth decade of life, is another significant causative factor.

Possible modes of bundle operation

The existence of dendrite bundles as morphological entities throughout the CNS can no longer be doubted. The sequence of maturational changes they follow, time-locked to the development of characteristic output patterns, is also well documented. The

394   ARNOLD B. SCHEIBEL

causal relationship we have inferred between the two is advanced on a basis that is, at present, largely intuitive. Yet the inference emerges from such time-honored postulates as (1) that structure and function are correlated and (2) that neuropil is the seat of information-processing in the nervous system and the ultimate wellspring of behavior. We have cited several cases illustrating the parallel development of dendrite bundles and particular species of behavior and one case in which an apparent decline in the efficacy of the latter coincides with deterioration of the former.

Several putative functional roles have been attributed to the dendrite bundle. These include (1) providing a substrate core to cortical cell columns (Peters and Walsh, 1972), (2) electrotonically summing events occurring in the associated elements (Fleischauer, Petsche, and Wittkowski, 1972), and (3) providing a site for central programs coding output patterns peculiar to the particular neural system (Scheibel and Scheibel, 1973, 1975a). The last of these has been based on the extended-membrane concept of Lehninger (1968) and Revel and Ito (1967). The dendrite bundle is conceived as providing a privileged space conducive to the development of ion-dependent molecular configurations that serve as representational analogs for output patterns.

The intrafascicular micromilieu is believed to be made up, at least in part, of extensions of the dendritic glycoprotein outer membranous zones—the glycocalyx (Rambourg and Leblond, 1967)—toward each other in an environment rich in hyaluronate and negatively charged polyelectrolyte (Katchalsky, 1969). Oligosaccharide and polysaccharide extensions of this greater membrane are capped by ganglioside–sialic acid moieties that compete for divalent cations, especially Ca^{2+} and Mg^{2+}, which are present throughout the extracellular compartment. These ions, particularly Ca^{2+}, exert a significant degree of control over the solubility and physicochemical characteristics of the acidic macromolecules (Tasaki, 1968). In addition, data exist to support the view that these ions affect the resistive impedance and total area of the extracellular compartment (Adey et al., 1969). We have suggested that cation-mediated linkages between adjacent oligosaccharide moieties composing this outer membrane may be stabilized in steric configurations, thereby encoding output patterns most characteristic of the neuronal system. The sheltered spaces between facing pairs or triads of dendritic membrane thus provide a unique setting where closely apposed systems of anionic polyelectrolytes and highly mobile divalent cations can develop a wide variety of tridimensional configurations

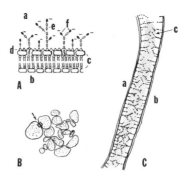

FIGURE 16 (A) Model of the extended membrane, modified slightly from Lehninger (1968). The neuronal membrane is conceived as a dynamic interface between the extraneuronal space (a) and the cellular cytoplasm (b). Its inner zone (c), a lipid-protein complex, bears a more diffuse, covalently linked outer zone composed of oligosaccharide chains (e) capped by negatively charged sialic-acid terminal moieties (f). (B) A cross section through a small dendrite bundle in cerebral cortex, based on tracing from electron micrographs. The arrow points to one interface between closely apposed dendrite membranes where no intervening membranes could be seen. (C) A hypothetical enlargement of the area between portions of the two dendrites, a and b, pictured in B. Oligosaccharide-sialic acid side chains are shown extending toward and interdigitating with each other, immersed in hyaluronate (shaded area) characterizing the extraneural space. (Modified slightly from Scheibel and Scheibel, 1973.)

spread longitudinally and representing an ordered sequence of neural output (Figure 16).

The entire system is dynamic and undoubtedly under continuous modulatory control of local processes, both electrical and chemical. While any of the cell-dendrite systems we have cited can serve as a model, we take as our final paradigm the Betz-cell system just described. We suggest that with each phasic volley that leaves the initial segment of a giant pyramid to propagate caudally, there are antidromically directed electrical gradients that, even in the absence of dendritic spike potentials (and none have so far been demonstrated in adult, healthy Betz cells), produce potent local, graded processes and field effects modulating threshold levels of polarization in adjacent neural elements (Schmitt, Dev, and Smith, 1976). Studies of Grinnell (1966) and Nelson (1966), among others, testify to the range and strength of such coupling potentials in the motoneuron pool of spinal cord. The unusual sensitivity of neuronal membrane to imposed voltage gradients up to ten orders of magnitude less than the potentials associated with spike-driven synaptic activity has been demonstrated by Adey (1975). Recently, Kreutzberg (1976) presented evidence of intradendritic transport and secretion of peptides and glycoprotein precursor moieties—another possible means by which large Betz-cell dendrites might affect their immediate surround, including the bundle systems of which they are a part.

Thus the Betz-cell pyramid can be conceived as serving two related functions whose mechanisms are time-locked but operationally very different. First, the characteristic early volley projected upon the large antigravity muscles conditions peripheral motor mechanisms for specific output sequences by producing an initial, partial lysis of antigravity tonus. Second, through their enormous dendritic systems, they generate field effects that are time-locked to the spike volley and that impinge on large numbers of adjacent pyramids and related dendrite systems. These electrical and chemical changes serve not only to synchronize the ensemble of Betz-cell volleys but also to condition large numbers of cortical pyramids that will be involved in ensuing motor sequences. The elaborate interrelationships generated in cortical neuropil by the dendritic elements of a comparative handful of giant Betz cells, the multiple mechanisms undoubtedly involved in their routine operation, and the profound functional changes that must obtain upon their deterioration and loss provide a useful model of neuropil in action. Possible patterns of partition and interaction within these cortical neuropil fields will be considered by John Szentágothai in the following chapter.

REFERENCES

ADEY, W. R., 1975. Evidence for cooperative mechanisms in the susceptibility of cerebral tissue to environmental and intrinsic electric fields. In *Functional Linkage in Biomolecular Systems*, F. O. Schmitt, D. M. Schneider, and D. M. Crothers, eds. New York: Raven Press, pp. 325–342.

ADEY, W. R., B. G. BYSTROM, A. COSTIN, R. T. KADO, and T. J. TARBY, 1969. Divalent cations in cerebral impedance and cell membrane morphology. *Exp. Neurol.* 23:29–50.

ANDERSEN, P., J. C. ECCLES, and T. A. SEARS, 1964. The ventrobasal complex of the thalamus: Types of cells, their responses and functional organization. *J. Physiol.* 174:370–399.

ASANUMA, H., and I. ROSEN, 1972. Topographical organization of cortical efferent zones projecting to distal forelimb muscles in the monkey. *Exp. Brain Res.* 14:243–256.

BALTHASAR, K., 1952. Morphologie der Spinalen-Tibialis-unde Peronaens-Kerne bei der Katze: Topographie, Architectonik, Axon- und Dentritenverlauf des Motoneurone und Zwischen-neurone in den Segmenten L6–S2. *Arch. Psychiatr. Nervenkr.* 188:345–378.

BARRON, D. H., 1953. In *The Spinal Cord*, J. L. Malcolm and J. A. B. Gray, eds. London: Churchill, p. 41.

BERITOFF, J. S., 1943. Transl. of the J. Bentashvili Physiologica Inst., no. 5, pp. XIV and 532. Tbilisi (Tiflis), Georgia, USSR (with abstracts in English). Quoted in C. J. Herrick, *The Brain of the Tiger Salamander*. Chicago: Univ. of Chicago Press, 1948.

BLAKEMORE, C., 1974. Developmental factors in the formation of feature extracting neurons. In *The Neurosciences: Third Study Program*. F. O. Schmitt and F. G. Worden, eds. Cambridge, MA: MIT Press, pp. 105–113.

BROWN, T. G., 1914. On the nature of the fundamental activity of the nervous centers together with an analysis of the conditioning of rhythmic activity in progression, and a theory of the evolution of function in the nervous system. *J. Physiol.* 48:18–46.

COGHILL, G. E., 1943. Flexion spasms and mass reflexes in relation to the ontogenetic development of behavior. *J. Comp. Neurol.* 79:463–486.

CONEL, J. L., 1939. *The Postnatal Development of the Human Cerebral Cortex.* vol. 1: *The Cortex of the Newborn.* Cambridge, MA: Harvard Univ. Press.

CONEL, J. L., 1959. *The Postnatal Development of the Human Cerebral Cortex.* vol. 6: *The Cortex of the Twenty-Four Month Infant.* Cambridge, MA: Harvard Univ. Press.

DAVIES, T. L., R. D. LINDSAY, M. E. SCHEIBEL, and A. B. SCHEIBEL, 1976. Ontogenetic development of somatosensory thalamus. II. Electrogenesis. *Exp. Neurol.* 52:13–29.

EVARTS, E. V., 1965. Relation of discharge frequency to conduction velocity in pyramidal tract neurons. *J. Neurophysiol.* 28:216–228.

EVARTS, E. V., 1967. Representation of movements and muscles by pyramidal tract neurons of the precentral motor cortex. In *Neurophysiological Basis of Normal and Abnormal Motor Activities*, M. D. Yahr and D. P. Purpura, eds. New York: Raven Press, pp. 215–253.

FERNÁNDEZ-MORÁN, H., 1954. The submicroscopic structure of nerve fibers. *Prog. Biophys.* 4:112–147.

FLEISCHAUER, K., H. PETSCHE, and W. WITTKOWSKI, 1972. Vertical bundles of dendrites in the neocortex. *Z. Anat. Entwichlungsgesch.* 136:213–223.

FOX, C. A., and J. W. BARNARD, 1957. A quantitative study of the Purkinje cell dendritic branchlets and their relationship to afferent fibers. *J. Anat.* 91:299–313.

FOX, M. W., O. R. IRMAN, and W. A. HIMWICH, 1967. The postnatal development of the spinal cord of the dog. *J. Comp. Neurol.* 130:233–240.

GLOBUS, A., and A. B. SCHEIBEL, 1967. Pattern and field in cortical structure: The rabbit. *J. Comp. Neurol.* 131:155–172.

GRINNELL, A. D., 1966. A study of the interaction between motoneurons in the frog spinal cord. *J. Physiol.* 182:612–648.

HERRICK, C. J., 1948. *The Brain of the Tiger Salamander*. Chicago: Univ. Chicago Press.

HILLMAN, D. E., 1969. Neuronal organization of the cerebellar cortex in amphibia and reptilia. In *Neurobiology of Cerebellar Evolution and Development*, R. Llinás, ed. Chicago: Inst. for Biomed. Res. AMA/ERF, pp. 279–325.

HUBEL, D. H., and T. N. WIESEL, 1970. The period of susceptibility to the physiological effects of unilateral eye closure in kittens. *J. Physiol.* 206:419–436.

KATCHALSKY, A., 1969. Polyelectrolytes and their biological interactions. In *Connective Tissue: Intercellular Macromole-*

cules (Proceedings of a symposium sponsored by the New York Heart Assoc.). Boston: Little, Brown, pp. 9–41.

KREUTZBERG, G. W., 1976. Transneuronal transfer: Inter- and extracellular pathways. *Neurosci. Res. Program Bull.* 14:275–293.

LANGWORTHY, O. R., 1929. A correlated study of the development of reflex action in fetal and young kittens and the myelinization of tracts in the nervous system. *Carnegie Inst. Contrib. Embryol.* 20:127–171.

LARUELLE, L., 1937. La structure de la moelle épinière en compes longitudinales. *Rev. Neurol.* 67:695–725.

LASSEK, A. M., 1954. *The Pyramidal Tract.* Springfield, IL: Charles C Thomas.

LEHNINGER, A. L., 1968. The neuronal membrane. *Proc. Natl. Acad. Sci. USA* 60:1055–1101.

LETTVIN, J. Y., H. R. MATURANA, H. R. McCULLOCH, and W. H. PITTS, 1959. What the frog's eye tells the frog's brain. *Proc. Inst. Radio Eng.* 47:1940–1951.

LIDDELL, E. G. T., and C. S. SHERRINGTON, 1924. Reflexes in response to stretch. *Proc. R. Soc. Lond.* B96:212–242.

LOHMAN, A. H. M., and G. M. MENTINK, 1969. The lateral olfactory tract, the anterior commissure and the cells of the olfactory bulb. *Brain Res.* 12:396–413.

LUNDBERG, A., 1969. *Reflex Control of Stepping.* Oslo: Universitetsforlaget, pp. 5–42.

LUNDBERG, A., and P. VOORHOEVE, 1962. Effects from the pyramidal tract on spinal reflex arcs. *Acta Physiol. Scand.* 56:201–219.

MacLEOD, P., 1971. Structure and function of higher olfactory centers. In *Handbook of Sensory Physiology,* 4/I. Berlin: Springer-Verlag, pp. 182–204.

MANNEN, H., 1960. "Noyau fermé" et "noyau ouvert." Contribution a l'étude cytoarchitectonique du tranc cérébral envisagée du point de vue du mode d'arborisation dendritique. *Arch. Ital. Biol.* 98:333–350.

MARSH, R. C., L. MATLOVSKY, and M. STROMBERG, 1971. Dendritic bundles exist. *Brain Res.* 33:273–277.

MATTHEWS, M. A., W. D. WILLIS, and V. WILLIAMS, 1971. Dendritic bundles in lamina IX of cat spinal cord: A possible source for electrical interaction between motoneurons. *Anat. Rec.* 171:313–328.

MINDERHOUD, J. M., 1971. An anatomical study of the efferent connections of the thalamic reticular nucleus. *Exp. Brain Res.* 12:435–446.

MOUNTCASTLE, V. B., 1957. Modality and topographic properties of single neurons of cat's somatosensory cortex. *J. Neurophysiol.* 20:408–434.

MOUNTCASTLE, V. B., 1961. Some functional properties of the somatic afferent system. In *Sensory Communication,* W. A. Rosenblith, ed. Cambridge, MA: MIT Press, pp. 403–436.

MOUNTCASTLE, V. B., G. F. POGGIO, and G. WERNER, 1963. The relations of thalamic cell response to peripheral stimuli varied over an intensive continuum. *J. Neurophysiol.* 26:807–834.

NELSON, D. G., 1966. Interaction between spinal motoneurons of the cat. *J. Neurophysiol.* 27:913–927.

OSHIMA, T., 1969. Studies of pyramidal tract cells. In *Basic Mechanisms of the Epilepsies,* H. Jasper et al., eds. Boston: Little, Brown, pp. 253–261.

PALADE, G. F., 1953. An electron microscope study of the mitochondrial structure. *J. Histochem. Cytochem.* 1:188–211.

PALAY, S. L., 1956. Synapses in the central nervous system. *J. Biophys. Biochem. Cytol.* 2 (Suppl.):193–202.

PEASE, D. C., 1955. Nodes of Ranvier in the central nervous system. *J. Comp. Neurol.* 103:11–15.

PERSSON, H. E., 1973. Development of somatosensory cortical functions. *Acta Physiol. Scand.* (suppl. 234): 5–64.

PETERS, A., and T. M. WALSH, 1972. A study of the organization of apical dendrites in the somatic sensory cortex of the rat. *J. Comp. Neurol.* 144:253–268.

POWELL, T. P. S., W. M. COWAN, and G. RAISMAN, 1965. The central olfactory connections. *J. Anat.* 99:791–813.

PURPURA, D. P., 1969. Interneuronal mechanisms in thalamically induced synchronizing and desynchronizing activities. In *The Interneuron,* M. A. B. Brazier, ed. Berkeley: Univ. California Press, pp. 467–496.

RAMBOURG, A., and C. P. LEBLOND, 1967. Electron microscope observations on the carbohydrate-rich cell coat present at the surface of cells in the rat. *J. Cell Biol.* 32:27–53.

RAMÓN Y CAJAL, S., 1909–1911. *Histologie du système nerveux de l'homme et des vertébrés,* 2 volumes. Paris: Maloine.

REVEL, J. P., and S. ITO, 1967. The surface components of the cell. In *The Specificity of Cell Surfaces,* B. D. Davis and L. Warren, eds. Englewood Cliffs, NJ: Prentice-Hall, pp. 211–234.

ROBERTSON, J. D., 1953. Ultrastructure of two invertebrate synapses. *Proc. Soc. Exp. Biol. Med.* 82:219–223.

ROMANES, G. J., 1946. Motor localization and the effects of nerve injury on the ventral horn cells of the cord. *J. Anat.* 80:117–131.

ROMANES, G. J., 1964. The motor pools of the spinal cord. In *Organization of the Spinal Cord,* J. C. Eccles and J. D. Schadé, eds. Amsterdam: Elsevier, pp. 93–119.

SCHEIBEL, M. E., T. L. DAVIES, R. D. LINDSAY, and A. B. SCHEIBEL, 1974. Basilar dendrite bundles of giant pyramidal cells. *Exp. Neurol.* 42:307–319.

SCHEIBEL, M. E., T. L. DAVIES, and A. B. SCHEIBEL, 1972. An unusual axonless cell in the thalamus of the adult cat. *Exp. Neurol.* 36:512–518.

SCHEIBEL, M. E., T. L. DAVIES, and A. B. SCHEIBEL, 1973. On thalamic substrates of cortical synchrony. *Neurology* 23:300–304.

SCHEIBEL, M. E., T. L. DAVIES, and A. B. SCHEIBEL, 1976. Ontogenetic development of somatosensory thalamus. I. Morphogenesis. *Exp. Neurol.* 51:392–406.

SCHEIBEL, M. E., R. D. LINDSAY, U. TOMIYASU, and A. B. SCHEIBEL, 1975. Progressive dendritic changes in aging human cortex. *Exp. Neurol.* 47:392–403.

SCHEIBEL, M. E., and A. B. SCHEIBEL, 1958. Structural substrates for integrative patterns in the brain stem reticular core. In *Reticular Formation of the Brain,* H. H. Jasper et al., eds. Boston: Little, Brown, pp. 31–55.

SCHEIBEL, M. E., and A. B. SCHEIBEL, 1966a. Patterns of organization in specific and nonspecific thalamic fields. In *The Thalamus,* D. Purpura and M. D. Yahr, eds. New York: Columbia Univ. Press, pp. 13–46.

SCHEIBEL, M. E., and A. B. SCHEIBEL, 1966b. The organization of the nucleus reticularis thalami: A Golgi study. *Brain Res.* 1:43–62.

SCHEIBEL, M. E., and A. B. SCHEIBEL, 1970a. Organization of spinal motoneuron dendrites in bundles. *Exp. Neurol.* 28:106 112.

SCHEIBEL, M. E., and A. B. SCHEIBEL, 1970b. Elementary

processes in selected thalamic and cortical subsystems—The structural substrates. In *The Neurosciences: Second Study Program*, F. O. Schmitt, ed. New York: Rockefeller Univ. Press, pp. 443–457.

SCHEIBEL, M. E., and A. B. SCHEIBEL, 1970c. Developmental relationship between spinal motoneuron dendrite bundles and patterned activity in the hind limb of cats. *Exp. Neurol.* 29:328–335.

SCHEIBEL, M. E., and A. B. SCHEIBEL, 1971a. Thalamus and body image—A model. *Biol. Psychiatry* 3:71–76.

SCHEIBEL, M. E., and A. B. SCHEIBEL, 1971b. Developmental relationship between spinal motoneuron dendrite bundles and patterned activity in the forelimb of cats. *Exp. Neurol.* 29:328–335.

SCHEIBEL, M. E., and A. B. SCHEIBEL, 1971c. Selected structural-functional correlations in postnatal brain. In *Brain Development and Behavior*, M. B. Sterman et al., eds. New York: Academic Press, pp. 1–21.

SCHEIBEL, M. E., and A. B. SCHEIBEL, 1972. Maturing neuronal subsystems: The dendrites of spinal motoneurons. In *Sleep and the Maturing Nervous System*, C. D. Clemente and D. P. Purpura, eds. New York: Academic Press, pp. 49–61.

SCHEIBEL, M. E., and A. B. SCHEIBEL, 1973. Dendrite bundles as sites for central programs: An hypothesis. *Int. J. Neurosci.* 6:195–202.

SCHEIBEL, M. E., and A. B. SCHEIBEL, 1975a. Dendrite bundles, central programs, and the olfactory bulb. *Brain Res.* 95:407–421.

SCHEIBEL, M. E., and A. B. SCHEIBEL, 1975b. Structural changes in the aging brain. In *Aging*, vol. 1, H. Brody et al., eds. New York: Raven Press, pp. 11–37.

SCHEIBEL, M. E., and A. B. SCHEIBEL, 1977. The dendritic structure of the human Betz cell. In *Architectonics of the Cerebral Cortex*, vol. 3, M. A. B. Brazier, ed. New York: Raven Press.

SCHEIBEL, M. E., A. B. SCHEIBEL, and T. L. DAVIES, 1972. Some substrates for centrifugal control over thalamic cell ensembles. In *Corticothalamic Projections and Sensorimotor Activities*, T. L. Frigyesi et al., eds. New York: Raven Press, pp. 131–156.

SCHEIBEL, M. E., U. TOMIYASU, and A. B. SCHEIBEL, 1977. The aging human Betz cell. *Exp. Neurol.* (in press).

SCHLAG, J., and M. WASZAK, 1971. Characteristics of unit responses in nucleus reticularis thalami. *Brain Res.* 21:286–288.

SCHMITT, F. O., P. DEV, and B. H. SMITH, 1976. Electrotonic processing of information by brain cells. *Science* 193:114–120.

SHEPHERD, G. M., 1967. The olfactory bulb as a simple cortical system: Experimental analysis and functional implications. In *The Neurosciences: Second Study Program*, F. O. Schmitt, ed. New York: Rockefeller Univ. Press, pp. 539–552.

SHERRINGTON, C. S., 1910. Flexion-reflex of the limb, crossed extension reflex, and reflex stepping and standing. *J. Physiol.* 40:28–121.

STERIADE, M., and P. WYZINSKI, 1972. Cortically elicited activities in thalamic reticularis neurons. *Brain Res.* 42:514–520.

SZENTÁGOTHAI, J., 1963. The structure of the synapse in the lateral geniculate body. *Acta Anat.* 55:166–185.

SZENTÁGOTHAI, J., 1967. Models of specific neuron arrays in thalamic relay nuclei. *Acta Morphol. Acad. Sci. Hung.* 15:113–124.

SZENTÁGOTHAI, J., 1971. Some geometrical aspects of neocortical neuropil. *Acta Biol. Acad. Sci. Hung.* 22:107–124.

SZENTÁGOTHAI, J., 1972. The basic neuronal circuit of the neocortex. In *Synchronization of EEG Activity in Epilepsies*, H. Petsche and M. A. B. Brazier, eds. Vienna, New York: Springer-Verlag, pp. 9–24.

TAKAHASHI, K., 1965. Slow and fast groups of pyramidal tract cells and their respective membrane properties. *J. Neurophysiol.* 28:908–924.

TASAKI, I., 1968. *Nerve Excitation: A Macromolecular Approach.* Springfield, IL: Charles C Thomas.

VALVERDE, F., 1964. The commissura anterior pars bulbaris. *Anat. Rec.* 148:406–407.

WASZAK, M., 1974. Firing patterns of neurons in the rostral and ventral part of the nucleus reticularis thalami during EEG spindles. *Exp. Neurol.* 43:38–59.

WINDLE, W. F., and A. M. GRIFFIN, 1931. Observations on embryonic and fetal movements of the cat. *J. Comp. Neurol.* 52:149–188.

YINGLING, C. D., and J. E. SKINNER, 1977. Gating of thalamic input to cerebral cortex by nucleus reticularis thalami. In *Cerebral Evoked Potentials in Man*, J. E. Desmedt, ed. Basel: S. Karger.

23 Local Neuron Circuits of the Neocortex

J. SZENTÁGOTHAI

ABSTRACT   The neocortex can be envisaged as a mosaic of *quasi*-discrete vertical columnar units of about 300 μm diameter, created primarily by arborization and specific convergence of corticocortical afferents. Another group of vertical columns, although not necessarily in register with the corticocortical columns, is caused by the termination of the specific subcortical afferents in flat tissue cylinders of similar diameters (in lamina IV) and a predominantly vertical relayed projection toward the upper and deeper layers of the cortex. The input to these large cortical columns appears to be rather widely distributed, and a selection mechanism for a much smaller group of output neurons has to be assumed for any combination of inputs. It is proposed that the selection mechanism is based on the interaction of local excitatory and inhibitory interneurons arranged in mutually interpenetrating space modules of definite sizes, shapes, and orientations. The diameters, mainly in the tangential direction, of these space modules may be one order of magnitude smaller than the main columns (~30 μm), and their combination may refine the selection of output neurons that can be activated in any given situation to small groups and even to individual cells. A substantial portion of the local interneurons and of the intracortical connectivity cannot be incorporated into this "selection concept" either because they are not neurons of the conventional histodynamically polarized type or because their intracortical spread is an order of magnitude larger (~3 mm) than the diameter of the main columns.

Introduction

THE NEOCORTEX must be considered a mosaic of relatively thin, vertically oriented, prismatic or columnar units that penetrate through the entire depth of the cortex. These prismatic or columnar units in both hemispheres are interconnected and have various subcortical targets and sources, according to some highly complex and specifically determined "wiring pattern." Anatomically, the size of the columnar units is determined primarily by the mode of arborization and convergence of corticocortical afferents. Strangely, the diameter of the columnar spaces established by the arborizations of the corticocortical fibers shows little variation from small rodents (rat) to monkey, and probably even up to man. More re-

markably still, the arborizations of individual corticocortical fibers (of both ipsilateral and callosal association) are within spaces of similar size and shape (Majorossy and Bodoky, 1977; Szentágothai, 1978) and have a tangential width of 100–300 μm. Only in the zonal layer of the cortex (lamina I) do the terminal branches of the ascending afferent fibers run for longer distances, so that a certain merging between neighboring columns is usually experienced.

In order to explain the characteristic columnar degeneration patterns (Grant, Landgren, and Silfvenius, 1975; Wolff and Záborszky, 1978) or the termination patterns defined by autoradiography of tritiated amino acids taken up by the nerve cells from intracortical injections (Goldman and Nauta, 1977), a convergence of the corticocortical afferents upon specific columnar spaces must be assumed. Otherwise there would be no explanation for the fact that the sizes and shapes of columns as defined by degeneration and autoradiography are virtually the same as those of individual axon arborizations. The individuality of the cortical column is strongly supported by the fact that the measured sizes of the columns are the same even if the cortical lesions or the injection sites of tritiated amino acids are relatively small (Grant, Landgren, and Silfvenius, 1975; Goldman and Nauta, 1977) or if a large part of the corpus callosum is transected (Wolff and Záborszky, 1978).

The termination of the specific subcortical afferents is less columnar than laminar; however, the horizontal spreads of both individual afferents (Szentágothai, 1973) and groups of afferents of common origin (Hubel and Wiesel, 1969; LeVay, Hubel, and Wiesel, 1975) are of the same order of magnitude, about 300 μm. It is therefore quite obvious that the organization into vertical columns of cells having similar receptive fields (Mountcastle, 1957; Hubel and Wiesel, 1959) can be explained only by an essentially vertical connectivity within the cortex that can transform the specific afferent input, delivered in laminar pattern, into the vertical columnar organization observed in the physiological experiments.

The crucial importance of the columns as the main local processors of the neocortex is also underscored by the quantitative data cited by Mountcastle (this

J. SZENTÁGOTHAI   1st Department of Anatomy, Semmelweis University Medical School, Tüzoltó u. 58, 1450 Budapest, Hungary

volume) on the relative stability, over a wide range of phylogeny, of cell numbers per surface area of the cortex (Rockel, Hiorns, and Powell, 1974). The basic similarity in neuron types and in their characteristic arborization patterns from mouse to man also seems to indicate that the neocortex must be visualized as a mosaic of "black boxes" of essentially similar build. The main change in mammalian phylogenesis is in the number and, consequently, in the complexity of interconnections between the individual black boxes.

This paper addresses itself primarily to the internal structure of the individual columns. The principal mental strategy to be pursued is determined by the fact that the size of the corticocortical columns—a diameter of 150–300 μm—makes them much too large to be really useful as processing units. We shall have to look for a selection mechanism that can choose from the total cell population under the relatively generalized input that apparently reaches each individual column (through the widely spread arborizations of the afferents) a small number of output cells in accordance with both the particular combination of active input channels and the antecedent activities of the column.

The main excitatory neuron chain

It has been implicit from the earliest studies of neural organization that neural centers are essentially devices for routing inputs toward outputs over chains of sequentially arranged neurons. Almost all textbooks from the various areas of neuroscience contain scores of diagrams based on this idea. Although the situation is much more complex in most of the higher centers, it is still worthwhile to try to gain insight into the relatively direct chains of neurons that might act as reflex arcs between afferents and efferents for the particular locus concerned. It is also evident that to understand the simplest reflex-arc neuron chains of the cortex, insight into the direct neuron chains connected with specific subcortical (sensory) afferents is desirable.

The complexity of neocortical structure, particularly the intricate intertwining of the dendrites of the many different cell types in any layer, make it extremely difficult to trace such neuron chains, even with the most advanced electron-microscopic degeneration or axoplasmic-transport methods. Although degeneration studies at the level of the electron microscope by Jones (1968), Colonnier and Rossignol (1969), and Jones and Powell (1970), followed by many others, made it clear that the specific subcortical afferents (at least in the primary sensory area) do establish synaptic contacts, usually with dendritic spines, this did not automatically solve the question of the immediate (monosynaptic) target cells of the specific afferents. First, the majority of synaptic sites in most parts of the cortex—particularly in lamina IV of the visual cortex (Garey and Powell, 1971)— are dendritic spines anyway. Second, degenerated synapses after lesion of the specific subcortical afferents have been found in contact with nonspine dendritic sites and also with dendrites that appear to be devoid of spines (Peters and Feldman, 1976). A random distribution of the terminals of the specific subcortical afferents in lamina IV, among all possible synaptic sites, would yield results not significantly different from what was actually found. These results thus do not yield much information on the most crucial question—whether specific subcortical afferents do or do not contact pyramidal cells, that is, cells that serve as immediate output elements.

This question is rather old. Indeed the assumption was already implicit in a diagram of Ramón y Cajal (1911, Figure 323) that showed specific afferents contacting the dendrites of pyramidal cells in the somatosensory area, the axons of which then returned to the main sensory (ventrobasal) nucleus of the thalamus. When the first workable degeneration methods for synapses became available, I tried—in the late thirties—to use them for the detection of the target cells of the visual afferents. The rationale at that time was that if the afferents associated themselves specifically with the apical dendrites or terminated selectively on cell bodies, this would be shown by the modified Bielschowsky stains I was then using (Schimert, 1938, 1939; Szentágothai-Schimert, 1941). As indicated by the Golgi pictures of specific afferents in Figure 1, and the parallel alignment of other terminal axons with pyramidal-cell apical dendrites, my assumption was not substantiated by the degeneration patterns of the specific sensory afferents, either with the early or with more recent degeneration methods.

A more direct approach, using sensory deprivation as an experimental model, seemed to indicate that the spines of the apical dendrites were in fact the main targets of the specific sensory input. This was thought to be reflected in a significant reduction of spines of the apical dendrites (Globus and Scheibel, 1966, 1967; Valverde, 1967) following sensory deprivation. But it was soon pointed out that the effect might be transneuronal, according to the experimental circumstances (Szentágothai, 1969). Nevertheless, the basal dendrites of the pyramidal cells and the side branches of the apical dendrites of deeper (lamina V

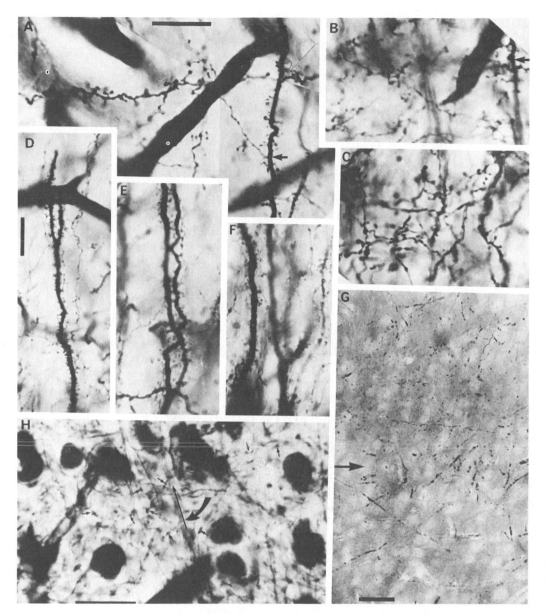

FIGURE 1   (A, B, C) Specific visual afferent terminations in cat area 17 in perfusion Golgi-Kopsch stain. (A) Large horizontal branch is at the border of laminae III and IV, where the ascending main branches turn characteristically back into lamina IV. (B, C) From the center of lamina IV; the main orientation of the terminal fibers is horizontal. No alignment to apical dendrites (arrows) is visible. (D, E, F) Typical parallel alignment of delicate terminal axons of local source to apical dendrites of pyramidal cells (rope-ladder phenomenon). (G) Nauta-Gygax stain of degener-ated visual afferents. Arrow indicates border between laminae IV and V, and the upper margin of the figure corresponds to the border between laminae III and IV. (H) Nonsuppressive stain of similar experiment from the late thirties. Degeneration fragments are indicated by small arrows and show that there is no alignment to the pale apical dendrite (curved arrow), the ascending direction of which is indicated by long slender arrow. All materials are from cat visual cortex; scale is the same (20 μm) for A, B, C, and H and for D, E, and F; it is 25 μm for G.

and VI) cells could not be excluded; and this was reflected in my earlier circuit diagrams (Figure 2-7 in Szentágothai, 1969).

This issue appeared in a radically different light when the presence of a large number of spiny inter-neurons in lamina IV of the primary sensory areas was recognized (Lund, 1973; Jones, 1975; Szentágo-thai, 1975). Such cells were known earlier (Ramón y Cajal, 1899) but were not clearly differentiated from other local interneurons or from pyramidal cells.

Many of these cells resemble ordinary pyramidal cells, but they are clearly distinguished by their axons, the main branch of which turns upwards and the few lower branches of which make direct synaptic contacts instead of issuing collaterals and becoming myelinated as true pyramidal neurons do. It was quite obvious that the axon-spine contacts found to degenerate following lesion of the subcortical relay nuclei could belong to these so-called spiny stellates of lamina IV. But this did not necessarily exclude the possibility of the pyramidal neurons also being the direct target neurons of the specific sensory afferents.

A new approach to this question was developed recently by Somogyi (1978), using reconstruction from a thin-section series of Golgi-stained neurons in the visual cortex following lesions of the lateral geniculate nucleus. Such studies are extremely laborious, and only bits of information are as yet available. Degenerated visual afferents established undoubted contacts with dendritic spines of both genuine pyramidal cells and of cells that on the basis of the standards mentioned in the preceding paragraph could be identified as spiny stellate cells (Figure 2A, B). Even more interestingly, the reconstructions from this section series of local axon arborizations showed that only about half of the Golgi-stained boutons established synapses with dendritic spines (Figure 2C); the other half had contacts with shafts of apparently nonspiny dendrites (Figure 2D). All of these contacts had postsynaptic membrane characteristics of excitatory synapses—the vesicles being invisible because of Golgi precipitates. No contacts of the degenerated specific afferents have as yet been ascertained on interneurons that might be assumed to be inhibitory. However, the fact that the axon branches of cells receiving specific afferent contacts did contact such a relatively large number of nonspiny dendrites indicates that inhibitory interneurons might be reached by specific afferents over one neuronal relay rather than monosynaptically. Unfortunately, the procedure of tracing three successive links of the cortical neuron chain, although most promising, is still in its infancy, so that nothing final can be said on various possibilities of direct neuron chains activated by the specific afferents. The issue is clear in only one respect: specific afferents directly contact at least some basal dendrites of pyramidal cells in lamina IV and deeper lamina III. The same could easily apply to the side branches of the apical dendrites of deeper-lamina (V, VI) pyramidal cells that are known to have very many side branches in lamina IV, where they might receive the specific afferents in abundance. The monosynaptic activation of subgennarian pyramidal cells (see

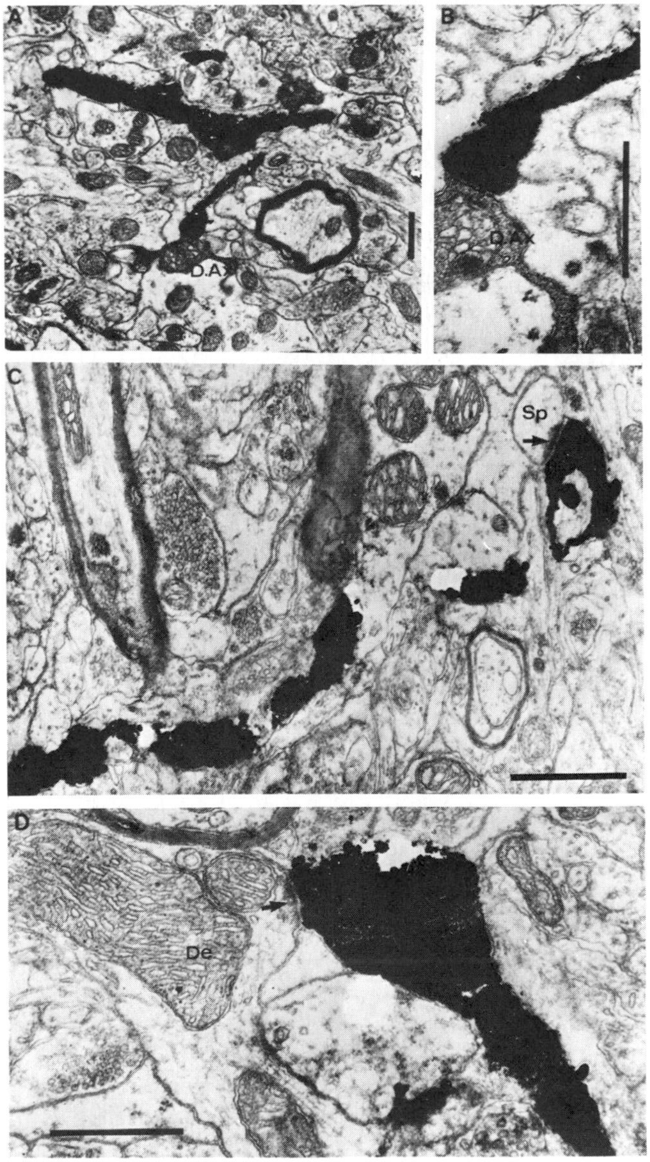

FIGURE 2 Identification of the synaptic contacts of a Golgi-stained spiny stellate neuron (of the type Sst shown in Figure 3) in an electron micrograph. (A) Spine belonging to Golgi-stained horizontal dendrite contacted by degenerated axon terminal (D.Ax), one day after lesion of lateral geniculate nucleus. (B) Detail of the contact in another section of the thin-section series. (C) A short side branch of the thin descending-axon collateral of the same cell terminates with small bouton on a dendritic spine (Sp). (D) Short sessile bulge of the same axon collateral contacts nonspiny part of dendrite (De). Although the internal structure of the axon terminals is not visible, due to the Golgi precipitate, the extended opacity under both postsynaptic membranes (arrows) is indicative of the AR (excitatory) nature of the contacts. Scale, 0.5 μm. (Material from the visual cortex of the rat, courtesy of P. Somogyi.)

Singer, this volume) by specific sensory afferents would clearly favor such a view.

Although this new information on the direct involvement of pyramidal neurons in the specific-afferent neuron chain opens the possibility of very short neuron circuits, relayed by a single synapse, it would be a mistake to overemphasize their significance, especially in view of what is known today both about the anatomical connections and about the method of impulse processing in the cortex. We know for certain that both spiny and nonspiny interneurons located in lamina IV have axonal arborizations that ascend into laminae III and II and descend into laminae V and VI. The strictly vertical orientation of the strands of terminal-axon branches given by these interneurons offer unique opportunities to establish large numbers of synapses between any given interneuron and apical dendrite(s) of one (or a few closely neighboring) pyramidal cell(s) (Szentágothai, 1969, 1973, 1975). Their synapses would thus resemble the mode of contact between a climbing fiber and its Purkinje cell, with probably the same consequence of a very powerful functional coupling. The similarities in general receptive-field properties of most cortical cells within a vertical column for inputs delivered largely in a single lamina (IV) would require the postulation of such a system of connections even if the corresponding anatomical data were not available.

The main excitatory neuron chain of the cortex for specific subcortical input must therefore be envisaged essentially in the form proposed ten years ago (Szentágothai, 1969, 1973, 1975) and summarized in Figure 3.

Inhibitory mechanisms

Attempts have been made in the past few years to identify putative inhibitory interneurons on the basis of two sets of criteria: (1) the fine-structural characteristics of the synaptic contacts; and (2) the local (short-axon) nature of the neurons.

First, however unlikely it seems, in view of the various types of known and/or assumed inhibitory and excitatory mediators, the vast majority of synapses in the CNS that can be assumed on a physiological basis to be excitatory have so-called asymmetric membrane specializations and a population of slightly larger spheroidal synaptic vesicles. Synapses that can be assumed on a physiological basis to be inhibitory have a more symmetric membrane attachment and a population of somewhat smaller ovoid or at least pleomorphic vesicles. The two main fine-

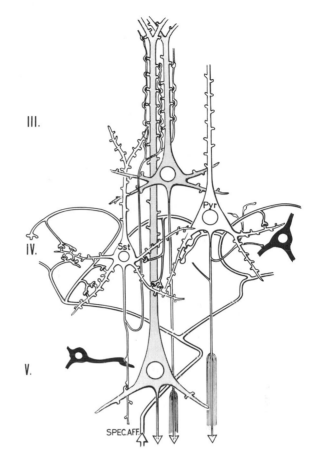

FIGURE 3   The direct excitatory neuron circuit of the specific (sensory) afferents, as deduced from the evidence so far available. Both spiny stellate (Sst, with ascending main axon) and true pyramidal (Pyr) cells are monosynaptically contacted. Inhibitory interneurons (black) may be contacted only disynaptically over the axon collaterals of the monosynaptic target cells. Apical dendrites of pyramidal cells (stippled) of laminae III and V are probably the main targets (over multiple climbing-type synapses) of the ascending axons of the spiny stellate cells.

structural criteria, the nature of the membrane specializations first recognized by Gray (1961), and the shape differences in the synaptic vesicles described by Uchizono (1965, 1967) show a rather good correlation in most synapses of known physiological nature. It is therefore with considerable confidence that we characterize synaptic contacts of the AR type (Asymmetric membrane specialization due to extended, thick postsynaptic opacity and having Round synaptic vesicles) as probably excitatory. The structural correlation with the known physiological nature of inhibitory synapses is even better, so that synaptic contacts of the SF type (Symmetric membrane specializations due to lacking or thin or patchy postsynaptic opacity and having at least partially Flattened

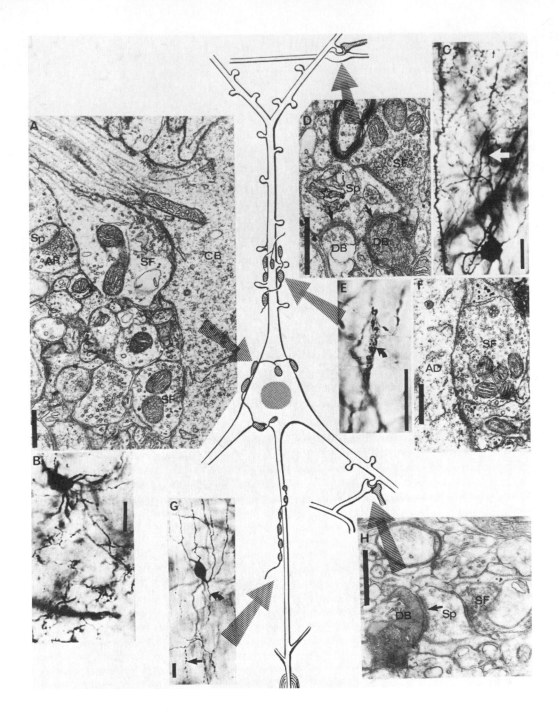

synaptic vesicles) are good candidates for inhibitory synapses. The situation, in fact, is not so simple, and many more types of snyapses can be distinguished. However, the above-mentioned fine-structural criteria can still be applied as a useful preliminary means of distinguishing between putative excitatory and inhibitory synapses.

Synapses of the two major types, AR and SF, have been distinguished routinely in the cortex since the first observations by Colonnier (1968). The differ-

ential localization of the two types is one of the major tools in attempts to identify putative, inhibitory interneurons.

The second criterion—being a local interneuron—is not useful by itself because many local interneurons are excitatory. Its usefulness lies in the fact that most of the long connections known so far, both afferent and efferent, are excitatory and have AR-type synapses. This statement is valid only for the conventional types of pathways (thalamic and corticocortical

FIGURE 4 Diagrammatic illustration of the modes by which and the sites on which a pyramidal neuron (center) can receive inhibitory synaptic contacts (hatched). The histological details and electron-microscopic evidence are presented in photographs A–H. Scale for the Golgi pictures is 20 μm; for the electron micrographs, 0.5 μm. Hatched arrows indicate the corresponding Golgi or EM evidence of the various types of synapses. (A) Persisting SF-type synapses on the surface of small pyramidal-cell body (CB) of lamina II in chronically isolated slab of visual cortex. Intact AR-type synapse contacts dendritic spine (Sp). (B) Small basket cell from the deeper layer of the cortex (see also Figure 6). (C) Axonal tufted cell of Ramón y Cajal from lamina II. The axonal trunk is indicated by a white arrow, delicate branches of the same axon by small arrows. (D) Dendritic spine (Sp) in lamina I (spine apparatus indicated by asterisk) of chronically isolated cortical slab with triple synaptic contact. Two of the boutons are in degeneration (DB); however, their AR nature is indicated by the still-visible postsynaptic opacity (arrows). The intact bouton is of SF type and is assumed to belong to the cell type shown in C. (E) Group of terminal boutons surrounding apical dendrite of a pyramidal cell. The delicate afferents of these boutons derive from the same axon of a "chandelier cell" (for histological information see Szentágothai, 1975, 1977). (F) SF-type persisting bouton in contact with apical dendrite (AD) of chronically isolated cortical slab. (G) Specific axoaxonic (inhibitory) interneuron. Main axon is indicated by curved arrow; vertical beaded terminal stretches (straight arrow) are characteristic for the axon endings of this cell type (see also Figure 5). (H) Double-spine synapses can also be found in the deeper layers of the cortex. In this case the degenerated bouton (Db) belongs to the visual afferent system and, as seen from the strong postsynaptic opacity (arrow) of the spine (Sp), was of AR type; the intact bouton is a characteristic SF-type terminal, probably also in contact with another spine to the right. (Courtesy of P. Somogyi.)

development of a concept of the modular architecture of the cortex within the larger columnar units.

It is unnecessary to dwell longer on the details, which have been described at several stages of their gradual development (Szentágothai, 1969, 1970, 1973, 1975, 1976). The modular concept will be dealt with more synthetically in the next section. Figure 4 summarizes the modes and the types of interneurons by which inhibitory influence can be exercised on a pyramidal cell. A similar diagram should be made for other types of interneurons, among them specific inhibitory ones. We do not yet have sufficient information for such an attempt, but we are confident that it will soon be available.

To summarize very briefly, the best candidates for specific inhibitory interneurons are obviously the basket cells, which can be subdivided into three distinct types: (1) large basket cells in laminae III–V with their parallel, flat, axonal arborization spaces, first recognized by Marin-Padilla (1970); (2) the small basket cells of lamina II (and also in the deeper layers; see Figure 4) that act at distances on the order of 100 μm and probably also on (small) pyramidals; (3) "columnar" basket cells, which appear to act on cell bodies arranged in vertical columns of 50–100 μm diameter and run vertically through several layers (see Figure 6, left–CBC). The next best candidate for inhibitory cells are the axonal tufted cells of lamina II (type 5 of Jones, 1975), which arborize mainly in the depth of lamina I and in lamina II and contact dendritic spines as one of the known double axon-spine synapses (Szentágothai, 1975). Similar cells may also exist in the deeper layers, as can be deduced from the fact that such double axon-spine synapses also occur in lamina IV, and even in combination with specific sensory afferents (see Figure 4H). There are undoubtedly also inhibitory cells that act on the apical dendritic shafts of pyramidal cells; a candidate for such an interneuron might be the so-called chandelier cell (Szentágothai, 1975).

But these are only the conventional types of putative inhibitory interneurons. More recently Somogyi (1977) observed a type of specific interneuron that differs from all others by acting over axoaxonic synapses and apparently specifically on the output of pyramidal cells. Synaptic contacts on the initial-axon segments of pyramidal cells had been described earlier (Palay et al., 1968; Peters, Proskauer, and Kaiserman-Abramof, 1968), but their origin remained unknown. The procedure used to trace the synaptic contacts of Golgi-stained specific cells yielded the unexpected observation that a hitherto occasionally seen Golgi type II interneuron with short, vertically ori-

afferents), and the situation is probably quite different for the monoaminergic afferents. Even so, the vast majority of the distant connections are excitatory, so that the restriction that an inhibitory neuron ought to be local reduces considerably the number of elements from which we must select. This was the main rationale for looking for putative inhibitory neurons in chronically isolated slabs (Szentágothai, 1965a,b).

What became really useful was a combination of the two criteria, that is, considering as candidates for inhibitory cells any local interneuron with an axon making SF-type synapses. This made the whole problem manageable technically and led to the identification of a fair number of good candidates for inhibitory interneurons. Most remarkably, the axons of all these candidates for inhibitory interneurons are distributed in tissue spaces of very definite shape, size, and orientation. This contributed significantly to the

ented terminal stretches of axon arborization specifically and exclusively makes synaptic contacts with initial-axon segments of pyramidal cells (Figure 5). The contacts are not the most characteristic examples

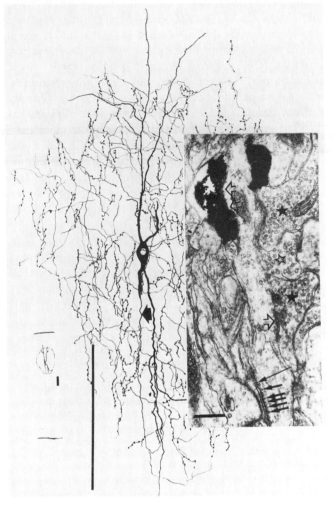

FIGURE 5 Specific axoaxonic interneuron of the rat visual cortex. Its position at the border of laminae II and III and the extension of its axonal arborization is shown at the left lower corner. The beaded vertical terminal stretches are characteristic for the axonal (arrow) arborization. Electron micrograph inset at right shows the termination of one of the stained terminals of this cell on an initial segment of pyramidal-cell axon. (No contact of this type of axon with any other structure has yet been identified.) The characteristic layered undercoat of the initial axonal segment is indicated by two different types of arrows in the lower part of the electron micrograph. Two nonstained terminals of the same type (black stars) show the typical flattened vesicles of these terminals; another terminal containing round vesicles has its contact at right with a dendritic profile. The mixed type of postsynaptic opacity in the axoaxonic synapses is indicated by outline arrows. Scales are 100 μm in the Golgi drawings and 0.25 μm in the electron micrograph. (Material courtesy of P. Somogyi; see Somogyi, 1977.)

of SF-type snyapses, but the vesicles of unstained synapses of this type are pleomorphic, and many are clearly ovoid (see the inset in Figure 5). From the number of stained and unstained synapses making contacts in regions where the axonal arborization of one cell of this type of apparently fully stained, it may be concluded that there is a convergence of about five beaded terminal-axon stretches on one initial-axon segment. In the monkey cerebral cortex, the dendritic tree of this axoaxonic interneuron type is particularly characteristic because of the rigid vertical orientation of the straight dendrites (Figure 4). This differentiates the cell from the chandelier cell (see Figure 5 in Szentágothai, 1975), which has a similar axonal arborization but in which cylindrically arranged groups of boutons (Figure 4E) are fed from separate, very delicate, branches of the same axon; in the axoaxonic cell, on the other hand, the rows of synaptic knobs are usually a single, vertical, beaded stretch of terminal-axon branches.

This observation shows the potential of tracing in thin-section series the whole dendritic and axonal arborization of neurons identified by Golgi staining. A great wealth of such new and probably unexpected information awaits us as this admittedly cumbersome technique comes to supersede the indirect method of unraveling the internal connectivity of the cerebral cortex. The research strategy available until recently, and exemplified by the results in Figures 1, 4, and 6, has probably run its course and will soon have to yield to the direct approach in reconstructing the synaptic contacts—both received and given—of identified cells. This will be done, partially, with the Golgi procedure (Somogyi, 1977, 1978) or, preferably, by some form of labeling after physiological identification.

The selection mechanism for output

It has already been mentioned that the anatomical size of the cortical column is so large that it is difficult to envisage it as a useful processor unit. This conclusion applies equally to the corticocortical connectivity columns, which really are columns, and to the specific subcorticocortical projection, which is more laminar but which, by the predominant vertical connectivity of the cortex, can be transformed secondarily (trans-synaptically) into a columnar pattern of about the same horizontal diameter ($\sim$300 μm) as its elements. The crucial bit of information leading to this conclusion is the wide distribution of individual afferents—mainly of the corticocortical but also of the specific subcorticocortical afferents—in spaces containing if not thousands then certainly hundreds of cells (Sholl, 1953, 1956; Szentágothai, 1973, 1978). It would thus be completely unrealistic to assume any major (multiple) connection between an individual afferent and any of the cortical neurons, that is, anything like a real one-to-one projection. Even massive lesions of the specific (sensory) subcortical nucleus cause only a small minority of the synapses on any given direct target neuron to degenerate (Somogyi, 1978).

Although a convergence of a specific set of afferents to any given cortical target cell may and perhaps even must be assumed, there is no way to avoid the conclusion that the input within the 200–300-μm-wide column is rather diffuse and generalized. No matter how strictly determined and specific the "wiring" may be—from subcortical sources to the main columns, between different columns, and from columns to subcortical targets—this could never satisfy the demands made by the known functional individuality of cortical neurons. A selection mechanism must therefore be postulated within each major column, according to the particular circumstances and, obviously, according to the antecedent history of the particular piece of neural tissue; this mechanism would be able to choose the few neurons that are activated as a result of the processing function of the larger unit. The columns of neurons having similar receptive-field properties may be an order of magnitude smaller than those established anatomically by individual or selectively grouped afferents—that is, they may sometimes be 20–30 μm instead of the 200–300 μm of the main anatomical columns. But even such tissue spaces would be too large for the individual properties of neurons that are often experienced in physiological experiments.

The anatomical bases of such a selection mechanism were first proposed rather tentatively (Szentágothai, 1967, 1969, 1970, 1973), and then with increasing confidence (Szentágothai, 1975, 1976, 1977b). Attempts at understanding the internal connectivity in terms of local interneuron arborizations, superimposed on the termination patterns of the afferents, led gradually and without premeditation to the concept of a *modular design* (Szentágothai and Arbib, 1974; Szentágothai, 1975) of the cortex. This concept required that cortical tissue—and in fact also the neuron network in many other neural centers—be envisaged as being built of repetitive and mutually interpenetrating spatial modules corresponding to the shapes and sizes of interneuron arborization spaces. The degree of overlap—or more correctly of interpenetration or sharing in space—is determined, obviously, by the density (number per unit space) of

the several cell types and the geometric parameters (particularly size) of their axon arborizations.

The modular design of neural centers is by no means a radically new concept, for it is implicit and a logical necessity in any structure assembled of a limited number of types of repetitively occurring elements that must fill a volume without leaving a substantial amount of "empty" space. This is exactly the case in neural centers, where the whole space is occupied—apart from the vessels, glial elements, and the narrow honeycomblike system of intercellular spaces—by the neural elements. Once a certain regularity in the axonal arborization spaces is recognized, as was the case in the neuropil of the brain stem reticular formation (Scheibel and Scheibel, 1958), the assumption of a modular architecture becomes almost a logical necessity. In the cortex, the regularity of the axonal arborizations is even more obvious, but the number of different types of elements made it difficult to put together a coherent picture of cortical architecture.

Envisaging the neural center as an assembly of a finite number of types of repetitive, mutually interpenetrating space modules has two advantages. First, it explains how a relatively high degree of specific connectivity can be achieved with a minimum of "genetic instruction" about what should be connected with what else (Szentágothai and Arbib, 1974). Second, it might serve as a selection mechanism to pick out a relatively few elements for activation from a large population of neurons having similar inputs.

If we assemble the available anatomical information on inputs and on putative excitatory and inhibitory interneurons in a synthetic diagram (Figure 6), it is immediately apparent that the columnar cell groups that come under the same general influence from extracortical input become an order of magnitude smaller, that is, 20–30 μm in diameter. By a suitable combination of inhibitory and excitatory interneurons, the individuality of the cells must become larger—in sensory projection areas—as one moves away from lamina IV toward lamina II and lamina VI, as is commonly experienced in physiological experiments. This diagram is on fairly safe ground concerning the putative inhibitory interneurons but is much more tentative with respect to excitatory ones, about which direct information is scanty. A number of arguments in favor of the existence of specific excitatory interneurons, in addition to the spiny stellates in lamina IV, have been given recently (Szentágothai, 1978) and need not be repeated here. The vast majority of interneuron terminal-axon branches are arranged in a way that is very suggestive of axon-

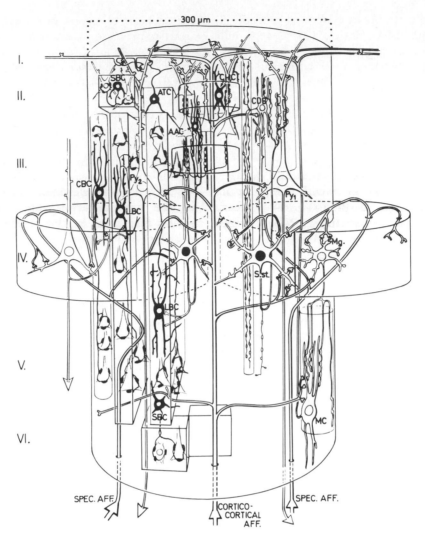

FIGURE 6 Diagrammatic (slightly stereoscopic) illustration of the internal connectivity of the neocortex. The main part of the diagram represents a corticocortical column 300 μm in diameter (internal details drawn in scale). The two halves of the diagram should be envisaged as showing assumed excitatory connections on the right (cells drawn in outlines) and putative inhibitory cells (in full black) and connections on the left. In addition, the two halves should be considered as mirror images, each containing everything that is indicated in the other side. Pyramidal cells Py_1 and Py_2 should be visualized as replicas of each other: the excitatory connections from a specific afferent over a spiny stellate (Sst) are shown in Py_1, whereas Py_2, at the left side, is assumed to escape through the inhibitory filter of large basket cells (LBCs), chandelier cells (CHCs), and axoaxonic cells (AACs) under the given circumstances. Excitatory ac-

tion is assumed to be conveyed further through *cellules à double bouquet* (CDBs) and, in descending direction (partially to Martinotti-type cells, MCs), microgliform interneurons (MGs). Inhibitory interneurons (black) are assumed in this diagram to be reached by specific afferents only disynaptically over the axon collaterals of monosynaptic target cells, either pyramids (at extreme left) or spiny stellates. Further inhibitory interneurons are columnar basket cells (CBCs) and small basket cells (SBCs) in the upper and lower layers and axonal tufted cells (ATCs) in lamina II. Modulelike spaces of axonal arborizations for various types of interneurons are indicated by delicate lines. The two flat cylinders in lamina IV correspond to the termination territory of a specific afferent, which is also about 300 μm in diameter but not necessarily in register with the corticocortical columns.

spine synapses. Since the vast majority of these synapses are of the AR type, it would be difficult to assume that many of the local neurons and connections are not excitatory. Because of the narrow vertically oriented strands of terminal-axon branches

given by many interneurons—for example, the *cellule à double bouquet* of Ramón y Cajal (1911)—and because of the common observation that such strands are closely associated with the spiny parts of apical dendrites (Szentágothai, 1969, 1971), the assumption

408   J. SZENTÁGOTHAI

of a powerful excitatory synaptic articulation of climbing-fiber type (of the cerebellum) was obvious. This concept is illustrated in the right half of Figure 6, which assumes a cascadelike excitatory selection mechanism. It should be kept in mind, however, that most of the information in this diagram is based on indirect reasoning and that methods are now available to base future diagrams on much more direct evidence. The left side of the diagram tries to illustrate the filtering effect exercised by the inhibitory interneurons; but one should keep in mind that the two mechanisms coexist in space and work together in time. In other words, each half of the diagram should be viewed mentally as if it also contained the mirror image of the other.

Nonconventional neurons and modes of connection

All the various types of neurons dealt with so far appear to be of the conventional type in that they conform to the basic tenets of classical neuron theory, including the principle of *histodynamic polarity*. Only the putative inhibitory specific axoaxonic cell described by Somogyi (1977) departs from the classical model by establishing synapses exclusively with initial-axon segments; such synapses, however, are known to occur in other neural centers—particularly in the cerebellar cortex—and seem not to differ otherwise in their basic functional properties from conventional synapses.

Since this Intensive Study Program addresses itself specifically to the problem of "local circuit neurons" and/or "local neuron circuits," it is reasonable to take a second look at the neocortical neuron network to see whether our present knowledge warrants application of the first mode of phrasing. "Local neuron circuits" can be arranged through entirely conventional types of neurons in an infinite variety, as shown in previous sections. Although it is not proposed here to enter into a discussion of semantics or definitions, it must be noted that the expression "local circuit neurons" conveys a radically different meaning; such neurons require elements, arrangements, and functions that would necessitate a complete reassessment of the principle of the histodynamic polarity of the neuron. There is no need, for the time being, to reconsider the neuron concept as the application of cell theory to the specific circumstances of the nervous system. The principle of histodynamic polarity never became a fundamental assumption of the neuron theory; but after the emergence of unit-level neurophysiology it did become—without being for-

mulated as such—practically the "central dogma" of all our reasoning about the structure and function of neural elements. It was also implicit, until very recently, in all diagrams trying to explain mechanisms by which nervous information is processed.

That there must be exceptions to this principle was generally accepted because of the existence of anaxonal cells, such as the amacrine cells of the retina, and also because the primary sensory neurons could not easily be integrated into the general concept. As this conference has discussed in great detail, there is ample—mainly structural—evidence to suggest that the view of the nervous system as built mainly of conventional histodynamically polarized neurons is no longer tenable. Although the nonconventional (that is, not simply histodynamically polarized) neurons are not necessarily anaxonal, as has occasionally been claimed, the principle of histodynamic polarity does not seem to hold for many (usually local inter-) neurons in many regions of the spinal cord, the brain stem, and the optic tectum. The examples available will probably increase when the reconstruction of synaptic articulations from thin-section series, especially of Golgi-stained or otherwise-labeled cells, becomes more common. There are many potential sites for presynaptic dendrites and dendritic synapses where the true identity of the synapsing elements can only be discovered through reconstruction, under the electron microscope.

For the neocortex the question arises whether the apparent lack of the usual signs of nonconventional neurons or modes of contacts—presynaptic dendrites, dendritic synapses, synaptic triads, reciprocal synapses—does or does not indicate that there are no such elements and/or arrangements. The apparent lack or rarity of such observations might be explained as well by assuming that—in contrast to the olfactory bulb, retina, and thalamic nuclei—the mentioned recognizable structural elements are not close in the cortex and are therefore unlikely to appear in the same section. All of the mentioned histological criteria of nonconventional synaptic arrangements are combinations of structural elements—for example, a presynaptic contact with accumulated vesicles established by a nerve-cell process that is obviously a dendrite (in that it contains ribosomes and is postsynaptic to some other process) or the presence of two (or more) synaptic contacts of reversed polarity between the same two profiles. If these elements were only a few microns apart, they would not show up in conventional electron-microscopic pictures; but they would be revealed in reconstructions of longer segments of nerve-cell processes from series of thin sections. For the time being, there is no direct evidence either way; the best that can be done is to approach the problem indirectly.

There are various types of local neurons in the cortex that do not quite fit the general pattern of conventional inhibitory or excitatory interneurons. First, there is a great wealth of neurogliform cells that have axons but have dendritic arborizations that look more axonal than dendritic in the Golgi picture (Figure 7A, C). The same is true in the geniculate nuclei, especially in the monkey, where very similar neurogliform local interneurons, albeit with recognizable axons, engage in presynaptic contacts of their dendrites (Pasik et al., 1973; Majorossy and Kiss,

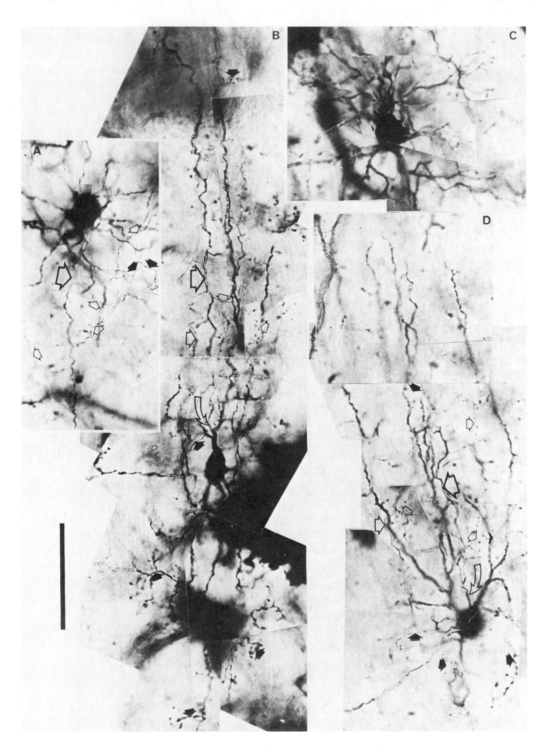

1976). Other types of interneurons arborize in vertically oriented columnar spaces and have secondary and tertiary dendritic branches that can hardly be differentiated from arborizations of the axon. Two such cells, also from the monkey cortex, are shown in Figure 7B, D; here the terminal branches belonging to the process that, according to the usual criteria, could be labeled as the axon are indicated separately from terminal branches belonging to processes that are undoubtedly dendrites. Although the arborization patterns of such neurons are by no means conclusive evidence for the occurrence of nonconventional neurons or neuronal connections, it is worth remembering that very similar terminal branches of dendrites are characteristic of almost all interneurons, from the spinal cord to the upper brain stem, in which the presynaptic engagements of such dendrites has been ascertained beyond doubt (see Ralston, this volume).

There is also evidence for synaptic contacts that are difficult to classify into any of the classical types. Scanning through electron micrographs of normal cortical tissue, the vast majority of synapses seem to be either AR-type contacts, predominantly with dendritic spines, or SF-type contacts generally established with the surface of a dendrite or of the soma. In isolated cortical slabs, by leaving sufficient time for the degeneration of the extraneous elements but not letting major sprouting or regeneration take place, contacts can be observed that do not fit into the main categories. This is especially true if the isolated slab is made with a diameter less than 1 mm and contains only laminae I, II, and a small portion of III. The situation is complicated in such material by the degeneration of dendritic elements whose cell bodies are separated by the cut. A selection of such elements is shown in Figure 8 and gives the impression that there are many intrinsic synaptic contacts in the cortex that cannot be classified into the major groups that, with greater or lesser justification are identified with one or the other type of classical connection.

This is, of course, not positive evidence for the existence of nonconventional connections of the types found in most lower centers, but it does indicate that we are still very far from having a complete inventory of local neurons and their connections in the neocortex. It has been claimed repeatedly, even by Ramón y Cajal (1911) himself, that the superior qualities in brain function on the higher phylogenetic levels depend on the larger number and diversity of local interneurons in the higher centers, particularly in the primates. No conclusive evidence for this has ever been presented; if anything, the opposite conclusion seems to emerge from the new quantitative data mentioned by Mountcastle (this volume; see Rockel, Hiorns, and Powell, 1974). What is striking when one compares Golgi architectonics of the cortex from mouse to man is the essential similarity in cell types and in the topology of arborization patterns, rather than the differences. It appears, however, that the arborizations of both dendrites and axons become more elaborate and more specific in the ascending phylogenetic scale, whereas the arborization spaces of single cells seem to become smaller. This is only a subjective impression, however, and no conclusions ought to be based on it.

Local connections at relatively longer distances

Intracortical connections that bridge larger distances than the diameter of the main anatomical columns are largely beyond the immediate concerns of this paper. Classical descriptions of cortical architecture already showed that there are relatively rich interconnections between the most superficial (laminae I, II) and the deeper (laminae V, VI) layers of the cortex. The relative abundance of surface parallel fibers in lamina I, ascending from cells located in laminae V and VI, was revealed by early studies on chronically isolated slabs of cortical tissue (Szentágothai, 1962, 1965a,b). What is not clearly known are the distances covered in a tangential direction by such fibers. After lesions to lamina I, degeneration of fibers can be traced up to distances of several millimeters. Assuming that fibers ascending from the deeper layers arborize upon arrival in lamina I, the

FIGURE 7 Local interneurons of the neocortex, in which the distinction of axonal and dendritic arborizations may become equivocal. Photomontages of four neurons of the parietal cortex of the monkey (*Cercopithecus aethiops aethiops*) from a perfusion Golgi-Kopsch series. The origin of the axon—if recognizable—is indicated by a curved arrow (B, D), and the main trunk of the assumed axon by a large outline arrow (A, B, D). Smaller branches that can be traced from the assumed axon are indicated by small outline arrows. Small, partially terminal branches that can be traced unequivocally from dendrites are indicated by small black arrows (A, B, D). The terminal branches of the dendrites are as delicate and beaded as the axon branches of the same size and show axonlike arborization patterns. (A) Microgliform neuron with descending axon in lamina IV. (B) Small neuron with vertically oriented columnar arborization of its processes; border between laminae II and III. (C) Neurogliform neuron from lamina V; no axon could be identified. (D) Vertically oriented small interneuron from lamina IV; note the short drumstick-shaped appendages of the major dendrites. Scale, 50 μm.

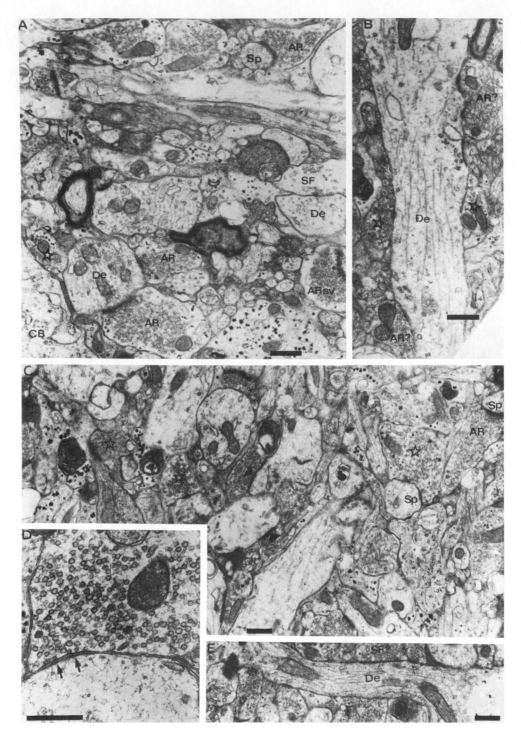

FIGURE 8 Details from the neuropil of a very small slab of cortical tissue (0.9 mm diameter, containing only laminae I, II, and a superficial stratum of III) isolated 3 days before. (Visual cortex of the cat; scale, 0.5 μm.) (A) Upper stratum of lamina III. (B) Middle stratum of lamina I. (C) Lamina II. (D) Deep stratum of lamina I. (E) Lamina II. Some of the persisting synapses with dendritic spines (Sp) or with dendrites (De) are of the usual (AR and SF) types. Many of the presynaptic profiles cannot be identified clearly, either because the round shape of the vesicles does not correspond to the small extension of the postsynaptic opacity (stars and the site indicated by arrows in D), the size of the vesicles is smaller (ARsv in A) than usual in the AR synapses, or the membrane contact is clearly asymmetric and the high density of the vesicles is unusual (black triangles in C). Few of the numerous presynaptic profiles contacting the dendrite (De) in E can be classified unequivocally.

total tangential spread of their arborizations could be calculated to be 5–6 mm if not more. Since the surface-parallel terminal-axon branches are running at relatively large angles (>45°) across their potential postsynaptic targets (the branches of the apical dendrites of pyramidal cells), it is unlikely that more than one or two synaptic contacts are established between any of the axons and dendrites (Szentágothai, 1971). It is difficult to imagine how such a synaptic system might work, apart from some mass action caused by electric stimulation.

The same considerations apply to another extensive connection system, the initial collaterals of the pyramidal cells. As can be deduced from many illustrations of the classical neurohistological literature, and particularly from a most elegant drawing of Scheibel and Scheibel (1970, Figure 7), the initial collateral system is very widely distributed within a vertical cylinder, cuts through virtually the entire depth of the cortex, and has a diameter close to 3 mm. In addition, the orientation of the collaterals is rather rigidly determined in most pyramidal neurons by the sequence of their origin. The first collaterals generally ascend almost vertically, while the courses of the ones that follow become more and more horizontal and eventually even descending (Figure 1 in Szentágothai, 1975). In such a rigidly determined arborization pattern, there is little room to specifically address the connections, apart from the possibility that the vertically ascending branches of the first collateral branches may have repeated contacts with the ascending apical dendrites of immediately neighboring pyramidal cells. Since the collaterals are distributed around such a large space, the few hundred presynaptic loci that can be estimated for the collaterals of each pyramidal cell on the basis of the number of their boutons and varicose thickenings must be distributed to almost as many different recipient cells. A very rough calculation (Szentágothai, 1977) indicates that there are about 17,000 pyramidal cells in the arborization space of the collaterals belonging to one pyramidal neuron. It had been assumed earlier that the majority of the pyramidal collateral synapses in layers I and II are established with dendritic spines of other pyramidal cells (Szentágothai, 1965b). Preliminary results of the reconstruction from thin-section series of Golgi-stained pyramidal-cell collateral arborizations seem to indicate (Szentágothai, 1978) that this assumption is correct. It does not apply to synapses given by the collaterals of the pyramidal cells that receive direct input from specific sensory afferents (Somogyi, 1978).

All this would indicate that both the system of the

main (200–300 μm) anatomical columns and the much smaller columns brought about by the modular arrangement illustrated in Figure 6 have superimposed a more diffuse connectivity system that is distributed in spaces at least an order of magnitude larger than the main columns (3 mm versus 300 μm diameter).

Conclusions

It seems relatively easy to envisage the neocortex as a mosaic of columnar processor units about 200–300 μm in diameter, connected with one another and with a number of subcortical sources and targets according to a very highly specific wiring blueprint. Both intuitively and on the basis of what we know about the function of cortical cells, it is probably acceptable to believe that the modular arrangement of excitatory and inhibitory interneurons can act as a mechanism for the selection of smaller specific groups, or even of individual cells, from the large population of the main column in accordance with the particular combination of active input channels and perhaps even according to what has happened in this column during its earlier history. The cells so selected would act as output cells toward other cortical columns, where such a selection mechanism would be repeated again and again. Some other cells would act as output cells toward subcortical targets. But the modular conception of local interneurons, however sophisticated, is probably not the whole story of local neuronal interaction. The rather vague data discussed above might suggest—in view of the great wealth of recent information in lower neural centers about nonconventional modes of interneuronal connections—that we need to keep our minds open for hitherto completely unknown local neuronal mechanisms (see also Schmitt, Dev, and Smith, 1976).

Probably the least acceptable aspects of cortical architecture are the relatively long-range and diffuse connectivity systems mentioned only briefly here but discussed in more detail recently (Szentágothai, 1977, 1978). Any suggestion of randomness, however insignificant in comparison with the immense specificity in most neural connections, is understandably repulsive to the neuroscientist of today. Some consideration, however, should be given to two aspects of this problem.

First, although the connections both to and from the main columns, and also those within the main anatomical columns, are largely unidirectional (with the exception of the callosal connections, which have some reciprocal character), the diffuse longer-range connections are almost completely symmetric and reciprocal; the same types and numbers of connections are given and received. There is generally some so-called reciprocity in neural connections, and this had been formulated as a general principle by Lorente de Nó (1933). However, this reciprocity is not symmetric, for the connections leading from A to B are basically different from those leading from B to A. We can observe something more like a circular chain of neurons consisting of a sequential arrangement that happens (partially) to return to itself. The definition given by Ramón y Cajal (1911) avoids the word *reciprocity* and so is probably better. Conversely, the diffuse connectivity system of the pyramidal-cell collaterals is really symmetrically reciprocal. It is highly debatable whether in a system of connectivity brought about by essentially nonreciprocal (unidirectional) connections—even if some of them are recurrent—the conditions for cooperativity, as postulated by Cragg and Temperley (1954), could be assumed to be satisfied on the macro (i.e., neuronal) level. (On the network level, it is entirely immaterial whether cooperativity exists on the molecular level.) Conversely, these conditions seem to be satisfied by a connectivity system with a high degree of reciprocity and symmetry.

Second, it is a general contention in systems theory applied to very complex systems that when the subsystems are well organized internally, the whole system can operate successfully and purposefully with a less well-organized—or less strictly determined—system of interconnections between the several subsystems.

I certainly do not mean to downgrade the importance of the extremely high degree of specific connectivity with which most of this paper has been concerned. What I hope to convey is the thought that the diffuse, not strictly addressed, connections that seem to exist in all parts of the nervous system are not necessarily the "flaw in the system"—or simply something arising from our meager understanding—but may be an essential part of the design.

REFERENCES

COLONNIER, M., 1968. Synaptic patterns on different cell types in the different laminae of the cat visual cortex. *Brain Res.* 9:268–287.

COLONNIER, M., and S. ROSSIGNOL, 1969. Heterogeneity of the cerebral cortex. In *Basic Mechanisms of the Epilepsies*, H. H. Jasper, A. A. Ward, and A. Pope, eds. Boston: Little, Brown, pp. 29–40.

CRAGG, B. G., and H. N. V. TEMPERLEY, 1954. The organization of neurones: A co-operative analogy. *EEG Clin. Neurophysiol.* 6:85–92.

GAREY, L. J., and T. P. S. POWELL, 1971. An experimental study of the termination of the lateral geniculo-cortical pathway in the cat and monkey. *Proc. R. Soc. Lond.* B179:41–63.

GLOBUS, A., and A. B. SCHEIBEL, 1966. Loss of dendritic spines as an index of presynaptic terminal pattern. *Nature* 212:463.

GLOBUS, A., and A. B. SCHEIBEL, 1967. Synaptic loci on visual cortical neurons of the rabbit: The specific afferent radiation. *Exp. Neurol.* 18:116–131.

GOLDMAN, P. A., and W. J. H. NAUTA, 1977. Columnar distribution of cortico-cortical fibers in the frontal association, limbic and motor cortex of the developing Rhesus monkey. *Brain Res.* 122:393–413.

GRANT, G., S. LANDGREN, and H. SILFVENIUS, 1975. Columnar distribution of U-fibres from the postcruciate cerebral projection area of the cat's group I-muscle afferents. *Exp. Brain Res.* 24:57–74.

GRAY, E. G., 1961. Ultra-structure of synapses of the cerebral cortex and certain specializations of neuroglial membranes. In *Electron Microscopy in Anatomy*, J. D. Boyd, F. R. Johnson, and J. D. Lever, eds. London: Edward Arnold, pp. 54–73.

HUBEL, D. H., and T. N. WIESEL, 1959. Receptive fields of single neurones in the cat's striate cortex. *J. Physiol.* 148:574–591.

HUBEL, D. H., and T. N. WIESEL, 1969. Anatomical demonstration of columns in the monkey striate cortex. *Nature* 221:747–750.

JONES, E. G., 1968. An electron microscopic study of the terminations of afferent fibre systems within the somatic sensory cortex of the cat. *J. Anat.* 103:595–597.

JONES, E. G., 1975. Varieties and distribution of nonpyramidal cells in the somatic sensory cortex of the squirrel monkey. *J. Comp. Neurol.* 160:205–268.

JONES, E. G., and T. P. S. POWELL, 1970. An electron microscope study of terminal degeneration in the neocortex of the cat. *Philos. Trans. R. Soc. Lond.* B257:29–43.

LEVAY, S., D. H. HUBEL, and T. N. WIESEL, 1975. The pattern of ocular dominance columns in macaque visual cortex revealed by a reduced silver stain. *J. Comp. Neurol.* 159:559–575.

LORENTE DE NÓ, R., 1933. Vestibulo-ocular reflex arc. *Arch. Neurol. Psychiatr.* 30:245–291.

LUND, J. S., 1973. Organization of neurons in the visual cortex area 17 of the monkey (*Macaca mulatta*). *J. Comp. Neurol.* 147:455–496.

MAJOROSSY, K., and M. BODOKY, 1977. Neuronal structure and intrinsic connections of the auditory cortex. *Acta Anat.* 99:292.

MAJOROSSY, K., and A. KISS, 1976. Types of interneurons and their participation in the neuronal network of the medial geniculate body. *Exp. Brain Res.* 26:19–37.

MARIN-PADILLA, M., 1970. Prenatal and early postnatal ontogenesis of the human motor cortex: A Golgi study, II. The basket-pyramidal system. *Brain Res.* 23:185–192.

MOUNTCASTLE, V. B., 1957. Modalities and topographic properties of single neurons of cat's sensory cortex. *J. Neurophysiol.* 20:408–434.

PALAY, S. L., C. SOTELO, A. PETERS, and P. M. ORKAND, 1968. The axon hillock and the initial segment. *J. Cell Biol.* 38:193–201.

PASIK, P., T. PASIK, J. HÁMORI, and J. SZENTÁGOTHAI, 1973. Golgi type II interneurons in the neuronal circuit of the monkey lateral geniculate nucleus. *Exp. Brain Res.* 17:18–34.

PETERS, A., and M. L. FELDMAN, 1976. The projection of the lateral geniculate nucleus to area 17 of the rat cerebral cortex. *J. Neurocytol.* 5:63–84.

PETERS, A., C. C. PROSKAUER, and I. R. KAISERMAN-ABRAMOF, 1968. The small pyramidal neuron of the rat cerebral cortex: The axon hillock and initial segment. *J. Cell Biol.* 39:604–619.

RAMÓN Y CAJAL, S., 1899. Estudios sobra la cortezza cerebral humana. *Rev. Trim. Microscopia* 4:1–63.

RAMÓN Y CAJAL, S., 1911. *Histologie du système nerveux de l'homme et des vertébrés,* vol. 2. Paris: Maloine.

ROCKEL, A. J., R. W. HIORNS, and T. P. S. POWELL, 1974. Numbers of neurons through full depth of neocortex. *J. Anat.* 118:371.

SCHEIBEL, M. E., and A. B. SCHEIBEL, 1958. Structural substrates for integrative patterns in the brain stem reticular core. In *Reticular Formation of the Brain*, H. H. Jasper, L. D. Proctor, R. S. Knighton, W. C. Noshay, and R. T. Costello, eds. Boston: Little, Brown, pp. 31–68.

SCHEIBEL, M. E., and A. B. SCHEIBEL, 1970. Elementary processes in selected thalamic and cortical subsystems— The structural substrates. In *The Neurosciences: Second Study Program*, F. O. Schmitt, ed. New York: Rockefeller Univ. Press, pp. 443–457.

SCHIMERT, J., 1938. Die Endigungsweise des Tractus vestibulospinalis. *Z. Anat. Enwicklungsgesch.* 108:761–767.

SCHIMERT, J., 1939. Das Verhalten der Hinterwurzelkollateralen im Rückenmark. *Z. Anat. Entwicklungsgesch.* 109:665–687.

SCHMITT, F. O., P. DEV, and B. H. SMITH, 1976. Electrotonic processing of information by brain cells. *Science* 193:114–120.

SHOLL, D. A., 1953. Dendritic organization in the neurons of the visual and motor cortices of the cat. *J. Anat.* 87:387–406.

SHOLL, D. A., 1956. *The Organization of the Cerebral Cortex.* New York: John Wiley.

SOMOGYI, P., 1977. A specific "axo-axonal" interneuron in the visual cortex of the rat. *Brain Res.* (in press).

SOMOGYI, P., 1978. The study of Golgi stained cells and of experimental degeneration under the electron microscope: A direct method for the identification in the visual cortex of three successive links in a neuron chain. *Neuroscience* 3:167–180.

SZENTÁGOTHAI, J., 1962. On the synaptology of the cerebral cortex. In *Structure and Function of the Nervous System*, S. A. Sarkissov, ed. Moscow: Medgiz, pp. 6–14. (In Russian.)

SZENTÁGOTHAI, J., 1965a. The synapse of short local neurons in the cerebral cortex. In *Modern Trends in Neuromorphology*, J. Szentágothai, ed. Budapest: Akadémiai Kiadó, pp. 251–276.

SZENTÁGOTHAI, J., 1965b. The use of degeneration methods in the investigation of short neuronal connections. In *Progress in Brain Research*, vol. 14: *Degeneration Patterns in the Nervous System*, M. Singer and J. P. Schadé, eds. Amsterdam: Elsevier, pp. 1–32.

SZENTÁGOTHAI, J., 1967. The anatomy of complex integrative units in the nervous system. In *Results in Neuroanatomy, Neurochemistry, Neuropharmacology and Neurophysiology*, K. Lissák, ed. Budapest: Akadémiai Kiadó, pp. 9–45.

SZENTÁGOTHAI, J., 1969. Architecture of the cerebral cortex. In *Basic Mechanisms of the Epilepsies*, H. H. Jasper, A. A. Ward, and A. Pope, eds. Boston: Little, Brown, pp. 13–28.

SZENTÁGOTHAI, J., 1970. Les circuits neuronaux de l'écorce cérébrale. *Bull. Acad. R. Med. Belg.* 10:475–492.

SZENTÁGOTHAI, J., 1971. Some geometrical aspects of the neocortical neuropil. *Acta Biol. Acad. Sci. Hung.* 22:107–124.

SZENTÁGOTHAI, J., 1973. Synaptology of the visual cortex. In *Handbook of Sensory Physiology*, VII/3B. R. Jung, ed. Heidelberg: Springer-Verlag, pp. 269–324.

SZENTÁGOTHAI, J., 1975. The "module-concept" in cerebral cortex architecture. *Brain Res.* 95:475–496.

SZENTÁGOTHAI, J., 1976. Die Neuronenschaltungen der Grosshirnrinde. *Verh. Anat. Ges.* 70:187–215.

SZENTÁGOTHAI, J., 1977. Specificity versus (quasi-) randomness in cortical connectivity. In *Architectonics of the Cerebral Cortical Connectivity*, M. A. B. Brazier and H. Petsche, eds. New York: Raven Press, pp. 77–97.

SZENTÁGOTHAI, J., 1978. The neuron network of the cerebral cortex: A functional interpretation. *Proc. R. Soc. Lond.* B201:219–248.

SZENTÁGOTHAI, J., and M. ARBIB, 1974. Conceptual models of neural organization. *Neurosciences Res. Program Bull.* 12:307–510. (Also available in book form from The MIT Press.)

SZENTÁGOTHAI-SCHIMERT, J., 1941. Die Endigungsweise der absteigenden Rückenmarksbahnen. *Z. Anat. Entwicklungsgesch.* 111:322–330.

UCHIZONO, K., 1965. Characteristics of excitatory and inhibitory synapses in the central nervous system of the cat. *Nature* 297:642–643.

UCHIZONO, K., 1967. Synaptic organization of the Purkinje cells in the cerebellum of the cat. *Exp. Brain Res.* 4:97–113.

VALVERDE, F., 1967. Apical dendritic spines of the visual cortex and light deprivation in the mouse. *Exp. Brain Res.* 3:337–352.

WOLFF, J. R., and L. ZÁBORSZKY, 1978. On the normal arrangement of fibres and terminals and limits of plasticity in the callosal system of the rat. In *Structure and Function of the Cerebral Commissures*, J. S. Russel and M. W. van Hof, eds. London: Macmillan.

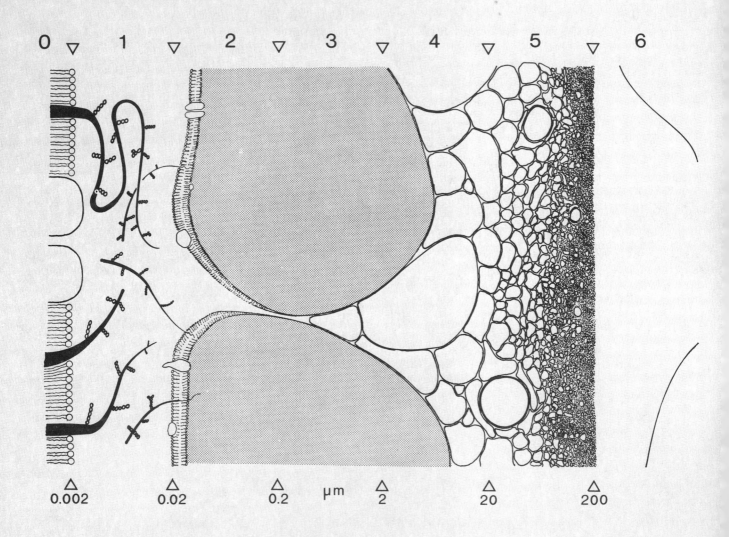

0 ▽ 1 ▽ 2 ▽ 3 ▽ 4 ▽ 5 ▽ 6

△
0.002

△
0.02

△
0.2

μm

△
2

△
20

△
200

GENERAL PRINCIPLES OF NEURONAL INTEGRATION

Brain-cell microenvironment from a logarithmic viewpoint. At the left one sees only the outer half of the lipid bilayer of a cell with embedded proteinaceous channel and glycoproteins extending into extracellular space. Moving to the right, the scale diminishes logarithmically; whole cells are encountered, then aggregates which merge into a mosaic that includes occasional blood vessels. Finally, the limiting surfaces of the brain are reached at the far right.

Introduction

RODOLFO LLINÁS

NEURONAL INTEGRATION is regarded today as an emergent property arising from the intimate superposition of morphological and functional characteristics of the neuron. In turn, the functional characteristics themselves represent an amalgam of the ohmic and capacitative properties of membranes and of the electrical nonlinearities introduced by voltage-dependent ionic conductances, themselves tempered by the nature of the intra- and extracellular ionic milieu. Given the central importance of the concept of neuronal integration in understanding the functional implications of local circuit neurons, we feel it timely to deal with it in full detail.

With this aim in mind we decided to bring together those aspects of morphology and function which we consider relevant to the present discussion and which may be novel, given that the concept of neuronal integration has undergone such a deep change recently. In years past, integration was considered to be fundamentally the simple algebraic summation of synaptic potentials at the soma and basal dendrites of neurons. However, the concept has become far more complex on several counts. First, it is now agreed that membrane potential across the soma and axon hillock is not exclusively modulated by the synapses located in their immediate vicinity. The assumption that "remote" dendritic segments were of no functional significance, due to their electrotonic distance from the soma, is now known to have been a serious misconception. In addition, the view of dendrites as simple inexcitable cables, whose main function is to channel synaptic potential (or more correctly, internal longitudinal current) centripetally toward the soma, has been completely revised. Indeed, not only can dendrites generate action potentials in their own right but, in addition, the properties of voltage summation are themselves quite complex. Furthermore, since such processes are not only sites of synaptic input but may be presynaptic to other structures, this simplified concept of neuronal integration has had to be abandoned. Since much of the local circuit aspect of this question has been covered in the first part of the study program, we shall approach the problem of neuronal integration from first principles.

In a most lucid presentation, the basic cable properties of cells are reviewed by Julian Jack who summarizes, from a theoretical and an experimental view, the techniques available for the study of cable properties and their strengths and limitations in understanding the electrophysiology of single cellular elements. One is reminded that neuronal function is irreversibly immersed in the neuronal parameters of form. These passive properties may truly be termed parameters of form as they are determined directly by the structure of the membrane and spatial organization of the cell as demonstrated by the brilliant work of Wilfrid Rall. It is indeed through the molding of electrotonic conduction that the membrane electric field can generate (like echoes in a cave) neuronal integration.

Frederick Dodge describes the nonlinear voltage-dependent properties that perform on the stage set by passive electronic conduction. This presentation emphasizes the integrative role of single and multiple spike initiation sites on normal and axotomized motoneurons. The problem of nonlinear summation of synaptic input is approached in conjunction with noncontinuous spike conduction in dendrites through the development of an elegant model.

Beyond the parameters of linear and nonlinear electrical properties of membrane, the second basic aspect of neuronal integration relates to the ionic driving forces that convert membrane ionic permeability into ionic conductance. While we are aware of the all-important ionic batteries generated by concentrational differences across membranes, it is often forgotten that, in a compact unstirred compartment such as the extracellular milieu, the activity of neurons leaves a wake of ionic turmoil that must modify its ionic gradients. Furthermore, in the sense that such ionic turmoil may be a constant rather than a transient state of affairs, the extracellular milieu is a truly active site of interaction between neurons and one that, rather than erratically fluctuating, must be firmly controlled.

The importance of this parameter in the function of local circuit neurons is difficult to overemphasize. This is especially so if one considers, for instance, the retina or the olfactory bulb. Here the extracellular system forms a three-dimensional continuous mosaic of ionic concentrational differences and of transmitter substances coexisting and interacting in a recip-

rocal way with the plasmalemmal surfaces that contain them. Charles Nicholson introduces the topic by considering the ways in which the properties of single cells are modified by the composition of the extracellular ionic milieu. His presentation emphasizes the *active regulation* of the brain cell elements by each other via the modulation of the ionic microcosm in which they are embedded. The use of ion-selective electrodes, combined with physiological paradigms ranging from local stimulation of the cerebellar cortex to spreading depression, is treated in detail as a method to study this extracellular ionic modulation and has shown a deep capacity for modulation of *all ions*. Of particular importance are what Nicholson calls the minority ions (K^+ and Ca^{++}), which he finds may change under some conditions by as much as half their normal concentration.

Having laid down the fundamental principles of neuronal integration, we turn our attention to the specific parameters governing these integrative properties. Dean Hillman analyzes the structural parameters which constitute neuronal form. The form of cells is envisaged as being brought about by interaction between intrinsic and extrinsic factors which reflect genetic invariances and epigenetic polymorphisms. The anatomical rationale on which branching power (and in fact all of the cable theory that Rall has developed over the last two decades) finds its counterpart in such morphometry.

A special case of integrative properties of the axonal terminal, the telodendrion, is presented by I. Parnas. His message is one dear to those who strive to relate structure to function. Axonal branches are capable of complex switching properties in some ways comparable to the "integration" seen at the soma to dendritic pole of nerve cells. He demonstrates the contribution of the linear and nonlinear electrical properties of membranes to the dynamics of information transmission. Equally important, these switching properties, by which the different branches of an axon may fire with their own rhythms, are determined by the neuronal variables outlined above and, in a dynamic sense, by the composition of the extracellular ionic milieu.

Beyond the question of integration by single cells is that of "integrative units" in the nervous system. In some cases this integrative unit may be a single cell; in others it may be a collection of such cells. The point arises quite clearly when nonspiking cells are considered. This formalism is introduced by William Calvin and Katherine Graubard, who also review the functional importance of repetitive firing in single units and small nerve nets. In addition, their contribution covers aspects such as presynaptic facilitation and inhibition and brings together many of the mechanisms discussed by the other participants regarding the functional properties of single cells.

Finally, in attempting to orchestrate the different aspects of neuronal function into the next level of complexity, that of the "sociological organization" of neurons, a powerful heuristic tool is required. Here again, as in the case of the analysis of single cell properties, mathematical models are indispensable. Thus, the concept of computer modeling in neurobiology is tackled by András Pellionisz, who presents a comprehensive review of the topic. His approach covers the vast area from single cells to the properties of neuronal circuits and their relation to certain types of behavior. As an example, a computer model developed from actual morphological and functional data is presented for the anuran cerebellum. The task at hand here is that of bringing together the myriads of cellular elements which compose any portion of our brain into something manageable by our intellect. This presentation reviews many of the fundamentals on which we must construct our modern view of brain function.

24 An Introduction to Linear Cable Theory

JULIAN JACK

ABSTRACT Cable theory is concerned with the mathematical methods that will give an accurate description of the flow of electric current both inside and outside cells. The usual assumptions made in formulating the equations are presented and assessed, as are the methods of solving the equations. Some features of the steady-state distribution of voltage are noted, and there is a discussion of the factors affecting the time course of a voltage waveform generated by transient injection of current (such as often characterizes synaptic potentials). The final section is concerned with four applications of the theory: (1) the importance of measuring the membrane resistance and the methods available; (2) a comparison of active versus passive propagation of voltage waveforms; (3) the apparent inadequacies in available models of the nerve cell; and (4) the problem of the "leak conductance" created by inserting a microelectrode into a cell.

Introduction

CABLE THEORY is a technique that can be used to quantify the description of electric current flow within and between cells. It will be obvious from this characterization that one of the principles adopted in the formulation of the theory is to model the cell(s) and surrounding fluid by an electric circuit. Before making any attempt to assess the validity of this description, it may be helpful to summarize the usual assumptions made. It is simplest to start by considering a segment of a cell that can be physically represented as a cylinder—for example, part of a process of the cell that is circular in cross section and uniform in diameter.

Figure 1 shows such a cylindrical segment and (below) the way it is represented as an equivalent electrical circuit. The choice of such a circuit is governed by the following considerations. All cells have a surface membrane, and there is quite good evidence that this may be given an adequate electrical description by representing it as a leaky capacitance (e.g., Cole, 1968; Jack, Noble, and Tsien, 1975). If only small

voltage displacements are considered, it is usually appropriate to describe the leak as a simple linear resistance in series with a battery (representing the resting membrane potential). Since one is primarily concerned with voltage deviations from the resting potential, this description may be simplified further by neglecting the battery; this yields the circuit for the membrane shown in Figure 1, with a resistance and capacitance in parallel. The symbols c_m and r_m denote the membrane capacitance and resistance per unit length of the cylinder. They are related to the more fundamental measures of capacitance (C_m) and resistance (R_m) per unit area of membrane by the simple formulas

$$c_m = \pi d C_m, \qquad r_m = \frac{R_m}{\pi d},$$

where d is the diameter of the cylinder.

In the cylinder of Figure 1, current can flow not only across the membrane but also longitudinally in the intracellular and extracellular compartments. Current flow through the intracellular fluid is assumed to be ohmic, and the flow of current within the cell is assumed to be in the longitudinal (axial) direction. If the cell is surrounded by a large volume

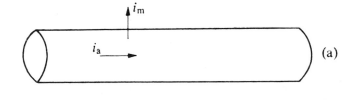

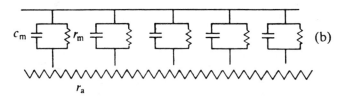

FIGURE 1 (a) A cylindrical segment of a cell. (b) Its equivalent electrical circuit. (From Jack, Noble, and Tsien, 1975.)

JULIAN JACK University Laboratory of Physiology, Oxford, England of fluid, the resistance to extracellular current flow is very small compared to the intracellular fluid, and it is convenient to treat it as negligible, as shown in Figure 1.

Given this electrical circuit, the basic equation for a linear cable can be obtained. The formulation and an explicit solution were first given in the physiological literature by Hodgkin and Rushton (1946) and Davis and Lorente de Nó (1947). All we need note here is that by the application of Ohm's law and Kirchoff's law (conservation of current) one finds

$$\frac{1}{r_a}\frac{\partial^2 V}{\partial x^2} = i_m, \tag{1}$$

where r_a is the intracellular resistance to axial flow of current ($= 4R_i/\pi d^2$, where R_i is the specific resistance of the intracellular fluid), V is the transmembrane voltage, x is distance along the cylinder, and i_m is the membrane current per unit length ($= \pi d I_m$, where I_m is the current per unit membrane area). The membrane current can be split into capacitative and resistive components as follows:

$$i_m = c_m\frac{\partial V}{\partial t} + \frac{V}{r_m}, \tag{2}$$

so that

$$\frac{1}{r_a}\frac{\partial^2 V}{\partial x^2} = c_m\frac{\partial V}{\partial t} + \frac{V}{r_m}, \tag{3}$$

where t denotes time. This is the basic differential equation of linear cable theory. It is commonly rearranged into the following form:

$$\frac{\partial^2 V}{\partial X^2} = \frac{\partial V}{\partial T} + V, \tag{4}$$

where

$$X = \frac{x}{\lambda}, \qquad \lambda = \sqrt{\frac{r_m}{r_a}} = \sqrt{\frac{R_m d}{4R_i}},$$

$$T = \frac{t}{\tau_m}, \qquad \tau_m = r_m c_m = R_m C_m.$$

Here λ is called the space constant and τ_m the membrane time constant.

Assumptions in the derivation

Several assumptions have been made in this derivation which are unlikely to be exactly, or generally, correct. Some of them are listed here and briefly discussed. A more detailed discussion of many of these points has been given by Scott (1972) and Jack, Noble, and Tsien (1975).

INTRACELLULAR CURRENT FLOW   The intracellular fluid appears to act as an ohmic resistance, but the representation in the equivalent circuit assumes that it presents a resistance only to axial flow of current and not, for example, to radial flow of current. A more accurate account would consider the flow in three dimensions (see Eisenberg and Johnson, 1970, for a review). It turns out that in most circumstances the simple assumption is sufficiently accurate, mainly because the diameter of the cylinder is sufficiently small to make, for example, the intracellular resistance to radial current negligibly small compared with the surface membrane resistance. Substantial inaccuracies may result in the immediate neighborhood of a source of current, particularly if one is considering very high frequencies of voltage variation (when the effective "resistance" of the membrane to current flow is relatively low because of the properties of the membrane capacitance).

EXTRACELLULAR CURRENT FLOW   In many parts of the nervous system the cell processes are closely packed together, so that the space between cells may be very small—as little as 200 Å in width. The assumption of a negligible extracellular resistance is clearly inappropriate. One obvious indication of this is that it is possible to record variations in membrane potential with extracellular electrodes. A finite extracellular resistance can, however, be accommodated very simply in the above formulation provided it is purely ohmic and takes a uniform value with distance. In this case the only modification to equation 4 is that

$$\lambda = \sqrt{\frac{r_m}{r_a + r_0}},$$

where r_0 is the extracellular resistance per unit length. The extracellular current may not be purely ohmic because, when one cell is a current source, some of the current may flow through other cells; hence the circuit should include the capacitance of the membrane of these cells as well as their resistance. Although this problem has been rarely assessed quantitatively (see Clark and Plonsey, 1970; Stein and Pearson, 1971), it is unlikely to be of significance except with rapidly varying current sources, that is, in just those circumstances where a three-dimensional (rather than one-dimensional) treatment of extracellular resistances is required. Some techniques for treating nonuniformity (with distance) of the extracellular resistance have been presented by Cole and Hodgkin (1939) and by Taylor (1963).

MEMBRANE PROPERTIES   The assumption that the membrane can be treated as a linear resistance and perfect capacitance in parallel is also not generally true. Many cells display a nonlinear current-voltage relation for even relatively small displacements from the resting potential, due to the properties of the ionic channels that are open in the resting state. Even if the effect of these open channels does lead to roughly linear resistive behavior, they may contribute an element to the membrane capacitance that is not linear. The reason for this is that in many excitable cells some of the resting membrane conductance is due to ionic channels with voltage-dependent gates. These gates possess charge and tend to move when the membrane potential changes ("gating" current: see Armstrong, 1974, and Schwarz, this volume, for reviews). Hodgkin (1975) has calculated that gating contributes approximately $0.2 \ \mu F/cm^2$ additional, nonlinear, capacitance to the membrane of the squid giant axon when it conducts an action potential (see also Adrian, 1975). Calculations have yet to be performed to assess the significance of this phenomenon for the purely passive spread of potential in a cable structure, but for smaller membrane potential changes the size of the capacitance change will be less.

NATURE OF THE CURRENT CARRIER   It is natural when presented with an electrical circuit to assume that current is primarily carried by electrons. In biological tissues, however, there is very strong evidence that most of the charge movement is by way of ions. Within the cell the predominant charge carrier will be potassium ions since potassium is in high concentration and has a diffusion coefficient similar to that in free solution (Hodgkin and Keynes, 1953). Outside the cell, in the extracellular space, the bulk of the charge movement will be due to sodium and chloride ions. Ion movements across the membrane, in response to small displacements of the membrane potential from the resting value, are usually due mainly to potassium (and perhaps chloride) ions. If a small membrane current is sustained for some time, there will inevitably be ion concentration changes both inside and outside the cell. The magnitude of such changes will depend on (1) the surface-volume ratios of both extracellular and intracellular spaces in relation to the membrane current density and (2) the response of ion pumps. The changes most likely to be of quantitative significance will occur in the space where the membrane current carrier is in low concentration (i.e., extracellular potassium and/or intracellular chloride concentration). Making allowance for these effects will lead to a much more complicated equation (Attwell, Cohen, and Eisner, in preparation) because one will need to treat not only the effect of the concentration change on the battery or batteries setting the resting membrane potential but also both the concentration dependence of the relevant conductance(s) and the longitudinal diffusion of the ion(s) in the relevant space.

It might be argued that the various qualifications mentioned above are relatively insignificant quantitatively. Evidence for this view comes from Hodgkin and Rushton's (1946) classical study of electrotonus in the crustacean axon. Their experimental results fitted closely those predicted from equation 4. There are, however, two ways in which this deduction could be wrong. The first is concerned with whether such an observation validates the particular electrical circuit selected. This is not so because quite different sets of electrical circuits can predict very similar behavior. A good example in the physiological literature illustrating this point is the classical study of Fatt and Katz (1951) on the passive spread of the endplate potential in frog skeletal muscle. They fit their data very successfully assuming the circuit model of Figure 1, although it is now known that the appropriate electrical circuit for frog skeletal muscle is much more complicated (Falk and Fatt, 1964; Schneider, 1970; Valdiosera, Clausen, and Eisenberg, 1974; Mathias, Eisenberg, and Valdiosera, 1977). There is, however, no evidence that the equivalent circuit for nerve cells should be modified to include internal membrane structures, as is appropriate for muscle.

The second way the deduction could be wrong pertains particularly to the last assumption discussed above. Hodgkin and Rushton studied their axons after dissecting them free from the nerve trunk. The exact size of the extracellular space in these axons is unknown, but it is quite possible that in this dissected preparation it is larger than, say, for nerve cell processes in the neuropil. There are several cases in the literature in which changes in extracellular potassium concentration have been observed following the passage of membrane current (e.g., Neher and Lux, 1973), so it remains likely that in some circumstances ignoring ion concentration changes during the spread of current is a serious quantitative error.

Solving the differential equation

In the derivation of the cable equation, a cylindrical segment of a cell process was treated. This simple geometry is adequate to describe an unbranching unmyelinated axon but may be inappropriate for describing a branching structure or the cell soma. One essential feature in obtaining an appropriate solution of the differential equation is therefore to incorporate into it the relevant "geometry"—more specifically, the "electrical geometry," by which is meant an electrical circuit representation of the actual geometry. Rall (1959, 1960, 1962) has provided a powerful formulation which applies to a large class of these problems. Three examples are considered here.

1. *Cell soma*: Although there is often some difficulty in defining the outline of the cell soma because of the way in which it gives off processes, it is commonly described by anatomists as spherical or ellipsoidal in shape. Rall (1959) has suggested that for most purposes it is appropriate to assume isopotentiality of the soma membrane potential, so that the whole soma surface membrane can be represented as a single resistance and capacitance in parallel.

2. *Termination of a cell process*: Cell processes are finite in length, and the most peripheral extension of a process is "sealed" by a continuous surface of the cell membrane. Rall (1959) has shown that this can be modeled quite accurately by assuming that the terminal disc of membrane is effectively of infinite resistance (the "open-circuit" termination). Mathematically this is equivalent to assuming that axial current i_a is zero (and hence $\partial V/\partial x = 0$) at the termination.

3. *Branching*: In most nerve cells, the individual dendrites undergo successive branching with increasing distance from the soma (see Hillman, this volume). The most general treatment of this problem is that given by Rall (1962; see also Rall and Rinzel, 1973; Rinzel and Rall, 1974). For one particular pattern of branching, a powerful simplification results. If there is a uniform diameter between each branch point and, at each branching,

$$d_0^{3/2} = d_1^{3/2} + d_2^{3/2}, \qquad (5)$$

where the subscripts 0, 1, and 2 indicate the parent and two daughter branches respectively, then the whole branching structure behaves, for peripheral spread of current (i.e., away from the soma), like a uniform-diameter cylinder. Rall (1962) has also shown that a wider class of dendritic branching patterns, involving tapering of the diameters with distance as well as branching, can also be treated as an equivalent cylinder for the purpose of analyzing the peripheral spread of current. In the latter cases the condition analogous to equation 5 can be formulated most simply when the diameters of the two daughter branches are equal; then it is

$$nd^{3/2} = \text{constant}, \qquad (6)$$

where n is the number of branches (changing with distance) and d changes continuously with distance (see also Jack, Noble, and Tsien, 1975, pp. 149–156).

Treatment of the central spread of current (i.e., toward the soma) is simple in principle but laborious in practice (see Rall, 1959; Rall and Rinzel, 1973). For that class of dendritic trees which can be represented as an equivalent cylinder, there is one useful generalization. The voltage recorded at the central termination of a particular dendrite (i.e., at the soma) is only dependent on the magnitude of the current and the (electrotonic) distance at which it is injected. It is independent of the proportion of dendritic branches into which the current is injected (providing current is injected at the same electrotonic distance in all these branches).

It should be noted that dendritic branching patterns other than those obeying equations 5 or 6 may still be tractable mathematically, but the form of the differential equation will be different (see Rall, 1962; Goldstein and Rall, 1974; Jack, Noble, and Tsien, 1975).

Application of the principles outlined in the three examples allows a complete description of the electrical geometry of a nerve cell. The soma is represented as a lumped resistive-capacitive element and each dendrite is treated as an equivalent cylinder of finite length, with an open-circuit termination. For the peripheral spread of current (or the soma voltage with central spread), Rall was able to establish a further simplification. If each of the equivalent cylinders (representing each dendrite) is of the same electrotonic length, then they can be treated collectively as a single, larger-diameter, equivalent cylinder. Figure 2 schematically illustrates the steps in this transformation. The final model is often called the Rall model of the nerve cell, but, as indicated above, the formulation given by Rall is much more general.

Apart from specifying the electrical geometry to be treated, further information is needed before a complete solution to the differential equation can be obtained, namely, the nature and site of the "excitation." Experimentally the common forms of excitation are the passage of current into the cell (the exact time course of the current must be specified) or the imposition of a constant displacement of the membrane potential (voltage clamp). Physiologically the form of excitation may be current injection (e.g.,

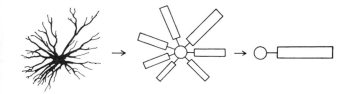

FIGURE 2 Transformations made in the development of the Rall model of the nerve cell. The nerve cell (left) is represented by a model with isopotential soma and each dendrite as an equivalent cylinder (middle). If each of these cylinders is of the same electrotonic length, a further transformation can be made lumping them all into a single equivalent cylinder. (From Jack, Noble, and Tsien, 1975.)

electrical synapses) or a change in the conductance of a patch of membrane (e.g., most chemically transmitting synapses—including most synaptic inhibition—and sensory transducers).

Various methods are available for solving the differential equation once all the above specifications (the boundary conditions to the equation) are provided. There is usually no difficulty in obtaining the steady-state solutions for the distribution of current and voltage in response to various forms of steady excitation. In this circumstance $\partial V/\partial T = 0$, so that the equation to be solved is a simple second-order ordinary differential equation, which has the general solution

$$V = Ae^{-X} + Be^{X}. \qquad (7)$$

Specific solutions are then obtained by incorporating the relevant boundary conditions. For example, if the geometry is an extended cable, one boundary condition is that the voltage displacement must become negligibly small a long distance away from its site of generation; hence $B = 0$. If the voltage displacement is produced by a voltage clamp (to V_0) at $X = 0$, then the specific solution becomes

$$V = V_0 e^{-X} \qquad (8)$$

since $V = V_0$ at $X = 0$.

The transient solutions are generally more difficult; three methods have been widely used. The only generally applicable one is to solve the equation by numerical methods. One convenient way of performing such calculations is by the compartmental method (Rall, 1964). The essence of this approach is to simplify the exact geometry into a series of interconnected regions, or compartments, treating each region as isopotential and linked to adjacent regions by a coupling resistance. The problem of solving the second-order partial differential equation then re-

duces to one of solving a set of coupled first-order equations. There is a likelihood of some quantitative inaccuracies in this method if the number of compartments chosen is small. This and several related problems have been explored recently by Perkel and Mulloney (1978a,b).

The other two methods have limited applicability but offer the advantage that they provide solutions in terms of exponentials, error functions, etc., where the individual variables, such as distance and time, do not have to be specified numerically. Particular solutions then generally require less complicated numerical calculations. Another advantage is that there is the possibility of deriving general relationships and/or approximations which describe various features of the transient response. So far these methods have only been successful with the simpler forms of excitation and electrical geometry.

The first of these analytical methods involves the use of the Laplace transform. The partial differential equation is converted, by this operation, into an ordinary differential equation; boundary conditions are then introduced in the same way as illustrated above for the steady-state solution, and thus a particular solution, in the Laplace transform domain, is obtained. The final step is to perform the inverse operation back out of the transform domain. (A more detailed exposition of this method is given in Jack, Noble, and Tsien, 1975, pp. 441–454.) The second method adopts a different strategy. A general solution to equation 4 is

$$V = (A_\alpha \sin \alpha X + B_\alpha \cos \alpha X) \exp (-(1 + \alpha^2)T), \quad (9)$$

where A_α, B_α, and α are constants determined by the boundary conditions. It is fairly straightforward to obtain a particular solution for α when the boundary conditions are uncomplicated (Rall, 1962, 1969; Iansek and Redman, 1973), but it is not so easy to determine A and B. Rall (1962, 1969) has indicated how this can be done, but full details have not yet been published. In general there is an infinite set of values of α (and associated values of A and B), so that the final solution takes the form

$$V = \sum_{n=0}^{\infty} (A_{\alpha_n} \sin \alpha_n X + B_{\alpha_n} \cos \alpha_n X) \times \exp(-(1 + \alpha_n^2)T). \quad (10)$$

As Rall (1969) has shown, it can be very useful to determine the values of α for a particular cable geometry, even if the values of A_α and B_α are not known, because this will give insight into the general form the transient response will take; and conversely, determining the values of α_0 and α_1 (the smallest values and hence the exponentials with the longest time constants) from an experimental transient provides some information about the specific electrical geometry.

Particular results

STEADY-STATE DISTRIBUTION OF VOLTAGE   The exponential decay of voltage with distance along an extended cylinder is a familiar result to all students of electrophysiology. What is the consequence of one side of the cylinder having a sealed end (open-circuit termination)? As mentioned earlier, this is equivalent, mathematically, to the axial current being zero at the end. One simple way to understand the effect of this condition is to imagine that the cylinder is infinitely extended and that the relevant boundary condition is "created" by having the actual axial current at the true end matched by an axial current of opposite direction and equal magnitude. Such an axial current can be readily produced by injecting a current equal to that injected in the true cylinder into the imaginary extension of the cylinder, at an equal distance from the true end as the actual current. By symmetry these two currents must create equal and opposite axial currents at the true end. Figure 3 illustrates this schematically; included in the figures are the voltages

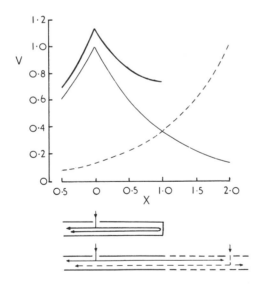

FIGURE 3   Steady-state voltage distribution in a semi-infinite cable. Current is injected into the cable one space constant from its sealed end. The thick line in the graph illustrates the voltage distribution. The thin and dashed lines represent the two components of voltage in a simulation of the sealed-end boundary condition in an infinite cable. The lower part of the figure is a schematic representation of the simulation.

produced by each of these current injections. The true voltage distribution in the real part of the cable is then simply the sum of these two voltages. It follows immediately that in a cylinder with an open-circuit termination at one end, the actual voltage at the end will be exactly double that predicted for an infinitely extended cylinder. In addition the voltage deviates less and less from that expected for an extended cylinder, the further (in electrotonic distance) one is from the end. More detailed accounts of the application of this technique, which is often called the method of images or the method of reflections to draw attention to the analogy with the behavior of light with a mirror, are given in Jack and Redman (1971a), Hodgkin and Nakajima (1972) and Jack, Noble, and Tsien (1975, Chapter 4). Multiple "reflections" must be considered if both ends of the cylinder are terminated. One familiar result for this latter circumstance is that when the total length of the cylinder is fairly short (e.g., less than half a space constant), and both ends have open-circuit terminations, the steady voltage distribution is fairly uniform, wherever the current is injected.

The steady-state distribution of voltage in complicated structures is a little more tedious to derive and calculate. For illustrations of the spread of voltage in branching structures the reader is referred to Rall (1959), Rall and Rinzel (1973), Barrett and Crill (1974b), Jack, Noble, and Tsien (1975, Chapter 7), and Graubard and Calvin (this volume). Strain and Brockman (1975) have calculated the steady voltage distribution for some examples in which the diameter of the cell process changes with axial distance.

Although this chapter is concerned only with linear cable theory, it may be worth noting that another consequence of axial current spread is the effect it has on the observed relationship between injected current and membrane voltage, when the membrane conductance is voltage-sensitive. In general, if current and voltage are recorded from the same point, the observed current-voltage relation will be more linear than the true membrane current-voltage relationship. Methods exist for correcting the observed steady-state current-voltage relationship so that the true current-voltage relation may be obtained. The principles of the method were originally given by Cole and Curtis (1941) and a review, with application to terminated cables, is given by Jack, Noble, and Tsien (1975, Chapters 9 and 12). A corollary of the result that the current-voltage relation is linearized when current injection and voltage recording are adjacent is that, when the voltage recording is made at some distance away from the current injection site, the observed relation may appear to be more nonlinear than the true (membrane) current-voltage relation.

THE VOLTAGE WAVEFORM IN RESPONSE TO A TRANSIENT INJECTION OF CURRENT

Many synaptic potentials are generated by a relatively brief current injection. The general pattern of the voltage response is thus a fairly brief rising phase, a peak, and then a gradual decline. A careful analysis of the exact time course of the voltage can be very informative about the time course of the injected current and/or the cable properties of the postsynaptic cell. A few generalizations will suffice here. At the site of current injection the duration of the rising phase is primarily set by the duration of the current injection. The peak amplitude reflects the time course and amplitude of the current as well as the cell's input impedance (*not* input resistance; see, for example, Redman, 1973). The time course of decay will be discussed below.

One reason for investigating the details of the voltage transient is to gain insight into the magnitude and time course of the effect produced by a synaptic action in other parts of a cell. In general, the further a synaptic potential spreads, the smaller its amplitude and the slower its time course becomes. Some details are listed here.

Peak amplitude The attenuation of the peak voltage with distance is much steeper than the attenuation of voltage when a steady current is injected. The briefer the time course of the injected current, the steeper the relative attenuation (see, for example, Figures 3.13, 4.7, 7.26, and 7.27 in Jack, Noble, and Tsien, 1975).

Area of the waveform Unlike the peak amplitude, the attenuation of the area with distance is independent of the time course of the injected current; it can be shown mathematically to be exactly the same as the steady-state attenuation for any electrical geometry (see Jack, Noble, and Tsien, 1975, pp. 187–188).

Propagation velocity In an electrical circuit consisting of only resistances and capacitances, the beginning of an electrical wave propagates at the speed of light. From a practical point of view, however, it is more useful to know when the waveform attains a significant amplitude. Several measures have been used in the literature: the "latency" (time to reach 10% of the peak value); the time to reach half amplitude in response to a step current excitation; and the time to peak (when the transient is produced by an instantaneous deposition of charge; this is mathematically equivalent to the inflection point time for a step of current). In an infinite cable geometry a

very rough estimate of these values is given by the following formulas:

Latency: $\quad T \approx 0.1\,X,$ (11)

Half-amplitude: $\quad T \approx 0.5\,(X + 0.5),$ (12)

Time to peak: $\quad T \approx 0.5\,(X - 0.5)$ (13)

(see Jack, Noble, and Tsien, 1975, Figures 3.6, 3.12, and 3.16). Note that in these formulas time and distance are normalized by the time constant and the space constant, respectively. It must be emphasized that the formulas only give order-of-magnitude estimates; the exact values depend on the time course of the current. The estimates tend to be least accurate for short distances. Iles (1977) has recently presented exact values for the latency of synaptic potentials generated in a model nerve cell.

Time course of decay Let us first consider the time course at the point of current injection. After cessation of current injection, the membrane potential decays passively. This can occur in two ways. Charge built up on the membrane capacitance at any point can discharge itself either through the local membrane conductance or by spread along the cell. The time course of decay of a transient is thus affected by the extent and time course of the axial spread of charge. There are three possibilities.

1. Negligible axial current throughout the whole time course: Axial current flows in response to differences in membrane potential between parts of the cell. If the cell is spherical or a cylinder of very small electrotonic length (e.g., < 0.2λ) with scaled ends, it becomes isopotential almost immediately. The only factor then setting the time course of decay is the local discharge of the membrane capacitance, so the time course of decay is exponential, with the rate of decay set by the membrane time constant.

2. Initial large axial currents, which become negligible after a time: Initially the time course of decay will be faster, but once the axial current becomes negligible the decay will be set by the membrane time constant, as above. This circumstance will apply to all finite cable structures with sealed ends. The time at which axial current becomes negligible is longer, the greater the electrotonic length of the cable. At early times the voltage decays in such a finite cable structure just as if it were infinitely extended, because there is a finite propagation time for the "reflections" to be generated by, and return from, the sealed ends.

3. Axial current flows throughout the whole decay time course: This occurs when the structure is effectively infinite (i.e., electrotonic lengths greater than

about four space constants) or, if finite, when the ends are not sealed. In this case the rate of decay at the point of current injection is always faster than that expected from the value of the membrane time constant. If the cable geometry is simply that of an infinitely extended cylinder, the time course of decay in response to very brief current injection is proportional to $e^{-t/\tau_m}/\sqrt{t}$.

When the voltage is recorded away from the site of current injection the explanation of the time course is a little more complicated because the direction of effect produced by axial current flow is different at early and late times. At early times axial current acts to *charge* the local membrane capacitance; hence the peak voltage occurs later than at the site of current injection. After the peak, axial current still continues to place charge on the membrane capacitance for a time whose duration increases with distance from the current injection site. In this period, then, the voltage decays more slowly than expected from the value of the membrane time constant. Subsequently the axial current acts to discharge the membrane capacitance, so that the rate of decay gradually becomes faster than expected.

Some applications

The whole point of cable theory is to provide a quantitative description of the spread of current in cells so that more sophisticated understanding can be gained of the process of signaling by electrical means. There are several reviews in the literature whose main aim has been to set out the implications of the cable properties of nerve-cell dendrites for the algebraic summation of synaptic effects (e.g., Rall, 1964, 1970; Jack, Noble, and Tsien, 1975, Chapter 7; Barrett, 1975; Redman, 1976). For this reason, some other aspects of cable theory will be discussed here.

MEASUREMENT OF R_m Clearly, the more specific the model selected the more precise are the theoretical predictions. It may be little help to the experimenter, however, to stipulate that the precise electrical geometry has to be determined before calculations can be performed. Even in the simplest geometry, an extended cable, exact determination of the values of R_m, R_i, and C_m requires, at the least, insertion of two microelectrodes a known distance apart as well as an accurate measurement of the diameter of the cylinder. But in most examples of recording from the neuropil, experimenters can count themselves lucky to make a secure penetration with a single microelec-

trode. Let us consider how much information can be gained in this circumstance.

It turns out that there are two important determinations to be made. The first is obvious; the actual geometry of the cell must be known. If the cell is an identified type, previous histological data may be adequate; otherwise the experimenter might determine it, for example, by filling the cell with a dye. The second requirement is an estimate of membrane resistance. In other words, it is reasonable to assume values for R_i and C_m, but not for R_m. This follows from a generalization that can be made about the results obtained for cells in which all three parameters have been measured. Once allowance is made for any membrane infoldings, etc., C_m is invariably close to 1 $\mu F/cm^2$. The value of R_i is always fairly close to the resistivity of the extracellular fluid in the same preparation; this depends on the electrolyte concentration and temperature, but is of the order of 100 Ω-cm. In contrast, the value of R_m has been observed to range from 1,000 Ω-cm^2 (squid giant axon) to nearly 10^6 Ω-cm^2 (*Aplysia* neuron).

These generalizations will be no surprise when the main factor in setting their value is recalled. All membranes are thought to be made up mainly of a bimolecular lipid sheet, so that the dielectric constant and thickness of the membrane is unlikely to vary a great deal; hence the relative constancy of the membrane capacitance. The intracellular fluid is thought to be predominantly an electrolyte solution, without significant restriction (for example, by ion binding) to the flow of those charge carriers that are in high concentration. Since the concentrations of electrolyte inside and outside the cell must be comparable, for osmotic reasons, so the resistivities should be comparable. The main factor setting R_m, however, is the density of membrane ion channels that are open in the resting state. A bimolecular lipid membrane without such channels may have a resistance greater than 10^8 Ω-cm^2, so that membrane resistances lower than this value are due to the presence of additional ion-carrying mechanisms. Their density could clearly vary, and there is good evidence, at least for the voltage-dependent sodium channels, that they do (see Ritchie, 1975).

The implications of such a wide variation in the value of R_m (in principle, over at least four orders of magnitude) are considerable. For example, the spatial spread of a steady voltage is set by the value of the space constant; the larger its value, the less attenuation there is with actual distance. A four-order-of-magnitude variation in R_m, for a given value of R_i, means a hundredfold difference in the space constant. For example, in a 0.4-μm-diameter extended cylinder, the space constant would be 10 μm if $R_i = 100$ Ω-cm and $R_m = 10^3$ Ω-cm², and 1,000 μm if $R_m = 10^7$ Ω-cm². Put another way, a steady voltage would, at a distance of 100 μm, be reduced to 0.005% or to 90% of its initial value. Obviously it would be most unwise to make deductions about the interactions between synaptic effects on a nerve cell solely on the basis of histological information.

There are two main ways to determine R_m if R_i and/or C_m are assumed. The first method depends on measuring the input resistance (R_{in}) at some site on the cell. The input resistance is defined from Ohm's law as the ratio of the membrane potential displacement to the current injected. In an infinite cylinder,

$$R_{in} = \sqrt{\frac{R_m R_i}{2\pi^2 d^3}}, \qquad (14)$$

so that, if the diameter d of the cylinder is known and R_i is assumed, R_m is obtained. Although straightforward in principle, there is a practical difficulty about this method when only one microelectrode can be inserted in the cell. The voltage recorded results from the passage of current through the resistance of the microelectrode as well as the cell's input resistance. It is common for the microelectrode resistance (R_{me}) to be much greater than R_{in}, so any error in the estimate of R_{me} will produce a relatively larger error in the derived value of R_{in}.

Another practical objection to this method arises when the geometry of the cell is complicated, as when one records from a cell body or a dendrite. Apart from the histological difficulties of measuring the geometry, as well as identifying the site of microelectrode penetration, the procedure for obtaining R_m from R_{in} is more complicated. Rall (1959) has presented the principles by which this may be done, and it is inescapably laborious.

For these reasons it may be more attractive to the experimenter to measure R_m by determining the membrane time constant ($\tau_m = R_m C_m$) of the cell. The method of preference is to pass a brief pulse of current through the microelectrode and record the subsequent changes in the membrane potential. The factors affecting the time course of decay of a transient potential have been set out in the previous section; by application of these principles the membrane time constant can be obtained. If it is unknown whether or not the structure is effectively finite, it will be necessary to plot both ln V and ln $(V\sqrt{t})$ against t to see which plot shows an exponential decay over its later time course (see Jack and Redman, 1971a,b).

Two qualifications should be mentioned. First, if the structure is effectively finite but the terminations are not an open circuit and/or the membrane time constant is not uniform, then the final decay on the plot of ln V against t will be exponential but its slope will not be proportional to the membrane time constant (see Jack and Redman, 1971a, Figure 17). Second, if the structure is effectively infinite but it is not accurate to represent any of its extensions as an equivalent cylinder (e.g., dendrites in which the branching pattern does not follow Equations 5 or 6), then, even if the plot of ln $(V\sqrt{t})$ against t shows a final exponential decay, the final time constant is not equal to the membrane time constant. Examples of these problems will be discussed later.

ACTIVE VERSUS PASSIVE PROPAGATION The classical account of the mode of signaling within a nerve cell is that there is active propagation (i.e., an action potential) along the axon, but the spread of current within the dendritic tree is by passive means. Recently it has become evident that this generalization is incorrect. Some nerve cells are apparently incapable of generating an action potential (see Ripley, Bush, and Roberts, 1968; Schmitt, Dev, and Smith, 1976; Pearson, this volume), and in others it is evident that action-potential propagation can be initiated in the dendritic tree (see Andersen and Lømo, 1966; Purpura, 1967; Kuno and Llinás, 1970; Llinás and Nicholson, 1971). Informed speculation about the functional significance of this diversity in the mode of signaling will doubtless depend on a fairly full understanding of the physiological role of the individual nerve cell, including the connections it receives and makes. As a preliminary to this it may be useful to consider some general features of active and passive propagation.

Conduction speed Some equations for propagation velocity of a passive potential have already been given. It is a common feature of the three quoted that dx/dt = constant; that is,

$$\frac{dx}{dt} \propto \frac{\lambda}{\tau_m} \propto \sqrt{\frac{d}{R_i R_m C_m^2}}. \qquad (15)$$

In other words the effective conduction speed of a passive potential is proportional to the square root of the fiber diameter and inversely proportional to the value of the membrane capacitance and to the square root of both the axoplasmic resistivity and membrane resistivity. If we assume that the membrane resistivity is the only one of these variables under physiological control (for a cell of a given size), then the cell can increase the speed of passive propagation by decreasing its membrane resistance.

How does this compare with active propagation? It is well known from cable theory analysis that the conduction velocity of an action potential in an unmyelinated fiber is, other things being equal, dependent on the fiber diameter and the axoplasmic resistivity in the same way as for passive propagation. It also depends on the rate constant for activation and the magnitude of the inward (sodium) current responsible for the regenerative depolarization. In order to gain quantitative insight into the additional factors, several workers have developed simplified models of the propagation process (see Hunter, McNaughton, and Noble, 1975). On one such model, which ignores recovery processes but realistically simulates the sodium conductance of the squid axon by a delayed activation process, Hunter, McNaughton, and Noble concluded that

$$\theta \propto d^{1/2} \, R_i^{-1/2} \, C_m^{-5/8} \, \tau^{-3/8} \, \overline{g_{Na}}^{1/8} \, , \qquad (16)$$

where θ is the conduction velocity, τ is the time constant for activation of the sodium conductance, $\overline{g_{Na}}$ is the maximum value of the sodium conductance, and the other symbols have their usual meaning. For present purposes the important point to note about this equation is that conduction velocity is independent of the value of the resting membrane resistance. [This prediction will not be true of real cells if the maximal sodium conductance is very small, but it does give a guide to the maximal conduction velocity attainable in an axon of a given size. On the other hand, this model neglects the effect of the "gating current," and its inclusion leads to the prediction that there will be an optimal magnitude of the maximal sodium conductance for achieving maximal conduction velocity (see Adrian, 1975; Hodgkin, 1975; Hunter, McNaughton, and Noble, 1975; Pickard, 1977). In the case of the squid axon, Adrian's computations with the full Hodgkin-Huxley model of the action potential showed that inclusion of gating current led to an approximately 20% reduction in the predicted velocity.]

The relative speeds of the two processes may be compared for the squid axon. The peak of a passive transient has a conduction velocity of approximately $2\lambda/\tau_m$. Taking $d = 476$ μm, $R_m = 1,000$ Ω-cm^2, $R_i = 35.4$ Ω-cm, and $C_m = 1$ μF/cm^2, a value of 11.6 m/sec is obtained. This may be compared with the action-potential propagation speed of 21.2 m/sec

measured by Hodgkin and Huxley (1952) for the same diameter axon.

Attenuation   The great advantage of an action potential is that it is invariant in size as it propagates along an axon. Passive potentials, by contrast, suffer severe attenuation in their peak amplitude. Even if one takes the area, rather than the peak amplitude, of a passive potential, there is still considerable attenuation. In an infinite cylinder the area of a synaptic potential at various distances is given by

$$A = Q \, \sqrt{\frac{R_m R_i}{\pi^2 d^3}} \cdot e^{-x/\sqrt{R_m d/R_i}}, \qquad (17)$$

where Q denotes the total charge injected at $x = 0$ (see Jack, Noble, and Tsien, 1975, p. 188). Thus the degree of attenuation is dependent on the value of R_m, being less the larger the value of R_m.

This result highlights the problem in using passive rather than active signaling. In order to avoid too much attenuation, it is desirable to increase R_m as much as possible, but when this is done, the speed at which the signal propagates is reduced. It is possible, therefore, that passive rather than active propagation is used in circumstances where it is not essential for the signal to be carried rapidly.

Time course   Another feature of passive propagation is that the time course of decay of a transient is much more prolonged than in an action potential, where the delayed increase in potassium conductance serves to restore the membrane potential back to near its resting level more rapidly than with passive decay. Rapid changes with time are thus more effectively signaled by using an action potential code.

Metabolic economy in the restitution of ionic gradients One possible reason for favoring passive propagation over an action-potential mechanism would arise if it proved more economical energetically. This would be so if the total inward charge required to produce a desired depolarizing effect at the end of a cell process were less for a passive mechanism. It turns out that passive propagation is not necessarily more efficient; but the higher the value of the membrane resistance the less charge is required (e.g., see equation 17). One difficulty about making general comparisons is that the charge required is also very sensitive to the particular electrical geometry. In addition, it is not clear that action-potential mechanisms are always equally efficient from an energetic point of view. In the squid giant axon the total amount of inward sodium movement is about four times the minimum required to achieve the amplitude attained; there is suggestive evidence that in smaller unmyelinated axons the peak amplitude of the sodium conductance per unit area is less and that this may have the consequence of a smaller net inward sodium movement per unit area per action potential (see Jack, 1975, 1976).

FINDING AN ADEQUATE MODEL OF THE NERVE CELL

The most systematically developed model of the nerve cell is that usually referred to as the Rall model. As outlined earlier, the cell soma is represented as an isopotential sphere and the dendrites as equivalent cylinders. The value of the membrane resistance is assumed to be the same over the whole cell surface.

The first careful testing of this model—as an adequate description of the cat motoneuron—was performed by Iansek and Redman (1973). They studied the voltage transients generated by very brief pulses of current, making the customary assumption that their microelectrode was inserted in the cell soma. They found that in approximately two-thirds of the cells, the voltage transients they recorded could not be simulated by the Rall model. The nature of the problem is illustrated in Figure 4; the experimental transients displayed, in their early time courses, a decay that was too rapid to be explained by any form of the conventional model. This type of result, for motoneurons, has also been obtained by Iles and Jack (unpublished).

There are two possible explanations for this result. Either the membrane resistance (or, more strictly, the membrane time constant) is not uniform over the whole cell surface, having a lower value near the site of microelectrode insertion, or axial current spreads away from the microelectrode at a rate faster than would be expected if the nerve cell were adequately represented by an equivalent cylinder. These suggestions arise from an understanding of the factors setting the time course of decay of a transient, which were presented earlier. The first point to note is that the deviation from the prediction of the model occurs at early times, when it would be expected that the voltage transient was not affected by the finite extent of the dendrites. Second, it is a prediction of the Rall model that, whatever the size of the cell body in relation to the sum of the dendritic diameters, the plot of ln $(V\sqrt{t})$ against t, at early times, will never show a rate of *decay* faster than that predicted by the membrane time constant and will gradually approach this rate of decay at later times (see Jack, Noble, and Tsien, 1975, Figure 7.17). [Two qualifications should be made about this last statement: (1) If the current is not brief, the early rate of decay may be faster (see

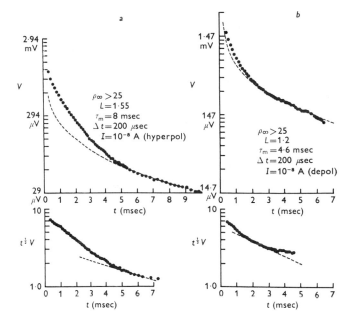

FIGURE 4 Two examples of experimental results that cannot be fit by the simplest Rall model of the nerve cell. The filled circles are the voltage responses to a brief pulse of current in two motoneurons (a and b). The upper half of the figure shows the relation between ln V and t. The dashed line on these graphs represents the best theoretical fit that could be obtained. Note the substantial deviation at early times. The lower half of the figure plots ln $(V\sqrt{t})$ against t. The accompanying dashed lines are straight lines with the same slopes as the final decay of the ln V curves above. As explained in the text, the standard circuit description of a nerve cell does not predict that there will be a more rapid decay on the ln $(V\sqrt{t})$ plot than the final decay on the ln V plot. Further details and discussion of these results are given in Iansek and Redman (1973), from which this figure is reproduced.

Jack and Redman, 1971b, Figure 7), but both Iansek and Redman (1973) and Iles and Jack (unpublished) were careful to avoid this difficulty. (2) Eventually the effect of the dendritic terminations will become evident. If they are open circuits, as suggested by Jack and Redman (1971b), the rate of decay will show a final decrease.] Thus, if we take a cylinder as our model of the nerve cell, the plot of ln $(V\sqrt{t})$ against t should be a straight line until the effect of the terminations becomes evident. Since the early part of this plot shows a faster decay, it follows that either there is a faster spread of axial current away from the recording site than expected for a cylinder or else the "local" membrane time constant at the recording site is shorter than in other parts of the cell.

There are several possible models that might yield the above result. I shall not attempt to be exhaustive in listing them but shall simply indicate some of the possibilities John Iles and I have considered because we find them the most plausible. First, the conventional Rall model may be correct, but the assumption that the microelectrode is inserted in the soma is not. If the microelectrode were in a proximal dendrite, the cell soma and other dendrites would act as a sink to attract axial current spread at a faster rate than in an equivalent cylinder. The plausibility of this alternative depends on the likelihood that a stable microelectrode recording is made in over half the cases from insertions into a proximal dendrite.

Another possibility is that the soma is not isopotential but might, for example, be better represented by a short cylinder to either end of which the larger-diameter equivalent cylinders for the dendrites are attached. But, according to our calculations, the soma in some cases would have to have an electrotonic length greater than 0.4λ. This is at odds with the known geometry.

Alternatively, it may be more correct to represent the dendrites not as equivalent cylinders but rather as processes whose overall diameter changes with distance away from the soma. In the limiting case of a very small soma, it can be shown that the time course of decay in such a model is given by

$$V \propto e^{-T[1+(K^2/4)]} \left[\frac{1}{\sqrt{\pi T}} - \frac{K}{2} \operatorname{exerfc}\left(\frac{K\sqrt{T}}{2}\right) \right], \quad (18)$$

where K expresses the degree of taper ($K < 0$, decreasing diameter with distance from soma) or flare ($K > 0$, increasing diameter) in the manner described by Rall (1962) and Goldstein and Rall (1974). When $K > 0$, the time course of decay is faster than for a cylindrical model; this is in accord with the intuition that axial current would flow away faster from the current injection site if the diameter increased with distance. But histological evidence does not support the suggestion of substantial flaring of the motoneuron dendritic tree (see Lux, Schubert, and Kreutzberg, 1970; Hillman, this volume). Indeed, Barrett and Crill (1974a) have suggested that tapering rather than flaring occurs.

Iansek and Redman (1973) favored the model in which the soma membrane time constant was lower than the time constant of the dendritic membrane. If this is the correct explanation of the form of the experimental transients, then it turns out from the calculations that John Iles and I have made that the soma membrane time constant must, in some cases, be as little as one-twentieth of the dendritic membrane time constant. This may seem a surprising difference, but there is one way in which it could readily

occur. When a microelectrode is inserted through the cell membrane, it inevitably creates a hole in the membrane. Although sealing of the membrane may occur, experimental measurements suggest that this sealing is not perfect and a substantial leak remains.

THE PROBLEM OF LEAK AROUND A MICROELECTRODE It has been well known, since the classic study of Nastuk and Hodgkin (1950), that insertion of a microelectrode into a cell can lead to a drop in the value of the resting potential. It may be presumed that this is caused by a leakage of ions around the electrode. if the reversal potential for this ionic current is assumed to be roughly 0 mV (i.e., all ions may be involved), then the relationship between the measured value of the resting potential (E_R^1) and the true value (E_R) is given by

$$E_R^1 = E_R \frac{G_{in}}{G_{in} + G_1}, \quad (19)$$

where G_{in} is the input conductance of the cell at the site of microelectrode insertion ($\equiv 1/R_{in}$, where R_{in} is the input resistance) and G_1 is the magnitude of the leak conductance around the microelectrode.

Two groups have made measurements of the value of G_1. Stefani and Steinbach (1969) reported an average value of 5×10^{-8} S (= 20 MΩ) and noted that it could be less if the microelectrodes had a high resistance and low value of tip potential, that is, in circumstances where one could presume that the tip diameter was particularly small. Hodgkin and Nakajima (1972) found values ranging between 0.1 and 2×10^{-7} S, with an average value of 10^{-7} S ($\equiv 10$ MΩ).

These values are not surprising when one considers the likely size of the gap between membrane and microelectrode (see also Lindemann, 1975). If one assumes that the microelectrode is circular at the tip with a diameter of 0.5 μm, that the fluid in the gap has a conductivity of 100 Ω-cm, and that the thickness of the membrane may be approximated as 100 Å, then the gap may be as little as 5 Å for a leak resistance of 10 MΩ.

The effects of such a leak conductance may be negligible or profound, depending on the ratio of G_1 to G_{in} (see equation 19). Apart from the reduction in the resting membrane potential, there will be the following consequences: (1) the measured R_{in} will be lower than its true value; (2) whatever technique is used to measure R_m, its value will be underestimated; and (3) if the membrane current-voltage relation is nonlinear, the measured current-voltage relation will be linearized and, because of the change in resting potential, the membrane resistance will not be uniform (assuming that it was before microelectrode penetration).

Let us consider some of these consequences in the circumstance of recording from the soma of a nerve cell such as the motoneuron. We shall assume that the cell has a geometry like that described by Rall (1959) and that, without microelectrode penetration, all the assumptions necessary for treating its electrical geometry as a standard Rall model are obeyed. Further, let us assume that $R_m = 10,000$ Ω-cm² (i.e., $\tau_m = 10$ msec), $E_R = -90$ mV, and $\rho_\infty = 40$. [Here ρ_∞ designates the dendrite-to-soma conductance ratio for infinitely extended dendrites (see Jack and Redman, 1971b). According to Rall's (1959) measurements of motoneuronal geometry, $\rho_\infty = 0.4 \sqrt{R_m}$.] When the microelectrode is inserted into the soma of the cell, it is assumed to create a leak conductance of 2×10^{-7} S ($\equiv 5$ MΩ), which is Hodgkin and Nakajima's worst case. If the cell has a true input resistance of 0.56 MΩ, its measured input resistance would be 0.5 MΩ and its measured resting potential -81 mV. With the above value of ρ_∞, the true conductance of the soma membrane would be 4.4×10^{-8} S, but after microelectrode penetration the soma conductance would increase to 24.4×10^{-8} S. In other words the ratio of dendritic membrane time constant to apparent soma membrane time constant would be 5.6. If the cell's dendrites were finite and had an electrotonic length of 1.5λ ($L = 1.5$), it can be calculated that the final time constant of decay on a ln V against t plot would be 9.3 msec rather than the true membrane time constant of 10 msec. Thus there would not be a serious error in the measurements of R_m. However, if the cell were smaller, the effect would be more serious. If the true input resistance were 3.3 MΩ, the measured input resistance would be 2 MΩ and the measured resting potential -54 mV. The ratio of dendritic to apparent soma membrane time constant would be 28.3, and the final exponential decay of a voltage transient would have a time constant of 7.5 msec (for $L = 1.5$). Furthermore, it would not be possible to fit the full time course of the transient using the Rall model of the nerve cell, the difficulty being as described in the previous section.

The above example indicates that it is important for experimenters, particularly those studying the cable properties of cells, to assess the effect of microelectrode leak. The most obvious initial guide to the possibility that this leak conductance is large relative to the input conductance at the recording site is the value of the recorded resting potential. If it is low (e.g., <70 mV internal negativity), then it is sensible

to assume that it may be a significant factor, although such a judgment has to take into account the concentration distributions of the ions important in setting the resting membrane potential. In general, the smaller the dimensions of the cell the more likely it is that the effect will be significant because of the expectation that input conductance will be loosely correlated (depending on the range of values of R_m) with cell size (see Hodgkin and Nakajima, 1972; Kuno, Miyata, and Muñoz-Martinez, 1974).

Is it possible to obtain a measure of the leak conductance when only one microelectrode can be inserted into the cell? In principle it is, but it may be a rather laborious procedure. In order to illustrate this, let us consider the simplest possible example: a microelectrode inserted into an infinite cable. The voltage response to a brief pulse of current is given by

$$V = \frac{Q_0}{\tau_m G_{in}} e^{-T} \left[\frac{1}{\sqrt{\pi T}} - a \text{ exerfc } (a\sqrt{T}) \right], \quad (20)$$

where $a = G_l/G_{ln}$.

A very simple method for obtaining both τ_m and a follows from this equation if adequate resolution of the time course of the voltage transient can be obtained for large values of $a\sqrt{T}$. Equation 20 then simplifies to

$$V \propto t^{3/2} e^{-T} \left[1 - \frac{3}{2a^2 T} + \frac{15}{8a^4 T^2} - \cdots \right], \quad (21)$$

so that the final time course of decay, at very large values of T, of a plot of ln $(Vt^{3/2})$ against t will decay exponentially at a rate set by the membrane time constant. Subtraction of this final exponential component from the curve will then allow the value of a^2, and hence of a, to be determined.

Unfortunately, although simple in principle, this may be difficult to do in practice, particularly when a is small. Equation 21 is only valid for large values of $a\sqrt{T}$, so that if $a = 0.5$, for example, measurements of V at very large values of T (> 20) are required. Information about the values of a and τ_m are, of course, given by the form of the voltage decay at early times, but I have not been able to devise a simple procedure for obtaining them. If this is not possible, it leaves the experimenter with a tedious curve-fitting task.

The obvious alternative is to devise means to reduce the value of the leakage conductance so that it may be safely ignored. Apart from a decrease in the tip diameter, "sealing" of the membrane might be encouraged by coating the external surface of the microelectrode with a lipophilic substance. R. F.

Miller (personal communication) has found considerable improvement in sealing when electrodes are dipped in dichloromethyl silane (4% in CCl_4). Technical advances of this kind may eventually help even with the smallest cells with the highest membrane resistance. It would certainly be desirable if this rather unfortunate feature of the electrical geometry could be made negligible, so that one could be confident that a cell penetrated by a microelectrode behaved just as it did before penetration.

ACKNOWLEDGMENTS   I would like to thank David Attwell and John Iles for their comments.

REFERENCES

ADRIAN, R. H., 1975. Conduction velocity and gating current in the squid giant axon. *Proc. R. Soc. Lond.* B189:81–86.

ANDERSEN, P., and T. LØMO, 1966. Mode of activation of hippocampal pyramidal cells by excitatory synapses on dendrites. *Exp. Brain Res.* 2:247–260.

ARMSTRONG, C. M., 1974. Ionic pores, gates and gating currents. *Q. Rev. Biophys.* 7:179–209.

BARRETT, J. N., 1975. Motoneuron dendrites: Role in synaptic integration. *Fed. Proc.* 34:1398–1407.

BARRETT, J. N., and W. E. CRILL, 1974a. Specific membrane properties of cat motoneurones. *J. Physiol.* 239:301–324.

BARRETT, J. N., and W. E. CRILL, 1974b. Influence of dendritic location and membrane properties on the effectiveness of synapses on cat motoneurones. *J. Physiol.* 239:325–345.

CLARK, J. W., and R. PLONSEY, 1970. A mathematical study of nerve fiber interaction. *Biophys. J.* 10:937–957.

COLE, K. S., 1968. *Membranes, Ions and Impulses.* Berkeley: Univ. California Press.

COLE, K. S., and H. J. CURTIS, 1941. Membrane potential of the squid giant axon during current flow. *J. Gen. Physiol.* 24:551–563.

COLE, K. S., and A. L. HODGKIN, 1939. Membrane and protoplasm resistance in the squid giant axon. *J. Gen. Physiol.* 22:671–687.

DAVIS, L., and R. LORENTE DE NÓ, 1947. Contribution to the mathematical theory of electrotonus. *Stud. Rockefeller Inst. Med. Res.* 131:442–496.

EISENBERG, R. S., and E. A. JOHNSON, 1970. Three-dimensional electric field problems in physiology. *Prog. Biophys. Mol. Biol.* 20:1–65.

FALK, G., and P. FATT, 1964. Linear electrical properties of striated muscle fibres observed with intracellular electrodes. *Proc. R. Soc. Lond.* B160:69–123.

FATT, P., and B. KATZ, 1951. An analysis of the end-plate potential recorded with an intracellular electrode. *J. Physiol.* 115:320–370.

GOLDSTEIN, S. S., and W. RALL, 1974. Changes of action potential shape and velocity for changing core conductor geometry. *Biophys. J.* 14:731–757.

HODGKIN, A. L., 1975. The optimum density of sodium channels in an unmyelinated nerve. *Phil. Trans. R. Soc. Lond.* B270:297–300.

HODGKIN, A. L., and A. F. HUXLEY, 1952. A quantitative description of membrane current and its application to conduction and excitation in nerve. *J. Physiol.* 117:500–544.

HODGKIN, A. L., and R. D. KEYNES, 1953. The mobility and diffusion coefficient of potassium in giant axons from squid. *J. Physiol.* 119:513–528.

HODGKIN, A. L., and S. NAKAJIMA, 1972. The effect of diameter on the electrical constants of frog skeletal muscle fibres. *J. Physiol.* 221:105–120.

HODGKIN, A. L., and W. A. H. RUSHTON, 1946. The electrical constants of a crustacean nerve fibre. *Proc. R. Soc. Lond.* B133:444–479.

HUNTER, P. J., P. A. McNAUGHTON, and D. NOBLE, 1975. Analytical models of propagation in excitable cells. *Prog. Biophys. Mol. Biol.*, 30:99–144.

IANSEK, R., and S. J. REDMAN, 1973. An analysis of the cable properties of spinal motoneurones using a brief intracellular current pulse. *J. Physiol.* 234:613–636.

ILES, J. F., 1977. The speed of passive dendritic conduction of synaptic potentials in a model motoneurone. *Proc. R. Soc. Lond.* B197:225–229.

JACK, J. J. B., 1975. Physiology of peripheral nerve fibres in relation to their size. *Br. J. Anaesth.* 47:173–182.

JACK, J. J. B., 1976. Electrophysiological properties of peripheral nerve. In *The Peripheral Nerve*, D. Landon, ed. London: Chapman & Hall, pp. 740–818.

JACK, J. J. B., D. NOBLE, and R. W. TSIEN, 1975. *Electric Current Flow in Excitable Cells.* Oxford: Clarendon Press.

JACK, J. J. B., and S. J. REDMAN, 1971a. The propagation of transient potentials in some linear cable structures. *J. Physiol.* 215:283–320.

JACK, J. J. B., and S. J. REDMAN, 1971b. An electrical description of the motoneurone, and its application to the analysis of synaptic potentials. *J. Physiol.* 215:321–352.

KUNO, M., and R. LLINÁS, 1970. Enhancement of synaptic transmission by dendrite potentials in chromatolysed motoneurones of the cat. *J. Physiol.* 210:807–821.

KUNO, M., Y. MIYATA, and E. J. MUÑOZ-MARTINEZ, 1974. Differential reaction of fast and slow α-motoneurones to axotomy. *J. Physiol.* 240:725–739.

LINDEMANN, B., 1975. Impalement artifacts in microelectrode recordings of epithelial membrane potentials. *Biophys. J.* 15:1161–1164.

LLINÁS, R., and C. NICHOLSON, 1971. Electrophysiological properties of dendrites and somata in alligator Purkinje cells. *J. Neurophysiol.* 34:532–551.

LUX, H. D., P. SCHUBERT, and G. W. KREUTZBERG, 1970. Direct matching of morphological and electrophysiological data in cat spinal motoneurones. In *Excitatory Synaptic Mechanisms*, P. Andersen and J. K. S. Jansen, eds. Oslo: Universitetsforlaget.

MATHIAS, R. T., R. S. EISENBERG, and R. VALDIOSERA, 1977. Electrical properties of frog skeletal muscle fibers interpreted with a mesh model of the tubular system. *Biophys. J.* 17:57–93.

NASTUK, W. L., and A. L. HODGKIN, 1950. The electrical activity of single muscle fibers. *J. Cell Comp. Physiol.* 35:39–73.

NEHER, E., and H. D. LUX, 1973. Rapid changes of potassium concentration at the outer surface of exposed single neurons during membrane current flow. *J. Gen. Physiol.* 61:385–399.

PERKEL, D. H., and B. MULLONEY, 1978a. Calibrating compartmental models of neurons. *Am. J. Physiol.* 235:R93–R98.

PERKEL, D. H., and B. MULLONEY, 1977b. Electrotonic properties of neurons: Steady-state compartmental model. *J. Neurophysiol.* 41:621–639.

PICKARD, W. F., 1977. The optimum density of sodium channels in an unmyelinated nerve: An analytic treatment. *Math. Biosci.* 34:23–34.

PURPURA, D., 1967. Comparative physiology of dendrites. In *The Neurosciences: A Study Program*, G. C. Quarton, T. Melnechuk, and F. O. Schmitt, eds. New York: Rockefeller Univ. Press, pp. 372–393.

RALL, W., 1959. Branching dendrite trees and motoneuron membrane resistivity. *Exp. Neurol.* 1:491–527.

RALL, W., 1960. Membrane potential transients and membrane time constant of motoneurons. *Exp. Neurol.* 2:503–532.

RALL. W., 1962. Theory of physiological properties of dendrites. *Ann. NY Acad. Sci.* 96:1071–1092.

RALL, W., 1964. Theoretical significance of dendritic trees for neuronal input-output relations. In *Neural Theory and Modelling*, R. F. Reiss, ed. Stanford: Stanford Univ. Press, pp. 73–79.

RALL, W., 1969. Time constants and electrotonic length of membrane cylinders and neurons. *Biophys. J.* 9:1483–1508.

RALL, W., 1970. Cable properties of dendrites and effects of synaptic location. In *Excitatory Synaptic Mechanisms*, P. Andersen and J. K. S. Jansen, eds. Oslo: Universitetsforlarget, pp. 175–187.

RALL, W., and J. RINZEL, 1973. Branch input resistance and steady attenuation for input to one branch of a dendritic neuron model. *Biophys. J.* 13:648–688.

REDMAN, S. J., 1973. The attenuation of passively propagating dendritic potentials in a motoneurone cable model. *J. Physiol.* 234:637–664.

REDMAN, S. J., 1976. A quantitative approach to integrative function of dendrites. In *International Review of Physiology: Neurophysiology II*, vol. 10, R. Porter, ed. Baltimore: University Park Press, pp. 1–35.

RINZEL, J., and W. RALL, 1974. Transient response in a dendritic neuron model for current injected at one branch. *Biophys. J.* 14:759–790.

RIPLEY, S. H., B. M. H. BUSH, and A. ROBERTS, 1968. Crab muscle receptor which responds without impulses. *Nature* 218:1170–1171.

RITCHIE, J. M., 1975. Binding of tetrodotoxin and saxitoxin to sodium channels. *Philos. Trans. R. Soc. Lond.* B270:319–336.

SCHMITT, F. O., P. DEV, and B. H. SMITH, 1976. Electrotonic processing of information by brain cells. *Science* 193:114–120.

SCHNEIDER, M. F., 1970. Linear electrical properties of the transverse tubules and surface membrane of skeletal muscle fibers. *J. Gen. Physiol.* 56:640–671.

SCOTT, A. C., 1972. Transmission line equivalent for an unmyelinated nerve axon. *Math. Biosci.* 13:47–54.

STEFANI, E., and A. B. STEINBACH, 1969. Resting potential and electrical properties of frog slow muscle fibres. Effect of different external solutions. *J. Physiol.* 203:383–401.

STEIN, R. B., and K. E. PEARSON, 1971. Predicted amplitude and form of action potentials recorded from unmyelinated nerve fibres. *J. Theor. Biol.* 32:539–558.

STRAIN, G. M. and W. H. BROCKMAN, 1975. A modified cable model for neuron processes with non-constant diameters. *J. Theor. Biol.* 51:475–494.

TAYLOR, R. E., 1963. Cable theory. In *Physical Techniques in Biological Research*, vol. 6: *Electrophysiological Methods*, part B, W. L. Nastuk, ed. New York: Academic Press, pp. 219–262.

VALDIOSERA, R., C. CLAUSEN, and R. S. EISENBERG, 1974. Circuit models of the passive electrical properties of frog skeletal muscle fibers. *J. Gen. Physiol.* 63:432–459.

25 The Nonuniform Excitability of Central Neurons as Exemplified by a Model of the Spinal Motoneuron

F. A. DODGE

ABSTRACT The parameters for a nonuniform cable model are set by the neuron's morphology and its input impedance. Regional densities of excitable ionic channels are found by comparing computed action potentials to electrophysiological data for different modes of excitation. The sodium conductance in the initial segment must be very high, as in the nodes of Ranvier, in order for the antidromic impulse to invade the soma. The sodium conductance of the soma is about an order of magnitude lower, and it is negligible in the dendrites of normal motoneurons. Simulation of nonlinear summation of synaptic potentials independently confirms the passive behavior of normal dendrites. In chromatolytic motoneurons the observation of partial dendritic spikes requires sufficient sodium conductance to propagate the action potential over the whole dendrite.

Introduction

WHEN A mathematical model of a neuron is made sufficiently realistic, it becomes a powerful tool for synthesizing different kinds of experimental data to yield new information and to make more precise, even novel, interpretations of old information. The first step in formulating such a model is to reconcile measurements of the input impedance of the neuron with its morphology in terms of parameters of a nonuniform electrical cable. We assume that each specific ionic permeability change that can be resolved by biophysical or pharmacological techniques represents a different ionic channel, and we distribute variable densities of each kind of channel along the cable. By requiring computed responses to match electrophysiological recordings for several different modes of excitation (e.g., antidromic, direct, and synaptic stimulation), we converge to a fairly definite distribution

of the average density of channels in different regions of the neuron. If we then make the dendrites branch with a realistic geometry, the model can be used to examine aspects of synaptic excitation that depend on the input impedance at different points in the dendrites.

Here I shall describe this procedure by modeling the spinal motoneuron of the cat. Mainly from the work of J. C. Eccles (1957, 1964) and his many collaborators, we have a great variety of detailed electrophysiological information for this neuron. More recently, intracellular staining techniques have been used to reconstruct the morphology of the motoneurons whose input impedance had been measured. With such precise data we can expect to put the strictest constraints on the parameters of a valid model.

The spinal motoneuron is a highly specialized projection neuron, and we must therefore exercise caution in extrapolating the results of this model to other central neurons. The manifest excitability of the dendrites of many central neurons is a particularly important difference. I shall for this reason model the generation of dendritic spikes in chromatolytic motoneurons, in order to set some general conditions on the distribution of excitable channels. Furthermore, we expect that the membrane characteristics of local circuit neurons will justify the use of one-dimensional cable theory. If so, these neurons can be modeled by the same procedure, and such models will thus contribute valuable insights into the relation between their structure and function.

The nonuniform-cable model

Under most conditions the distribution of membrane potential along the cylindrical neural process is ac-

F. A. DODGE IBM Corporation, T. J. Watson Research Center, P.O. Box 218, Yorktown Heights, NY 10598

curately described by the one-dimensional cable equation of the form

$$\frac{a}{2R_i} \frac{\partial^2 V}{\partial t^2} = I_m = C_m \frac{\partial V}{\partial t} + I_i,$$ (1)

which says that the local value of the membrane current density I_m is given by the local difference in longitudinal current (left side). But I_m also depends on the local electrical properties of the membrane (right side), which is, in general, the sum of a capacitative displacement current and the movement of ions through the membrane (I_i). In equation 1, the membrane potential V is measured relative to its stable resting value, a is the local value of the fiber radius, and R_i is specific resistance of the axoplasm, which we assume has the constant value of 100 Ω-cm. We have also assumed that the extracellular voltage differences are negligibly small.

The cell membrane consists of a lipid bilayer stabilized by a layer of proteins on each surface. The lipid bilayer gives the membrane a capacitance (C_m) of 1.0 $\mu F/cm^2$. A higher effective capacitance is measured if the neuronal surface is wrinkled or invaginated. Conversely, the capacitance is reduced in the myelin-covered regions of the axon by a factor equal to the number of layers of Schwann-cell membrane that wrap the axon.

From studies of artificial membranes, we believe that the lipid bilayer is quite impermeable to ions, but that ions do move through various kinds of channels which are discrete macromolecules perforating the membrane. At this time we do not have direct molecular characterizations of the various channels, but we identify and describe them in terms of the variables that control their opening and closing. In the case of channels that are activated by synaptic transmitters, we know by direct measurement that they are typically localized in the subsynaptic membrane. In the case of the sodium and potassium ionic channels that underlie excitation and propagation of the action potential, we know only that they cannot be distributed uniformly. The present model includes only four different channels: the nonlinear sodium and potassium ionic channels of the excitable membrane; the linear "leakage" channels that determine the resting state; and the channels that are opened by excitatory synaptic actions. Accordingly, the local value of I_i will be given by

$$I_i = g_{Na}(V - V_{Na}) + g_K(V - V_K) + g_l(V - V_l) + g_e(V - V_e),$$ (2)

where the terms in parentheses are the electrochemical driving force of the ions flowing through a par-

ticular channel and the local density of open channels is measured in terms of membrane conductance variables.

For small perturbations of the membrane potential from its stable resting value, the neuronal membrane typically behaves as if it were passive; that is, $I_i = V/R_m$. In our model the resting state is dominated by the leakage channels, a very small fraction of the potassium channels are open, and all of the sodium and synaptic channels are closed. For such a passive cable we can define several quantities that are useful in determining values for model parameters from experimental measurements. These are the membrane time constant,

$$\tau_m = R_m C_m,$$ (3)

the electrical characteristic length,

$$\lambda = \sqrt{a R_m / 2R_i},$$ (4)

and the input resistance looking into one end of a uniform cable of length L whose other end is sealed,

$$R_N = \frac{\lambda R_i}{\pi a^2} \coth\left(\frac{L}{\lambda}\right).$$ (5)

EQUIVALENT-CYLINDER REPRESENTATION OF THE DENDRITES The theoretical breakthrough that made practical the quantitative interpretation of the electrical signals in the motoneuron was Rall's (1959) discovery that the electrical characteristics of its branching dendritic tree could be represented by an equivalent uniform cable. The physical basis of this representation is that at each bifurcation the electrical load of the two daughter branches (radii a_1 and a_2) should match that of an equivalent length of the parent branch (radius a_0). This condition is met when $a_1^{3/2} + a_2^{3/2} = a_0^{3/2}$, which follows directly from equation 5. Rall (1962, 1967, 1969, 1970) has extensively developed the mathematical analysis of current flow in dendritic trees, particularly with respect to the measurement of membrane constants and to the effect of the location of a synapse on the waveform of its synaptic potential.

Applying Rall's (1969) methods to measurement of the input impedance of cat spinal motoneurons, Nelson and Lux (1970) found as typical values $\tau_m = 6$ msec and $L = 1.5\lambda$. Burke and tenBruggencate (1971) confirmed these values for motoneurons of widely varying size, that is, neurons whose input resistance ranged from 0.5 to 3.5 MΩ. Using different intracellular staining techniques, Lux, Schubert, and Kreutzberg (1970) and Barrett and Crill (1971, 1974a) reconstructed the morphology of neurons on which electrical measurements had been made. These studies generally found excellent agreement between the morphological and electrical estimates of the equivalent length of the dendrites, and they provide the most reliable values for the specific membrane constants.

In constructing our model (Figure 1) we rely primarily on the measurements of Lux, Schubert, and Kreutzberg (1970). We simulate a large motoneuron with an input resistance of 1 MΩ, $\tau_m = 6$ msec, and $L = 1.5\lambda$. We lump the soma and tapered stumps of the proximal dendrites together into a single compartment that contains 6.5% of all the soma dendritic membrane. Taking $C_m = 2$ μF/cm^2, τ_m fixes R_m at 3,000 Ω-cm^2. The input resistance sets the radius of the dendritic equivalent cylinder to 23 μm and its length to 2,800 μm. We arbitrarily make the radius of soma compartment twice as large so that there will be a negligible voltage drop along that compartment.

As pointed out by Lux, Schubert, and Kreutzberg

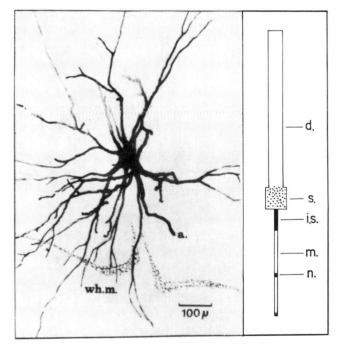

FIGURE 1 *Left*: Morphological reconstruction of a large spinal motoneuron by Lux, Schubert, and Kreutzberg (1970). The axon (a.) and boundary of the white matter (wh.m.) are identified. *Right*: Representation of the electrical characteristics of a motoneuron by a nonuniform cable divided into regions that have the surface area of corresponding regions of the neuron. These are the dendrites (d.), which are lumped together as an equivalent cylinder, the soma (s.), the initial segment of the axon (i.s.), myelinated internode (m.), and the nodes of Ranvier (n.). The density of stippling is meant to suggest the density of sodium channels in that region of a normal motoneuron.

(1970), the axon comes out of the soma as a uniform cylinder. In our model the axon has a diameter of 10 μm, the unmyelinated initial segment has a length of 100 μm, and C_m is taken as 1 μF/cm^2. The first node of Ranvier is connected by a myelinated segment 230 μm long, in which the myelin is represented by a passive membrane with $C_m = 0.01$ μF/cm^2 and $R_m = 0.1$ MΩ-cm^2. Another myelinated segment and another node of Ranvier are used to move an antidromic stimulus away from the initial segment. (The dimensions of this equivalent cylinder differ somewhat from that of Dodge and Cooley, 1973, who used $C_m = 1$ μF/cm^2 for a neuron with the same input impedance.)

CURRENT-VOLTAGE RELATIONS OF THE EXCITABLE MEMBRANE The highly nonlinear sodium and potassium conductances are given a kinetic description by equations of the form developed by Hodgkin and Huxley (1952) for the squid axon, but whose empirical constants were modified to fit voltage-clamp data from vertebrate nerve fibers (Dodge and Frankenhaeuser, 1958).

Coombs, Curtis, and Eccles (1957) postulated that the somatodendritic membrane has a voltage threshold about 10 mV higher than that of the initial segment to explain their observation that the action potential starts in the initial segment even when the somatodendritic membrane is more depolarized by synaptic excitation. This difference in voltage threshold was confirmed by Araki and Terzuolo (1962) who applied the voltage-clamp technique to the motoneuron soma and observed that action potentials were stimulated in the axon over a range of depolarizations that were subthreshold for the generation of current by the soma. We do not believe that this difference in threshold implies that there are two different kinds of sodium channels in the initial segment and soma membranes. Instead, we believe that the same kind of channel sees a different local fixed-charge environment, as is postulated to explain the effect of divalent ions on the threshold of axons (Frankenhaeuser and Hodgkin, 1957). Hence in our model we take account of this difference in threshold by putting a voltage shift on the rate constants for the somatodendritic membrane.

The membrane currents measured by a voltage clamp on the soma are so severely contaminated by current flow from the dendrites and axon, where the voltage is not controlled, that they cannot be used to formulate kinetic equations. Nonetheless, they do give some very important specifications for our model. Araki and Terzuolo (1962) measured a maximum inward current of about 0.5 nA for a neuron with 1.2 MΩ input resistance. Their measurements of the current-voltage relations for the peak of the transient inward current and the late outward current suggest that the ratio of the maximum sodium conductance to the maximum potassium conductance of the soma is similar to that observed in peripheral axons. Accordingly, we have arbitrarily assumed in our model that this ratio is fixed when the density of channels is varied. See Dodge and Cooley (1973) for details of the kinetic equations.

COMPUTATIONAL METHODS   To simulate the electrical responses of the motoneuron, we must solve the nonlinear partial differential equation (equation 1) in which the radius and several membrane parameters vary with distance along the cable. We derived a finite-difference approximation (Dodge and Cooley, 1973) by dividing the cable into numerous short segments, evaluating the membrane current assuming uniform membrane potential over each segment, and evaluating the longitudinal current between adjacent segments as the ratio of the potential difference to the resistance between the midpoints of the segments. The membrane current of each segment is described by four differential equations like those of the Hodgkin-Huxley model. This system of equations is solved numerically by the same procedure that we developed for simulating the squid axon (Cooley and Dodge, 1966). In the latter case we demonstrated the accuracy of our spatial difference approximation by comparing our computations to the uniformly propagating impulse that can be computed precisely by a different method.

Excitability of the normal motoneuron

THE SOMA HAS A LOW DENSITY OF SODIUM CHANNELS   If we represent the input impedance of the motoneuron by a lumped equivalent circuit consisting of a 0.025 μF capacitor shunted by a 1 MΩ resistor, we find that the amount of sodium conductance measured by Araki and Terzuolo (1962) is not sufficient to generate an action potential. On the other hand, if we spread that amount of sodium conductance uniformly over the soma compartment of the equivalent-cylinder model, we do get a 90 mV action potential with a maximum rate of rise of 250 V/sec, which agrees well with experimental values. This result clearly demonstrates the importance of treating the neuron as a distributed system for a quantitative interpretation of electrical measurements.

In this case the sodium conductance is 140 mmho/cm^2 on the soma and zero in the dendrites. But we cannot conclude that this is the normal distribution. We get an equally good action potential if we make the somatodendritic membrane uniformly excitable with g_{Na} = 100 mmho/cm^2. Moreover, simulation of a voltage clamp at the soma gave about the same peak inward current since the clamp cannot control the potential for more than about 0.1λ out on the dendrite. We shall consider the problem of dendritic excitability later after adding the motor axon to the model.

THE INITIAL SEGMENT HAS A HIGH DENSITY OF SODIUM CHANNELS   From voltage-clamp measurements on single nodes of Ranvier (Dodge and Frankenhaeuser, 1958), we know that the nodal membrane has a very high sodium conductance—using the conservative estimate of the nodal area of 100 μm^2, g_{Na} is greater than 1,000 mmho/cm^2. Having fixed the axon diameter at 10 μm, we set the length of the first myelin segment so that an antidromic action potential generated by the node will give a 2 mV spike in the soma when invasion of the initial segment is blocked by hyperpolarization (Coombs, Eccles, and Fatt, 1955).

Eccles (1957) cites the dimensions of the initial segment of a representative motoneuron as 80 μm long for a diameter of 8 μm. We have kept the same proportions, setting the length at 100 μm for our somewhat larger neuron. Figure 2 illustrates the effect of varying g_{Na} of the initial segment. The plots of the rate of change of the soma potential show more clearly the characteristic inflection on the rising phase caused by the severe electrical load of the somatodendritic membrane on the initial segment (Coombs, Eccles, and Fatt, 1955). Comparing the simulations of Figure 2 to typical experimental observations (e.g., Coombs, Curtis, and Eccles, 1957), we find few examples of delays between the initial-segment and soma spikes as long as that of curve c, and curves a and b are more typical. Thus we can conclude that g_{Na} = 600 mmho/cm^2 is a lower bound, and a value of 1,000 mmho/cm^2 is more probable. In other words, the fact that we observe an antidromic impulse invading the soma means that the initial segment has a high density of sodium channels. In fact, the density is nearly the same as that of nodes of Ranvier.

THE DENDRITES ARE INEXCITABLE   Now that the action potential of our model is initiated in the initial segment, we can return to the question of dendritic excitability. The basis for answering this ques-

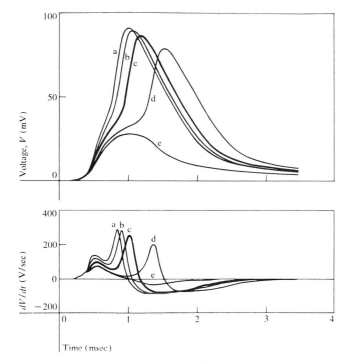

FIGURE 2 Determination of the density of sodium channels in the membrane of the initial segment of the axon. Responses to an antidromic impulse computed for sodium conductances of (a) 1,000, (b) 800, (c) 600, (d) 500, and (e) 400 mmho/cm². Lower curves are first derivatives of the upper curves. (From Dodge and Cooley, 1973.)

tion is the response of the neuron to synaptic stimulation. Figure 3 shows the two extreme cases: in a the dendrites are passive and the soma has g_{Na} = 140 mmho/cm²; in b the somatodendritic membrane is uniformly excitable with g_{Na} = 100 mmho/cm². Both cases show a prominent inflection on the rising phase of the antidromic spike (curves a). We simulated synaptic excitation by applying a 0.5 msec rectangular pulse of current at a point 0.4λ out on the dendrites. For a threshold stimulus (curves b) we see an inflection which signals the prior excitation of the initial segment in both cases. Here the somewhat greater depolarization does not overcome the effect of the lower threshold of the initial-segment membrane. But if the synaptic current is 25% greater (curves c), then in the case of uniform excitability (b) we find the action potential initiated in the dendrite, and our recording shows the sudden loss of the inflection and a dramatic increase in the rate of rise of the soma spike. In the case of inexcitable dendrites, there is little change in the spike waveform. Normal adult motoneurons behave only in the manner of Figure 3a. On the other hand, chromatolytic motoneurons typically have excitable dendrites, and responses like

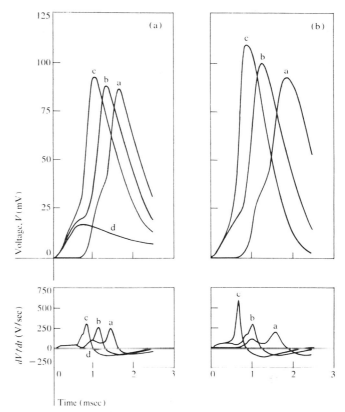

FIGURE 3 Comparison of the responses of a motoneuron model with passive dendrites (a) and with uniform weak excitability of both the soma and dendritic membranes (b) to different modes of excitation. For both cases curve a is antidromic excitation, b is threshold synaptic excitation, and c is suprathreshold (× 1.25) synaptic excitation. Lower curves are first derivatives of the upper curves. (From Dodge and Cooley, 1973.)

Figure 3b are observed (Eccles, Libet, and Young, 1958). We shall investigate dendritic excitability of chromatolytic motoneurons below.

The preceding results clearly suggest that the density of sodium channels in the dendrites is much lower than in the soma, but they cannot give a good estimate of how much lower. A much more sensitive test is obtained by asking how dendritic excitability would affect the excitatory postsynaptic potential (EPSP). The EPSP is generated by a brief conductance change that opens channels whose equilibrium potential is some 50–70 mV depolarized from the normal resting potential (Eccles, 1964). If an action potential propagates out the dendrite, and if we time a test stimulus so that the excitatory conductance occurs near the peak of the action potential, we would expect to see the EPSP greatly diminished or even reversed. In Figure 4 we simulate such an experiment for two cases: in A the dendrites are passive (g_{Na} = 0);

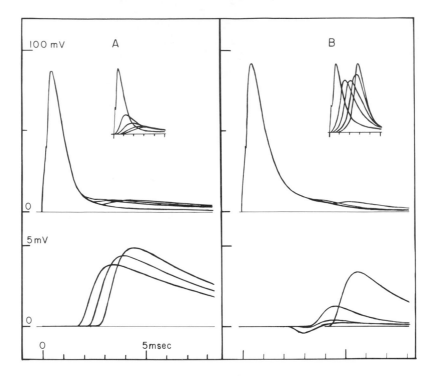

FIGURE 4 Simulation of an experiment to measure the spread of an action potential into the dendrites using the waveform of the EPSP generated at a remote site. We consider two motoneuron models: A has passive dendrites and B has weakly excitable dendrites. We assume that the synaptic terminations are clustered at 0.8λ from the soma and that they are stimulated at various times (1.5–4.0 msec) after the soma has been excited by a brief electrical pulse. Lower curves are the differences between a test record and the record of the action potential displayed at higher gain. The insets show how the action potential spreads into dendrites by superimposing the computed membrane potential at the soma and points 0.5, 0.8, 1.1, and 1.4λ along the dendrite.

in B there is a very low density of sodium channels ($g_{Na} = 30$ mmho/cm²); in both cases $g_{Na} = 140$ mmho/cm² in the soma. The insets show how the action potential spreads into the dendrite. At a point in the dendrites 0.8λ from the soma, the maximum depolarization is 13 mV at 1.1 msec after the peak of the soma spike in A, but it is 65 mV at 1.5 msec in B. With the kinetic equations that we use to describe the sodium conductance of the dendrites, a long uniform cylinder with $C_m = 2$ μF/cm² requires g_{Na} to be greater than 32 mmho/cm² in order to propagate an action potential at uniform velocity. Thus in the inset of Figure 4B, we see that the antidromic impulse decrements as it propagates into the equivalent cylinder of the dendrites. But as the impulse approaches the sealed end of the equivalent cylinder, the active region sees a smaller electrical load, which allows the action potential to speed up and grow in amplitude.

For this simulation we have assumed that the excitatory synapses are clustered at a distance of 0.8λ from the soma, that the equilibrium potential of the EPSP (V_e) is 50 mV, and that the duration of the excitatory conductance is much shorter than τ_m. We excite the soma spike by a brief current pulse, and then with varying delay we apply the excitatory conductance. We illustrate the potential changes recorded at the soma and then subtract the soma action potential from each record in order to display the EPSP at higher gain. As expected, in Figure 4B there is a critical interval in which the early part of the EPSP is reversed, corresponding to the maximal depolarization of the synaptic site by the dendritic action potential. Since the brief synaptic current is monophasic, it was rather surprising to see a biphasic reversed EPSP, which is a consequence of the synaptic potential affecting propagation of the dendritic spike. In the case of passive dendrites, the EPSP suffers only partial attenuation.

Eccles (1957, Figure 12) has done this experiment, but for quite a different reason. His results are fully consistent with Figure 4A, differing slightly because his synapses were located more proximal to the soma. In our simulation there is the untested assumption that the excitatory synapses were concentrated at a particular distance out on the dendrite, but it will be shown below that this is often a good approximation of the real situation. We conclude that the density of sodium channels in the dendrites of normal spinal motoneurons is so low that the membrane is essentially passive.

SOME INADEQUACIES OF THIS MODEL   The response of our model differs from that of real motoneurons in two important respects. First, it neglects the slow potassium channels that generate the 50–100 msec hyperpolarization that follows a soma spike. Second, because we use kinetic equations derived from peripheral nerve, our model does not give tonic repetitive firing in response to maintained depolarization, as do most motoneurons. The qualitative features of repetitive firing are obtained by slight adjustment of the kinetics of the sodium conductance to reduce accommodation and by adding the slow potassium channels (Kernell and Sjöholm, 1973). Traub and Llinás (1977) have recently put these modifications into a distributed motoneuron model, and their simulations established the particularly important point that the slow potassium channels are localized to the dendrites, achieving appreciable density only beyond 0.3λ from the soma. Traub (1977) has shown that the kinetics of the slow potassium channels must vary systematically with cell size in order to match the observed dependence of the rate on stimulus intensity.

A general limitation of the equivalent-cylinder representation is that it is not physically realistic for processes that depend on the input impedance of the dendrite: for example, the nonlinear summation of synaptic potentials, and the orthodromic propagation of dendritic spikes in neurons that have excitable dendrites. Fortunately, our computational technique can be applied to a branching cable, and we shall consider such questions in the following sections.

Synaptic interactions on a branching dendrite

STATEMENT OF THE PROBLEM   Burke (1967) investigated the summation of EPSPs by stimulating the Ia fibers of two separate muscle nerves. In 60% of the test he observed nearly perfect summation, but in the remainder the response to stimulating both nerves was always less than the sum of the two components. He attributed these results to the nonlinear summation expected when the EPSP at the synaptic site is large enough to diminish its driving force. For branching dendrites, measurable nonlinear summa-

tion would occur only between synapses that are electrically close and are located on thin dendritic shafts so that the input impedance at the synapse is relatively high.

A quantitative treatment of Burke's observations gives us another test of our conclusion that the dendrites are passive and suggests some profound hypotheses about the distribution of Ia innervation. But to do this we must first put a branching dendrite on our model motoneuron and then appeal to other experimental studies to estimate the number and location of Ia synapses.

A BRANCHING DENDRITE MODEL   Lux, Schubert, and Kreutzberg (1970) observed that the number of main dendrites arising from the soma vary in the range 9–15. For our model we let the cable bifurcate at the soma so that the branching dendrite has one-twelfth of the total dendritic conductance, while all the other dendrites are lumped together in a single cylinder. The diameter of this dendrite is 8.8 μm. We use a branching pattern (Figure 5A) that is electrically re-

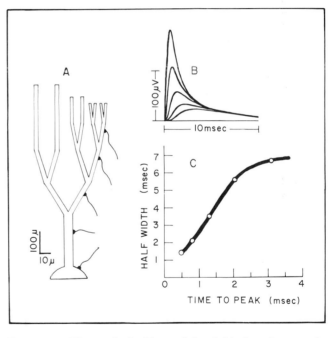

FIGURE 5   Theoretical effect of dendritic location on the amplitude and waveform of a quantal EPSP measured at the soma. (A) We assume an idealized, regularly branching dendrite that has one-twelfth of the total surface and bifurcates with equal diameter branches every 0.3λ. (B) Computed waveforms of a quantal EPSP showing diminution of amplitude and slowing of rise time as the synaptic site is moved from the soma to the points shown in A. (C) The shape-index plot for the quantal EPSP.

alistic, although it idealizes the morphology somewhat. We assume that the dendrite bifurcates at points 0.3λ apart and that the two branches have the same diameter—0.630 times the diameter of the preceding branch. Approximately equal branching is typically observed in motoneurons, but the equivalent distances between branch points appears to be highly variable (Lux, Schubert, and Kreutzberg, 1970; Barrett and Crill, 1974b).

QUANTAL COMPONENTS OF THE EPSP The EPSPs evoked by repeated firing of the same Ia afferent fluctuate greatly in size and sometimes fail. Katz and Miledi (1963), Kuno (1964), Burke (1967), and Kuno and Miyahara (1969) have measured amplitude distributions and have interpreted their data as resolving quantal components of the EPSP, analogous to the miniature endplate potentials of the myoneural junction (del Castillo and Katz, 1954). Even in the same motoneuron, different Ia fibers evoked EPSPs of widely different shape, but these shapes could be explained entirely by assuming different synaptic locations (Rall, 1967). Indeed, Rall's (1967) compartmental model established the shape index, a plot of the time to peak against the duration at half amplitude, as a very sensitive measure of the electrical separation of the synapse from the soma.

The dependence of the size and shape of the quantal EPSPs on synaptic location is illustrated in Figure 5. For these computations the quantal synaptic conductance is fixed to a brief transient given by

$$g_0(t) = \alpha T \exp(-T),$$

where $T = t/0.2$ msec and $\alpha = 5 \times 10^{-8}$ mho. This transient was chosen so that the quantal EPSP generated by a somatic synapse has a rise time of 0.5 msec and a peak amplitude of 0.17 mV (Kuno, 1964). In Figure 5B are records of the EPSP measured at the soma as the synapse is moved out along the dendrite to the points shown in Figure 5A. The integral of a quantal EPSP generated by a synapse on the most remote dendrite is about 25% that of the somatic EPSP, illustrating the point that remote synapses are quite effective in depolarizing the neuron (Barrett and Crill, 1974b). At that remote synapse the input impedance of the 1.4 μm diameter dendrite is so high that the driving force of the quantal synaptic potential is reduced to a point where only about half as much charge is injected there as at a somatic synapse. About half of that charge is dissipated along the passive dendrite before the remainder acts to

depolarize the soma. Figure 5C shows the shape-index plot for these quantal EPSPs.

Kuno and Miyahara (1969) observed that the quantum content estimated from the coefficient of variation of the amplitude fluctuations was generally smaller than the quantum content estimated by the failure rate, and they attributed this effect to nonlinear summation of the quantal components. They used this discrepancy to measure the degree of nonlinear summation in terms of the parameter k defined as the ratio of the effective quantal potential at the synapse to the equilibrium potential. They found that k ranged from zero (somatic synapses) to 0.2, with 0.07 being the most representative value.

Since the coefficient k depends on the input impedance at the synapse, its value depends strongly on the diameter of dendrite on which the synapse is located, and to a lesser extent on how close the synapse is to the proximal bifurcation. Even in a mathematical model the simplest way to evaluate k is to do a computational experiment. If we denote the EPSP generated by n quanta by V_n and the quantal EPSP as V_0, then theory says

$$\frac{V_n}{V_0} = \frac{n}{1 + k(n - 1)}$$

if the dendritic membrane is passive. For our model dendrite (Figure 5A), we find $k = 0.14$ at 1.1λ from the soma, $k = 0.076$ at 0.8λ, and $k = 0.028$ at 0.35λ. But if the synapse were located on a smaller than average dendrite, k would be larger at a given distance. For example, if the diameter of the primary dendrite were 5 μm, we would have $k = 0.065$ at 0.35λ. Thus we should not be surprised to find that some synapses show appreciable nonlinear summation even though their waveforms indicate that they are close to the soma. If Ia synapses are found anywhere on the dendritic surface, then these results are fully consistent with Kuno and Miyahara's data with respect to the distribution of values of k.

In the preceding simulations we measured nonlinear summation of several quanta acting at one point. But suppose a single Ia fiber had several terminations; then we should ask how close they must be in order to sum nonlinearly. We simulated the case of four quanta acting at the same point 0.8λ from the soma to generate an EPSP that is about 82% of the linear sum. But we get perfectly linear summation if we put one quantum on each of the four third-order dendritic branches at the same electrotonic distance. A rough answer to the question posed is that only those terminations that lie on the same dendritic shaft can interact nonlinearly.

At this point the reader might be cautioned that the interpretation of the Ia EPSP in terms of quantal conductance changes is not universally accepted. Edwards, Redman, and Walmsley (1976a,b,c) used a very sophisticated deconvolution technique to extract EPSPs from noise and found that the charge fluctuation was not as predicted by the quantal hypothesis, but more like that expected for random failure of excitation of boutons that transmit in an all-or-none manner. Since they were also unable to reverse presumably somatic EPSPs by injected current, they concluded that the mechanism of charge injection is more complicated than a quantal conductance change. Our mathematical model does not have anything to say about the possible validity of these conclusions, but it does test the consistency of the quantal hypothesis with different kinds of data and also provides a more precise interpretation of some previous experiments.

ON THE TERMINATION OF Ia AFFERENTS   Anatomical and physiological data combine to suggest that if a motoneuron is innervated by a particular Ia afferent fiber, there is a high probability (about 0.9) that only one terminal branch of one collateral of that fiber makes the synaptic contact. We reach this conclusion from the fact that the number of target neurons is approximately equal to the probable number of terminations of a single afferent. Although the evidence is necessarily quite indirect, this conclusion is supported by several other observations.

Mendell and Henneman (1968, 1971) measured computer-averaged EPSPs generated by single Ia afferents from the medial gastrocnemius muscle in motoneuron of the medial (homonymous) and lateral (heteronymous) gastrocnemius pools. Their data indicate that a single Ia fiber would probably innervate 93% of the 300 homonymous motoneurons and about 65% of the like number of heteronymous motoneurons. Since this neuron will likewise innervate soleus and some other synergists, we conservatively estimate the number of target motoneurons to be more than 600.

The anatomical basis for such extensive projections of Ia terminations has been elucidated by Scheibel and Scheibel (1969), using Golgi-stained cat spinal cord. Some details of their results are illustrated in Figure 6. The Ia afferent fiber in the dorsal column gives off collaterals as frequently as every 100 μm for several millimeters adjacent to its dorsal-root entry.

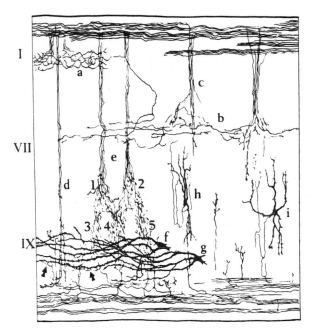

FIGURE 6   Some observations on primary afferent innervation of cat spinal motoneurons by Scheibel and Scheibel (1969) using Golgi stain. In this sagittal section we see the myelinated collateral branches of several afferents collect together to form microbundles (d, e) that drop straight down to the ventral horn. There each collateral branches several times, spreading in the plane perpendicular to the spinal axis, to make terminations on the dendrites of many different motoneurons (f, g) at differing electrotonic distances. (Courtesy of *Brain Research*.)

Collaterals from as many as ten fibers collect to form "microbundles," which drop straight down to the ventral horn where the collaterals give off fine terminal branches. The terminal branches extend predominantly in the plane perpendicular to the spinal axis where they contact the longitudinally oriented dendrites of different motoneurons. Scheibel and Scheibel (1969) observed that the number of terminal branches given off by a collateral is highly variable, but they estimated that an average of nine motoneurons receive synapses from a collateral. Since the longitudinal extent of the gastrocnemius pools is about 6 mm (Mendell and Henneman, 1971), we would expect that an average Ia fiber from the medial gastrocnemius might give off about 60 collaterals and so make about 540 synaptic contacts. That is in the same range as the number of target neurons estimated above.

Iles (1976) studied Ia terminations using the cobalt stain technique. He found that the very thin unmyelinated axon often made one or more boutons *en passant* in addition to its terminal bouton. Although as many as six boutons were found, the distribution of number of boutons per axon is markedly skewed toward small numbers, with 1.85 as the mean value. Using different anatomical information, Jack et al. (1971) calculated that on the average only two boutons connect an Ia afferent and a motoneuron. Iles's results imply that these two boutons arise from the same terminal axon.

A few motoneurons probably receive more than one termination from a particular Ia fiber. Mendell and Henneman (1971) illustrated two cases (out of 160) in which the EPSP waveform had double peaks, which implies that the synaptic loci differ greatly in their electrical distance from the soma. The distribution of mean quantal contents measured by Kuno and Miyahara (1969, Figure 2) is greatly skewed toward small values. The average quantum content is about 2.0, and the distribution is similar to the distribution of number of boutons per termination measured by Iles (1976, Figure 5). Thus, if our conjecture that typically there is only one termination of a Ia fiber on a motoneuron is true, we can conclude that the observed variability in quantum content is entirely explained by variability in the structure of the termination. Iles (1976) found the average area of synaptic content to be 12.3 μm^2, hence the density of quantal release is about 0.16 μm^2. This density is curiously similar to that of the frog endplate, where we can get approximately 500 quanta released at a large junction where the terminal axon is perhaps 1600 μm long and 1.5 μm in diameter (Dodge and Rahamimoff, 1967).

The quantitative measurement of the waveform and the amplitude of EPSPs of single Ia afferents conform well to the idea of a single termination. Mendell and Henneman (1971, Figure 9) found that the shape index measured on many different average waveforms fell close to Rall's theoretical curve, implying a single, compact source of the synaptic current. Jack et al. (1971) studied EPSP waveforms in neurons whose cable properties had also been measured and found generally good agreement with the assumption of a single synaptic source. Because the amplitude of an EPSP is affected by the highly variable structure of the termination and the size of the motoneuron, as well as the synaptic location, there is very little correlation between amplitude and waveform. Mendell and Henneman (1971, Figure 12) plotted their observations of amplitude against rise time, which we can compare to the predictions of our model. We find that about two-thirds of their points fall below the theoretical curve for a quantum content

of 2, and nearly all fall below the curve for a quantum content of 3. Since our value for the quantal conductance had been fixed by completely independent data, we judge these results to agree very well with the skewed distribution of mean quantal contents (Kuno and Miyahara, 1969).

STRUCTURAL IMPLICATIONS OF NONLINEAR SUMMATION Simulation of Burke's (1967) experiment proceeds in two steps. For each muscle nerve we must find a spatial distribution of synapses such that the theoretical EPSP matches the experimental. Then in the region of overlap of the distributions we find how many synapses of one nerve must be associated with synapses of the other nerve in order to match the observed degree of nonlinear summation. Here association means location of the two synapses within, say, 0.1λ of each other on the same branch. This somewhat arbitrary definition is based on our previous result that nonlinear interaction decreases rapidly with separation of the synapses.

As the most stringent test of our model, we have attempted to simulate the greatest degree of nonlinear summation observed by Burke (1967). His experimental records are reproduced in Figure 7A. The two component EPSPs have quite different waveforms, and their respective shape-index points lie well above the quantal shape-index curve, indicating that both are composite waveforms with synapses at different electrotonic distances from the soma. Our experience with computing composite waveforms has shown that the half-width correlates well with the average distance of the synapses (Figure 7C), but that the rising phase is dominated by the most proximal synapses. The distributions of synapses shown in Figure 7B, where each termination has a quantum content of four, give waveforms (Figure 7D) that fairly well match the experimental ones. If we associate all the terminations available from these distributions, then the EPSP obtained by stimulating both nerves is only 83% of the sum of the two components, which is about the same as the maximal degree of nonlinear summation observed by Burke (1967). For this simulation we put all the terminations on the same dendrite only for computational convenience. However, because synapses that are located 0.3λ apart do have a little interaction, we must expect somewhat less nonlinear summation if we distribute these associated synapses among several dendrites. The important conclusion that can be drawn from this simulation is that, in order to account for the maximum observed nonlinear summation, at least half the terminations

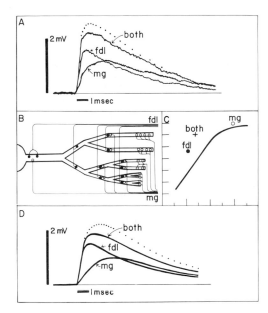

FIGURE 7 Simulation of Burke's (1967) observation of nonlinear summation of Ia EPSPs from different nerves. (A) Tracings of computer-averaged EPSPs (25 records each) evoked by electrical stimulation of nerves to flexor digitorum longus (fdl) and to medial gastrocnemius (mg). Stimulation of both nerves gave an EPSP only 83% as large as the sum of the two components (dotted curve). (B) A distribution of synaptic terminations whose computed EPSPs show about the same degree of nonlinear summation as the experiment. (C) Shape index plots of the composite EPSPs computed for this distribution. (D) Waveforms of the computed EPSPs.

of one nerve must be associated with a termination of the other.

Having illustrated the principles by simulation of a particular distribution of synapses, we can confirm this conclusion by a simple formal argument. Let us consider a single associated synapse and assume that the terminations are close enough that we can treat them as acting at the same point. Depending on the distance of the synapse from the soma, a certain fraction of the charge injected at the synapse will reach the soma, where we can measure it by dividing the area under the EPSP by the input resistance of the neuron. Denoting the amount of charge by q, subscripted according to the number of quanta acting at the synapse, the summation of n quanta is given by

$$q_n = \frac{nq_1}{1 + k(n - 1)} \qquad (6)$$

as above. It can be shown from equation 6 that for a fixed total number of quanta, the nonlinear summation is maximum when these two components are

the same size; hence we shall specialize our argument to this case. Equation 6 gives a particularly simple relation if we measure the relative amount of charge lost by nonlinear summation of two associated terminations each releasing n quanta, namely

$$1 - \frac{q_{2n}}{2q_n} = \frac{nk}{1 + k(2n - 1)}. \qquad (7)$$

We shall first use this equation to estimate the maximal degree of nonlinear summation. From the shape index of the two component EPSPs, we argue that the average distance of the associated synapses would probably be about 1.0λ, at which point $k = 0.08$ in our model. Assuming that the average quantum content is four and the associated synapses are dispersed over many dendrites, then equation 7 says we can expect only 20.5% loss of charge even if all terminations were associated. Thus in order to get as much as 17%, which was observed in Burke's experiment, we have the improbable result that over three-quarters of the total synaptic current must have been generated by associated synapses. It is more likely that the average value of k was higher in the real neuron, as would occur if $n = 2$, reflecting a much higher input resistance than our model.

On the other hand, equation 7 can be interpreted as showing how improbable it would be to observe nonlinear summation even if there were a high degree of association. For the dendritic branching and input resistance of our model, k falls below 0.03 as the synaptic site is moved more proximal than 0.35λ from the soma. The fact that Burke (1967) observed a charge loss greater than 5% in about a quarter of his tests suggests that some degree of association between terminations of synergistic nerves may be a general rule. Certainly we should ask if there is much association between subsets of the same nerve. What is the morphological basis of such associations? Are there clusters of Ia terminations in which the local density greatly exceeds the average density? Or could the "microbundles" of collateral branches described by Scheibel and Scheibel (1969) be sufficient to organize the nonrandom distributions implied by association? These questions must be left for future experimental, as well as theoretical, investigation.

Before we leave this simulation, we shall use it to reexamine the density of sodium channels in the dendrites. The mechanism of nonlinear summation requires large depolarization at the synapses; hence any nearby sodium channels must be excited. If we put a sodium conductance of only 15 mmho/cm² uniformly over the dendritic surface, we find that the

EPSP evoked by simultaneous stimulation of both nerves always exceeds the sum of the separate EPSPs. The fact that this was not observed by Burke (1967) strongly supports the assumption that the dendrites of normal spinal motoneurons are passive.

Dendritic excitability of chromatolytic motoneurons

When a motoneuron reacts to regenerate its severed axon, there is a great elaboration of the biochemical machinery for synthesis of macromolecules (chromatolysis). During the period of axonal growth the somatodendritic membrane becomes much more excitable, often to the point where action potentials can be generated in the dendrites. In this section we shall examine how the normal distribution of sodium channels must be modified to explain the characteristic electrical responses of chromatolytic motoneurons, as described by Eccles, Libet, and Young (1958) and by Kuno and Llinás (1970a,b). Here our model will show that the geometry of dendritic branching of a spinal motoneuron severely limits the amplitude of dendritic spikes measured from the soma. This situation is in marked contrast to that of the cerebellar Purkinje cell, in which excitability of the dendrites contributes major components to the spike (Llinás and Nicholson, 1971). Recently Pellionisz and Llinás (1977) have modeled the Purkinje cell, demonstrating that the different dendritic morphology greatly alters the electrical behavior of the neuron (see also Pellionisz, this volume).

INCREASED SODIUM CONDUCTANCE IN THE SOMA MEMBRANE The unfailing concomitant of chromatolysis is a marked increase in the safety factor for invasion of the soma by an antidromic action potential. In a normal motoneuron the connection between the initial segment and soma is a point of low safety factor, as shown by the fact that it is easy to block only the soma spike by relative refractoriness or by slight hyperpolarization, and as confirmed by our simulations (Figure 2). In a chromatolytic motoneuron such gentle conditions are quite ineffective, and more drastic conditions typically cause block of the initial-segment spike. Although the waveform of the antidromic spike (Figure 8A) appears normal to a casual glance, the differentiated record shows that the delay between the onset of the initial-segment spike and the soma spike is greatly reduced. Moreover, chromatolytic motoneurons have a significantly lower rheobase for direct stimulation. Since no significant differences in the input impedance were found, we

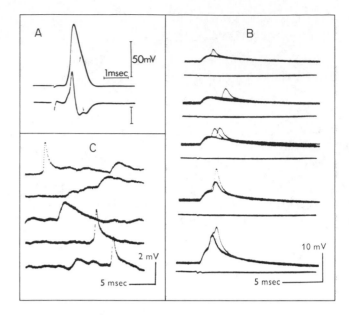

FIGURE 8 Some characteristic features of the altered excitability of chromatolytic motoneurons. (A) Antidromic spike and its first derivative show typically faster rise rate (calibration is 200 V/sec) and an inflection (marked by arrows) on the falling phase. (From Llinás, 1975.) (B, C) Recruitment of a few different partial spike responses with increasing intensity of electrical stimulus to triceps surae nerve (dorsal-root volley recorded on the second sweep). (B and C from Kuno and Llinás, 1970, courtesy of the *Journal of Physiology*.)

must ascribe all these differences to a marked alteration of the excitability of the soma membrane.

If we measure published recordings of the soma spike elicited by antidromic stimulation, we find a typical value for the maximum rise rate to be 400 V/sec for a chromatolytic motoneuron as compared to a typical value of 200 V/sec for normal motoneurons. To get the faster rise rate in our model we must increase the density of sodium conductance in the soma membrane by about the same factor. Eccles, Libet, and Young (1958) observed that with direct stimulation of chromatolytic motoneurons the separation between the initial-segment spike and soma spike virtually disappears. This observation becomes sufficient evidence for a shift in the voltage dependence of the sodium channels in the soma membrane to a smaller depolarization characteristic of channels in the axon membrane when comparison is made to simulations of direct stimulation (Figure 6 in Dodge and Cooley, 1973). Thus, in order to mimic representative waveforms of chromatolytic motoneurons (as in Figure 8A), we must make both changes in our model, doubling the density of sodium conductance in the soma membrane and shifting its voltage dependence by about 8 mV toward a lower threshold.

ACTION POTENTIALS IN THE DENDRITES   The somewhat less regular concomitant of chromatolysis is the insertion of enough sodium channels into the dendritic membrane to permit excitation and propagation of an action potential. This condition is manifested by small, spikelike, partial responses superimposed on the EPSP (Figure 8B). Partial responses typically behave in an all-or-none manner when the EPSP is graded with the intensity of the afferent stimulus, or when they are suppressed by strong hyperpolarization of the soma (Eccles, Libet, and Young, 1958). The partial responses of different motoneurons have different amplitudes, generally in the range 1–5 mV, but rarely as large as 10 mV. Often several partial responses of different sizes are observed in the same chromatolytic neuron (e.g., Figure 8B). In such cases the different partial responses behave independently, although a full-sized soma spike makes the neuron refractory to the generation of partial responses (Kuno and Llinás, 1970).

Electrophysiological evidence convincingly established the dendritic origin of the partial responses. Eccles, Libet, and Young (1958) showed that no axon spike was associated with partial responses, and Kuno and Llinás (1970) showed that partial responses persisted when the soma was kept more polarized than its resting potential but were easily suppressed by dendritic inhibition. The waveform of the partial response that has a sharp rising phase and a briefer duration than the EPSP implies that it must be generated at a point on the dendrite electrically close to the soma. Sometimes partial responses appear spontaneously (Figure 8C), and they are often elicited by very small, slow EPSPs. These observations imply a remote dendritic origin and orthodromic propagation of the action potential to a point near the soma where it is blocked. Because the safety factor for antidromic propagation into a branching dendritic tree must be substantially greater than that for orthodromic propagation, we argue that the partial response is an action potential that spreads over the whole tree served by a primary dendrite. We can test the validity of this argument most easily by simulating partial responses with our mathematical model.

Because chromatolytic motoneurons sometimes show prior firing of the initial-segment spike with threshold synaptic excitation (Eccles, Libet, and Young, 1958), we give the dendrites of our model neuron a higher threshold by using rate equations with the same voltage dependence as we use for the normal soma. As cited above, uniform propagation requires a sodium conductance greater than 32 mmho/cm².

In Figure 9 we examine what sodium conductance is required to allow propagation of an orthodromic impulse in a branching dendrite. For the cases where excitation occurs at a single remote synapse, we find that with a sodium conductance of 80 mmho/cm² the action potential invades the primary dendrite and consequently spreads over the entire dendrite. With 70 mmho/cm² the orthodromic impulse blocks at the bifurcation of primary dendrite, and with 60 mmho/cm² the orthodromic impulse fails at the bifurcation of the secondary dendrite. These results are easily explained by considering the electrical load seen by the advancing impulse. By design of the branching geometry a bifurcation is invisible to an antidromic impulse—but to an orthodromic impulse each bifurcation presents an electrical load three times larger than characteristic loading of the active branch. On this basis we would expect to get a full partial response with a low density sodium conductance if, as in Figure 9D, synapses of a given muscle nerve are distributed among the remote branches of

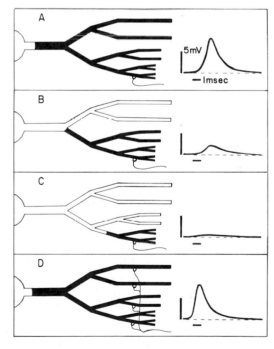

FIGURE 9   Theoretical dependence of the generation of partial spike responses on the average density of sodium channels. For these computations we assume uniform densities of g_{Na} = 80 mmho/cm² in A, 70 in B, and 60 in C and D. A full partial spike is generated in D if the synaptic terminations are distributed over enough of the remote branches.

the same dendritic tree in such a way that excitation occurs in several branches simultaneously.

Propagation of the orthodromic impulse is slow because excitation is delayed at each bifurcation. In Figure 10 we illustrate how the active region spreads over the dendritic tree when the sodium conductance is sufficient (90 mmho/cm²) to support orthodromic propagation. It takes about 2.4 msec for excitation to spread from the remote synapse to the primary dendrite, but only about 1.0 msec for antidromic propagation to spread over the remainder of the dendrite. The peak of the partial response occurs here about 3 msec after the excitatory conductance change. As a consequence of slow orthodromic propagation, a partial response triggered at a remote synapse would appear well after the peak of the EPSP whose waveform is dominated by proximal synapses. On the

other hand, partial responses that are locked to the rising phase of an EPSP imply a proximal site of initiation and a clustering of synapses on the same dendrite sufficient to excite an action potential at that site. Indeed, a careful study of chromatolytic motoneurons might answer the outstanding question whether the Ia synapses from a given nerve tend to go to the same dendrite. For example, we might ask if different muscle nerves excite different (noninteracting) partial responses. To what extent is the threshold for exciting a partial response with one nerve reduced by stimulating another?

Our simulations contribute a more detailed interpretation of observed partial responses. The amplitude of a partial response depends strongly on two factors: the input impedance of the neuron and the diameter of the dendritic branch where the ortho-

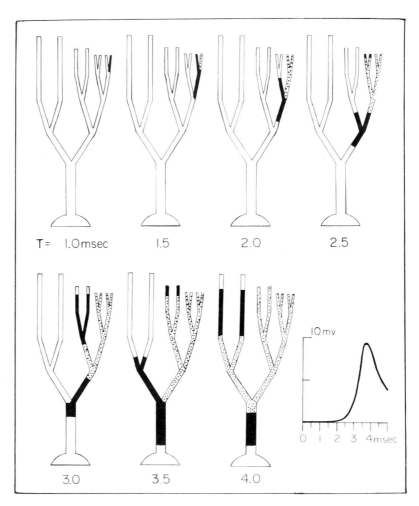

FIGURE 10   Time course of action-potential propagation over the dendrite during generation of a partial spike response. Here the uniform excitability is sufficient (g_{Na} = 90 mmho/cm²) for orthodromic propagation following exci-

tation by a quantal conductance change at a remote synapse. The filled area of each diagram marks the active region where the inward membrane current exceeds 0.1 mA/cm².

dromic impulse is blocked. (Clearly our model dendrite is unrealistically large; but since the amplitude should vary as the 3/2 power of the diameter, we do not believe there is any appreciable discrepancy with the known morphology of the neuron.) We are confident that all of the dendritic tree distal to the point of block has been excited. Because a degree of dendritic excitability that allows spontaneous partial responses (Kuno and Llinás, 1970) is relatively rare, we conclude that the average sodium conductance in the dendrites of chromatolytic motoneurons is typically less than 80 mmho/cm². But we expect that it is often as high as 60 mmho/cm² since the recruitment of one or more partial responses with increasing afferent stimulus size is commonly observed.

In our simulation we have spread the sodium channels over the dendritic membrane with uniform density. There is good evidence that this assumption is untrue. The antidromic spike of a chromatolytic motoneuron shows a hump on the falling phase (marked by an arrow in Figure 9A) that is absent in a normal spike. Traub and Llinás (1977) have shown that such a hump occurs only if there is a region of lowered safety factor between the soma and the excitable dendrites. For the rate equations used here this region must be about 0.2λ long to reproduce the illustrated hump. But if the sodium channels in fact concentrated into patches, then numerous patches must be distributed along the dendrite since the orthodromic impulse must pass several bifurcations. The estimates of sodium conductance derived from the simulations above must therefore be interpreted as average values for an unknown spatial distribution.

On the nonuniform distribution of sodium channels

Eccles (1957) has pointed out that an important principle for understanding the integrative function of the motoneuron is that all synaptic influences are combined before acting on the single point that determines the output, namely, the initial segment. At the level of membrane parameters, our mathematical model has shown that the design is implemented by varying the density of sodium channels in different regions of the neuron and especially by the essential exclusion of sodium channels from the dendritic membrane.

The fact that motoneurons of newborn kittens have excitable dendrites (Kellerth, Mellström, and Skoglund, 1971) indicates that differentiation of the motoneuron involves some mechanism for eliminating sodium channels from the dendrites. The reappearance of dendritic excitability during chromatolysis shows that the normal differentiated state is not an irreversible change in membrane structure, but suggests that it is maintained by competing dynamic processes.

There is accumulating evidence that a discrete macromolecular entity, a channel built of proteins, underlies each specific ionic permeability change (see reviews by Hille, 1970; Armstrong, 1975). We do not know the lifetime of a sodium channel in the membrane by direct experiment, but a value of about a month is suggested from a study of the effect of denervation of amphibian slow muscle. Miledi, Stefani, and Steinbach (1971) observed that this normally passive fiber becomes electrically excitable a few days after nerve section, and that excitability is lost about 45 days after reinnervation by the correct nerve fiber. On the assumption that reinnervation promptly stops synthesis of sodium channels, this observation sets an upper bound on their lifetime in the membrane.

If we assume that axon sodium channels have a comparable lifetime, we can immediately identify two processes that influence their distribution: the synthesis of macromolecules in the nucleus and the axoplasmic transport of new channels to the sites where worn-out ones must be replaced. There are strong suggestions that the axoplasmic transport of polypeptide products is an essential component of the feedback control of the rate of macromolecular synthesis. Chemicals that stop axoplasmic transport induce chromatolysis (see, e.g., Purves, 1976), but retrograde transport of nerve growth factor applied to the cut end of an axon prevents chromatolysis (West and Bunge, 1976). Since the chromatolytic state arises from a vastly higher rate of protein synthesis, we might be tempted to explain its associated excitability changes as simply the spillover of excess sodium channels. But this begs the hard question, namely, what mechanisms discriminate against insertion of sodium channels into the dendritic membrane of normal motoneurons? Certainly there must be newly synthesized sodium channels in the axoplasm, and other kinds of channels such as those associated with synaptic responses must get to the most remote dendrites.

One candidate for such a discriminatory mechanism is suggested by observations on the localization of sodium channels in the myelinated axon. Studies of acute demyelination suggest that the axonal membrane under the myelin is inexcitable (Rasminsky and Sears, 1972). During voltage-clamp experiments on isolated nodes of Ranvier it is frequently observed that the capacitance of the node increases continuously, and this is undoubtedly caused by the myelin lifting away from the adjacent axonal membrane (Hille, 1967). Although the nodal area (capacitance) can increase more than a factor of ten, there is no increase in ionic currents (Dodge and Frankenhaeuser, 1958), and we conclude that there are no ionic channels in the axonal membrane that had been tightly wrapped by myelin. A recent ultrastructural study of nodes shows that large intramembranous particles (sodium channels?) are excluded whenever the axonal and myelin membranes are opposed (Rosenbluth, 1976). We suggest that a tight glial wrapping of a dendrite might operate to inhibit insertion of sodium channels. Perhaps it is not just coincidence that neurons in tissue culture typically lack glia and have excitable dendrites (Fischbach and Dicter, 1974).

Another candidate mechanism for regulating dendritic excitability might be found among the trophic effects of synaptic connections. Since the nerve terminal organizes the dendritic membrane so that macromolecules responding to its transmitter are localized in apposition to the terminal, perhaps its influence spreads to adjacent membrane. The plausibility of this idea is supported experimentally if—as asserted by Nastuk (personal communication)—a locally higher density of sodium channels is the only explanation for the observation that a remotely stimulated action potential propagates through the endplate region of a frog muscle fiber with higher velocity and rise rate than elsewhere along the fiber (Nastuk and Alexander, 1973).

In conclusion, we note that the computational techniques we have applied are applicable to neurons of arbitrary geometry. Starting with a realistic geometry, comparison of computed responses with measurement of the input impedance should fix the resting membrane parameters within a reasonable tolerance. Testing responses to arbitrary distributions of excitability and of synapses against electrophysiological observations should greatly enhance the precision with which we can interpret the relation between structure and function in neurons.

REFERENCES

ARAKI, T., and C. A. TERZUOLO, 1962. Membrane currents in spinal motoneurons associated with the action potential and synaptic activity. *J. Neurophysiol.* 25:772–789.

ARMSTRONG, C. M., 1975. Ionic pores, gates, and gating currents. *Q. Rev. Biophys.* 7:179–209.

BARRETT, J. N., and W. E. CRILL, 1971. Specific membrane resistance of dye-injected cat motoneurons. *Brain Res.* 28:556–561.

BARRETT, J. N., and W. E. CRILL, 1974a. Specific membrane properties of cat motoneurones. *J. Physiol.* 239:301–324.

BARRETT, J. N., and W. E. CRILL, 1974b. Influence of dendritic location and membrane properties on the effectiveness of synapses on cat motoneurones. *J. Physiol.* 293:325–345.

BURKE, R. E., 1967. Composite nature of the monosynaptic excitatory postsynaptic potential. *J. Neurophysiol.* 30:1114–1137.

BURKE, R. E., and G. TEN BRUGGENCATE, 1971. Electrotonic characteristics of alpha motoneurones of varying size. *J. Physiol.* 212:1–10.

COOLEY, J. W., and F. A. DODGE, 1966. Digital computer solutions for excitation and propagation of the nerve impulse. *Biophys. J.* 6:583–599.

COOMBS, J. S., D. R. CURTIS, and J. C. ECCLES, 1957. The generation of impulses in motoneurones. *J. Physiol.* 139:232–249.

COOMBS, J. S., J. C. ECCLES, and P. FATT, 1955. The electrical properties of the motoneuron membrane. *J. Physiol.* 130:291–325.

DEL CASTILLO, J., and B. KATZ, 1954. Quantal components of the end-plate potential. *J. Physiol.* 124:560–573.

DODGE, F. A., and J. W. COOLEY, 1973. Action potential of the motorneuron. *IBM J. Res. Dev.* 17:219–229.

DODGE, F. A., and B. FRANKENHAEUSER, 1958. Membrane currents in isolated frog nerve fiber under voltage-clamp conditions. *J. Physiol.* 143:76–90.

DODGE, F. A., and R. RAHAMIMOFF, 1967. Co-operative action of calcium ions in transmitter release at the neuromuscular junction. *J. Physiol.* 193:419–432.

ECCLES, J. C., 1957. *The Physiology of Nerve Cells.* Baltimore: The Johns Hopkins Press.

ECCLES, J. C., 1964. *The Physiology of Synapses.* New York: Academic Press.

ECCLES, J. C., B. LIBET, and R. R. YOUNG, 1958. The behaviour of chromatolysed motoneurones studied by intracellular recording. *J. Physiol.* 143:11–40.

EDWARDS, F. R., S. J. REDMAN, and B. WALMSLEY, 1976a. Statistical fluctuations in charge transfer at Ia synapses on spinal motoneurones. *J. Physiol.* 259:665–688.

EDWARDS, F. R., S. J. REDMAN, and B. WALMSLEY, 1976b. Non-quantal fluctuations and transmission failures in charge transfer at Ia synapses on spinal motoneurones. *J. Physiol.* 259:689–704.

EDWARDS, F. R., S. J. REDMAN, and B. WALMSLEY, 1976c. The effect of polarizing currents on unitary Ia excitatory post-synaptic potentials evoked in spinal motoneurones. *J. Physiol.* 259:705–723.

FISCHBACH, G. D., and M. A. DICTER, 1974. Electrophysiologic and morphologic properties of neurons in dissociated chick spinal cord cell cultures. *Dev. Biol.* 37:110–116.

FRANKENHAEUSER, B., and A. L. HODGKIN, 1957. The action of calcium ions on the electrical properties of squid axons. *J. Physiol.* 137:218–244.

HILLE, B., 1967. The selective inhibition of delayed potassium currents in nerve by tetraethylammonium ion. *J. Gen. Physiol.* 50:1287–1302.

HILLE, B., 1970. Ionic channels in nerve membrane. *Prog. Biophys. Mol. Biol.* 21:1–20.

Hodgkin, A. L., and A. F. Huxley, 1952. A quantitative description of membrane current and its application to conduction and excitation in nerve. *J. Physiol.* 117:500–544.

Iles, J. F., 1976. Central terminations of muscle afferents on motoneurones in the cat spinal cord. *J. Physiol.* 262:91–117.

Jack, J. J. B., S. Miller, R. R. Porter, and S. J. Redman, 1971. The time course of minimal excitatory post-synaptic potentials evoked in spinal motoneurones by group Ia afferent fibres. *J. Physiol.* 215:353–380.

Katz, B., and R. Miledi, 1963. A study of spontaneous miniature potentials in spinal motoneurones. *J. Physiol.* 168:389–422.

Kellerth, J.-O., A. Mellström, and S. Skoglund, 1971. Postnatal excitability changes of kitten motoneurones. *Acta Physiol. Scand.* 83:31–41.

Kernell, D., and H. Sjöholm, 1973. Repetitive impulse firing: Comparisons between neurone models based on "voltage clamp equations" and spinal motoneurones. *Acta Physiol. Scand.* 87:40–56.

Kuno, M., 1964. Quantal components of excitatory synaptic potentials in spinal motoneurones. *J. Physiol.* 175:81–99.

Kuno, M., and R. Llinás, 1970a. Enhancement of synaptic transmission by dendritic potentials in chromatolysed motoneurones of the cat. *J. Physiol.* 210:807–821.

Kuno, M., and R. Llinás, 1970b. Alterations of synaptic action in chromatolysed motoneurones of the cat. *J. Physiol.* 210:823–838.

Kuno, M., and J. T. Miyahara, 1969. Non-linear summation of unit synaptic potentials in spinal motoneurones of the cat. *J. Physiol.* 201:465–477.

Llinás, R., 1975. Electroresponsive properties of dendrites in central neurons. In *Advances in Neurology*, vol. 12: *Physiology and Pathology of Dendrites*, G. W. Kreutzberg, ed. New York: Raven Press, pp. 1–13.

Llinás, R., and C. Nicholson, 1971. Electrophysiological properties of dendrites and somata in alligator Purkinje cells. *J. Neurophysiol.* 34:532–551.

Lux, H. D., P. Schubert, and G. W. Kreutzberg, 1970. Direct matching of morphological and electrophysiological data in cat spinal motoneurones. In *Excitatory Synaptic Mechanisms*, P. Andersen and J. Jansen, eds. Oslo: Universitetsforlaget, pp. 175–187.

Mendell, L. M., and E. Henneman, 1968. Terminals of Ia fibers: Distribution within a pool of 300 homonymous motor neurons. *Science* 160:96–98.

Mendell, L. M., and E. Henneman, 1971. Terminals of single Ia fibers: Location, density, and distribution within a pool of 300 homonymous motoneurons. *J. Neurophysiol.* 34:171–187.

Miledi, R., E. Stefani, and A. B. Steinbach, 1971. Induction of the action potential mechanism in slow muscle fibres of the frog. *J. Physiol.* 217:737–754.

Nastuk, W., and J. T. Alexander, 1973. Non-homogeneous electrical activity in single muscle fibers. *Fed. Proc.* 32:333.

Nelson, P., and H. D. Lux, 1970. Some electrical measurements of motoneuron parameters. *Biophys. J.* 10:55–73.

Pellionisz, A., and R. Llinás, 1977. A computer model of the cerebellar Purkinje cells. *Neuroscience* 2:37–48.

Purves, D., 1976. Functional and structural changes in mammalian sympathetic neurones following colchicine application to post-ganglionic nerves. *J. Physiol.* 259:159–175.

Rall, W., 1959. Branching dendritic trees and motoneuron membrane resistivity. *Exp. Neurol.* 1:491–527.

Rall, W., 1962. Theory of physiological properties of dendrites. *Ann. NY Acad. Sci.* 96:1071–1092.

Rall, W., 1967. Distinguishing theoretical synaptic potentials computed for different soma-dendritic distributions of synaptic input. *J. Neurophysiol.* 30:1138–1168.

Rall, W., 1969. Time constants and electrotonic length of membrane cylinders and neurons. *Biophys. J.* 9:1483–1508.

Rall, W., 1970. Cable properties of dendrites and effects of synaptic location. In *Excitatory Synaptic Mechanisms*, P. Andersen and J. Jansen, eds. Oslo: Universitetsforlaget, pp. 175–187.

Rasminsky, M., and T. A. Sears, 1972. Internodal conduction in undissected demyelinated nerve fibres. *J. Physiol.* 227:323–350.

Rosenbluth, J., 1976. Intramembranous particle distribution of the node of Ranvier and adjacent axolemma in myelinated axons of the frog brain. *J. Neurocytol.* 5:731–745.

Scheibel, M. E., and A. B. Scheibel, 1969. Terminal patterns in cat spinal cord. III. Primary afferent collaterals. *Brain Res.* 13:417–443.

Traub, R. D., 1977. Motorneurons of different geometry and the size principle. *Biol. Cybernetics* 25:163–176.

Traub, R. D., and R. Llinás, 1977. The spatial distribution of ionic conductances in normal and axotomized motorneurons. *Neuroscience* (in press).

West, N. R., and R. P. Bunge, 1976. Prevention of the chromatolytic response in rat superior cervical ganglion neurons by nerve growth factor. *Society for Neurosci. Abstr.* 1499.

26 Brain-Cell Microenvironment as a Communication Channel

C. NICHOLSON

ABSTRACT The brain-cell microenvironment is not simply a saline-filled space around neurons but rather a complex medium capable of transmitting information between nerve cells. This viewpoint forces new interpretations of the spatial organization of brain-cell ensembles in terms of proximity of elements as well as network properties.

The microenvironment is depicted as a sequence of logarithmically scaled zones extending from the cell membrane. The properties of electric and ionic fields within the microenvironment have been clarified through the use of new techniques, including ion-selective micropipettes. Such investigations show that the minority ions, K^+ and Ca^{2+}, can be modulated during typical brain activity. Under traumatic conditions, such as spreading depression or anoxia, large changes also occur in Na^+ and Cl^-. The multimodality of electrochemical interaction within the brain-cell microenvironment poses novel problems and possibilities for interneuronal communication.

IT IS EVIDENT that the milieu surrounding a cell plays a vital role in cellular function. The cell imposes a local structure on its environment and is coupled to it through the interface at the cell membrane. When cells aggregate, as in the brain, a highly organized microenvironment can ensue which then acquires the potentiality for being a communication channel.

Until quite recently the brain was considered primarily as a network—a vast telephone system receiving signals via synapse and dendrite, processing them within the confines of the neuron, and dispatching them through the axon. Speculation about other modes of information transfer arose from time to time but remained largely unsubstantiated. Now new techniques are enabling us to explore both the structural and functional potential of the extracellular environment. The result has been a radical change in our understanding of the functional significance of the three-dimensional cytoarchitecture of the brain. Because the spatial relationships of neurons define the structure of the microenvironment, viewing this environment as a communication channel necessitates a new physiological interpretation of the spatial disposition, in terms of proximity, of neuronal elements.

Our knowledge has not yet progressed to a point where we can display elegant examples of communication via the microenvironment. It is now possible, however, to indicate some of the ways in which the environment is modulated and, perhaps even more importantly, to suggest the novel conceptual changes that such data are forcing upon us.

What is the brain-cell microenvironment?

A good way to envisage the microenvironment of a neuron is to consider the relative significance of structures as one travels outward from the membrane (plane 0, Figure 1).

Most significant is the region adjacent to the cell membrane. I call this zone 1 and define it to extend from the fluid mosaic membrane of the cell outward about 200 Å or 20 nm. This zone contains, first, the cell coat or glycocalyx consisting of long filamentous sugar molecules anchored in the lipid membrane of the cell and, second, a bathing medium consisting of dilute aqueous salt solution with a few organic molecules. The profound role of the ionized salts in this solution will be the subject of much of this paper. The region narrows at sites of chemical synapses and is obliterated altogether at gap junctions, but these features are rare compared to the vast expanse of normal membrane and will not be a focus of this paper. One can conclude that zone 1, often called the extracellular space (ECS) of the brain, is the most critical region for discussion of the microenvironment.

Zone 2 takes us from 200 Å to 2,000 Å (20 nm to 0.2 μm) out from the neuronal membrane; 0.2 μm is about the resolution limit of the light microscope. As one traverses zone 2, the cell coats of other cells, interdigitating with those of zone 1, are encountered; then the membranes of other cells appear. These membranes represent both complex barriers and

C. NICHOLSON Department of Physiology and Biophysics, New York University Medical Center, New York, NY 10016

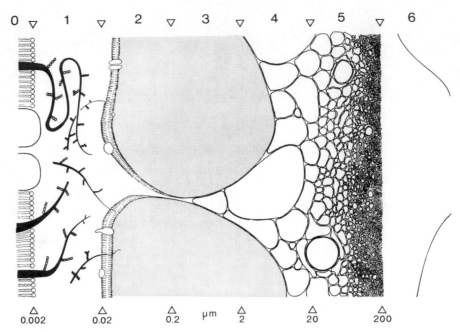

FIGURE 1 Brain-cell microenvironment. Figure is scaled logarithmically in the horizontal direction. Scale indicated below, zone number above. Plane 0 is part of the membrane of a single cell with a proteinaceous pore in the bilipid layer and several glycoprotein and glycolipid molecules (black) extending into zone 1. Zone 1 is the conventional 200 Å gap between cells. It contains the glycoproteins and glycolipids of adjacent cell membranes and the ionic milieu that permeates the extracellular space. Zone 2 includes the membrane of nearest-neighbor cells to plane 0. Intracellular region indicated by shading. Several proteins are embedded in the bilipid layer of the membrane. Zones 3 and 4 contain more cells and extracellular space. Mosaic pattern begins to emerge. Zone 5 is on a yet smaller scale; two blood vessels are apparent in this zone. Zone 6 is on such a minute scale that detail cannot be depicted. Pial and ventricular surfaces finally delimit brain.

transducers for the information carriers of the microenvironment. The ionic environment on the inside of the membranes is very different from that on the outside, thus enabling electric fields and ion fluxes to be generated across the membrane. (Identical properties exist, of course, in the primary cell, plane 0.)

Transactions are carried out in these regions between cells. The signals are electric fields, water, simple ions, organic molecules, and dissolved gases, mainly O_2 and CO_2. The transducers for the signals are associated with the cell membranes and comprise the molecules of the cell coat, membrane channels, active transmembrane transport, and endo- and exocytosis.

Zone 3 extends from 0.2 μm to 2 μm and encompasses an increasing amount of juxtamembranous intracellular apparatus. It is important to appreciate that this intracellular region constitutes a part of the extracellular environment of the primary cell, since ions, electric fields, and dissolved gases permeate this region to varying degrees.

Zone 4, from 2 to 20 μm, traverses whole neuronal elements—that is, dendrites, axons, and somata of moderate size. Cellular elements are generally recognizable at this level in both electron and light microscopy, and they can be classified at the functional level into neurons and glia. This classification, which of course extends to the membrane-related elements of zones 2 and 3, appears very important for discussing the microenvironment.

Zone 5, from 20 to 200 μm, includes all the elements on a smaller scale; most of the space is by necessity intracellular. One new structure is encountered with a spacing of 30–50 μm or so: the blood vessel. This element is surrounded by the (partly conceptual) blood-brain barrier. Zone 5 is approximately one electrotonic length constant in width; thus current flows from sources to sinks take place largely on a scale of this dimension.

Beyond zone 5 more regions could be defined that are of less significance. Typically in the next zone are the pia-arachnoid-dura of the outer brain surface or the inner ventricular surface. These macroscopic interfaces, together with the blood-brain barrier, are the final determinants of the extracellular ionic environment of the brain cell, the ultimate reference point for the system.

It will be apparent by now that the zones are scaled logarithmically; such a scaling seems the most intuitively clear way to represent the relative influence of increasingly remote regions. Obviously, as one gets further from the primary cell, individual influences wane and collective effects predominate. I shall now describe more fully the nature of the most important zones.

THE FIRST ZONE   Our present concept of the membrane is as an oil-like fluid in which are embedded proteins of many different types (Singer and Nicolson, 1972). It is now apparent that some of the proteins and lipids have long sugar molecules extending outward from the surface (glycoproteins and glycolipids) (Luft, 1976). Some of the glycoproteins belong to a special class known as mucopolysaccharides (polysaccharides containing amino sugars). The filamentous sugar molecules constitute a cell coat typically some 100–200 Å thick. This coat now seems to be present on most cell types and may have many different functions. In addition to being called a cell coat, it has been variously and descriptively termed "the outer zone of the membrane," the "glycocalyx," the "fuzz," and a "macromolecular jungle." Our present knowledge of the cell coat, as revealed by histological and histochemical techniques, has been reviewed by Luft (1976), and the cell coats of neurons have been discussed by Schmitt and Samson (1969) and more recently by Watson (1976). It seems that the neuronal cell coat consists mainly of hyaluronic acid, chondroitin-4-sulfate and chondroitin-6-sulfate. Some heparin sulfate and dermatan sulfate are also present (Watson, 1976). Many of the glycoproteins contain acidic components such as sialic acid and have a negative charge. Furthermore, some of them are extremely long (e.g., hyaluronic acid) and thus cannot be linearly extended in the approximately 200 Å space between neuronal elements. Thus the first chemical entity apparent in zone 1 is a negatively charged jungle of filamentous sugar molecules.

This jungle is permeated by an aqueous salt solution whose composition is very close to that of cerebrospinal fluid (Table I). We can distinguish two classes of ion, the majority species, Na^+ and Cl^-, and the minorities, K^+, Ca^{2+}, Mg^{2+}, and HCO_3^-. This distinction is very important since information transfer in the microenvironment is achieved through modulation of the minority ions. Only under pathological conditions do functionally significant changes of the majority ions occur. Some organic molecules, both charged and uncharged, also move through this

TABLE I

Concentrations of various solutes (mEq/kg water) in plasma and lumbar cerebrospinal fluid (CSF) of human subjects

Substance	Plasma	CSF
Na	150	147
K	4.63	2.86
Mg	1.61	2.23
Ca	4.70	2.28
Cl	99	113
HCO$_3$	26.8	23.3

Source: After Davson (1976)

space. One obvious class is chemical transmitter molecules, but many other types probably exist and act in a neurohumoral role. Direct measurement of these chemicals is mostly beyond our technology at present, so discussion of these entities will be largely omitted from this paper. Discussion of metabolic substrates and products, such as glucose, lactate, O_2, and CO_2, will also be omitted for the most part, although they may come to be regarded as long-term information carriers. Thus the chemical signals of zone 1, that is, the mobile carriers of information, are water, inorganic ions, organic molecules, and dissolved gases.

One other major information-transmitting modality of zone 1 is the electric field. The fact that membranes generate electric fields and that both ions and mucopolysaccharides are charged means that our final synthesis of the properties of this region will be in the realm of the electrochemistry of polyelectrolytes.

The actual dimensions of zone 1, either as a separation distance between cells or as a percentage of brain volume, have been the subject of much controversy. Electron-microscopic practices that were considered to yield "good fixation" (i.e., many clearly delineated ultrastructural details) often suggested very little space between neurons. Fixation techniques that attempted to retain the spatial relations believed to exist in life (Van Harreveld, 1972) revealed much larger spaces between cells but did not give such aesthetically pleasing pictures of the cytology. Gradually the weight of evidence from extracellular markers (Davson and Welch, 1971; Van Harreveld, 1972; Fenstermacher and Patlak, 1975) and impedance measurements (Van Harreveld, 1972) confirmed that the extracellular space is quite large, about 12–25% of the brain volume, and that many fixation procedures can result in an apparent change in the space between brain cells (Nevis and Collins, 1967).

If a brain element has a volume V, a surface area S, and a layer of extracellular region of thickness d

associated with every surface element, then the volume of the extracellular region is Sd and the fraction of the total volume is $Sd/(Sd + V)$ or $d/(d + R)$, where $R = V/S$. If the extracellular volume is 20% of the total volume, then $d = R/4$—that is, the mean distance between cellular elements, $2d$, is half the volume-to-surface ratio of the elements. If the brain were packed with cubes of side x, then R would be $x/6$ and for $2d = 200$ Å, x would be approximately 0.24 μm. Thus our present concepts of extracellular volume imply a very small volume-to-surface ratio for brain-cell elements, a conclusion that is qualitatively supported by electron microscopy.

Using ion-selective electrodes, as described later in this paper, recent measurements of K^+ ion diffusion in the brain extracellular space have suggested that these ions move with a diffusion coefficient that is reduced relative to that of aqueous solution of similar concentration (Lux and Neher, 1973; Fisher, Pedley, and Prince, 1976).

Regional variations are to be expected, and even in a single location ions may move slightly differently in different directions, as evidenced by measurement of the conductivity tensor (Yedlin et al., 1974; Nicholson and Freeman, 1975).

Physically the ionic concentrations of the brain imply that, on average, there is but one ion pair in a volume 25 Å on edge, assuming ionic strength 0.15 (Schmitt and Samson, 1969). This refers primarily to the majority ions; for the minority ions the volume would be about 50 times greater.

THE SECOND ZONE   Moving through the second zone we encounter the cell coats of adjacent cells, which interdigitate and may even interact with the coat of the primary cell. Since enormous variety is possible in the structure of glycoproteins, it is conceivable that each cell has a distinguishable coat; thus cells "may resemble calico cats in more ways than one" (Luft, 1976). The functional implications of this are yet to be assessed.

The membranes of adjacent cells are of immense significance in describing the microenvironment. Through these membranes move fluxes of water, ions, and organic molecules. The membranes are the chemical control surfaces of the microenvironment, translating the major electric fields of the brain that lie across the cell membranes into streams of ions. The magnitude is governed by three factors: the difference in ionic species concentration across the membrane, the relative selectivity of the membrane to different ions, and the small thickness of the membrane (50 Å or less). Thus a potential difference of

70 mV across the membrane creates a field of 150,000 V/cm. By comparison extracellular fields are of the order of 0.1 V/cm. Modulation of intramembrane electric fields is brought about mainly by molecular permeability changes caused by changes in field conditions in adjacent membranes (action potentials) or the local action of organic molecules (synaptic transmission). Changes in ionic concentration are a second means of influencing transmembrane electric fields and will be discussed later.

Membranes of the nervous system can be assigned to two categories: those belonging to neurons and those belonging to glial cells. While our knowledge of neuronal membranes is quite extensive, glia remain an enigma, largely due to the difficulties of making accurate in situ measurements. The following facts seem indisputable, however. The fundamental distinction between neuron and glia is that transmembrane electric fields of neurons are controlled by electric and chemical mechanisms (as described above) whereas those of glia are controlled by ionic concentrations. It is generally accepted that the major permeant ion for the glial membrane is K^+, and thus the potential is governed by the Nernst equation for that ion, even in mammalian glia with extracellular potentials taken into account (Somjen, 1975). Glial properties have been the subject of several recent reviews (Orkand, 1977; Somjen, 1975; Watson, 1974; Kuffler and Nicholls, 1966).

THE REMAINING ZONES   Only a few features will be discussed here. As one views larger and larger areas of the brain, the distinct cellular morphology becomes apparent and neurons can be distinguished from glia. Neurons have distinct, treelike processes providing receptive surfaces for synaptic inputs. Some glia have fine filamentous sheetlike processes; teleologically these seem optimized for maximum surface-to-volume ratio, underlining once again their potentiality for maximizing transmembrane ion movement and possibly glia-glia contact.

The other evident feature is the blood vessel. It has been estimated that the average spacing of blood vessels in the cerebral cortex is less than 50 μm (Purves, 1972). This is sufficient to ensure adequate oxygenation under normal conditions. The movement of substances between blood and brain is controlled by the blood-brain barrier, believed to reside in a layer of tightly coupled cells surrounding the vessel, although local glia may also contribute (Davson and Welch, 1971; Davson, 1976; Rapoport, 1976). Because of this barrier, brain electrolyte solutions are in equilibrium not with the plasma (Table

I) but rather with the cerebrospinal fluid (CSF) that permeates ventricles and subarachnoid space. These gross interfaces provide for exchange between CSF and brain.

Electric fields in the microenvironment

At any instant potential differences exist between different locations in the microenvironment. These potentials are usually generated by neurons. When two regions of a neuronal membrane are at a different potential, a current flow occurs inside the cell and a return current flows outside the cell in the microenvironment. The size of the current is almost entirely determined by the membrane resistance of the neuron, since this is large in comparison to the resistance of the extracellular environment, and thus the cell appears as a current generator and absorber (i.e., a source and sink) when viewed from the microenvironment (Nicholson and Llinás, 1971; Nicholson, 1973; Llinás and Nicholson, 1974). As the current traverses the microenvironment, it establishes a potential difference across the resistance of the medium.

Typical potentials are shown in Figure 2B, as recorded in the cerebellum in response to a local surface stimulus. They have maximum amplitudes in the range 1–10 mV. The potential at any point is an algebraic summation of the potentials generated by all the active sources and sinks. Some of these sources and sinks may be remote from the recording location, and it is impossible to say that a given potential is simply the product of current generators in its immediate vicinity (Llinás and Nicholson, 1974). By making appropriate measurements of the potential in three dimensions it is possible to compute the local current source density (CSD), a quantity directly related to synaptic and action currents (Figure 2A, C; see Nicholson and Freeman, 1975; Freeman and Nicholson, 1975; Nicholson and Llinás, 1975). This provides more useful information than the potentials and also relates directly to questions of ionic movement. Potential differences could also be generated by differences in ionic concentrations (liquid junction potentials), but such potentials are likely to be extremely small unless the mobility of some ionic species in the microenvironment differs greatly from that in free solution (Somjen, 1973). Extracellular potentials and CSDs are very useful indicators of neuronal activity, especially in regions where intracellular recording is impossible, as in fine dendrites.

It has long been speculated that the extracellular electric fields may be functionally significant in neu-

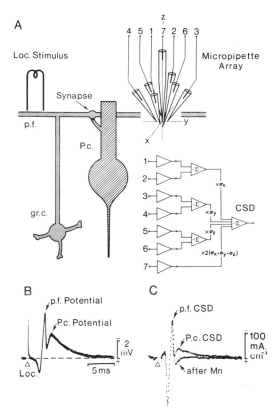

FIGURE 2 Extracellular field potentials and current source density (CSD) evoked by cerebellar stimulation in cat. (A) Basic cerebellar circuit consisting of granule cells (gr.c.) and their axons, the parallel fibers (p.f.), which make synaptic contact with the dendrites of Purkinje cells (P.c.). Local (Loc.) surface stimulation evokes a volley of action potentials in parallel fibers and subsequent postsynaptic potentials in the Purkinje cells. Microelectrodes in the extracellular space record the field potentials due to the currents generated by the neuronal events (B). By using an array of recording electrodes (A) and suitable electronic processing, the CSD proportional to the actual transmembrane currents can be computed (C). (B) Pre- and postsynaptic potentials recorded from ECS just under the pial surface. (C) Superimposed CSDs in a similar location before and after the application of the synaptic blocking agent manganese. This enables the pre- and postsynaptic components to be verified. Time scales in B and C are the same. Recording position just below cerebellar surface.

ronal ensembles. One of the first attempts to quantify such effects experimentally was by Katz and Schmitt (1940), who showed that activity in one crab nerve of an adjacent pair was insufficient to fire the inactive fibers. The activity, however, could induce spike-conduction synchronization if spikes were occurring in the second fiber. Arvanitaki (1942) coined the word *ephapse* to describe such influences between contiguous but not structurally linked neuronal elements. Among recent studies Bullock and Horridge (1965) discussed the question in light of the available data and Nelson (1966) showed that antidromic invasion of motoneuron axons is influenced by large-scale activation of surrounding fibers. The theoretical basis of ephaptic influences has been explored by Clark and Plonsey (1970). Recently the discovery of dendritic bundles has encouraged further speculation about ephaptic interactions (Petsche et al., 1975; Scheibel and Scheibel, 1975). One of the very few cases where a type of ephaptic mechanism operates is in the neuronal circuitry surrounding the Mauthner cell (Korn, this volume).

Mostly it has been difficult to establish a clear-cut case of functional ephaptic transmission. One of the

problems is that the electric-field changes are inevitably accompanied by ionic changes that may themselves influence neighboring neuronal elements. Some evidence for this has been presented by Kaczmarek and Adey (1974) and Bawin and Adey (1976); these results are hard to interpret at present. The question of the multimodality of information transfer in the microenvironment will be discussed at the end of this paper.

Modulation of the ionic milieu

In discussing our rapidly expanding knowledge of the ionic aspects of the microenvironment, it is useful to consider three levels of ionic state. The first level is the resting state, which is obviously actively maintained. Stability here is essential if meaningful modulation is to occur. The second level comprises ionic modulation, defined here as changes within the expected range of normal brain activity. It involves mainly shifts in the minority ions, K^+ and Ca^{2+}, and is the topic of this section. The third level is that of large-scale ionic changes of a pathological or traumatic type. Here both minority and majority ions radically change their concentrations. It is very plausible that water movements are also induced at this level.

MODULATION OF $[K^+]_0$ The recent invention of a fast, stable, and easily fabricated ion-selective micropipette (ISM) using a liquid membrane (Orme, 1969) is leading to profound changes in our concept of the brain-cell microenvironment. The first practical ISMs were K^+-selective (Walker, 1971), and most subsequent work and development (e.g., Lux, 1974a) has centered on this type (Figure 3A). Many conjectures have arisen concerning the role of $[K^+]_0$ changes in

FIGURE 3 $[K^+]_0$ increase evoked by repetitive local stimulation of cat cerebellum. (A) Double-barrelled micropipette containing ion-exchanger for K^+ on one side and NaCl for reference on the other. The electronic circuit subtracts the potential component from the ion signal to give an output proportional to the logarithm of $[K^+]_0$. Cerebellar elements same as in Figure 2. (B) $[K^+]_0$ rise caused by 30 sec repetitive local surface stimulation at 5, 10, and 20 Hz. Left-hand sequence under normal conditions; right-hand sequence follows superfusion of the cerebellum with 2.0 mM $MnCl_2$. Lowest records show CSDs computed with a seven-electrode array. In this experiment the center electrode was also a K^+ ISM. CSDs reveal that the postsynaptic response is abolished by Mn (same records as Figure 2C). Thus much of the K^+ increase during stimulation is evoked from the presynaptic component. Note the undershoot in $[K^+]_0$ following stimulus cessation. Recording position just below cerebellar surface.

neuronal function. Before reviewing some of these I shall illustrate salient results from recent work with K^+ ISMs. A K^+ ISM cannot accurately record K^+ in the 200–400 Å space around a single cell. The electrode probably creates a space of not more than 15 μm around it (Hertz, Zieglgänsberger, and Färber, 1969; Lux and Neher, 1973), with which the true ECS equilibrates. So long as a population of cells is active, thus creating a large spatial K^+ source around the electrode, and sufficient time is allowed for equilibration (8–70 msec; Lux and Neher, 1973), these measurements should be accurate.

The cerebellum is an excellent area of the brain in which to study basic relationships between neuronal elements and ionic signals. Surface stimulation of the parallel fibers (Figures 2, 3) excites a very simple circuit consisting of presynaptic parallel fibers and postsynaptic Purkinje-cell dendrites (Eccles, Llinás, and Sasaki, 1966). Interneurons are also activated, but their contributions to extracellular potentials and ion changes are insignificant compared to those of the vastly more numerous parallel fibers and Purkinje cells. The pre- and postsynaptic responses can be clearly seen in extracellular field potentials and more precisely in current source density analysis (Figure 2). The $[K^+]_o$ increase associated with such activation is shown in Figure 3B. These records and those in Figure 5 were taken from a series of experiments carried out in collaboration with Prof. G. ten Bruggencate and coworkers on the cerebellum of the cat (Nicholson et al., 1978). Here the local stimulation was repeated at different frequencies for a period of 30 sec. Repeated stimulation is used because the $[K^+]_o$ increase due to a single stimulus is small. $[K^+]_o$ rises slowly to a plateau, stays at this level until the stimulus train ends, then decays toward its baseline value, which it undershoots before slowly returning to the resting level.

The summation of responses and slow rise rate show that each stimulus generates a $[K^+]_o$ increment whose duration exceeds the stimulus interval; that is, it lasts several hundred milliseconds. Similar $[K^+]_o$ responses have been reported by other investigators in, for example the cortex (Figure 4A) and spinal cord (Figure 4C). The plateau level is a function of stimulus frequency, often linear, up to about 10 mM. At that level a ceiling is reached in the cerebellum and all other regions so far examined in mature animals (Kříž, Syková, and Vyklický, 1975; Moody, Futamachi, and Prince, 1974; Sypert and Ward, 1974; Heinemann and Lux, 1977). Apparently this ceiling is only exceeded during spreading depression, anoxia, and death (see below).

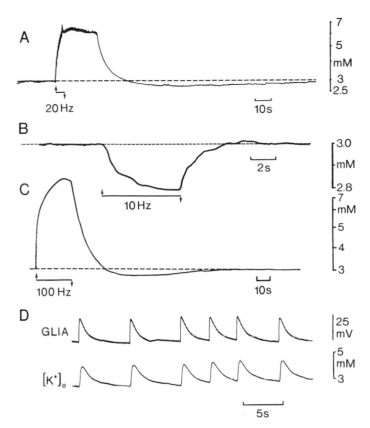

FIGURE 4 Examples of potassium signals recorded from different regions of central nervous system. (A) $[K^+]_o$ increase recorded at a depth of 900 μm in the cerebral cortex of cat following direct cortical stimulation at 20 Hz (after Heinemann and Lux, 1975). (B) Decrease in $[K^+]_o$ without preceding rise (a primary undershoot) recorded at 700 μm depth from cerebral cortex of cat following 10 Hz pyramidal-tract stimulation (Heinemann and Lux, 1975). (C) $[K^+]_o$ increase in spinal cord of cat evoked by 100 Hz stimulation of posterior tibial nerve (after Kříž, Syková, and Vyklický, 1975). (D) Intracellular glial potential and $[K^+]_o$ signal recorded simultaneously during interictal seizure (after Futamachi and Pedley, 1976). Intracellular electrode is 30–70 μm from the K^+ recording electrode and reference. Electrodes at 1,750 μm depth in pericruciate cortex of cat. Note that $[K^+]_o$ rises and falls slowly, does not exceed about 7 mM, and frequently exhibits small undershoot of less than 0.5 mM (cf. Figures 3 and 5).

The origin of some of the $[K^+]$ elevation can be demonstrated in the cerebellum by superfusing the cortex with Ringer's solution containing manganese. Under these conditions synaptic transmission is abolished (Figures 2C, 3B) but the average potassium release is reduced by not more than 50%. Thus at least half the K^+ comes from the action potentials of the presynaptic fibers, which are unaffected by the manganese. These action potentials are apparently conventional Na^+-K^+ spikes since they are abolished by tetrodotoxin (Llinás and Hess, 1976). The remaining $[K^+]_0$ increase is apparently associated with synaptic transmission and postsynaptic events.

One additional observation is that "primary undershoots" can occur without a preceding rise in $[K^+]_0$ (Figure 4B). These may be mediated by the activation of inhibitory interneurons.

$[K^+]_0$ rises can of course be evoked by stimuli remote from the site of recording, including distant nerves, other brain regions, and visual stimuli (Singer and Lux, 1973, 1975; Oakley and Green, 1976; Karwoski and Proenza, 1977). $[K^+]_0$ rises also occur during epileptic seizures (Figure 4D), as described below.

RESTORATION OF NORMAL $[K^+]_0$ LEVELS   The data described above show that $[K^+]_0$ can be elevated by 200% or more during neuronal activity. It is important therefore to ask how the normal $[K^+]_0$ level is restored. This question is not entirely answered at the present time, but at least five mechanisms may contribute. These are: diffusion in the ECS, active K^+ uptake by the Na-K pump in neurons, dispersal across the blood-brain barrier, passive dissipation via glial cells, and active removal by glial cells.

Diffusion in the ECS clearly takes place whenever a concentration gradient is established; K^+ will then migrate, and a 200 Å separation between neurons is adequately large to permit relatively unobstructed passage of hydrated K^+ ions (Kuffler and Nicholls, 1966). Of course the glycoproteins, glycolipids, and fixed negative charges may affect migration. Experiments using a point source of K^+ (Lux and Neher, 1973) or a semi-infinite source (Fisher, Pedley, and Prince, 1976) and K^+ ISMs have shown K^+ changes that are well described by the diffusion equation based on Fick's Law, but with a reduction of the apparent free diffusion coefficient by about one-sixth. These data were interpreted to mean that the migrating K^+ remained largely in in the ECS. This simple explanation has been questioned by Katzman (1976) in the light of earlier work (Pape and Katzman, 1972), using labeled K^+, which showed that a large amount of the applied K^+ would enter cells under the conditions of the experiments of both Lux and Fisher. If this were so, both the brain volume accessible to K^+ and the kinetics of transmembrane movement could influence the apparent diffusion constant. Recent experiments (Nicholson, Phillips, and Gardner-Medwin, unpublished) have confirmed that K^+ migration is anomalous relative to ions such as the tetraalkylammonium series, which are confined to the ECS.

The relative role of diffusion is further complicated by the fact that under normal circumstances $[K^+]_0$ is elevated by neuronal activity that involves action potentials and the entry of Na^+ into cells. This will trigger the Na-K pump, which will reabsorb some of the K^+ released by the action potentials. The pump will be controlled by the elevation of intracellular Na, so that pumping may continue even after $[K^+]_0$ has been reduced to its baseline value because some of the released K^+ will be simultaneously dissipated by diffusion in the ECS. Consequently transient undershoots in $[K^+]_0$ may be seen following prolonged activity. These have been reported frequently (see Figures 3, 4, 5) and discussed in detail (Heinemann and Lux, 1975; Krnjević and Morris, 1975b; Lewis and Schuette, 1975b). Such undershoots are sensitive to lowered blood pressure (Kříž, Syková, and Vyklický, 1975; Krnjević and Morris, 1975b) and cardiac glycosides, which block the Na-K pump (Krnjević and Morris, 1975b). Analysis of the falling phrase of $[K^+]_0$ after stimulation has indicated that passive diffusion is inadequate to account for the abbreviated time course (Krnjević and Morris, 1974, 1975b; Vern, Schuette, and Thibault, 1977) and that some form of active K^+ absorption must be postulated under conditions of stimulated K^+ release.

Three other mechanisms are more speculative. K^+ dissipation across the blood-brain barrier is obviously conceivable and was demonstrated by Bradbury and Stulcová (1970), but the relative magnitude of the contribution is hard to assess. A more controversial question is the role of glia. Kuffler and Nicholls (1966) discussed a model based on glial depolarization due to elevated $[K^+]_0$ which would drive K^+ into the glial cell at the site of depolarization and out at remote sites. Lux and Neher (1973) claimed that such a mechanism was unlikely, based on estimated glial membrane parameters for the central nervous system. Recent experiments (Gardner-Medwin, 1977, Gardner-Medwin and Nicholson, 1978) have shown, however, that when current is passed through the brain, K^+ has a higher transport number in the brain than would be anticipated from its relative concentration in the ECS. This shows that under these conditions much of the migrating K^+ moves via intracellular compartments, which would be either glial cells or neurons. A second type of proposed glial mechanism is the active uptake of K^+ by glia. Some evidence for this exists (e.g. Henn, Haljamäe, and Hamberger, 1972; Bourke et al., 1970, 1975; Hertz and Schousboe, 1975; Mori, Miller, and Tomita, 1976), but it is difficult to interpret. Differences may also exist between glia that have been well studied (packet cells of the leech and glial cells of the optic nerve of *Necturus*) and those found in the mammalian brain (Hertz and Nissen, 1976). Indeed K^+ removal seems to have a Q_{10} of 1.56 in the *Necturus* preparation (Bracho and Orkand, 1972) but a value of 2.08 in the cortex (Lewis and Schuette, 1975a); in the latter case, of course, this may not simply reflect glial activity. Thus the role of glia continues to be an enigma.

Two other facts deserve mention in this context. The first is that under a wide range of stimulus conditions, and even in seizure activity, $[K^+]_0$ does not exceed about 12 mM (see Heinemann and Lux, 1977). Only under such pathological conditions as spreading depression (see later) and anoxia is this ceiling exceeded. $[K^+]_0$ levels then rise to 30 mM or more. Thus powerful and stable mechanisms normally operate to restrict $[K^+]_0$ increases. The second fact is the well-documented (see Hertz and Schousboe, 1975) increase in O_2 consumption and other changes that occur in cells when $[K^+]_0$ exceeds 20 mM. This suggests that additional cellular mechanisms may be triggered when $[K^+]_0$ exceeds this level.

FUNCTIONAL IMPLICATIONS OF $[K^+]_0$ MODULATION $[K^+]_0$ plays a dominant role in establishing the resting potentials of brain cells and is also an ion of major importance in action potentials and synaptic polarization. Many conjectures have been made regarding its functional potentialities. The afterhyperpolarization of an action potential is caused by the increased K^+-permeability of the membrane at that time and a K^+ equilibrium potential more negative than the resting level. Thus it might be expected that this phase of the action potential would be sensitive to $[K^+]_0$ changes, particularly those induced by a train of spikes in the neuron itself. This was elegantly demonstrated by Frankenhaeuser and Hodgkin (1956) for the squid axon. These authors deduced that the ECS of the axon was about 300 Å wide, being bounded by the enveloping Schwann cell. The calculated rise in $[K^+]_0$ during an action potential, in this space, was 1.6 mM, and decay was exponential with a time constant of 30–100 msec. Subsequently extensive studies were undertaken to incorporate these and other findings into the Hodgkin-Huxley equations (Adelman and Palti, 1969; Adelman, Palti, and Senft, 1973).

The change in spike afterhyperpolarization has also been used to study $[K^+]_0$ in leech ganglia. Baylor and Nicholls (1969a,b) estimated a value of 0.8 mM for the increase in $[K^+]_0$ and a decay constant of 100 msec. A significant conclusion was that the release of K^+ by neurons could influence the behavior of neighboring cells. Recently similar interneuronal ionic

communication was postulated for Rhohon-Beard cells of the tadpole (Spitzer, 1976).

The possible influence of $[K^+]_0$ increases on synaptic transmission in the squid stellate ganglion has recently been discussed by Erulkar and Weight (1977) and by Weight and Erulkar (1976). These authors conjectured that some of the reduction in synaptic efficacy during repetitive synaptic activation could be accounted for by intrinsic $[K^+]_0$ increases, though this could not account for all the reduction during repeated orthodromic activation affecting the presynaptic spike amplitude (Erulkar and Weight, 1977). These results are in agreement with the effect of raised extrinsic K^+ in lowering the synaptic transfer function in the squid synapse (Kusano, 1970).

A combination of specialized geometry and intrinsic $[K^+]_0$ increase has been postulated as a partial explanation of spike frequency modulation in the giant axon of the cockroach (Parnas, this volume). It was found difficult to account entirely for the phenomenon on this basis.

The role of $[K^+]_0$ changes in neuronal aggregates has not been analyzed in detail because of difficulties in obtaining data. One exception is the theoretical study on neuronal and glial interactions via $[K^+]_0$ changes by Lebovitz (1970).

In all of the above work the role of $[K^+]_0$ modulation has been conjectured on the basis of indirect, though often excellent, evidence. With the advent of the K^+ ISM it has become possible to test some of these conjectures. I shall discuss here two examples of the use of K^+ ISMs to clarify existing concepts: the problem of presynaptic inhibition, and that of epileptic seizures.

The monosynaptic excitatory postsynaptic potentials of spinal motoneurons can exhibit a long-lasting depression that is ascribed to some form of presynaptic inhibition associated with a depolarization of primary afferent terminals (primary afferent depolarization, PAD) (for reviews see Schmidt, 1971; Burke and Rudomin, 1977). One of the earliest conjectures about this phenomenon was that it involved a $[K^+]_0$ increase around the presynaptic terminals (Barron and Matthews, 1938). A later alternative explanation was that the presynaptic terminals were themselves subject to inhibition by gamma-aminobutyric acid (GABA) (Eccles, Eccles, and Magni, 1961). Since the concept of presynaptic inhibition is widely applicable (Schmidt, 1971), a resolution of these alternative mechanisms is important, and this should be possible using the K^+ ISM.

Several groups of investigators have used K^+ ISMs to show that PAD is correlated with a rise in

[K$^+$]$_0$ (Syková et al., 1976; Kříž et al., 1974; Kříž, Syková, and Vylický, 1975; Lothman and Somjen, 1975; ten Bruggencate, Lux, and Liebl, 1974; Krnjević and Morris, 1972, 1975a; Deschenes and Feltz, 1976). In no case, however, has a precise correlation been obtained between the potentials representing the presynaptic inhibition and the potassium rise.

One should note that a disagreement between the time course of a potential and an ion signal does not automatically imply that the two have different origins. Due to the low electrical capacity of the microenvironment, electric fields are established virtually instantaneously (their time course governed by the time courses of the sources and sinks), whereas an ionic signal always involves a time delay due to the diffusion process. When these basic differences are summed over an extended population of generating elements, it requires some theoretical sophistication to decide whether the resulting ionic and electric signals are generated by the same or different neuronal populations. More significantly, a pharmacological dissociation of the PAD and [K$^+$]$_0$ changes was obtained by ten Bruggencate, Lux, and Liebl (1974). Thus it appears that a change in [K$^+$]$_0$ cannot be the entire mediator of the presynaptic inhibition, and the complete mechanism remains unresolved (Burke and Rudomin, 1977).

A second phenomenon that has been extensively investigated with K$^+$ ISMs is seizure activity. It was variously postulated that increases in [K$^+$]$_0$ could be responsible for the initiation, maintenance, or abolition of seizure activity (Green, 1966; Fertziger and Ranck, 1970). [K$^+$]$_0$ changes have subsequently been measured in a variety of animal models of seizure (Moody, Futamachi, and Prince, 1974; Mutani, Futamachi, and Prince, 1974; Futamachi, Mutani, and Prince, 1974). A rise in [K$^+$]$_0$ is usually seen during seizure (Figure 4D), but the levels do not exceed the 12 mM ceiling described above. It is now generally concluded, however, that none of the phases of seizure activity are necessarily accompanied by [K$^+$]$_0$ changes, and thus [K$^+$]$_0$ cannot be the sole determinant of any particular aspect of epileptic activity (Pedley et al., 1976; Fisher et al., 1976; Lux, 1974b). An interesting feature revealed in Figure 4D is the well-known close correlation of intracellular glial potentials with changes in [K$^+$]$_0$ (see Somjen, 1975). In contrast, neurons are probably insensitive to [K$^+$]$_0$ changes in the neighborhood of baseline values (Hodgkin, 1951). This suggests that [K$^+$]$_0$ may have to rise by several millimoles before neuronal activity is significantly modulated by depolarization.

Thus at present it must be concluded that no direct demonstration has been given of [K$^+$]$_0$ as a sole causal agent in any phenomenon.

MODULATION OF [Ca^{2+}]$_0$ The second minority ion of obvious interest is Ca^{2+}. Changes in [Ca^{2+}]$_0$ are known to affect axonal excitability (Frankenhaeuser and Hodgkin, 1957) and synaptic transmission (Katz, 1969), excitability increasing and transmission decreasing with a lowering of [Ca^{2+}]$_0$.

The recent development of a highly selective Ca^{2+} ISM (Oehme, Kessler, and Simon, 1976), based on a neutral carrier liquid membrane (Ammann et al., 1975), has enabled a direct demonstration of intrinsic [Ca^{2+}]$_0$ changes in the cerebellum (Nicholson et al., 1976, 1977). Changes of similar magnitude have been confirmed in the cerebral cortex during seizure (Heinemann, Lux, and Gutnick, 1977) and have been further characterized in the cerebellum (Nicholson et al., 1978).

The nature of [Ca^{2+}]$_0$ modulation in the brain is most clearly illustrated by simultaneous laminar analysis of both [Ca^{2+}]$_0$ and [K$^+$]$_0$ in the cerebellar cortex (Figure 5). In this experiment both Ca^{2+} and K$^+$ ISMs were used with tip separation about 50 μm. Field potential observation confirmed that both electrodes were at the same depth and recorded similar responses. As in the experiment depicted in Figure 3, 30-sec stimulation at different frequencies was used to evoke the ion changes; 20-Hz results are shown in Figure 5. It is seen at once that [Ca^{2+}]$_0$ falls during stimulation, in contrast to [K$^+$]$_0$ which, of course, rises. At 20 Hz, [Ca^{2+}]$_0$ falls by as much as 0.4 mM just under the pial surface. On stimulus cessation, [Ca^{2+}]$_0$ returns to baseline and sometimes shows a small, long-lasting overshoot. The [Ca^{2+}]$_0$ change becomes negligible below 250 μm. This is in marked contrast to the [K$^+$]$_0$ increase, which persists to some extent at all depths. The relative migration properties of K$^+$ and Ca^{++} in the brain await detailed analysis, but preliminary superfusion experiments indicate fairly similar rates of penetration of the ions. Thus, the differences in spatial distribution of ions are probably due to differences in the location of sites of transmembrane flux. [Ca^{2+}]$_0$ decreases seem localized to the region of synaptic bombardment, whereas [K$^+$]$_0$ increases appear throughout the length of the Purkinje cells (Nicholson et al., 1978). This supports the idea that the Ca^{2+} decrease is associated with synaptic transmission, although other mechanisms are possible (see below). [K$^+$]$_0$ increases probably have multiple origins, the major source being action currents of presynaptic fibers but with significant con-

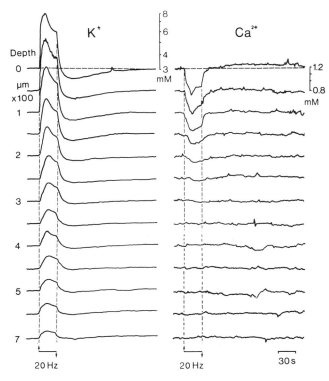

FIGURE 5 Laminar analysis of $[K^+]_o$ increase and $[Ca^{2+}]_o$ decrease recorded simultaneously in cat cerebellum. Twin double-barreled ISMs were used with a tip spacing of 25 μm. Ion changes evoked by 20 Hz local stimulation for 30 sec. Ion changes are largest in the region of maximum stimulation, close to the surface, but some $[K^+]_o$ increase persists at all depths. In contrast, the $[Ca^{2+}]_o$ fall is restricted to a superficial region, the area of synaptic activation. Note undershoot in $[K^+]_o$ and overshoot in $[Ca^{2+}]_o$ following stimulus cessation. Recording depth below cerebellar surface indicated at left.

tributions also coming from postsynaptic elements, including deep passive sources due to return of electrotonic current through vertical core conductors such as Purkinje cells.

FUNCTIONAL IMPLICATIONS OF $[Ca^{2+}]_o$ MODULATION

At the outset the possible mechanisms for $[Ca^{2+}]_o$ reduction should be amplified. It is now established that transmembrane flux of Ca^{2+} is a crucial step in the release of transmitter at a chemical synapse (Llinás and Nicholson, 1975). The Ca^{2+} entry is triggered by the opening of channels through neuronal depolarization; Ca^{2+} then moves inward down its electrochemical gradient, since intracellular Ca^{2+} is of the order of 1 μm or less (Baker, 1972). Thus the presence of vast numbers of active synaptic terminals in the cerebellum suggests this as a prime mechanism for the observed $[Ca^{2+}]_o$ reduction. Some Ca^{2+} may also enter the subsynaptic region of the postsynaptic element (Kusano, Miledi, and Stinnakre, 1975). On the other hand, little Ca^{2+} probably enters the presynaptic fibers. In the squid axon only a minute Ca^{2+} entry is associated with the Na^+-mediated action potential (Baker, 1972). Since parallel fibers are blocked by tetrodotoxin (Llinás and Hess, 1976), it is assumed that Na^+ is the main inward current carrier. Moreover, manganese in low concentrations does not affect the presynaptic volley (Figures 2, 3), but experiments show that it drastically reduces the $[Ca^{2+}]_o$ decrease (Nicholson et al., 1978).

$[Ca^{2+}]_o$ may also be reduced by local dendritic action potentials in the Purkinje cells. It is known that the Purkinje cells in some species (Nicholson and Llinás, 1971; Llinás and Nicholson, 1971; Llinás and Hess, 1976) produce dendritic spikes and that these spikes involve Ca^{2+} movement (Llinás and Hess, 1976; Llinás, this volume). Although dendritic spikes are not prominent in the cat cerebellum, some local responses may occur in the area of intense, synaptically induced depolarization. Such Ca^{2+} spikes could have wider implications, since it has recently been shown that a coupling exists between Ca^{2+} entry and outward K^+ fluxes in some molluscan cells (Meech and Standen, 1975; Heyer and Lux, 1976; Lux and Heyer, this volume) and in vertebrate motoneurons (Barrett and Barrett, 1976).

A further mechanism deserving consideration is the possibility that Ca^{2+} is transiently bound to some of the membrane macromolecules that constitute the cell coat (Adey et al., 1969; Adey, 1971). This has not yet been demonstrated, and the theoretical consequences are far from clear; nevertheless it has potential as a means of modulating the microenvironment.

Two major effects of $[Ca^{2+}]_o$ modulation on neuronal elements can be described. First, a reduction in the Ca^{2+} available for synaptic transmission obviously reduces the release of transmitter. The kinetics for elements of the central nervous system are unknown, but in the giant synapse of the squid a power law has been described (Katz and Miledi, 1970). Recently Hackett (1976) has shown that synaptic transmission in the isolated frog cerebellum is greatly reduced by lowering the $[Ca^{2+}]_o$ level.

An effect opposite to that involving synaptic transmission is seen when the influence of reduced $[Ca^{2+}]_o$ is examined in axonal preparations. Here reduced $[Ca^{2+}]_o$ leads to an increase in excitability (Frankenhaeuser and Hodgkin, 1957), due to modification of the electric field of the membrane by the divalent ions. The excitability changes are exponentially equivalent to depolarizing steps of membrane potential (Frankenhaeuser and Hodgkin, 1957). Lowered $[Ca^{2+}]_o$ effects have not been conclusively demonstrated in the central nervous system, but raising local $[Ca^{2+}]_0$ by local iontophoresis has been shown to depress neuronal excitability (Kato and Somjen, 1969; Kelly, Krnjević, and Somjen, 1969).

Further studies using the Ca^{2+} ISM should aid greatly in describing the role of $[Ca^{2+}]_0$ modulation.

Large ionic changes in the microenvironment

The ionic changes considered so far have consisted of small modulations that might be encountered during normal brain activity. These ion changes have been reflected in variations of the minority ions. $[K^+]_0$ increases did not exceed 12 mM, and $[Ca^{2+}]_0$ decreases were seen to be 0.4 mM or less. Comparable excursions undoubtedly occur in $[Na^+]_0$ or $[Cl^-]_0$ or both to preserve electroneutrality, but they are difficult to detect against the high resting levels of these majority ions.

There are conditions under which much larger changes in $[K^+]_0$ and $[Ca^{2+}]_0$ occur, and in these cases huge movements of $[Na^+]_0$ and $[Cl^-]_0$ can be seen. These changes differ from the small modulations in that, first, they are associated with pathological brain states and, second, it is almost certain that a bulk flow of water across membranes occurs in response to osmotic gradients created by the ion shifts. In fact, this feature of water movement may be a defining characteristic of this class of ion changes. These changes occur, for example, during spreading depression, ischemia, and anoxia. Since we have been studying spreading depression for some time, I shall use this as a model system.

SPREADING DEPRESSION AS A MODEL FOR LARGE-SCALE ION CHANGES   Spreading depression (SD) is a curious phenomenon, first described by Leão (1944) in the cerebral cortex of the rabbit. It consists of a complete extinction of all neuronal activity in a region of the cortex. This depression spreads as a wave at about 3 mm/min; subsequently affected areas recover and remain refractory to SD for periods of several minutes. It was later discovered that SD is accompanied by a large negative excursion of the extracellular potential (20 mV or more). SD is not normally found in the cortex, or elsewhere in brain, but under suitable conditions it can be evoked by a variety of stimuli such as strong direct stimulation and local application of hypertonic KCl. The phenomenon has recently been reviewed in depth by Bureš, Burešová, and Křivánek (1974).

Two major hypotheses have been advanced to account for SD. The first is due to Grafstein (1956) and

postulates that excessive neuronal activity leads to the accumulation of K^+ in the extracellular space, which in turn triggers the release of more K^+ due to neuronal depolarization. This establishes a positive feedback cycle that finally ceases due to sodium inactivation. Propagation occurs through both the diffusion of K^+ and activity in nerve fibers (Grafstein, 1963). This theory is attractive but does not directly account for two concomitant features of SD: brain swelling and increase in impedance. An alternative theory by Van Harreveld (1959) proposed that a release of endogenous glutamate from cells produced an increase in sodium permeability of local membranes leading to the entry of sodium and chloride, as counter-ion, into cellular elements. Water would follow to restore the osmotic balance and cells would swell, compressing the extracellular space and increasing brain impedance. Potassium release would occur as a secondary phenomenon during the inevitable cellular depolarization. This theory has attractive features also, but the crucial step—glutamate release—has never been conclusively demonstrated. Recently Van Harreveld has suggested that both the K^+ and glutamate mechanisms operate (Van Harreveld and Fifkova, 1973; Van Harreveld, 1977).

With this preamble, the recent ISM studies can be appreciated. R. P. Kraig and I have studied SD in the cerebellum of the catfish. The basic features of SD—cessation of evoked responses, large negative swing in the extracellular potential, and subsequent recovery—are shown in Figure 6. Figure 7 shows that large

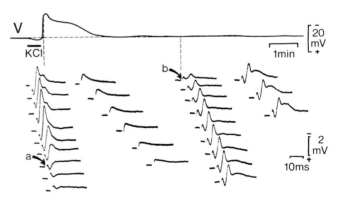

FIGURE 6   Spreading depression (SD) in catfish cerebellum. SD initiated by local microinjection of KCl and manifested by slow, predominantly negative wave, V (upper trace) and cessation of evoked field potentials (lower records). Field potentials evoked every 5 sec and recorded from same potential-sensing micropipette as used to register slow potential. Stimulus on each evoked response corresponds in time to the point directly above on the slow potential; otherwise note the difference in time scale. Most of the evoked response is depressed at arrow a and returns at arrow b. Recording position just below cerebellar surface.

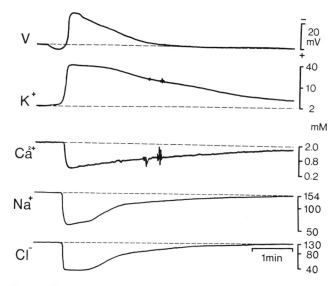

FIGURE 7 Ion changes during spreading depression in catfish cerebellum. A rise in K+ accompanies the slow negative potential *V*, but Ca²⁺, Na⁺, and Cl⁻ all fall. Note different baseline values for minority ions K⁺ and Ca²⁺, compared with the majority ions Na⁺ and Cl⁻. Because of this and the logarithmic response of the electrodes, the waveforms represent very different ionic excursions. *V*, K⁺, and Ca²⁺ records were made simultaneously in one experiment; Cl⁻ and Na⁺ simultaneously in another experiment. Recording positions just below cerebellar surface.

increases in $[K^+]_0$ occur during SD, of the order of 20–40 mM. Similar and even larger $[K^+]_0$ increases have been reported by others (Vyskočil, Kříž, and Bureš, 1972; Prince, Lux, and Neher, 1973; Futamachi, Mutani, and Prince, 1974; Morris and Krnjević, 1974; Sugaya, Takato, and Noda, 1975; Mori, Miller, and Tomita, 1976). In addition, earlier radiotracer studies had indicated the existence of this K⁺ efflux (Brinley, Kandel, and Marshall, 1960; Křivánek and Bureš, 1960). These findings support Grafstein's hypothesis, but Sugaya, Takato, and Noda (1975) showed that SD occurs in the presence of tetrodotoxin, thus indicating that the normal Na⁺-K⁺ spike mechanism was not necessary. Further evidence of the need for a more complex theory has come from our own measurements of ions other than K⁺ during SD. Using a Cl⁻ ISM we showed that a dramatic fall in $[Cl^-]_0$—about 100 mM—accompanies SD (Nicholson and Kraig, 1975). This raised the question of how electroneutrality was preserved and required the measurement of $[Na^+]_0$. To do this we developed a fast-responding Na⁺ ISM (Kraig and Nicholson, 1976). We showed that the Cl⁻ shift was accompanied by a large drop in $[Na^+]_0$. In fact it seems, within the limits of experimental error, that the changes in Na⁺ and Cl⁻ have the same magnitude and time course

(Kraig and Nicholson, 1978). The movement of so much NaCl should set up osmotic gradients that would lead to a water movement. Our findings therefore agree with aspects of Van Harreveld's hypothesis but throw no light on the crucial glutamate mechanism.

A surprising finding concerned $[Ca^{2+}]_0$ changes during SD. We found that $[Ca^{2+}]_0$ dropped to about 10% of the resting value at the peak of SD in the rat cerebellum (Nicholson et al., 1977). This type of change has been confirmed in the catfish cerebellum (Kraig and Nicholson, 1978; Figure 7).

Taken together the changes in the four measured ions during SD indicate that all these extracellular ions move toward their intracellular concentrations. Since intracellular space is some five times the extracellular space in volume, this observation may be most simply explained by envisioning the transient appearance of "holes" in membranes during SD, of sufficient size to allow the passage of all the observed ions. What triggers the opening and closing of such channels, if they exist, remains unknown. It also cannot be ruled out that ions do not simply move between intra- and extracellular compartments but are bound to extracellular sites or traverse the blood-brain barrier and meninges. Our measurements simply reveal the change of activity in the extracellular compartment. Somewhat similar ion changes probably occur during many histological fixation procedures (Nevis and Collins, 1967; Van Harreveld, 1972).

Large shifts in $[K^+]_0$ and $[Ca^{2+}]_0$ can also be induced in the cerebellum by superfusing with Ringer's containing aminopyridine before stimulation (Nicholson, ten Bruggencate, and Senekowitsch, 1976; Nicholson et al., 1976). These shifts can resemble those of SD in magnitude, but they are very localized. What is surprising is that aminopyridine blocks the voltage-dependent K⁺ conductance change associated with other preparations (Pelhate and Pichon, 1974; Yeh, Oxford, and Narahashi, 1976). Thus, apparently, an agent that normally prevents K⁺ efflux promotes large increases in $[K^+]_0$. This effect can also be seen with barium superfusion (Nicholson, ten Bruggencate, and Senekowitsch, 1976), which again blocks K⁺ currents. The facts that a large $[Ca^{2+}]_0$ decrease also accompanies the $[K^+]_0$ increase and that the phenomenon does not occur when $[Ca^{2+}]_0$ is reduced with citrate (Nicholson et al., 1976) suggest that Ca²⁺ may play a role. This could occur, for example, if Purkinje-cell dendrites possessed two distinct K⁺ channels. The first channel would be blocked by established K⁺ blockers such as aminopyridine, barium, or tetraethylammonium, and the second would be insensitive to these compounds but activated through an inward Ca^{2+} flux. Such channels have been demonstrated in other preparations (Meech and Standen, 1975; Barrett and Barrett, 1976; Heyer and Lux, 1976; Thompson, 1977; Lux and Heyer, this volume). By blocking the first K^+ channel, the Ca^{2+} current could become fully expressed instead of being terminated by repolarization, and the second K^+ flux would be activated. This is consistent with the apparent enhancement of dendritic spikes (Llinás and Hess, 1976) and postsynaptic field potential components (Nicholson, ten Bruggencate, and Senekowitsch, 1976) in the presence of aminopyridine in the cerebellum. The existence of Ca^{2+}-activated K^+ channels in dendrites could also account for some of the Mn-sensitive $[K^+]_0$ increase described above and perhaps even for some features of SD (Nicholson et al., 1978).

It is interesting that once again the use of ISMs has clarified the phenomenology of SD but has failed to confirm in detail preexisting hypotheses of ionic mechanisms.

Energy and the microenvironment

The short-term fluxes of ions during synaptic events and action potentials are generated by ions moving passively down their electrochemical gradients. The long-term maintenance of these gradients involves the expenditure of energy, which is reflected in the metabolic rate of the brain.

The brain accounts for about 20–25% of the oxygen consumption of the body (McIlwain and Bachelard, 1971), indicating a large energy consumption; most of this energy is probably used by the Na-K pump (Lowry, 1975; Bachelard, 1975). Of course other transport systems exist, but in some cases an exchange diffusion with Na may be the mechanism (Baker, 1972; MacKnight and Leaf, 1977), indicating once again the primary role of the Na-K pump. The pump derives its energy from ATP, which is mostly produced in the tricarboxylic acid cycle (DeWeer, 1975; Thomas, 1972; Glynn and Karlish, 1975).

An extensive literature using a wide variety of techniques has been compiled concerning the metabolism of the brain and its cells; recent reviews include Siesjö and Sørenson (1971), Ingvar and Lasson (1975), and Hertz and Schousboe (1975). Here I shall briefly mention several studies that directly relate to ion modulation and large-scale ion changes.

During the past few years the techniques of spectroscopy and spectrofluorometry have been used to directly monitor the oxidation of NADH to NAD and redox changes in the cytochromes (Jöbsis et al., 1975; Somjen et al., 1976; Lewis and Schuette, 1975b, 1976). In many cases these studies have been combined with the use of K^+ ISMs. A linear relation between the logarithm of $[K^+]_0$ rise and NADH oxidation has been seen during ionic modulation at levels that might occur during normal neuronal activity (Lothman et al., 1975). During epileptic seizure, however, NADH oxidation rises above the level predicted by the linear relation. A similar level of oxidation is reached during SD, but in this case the $[K^+]_0$ levels become very high, again violating the linear relationship. Older evidence indicates that a substantial metabolic deficit accrues during repeated SD (Bureš, Burešová, and Křivánek, 1974). During anoxia, complete reduction of NADH occurs (Jöbsis et al., 1975); thus epilepsy and SD are not caused by anoxia. The Na-K ATPase inhibitor, ouabain, blocks the Na-K pump and slows but does not abolish the NADH oxidation (LaManna and Rosenthal, 1975; Rosenthal and LaManna, 1975). It is assumed that the NADH oxidation takes place mainly in mitochondria, the major site of ATP production via the tricarboxylic acid cycle. Other mechanisms of ATP production, not involving NADH oxidation, will not be monitored by the fluorometric technique but are assumed to be small.

Measurements of the cytochromes have been less extensive but have generally agreed with the NADH oxidation determinations; they also suggest that the normal brain is maintained in a slightly hypoxic state (Rosenthal et al., 1976).

We conclude that the ionic changes in the microenvironment can trigger metabolically driven clearance mechanisms, probably mainly the Na-K pump. More than one mechanism may exist, however, particularly at high $[K^+]_0$ levels (Jöbsis et al., 1975). This conclusion is supported by much of the older data on the dramatic swelling and increase in metabolism exhibited by brain tissue when $[K^+]_0$ reaches 20 mM or more (Hertz and Schousboe, 1975), as mentioned earlier in this paper.

Finally, it is worth recalling that a major distinction between plant and animal cells is that animal cells have no rigid walls (MacKnight and Leaf, 1977). Volume depends on water movement and thus on the maintenance of ionic concentrations across the membrane. This balance is brought about by the continued action of the Na-K pump. Thus nerve cells, and indeed all animal cells, constitute dissipative structures (Katchalsky, Rowland, and Blumenthal, 1974) whose integrity is only maintained by the continued expenditure of energy. Since it is the aggregate of neurons that forms the brain-cell microenvironment, it follows that the microenvironment is also a dissipative structure dependent on the continuous expenditure of energy for its existence.

Brain-cell microenvironment: A new dimension in neuronal communication

This survey has focused on recent data about the extracellular microenvironment acquired through the use of new techniques. Some of the major results of recent research into ion fluctuation in the brain-cell microenvironment are illustrated in Figure 8, which indicates the total number of Na^+ and K^+ ions in a cube of side 200 Å (the probable separation of brain-cell membranes) in three states. If this cube were bounded on four sides by surface membranes, it would have a membrane area of 0.0016 μm^2. Since the mean density of Na^+ channels is perhaps 16 per μm^2 (Hille, 1977), there would only be a probability of 0.03 of finding one on the wall of the 200 Å cube.

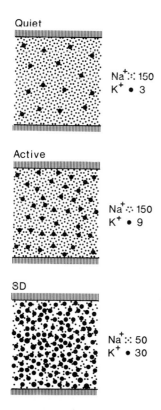

Quiet

Na^+ :: 150
K^+ • 3

Active

Na^+ :: 150
K^+ • 9

SD

Na^+ :: 50
K^+ • 30

FIGURE 8 Representation of ionic concentrations in ECS in quiescent, active, and SD states. Each diagram shows total number of Na^+ and K^+ ions contained within a cube of side 200 Å of the ECS. Concentrations shown in millimoles beside each diagram. Ion dimensions not to scale, and volume changes in ECS not shown.

Potassium channels could be 100 times more numerous than Na channels (Hille, 1977); this would give a density of 2.6 on the cube. Na-K pump sites may average about 1,000 per μm^2 (Cohen and DeWeer, 1977), giving a density of 1.6 on the cube. Thus at these dimensions both ions and membrane transduction sites are quite sparse.

This survey is certainly incomplete. For example, nothing has been said about variations in H^+, HCO_3^-, or Mg^{2+}, all of which could be expected to have significant functional roles. At present our techniques do not enable us to monitor these variables unambiguously in the microenvironment, and without such data discussion has limited value. The results that have been discussed are sufficient to challenge our traditional concepts of the microenvironment as simply an uninteresting salt solution. Beyond that, the new information shows that some of our ways of thinking about causes and effects are in need of revision.

The new techniques have been effective in revealing new phenomena, but they have not unambiguously confirmed any of the hypotheses about the role of ions, or of electric fields, formulated prior to the measurements. Thus in the true sense of information theory, these experiments have been very informative, notwithstanding that the practicing neurobiologist would doubtless have preferred a higher success rate in verifying his prior conceptions. What has been shown is that there is a correlation between different types of events. This could mean that one causes another, but it could also mean that both are caused by a third, undetected event. Causality implies that one event is prior to another, but the existence of feedback mechanisms between phenomena weakens the notion of priority. It is also evident that we are dealing with multiparameter events. For example, one might predict that either raising $[K^+]_0$ or lowering $[Ca^{2+}]_0$ would increase neuronal excitability. If both ion changes occur and excitability changes, it is difficult to ascribe the effect to either ion species alone. Indeed I suggest that in repeated trials the relative influence of the two ions may fluctuate, thus requiring a stochastic element in our thinking. An effect can have different causes on different occasions. There is a real possibility of multiple routes to the same goal; indeed redundancy is the key to efficient communication in a noisy environment.

We should also be aware that we are judging processes by particular effects. For example, we might seek ionic modulation in the variation in firing pattern of a neuron, but neurons do not necessarily transmit all their information by this means. It is conceivable, though not clearly demonstrated, that the response to a change in the ionic environment may be, for example, the release of peptides into the surrounding milieu. This, in turn, could lead to further ionic modulation by receptive neighboring neuronal elements. Again, effects ascribed to ephaptic transmission might actually be an expression of a change in the ionic signal modality of the neuron rather than in the electrical modality.

Our view of neurons as predominantly devices for dispatching electrical signals is too narrow. We must begin to see the electrical signals and their communication network as a fast control system for ionic and molecular fluxes, rather than the other way around. What we are beginning to appreciate is that neurons are actually a form of biological cell and not merely nonlinear electrical elements. Thus nerve cells have available to them most of the complex and fascinating communication modalities of nonneuronal cells, and it would be surprising if these modalities were not used. Some of our problems may represent a failure on our part to adequately conceptualize the nature of communication, rather than a failure of neurons to communicate via the brain-cell microenvironment.

Once the microenvironment is seen as a communication channel, the potential subtlety is awesome. A unique medium is available in which every element of a three-dimensional continuum can function as an emitter, absorber, or transmitter of chemical signals. This continuum can be dynamically structured by the electrical impulses of the intrinsic neuronal networks and more long-term neurohumoral influences. This potentiality for total three-dimensional modulation finally ascribes significance to the overwhelming predominance of complex electrochemical interfaces that constitutes the brain cell.

ACKNOWLEDGMENTS   I am indebted to G. ten Bruggencate, R. P. Kraig, R. Senekowitsch, R. Steinberg, and H. Stöckle for their collaboration in some of the research described here. The work was supported by U.S. Public Health Service Research Grant NS-13742, Deutsche Forshungsgemeinshaft Grant Br 242/12, and the Alexander von Humboldt Foundation. Figures 4A, B, D are reproduced (with modifications) with permission of Elsevier/North-Holland Biomedical Press and Figure 4C by permission of the *Journal of Physiology*.

REFERENCES

ADELMAN, JR., W. J., and Y. PALTI, 1969. The influence of external potassium on the giant axon of the squid, *Loligo pealei. J. Gen. Physiol.* 53:685–703.

ADELMAN, JR., W. J., Y. PALTI, and J. P. SENFT, 1973. Potassium ion accumulation in a periaxonal space and its effect on the measurement of membrane potassium ion conductance. *J. Membrane Biol.* 13:387–410.

ADEY, W. R., 1971. Evidence for cerebral membrane effects of calcium derived from direct current gradient, impedance and intracellular records. *Exp. Neurol.* 30:78–102.

ADEY, W. R., B. G. BYSTROM, A. COSTIN, R. T. KADO, and T. TARBY, 1969. Divalent cations in cerebral impedance and cell membrane morphology. *Exp. Neurol.* 23:29–50.

AMMANN, D., M. GÜGGI, E. PRETSCH, and W. SIMON, 1975. Improved calcium ion-selective electrode based on a neutral carrier. *Anal. Lett.* 8:709–720.

ARVANITAKI, A., 1942. Effects evoked in an axon by the activity of a contiguous one. *J. Neurophysiol.* 5:89–108.

BACHELARD, M. S., 1975. Energy utilized by neurotransmitters. In *Brain Work*, D. H. Ingvar and N. A. Lassen, eds. Copenhagen: Munksgaard, pp. 79–81.

BAKER, P. F., 1972. Transport and metabolism of calcium ions in nerve. *Prog. Biophys. Mol. Biol.* 24:177–223.

BARRETT, E. F., and J. N. BARRETT, 1976. Separation of two voltage-sensitive potassium currents, and demonstration of a tetrodotoxin-resistant calcium current in frog motoneurons. *J. Physiol.* 255:737–774.

BARRON, D. H., and B. M. C. MATTHEWS, 1938. The interpretation of potential changes in the spinal cord. *J. Physiol.* 92:276–321.

BAWIN, S. M., and W. R. ADEY, 1976. Sensitivity of calcium binding in cerebral tissue to weak environmental electric fields oscillating at low frequency. *Proc. Natl. Acad. Sci. USA* 73:1999–2003.

BAYLOR, D. A., and J. G. NICHOLLS, 1969a. Changes in extracellular potassium concentration produced by neuronal activity in the central nervous system of the leech. *J. Physiol.* 203:555–569.

BAYLOR, D. A., and J. G. NICHOLLS, 1969b. After effects of nerve impulses on signalling in the central nervous system of the leech. *J. Physiol.* 203:571–589.

BOURKE, R. S., H. K. KIMELBERG, C. R. WEST, and A. M. BREMER, 1975. The effect of HCO_3^- on the swelling and ion uptake of monkey cerebral cortex under conditions of raised extracellular potassium. *J. Neurochem.* 25:323–328.

BOURKE, R. S., K. M. NELSON, R. A. NAUMANN, and O. M. YOUNG, 1970. Studies of the production and subsequent reduction of swelling in primate cerebral cortex under isosmotic conditions *in vivo. Exp. Brain Res.* 10:427–446.

BRACHO, M., and R. K. ORKAND, 1972. Neuron-glia interaction: Dependence on temperature. *Brain Res.* 36:416–419.

BRADBURY, M. W. B., and B. STULCOVÁ, 1970. Efflux mechanism contributing to the stability of the potassium concentration in cerebrospinal fluid. *J. Physiol.* 208:415–430.

BRINLEY, JR., F. J., E. R. KANDEL, and W. MARSHALL, 1960. Potassium outflux from rabbit cortex during spreading depression. *J. Neurophysiol.* 23:246–256.

BRUGGENCATE, G. TEN, H. D. LUX, and L. LIEBL, 1974. Possible relationships between extracellular potassium activity and presynaptic inhibition in the spinal cord of the cat. *Pflügers Arch.* 349:301–317.

BULLOCK, T. M., and G. A. HORRIDGE, 1965. *Structure and Function in the Nervous Systems of Invertebrates*, vol. I, San Francisco: W. H. Freeman.

BUREŠ, J., O. BUREŠOVÁ, and J. KŘIVÁNEK, 1974. *The mechanism and Applications of Leão's Spreading Depression of*

Electroencephalographic Activity. New York: Academic Press.

BURKE, R. E., and P. RUDOMIN, 1977. Spinal neurons and synapses. In *Handbook of Physiology: The Nervous System*, J. M. Brookhart and V. B. Mountcastle, eds. Bethesda: Am. Physiol. Soc., section 1, vol. I, pp. 877–944.

CLARK, J. W., and R. PLONSEY, 1970. A mathematical study of nerve fiber interaction. *Biophys. J.* 10:937–957.

COHEN, L. B., and P. DEWEER, 1977. Structural and metabolic processes directly related to action potential propagation. In *Handbook of Physiology: The Nervous System*, J. M. Brookhart and V. B. Mountcastle, eds. Bethesda: Am. Physiol. Soc., section 1, vol. I. pp. 137–159.

DAVSON, H., 1976. The blood brain barrier. *J. Physiol.* 255:1–28.

DAVSON, H., and K. WELCH, 1971. The relations of blood, brain and cerebrospinal fluid. In *Ion Homeostasis of the Brain*, B. K. Siesjö and S. C. Sørenson, eds. Copenhagen: Munksgaard, pp. 9–12.

DESCHENES, M., and P. FELTZ, 1976. GABA-induced rise of extracellular potassium in rat dorsal root ganglia: An electrophysiological study in vivo. *Brain Res.* 118:494–499.

DEWEER, P., 1975. Aspects of neuronal recovery processes in nerve. In *MTP International Review of Science: Neurophysiology*, series 1, vol. 3, A. C. Guyton, ed. London: Butterworths, pp. 1–48.

ECCLES, J. C., R. M. ECCLES, and F. MAGNI, 1961. Central inhibitory action attributable to presynaptic depolarization produced by muscle afferent volleys. *J. Physiol.* 159:147–166.

ECCLES, J. C., R. LLINÁS, and K. SASAKI, 1966. Parallel fiber stimulation and the responses induced thereby in the Purkinje cells of the cerebellum. *Exp. Brain Res.* 1:17–39.

ERULKAR, S. D., and F. F. WEIGHT, 1977. Extracellular potassium and transmitter release at the giant synapse of squid. *J. Physiol.* 266:209–218.

FENSTERMACHER, J. D., and C. S. PATLAK, 1975. The exchange of material between cerebrospinal fluid and brain. In *Fluid Environment of the Brain*, H. F. Cserr, J. D. Fenstermacher, and V. Fencl, eds. New York: Academic Press, pp. 201–214.

FERTZIGER, A. P., and J. B. RANCK, JR., 1970. Potassium accumulation in interstitial space during epileptiform seizures. *Exp. Neurol.* 26:571–585.

FISHER, R. S., T. A. PEDLEY, and D. A. PRINCE, 1976. Kinetics of potassium movement in normal cortex. *Brain Res.* 101:223–237.

FISHER, R. S., T. A. PEDLEY, W. J. MOODY, and D. A. PRINCE, 1976. The role of extracellular potassium in hippocampal epilepsy. *Arch. Neurol.* 33:76–83.

FRANKENHAEUSER, B., and A. L. HODGKIN, 1956. The after effects of impulses in the giant nerve fibers of *Loligo*. *J. Physiol.* 131:341–376.

FRANKENHAEUSER, B., and A. L. HODGKIN, 1957. The action of calcium on the electrical properties of squid axon. *J. Physiol.* 137:218–244.

FREEMAN, J. A., and C. NICHOLSON, 1975. Experimental optimization of current source density technique for anuran cerebellum. *J. Neurophysiol.* 38:369–382.

FUTAMACHI, K. J., R. MUTANI, and D. A. PRINCE, 1974. Potassium activity in rabbit cortex. *Brain Res.* 75:5–25.

FUTAMACHI, K. J., and T. A. PEDLEY, 1976. Glial cells and extracellular potassium: Their relationship in mammalian cortex. *Brain Res.* 109:311–322.

GARDNER-MEDWIN, A. R., 1977. The migration of potassium produced by electric current through brain tissue. *J. Physiol.* 269:32P–33P.

GARDNER-MEDWIN, A. R., and C. NICHOLSON, 1978. Measurements of extracellular potassium and calcium concentration during passage of current across the surface of the brain. *J. Physiol.* 275:66–67P.

GLYNN, I. M., and S. J. O. KARLISH, 1975. The sodium pump. *Annu. Rev. Physiol.* 37:13–55.

GRAFSTEIN, B., 1956. Mechanism of spreading cortical depression. *J. Neurophysiol.* 19:154–171.

GRAFSTEIN, B., 1963. Neuronal release of potassium during spreading depression. In *Brain Function*, M. A. B. Brazier, ed. Berkeley: Univ. California Press, pp. 87–124.

GREEN, J. O., 1966. The hippocampus. *Physiol. Rev.* 44:501–608.

HACKETT, J. T., 1976. Calcium dependency of excitatory chemical synaptic transmission in the frog cerebellum in vitro. *Brain Res.* 114:35–46.

HEINEMANN, U., and H. D. LUX, 1975. Undershoots following stimulus induced rises of extracellular potassium concentration in cerebral cortex of cat. *Brain Res.* 93:63–76.

HEINEMANN, U., and H. D. LUX, 1977. Ceiling of stimulus induced rises in extracellular potassium concentration in cerebral cortex of cat. *Brain Res.* 120:231–249.

HEINEMANN, U., H. D. LUX, and M. J. GUTNICK, 1977. Extracellular free calcium and potassium during paroxysmal activity in the cerebral cortex of the cat. *Exp. Brain Res.* 27:237–243.

HENN, F. A., H. HALJAMÄE, and A. HAMBERGER, 1972. Glial cell function: Active control of extracellular K^+ concentration. *Brain Res.* 43:437–443.

HERTZ, L., and C. NISSEN, 1976. Differences between leech and mammalian nervous systems in metabolic reaction to K^+ as an indication of differences in potassium homeostasis mechanisms. *Brain Res.* 110:182–188.

HERTZ, L., and A. SCHOUSBOE, 1975. Ion and energy metabolism of the brain at the cellular level. *Int. Rev. Neurobiol.* 18:141–211.

HERZ, A., W. ZIEGLGÄNSBERGER, and G. FÄRBER, 1969. Microelectrophoretic studies concerning the spread of glutamic acid and GABA in brain tissue. *Exp. Brain Res.* 9:221–235.

HEYER, C. B., and H. D. LUX, 1976. Control of the delayed outward potassium currents in bursting pace-maker neurones of the snail, *Helix pomatia*. *J. Physiol.* 262:349–382.

HILLE, B., 1977. Ionic basis of resting potential. In *Handbook of Physiology: The Nervous System*, J. M. Brookhart and V. B. Mountcastle, eds. Bethesda: Am. Physiol. Soc., section 1, vol. I, pp. 99–136.

HODGKIN, A. L., 1951. The ionic basis of electrical activity in nerve and muscle. *Biol. Rev.* 26:339–409.

INGVAR, D. H., and N. A. LASSEN, 1975. *Brain Work*. Copenhagen: Munksgaard.

JÖBSIS, F., M. ROSENTHAL, J. LAMANNA, E. LOTHMAN, G. CORDINGLY, and G. SOMJEN, 1975. Metabolic activity in epileptic seizures. In *Brain Work*, D. H. Ingvar and N. A. Lassen, eds. Copenhagen: Munksgaard, pp. 185–196.

KACZMAREK, L. K., and W. R. ADEY, 1974. Weak electric gradients change ionic and transmitter fluxes in cortex. *Brain Res.* 66:537–540.

KARWOSKI, C. J., and L. M. PROENZA, 1977. Relationship between Müller cell responses, a local transretinal potential, and potassium flux. *J. Neurophysiol.* 40:244–259.

KATCHALSKY, A. K., V. ROWLAND, and R. BLUMENTHAL, 1974. Dynamic patterns of brain cell assemblies. *Neurosci. Res. Program Bull.* 12:1–187. (Also available in book form from The MIT Press.)

KATO, G., and G. G. SOMJEN, 1969. Effects of micro-iontrophoretic administration of magnesium and calcium on neurons in the central nervous system of cats. *J. Neurobiol.* 1:181–195.

KATZ, B., 1969. *The Release of Neural Transmitter Substances.* Liverpool: Liverpool Univ. Press.

KATZ, B., and R. MILEDI, 1970. Further study of the role of calcium in synaptic transmission. *J. Physiol.* 207:789–801.

KATZ, B., and O. H. SCHMITT, 1940. Electrical interaction between two adjacent nerve fibres. *J. Physiol.* 97:471–488.

KATZMAN, R., 1976. Maintenance of a constant brain extracellular potassium. *Fed. Proc.* 35:1244–1247.

KELLY, J. S., K. KRNJEVIĆ, and G. G. SOMJEN, 1969. Divalent cations and electrical properties of cortical cells. *J. Neurobiol.* 1:197–208.

KRAIG, R. P., and C. NICHOLSON, 1976. Sodium liquid ion exchanger microelectrode used to measure large extracellular sodium transients. *Science* 194:725–726.

KRAIG, R. P., and C. NICHOLSON, 1978. Extracellular ionic variations during spreading depression. *Neurosciences* (in press).

KŘIVÁNEK, J., and J. BUREŠ, 1960. Ion shifts during Leão's spreading cortical depression. *Physiol. Bohemoslov.* 9:494–503.

KŘÍŽ, N., E. SYKOVÁ, E. UJEC, and L. VYKLICKÝ, 1974. Changes of extracellular potassium concentration induced by the neural activity in the spinal cord of the cat. *J. Physiol.* 238:1–15.

KŘÍŽ, N., E. SYKOVÁ, and L. VYKLICKÝ, 1975. Extracellular potassium changes in the spinal cord of the cat and their relation to slow potentials, active transport and impulse transmission. *J. Physiol.* 249:167–182.

KRNJEVIĆ, K., and M. E. MORRIS, 1972. Extracellular K^+ activity and slow potential changes in spinal cord and medulla. *Can. J. Physiol. Pharmacol.* 50:1214–1217.

KRNJEVIĆ, K., and M. E. MORRIS, 1974. Extracellular accumulation of K^+ evoked by activity of primary afferent fibers in the cuneate nucleus and dorsal horn of cats. *Can. J. Physiol. Pharmacol.* 52:852–871.

KRNJEVIĆ, K., and M. E. MORRIS, 1975a. Correlation between extracellular focal potentials and K^+ potentials evoked by primary afferent activity. *Can. J. Physiol. Pharmacol.* 53:912–922.

KRNJEVIĆ, K., and M. E. MORRIS, 1975b. Factors determining the decay of K^+ potentials and focal potentials in the central nervous system. *Can. J. Physiol. Pharmacol.* 53:923–934.

KUFFLER, S. W., and J. G. NICHOLLS, 1966. The physiology of neuroglial cells. *Ergebn. Physiol.* 57:1–90.

KUSANO, K., 1970. Influence of ionic environment on the relationship between pre and post-synaptic potential. *J. Neurobiol.* 1:435–457.

KUSANO, K., R. MILEDI, and J. STINNAKRE, 1975. Post-synaptic entry of calcium induced by transmitter action. *Proc. R. Soc. Lond.* B189:49–56.

LaMANNA, J. C., and M. ROSENTHAL, 1975. Effect of ouabain and phenobarbital on oxidative metabolic activity associated with spreading cortical depression in cat. *Brain Res.* 88:145–169.

LEÃO, A. A. P., 1944. Spreading depression of activity in the cerebral corex. *J. Neurophysiol.* 7:359–390.

LEBOVITZ, R. M., 1970. A theoretical examination of ionic interactions between neural and non-neural membranes. *Biophys. J.* 10:423–444.

LEWIS, D. V., and W. K. SCHUETTE, 1975a. Temperature dependence of potassium ion clearance in the nervous system. *Brain Res.* 99:175–178.

LEWIS, D. V., and W. K. SCHUETTE, 1975b. NADH fluorescence and $[K^+]_0$ changes during hippocampal electric stimulation. *J. Neurophysiol.* 38:405–417.

LEWIS, D. V., and W. K. SCHUETTE, 1976. NADH fluorescence, $[K^+]_0$ and oxygen consumption in a cerebral cortex during direct cortical stimulation. *Brain Res.* 110:523–535.

LLINÁS, R., and R. HESS, 1976. Tetrodotoxin-resistant dendritic spikes in avian Purkinje cells. *Proc. Natl. Acad. Sci. USA* 73:2520–2523.

LLINÁS, R., and C. NICHOLSON, 1971. Electrophysiological properties of dendrites and somata in alligator Purkinje cells. *J. Neurophysiol.* 34:532–551.

LLINÁS, R., and C. NICHOLSON, 1974. Analysis of field potentials in the central nervous system. In *Handbook of Electroencephalography and Clinical Neurophysiology,* part B, vol. 2, A. Rémond, ed., Amsterdam: Elsevier, pp. 61–83.

LLINÁS, R., and C. NICHOLSON, 1975. Calcium role in depolarization-secretion coupling: An aequorin study in squid giant synapse. *Proc. Natl. Acad. Sci. USA* 72:187–190.

LOTHMAN, E., J. LaMANNA, E. CORDINGLY, M. ROSENTHAL, and G. G. SOMJEN, 1975. Responses of electrical potential, potassium levels and oxidative metabolic activity of the cerebral neocortex of cats. *Brain Res.* 88:15–36.

LOTHMAN, E., and G. G. SOMJEN, 1975. Extracellular potassium activity, intracellular and extracellular potential responses in the spinal cord. *J. Physiol.* 252:115–136.

LOWRY, O. H., 1975. Energy metabolism in brain and its control. In *Brain Work,* D. H. Ingvar and N. A. Lassen, eds. Copenhagen: Munksgaard, pp. 48–63.

LUFT, J. H., 1976. The structure and properties of the cell surface coat. *Int. Rev. Cytol.* 45:291–382.

LUX, H. D., 1974a. Fast recording ion specific microelectrodes: Their use in pharmacological studies in the CNS. *Neuropharmacology* 13:509–517.

LUX, H. D., 1974b. The kinetics of extracellular potassium: Relation to epileptogenesis. *Epilepsia* 15:375–393.

LUX, H. D., and E. NEHER, 1973. The equilibration time course of $[K^+]_0$ in cat cortex. *Exp. Brain Res.* 17:190–205.

McILWAIN, H., and M. S. BACHELARD, 1971. *Biochemistry and the Central Nervous System.* Edinburgh and London: Churchill, Livingstone.

MacKNIGHT, A. D. C., and A. LEAF, 1977. Regulation of cellular volume. *Physiol. Rev.* 57:510–573.

MEECH, R. W., and N. B. STANDEN, 1975. Potassium activation in *Helix aspersa* neurons under voltage clamp: A component mediated by calcium influx. *J. Physiol.* 249:211–239.

MOODY, W. J., K. J. FUTAMACHI, and D. A. PRINCE, 1974.

Extracellular potassium activity during epileptogenesis. *Exp. Neurol.* 42:248–263.

MORI, S., W. M. MILLER, and T. TOMITA, 1976. Müller cell function during spreading depression in frog retina. *Proc. Natl. Acad. Sci. USA* 73:1351–1354.

MORRIS, M. E., and K. KRNJEVIĆ, 1974. Some measurements of extracellular potassium activity in the mammalian central nervous system. In *Ion Selective Microelectrodes*, H. J. Berman and N. C. Herbert, eds. New York: Plenum, pp. 129–141.

MUTANI, R., K. J. FUTAMACHI, and D. A. PRINCE, 1974. Potassium activity in immature cortex. *Brain Res.* 75:27–39.

NELSON, P., 1966. Interactions between spinal motoneurons of the cat. *J. Neurophysiol.* 29:275–287.

NEVIS, A. H., and G. H. COLLINS, 1967. Electrical impedance and volume changes in brain during preparation for electron microscopy. *Brain Res.* 5:57–85.

NICHOLSON, C., 1973. Theoretical analysis of field potentials in anisotropic ensembles of neuronal elements. *IEEE Trans. Biomed. Eng.* BME 20:278–284.

NICHOLSON, C., and J. A. FREEMAN, 1975. Theory of current-source density analysis and determination of conductivity tensor for anuran cerebellum. *J. Neurophysiol.* 38:356–368.

NICHOLSON, C., and R. P. KRAIG, 1975. Chloride and potassium changes measured during spreading depression in catfish cerebellum. *Brain Res.* 96:384–389.

NICHOLSON, C., and R. LLINÁS, 1971. Field potentials in the alligator cerebellum and theory of their relationship to Purkinje cell dendritic spikes. *J. Neurophysiol.* 34:509–531.

NICHOLSON, C., and R. LLINÁS, 1975. Real time current-source density analysis using multi-electrode array in cat cerebellum. *Brain Res.* 100:418–424.

NICHOLSON, C., R. STEINBERG, H. STÖCKLE, and G. TEN BRUGGENCATE, 1976. Calcium decrease associated with aminopyridine-induced potassium increases in cat cerebellum. *Neurosci. Lett.* 3:315–319.

NICHOLSON, C., G. TEN BRUGGENCATE, and R. SENEKOWITSCH, 1976. Large potassium signals and slow potentials evoked during aminopyridine or barium superfusion in cat cerebellum. *Brain Res.* 113:606–610.

NICHOLSON, C., G. TEN BRUGGENCATE, R. STEINBERG, and H. STÖCKLE, 1977. Calcium modulation in brain extracellular microenvironment demonstrated with ion-selective micropipette. *Proc. Natl. Acad. Sci. USA* 74:1287–1290.

NICHOLSON, C., G. TEN BRUGGENCATE, H. STÖCKLE, and R. STEINBERG, 1978. Calcium and potassium changes in extracellular microenvironment of cat cerebellum. *J. Neurophysiol.* 41:1026–1039.

OAKLEY II, B., and D. G. GREEN, 1976. Correlation of light-induced changes in retinal extracellular potassium concentration with c-wave of the electroretinogram. *J. Neurophysiol.* 39:1117–1133.

OEHME, M., M. KESSLER, and W. SIMON, 1976. Neutral carrier Ca^{2+}-microelectrode. *Chimia* 30:204–206.

ORKAND, R. K., 1977. Glial cells. In *Handbook of Physiology: The Nervous System*, J. M. Brookhart and V. B. Mountcastle, eds. Bethesda: Am. Physiol. Soc., section 1, vol. I, pp. 855–875.

ORME, F. W., 1969. Liquid ion exchanger microelectrode. In *Glass Microelectrodes*, M. Lavallee, O. F. Schanne and N. C. Herbert, eds. New York: Wiley, pp. 376–395.

PAPE, G. P., and R. KATZMAN, 1972. K^{42} distribution in brain during simultaneous ventriculocisternal and subarachnoid perfusion. *Brain Res.* 38:49–69.

PEDLEY, T. A., R. S. FISHER, K. J. FUTAMACHI, and D. A. PRINCE, 1976. Regulation of extracellular potassium concentration in epileptogenesis. *Fed. Proc.* 35:1254–1259.

PELHATE, M., and Y. PICHON, 1974. Selective inhibition of potassium current in the giant axon of the cockroach. *J. Physiol.* 242:90P–91P.

PETSCHE, M., O. PROMASKA, P. RAPPELSBERGER, and R. VOLLMER, 1975. The possible role of dendrites in EEG synchronization. *Adv. Neurol.* 12:53–70.

PRINCE, D. A., H. D. LUX, and E. NEHER, 1973. Measurement of extracellular potassium activity in cat cortex. *Brain Res.* 50:489–495.

PURVES, M. J. 1972. *The Physiology of the Cerebral Circulation*. Cambridge: Cambridge Univ. Press.

RAPOPORT. S. I., 1976. *Blood Brain Barrier in Physiology and Medicine*. New York: Raven Press.

ROSENTHAL, M., and J. C. LaMANNA, 1975. Effect of ouabain and phenobarbital on the kinetics of cortical metabolic transients associated with evoked potentials. *J. Neurochem.* 24:111–116.

ROSENTHAL, M., J. C. LaMANNA, F. F. JÖBSIS, J. E. LEVASSEUR, N. E. KONTOS, and J. L. PATTERSON, 1976. Effects of respiratory gases on cytochrome a in intact cerebral cortex: Is there a critical pO_2? *Brain Res.* 108:143–154.

SCHEIBEL, M. E., and A. B. SCHEIBEL, 1975. Dendrites as neuronal couplers: The dendrite bundle. In *Golgi Centennial Symposium Proceedings*, M. Santini, ed. New York: Raven Press, pp. 347–354.

SCHMIDT, R. F., 1971. Presynaptic inhibition in the vertebrate central nervous system. *Ergebn. Physiol.* 63:20–101.

SCHMITT, F. O., and F. E. SAMSON, JR., 1969. Brain cell microenvironment. *Neurosci. Res. Program Bull.* 7:277–417.

SIESJÖ, B. K., and S. C. SØRENSON, 1971. *Ion Homeostasis of the Brain*. Copenhagen: Munksgaard.

SINGER, S. J., and G. L. NICOLSON, 1972. The fluid mosaic model of the structure of cell membrane. *Science* 175:720–731.

SINGER, W., and H. D. LUX, 1973. Presynaptic depolarization and extracellular potassium in the cat lateral geniculate nucleus. *Brain Res.* 64:17–33.

SINGER, W., and H. D. LUX, 1975. Extracellular potassium gradients and visual receptive field in the cat striate cortex. *Brain Res.* 96:378–383.

SOMJEN, G. G., 1973. Electrogenesis of sustained potentials. *Prog. Neurobiol.* 1:201–257.

SOMJEN, G. G., 1975. Electrophysiology of neuroglia. *Annu. Rev. Physiol.* 37:163–190.

SOMJEN, G. G., M. ROSENTHAL, G. CORDINGLY, J. LaMANNA, and E. LOTHMAN, 1976. Potassium, neuroglia and oxidative metabolism in cerebral gray matter. *Fed. Proc.* 35:1266–1271.

SPITZER, N. C., 1976. The ionic basis of the resting potential and a slow depolarizing response in Rhohon-Beard neurones of *Xenopus* tadpole. *J. Physiol.* 255:105–135.

SUGAYA, E., T. TAKATO, and Y. NODA, 1975. Neuronal and glial activity during spreading depression in cerebral cortex of cat. *J. Neurophysiol.* 38:822–841.

Syková, E., B. Shirayev, N. Kříž, and L. Vyklický, 1976. Accumulation of extracellular potassium in the spinal cord of frog. *Brain Res.* 106:413–417.

Sypert, E. W., and A. A. Ward, Jr., 1974. Changes in extracellular potassium activity during neocortical propagated seizures. *Exp. Neurol.* 45:19–41.

Thomas, R. C., 1972. Electrogenic sodium pump in nerve and muscle cells. *Physiol. Rev.* 52:563–594.

Thompson, S. H., 1977. Three pharmacologically distinct potassium channels in molluscan neurones. *J. Physiol.* 265:465–488.

Van Harreveld, A., 1959. Component of brain extracts causing spreading depression of cerebral cortical activity and crustacean muscle. *J. Neurochem.* 3:300–315.

Van Harreveld, A., 1972. The extracellular space in the vertebrate central nervous system. In *The Structure and Function of Nervous Tissue*, G. H. Bourne, ed. New York: Academic Press, pp. 449–511.

Van Harreveld, A., 1977. Two mechanisms of spreading depression in chicken retina. *Soc. Neurosci.* 3:325 (abstract).

Van Harrveveld, A., and E. Fifkova, 1973. Mechanism involved in spreading depression. *J. Neurobiol.* 4:375–387.

Vern, B. O., W. H. Schuette, and L. E. Thibault, 1977. [K]$_0$ clearance in cortex: A new analytical model. *J. Neurophysiol.* 40:1015–1023.

Vyskočil, F., N. Kříž, and J. Bureš, 1972. Potassium-selective microelectrode used for measuring the extracellular brain potassium during spreading depression and anoxic depolarization in rats. *Brain Res.* 39:255–259.

Walker, Jr., J. L., 1971. Ion specific liquid ion exchanger microelectrodes. *Anal. Chem.* 43:89A–93A.

Watson, W. E., 1974. Physiology of neuroglia. *Physiol. Rev.* 54:245–271.

Watson, W. E., 1976. *Cell Biology of Brain*. London: Chapman and Hall.

Weight, F. F., and S. D. Erulkar, 1976. Modulation of synaptic transmitter release by repetitive postsynaptic action potentials. *Science* 193:1023–1025.

Yedlin, M., H. Kwan, J. T. Murphey, H. Nguten-Huu, and T. C. Wong, 1974. Electrical conductivity in cat cerebellar cortex. *Exp. Neurol.* 43:555–569.

Yeh, J. Z., G. S. Oxford, and T. Narahashi, 1976. Interaction of aminopyridines with potassium channels of squid axon membranes. *Biophys. J.* 16:77–81.

27 Neuronal Shape Parameters and Substructures as a Basis of Neuronal Form

D. E. HILLMAN

ABSTRACT   Computer technology has provided a means to record neuronal arborizations in three dimensions and to analyze the data for fundamental parameters of neuronal shape. Quantitative values for the elements comprising the cytoskeleton correlate with the parameters of shape and subcellular structure.

Seven parameters are needed to define the fundamental aspects of dendritic shape. The basis for this assumption is that the cross-sectional area of a process that emerges from the soma is divided successively by branching until a limiting terminal diameter is reached. Branch points serve to define segment length, branch power, daughter-branch ratio, and segment orientation. Tapering may occur between branch points.

Underlying neuronal shape are prominent structural components of arborizations (tubules and filaments) comprising a cytoskeleton that may be involved in maintaining the diameter of dendrites. This is evident in some neuronal types where microtubule density is constant throughout the arbor and the branch power equals two (cross-sectional area is preserved along the extent of the arbor). In motoneurons the branch power equals 3/2. Here both filaments and tubules shape the dendritic processes. Filaments produce a geometrical tapering of the tree (beginning at the soma, the cross-sectional area is decreased at and between branch points).

The determinants of form are discussed in relation to the variability of the fundamental parameters. It is shown that stem diameter, segment length, daughter-branch ratio, and orientation are considerably variable and thus are most likely determined through interactive influences during development. Total stem diameters arising from soma, branch power, segment taper, and terminal diameters are much more tightly constrained and may be largely determined by the intrinsic influences acting through the subcellular components of the cell.

Introduction

OUR PRESENT concepts regarding neuronal form have evolved over the last 150 years and have been largely dependent on the development of microscopic techniques. In particular, new staining methods and refinements in light optics ushered in a morphological revolution in the latter part of the nineteenth century. At this time, using cerebellar tissue, neuronal cell bodies were first seen with the light microscope (Purkinje, 1837). Later, groups of cell bodies were found in various regions (Deiters, 1865). Although the subsequent visualization of a network of processes lacing throughout the brain (Schulze, 1871) was instrumental to the development of a concept of the form of neurons, the key development was the discovery of the Golgi technique, which first allowed visualization of individual neuronal somata together with their processes (Golgi, 1874).

An early concept, held by the reticularists, viewed the nervous system as composed of a syncytium of cells and fibers. This concept was largely due to the development of the reduced silver reaction, which revealed within the cell processes fibrillar material that appeared to form a continuous meshwork connecting the various neuronal elements (Apáthy, 1897; Bielschowsky, 1902).

It was not until the Golgi technique had been applied to numerous areas of the nervous system that a compelling case was made for the existence of neurons as independent cellular elements (Ramón y Cajal, 1909, 1911). This view was initially stated by Waldeyer (1891) and Kölliker (1891) as the neuron doctrine. The strongest support for this concept came from the work of Ramón y Cajal (1911), who demonstrated not only that the nervous system was composed of several cell types, but that particular types of neurons were characteristic of given regions of the nervous system. This work also revealed that the meshwork previously described actually consisted of an overlapping of many orderly, treelike processes emerging from the cell bodies.

D. E. HILLMAN   Department of Physiology and Biophysics, New York University Medical Center, New York, NY 10016

The final demonstration that the nervous system was composed of individual neurons and was not a continuous network came with the advent of the electron microscope. The high resolution of this instrument revealed that each neuron was a separate cellular entity and that "contact sites" were actually separated by extracellular space or synaptic clefts without continuity of the neurofibrillar material (Palay, 1956). Throughout this history, a vast amount of information has been collected regarding the different neuronal processes and the circuits they generate.

Neurons and neuronal circuits were initially understood and displayed in drawings by such people as Purkinje (1837), Golgi (1874), Kölliker (1891), Ramón y Cajal (1909, 1911), and Lorente de Nó (1934). Although drawings remain a principal way to depict neurons, this method has obvious drawbacks (Figure 1). For example, a true three-dimensional image cannot be obtained, and the size of the cells can only be approximated. Methods have therefore been developed to describe nerve cells quantitatively (Bok, 1936a; Sholl, 1953) and to display these constructs in three dimensions (Mannen, 1966).

An important advance along these lines was made when computer technology was applied to the analysis of neuronal morphology (Glaser and Van der

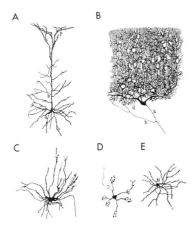

FIGURE 1 Illustrations of neuronal dendritic arborizations by Ramón y Cajal. (A) Pyramidal cells are multipolar with a single apical dendrite (b), which gives rise to branching patterns that differ from basal arbors (a). (B) The human Purkinje cell has two major trunks (other mammalian forms usually have only one). An elaborate arborization that spreads in a single plane through the molecular layer of the cerebellum has more numerous terminals and branch points than pyramidal cells. (C) Motoneuron dendrites have large stems and few branch points. (D) The small cerebellar granule cell usually has only 3–6 dendrites, which end in clawlike formations. (E) The stellate cell has long terminal dendritic segments. (From Ramón y Cajal, 1909; Figures 8, 9, and 129; Ramón y Cajal, 1911: Figures 23 and 24.)

Loos, 1965). Many nerve cells could be reconstructed in the computer and rotated and displayed from any viewpoint; dissimilarities as well as consistencies in the shape of neurons could then be fully appreciated. Even here, however, the need to view neuronal circuits in three dimensions—as in holograms—became apparent. Thus, as the tools we have for "seeing" neurons improve, what we see changes because our concept of neuronal form changes.

Although the term "form" is often used by morphologists, what is usually meant is "shape." However, in this paper "shape" is used in a geometric sense and refers to the three-dimensional outline of each cell including its processes. Shape is independent of content and size. "Form" is used in an architectural sense and refers to the combination of shape with structure (form is also independent of size). I introduce these definitions here because, with the refinement of techniques, the quantification of neuronal shapes and their underlying cytoskeletal elements is now possible; thus, for the first time, we can truly speak of neuronal *form*. Developmental studies (Rakic, 1974; Berry and Bradley, 1976b) show, however, that the shape of nerve cells is influenced not only by intracellular structural elements but also by the environs of the neurons during development; that is, a study of neuronal form must consider ontogenetic influences.

Thus, with a quantitative description of neurons in hand, we can proceed to explore both the ultrastructural and the developmental basis for cell shape. Following this thought, this paper has been organized in three parts. First, from the mass of quantitative information available on cell shape, the fundamental parameters of form are extracted (i.e., those measurements essential to providing a complete description of a neuron). Next, the number and distribution of the subcellular structures underlying these parameters are determined. Finally, this information is used to establish which factors in ontogeny determine the values of the various parameters, utilizing a quantitative determination of variance within the parameters. The amount of *variability* is used as a key, together with the vast amount of information concerning the developmental process, to establish (although tentatively) which of these parameters may be determined by intrinsic and which by interactive (extrinsic) factors.

Quantitation of neuronal morphology

Although the polymorphic character of neuronal arborizations has long been known, the quantitative analysis of these elements has been attempted only recently. Among the first to develop techniques for the quantitation of neurons were Bok (1936a) and Sholl (1953). These early methods were modified and used extensively in studies concerning the effects of various perturbations on neuronal shape (Eayrs, 1955; Clendinnen and Eayrs, 1961; Schadé and Groenigen, 1961; Coleman and Riesen, 1968; Schadé and Caveness, 1968) and have since been altered to eliminate certain artifactual results (Colon and Smit, 1970, 1971; Berry, Anderson, Hollingworth, and Flinn, 1972). A recent advance has been the use of computer methods to record and analyze neurons; following the pioneering work of Glaser and Van der Loos (1965), these methods have been elaborated and a number of approaches developed (see Brown, 1976; Lindsay 1977a). Network analysis, an entirely different and very fruitful approach, has been used by Berry et al. (1975) to define branch patterns and their progressive change (e.g., during development).

The application of these techniques has generated a large literature in which neuronal shape has been measured in multiple ways. In an attempt to unify some of these results, a set of parameters has been established. The criteria are that each parameter must (1) be easily measurable, (2) be consistent with and meaningful to the development of electrophysiological models, (3) be useful for comparing different types of arborizations, and (4) be nonredundant. Finally, the full set of parameters must be sufficient to describe the shape of neurons. These parameters would then serve as a fundamental basis for analyzing and evaluating numerous more complex aspects of neuronal morphology.

In the following section, each of the parameters will be defined and the techniques utilized to obtain them described. Then the distribution of these parameters in several cell types will be presented.

Parameters of Neurite Shape   From an analysis of the length, diameter, and spatial orientation of the dendritic trees (see Figures 1 and 2), the following fundamental parameters have been abstracted:
  1. stem diameter (D),
  2. terminal-segment diameter (T),
  3. segment taper (ΔA),
  4. segment length (L),
  5. branch power (n),
  6. ratio between cross-sectional areas of daughter branches (R),
  7. spatial orientation of segments (including branch angle).

FUNDAMENTAL PARAMETERS OF NEURITE SHAPE

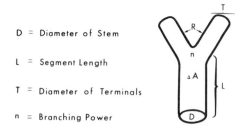

D = Diameter of Stem

L = Segment Length

T = Diameter of Terminals

n = Branching Power

R = Ratio of Daughter Branch Diameters

ΔA = Segment Taper

Spatial Orientation of Stem and Branch Segments

Distribution for Variation of the Fundamental Parameters

Figure 2 Neuronal shapes can be defined by seven variable parameters that describe the form of neuronal arborizations. Variations in the distribution of these fundamental parameters over the tree produce differences in tree types as well as the individual characteristics of neurites.

These parameters describe dendritic trees in the following way. The base of the tree, the *stem segment* (with diameter D), is divided at the first branch point. Here the stem length is determined and two daughter branches formed. (Trifurcation sites occur, but so infrequently that they will not be considered here; see Berry and Bradley, 1976a.) At each successive branch site, *segment lengths* (L) are determined, and the diameter is reduced until the *terminal diameter* (T) is reached. The division of the cross-sectional area of a parent segment into daughter branches is described by two parameters, the *branch power* (n) and the *daughter-branch ratio* (R). Branch power relates the cross-sectional area of the parent segment to the total cross-sectional area of the daughter segments. The daughter-branch ratio is the ratio of the cross-sectional area of the two daughter branches. Between branch points, the diameter may decrease as a *segment taper* (ΔA). Also at branch points the three-dimensional *orientation* of the segments is defined by the direction of the segments with respect to the soma.

The size of the dendritic tree is governed by the stem and terminal diameters, branch power, segment taper, and segment lengths; shape is defined by all seven parameters. Variations in these parameters contribute to the variety and complexity of neuronal arborizations.

Three-Dimensional Reconstruction and Parameter Extraction   Three major approaches are currently in use for tracking neurites in dye-injected or Golgi-impregnated neurons. The first, designed by Glaser and Van der Loos (1965) and adopted by Wann et al. (1973), employs a fixed cursor located in the center of the microscopic field while the X, Y, and Z coordinates are obtained by operator-controlled stage movements and focusing. The second approach employs a movable cursor in conjunction with stage displacements. This method facilitates the manual tracking operations (Llinás and Hillman, 1975; Hillman, Llinás, and Chujo, 1977; Paldino and Harth, 1977a; Lindsay, 1977b) and was used to develop a semiautomatic method (Garvey et al., 1973; Coleman, West, and Wyss, 1973; Coleman et al., 1977). The last approach records the structures by interactive or automatic extraction of the perimeters from profiles of neurons and their processes in serially sectioned preparations (Levinthal and Ware, 1972; Reddy et al., 1973; Selverston, 1973; Levinthal, Macagno, and Tountas, 1974; Glasser et al., 1977; Hillman, Llinás, and Chujo, 1977). This modern version of the wax sheet reconstruction method (Born, 1883) not only allows viewing from every perspective (Hillman, Llinás, and Chujo, 1977), but also provides the necessary data base for an analysis of global parameters such as surface area, volume, and process lengths (Glasser et al., 1977; Hillman, Llinás, and Chujo, 1977).

In our approach, the Cartesian coordinates and diameters of neuronal somata and their processes were recorded with the aid of a graphics computer interfaced to a light microscope (Llinás and Hillman, 1975; Hillman, Llinás, and Chujo, 1977). The system has been specifically configured to provide maximum resolution, 0.2–0.4 μm, in X and Y. Data points are defined for the origin of the dendrites (at the soma), changes in the course of the process, branching sites, terminals, and cut ends (for alignment to subsequent sections).

The data consist of the soma diameter and the length, diameter, and spatial orientation of each dendritic segment. Analysis programs extract and compare values from the data file for parameters of different cells and cell types and compute values for the global parameters of arborizations (e.g., total length, volume, and surface area). Finally, this information is displayed as bar graphs or point plots. The examples included in this paper were obtained from an analysis of rat and cat cerebral pyramidal cells, cerebellar Purkinje, stellate, and granular cells, and motoneurons (see Figure 1). Analysis at the light-microscopic level was based on Golgi material, while subcellular structures were studied from electron micrographs. In ultrastructural studies, the entire regions of the dendritic fields of Purkinje cells, motoneurons, and pyramidal cells were analyzed for microtubules and neurofilaments. These records were quantitated on an image-analysis computer and recorded with reference to the diameter of the respective dendritic profile.

THE FUNDAMENTAL SHAPE PARAMETERS

Stem diameter (D) The diameters of stem dendrites range from over 10 μm to less than 1 μm. This range is largely due to the variable diameters of individual primary dendrites in multipolar neurons (Bok 1936a,b; Haggar and Barr, 1950; Chu, 1954; Bok, 1959; Balthasar, 1962). The sum of these diameters shows little variability (Table I). Furthermore, for a number of multipolar cell types, this summed cross-sectional area was found to bear a consistent relationship to soma size (Figure 3). This is in agreement with Rall (1959), who found that motoneuron stem diameters (represented by the sum of their diameters to the 3/2 power "combined trunk parameter") correlated well with soma surface area. The significance of this finding lies in the relationship between the summed stem cross-sectional area and the volume of the dendritic tree (see below). The diameters of cells with only one stem dendrite are less variable (e.g., see Purkinje cells, Table I); although this parameter has a similar correlation with soma size, the dendritic cross-sectional area is somewhat smaller.

Terminal diameter (T) As illustrated in Figure 4, the minimum diameter of terminal segments is sharply delineated (there are very few segments smaller than 0.5 μm). Furthermore, although terminal diameter is the least variable parameter (Table I), two groups are found, the first with a mean diameter of 1.1 μm, the second with a mean of 0.76 μm.

Segment taper (ΔA) In a number of cell types, the

FIGURE 3 The sum of cross-sectional areas of all stem dendrites that arise from the soma shows a correlation to the soma diameter. Granule cells, pyramidal cells, and motoneurons form a series of somas with increasing diameter, and when plotted as the square with the cross-sectional area for the sum of emerging dendrites, a strict correlation is found. The slope of this relationship (a) is 3/2, indicating that this dendritic cross-sectional area is proportional to a spherical volume related to the soma. A second parallel slope (b) is formed by Purkinje cells. Thus multipolar neurons have more cross-sectional area emerging from a soma of particular size than do unipolar cells of comparable size. These data are consistent with the relationship of the "combined trunk parameter" to soma surface area (Rall, 1959). Soma and stem diameters obtained by computerized interactive recording of Golgi preparations. (Unpublished results.)

TABLE I

Parameters of form

| Cell type | Cross-sectional area (μm²) | | Diameter of terminal segments* (μm) | Length (μm) | | Branch power | Taper | Daughter-branch ratio |
	Individual stem dendrites	All stem dendrites		Terminal segments	All segments			
Pyramidal	12.8 ± 13 (100)[a]	76.8 ± 21 (26)	1.17 ± 0.34 (29)	120 ± 59 (49)	70.8 ± 65 (91)			
Apical dendrites						1.99 ± 0.79 (40)	marked[b]	2–6
Basal dendrites			1.11 ± 0.33 (29)			2.28 ± 0.89 (39)	not evident	<2
Purkinje	109.3 ± 14 (13)	109 ± 14 (13)	1.04 ± 0.30 (29)	15.2 ± 10 (79)	11.6 ± 9.2 (79)	2.36 ± 1.2 (51)	none (except stem)	low and high
Granule	1.51 ± 0.79 (52)	5.48 ± 0.94 (17)	0.66 ± 0.25 (38) 0.76 ± 0.29 (32)	4.58 ± 3.7 (81)	10.7 ± 8.4 (78)	2.58 ± 1.8 (71)	not evident	low
Stellate	2.75 ± 1.35 (49)	11.0 ± 3.4 (31)	0.73 ± 0.30 (41)	23.9 ± 29 (100)[a]	31.7 ± 23 (72)	2.24 ± 1.2 (53)	not evident	low
Moto-neuron	88.4 ± 56 (64)	886 ± 71 (11)	—	—	—	1.69 ± 0.48 (28)	marked[c]	low

Mean values ± S.D. Numbers in parentheses are coefficients of variation, defined as the standard deviation as a percentage of the arithmetic mean.

* As measured near the final branch point.

[a] Test assumes a normal distribution and is actually inappropriate for these skewed distributions.

[b] Unpublished observations.

[c] See Barrett and Crill (1974a) and Lux, Schubert, and Kreutzberg (1970).

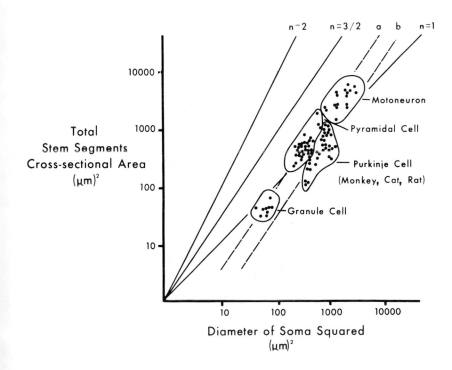

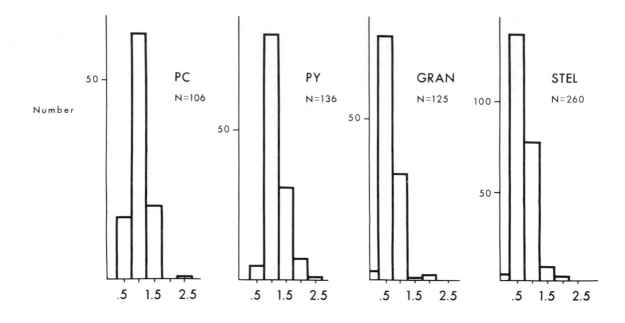

Number

PC
N=106

PY
N=136

GRAN
N=125

STEL
N=260

Terminal Diameter (μm)

FIGURE 4   Diameters of terminal segments are consistently constrained by minimal and maximal limits. Purkinje (PC) and pyramidal (PY) cells tend to have somewhat larger terminal diameters than do granule (GRAN) and stellate (STEL) cells. These differences may be related to the fact that Purkinje and pyramidal cells have numerous spines along their course while granule and stellate cells for the most part lack spinelike structures. The diameter was recorded on Golgi-impregnated neurons near the final bifurcation. (Hillman, Llinás, and Iberall, unpublished results.)

diameter of the dendritic process decreases between branch points. Taper varies between cell types; a marked taper has been found in some cells while others show none (see Table I; Lux, Schubert, and Kreutzberg, 1970; Barrett and Crill, 1974a).

Segment length (L)   Marked variations are found in the length of dendritic segments (Table I; Figure 5; see also Smit, Uylings, and Vledmaat-Wansink, 1972; Berry and Bradley, 1976b; Lindsay, 1977c). The shortest segments result from trichotomous branching in which the daughter branches arise very close together (Berry and Bradley, 1976a). In contrast, terminal segments can reach from 30 μm to over 200 μm (Bok, 1936a; Peters and Bademan, 1963). Intermediate and stem segments have a smaller group range. Pyramidal cells are unusual in that their terminal-segment length is drastically different from that of other segments.

Since the distribution of segment lengths over the tree varies widely, this factor no doubt contributes to the range of shapes as well as sizes of dendritic trees.

Branch power (n)   Tree shape is influenced by changes in the cross-sectional area at branch points. One way to assess if such a change has occurred is to determine the branch power n, defined as the exponent that satisfies

$$D^n = \sum_j d_j^n , \qquad (1)$$

where D is the diameter of the parent dendrite and d_j is the diameter of the jth daughter dendrite (Figure 6). This equation describes a geometric relationship between tree branches and has been found to be of great importance in describing the cable properties of neurons when both *geometric* and *electric* factors must be brought together (Rall, 1959).

A first step in developing the equation for branch power is to determine the input conductance of an individual dendritic segment. When considering elec-

FIGURE 6   Two branch power rules: $n = 3/2$ and $n = 2$. The 3/2 power law, postulated by Rall (1959), was believed to be important for conservation of electrical charge for electronic spread from distal parts of the dendritic tree. In contrast, a conservation of cross-sectional area results from a square law when the volume remains constant throughout the dendritic tree. The equivalent volume and equivalent electrical cylinders are illustrated for each rule. Surface area (not shown) would be considerably increased.

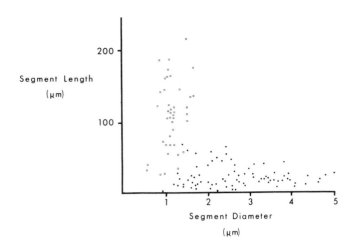

FIGURE 5 Segment lengths are variable within dendritic trees; however, there are characteristic limitations on the maximum lengths. Here in an example of pyramidal-cell dendrites, stem segments and intermediate segments extend up to 50–60 μm (dots) while terminal segments (squares) exceed 200 μm. Note the constrained diameter range of the terminal segments. The diameters were recorded near the final branch point, and the terminal segments were defined by the Strahler ordering method.

trotonic properties of neurons, it is common practice to idealize axons and, therefore, dendritic segments as uniform cylinders.

The input conductance G of a cylinder is proportional to the 3/2 power of the diameter d:

$$G \propto (R_\mathrm{m}R_\mathrm{i})^{-1/2}d^{3/2}, \tag{2}$$

where R_m is the resistance across a unit area of membrane and R_i is the specific resistance of the internal medium.

In order to facilitate the treatment of electrotonus in dendrites, the tree was collapsed into a uniform cylinder. In order to perform this simplification, however, passive electrical properties of cables dictate that the input conductances on each side of a branch point must be the same, so that charge is not lost. Thus

$$G_\mathrm{parent} = \Sigma\, G_\mathrm{daughters}. \tag{3}$$

Combining Equations 2 and 3,

$$(R_\mathrm{m}R_\mathrm{i})^{-1/2}D^{3/2} = (R_\mathrm{m}R_\mathrm{i})^{-1/2}\sum_j d_j^{3/2}, \tag{4}$$

so that

$$D^{3/2} = \sum_j d_j^{3/2}. \tag{5}$$

This has come to be known as the 3/2 power rule.

On the basis of published photographs of Golgi-impregnated motoneurons, Rall (1959) found that the 3/2 power rule, derived from theoretical consideration, did indeed hold for this cell type. More recently, Lux, Schubert, and Kreutzberg (1970), Barrett and Crill (1974a,b), and our own studies (Figure 7) have verified these first measurements.

Similar measurements for branching in pyramidal and Purkinje cells do not support the 3/2 power rule

Branch Power Rules

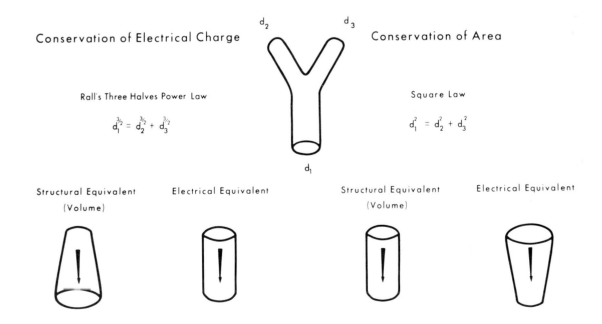

Conservation of Electrical Charge

Rall's Three Halves Power Law

$$d_1^{3/2} = d_2^{3/2} + d_3^{3/2}$$

Conservation of Area

Square Law

$$d_1^2 = d_2^2 + d_3^2$$

Structural Equivalent (Volume)   Electrical Equivalent

Structural Equivalent (Volume)   Electrical Equivalent

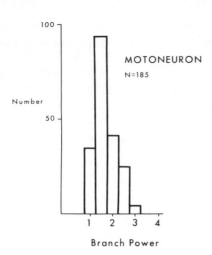

FIGURE 7 Histogram for branch power in motoneurons. The values of branch power for individual motoneuron branches cluster near 3/2. Branch power was obtained by solving the branch power equation by successive approximation (Newton-Raphson algorithm). The spread for the smaller population of the branch powers is primarily due to the sensitivity of the method for very large daughter-branch ratios. Data recorded from Golgi preparations of rat spinal cord.

(Table I; Figure 8), but rather approximate a square rule. In these cells charge is not conserved across branch points. The important point to be considered here, however, is that in cells following the 3/2 power rule, cross-sectional area is reduced at branch points, but in those following the square rule, cross-sectional area is conserved. The functional significance of these power rules is beyond the scope of this paper. (For a detailed discussion see Jack, this volume.)

Daughter-branch ratio (R) The ratio of the diameters of daughter-branch processes at each bifurcation defines the daughter-branch ratio R (the usual range is 1–10). Equal daughter branch diameters ($R = 1$) are seldom observed; values of 1.5–4 are more often found. Clearly this parameter (together with branch power) alters tree shape at branch points. For example, at a bifurcation having a daughter ratio of 4, the larger-diameter daughter branch will require many further bifurcations to reach the terminal diameter than will the smaller daughter branch. If this disparity is common, the entire pattern of branch distribution is affected. From this relationship alone it is evident that daughter-branch ratio can have a deep influence on tree shape. Specifically, pyramidal-cell apical dendrites have very high (2–6) daughter-branch ratios and therefore have numerous unequal bifurcations. This produces a relatively narrow tree growing from a single thick trunk. In contrast, the basal dendrites have a daughter ratio less than two,

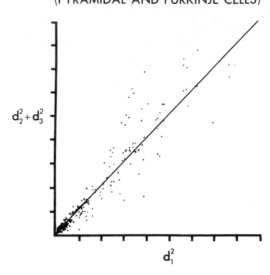

BRANCH POWER
(PYRAMIDAL AND PURKINJE CELLS)

FIGURE 8 In pyramidal and Purkinje cells, branch power was determined by a graphic method for solving the power equation. Plots were made for a 3/2 power and for a power of 2. It was found that, on average, a least-squares fit, for a power of 2, had a slope of one (this illustration). Thus $d_1^2 = d_2^2 + d_3^2$, where d_1 is the diameter of a parent and d_2 and d_3 are the diameters of its daughter branches. (Rat pyramidal and Purkinje cells.)

and the branching number at each level is almost constant from the stem to the terminal segments (Figure 9B). Thus a "bushy" tree is produced (compare Figures 1A, B and 9).

Although mammalian Purkinje cells also have close to equal bifurcations throughout the tree, numerous smaller daughter branches are also found on large dendrites. This interspersion of small-diameter branches ($R > 2$) results in a very dense arbor.

Spatial orientation A complete description of dendritic trees requires defining the tridimensional orientation of each segment. Of the many schemes developed toward this end, two are particularly useful: the application of principal-component analysis (Brown, 1977) and the use of polar coordinates (Paldino and Harth, 1977b). Other methods in use only approximate or describe limited aspects of the three-dimensional relationship of processes (see, for example, Uylings and Smit, 1975; Lindsay, 1977d). We have instituted a simplified spherical coordinate system very similar to that used by Paldino and Harth (1977b). This system is capable of defining spatial relationships with sufficient accuracy to catalog the position of individual segments and is at the same time flexible enough to be used to define the position

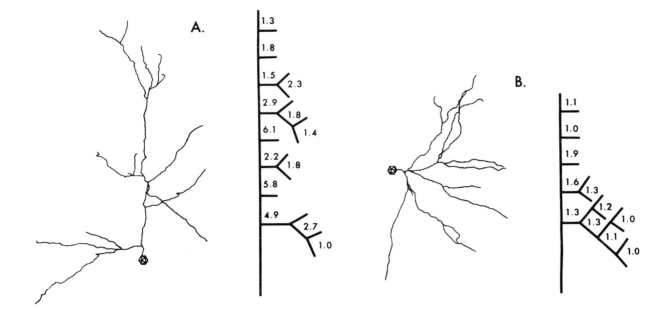

Apical Dendrite   Basal Dendrite

FIGURE 9 Daughter-branch ratios vary consistently over various tree types. Topological patterns are displayed according to Berry et al. (1975) for each reconstructed dendrite. The numbers at the bifurcations are daughter-branch ratios. In apical dendrites of pyramidal cells (A) the bifurcations of the main stem have very high daughter-branch ratios (2–6). Basal dendrites (B), on the other hand, have daughter-branch ratios less than two. We believe that this factor is most important in determining topological type in neuronal form.

"Topological type" refers to branching patterns irrespective of length, diameter, and orientation. According to the dendritic model this relationship in neurites can be modified by four fundamental parameters: branch power, segment taper, terminal diameter, and daughter-branch ratio. The most marked influence is that of the daughter-branch ratio; the other three parameters are relatively consistent within cell types and thus do not significantly alter the number of branch levels necessary to reach the terminal diameter.

of an entire neuron including its dendrites, soma, and axon. Thus the location and extent of a great number of neurons can be compiled for comparative analysis. (This method is discussed below.)

GLOBAL PARAMETERS The combination of certain of these fundamental parameters (e.g., segment length and diameter) forms a new set, that of global parameters. These parameters are important because they go beyond specific aspects of shape to provide information about the size and orientation of trees. It is at the level of global parameters that cell form is most clearly related to function.

Volume Volume is a measure of the size of the dendritic tree and has a close correlation to soma size (Mannen, 1966). In fact, all measurable global parameters (surface area, summed segment length, maximum continuous length) are correlated with soma size (Sholl, 1955; Mannen, 1966; Gelfan, Kara, and Ruchkin, 1970). Likewise, we have found that the volume of each individual dendritic tree is cor-

related with the diameter of its stem (Figure 10B). Thus the distribution of each of these parameters among individual dendrites can be discerned by measuring the diameters of the stem dendrites. The correlation of global parameters with soma size is to be expected as all these parameters ultimately reflect the amount of cytoplasm and membrane in the dendrites. These are composed of molecular entities which must be maintained by the machinery of the cell factories located, for the most part, in the cell soma (Llinás and Iberall, 1977).

Surface area The dendritic surface area is the largest interactive part of the cell, comprising more than 80% of the surface in some neurons (Mannen, 1966). Furthermore, dendrites have recently been recognized as having presynaptic (Shepherd, this volume) as well as postsynaptic and nonsynaptic (Kreutzberg, this volume) interactions. The surface area then reflects the capacity of a cell to receive (Rall, 1970) and, in many cells, to contribute inputs.

Length The length of dendritic processes has been

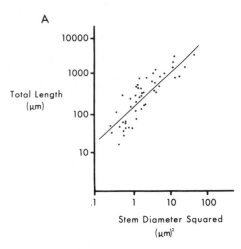

FIGURE 10 Correlation for stem diameter with total length and volume of individual dendritic trees. Each point rep-resents a single tree from a granule, stellate, or pyramidal cell. (Unpublished results.)

measured in a number of ways (Sholl, 1953; Fox and Barnard, 1957; Schadé and Van Groenigen, 1961; Glaser and Van der Loos, 1965; Mannen, 1966; Gelfan, Kara, and Ruchkin, 1970; Wann et al., 1973; Hillman, Chujo, and Llinás, 1974; Lindsay and Scheibel, 1974). One of the most useful measurements is the maximum continuous dendritic length (Gelfan, Kara, and Ruchkin, 1970) since, when this value is combined with the process direction (with reference to the soma), the vector quantity *spread* is formed. Information is then available concerning how far and in which direction a cell sends its dendrites. Used in this way, length is the only global parameter to combine size with another aspect of neuronal morphology. Furthermore, when length and diameter are combined with orientation (see below), a complete description of the shape and size of a cell emerges.

Orientation Orientation, as a fundamental parameter (see above), describes the location of dendritic segments and processes with respect to each other and to the soma. As a global parameter, orientation first places the neuron with reference to major brain landmarks (e.g., hippocampus, corpus callosum) and then in the context of neighboring structures (e.g., other neurons, glia, blood vessels). From a functional viewpoint, the most important of these structures are the neighboring neurons, for these comprise the circuit in which the cell functions.

There is an extensive literature demonstrating the specificity of cell orientation in both laminar and nuclear structures (e.g., Ramón y Cajal, 1909, 1911; Lorente de Nó, 1934; Palay and Chan-Palay, 1974). Other studies have been most valuable in determining precise shifts in dendritic projections following

perturbations (Clendinnen and Eayrs, 1961; Schadé and Van Groenigen, 1961; Peters and Bademan, 1963; Colonnier, 1964; Mungai, 1967; Wong, 1967; Schadé and Caveness, 1968; Smit, Uylings, and Vledmaat-Wansink, 1972; Smit and Uylings, 1975; Coleman et al., 1977; Lindsay, 1977d; Paldino and Harth, 1977b). Despite the important contributions of this recent work, a universal method capable of defining spatial relationships with sufficient accuracy to catalog and compare neurons and their locations has not been developed. We have instituted a simplified spherical coordinate system, similar to that recently used by Paldino and Harth (1977b), which may meet this need (cf. Peterson, 1955).

According to this scheme, the primary reference point is the soma center, around which an imaginary sphere is drawn. The intersection of a dendritic process with the surface of the sphere is defined by latitudinal (range 0 to 180 degrees) and longitudinal (range 0 to 360 degrees) coordinates. The application of this system to a cortical pyramidal cell is illustrated in Figure 11. In this example latitudinal coordinates greater than 90° indicate that the dendrite projects away from the pial-glial surface (Figure 11B). Longitudinal coordinates less than 180° indicate that the processes project caudally.

Essentially this method utilizes two common references to yield two coordinate points for each site of interest. The orientation of dendritic stem segments and segments at branch points can be defined, thus facilitating descriptive comparisons and cataloging of spatial orientation. (The cell body itself is located on a three-dimensional Cartesian coordinate system which is fixed for a given brain or region.)

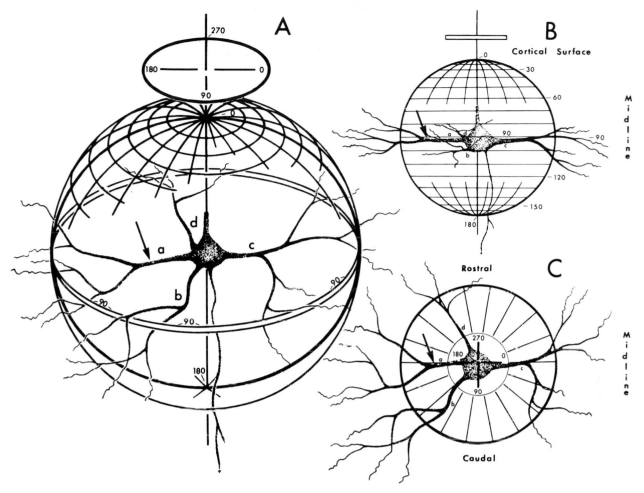

FIGURE 11 A spherical-coordinate method for defining orientation and comparing dendritic branching. Two reference axes are established in order to limit the number of coordinates to two for each segment. One reference is an axis that might, for example, extend from a surface of a laminar structure perpendicularly into the depth of the nervous tissue. This axis passes through the center of the soma, tree base, or branch point and represents the center of the sphere (A). The orientation of the dendritic segments relative to this axis is defined by two coordinates: First, a latitudinal (La) coordinate extends from 0 to 180°, representing a north-south relationship (B), where north is the surface of a laminar structure in the brain. A dendrite that extends above the equatorial zone, 90°, projects toward the surface and has an (La) angle within the 0–90° range. Those below the equatorial zone have angles between 90° and 180°. Second, the orientation of these dendrites around this north-south axis are made by longitudinal (Lo) coordinates that range from 0° to 360° (C). The zero reference for the longitudinal coordinates is related to another common landmark such as an afferent, efferent, or identifiable dendrite that is consistently limited to the same side of this north-south axis. It is important that this reference reflect the convolution and the curvature of the cortex so that accurate comparisons can be made between the cells.

Topological types Each dendritic tree can be categorized according to its topological type (Berry et al., 1975). The assignment of a tree to a particular category depends on the patterning of its segments and is independent of their length, diameter, or orientation (Hoopen and Reuver, 1970). The four fundamental parameters determining the number of branch points (stem diameter, terminal diameter, branch power, daughter-branch ratio) influence these patterns. The most variable of these (next to stem diameter), daughter-branch ratio, makes the most significant contribution and plays a major role in determining the topological type of a dendritic tree.

This approach to categorizing neuronal trees has been used to compare the probability for the occurrence of particular branching patterns in normal adults (Berry et al., 1975) with the probability of their occurrence in animals at various stages of development (Berry and Bradley, 1976b) or following alterations to the adult nervous system (McConnell and Berry, 1978).

Arborizational taper Taper in neuronal branches is extremely important because of its significance in electrotonus (Rall, 1959, 1962). A means of evaluating this factor is to determine the power relationships for each arborization. This parameter expresses both branch power and segment taper as a power for the entire dendritic tree and is given by the relationship

$$D_s^n = d_{t_1}^n + d_{t_2}^n + \cdots + d_{t_N}^n = \sum_j d_{t_j}^n,$$

where D_s is the diameter of the stem and d_{t_j} is the diameter of the jth tree terminal. The approach is a modification of Rall's (1959, 1962) branch-power equation and is a means of approximating changes in cross-sectional area for the entire tree. The solution of the power equation is generated by software for a method of successive approximation. Furthermore, the difference in cross-sectional area between the stem and the sum of the terminals can be combined with length to establish tree taper. Hillman and Gelbfish (unpublished observations) have determined the arborizational taper of basal dendrites of pyramidal cells and produced encouraging results. Further work will determine its usefulness.

Structural components of neuronal form

Having established basic parameters of neuronal shape, we can ask what intra- or extracellular elements provide the structural basis for neuronal form. The most general hypothesis is that of Porter and Tilney (1965), who suggested that the subcellular elements form a structural core underlying the shape of cells. Basically it is assumed that cell shapes deviating from a sphere require an intracellular scaffold or framework. Thus elongation of cells would require the support of a cytoskeleton composed of specific subcellular organelles (Tilney and Porter, 1967; Yamada, Spooner, and Wessells, 1970). Following the ultrastructural identification of microtubules and neurofilaments by Schmitt and Geren (1950), investigators have suggested that these elements may be the principal components of this cytoskeleton.

SUBCELLULAR STRUCTURES   Quantitative analysis of neuronal ultrastructure has been limited, for the most part, to the soma and axon. Studies determining soma size and the nucleus-to-cytoplasm ratio are the most numerous (Bok, 1936b, 1959; Sholl, 1955; Gelfan, Kara, and Ruchkin, 1970). Little information has

been forthcoming regarding subcellular structures that may be correlated to nuclear or somatic size.

In axons, microtubules and neurofilaments have been the primary focus for analysis (see Schmitt, 1968; Wuerker and Kirkpatrick, 1972). Most quantitative studies of these structures have been limited to correlating tubule and filament number to axon diameter (Friede and Samorajski, 1970; Zenker, Mayr, and Gruber, 1973). However, there have been two attempts to determine whether axonal tubules branch or are lost, after they leave the soma, by comparing the number of tubules in the axon after it emerges from the central nervous system with the number in the telodendron (Weiss and Mayr, 1971; Zenker and Hohberg, 1973). These studies are not in agreement, and further investigation is needed.

Qualitative descriptions of filaments and tubules in dendrites of pyramidal and Purkinje cells (Wuerker and Kirkpatrick, 1972), cerebral cortical cells (Peters, 1968, 1971), motoneurons (Wuerker and Palay, 1969), and Clark's column cells (Smith, 1973) have found that when dendrites are viewed in cross section, tubules are evenly dispersed but filaments are usually found in groups (Figure 12). Also, the densities of these elements vary among cell types.

In studies counting both filaments and tubules, we have verified these findings for three cell types (Figure 13A, C; Table II). Specifically, pyramidal- and Purkinje-cell dendrites maintain a constant microtubular density (Figure 13A), whereas a second pattern is found in motoneurons. Here the tubule density decreases sharply toward the base of the tree while the smallest branches have concentrations close to those found in pyramidal-cell dendrites of similar diameter (Figure 13C).

The distribution of neurofilaments also depends on cell type. Motoneurons and pyramidal cells have a relatively constant filament density. In fact, in most motoneuron processes, filament density surpasses tubule density (see Figure 13A, B). Purkinje cells, for the most part, lack neurofilaments.

TABLE II
Density of cytoskeletal structures

Cell type	Microtubules (μm^2)	Neurofilaments (μm^2)	T/F ratio
Pyramidal	70.8	4.99	14:1
Purkinje	28.4	1	–
Motoneuron		38.6	
base	31.9		1:1
terminals	100		2.5:1

T, microtubules; F, neurofilaments.

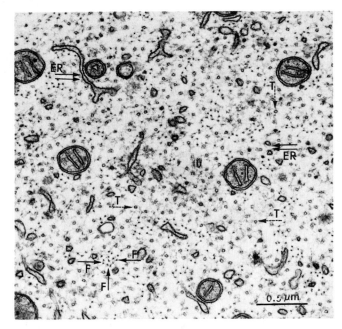

FIGURE 12 Distribution of tubules and filaments in a motoneuron dendrite. Here an electron micrograph from the ventral horn of the spinal cord demonstrates the general distribution of microtubules and neurofilaments in cross section. Preparation stained with uranyl acetate and lead citrate. (T, tubules; F, filaments; ER, smooth endoplasmic reticulum.)

CORRELATIONS BETWEEN SHAPE PARAMETERS AND SUBCELLULAR COMPONENTS One of the major questions generated by these findings is whether microtubules and neurofilaments, or indeed other cellular organelles, represent components of a structural framework that helps define the shape of neuronal somata and processes. This is a problem we are just beginning to explore, and the following results are the first from an approach that promises to play an important part in our study of neuronal form.

Stem diameter The clearest correlation between cytoskeletal structures and parameters of form is found with stem diameter. In fact, this is true for the diameter not just of the stem, but of all segments. For this reason all segments, including stem and terminal segments, will be considered here. There is a clear correlation between number of microtubules and neurofilaments and segment diameter in Purkinje cells (Figure 12), pyramidal cells (Figure 13A), and motoneurons (Figure 13C). In order to understand the relationship of microtubules and neurofilaments to segment diameter, one must consider not only the increase in the *number* of these elements with increases in diameter, but also (1) changes in the *density* of these elements and (2) the *ratio* of microtubule to neurofilament density (Table II). The three cell types

studied will be considered sequentially, beginning with the simplest case—the Purkinje cell.

In Purkinje cells, microtubule numbers increase with segment diameter and maintain a constant, although relatively low, density ($28/\mu m^2$). This cell contains almost no neurofilaments; therefore the tubules are clearly correlated with and may play a major role in establishing segment diameter (Figure 13B). Pyramidal cells have a higher density of tubules ($71/\mu m^2$) and also contain neurofilaments. Although the tubule-to-filament ratio is 14:1, the filament density is fairly constant, and both these elements doubtless contribute to determining the segment diameter in this cell type (Figure 13B).

The most complicated case is the motoneuron. Here tubule density decreases with increased segment diameter, but there is a significant number of filaments and their density is constant (Figure 13D). Again, at least one element, the neurofilament, can be clearly correlated with diameter.

This correlation between segment diameter and cytoskeletal elements suggests that these structures may provide the framework for dendritic processes and so may contribute significantly to determining the diameter of the branches of dendritic trees. While the observation that the total stem cross-sectional area is proportional to soma volume is intriguing (see Figure 3), very little can be said about this relationship since little is known about the ultrastructural basis of soma size.

Terminal diameter There are two aspects of terminal-segment diameter that bear further consideration: (1) the sharp lower size limit, and (2) the difference between terminal segments with spiny branches and those without. First, the clear and consistent relationship between segment diameter and tubule number suggests that the smallest diameters' may, in fact, reflect the space needed to contain a certain number of tubules—the number required to maintain the process. This suggestion finds support in the observation that terminals bearing spines are wider. Preliminary studies of electron micrographs indicate that these processes do not contain more tubules but have more endoplasmic reticulum than do the narrower terminal processes.

Segment taper Although the tapering between branch points decreases the process surface area, it reduces the process volume even more. Thus, as a segment tapers either the *density* of the cytoskeletal elements must increase or their *number* must decrease. These results suggest that the latter may be the case and that tapering is associated with a decrease in neurofilament number. Although this re-

PURKINJE AND PYRAMIDAL CELL DENDRITES

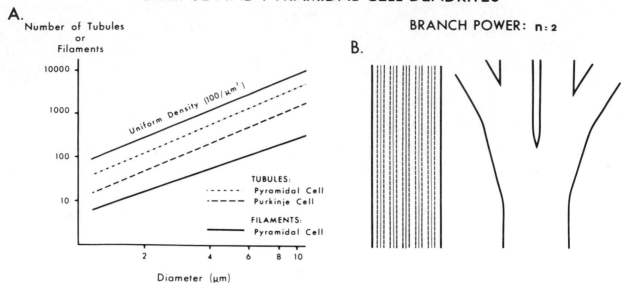

A.

Number of Tubules
or
Filaments

BRANCH POWER: n=2

B.

TUBULES:
.... Pyramidal Cell
— — — Purkinje Cell

FILAMENTS:
———— Pyramidal Cell

Diameter (μm)

MOTONEURON DENDRITES

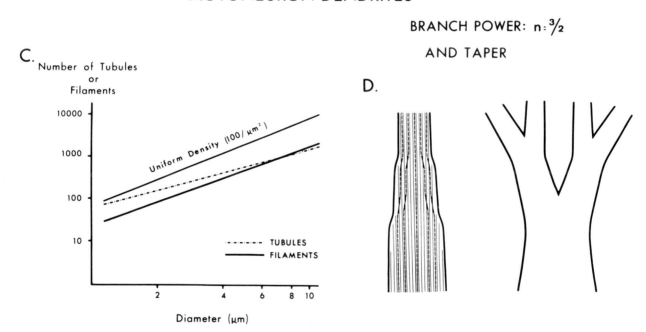

C.

Number of Tubules
or
Filaments

BRANCH POWER: n=³⁄₂

AND TAPER

D.

.... TUBULES
———— FILAMENTS

Diameter (μm)

quires further investigation, I have found that while cells with the most marked taper—motoneurons—contain the highest density of filaments ($38.6/\mu m^2$), this density remains constant as the diameter of processes decreases.

The ultrastructural basis for the unusually large taper seen in motoneuron (Barrett and Crill, 1974a) and pyramidal-cell stem segments is different. In these instances the stem taper is correlated with the extension of Golgi complex and rough endoplasmic reticulum (see Peters, Palay, and Webster, 1976) into the base of the arbor.

Branch power The finding of cell types obeying the 3/2 power rule (motoneurons) and the square power rule (pyramidal and Purkinje cells) is especially interesting if one considers the distribution of microtu-

490   D. E. HILLMAN

FIGURE 13 Microtubule and filament densities and their correlation to branch power. (A) Tubules (broken lines) within Purkinje- and pyramidal-cell dendritic trees follow a constant density throughout the range of cross-sectional profiles for different parts of the arbor. Pyramidal-cell tubules have the highest density while Purkinje cells are somewhat less concentrated. Filament density (solid lines) in pyramidal cells is nearly uniform. The Purkinje-cell filaments are not prominent or lacking and thus could not be quantitated. (Compiled from data by Hillman, Gelbfish, Llinás, and Iberall.) (B) The diameter of a bifurcating tree (right) and an equivalent cylinder (left) are illustrated for a branch power of 2 (e.g., pyramidal and Purkinje cells). Note that as the segments bifurcate, the diameter decreases while the equivalent cylinder maintains the same diameter over the tree; thus cross-sectional area is conserved. The subcellular filaments (solid lines) and microtubules (broken lines) maintain uniform tubule and filament concentrations. (C) Filaments (solid lines) in motoneurons have a uniform density throughout the extent of cross-sectional profiles for dendrites of different diameters. In contrast, the microtubules in the same profiles decreased in density for profiles with larger diameters. Note that in the larger profiles, the densities of filaments and tubules are nearly equal. It appears that filaments take over the role of maintaining diameter for the base of the tree. The subcellular structures were quantitated in the ventral horn of the rat spinal cord. (Compiled from unpublished data by Hillman and Gelbfish.) (D) The diameter of a bifurcating arbor having a 3/2 power and taper (right) and its equivalent cylinder (left). The reduction in diameter at each bifurcation for branch power 3/2 is significantly greater than that which occurs for branching with a power of two (B above). In the equivalent cylinder each branch point results in a decrease in diameter and thus in cross-sectional area. For the two branches illustrated, the first level represents the diameter for a cross-sectional area from two daughters, while the second represents this equivalent diameter for four daughters. As shown in C, filament density remains constant, thus they end (D, solid lines) or condense into fewer structures for each branch level. Tubules (broken lines), on the other hand, converge centripetally or, conversely, decrease their density toward the base.

bules and neurofilaments, and their relationship to diameter, in these neurons.

Consider first Purkinje and pyramidal cells. Since the cross-sectional area is maintained throughout the arborizations ($n = 2$), the trees can be modeled as simple, uniform cylinders (Figure 13B). (The simplifying assumption that branch power is constant throughout the tree has been made. Our data show a large amount of variability—see Table I and Figures 7 and 8—but this is probably due to the technical difficulties encountered in determining the diameters of small segments.) This finding, coupled with the observation that the microtubules, the major dendritic cytoskeletal elements in these cells, maintain a constant density throughout the tree, supports the hypothesis that microtubules (together with neurofilaments in pyramidal cells) are important determinants not only of process diameter but ultimately of branch power and dendritic volume.

Motoneurons present a more complex case in that neurofilaments and microtubules must both be considered. Because these cells have a branch power of 3/2, the cross-sectional area and volume of each process are reduced at branch points; that is, the dendritic tree must be represented as a tapering cylinder (Figure 13D). (Note that this is a geometric rather than an electrical representation of the cell. Furthermore, the total membrane surface area increases toward the dendritic terminals; thus volume and surface area must be considered separately.) Neurofilaments probably determine this taper, since their numbers must decrease toward the periphery if their density is to be kept constant. The filament number is probably reduced gradually between branch points, and this is reflected in the taper found in the individual segments of these cells (see Lux, Schubert, and Kreutzberg, 1970; Barrett and Crill, 1974a).

In motoneurons the findings that the microtubule density is increased at branch points and that $n = 3/2$ (i.e., the volume decreases at branches) support the view that the number of microtubules is constant in this cell type. This proposal finds support in the work of Weiss and Mayr (1971) who studied microtubule numbers in sensory and motoneuron axons and found that tubule numbers were constant across branch points. They concluded that tubules begin at the soma and extend to the terminals without branching or being lost (this may not be the case in all motoneuron axons: see Zenker and Hohberg, 1973). Hence, our results suggest that tubule numbers are constant in the dendrites of motoneurons and pyramidal and Purkinje cells (in the last two cell types, tubule density and process volume are both constant).

Thus both those cells in which the dendritic volume can be modeled as a uniform cylinder (pyramidal and Purkinje) and those in which it is best modeled as a tapering cylinder (motoneurons) have cytoskeletal elements whose density is constant throughout the dendritic tree: tubules in the former case, filaments in the latter. Cytoskeletal elements can therefore be closely correlated with the diameter of dendritic processes and with their volume. In fact, although there is no direct evidence that these structures "determine" the size of dendrites, I would support this viewpoint rather than its converse (i.e., that the size of the dendrites determines their contents).

Finally, I would propose that the reason *filament* density (not tubule density) is maintained in tapering trees is that microtubule numbers are held constant in dendritic trees and therefore cannot serve alone as the shaping scaffold of tapering processes (although they can provide structural support).

Daughter-branch ratio This parameter is essentially one of diameter (daughter-branch ratio is a ratio of diameters); thus the arguments for the ultrastructural basis for segment diameter are applicable. The relevant question here is whether the cytoskeletal elements contribute to establishing the ratio itself. Although Weiss and Mayr (1971) determined the distribution of these components between daughter branches, they did not report the diameters of the branches, and their data do not shed any light on this problem. There is, in fact, reason to believe that ultrastructural elements contribute to the cytoskeleton as an underlying base for the daughter-branch ratio. This question bears further study.

Segment length and orientation The orientation and length of dendritic segments are both parameters for which there are, at this time, no direct ultrastructural correlates.

Developmental determinants of the fundamental parameters of shape

The ontogenetic process that gives rise to form in the CNS has been studied extensively for over 100 years (Boll, 1873). From more recent studies it has been proposed that the major factors operating during development fall into two classes, those controlled directly by the genome of each cell (intrinsic factors) and those arising from interactions between cells (extrinsic factors) (see Rakic, 1974, 1975; Berry and Bradley, 1976a,b; Lash and Burger, 1977). In neurons, *intrinsic factors* control cell division and the elongation of the cytoplasmic structures and membrane into elaborate ramifications. As shown in culture, isolated neurons and neuroblasts branch and form arborizations characteristic of neurons (Bray, 1970, 1973). *Extrinsic factors* arise from the specific interactive properties of glia (Guillery, Sobkowicz, and Scott, 1970; Rakic, 1971, 1974) and nerve cells. Of particular importance is the arrival of the afferent plexus (Morest, 1969a,b) and the subsequent formation of synapses (Skoff and Hamburger, 1974; Vaughn, Henrikson, and Grieshaber, 1974). In addition, fiber bundles, blood vessels, and brain surface areas passively influence the shape of developing neurons.

A major question here is whether correlations can be found between the parameters of form and the intrinsic or extrinsic developmental factors. Certainly shape parameters will not be determined entirely by intrinsic or by extrinsic factors but will, rather, result from their cooperative interaction. Nevertheless, certain parameters may be dominated by one or another of these factors.

Because consistent aspects of cell shape are likely to be controlled by the genome (for example, through the synthesis of subcellular components), one expects that cytoskeletal elements and those shape parameters that they influence will be determined largely by intrinsic factors. One approach to testing this reasoning is to search for invariances or constraints in shape parameters within cell types. On the other hand, variable parameters are more likely to be dominated by extrinsic factors and would reflect the lack of uniformity usually found in the environment immediately surrounding each developing cell. In this type of analysis one must keep in mind that a uniform external field (such as is found in the cerebellum) can be responsible for the consistent spatial orientation found in some cell types (for example, the planar character of the Purkinje-cell dendritic tree).

In pursuit of this line of thought I have included (when appropriate) the variance of the values obtained for the fundamental parameters of shape (see Table I). I would suggest that those aspects of cell shape that show the least variability (e.g., sum of cross-sectional areas of stem dendrites, terminal-segment diameter, branch power) are controlled by intrinsic factors and that those that vary widely (e.g., segment length and orientation) are controlled by extrinsic factors. Some support for this hypothesis can be found in the published studies of neuronal development that are described below.

PARAMETERS DOMINATED BY INTRINSIC FACTORS These and other investigations (Rall, 1959; Lux, Schubert, and Kreutzberg, 1970; Barrett and Crill, 1974a) have demonstrated that some parameters of form show little variability.

Although the size and shape of the soma are two of the most constant features of cells (Bok, 1936b, 1959) and represent the basis of cytoarchitectonic classifications (Campbell, 1905), the underlying ultrastructural basis for soma size is, to date, unknown.

Although neuronal processes are not as constant as the soma, there are three aspects that are relatively invariant and about whose ultrastructural basis some speculations can be made. The factors are (1) the sum of the cross-sectional areas of the stem processes, (2) the terminal-segment diameter, and (3) branch power. These three parameters of tree shape, and segment taper as well, are all measurements of diameter and thus probably depend ultimately on the number of cytoskeletal elements such as neurotubules and neurofilaments whose synthesis and organization into a cytoskeleton is presumably controlled by the genome of each cell and little influenced by external factors.

Studies by Yamada and co-workers (1970) showed that microtubules were essential to neurite lengthening. When microtubule formation was stopped by application of colchicine, all processes failed to extend and some retracted. Thus the microtubules were believed to form a structural framework which was necessary for the elongation and stabilization of newly formed processes.

The role of microtubules in determining the three parameters listed above has not been addressed. One might speculate how the volume of a cell dendritic tree may be established genetically through limiting the number of tubules, filaments, or other cytoskeletal elements. In the simplest case, tubules alone are considered. One may propose that a cell generates a given number of tubules (composed of a fixed amount of tubulin) which continue to the terminals without dividing. If a constant tubule density is maintained, then regardless of the topology of the dendritic tree, the total volume of the tree is predetermined by the number of stem microtubules and their density. The conditions listed above are not unrealistic, for our results indicate that they are met in at least one cell type—the pyramidal-cell basal dendrites. In light of this suggestion, it is not surprising that the sum of the stem segments is correlated to soma size (Figure 3), since the stem-segment diameters merely reflect the number and density of their microtubules.

PARAMETERS DOMINATED BY EXTRINSIC FACTORS
There are four fundamental parameters of form that show considerable variability: (1) the number of dendritic stems emerging from the soma, (2) segment length, (3) segment orientation, and (4) daughter-branch ratio. These parameters are determined by the interactive influence (extrinsic) of properties of the interacting elements. Added to these influences are passive factors.

Stem diameter The diameter of individual stem segments and their distribution over the soma surface vary considerably from cell to cell. There is some support for the proposal that this feature is determined by the interaction of the developing cells with the environment. For example, although mammalian Purkinje cells show a marked potential to form more than one dendrite (as demonstrated by the appearance of numerous filopodia), adult cells have but one dendritic tree (Ramón y Cajal, 1911, 1929). This single tree may result from the strong influence of a climbing fiber (Kornguth and Scott, 1972). Following the capping of one pole of the soma by this afferent (Ramón y Cajal, 1911, 1929; Bradley and Berry, 1976), the only successful process extends from this pole. Subsequently all available microtubules and neurofilaments have but two pathways—the single dendrite and the axon.

In contrast, pyramidal cells migrate away from their strong afferent (and in doing this, away from the cortical surface) (Ramón y Cajal, 1929; Rakic, 1972). In this process the soma moves "downward," leaving the future apical dendritic process in its wake (Rakic, 1972). After arriving at its destined cortical level, multiple afferents interact with certain filopodia to direct the basal dendrites (see Schadé and Van Groenigen, 1961; Figures 4 and 5).

In the same way, cells developing in a completely isotropic field (e.g., the spiny cells of the caudate nucleus and central inferior olivary cells) have spherically radiating dendritic trees (Scheibel and Scheibel, 1955; Fox et al., 1971).

Segment length There is also some evidence from developmental studies that segment length is largely determined by extrinsic influences (Berry and Bradley, 1976b; Bradley and Berry, 1976). Developing cells express the potential to branch by producing numerous filopodia; however, the establishment of one of these mobile fingers into a stable process, with its own growth cone (see Tennyson, 1970), is dependent on its successful interaction with surrounding structures (Vaughn, Henrikson, and Grieshaber, 1974). Once process status is achieved, the length of each segment depends on the sites at which one or more filopodia are again stabilized as processes, and these then extend further, each with a growth cone. This continues until a mature neuron is formed. Thus the selection of filopodia determines the initial-segment length, the number of daughters at each branch point (Berry and Bradley, 1976b), and ultimately the orientation (see below) of each segment. These initial-segment lengths are not fixed (Berry and Bradley, 1976b), but can be altered as other developing processes enter the area (e.g., afferents and the dendrites of surrounding neurons). Under the influence of these processes the segment lengthens, largely, it seems, to provide room for these fibers. The interaction between the filopodia and the surround occurs through induction from synaptic afferents (Morest, 1969a,b; Vaughn, Henrikson, and Grieshaber, 1974) and by surface recognition of filopodia by other surrounding structures (see Guillery, Sobkowicz, and Scott, 1970; Rakic, 1974, 1975; Berry and Bradley, 1976a,b).

Spatial orientation The spatial orientation of segments, and ultimately of the entire arborization, seems to be dominated by extrinsic factors. In this context the selection of filopodia determines the direction of successful processes (although certain preferences may be provided intrinsically). For example, the highly restricted directional growth of the Purkinje-cell dendritic tree (Figure 1) is largely controlled by its interaction with parallel fibers to form synapses (Rakic, 1974). Similarly, tissue-culture studies indicate that the achievement of the unique shapes of nerve cells, which we recognize as dendritic and axonal trees, are highly dependent on the external interactions of the cells during development. Although some studies show that there is a tendency for branching in the absence of specifically organized afferents (Pomerat et al., 1967; Privat and Drian, 1976) and that isolated cells form characteristic arborizations (Bray, 1970, 1973), forms typical of the area of origin of these cells do not occur unless their normal afferents are present (Wolf and Dubois-Dalaq, 1970; Privat and Drian, 1976).

Daughter-branch ratio Little work has been directed toward understanding the determinants of daughter-branch ratios. The selection of the dominant filopodium is determined by developmental interactions with the surrounding field (the influence of afferent fibers is especially marked: see Morest, 1969a,b; Berry and Bradley, 1976b), and this seems to be a promising direction in which to look for the determinants of this parameter.

Conclusion and summary

Utilizing computerized three-dimensional recording and analysis, I have described the shapes of arborizations in the nervous system by means of seven fundamental parameters. The basis of this model is that the stem and succeeding segments are successively divided by bifurcations until a limiting (terminal) diameter is reached. Thus stem diameter and terminal diameter are two fundamental parameters. A third parameter, segment length, is the distance between branch points. Three other parameters are related to branch points. First, branch power measures any change in the cross-sectional area across branch points. Second, daughter-branch ratio (the ratio of the diameters of the daughter branches) represents the distribution of cross-sectional areas between daughter branches. Third, the orientation of these

segments is a measure of the angle and direction of each segment at the branch point. An additional parameter, segment taper, is needed in those neurons exhibiting a decrease in segment diameter between branch points.

Variations in neuronal form (characterized by differences in the shape of the soma and of dendritic arborizations) result from shifts in underlying intracellular structures. These structures compose a cytoskeleton that stabilizes elongation and provides a structural base for dendritic diameter. Microtubules are a fundamental component of this cytoskeletal core and extend, without branching, from their origin at the soma to the dendritic terminals. Furthermore, by maintaining tubule density, the total cross-sectional area (volume) remains constant from the stem through all the terminals. In some cell types this volume decreases toward the terminals. Here filaments in high density appear to increase the cross-sectional area at the base of the tree. This decreases the tubule density for the same region, yet the filament concentration remains constant (filaments are lost progressively as the total dendritic volume decreases distally).

During development, the sculpturing of this cytoskeletal core into arborizations takes place through an interplay between intrinsic influences provided through the subcellular structures and interactive influences that occur between the neuron and its surround. The following summary is presented to bring together some current thinking on neuronal form.

Three fundamental parameters (sum of the stem diameters, branch power, terminal diameter) show little variation and are believed to be primarily controlled by intrinsic factors during development. These parameters have a strong correlation with subcellular structures. Segment taper is probably also a member of this category. In contrast, individual stem diameter, segment length, daughter-branch ratio, and segment orientation all show significant variability. The developmental process that organizes the subcellular components into the cytoskeleton according to these four parameters is predominantly controlled by interactive (extrinsic) influences.

Soma volume reflects subcellular structures whose number is determined by the genome, which in turn constrains the total available volume of all dendritic structures of a cell. This volume is constrained by components of the cytoskeleton, basically tubules. The stem diameter of each dendrite is determined by tubule numbers, possibly from a total pool (in some cells filaments are an added factor). The distribution of this cross-sectional area between individual dendrites on a soma is largely controlled by the "strength" of the interaction with surrounding structures. This selection process determines the number of tubules within each stem. The volume of the individual tree follows as a dependence on the numbers of tubules and filaments that compose the stem diameter while the length of segments distributes the volume.

In arborizations, the cross-sectional area of the stem is reduced by the generation of daughter branches. The first branch point defines the initial-segment length, which may increase with interspersion of additional neuropil (Berry and Bradley, 1976a). At each branch point the tubules of the core are divided between the daughters according to the "strength" of interactions (filopodial selection), thus giving rise to variations in the daughter-branch ratio. The branch power is determined by the properties of the core. For example, when tubules are the principal component, the cross-sectional area remains constant. If high concentrations of filaments are present, the cross-sectional area is reduced across the branch point and along segments. Finally, the branch point serves to determine the orientation for the subsequent daughter segments. This is also governed through filopodial selection (extrinsic factors). The bifurcation process is probably complete when the tubule number is reduced to a level such that a further division is insufficient to form two additional processes (each with at least a minimal complement). Further lengthening of terminal segments is possible even if division is not. (Thus terminal segments can be longer than other segments: see Berry and Bradley, 1976a,b.)

ACKNOWLEDGMENTS I am very appreciative of the expert technical assistance provided by S. Chen, S. Cuccio, and J. Gelbfish and the computer programming provided by M. Chujo and J. Gelbfish. Research was supported by USPHS grants HD-10934 from the National Institute of Child Health and Human Development and NS-13742 from the National Institute of Neurological and Communicative Disorders and Stroke.

REFERENCES

APÁTHY, S., 1897. Das leitende Element des nervensystems und seini topographischen Beziehungen zu den Zellen. *Mitth. Zool. Sta. Neapel.* 12:495–748.

BALTHASAR, K., 1962. Morphologie der spinalen Tibialis—und Peronaeus—Kerne bei der Katze: Topographie, Architektonik, Axon—und Dendritenverlauf der motoneurone und Zwischenneurone in den Segmenten L₆-S₂. *Arch. Psychiatr. Neurol.* 188:345–378.

BARRETT, J. N., and W. E. CRILL, 1974a. Specific membrane properties of cat motoneurons. *J. Physiol.* 239:301–324.

BARRETT, J. N., and W. E. CRILL, 1974b. Influence of dendritic location and membrane properties on the effectiveness of synapses on cat motoneurons. *J. Physiol.* 239:325–345.

BERRY, M., E. M. ANDERSON, T. HOLLINGWORTH, and R. M. FLINN, 1972. A computer technique for the estimation of the absolute three-dimensional array of basal dendritic fields using data from projected histological sections. *J. Microsc.* (Oxford) 95:257–267.

BERRY, M., and P. BRADLEY, 1976a. The application of network analysis to the study of branching patterns of large dendritic fields. *Brain Res.* 109:111–132.

BERRY, M., and P. BRADLEY, 1976b. The growth of the dendritic trees of Purkinje cells in the cerebellum of the rat. *Brain Res.* 112:1–35.

BERRY, M., T. HOLLINGWORTH, E. M. ANDERSON, and R. M. FLINN, 1975. Application of network analysis to the study of the branching patterns of dendritic fields. *Adv. Neurol.* 12:217–245.

BERRY, M., T. HOLLINGWORTH, R. M. FLINN, and E. M. ANDERSON, 1972. Dendritic field analysis: A reappraisal. *T.-I.T. J. Life Sci.* 2.129–140.

BIELSCHOWSKY, M., 1902. Die Silberimprägnation dei Axencylinder. *Neurol. Zentrabl.* 21:579–584.

BOK, S. T., 1936a. The branching of the dendrites in the cerebral cortex. *Verh. Kon. Med. Akad. Wetenshap.* 39:1209–1218.

BOK, S. T., 1936b. A quantitative analysis of the structure of the cerebral cortex. *Verh. Kon. Med. Akad. Wetenshap.* 35:1–55.

BOK, S. T., 1959. *Histonomy of the Cerebral Cortex.* Amsterdam: Elsevier.

BOLL, F., 1873. Die Histologie und Histiogenese der nervösen Centralorgane. *Arch. Psychiatr.* (Berlin) 4:1–138.

BORN, G., 1883. Die Plattenmodelliermethode. *Arch. Mikrosk. Anat.* 22:584–599.

BRADLEY, P. M., and BERRY, M., 1976. The effects of reduced climbing and parallel fibre input on Purkinje cell dendritic growth. *Brain Res.* 109:133–151.

BRAY, D., 1970. Surface movements during the growth of single explanted neurons. *Proc. Natl. Acad. Sci. USA* 65:905–910.

BRAY, D., 1973. Branching patterns of individual sympathetic neurons in culture. *J. Cell. Biol.* 56:702–712.

BROWN, C., 1977. Neuron orientations: A computer application. In *Computer Analysis of Neuronal Structures,* R. D. Lindsay, ed. New York and London: Plenum, pp. 177–188.

BROWN, P. B., 1976. *Computer Technology in Neurosciences.* Washington and London: Hemisphere.

CAMPBELL, A. W., 1905. *Histological Studies on the Localisation of Cerebral Function.* New York: Cambridge Univ. Press.

CHU, L. W., 1954. A cytoskeletal study of anterior horn cells isolated from human spinal cord. *J. Comp. Neurol.* 100:381–416.

CLENDINNEN, B. G., and J. T. EAYRS, 1961. The anatomical and physiological effects of prenatally administered somatropin on cerebral development in rats. *J. Endocrinol.* 22:183–193.

COLEMAN, P., C. GARVEY, J. YOUNG, and W. SIMON, 1977. Semi-automatic tracking of neuronal processes. In *Computer Analysis of Neuronal Structures,* R. D. Lindsay, ed. New York and London: Plenum, pp. 91–110.

COLEMAN, P. D., and A. H. RIESEN, 1968. Environmental effects on cortical dendritic fields. I. Rearing in the dark. *J. Anat.* 102:363–374.

COLEMAN, P. D., M. J. WEST, and R. WYSS, 1973. Computer-aided quantitative neuroanatomy. In *Digital Computers in the Behavioral Lab.*, B. Weiss, ed. New York: Appleton-Century-Crofts, pp. 379–426.

COLON, E. J., and G. J. SMIT, 1970. Quantitative analysis of the cerebral cortex. II. A method for analyzing basal dendritic plexuses. *Brain Res.* 22:363–380.

COLON, E. J., and G. J. SMIT, 1971. A quantitative analysis of dendritic patterns in the cerebral cortex. *Acta Morphol. Neerl. Scand.* 9:21–39.

COLONNIER, M., 1964. The tangential organization of the visual cortex. *J. Anat.* 98:327–344.

DEITERS, O., 1865. *Untersuchungen über Gehirn und Rückenmark des menschen und der Saügetiere.* Braunschweig.

EAYRS, J. T., 1955. The cerebral cortex of normal and hypothyroid rats. *Acta Anat.* 25:160–183.

FOX, C. A., and J. W. BARNARD, 1957. A quantitative study of Purkinje cell dendritic branchlets and their relationship to afferent fibers. *J. Anat.* 91:299–313.

FOX, C. A., A. N. ANDRADE, D. E. HILLMAN, and R. C. SCHWYN, 1971. The spiny neurons in the primate striatum: A Golgi and electron microscopic study. *J. Hirnforschung.* 13:181–201.

FRIEDE, R. L., and T. SAMORAJSKI, 1970. Axon caliber related to neurofilaments and microtubules in sciatic nerve fibers of rats and mice. *Anat. Rec.* 167:379–388.

GARVEY, C. F., J. H. YOUNG, P. D. COLEMAN, and W. SIMON, 1973. Automated three-dimensional dendrite tracking system. *EEG Clin. Neurophysiol.* 35:199–204.

GELFAN, S., G. KARA, and D. S. RUCHKIN, 1970. The dendritic tree of spinal neurons. *J. Comp. Neurol.* 139:385–412.

GLASER, E. M., and H. VAN DER LOOS, 1965. A semi-automatic computer microscope for the analysis of neuronal morphology. *IEEE Trans. Biomed. Eng.* 12:22–31.

GLASSER, S., J. MILLER, N. G. YOUNG, and A. SELVERSTON, 1977. Computer reconstruction of invertebrate nerve cells. In *Computer Analysis of Neuronal Structures*, R. D. Lindsay, ed. New York and London: Plenum, pp. 21–58.

GOLGI, C., 1874. Sulla fina anatomia del cervelletto umano. Reprinted in *Opera Omnia*, vol. 1: *Istologia normale, 1870–1883.* Milan: Ulrico Hoepli (1903), pp. 99–111.

GUILLERY, R. W., H. M. SOBKOWICZ, and G. L. SCOTT, 1970. Relationships between glial and neuronal elements in the development of long term cultures of the spinal cord of the fetal mouse. *J. Comp. Neurol.* 140:1–34.

HAGGAR, R. A., and M. L. BARR, 1950. Quantitative data on the size of synaptic end bulbs in the cat's spinal cord. *J. Comp. Neurol.* 93:17–36.

HILLMAN, D. E., M. CHUJO, and R. LLINÁS, 1974. Quantitative computer analysis of the morphology of cerebellar neurons. *Anat. Rec.* 178:375 (abstract).

HILLMAN, D. E., R. LLINÁS, and M. CHUJO, 1977. Automatic and semi-automatic analysis of nervous system structure. In *Computer Analysis of Neuronal Structures*, R. D. Lindsay, ed. New York and London: Plenum, pp. 73–89.

HOOPEN, M. TEN, and H. A. REUVER, 1970. Probabilistic analysis of dendritic branching patterns of cortical neurons. *Kybernetik* 6:176–188.

KÖLLIKER, A. V., 1891. Die Lehrer von den Beziehungen der nervösen Elemente zu einander. *Anat. Anz. Ergazungshftr.* 1891:5–20.

KORNGUTH, S. E., and G. SCOTT, 1972. The role of climbing fibers in the formation of Purkinje cell dendrites. *J. Comp. Neurol.* 146:61–82.

LASH, J. W., and M. M. BURGER, eds., 1977. *Cell and Tissue Interactions.* New York: Raven Press.

LEVINTHAL, C., E. MACAGNO, and C. TOUNTAS, 1974. Computer-aided reconstruction from serial sections. *Fed. Proc.* 33:2326–2340.

LEVINTHAL, C., and R. WARE, 1972. Three-dimensional reconstruction from serial sections. *Nature* 236:207–210.

LINDSAY, R. D., ed., 1977a. *Computer Analysis of Neuronal Structures.* New York and London: Plenum.

LINDSAY, R. D., 1977b. The video computer microscope and A.R.G.O.S. In *Computer Analysis of Neuronal Structures*, R. D. Lindsay, ed. New York and London: Plenum, pp. 1–19.

LINDSAY, R. D., 1977c. Tree analysis of neuronal processes. In *Computer Analysis of Neuronal Structures*, R. D. Lindsay, ed. New York and London: Plenum, pp. 149–164.

LINDSAY, R. D., 1977d. Neuronal field analysis using Fourier series. In *Computer Analysis of Neuronal Structures*, R. D. Lindsay, ed. New York and London: Plenum, pp. 165–175.

LINDSAY, R. D., and A. B. SCHEIBEL, 1974. Quantitative analysis of the dendritic branching pattern of small pyramidal cells from adult rat somesthetic and visual cortex. *Exp. Neurol.* 45:424–434.

LLINÁS, R., and D. E. HILLMAN, 1975. A multipurpose tridimensional reconstruction computer system for neuroanatomy. In *Golgi Centennial Symposium: Perspectives in Neurobiology*, M. Santini, ed. New York: Raven, pp. 519–528.

LLINÁS, R., and A. IBERALL, 1977. A global model of neuronal command-control systems. *BioSystems* 8:233–235.

LORENTE DE NÓ, R., 1934. Studies on the structure of the cerebral cortex. II. Continuation of the study of the ammonic system. *J. Psychol. Neurol.* (Leipzig) 46:113–177.

LUX, H. D., P. SCHUBERT, and G. W. KREUTZBERG, 1970. Direct matching of morphological and electrophysiological data in cat spinal motoneurons. In *Excitatory Synaptic Mechanisms*, P. Anderson and J. K. I. Jansen, eds. Oslo: Universitetsforlaget.

McCONNELL, P., and M. BERRY, 1978. The effect of undernutrition on Purkinje cell dendritic growth in the rat. *J. Comp. Neurol.* 177:159–172.

MANNEN, H., 1966. Contribution to the quantitative study of the nervous tissue: A new method for measurement of the volume and surface area of neuron. *J. Comp. Neurol.* 126:75–90.

MOREST, D. K., 1969a. The differentiation of cerebral dendrites: A study of the post-migratory neuroblast in the medial nucleus of the trapezoid body. *Z. Anat. Entwicklungsgesch.* 128:271–289.

MOREST, D. K., 1969b. The growth of dendrites in the mammalian brain. *Z. Anat. Entwicklungsgesch.* 128:290–317.

MUNGAI, J. M., 1967. Dendritic patterns in the somatic sensory cortex of the cat. *J. Anat.* 101:403–418.

PALAY, S., 1956. Synapses in the central nervous system. *J. Biophys. Biochem. Cytol.* 2:193–201.

PALAY, S. L., and V. CHAN-PALAY, 1974. *Cerebellar Cortex: Cytology and Organization.* New York: Springer-Verlag.

PALDINO, A., and E. HARTH, 1977a. A measuring system for analyzing neuronal fiber structure. In *Computer Analysis of Neuronal Structures,* R. D. Lindsay, ed. New York and London: Plenum, pp. 59–72.

PALDINO, A., and E. HARTH, 1977b. A computerized study of Golgi impregnated axons in rat visual cortex. In *Computer Analysis of Neuronal Structures,* R. D. Lindsay, ed. New York and London: Plenum, pp. 189–207.

PETERS, A., 1968. Characterization of microtubules, neurofilaments and cross bridges in various neuronal types. *Neurosci. Res. Program Bull.* 6:162–188.

PETERS, A., 1971. Stellate cells in the rat parietal cortex. *J. Comp. Neurol.* 141:345–374.

PETERS, H. G., and H. BADEMAN, 1963. The form and growth of stellate cells in the cortex of the guinea pig. *J. Anat.* 97:111–117.

PETERS, A., S. PALAY, and H. WEBSTER, 1976. *The Fine Structure of the Nervous System: The Neurons and Supporting Cells.* Philadelphia: W. B. Saunders.

PETERSON, T. S., 1955. *Analytic Geometry and Calculus.* New York: Harper and Brothers, p. 410.

POMERAT, C. M., W. J. HENDELMAN, C. W. RAIBORN, and J. F. MASSEY, 1967. Dynamic activities of nervous tissue *in vitro.* In *The Neuron,* H. Hydén, ed. New York: Elsevier, pp. 119–178.

PORTER, K. R., and L. G. TILNEY, 1965. Microtubules and intracellular motility. *Science* 150:382.

PRIVAT, A., and M. J. DRIAN, 1976. Postnatal maturation of rat Purkinje cells cultivated in the absence of two afferent systems: An ultrastructural study. *J. Comp. Neurol.* 166:201–244.

PURKINJE, J. E., 1837. Bericht über die Versammlung deutscher Naturforscher und Ärzte (Prag). *Anat. Physiologische Verhandlungen* 3:177–180.

RAKIC, P., 1971. Neuron-glia relationships during granule cell migration in developing cerebellar cortex. A Golgi and electronmicroscope study in *Macacus rhesus. J. Comp. Neurol.* 141:283–312.

RAKIC, P., 1972. Mode of cell migration to the superficial layers of fetal monkey neocortex. *J. Comp. Neurol.* 145:61–84.

RAKIC, P., 1974. Intrinsic and extrinsic factors influencing the shape of neurons and their assembly into neuronal circuits. In *Frontiers in Neurology and Neuroscience Research,* P. Seeman and G. M. Brown, eds. Toronto: Univ. Toronto Press, pp. 112–132.

RAKIC, P., 1975. Role of cell interaction in development of dendritic patterns. *Adv. Neurol.* 12:117–134.

RALL, W., 1959. Branching dendritic trees and motoneuron membrane resistivity. *Exp. Neurol.* 1:491–527.

RALL, W., 1962. Electrophysiology of a dendritic neurone model. *Biophys. J.* 2:145–167.

RALL, W., 1970. Cable properties of dendrites and effects of synaptic location. In *Excitatory Synaptic Mechanisms,* P. Andersen and J. K. S. Jansen, eds. Oslo: Universitetsforlaget.

RAMÓN Y CAJAL, S., 1909. *Histologie du système nerveux de l'homme et des vertébrés,* vol. I. Paris: Maloine.

RAMÓN Y CAJAL, S., 1911. *Histologie du système nerveux de l'homme et des vertébrés,* vol. II. Paris: Maloine.

RAMÓN Y CAJAL, S., 1929. *Studies on Vertebrate Neurogenesis.* Springfield, IL: Thomas.

REDDY, D. R., W. J. DAVIS, R. B. OHLANDER, and D. J. BIHARY, 1973. Computer analysis of neuronal structures. In *Intracellular Staining in Neurobiology,* S. B. Kater and C. Nicholson, eds. New York: Springer-Verlag, pp. 227–253.

SCHADÉ, J. P., and W. F. CAVENESS, 1968. Pathogenesis of X-irradiation effects in the monkey cerebral cortex. IV. Alteration in dendritic organization. *Brain Res.* 7:59–84.

SCHADÉ, J. P., and W. B. VAN GROENIGEN, 1961. Structural organization of the human cerebral cortex. I. Maturation of the middle frontal gyrus. *Acta Anat.* 47:74–111.

SCHEIBEL, M. E., and A. B. SCHEIBEL, 1955. The inferior olive—A Golgi study. *J. Comp. Neurol.* 102:77–132.

SCHMITT, F. O., 1968. The molecular biology of neuronal fibrous proteins. *Neurosci. Res. Program Bull.* 6:119–144.

SCHMITT, F. O., and B. B. GEREN, 1950. The fibrous structure of the nerve axon in relation to the localization of "neurotubules." *J. Exp. Med.* 91:499–507.

SCHULZE, M., 1871. Allgemeines über die Structurelemente des Nerven Systems. In *Handbüch der Lehre von den Geweben,* S. Stricker, ed. Leipzig.

SELVERSTON, A. L., 1973. The use of intracellular dye injections in the study of small neural networks. In *Intracellular Staining in Neurobiology,* S. B. Kater and C. Nicholson, eds. New York: Springer-Verlag, pp. 255–280.

SHOLL, D. A., 1953. Dendritic organization in the neurons of the visual and motor cortices of the cat. *J. Anat.* 87:387–406.

SHOLL, D. A., 1955. The surface area of cortical neurons. *J. Anat.* 89:571–572.

SHOLL, D. A., 1956. *The Organization of the Cerebral Cortex.* London: Methuen.

SKOFF, R. P., and V. HAMBURGER, 1974. Fine structure of dendritic and axonic growth cones in embryonic chick spinal cord. *J. Comp. Neurol.* 153:107–148.

SMIT, G. J., and H. B. UYLINGS, 1975. The morphometry of the branching pattern in the dendrites of the visual cortex pyramidal cells. *Brain Res.* 87:41–53.

SMIT, G. J., H. B. UYLINGS, and L. VLEDMAAT-WANSINK, 1972. The branching pattern in dendrites of cortical neurons. *Acta Morphol. Neerl. Scand.* 9:253–274.

SMITH, D. E., 1973. The location of neurofilaments and microtubules during the postnatal development of Clarke's nucleus in the kitten. *Brain Res.* 55:41–53.

TENNYSON, V. M., 1970. The fine structure of the axon and growth cone of the dorsal root neuroblast of the rabbit embryo. *J. Cell. Biol.* 44:62–79.

TILNEY, L. G., and K. R. PORTER, 1967. Studies on the microtubules in heliozoa. II. The effect of low temperature on these structures in the formation and maintenance of the axopodia. *J. Cell. Biol.* 34:327–343.

UYLINGS, H. B., and G. J. SMIT, 1975. Three-dimensional branching structure of pyramidal cell dendrites. *Brain Res.* 87:55–66.

VAUGHN, J. E., C. K. HENRIKSON, and J. A. GRIESHABER, 1974. A quantitative study of synapses on motoneuron dendritic growth cones in developing mouse spinal cord. *J. Cell. Biol.* 60:664–672.

WALDEYER, W., 1891. Über einige neurere Forschungen im Gebrete der Anatomie des Central Nerven Systems. *Berl. Klin. Wchnschr.* 28:691.

WANN, D. F., T. A. WOOLSEY, M. L. DIERKER, and W. M. COWAN, 1973. An on-line digital-computer system for the semi-automatic analysis of Golgi impregnated neurons. *IEEE Trans. Biomed. Eng.* 20:233–247.

WEISS, P. A., and R. MAYR, 1971. Neuronal organelles in neuroplasmic ("axonal") flow. II. Neurotubules. *Acta Neuropathol.* (Berlin) Suppl. 5:198–206.

WOLF, M. K., and M. DUBOIS-DALAQ, 1970. Anatomy of cultured mouse cerebellum. I. Golgi and electron microscopic demonstrations of granule cells, their afferent and efferent synapses. *J. Comp. Neurol.* 140:261–280.

WONG, W. C., 1967. The tangential organization of dendrites and axons in three auditory areas of the cat's cerebral cortex. *J. Anat.* 101:419–433.

WUERKER, R. B., and J. B. KIRKPATRICK, 1972. Neuronal microtubules, neurofilaments and microfilaments. *Int. Rev. Cytol.* 33:45–75.

WUERKER, R. B., and S. PALAY, 1969. Neurofilaments and microtubules in anterior horn cells of the rat. *Tissue & Cell* 1:387–402.

YAMADA, K. M., B. S. SPOONER, and N. K. WESSELLS, 1970. Axon growth: Roles of microfilaments and microtubules. *Proc. Natl. Acad. Sci. USA* 66:1206–1212.

ZENKER, W., and E. HOHBERG, 1973. A α-nerve-fibre: Number of neurotubules in the stem fibre and in the terminal branches. *J. Neurocytol.* 2:143–148.

ZENKER, W., R. MAYR, and H. GRUBER, 1973. Axoplasmic organelles: Quantitative differences between ventral and dorsal root fibres of the rat. *Experientia* 29:77–78.

28 Propagation in Nonuniform Neurites: Form and Function in Axons

I. PARNAS

ABSTRACT   This paper considers the mechanisms and effects of differential conduction of trains of action potentials in axons. Effects of diameter changes and changes in synaptic input are examined in the case of the giant abdominal axon of the cockroach, which tapers from 60 μm at the posterior end of ganglion T_3 to 30 μm as it passes through the ganglion, where it receives a number of synaptic inputs, and then spreads to about 45 μm at the anterior end. Effects of the geometrical ratio and of extracellular potassium concentration on conduction in branching axons are explored in the case of a branching excitatory axon innervating the extensor muscles in the abdomen of the lobster, a preparation with a geometrical ratio of about one. It is concluded that the complex arborizations of nerve cells cannot be considered simply as transmission lines but must be treated as active elements capable of modulating the flow of impulses from one region to another.

Introduction

Since the finding of "all-or-none" conduction of action potentials (Adrian, 1914), there has been a tendency to minimize the role of axons in nervous integration. Axons have been regarded as simple transmission lines conducting impulses rapidly and accurately into all their branches. Differential conduction along divergent pathways has been assumed for the most part to be controlled exclusively by synaptic mechanisms (Kuffler and Nicholls, 1976; Kandel, 1976).

The concept that different branches of the same neuron might carry activity independently was introduced by Bullock and Terzuolo (1957) and by Hagiwara and Bullock (1957). Recording from the soma of a branching neuron, they observed fast-rising potentials of two amplitudes. These originated from action potentials in two different branches which had spread electronically through an inexcitable region into the soma. No "cross talk" between the two branches was found (Friesen, 1975); thus these two branches can be looked upon as two separate neurons

I. PARNAS   Neurobiology Unit, The Hebrew University, Jerusalem, Israel

supported metabolically by one soma. The possibility of differential conduction was not pursued further, however; it was assumed that action potentials or trains of action potentials propagated unfailingly along all the ramifications of each branch.

In recent years data have accumulated indicating that in certain regions axons are able to modulate the pattern of trains of action potentials and, at branch points, may even conduct action potentials differentially into two branches (Tauc and Hughes, 1963; Chung, Raymond, and Lettvin, 1970; Parnas, 1972; Grossman, Spira, and Parnas, 1973; for reviews see Waxman, 1972, 1975). Moreover, since the ability of an axon to modulate conduction varies with activity (Calvin and Hartline, 1977), differential propagation can depend on the past history of the axon (Spira, Yarom, and Parnas, 1976).

In this chapter emphasis will be placed on this modulation of impulse propagation through regions of special geometry along axons and on the mechanisms underlying this behavior.

Effects of diameter changes on conduction

An action potential can be propagated through a region of increasing axonal diameter with a lower safety factor (Khodorov et al., 1969; but see Dodge, this volume). One example of such a case is the antidromic invasion of action potentials into the soma (Coombs, Curtis, and Eccles, 1957; Khodorov et al., 1969). In some instances, despite the excitability of the soma membrane, the action potential fails to invade the soma actively, and only a decremental response is observed.

An interesting system in which changes in axonal diameter affect conduction in a physiological pathway is the abdominal giant axon of the cockroach. The giant axons originate at the sixth abdominal ganglion (A_6) and ascend without interruption along the ventral nerve cord through the abdomen and thorax (Farley and Milburn, 1969; Parnas et al., 1969; Spira, Parnas, and Bergman, 1969a,b). For many years, the giant axons were thought to terminate in the meta-thoracic ganglion (T_3) and to form there synapses on ascending interneurons that completed the pathway through the thorax (Roeder, 1948). In fact, the giant axons are constricted while passing through the me-tathoracic ganglion, and the physiological conse-quences of this change in diameter were misinter-preted as evidence for an interposed synapse. For example, the conduction time across ganglion T_3 is longer, and the delay is not constant but shows fluc-tuations at higher frequencies of stimulation. Second, the minimum interval at which two impulses propa-gate through the ganglion is longer than the refrac-tory period (Parnas et al., 1969). Third, nicotine, which is known to be a depolarizing synaptic blocker in insects (Roeder, 1948; Callec, 1972), blocks con-duction of the giant axons in T_3 but not in the first to fifth abdominal ganglia (A_1–A_5). Finally, after the connectives at A_5–A_6 had been severed, degeneration of the giant axons was seen to proceed up to ganglion T_3 but not rostral to it (Hess, 1958; but see Spira, Parnas, and Bergman, 1969b). These data were con-sidered sufficient to establish the existence of a syn-apse in ganglion T_3 along a pathway in which it was technically difficult to record synaptic potentials from the postsynaptic cell. However, direct experiments, in which intracellular injection of cobalt was used to reveal the full extent of the giant axons, confirmed that the giants cross ganglion T_3 without interruption but are constricted by about 50% as they pass through the ganglion (Figure 1 and Castel et al., 1976). All of the findings that suggested the presence of a synapse in the giant axon pathway were finally shown to be a consequence of this diameter change and of the presence of synaptic inputs on the giant axons in this region (Spira, Yarom, and Parnas, 1976).

The region of the giant axon passing through gan-glion T_3 is thus a convenient system in which to study

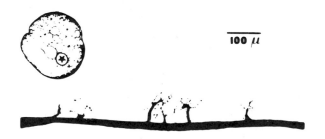

FIGURE 1   A giant axon injected with cobalt in the meta-thoracic ganglion. The axon was injected at the caudal base of the ganglion. Shown are a cross section through the connective at T_3–A_1 (the injected axon is marked by a star) and the same axon photographed in whole mount. (From Castel et al., 1976.)

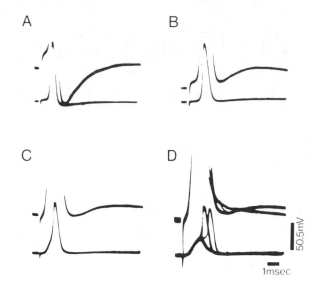

FIGURE 2   Effects of high-frequency stimulation on con-duction of action potentials in the giant axons in the region of the metathoracic ganglion. Recordings were made at the caudal base of the ganglion, and the connectives were stim-ulated at T_2–T_3. The two sweeps show the same events at low and high gains. Stimulation rate was 50/sec. (A) Re-sponses after 1 sec of stimulation. (B) After 24 sec. (C) After 42 sec. (D) After 50 sec. In the lower sweep in D note the development of a prepotential, a change in conduction velocity, and a block of conduction. (Modified from Spira, Yarom, and Parnas, 1976.)

effects of diameter changes on conduction. More-over, while the diameter of the giant axon at the posterior end of ganglion T_3 is 60–70 μm, it narrows to 25–30 μm as it passes through the ganglion and widens at the anterior end to 40–45 μm. Because this region of the axon is not symmetrical, it is possible, by comparing conduction in both directions, to study effects of different diameter changes on conduction using a single axon.

When a giant axon is impaled at the posterior end of ganglion T_3 and the anterior connectives are stim-ulated at high frequency, the following changes are observed. Although single action potentials propa-gate well (Figure 2A), at 50 Hz conduction becomes slower, a prepotential appears (Figure 2C), and the action potential is reduced in amplitude. The delay across the ganglion is nonconstant (Figure 2D), and conduction rapidly fails (Figure 2D). In addition, the afterhyperpolarization becomes smaller and the membrane is depolarized by about 14 mV (not shown; see Spira, Yarom, and Parnas, 1976). The cell depolarization and the reduction in size of the after-hyperpolarization suggest an increase in extracellular potassium concentration (Frankenhaeuser and Hodgkin, 1956). It was therefore proposed (Spira,

Yarom, and Parnas, 1976) that during repetitive stimulation potassium accumulates in the periaxonal space to produce membrane depolarization and sodium inactivation (Hodgkin and Huxley, 1952; Adelman and Palti, 1969a,b). Indeed, when the membrane of a stimulated axon was hyperpolarized by inward current injection, conduction was restored even with high-frequency stimulation (Figure 7 of Spira, Yarom, and Parnas, 1976). Ultrastructural studies reveal that the giant axons are surrounded by glial cells with a periaxonal space of about 200 Å (Castel et al., 1976). In such a space the increase in potassium concentration can be in the range of several mM after a few impulses at 50–100 Hz (Frankenhaeuser and Hodgkin, 1956).

Figure 3 compares ascending and descending propagation through ganglion T_3. In general, it can be stated that conduction in the anterior-to-posterior direction ($45 \rightarrow 30 \rightarrow 60$ μm) is more vulnerable than that in the opposite direction ($60 \rightarrow 30 \rightarrow 45$ μm): a lower frequency or a shorter period of stimulation at a given frequency is needed to block conduction in the anterior-to-posterior direction. An additional change with high-frequency stimulation can be seen by recording in the wide region of the axon

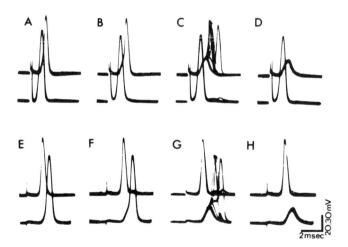

FIGURE 3 Block of conduction in the giant axons in the metathoracic ganglion. Simultaneous recording of action potentials from the same giant axon on both sides of ganglion T_3 during stimulation at 50/sec. The upper and lower traces show responses recorded at the caudal and rostral bases of ganglion T_3, respectively. (A–D) Stimulation of the connectives at T_2–T_3. Note on continued stimulation the development of a prepotential at the posterior base (upper trace in C) and the appearance of a reflection potential at the anterior end of the ganglion. (E–H) Stimulation at A_4–A_5. Note the delay in the action potentials at the anterior end of the ganglion and the appearance of a reflection potential at the posterior base of the ganglion (G). (From Spira, Yarom, and Parnas, 1976.)

on the same side of the ganglion as the stimulating electrode. In this case, as conduction through the ganglion is delayed, a small depolarizing "hump" or reflection potential appears after the action potential (Figure 3C,G). Block of conduction is associated with the disappearance of this reflection potential, indicating that it represents the electrotonic spread of the late-arising action potential back up the axon toward the stimulating electrode. The appearance of a reflection potential was predicted theoretically for a single action potential approaching a wider region (Khodorov et al., 1969) or for repetitive firing (Parnas, Hochstein, and Parnas, 1976). The role of these reflection potentials in modulating conduction is treated below (see also Calvin and Hartline, 1977).

Effects of synaptic inputs on conduction in the giant axons

As demonstrated above, the conduction of action potentials in the giant axons across ganglion T_3 has a low safety factor because of the anatomical organization. The current produced by an action potential in the narrow region is barely sufficient to depolarize the wider region to bring it to threshold. Any mechanism that will produce shunting of current in the narrow region will lower the safety factor further; and if shunting is substantial, conduction will be blocked.

The giant axons receive a variety of synaptic inputs in ganglion T_3, and activation of these inputs modulates the pattern of action potentials (Spira, Yarom, and Parnas, 1976). For example, Figure 4 shows activity recorded from a giant axon at the posterior end of ganglion T_3. The ipsilateral connective was stimulated anterior to the ganglion. Trains of four action potentials 4 msec apart were produced at a rate of 3/sec. At this stimulation rate all four action potentials could be conducted for long periods (Figure 4A). When the contralateral connective was stimulated to produce a synaptic potential (not visible under these recording conditions), the pattern of signaling through the ganglion was altered (Figure 4B,C). The effects of the synaptic potentials were long-lasting and cumulative, but a few minutes after cessation of the synaptic input all four action potentials propagated through the ganglion (Figure 4D).

Theoretical computation for conduction across a region with an increase in diameter

The original Hodgkin-Huxley (1952) equations were solved for a homogeneous axon (a long cylinder) for

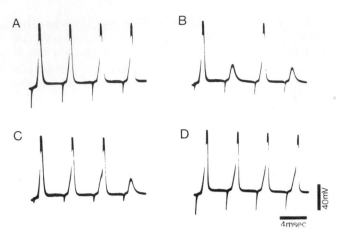

40mV

4msec

FIGURE 4 Effect of synaptic activation on conduction of action potentials in a giant axon across the metathoracic ganglion. (A) As a control, four action potentials separated by 4 msec were elicited by stimulation of the ipsilateral connective at T_2–T_3 and recorded at the caudal base of ganglion T_3. Repetition rate was 3/sec. At this rate of stimulation the four action potentials were conducted faithfully for long periods (30 minutes). (B,C) The contralateral connective was stimulated to elicit a synaptic input which preceded each train by 1.1 msec (the synaptic potentials are not seen at this gain of recording). (B) Two seconds after the synaptic input was activated the fourth action potential was blocked. (C) Five seconds later the second and fourth action potentials were blocked. (D) Ten minutes after the removal of the synaptic input the burst recovered. (Modified from Spira, Yarom, and Parnas, 1976.)

the space-clamp condition or under the assumption of a constant conduction velocity. Neither of these assumptions can be applied to regions where the axon diameter changes. Nor do the Hodgkin-Huxley equations take into account the changes in extracellular and intracellular ion concentrations that occur during repetitive activity. Khodorov et al. (1969) therefore used the numerical method of Cooley and Dodge (1966) for a nonhomogeneous axon with a step increase in fiber diameter. They were the first to show that a single action potential could propagate through a region with a fivefold increase in diameter, though with a delay. When the increase in diameter was sixfold, conduction was blocked.

Since then several theoretical computations considering different axonal shapes and changes in excitability have been published. For a detailed description of the numerical methods and the equations describing conduction through a step or gradual increase in fiber diameter the reader should consult the papers of Cooley and Dodge (1966), Dodge and Cooley (1973), Khodorov et al. (1969), and Parnas, Hochstein, and Parnas (1976). The latter paper shows that an increase in extracellular potassium concentration

is, by itself, sufficient to produce a conduction block in a region where the fiber diameter is increased. The changes in shape of the computed action potentials under repetitive firing resemble those seen experimentally.

Of course, a step change in fiber diameter does not occur in nature. This restriction was made to simplify the equations, under the rationale that the space constant of an axon at frequency components of the action potential is relatively long in comparison to the region over which the diameter changes. However, the slope at which the diameter expansion occurs may be an important factor in the modulation of conduction. Figures 5, 6, and 7 show results of computations in which the same increase in diameter (fivefold) is taken over the same length of the axon (five segments), but the size of the individual steps is different. In this simulation, a train of six impulses is initiated at the extreme left end of the axon and records of membrane potential versus time are computed for various positions along the axon. It is clear that small variations in the rate of change of axon diameter give rise to markedly different patterns of signaling. In Figure 5 all six impulses propagate through the region of axon expansion. In Figure 6 propagation fails after only two impulses. In Figure 7 the conduction of every third impulse is blocked, producing an obvious recoding of the pattern of the action potential train. To understand how this recoding comes about it is convenient to look at the responses in the 35th segment (Figure 7). This response is composed of only four action potentials, each with a reflection potential. The reflection potentials following the second and fourth action potentials are sufficiently large that they initiate new action potentials (Figure 7, segment 20) and render the membrane refractory to the third and sixth stimuli in the original train, blocking their further propagation (Parnas, Hochstein, and Parnas, 1976). The role of reflection potentials in producing extra spikes in a train is treated by Calvin and Hartline (1977) and Calvin and Sypert (1976).

Propagation of action potentials in branching axons

THEORETICAL COMPUTATIONS   Goldstein and Rall (1975) computed that the conduction of an action potential through a branch point depends on the geometrical ratio (GR):

$$GR = \sum_i d_i^{3/2} / d_a^{3/2} ,$$

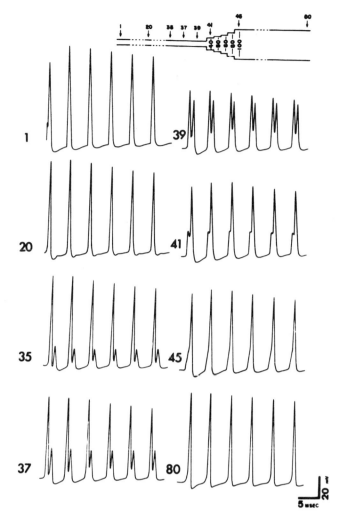

parent into the daughter branches has the same safety factor as conduction along an unbranched axon of the same diameter as the parent axon (independent of the diameter of the branches). When GR > 1, the safety factor will be lower, as in a region with an increase in diameter; and when GR < 1, the safety factor will be higher, as in the case of a decrease in fiber diameter (Figure 8).

Extending the numerical methods of Cooley and Dodge (1966) and Parnas, Hochstein, and Parnas (1976) for branching axons to include changes in extracellular potassium concentration, Parnas and Segev (in preparation) and Segev (1976) obtained the following results:

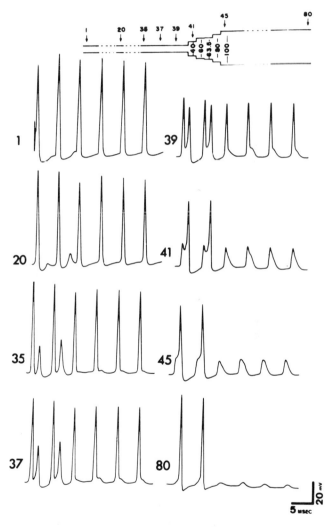

FIGURE 5 Computer simulation of a train of action potentials propagating over a sloped region. See inset for the shape of the axon and change in diameter. A fivefold increase in diameter over a distance of 500 μm was assumed. Sites of "recordings" and segment diameters are shown in the inset. The interval between action potentials was 5 msec. Note the change in the shape of the action potentials in the train as they approach and cross the sloped region. The diameter of the axon in segments 1–39 was 20 μm. Diameters of the following five segments in the sloped region were 40, 50, 60, 80, and 100 μm. Diameter of the axon after the slope was taken as 100 μm. The length of each segment Δx was taken as 100 μm. The time interval for integration was $\Delta t = 0.02$ msec; the periaxonal space θ, in which changes in potassium concentration during firing were assumed, was taken as 600 Å. The time constant for recovery processes for excess potassium was taken as 20 msec. (From Parnas, Hochstein, and Parnas, 1976.)

where d_a is the diameter of the parent branch and d_i is the diameter of the daughter branch i. The derivation is based on the assumption that the membrane properties are the same for all branches at rest and during activity. When GR = 1, conduction from the

FIGURE 6 Same conditions as in Figure 5, but with different segment diameters in the sloped region (given in the inset). Note that now only the first two action potentials propagated beyond segment 45, and that reflection potentials, in the region before the slope, are seen only for the first two action potentials. Diameters of segments in the slope were 40, 60, 63.5, 80, and 100 μm.

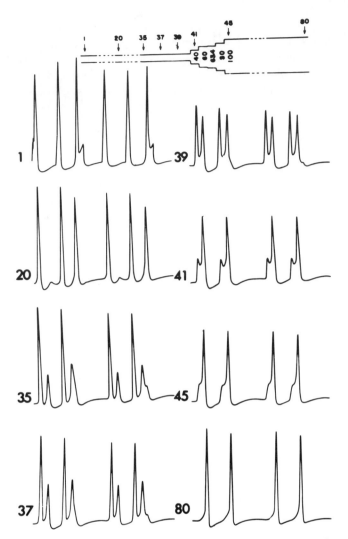

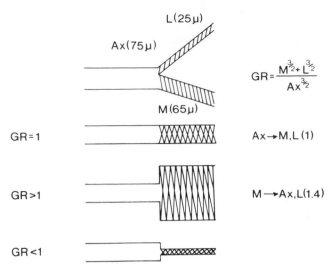

$$GR = \frac{M^{\frac{3}{2}} + L^{\frac{3}{2}}}{Ax^{\frac{3}{2}}}$$

GR = 1   Ax→M,L (1)

GR > 1   M→Ax,L(1.4)

GR < 1

FIGURE 8 A scheme of a branching axon and the equivalent cylinder (shaded areas) for conduction when the geometrical ratio is one, greater than one, and smaller than one. The diameters given are approximately those found in the common excitatory axon innervating the deep abdominal extensor muscles. (Ax, the parent branch; M and L, the daughter branches.) The geometrical ratio for conduction from Ax into M and L is one; from M into Ax and L, 1.4.

FIGURE 7 Same conditions as in Figures 5 and 6, but the diameter of segment 43 was reduced by 0.1 μm to 63.4 μm. In segment 35, note the large second and fourth reflection potentials. In segment 20, these reflection potentials spread backwards and initiated new action potentials; six action potentials are thus seen. Note that the intervals between the first and second original spikes and second and third extra spikes are not the same. The third and sixth extra spikes in segment 1 rendered the membrane refractory to the third and sixth original stimuli. Note the difference in train pattern in segment 1 and segment 80.

1. When GR = 1, conduction into the two branches is independent of branch diameter (even to a ratio of 1:1,000). When potassium accumulation is taken into account, conduction is blocked at the same instant in the parent axon and daughter branches.

2. When GR > 1 and potassium is allowed to accumulate extracellularly, impulses fail to propagate into both branches at the same time when conduction block occurs at the branch point.

3. Differential conduction into the two branches can be obtained when different periaxonal spaces around the two branches or different time constants for recovery processes are assumed, so that potassium accumulation around the two branches is not the same.

Figure 9 is an example of such a computation. A branching axon was stimulated at the parent branch to produce a train of four action potentials. Action potentials (lower traces) and potassium accumulations in the periaxonal space were computed along the parent branch (10A), the small branch (52S), and the large branch (52B). The time constant for recovery processes was the same for all branches, but the periaxonal space around the large branch was smaller (200 Å as compared to 600 Å in the small and parent branches). The result was a larger accumulation of potassium in the periaxonal space of the large branch, resulting in block of conduction in this branch (compare 52S and 52B).

EXPERIMENTAL FINDINGS An excitatory axon innervating the extensor muscles in the abdomen of the lobster (Parnas and Atwood, 1966) branches as it approaches the muscles into one large and one small daughter axon. The axons are easy to identify and record from and the geometrical ratio is close to one,

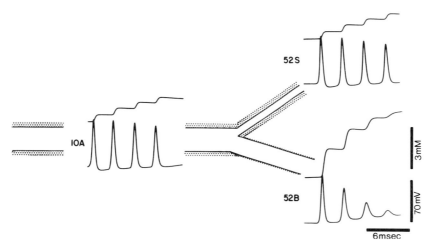

FIGURE 9 Computer simulation of a train of action potentials propagating in a branching axon with GR = 1. Potassium accumulation during the activity was assumed. The periaxonal space around the parent branch and small daughter branch were taken as 600 Å. The periaxonal space around the thick branch was taken as 200 Å. Time constant for recovery was taken as 20 msec for all branches. The upper traces indicate the change in potassium concentration in the periaxonal space. The lower traces show action potentials. Under these conditions, differential conduction is obtained.

making this an ideal preparation in which to study propagation of action potentials in a branching axon. Intracellular microelectrodes were used to record activity before (Ax) and after (M) the branch point and extracellular electrodes to record potentials along the two branches, M and L (see insert in Figure 10). As predicted theoretically, single action potentials propagated into both branches (Figure 10A). During high-frequency stimulation, however, the M action potential became smaller and its rise time became prolonged (Figure 10B), and then conduction into branch M failed, although action potentials still prop-

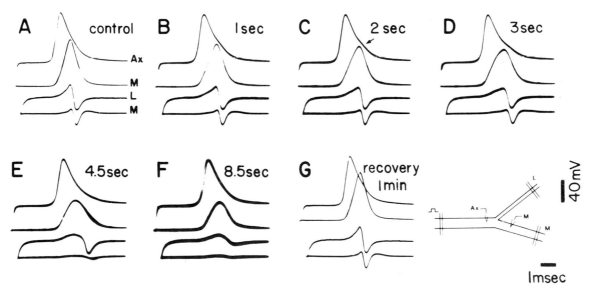

FIGURE 10 Differential conduction block at the M and L branches. The experimental setup is shown in the inset. *Top two traces*: intracellular recording at Ax and M. *Bottom two traces*: extracellular recording at M and L, 3 mm after the branch point. (A) Control; note the slower rise time in the M action potential. (B–F) Stimulation at 50 Hz at Ax. Time of stimulation is indicated above traces. Exposures composed of five superimposed sweeps. (C) After 2 sec of stimulation note hump (arrow) on falling phase of Ax action potential. (E) When conduction into M was blocked, the hump on the falling phase of the Ax action potential was missing. (F) Conduction block in both the M and L branches. (G) Recovery after rest.

agated into branch L (Figure 10C). With further stimulation, impulses failed to invade the L branch as well (Figure 10D). Two aspects of these results are at variance with the theoretical predictions: first, propagation into the two daughter branches did not fail at the same time; second, conduction failed only at the branch point and not along the parent and daughter axons as well.

In the lobster axons, the block of conduction was not associated with a marked membrane depolarization as was the case in the cockroach giant axons discussed above. However, although there was only a slight depolarization at the time of the block, the membrane resistance dropped by about 15%. It is clear that in this case the simple assumption of potassium accumulating in the periaxonal space to produce membrane depolarization, and consequently sodium inactivation, is not sufficient. For example, if the axon is directly depolarized by outward current injections, even by as much as 8–10 mV for prolonged periods (30 seconds), membrane resistance does not change and conduction is not blocked (Grossman, 1976).

A striking finding is that at the time of conduction block the electrotonic potential of 45 mV that passively spreads from Ax to M is not sufficient to initiate an action potential in M (Figure 10C). This suggests a marked increase in threshold in the M branch. Indeed, compared to controls, after high-frequency stimulation a fourfold increase in current is required

to stimulate branch M to produce an action potential (Grossman, 1976).

The theoretical analysis predicts block of conduction after high-frequency stimulation at the same instant in both the parent and the daughter branches. The experimental results, however, show not only differential conduction into the two daughter branches, but also that the block occurs at the branch point per se. Figure 11 shows activity recorded by microelectrodes at Ax and M when the axon was stimulated at both ax (orthodromically) and m (antidromically) at 50 Hz. Stimulation at ax preceded that at m in such a way that the two action potentials collided in branch m distal to the M microelectrode (A-C hatched area). In Figure 11A, therefore, only the action potentials initiated by stimulation at ax are seen. As soon as conduction from ax into m was blocked (Figure 11B,C), an antidromic action potential was recorded in M but not in Ax. Obviously, at the time of the block, collision could not take place, and the m action potential propagated antidromically to the M microelectrodes but could not cross the branch region into Ax. These results show that conduction was blocked across the branch point (in both directions) and that branch m was still excitable at that time. They also show that the safety factor for propagation of action potentials at high frequency from ax into m, or m into ax, is lower than for conduction in either ax or m.

What mechanisms allow differential conduction

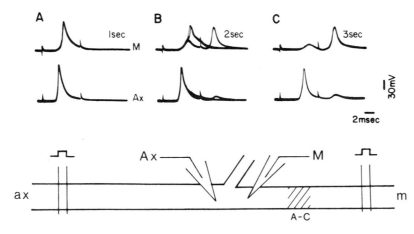

FIGURE 11 Collision experiment showing that conduction block at high frequency occurs at the branch point. The experimental setup is shown at bottom. The axon was stimulated with extracellular electrodes at both ax and m. Action potentials were recorded intracellularly at Ax and M. In A–C, ax stimulation preceded m stimulation with an interval such that the orthodromic and antidromic action potentials collided distally to the M microelectrode (hatched area). Therefore, in the control (A), the two microelectrodes Ax and M recorded only the orthodromic potential. (B) After two seconds of stimulation at 50 Hz, the action potential failed to invade from Ax into M (upper trace), and at the same instant the M electrode recorded the antidromic potential (upper trace right), which failed to invade the Ax region.

into branches of an axon when the geometrical ratio is one, and why does conduction fail only at the branch point? Attempts to answer these questions were made by assuming different densities of sodium channels in the different branches near the bifurcation (Zeevi, 1972, and personal communication). However, no experimental evidence to support such an assumption is available. On the contrary, data from patch-clamp experiments indicate that the peak inward current densities measured in Ax, M, and L either near the bifurcation or along Ax and the branches do not show significant differences (Grossman, 1976). In all three branches, the current density varied between 1.5 and 1.6 $\mu A/cm^2$. It is quite possible that the method of measuring current was not sensitive enough to show fine temporal or spatial differences; but as shown in Figure 12B, a decrease in peak inward current amplitude of more than 50% would be necessary to block conduction along Ax. Therefore, differences in the density of sodium channels do not appear to be large enough to account for the differential conduction of action potentials into the M and L branches. The remainder of this chapter will describe experiments aimed at explaining why conduction is blocked and why propagation into M fails before that into L.

During repetitive activation of an axon, changes in intracellular (sodium, calcium) as well as extracellular (potassium) ion concentrations take place (Hodgkin and Huxley, 1952; Frankenhaeuser and Hodgkin, 1956, 1957; Heyer and Lux, 1976a,b). The effects of similar changes in extracellular and intracellular ion concentrations on conduction, specifically those effects not directly attributable to changes in the resting potential or driving forces, were pursued by Grossman (1976). The question was whether a small increase in potassium concentration in the periaxonal space might cause conduction block by some mechanism not dependent on the slight membrane depolarization produced.

Figure 12 shows that this is in fact the case. Intracellular microelectrodes were inserted before and after the branch point, and extracellular electrodes were placed at branches M and L for recording and at Ax for stimulation. In addition, a patch-clamp electrode recorded membrane current at Ax (see inset to Figure 12 for details). About 10 minutes after the extracellular potassium concentration was increased by only 2.5 mM, the membrane was depolarized by about 2–3 mV and conduction was blocked; this occurred at the same instant in both the M and L branches and not differentially as seen after high-frequency stimulation. It is interesting that the peak

inward membrane current in Ax was reduced by about 50% and yet conduction along Ax was not blocked, showing again that the safety factor for conduction along Ax is higher than for that across the bifurcation. If at this stage the membrane was hyperpolarized back to its control level for 30 seconds, conduction into the M and L branches was not restored (Figure 12C), confirming that the small membrane depolarization itself did not cause propagation across the branch point to fail. However, a sufficiently strong hyperpolarization (14 mV for 5 seconds) could transiently restore conduction into the M and L branches (Figure 12D). In this experiment, recovery lasted for 11 seconds, after which conduction failed again (Figure 12E,F). After a washing with normal saline, conduction recovered at the same time in both branches. One conclusion from this experiment is that potassium, in addition to producing membrane depolarization, affects membrane excitability by some other mechanism. Additional support for this conclusion stems from the finding that small increases in extracellular potassium concentration produce membrane depolarizations greater than expected from the Nernst equation and reduce membrane resistance more than expected from the delayed rectification (Grossman, 1976).

The effects seen after high-frequency stimulation are similar to those occurring after the extracellular potassium concentration has been increased by 2.5 mM. These include a 10–20% reduction in effective membrane resistance, an approximately 15% reduction in the amplitude of the action potential in Ax, and a 2–5 mV membrane depolarization. In both cases a 10–15 mV hyperpolarization produces a temporary relief of the block. These similarities suggest that the main reason for the conduction block after stimulation at high frequency is the accumulation of potassium in the periaxonal space.

What mechanism can be responsible for the effects of such small increases in extracellular potassium concentrations? Adelman and Palti (1969a,b) showed in the squid giant axon, under voltage-clamp conditions, that when extracellular potassium concentration was increased by 25–100 mM, sodium inactivation was increased. Furthermore, by hyperpolarizing the membrane to −120 mV they could cancel the direct effects of potassium on sodium inactivation, probably through a reduction in the concentration of extracellular potassium in the periaxonal space. It is possible that extracellular potassium produces sodium inactivation in the case of the lobster axon also, and by a similar process a 15 mV hyperpolarization was sufficient to reduce transiently the small increase

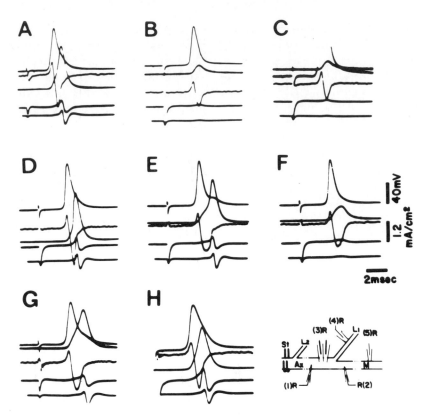

FIGURE 12 Effect of increase in extracellular potassium concentration on conduction. The experimental setup is shown in the inset. Intracellular recordings were made in Ax and M before and after the branch point (electrodes 1, 2). Membrane current was recorded at Ax (electrode 3), and extracellular recording electrodes were placed at M and L (electrodes 4, 5). (A) Control, after a single impulse at Ax. (B) About 10 min after extracellular potassium concentration was increased by 2.5 mM (normal concentration 12 mM), the membrane was depolarized by 2.5 mV and conduction into M and L was blocked. Note that despite the reduced membrane current in Ax it continued to con-duct action potentials. (C) Although the membrane was hyperpolarized by 2.5 mV to the control level, conduction was not restored. Between C and D the membrane was hyperpolarized by 12 mV for 5 sec. When the current injection was stopped, conduction into both M and L was restored (D), and the membrane current in Ax is almost the same as in the control. (E) Nine seconds later a slower rise time is observed in the M response. (F) After two more seconds, conduction was blocked again at the same instant in both branches. (G, H) Recordings after 15 and 18 min of wash in normal Ringer's.

(2.5 mM) in extracellular potassium. The time to restoration of block after the hyperpolarization (a few seconds) agrees well with the second time constant of sodium inactivation of Adelman and Palti (1969a,b). This increase in sodium inactivation is not sufficient to explain the reduction in effective membrane resistance and the differential block seen after high-frequency stimulation, and additional mechanisms should be sought. However, the striking finding from the experiment described above is that a small change in potassium concentration (2.5 mM) that is known to occur following a few impulses at high frequency (Frankenhaeuser and Hodgkin, 1956) produced conduction block.

Assuming that potassium accumulation is responsible for the failure of propagation across the bifur-cation, how can the differential block seen after high-frequency stimulation be explained? The increase in extracellular potassium concentration after high-frequency stimulation should not depend on branch diameter if the width of the periaxonal space around the two branches is the same. For this reason, conditions that allow for differential accumulation of potassium around the two branches were looked for. Such differential accumulation is possible if there are differences in the ultrastructure of the branches (width of periaxonal space, diffusion pathways, etc.), in their recovery processes (electrogenic pumps, uptake by other elements, diffusion pathways), or in the net efflux of potassium per impulse per unit area. These possibilities will be examined in turn in the following sections.

Ultrastructural studies

By the use of lanthanum and horseradish peroxidase as extracellular markers, it has been shown that there are no apparent differences in the widths of the periaxonal spaces around the parent and daughter branches, in the surrounding glial layers, or in the diffusion pathways (Grossman, 1976). Figure 13 shows the giant axon surrounded by a glial element with a periaxonal space of 200 Å. A network resembling sarcoplasmic reticulum is seen to traverse the glial cells (ER). That these networks are open to the extracellular space can be shown by the penetration of lanthanum through them (Figure 14). Thus there are no obvious differences in ultrastructure between the two branches that could give rise to a differential increase in extracellular potassium concentration.

Electrogenic pump

Different rates of recovery in the two branches might be a factor in a differential accumulation of potassium. One important recovery mechanism is the sodium-potassium pump (Thomas, 1972). Activation of

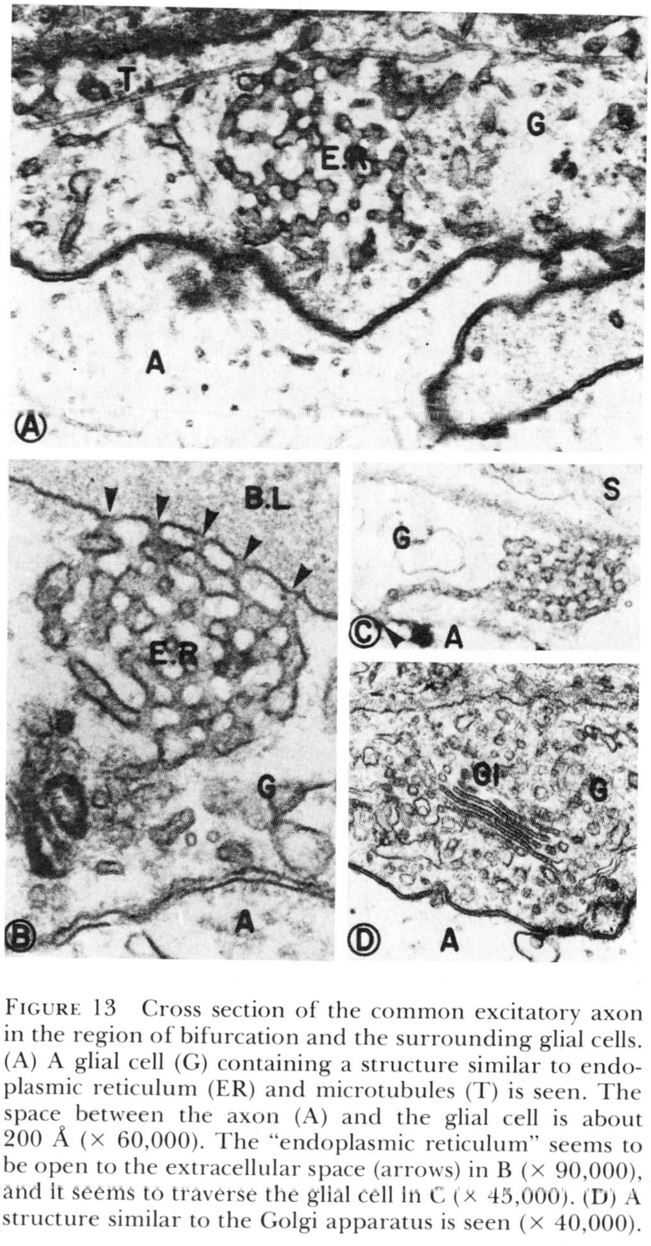

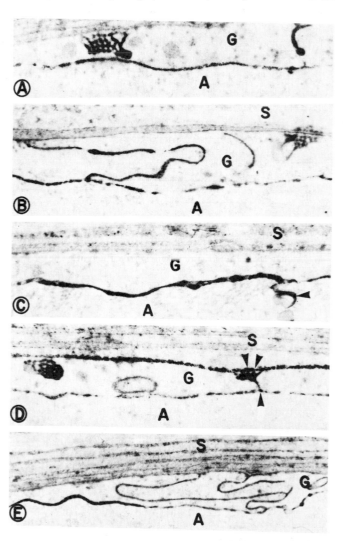

FIGURE 13 Cross section of the common excitatory axon in the region of bifurcation and the surrounding glial cells. (A) A glial cell (G) containing a structure similar to endoplasmic reticulum (ER) and microtubules (T) is seen. The space between the axon (A) and the glial cell is about 200 Å (× 60,000). The "endoplasmic reticulum" seems to be open to the extracellular space (arrows) in B (× 90,000), and it seems to traverse the glial cell in C (× 45,000). (D) A structure similar to the Golgi apparatus is seen (× 40,000).

FIGURE 14 By using lanthanum as an extracellular marker it can be seen that the "endoplasmic reticulum" and the periaxonal space are open to the extracellular space. All sections are from the same axon. A and B show sections in Ax; C, D, and E, sections in M. (A, axon; G, glia; S, interstitial tissue.) Arrows point to the opening of an "endoplasmic reticulum" to the periaxonal and extracellular spaces. Lanthanum penetrated well into the space between two adjacent glial cells.

a sodium pump after high-frequency stimulation has been demonstrated in several cases (Thomas, 1972; Van Essen, 1973; Jansen and Nicholls, 1973), and an electrogenic pump is present in lobster axons (Sokolov and Cooke, 1971; Grossman, 1976). A variety of experiments were done to determine how propagation through the branch point was affected by the activity of an electrogenic sodium pump. The most significant result was that after the pump was blocked with ouabain the time required for conduction failure during high-frequency stimulation was shortened. Since ouabain treatment causes a 5–8 mV depolarization, control experiments were done in which prolonged depolarization of 5–8 mV was produced by outward current injections. This shortened the time to conduction block by about 20%. In the ouabain-treated axons, the time required for block at the same frequency was shortened by 30–50%.

Thus it is possible that an electrogenic pump plays a role in the differential conduction at high frequency in the two branches. At high frequency, sodium ions will build up sooner in the thin branch. The increased intracellular sodium will trigger the electrogenic pump, producing two effects: (1) hyperpolarization, which by itself improves conduction at high frequency, and (2) a lowering of the potassium concentration around the thin branch, reducing or eliminating its effects on excitability.

Effect of Ca^{++} ions

Another factor that might prevent or delay the appearance of conduction block is an increase in the intracellular concentration of Ca^{++} ions. During the period of the action potential, Ca^{++} ions enter the axon (Baker, Hodgkin, and Ridgeway, 1971; Stinnakre and Tauc, 1973; Heyer and Lux, 1976a,b); and at high frequency intracellular Ca^{++} ions should reach higher levels in the thin branch than in the thick branch. To determine whether a difference in calcium accumulation might also be a factor in the differential conduction block, Ca^{++} was injected intracellularly (30 nA for 10 sec between two intracellular electrodes) into the axon at Ax. As a result, the duration of high-frequency stimulation required to produce a block was increased by a factor of 3–5. In addition, in cases where conduction from Ax to M was already blocked, Ca^{++} injection (30 nA for 10 sec) restored conduction for a period of 8–10 sec. Thus an increase in intracellular Ca^{++} concentration prevents or delays conduction block during high-frequency stimulation. The mechanism of Ca^{++} action is not known. It is possible that it triggers mechanisms

such as the electrogenic pump or that it reduces the net influx of potassium (as suggested by Heyer and Lux, 1976a,b).

Differential block

The results described so far suggest that the differential conduction of action potentials into two branches arises in the following way. During activity at high frequency there is an efflux of potassium into the periaxonal space and an influx of sodium and calcium into the axon. The ultrastructure of the axon and its branches, including the periaxonal space (200 Å) and glial sheaths, is the same at Ax as in the two branches M and L. Therefore, potassium accumulation around the axons should be the same, assuming that the membrane in the three branches has the same properties. On the other hand, due to the difference in surface-to-volume ratio in the two branches, during high-frequency stimulation intracellular sodium and calcium concentrations will rise faster in the thin branch, triggering the sodium pump and calcium-dependent mechanisms. This will lower the potassium concentration around the thin branch, resulting in a net difference in the accumulation of potassium around the two branches. The higher concentration of potassium around branch M will reduce its excitability, so that conduction of an action potential arriving from the parent branch Ax will be blocked.

Similar mechanisms seem to be involved in producing a conduction block in the two systems described in this article. In the cockroach, the geometrical organization of the axon is such that the safety factor for conduction is lowered in one region. A depolarization of 10 mV produces sufficient sodium inactivation to lower the safety factor further and block conduction; the increase in extracellular potassium was considered the main mechanism for producing the conduction block (Spira, Yarom, and Parnas, 1976; Parnas, Hochstein, and Parnas, 1976).

In the branching axon of the lobster, geometrical considerations again are important for differential conduction at high frequency. The accumulation of potassium, which reduces excitability more than expected from membrane depolarization alone (Adelman and Palti, 1969a,b; Grossman, 1976), is slowed around the thin branch by the earlier activation of the sodium pump and the increase in intracellular Ca^{++} concentration.

Conduction failure has been studied in other invertebrates. In the common excitatory axon innervating the opener and stretcher muscles in the legs of crayfish, Hatt and Smith (1975) suggested that in a certain region in the branch innervating the opener muscles, the enveloping sheath structure is denser, thus restricting potassium diffusion so that potassium accumulates more rapidly. They did not study whether potassium exerts effects on excitability beyond those expected from the associated change in resting potential. It is interesting that for the same axon of the crab (*Ocypoda cursor*) Benshalom and Parnas (1973) were unable to produce a conduction block, and the opener and stretcher muscles (and axon branches) followed activity even at 200 Hz.

In other branching neurons such as those of the leech (Van Essen, 1973; Jansen and Nicholls, 1973; Yau, 1976), the geometrical ratio can be greater than one. Propagation from the thin branch into the main branch of the touch-sensitive mechanosensory cell (GR ≈ 5) again has a low safety factor. In this system, it was suggested that activation of an electrogenic sodium-potassium pump produces such a strong hyperpolarization that the amplitude of the approaching action potential in the smaller branch is not sufficient to bring the main branch to threshold; thus conduction is blocked. Whether the activation of this pump occurs sooner in the thin branches was not determined.

Physiological significance

It is not clear whether the differential channeling of action potentials in these systems has behavioral significance. In the cockroach, the giant axons fire at high enough frequencies for sufficient lengths of time to produce conduction block (Spira, Yarom, and Parnas, 1976). The same was found to be true for the branching axon of the lobster (Grossman, 1976).

In the leech, natural activation of the touch sensory neuron is possible by touching the skin. At low frequencies, the touch cell can be stimulated from skin in its own segment as well as from skin in the anterior and posterior segments. With a strong touch, stimulation of the touch cells is sufficiently intense to block conduction from the adjacent segments.

In conclusion, several examples of conduction modulation in regions with special geometry have been demonstrated. The case of differential conduction at high frequency in a branching axon with a geometrical ratio of one should call for an extension of the Goldstein and Rall (1975) model to include *dynamic* changes that take place during high-frequency stimulation. In addition, the question remains open of why conduction block following high-frequency stimulation or the application of potassium occurs at the branch points even though the geometrical ratio is one. Clearly the complex arborizations of nerve cells cannot be considered simply as transmission lines but must be treated as active elements capable of modulating the flow of impulses from one region to another.

ACKNOWLEDGMENTS It is a pleasure to thank Dr. Bruce Wallace for his critical and constructive comments on the manuscript. The work was supported by Grant 741 from the United States–Israel Binational Science Foundation and by Grant AZ 11 1955 from Stiftung Volkswagenwerk.

REFERENCES

ADELMAN, W. J., JR., and Y. PALTI, 1969a. The influence of external potassium on the inactivation of sodium currents in the giant axon of the squid *Loligo pealei. J. Gen. Physiol.* 53:685–703.

ADELMAN, W. J., JR., and Y. PALTI, 1969b. The effects of external potassium and long duration voltage conditioning on the amplitude of sodium currents in the giant axon of the squid *Loligo pealei. J. Gen. Physiol.* 54:589–606.

ADRIAN, E. D., 1914. The all-or-none principle in nerve. *J. Physiol.* 47:460–474.

BAKER, P. F., A. L. HODGKIN, and E. B. RIDGEWAY, 1971. Depolarization and calcium entry in squid giant axon. *J. Physiol.* 218:705–755.

BENSHALOM, G., and I. PARNAS, 1973. Conduction of information in a motor axon innervating two muscles in different segments of the crab leg. *Israel J. Med. Sci.* 9:681–682.

BULLOCK, T. H., and C. A. TERZUOLO, 1957. Diverse forms of acivity in the somata of spontaneous and integrating ganglion cells. *J. Physiol.* 138:341–364.

CALLEC, J. J., 1972. Etude de la transmission synaptique dans le système nerveux central d'un insecte (*Periplanete americana*). Ph.D. thesis, Université de Rennes, Rennes, France.

CALVIN, W. H., and D. K. HARTLINE, 1977. Retrograde invasion of lobster stretch receptor somata in control of firing rate and extra spike patterning. *J. Neurophysiol.* 40:106–118.

CALVIN, W. H., and G. W. SYPERT, 1976. Fast and slow pyramidal tract neurons: An intracellular analysis of their contrasting repetitive firing properties in the cat. *J. Neurophysiol.* 39:420–433.

CASTEL, M. E., I. SPIRA, I. PARNAS, and Y. YAROM, 1976. Ultrastructure of region of a low safety factor in inhomogeneous giant axon of the cockroach. *J. Neurophysiol.* 39:900–908.

CHUNG, S., S. A. RAYMOND, and J. Y. LETTVIN, 1970. Multiple meaning in single visual units. *Brain Behav.* 3:72–101.

COOLEY, J. W., and F. A. DODGE, 1966. Digital computer solutions for excitation and propagation of the nerve impulse. *Biophys. J.* 6:583–599.

COOMBS, J. S., D. R. CURTIS, and J. C. ECCLES, 1957. The interpretation of spike potentials of motoneurons. *J. Physiol.* 139:198–231.

DODGE, F. A., and J. W. COOLEY, 1973. Action potential of the motoneuron. *IBM J. Res. Develop.* 17:219–229.

FARLEY, R. D., and N. S. MILBURN, 1969. Structure and function of the giant fiber system in the cockroach *Periplaneta americana. J. Insect. Physiol.* 15:457–476.

FRANKENHAEUSER, B., and A. L. HODGKIN, 1956. The aftereffects of impulses in the giant nerve fibre of *Loligo. J. Physiol.* 131:341–376.

FRANKENHAEUSER, B., and A. L. HODGKIN, 1957. The action of calcium on the electrical properties of squid axons. *J. Physiol.* 137:218–244.

FRIESEN, O. W., 1975. Physiological anatomy and burst pattern in the cardiac ganglion of the spiny lobster *Panulirus interruptus. J. Comp. Physiol.* 101:173–189.

GOLDSTEIN, S., and W. RALL, 1975. Changes of action potential shape and velocity changing core conduction geometry. *Biophys. J.* 14:731–757.

GROSSMAN, Y., 1976. Conduction of action potentials along bifurcating axons. Ph.D. thesis, The Hebrew University, Jerusalem, Israel.

GROSSMAN, Y., M. E. SPIRA, and I. PARNAS, 1973. Differential flow of information into branches of a single axon. *Brain Res.* 64:327–386.

HAGIWARA, S., and T. H. BULLOCK, 1957. Intracellular potentials in pacemakers and integrative neurons of the lobster cardiac ganglion. *J. Cell. Comp. Physiol.* 50:25–47.

HATT, H., and D. O. SMITH, 1975. Axon conduction block: Differential channeling of nerve impulses in the crayfish. *Brain Res.* 87:85–88.

HESS, A., 1958. Experimental anatomical studies of pathways in the severed central nerve cord of the cockroach. *J. Morphol.* 103:479–499.

HEYER, C. B., and H. D. LUX, 1976a. Properties of a facilitating calcium current in pacemaker neurons of the snail *Helix pomatia. J. Physiol.* 262:319–348.

HEYER, C. B., and H. D. LUX, 1976b. Control of the delayed outward potassium currents in bursting pacemaker neurons of the snail *Helix pomatia. J. Physiol.* 262:349–382.

HODGKIN, A. L., and A. F. HUXLEY, 1952. A quantitative description of membrane current and its application to conduction and excitation in nerve. *J. Physiol.* 117:500–544.

JANSEN, J. K. S., and J. G. NICHOLLS, 1973. Conductance changes, an electrogenic pump and the hyperpolarization of leech neurons following impulses. *J. Physiol.* 229:635–655.

KANDEL, E. R. 1976. *Cellular Basis of Behavior: An Introduction to Behavioral Neurobiology.* San Francisco: W. H. Freeman.

KHODOROV, B. I., YE. N. TIMIN, S. YA. VILENKIN, and F. B. GUL'KO, 1969. Theoretical analysis of the mechanisms of conduction of a nerve pulse over an inhomogeneous axon. I. Conduction through a portion with increased diameter. *Biofisika* 14:304–315.

KUFFLER, S. N., and J. G. NICHOLLS, 1976. *From Neuron to Brain: A Cellular Approach to the Function of the Nervous System.* Sunderland, MA: Sinauer Associates.

PARNAS, I., 1972. Differential block at high frequency of branches of a single axon innervating two muscles. *J. Neurophysiol.* 35:903–914.

PARNAS, I., and H. L. ATWOOD, 1966. Phasic and tonic neuromuscular system of the crayfish and rock lobster. *Comp. Biochem. Physiol.* 18:701–723.

PARNAS, I., S. HOCHSTEIN, and H. PARNAS, 1976. Theoretical analysis of parameters leading to frequency modulation along an inhomogeneous axon. *J. Neurophysiol.* 39:909–923.

PARNAS, I., M. E. SPIRA, R. WERMAN, and F. BERGMAN, 1969. Nonhomogeneous conduction in giant axons of the nerve cord of *Periplaneta americana. J. Exp. Biol.* 50:635–649.

ROEDER, K. D., 1948. Organization of the ascending giant fiber system of the cockroach *Periplaneta americana. J. Exp. Zool.* 108:243–262.

SEGEV, I., 1976. A mathematical model for the propagation of action potentials along a bifurcating axon. M. S. thesis, The Hebrew University, Jerusalem, Israel.

SOKOLOV, P. G., and I. M. COOKE, 1971. Inhibition of impulse activity in a sensory neuron by an electrogenic sodium pump. *J. Gen. Physiol.* 57:125–163.

SPIRA, M. E., I. PARNAS, and F. BERGMAN, 1969a. Organization of the giant axons of the cockroach *Periplaneta americana. J. Exp. Biol.* 50:615–627.

SPIRA, M. E., I. PARNAS, and F. BERGMAN, 1969b. Histological and electrophysiological studies on the giant axons of the cockroach *Periplaneta americana. J. Exp. Biol.* 50:629–634.

SPIRA, M. E., Y. YAROM, and I. PARNAS, 1976. Modulation of spike frequency by regions of special axonal geometry and by synaptic inputs. *J. Neurophysiol.* 39:882–899.

STINNAKRE, J., and L. TAUC, 1973. Calcium influx in active *Aplysia* neurons detected by injected aequorin. *Nature New Biol.* 242:113–115.

TAUC, L., and G. M. HUGHES, 1963. Modes of initiation and propagation of spikes in branching axon of molluscan central neurons. *J. Gen. Physiol.* 46:533–549.

THOMAS, R. C., 1972. Electrogenic sodium pump in nerve and muscle cells. *Physiol. Rev.* 52:563–594.

VAN ESSEN, D. C., 1973. The contribution of membrane hyperpolarization to adaptation and conduction block in sensory neurons of the leech. *J. Physiol.* 230:509–534.

WAXMAN, S. G., 1972. Regional differentiation of the axon: A new review with special reference to the concept of the multiplex neuron. *Brain Res.* 47:209–288.

WAXMAN, S. G., 1975. Integrative properties and design principles of axons. *Int. Rev. Neurobiol.* 18:1–40.

YAU, KING-WAI, 1976. Receptive fields, geometry and conduction block of sensory neurons in the control nervous system of the leech. *J. Physiol.* 263:513–538.

ZEEVI, Y. Y., 1972. Ph.D. dissertation, University of California, Berkeley.

29 Styles of Neuronal Computation

WILLIAM H. CALVIN and KATHERINE GRAUBARD

ABSTRACT Neurons seldom serve as relay stations; they typically transform their inputs in some manner to produce a new output function. A conventional processing path within a neuron includes a cascaded series of steps, each capable of contributing characteristic styles of computation: passive spread of PSPs to a spike trigger zone, spike initiation and repetitive firing, spike propagation, and ultimately synaptic output. We now know of many neurons where this one-way cascade must be supplemented with additional processes, such as intermittent conduction or dendritic spikes. There are also simpler cases, such as the passive-to-synaptic cascade of spikeless neurons. Styles of computation (e.g., arising from transient or sustained responsiveness, from high or low thresholds, and so forth) may be contributed by different stages of the cascade (e.g., from spike initiation regions, from conduction in axons, from synaptic input-output processes). Processing may thus differ among the various presynaptic regions of the same neuron.

Introduction

HOW DO NEURONS transform their input to produce something new? This is accomplished partly by wiring (the hierarchical arrangement of receptive fields in the nervous system provide an example: see Hubel and Wiesel, 1977) and partly by the intrinsic properties of the neurons. Here we shall be concerned only with how transformations occur *intra*neuronally; in particular, we shall be concerned with the processing pathway through the neuron and how its cascaded stages each contribute characteristics that determine the various overall styles of neuronal computation.

An example of the processing pathway comes from the "conventional neuron" commonly described in textbooks, where there is a one-way cascade of processes by which the synaptic inputs (confined to the soma-dendritic region) communicate with the synaptic outputs on the axon terminals. After the transmitter produces a synaptic current, the current spreads passively to the spike trigger zone (e.g., the axon's initial segment) rather than producing a local spike. The low threshold trigger zone summates positive and negative currents from a multitude of excitatory and inhibitory synaptic inputs. A decision made at this single site determines whether or not a spike will be produced. Once a spike is initiated, it propagates more or less faithfully to the output synapses on the far end of the axon. A standard amount of transmitter is then released by the spike, although some historical effects such as facilitation, depression, or potentiation are allowed in this conventional view; indeed the synapse would be the major candidate for plasticity since the rest of the neuron seems rather rigid.

The processing path thus includes a number of discrete, cascaded stages: passive spread, spike initiation, spike propagation, and synaptic transfer. Yet this description of the birth and death of a single spike is misleading; for most neurons, processing varies over time in several stages of the cascade. *Spike trains* are initiated, they propagate through regions with varying safety factors, and the synaptic release varies for the spikes that do reach the terminals. Thus even in the conventional neuron the input-output characteristics of the various stages give rise to several styles of computation: a sustained input may give rise to either sustained or transient responses; output may decline or build up during a sustained input; near coincidence in time by several large inputs may be required to produce an output; output may grade smoothly with the net sum of many inputs; and so forth. The style of computation need not remain fixed; it can vary over time as a result of such extrinsic influences as synaptic inputs or hormones, besides any intrinsic time or use dependencies.

There is also a story within a story: there are neurons in which some synaptic outputs act semi-independently of other synaptic outputs—that is, there are multiple processing paths within one neuron. While the anatomical unity of the neuron is unquestioned (Peters, Palay, and Webster, 1976), whether the single neuron is always a single functional entity has been questioned for decades (Bullock, 1959; Shepherd, 1972; Graubard and Calvin, this volume) as the conventional neuron model has become increasingly inadequate. The existence of spikeless neurons and of synaptic outputs intermixed with syn-

WILLIAM H. CALVIN and KATHERINE GRAUBARD Departments of Neurological Surgery and Zoology, University of Washington, Seattle, WA 98195

aptic inputs (e.g., dendrodendritic and axoaxonic arrangements) are of particular concern. In Table I we contrast some of the major features of the conventional neuron with some of the analogous disturbing features. While one cannot replace the conventional neuron with a modern view of equal simplicity, we shall attempt to show that the processing path itself can serve as a substitute concept for the elementary computing entity. When there is only one processing path within a neuron, the neuron will function as a unit; if there are multiple paths, it may not.

Black boxes vs. the experimental situation

We can never measure the actual quantities of transmitter received by the neuron membrane and compare this input with the actual output of transmitter from the distant axon terminals. As in Figure 1, the neurophysiological study of neuronal properties often involves two neurons at a time, for example, an electrode in the soma of one neuron and another electrode in the soma of a downstream neuron. This *transneuronal input-output function* taps into the cascade at a similar place in each cell and thus represents one neuron's worth of cascaded processes. We tend to translate this transneuronal input-output relation into a *neuronal input-output function*, considering it as if all of the cascaded processes were within a single neuron so that the usual black-box boundaries cor-

responded to the cell membrane. It is for this reason that we speak here of *input synapses* and *output synapses*. The input synapse is the postsynaptic element of the synapse as seen in the electron microscope. The output synapse of the same neuron corresponds to a presynaptic terminal. We thus reference our terminology all within one neuron and avoid the entanglements ("postsynaptic to the presynaptic neuron") involved with multiple-neuron terminology.

The simplest black box has many inputs but only one output (Figure 2A). If the black box is separated into a cascaded series of boxes, it is recognizably the processing path of the conventional neuron (Figure 2B). When a neuron has two semi-independent outputs (Figure 2C), one attempts to take apart the black box to show the stages in the processing path for each output (Figure 2D). These graphical representations can be pursued with mathematical elaborations, but we shall treat the subject here at the phenomenological level suitable to the present level of knowledge in cellular neurophysiology.

In some cases, the passive-to-excitable-to-synaptic cascade of the conventional neuron is augmented with additional stages. We begin, however, with a simpler case than the conventional neuron: the spikeless neuron, having only passive and synaptic stages in its processing path. Later the passive assumption about the membrane will be made more realistic. Excitability will be treated in the context of both den-

TABLE I

Conventional view of the neuron and aspects which, when seen in addition to (or substituted for) the corresponding aspects of the conventional neuron, raise questions about whether a single neuron can simultaneously produce different outputs

The Conventional Neuron	Additions or Substitutions
long axon	short axon, perhaps no axon
segregated input and output synapses	intermingled input and output synapses (e.g., dendrodendritic, axoaxonic)
spikes	spikeless neurons
all-or-none threshold decisions	graded firing rates, graded spikeless synaptic release
voltages as common currency	second messengers; metabolic modulation; indirect effects on pacemakers
a single decision-making site (e.g., initial-segment trigger zone)	multiple trigger zones; different decisions possible from different output synapses
faithful conduction of spikes	intermittent conduction: activation of normally silent branches?
standard amount of transmitter released by spike, or only minor historical effects	historical effects (e.g., facilitation, depression, potentiation), different at different output synapses from same cell.
taken together, suggest that neuron is a single functional "unit"	*suggest that each output synapse has the potential for semi-independent function*

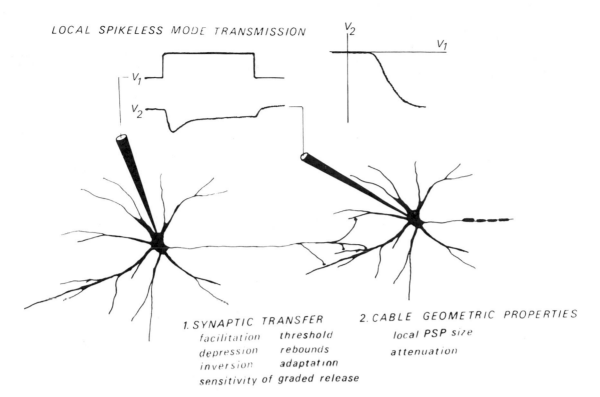

LOCAL SPIKELESS MODE TRANSMISSION

1. SYNAPTIC TRANSFER

facilitation   threshold
depression   rebounds
inversion   adaptation
sensitivity of graded release

2. CABLE GEOMETRIC PROPERTIES

local PSP size
attenuation

FIGURE 1 Cascade of intraneuronal processes in local spikeless computation. Since the reception and release of transmitter from a single neuron cannot be directly measured to obtain a true neuronal input-output relation, one works from the soma of one neuron to the soma of a downstream neuron and plots a transneuronal input-output curve (top). In spikeless cases, there may be only two stages to the cascade: passive spread and the synaptic transfer characteristics, sometimes supplemented by subexcitable phenomena such as rebounds.

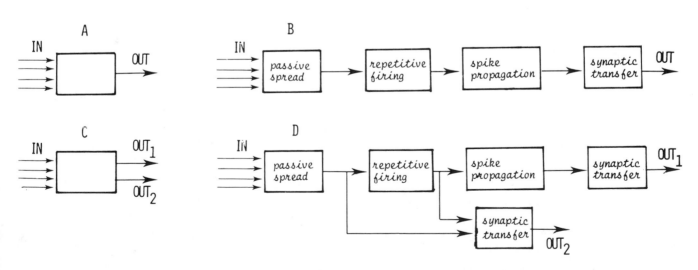

FIGURE 2 (A) The simplest neuronal input-output relation involves only a single output, which is a function of time and the inputs. (B) Decomposing the black box into the intraneuronal cascade of the "conventional neuron." (C) A case in which a neuron produces two semi-independent outputs that are differing functions of time and the inputs. (D) An example in which C can be decomposed into a conventional neuron cascade plus an output synapse operating on both spike trains and the passive spread of input currents.

dritic-spike "booster stations" and the properties of axon trigger zones. Repetitive firing, and the conduction of the spike train through intermittently conducting regions of the axon, will be examined for their characteristics. Finally, synaptic input-output processes and their interaction with presynaptic inhibition and facilitation will be considered for their contributions to the last step of the cascade.

Processing in the spikeless neuron

The transneuronal input-output function for a spikeless neuron is primarily determined by (1) the weighting of the input PSPs, as seen at an output synapse (determined by cable-geometric factors) and (2) the synaptic input-output relation itself. Thus the various output synapses from such a neuron could differ from each other by nonuniformity in either aspect.

The weighting of input PSPs depends strongly on the neuron's geometry and the location of the output synapse within this geometry (see Graubard and Calvin, this volume). Two output synapses located on the distal portions of different dendrites will be especially likely to differ from one another (provided that randomness of synaptic input locations does not obscure the intrinsic capability to emphasize one set of inputs and attenuate another). Two proximal dendritic or somatic output synapses are unlikely to differ significantly in the input weighting perceived.

The synaptic input-output properties could differ between the various output synapses from a given neuron. The release threshold (see Figure 3 in Graubard and Calvin, this volume) might differ, or perhaps the extent to which the output synapse adapts to a sustained depolarization. (The term "threshold" is, of course, a descriptive convenience; Llinás discusses the actual S-shaped relation elsewhere in this volume.) There is no indication that all of the outputs from a given neuron behave uniformly in synaptic transfer properties.

Were all of the output synapses to be segregated onto one process (an "axon") in a spikeless neuron, they would all receive the same *relative* weightings of the input PSPs. This is due to all of the passive spread being funneled through the bottleneck at the beginning of the axon. The only differences between such output sites would be greater attenuation and a lower frequency response for more distant terminals. Were all of these segregated output synapses to have uniform synaptic input-output properties, the spikeless neuron would then resemble the conventional neuron in that it could act as a "unit." It is the segregation

of output synapses onto a process different from the ones that receive input PSPs that is especially important for the "unitary" picture of neuronal computation, not spikes.

Adding complexity to the passive cable model

Two synapses active at the same time do not necessarily add their PSPs together linearly (e.g., 2 + 2 = 3). The simplest case of interaction is shunting (e.g., 2 + 0 = 1), where the second input produces a conductance increase but no voltage change because the reversal potential of that input is the same as the cell's resting potential. The conductance increase of this second synapse decreases the size of the first PSP by increasing the input conductance at the first synapse. This reduces the local size of the PSP as well as its size in the soma or at the spike trigger zone. Should an output synapse be located on the same process as the shunting input, its sensitivity to local and distant inputs would be reduced (see Calvin and Graubard, 1977).

Some synapses do not cause conductance increases but instead decrease membrane conductance (Weight, 1974; Carew and Kandel, 1976; but see Parnas, Rahamimoff, and Sarne, 1975); thus activity at an input synapse could increase the sensitivity of a neighboring output synapse to still other synaptic inputs. These sensitivity alterations are in addition to the effects of any synaptic current produced by the synaptic conductance changes when synaptic reversal potentials are not at the resting potential.

Second messengers such as cAMP, cGMP, and Ca^{++} (see Greengard, 1978) introduce a whole new realm of nonelectrical modulation. Should the internal calcium ion concentration be modulated near an output synapse by input synapse activity, one could have a modulation of the synaptic release function. Such calcium modulation might be secondary to synaptic activity or might arise from calcium entry because of a membrane conductance with voltage sensitivity (e.g., calcium spikes).

This raises the problem of changes in passive membrane properties that affect the cable properties: membrane resistivity, for example, may change severalfold within a physiological range of variation of voltage about the resting potential, thus changing the local PSP size and its attenuation with distance.

Rebound phenomena are also seen in spikeless cells (Graubard, 1978). Upon the removal of a hyperpolarizing current, the membrane potential may overshoot the resting potential. If the rebound is large enough, it can cross the release threshold, just as rebounds in spiking neurons sometimes cross the spike threshold.

Excitability, the regenerative property whereby depolarization begets more depolarization, provides a nonlinear amplification of input PSPs. In some cells, spikes arise locally in the dendrites; such dendritic spikes (see, e.g., Kuno and Llinás 1970) often have poor safety factors and only spread passively into the central regions of the neuron. From the standpoint of central decision-making processes, they may serve as boosters for certain combinations of input synapses. They could cause a large increment in release from output synapses near their sites of origin.

In a short-axon neuron, axon terminal output synapses could operate upon a combination of passively spread PSPs and spikes (see Figure 4 in Graubard and Calvin, this volume). As the axon becomes longer, the passively spread PSPs would become quite small but the height of an actively propagating spike would stay the same. Graded synaptic transfer characteristics (where threshold and graded release are key factors in determining transneuronal input-output properties) would decline in importance as standard-sized spikes came to provide the sole drive upon the presynaptic terminal. Decision-making would thus shift from emphasizing synaptic characteristics (as in Figure 1) to emphasizing those of the spike trigger zone at the beginning of the axon (as in Figures 3 and 4). Synaptic input-output curves have characteristics such as an apparent release threshold, a graded release region with an associated sensitivity, adaptation, rebounds, and historical factors such as facilitation/depression. When the actual output synapses are merely repeating decisions made elsewhere, one must ask what are the relevant characteristics of the spike production processes.

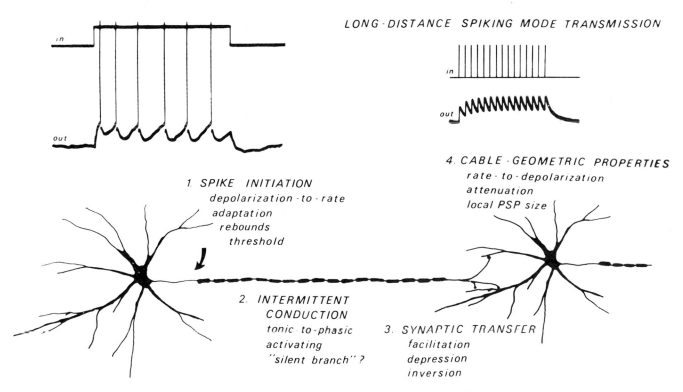

LONG-DISTANCE SPIKING MODE TRANSMISSION

1. SPIKE INITIATION
   depolarization-to-rate
   adaptation
   rebounds
   threshold

2. INTERMITTENT CONDUCTION
   tonic-to-phasic
   activating
   "silent branch"?

3. SYNAPTIC TRANSFER
   facilitation
   depression
   inversion

4. CABLE-GEOMETRIC PROPERTIES
   rate-to-depolarization
   attenuation
   local PSP size

FIGURE 3   Cascade of intraneuronal processes in long-distance transmission utilizing spike trains. The net depolarizing current in the initial segment of the axon produces a spike train whose rate varies with depolarization, as shown in Figure 4. Intermittent conduction may occur between the spike trigger zone and the output synapses, modifying the characteristics contributed by the spike-initiation process. The synaptic process itself contributes fewer features than in the spikeless case (Figure 1) if it is merely driven by standard-sized spikes. The passive characteristics of the dendritic tree of the downstream neuron are similar to the spikeless case, but the temporal summation of spike-evoked postsynaptic potentials tends to produce an average depolarization proportional to the spike rate (and hence to the original depolarization that produced the spike train in the upstream neuron, provided there is no modification by intermittent conduction or facilitation/depression).

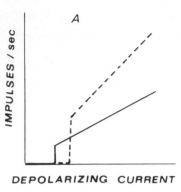
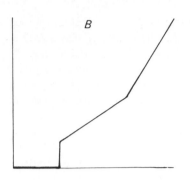
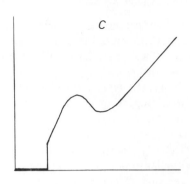

IMPULSES / sec

A

B

C

DEPOLARIZING CURRENT

FIGURE 4 Spike-initiation regions produce repetitive firing with various input-output characteristics. Typically there is minimum depolarization required to produce sustained rhythmic firing (A, solid line). The neuron then begins firing at its minimum rhythmic firing rate (e.g., 20/sec in a neuron with an afterhyperpolarization lasting 50 msec). The firing rate grades smoothly with additional depolarizing current with a certain sensitivity. In some neurons, the minimum depolarization, the minimum rhythmic firing rate, and the sensitivity are all greater (A, dashed curve). In some neurons, the depolarization-to-rate curve exhibits increases in sensitivity at intermediate currents (B).

This may be due either to alterations in the rhythmic firing oscillator process (as in the "secondary range" of cat spinal motoneurons) or to extra spikes (two-spikes-for-the-price-of-one, as in cat pyramidal-tract neurons). In some neurons, extra spikes are seen only at low depolarizing currents and gradually disappear as current is increased (e.g., cat and human spinal motoneurons). This may lead to a paradoxical drop in average firing rate as depolarization increases, and thus to a negative sensitivity region (C). As in Figures 1 and 3, the "data" shown is diagrammatic but based on recognized response types.

Production of spike trains

Spikes tend to originate from discrete sites called *trigger zones*; the initial segment of the axon is often the sole site from which spikes are initiated (although some cells utilize multiple trigger zones: see Iggo and Muir, 1969; Calabrese and Kennedy, 1974). It is the weighting of the PSPs at such a *virtual output site* that controls synaptic output at the far end of the axon. Central structures such as the soma and the initial segment often exhibit roughly equal weightings of input PSPs, with distal inputs being only 10–40% less effective than somatic inputs in their contribution to a steady depolarization level (unless extremely long, thin dendrites are involved; compare Figures 9–11 of Graubard and Calvin, this volume). Certainly the 35-fold range of relative weightings seen at some distal dendrodendritic synaptic sites is not characteristic of spike trigger zones (unless rapid transients in voltage are especially important, in which case somatic synapses are many times more effective: see Rinzel and Rall, 1974).

Besides weighting, one must consider the transfer characteristics of the spike production process. The conventional view of the neuron, which focuses on how a quiescent cell initiates a single spike, lends itself to the notion of a PSP standing on the shoulder of another PSP in order to reach the spike threshold. This "AND gate" view of neuronal computation may

be valid for some neurons in which the spike-evoked PSP from a single upstream neuron is very large, (e.g., 50% of the distance from the resting potential to the spike threshold). Most synaptic inputs to most neurons (see Calvin, 1975, for a review) are probably smaller than this by one or two orders of magnitude. Their pitter-patter integrates to create a graded shift in the membrane potential. It is the area beneath a spike-evoked PSP that determines its contribution to the net shift, not its peak value (Calvin, 1975). Suprathreshold shifts often produce a sustained train of spikes at the trigger zone, just as if the neuron were a pacemaker that only required some depolarizing bias to begin producing a rhythmic train of spikes.

REPETITIVE FIRING PROPERTIES The relationship between depolarizing current and average rhythmic firing rate has been studied in many types of neurons, typically by injecting current steps through the intrasomatic recording microelectrode to mimic a steady asynchronous synaptic bombardment. Figure 4A shows a typical current-to-rate curve (usually called a "frequency-current" or "f-I" curve). It exhibits a threshold current for the production of a sustained spike train. At this minimum current, the firing rate jumps up to a nonzero minimum rhythmic firing rate (e.g., 20/second). With more current, the firing rate increases in a graded manner; the slope of this relationship is called the *sensitivity*. Such properties are often a function of cell size (as inferred from axon conduction speed): "fast" neurons can have a higher minimum current requirement than "slow" ones, as well as a higher minimum rhythmic firing rate and a higher sensitivity (Figure 4A, dashed line; see Kernell, 1966; Koike et al., 1970; Calvin and Sypert, 1976).

Another feature of current-to-rate conversions is sometimes an alteration in sensitivity (Calvin, 1978a), such as the sudden increase in sensitivity shown in Figure 4B. In cat spinal motoneurons, these are called *primary* and *secondary ranges* (Granit, Kernell, and Lamarre, 1966) and are due to a marked alteration in the properties of the pacemaker-like oscillator process at the transition point (Schwindt and Calvin, 1972; Heyer and Llinás, 1977).

In some other cases, the rhythmic nature of the repetitive firing is interrupted by "extra" spikes occurring several msec after an "expected" rhythmic spike (Calvin, 1975, 1978a,b); the trigger zone is reexcited by depolarization from the antecedent spike. This two-for-the-price-of-one phenomenon can double the sensitivity of the current-to-rate curve, although compensatory processes may prevent the doubling in some cases (Calvin, 1978a). Sometimes this doubling of sensitivity occurs at the high end of the curve, as in Figure 4B; in other neurons, it occurs at the low end of the curve, with the extra spikes dropping out as current increases. The dropout can create a negative sensitivity region (Figure 4C; see Calvin and Hartline, 1977). Of course, the patterning of the spike train may carry a special significance beyond whatever changes it produces in the average firing rate; facilitation or potentiation at the output synapses may mean that extra spikes release much more transmitter.

Extra spikes and other phenomena altering the sensitivity are thought to be controlled by alterations in the retrograde invasion of the spike into the soma-dendritic region (Calvin, 1978a,b); for example, the retrograde invasion may actively involve the dendrites in some cases but only passively spread into the dendrites in other cases (see Heyer and Llinás, 1977).

Intrinsic Properties Controlling Repetitive Firing There are some cells, usually called *pacemakers*, that have intrinsic biases upon the repetitive firing processes. Some pacemakers burst; there are time-varying intrinsic currents which provide rhythmic depolarizing waves and periodically drive the cell up its depolarization-to-rate curve. Cells may be observed to shift from rhythmic pacemaker activity to bursting pacemaker activity (see Chalazonitis and Boisson, 1978). In some cases, synaptic (Parnas and Strumwasser, 1974) and hormonal (Barker and Smith, 1977) influences provide long-lasting activation of pacemaker activity and shifts from "pacing" to bursting. Some neurons "latch up," producing bursts that continue after a brief depolarization (Kandel and Spencer, 1961; Russell and Hartline, 1977); extra spikes can also be strongly influenced by recent history (Calvin and Hartline, 1977).

In addition, most neurons exhibit adaptation, that is, a decline in firing rate during a sustained depolarization. In some cases, this is due to electrogenic pumps providing a hyperpolarizing bias current (Nakajima and Takahashi, 1966); in other cases, the sensitivity of the depolarization-to-rate conversion declines (see, e.g., Schwindt and Calvin, 1972). In cells with extra spikes, the probability of extra spikes occurring may decline with time (Calvin and Sypert, 1976). When the minimum rhythmic firing rate is approached, the firing may shut off despite the sustained depolarizing drive. "Phasic" neurons are those with pronounced tendencies to shut down; this produces, of course, a distinct computational style.

As inputs fluctuate, one expects to see the spike rate vary along the current-to-rate curve, with time-locking to the input PSPs more noticeable when the input PSPs are individually large. As inputs fluctuate, the output patterning will change, reflecting not only the changing input but also any altered probabilities for producing extra spikes or bursts. As inputs fluctuate, adaptation will be reset.

Input-Output Characteristics of Repetitive Firing The overall characteristics of the spike production process may be briefly summarized as including a threshold, a region of graded response, adaptation, and rebounds from hyperpolarization. Thus the virtual output site has acquired the main features of spikeless synaptic processing, but it also has additional features (jumps to minimum output levels, distinct "ranges," of differing sensitivities) not yet observed in synaptic input-output curves.

Intermittent conduction

Even if the repetitive firing process sends a long train of spikes down the axon, only a brief train may reach some terminals; this can be one result of intermittent conduction, described elsewhere in this volume by Parnas. In this sense, the process may be descriptively similar to the adaptation process, producing a tonic-to-phasic conversion from the standpoint of some axon terminals. Conversely, some axon branches may be normally silent, so that a sustained train (or a burst, or some combination of factors) is required for spikes to begin invading these terminals (Waxman, 1975). Wall (1977) has described "ineffective synapses" in cat spinal cord and some of the circumstances that serve to unmask them; intermittent conduction and/or presynaptic inhibition changes are natural candidates for the underlying mechanisms.

Synaptic input-output properties: Basics and complications

The basic input-output features of a conventional neuron's synapse are essentially those of the transneuronal input-output curve in Figure 1. There is an apparent threshold presynaptic voltage which must be attained before there is any significant release. There is a suprathreshold region which is S-shaped, providing a roughly linear region, perhaps followed by a saturation region. Thus, for spike-evoked release, there is a standard-sized jump in release for a brief moment. For graded inputs, there can be graded output.

There are many phenomena associated with changes in synaptic input-output properties: facilitation, depression, and posttetanic potentiation are all historic effects known at many types of synapses. Parnas (1972) and Muller and Nicholls (1974) have noted that the extent of facilitation need not be identical at two different output synapses from the same cell and suggest that the differences lie in the presynaptic terminals.

The postsynaptic side of the synapse can also produce diversity in synaptic input-output properties. A single transmitter from a single presynaptic neuron can cause postsynaptic conductance changes that are brief or long-lasting, that increase or decrease, that affect different ions, and that selectively desensitize, all depending on the choice of postsynaptic receptor (see Kandel, 1976).

PRESYNAPTIC INHIBITION AND FACILITATION   Foremost among the possibilities for producing diversity at output synapses is presynaptic inhibition. Presynaptic inhibition (or facilitation) is the modulation in the size of a *mono*synaptic PSP subsequent to activation of a second pathway which itself produces no (or little) effect on the postsynaptic cell. Many mechanisms have been proposed to explain this phenomenon, and it is likely that there are, in fact, a number of ways to produce it.

Decreases in spike-evoked PSPs in a monosynaptic

pathway can often be observed if one can activate other neurons that will somehow depolarize the presynaptic terminals of the monosynaptic pathway. This physiological phenomenon is often associated with the anatomical finding of axoaxonic synapses, and it is thought that such input synapses near output synapses somehow condition spike-evoked release.

Depolarizing conditioning can produce alterations in synaptic input-output curves which reduce the release from a standard-sized stimulus (Hagiwara and Tasaki, 1958; Bloedel et al., 1966). Hyperpolarizing conditioning of cells also reduces spike-evoked release, as has now been demonstrated in arthropods, molluscs, and annelids (Maynard and Walton, 1975; Shimahara and Tauc, 1975; Wallace and Nicholls, 1977).

Another possible mechanism for presynaptic inhibition is a reduction in spike size in the presynaptic terminal, thus varying the "standard-sized" stimulus to synaptic release. This line of evidence, from crustacea (Dudel, 1965; Kennedy, Calabrese, and Wine, 1974), suggests that axoaxonic synapses produce sufficient conductance changes in the terminal as to cause a reduction in safety factor. If the active propagation of the spike ceases upstream from the terminal at various distances (intermittent conduction), the passive spread of the spike into the terminal should vary in size and hence vary the stimulus to synaptic release.

Other variations upon the intermittent-conduction theme are consistent with the results of Kuno (1974) in cat spinal cord, whose reductions in mean quantal content during presynaptic inhibition may be the result of the complete failure of spike-evoked release from some terminals contributing to a composite PSP. Recent investigations of "synaptic" facilitation and depression (e.g., Hatt and Smith, 1976) have uncovered a role of intermittent conduction well upstream from the axon terminals; while nonsynaptic factors such as extracellular potassium accumulation in critical regions of low safety factor are an identifiable mechanism (see Parnas, this volume), the influence of an axoaxonic synapse could likewise be well upstream of the actual output synapses at the axon terminals.

Presynaptic facilitation may be generated in the same manner as presynaptic inhibition, by activating a pathway that modulates spike-evoked transmitter release from the presynaptic neuron while itself causing little or no postsynaptic effect. In *Aplysia*—so far the only example (Castellucci and Kandel, 1976)— the mechanism is thought to involve a neuron synapsing on the presynaptic cell and causing an increase in cyclic AMP (and thus of internal Ca^{++}, which results in enhanced transmitter release). Unlike presynaptic inhibition, there is as yet no evidence that any particular synaptic geometry is involved in presynaptic facilitation or that the enhancement of release is selective in the output synapses it affects.

One need not view axoaxonic synaptic arrangements solely in the context of conditioning spike-evoked release, however. The small axon terminals are analogous to the distal dendritic tips in our prior discussion of dendritic geometry (Graubard and Calvin, this volume), and the input synapse may well produce a large local PSP, perhaps itself capable of stimulating release or modulating tonic release (Parnas, Rahamimoff, and Sarne, 1975).

RETROGRADE EFFECTS UPON PRESYNAPTIC TERMINALS? Could the postsynaptic neuron exert an influence over its own inputs? A direct retrograde influence of postsynaptic dendrite upon presynaptic axon has been sought for decades. Recently Erulkar and Weight (1977) utilized the squid giant synapse and showed significant decreases in spike-evoked EPSPs after conditioning by a train of *post*synaptic spikes. They found that increases in extracellular potassium could also produce such decreases in spike-evoked PSPs, suggesting that the release of potassium by the postsynaptic neuron "conditions" the spike-evoked release from the presynaptic terminal.

Discussion

The conventional neuron seemed rigid, lacking in major opportunities for plasticity except at the synapse itself. The present "complications" (summarized in Table II) point up the possibilities for flexible styles of computation elsewhere in the neuron. Now we have passive properties that might change (e.g., at the dendritic spine: Rall and Rinzel, 1971; Fifkova and Van Harreveld, 1977), excitable mechanisms influenced by more than just synaptic currents, and repetitive firing and intermittent conduction mechanisms with historic effects—all quite in addition to the promise of the synapse itself for plasticity.

Anatomists divide the neuron into morphologically characteristic regions; physiologists attempt to identify functional subdivisions and relate them to the anatomical ones. In the search for the elementary computing unit, how should one partition the neuron? Certainly not a priori along classical anatomical lines: outputs may occur from dendrites, while inputs may occur upon axon terminals. The usual physiological subdivisions of passive and excitable do not

TABLE II
Variations in neurons that affect input-output properties

1. Neurons can be organized with dendritic and axonal regions or they may lack all or part of this arrangement.

2. Synaptic inputs may be on dendrites, the soma, the initial segment of the axon, axon spines, or axon terminals.

3. A presynaptic neuron may distribute its output sites onto a single postsynaptic cell in a single restricted region, over several regions, or uniformly over the cell's synaptic surface.

4. Receptors for particular transmitters and conductance mechanisms may be uniformly distributed over the synaptic surface of the neuron or they may be regionally segregated.

5. Transmitter arriving at an input synapse may cause postsynaptic conductance changes that are brief or long-lasting, that increase or decrease, that affect different ions, or that selectively desensitize, all depending on the postsynaptic receptors.

6. For conductance-increasing synaptic inputs, two simultaneous inputs will produce a PSP that may be equal to, but is often less than, the sum of the individual input PSPs.

7. For conductance-decreasing synaptic inputs, two simultaneous inputs will produce a PSP that may be equal to, but could be greater than, the sum of the individual PSPs.

8. PSPs from single inputs may be very small, or their height may be an appreciable fraction of the excursion from the resting potential either to the spike threshold or to the threshold for graded transmitter release.

9. Passive spread may weight inputs equally or may strongly emphasize local inputs.

10. Passive spread could be affected by changes in membrane resistance with voltage (e.g., anomalous or delayed rectification).

11. Depolarizing "rebound" following the removal of hyperpolarization may be large or small and may vary in different parts of the neuron.

12. Action potentials can occur in dendrites, the cell soma, the axon and its terminals.

13. Spikes may propagate actively without decrement or spread passively with decrement in any part of the neuron.

14. Neurons may have a single low-threshold spike trigger zone, or there may be multiple trigger zones for initiating spikes.

15. Spike threshold may be lower if a rapid voltage change is used to approach it.

16. Slow approaches to spike threshold may never succeed in spike initiation, or they may always evoke a spike when a "ceiling" is reached beyond which accommodation no longer occurs.

TABLE II (continued)

17. Sustained depolarizations may evoke either a sustained or a transient train of spikes.

18. Adaptation may lower spike production rates, settling to a steady state in many seconds, within a few spikes, or instantly.

19. The minimum input current for producing a sustained spike train may be high or low (or zero for pacemakers), often depending on whether the cell is large or small.

20. The minimum rate at which a neuron will fire rhythmically can be low or high (usually depending on whether the spike afterhyperpolarization is long or short).

21. The curve relating depolarizing current strength to spike firing rate can bend over gradually, be linear, be piecewise linear, or exhibit hysteresis.

22. The sensitivity of the current-to-rate curve may be high or low (sometimes depending on whether the cell is large or small).

23. A sustained spike train evoked by a depolarizing current step may be rhythmic, irregular, rhythmic with occasional "extra spikes," or bursty.

24. Extra spikes following the expected spikes in a rhythmic discharge may increase the sensitivity of the current-to-rate curve, or compensation may occur by lengthening of the interval to the next expected spike.

25. Augmentation of current-to-rate sensitivity by extra spikes can occur at the high end of the curve or only at the low end (creating a "negative sensitivity region" at intermediate currents where extra spikes fail to occur).

26. Extra spikes may be augmented by fatigue or by lack of preceding activity.

27. Extra spikes may themselves reexcite the spike trigger zone to create another extra spike, or extra spikes may fail to create the conditions necessary for reexcitation.

28. Reexcitation may create extra spikes initiating from the axon trigger zone due to a delay, a change in conduction speed, or a prolongation of the retrograde invasion of the soma-dendritic region by the preceding spike.

29. Adaptation in spike rate during sustained depolarizations may be due to hyperpolarizing bias currents developing from a change in the sensitivity of the current-to-rate process or from a decreasing probability of extra spikes occurring.

30. Bursts of spikes may occur from reexcitation or from an underlying depolarizing drive upon the current-to-rate process.

31. Hormones or second messengers can modulate cell metabolism and ionic conductances and thus change the firing properties of the cell.

32. Spikes may propagate faithfully or may conduct only intermittently through some regions.

33. Spike conduction may begin to fail after only a few spikes, or only after many minutes, or never.

34. Synaptic outputs may be from distal or proximal dendrites, the soma, axon spines, axon swellings (en passage), or terminals and from almost any combination of regions.

35. Output synapses may be segregated from, or intermixed with, input synapses.

36. Synaptic release may be stimulated by spikes, graded PSPs, or a combination of both.

37. Hormones or second messengers may modulate synaptic release.

38. The synaptic input-output curve may be the same, or different, at the various output synapses from a given neuron.

39. The synaptic release threshold may be high or low.

40. Tonic release of transmitter from output synapses may be large or small, occasional or continuous.

41. Sensitivity (the slope of the synaptic input-output curve) may be high or low, positive or negative.

42. Synaptic release may increase or decline during long-lasting depolarizations.

43. Synaptic release during a sustained spike train may increase (facilitate), depress (antifacilitate), or remain the same with successive spikes.

44. Synaptic release may be potentiated, following a conditioning train of spikes, for a short time or for many days.

45. Facilitation may be the same or different, in magnitude and time course, at various output synapses from a given neuron.

46. Conditioning pathways may decrease (presynaptic inhibition) or increase (presynaptic facilitation) spike-evoked transmitter release from output synapses.

47. Presynaptic inhibition may be caused by conditioning depolarization or hyperpolarization of presynaptic terminals or by a conductance increase in the terminal region.

48. Tonic and spike-evoked release of transmitter may be modified by the ionic milieu, and thus perhaps by spike activity in the postsynaptic neuron.

allow for the array of subexcitable phenomena such as resistivity changes and rebounds. Graded and all-or-none regions were once useful divisions, but the extension of graded properties to spike generators and spikeless synapses has left only the middle of an axon with nominal all-or-none properties. One might try dividing the neuron into regions that compute (have thresholds and sensitivity, adaptation, and so forth) and those that merely conduct, but intermittent conduction in the middle of an axon can be viewed as creative failure, causing a tonic-to-phasic style just as surely as if the spike-initiating process had done it. Trying to divide the neuron into computing units is even harder: if one cannot define the boundaries of the elementary computing unit, or tell how many are contained within a single neuron, should we simply revert to the syncytium and give up in our attempt to define the most elementary building blocks with which the computing machine of the brain is built?

Difficult though it may be to delimit the boundaries of the computing unit, one can usefully trace the processing path through the cascade of intraneuronal processes linking the input synapses with the output synapses. We have seen both local and long-distance versions of this processing path, and it is apparent that an obvious candidate, upon which to base an elementary computing unit, is the processing path leading to an individual output synapse. Must one therefore treat a neuron with 100 separate output synapses as containing 100 elementary computing units? Not necessarily.

It is clear that we shall be able to view many CNS neurons as "units" much of the time. For example, cat spinal motoneurons are not reported to possess dendrodendritic synapses, and their various axon terminals are not known to differ functionally from one another in a manner that might segregate messages. Some neurons are perhaps "dual," such as the class of retinal horizontal cells studied by Nelson et al. (1975). These have two regions of extensive arborization, each with input and output synapses; one region synapses with rods, the other with cones. The two regions are connected by a long, thin axon that should severely attenuate PSPs. The cells seem to be spikeless. All of this suggests a neuron with two independent regions, almost as if it were two neurons (at least). In other cases, such as a superior colliculus horizontal cell (see Figure 11 in Graubard and Calvin, this volume), each output synapse along a long, thin dendrite might favor local inputs, with input effectiveness falling off with distance. Thus a dozen output synapses from one neuron might accomplish the job that otherwise would require a dozen neurons with more restricted dendritic trees.

Just as anatomists have long classified neurons by the shapes of their dendritic trees, so cellular neurophysiologists may come to recognize classes of neuronal computation styles. In the absence of the kind of analysis that has been partially done for a few cell types, can one use spiking/nonspiking as a major clue? This seems unlikely. Both spiking and nonspiking neurons can, under some conditions, function as elementary computing units; both types can also have diverse outputs, with regional influences superimposed upon central influences. Spike trigger zones do tend to provide strong central influences which, in the absence of additional processing between the trigger zone and the output synapses, will force all output synapses to act briefly as a unit. Combinations of Table I features such as "spikeless" and "intermixed input and output synapses" do make one suspect multiple computational units in such neurons. Until functional types of neurons are more clearly established by examining how they combine features such as those in Table II, the modern view of neuronal computation will be complicated by the necessity of examining each output synapse from a single neuron for the possibility that it is sometimes, in some sense, an elementary computing unit.

ACKNOWLEDGMENTS We thank T. H. Bullock for helpful suggestions. This research was supported by grants NS 09677 and NS 04053 from NINCDS/USPHS. K.G. was the recipient of postdoctoral research service award NS 05060 from NINCDS/USPHS.

REFERENCES

BARKER, J. L., and T. G. SMITH, JR., 1977. Peptides as neurohormones. *Soc. Neurosci. Symp.* 2:340–373.

BLOEDEL, J. R., P. W. GAGE, R. LLINÁS, and D. M. J. QUASTEL, 1966. Transmission across the squid giant synapse in the presence of tetrodotoxin. *J. Physiol.* 188:52P–53P.

BULLOCK, T. H., 1959. Neuron doctrine and electrophysiology. *Science* 129:997–1002.

CALABRESE, R. L, and D. KENNEDY, 1974. Multiple sites of spike initiation in a single dendritic system. *Brain Res.* 82:316–321.

CALVIN, W. H., 1975. Generation of spike trains in CNS neurons. *Brain Res.* 84:1–22.

CALVIN, W. H., 1978a. Setting the pace and pattern of discharge: Do CNS neurons vary their sensitivity to external inputs via their repetitive firing processes? *Fed. Proc.* 37:2165–2170.

CALVIN, W. H., 1978b. Re-excitation in normal and abnormal repetitive firing of CNS neurons. In *Abnormal Neuronal Discharges*, N. Chalazonitis and M. Boisson, eds. New York: Raven Press, pp. 49–61.

CALVIN, W. H., and K. GRAUBARD, 1977. Dendritic geometry and spikeless neuronal computation. *Neurosci. Abstr.* 3:1236.

CALVIN, W. H., and D. K. HARTLINE, 1977. Retrograde invasion of lobster stretch receptor somata in control of firing rate and extra spike patterning. *J. Neurophysiol.* 40:106–118.

CALVIN, W. H., and P. C. SCHWINDT, 1972. Steps in production of motoneuron spikes during rhythmic firing. *J. Neurophysiol.* 35:297–310.

CALVIN, W. H., and G. W. SYPERT, 1976. Fast and slow pyramidal tract neurons: An intracellular analysis of their contrasting repetitive properties in the cat. *J. Neurophysiol.* 39:420–434.

CAREW, T. J., and E. R. KANDEL, 1976. Two functional effects of decreased conductance EPSPs: Synaptic augmentation and increased electrotonic coupling. *Science* 192:150–153.

CASTELLUCCI, V., and E. R. KANDEL, 1976. Presynaptic facilitation as a mechanism for behavioral sensitization in *Aplysia. Science* 194:1176–1178.

CHALAZONITIS, N., and M. BOISSON, eds., 1978. *Abnormal Neuronal Discharges.* New York: Raven Press.

DUDEL, J., 1965. The mechanism of presynaptic inhibition at the crayfish neuromuscular junction. *Pflügers Arch.* 284:66–80.

ERULKAR, S. D., and F. F. WEIGHT, 1977. Extracellular potassium and transmitter release at the giant synapse of squid. *J. Physiol.* 266:209–218.

FIFKOVA, E., and A. VAN HARREVELD, 1977. Long-lasting morphological changes in dendritic spines of dentate granular cells following stimulation of entorhinal area. *J. Neurocytol.* 6:211–230.

GRANIT, R., D. KERNELL, and Y. LAMARRE, 1966. Synaptic stimulation superimposed on motoneurones firing in the 'secondary range' to injected current. *J. Physiol.* 187:401–415.

GRAUBARD, K., 1978. Synaptic transmission without action potentials: Input-output properties of non-spiking presynaptic neuron. *J. Neurophysiol.* 41:1014–1025.

GREENGARD, P., 1978. Phosphorylated proteins as physiological effectors. *Science* 199:146–152.

HAGIWARA, S., and I. TASAKI, 1958. A study on the mechanism of impulse transmission across the giant synapse of the squid. *J. Physiol.* 143:114–137.

HATT, H., and D. O. SMITH, 1976. Synaptic depression related to presynaptic axon conduction block. *J. Physiol.* 259:367–393.

HEYER, C. B., and R. LLINÁS, 1977. Control of rhythmic firing in normal and axotomized cat spinal motoneurons. *J. Neurophysiol.* 40:480–488.

HUBEL, D. H., and T. N. WIESEL, 1977. Functional architecture of macaque visual cortex. *Proc. R. Soc. Lond.* B198:1–59.

IGGO, A., and A. R. MUIR, 1969. The structure and function of a slowly adapting touch corpuscle in hairy skin. *J. Physiol.* 200:763–796.

KANDEL, E. R., 1976. *Cellular Basis of Behavior.* San Francisco: W. H. Freeman.

KANDEL, E. R., and W. A. SPENCER, 1961. Electrophysiology of hippocampal neurons. II. Afterpotentials and repetitive firing. *J. Neurophysiol.* 24:243–259.

KENNEDY, D., R. L. CALABRESE, and J. J. WINE, 1974. Presynaptic inhibition: Primary afferent depolarization in crayfish neurons. *Science* 186:451–454.

KERNELL, D., 1966. Input resistance, electrical excitability and size of ventral horn cells in cat spinal cord. *Science* 152:1637–1639.

KOIKE, H., N. MANO, Y. OKADA, and T. OSHIMA, 1970. Repetitive impulses generated in fast and slow pyramidal tract cells in intracellularly applied current steps. *Exp. Brain Res.* 11:263–281.

KUNO, M., 1974. Factors in efficacy of central synapses. In *Synaptic Transmission and Neuronal Interaction*, M. V. L. Bennett, ed. New York: Raven Press, pp. 79–85.

KUNO, M., and R. LLINÁS, 1970. Enhancement of synaptic transmission by dendritic potentials in chromatolysed motoneurones of the cat. *J. Physiol.* 210:807–821.

MAYNARD, D. M., and K. D. WALTON, 1975. Effects of maintained depolarization of presynaptic neurons on inhibitory transmission in lobster neuropil. *J. Comp. Physiol.* 97:215–243.

MULLER, K. J., and J. G. NICHOLLS, 1974. Different properties of synapses between a single sensory neurone and two different motor cells in the leech CNS. *J. Physiol.* 238:357–369.

NAKAJIMA, S., and K. TAKAHASHI, 1966. Post-tetanic hyperpolarization and electrogenic Na pump in stretch receptor neurone of crayfish. *J. Physiol.* 187:105–127.

NELSON, R., A. V. LÜTZOW, H. KOLB, and P. GOURAS, 1975. Horizontal cells in cat retina with independent dendritic systems. *Science* 189:137–139.

PARNAS, I., 1972. Differential block at high frequency of branches of a single axon innervating two muscles. *J. Neurophysiol.* 35:903–914.

PARNAS, I., R. RAHAMIMOFF, and Y. SARNE, 1975. Tonic release of transmitter at the neuromuscular junction of the crab. *J. Physiol.* 250:275–286.

PARNAS, I., and F. STRUMWASSER, 1974. Mechanisms of long-lasting inhibition of a bursting pacemaker neuron. *J. Neurophysiol.* 37:609–620.

PETERS, A., S. L. PALAY, and H. deF. WEBSTER, 1976. *The Fine Structure of the Nervous System: The Neurons and Supporting Cells.* Philadelphia: Saunders.

RALL, W., and J. RINZEL, 1971. Dendritic spines and synaptic potency explored theoretically. *Int. Cong. Physiol. Sci. Proc.* 9:1384.

RINZEL, J., and W. RALL, 1974. Transient response in a dendritic neuron model for current injected at one branch. *Biophys. J.* 14:759–790.

RUSSELL, D. F., and D. K. HARTLINE, 1977. Inputs to the lobster stomatogastric ganglion unmask bursting properties in many of its motorneurons. *Neurosci. Abstr.* 3:1227.

SCHWINDT, P. C., and W. H. CALVIN, 1972. Membrane-potential trajectories between spikes underlying motoneuron firing rates. *J. Neurophysiol.* 35:311–325.

SHEPHERD, G. M., 1972. The neuron doctrine: A revision of functional concepts. *Yale J. Biol. Med.* 45:584–599.

SHIMAHARA, T., and L. TAUC, 1975. Multiple interneuronal afferents to the giant cells in *Aplysia. J. Physiol.* 247:299–317.

WALL, P. D., 1977. The presence of ineffective synapses and the circumstances which unmask them. *Phil. Trans. R. Soc. Lond.* B278:361–372.

WALLACE, D. G., and J. NICHOLLS, 1977. Modulation of transmitter release at an inhibitory synapse on the CNS of the leech. *Neurosci. Abstr.* 3:1665.

WAXMAN, S. G., 1975. Integrative properties and design principles of axons. *Int. Rev. Neurobiol.* 18:1040.

WEIGHT, F. F., 1974. Physiological mechanisms of synaptic modulation. In *The Neurosciences: Third Study Program*, F. O. Schmitt and F. G. Worden, eds. Cambridge, MA: MIT Press, pp. 929–941.

30 Modeling of Neurons and Neuronal Networks

ANDRÁS PELLIONISZ

ABSTRACT Neuronal systems have been investigated at the molecular, membrane, cellular, network, and system levels, and a multitude of experimental techniques have been used at each level. Due to the complexity of neuronal systems, however, it is often impossible to account for holistic properties at any level on the basis of detailed components. The task of synthesizing all essential data into a self-consistent framework is made harder by the fact that data are often obtained from different levels and with different methodologies.

Using the cerebellum as an example, it is shown that neuronal modeling, as a conceptual representation of data, can be an effective tool to bridge these gaps, especially if the quantitative methodology is aided by computers. A computer model of the cerebellum is presented, based on current morphological and physiological data. It accounts for structurofunctional properties of single neurons (e.g., the so-called complex spike of Purkinje cells) and of the entire cerebellar cortex (e.g., gross spatial distribution and individual dynamical properties of activated cells within the structure of 1.68 million neurons). Finally, the expanded model also encompasses global cerebellar systems (e.g., fundamental characteristics of vestibulocerebellum and the cerebellar coordination of locomotion).

Introduction

NEUROSCIENCE, in its relatively short history, has amassed such a formidable body of data that unifying approaches are becoming necessary to assess the functional implications of new results. The problem is twofold. First, as the body of data grows it is increasingly difficult, due to sheer volume, to establish the relative significance of a given datum. Furthermore, it is not uncommon to have some knowledge of the overall properties of a system and some particular details of the system, with large gaps between the two sets of information. Second, because experimental observations are sometimes obtained in the absence of a general concept, their ultimate use is often quite limited. These problems threaten the continuing synthesis of experimental findings into general concepts.

It is clear that to overcome these problems a quantitative methodology is needed that can provide a self-consistent framework for the handling of complex data. One such methodology is neuronal modeling, which has become a powerful tool with the advent of computers. This has the additional merit of bridging the gap between experimentalists and theoreticians and thus promoting dialogue.

This paper will outline some aspects of neuronal modeling. Then, with the cerebellum as an example, computer modeling of individual neurons and neuronal networks will be discussed.

Outline of neuronal modeling

Although the word *model* from the Latin *modulus* (small measure) is usually taken to mean an "illustration," "prototype," or "standard," in this paper the term *neuronal model* refers to a conceptual representation of data concerning neurons or neuronal systems. If the underlying principle is hypothetical, then the model provides the methodology by which it may be determined whether the hypothesis is consistent with the available data in a systematic quantitative manner. As a body of data grows in complexity, confirmation or falsification of hypotheses becomes increasingly crucial, and thus modeling becomes an indispensable tool.

Models have three important characteristics. First, they are powerful in organizing and simplifying the body of data, since they dictate, by definition, the class of data to be included. Second, modeling is an important heuristic tool that helps us gain insight into how the data are related to underlying concepts. Such insights and the deeper understanding that the modeling yields often lead to new hypotheses. Third, properly designed models are predictive, that is, they reveal previously unseen conclusions that are often testable experimentally.

Neuronal modeling is used in neurobiology as well

ANDRÁS PELLIONISZ Department of Physiology and Biophysics, New York University Medical Center, New York, NY 10016

as in artificial-intelligence research, but it is used for different purposes in each discipline. In artificial intelligence the aim is the design of machines capable of performing particular brainlike functions, even though their working principle may be totally different from that of brain. Consequently the role of neuronal modeling in artificial intelligence is limited to the representation of data that fit into a scheme (often biologically unrealistic) of a particular brain function such as pattern recognition.

In contrast, neurobiology seeks to understand how the nervous system itself works. Since there can be no a priori decision concerning which particular function or functional unit is the key to understanding the basic principles of its operation, neuroscience adopted an all-out strategy: the nervous system has been studied stimultaneously at *all* levels of complexity and by *all* available experimental techniques. As a result, the body of available data is as unwieldy as its interpretation is diverse. In neurobiology, modeling should therefore serve as a tool for synthesis. This crystallization of data starts at several points

simultaneously, by a cementing together of smaller groups of experimental evidence. Accordingly, neuronal modeling has developed along several lines that were at times independent of one another, and at times quite intertwined. The main evolutionary lines in neuronal modeling are illustrated in Table I. A rough chronology also gives perspective, although sometimes a digression in time may be necessary to reconstruct a particular line of models from its conception.

For the early history of neuronal modeling the reader is referred to the excellent reviews of Harmon and Lewis (1966) and Cole (1972). Modern neuronal modeling stems from three roots: efforts were made (1) to interpret the nervous electrical phenomena, (2) to abstract the principles of functional organization of neuronal assemblies, and (3) to relate morphology to function in the central nervous system.

Electrophysiology began its development with Helmholtz (1853), who realized that some fundamental electrical properties of the nerve, such as its slow conduction velocity, could not be interpreted in terms

TABLE I

Main evolutionary lines in the modeling of neurons and neuronal networks.

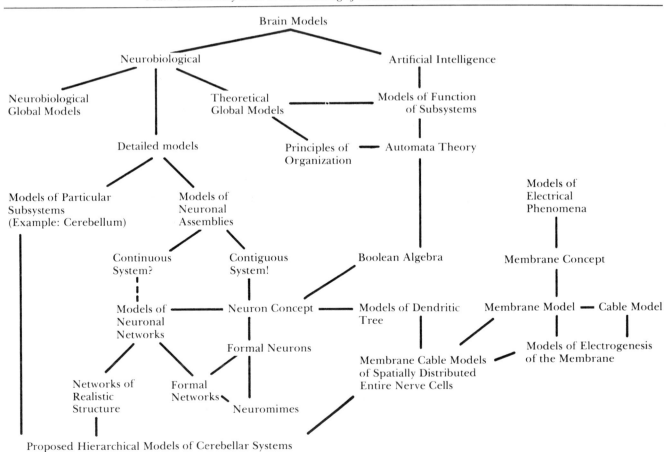

ANDRÁS PELLIONISZ

of the electrical properties of known conductors. Equally important was Bernstein's hypothesis that neurons are encompassed by a membrane that governs the different ionic milieus across the cell (Bernstein, 1902).

Although "global" concepts for brain function such as the reflex-schools of Sherrington (1906) and Pavlov (1927) gave great impetus to neurobiology, only recently has this kind of global approach been developed into a theoretical model of the organization of the brain. The best-known examples of these efforts are those of Ashby (1952), Young (1964), and, in a different light, von Neumann (1959), who pointed out the fundamental differences between brains and computers. Von Neumann's essay had a most salutory effect since the prevailing neuron model gave a misleading impression that the two systems (computers and brains) had a common basis in Boolean algebra (see below).

The idea that the morphology of neuronal assemblies reflects their function prompted a "mapping" of circuitries, resulting in a vast amount of detail (see Ramón y Cajal, 1911). The pursuit of the meaning of neuronal form not only diversified the body of data but also led to controversies. For example, did the neuronal assemblies constitute a continuous net or a set of contiguous units? This question was first answered with the help of light-microscopic methods, and the consequent neuron concept blossomed in the classical work of Ramón y Cajal (1911). Final consolidation of the neuron doctrine was later achieved with the help of electron-microscopic techniques (see Szentágothai, 1975).

Another open question was whether understanding the properties of single neurons and neuronal networks was a sequential task. One may contend that in order to understand circuits, the function of their elements must first be known. Then again, it may be impossible to understand the properties of elements without first knowing the principles by which they are organized into networks. Neurobiologists adopted the only practical strategy—simultaneous exploration of both the properties of networks and single neurons. As a result, neuronal modeling has been plagued by an obvious ambivalence, pursuing networks and single neurons, sometimes separately, sometimes jointly, with varying degrees of emphasis on one or the other. [Recently new considerations have influenced this matter: (1) Results showing that assemblies of neurons can be directly affected through the interneuronal ionic medium (see Nicholson, this volume) lessen the emphasis on the axonal "wiring" among neurons of a network. (2) The dom-

inance of axonal wiring in the organization of a circuit is seriously brought into question by the existence of dendritic interactions via local circuit neurons (see Shepherd, this volume).]

ABSTRACT FUNCTIONAL MODELS: FORMAL NEURONS
Once the neuron doctrine was accepted, the morphological investigation of different kinds of neurons and neuronal networks rapidly became a major field of research. From a functional viewpoint, the mechanisms underlying the working of single neurons was tackled rather early. McCulloch and Pitts (1943) proposed the so-called formal-neuron model, which equates a neuron to a decision-making unit that performs logical threshold functions on its inputs and, as a result, generates a binary output. Boolean algebra was thus applicable to formal neurons, so that the function of even networks of neurons could be handled, although the structures of the circuits studied were largely arbitrary. The formal-neuron model was of interest because it linked single neurons to neuronal networks, but the main reason for the popularity of the McCulloch-Pitts view was that it tied brain theories to the rapidly developing field of computer science. By equating neurons to electronic flip-flops and neuronal networks to finite-state automata and to computers, the misconception was established that the success by brain research and that of computer science were directly coupled. In spite of the disillusionment of von Neumann (1959), the field of formal-neuron modeling expanded rapidly, and some of its adherents are still to be found making analogies between computers and brains or representing a single neuron as a set of several decision-making elements.

Formal-neuron modeling diverged in three directions. One direction was the exploration of events occurring in arbitrary neuronal nets. Discrete computer models of networks by Rochester et al. (1956) and Farley and Clarke (1961) and continuous mathematical models by Beurle (1956) are prominent examples of this approach. Boolean algebra provided a second avenue for handling assemblies of formal neurons and interpreting their potential function. This theoretical approach overlapped with abstract automata theory (and this field therefore linked neuronal modeling to artificial intelligence and to computer science). The works of Turing (1950), Kleene (1956), Uttley (1959), Arbib (1969), and the school of Caianello (1968) are typical of this approach (see also Griffith, 1971, and Reiss, 1964). The third approach was the physical representation of highly simplified neurons by small electrical circuits (so-called neuromimes: see Harmon, 1959; McGrogan, 1961; Jenik, 1962; Lewis, 1964). Although this approach received a great impetus from the widespread acceptance of the McCulloch-Pitts concept, it is actually rooted in an idea of Schmitt (1937), who created the binary-output electrical circuit that realizes threshold function (the Schmitt trigger).

These artificial neurons were meant to be used for analysis of the salient properties of simple networks. For example, this approach was combined with a simple arrangement of spinal motoneurons to provide a cyclic firing pattern similar to the spinal pattern generator for locomotion in *Urodela* (Székely, 1965) and led to the use of mathematical methods to describe abstract properties of cyclic nets of formal neurons (Ádám, 1968). This latter approach represented a departure from arbitrary networks of highly simplified neurons and moved toward a more realistic representation of neuronal activity. Moving in the opposite direction (toward abstraction via automata theory), the formal-neuron concept was implicitly utilized to interpret the overall function of subsystems of the nervous system (Rosenblatt, 1962).

DIVERSITY IN MODELING: CEREBELLAR MODELS Research on the cerebellum can be divided into two main lines. The first seeks a theoretical explanation of overall function based on a single hypothesis with little concern for other functional details. One example is the model of Braitenberg (1961), which suggests that the cerebellar cortex is a timing device that utilizes the delays provided by the conduction time in parallel fibers. Another example shows rather clearly how an abstract idea can develop into a "theory": The hypothesis of modifiable synapses by Hebb (1949) was gradually turned into a theory for motor learning in the cerebellum (Brindley, 1964) and was further elaborated by Marr (1969) and Albus (1971) but failed to gain experimental support (see Eccles, 1973).

The second line provides a complementary approach: the generation of realistic models of detailed functioning. These phenomenological models can be further grouped into two categories according to whether they bypass or follow the neuron concept. If the representation of single neurons is bypassed in a cerebellar model, the system can be significantly simplified and treated linearly (Calvert and Meno, 1972). Similarly it may be viewed from a system-theoretical point of view without taking into consideration details of cerebellar structure and function (Arbib, Franklin, and Nilsson, 1968). Other approaches treat larger assemblies of neurons as units (Mortimer, 1970) or

emphasize the dynamics of the operation of circuitry (Boylls, 1975). In the second category of phenomenological models, the integral components of neural assemblies are single neurons. As mentioned before, neuronal networks have proved not to be continuous in structure. Still the idea held that the structure of the networks bears direct relevance to their function. In the special case of the cerebellum, this structuro-functional approach to neuronal networks was firmly established by Szentágothai (1963, 1968, 1975). The idea of deducing the basic functional properties of a system from morphological structure required systematic quantitative morphological models of circuitry (Palkovits, Magyar, and Szentágothai, 1971a,b,c, 1972). On this basis, phenomenological models containing McCulloch-Pitts-type neurons were constructed (Pellionisz, 1970). Later single units featuring some aspects of dendritic neuronal models were used (Pellionisz and Szentágothai, 1973, 1974). A similar approach to cerebellar modeling has been used by Mittenthal (1974).

The above approach has been applied to the visual cortex by von der Malsburg (1973). A review of current conceptual models of neuronal organizations (including the cerebellum) is provided by Szentágothai and Arbib (1974).

MODELING OF NEURONAL ELECTRICAL PHENOMENA The first significant theories developed to explain electrophysiological phenomena focused on the role of the cellular membrane and were based on the concepts of Bernstein (1902). Rashevsky (1933) and Hill (1936) used differential equations to develop an empirical description of the membrane potential in an active nerve, based on the idea that two opposing forces lie behind the dynamism of the rising and falling phases of an action potential. The pursuit of the phenomena underlying the genesis of action potential was greatly advanced by the development of sophisticated electrophysiological techniques, especially the powerful method of voltage clamping (see reviews by Katz, 1966, and Cole, 1972).

Probably the single most important development in the modeling of neuronal electrical phenomena was that of Hodgkin and Huxley (1952). They provided an empirical description of the electrogenesis of regenerative membrane discharge. In this model, the constants for a set of differential equations were established by fitting theoretical curves to the data obtained by voltage clamping the squid giant axon. This model is based on the notion that the sodium and potassium ion channels of the membrane have a time- and voltage-dependent permeability. That is, the dynamics of the permeability is responsible for the characteristic shape of the observed action potentials. The strength of this model is that it is a quantitative elaboration of Bernstein's ionic membrane theory. Thus the solution of the Hodgkin-Huxley equations could be related directly to a variety of electrophysiological recordings. The predictive power of the model has provided a stimulus for a vast array of investigations (for reviews see Cole, 1972; Adelman, 1971; Jack, Noble, and Tsien, 1975).

Despite its obvious strengths, the model has several conceptual limitations. For example, the only question the Hodgkin-Huxley model asks is, "How does the dynamics of ion permeabilities explain the shape of the active membrane potential?" Also, the relevance of the original model was limited to a spatially homogeneous segment of an axon.

The Hodgkin-Huxley model has proven to be very flexible since it was formulated a quarter of a century ago. For example, the parameters of equations have been adapted to preparations other than the squid giant axon (for the sciatic nerve of frog see Frankenhaeuser and Huxley, 1964).

The differential equations made the quantitative handling of the Hodgkin-Huxley model cumbersome before the advent of digital computers. In fact, digital computers were probably the most important determinant in the widespread applications of this model (FitzHugh, 1955; FitzHugh and Antosiewicz, 1959; Cooley and Dodge, 1966; Adelman and Fitzhugh, 1975). As stated above, by combining the original Hodgkin-Huxley equations with the cable equations, (which were originally applied to transatlantic telegraph lines by Lord Kelvin (1855) and then to excitable cells by Weber (1873), the Hodgkin-Huxley model is capable of explaining spatially distributed electrical phenomena. This allows mathematical treatment of the propagation of a spike along the axon (Joyner, Moore, and Ramon, 1975; Hardy, 1973). Recent techniques permit the computation of action-potential propagation even along spatially inhomogeneous axons (see Parnas, this volume).

The differences between the fully developed formal-neuron models and the Hodgkin-Huxley cable models are clear. Formal-neuron models address themselves to the ultimate function of neurons. The Hodgkin-Huxley model is concerned with the precise description of the shape of the output signal. It follows from this fundamental difference that for formal-neuron models the "wiring" of axonal connections is crucial, whereas for the Hodgkin-Huxley model only the membrane properties of the axon are important.

Such basic theoretical questions as the nature of neuronal coding or of neuronal information processing are not directly addressed by the Hodgkin-Huxley model, but they are amenable to study by successors of formal-neuron models (von Neumann, 1956; Perkel, 1970; Bullock, 1970). As for neuronal integration, formal neurons provided a simple abstraction stating that integration is a threshold function. The unsatisfactory character of such a solution to this basic question became increasingly evident through the years as a result of morphological and electrophysiological findings and theoretical studies. If nothing else, the impressive polymorphic appearance of dendritic trees made a simple threshold function unlikely, even from a teleological point of view. Further, detailed studies of the electroresponsiveness of dendritic trees strongly suggested that the concept of neurons being simple decision-making units was at best an oversimplification (see Llinás and Nicholson, 1971).

The question of how synaptic inputs arriving at various locations on a passive dendritic tree might propagate electrotonically to the soma has been studied in great detail by Rall (1959, 1962, 1964; for review see Rall, 1977). The idealization of dendritic trees into uniform equivalent cylinders simplified the analysis of the contribution of dispersed inputs to the passive steady-state membrane potential in the dendrites. Although this technique provided an excellent approach to relating dendritic electrotonic phenomena to cable properties (Calvin, 1969; for review see Jack, Noble, and Tsien, 1975), it was only recently combined with the Hodgkin-Huxley equations to model a motoneuron (Dodge and Cooley, 1973). This modeling technique was carried one step further in order to treat neurons with complex morphologies. This was accomplished through multicompartmental Hodgkin-Huxley cable models in which each spatial compartment quantitatively represents both the particular structural properties of the neuron and the electrical parameters of its membrane. The model incorporated functional inhomogeneities throughout the entire neuron. Such a mathematical model (Pellionisz and Llinás, 1975, 1977a) was shown to be capable of synthesizing a single-unit morphology with detailed electrophysiological findings and of providing a means for the analysis of complex membrane properties, such as the role of multiple sites of spike initiation in the integrative properties of single neurons. A similar model for the motoneuron was recently developed by Traub and Llinás (1978), and by Dodge (this volume).

It is conceivable that by including the dynamics of

calcium ion membrane conductance in the Hodgkin-Huxley model (see Llinás, this volume), it will become possible to analyze the role played by calcium currents in the integrative properties (and eventually in the neuronal coding mechanism) of nerve cells.

Neuronal modeling in cerebellar research

The most striking feature of diversity of cerebellar research is the multitude of simultaneous levels of approach. This is due in part to the limits of applicability of the various methods. For example, electron-microscopic techniques are most suitable for studying spatial relationships between synaptic structures, while microelectrode techniques are well suited to single-unit analysis. The pluralistic approach is also a result of the divergent basic considerations that guide this research. For example, the network approach led to investigations of neuronal assemblies, while the membrane theory stressed the importance of investigations at the membrane level.

In this section, cerebellar research will be used as an example of the role of modeling in bringing apparently divergent data together. It will be shown that within a hierarchy of complexities on several levels there are data available concerning both the details of the machinery and the overall properties that emerge from the details. Still, the complexity of the unit under investigation masks the relationship between the parts and the whole. By creating a common basis, a model allows the data to be synthesized and allows us to establish how the complex system is more than the simple sum of its components.

MODELING SINGLE CEREBELLAR NEURONS   As in other areas of neurobiology, the main thrust of cerebellar research is at the level of single cells. These investigations are especially fruitful because at this level there is a convergence of several basic considerations: (1) neuronal form reflects function; (2) the neuron is the unit of activity; and (3) networks of single cells should be studied from a structurofunctional viewpoint. Further, several experimental methods, including light and electron microscopy and intra- and extracellular electrophysiology, are applicable at single-neuron level.

This section presents a computer model of the Purkinje cell (Pellionisz and Llinás, 1975, 1977a). The goal of this model is to account for the functional properties of the total neuron from its morphological and functional details. This will enable us to synthesize electrophysiological recordings (which reflect the electrogenesis of the whole, spatially distributed cell)

from details of morphological structure and membrane properties. Explanations will thus be given for different characteristic intracellular recordings, such as the hitherto ambiguously interpreted "complex spike" of Purkinje cells.

Why should we concentrate our efforts on this particular type of neuron of the cerebellar cortex? There are two reasons. First, the cerebellar cortex is of special interest because it is morphologically unique. Its regular, almost crystalline cytoarchitecture is constructed from only a handful of types of neurons. It has but two input systems: the mossy-fiber/granule-cell/parallel-fiber path and the climbing-fiber input. These afferents converge on the only output elements, the Purkinje cells (for details see Eccles, Ito, and Szentágothai, 1967; Llinás, 1969; Palay and Chan-Palay, 1974). Moreover, it apparently lacks internal loops that could perpetuate reverberations; the interneuron systems (comprised of Golgi, basket, and stellate cells) are not only entirely inhibitory but are a superposition onto the so-called "basic circuit" of lower species such as amphibians (see Llinás, 1969).

Second, the single Purkinje cell is a center of interest because (1) it is the sole output neuron, (2) the two input systems converge on it, and (3) the convergence is extreme (as many as 400,000 parallel fibers may contact one Purkinje cell in the cat: see Palkovits, Magyar, and Szentágothai 1971a). On the other hand, there is one and only one climbing fiber per Purkinje cell, but they form a large number of contacts (in frog, 200–300 synapses; see Hillman, 1969a). Finally, (4) the Purkinje cell is remarkable in both its size and its anisotropic dimensions: it has an almost planar dendritic tree (measuring about 250 × 250 × 8 microns; see Figure 5A).

There is a wealth of morphological data available for cerebellar Purkinje cells (see Hillman, 1969a; Llinás, 1969). Moreover, using quantitative three-dimensional stereological methods (especially computer-aided methods) the morphological features of this cell can be established to an unprecedented degree of precision and completeness (Hillman, Chujo, and Llinás, 1974; Somogyi and Hámori, 1976).

The details of the generation of electrical signals in this cell are also well understood, especially since all of our basic knowledge of membranes (the Hodgkin-Huxley model, cable theory, and methods for modeling electrotonic signal propagation) should be applicable to this kind of neuron. In addition to a wealth of morphological and physiological details concerning the machinery of the Purkinje cell, considerable information is available on the overall properties emerging from the entire cell. This latter knowledge is provided largely through single-unit electrophysiology, for which the Purkinje cell is an ideal target since it has a large soma (about 15 μm in diameter even in the frog: Hillman, 1969a) and it can be activated in three distinctly different ways: (1) orthodromically by parallel fibers, both naturally and by artificial electrical stimulation (Eccles, Llinás, and Sasaki, 1966a), (2) antidromically by artificially evoking a backward invasion of the neuron via stimulation of the outgoing axon in the white matter of the cerebellar cortex (Llinás, Bloedel, and Roberts, 1969), and (3) orthodromically by the climbing fiber of the Purkinje cell (Eccles, Llinás, and Sasaki, 1966b; Martinez, Crill, and Kennedy, 1971). While all three activations result in markedly different waveforms of the action potential, the climbing-fiber-evoked response (CFR) stands out with its complicated pattern of wavelets; it is appropriately called a "complex spike" (see Figure 5).

Details and overall properties of the Purkinje cell are shown in Figure 1. An intracellular recording of an antidromically evoked spike in frog cerebellum is shown in Figure 1B. Coupling the information available on both the structural and functional details (electroresponsive properties of membrane) would, in theory, allow one to account directly for such overall properties as the characteristic waveform of antidromic response (note the prolonged afterdepolarization in Figure 1B). However, the complexity of even one cell is too great to be penetrated by intuitive reasoning. Therefore, while such a rather simple response as the antidromically evoked action-potential waveform can be speculated about with relative ease and with some confidence, for the interpretation of more complex phenomena such as the climbing-fiber response of Purkinje cells, a systematic methodology is needed. Elaborating such a technique for Purkinje cells offers an advantageous opportunity since the threefold challenge of markedly different responses to parallel-fiber-evoked orthodromic, artificial antidromic, and climbing-fiber-evoked orthodromic stimulations provides a reasonable guarantee that if the model produces all these different responses accurately, then it must represent the Purkinje cell realistically.

In order to synthesize the morphological, membrane biophysical, and electrophysiological data into a meaningful whole, a model of the Purkinje cell was developed (Pellionisz and Llinás, 1975, 1977a; see Figure 2). This model combines the Hodgkin-Huxley membrane model and cable theory with the electrotonic propagation of dendritic signals. Specifically, morphological knowledge of a particular dendritic

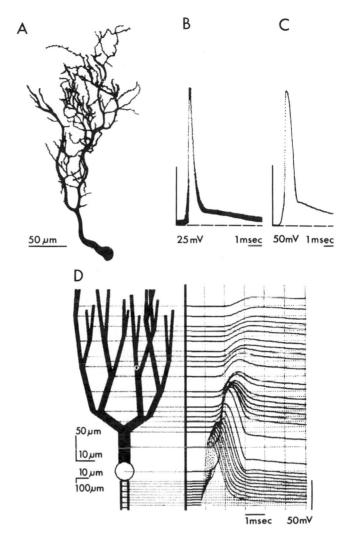

FIGURE 1 Structurofunctional model of the Purkinje cell. A: Golgi-impregnated Purkinje cell of the frog (after Hillman, 1969a). B: Intracellular recording of the Purkinje cell response to antidromic stimulation (courtesy of Llinás and Sugimori). C: Comparable output of the computer model: somatic membrane potential response to antidromic stimulation (from D). D: Computer model synthesizing morphological and electrophysiological data to provide an explanation for the electrogenesis of antidromic response throughout the model Purkinje cell. To the left is the model neuron composed of 62 compartments with individual morphological and physiological variables. All dendritic compartments are passive. To the right are the membrane potential waveforms at different compartments. (From Pellionisz and Llinás, 1975, 1977a.)

tree and the somatoaxonal area is merged with electrophysiological data. The model directly relates the two sets of information and could provide the needed explanation for the waveform of the antidromically evoked action potential (as shown in Figure 1C, D). An outline of this modeling method is given below.

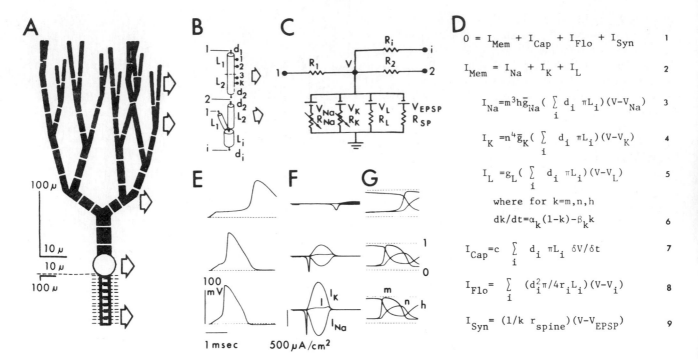

FIGURE 2   Scheme of the model of Purkinje cell with particular setting of structural and functional parameters of each compartment. A: Structure of compartmentalization (62 compartments: 31 dendritic branches, 15 bifurcation points, soma, initial segment, and 7 nodes with 7 myelinated segments). B: Single compartment with individual values for length (L_i) and diameter (d_i). C: Equivalent circuit for one compartment. All functional parameters (including Na and K excitability) are individually set. D: Equations governing the membrane electrogenesis for each compartment. The membrane potential (V) is determined by four currents: transmembrane (eq. 2; as described by the Hodgkin-Huxley equations 3–6), capacitive (eq. 7), longitudinal (eq. 8), and synaptic (eq. 9). E–G: Solutions by numerical integration of the Hodgkin-Huxley equations (as a function of time following a brief current injection) for three compartments. *Upper row*: Dendritic branching (low excitability). *Middle row*: Soma. *Lower row*: Node of Ranvier (high excitability). E: Membrane potential. F: Transmembrane currents. G: Hodgkin-Huxley *m, n, h* variables. (After Pellionisz and Llinás, 1975, 1977a.)

In this approach the entire neuron (dendritic tree, soma, initial segment, and axon) is constructed of cylindrical segments of specific lengths and diameters. The ability to assign values to each segment individually is especially important because the abstraction of real dendritic trees into equivalent cylinders is permitted only for trees following the 3/2 constraint of branching power (Rall, 1959, 1962, 1964); apparently, Purkinje cells do not obey this rule (Hillman, this volume). Another important advantage of modeling particular cells is that the electrical properties of each compartment are also determined individually. Therefore, each compartment can be set to conform electrically with either a passive (resistor-capacitor) or an active equivalent circuit (with individualized setting of Hodgkin-Huxley excitability parameters). In this way the model can be used to investigate the functional implications of a partially or totally active dendritic tree, even one that elicits dendritic spikes (Purpura, 1967; Nicholson and Llinás, 1971; Czéh, 1972; Llinás and Hess, 1976).

In modeling the antidromically evoked response of Purkinje cell the dendritic compartments were initially assumed to be passive resistor-capacitor cables. Application of a brief (<0.05 msec) current injection of 10 nA to the lowermost axonal compartment evoked an antidromically propagated axonal spike and a response at the soma level comparable to electrophysiological recordings (Figure 1B, C). The display of the intracellular voltage across the different dendritic segments reveals a rapid reduction of membrane potential with distance from the soma. For dendritic trees, reduced to equivalent cylinders, the attenuation of the electrotonic invasion in response to a given spike waveform could also be described by the theory of passive cables (see Jack, this volume). This attenuation in the Purkinje-cell dendritic tree is in good agreement with conclusions drawn from field-potential analysis (Llinás, Bloedel, and Roberts, 1969; Freeman and Nicholson, 1975).

Orthodromic activation of Purkinje cells by parallel-fiber stimulation via surface electrodes has been thoroughly investigated (Eccles, Llinás, and Sasaki, 1966a), and theoretical consideration has also been given to the possible implications of differences in integration as a result of different spatial patterns of parallel-fiber input (Llinás, 1970). This type of Purkinje-cell activity was modeled by current injections into dendritic spines distributed over the dendritic arborization (Pellionisz and Llinás, 1975, 1977a; see Figure 2B).

Spatially different orthodromic activations, assuming a passive dendritic tree, are modeled as shown in Figure 3. If the tree is stimulated through parallel fibers in a horizontal strip along the uppermost dendritic branches via a brief (0.5 msec) current pulse, the depolarization propagates electrotonically in much the same way as expected from Rall's studies (1964), and the stimulus remains subthreshold (Figure 3B). However, if the current injection is applied 0.05 msec longer, then after a delay of 2 msec a spike is generated which propagates along the axon and produces an attenuated electrotonic invasion of the upper dendrites.

By comparison, vertical application of a synaptic input of equal strength and duration as in Figure 3C results in a markedly different response (Figure 3D, E). Thus vertical integration produces an amply suprathreshold depolarization, resulting in a short "burst" of two propagating spikes.

Beyond the analysis of passive cable properties of particular arborizations, this model also yields a powerful method with which to explore effects of different variables of the machinery on the overall electrogenesis. Perhaps its most important use is in analyzing the significance of partially active dendritic trees in the integrative properties of the whole cell. This work has just begun for the Purkinje cell (Pellionisz and Llinás, 1975) and motoneurons (Traub and Llinás, 1978; Dodge, this volume). Since in the model presented here all structural and functional properties of the compartments are set individually, it is easy to experiment with "mosaic patterns" of ion permeabilities over the dendrites.

Orthodromic activation of the Purkinje-cell model, capable of firing dendritic spikes, is studied in close connection with electrophysiological recordings (Llinás, this volume). In the case shown in Figure 4, the branching compartments of the tree were considered active; sodium and potassium conductance values

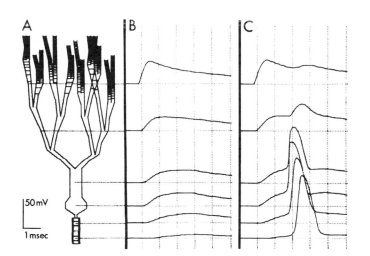
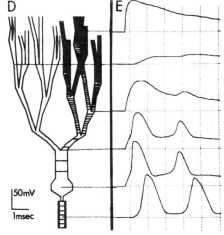

FIGURE 3 Numerical solutions for membrane potential responses to spatially different orthodromic stimulation in a passive dendritic tree (after Pellionisz and Llinás, 1975, 1977a). A: Orthodromic activation of the model Purkinje cell by injecting a square pulse of synaptic current into the uppermost dendritic branches. Hatching is proportional to the depolarization at 0.5 msec after the onset of input. B: Five representative recordings from the computed responses of 62 compartments. The current pulse is just subthreshold; therefore the dendritic compartments show only a passive electrotonic propagation of the depolariza-tion, and no spike is generated at the soma. C: Same as B, but the stimulus is suprathreshold. D: Model of vertical integration. Synaptic current pulse (identical in overall strength and duration to the case in C) was applied to the right half of the dendritic tree. The hatching shows the membrane depolarization computed at 3.0 msec. Note that in case of vertical integration the input evokes a burst of two spikes starting at only 0.3 msec latency. The somatic action potentials electrotonically invade the left side of dendritic tree, which was not stimulated by current injection.

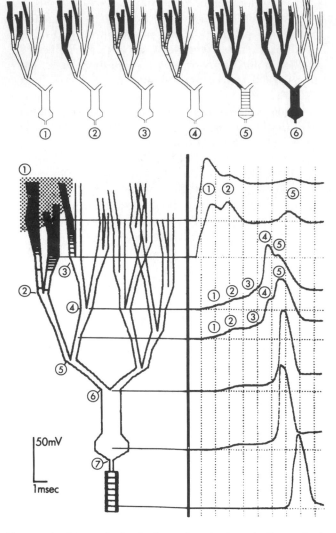

FIGURE 4 Numerical solution of orthodromically evoked action potential in a Purkinje-cell model capable of firing dendritic spikes. Dendritic branching compartments are active. Upper row of schematic dendritic trees provides a phase diagram of the sequence of dendritic spikes. (Hatching is proportional to the computed membrane depolarizations.) Lower part of the figure is a spatiotemporal display of the computed response. To the left, the spatial scheme of the Purkinje cell is shown. The dendritic tree was stimulated by synaptic current injection at the dotted area. This triggers a sequence of the firing of bifurcation zones (follow the numbering). To the right, a temporal display is given of seven representative membrane potential waveforms of the computed responses of 62 compartments.

were 10–30% of those of the initial segment and decreased with the distance between the soma and branching compartment. Also, a higher longitudinal resistance of the dendritic branches was assumed (the branching power was taken as 2.0; see Hillman, this volume). For other details see the model in Pellionisz

and Llinás (1977a). A brief (<0.3 msec) current pulse was applied to the upper dendritic branches at the left (see dotted area in Figure 4) and evoked dendritic spikes at the uppermost branching regions. The sequence of six dendritic spikes and the seventh firing (of the soma) can be followed by the numbering in Figure 4. Dendritic spikes 1 and 2 produce a prolonged depolarization at somatic level but do not bring it to firing. However, the even weaker corollary stimulation of the neighboring branch (at 3) triggers another sequence (3 and 4) which provides a late contribution to the somatic depolarization. Thus a propagated firing emerges (5, 6, and 7). At midlevel of the dendritic tree the ortho- and antidromically propagating dendritic and generalized spikes produce a characteristic cascaded waveform of membrane potential (see, e.g., 4 in Figure 4; see also Llinás, this volume).

The most stringent test of the accuracy of the Purkinje-cell model is that it ought to yield not only realistic antidromic and orthodromic responses but also the complicated, but still highly stereotyped, "complex-spike" response (or CFR). This response is evoked by the climbing fiber that injects currents through its numerous synapses over most of the dendritic tree of the Purkinje cell (see the classical figure of Ramón y Cajal, reproduced in Figure 5A). The overall response of the whole neuron to this massive electrotonic event is known by intracellular recordings from several different preparations (see Figure 5B, C). Precisely because the entire neuron is involved in this response, however, speculations as to how this characteristic waveform is generated have remained obscure and ambiguous. Two basic and equally compelling suggestions were that the wavelets in CFR emerge either from the dendrites or from the axon (Eccles, Llinás, and Sasaki, 1966b; Martinez, Crill, and Kennedy, 1971). A clarification of this point was required, not only to resolve this dilemma, but also because it was expected that a deeper understanding of the electrogenesis of CFR could provide important insights into the operation of the cerebellar cortex itself.

First, using an entirely passive dendritic tree, it was asked whether the model would yield a realistic CFR without including the possibility of dendritic spikes. As shown in Figure 5D, E, the output of the model to brief but massive current injection into the dendrites (which simulates climbing-fiber activation) is comparable to the electrophysiological recordings. Note that not only is the overall pattern of the prolonged waveform reproduced, but the intriguing double twin wavelets are also present.

It is noteworthy that, at least in this particular case, by putting already known details into the model we can generate information that was not known before; that is, we can determine where the multiple wavelets are generated. From Figure 5E it is apparent that the twin wavelets recorded at the soma are generated by the repetitive firing of the axon initial segment. Figure 5E also suggests that the repetitive firing of the initial segment is caused by a basically rather simple chain of events: The climbing-fiber synapses inject a large amount of current into the entire dendritic tree, resulting in a virtually homogeneous, massive depolarization. Repolarization of the dendritic compartments is impeded because the neighboring compartments, being similarly depolarized, cannot drain charges away rapidly enough. Repolarization therefore depends largely on the leakiness of the dendritic cable. During this prolonged process the highly active somatic and axonal compartments not only repolarize, but fire repetitively.

Some corollary results of the modeling of CFR are also worth mentioning. First, it was considered a promising initial result that the model could reproduce a CFR with a passive dendritic tree. The next problem was to determine how robust this response was, that is, to establish if the characteristic waveform was consistent with a partially active dendritic tree. Using the active dendritic tree shown in Figure 4, the repolarization of dendrities during CFR was faster, but the active compartments at branching points boosted the repeated action of the initial segment. As a result of these balancing differences, the pattern of CFR was remarkably retained. (The main difference was that because of the increased firing rate the last two spikes of the initial segment merged into one propagated spike. This may explain the variation in propagating spikes of a CFR found by Ito and Simpson (1971).) The studies described above suggest that the proven existence of dendritic spikes in Purkinje cells of several species is immaterial, as regards the CFR waveform.

Second, the robustness of modeled CFR to other variations of structural and functional parameters was also found satisfactory. For example, it was demonstrated that, in very good agreement with electrophysiological recordings (Llinás and Volkind, 1972;

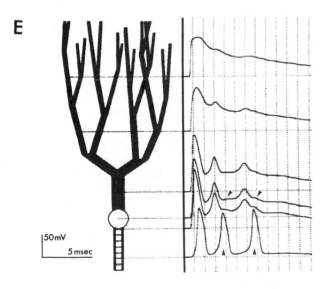

FIGURE 5 An explanation by computer modeling of the climbing-fiber-evoked complex spike (CFR) of the Purkinje cell. A: Golgi-impregnated Purkinje cell (b) and its climbing fiber (a) in cat (after Ramón y Cajal, 1911, Fig. 47). B: Six superimposed intracellular recordings of the Purkinje-cell response to climbing-fiber stimulation (CFR, as recorded in the soma), in cat. Arrows point to the two most delicate wavelets of the largely stereotypic response. (After Llinás and Volkind, 1972.) C: Intracellular recording of CFR in frog. Note the remarkable similarity of the double twin wavelets of CFR in frog and cat, although the structural features of the Purkinje cell are different in these species (compare Figures 5A and 1A). (After Llinás, Bloedel, and Hillman, 1969.) D: Output of the computer model of Purkinje cell of frog (compare with E). Note that the model provides a comparable somatic membrane potential waveform of CFR, including the double twin wavelets (arrows). E: Computer model that synthesizes morphological and electrophysiological data to provide an explanation for the electrogenesis of the CFR. To the left is a model neuron composed of 62 compartments with passive dendritic tree. To the right are six representative recordings from the computed responses of 62 compartments. Note that the double twin wavelets in CFR are produced by the repetitive firing of the axon initial segment, each spike followed by an antidromic invasion (arrows) evoked by the propagating axonal spike (arrows). (After Pellionisz and Llinás, 1975, 1977a.)

see Figure 5B), it is the last wavelet of the CFR that is most vulnerable to variations. Reversal of the climbing-fiber-evoked EPSP by depolarizing the soma was modeled in accordance with the data as well. (For the detailed studies see Pellionisz and Llinás, 1977a.)

Third, beyond providing an explanation for a complex phenomenon, this model also led to a novel, though rather speculative, line of thought that may be worth mentioning to illustrate its heuristic power. The idea concerns the possible role of climbing-fiber activation of Purkinje cells. In view of the massive overall depolarization of even the uppermost regions of dendritic tree during the CFR (see Figure 5E), it is conceivable that the primary function of climbing-fiber activation is not to elicit a burst of spikes, but to generate this deep and prolonged depolarization of the entire dendritic tree. It has been hypothesized that the CFR modifies ("shapes") the dynamism of the Purkinje-cell spike-producing membrane mechanism (Pellionisz, 1976). This notion of physiological tuning (Pellionisz, 1976, 1978), which is in contrast to the modification of synaptic efficacy (Marr, 1969), may shed new light on the operation of the cerebellar cortex. (It has also been pointed out that the basic functioning of neurons, in general, may be based on the plasticity of their spike-generating properties: see Pellionisz, 1976; Traub and Llinás, 1977.)

The described single-unit model illustrates that, if hitherto isolated fields of research (in this case single-cell morphology and electrophysiology) are integrated by computer modeling, even highly complex phenomena such as the CFR may be explained on the basis of already known details. Such modeling of particular neurons may therefore become a fruitful area in the future since there are many sets of corresponding electrophysiological and morphological data available for specific neurons that await mutual explanation by such synthesis.

It should be stressed that the approach of investigating the cerebellum at the single-neuron level is a rather "close view" of the cerebellar system. Although without the help of computers even one Purkinje cell is much too complex to allow us to directly interrelate morphological and physiological details, it is inevitable that we proceed to consider single cells from a broader, "more general" perspective, that is, from the point of view of the role they might play in the cerebellar cortex. In making this attempt, the obvious problem is that even an "overall" phenomenon of a single neuron (e.g., the CFR) is only an element in the functioning of the circuitry of cerebellar cortex. However, at this higher level in the hierarchy of complexities, the situation that was seen at the single-neuron level repeats itself: we know many of the overall features and also various details of the cerebellar cortex, but the two need to be interrelated in some systematic way. It is therefore reasonable to turn to the already proven method of computer modeling at this higher level of complexity.

MODELING LOCAL CEREBELLAR NETWORKS The cytoarchitecture and electrophysiology of the elements of the cerebellar cortex are well known (Eccles, Ito, and Szentágothai, 1967; Llinás, 1969; Palay and Chan-Palay, 1974; Palkovits, Magyar, and Szentágothai, 1971a,b,c, 1972). Combining these separate sets of information concerning the individual elements in order to achieve an understanding of the function of this cortex has only just begun. Early attempts to synthesize data concerning both single cells and large networks of cerebellar circuits (not the entire cortex) met with many difficulties (see, e.g., Szentágothai, 1963; Eccles, Ito, and Szentágothai, 1967; Eccles, 1973). This was due mainly to a lack of adequate techniques to handle the complex body of data that it takes to describe tens of thousands of neurons. Computer methods have since been introduced that can provide phenomenological models for the possible events of a "functional block" (i.e., a small piece of cerebellar cortex that can be interpreted as an unbroken self-contained network). The first cerebellar computer models (Pellionisz, 1970) treated the neurons as either excitatory or inhibitory McCulloch-Pitts-type elements, connected as the elements are known to be in the real circuit. Subsequent computer simulation (Pellionisz and Szentágothai, 1973, 1974) studied the patterns of excitation and inhibition that emerged from these neuronal assemblies. These models suggest, for example, that the original assumption (Szentágothai, 1963) that the activity of Purkinje cells is characterized by simultaneous excitation of rows of Purkinje cells along a parallel-fiber beam may, in fact, need to be modified to include the isolated firings of single Purkinje cells. This modeling led to a newly established functional interpretation of the individual character of firing (see Pellionisz and Llinás, 1978, 1979).

In problems concerning the whole cerebellar cortex, the contribution of such studies on restricted segments of circuitry is limited. For example, activity following vestibular stimulation is a good example of a feature that emerges from the *entire* circuitry of cerebellar cortex. Activity in the frog cerebellum following angular acceleration is characterized by a marked spatial distribution of Purkinje-cell activities involving the whole cerebellar cortex. Precht and Llinás (1969) showed that Purkinje cells with type I and type III firing patterns (see below and Figure 9) are distributed in different areas of the cerebellum. These features of the total cerebellar cortex are obviously related both to the structural organization of the entire cerebellum ("how an input to the cerebellar cortex is conducted through the circuitry to reach certain Purkinje cells") and to single-unit activity ("how the single Purkinje neuron processes that information"). Thus our knowledge of morphology and single-cell activity offers no direct explanation for the spatial distribution of the firing patterns in the model *unless* the two are interpreted within a single, self-consistent framework. This dictates that the hierarchy of models be extended to include modeling of the entire cerebellar cortex.

MODELING THE ENTIRE CEREBELLAR CORTEX   In an attempt to bridge the described gap in our understanding, a computer model based on morphological structure was developed (Pellionisz, Llinás, and Perkel, 1977). The model simulates the morphogenesis of the entire frog cerebellar cortex. What makes this approach possible is the relative simplicity of the amphibian cerebellum. It is a good model of the "basic cerebellar circuit": it has practically no inhibitory interneurons, its overall structure is limited to only one transverse folium, and the total number of neurons is only on the order of 1–2 million (Hillman, 1969a,b; Llinás, 1969, 1977).

The model "grows" the circuitry; that is, it generates mossy fibers, Purkinje cells, and parallel fibers by simulating the ontogenetic development. The same programs that generate these neuronal elements can be used to set up any particular configuration of activated neuronal elements of the circuitry. Thus, although the programs are capable of generating the total circuitry of the cerebellar cortex, the computer must deal with only those sections that are actually activated (Pellionisz, Llinás, and Perkel, 1977). This appeared to be the only reasonable approach for handling a circuit containing over a million neurons.

The morphogenesis programs are based on the assumption that the growth of neuronal elements is probabilistic. Thus probability distributions were set up for the key parameters of different cells from the available morphological data. Then the actual parameter values for every neuron were drawn at random from these probability distributions. The morphological structure of the computer model of frog cerebellum is shown in Figure 6. The overall body of the cerebellum is represented by a curved three-layered lattice structure containing 1.68 million cell locations. Mossy fibers project into the granular layer through the two peduncles. A straight trunk of mossy fibers forms the basis for a triangular "fan" on which the endings lie. (The fan takes off from the trunk by pitch, roll, and yaw angles that are drawn from standard distributions.) It is assumed that a spatiotemporally coincident excitation of mossy-fiber endings is required for activation of a granule cell. Granule cells are located at three-dimensional lattice points in the granular layer. Their axons, the parallel fibers, ascend into the molecular layer where they make a T-shaped bifurcation. The parallel fibers run transversely through the planar dendritic trees of Purkinje cells, whose bodies lie on the middle Purkinje-cell layer (each dot of the Purkinje layer in Figure 6C represents one of 8,285 cell body locations). Dendritic trees are generated with different arborization patterns in order to provide a variance in their parallel-fiber input. This comprehensive model enables us to tackle questions relating to the functioning of the entire cerebellar cortex.

Partial activation of the circuitry was used to analyze such problems as the spatial distribution of excitation in populations of granule and Purkinje cells. Such localized activation of mossy-fiber inputs is triggered, for example, by vestibular input evoked by angular acceleration. (See the schematic diagram in Figure 7.) This activation has been thoroughly investigated by both anatomical (Hillman, 1977) and physiological (Llinás and Precht, 1972) methods. The model simulates this case as shown in Figures 6 and 7. A cluster of such incoming mossy fibers activates a "spindle" of granule cells that, in turn, excites a rather tight bundle of parallel fibers. Accordingly, a column of Purkinje cells select their inputs from a basically identical set of activated parallel fibers (although Purkinje cells are not totally "in register"; in the cat they show a staggered arrangement: see Palkovits, Magyar, and Szentágothai, 1971a).

One striking structural feature of the model cerebellum is a tendency to form spindles of activated parallel fibers (see Figure 6). This property of the model of the frog's cerebellum was shown to be a very robust feature, in two ways. First, even with a large variance (more than doubling the standard deviation) of pitch, yaw, and roll angles between the trunk and the fan of mossy fibers, the "beams" of activated granule cells were retained (Pellionisz, Llinás, and Perkel, 1977). Second, it was expected that separated mossy-fiber systems, when they project into the cerebellum, would give a combined action on certain Purkinje cells that are in the spatial overlap

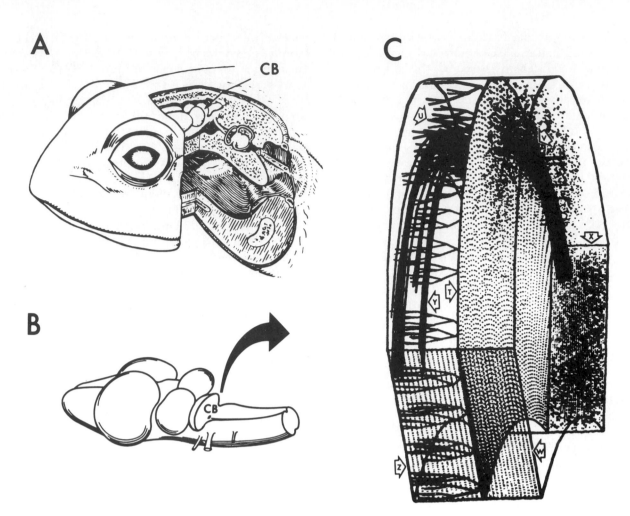

FIGURE 6   The morphological basis of the computer model of the frog cerebellar cortex. A: Cutaway illustration of a frog head showing the cerebellum (CB) and its connection with left vestibular labyrinth (after Precht, Llinás, and Clarke, 1971). B: Diagram of a frog brain with the single-folium cerebellum (after Hillman, 1969). C: Structure of the model. The mossy fibers entering the cerebellar peduncle are indicated only by their entry points (X), except for a cluster of 100 vestibular mossy fibers. These are illustrated by their trunks and 2% of their endings (V). This cluster triggers granule cells (depending on their threshold to mossy-fiber stimulation). For illustrative purposes the threshold is high (6) and only 56 granule cells are activated. The parallel fibers (Y) arising from these granule cells protrude from the granule layer (W) into the molecular layer (Z). This activated "beam" of parallel fibers traverses the Purkinje cells (U) whose somata are found in the Purkinje-cell layer (T). For a fuller description see Pellionisz, Llinás, and Perkel (1977).

of the two populations of excited mossy-fiber terminals. These neurons would then "integrate" the information coming from separate inputs. This assumption was tested by the model. Figure 8 shows the effect of the spatial localization of incoming mossy fibers on the spatial distribution pattern of activated granule cells. In the first case, two separated clusters of mossy fibers enter the peduncle (upper part of Figure 8A). In the second, the activated mossy fibers (which may be coming from different sources) are scattered at random over a quarter of the peduncle (lower part of Figure 8B). In both cases, the activated mossy-fiber endings cover almost the entire granular layer (Figure 8B). Thus, in terms of mossy fiber endings, the model seems to support the expectation that Purkinje cells over the center of the activated region would be of the integrative type. However, as shown in Figure 8, in spite of the apparent loss of spatial specificity of mossy fibers, the activated granule cells form spindles. In the first case, these appear in the form of remarkably separated clusters (upper part of Figure 8C), each carrying information that comes from one or the other mossy-fiber input. More interestingly, the other, similarly massive "cloud" of activity created by the scattered input forms three small spindles (lower part of Figure 8C). In the latter case,

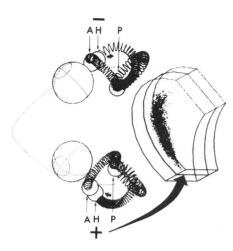

FIGURE 7 Schematic diagram of the asymmetrical spatial input to the cerebellum in the case of angular acceleration in yaw (horizontal rotation counterclockwise). The two sets of semicircular canals of the labyrinth are shown magnified. The horizontal (H), anterior (A), and posterior (P) semicircular canals are represented in the form of "coil springs" to visualize the "pushing and pulling" inertial forces in response to angular acceleration. In horizontal accelerating rotation only the horizontal semicircular canals are activated. In the left labyrinth the inertia exerts a force towards the ampulla (see small arrow) that evokes excitation (+). At the right labyrinth the inertia is "pulling away" from the ampulla (see small arrow) and reduces the spontaneous firing (−). The resulting asymmetrical input to cerebellum (from left labyrinth, see big arrow) is shown by the inset, indicating the "spindle" of activated granule cells.

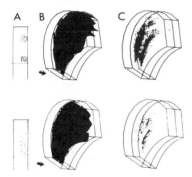

FIGURE 8 The spatial distribution over the cerebellar cortex of clusters of activated mossy fibers. A: A cross section of the cerebellar peduncle. The entry points of mossy fibers are shown by dots. In the upper row two clusters of 100 mossy fibers project into the cerebellum. In the lower row 100 mossy fibers are scattered randomly over one-quarter of the peduncle. B: Spatial distribution in the cortex of these mossy fibers and their endings. In both cases the activated mossy fiber endings cover most of the cortex. C: The spatial distribution of activated granule cells. Note the remarkable separation of the activated granule cells into two spindles (upper row) and the three smaller but separated spindles of granule cells that emerge as a result of the scattered mossy-fiber activation. (After Pellionisz, Llinás, and Perkel, 1977.)

the granule cells in one spindle receive mossy-fiber information from both mossy-fiber inputs. In either case, the result of activation is a bombardment of a set of Purkinje cells by basically the same parallel-fiber spindle.

This feature of the model suggests that the anuran cerebellum has a natural ability to extract transverse spindles of granule-cell activities with a strikingly limited dorsoventral integration. This, in fact, may be a general property that is further refined in high vertebrates by the lateral inhibition produced by the basket cells.

With the help of the model we can now attempt to explain the spatial distribution of type I and type III Purkinje cells (those that are activated by only one direction of rotation or by both, respectively), as observed in experimental vestibular stimulation (Figure 9A). Since these cells differ in their individual spike pattern response (and their spatial distribution covers the entire cortex), it is obvious that the above experimental results cannot be accounted for without combining the structural model of the entire cerebellar cortex with functional models of single Purkinje cells. In the case of ipsi- and contralateral horizontal angular acceleration, mossy fibers from the horizontal semicircular canal are carried in the eighth nerve and project into the cerebellum through the peduncle (Hillman, 1969b; Precht, Llinás, and Clarke, 1971; Hillman, 1977). Ipsi- and contralateral angular acceleration is modeled, therefore, by the activation of a cluster of mossy fibers, projecting from either the ipsi- or contralateral side (compare Figure 7). This activation creates a beam of excited mossy-fiber terminals (as shown in Figure 6).

A map of Purkinje cells receiving a suprathreshold (>30) number of activated parallel fibers is shown in Figure 9C–E. By varying this arbitrary threshold the spatial distributions of type I and type III cells are revealed. Type I cells are shown for ipsilateral (Figure 7C) and contralateral (Figure 9D) activation. Type III cells are also shown (Figure 9E). By a tenfold increase in the threshold one may localize those areas in which the input to Purkinje cells is maximal (i.e., those areas having the highest probability of containing type I cells). The model predicts that these regions are not directly at the peduncles, as one might expect intuitively, but are about one-third of the folium away from the peduncle transversely along the parallel fibers. Recent experimental observations confirm this prediction (Amat, personal communication).

At this level of modeling, it is possible to relate electrophysiological recordings for single Purkinje cells to the microstructure of the entire cerebellar

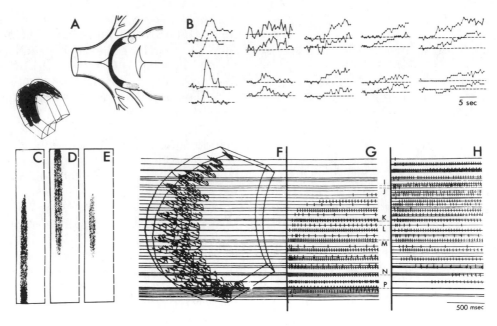

FIGURE 9 Comparison of experimental and modeled spatial distribution of single-unit activities of Purkinje cells in response to vestibular input. Parts A and B show experimental data; C–H show output from the model. A: Schematic diagram of frog brain stem and cerebellum (top view). Type III Purkinje cells are found on the dorsal rim of the cerebellum (dark area). Type I cells are found in the two lateral dotted areas. B: Frequency responses of ten type III cells, following a ramp increase of horizontal angular acceleration. Although each cell shows individual dynamism, the twin sets of recordings in both rows are almost identical pairs of responses of the cell to ipsi- and contralateral rotation. Note the wide spectrum of phasic-to-tonic dynamism of individual Purkinje cells. These rotations correspond in the model to the activation of clusters of mossy fibers (see insert at left and Figures 4 and 5). Purkinje cells receiving a suprathreshold number of activated parallel fibers (>30) are shown for ipsilateral (C) and contralateral (D) rotation. Their spatial overlap (E) contains cells responding to both directions of rotation (type III). F, G and H show spike trains of randomly selected Purkinje cells at different locations, responding to the modeled asymmetrical mossy-fiber input. Cells I, J, and P are type I cells; K, L, M, and N are type III. Note the variety of firing patterns. (Part A after Precht and Llinás, 1969; part B after Llinás, Precht, and Clarke, 1971; parts C–E from Pellionisz, Llinás, and Perkel, 1977; parts F–H from Pellionisz and Llinás, 1977b.)

cortex. This is done by combining the single-Purkinje-cell model with that of the whole circuit in the following way. The morphogenesis provides the spatial distribution of activated Purkinje cells for a given mossy-fiber input, and the resulting parallel-fiber activation is then applied to single Purkinje cells (Pellionisz and Llinás, 1977b).

One intriguing finding that has to be accounted for by this approach is the extreme variance of dynamical properties of type III Purkinje cells recorded at various locations over the cortex. Different Purkinje cells exhibit a remarkably wide spectrum of phasic-to-tonic dynamics of spike-train responses to identical vestibular input (Figure 9B). Moreover, the phasic or tonic character of the dynamics of one cell is maintained for both ipsi- and contralateral angular acceleration. This finding was accounted for in the model as follows. In order to simulate the microelectrode penetration of cells at various loci over the cerebellar cortex, the parallel-fiber beam that is activated by ipsi-

or contralateral mossy-fiber cluster input was applied to quasi-randomly selected Purkinje cells (Figure 9F). At all "probed" locations the activated or nonactivated parallel fibers represent two-dimensional matrices. Purkinje cells, by their modeled dendritic arborization pattern, contact a sample of the total number of encountered parallel fibers. These samples vary, since Purkinje cells are staggered and also differ in their dendritic patterns (some having partially overlapping dendritic trees). This difference is most significant for Purkinje cells at different dorsoventral positions. Some will be "on-line" and others "off-line" with regard to the parallel-fiber beam.

The model shown in Figure 9 involves the activity of several Purkinje cells over many tens of milliseconds. For this reason a simplified single-unit model of the Purkinje cells was used instead of the full multicompartmental Hodgkin-Huxley model. It was assumed that the threshold of Purkinje cells increases after every spike and then returns exponentially to its original resting value. This is necessary to provide a phasic-to-tonic firing response following an input that increases linearly and then saturates. In order to study the variance that is provided solely by the difference in parallel-fiber input to Purkinje cells, the algorithm of firing was held strictly identical for all Purkinje cells (i.e., no individuality was allowed). Then the parallel-fiber beam generated by the ipsi- and then contralateral mossy-fiber cluster was applied to a sample of Purkinje cells selected at random from the entire body of cerebellar cortex. The spatial distribution of overall activation and the individual dynamic properties arising from the spatial dispersion of parallel-fiber activation emerges from the model as shown in Figures 9G and H. This result illustrates the extent to which the observed phenomena can be explained on the basis of a knowledge of the structure of circuitry. The network provides a spatial variance in transmitting mossy-fiber inputs through parallel fibers to Purkinje cells. As seen in Figure 9G and H, the overall spatial distributions of the type I and type III activities are adequately explained. Also, it can be concluded that a wide variety of dynamic patterns of Purkinje cells may arise solely from the variance of the parallel-fiber input. However, the consistent characteristic of phasic or tonic firing for both ipsi- and contralateral rotation does not emerge from this model because it excludes individuality. The model thus suggests that the individual character of the activity of Purkinje cells is more likely to originate from individual differences of the electroresponsive properties of Purkinje cells than from their varied parallel-fiber inputs.

This conclusion is important when considering that these sets of Purkinje-cell output patterns do not merely represent an envelope of spike trains with various dynamics but probably reflect some fundamental principles regarding the organization of the functional output of the cerebellar cortex (for a recent hypothesis utilizing this individual Purkinje-cell dynamics see Pellionisz, 1976, 1978). Presently completed models (Pellionisz and Llinás, 1978, 1979) have provided a meaningful functional interpretation of such varied Purkinje-cell activities: they act as a spatially distributed Taylor series expansion, yielding prediction. Tackling such questions requires that the cerebellar output (in the form of Purkinje-cell activities) be put in the context of a total cerebellar control system. Thus a still higher level of complexity needs to be considered.

MODELING THE CEREBELLAR CONTROL SYSTEM It is generally accepted that it may be impossible to understand the function of the cerebellum without considering the cerebellar control system as a whole. Beyond this consideration, it is on the *system level* that some global functions of the cerebellum present themselves in the form of the coordination of motor activities. Skilled locomotion, balanced posture, and coordinated head and eye movements are a few prominent final results to which the cerebellar control system contributes (see Dow and Moruzzi, 1958). These functions can be directly observed and have been studied at the phenomenological level in great detail (for a review on locomotion and posture see Stein et al., 1973; on head and eye coordination see Bach-y-Rita, Collins, and Hyde, 1971).

It is important to realize that in order to meet the ultimate challenge of explaining such emergent properties as, for example, a coordinated gait, a methodology must be prepared that can handle such complex phenomena on the basis of known details of the functioning of the underlying neuronal machinery. From the perspective of this highest level of complexity, even the overall spatial distribution of the Purkinje-cell output of the cerebellar cortex represents only a small detail. A number of other isolated experimental findings also appear as details: the structural and functional features of the peripheral vestibular apparatus, vestibular and cerebellar nuclei, olivary system, or skeletal and eye musculature. The degree of complexity of any of the above systems is high, and the amount of factual information abundant. It is essential, therefore, to generate realistic conceptual representations that both synthesize these data and penetrate the complexity of the system. Within the hierarchy of computer models of the cerebellum, spanning several levels of complexity, techniques are being developed for representing the overall outputs of the system, such as locomotion and eye and head movements.

As a first step in putting this hierarchical modeling in perspective, a computer representation of the skeleton of bullfrog was established (Figure 10). Lengths and three-dimensional angles of the major elements of the skeleton are handled in the model as vectors in successive three-dimensional polar coordinate systems. For example, the radio-ulna bone is oriented in its own polar coordinate system fixed to the humerus. As long as the elbow joint is not moved, the radio-ulna moves with the humerus, keeping its own θ and ϕ coordinates representing the flexion and rotation, respectively. The frog's head and eyes are also shown schematically. The three-dimensional positions and movements of all these elements are handled by the computer and displayed graphically (Fig-

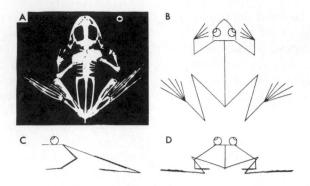

FIGURE 10 Computer representation of the skeleton of bullfrog. A: Top view of skeleton. B: Top view of the model, showing major skeletal bones and schematic head and eyes. C: Side view. D: Front view.

ures 10 and 11). Further, eye and head movements can be analyzed in relation to each other, as well as to the body. Since all joints of the skeleton model are movable, by varying the θ and ϕ angles, the model can display movements such as uncoordinated or coordinated locomotion. Thus the basic characteristics of eye, head, and limb movements can be displayed and analyzed separately as well as simultaneously. The graphic display enables direct observation of their combined result and makes it easier to relate this to the experimental findings. This ability to represent overall emergent phenomena ends the hierarchy of interconnected computer models spanning the range from membranes to the overall input-out-

put function of angular accelerations and correlated body movements. It is therefore expected that with the help of this framework accommodating both the details and the overall features of the system, it will become possible to account for emergent phenomena on the basis of details (as the model of a single Purkinje cell made it possible to explain the waveform of a complex spike).

The methodology offered by these models might be used, for example, to study the following problem. Vestibular stimulation of a frog in the dark results largely in head nystagmus, while optokinetic input without vestibular stimuli evokes eye nystagmus (Grüsser and Grüsser-Cornehls, 1977; Precht, 1977). In the case of combined vestibular and optokinetic stimulation, the response of the total system is a combined response of head and eye movements. However, these two systems are far from being independent (they are coupled both physically and through the visual field) and are both under cerebellar control (Grüsser and Grüsser-Cornehls, 1977). It is important, therefore, to be equipped to study them together and in connection with the cerebellar model.

Although locomotor movements of the limbs themselves raise many questions that await explanation, our particular interest is in how coordination of locomotion is achieved. Coordination is both intrinsic and extrinsic. In an intrinsic sense it concerns how the activations of different major muscles are related to one another. This coordination results in an overall

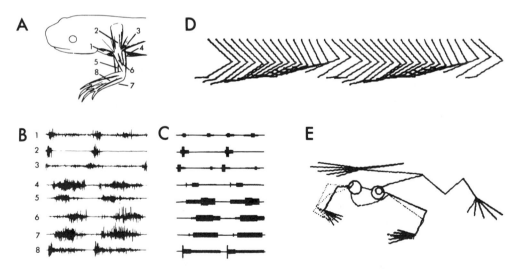

FIGURE 11 Computer techniques for the representation of locomotor movements. A: Anatomical positions of eight major forelimb muscles used for electromyogram recordings during locomotion: 1, acromialis; 2, dorsalis scapulae; 3, latissimus; 4, pectoralis; 5, brachialis; 6, extensor ulnae; 7, (hidden) flexor digitorum; 8, extensor digitorum. (Modified from Székely, Czéh, and Vörös, 1969.) B: Myochron-

ograms recorded from the forelimb of an intact *Triturus* (modified from Székely and Czéh, 1977). C: Computer representation of myochronograms. D: Phase diagram of two step cycles of the left forelimb (side view), as reconstructed from C by the computer model. E: Diagram of the computer model of frog skeleton to illustrate the display of reconstructed locomotor movements of forelimbs.

542   ANDRÁS PELLIONISZ

locomotor activity that is functionally superior to the simple sum of the elementary muscle contractions. In an extrinsic sense, it is important to be able to analyze how locomotor movements are coordinated to resist external disturbances of the total system (such as, for example, angular acceleration during locomotion). An understanding of the principles of these extrinsic and intrinsic aspects of motor coordination (and of the role of cerebellum) is needed to account for such extremely complex emergent properties as walking. (For a newly developed tensorial interpretation of coordination as a distributed property, see Pellionisz and Llinás, 1978, 1979.)

As a first approach to the development of a methodology for handling these complex phenomena, the computer model of the frog skeleton was used to directly observe the overall effects of elementary locomotor muscle contractions. Electromyograms recorded from freely moving salamanders are available in the form of "electromyocronograms" (Czéh and Székely, 1971; Székely and Czéh, 1977; see Figure 11A). The amplitude and time sequence of the activation of eight major forelimb muscles was deduced from these recordings (Figure 11B). These data were used to alter the three-dimensional angles of the joint vectors (representing skeletal bones). By computer display and cinematographic animation of the skeletal model, these data emerge as a crude pattern of locomotor limb movements (see Figure 11C).

In order to coordinate this crude form of locomotor movements, to allow the model to accommodate external disturbances (such as angular acceleration), the outputs of Purkinje cells of the cerebellar cortex have to be incorporated into the full model of motor control. This requires further information, especially about the structural and functional features of the cerebellar nuclei and of the olivary system. While important new anatomical findings (Palkovits et al., 1977; Chan-Palay, 1977), overall functional observations (Llinás et al., 1975), and basical electrophysiological knowledge (Ito et al., 1970) are available for these systems, it is crucial that, for further advancement of this modeling, a concept be developed for the role of these systems in cerebellar coordination. Any such proposal is the more useful if it can interpret single-neuron events as well as phenomena at the system level; but it is very difficult to envisage the evolution of a new scheme capable of integrating such an enormous span of details without the working tool of hierarchical computer modeling such as described in this paper.

This goal of promoting a dialogue between concepts and data on any and all levels is the ultimate reason for modeling. If interconnected computer models within a coherent framework succeed in encompassing the data on neuronal membranes, single neurons, populations of cells in the cerebellar cortex, the structure of the cerebellum, the spatial distribution properties of single-unit activities in the cerebellar cortex, and overall emergent phenomena, we hope it will help to achieve a breakthrough in the understanding of the function of the cerebellum.

Computer modeling of cerebellar neurons and networks is only one example of efforts in recent years to develop methods that can bring together, in a supradisciplinary manner, a heterogeneous and diffuse body of data. Since this trend must counterbalance spontaneous "centrifugal" tendencies (that the empirical basis of scientific fields scatters and proliferates into increasingly unwieldy agglomerations of data), it is expected that computer modeling will become indispensable in the coming years not only in neuroscience, but in all fields requiring the handling and interpreting complex systems.

ACKNOWLEDGMENT This research was supported by U.S.P.H.S. research grant NS-13742 from the National Institute of Neurological and Communicative Disorders and Stroke.

REFERENCES

ÁDÁM, A., 1968. Simulation of rhythmic nervous activities. II. Mathematical models for the function of networks with cyclic inhibition. *Kybernetik* 5:103–109.

ADELMAN, W. J., 1971. *Biophysics and Physiology of Excitable Membranes.* New York: Van Nostrand Reinhold.

ADELMAN, W. J., and R. FITZHUGH, 1975. Solutions of the Hodgkin-Huxley equations modified for potassium accumulation in a periaxonal space. *Fed. Proc.* 34:1322–1329.

ALBUS, J. S., 1971. A theory of cerebellar function. *Math. Biosci.* 10:25–61.

ARBIB, M. A., 1969. *Theories of Abstract Automata.* Englewood Cliffs, NJ: Prentice-Hall.

ARBIB, M. A., G. G. FRANKLIN, and N. NILSSON, 1968. Some ideas on information processing in the cerebellum. In *Neural Networks,* E. R. Caianello, ed. New York: Springer-Verlag, pp. 43–58.

ASHBY, W. R., 1952. *Design for a Brain.* New York: John Wiley.

BACH-Y-RITA, P., C. C. COLLINS, and J. E. HYDE, 1971. *The Control of Eye Movements.* New York: Academic Press.

BERNSTEIN, J., 1902. Untersuchungen zur Thermodynamik der bioelektrischen Ströme. I. *Arch. Ges. Physiol.* 92:521–562.

BEURLE, R. L., 1956. Properties of a mass of cells capable of regenerating pulses. *Trans. R. Soc. Lond.* B240:55–94.

BOYLLS, C. C., 1975. A theory of cerebellar function with application to locomotion. I. The physiological role of climbing fiber inputs in anterior lobe operation. *COINS*

Technical Report 75C-6. Univ. Massachusetts, Amherst, MA.

BRAITENBERG, V., 1961. Functional interpretation of cerebellar histology. *Nature* 190:539–540.

BRINDLEY, G. S., 1964. The use made by the cerebellum of the information that it receives from sense organs. *IBRO Bull.* 3:80.

BULLOCK, T. H., 1970. The reliability of neurons. *J. Gen. Physiol.* 55:563–584.

CAIANELLO, E. R., ed., 1968. Proceedings of the school on neural networks. In *Neural Networks*, E. R. Caianello, ed. New York: Springer-Verlag.

CALVERT, T. W., and F. MENO, 1972. Neural systems modeling applied to the cerebellum. *IEEE Trans. Systems, Man, Cybernetics* SMC-2 3:363–374.

CALVIN, W. H., 1969. Dendritic synapses and reversal potentials: Theoretical implications of the view from the soma. *Exp. Neurol.* 24:248–264.

CHAN-PALAY, V., 1977. *The Morphology of the Deiters Nucleus of Cerebellum*. New York: Springer-Verlag.

COLE, K. S., 1972. *Membranes, Ions and Impulses*. Berkeley: Univ. California Press.

COOLEY, J. W., and F. A. DODGE, 1966. Digital computer solutions for excitation and propagation of the nerve impulse. *Biophys. J.* 6:583–599.

CZÉH, G., 1972. The role of dendritic events in the initiation of monosynaptic spikes in frog motoneurons. *Brain Res.* 39:505–509.

CZÉH, G., and G. SZÉKELY, 1971. Muscle activities recorded simultaneously from normal and supernumerary forelimbs in ambystoma. *Acta Physiol. Acad. Sci. Hung.* 40:287–301.

DODGE, F. A., and J. W. COOLEY, 1973. Action potential of the motoneuron. *IBM J. Res. Develop.* May:219–229.

DOW, R. S., and G. MORUZZI, 1958. *The Physiology and Pathology of the Cerebellum*. Minneapolis: Univ. Minnesota Press.

ECCLES, J. C., 1973. The cerebellum as a computer: Patterns in space and time. *J. Physiol.* 229:1–32.

ECCLES, J. C., M. ITO, and J. SZENTÁGOTHAI, 1967. *The Cerebellum as a Neuronal Machine*. Berlin, Heidelberg, New York: Springer-Verlag.

ECCLES, J. C., R. LLINÁS, and K. SASAKI, 1966a. Parallel fibre stimulation and the responses induced thereby in the Purkinje cells of the cerebellum. *Exp. Brain Res.* 1:17–39.

ECCLES, J. C., R. LLINÁS, and K. SASASKI, 1966b. The excitatory synaptic action of climbing fibers on the Purkinje cells of the cerebellum. *J. Physiol.* 182:268–296.

FARLEY, B. G., and W. A. CLARKE, 1961. Activity in networks of neuron-like elements. In *Information Theory (Fourth London Symposium)*, C. Cherry, ed. London: Butterworths, pp. 242–251.

FITZHUGH, R., 1955. Mathematical models of threshold phenomena in the nerve membrane. *Bull. Math. Biophys.* 17:257–278.

FITZHUGH, R., and H. A. ANTOSIEWICZ, 1959. Automatic computation of nerve excitation: Detailed corrections and additions. *J. Soc. Ind. Appl. Math.* 7:447–458.

FRANKENHAEUSER, B., and A. F. HUXLEY, 1964. The action potential in the myelinated nerve fibre of *Xenopus laevis* as computed on the basis of voltage clamp data. *J. Physiol.* 171:302–315.

FREEMAN, J. A., and C. NICHOLSON, 1975. Experimental optimization of current source-density technique for anuran cerebellum. *J. Neurophysiol.* 38:369–382.

GRIFFITH, J. S., 1971. *Mathematical Neurobiology*. New York: Academic Press.

GRÜSSER, O. J., and U. GRÜSSER-CORNEHLS, 1977. Neurophysiology of the anuran visual system. In *Frog Neurobiology*, R. Llinás and W. Precht, eds. New York: Springer-Verlag, pp. 297–385.

HARDY, W. L., 1973. Propagation speed in myelinated nerve. II. Theoretical dependence on external Na^+ and on temperature. *Biophys. J.* 13:1071–1089.

HARMON, L. D., 1959. Artificial neuron. *Science* 129:962–963.

HARMON, L. D., and E. R. LEWIS, 1966. Neural modeling. *Physiol. Rev.* 3:513–590.

HEBB, D. O., 1949. *The Organization of Behavior*. New York: John Wiley.

HELMHOLTZ, H., 1853. Über einige Gesetze der Vertheilung elektrischer Ströme in körperliche Leitern, mit Anwendung auf die thierischen elektrischen Versuche. *Ann. Physik Chem.* (Ser. 2) 89:211–233.

HILL, A. V., 1936. Excitation and accommodation in nerve. *Proc. R. Soc. Lond.* B119:305–355.

HILLMAN, D. E., 1969a. Morphological organization of frog cerebellar cortex: A light and electron microscopic study. *J. Neurophysiol.* 32:818–846.

HILLMAN, D. E., 1969b. Light and electron microscopical study of the relationships between the cerebellum and the vestibular organ of the frog. *Exp. Brain Res.* 9:1–15.

HILLMAN, D. E., 1977. Morphology of peripheral and central vestibular systems. In *Frog Neurobiology*, R. Llinás and W. Precht, eds. New York: Springer-Verlag, pp. 452–480.

HILLMAN, D. E., M. CHUJO, and R. LLINÁS, 1974. Quantitative computer analysis of the morphology of cerebellar neurons. I. Granule cells. *Anat. Rec.* 178:375 (abstract).

HODGKIN, A. L., and A. F. HUXLEY, 1952. A quantitative description of membrane current and its application to conduction and excitation in nerve. *J. Physiol.* 117:500–544.

ITO, M., K. YOSHIDA, K. OBATA, N. KAWAI, and M. UDO, 1970. Inhibitory control of intracerebellar nuclei by the Purkinje cell axons. *Exp. Brain Res.* 10:64–80.

ITO, M., and J. I. SIMPSON, 1971. Discharges in Purkinje cell axons during climbing fiber activation. *Brain Res.* 31:215–219.

JACK, J. J. B., D. NOBLE, and R. W. TSIEN, 1975. *Electric Current Flow in Excitable Cells*. Oxford: Clarendon Press.

JENIK, F., 1962. Electronic neuron models as an aid to neurophysiological research. *Erg. Biol.* 25:206–245.

JOYNER, R. W., J. W. MOORE, and F. RAMON, 1975. Axon voltage-clamp simulation. III. Postsynaptic region. *Biophys. J.* 15:37–69.

KATZ, B., 1966. *Nerve, Muscle and Synapse*, New York: McGraw-Hill.

KELVIN, W. T., 1855. On the theory of the electric telegraph. *Proc. R. Soc. Lond.* 7:382–399.

KLEENE, S. C., 1956. Representation of events in nerve nets and finite automata. In *Automata Studies*, C. E. Shannon and J. McCarthy, eds. Princeton, NJ: Princeton Univ. Press, pp. 3–41.

LEWIS, E. R., 1964. An electronic model of the neuron

based on the dynamics of potassium and sodium ion fluxes. In *Neural Theory and Modeling,* R. F. Reiss, ed. Stanford, CA: Stanford Univ. Press, pp. 154–173.

LLINÁS, R., ed., 1969. *Neurobiology of Cerebellar Evolution and Development.* Chicago: American Medical Association.

LLINÁS, R., 1970. Neuronal operations in cerebellar transactions. In *The Neurosciences: Second Study Program,* F. O. Schmitt, ed. New York: Rockefeller Univ. Press, pp. 409–423.

LLINAS, R., 1977. Cerebellar physiology. In *Frog Neurobiology,* R. Llinás and W. Precht, eds. New York: Springer-Verlag, pp. 892–923.

LLINÁS, R., J. R. BLOEDEL, and W. ROBERTS, 1969. Antidromic invasion of Purkinje cells in frog cerebellum. *J. Neurophysiol.* 32:881–891.

LLINÁS, R., J. R. BLOEDEL, and D. E. HILLMAN, 1969. Functional characterization of neuronal circuitry of frog cerebellar cortex. *J. Neurophysiol.* 32:847–870.

LLINÁS, R., and R. HESS, 1976. Tetrodotoxin-resistant dendritic spikes in avian Purkinje cells. *Proc. Natl. Acad. Sci. USA* 73:2520–2523.

LLINÁS, R., and C. NICHOLSON, 1971. Electrophysiological properties of dendrites and somata in alligator Purkinje cells. *J. Neurophysiol.* 34:532–551.

LLINÁS, R., and W. PRECHT, 1972. Vestibulocerebellar input: Physiology. *Prog. Brain Res.* 37:341–359.

LLINÁS, R., W. PRECHT, and M. CLARKE, 1971. Cerebellar Purkinje cell responses to physiological stimulation of the vestibular system in the frog. *Exp. Brain Res.* 13:408–431.

LLINÁS, R., and R. A. VOLKIND, 1972. Repetitive climbing fiber activation of Purkinje cells in the cat cerebellum following administration of harmaline. *Fed. Proc.* 31:377 (abstract).

LLINÁS, R., K. WALTON, D. E. HILLMAN, and C. SOTELO, 1975. Inferior olive: Its role in motor learning. *Science* 190:1230–1231.

MCCULLOCH, W. S., and W. PITTS, 1943. A logical calculus of the ideas imminent in nervous activity. *Bull. Math. Biophys.* 5:115–133.

MCGROGAN, E. P., 1961. Improved transistor neuron models. In *Proceedings of the National Electronics Conference,* Chicago, vol. 17, pp. 302–310.

MALSBURG, C. VON DER, 1973. Self-organization of orientation sensitive cells in the striate cortex. *Kybernetik* 14:85–100.

MARR, D., 1969. A theory of cerebellar cortex. *J. Physiol.* 202:437–470.

MARTINEZ, F. E., W. E. CRILL, and T. T. KENNEDY, 1971. Electrogenesis of cerebellar Purkinje cell response in cats. *J. Neurophysiol.* 34:3.

MITTENTHAL, J. E., 1974. Reliability of pattern separation by the cerebellar mossy fiber granule cell system. *Kybernetik* 16:93–101.

MORTIMER, J. A., 1970. A cellular model for mammalian cerebellar cortex. Technical report, Univ. Michigan.

NEUMANN, J. VON, 1956. Probabilistic logics and the synthesis of reliable organisms from unreliable components. In *Automata Studies,* C. E. Shannon and J. McCarthy, eds. Princeton, NJ: Princeton Univ. Press, pp. 43–98.

NEUMANN, J. VON, 1959. *The Computer and the Brain.* New Haven, CT: Yale Univ. Press.

NICHOLSON, C., and R. LLINÁS, 1971. Field potentials in the

alligator cerebellum and theory of their relationship to Purkinje cell dendritic spikes. *J. Neurophysiol.* 34:509–531.

PALAY, S. L., and V. CHAN-PALAY, 1974. *Cerebellar Cortex: Cytology and Organization.* Berlin, Heidelberg, New York: Springer-Verlag.

PALKOVITS, M., P. MAGYAR, and J. SZENTÁGOTHAI, 1971a. Quantitative histological analysis of the cerebellar cortex in the cat. I. Number and arrangement in space of the Purkinje cells. *Brain Res.* 32:1–13.

PALKOVITS, M., P. MAGYAR, and J. SZENTÁGOTHAI, 1971b. Quantitative histological analysis of the cerebellar cortex in the cat. II. Cell numbers and densities in the granular layer. *Brain Res.* 32:15–30.

PALKOVITS, M., P. MAGYAR, and J. SZENTÁGOTHAI, 1971c. Quantitative histological analysis of the cerebellar cortex in the cat. III. Structural organization of the molecular layer. *Brain Res.* 34:1–18.

PALKOVITS, M., P. MAGYAR, and J. SZENTÁGOTHAI, 1972. Quantitative histological analysis of the cerebellar cortex in the cat. IV. Mossy fiber–Purkinje cell numerical transfer. *Brain Res.* 45:15–29.

PALKOVITS, M., E. MEZEY, J. HÁMORI, and J. SZENTÁGOTHAI, 1977. Quantitative histological analysis of the cerebellar nuclei in the cat. I. Numerical data on cells and on synapses. *Exp. Brain. Res.* 28:189–209.

PAVLOV, I. P., 1927. *Conditioned Reflexes: An Investigation of the Physiological Activity in the Cerebral Cortex.* New York: Dover.

PELLIONISZ, A., 1970. Computer simulation of the pattern transfer of large cerebellar neuronal fields. *Acta Biochim. Biophys. Acad. Sci. Hung.* 5:71–79.

PELLIONISZ, A., 1976. Proposal for shaping the dynamism of Purkinje cells by climbing fiber activation. *Brain Theory Newsletter* 2:2–6.

PELLIONISZ, A., 1978. Cerebellar control theory. In *Recent Developments of Neurobiology in Hungary,* vol. 8, K. Lissák, ed. Budapest: Akadémiai Kiadó (in press).

PELLIONISZ, A., and R. LLINÁS, 1975. Simple and complex spike generation in a computer model of cerebellar Purkinje cells. *Soc. Neurosci. Abst.,* 1:31.

PELLIONISZ, A., R. LLINÁS, and D. H. PERKEL, 1977. A computer model of the cerebellar cortex of the frog. *Neuroscience* 2:19–35.

PELLIONISZ, A., and R. LLINÁS, 1977a. A computer model of the cerebellar Purkinje cells. *Neuroscience* 2:37–48.

PELLIONISZ, A., and R. LLINÁS, 1977b. Analysis of spatial distribution of Purkinje cells with individual dynamisms activated by vestibular input: A computer simulation study. In *Neuron Concept Theory,* J. Szentágothai, J. Hámori, and E. S. Vizi, eds. Tihany, Budapest: Publishing House of the Hungarian Academy of Science, p. 282.

PELLIONISZ, A., and R. LLINÁS, 1978. A formal theory for cerebellar function: The predictive distributed property of the corticonuclear cerebellar system as described by tensor network theory and computer simulation. *Soc. Neurosci. Abst.* 4:68.

PELLIONISZ, A., and R. LLINÁS, 1979. Brain modeling by tensor network theory and computer simulation. The cerebellum: distributed processor for predictive coordination. *Neuroscience* (in press).

PELLIONISZ, A., and J. SZENTÁGOTHAI, 1973. Dynamic single unit simulation of a realistic cerebellar network model. *Brain Res.* 49:83–99.

PELLIONISZ, A., and J. SZENTÁGOTHAI, 1974. Dynamic single unit simulation of a realistic cerebellar network model. II. Purkinje cell activity within the basic circuit and mmdified by inhibitory systems. *Brain Res.* 68:19–40.

PERKEL, D. H., 1970. Spike trains as carriers of information. In *The Neurosciences: Second Study Program*, F. O. Schmitt, ed. New York: Rockefeller Univ. Press, pp. 587–597.

PRECHT, W., 1977. Physiology of the peripheral and central vestibular systems. In *Frog Neurobiology*, R. Llinás and W. Precht, eds. New York: Springer-Verlag, pp. 481–512.

PRECHT, W., and R. LLINÁS, 1969. Comparative aspects of the vestibular input to the cerebellum. In *Neurobiology of Cerebellar Evolution and Development*, R. Llinás, ed. Chicago: American Medical Association, pp. 619–627.

PRECHT, W., R. LLINÁS, and M. CLARKE, 1971. Physiological responses of frog vestibular fibers to horizontal angular rotation. *Exp. Brain Res.* 13:378–407.

PURPURA, D. P., 1967. Comparative physiology of dendrites. In *The Neurosciences: A Study Program*, G. C. Quarton, T. Melnechuk, and F. O. Schmitt, eds. New York: Rockefeller Univ. Press, pp. 372–393.

RALL, W., 1959. Dendritic current distribution and whole neuron properties. *Naval Med. Res. Inst. Res.*, Report NM 01-05-00.01.02, pp. 479–526.

RALL, W., 1962. Electrophysiology of a dendritic neuron model. *Biophys. J. (Suppl.)* 2:145–167.

RALL, W., 1964. Theoretical significance of dendritic trees for neuronal input-output relations. In *Neural Theory and Modeling*, R. F. Reiss, ed. Stanford, CA: Stanford Univ. Press, pp. 73–97.

RALL, W., 1977. Core conductor theory and cable properties of neurons. In *Handbook of Physiology: The Nervous System I*, E. R. Kandel, ed. Bethesda, MD: American Physiological Society, pp. 39–97.

RAMÓN Y CAJAL, S., 1911. *Histologie du système nerveux de l'homme et des vertébrés*, 2 volumes. Paris: Maloine.

RASHEVSKY, N., 1933. Outline of a physico-mathematical theory of excitation and inhibition. *Protoplasma* 20:42–56.

REISS, R. F., ed., 1964. *Neural Theory and Modeling*. Stanford, CA: Stanford Univ. Press.

ROCHESTER, N., J. H. HOLLAND, L. H. HAIBT, and W. L. DUDA, 1956. Tests on a cell assembly theory of the action of the brain, using a large digital computer. *IRE Trans. Inf. Theory* IT-2 (3):80–93.

ROSENBLATT, F., 1962. *Principles of Neurodynamics: Perceptrons and the Theory of Brain Mechanisms*. Washington: Spartan Books.

SCHMITT, O. H., 1937. Mechanical solution of the equations of nerve impulse propagation. *Am. J. Physiol.* 119:399–400.

SHERRINGTON, S. C., 1906. *The Integrative Action of the Nervous System*. New Haven, CT: Yale Univ. Press.

SOMOGYI, P., and J. HÁMORI, 1976. A quantitative electron microscopic study of the Purkinje cell axon initial segment. *Neuroscience* 1:361–365.

STEIN, W. B., K. G. PEARSON, R. S. SMITH, and J. B. REDFORD, 1973. *Control of Posture and Locomotion*. New York: Plenum Press.

SZÉKELY, GY., 1965. Logical network for controlling limb movements in *Urodela*. *Acta Physiol. Acad. Sci. Hung.* 27:285–289.

SZÉKELY, GY., A. CZÉH, and A. VÖRÖS, 1969. The activity pattern of limb muscles in freely moving normal and deafferented newts. *Exp. Brain Res.* 9:53–62.

SZÉKELY, GY., and A. CZÉH, 1977. Organization of locomotion. In *Frog Neurobiology*, R. Llinás and W. Precht, eds. New York: Springer-Verlag, pp. 765–792.

SZENTÁGOTHAI, J., 1963. Ujabb adatok a synapsis funkcionális anatómiájához. *MTA Biol. Tud. Oszt. Közl.* 6:217–227.

SZENTÁGOTHAI, J., 1968. Structuro-functional considerations of the cerebellar neuron network. *Proc. IEEE* 56 (6):960–968.

SZENTÁGOTHAI, J., 1975. From the last skirmishes around the neuron theory to the functional anatomy of neuron networks. In *The Neurosciences: Paths of Discovery*, F. G. Worden, J. P. Swazey, and G. Adelman, eds. Cambridge: MIT Press, pp. 103–120.

SZENTÁGOTHAI, J., and M. A. ARBIB, 1974. Conceptual models of neural organization. *Neurosci. Res. Program Bull.* 12:307–510.

TRAUB, R. D., and R. LLINÁS, 1977. Spatial distribution of ionic conductances in normal and axotomized motoneurons. *Neuroscience* 2:829–849.

TURING, A. M., 1950. Computing machinery and intelligence. *Mind* 59:433–460.

UTTLEY, A. M., 1959. Conditional probability computing in a nervous system. In *Mechanization of Thought Processes*. London: Her Majesty's Stationery Office, vol. 1, pp. 119–132.

WEBER, H., 1873. Über die stationären Strömungen der Electricität in Cylindern. *J. Reine Angew. Math.* 76:1–20.

YOUNG, J. Z., 1964. *A Model of the Brain*. London: Oxford Univ. Press.

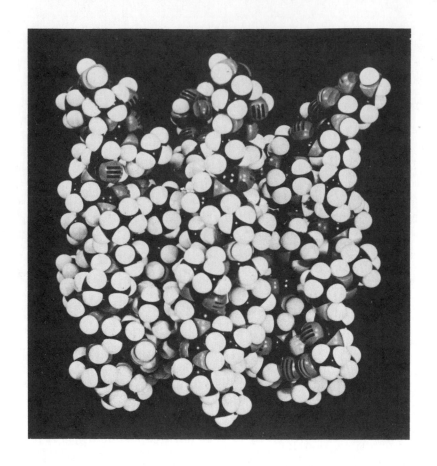

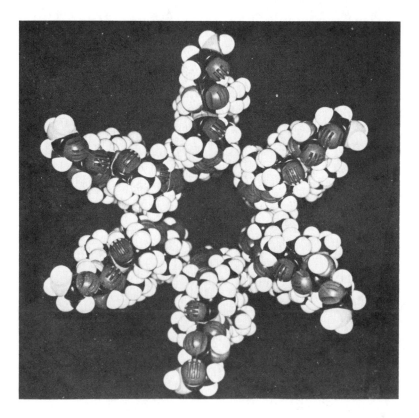

HIGH-SENSITIVITY
TRANSDUCTION

Hypothetical molecular model of a membrane channel formed by the aggregation of six alamethicin molecules. The peptide chain is folded into a hairpin loop with one side in β configuration, the other containing four residues in α-helix configuration. Top: *Side view, parallel to the membrane plane. The nonpolar groups, facing outward, interact with the lipid hydrocarbon chains.* Bottom: *View into the channel normal to the membrane plane. The carbonyl groups of the β chain face inward, forming a hydrophilic channel interior. (From G. Baumann and P. Mueller, A molecular model of membrane excitability* Journal of Supramolecular Structure 2:538-557, 1974.)

Introduction

RODOLFO LLINÁS

THE POSSIBILITY that neurons may interact other than synaptically and through means other than action potentials has been considered since the time of Ramón y Cajal. Indeed his retinal "amacrine" (or axonless) cells suggested to him that "unusual" forms of connectivity could exist between these cells. Nowadays such specialized connectivity is understood to be quite common and, in fact, to form the basis for what are referred to as local circuit interactions.

The concept of local circuit neurons has gained vigorous support from morphological and functional studies in vertebrates and invertebrates, but the possibility of truly local interactions between neuronal elements was in fact born out of theoretical considerations of the molecular properties of neuronal membranes (cf. Schmitt, Dev, and Smith, 1976). This is not altogether surprising since many significant insights into the functional properties of nerve cells have derived from membrane biophysics. Although the treatment of neuronal cable properties continues to be central to the understanding of nerve conduction, a true conception of the nature of electroresponsiveness can only result from superimposing upon these passive properties voltage- and chemical-dependent ionic membrane conductance changes. The voltage-dependent changes were basically clarified by the now-classical contribution of Hodgkin and Huxley. Also of great significance was the realization that the dielectric properties of membranes reside in the lipid bilayer, as postulated by Danielli and Davson, and as a corollary that, given an effective dielectric thickness of 50 Å and a resting potential on the order of -70 mV, an electric field of 140 kV/cm is present across the membrane interphases. Further insight was reached through the realization that macromolecules may actually span the thickness of the membrane and thus be said to "see" this large transmembrane field. At this present stage, then, electrophysiology, ultrastructure, and molecular biology are undergoing a process of conceptual interlacing out of which a more realistic view of membrane biophysics has begun to emerge. Indeed we are becoming accustomed to thinking in terms of transmembrane macromolecular conformation, electrostatic equivalents (Debye), dipole moments and torques, and membrane fluidity, to name only a few. Beyond this, ionic specificity and charge displacement, and their relation to chemical structure, are all part of the general approach.

These aspects of membrane biophysics are treated by two main themes in this section. First, the relations between specific ionic conductances (in particular, those for calcium) are considered with regard to different aspects of neuronal function. Second, the properties of transmembrane electric fields and their action on membrane-bound macromolecules are explored.

In the first paper, I review some of the kinetic properties of voltage-dependent calcium conductance changes and their relationship to both transmitter release in presynaptic terminals and neuronal integration via calcium-dependent dendritic spikes. A general hypothesis of the role played by such calcium currents in neuronal function is presented. The main emphasis of the hypothesis is on the similarities between synaptic release and neuronal plasticity, as exemplified by the concept of isometric growth.

A detailed analysis of the actual process of transmitter release as seen from a rapid-freezing ultrastructural point of view is introduced by John Heuser and Thomas Reese. Their paper summarizes most of what we now know of the process of exocytosis and the mechanism for vesicular recycling. Using such drugs as 4-aminopyridine, which are known to block potassium conductance, Heuser and Reese have increased the magnitude and duration of the synaptic release and thus demonstrated many morphological aspects of vesicular exocytosis.

Another aspect of calcium regulation of neuronal integration is reviewed by H. D. Lux and C. B. Heyer. They analyze the voltage-dependent properties of the slow calcium current in the somata of molluscan neurons and relate them to the calcium-dependent potassium current $I_{K(Ca)}$ and the process of calcium current facilitation by repetitive stimulation. The authors underline the importance of this mechanism in neu-

ronal integration, as well as many of the comparative aspects of this ion-dependent ionic conductance change.

The problem of calcium as a general modulator and as a second messenger in eukaryotic cells is considered by Robert Kretsinger. His views are based on the structural characteristics of calcium-modulated proteins, which he assumes to be homologous throughout phylogeny. Kretsinger presents a very compelling argument based on the similarities of such calcium-binding molecules in different biological systems and on the importance of the so-called EF hand binding sites (consisting of a helix, a calcium-binding loop, and then another helix), which he assumes to be the molecular basis for the calcium-specific functions in the cellular economy.

In the second portion of this section, E. Neher and C. F. Stevens, Gerhard Schwarz, and Paul Mueller discuss different aspects of field-dependent modifications on membrane-bound macromolecules, and P. Gräber and H. T. Witt approach the problem of membrane field as a source for ATP synthesis.

Neher and Stevens analyze the kinetic basis for molecular gating, using the neuromuscular acetylcholine receptor as a model. They approach the question of energy profile for given macromolecular configurations and the rate of conformational change at different energy levels. They conclude that the electric field is indeed capable of producing conformational change in the postsynaptic receptor moiety by modifying the equilibrium dipole moment for the open and closed conformations of this channel.

Continuing with this theme, Schwarz examines in detail the effect of electric fields on the membrane-bound macromolecules. He emphasizes that, in addition to the purely mechanical force exerted on the macromolecular dipole by the membrane field, the displacement of chemical equilibrium within the macromolecule itself may be decisive in the field-gating process. He proposes that if interactions between macromolecular compartments can be organized in a cooperative manner, a strongly interacting chemical subunit will ensue, which may be a better model for conformational changes than the purely physical view of molecular reorientation across the membrane.

Mueller, on the other hand, presents a very elegant physical model for electrical excitability in artificial lipid bilayers. Going beyond the classical view that intramolecular conformational change produces a transmembrane channel, he examines the possibility that a channel may actually be formed across the membrane by modulation of the membrane field. In particular, experimental evidence on the properties of lipid bilayers in the presence of alamethicin and related compounds suggests that the field itself may produce a flip-flop effect on molecules lying on the surface of the membrane, so that they are forced to span the thickness of the membrane. Several such molecules may then aggregate to form ionic channels. This insertion aggregation model is viewed as capable of reproducing all of the electrophysiological phenomena observed in nerve.

Gräber and Witt approach the problem of electric fields from a different angle. They have determined that the photosynthetic process of chloroplasts generates an electric field across the membrane. However, rather than utilize the photosynthetic abilities of these cellular systems to generate electrical changes across membranes, they have used the system backwards by modifying the membrane potential via an external electric field. The action of the electric field can thus be isolated from the photosynthetic step. Using this methodology, the authors demonstrate that membrane field changes themselves are capable of activating a membrane-bound ATPase, which in turn allows a transmembrane proton movement and through it the synthesis of ATP. In this case, rather than the activation of a conductance change, we see the membrane potential per se triggering ATP synthesis.

All in all, the molecular mechanisms necessary to modulate cell function, from action potentials to subtle chemical changes, seem to be present in great abundance. The point at hand, however, is whether there is a common level of complexity, a basic coinage to all the electrophysiological events that underlie brain function. The data presented here seem to indicate clearly that this common level is not the neuron or the synapse; instead, we seem to have irreversibly risen to the molecular phase of our quest!

REFERENCE

SCHMITT, F. O., P. DEV, and B. H. SMITH, 1976. Electronic processing of information by brain cells. *Science* 193:114–120.

31 The Role of Calcium in Neuronal Function

RODOLFO LLINÁS

ABSTRACT Different aspects of calcium-dependent neuronal functions are discussed, with particular emphasis on synaptic transmission and dendritic spikes. In regard to synaptic transmission, quantitative parameters relating presynaptic depolarization to transmitter release are presented. A set of kinetic equations derived from presynaptic voltage-clamp studies is used to develop a comprehensive mathematical model for synaptic transmission. Next the role of calcium conductance in dendritic electroresponsiveness is considered. Evidence is presented that, besides being a current carrier, calcium may have other functions relating to general neuronal economy. The possibility that a calcium current modulates dendritic release of synaptic transmitters, peptides, and hormones and the possible role of calcium in dendroplasmic flow and genome expression are discussed.

The presynaptic and dendritic actions of calcium conductance are then unified into a single hypothesis, which proposes that dendritic spiking and synaptic transmission may be part of a more general calcium action (i.e., the regulation of growth). Such growth is termed "isometric," implying that its main purpose is not to increase the cell surface but rather to serve, through exocytosis and related mechanisms, as a vehicle for the release of intracellular substances and for the insertion of new membrane and new membrane-bound proteins onto the plasmalemmal surface. The paper concludes by suggesting that some aspects of synaptic transmission and neuronal plasticity are, in fact, vestigial growth-cone properties.

THE ROLE of calcium as a regulator of cell biological properties has been the subject of a great many research papers, reviews, and symposia over the last ten years (see, e.g., Cuthbert, 1970; Rubin, 1974; Smellie, 1974; Baker and Reuter, 1975; Blaustein, 1976a,b; Duncan, 1976). From the neurobiological point of view, calcium is currently regarded as one of the key factors in the operation of nerve cells, not only through its mediation of synaptic transmission but also, and in a deeper sense, in the maintenance of long-term neuronal viability.

Historically the role of calcium in neuronal func-

RODOLFO LLINÁS Department of Physiology and Biophysics, New York University Medical Center, New York, NY 10016

tion was seen mainly as a stabilizing factor for membrane electroresponsiveness (Frankenhaeuser and Hodgkin, 1957; cf. Shanes, 1958). For many years it was considered of minor importance, especially with respect to neuronal integration and nerve conduction. This was, however, not the case regarding its role in synaptic transmission. The fact that calcium is required for transmission at the neuromuscular junction was determined almost a century ago (Locke, 1894) and has been championed for more than two decades by Katz and colleagues at University College, London (see Katz, 1969). More recent developments in our knowledge of the role of this ion in synaptic release will be discussed at some length here.

It is my own feeling, shared with many colleagues, that calcium plays a more far-reaching role in neuronal function than may be apparent from its action as membrane stabilizer, trigger of transmitter release, or transmembrane charge carrier. In this paper I shall summarize certain aspects of calcium action at the single-cell level and propose a general hypothesis for its role in neuronal function.

Calcium in synaptic transmission

It is now agreed that the triggering of synaptic transmitter release is produced by an inward calcium current across the presynaptic terminal and that such release is, fundamentally, a variation on the general theme of cellular secretion (Rubin, 1970, 1974; cf. Douglas, 1976). Thus a number of common denominators in the so-called depolarization-secretion coupling seem to be emerging, among them: (1) its calcium dependence, which is often itself voltage-dependent (Douglas, 1974; Rubin, 1974; Mackie, 1975, 1976; Llinás and Heuser, 1977); (2) the antagonism between calcium and magnesium (Rubin, 1974); and (3) the blockage of secretion by substances that block calcium permeability (Dean and Mathews, 1970; Rubin, 1974).

From the viewpoint of synaptic transmission, the role of calcium has been investigated directly in the

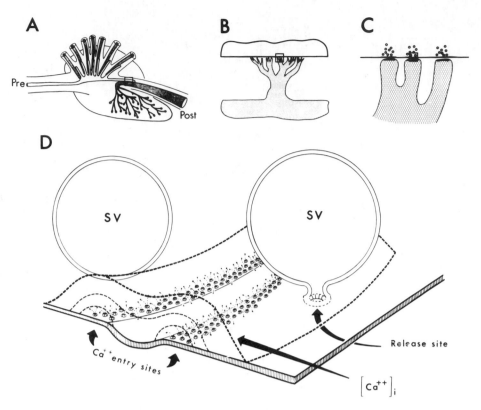

FIGURE 1 Schematic diagram of the morphology of the giant synapse in squid stellate ganglion. (A) The presynaptic axon (Pre) generates eight terminals in contact with their respective postsynaptic (Post) axons. (B) The small area marked in A by a square is enlarged, illustrating that the junction between the pre- and postsynaptic fiber takes place via dendritelike processes from the postsynaptic axon. (C) The synapse is actually made between a flat presynaptic terminal and spinelike projections at the tips of the postsynaptic processes. Typical synaptic specializations containing pre- and postjunctional thickenings and synaptic vesi-cles are indicated. (D) Diagram of the active zone, modeled after freeze-fracture micrographs of the active zone in the neuromuscular junction. The voltage-dependent calcium current is assumed to enter the terminal through channels believed to be the intramembranous particles seen in freeze-fracture (calcium entry sites). Broken lines illustrate the hypothetical distribution of intracellular calcium, $[Ca^{++}]_i$, and its relation to the synaptic release sites. Calcium current is assumed to generate a well-localized change in calcium concentration in the vicinity of the active zone, triggering vesicle (SV) opening at that location.

squid stellate ganglion (Young, 1939), in which the presynaptic and postsynaptic elements are large enough (Figure 1) to be intracellularly impaled by several electrodes simultaneously (Bullock and Hagiwara, 1957; Hagiwara and Tasaki, 1958; Takeuchi and Takeuchi, 1962; Miledi and Slater, 1966). Qualitatively the most salient point in recent studies of this synapse has been the demonstration that an increase in intracellular calcium concentration, $[Ca^{++}]_i$ (or better still, calcium activity), is the necessary and sufficient condition to trigger transmitter release. This increase in $[Ca^{++}]_i$ usually is produced by a voltage-dependent calcium conductance change, but any other mechanism capable of producing an equivalent increase in $[Ca^{++}]_i$ (at the appropriate site) would be equally effective. Three kinds of experiments support this conclusion.

1. As shown in Figure 2A–C even with pharmacological blockage of the voltage-dependent sodium and potassium permeabilities in the squid presynaptic terminal, synaptic transmitter may still be released by direct depolarization of the terminal (Bloedel et al., 1966; Katz and Miledi, 1967, 1970; Kusano, Livengood, and Werman, 1967; Kusano, 1970; Llinás and Nicholson, 1975) if the calcium conductance has not been blocked by other means (see below).

2. Synaptic transmission is accompanied by an inward calcium current. This was strongly suggested by the discovery of tetrodotoxin-insensitive presynaptic spikes (Katz and Miledi, 1969) and was directly demonstrated by injecting aequorin, a calcium-dependent, light-emitting protein (Shimomura and Johnson, 1970; Blinks, Prendergast, and Allen, 1976), into the presynaptic terminal. It was shown that under these

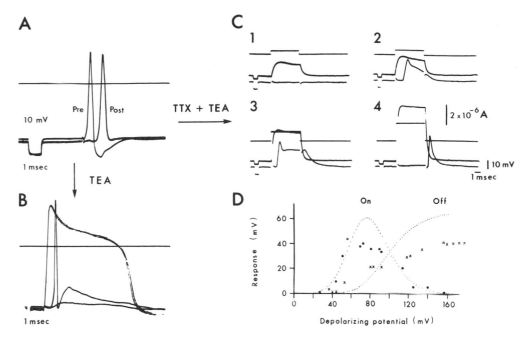

FIGURE 2 Synaptic transmission following blockage of sodium and potassium conductance at the squid synapse. (A) Simultaneous pre- and postsynaptic recording during synaptic transmission. (B) Same as A but following presynaptic intracellular injection of TEA, which prolongs the presynaptic spike and thus the postsynaptic response. (C) Same as B but, in addition, sodium conductance is blocked by TTX. The relationship between presynaptic depolarization (middle trace) and postsynaptic response (lower trace) is illustrated. The upper trace marks amplitude and duration of presynaptic current injection. In C4 presynaptic depolari-zation reaches suppression potential, so that only an "off" response is observed postsynaptically at the end of the current pulse. (From Llinás and Nicholson, 1975.) (D) Plot of the relationship between presynaptic depolarization and postsynaptic potential for the "on" and "off" responses. Experimental values are shown as filled circles (on) and crosses (off); dotted lines correspond to the numerical solution for equations derived from voltage-clamp experiments. (From Llinás, Steinberg, and Walton, 1976.) In this and subsequent figures, the voltage, current, and time calibrations are as indicated.

conditions synaptic transmission is accompanied by light emission, demonstrating an increase in $[Ca^{++}]_i$ (Llinás, Blinks, and Nicholson, 1972). A subsequent study showed that the magnitude of light emission is a complex nonlinear function of the presynaptic potential (Llinás and Nicholson, 1975) quite similar to that observed between presynaptic depolarization and transmitter release (see Figure 2D) (Katz and Miledi, 1967; Kusano et al., 1967; Llinás and Nicholson, 1975).

The level of depolarization at which synaptic transmitter release is blocked is now known as the "suppression potential" (Katz and Miledi, 1967). In agreement with Katz and Miledi's assumption, the aequorin study indicated that this suppression is produced by the abolition of inward calcium current as the membrane potential reaches the calcium equilibrium level (E_{Ca}) (Llinás and Nicholson, 1975). A similar "off" calcium current had been previously observed, with aequorin, in *Aplysia* cell bodies depolarized to E_{Ca} (Stinnakre and Tauc, 1973).

3. Further evidence for a calcium-dependent re-lease was obtained by injecting calcium into the stellate ganglion preterminal (Miledi, 1973) or by the increased presynaptic $[Ca^{++}]_i$ following release from intracellular stores at the neuromuscular junction (Glagoleva, Lieberman, and Khashayev, 1970; Katz and Edwards, 1973; Alnaes and Rahamimoff, 1975).

Voltage-clamp studies

Recently the question of the role of calcium in synaptic transmission has been tackled in a more quantitative fashion, with a voltage-clamp approach used to determine the voltage and time dependence of the ionic presynaptic currents during transmission (Llinás, Steinberg, and Walton, 1976; cf. Llinás, 1977). In preparations where sodium conductance is blocked by tetrodotoxin (TTX) (Narahashi, Moore, and Scott, 1964) and potassium conductance by 3- or 4-aminopyridine (3- or 4-AmP) (Pelhate and Pichon, 1974; Llinás, Walton, and Bohr, 1976) or tetraethyl-ammonium (TEA) (Armstrong and Binstock, 1965), rapid depolarization steps using a voltage-clamp technique (Adrian, Chandler, and Hodgkin, 1970) may be accomplished at the presynaptic terminal. This step depolarization is shortly followed by a calcium-dependent inward current, which may be blocked by removing calcium from the extracellular medium or by the addition of manganese 50 mM or cadmium chloride 1 mM (Llinás, 1977), as shown previously for other voltage-dependent calcium currents (Hagiwara and Takahashi, 1967; Baker, Hodgkin, and Ridgway, 1971; Baker, 1972; Baker, Meves, and Ridgway, 1973; Reuter, 1973; Baker and Glitsch, 1975; cf. Meves, 1975; Kostyuk and Krishtal, 1977). The voltage-clamp results have revealed a number of interesting points, which will be discussed sequentially.

VOLTAGE AND TIME DEPENDENCE OF THE CALCIUM CONDUCTANCE CHANGE   Following the onset of a sustained presynaptic depolarization, the membrane permeability to calcium increases rather slowly compared to that of sodium (Hodgkin and Huxley, 1952) and reaches a peak whose amplitude varies with the level of depolarization (Figure 3B). This S-shaped onset function is followed by a plateau of calcium current, indicating that the calcium permeability does not inactivate, at least for pulses of up to 30 msec in duration. At the end of the pulse, a calcium tail current is apparent and is followed by a secondary transmitter release, the "off-response."

The relationship between membrane depolarization and the calcium current is seen in Figure 3B. Here a set of experimental points are superimposed on a continuous line obtained as a numerical solution to a set of mathematical equations derived from these voltage-clamp experiments (Llinás, Steinberg, and Walton, 1976; see below). Given that the voltage de-

pendence of this inward current parallels that observed for synaptic release under current-clamp conditions (Figures 2D and 6G), transmitter release must be approximately linearly related to the inward calcium current, at least at the calcium concentrations studied in these experiments (5, 10, 20, and 40 mM). The relationship between calcium current and transmitter release is shown in Figure 3C in a double log plot with a slope of 1.25, indicating an almost linear relationship between these two variables. The significance of these findings to the process of release will be discussed later in more detail. It suffices to say at this stage that the magnitude of the calcium currents in these experiments suggests that a large number of calcium ions move into the presynaptic terminal prior to and during transmitter release. Thus the prevalent idea that only a few calcium ions move across the membrane for each vesicle release seems unwarranted. This is not to say, however, that the actual opening of a given vesicle may require interaction with only one or a few calcium ions.

The second important variable determining calcium conductance is the time dependence of this permeability change. As shown in Figure 3A, after a rapid step depolarization of the preterminal, there is a delay in the onset of the calcium current (I_{Ca}) of 600–700 μsec at depolarization levels on the order of 35 mV. The tail current, on the other hand, has a virtually instantaneous onset, the presence of any delay being related almost exclusively to the speed of the voltage-clamp step.

SYNAPTIC DELAY: TWO COMPONENTS   Another interesting result obtained from these voltage-clamp studies relates to the nature of synaptic delay. As discussed in previous papers (e.g., Llinás, 1977) and

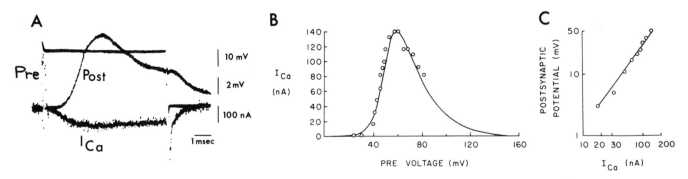

FIGURE 3   Presynaptic voltage clamp in the squid synapse. (A) Records obtained by voltage clamping a presynaptic terminal (Pre) by 35 mV (from a resting potential of −70 mV). Inward calcium current (I_{Ca}) is seen as a downgoing deflection with a slow onset and tail current. Postsynaptic

response (Post) shows an "on" response and small "off" potential. (From Llinás, 1977.) (B) Plot of I_{Ca} against presynaptic voltage. (C) Plot of postsynaptic potential against I_{Ca} (note the double log scale).

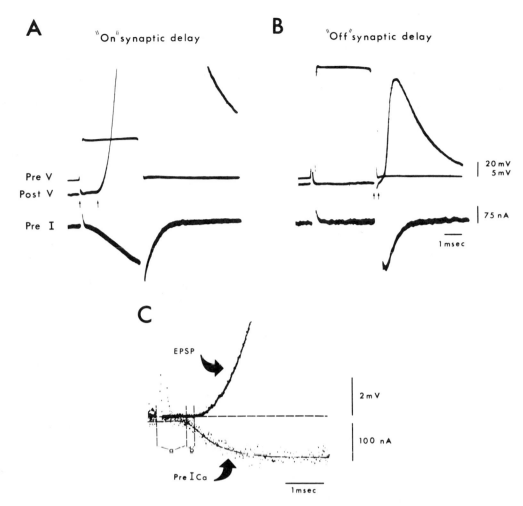

A "On" synaptic delay

Pre V
Post V
Pre I

B "Off" synaptic delay

20 mV
5 mV

75 nA

1 msec

C

EPSP

2 mV

100 nA

Pre I Ca

1 msec

FIGURE 4 Synaptic delay. (A) The "on" response is shown for a voltage step of 60 mV from resting (upper trace). Postsynaptic potential shows a synaptic delay (arrows) of 1 msec. The presynaptic current shows a slow onset and a sharp tail current. (B) The "off" delay (about 200 μsec, marked by arrows) following a depolarization to the suppression potential (140 mV from resting) and the associated tail current. (Llinás and Walton, unpublished results.) (C) Records showing the delay (a) for the onset of the calcium current (Pre I_{Ca}) and the delay (b) between onset of the calcium current and onset of the postsynaptic response. (From Llinás, 1977.)

illustrated in Figure 4, the temporal relationship between depolarization and transmitter release may be divided into two parts, which we have called a and b. The first component of this delay, a, is related to the time required for opening of the calcium channels, while the b portion relates to the time between entry of calcium and release of transmitter substance. Examples of these two components of delay can be obtained by comparing the on- and off-release as shown in Figure 4A and 4B. In record A, a 60 mV presynaptic voltage-clamp step (from 70 mV holding potential) demonstrates a characteristic 1 msec delay for the on-response. The record in B, taken at the suppression potential, illustrates the "off" calcium tail current and the synaptic potential generated by this short (300–400 μsec time constant) inward surge of calcium (Llinás, Walton, and Sugimori, 1977 and unpublished results). In this case the synaptic delay is quite short (in the vicinity of 200 μsec). The actual synaptic delay may, in fact, be slightly shorter since the falling phase of the pulse is not instantaneous. In Figure 4C (same experiment as shown in Figure 3A) the a and b synaptic delays can be seen directly at higher gain and sweep speed. Here the presynaptic depolarization was smaller than that in A, allowing a clear visualization of the a delay. A direct measurement for these two components was obtained (Llinás, 1977) by comparing the time of onset of the voltage-clamp pulse with the first sign of inward calcium current (a in Figure 4C) and then the delay between the current onset with the initiation of transmitter release (*b* in Figure 4C).

Among these measurements, the short delay between calcium current and transmitter release is apparently the most significant. The brevity of the delay indicates that the site of calcium entry must be strategically located quite near the site of release, as shown in Figure 1D. This view has been analyzed theoretically by Parsegian (1977; see also Llinás and Heuser, 1977). Indeed, based on this short latency, it has been proposed that the intramembranous particles observed at the neuromuscular active zone (Couteaux and Pécot-Dechavassine, 1970) and in CNS synapses by freeze-fracture are the actual calcium channels (Reese, in Llinás and Heuser, 1977; see also Venzin et al., 1977). Furthermore, in a preliminary set of measurements Heuser (personal communication) has calculated that the number of such active-zone intramembranous particles at the neuromuscular junction is almost $150/\mu m^2$, comparable to the number recently measured in squid synapses (Pumplin, Reese, and Llinás, in preparation). Using this hypothesis, we have estimated that since calcium current density during an action potential is 35 $\mu A/cm^2/sec$, an average of 8 calcium ions may move per channel per action potential (Llinás, 1977). Assuming that only about 10 percent of the channels actually "open" during the spike, the total number of ions moving per channel would be 80; this is equivalent to a conductance per channel of approximately $10^{-14}S$, a figure very similar to that obtained for calcium noise in *Aplysia* neurons by Brown, Akaike, and Lee (1978). Finally, most of the voltage-clamp experiments reported here were performed at 18°C. At lower temperatures and in agreement with previous work (Lester, 1970; Weight and Erulkar, 1976), the synaptic delay is enhanced. This is partly due to the slowing of calcium current kinetics (Llinás, Walton, and Sugimori, 1978) and partly due to slowing of the release process, probably caused, among other parameters, by a change in lipid bilayer fluidity.

In short, while this hypothesis is far from being demonstrated, it is attractive to suppose that the rows of intramembranous particles observed at the neuromuscular junction (Dreyer et al., 1973; Dreifuss et al., 1973; cf. Heuser and Reese, 1977) and those in central synapses of vertebrates and invertebrates (Pfenninger et al., 1971, 1972; Venzin et al., 1977) may be the actual calcium channels. Beyond the question of synaptic transmission, this arrangement suggests that calcium channels are distributed in a nonrandom manner on the axolemmal surface, probably in relation to intracellular structures involved in transmitter release or, as we shall see later, to other cellular functions.

MATHEMATICAL MODEL FOR SYNAPTIC TRANSMITTER RELEASE   Based on the above results, Steinberg, Walton, and I developed a kinetic model for the relation between presynaptic depolarization and calcium current and between calcium current and transmitter release (Llinás, Steinberg, and Walton, 1976). The model indicates: (1) that the calcium conductance change follows fifth-order Michaelis-Menten kinetics; and (2) that the opening of the channel is probably accompanied by a gating current (Armstrong and Bezanilla, 1973; Keynes and Rojas, 1974) of five charges—assuming that the fifth-order kinetics corresponds to five noncooperative conformational changes occurring prior to the channel opening. These conformational changes, which are voltage- and time-dependent, are thought to be governed, as in the Hodgkin and Huxley model (1952), by forward and backward rate constants between the active and inactive states of the subunits in the channels. Based on these assumptions, a numerical solution for I_{Ca}^{∞} was calculated and is illustrated in Figure 3B (continuous line).

These equations have also allowed Pellionisz and myself to determine the calcium conductance in the presynaptic terminal (Figure 5). The presynaptic terminal was modeled as a one-compartment cable. Sodium and potassium currents (I_{Na} and I_K) were calculated, using Hodgkin and Huxley's equations (1952) and calcium current (I_{Ca}) from equation 8 in Llinás, Steinberg, and Walton (1976). The sodium, potassium, and calcium conductance changes for an action potential are illustrated in Figure 5A, in which it is assumed that the sodium and potassium currents in the terminal are comparable to those of the postsynaptic axon. Permeability curves shown in Figure 5A suggest that calcium permeability (g_{Ca}) during an action potential is rather small and has a late onset with respect to both sodium and potassium (g_{Na} and g_K, respectively). The current carried by these three ions during an action potential is shown in the lower record and indicates that I_{Ca} is approximately twenty times smaller than I_{Na}.

The remaining steps leading to synaptic transmission were modeled by assuming a linear relationship between calcium current and transmitter release and a constant delay of 200 μsec between the onset of calcium current and the postsynaptic response. Thus, as illustrated in Figure 5B, an experimentally obtained action potential was utilized to obtain (via equations 5 and 8 from our paper) the time courses

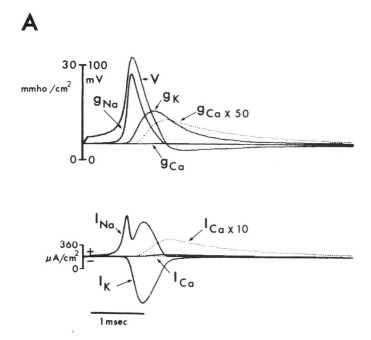

A

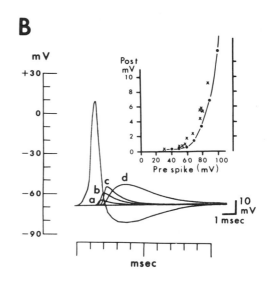

B

FIGURE 5   Theoretical solution for propagating action potential in the presynaptic terminal and related steps in synaptic transmission. (A) Ionic conductances and currents associated with the activation of the presynaptic terminal following the Hodgkin-Huxley (1952) equations for sodium (g_{Na}) and potassium (g_K) conductances. The calcium conductance (g_{Ca}) was derived from equation 8 of Llinás, Steinberg, and Walton (1976) and is shown at unity and on an expanded (×50) scale to illustrate the time course. The lower trace shows currents for the three ions during the presynaptic action potential (I_{Ca} at unity and × 10 scale).

(Llinás and Pellionisz, unpublished results.) (B) Reconstruction of events during synaptic transmission, based on equations 5 and 8 of Llinás, Steinberg, and Walton (1976). (a) Calcium channel formation, (b) calcium current, (c) synaptic current, and (d) synaptic potential. The insert to the right shows the changes in the amplitude of the postsynaptic potential in millivolts against the presynaptic amplitude obtained experimentally by Takeuchi and Takeuchi (1962; crosses) and the results obtained from the model (filled circles), on an arbitrary scale. (From Llinás, Steinberg, and Walton, 1976.)

of (a) the calcium-channel formation, (b) the calcium current, (c) the postsynaptic current, and (d) the postsynaptic potential. The characteristics of these variables (especially those of c and d) are amenable to comparison with actual records and resemble typical experimental results (Llinás, 1977) quite closely. Furthermore, when the amplitude of the action potential is varied from 40 to 100 mV (inset in Figure 5B), the results obtained by the mathematical model (circles) closely resemble the experimental results (crosses) of Takeuchi and Takeuchi (1962). The data reviewed here thus suggest that the kinetics of the voltage-dependent calcium conductance change in the presynaptic terminal go a long way toward explaining some of the properties of synaptic release.

One interesting detail clarified by this model is the fact that transmitter release by an action potential is mainly an "off" release, since, given the time course of the action potential, I_{Ca} normally occurs at the falling phase of the spike. It is interesting that the onset of g_{Ca} occurs while the membrane potential is

returning to its resting level; thus the ionic conductance change occurs at a high calcium EMF. Furthermore, since g_{Ca} lasts for several milliseconds, it actually overlaps with the afterhyperpolarization, which further increases calcium EMF.

High- and low-gain synapses

As stated at the beginning of this paper, it is now believed that a common mechanism exists for the release process in all chemical synapses. Of central interest in the present volume is an attempt to understand the depolarization-release properties of different chemical junctions. This is especially important since many morphological details in CNS synapses (see Shepherd, this volume) suggest that transmission may involve several varieties of junctions and may in some cases occur in the absence of action potentials. The term *high- and low-gain synapses* refers here to the relationship between presynaptic depolarization and transmitter release. Low-gain synapses are most often subserved by presynaptic action potentials and produce transient release of transmitter substances. This is the most common type of synapse in the central nervous system (e.g., Ia input to motoneurons, climbing-fiber/Purkinje-cell synapse). In this case synaptic release may require presynaptic action potentials of at least 40 mV amplitude (see insert in Figure 5B). In high-gain synapses, on the other hand, minute changes in presynaptic membrane potential may produce a rather large response in the postsynaptic cells (on the order of 1 mV in Figure 6H), as shown by Bennett (1967) in the electroreceptor. In fact, some of these systems seem to have a maximum range of about 1 mV from either side of the basic firing level. Such high-gain synaptic release is now known to occur in peripheral systems besides electroreceptors, for example, in vestibular receptors (Benshalom and Flock, 1977) and retinal circuits (Dowling, this volume), as well as in the CNS of invertebrates (Pearson, this volume; Graubard and Calvin, this volume).

The question, then, is whether high-gain synaptic transmission represents a special category or simply a variation on the general theme. To study the problem in another light, we proceeded to determine whether synaptic transmission in the squid synapse has a threshold (i.e., whether the preterminal must be depolarized to a given level before transmitter release is observed). It was found (Llinás and Walton, unpublished observations) that following TTX and 3-AmP it is possible to measure a synaptic transmitter release with depolarizations as small as 6 mV (Figure 6F). Here, rather than applying a fast transient pulse, long pulses of small amplitude were applied presynaptically. The postsynaptic responses were amplified enough to observe miniature potentials (Miledi, 1967; Mann and Joyner, 1976; Llinás and Walton, unpublished observations). As shown in Figure 6A–E, the results clearly indicate that release is an almost continuous function of voltage; in this respect, low- and high-gain synapses are similar. Moreover, Charlton and Atwood (1977) have found that presynaptic depolarizations as small as 3 mV may be sufficient to release transmitter, in this synapse, if the pulses are long enough (1–4 sec). Two factors must then be considered: (1) voltage sensitivity and (2) time dependence.

Close analysis of the voltage sensitivity of these two forms of transmission indicates that the difference, as suggested by Bennett (1968), may depend in part on the biasing of the voltage-dependent properties of the calcium channel by the membrane potential. That is, the rather sensitive property of the high-gain synapse may be reproduced in the squid synapse if,

rather than a resting potential close to −70 mV, the system is held at, let us say, −30 mV. In this case, since the voltage dependence of the calcium channel would be located in the steepest part of the release curve (see Figure 6G), the sensitivity of this system could, in principle, be comparable to that of the high-gain synapse. In fact, we find an *e*-fold calcium-current increase every 6 mV of predepolarization (Llinás, 1977), which is comparable to that found in the transmission between the nonspiking stretch receptor to the motoneuron synapse in the crab (Blight and Llinás, unpublished observations) and in high-gain systems in other invertebrates (K. Graubard, personal communication) as well as in the squid giant axon (Baker, Hodgkin, and Ridgway, 1971).

One of the problems in trying to reproduce the properties of high-gain synapses with a low-gain system is that low-gain synapses fatigue quite easily when depolarization is maintained. Thus continuous release cannot be obtained, and depletion of transmitter substance quickly ensues. High-gain synapses, then, may be different from low-gain synapses mainly in the mechanism of vesicle turnover and transmitter synthesis, rather than in the voltage-dependent mechanism. There is some evidence for this in the morphological differences between the synapses usually found in the CNS and the high-gain synapses observed, for instance, in the retina, where the presence of ribbon junctions (Sjoestrand, 1958) already suggests a facilitated turnover of vesicle membrane (see Dowling, this volume).

Calcium currents in regions other than presynaptic terminals

Voltage-dependent calcium conductance changes large enough to be regenerative have been observed in a number of preparations: egg (Miyazaki, Takahashi, and Tsuda, 1974; Okamoto, Takahashi, and Yoshii, 1976; Ohmori and Yoshii, 1977); muscle (Fatt and Ginsborg, 1958; Kidokoro, 1973, 1975; Di Polo, 1974; Hagiwara, Fukuda, and Eaton, 1974); gland (Rubin, 1974; Mackie, 1975, 1976; Douglas, 1977; Kater, 1977); and protozoa (e.g., paramecium: Kung and Eckert, 1972; Naitoh, Eckert, and Friedman, 1972; Kung and Naitoh, 1973; Satow and Kung, 1974, 1976; Schein, Bennett, and Katz, 1976). (See also Hagiwara, 1973; Reuter, 1973.) Most of the work, however, utilized invertebrate neurons (Geduldig and Junge, 1968; Geduldig and Gruener, 1970; Wald, 1972; Kostyuk, Krishtal, and Doroshenko, 1974a,b; Kleinhaus and Prichard, 1975; Standen, 1975a,b; Eckert and Lux, 1976; Horn, 1977; Kostyuk

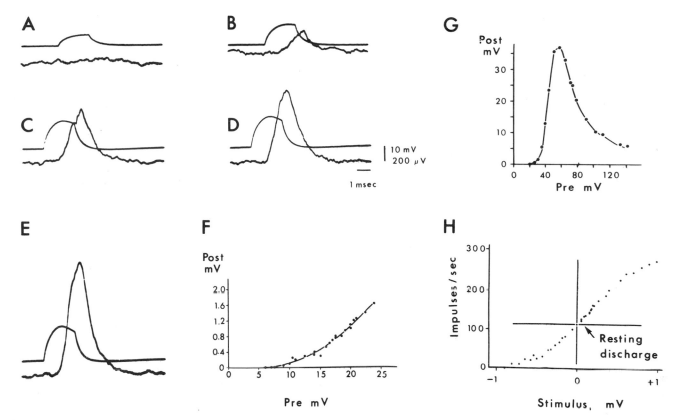

FIGURE 6   Gain properties of synapses. (A–E) Relationship between small presynaptic depolarizations and postsynaptic potential (at high amplification) in the squid synapse. (F) Plot of experimental results. (G) A continuation of the plot in F, with lower postsynaptic amplification showing the steep relationship between depolarization and release for voltages between 30 and 50 mV. (Llinás and Walton, unpublished observations.) (H) Relationship between stimuli in millivolts (abscissa) to impulses per second in electroreceptors, showing also an S-shaped onset. (Modified from Bennett, 1968.)

and Krishtal, 1977). In vertebrates, action potentials may be observed in several types of central and peripheral neurons (Koketsu and Nishi, 1969; Hirst and Spence, 1973; Dichter and Fischbach, 1977; Moolenaar and Specter, 1977) in addition to the receptor sites discussed previously. The rule of thumb concerning the site of this inward calcium current has been that the soma and the presynaptic terminals show calcium spikes, while the axon is for the most part devoid of such activity. Recently an exception to this rule has been found (Horn, 1977). The question of whether a voltage-dependent calcium conductance change exists at all in most axons and that of how it relates to calcium-dependent spikes are really two separate issues. Thus, in the squid giant axon, a voltage-dependent calcium conductance change may be observed with aequorin under voltage-clamp conditions (Baker, Hodgkin, and Ridgway, 1971); however, the current is so small that the system is far from being self-regenerative.

DENDRITIC ELECTRORESPONSIVENESS   Several points regarding the electroresponsiveness of the different neuronal processes deserve comment here. It is now agreed that electroresponsiveness is not limited to the soma and axon but also occurs in the dendritic tree (Spencer and Kandel, 1961; cf. Purpura, 1967; Llinás, 1975). Examples of direct dendritic recordings in Purkinje cells are given in Figure 7. Here the difference between action potentials recorded at somatic and dendritic levels is evident. At the somatic level, action potentials have well-known properties: they last for approximately 1 msec and, in some cases (when the orthodromic stimulation is large enough), afterdepolarizations of varying duration and complexity may be seen. That the action potentials recorded at this level are actually generated across the membrane of the soma can be demonstrated by artificially hyperpolarizing the membrane, which prevents spike generation near the site of recording. This technique was initially utilized to demonstrate

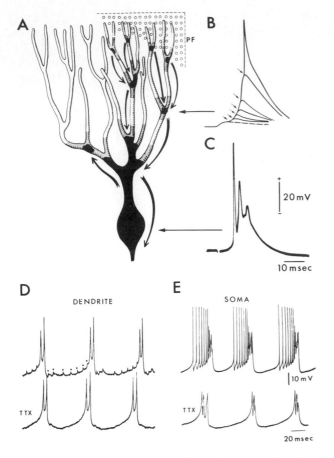

FIGURE 7 Dendritic and somatic action potentials from Purkinje cells. (A) Diagram of dendritic spike generation. Each all-or-none dendritic spike component (B, arrow) is generated by a different hot spot, probably at or near dendritic bifurcations (dark areas in A). Somatic spikes (C) are activated by electrotonically conducted dendritic spikes and synaptic potentials. Dendritic spikes are largely calcium-dependent. Intradendritic spikes from in vitro mammalian Purkinje cells (D) are not blocked by TXX (lower record), while fast somatic spikes (E) are abolished (lower record). (Somatic spikes are passively conducted into dendrites—dots in D—and are blocked by TXX.) Similar results are found after removing sodium from the bathing solution (Llinás and Sugimori, unpublished observations).

the IS and SD components of the somatic action potentials in motoneurons (Eccles, 1957).

Intracellular recording from the dendrites differs from that at the soma in that the action potentials are generally prolonged and are composed of several voltage steps (Llinás and Nicholson, 1971; Nicholson and Llinás, 1971; see also Figure 20 in Pellionisz, this volume). In the case illustrated, seven different spike-initiating sites can be observed by hyperpolarizing the membrane through the recording electrode (a composite of these is shown in Figure 7B). Hyperpolari-

zation of the dendrite, as described above, produces a blockage such that the larger spike components disappear first, indicating their proximity to the recording site. As the hyperpolarization progresses, the spikes blocked are increasingly smaller; that is, they are generated at greater electrotonic distances from the recording site. This kind of electrophysiological datum reminds us that nerve cells are far from being simple algebraic summators of synaptic potentials.

More relevant to the present discussion is the fact that dendritic spikes are now known to be generated not only by sodium, but also by calcium current. In fact, dendritic calcium-dependent spikes have recently been demonstrated by direct somatic and dendritic recording from Purkinje (Llinás and Hess, 1976; Llinás, Sugimori, and Walton, 1977) and hippocampus pyramidal cells (Schwartzkroin and Slawsky, 1977; Wong and Prince, 1977). Calcium-dependent dendritic spikes in Purkinje cells have also been demonstrated in rat and guinea pig in in vitro cerebellar slices. These spikes are not blocked by TTX or by removal of extracellular sodium. They are blocked, however, by cadmium chloride 1 mM or by removal of extracellular calcium (Llinás and Sugimori, 1978 and unpublished observations). As indicated in Figure 7A, somatic spikes do not invade the dendritic tree antidromically (see left dendrite). This is shown in D where the large intradendritic calcium spikes are recorded together with the small somatic spikes (dots). It is also clear from D and E that the Purkinje cell "bursting" is not modified by addition of TTX to the medium, indicating that this voltage-dependent bursting (blocked by hyperpolarization) is calcium-dependent. The hyperpolarization that follows each spike is most probably due to the calcium-dependent potassium conductance change (cf. Lux and Heyer, this volume) since both the calcium spiking and the afterhyperpolarization are blocked by cadmium chloride or by removal of extracellular calcium.

POSSIBLE ROLES OF DENDRITIC CALCIUM SPIKES   The entry of calcium into dendrites can serve many biological functions: first and most obviously, as Figures 7 and 8 show, it is a charge carrier system. Indeed in the records shown it is clear that calcium spikes do occur and that their presence must change the electrical properties of nerve cells. In fact, Traub and Llinás (1977) have demonstrated that the magnitude and precise distribution of calcium conductances is a significant variable in the integrative properties of nerve cells (see also the papers by Dodge and by Pellionisz, this volume). In addition to the actual

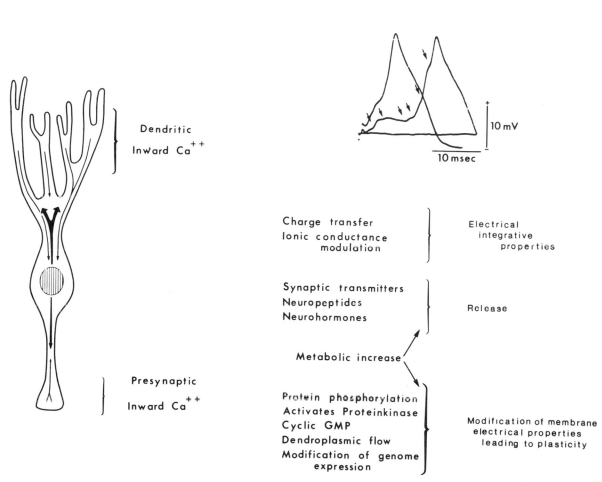

FIGURE 8 Dendritic calcium spikes. (A) Dendritic and pre-synaptic calcium currents are assumed to activate a set of events leading to a modification of genome expression (centripetal arrows). The product of nuclear transcription is envisaged as distributed centrifugally via axoplasmic and dendroplasmic flow back to the somatic, dendritic, axonic, and presynaptic plasmalemmal membrane (thick arrows). (B) Purkinje-cell dendritic calcium spikes following blockage of sodium currents with TTX. Note the presence of multiple sites for spike origin (arrows). The table suggests different actions of calcium spikes in cell function.

movement of calcium itself, this current can activate calcium-dependent potassium conductance changes (Krnjević and Lisiewicz, 1972; Meech, 1972, 1974; Jansen and Nicholls, 1973; Nishi and North, 1973; Clusin, Spray, and Bennett, 1975; Lux and Schubert, 1975; Meech and Standen, 1975; Barrett and Barrett, 1976; Heyer and Lux, 1976; Lux and Heyer, this volume) that produce very significant changes in the electrophysiological properties of neurons.

Beyond its charge carrier function, calcium may be regarded as triggering the release of intracellular substances from dendrites; it thus becomes a central issue in the problem of local circuit function. That calcium does trigger transmitter release from den-drites, as it does from the presynaptic terminal, is indicated by the work of Iversen (this volume) and Glowinski (this volume). In addition, it is possible that calcium plays a role in the release from dendrites of substances other than transmitter, for example, peptides and neurohormones (see Barker and Smith, 1977; Kreutzberg and Schubert, this volume). The functional advantage of this scheme is that such release would be actively regulated by the functional state of the dendrites themselves and would not necessarily depend on somatic or axonic firing. From this viewpoint, brain regulation would transcend its information-transaction functions and the brain would also be considered an endocrinelike system capable of producing *Hirnstoffs* (peptides) important to the overall maintenance of the organism. It is also quite possible that calcium influences the metabolic level of the cell (see the table in Figure 8; Landowne and Ritchie, 1971; Kretsinger, 1976), which would be important to the maintenance of dendritic release and to the possible plastic effects subserved by electrical activity.

Calcium probably plays a role in dendrites similar to the role it plays in peripheral nerve with respect to axoplasmic flow. It is apparent from various studies (Ochs, 1970; Edstrom, 1974; Dravid and Hammerschlag, 1975; Hammerschlag, Dravid, and Chiu, 1975; Hammerschlag, Chiu, and Dravid, 1976; Dravid, 1977; Hammerschlag et al., 1977; Ochs, Worth, and Chan, 1977) that calcium regulates axoplasmic flow. It seems reasonable, therefore, to propose that dendroplasmic flow (Kreutzberg et al., 1973; Kreutzberg and Schubert, this volume) may also be regulated to some extent by a similar mechanism; that is, the speed with which substances flow along the intradendritic compartment may be modulated, as it is in axons (Badr and McLean, 1975), by the membrane's electric field via the voltage-dependent inward calcium current. Inasmuch as calcium is now being considered as a trigger for cyclic nucleotide synthesis—in particular, cyclic GMP (Rasmussen, 1970; Schultz et al., 1973; Bloom, 1975; Guidotti, Biggio, and Costa, 1975; Ferendelli, Rubin, and Kinscherf, 1976; Rasmussen and Goodman, 1977; Greengard, 1978)—the possibility that synaptic input, through either direct or voltage-dependent calcium inflow, may be part of the second messenger system is very attractive (see Berridge, this volume).

Very recently a more direct calcium action has been indicated by Schulman and Greengard (1978), who have shown that this ion can produce phosphorylation directly and can activate protein kinases independent of its influence on cyclic GMP. This very significant finding may imply, among other possibilities, the existence of several second messenger systems operating in parallel. Further, if we consider that calcium conductance is restricted to strategically significant "hot spots" in the plasmalemmal membrane—as suggested by its presynaptic and dendritic distribution—an intracellular organization is implied whose complexity may ultimately rival that of the brain circuits. The possibility of a coexistent set of second messenger systems is intriguing, since in principle each system could regulate different but parallel regimes. The concept of membrane inhomogeneity, implying intracellular compartmentalization, is particularly attractive with respect to calcium as, due to

the avidity with which it is taken up by the intracellular environment (Baker, 1972; cf. Rubin, 1974; Brinley et al., 1977), calcium will always have a short intracellular range.

Finally, and most excitingly, one can assume that this voltage-dependent calcium entry into dendrites is important in modulating the long-term excitability of cells, since electrical activity must produce neuronal changes in order to generate, for instance, memory. The most far-reaching possibility, of course, is that calcium, by acting as a second messenger and in conjunction with the other properties mentioned above, may modify transcription by altering genome expression, as recently shown for cartilage (Rodan, Bourret, and Norton, 1978); it could thus serve as a feedback system regulating the nuclear production of membrane proteins. In this sense, then, the system would work in the manner envisaged by Palade (1975) for the generation of gamma globulin or, in more direct relation to the present problem, in the manner envisaged by Fambrough and Devroetes (1978), who have shown that ACh receptors are found at the perinuclear Golgi apparatus before they are inserted in the membrane. Although the above scheme (Llinás and Iberall, 1977) is still very conjectural, it belongs to the realm of promising topics for study in years to come, since mechanisms such as these must ultimately underlie the molecular and cell-biological basis for plasticity and thus for memory. With reference to plasticity, Kandel has suggested, in his 1977 Neuroscience Grass Lecture, that the modification of presynaptic calcium conductance may be the mechanism for the behavioral dishabituation in *Aplysia* brought about by serotonin. Beyond the examples of presynaptic somatic and dendritic calcium conductances, one imagines that there may be a more basic theme underlying these phenomena. I would like to offer this as a general hypothesis regarding the role of calcium in neuronal function.

General hypothesis

SYNAPTIC TRANSMISSION AND PLASTICITY AS DIFFERENT ASPECTS OF "ISOMETRIC CALCIUM-DEPENDENT GROWTH" As stated by Kretsinger in his elegant paper in this volume, calcium has a long evolutionary history as a cell regulator; for that reason the functional themes in which calcium may be involved are probably diverse and may involve many levels of organization. Moving from the specific to the general, I would like to emphasize that, for the reason given by Kretsinger—that an intracellular machinery would have developed to use calcium as a regulating factor—it seems reasonable to suppose that the calcium actions described here may be incorporated into a global scheme. My own bias is for the view that calcium, which regulates cell motility from muscle to protozoa (Porter, 1976), would, through this action, regulate growth. The actual mechanism could be one in which calcium controls the rate of addition of new membrane, as probably occurs in growth cones; in this way newly minted proteins would be inserted into the plasmalemmal membrane. The teleology behind this view, assuming that growth cones do have a high (probably voltage-dependent) calcium conductance, is that calcium would (1) reduce intracellular viscosity by regulating the fluidity of the axoplasm (Hodgkin and Katz, 1949) or dendroplasm, (2) activate axoplasmic or dendroplasmic flow, probably by acting on the endoskeletal filamentous structures (Droz, Rambourg, and Koenig, 1975; Mannherz and Goody, 1976) or on the smooth membrane cisternae (Wood, McLaughlin, and Barber, 1974; Wood and McLaughlin, 1976), and (3) stimulate synthesis of new protein. This would allow the high mobility a growth cone is known to possess.

It follows that synaptic terminals may be regarded as a modified growth cone in which growth is largely subdued and actually becomes isometric; in other words, membranes are introduced into the plasmalemma by synaptic vesicles, only to be taken up again by a recycling mechanism such as that postulated by Heuser and Reese (1973; this volume). That an actual increase in the surface area of synaptic terminals occurs with synaptic release has been shown by Frontali et al. (1976) in the neuromuscular junction and by Schaeffer and Raviola (1975) and Ripps, Shakib, and MacDonald (1977) in the retina.

Furthermore, dendrites may have such properties as well. One may assume that the growth cone that generates the dendrite is vestigially represented by a membrane turnover for the release of intracellular substances and as a mechanism to introduce new proteins into surface membrane. In this respect, presynaptic terminals and dendritic arborizations (especially the remote dendrites) may be modified growth cones and plasticity nothing more than a modification of the general growth theme.

In the final analysis, local circuits, synaptic transmission, and plasticity may be related to each other and may represent the level at which most of the complexity of the CNS resides. It is, in fact, at this level that the themes covered in this volume (e.g., spikeless interactions, molecular cooperativity, field sensing, and the modulation of the all-important extracellular milieu) merge to give us an initial glimpse into the nature of concerted brain functions.

ACKNOWLEDGMENT This research was supported by U.S. Public Health Service Research Grant NS-13742 from the National Institute of Neurological and Communicative Disorders and Stroke.

REFERENCES

ADRIAN, R. H., W. K. CHANDLER, and A. L. HODGKIN, 1970. Voltage clamp experiments in striated muscle fibers. *J. Physiol.* 208:607–644.

ALNAES, E., and R. RAHAMIMOFF, 1975. On the role of mitochondria in transmitter release from motor-nerve terminals. *J. Physiol.* 248:285–306.

ARMSTRONG, C. M., and F. BEZANILLA, 1973. Currents related to movement of the gating particles of the sodium channels *Nature* 242:459–461.

ARMSTRONG, C. M., and L. BINSTOCK, 1965. Anomalous rectification in the squid giant axon injected with tetraethylammonium chloride. *J. Gen. Physiol.* 48:859–872.

BADR, G. G., and W. G. MCLEAN, 1975. The effect of electrical stimulation on the distribution of labelled proteins in isolated segments of rabbit vagus nerve. *J. Neurochem.* 25:921–923.

BAKER, P. F., 1972. Transport and metabolism of calcium ions in nerve. *Prog. Biophys. Mol. Biol.* 24:177–223.

BAKER, P. F., and H. G. GLITSCH, 1975. Voltage-dependent changes in permeability of nerve membranes to calcium and other divalent cations. *Philos. Trans. R. Soc. Lond.* B270:389–408.

BAKER, P. F., A. L. HODGKIN, and E. G. RIDGWAY, 1971. Depolarization and calcium entry in squid giant axons. *J. Physiol.* 218:709–755.

BAKER, P. F., H. MEVES, and E. B. RIDGWAY, 1971. Phasic entry of calcium in response to depolarization of giant axons of *Loligo. J. Physiol.* 216:70–71P.

BAKER, P. F., H. MEVES, and E. B. RIDGWAY, 1973. Effects of manganese and other agents on the calcium uptake that follows depolarization of squid axons. *J. Physiol.* 231:511–526.

BAKER, P. F., and H. REUTER, 1975. *Calcium Movement in Excitable Cells.* Oxford: Pergamon.

BARKER, J. L., and T. G. SMITH, JR., 1977. Peptides as neurohormones. In *Society for Neuroscience Symposia,* vol. 2, W. M. Cowan and J. A. Ferendelli, eds. Bethesda, MD: Society for Neuroscience, pp. 340–373.

BARRETT, E. F., and J. BARRETT, 1976. Separation of two voltage-sensitive potassium currents, and demonstration of a tetrodotoxin-resistant calcium current in frog motoneurones. *J. Physiol.* 255:737–774.

BENNETT, M. V. L., 1967. Mechanisms of electroreception. In *Lateral Line Detectors,* P. Cahn, ed. Bloomington: Indiana Univ. Press, pp. 313–393.

BENNETT, M. V. L., 1968. Similarities between chemically and electrically mediated transmission. In *Physiological and Biochemical Aspects of Nervous Integration,* F. D. Carlson, ed. Englewood Cliffs, NJ: Prentice-Hall, pp. 73–128.

BENSHALOM, G., and A. FLOCK, 1977. Calcium-induced electron density in synaptic vesicles of afferent and efferent synapses on hair cells in the lateral line organ. *Brain Res.* 121:173–178.

BLAUSTEIN, M. P., 1976a. The ins and outs of calcium transport in squid axons: Internal and external ion activation of calcium efflux. *Fed. Proc.* 35:2574–2578.

BLAUSTEIN, M. P. 1976b. Sodium-calcium exchange and the regulation of cell calcium in muscle fibers. *Physiologist* 19:525–540.

BLINKS, J. R., F. G. PRENDERGAST, and D. G. ALLEN, 1976. Photoproteins as biological calcium indicators. *Pharmacol. Rev.* 28:1–93.

BLOEDEL, J. R., P. W. GAGE, R. LLINÁS, and D. M. J. QUASTEL, 1966. Transmission across the squid giant synapse in the presence of tetrodotoxin. *J. Physiol.* 188:52–53P.

BLOOM, F. E., 1975. The role of cyclic nucleotides in central synaptic function. *Rev. Physiol. Biochem. Pharmacol.* 74:1–103.

BRINLEY, F. J., JR., T. TIFFERT, A. SCARPA, and L. J. MULLINS, 1977. Intracellular calcium buffering capacity in isolated squid axons. *J. Gen. Physiol.* 70:355–384.

BROWN, A. M., N. AKAIKE, and K. S. LEE, 1978. Calcium conductance of neurons. *Ann. NY Acad. Sci.* (in press).

BULLOCK, T. H., and S. HAGIWARA, 1957. Intracellular recording from the giant synapse of the squid. *J. Gen. Physiol.* 40:565–577.

CHARLTON, M. P., and H. L. ATWOOD, 1977. Slow release of transmitter at the squid giant synapse. *Neurosci. Lett.* 286.

CLUSIN, W., D. C. SPRAY, and M. V. L. BENNETT, 1975. Activation of a voltage-insensitive conductance by inward calcium current. *Nature* 256:425–427.

COUTEAUX, R., and M. PÉCOT-DECHAVASSINE, 1970. Vésicules synaptiques et poches au niveau des zones actives de la jonction neuromusculaire. *C. R. Acad. Sci. Paris [D]* 271:2346–2349.

CUTHBERT, A. W., ed., 1970. *A Symposium on Calcium and Cellular Function.* New York: St. Martin's Press (Macmillan).

DEAN, P. M., and E. K. MATHEWS, 1970. Electrical activity in pancreatic islet cells: Effect of ions. *J. Physiol.* 210:265–275.

DICHTER, M. A., and G. D. FISCHBACH, 1977. The action potential of chick dorsal root ganglion neurones maintained in cell culture. *J. Physiol.* 267:281–298.

DI POLO, R., 1974. Sodium-dependent calcium influx in dialyzed barnacle muscle fibers. *Biochim. Biophys. Acta* 298:279–283.

DOUGLAS, W. W., 1974. Involvement of calcium in exocytosis and the exocytosis-vesiculation sequence. In *Calcium and Cell Regulation*, R. M. S. Smellie, ed. London: Biochemical Society, pp. 1–28.

DOUGLAS, W. W., 1976. The role of calcium in stimulus-secretion coupling. In *Stimulus-Secretion Coupling in the Gastrointestinal Tract*, R. M. Case and H. Goebell, eds. Baltimore, MD: University Park Press, pp. 17–48.

DOUGLAS, W. W., 1977. Stimulus-secretion coupling: Variations on the theme of calcium-activated exocytosis involving cellular and extracellular sources of calcium. In *Respiratory Tract Mucus* (CIBA Foundation Symposium no. 54). New York: Elsevier.

DRAVID, A. R., 1977. Role of calcium in the initiation of fast axonal transport of protein: Effects of divalent cations. *J. Neurobiol.* 8:439–451.

DRAVID, A. R., and R. HAMMERSCHLAG, 1975. Axoplasmic transport of proteins *in vitro* in primary afferent neurons of frog spinal cord: Effect of Ca^{2+}-free incubation conditions. *J. Neurochem.* 24:711–718.

DREIFUSS, J. J., K. AKERT, C. SANDRI, and H. MOOR, 1973. Specific arrangements of membrane particles at sites of exo-endocytosis in the freeze-etched neurohypophosis. *Cell Tiss. Res.* 165:317–325.

DREYER, F., K. PEPER, K. AKERT, C. SANDRI, and H. MOOR, 1973. Ultrastructure of the "active zone" in the frog neuromuscular junction. *Brain Res.* 62:373–380.

DROZ, B., A. RAMBOURG, and H. L. KOENIG, 1975. The smooth endoplasmic reticulum: Structure and role in the renewal of axonal membrane and synaptic vesicles by fast axonal transport. *Brain Res.* 93:1–13.

DUNCAN, C. J., ed., 1976. *Calcium in Biological Systems.* New York: Cambridge Univ. Press.

ECCLES, J. C., 1957. *Physiology of Nerve Cells.* Baltimore: Johns Hopkins Press.

ECKERT, R., and H. D. LUX, 1976. A voltage-sensitive persistent calcium conductance in neuronal somata of *Helix. J. Physiol.* 254:129–151.

EDSTRÖM, A., 1974. Effects of Ca^{2+} and Mg^{2+} on rapid axonal transport of proteins *in vitro* in frog sciatic nerves. *J. Cell Biol.* 61:812–818.

FAMBROUGH, D. M., and P. N. DEVREOTES, 1978. Newly synthesized acetylcholine receptors are located in the Golgi apparatus. *J. Cell Biol.* 76:237–244.

FATT, P., and B. L. GINSBORG, 1958. The ionic requirements for the production of action potentials in crustacean muscle fibres. *J. Physiol.* 142:516–543.

FERENDELLI, J. A., E. H. RUBIN, and D. A. KINSCHERF, 1976. Influence of divalent cations on regulation of cyclic GMP and cyclic AMP levels in brain tissue. *J. Neurochem.* 26:741–748.

FRANKENHAEUSER, B., and A. L. HODGKIN, 1957. The action of calcium on the electrical properties of squid axons. *J. Physiol.* 137:218–244.

FRONTALI, N., B. CECCARELLI, A. GORIO, A. MAURO, P. SIEKEVITZ, M.-C. TZENG, and W. P. HURLBUT, 1976. Purification from black widow spider venom of a protein factor causing the depletion of synaptic vesicles at neuromuscular junctions. *J. Cell Biol.* 68:462–479.

GEDULDIG, D., and R. GRUENER, 1970. Voltage clamp of the *Aplysia* giant neurone early sodium and calcium currents. *J. Physiol.* 211:217–244.

GEDULDIG, D., and D. JUNGE, 1968. Sodium and calcium components of action potentials in the *Aplysia* giant neurone. *J. Physiol.* 199:347–365.

GLAGOLEVA, I. M., E. A. LIEBERMAN, and Z. KHASHAYEV, 1970. Effect of uncoupling agents of oxidation phosphorylation on the release of acetylcholine from nerve endings. *Biofizika* 15:76–83.

GREENGARD, P., 1978. Phosphorylated proteins as physiological effectors. *Science* 199:146–152.

GUIDOTTI, A., G. BIGGIO, and E. COSTA, 1975. 3-Acetylpyridine: A tool to inhibit the tremor and the increase of cGMP content in cerebellar cortex elicited by harmaline. *Brain Res.* 96:201–205.

HAGIWARA, S., 1973. Calcium spikes. *Adv. Biophys.* 4:71–102.

HAGIWARA, S., J. FUKUDA, and D. C. EATON, 1974. Membrane currents carried by Ca, Sr and Ba in barnacle muscle fiber during voltage clamp. *J. Gen. Physiol.* 63:564–578.

HAGIWARA, S., and K. TAKAHASHI, 1967. Surface density of calcium binding sites in the barnacle muscle fiber membrane. *J. Gen. Physiol.* 50:583–601.

HAGIWARA, S., and I. TASAKI, 1958. A study of the mechanism of impulse transmission across the giant synapse of the squid. *J. Physiol.* 143:114–137.

HAMMERSCHLAG, R., C. BAKHIT, A. Y. CHIU, and A. R. DRAVID, 1977. Role of calcium in the initiation of fast axonal transport of protein: Effects of divalent cations. *J. Neurobiol.* 8:439–451.

HAMMERSCHLAG, R., A. Y. CHIU, and A. R. DRAVID, 1976. Inhibition of fast axonal transport of ^{3}H protein by cobalt ions. *Brain Res.* 114:353–358.

HAMMERSCHLAG, R., A. R. DRAVID, and A. Y. CHIU, 1975. Mechanism of axonal transport: A proposed role for calcium ions. *Science* 188:273–275.

HEUSER, J. E., and T. S. REESE, 1973. Evidence for recycling of synaptic vesicle membrane during transmitter release at the frog neuromuscular junction. *J. Cell Biol.* 57:315–344.

HEUSER, J. E., and T. S. REESE, 1977. Structure of the synapse. In *Handbook of Physiology,* vol. 1: *The Nervous System,* E. Kandel, ed. Bethesda, MD: American Physiological Society.

HEYER, C. B., and H. D. LUX, 1976. Properties of a facilitating calcium current in bursting pacemaker neurons of the snail, *Helix pomatia. J. Physiol.* 262:319–348.

HIRST, G. D. S., and I. SPENCE, 1973. Calcium action potentials in mammalian peripheral neurons. *Nature* 243:54–56.

HODGKIN, A. L., and A. F. HUXLEY, 1952. A quantitative description of membrane current and its application to conduction and excitation in nerve. *J. Physiol.* 117:500–544.

HODGKIN, A. L., and B. KATZ, 1949. The effect of calcium on the axoplasm of giant nerve fibres. *J. Exp. Biol.* 26:292–294.

HORN, R., 1977. Tetrodotoxin-resistant divalent action potentials in an axon of *Aplysia. Brain Res.* 133:177–182.

JANSEN, J. K. S., and J. G. NICHOLLS, 1973. Conductance changes, an electrogenic pump and the hyperpolarization of leech neurones following impulses. *J. Physiol.* 229:635–655.

KATER, S. B., 1977. Calcium electroresponsiveness and its relationship to secretion in molluscan exocrine gland cells. In *Society for Neuroscience Symposia,* vol. 2, W. M. Cowan and J. A. Ferendelli, eds. Bethesda, MD: Society for Neuroscience, pp. 195–211.

KATZ, B., 1969. *The Release of Neural Transmitter Substances.* Springfield, IL: Charles C Thomas.

KATZ, B., and R. MILEDI, 1967. A study of synaptic transmission in the absence of nerve impulses. *J. Physiol.* 192:407–436.

KATZ, B., and R. MILEDI, 1969. Tetrodotoxin-resistant electric activity in presynaptic terminals. *J. Physiol.* 203:459–487.

KATZ, B., and R. MILEDI, 1970. Further study of the role of calcium in synaptic transmission. *J. Physiol.* 207:789–801.

KATZ, N. L., and C. EDWARDS, 1973. Effects of metabolic inhibitors on spontaneous and neurally evoked transmitter release from frog motor nerve terminals. *J. Gen. Physiol.* 61:259.

KEYNES, R. D., and E. ROJAS, 1974. Kinetics and steady state properties of the charged system controlling sodium conductance in the squid giant axon. *J. Physiol.* 239:393–434.

KIDOKORO, Y., 1973. Development of action potentials in a clonal rat skeletal muscle cell line. *Nature* 241:158–159.

KIDOKORO, Y., 1975. Sodium and calcium components of the action potential in a developing skeletal muscle cell line. *J. Physiol.* 244:145–159.

KLEINHAUS, A. L., and J. W. PRICHARD, 1975. Calcium dependent action potentials in leech Retzius cells by tetraethylammonium chloride. *J. Physiol.* 246:351–361.

KOKETSU, K., and S. NISHI, 1969. Calcium and action potentials of bullfrog sympathetic ganglion cells. *J. Gen. Physiol.* 53:608–623.

KOSTYUK, P. G., and O. A. KRISHTAL, 1977. Separation of sodium and calcium currents in the somatic membrane of mollusc neurones. *J. Physiol.* 270:545–568.

KOSTYUK, P. G., O. A. KRISHTAL, and P. A. DOROSHENKO, 1974a. Calcium currents in snail neurones. I. Identification of calcium current. *Pfluegers Arch.* 348:83–93.

KOSTYUK, P. G., O. A. KRISHTAL, and P. A. DOROSHENKO, 1974b. Calcium currents in snail neurones. II. The effect of external calcium concentration on the calcium inward current. *Pfluegers Arch.* 348:95–104.

KRETSINGER, R. H., 1976. Calcium-binding proteins. *Ann. Rev. Biochem.* 45:239–266.

KREUTZBERG, G. W., P. SCHUBERT, L. TÓTH, and E. RIESKE, 1973. Intradendritic transport to postsynaptic sites. *Brain Res.* 62:399–404.

KRNJEVIĆ, K., and A. LISIEWICZ, 1972. Injections of calcium ions into spinal motoneurones. *J. Physiol.* 225:363–390.

KUNG, C., and R. ECKERT, 1972. Genetic modification of electric properties in an excitable membrane. *Proc. Natl. Acad. Sci. USA* 69:93–97.

KUNG, C., and Y. NAITOH, 1973. Calcium-induced ciliary reversal in the extracted models of "pawn," a behavioral mutant of paramecium. *Science* 179:195–196.

KUSANO, K., 1970. Influence of ionic environment on the relationship between pre- and postsynaptic potentials. *J. Neurobiol.* 1:437–457.

KUSANO, K., D. R. LIVENGOOD, and R. WERMAN, 1967. Correlation of transmitter release with membrane properties of the presynaptic fiber of the squid giant synapse. *J. Gen. Physiol.* 50:2579–2601.

LANDOWNE, D., and J. M. RITCHIE, 1971. On the control of glycogenolysis in mammalian nervous tissue by calcium. *J. Physiol.* 212:503–517.

LESTER, H. A., 1970. Transmitter release by presynaptic impulses in the squid stellate ganglion. *Nature* 227:493–496.

LLINÁS, R., 1975. Electroresponsive properties of dendrites in central neurons. In *Physiology and Pathology of Dendrites* (Advances in Neurology, vol. 12), G. W. Kreutzberg, ed. New York: Raven Press, pp. 1–13.

LLINÁS, R. R., 1977. Calcium and transmitter release in squid synapse. In *Society for Neuroscience Symposia,* vol. 2, W. M. Cowan and J. A. Ferendelli, eds. Bethesda, MD: Society for Neuroscience, pp. 139–160.

LLINÁS, R., J. R. BLINKS, and C. NICHOLSON, 1972. Calcium transient in presynaptic terminal of squid giant synapse:

Detection with aequorin. *Science* 176:1127–1129.

LLINÁS, R., and R. HESS, 1976. Tetrodotoxin-resistant dendritic spikes in avian Purkinje cells. *Proc. Natl. Acad. Sci. USA* 73:2520–2523.

LLINÁS, R., and J. R. HEUSER, 1977. Depolarization-release coupling systems in neurons. *Neurosci. Res. Program Bull.* 15:557–687.

LLINÁS, R., and A. IBERALL, 1977. A global model of neuronal command-control systems. *BioSystems* 8:233–235.

LLINÁS, R., and C. NICHOLSON, 1971. Electrophysiological properties of dendrites and somata in alligator Purkinje cells. *J. Neurophysiol.* 34:532–551.

LLINÁS, R., and C. NICHOLSON, 1975. Calcium role in depolarization-secretion coupling: An aequorin study in squid giant synapse. *Proc. Natl. Acad. Sci. USA* 72:187–190.

LLINÁS, R., I. Z. STEINBERG, and K. WALTON, 1976. Presynaptic calcium currents and their relation to synaptic transmission: Voltage clamp study in squid giant synapse and theoretical model for the calcium gate. *Proc. Natl. Acad. Sci. USA* 73:2918–2922.

LLINÁS, R., and M. SUGIMORI, 1978. Dendritic calcium spiking in mammalian Purkinje cells: *In vitro* study of its function and development. *Soc. Neurosci. Abst.* 4:66.

LLINÁS, R., M. SUGIMORI, and K. WALTON, 1977. Calcium dendritic spikes in the mammalian Purkinje cells. *Soc. Neurosci. Abstr.* 3:58.

LLINÁS, R., K. WALTON, and V. BOHR, 1976. Synaptic transmission in squid giant synapse after potassium conductance blockage with external 3- and 4-aminopyridine. *Biophys. J.* 16:83–86.

LLINÁS, R., K. WALTON, and M. SUGIMORI, 1977. Presynaptic calcium currents in squid stellate ganglion: A voltage clamp study using TTX and TEA. *Biol. Bull.* 153:436–437.

LLINÁS, R., K. WALTON, and M. SUGIMORI, 1978. Voltage-clamp study of the effects of temperature on synaptic transmission in the squid. *Biol. Bull.* 155:454.

LOCKE, F. S., 1894. Notiz ueber den Einfluss physiologischer Koch-salzloesung auf die elektrische Erregbarkeit von Muskel und Nerve. *Zentrabl. Physiol.* 8:166–167.

LUX, H. D., and P. SCHUBERT, 1975. Some aspects of the electroanatomy of dendrites. In *Physiology and Pathology of Dendrites* (Advances in Neurology, vol. 12), G. W. Kreutzberg, ed. New York: Raven Press, pp. 29–44.

MACKIE, G. O., 1975. Spike propagation through coupled gland cells and secretion release. *J. Cell Biol.* 67:254.

MACKIE, G. O., 1976. Propagated spikes and secretion in a coelenterate glandular epithelium. *J. Gen. Physiol.* 68:313–325.

MANN, D. M., and R. W. JOYNER, 1976. Quantal transmission at the squid giant synapse. *Soc. Neurosci. Abstr.* 2:1008.

MANNHERZ, H. G., and R. S. GOODY, 1976. Proteins of contractile systems. *Annu. Rev. Biochem.* 45:428–465.

MEECH, R. W., 1972. Intracellular calcium injection causes increased potassium conductance in *Aplysia* nerve cells. *Comp. Biochem. Physiol.* 42A:493–499.

MEECH, R. W., 1974. Sensitivity of *Helix aspersa* neurons to injected calcium ions. *J. Physiol.* 237:259–277.

MEECH, R. W., and N. B. STANDEN, 1975. Potassium activation in *Helix aspersa* neurones under voltage clamp: A component mediated by calcium influx. *J. Physiol.* 249:211–239.

MEVES, H., 1975. Calcium currents in squid giant-axon. *Philos. Trans. R. Soc. Lond.* B270:377–387.

MILEDI, R., 1967. Spontaneous synaptic potentials and quantal release of transmitter in the stellate ganglion of the squid. *J. Physiol.* 192:379–406.

MILEDI, R., 1973. Transmitter release induced by injection of calcium ions into nerve terminals. *Proc. R. Soc. Lond.* B183:421–425.

MILEDI, R., and C. R. SLATER, 1966. The action of calcium on neuronal synapses in the squid. *J. Physiol.* 184:473–498.

MIYAZAKI, S., K. TAKAHASHI, and K. TSUDA, 1974. Electrical excitability in the egg cell membrane of the tunicate. *J. Physiol.* 238:37–54.

MOOLENAAR, W. H., and I. SPECTOR, 1977. Membrane currents examined under voltage clamp in cultured neuroblastoma cells. *Science* 196:331–336.

NAITOH, Y., R. ECKERT, and K. FRIEDMAN, 1972. A regenerative calcium response in paramecium. *J. Exp. Biol.* 56:667–681.

NARAHASHI, T., J. W. MOORE, and W. R. SCOTT, 1964. Tetrodotoxin blockage of sodium conductance increase on lobster giant axons. *J. Gen. Physiol.* 47:965–974.

NICHOLSON, C., and R. LLINÁS, 1971. Field potentials in the alligator cerebellum and theory of their relationship to Purkinje cell dendritic spikes. *J. Neurophysiol.* 34:509–531.

NISHI, S., and R. A. NORTH, 1973. Intracellular recording from the myenteric plexus of the guinea-pig ileum. *J. Physiol.* 231:471–491.

OCHS, S., 1972. Fast transport of material in mammalian nerve fibers. *Science* 176:252–260.

OCHS, S., R. M. WORTH, and S.-Y. CHAN, 1977. Calcium requirement for axoplasmic transport in mammalian nerve. *Nature* 270:748–750.

OHMORI, H., and M. YOSHII, 1977. Surface potential reflected in both gating and permeation mechanisms of sodium and calcium channels of the tunicate egg cell membrane. *J. Physiol.* 267:429–463.

OKAMOTO, H., K. TAKAHASHI, and M. YOSHII, 1976. Membrane currents of the tunicate egg under the voltage clamp condition. *J. Physiol.* 254:607–638.

PALADE, G., 1975. Intracellular aspects of the process of protein synthesis. *Science* 189:347–358.

PARSEGIAN, V. A., 1977. Considerations in determining the mode of influence of calcium on vesicle-membrane interaction. In *Society for Neuroscience Symposia*, vol. 2, W. M. Cowan and J. A. Ferendelli, eds. Bethesda, MD: Society for Neuroscience, pp. 161–171.

PELHATE, M., and Y. PICHON, 1974. Selective inhibition of potassium current in the giant axon of the cockroach. *J. Physiol.* 242:90–91P.

PFENNINGER, K., K. AKERT, H. MOOR, and C. SANDRI, 1971. Freeze-fracturing of presynaptic membranes in the central nervous system. *Philos. Trans. R. Soc. Lond.* B261:387–388.

PFENNINGER, K., K. AKERT, H. MOOR, and C. SANDRI, 1972. The fine structure of freeze-fractured presynaptic membranes. *J. Neurocytol.* 1:129–149.

PORTER, K. R., 1976. Motility in cells. In *Cell Motility*, vol. 3, R. Goldman, T. Pollard, and J. Rosenbaum, eds. Cold Spring Harbor, NY: Cold Spring Harbor Laboratory, pp. 1–28.

PURPURA, D. P., 1967. Comparative physiology of dendrites. In *The Neurosciences: A Study Program*, G. C. Quarton, T. Melnechuk, and F. O. Schmitt, eds. New York: Rockefeller Univ. Press, pp. 372–393.

PUTNEY, J. W., JR., 1977. Muscarinic, alpha-adrenergic and peptide receptors regulate the same calcium influx sites in the parotid gland. *J. Physiol.* 268:139–149.

RASMUSSEN, H., 1970. Cell communication, calcium ion and cyclic adenosine monophosphate. *Science* 170:404–412.

RASMUSSEN, H., and D. B. P. GOODMAN, 1977. Relationships between calcium and cyclic nucleotides in cell activation. *Physiol. Rev.* 57:421–509.

REUTER, H., 1973. Divalent cations as charge carriers in excitable membranes. *Prog. Biophys. Mol. Biol.* 26:1–43.

RIPPS, H., M. SHAKIB, and E. D. MacDONALD, 1977. On the fate of synaptic vesicle membrane in photoreceptor terminals of the skate retina. *Biol. Bull.* 153:443–444.

RODAN, G. A., L. A. BOURRET, and L. A. NORTON, 1978. DNA synthesis in cartilage cells is stimulated by oscillating electric fields. *Science* 199:690–692.

RUBIN, R. P., 1970. The role of calcium in the release of neurotransmitter substances and hormones. *Pharmacol. Rev.* 22:389–428.

RUBIN, R. P., 1974. *Calcium and the Secretory Process.* New York: Plenum.

SATOW, Y., and C. KUNG, 1974. Genetic dissection of the active electrogenesis in *Paramecium aurelia. Nature* 247:67–71.

SATOW, Y., and C. KUNG, 1976. Mutants with reduced calcium activation *Paramecium aurelia. J. Membrane Biol.* 28:277–294.

SCHAEFFER, S. F., and E. RAVIOLA, 1975. Ultrastructural analysis of functional changes in the synaptic endings of turtle cone cells. *Cold Spring Harbor Symp. Quant. Biol.* 40:521–528.

SCHEIN, S. J., M. V. L. BENNETT, and G. M. KATZ, 1976. Altered calcium conductance in pawns, behavioral mutants of *Paramecium aurelia. J. Exp. Biol.* 65:699–724.

SCHULMAN, H., and P. GREENGARD, 1978. Stimulation of brain membrane protein phosphorylation by calcium and an endogenous heat-stable protein. *Nature* 271:478–479.

SCHULTZ, G., J. G. HARDMAN, K. SCHULTZ, C. E. BAIRD, and E. W. SUTHERLAND, 1973. The importance of calcium ions for the regulation of guanosine 3′,5′-cyclic monophosphate levels. *Proc. Natl. Acad. Sci. USA* 70:3889–3893.

SCHWARTZKROIN, P. A., and M. SLAWSKY, 1977. Probable calcium spikes in hippocampal neurons. *Brain Res.* 135:157–161. j

SHANES, A. M., 1958. Electrochemical aspects of physiological and pharmacological action in excitable cells. II. The action potential and excitation. *Pharmacol. Rev.* 10:165–273.

SHIMOMURA, O., and F. H. JOHNSON, 1970. Calcium binding, quantum yield and emitting molecule in aequorin bioluminescence. *Nature* 227:1356–1357.

SJOESTRAND, F. S., 1958. Ultrastructure of retinal rod synapses of the guinea pig eye as revealed by three-dimensional reconstruction from serial sections. *J. Ultrastruct. Res.* 2:122–170.

SMELLIE, R. M. S., ed., 1974. *Calcium and Cell Regulation.* London: Biochemical Society.

SPENCER, W. A., and E. R. KANDEL, 1961. Electrophysiology of hippocampal neurons. IV. Fast prepotentials. *J. Neurophysiol.* 24:272–285.

STANDEN, N. B., 1975a. Calcium and sodium ions as charge carriers in the action potential of an identified snail neurone. *J. Physiol.* 249:241–252.

STANDEN, N. B., 1975b. Voltage-clamp studies of the calcium inward current in an identified snail neurone: Comparison with the sodium inward current. *J. Physiol.* 249:253–268.

STINNAKRE, J., and L. TAUC, 1973. Calcium influx in active *Aplysia* neurones detected by injected aequorin. *Nature* 242:113–115.

TAKEUCHI, A., and N. TAKEUCHI, 1962. Electrical changes in pre- and postsyhaptic axons of the giant synapse of *Loligo. J. Gen. Physiol.* 45:1181–1193.

TRAUB, R. D., and R. LLINÁS, 1977. Spatial distribution of ionic conductances in normal and axotomized motoneurons. *Neuroscience* 2.

VENZIN, M., C. SANDRI, L. AKERT, and U. R. WYSS, 1977. Membrane associated particles of the presynaptic active zone in rat spinal cord: A morphometric analysis. *Brain Res.* 130:393–404.

WALD, F., 1972. Ionic differences between somatic and axonal action potentials in snail giant neurones. *J. Physiol.* 220:267–281.

WEIGHT, F. F., and S. D. ERULKAR, 1976. Synaptic transmission and effects of temperature at the squid giant synapse. *Nature* 261:720–722.

WONG, R. K. S., and D. A. PRINCE, 1977. Burst generation and calcium mediated spikes in hippocampus neurons. *Soc. Neurosci. Abstr.* 3:148.

WOOD, J. G., and B. J. McLAUGHLIN, 1976. Cytochemical studies of lectin sites in smooth membrane cisternae of rat brain. *Brain Res.* 118:15–26.

WOOD, J. G., B. J. McLAUGHLIN, and R. P. BARBER, 1974. Visualization of concanavalin A binding sites in Purkinje cell somata and dendrites of rat cerebellum. *J. Cell Biol.* 63:541–549.

YOUNG, J. Z., 1939. Fused neurones and synaptic contacts in the giant nerve fibres of cephalopods. *Philos. Trans. R. Soc. Lond.* B229:465–503.

32 Synaptic-Vesicle Exocytosis Captured by Quick-Freezing

JOHN E. HEUSER and THOMAS S. REESE

ABSTRACT Exocytosis of synaptic vesicles has been captured by quick-freezing frog neuromuscular junctions at the precise moment of transmitter release, and the abundance of exocytosis has been correlated with the number of quanta that are discharged, at several different levels of release produced by stimulation in different doses of 4-aminopyridine. This strongly supports Katz's original vesicle hypothesis. Quick-freezing has also been used to observe the behavior of discharged vesicles in the first few milliseconds after transmitter release, at which time they can be seen to collapse and mix their membrane with the presynaptic membrane. In the succeeding seconds, equivalent amounts of membrane are retrieved from the presynaptic membrane by two different forms of endocytosis, which operate on different time scales and with different degrees of selectivity. One, the formation of large vesicles by direct invagination of the presynaptic membrane, is nonselective and occurs in the first one or two seconds after stimulation. The other, formation of coated vesicles, occurs more slowly but appears to be highly selective in that it retrieves from the presynaptic membrane large intramembranous particles that look like those in synaptic vesicles' membranes. Together, these two forms of endocytosis compensate for the expansion of the presynaptic membrane that accompanies synaptic-vesicle endocytosis and allow for the recycling of membrane into new generations of synaptic vesicles, as we originally hypothesized to occur at the synapse.

WE AND OTHER researchers have published a number of electron micrographs that appear to show synaptic vesicles caught in the act of exocytosis (Couteaux and Pécot-Dechavassine, 1970; Heuser, Reese, and Landis, 1974; Peper et al., 1974). These micrographs fit in well with the idea that transmitter is discharged in quanta because it is released from within synaptic vesicles (Katz, 1969, 1971). However, all the micrographs published so far have been obtained from nerves that were fixed with chemical cross-linking

JOHN E. HEUSER and THOMAS S. REESE Department of Physiology, School of Medicine, University of California, San Francisco, CA 94143; Laboratory of Neuropathology and Neuroanatomical Sciences, NINCDS, National Institutes of Health, Bethesda, MD 20014

agents to capture the structural changes associated with quantal transmitter release. Such chemicals fix very slowly, compared to the speed of transmitter release from the nerve. As a consequence, it has been impossible to use fixed tissues to establish a firm correlation between the abundance of electron-microscopic images of exocytosis and the physiological rate of quantal release measured in the final moments before fixation. In fixed tissues, the electron-microscopic images of synaptic-vesicle exocytosis are usually much more abundant than might be expected from the physiological measurements; this suggests that the exocytotic event lasts far longer than we would expect if it represented a fusion between two fluid membranes (Heuser, Reese, and Landis, 1974; Heuser, 1976). Thus electron micrographs of chemically fixed tissues have failed to provide accurate information about the basic molecular processes that occur when calcium acts to trigger the fusion between synaptic vesicles and the plasma membrane in the process of exocytosis.

In an effort to avoid problems with chemical fixation, we have developed a machine that allows us to capture synaptic-vesicle exocytosis at precise times during synaptic transmission by freezing completely fresh, unfixed nerve-muscle preparations against an ultracold block of copper or silver (Heuser, Reese, and Landis, 1976). The design and operation of our freezing machine, which is derived from a type originally devised by Van Harreveld (Van Harreveld and Crowell, 1964), is shown in Figure 1. We use frog cutaneous pectoralis muscles, which we first expose to 4-aminopyridine (4-AmP) in order to augment the amount of transmitter released in response to each nerve stimulus. This allows us to capture so many images of synaptic-vesicle exocytosis that we can conveniently: (1) map the distribution of synaptic-vesicle exocytosis in the presynaptic membrane; (2) measure the abundance of exocytosis and relate this to physiological output recordings; and (3) observe the evolution of presynaptic membrane changes that occurs before and after exocytosis.

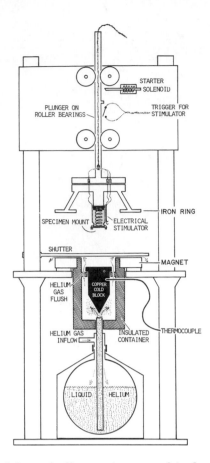

FIGURE 1 Schematic diagram (not to scale) of our current design for a machine that quick-freezes living muscles by pressing them against a block of ultrapure copper cooled to the temperature of liquid helium (4°K). Delicate cutaneous pectoralis nerve-muscles are dissected from the smallest *Rana pipiens* available and placed on the cushioned specimen mount; the nerves are draped over two stimulating wires. The specimen mount is plugged into the end of a long plunger suspended directly above the copper block. Just before this is done, the copper block is cooled by spraying liquid helium against its lower surface. (The liquid helium is delivered through a vacuum-insulated line from a 25 liter Dewar located beneath the freezing machine. About 1 liter of liquid helium is needed to cool the copper block down to 4°K; the cost is thus around $3 to freeze each muscle.) When a thermocouple plugged into the copper block registers approximately 4°K, the operator presses a button that simultaneously releases the plunger into free fall and opens a shutter that until then has covered the top of the copper block (to prevent air or water from condensing on its cold surface). Once the tissue strikes the copper block, the continuing downward momentum of the plunger is absorbed by the spring mounted under the specimen mount, and it is prevented from bouncing back up by a strong electromagnet that grabs the iron ring around the specimen mount. The frozen muscle is quickly transferred to liquid nitrogen for storage and kept there until it can be freeze-fractured or freeze-substituted. (From Heuser et al., 1979.)

The details of these results and our experimental techniques are published elsewhere (Heuser et al., 1979; Heuser and Reese, 1979); they are reviewed here as a basis for a general review of our current concept of synaptic-vesicle exocytosis and recycling. First, it will help to consider how 4-AmP augments transmitter release, and why it might distort the normal process of vesicle exocytosis somewhat by forcing it to be so abundant.

The action of 4-aminopyridine

When applied in millimolar amounts, 4-AmP substantially increases the amount of acetylcholine (ACh) that each nerve terminal releases when it is invaded by an action potential. Typically the increase in output is so great that a muscle bathed in fifty times the dose of curare normally needed to paralyze it will begin to twitch again when 1 mM 4-AmP is added. The magnitude of this increase in evoked transmitter output can be measured by recording endplate potentials with intracellular micropipettes, as in Figure 2. In this experiment, M. Dennis, L. Jan, and Y. Jan bathed a frog cutaneous pectoralis muscle in an unusually high dose of curare and recorded the diminished endplate potential (lower trace) from one of its muscle fibers. Then they added 1 mM 4-AmP to the same curare-loaded bath; after about fifteen minutes, they impaled the same fiber they had recorded before and photographed its new endplate potential (upper trace). The dramatic increase in endplate potential amplitude shown in this figure was typical of the results obtained from more than fifty individually identified muscle fibers from five different muscles. The average increase in endplate potential amplitude with 1 mM 4-AmP was fiftyfold.

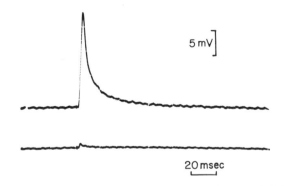

FIGURE 2 Intracellular endplate potentials recorded from a single identified muscle fiber in 10^{-4} M curare, before (below) and after (above) exposure to 1 mM 4-AmP. The increase of transmitter output produced by 4-AmP is about fiftyfold. (From Heuser et al., 1979.)

It is not entirely clear how 4-AmP produces this effect. In squid axons it is known to block the voltage-sensitive potassium channels that open to turn off the action potential (Meves and Pichon, 1975; Pelhate and Pichon, 1974; Yeh et al., 1976); it probably prolongs the action potential in the frog motoneuron terminal as well. We would expect this to cause an abnormally long-lasting influx of calcium across the presynaptic membrane and thus to generate an abnormally great stimulus for secretion (Katz and Miledi, 1967; Llinás, Steinberg, and Walton, 1976; Llinás, Walton, and Bohr, 1976). Katz and Miledi (1977) have shown that similar "giant" endplate potentials occur in frog muscles bathed in tetraethylammonium (TEA) ions, which are also known to prolong the nerve action potential by blocking its voltage-sensitive potassium channels (Armstrong, 1967, 1969) and thus presumably act in the same way as 4-AmP.

Unfortunately, frog nerve terminals are too small to impale with microelectrodes, so one cannot record such a prolongation of the action potential. Nor was M. Dennis able to observe any prolongation of the extracellular currents that accompany the action potential in 4-AmP. His extracellular recordings, made with a blunt microelectrode pushed against a motoneuron terminal (as in Figure 3), are sensitive only to fast current changes and probably would not reveal a prolongation of the action potential if it did occur in 4-AmP. The recording in Figure 3 reveals at least that the rising phase of the endplate current is prolonged. This postsynaptic current is a measure of the number of postsynaptic receptor channels opened by ACh at any moment and thus is a direct measure of the instantaneous rate of ACh release from the nerve (Steinbach and Stevens, 1976). It illustrates that ACh secretion in 4-AmP begins after the normal synaptic delay that follows the nerve impulse (during which time calcium channels are opening in response to the presynaptic depolarizaton that accompanies the action potential); and it illustrates that secretion increases progressively for the next several milliseconds. Unlike the endplate current in normal Ringer's, which reaches its maximum after only 1 msec and then promptly declines, the current in 1 mM 4-AmP continues to rise for more than 3 msec and does not decline back to baseline until 8–9 msec after it began. This presumably indicates that the calcium channels are indeed held open longer in 4-AmP, which fits with the possibility that 4-AmP prolongs the action potential. Prolonged calcium current would, of course, be expected to lead to a greater accumulation of calcium inside the nerve.

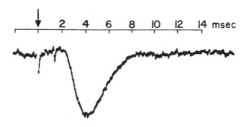

FIGURE 3   Extracellular recording from a curarized neuromuscular junction bathed in 1 mM 4-AmP and given single electrical stimulus at the arrow. The tiny biphasic blip about 1.5 msec after the stimulus represents the arriving nerve action potential. The large downward deflection that begins 1 msec later represents the postsynaptic endplate current evoked by ACh discharged from the nerve. This trace reveals that ACh discharge is not only much more massive in 4-AmP, but that it peaks later and lasts longer. This suggests that in 4-AmP the calcium channels in the presynaptic membrane are held open longer than usual. (From Heuser et al., 1979.)

Exocytosis associated with secretion in 4-aminopyridine

Traces such as those in Figure 3 illustrate that the ideal time to catch exocytosis in frozen nerves ought to be 4–6 msec after the nerve impulse, when the endplate current—and thus the rate of ACh release—is near its peak. Freezing can be accomplished during this interval by attaching a simple timing circuit to the freezing machine to trigger the delivery of a 0.3 msec, 2 V shock to the nerve at precise times before the muscles are frozen. After freezing, the frog muscles are fractured open in a Balzers vacuum evaporator, and a platinum-carbon shadow casting is made of their fractured surfaces. The platinum-carbon replica can then be separated from the tissue and viewed in the electron microscope with standard techniques (Moor and Muhlethaler, 1963).

Viewing nerve terminals in such freeze-fracture replicas, we can compare muscles frozen at various times before and after stimulation and determine the structural changes that accompany secretion of ACh. Figures 4 and 5, for example, compare the typical freeze-fracture appearance of individual "active zones" on nerve frozen 3 msec and 5 msec after receiving a shock in 1 mM 4-AmP. The active zone frozen at 3 msec (Figure 4) looks exactly like those found on resting or unstimulated nerves fixed with chemical fixatives (Heuser, Reese, and Landis, 1974). It can be identified as an active zone by two characteristic double rows of large intramembranous particles that appear to pile up against a central ridge in

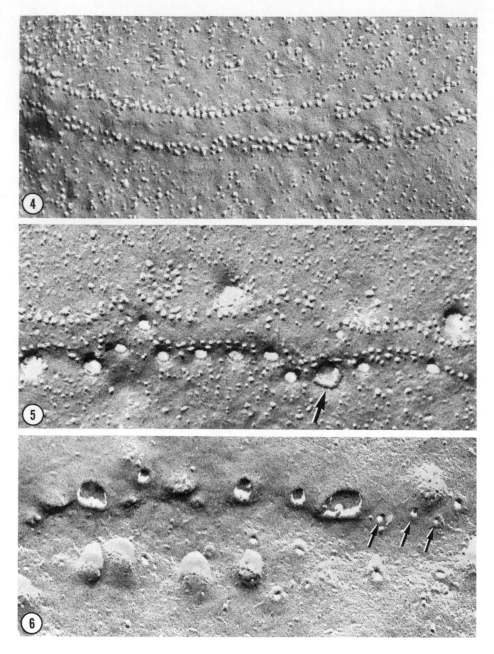

FIGURE 4   High-magnification view of one active zone from a frog neuromuscular junction soaked in 1 mM 4-AmP and frozen 3 msec after stimulation—too early to catch any exocytosis of synaptic vesicles. This and all subsequent micrographs—except Figure 6—are views of the inner leaflet of the fractured presynaptic membrane as it looks from a vantage point outside the nerve, called the P-face (Branton et al., 1975). In the absence of exocytosis, the active zone can be recognized simply by the alignment of large intramembranous particles, which persists regardless of the functional state of the nerve. These large particles might be the calcium channels in the presynaptic membrane (Heuser, Reese, and Landis, 1974; Llinás and Heuser, 1977).

FIGURE 5   An active zone 5 msec after stimulation in 1 mM 4-AmP, when exocytosis of synaptic vesicles is abundant. In this P-face view of the inner leaflet of presynaptic membrane, vesicle openings look like depressions or dimples. They occur in a variety of sizes. One of the larger openings displays a very distinct rim (arrow), but most of the smaller ones have such rims as well (see Figure 7).

FIGURE 6   A view of synaptic-vesicle exocytosis that is complementary to Figure 5. Here the outer leaflet of the presynaptic membrane is viewed from a vantage point inside the nerve, known as the E-face (Branton et al., 1975). Exocytotic synaptic vesicles look either like dome-shaped elevations or, if they were evulsed during the fracture procedure, like craters with elevated rims. Some of these craters are extremely small (arrows).

the presynaptic membrane, which has very few intramembranous particles and looks very similar to the attachment zones or zonula adherentes seen in other epithelia (McNutt and Weinstein, 1973). There is no sign at such active zones of any physical interaction between the presynaptic membrane and the synaptic vesicles that must underlie it.

This result confirms our earlier claim that synaptic vesicles do not form persistent attachments with the presynaptic membrane in the absence of nerve stimulation (Heuser, Reese, and Landis, 1974); this has been a point of contention (Akert et al., 1972; Peper et al., 1974) and has been difficult to prove in chemically fixed tissues because of the danger that chemical fixatives might affect nerve structure adversely during the final moments of physiological activity. As long as fixation was required to prepare nerves for freeze-fracture, the only way we could be sure to obtain a resting appearance was to dissect nerve-muscle preparations from the frog and bathe them in calcium free Ringer's containing magnesium—to prevent secretion from occurring during the inevitable depolarization produced by the fixative (Heuser, Reese, and Landis, 1974).

Finally, Figure 4 illustrates that 4-AmP alone does not produce any of the structural changes seen to occur on nerves frozen a bit later after stimulation, near the peak of the endplate potential (as in Figure 5). This figure shows the active zone of a nerve stimulated 5 msec before it was frozen. This nerve's appearance is typical of most of those found in muscles frozen after this time interval. Invariably, a few of the nerves in each muscle showed no structural differences at all from Figure 4; there was reason to suspect that they failed to receive a nerve impulse because their axons were cooled prematurely from too close proximity to the freezing block at the moment of stimulation. Five milliseconds before impact they were less than 5 mm from the freezing block.

The active zone in Figure 5 differs from that in Figure 4 in being bordered by rows of depressions or dimples of characteristic size and shape. Most of these structures are typical examples of the freeze-fracture view of exocytosis as it looks from outside the cell after the outer half of the membrane has been split away and the inner half or "P-face" (Branton et al., 1975) of the membrane has been replicated with platinum and carbon. At each depression the presynaptic membrane curves down onto a broken membrane rim, which represents the point at which the fracture plane could no longer follow such a deep invagination of the presynaptic membrane and broke across the invagination's open neck. Complementary

views of outer membrane halves that are broken away from these depressions, seen in Figure 6, reveal even more clearly these perturbations in the presynaptic membrane. What look like depressions in the P-face view of Figure 5 naturally look like elevations in the complementary E-face views. In this replica each elevation appears to be crater-shaped because its apex has been etched away by subliming water off the surface of the fractured nerve into the vacuum before replicating it with platinum and carbon. Such etching of the apex of the freeze-fracture deformity illustrates that the fracture jumped across the open neck of some sort of invagination, which we presume to be an exocytotic synaptic vesicle. (We suppose that such invaginations represent exocytotic vesicles because they appear at the precise time when quanta of ACh are released.) Figure 7 summarizes how these complementary images are produced during the freeze-fracture procedure.

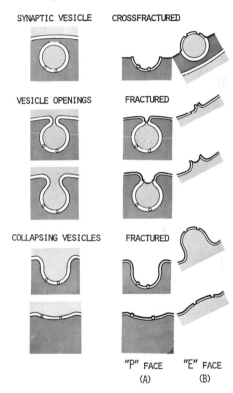

FIGURE 7 Diagram illustrating how the various stages of synaptic-vesicle exocytosis caught by quick-freezing (left) produce characteristic electron-microscopic images when the presynaptic membrane is split and replicated with platinum (right). Early stages of vesicle openings fracture through the narrow necks of the vesicles and produce the characteristic rimmed depressions and elevations on the P-face and E-face, respectively. In contrast, the fracture plane passes continuously along later-stage vesicles that are more wide open, thereby producing smooth pockets or domes in the respective faces.

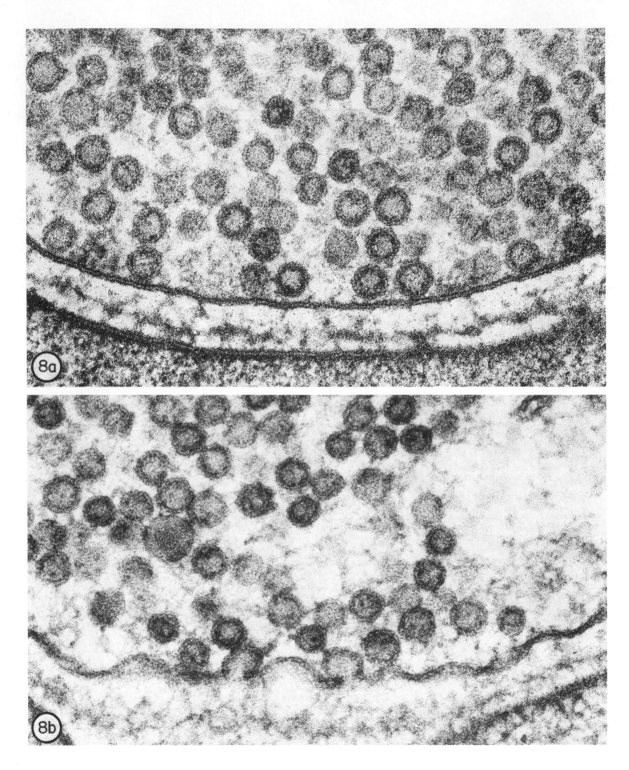

FIGURE 8   High-magnification views of freeze-substituted nerve terminals that were quick-frozen while resting in normal Ringer's (above) or immediately after one shock in 1 mM 4-AmP (below). In the absence of stimulation, a number of synaptic vesicles lie very close to the presynaptic membrane, and the presynaptic membrane is unperturbed. After one shock in 4-AmP, the vesicles close to the presynaptic membrane are replaced by omega figures and other, more gentle, campanulate perturbations in the presynaptic membrane which presumably represent thin-section views of different stages in synaptic-vesicle collapse after exocytosis. (From Heuser and Reese, 1979.)

Another reason to think that the freeze-fracture structures are examples of synaptic-vesicle exocytosis comes from parallel thin-section studies of muscles quick-frozen at the same moment of peak ACh secretion. Such muscles are prepared for thin-sectioning by the process known as freeze-substitution (Feder and Sidman, 1958): they are warmed in a mixture of acetone and osmium tetroxide and then embedded in plastic so that they can be thin-sectioned and viewed (see Figure 8). High magnifications of nerves given one shock in 4-AmP about five msec before being frozen display omega forms, such as those in Figure 9, which look even more like fused synaptic vesicles than the original images of plasmalemmal pockets that Couteaux and Pécot-Dechavassine (1970) described in the paper that first identified and defined the active zones of this synapse.

The trouble with Couteaux and Pécot-Dechavassine's views, however, was that they were obtained from aldehyde-fixed nerves. Thus these observers could not know the exact functional history of their nerves and could not be sure that the plasmalemmal pockets they saw represented sites of synaptic-vesicle exocytosis. It could have been argued that their pockets represented the formation of synaptic vesicles by some sort of micropinocytosis of the presynaptic membrane

Capturing these pockets by quick-freezing provides several new reasons for believing that they do represent exocytosis of synaptic vesicles and that exocytosis is the structural basis of ACh release. First and most important, these pockets appear only during moments of transmitter release. Comparing Figure 4 with Figure 5 illustrates that they are not present immediately preceding transmitter release and that they are not brought on simply by some deleterious action of 4-AmP. Second, the abundance of these images of vesicle fusion fits—as well as can be determined—with the number of quanta discharged by one nerve impulse in 4-AmP (see Figure 10). This has been a difficult correlation to make with any accuracy because of problems involved in measuring the physiological quantal contents of such large endplate potentials. The correlation will not be further substantiated here; all of the evidence that one vesicle equals one quantum is considered in more detail by Heuser et al. (1979).

The third reason for believing that these plasmalemmal pockets represent exocytosis rests on the basis of exclusion—that is, the evidence that they do not represent micropinocytosis. One can imagine that the release of ACh might activate some sort of rapid

micropinocytosis involved in retrieving transmitter or other materials from the synaptic cleft when synaptic transmission is over. Indeed, in some sorts of aminergic synapses, retrieval of transmitter may be an important means of stopping the transmitter action (Wolfe et al., 1962; Axelrod, 1971). Nonetheless, there are several reasons for believing that the vesicle openings caught by freezing during the endplate potential do not represent such endocytosis. For one thing, if they did, we would have found extracellular tracers such as horseradish peroxidase (HRP) taken up into vesicles around the active zones immediately after stimulation. But we have already established that HRP is rarely found in the vesicles around the active zone in the early moments of tracer uptake (Heuser and Reese, 1973). This observation did not completely settle the matter, however, because to determine the location of HRP in the electron microscope we had to follow the usual histochemical procedure (Graham and Karnovsky, 1966), which meant that nerves had to be fixed first in the traditional way with aldehyde. So the usual problems involved in

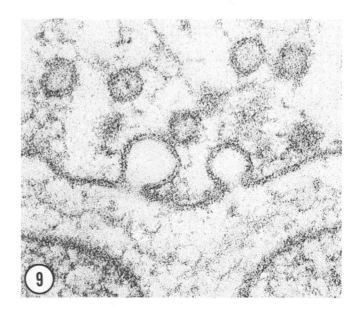

FIGURE 9 High magnification of an extremely thin section through one active zone on a nerve that was quick-frozen 5.1 msec after receiving one shock in 1 mM 4-AmP. This shows clearly how synaptic vesicles fuse with the plasma membrane as neurotransmitter is discharged. (From Heuser, 1976.)

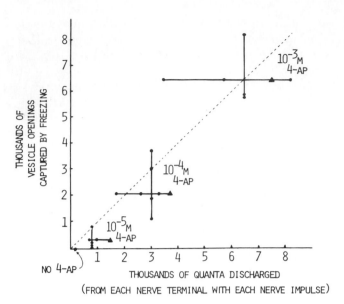

FIGURE 10 Correlation at different doses of 4-AmP between the number of vesicle openings counted on frozen nerve terminals and physiological estimates of the number of quanta discharged. To do the vesicle counts for each muscle, 50–150 active zones were photographed from freeze-fracture replicas of several different neuromuscular junctions, and the average number of vesicle openings per active zone was determined. This number was multiplied by 500, which is approximately the number of active zones per nerve terminal, to give the values shown on the graph. To estimate the number of quanta for each muscle, end-plate potential amplitudes were measured at 5–10 identified neuromuscular junctions before and after 4-AmP, and the degree of augmentation was calculated from (amplitude after/amplitude before). This value was multiplied by 125 quanta—which is the mean number of quanta to discharge normally from such small frog neuromuscular junctions—to give the values shown on the abscissa. The horizontal and vertical bars plot the full range of average values obtained from each of the muscles studied at each dose of 4-AmP; the points of intersections of these bars represent the overall mean number of vesicles and quanta for each dose of 4-AmP. If one vesicle equaled one quantum, the means should fall exactly on the 45° line going through the origin. Except at the highest dose of 4-AmP, however, the number of vesicle openings we saw was somewhat less than the number of quanta that should have discharged. (From Heuser et al., 1979.)

using aldehydes to catch exocytosis were present. The slow rate of chemical fixation might have allowed enough time for a fast micropinocytosis to subside and for vesicles newly formed at the active zone to escape, with their charge of HRP, into the axoplasm at large. If so, such fast micropinocytosis would have escaped undetected in aldehyde-fixed tissues.

Quick-freezing can now be used to stop the action at the synapse much more quickly, confirming that the omega forms that appear during the peak of the action potential *do not* represent micropinocytosis. This is done using ferritin as an extracellular tracer.

Restriction of exocytosis to active zones

Perhaps the most impressive fact about the images of synaptic-vesicle exocytosis provided by quick-freezing is that they fully confirm Couteaux and Pécot-Dechavassine's original claim that the dense bands of cytoplasmic fuzz, which are the thin-section equivalent of the intramembranous particles seen in freeze-fracture, do indeed mark the active secretory zones of this synapse (Couteaux and Pécot-Dechavassine, 1970, 1973). Invariably, images of synaptic-vesicle fusion, such as those in Figures 5 and 6, are found lined up beside these zones. Rarely is a vesicle opening observed as far as 500 Å away. In fact, the localization of exocytosis in quick-frozen nerves is even more strict than had appeared in our earlier micrographs of nerves fixed while being stimulated (Heuser, Reese, and Landis, 1974). This was probably because in fixed nerves some of the openings that occur a bit farther from the active zone were actually instances of endocytosis. (We should have expected endocytosis to have been provoked in these fixed nerves because they received several seconds of stimulation before the fixative had time to act; by then endocytosis should have started up to compensate for all the exocytosis.)

At the moment there is no explanation for why exocytosis is so strictly localized to active zones at the frog neuromuscular junction. It may be because the calcium channels in the plasma membrane are located in these areas and the calcium entering them does not have enough time to diffuse very far into the axoplasm before it triggers exocytosis (Llinás and Heuser, 1977). However, if one were to imagine that exocytosis is localized to active zones because inward calcium currents are localized there, one would predict that drugs that stimulate transmitter release by increasing the concentration of free calcium throughout the whole axoplasm ought to produce exocytosis of synaptic vesicles all over the nerve—not just at the active zones. This has not been shown so far, although it has not been disproven either. The problem with using quick-freezing to study *where* exocytosis occurs during such drug treatments is that the instantaneous rate of secretion never reaches high enough levels so that one could hope to capture enough of it. For example, even during the intense burst of secretion that occurs in black-widow-spider venom (Clark, Hurlbut, and Mauro, 1972) or in lanthanum (Heuser and Miledi, 1971), miniature end-plate potential frequency rarely reaches more than about 1,000/sec. This would translate to one vesicle opening per millisecond. But if each opening lasted less than 10 msec (as we shall illustrate below), we would expect to capture fewer than ten openings at a time if we quick-froze the nerve during such stimulation. And since these ten openings would be spread over a wide area of the nerve terminal, we are very unlikely to find them in the fragmentary views obtained in freeze-fracture. In contrast, the abundant exocytosis found after one shock in 4-AmP represents the "catch" from a single discharge of 5,000 quanta in less than 5 msec. This rate of release would translate to 10^6 quanta/sec if it could go on continuously—three orders of magnitude greater than the maximum rate of release one can expect with calcium-perturbing drugs or toxins! Thus it remains to be seen whether exocytosis must always occur at the active zone.

If it does always occur at the active zone, even when intracellular calcium is elevated diffusely throughout the nerve terminal, then we should look more carefully at the detailed spatial relationships that synaptic vesicles establish with the presynaptic membrane in the first place, before stimulation. Couteaux and Pécot-Dechavassine (1974) have demonstrated that the vesicles on either side of the dense cytoplasmic fuzz that identifies the active zone in thin sections lie particularly close to the plasma membrane. This observation was made on fixed tissue, and we can confirm it with thin-section views of quick-frozen nerves (as in Figure 8). Such active-zone vesicles are found exactly where exocytosis occurs, and so it is natural to assume that their location favors exocytosis. Thus one could envision an inhomogeneous distribution of synaptic vesicles inside the nerve—characterized by clusters of vesicles around active-zone densities—to explain why exocytosis is so localized at the active zones. There need be nothing special about presynaptic membrane at the active zone, nor any special calcium currents there. Instead, exocytosis would occur only

at the active zone simply because this is the only area supplied with vesicles in high concentrations.

Once we know more about the forces that act on synaptic vesicles and about how vesicles move about in the axoplasm and end up at the active zone, we may begin to understand why exocytosis is confined to these zones. But already we see one important consequence of our finding from the frog neuromuscular junction, and it is probably true for CNS synapses as well: namely, that the number of quanta a synapse can release is limited by the area of its active zone and by the number of spaces it provides for synaptic vesicles in that area. For example, at our frog neuromuscular junction, the maximum number of quanta that can be released in one burst, by optimal levels of 4-AmP and high calcium, is about 15,000. Katz and Miledi (1977) observed about the same maximum after stimulation in TEA ions. This is close to the maximum number of vesicle openings that we can find on nerves frozen after one shock in 1 mM 4-AmP. Correspondingly, the maximum number of vesicles that can line up beside the active zones in any particular nerve terminal is about 20,000—assuming there are 500 one-micron-long bands of active zone in each frog nerve terminal and that each band can become surrounded by forty closely packed synaptic vesicles (Heuser, 1976). Since exocytosis appears never to occur away from the active zone, it would have to draw entirely from this population of 20,000 vesicles.

Clearly, in 4-AmP the nerve impulse is able to trigger discharge of nearly all 20,000 of these vesicles at once. Under normal conditions, however, each action potential releases about 200 quanta, only about 1 percent of this population of vesicles. The rest of the vesicles may provide a backup to sustain exocytosis during a volley of action potentials, which is undoubtedly how motoneurons fire during actual movements of the living frog. Such considerations will become clear only when we know how fast synaptic vesicles can move about in the axoplasm; we should be able to learn this from observing how fast vesicles restock the active zone after one shock in 4-AmP.

Presumably the upper limit on exocytosis in CNS synapses will turn out to be the number of vesicles that can be packed into their presynaptic grids of dense projections (Akert, 1973; Akert et al., 1972). How many vesicles discharge normally will then be determined by this immediate supply of vesicles, as well as by the subtle variations in calcium levels brought about by modulation of the frequency of action potentials activating them from afar or by modulation of the local currents spreading into them passively from nearby synapses.

Random distribution of exocytosis within individual active zones

With this evidence that quick-freezing reveals the exocytosis of synaptic vesicles that underlies transmitter release and with the observation that exocytosis occurs only beside the active zone, we can begin to examine the distribution of vesicle openings along each active zone and the relative abundance of vesicle openings from active zone to active zone. Such information may help to elucidate how calcium acts to trigger synaptic-vesicle exocytosis.

The distribution of vesicle openings along the length of each individual active zone appears to be random. When the openings are infrequent, they can be located anywhere along an active zone; they are found as frequently near the center of the zone as toward its edges. This is equally true (1) when the nerves are frozen at early moments of transmitter release in high doses of 4-AmP, at which time the first vesicles are opening up but the endplate potential has not yet reached its maximum, or (2) when nerves are frozen after one shock in lower doses of 4-AmP, under which conditions quantal discharge is less abundant and vesicle openings are rare at all times during the endplate potential (Figure 10). There thus appears to be no particular locus along the individual active zone that is specialized for exocytosis; the whole edge seems equally special.

In the two situations in which vesicle exocytosis is infrequent, it is also clear that vesicle openings occur singly and not in any obvious association with neighboring openings. At least we never find short rows of several openings located close together. There is no visible indication that several vesicle openings occur together, linked in time or in space, as they might if they were responding to the same calcium signal. For example, if calcium entered the active zone only at one point along the presynaptic membrane, we might have expected to find that, when exocytosis was rare, it would always be located at that spot; correspondingly, when 4-AmP was present and the calcium influx through that point was prolonged, many vesicle openings would be found in the immediate vicinity of this calcium entry point.

We wanted to look for evidence in favor of a single point source of calcium at each active zone because it would be a ready explanation for why each zone might normally discharge no more than one vesicle in response to each action potential, which is thought to be the way the system works (Heuser, 1976; Martin, 1977). In that case one could simply imagine (1) that only one vesicle could be in close proximity to each active zone's single point of calcium entry at any given moment; and (2) that only one vesicle has time to open up at that spot during a normal-sized endplate potential. Unfortunately the randomness with which vesicle openings distribute themselves along active zones (see Figure 11) does not fit this simple model. All the vesicles that lie along the edge of the active zone appear to have an equal chance of opening.

We could have concluded the foregoing from our earlier observations of the widespread, uniform distribution of vesicle openings along active zones on stimulated nerves chemically fixed with aldehydes (Heuser, Reese, and Landis, 1974). We showed that weak or dilute fixatives characteristically produced an exaggerated overabundance of such openings. (Probably they prevent the open vesicles from collapsing before they stop additional vesicles from opening, so that vesicle openings accumulate during the final moments of stimulation.) From such chemically fixed nerves we obtained many examples of active zones bordered by confluent rows of exocytotic openings along their entire length. These were stimulated in normal Ringer's, so there was no doubt that the normal entry of calcium was able to trigger release of vesicles all along the active zone. Now we often find almost confluent rows of exocytotic openings in nerves quick-frozen during the giant endplate potential produced by one shock in 4-AmP (Figures 5 and 13). These, too, extend from one end of each active zone to the other, as was the case in the chemically fixed nerves. In such cases we never find that the rows of vesicle openings stop short of the ends of the rows of intramembranous particles that mark the active zone in freeze-fracture. The whole differentiated membrane zone displays the ability to support exocytosis; thus it is not surprising that the entire active zone is normally backed by confluent rows of synaptic vesicles at rest, as Couteaux's pictures originally showed.

We can see these rows of vesicles quite clearly in micrographs of freeze-substituted nerves such as Figure 8. But even though quick-freezing must stop almost instantaneously whatever natural Brownian movement the vesicles may have (and thus ought to reveal the vesicles' true locations in life), we cannot make out any consistent differences among the vesicles—differences such as distance away from the pre-

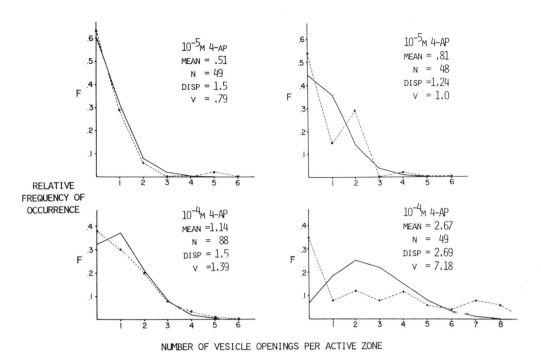

RELATIVE FREQUENCY OF OCCURRENCE

NUMBER OF VESICLE OPENINGS PER ACTIVE ZONE

FIGURE 11 Tests for the independence of synaptic-vesicle exocytosis. Each graph displays the distribution of synaptic-vesicle exocytosis along a single nerve terminal, from experiments in which exocytosis was relatively rare because only low doses of 4-AmP were applied. In these situations, if each vesicle discharged independently of its neighbor, there should have been no tendency for vesicle openings to group together along particular active zones. To test this we counted the number of vesicle openings at each active zone and determined the mean number of openings per active zone for each muscle. From this mean value we calculated how many active zones ought to display 0, 1, 2,

... openings if they occurred independently, as predicted by Poisson's theorem. We then compared the Poisson prediction (solid line) with the actual distribution of vesicle openings observed (dotted line). The fit was good for the two terminals on the left, indicating that the distribution of vesicle exocytosis was random in them. The fit was very poor for the terminal on the lower right, largely because there were too many active zones with no vesicle openings, although there may have been a few multiple occurrences as well. (N, the number of active zones observed; DISP, the coefficient of dispersion, which equals variance/mean; V, variance.)

synaptic membrane—that would cause one out of forty of them to be much more likely to discharge than its neighbors.

It was important to look for such differences because the most recent statistical analyses of transmitter release from this synapse have suggested that quanta are discharged from a pool or store of only a few hundred vesicles inside the nerve (Wernig, 1975). Such statistical analyses have traditionally been based on the assumption that a discrete pool of vesicles, all with equally high probability of being discharged, exists inside the nerve. But recently it has become clear that this need not be true, even though the statistics suggest it is. The statistics could fit equally well with the assumption that all synaptic vesicles have continuously varying probabilities of release, each different from the other, as they might if they were continuously wandering, sometimes closer to sometimes farther from the presynaptic membrane

(Barton and Cohen, 1977; Brown, Perkel, and Feldman, 1976; Hatt and Smith, 1976; Zucker, 1977). In that case there would be no discrete pool of several hundred vesicles to be singled out as the ones uniquely ready for release. We would still, of course, need to explain why transmitter release behaves as if there were a few hundred vesicles with an especially high probability of release at any one moment.

The reason this number seems to be so small remains a mystery. It is close to the number of active zones at an individual synapse, which at first led us to wonder whether each active zone could discharge only one vesicle with each nerve impulse. We looked to see whether there was only one special spot on each active zone where exocytosis occurred (Heuser, 1976, 1977). This clearly is not the case, however, so we must seek elsewhere for an explanation of the statistical results. Later in this chapter we describe one way in which the discharge of one vesicle could alter the presynaptic membrane almost instantaneously, so that no further vesicles would discharge in the vicinity of the first until some propagated molecular disturbance in the presynaptic membrane had had time to "clear." One could imagine that the rate of accumulation and clearance of such presynaptic membrane disturbances would determine the kinetics of transmitter release from individual active zones and would produce the overall fatigue in quantal transmitter release that is seen during rapid tetanic stimulation.

A subtle type of nonrandomness did emerge from counting vesicle openings per micron of active zone and then comparing the counts from one active zone to the next; it was found that the relative abundance of vesicle openings can vary in a slightly nonrandom way along the length of any individual nerve terminal branch. That is, we found regions in which several active zones in a row had a higher mean number of vesicle openings alternating with regions in which several active zones had fewer vesicle openings or even none at all (see Figure 12). Such variations along the length of individual branches were markedly fewer, however, than the variations in mean vesicle openings seen from one whole endplate to the next in the same muscle.

We do not know the source of this variation in either case. It may reflect a natural variation in amount of transmitter being put out at the moment of freezing because of such internal variations in the nerve terminal's physiological condition as background level of ionized calcium and stock of synaptic vesicles. Alternatively it may reflect an unnatural variation introduced by the experimental conditions necessary for quick-freezing. With our current method, there is a serious possibility of nerves being damaged during the dissection and mounting of the muscle. Such damage is greatly worsened by exposure to 4-AmP. There is also considerable risk that an exposed muscle will dry out or be chilled in the last moments before it is frozen. Because we see less and less of it as we improve our experimental techniques, we at-

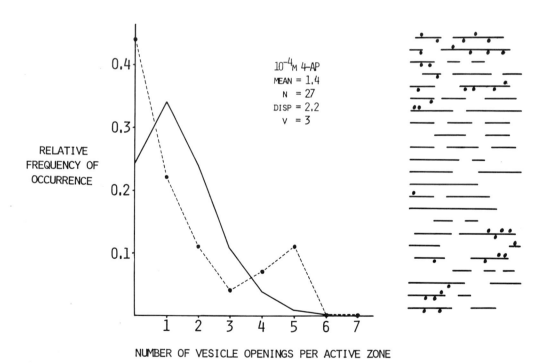

10^{-4} M 4-AP
MEAN = 1.4
N = 27
DISP = 2.2
V = 3

RELATIVE FREQUENCY OF OCCURRENCE

NUMBER OF VESICLE OPENINGS PER ACTIVE ZONE

FIGURE 12 One nerve terminal in which an explanation was found for why the observed distribution of vesicle openings (dotted line) did not fit the Poisson prediction (solid line). To the right is a foreshortened diagram of this nerve terminal, in which its active zones are displayed as straight lines (with a typical degree of interruption) and the vesicle openings caught by freezing are displayed as black dots. The diagram illustrates quite clearly that the deviation from randomness—expressed by a dispersion coefficient of 2.2—is due not so much to a local clumping of synaptic-vesicle openings, but rather to the large inactive area that happened to be included in the center of this particular freeze-fracture replica. This brought the mean number of vesicle openings down from 4 per active zone, the usual number in 10^{-4} M 4-AmP (Figure 10), to 1.4 per active zone and gave a spurious prediction from the Poisson equation.

tribute much of the variation to these unnatural causes. How much natural variation there is in the abundance of exocytosis from nerve to nerve and along individual nerve branches remains to be determined.

Freeze-fracture data on the mechanism of exocytosis

Close scrutiny of the exocytotic openings seen on frozen nerves provides some information about exactly how vesicle and plasma membranes fuse with each other, which bears further on the problem of how calcium triggers such membrane fusion. First, it is clear from the figures shown so far that exocytotic openings occur in a variety of sizes (cf. Figures 5 and 6). Presumably this reflects the fact that all the openings did not occur at exactly the same moment and that freezing has caught them at different stages in their life history. For example, Figure 13 shows again that at 5 msec most openings appear as narrow necks connected to underlying omega vesicles. Some necks are more wide open; one is open so wide that the fracture entered it and scooped out the whole internal leaflet of the vesicle membrane.

Since such wide open forms are rare at early times but become more abundant 20-50 msec after the nerve impulse (Figure 13), we assume that they represent a later stage of exocytosis. We can envision vesicles that pass through such a sequence of opening wider and wider after exocytosis as then collapsing into the presynaptic membrane (as in Figure 7). But a few static images of vesicles caught in the act of collapsing do not reveal what fraction of all exocytosed vesicles suffer this fate. To know that, we would have to watch several individual vesicles go through the whole process in a living synapse, rather than using quick-freezing to take snapshots of large groups of vesicles going through the process slightly out of synchrony with each other. Nevertheless, it is not unreasonable to conclude from micrographs such as the one in the middle of Figure 13—showing exocytosis after 20 msec—that a significant proportion of the vesicles in the field were, in fact, in the process of collapsing when they were frozen.

Figure 13 also shows that the total number of vesicle openings at 20 msec is fewer than is typically found 5 msec after stimulation in the same dose of 4-AmP. By averaging all our 20 msec images, we found that the mean number of vesicle openings was 5 per micron of active zone. This was significantly fewer than the mean of 10 vesicle openings per micron of active zone that we counted at 5 msec. Thus

some vesicle openings apparently have come and gone completely in the 20 msec interval since secretion began; and one must wonder whether they all go by collapsing completely into the presynaptic membrane or whether some "pinch off" from the plasma membrane of the nerve terminal immediately after exocytosis.

If vesicles could pinch off that fast, we would expect to find extracellular tracers entering a few of the vesicles near the active zones right after exocytosis. As mentioned earlier, however, we found, using HRP as an extracellular tracer, that the active-zone vesicles do not become selectively labeled during the early moments of stimulation. Still, we might have missed the earliest uptake or we might have perturbed uptake by the aldehyde fixative that we applied in preparation for HRP histochemistry. We can no longer use HRP as a tracer in tissues that are frozen and freeze-substituted because the osmium tetroxide fixative used in the substitution fluid destroys HRP's enzymatic activity. We can use ferritin as an extracellular tracer, however, and count exactly how many vesicles near the active zones contain ferritin in nerves frozen, for example, 1 sec after stimulation. These counts reveal how many synaptic vesicles pinch off from the presynaptic membrane in the early moments after stimulation. (By 1 sec after stimulation, very few images of any sort of vesicle opening remain on the presynaptic membrane, so they must have all disappeared, either by collapsing or by pinching off.)

We recently completed counts on six endplates from three different muscles that were soaked in 40% ferritin and 1 mM 4-AmP for one hour before being stimulated with one shock and frozen 0.5-1 sec afterward. In all, some 175 active zones were sectioned, but only 21 examples of ferritin-labeled vesicles were found in the vicinity of these active zones. This is about 1% of the number of vesicles that should have popped open and then disappeared (mean vesicle openings of 10 per active zone multiplied by 175 active zones). So it would appear that very few vesicles pinch off from the presynaptic membrane so soon (1 sec) after stimulation. Those that do—that is, those that become loaded with ferritin in these experiments—do not look like normal synaptic vesicles in any case. Most, like the ones in Figure 14, are larger in diameter, and their membrane looks in freeze-fracture exactly like plasma membrane in terms of the number of large and small intramembranous particles displayed. Their membrane is quite unlike synaptic-vesicle membrane, which possesses a high concentration of unusually large intramembranous particles. Thus quick-forming, oversized endocytotic

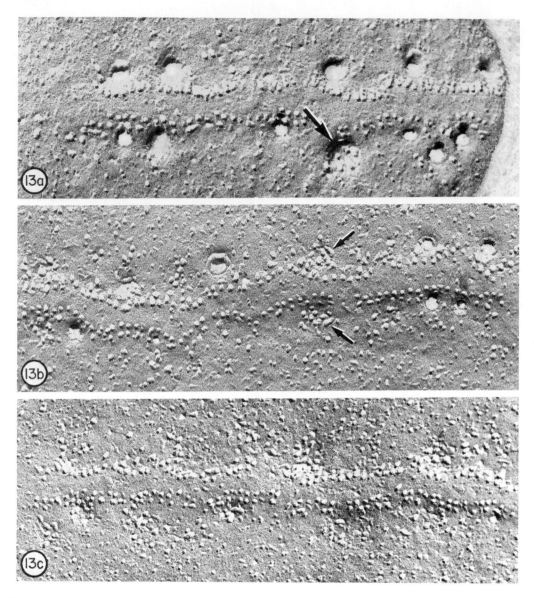

FIGURE 13   High-magnification views of active zones quick-frozen 5, 20, and 50 msec after receiving one shock in 1 mM 4-AmP. At 5 msec vesicle openings are most abundant and assume a variety of sizes and shapes; a few are wide open and reveal several intramembranous particles in their depths (arrow). By 20 msec vesicle openings are only half as abundant as at 5 msec, but in their place can be found a number of more or less discrete clusters of large intra-membranous particles, some of which are even larger than the intramembranous particles that demarcate the active zone (arrows). Finally, 50 msec after exocytosis began, vesicle openings are rare, but the shallow depressions bearing large intramembranous particles have become plentiful. Presumably these represent the final stage of vesicle collapse illustrated in Figure 7. (From Heuser and Reese, 1979.)

vesicles look rather like simple abscissions of the plasma membrane.

We had previously seen similar membrane forms in chemically fixed nerves; but then they were often so distorted in shape that we called them cisternae (for "flattened sacs") (Heuser and Miledi, 1971). Using HRP as a tracer we saw such cisternae formed by endocytosis from the plasma membrane less than a minute after starting a tetanic stimulation in normal Ringer's. It now seems that we misinterpreted the HRP uptake data from chemically fixed nerves. We saw so few examples of cisternae still connected to the plasma membrane and so many coated vesicles attached to cisternae that we proposed a recycling scheme in which coated vesicles do all the work of pinching membrane off the plasma membrane and

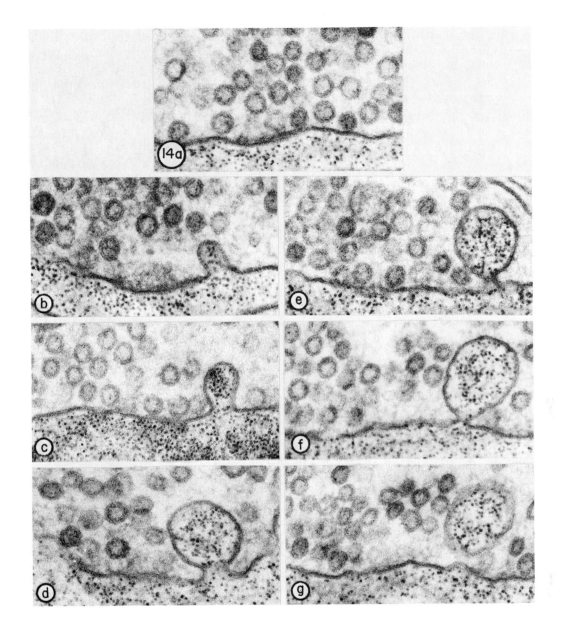

FIGURE 14 Several views of freeze-substituted active zones from nerves soaked in 40% ferritin in frog Ringer's containing 1 mM 4-AmP and then stimulated once, 1 sec before quick-freezing. Ferritin can be seen scattered throughout the synaptic cleft in the lower portion of each figure and also in the large vesicles or vacuoles that appear to have been caught in the act of budding off from the presynaptic membrane in b–g.

then deliver it secondarily to cisternae. This now appears to be incorrect. Several investigators have since observed deep plasma-membrane invaginations that could be cisternae caught in the act of forming during stimulation (Bennett, Model, and Highstein, 1976; Clark, Hurlbut, and Mauro, 1972; Rutherford, Nastuk, and Gennaro, 1976). Now quick-freezing with a ferritin tracer demonstrates that oversized vesicles can pinch off directly from the plasma membrane less than a second after stimulation (Figure 14). We should have paid more attention to how quickly cis-

ternae formed in our old HRP uptake studies; and we should have realized that coated vesicles probably could not pinch off fast enough to form cisternae that quickly.

But exactly how these cisternae form is perhaps a minor point, not worth stressing or correcting ourselves. After all, very few oversized vesicles or cisternae are found in most synapses when they are fixed during their natural ongoing activity in the intact animal. Cisternae become plentiful only when synapses are forced in the laboratory to secrete at abnormally high rates (as in 4-AmP) or for abnormally long periods of continuous stimulation (say 15 minutes at 10 Hz). In such cases cisternae are in a sense an artifact of the excessive amount of exocytosis that has occurred and the excessive demands for some sort of compensatory endocytosis. Quick-freezing has now shown clearly that such endocytosis is by direct invagination and abscission of random bites of plasma membrane and that coated vesicles are not involved.

We still believe that the normal way in which synaptic-vesicle membrane is retrieved from the plasma membrane after exocytosis, when release rates are not so abnormally high, is by the more leisurely process of coated-vesicle formation. These two independent pathways of retrieval are clearly distinguishable in Figure 15.

Figure 16 shows what coated-vesicle formation

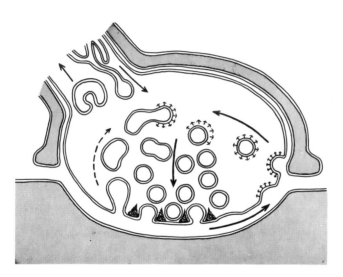

FIGURE 15 Summary of our current view of synaptic-vesicle recycling at the frog neuromuscular junction, based on the new quick-freezing data reviewed in this report. After synaptic vesicles undergo exocytosis and collapse into the presynaptic membrane, two different sorts of compensatory endocytosis can occur. Normally, during moderate rates of synaptic activity, the more leisurely pathway on the right is operative. In it, coated vesicles selectively retrieve specific vesicle components from the presynaptic membrane and directly produce new synaptic vesicles. On the other hand, when secretion is driven to unusually high levels experimentally, the dotted pathway on the left also comes into play. (Whether these conditions and this pathway ever occur in vivo is not known.) Large vacuoles composed of random bites of membrane pinch off rapidly from the presynaptic membrane and gather inside the nerve terminal. How these give rise to new synaptic vesicles is not known. They may simply divide down to vesicle size again; or coated vesicles may pinch off from them, exactly as if they were still part of the presynaptic membrane.

looks like on the surface of freeze-fractured nerves. These are fractures through the plasma membranes of nerves that were exposed to β-bungarotoxin (β-BTX) and stimulated 5 min before fixation, a treatment that invariably produces an abnormal accumulation of "coated pits" such as those in Figure 18. Elsewhere we explain that this accumulation of coated pits represents a block of coated-vesicle formation by the β-BTX (Lassignal and Heuser, 1977). This is not important here; but the advantage of this effect of β-BTX is that it allows one to produce so many coated pits that it becomes easy to recognize them, in freeze-fractures such as Figure 16, by their cluster of unusually large intramembranous particles. Comparing Figure 16 with Figure 17 illustrates that the particles are the same size as the large ones found in synaptic-vesicle membranes; like the vesicle particles, they are even a bit larger than the particles that line up alongside each active zone on the presynaptic membrane. Figure 19 summarizes how the freeze-fracture and thin-section images of coated pits can be correlated.

If we could conclude on the basis of their similar size that large particles in synaptic vesicles and in coated pits are the same, we would have a ready explanation for why coated pits possess a cluster of such large particles. We could reason as follows. We have shown in earlier HRP tracer studies that stimulation of transmitter release leads to the formation of many coated vesicles from the plasma membrane (Heuser and Reese, 1973). We have argued that such coated-vesicle formation is a compensatory endocytosis coupled to exocytosis (see Figure 15), as it is believed to be in many other secretory cells (Nagasawa and Douglas, 1972; Douglas, 1973; Benedeczy and Smith, 1972). We realized that if endocytosis of coated vesicles were supposed to be able to compensate completely for exocytosis at the nerve terminal, it would have to retrieve from the plasma membrane not only just as much membrane as was added to it by exocytosis, but also the right type of membrane, in order to maintain the biochemical individuality of the vesicle and plasma membranes.

Formation of coated vesicles is in fact thought to be a specific membrane-uptake process in several other types of cells (Fawcett, 1964). Examples range from human fibroblasts, which selectively internalize their surface low-density lipoprotein receptors (Anderson, Goldstein, and Brown, 1976), to insect oocytes, which pinocytose specific proteins from their yolk (Roth and Porter, 1964; Roth, Cutting, and Atlas, 1976). The observation that coated vesicles sequester certain characteristic intramembranous par-

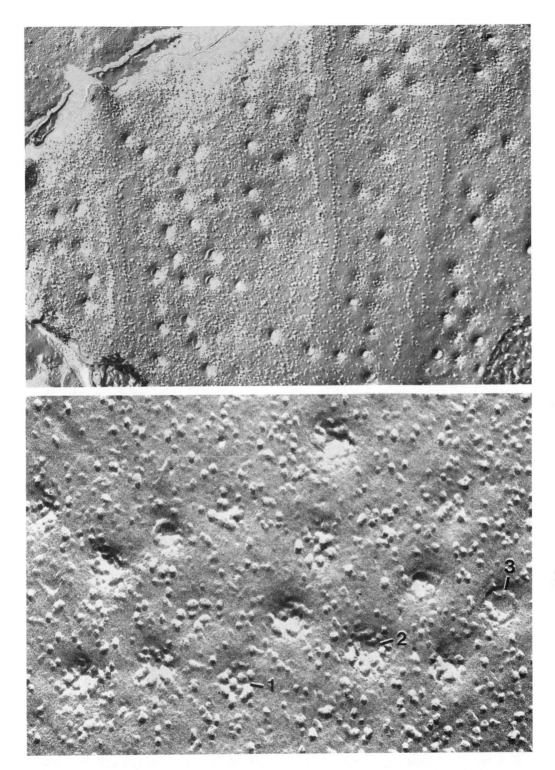

FIGURE 16   Freeze-fracture appearance of the coated pits that form in the presynaptic membrane to compensate for synaptic-vesicle exocytosis. In these nerves, coated pits were made more abundant than normal by soaking frog muscles in 2 μg/ml β-BTX for 45 min at 22°C, then stimulating them for 5 min at 10 IIz, and finally quick-freezing them The upper figure shows that coated pits can form anywhere on the presynaptic membrane except in the immediate vicinity of the active zones where exocytosis occurs. The lower figure illustrates the earliest stages of this type of endocytosis: (1) clustering of large intramembranous particles; (2) dimpling of the particle clusters; and (3) invagination of the plasma membrane to such a depth that the fracture plane can no longer follow the budding vesicle.

ticles—which look like they belong to synaptic-vesicle membranes—could be taken as an indication that coated vesicles do indeed retrieve the right type of membrane from the plasma membrane in that they "select" vesicle components in particular. Eventually this possibility could be substantiated by biochemical comparison of the proteins in coated vesicles and synaptic vesicles to show whether the two types of presynaptic organelles are formed from the same membrane components. The data so far fit in with the idea that both are composed of the same proteins and that neither synaptic vesicles nor coated vesicles contain certain characteristic plasma-membrane proteins (Kadota and Kadota, 1973, 1975; Tanaka, Takeda, and Jaimovich, 1976; Blitz, Fine, and Toselli, 1977). If this is true, the coated vesicles must form out of components of synaptic-vesicle membrane that they pull out of the plasma membrane. The collections of large intramembranous particles we observe in their coated-pit stages may thus represent one step, prior to reuptake, in the sequestration of synaptic-vesicle components from the rest of the plasma membrane.

Quick-freezing promises to be a means of observing the complete time course of this endocytotic process. Chemical fixation has been useless because it usually fails to arrest the process in a sufficiently early stage of vesicle formation to reveal the clusters of large intramembranous particles in the coated pits. It catches only the late stages, which are too deeply invaginated for the freeze-fracture plane to follow and which look deceptively like the broken necks of exocytotic vesicles. Quick-freezing, however, catches all stages indiscriminately and thus in a relative abundance that depends only on their relative lifetimes during the ongoing process of coated-vesicle formation. In fact, it catches a particularly large fraction of coated pits at very early stages, when clusters of large intramembranous particles are just beginning to be evident and the plasma membrane is only slightly indented (Figure 16). These stages must proceed relatively slowly, and they must persist a long time com-

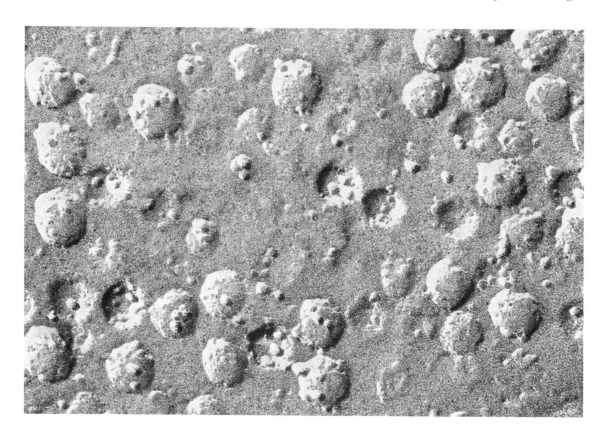

FIGURE 17 A cross-fracture through the axoplasm of a quick-frozen nerve, which exposed its complement of synaptic vesicles in two different views. The convex profiles of vesicles reveal the luminal half of their membrane, or their E-faces. The concave profiles reveal the cytoplasmic half of their membrane, or their P-faces. On such concave P-face hemispheres appear one or more large intramembranous particles, indicating that vesicle membrane has a very high concentration of such particles. (From Heuser and Reese, 1979.)

pared to the subsequent steps in coated-vesicle abscission from the plasma membrane.

Quick-freezing also helps to distinguish exocytosis from endocytosis in another way, by revealing the different time courses of the two processes. To accomplish this, nerves are frozen at various times after a single shock in 4-AmP or at various times after the start of a tetanus. Upon freeze-fracture of such stimulated nerves, very few examples of coated pits can be found until more than 5 sec after a single giant endplate potential in 4-AmP. This type of endocytosis does not become plentiful until 15–20 sec after the onset of tetanic stimulation. By this time it is not uncommon to find as many as ten coated pits in the vicinity of each active zone, although five is more typical. The freeze-fracture images of coated pits continue to be more abundant than on resting nerves for at least a minute or two after stimulation ceases. These quick-freezing data fit in with the abundance of coated pits observed in thin sections of nerves subjected to 15 min of continuous tetanic stimulation, after which coated pits continue to be more abundant than normal for at least half an hour (Heuser and Reese, 1973).

At such late times, when coated pits are abundant on quick-frozen nerves and exocytosis at the active zone is finished and gone, one can appreciate most clearly where on the nerve this sort of endocytosis occurs. On the basis of older thin-section data, we originally said that coated vesicles form mostly where the plasma membrane is opposite a Schwann-cell process. Quick-freezing shows this is incorrect; coated pits can be found anywhere on the presynaptic membrane, and their abundance is only occasionally greater under Schwann-cell processes. We have no explanation for this apparent discrepancy; but we favor the quick-freezing data because they are based on many broad, expansive views of the plasma membrane, rather than on the narrow perimeters to which we were restricted in thin sections of fixed tissues.

The very fact that synaptic-vesicle exocytosis and coated-vesicle endocytosis do not occur in the same places on the presynaptic membrane has led many observers to doubt that coated vesicles could be centrally involved in retrieving synaptic-vesicle membrane from the surface. For how could synaptic-vesicle membrane move from where it is added to the plasma membrane at the active zone to where the coated vesicles could retrieve it, which is typically 0.25 μm away? Of course, if the presynaptic membrane were sufficiently fluid—for example, like olive oil, which has a viscosity of 100 cP—components of the vesicle membrane would be able to diffuse over this

0.25 μm in a relatively short period. One could predict, for example, from Einstein's equation for random Brownian movement, $\sqrt{X^2} = \sqrt{(2Dt)}$ that if the vesicle's proteins and phospholipids moved freely as independent entities, their phospholipids would diffuse that distance in an average of 30 msec (assuming their radius is 10 A and their diffusion coefficient is 10^{-8} cm^2/sec); the proteins would diffuse that far in less than 3 sec (assuming their radius is 100 A and their diffusion coefficient is 10^{-10} cm^2/sec). Thus after a single nerve impulse the large intramembranous particles released from synaptic vesicles ought to have time to reach the regions of the nerve terminal where endocytosis occurs well before this process begins.

Again, quick-freezing offers a way to observe directly such a diffusion of vesicle membrane. If attention is focused on the large intramembranous particles found in synaptic vesicles (Figure 17), which appear in the depths of the vesicle openings after they fuse with the presynaptic membrane (Figure 13), one can—by freezing nerves at various times after one shock in 1 mM 4-AmP—simply watch what happens to the particles at various times after they have become incorporated into the presynaptic membrane. (It would not be possible to do this with chemically fixed tissues because the particles in question, if they were able to diffuse at all, would have many seconds or even minutes in which to get away from their natural distribution before the fixative immobilized them; see McIntyre, Gilula, and Karnovsky, 1974.) Of course, it is not possible to be sure that the large particles one discerns among other particles on the presynaptic membrane are really the same molecules that produce the characteristic vesicle particles. For the moment that is only an assumption; it seems reasonable, however, if only because the pattern of distribution of such large particles at various times after stimulation looks as though they are diffusing away from sites of insertion along the active zones (Figure 20).

We have seen in Figure 13 that such large intramembranous particles first appear in the depth of plasmalemmal pockets along the active zone; these pockets look like wide open synaptic vesicles. By 20 msec a large fraction of all the vesicle openings are wide open, and many appear to have collapsed almost completely. However, they can still be recognized as patches of synaptic-vesicle membrane by the 2–4 large intramembranous particles they bear. By 50 msec nearly all vesicles have collapsed, but most active zones still are bordered by several small clusters of 2–4 large intramembranous particles. By 100 msec such clusters of intramembranous particles are no

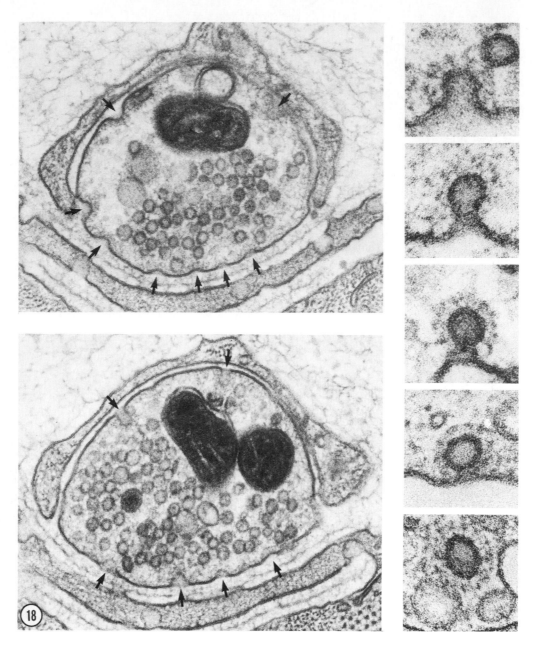

FIGURE 18 Thin-section appearance of coated pits in the plasma membrane. On the left are two views of a nerve that was quick-frozen after stimulation at 10 Hz for 5 min in 20 μg/ml β-BTX, a treatment that produces an unusual abundance of coated pits (arrows). On the right are five examples at higher magnification of coated pits and vesicles found in freeze-substituted nerves and arranged in a hypothetical sequence of endocytosis. Although not perfectly preserved by freeze-substitution, their coat appears to consist of a corona of delicate filaments and dots around the invaginated membrane. This corona is presumably a flat image of the delicate polygonal basketwork of clathrin that surrounds these membranes in three dimensions (Crowther, Finch, and Pearse, 1976; Kanaseki and Kadota, 1969). (From Lassignal and Heuser, 1977.)

longer apparent, and the overall concentration of these particles in the presynaptic membrane has more than doubled in the areas up to 0.25 μm away from the active zone. [The plasma membrane always contains about 25 such large particles per square micron, regardless of its functional history, so the concentration increase at 100 msec represents the addition of about another 50 particles per square micron to an area about 1 μm × 0.5 μm (considering both sides of the active zone) or 25 particles per active zone. If

592   JOHN E. HEUSER AND THOMAS S. REESE

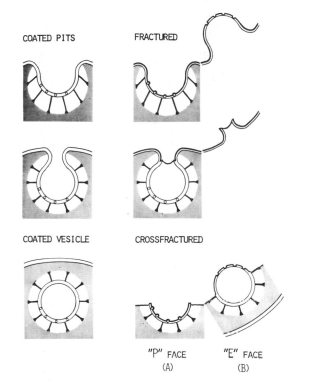

COATED PITS FRACTURED

COATED VESICLE CROSSFRACTURED

"P" FACE "E" FACE
(A) (B)

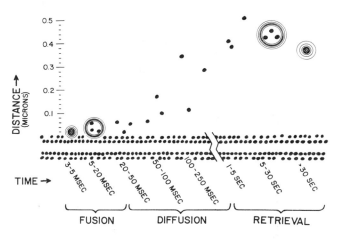

FIGURE 20 Summary of the intramembranous particle changes seen in the presynaptic membrane of the frog neuromuscular junction at various times after one shock in 1 mM 4-AmP. Black dots represent only the largest particles found in the presynaptic membrane. The two double rows of particles are present at all times and delineate the active zone of this synapse even when it is not secreting. At 3–5 msec after stimulation, synaptic-vesicle exocytosis (represented as a hole surrounded by small concentric circles) can be seen to occur in the immediate vicinity of the rows of particles. In the next few msec the exocytotic vesicle collapses into the presynaptic membrane and deposits three or more additional intramembranous particles at the active zone—particles that presumably originated in the vesicle membrane itself. Unlike the large particles, which always remain lined up beside the active zone, these new vesicle particles appear to be free to diffuse away from the spot where they were added, for at later times following exocytosis they are found at progressively greater distances from the active zone. Their speed—averaging 0.25 μm in 1 sec—indicates that their diffusion coefficient is about 2×10^{-10} cm²/sec, intermediate between membrane proteins that float free in the bilayer, such as rhodopsin ($D = 3.5 \times 10^{-9}$ cm²/sec), and membrane proteins whose movement is restricted by linkage to internal or external structures, such as the antibody and lectin receptors on lymphocytes ($D = 5 \times 10^{-11}$ cm²/sec). At still later times, starting several seconds after exocytosis, large particles of this sort begin to be found in small clusters, often in areas midway between active zones. These particle clusters appear to be incorporated into coated pits as they form in the plasma membrane—shown diagrammatically by the concentric circles around a particle cluster at 5–30 sec. They are then internalized when a complete vesicle pinches off the surface, designated by the hole surrounded by concentric circles later than 30 sec (this is meant to indicate that abscission can take place at any time up to several minutes after exocytosis). (From Heuser and Reese, 1979.)

FIGURE 19 Diagrammatic summary of the stages of coated-vesicle formation that are captured by quick-freezing, reconstructed from freeze fracture and thin-section views. Coated pits first become obvious in freeze-fracture when they assume the form of shallow pockets in the presynaptic membrane and are laden with three or more large intramembranous particles. Subsequent flask-shaped stages fracture across their narrow necks. Such fractures do not reveal the intramembranous particles collected by the coated vesicles; instead they look very much like the craters produced by discharging synaptic vesicles. (They can only be distinguished from such exocytosis by certain differences in when and where they occur.) For the sake of completeness, the lower panel shows how a cross-fractured coated vesicle lying wholly in the axoplasm ought to display the same intramembranous particles that characterize coated pits still connected to the presynaptic membrane. Such cross-fractured coated vesicles probably could not be distinguished from cross-fractured synaptic vesicles.

each exocytotic vesicle contributed 2 or 3 particles, this would imply that 10–12 vesicles discharged per active zone, which is close to the number of vesicle openings we see at such early times as 5 msec after stimulation.]

By 1 sec the concentration of large intramembranous particles has more than doubled in an area up to 0.32 μm from the active zone. If we assume that all these particles were added to the active zone 1 sec earlier and were then free to diffuse away by random Brownian movement, we can measure their root-mean-square displacement from the active zone

$\sqrt{\bar{X}^2}$ (it turns out to be nearly 0.25 μm); from that we can calculate the diffusion coefficient D from $\sqrt{\bar{X}^2} = \sqrt{(2Dt)}$, where $t = 1$ sec. This gives a D for the vesicle particles of 2×10^{-10} cm²/sec, which is fast compared to most membrane proteins—which have a D of about 5×10^{-11} cm²/sec (Schlessinger et al.,

1976)—but is slower than the D of rhodopsin molecules in photoreceptor membranes (3.5×10^{-9} cm²/sec: see Poo and Cone, 1974). Now, diffusion coefficients of most membrane proteins are slower than would be predicted by the Einstein-Sutherland diffusion equation ($D = kT/6\pi a\eta$, where k is the Boltzmann constant, T is absolute temperature, a is the radius of the protein, and η is the viscosity of the membrane). This equation would apply if the proteins floated freely in an isotropic sea of fluid phospholipids. Because it does not, in fact, fit, it would appear that most membrane proteins must be restricted in their diffusion, possibly by attachments to stable structures outside the membrane or to structures inside, in the cell cortex. In contrast, vesicle particles appear to diffuse more quickly, so they may not be restricted and Einstein's equation may well apply to them. If so, a D of 2×10^{-10} cm²/sec would indicate that the fluidity of the presynaptic membrane was about 100 cP, close to that of olive oil.

The sequence of large-particle diffusion that can thus be reconstructed from freezing at 5, 20, 50, 100, and 250 msec, as summarized in Figure 20, suggests that synaptic vesicles and plasma membranes mingle intimately at the molecular level after exocytosis. Moreover, it appears that large intramembranous particles from the synaptic vesicles eventually spread over the surface of the nerve. We reported elsewhere that when tetanic stimulation was applied for 1–3 min, a fourfold increase in the concentration of such large intramembranous particles was found all over the presynaptic membrane, even in chemically fixed tissues (Heuser and Reese, 1975). Recently Akert and co-workers observed a similar increase in large intramembranous particles when comparing stimulated to anesthetized CNS synapses after chemical fixation, although they did not consider the possibility that discharging vesicles could be the source of these particles (Venzin et al., 1977).

The greatest increase in large particles we have seen in a presynaptic membrane occurred after prolonged lanthanum stimulation, which discharged all the vesicles and eventually left frog nerve terminals almost empty (Heuser and Miledi, 1971). Here all of the vesicle membrane must have merged with the presynaptic membrane. One can express this quantitatively by remembering that the total area of all the vesicle membrane in a typical frog nerve terminal is roughly equal to the area of the plasma membrane (Heuser and Reese, 1973); thus discharging all the vesicles during lanthanum stimulation should approximately double the area of the plasma membrane and raise its concentration of large intramembranous particles halfway to the concentration found in synaptic-vesicle membrane to begin with, which is nearly ten times the normal concentration of large intramembranous particles in the presynaptic membrane. This plasmalemmal expansion and increase in intramembranous particles is found after various other types of prolonged stimulation (Damassa et al., 1976); thus the freeze-fracture and thin-section data go hand in hand to show that synaptic-vesicle membrane is indeed added to plasma membrane as a consequence of exocytosis.

Such evidence that synaptic-vesicle particles appear on the plasma membrane after exocytosis and diffuse freely would at first sight seem to contradict the evidence that such particles later regroup into clusters and get hauled back inside by coated vesicles. For how could vesicle particles first diffuse randomly throughout the plasma membrane, then move into the very nonrandom clusters that develop in coated pits? Perhaps the simplest explanation is that these particles stop moving randomly when they become attached to an element in the filamentous ectoplasm beneath the plasma membrane. The "coat" of clathrin (Pearse, 1975, 1976), which appears in the areas where particles cluster (see Figure 18) may be just such a device for attaching membrane proteins to the ectoplasm and drawing them inside. This could well be the mechanism by which coated vesicles achieve their specificity of uptake in all cases. If so, it will be necessary to show that clathrin has an affinity for the particular membrane proteins selected for uptake in each case and that clathrin binds to them specifically where they are exposed to the underlying cytoplasm. (Several questions might come up in this connection. Will clathrin bind membrane proteins only when they are in a particular allosteric configuration? Or only when they are clustered into groups? Will this be controlled by prior binding of these membrane proteins to external proteins?) It will also be necessary to determine how clathrin associates with the filamentous components of the ectoplasm and how it draws the membrane into a coated vesicle. These are problems for a very general cell-biological inquiry, but they are essential to our understanding of the neurobiology of synaptic transmission as well because, if coated-vesicle formation does turn out to be the synapse's major means of retrieving synaptic-vesicle membrane after exocytosis, this could limit the synapse's ability to recycle synaptic-vesicle membrane and could thereby limit the synapse's long-term secretory capabilities.

Possibly this is why one observes such differences in the relative abundance of coated vesicles in different types of synapses. Coated vesicles are relatively rare in synapses that fire only intermittently and have a large stock of synaptic vesicles, such as the neuromuscular junctions on phasic muscles we have been considering here. On the other hand, coated vesicles appear to be more numerous in neuromuscular junctions driving tonic muscles, and they are particularly abundant in synapses that secrete continuously such as photoreceptors and electroreceptors, which also possess presynaptic "ribbons" that help guide vesicles down to their active zones (Gray and Pease, 1971; Hama and Saito, 1977; Heuser and Reese, 1977). Considering these natural differences, one might imagine that if a synapse were to "learn" to secrete more quanta and to secrete more over a long period, it would have to hypertrophy its machinery for forming coated vesicles to keep up with the increased demand for new synaptic vesicles. Eventually it should be possible for electron microscopists to predict a synapse's long-term secretory capabilities (1) by counting the number of coated vesicles and coated pits it has under different functional conditions and (2) by mapping by immunocytochemistry the extent and distribution of all the clathrin "coat protein" it contains.

Problems

So far this account has glossed over the problems involved in using freezing to capture membrane fusion and recycling. The most fundamental problem is that our method of freezing does not seem to be fast enough to capture the very earliest changes associated with exocytosis. How fast these changes are can be appreciated from our earlier comparison of nerves frozen at 3 msec and at 5 msec. At 3 msec no vesicle openings were present at all; yet by 5 msec the openings were captured at several different stages, including a few that were in very late stages of vesicle collapse. Presumably none of these openings would have been visible if this nerve had been frozen at 3 msec instead of 5 msec, so they must have progressed that far in 2 msec! Freezing captured them, but did it miss others that lasted less than 2 msec? We suspect that it did. At the moment we have no other explanation for the fact that we see so few vesicle openings in normal muscles frozen after one shock in normal Ringer's without 4-AmP (Heuser, Reese, and Landis, 1976). And even when 4-AmP is used, vesicle openings do not become abundant until the dose is raised to 10^{-4}M, even though 10^{-5}M 4-AmP increases frog endplate potentials more than fourfold, to a quantal content of at least 1,000 per nerve impulse. Why are vesicle openings rare unless quantal contents are higher than 1,000? At that level of release we would expect to find about 2 vesicle openings at each active zone, but often we saw none (see Figure 10). We suspect that they did occur but that they "got away"; that is, they collapsed into the presynaptic membrane in less than 2 msec and thus eluded the freezing. At even higher levels of release we assume that the first 1,000 vesicle openings get away in the same way, but that subsequent vesicle openings brought on by the greatly prolonged action potential and prolonged calcium entry—which can often total more than 10,000 quanta—dissipate more slowly and thus can be caught by our freezing technique.

If this is so, it means that our freezing is not fast enough to catch events that last less than 2 msec. And we cannot correct this problem simply by shortening the interval between stimulation and freezing. In order to do so, we would have to deliver the stimulation at a time when the muscle is so close to contact with the $-270°C$ block that its surface would have already cooled substantially. Delicate thermocouples placed on the muscle surface record at least a $10°$ drop during the last few milliseconds before impact against the copper freezing block. Our machine is not designed to protect the muscles from such precooling, and as a consequence we must leave an interval between stimulation and impact long enough for the nerve impulse to travel into the synapse and initiate the endplate potential. But by then the exocytosis is over (in less than 2 msec) and, apparently, the membrane has not yet frozen.

We have attempted to record the rate of freezing at various times after impact by observing the change in capacitance of the tissue, using a circuit that measures the transmission of a 100 kHz oscillating potential through the tissue at various times after it hits the copper (Figure 21). The decline of this signal shows the rate of conversion of tissue water (which has a high dielectric constant), into ice (which has a very low dielectric constant). Assuming that an ice front grows into the tissue as a plane, parallel to the freezing block, one can view the tissue at any time during freezing as two equal-sized capacitors in series, one filled with water and one filled with ice. Fitting our data to this model gives the experimental points shown in Figure 22.

We do not know why these measurements deviate at small distances from the rapid rates of cooling predicted by the classical diffusion equations of Carslaw and Jaeger (1947) for this situation. Possibly the deviation is due to confusing nonlinear transients in our electrical circuit or inaccuracies in our calibra-

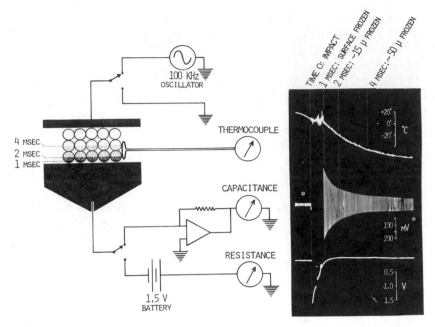

FIGURE 21 Diagram of the various circuits that can be used to measure the rate of freezing of the muscle (shown schematically as the circles between the wedge-shaped copper freezing block below and the flat aluminum specimen mount above). The simplest circuit is a thermocouple in contact with the surface of the muscle; but no commercially available thermocouple is small enough to record what happens in the first 10–20 μm where the freezing is best. Alternatively a simple battery circuit can be used to pass current through the muscle once it has contacted the copper block so that its resistance can be measured. As soon as the thinnest layer of ice has formed on the muscle surface, however, its resistance is so high that the circuit is essentially broken. This happens in less than 1 msec. A better index is the change in muscle capacitance that occurs during freezing, which can be measured by applying a 100 kHz oscillating signal to the muscle mount and recording its transmission through the muscle with a virtual ground plugged into the copper block. When the surface has frozen and the relatively large resistive current flow is over, the decline in capacitance is a direct measure of the subsequent growth of ice into the muscle. (From Heuser et al., 1979.)

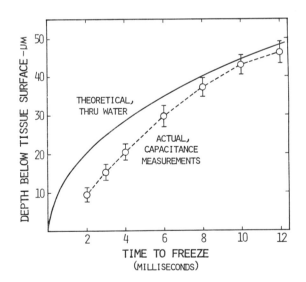

FIGURE 22 Comparison of the rates of freezing actually measured by the capacitance circuit shown in Figure 21, with the rate calculated from Carslaw and Jaeger's theoretical equations for the conduction of heat. The rate of freezing predicted by theory depends critically on whether

tions for especially thin layers of low-dielectric material. (We calibrate this circuit by sandwiching thin layers of cellophane between the tissue and copper block when it is at room temperature and measuring the steady-state change in capacitance.) Alternatively, the deviation may be real, and we should conclude that nothing in the tissue freezes faster than 0.5 msec. This may be the minimum time required to bring about the phase change from liquid to solid water; this conclusion is, however, inconsistent with the resistance changes, which indicate that the surface at

we imagine that heat must be drawn out of the muscle entirely through water, or whether it is drawn out through an advancing ice front; the latter would be much faster because ice has a thermal capacity four times higher than water. The mean values from freezing three muscles (vertical bars are standard errors) approximate the slower prediction for heat removal through water, although they deviate significantly toward lower freezing rates at depths up to 20 μm; these are the most interesting depths because it is in this region that we find well-frozen nerve terminals.

least freezes in less than a millisecond (Figure 21). But even if the rate of phase change is the limiting factor, this would not fully explain why we cannot catch whatever exocytosis dissipates in less than 2 msec after impact, because the theoretical cooling curves would still predict that the surface of the tissue should become supercooled long before it freezes. One would have thought that supercooling ought to stop exocytosis just as well as freezing; but perhaps it does not once membrane fusion has begun. In any case, the measurements to date illustrate that even our fastest freezing technique may be slow compared to the events we are trying to catch. In particular, it may not be fast enough to catch the first thousand or so vesicles that open during each endplate potential.

But why would the vesicles that open *later* collapse *more slowly?* One reason we have proposed is that these vesicles are opening into a plasma membrane that is already expanded to its limit from the vesicles that have already fused with it and thus resists further vesicle collapse (Heuser, 1977). This statement must represent an oversimplification. Each entering synaptic vesicle should add a 1,000-Å-diameter patch of phospholipids. This patch would expand the adjoining presynaptic membrane by only about 1%; but it might be expected to expand the inner leaflet more than the outer leaflet because the vesicle's extreme curvature means that it has many more phospholipids in its inner than in its outer leaflet to start with. Generating such asymmetry of phospholipid distribution may well affect how the membrane accommodates curves such as vesicle pockets (Sheetz and Singer, 1974, 1977), but the exact mechanism remains to be determined.

One sign that the plasma membrane does indeed become overstuffed with synaptic-vesicle membrane during the giant endplate potentials produced in 4-AmP is that it begins to pinch off cisternae under these conditions (as in Figure 14). The driving force behind this type of invagination and rapid abscission of random bites of membrane may well have something to do with the excess of membrane area and the asymmetric distribution of phospholipids produced by the collapsing synaptic vesicles.

One clear indication that an excess of plasma membranes does inhibit vesicle collapse comes from our new observations on vesicle exocytosis after hypertonic stimulation. Ringer's solutions that are made 50% hypertonic with sucrose are known to stimulate spontaneous transmitter secretion to levels as high as a few hundred quanta per second (Furshpan, 1956; Kita and Van der Kloot, 1977). This degree of stimulation is nothing, however, compared to the level of discharge during a normal endplate potential, when more than 100 quanta are released in about a millisecond. Nevertheless, it is quite easy to find examples of synaptic-vesicle exocytosis on nerves that are quick-frozen 5 min after immersion in 50% hypertonic Ringer's. Some 180 active zones have been located in these muscles so far, and overall they display a mean of one vesicle opening per running micron of active-zone length or 500 total openings on the average nerve terminal (since each terminal typically has 500 μm of active zone). Now the average nerve terminal should have been discharging around 100 quanta per second at the moment it was frozen; if 500 vesicles were open at that moment, then each vesicle opening must last about 5 sec in 50% hypertonic Ringer's. Thus, under these conditions, vesicle collapse would appear to be at least 100 times slower than even the slowest vesicles in 4-AmP, which collapse in 20–50 msec, and more than a thousand times slower than during a normal endplate potential in normal Ringer's, when we believe vesicles collapse in less than 2 msec and so are impossible to catch at all. (In this degree of hypertonic Ringer's the nerve terminal becomes quite shrunken. As a result its surface membrane becomes too large in area relative to its volume, and the membrane wrinkles up into a variety of distortions that take up the excess. So it should not surprise us to find that the plasma membrane appears to resist the addition of more membrane, as would result from the collapse of discharged synaptic vesicles.)

The consequences of nerve-terminal shrinkage with hypertonic Ringer's may thus be an extreme example of a plasma-membrane change that could also result from the collapse of a thousand vesicles or so at one time, which could explain why vesicle collapse is somewhat slowed in 4-AmP.

Summary and Conclusions

1. Quick-freezing allows one to capture synaptic-vesicle exocytosis with a new degree of naturalness. It reveals that synaptic vesicles discharge at certain easily recognized active zones on the nerve-terminal plasma membrane, beneath which discrete clusters of synaptic vesicles queue up in the interstices of the characteristic presynaptic densities.

2. Within each active zone, vesicles can apparently discharge anywhere, independent of neighboring vesicles in the same cluster.

3. The earliest moments of discharge still escape detection, even with quick-freezing; but the first vesicle openings that appear in the plasma membrane

illustrate that fusion between vesicles and plasma membrane begins at the tiny spot where the vesicle first touches the plasma membrane and that membrane fusion proceeds to completion in less than a millisecond. Thereafter the vesicle opening enlarges progressively until the vesicle has collapsed flat into presynaptic membrane.

4. The rate at which vesicles collapse depends on whether the plasma membrane can accommodate the added vesicle membrane. Usually it has no trouble accommodating the number of vesicles that discharge in normal transmission, and the vesicles are free to collapse in less than 2 msec. But the number of vesicles that discharge in 4-AmP is so large that the plasma membrane cannot accommodate all of them; in this case the collapse of many vesicles is slowed to 20–50 msec or longer. Vesicle collapse can be slowed even further—so that it takes several seconds for the vesicle opening to disappear after exocytosis—by shrinking nerves with hypertonic solutions until their plasma membrane becomes folded or convoluted and resists further expansion.

5. Quick-freezing nerves at various times after stimulation shows not only that vesicles collapse after exocytosis, but also that components of their membrane mix intimately with the plasma membrane. Three or more unusually large intramembranous particles characterize the membrane of each fractured synaptic vesicle. After vesicles fuse with the plasma membrane and collapse into it, these particles can be seen diffusing away from the active zone. After long periods of stimulation, these particles appear to become distributed uniformly over the plasma membrane.

6. Under conditions of plasma-membrane excess, such as after exocytosis in 4-AmP, the nerve displays a tendency to invaginate and pinch off vacuoles. These can be distinguished from synaptic vesicles because they are larger and are composed of membrane with a freeze-fracture particle complement that looks like a random bite of plasma membrane, not like a particle-rich vesicle membrane. These are the endocytotic structures we formerly called cisternae, which we saw becoming progressively more abundant during prolonged periods of unusually intense stimulation.

7. Under more normal conditions of stimulation, when the rate of addition of synaptic-vesicle membrane to the plasma membrane is not so excessive, coated vesicles are pinched off the plasma membrane in considerable abundance by a slower process of endocytosis that can be caught by quick-freezing at several different stages. Freeze-fracture of the earlier stages reveals that this process selects, from the random mixture of particles in the presynaptic membrane, certain particles that look like the ones found in synaptic-vesicle membrane (they also resemble the particles found in the vicinity of the active zones immediately after exocytosis occurs there, and we believe they are one and the same). Thus the formation of coated vesicles appears to mediate a selective retrieval of synaptic-vesicle membrane components from the plasma membrane, which is essential for the local recycling of synaptic vesicles in the nerve terminal.

REFERENCES

AKERT, K., 1973. Dynamic aspects of synaptic ultrastructure. *Brain Res.* 49:511–518.

AKERT, K., K. PFENNINGER, C. SANDRI, and H. MOOR, 1972. Freeze-etching and cytochemistry of vesicles and membrane complexes in synapses of the central nervous system. In *Structure and Function of Synapses*, G. D. Pappas and D. P. Purpura, eds. New York: Raven Press, pp. 67–86.

ANDERSON, R. G. W., J. L. GOLDSTEIN, and M. S. BROWN, 1976. Localization of low density lipoprotein receptors on plasma membrane of normal human fibroblasts and their absence in cells from a familial hypercholesterolemia homozygote. *Proc. Natl. Acad. Sci. USA* 73:2434–2438.

ARMSTRONG, C., 1967. Time-course of TEA-induced anomalous rectification in squid giant axons. *J. Gen. Physiol.* 50:491–503.

ARMSTRONG, C., 1969. Inactivation of the potassium conductance and related phenomena caused by quaternary ammonium ion injection in squid axons. *J. Gen. Physiol.* 54:553–573.

AXELROD, J., 1971. Noradrenaline: Fate and control of its biosynthesis. *Science* 173:598–606.

BARTON, S. B., and I. S. COHEN, 1977. Are transmitter release statistics meaningful? *Nature* 268:267–268.

BENEDECZKY, I., and A. D. SMITH, 1972. Ultrastructural studies on the adrenal medulla of golden hamster: Origin and fate of secretory granules. *Z. Zellforsch.* 124:367–386.

BENNETT, M. V. L., P. G. MODEL, and S. M. HIGHSTEIN, 1976. Stimulation-induced fatigue of transmission and recovery processes at a vertebrate central synapse. *Cold Spring Harbor Symp. Quant. Biol.* 40:25–35.

BLITZ, A. L., R. E. FINE, and P. A. TOSELLI, 1977. Evidence that coated vesicles isolated from brain are calcium-sequestering organelles resembling sarcoplasmic reticulum. *J. Cell Biol.* 75:135–147.

BRANTON, D., et al., 1975. Freeze-etching nomenclature. *Science* 190:54–56.

BROWN, T. H., D. H. PERKEL, and M. W. FELDMAN, 1976. Evoked neurotransmitter release: Statistical effects of nonuniformity and nonstationarity. *Proc. Natl. Acad. Sci. USA* 73:2913–2917.

CARSLAW, H. S., and J. C. JAEGER, 1947. *Conduction of Heat in Solids.* Oxford: Clarendon Press.

CLARK, A. W., W. P. HURLBUT, and A. MAURO, 1972. Changes in the fine structure of the neuromuscular junction of the frog caused by black widow spider venom. *J. Cell Biol.* 57:1–14.

COUTEAUX, R., and M. PÉCOT-DECHAVASSINE, 1970. Vésicules synaptiques et poches au niveau des zones actives de la jonction neuromusculaire. *C. R. Acad. Sci. Paris* [D] 271:2346–2349.

COUTEAUX, R., and M. PÉCOT-DECHAVASSINE, 1973. Données ultrastructurales et cytochimiques sur le mécanisme de libération de l'acetylcholine dans la transmission synaptique. *Arch. Ital. Biol.* 3:231–262.

COUTEAUX, R., and M. PÉCOT-DECHAVASSINE, 1974. Les zones specialisées des membranes présynaptiques. *C. R. Acad. Sci. Paris* 280:299–301.

CROWTHER, R. A., J. T. FINCH, and B. M. F. PEARSE, 1976. On the structure of coated vesicles. *J. Mol. Biol.* 103:785–798.

DAMASSA, D. A., T. L. DAVIS, D. M. SHOTTON, J. E. HEUSER, D. PUMPLIN, and T. S. REESE, 1976. Structure of nerve terminals in frog muscle after prolonged treatment with black widow spider venom. *Biol. Bull.* 151:406–407.

DOUGLAS, W. W., 1973. Mechanism of release of neurohypophysial hormones: Stimulus-secretion coupling. In *Handbook of Physiology*, section 7: *Endocrinology*, vol. 4. Bethesda, MD: American Physiological Society, pp. 191–224.

FAWCETT, D. W., 1964. Surface specializations of absorbing cells. *J. Histochem. Cytochem.* 13:75–89.

FEDER, N., and R. L. SIDMAN, 1958. Methods and principles of fixation by freeze-substitution. *J. Biophys. Biochem. Cytol.* 4:593–600.

FURSHPAN, E. J., 1956. The effects of osmotic pressure changes on the spontaneous activity at motor nerve endings. *J. Physiol.* 134:689–697.

GRAHAM, JR., R. C., and M. J. KARNOVSKY, 1966. The early stages of absorption of injected horseradish peroxidase in the proximal tubules of mouse kidney: Ultrastructural cytochemistry by a new technique. *J. Histochem. Cytochem.* 14:291–302.

GRAY, E. G., and H. L. PEASE, 1971. On understanding the organization of the retinal receptor synapses. *Brain Res.* 35:1–15.

HAMA, K., and K. SAITO, 1977. Fine structure of the afferent synapse of the hair cells in the saccular macula of the goldfish, with special reference to anastomosing tubules. *J. Neurocytol.* 6:361–373.

HATT, H., and D. O. SMITH, 1976. Non-uniform probabilities of quantal release at the crayfish neuromuscular junction. *J. Physiol.* 259:395–404.

HEUSER, J. E., 1976. Morphology of synaptic vesicle discharge and reformation at the frog neuromuscular junction. In *Motor Innervation of Muscle*, S. Thesleff, ed. London: Academic Press, pp. 51–115.

HEUSER, J. E., 1977. Synaptic vesicle exocytosis revealed in quick-frozen frog neuromuscular junctions treated with 4-aminopyridine and given a single electrical shock. In *Society for Neuroscience Symposia*, vol. 2, W. M. Cowan and J. A. Ferendelli, eds. Bethesda, Md.: Society for Neuroscience, pp. 215–239.

HEUSER, J. E., and R. MILEDI, 1971. Effect of lanthanum ions on function and structure of frog neuromuscular junctions. *Proc. R. Soc. Lond.* B179:247–260.

HEUSER, J. E., and T. S. REESE, 1973. Evidence for recycling of synaptic vesicle membrane during transmitter release at the frog neuromuscular junction. *J. Cell Biol.* 57:315–344.

HEUSER, J. E., and T. S. REESE, 1975. Redistribution of intramembranous particles from synaptic vesicles: Direct evidence for vesicle recycling. *Anat. Rec.* 181:374.

HEUSER, J. E., and T. S. REESE, 1977. The structure of the synapse. In *Handbook of Physiology*, section 1: *The Nervous System*, vol. 1, E. Kandel, ed. Bethesda, MD: American Physiological Society.

HEUSER, J. E., and T. S. REESE, 1979. Fate of synaptic vesicle membrane after exocytosis. *J. Cell Biol.* (submitted).

HEUSER, J. E., T. S. REESE, and D. M. D. LANDIS, 1974. Functional changes in frog neuromuscular junctions studied with freeze-fracture. *J. Neurocytol.* 3:109–131.

HEUSER, J. E., T. S. REESE, and D. M. D. LANDIS, 1976. Preservation of synaptic structure by rapid freezing. *Cold Spring Harbor Symp. Quant. Biol.* 40:17–24.

HEUSER, J. E., T. S. REESE, M. J. DENNIS, Y. JAN, L. JAN, and L. EVANS, 1979. Exocytosis of synaptic vesicles captured by quick-freezing. *J. Cell Biol.* (in press).

KADOTA, K., and T. KADOTA, 1973. A nucleoside diphosphate phosphohydrolase present in a coated-vesicle fraction from synaptosomes of guinea-pig whole brain. *Brain Res.* 56:371–376.

KADOTA, K., and T. KADOTA, 1975. Isolation of coated vesicles, plain synaptic vesicles and fine particles from synaptosomes of guinea pig whole brain. *J. Electron Microsc.* 22:91–98.

KANASEKI, T., and K. KADOTA, 1969. The "vesicle in a basket." *J. Cell Biol.* 42:202–220.

KATZ, B., 1969. *The Release of Neural Transmitter Substances*. Liverpool: Liverpool University Press.

KATZ, B., 1971. Quantal mechanism of neural transmitter release. *Science* 173:123–126.

KATZ, B., and R. MILEDI, 1967. The release of acetylcholine from nerve endings by graded electrical pulses. *Proc. R. Soc. Lond.* B167:23–36.

KATZ, B., and R. MILEDI, 1977. Suppression of transmitter release at the neuromuscular junction. *Proc. R. Soc. Lond.* B196:465–469.

KITA, H., and W. VAN DER KLOOT, 1977. Time course and magnitude of effects of changes in tonicity on acetylcholine release at frog neuromuscular junction. *J. Neurophysiol.* 40:212–224.

LASSIGNAL, N. L. and J. E. HEUSER, 1977. Evidence that β-bungarotoxin arrests synaptic vesicle recycling by blocking coated vesicle formation. *Neurosci. Abstr.* 3:373.

LLINÁS, R., and J. E. HEUSER, 1977. Depolarization-release coupling. *Neurosci. Res. Program Bull.* 15:557–687.

LLINÁS, R., I. Z. STEINBERG, and K. WALTON, 1976. Presynaptic calcium currents and their relation to synaptic transmission: Voltage clamp study in squid giant synapse and theoretical model for the calcium gate. *Proc. Natl. Acad. Sci. USA* 73:2918–2922.

LLINÁS, R., K. WALTON, and V. BOHR, 1976. Synaptic transmission in squid giant synapse after potassium conductance blockage with external 3- and 4-aminopyridine. *Biophys. J.* 16:83–86.

MCINTYRE, J. A., N. B. GILULA, and M. J. KARNOVSKY, 1974. Cryoprotectant-induced redistribution of intramembranous particles in mouse lymphocytes. *J. Cell Biol.* 60:192–203.

McNutt, N. S., and R. S. Weinstein, 1973. Membrane ultrastructure at mammalian intercellular junctions. *Prog. Biophys. Mol. Biol.* 26:45–101.

Martin, A. R., 1977. Junctional transmission. II. Presynaptic mechanisms. In *Handbook of Physiology,* section 1: *The Nervous System,* vol. 1, E. Kandel, ed. Bethesda, MD: American Physiological Society.

Meves, H., and Y. Pichon, 1975. Effects of 4-aminopyridine on the potassium current in internally perfused giant axons of the squid. *J. Physiol.* 251:60P–61P.

Moor, H., and K. Muhlethaler, 1963. Fine structure in frozen-etched yeast cells, *J. Cell Biol.* 17:609–627.

Nagasawa, J., and W. W. Douglas, 1972. Thorium dioxide uptake into adrenal medullary cells and the problem of recapture of granule membrane following exocytosis. *Brain Res.* 37:141–145.

Pearse, B. M. F., 1975. Coated vesicles from pig brain: Purification and biochemical characterization. *J. Mol. Biol.* 97:93–98.

Pearse, B. M. F., 1976. Clatherin: A unique protein associated with intracellular transfer of membrane by coated vesicles. *Proc. Natl. Acad. Sci. USA* 73:1255–1259.

Pelhate, M., and Y. Pichon, 1974. Selective inhibition of potassium current in the giant axon of the cockroach. *J. Physiol.* 242:90P–91P.

Peper, K., F. Dryer, C. Sandri, K. Akert, and H. Moor, 1974. Structure and ultrastructure of the frog motor endplate. A freeze-etching study. *Cell Tiss. Res.* 149:437–453.

Poo, M., and R. A. Cone, 1974. Lateral diffusion of rhodopsin in the photoreceptor membrane. *Nature* 247:438–441.

Roth, T. F., J. A. Cutting, and S. B. Atlas, 1976. Protein transport: A selective membrane mechanism. *J. Supramol. Struct.* 4:527–548.

Roth, T. F., and K. R. Porter, 1964. Yolk protein uptake in the oocyte of the mosquito *Aedes aegypti. J. Cell Biol.* 20:313–332.

Rutherford, D. T., W. L. Nastuk, and J. F. Gennaro, 1976. Reversible depletion of synaptic vesicles in K+ depolarized junctions. *J. Cell Biol.* 70:375a.

Schlessinger, J., D. E. Koppel, D. Axelrod, K. Jacobson, W. W. Webb, and E. L. Elson, 1976. Lateral transport on cell membranes: Mobility of concanavalin A receptors on myoblasts. *Proc. Natl. Acad. Sci. USA* 73:2409–2413.

Sheetz, M. P., and S. J. Singer, 1974. Biological membranes as bilayer couples: A molecular mechanism of drug-erythrocyte interactions. *Proc. Natl. Acad. Sci. USA* 71:4457–4461.

Sheetz, M. P., and S. J. Singer, 1977. On the mechanism of ATP-induced shape changes in human erythrocyte membranes. I. The role of the spectrin complex. *J. Cell Biol.* 73:638–646.

Steinbach, J. H., and C. F. Stevens, 1976. Neuromuscular transmission. In *Frog Neurobiology,* R. Llinás and W. Precht, eds. Berlin: Springer-Verlag, pp. 33–92.

Tanaka, R., M. Takeda, and M. Jaimovich, 1976. Characterization of ATPases of plain synaptic vesicle and coated vesicle fractions isolated from rat brains. *J. Biochem.* 80:831–837.

Van Harreveld, A., and J. Crowell, 1964. Electron microscopy after rapid freezing on a metal surface and substitution fixation. *Anat. Rec.* 149:381–386.

Venzin, M., C. Sandri, K. Akert, and U. R. Wyss, 1977. Membrane-associated particles of the presynaptic active zone in rat spinal cord: A morphometric analysis. *Brain Res.* 130:393–404.

Wernig, A. 1975. Estimates of statistical release parameters from crayfish and frog neuromuscular junctions. *J. Physiol.* 244:207–221.

Wolf, D. E., L. T. Potter, K. C. Richardson, and J. Axelrod, 1962. Localizing tritiated norepinephrine in sympathetic axons by electron microscopic autoradiography. *Science* 138:440–442.

Yeh, T. A., G. S. Oxford, C. H. Wu, and T. Narahashi, 1976. Dynamics of aminopyridine block of potassium channels in squid axon membrane. *J. Gen. Physiol.* 68:519–535.

Zucker, R. S., 1977. Synaptic plasticity at crayfish neuromuscular junctions. In *Identified Neurons and Behavior of Arthropods,* G. Hoyle, ed. New York: Plenum Press.

33 A New Electrogenic
Calcium-Potassium System

H. D. LUX and C. B. HEYER

ABSTRACT   Ionic currents in somata of molluscan neurons can differ significantly from those described previously in axonal membranes. A slow inward calcium current, found in certain identified neurons, does not inactivate completely with sustained depolarizations and in fact facilitates (i.e., increases with repeated depolarizing voltage-clamp pulses). Furthermore, in cells with proportionately large Ca currents, a major component of the delayed outward K current ($I_{K(Ca)}$) is directly controlled by Ca ions and can be separated pharmacologically from the primarily voltage-dependent delayed outward K current ($I_{K(V)}$). $I_{K(Ca)}$ is transiently activated by the Ca current and is depressed by increases in [Ca]$_i$ resulting from depolarization or injection. Both activation and depression are complex functions of time and voltage and are unlike those found for $I_{K(V)}$ or currents in axonal membranes under normal voltage-clamp conditions. The concept of a coupled Ca-K system is described, and possible roles for the slow inward Ca and Ca-mediated K currents in vertebrates are discussed.

Introduction

Early studies on the squid giant axon established the primary role of a voltage-sensitive sodium entry in the regenerative depolarization of action potentials. The importance of this work has been emphasized by many subsequent studies in which the time- and voltage-dependent parameters of such sodium conductances described in a number of systems could be fit into similar schemes (for reviews see Noble, 1966; Cole, 1968). More recently Ca has been found to be the major component of voltage-sensitive inward currents in some neuron and muscle membranes (for review see Reuter, 1973; Baker and Glitsch, 1975); and it is not surprising that initial attempts to explain the behavior of these Ca ions as current carriers were modeled on properties of the Na system (e.g., Reuter, 1973). Indeed, in the squid axon, part of the Ca influx (as shown by its tetrodotoxin sensitivity) occurs through the so-called Na channels (Baker, Hodgkin, and Ridgway, 1971). However, many Ca currents,

including a component in the squid axon, are not tetrodotoxin (TTX)-sensitive and do not appear to go through Na channels (Katz and Miledi, 1971; Baker, Hodgkin, and Ridgway, 1971; see also Baker, 1972), suggesting that these "late" Ca currents may have properties that differ from those of fast sodium currents. It has been difficult to study properties of the late Ca system and to determine its function in squid axon because, compared with other currents in the axon, it is small and results in the entry of very few Ca ions (Hodgkin and Keynes, 1957; see also Baker and Glitsch, 1975). However, the late system is proportionately larger in other membranes, particularly in the somata of identified molluscan pacemaker cells (Lux and Eckert, 1974; Eckert and Lux, 1975, 1976). These cells still present a problem for analysis because the inward current overlaps in time with delayed outward K currents. By combining techniques, however, it has been possible to determine some properties of the slow Ca current (Heyer and Lux, 1976a); these clearly differ from those of fast axonal Na currents.

In the absence of a unifying theory for membrane Ca conductivities, we feel that it would be useful at this point to outline the characteristics of one such slow Ca current, not only because of the unusual properties of the conductances that appear to underlie it, but also because the Ca ions can, in turn, play a much more important role in controlling the behavior of neurons than is normally attributed to the entry of Na ions. Of particular importance to the electrical properties of the neuron is the fact that a large component of the K current is directly controlled by Ca (Heyer and Lux, 1976b). Again, because the behavior of this Ca-mediated K current differs from that of more frequently considered K currents and because it can constitute a major part of the total K current, at least in some molluscan neurons, we feel that a preliminary description of its properties is relevant now. Indeed, increasing evidence for the existence of slow Ca currents and associated K currents in vertebrate neurons emphasizes the necessity

H. D. LUX and C. B. HEYER   Department of Neurophysiology, Max Planck Institute for Psychiatry, Kraepelinstrasse 2, D-8000 Munich 40, Federal Republic of Germany

for understanding the properties of Ca ion movements and the responses of the K currents controlled thereby. Possible roles for the slow Ca and Ca-mediated K currents in producing output patterns in bursting molluscan pacemakers have been discussed (Eckert and Lux, 1976; Heyer and Lux, 1978). Of course, we do not know how similar Ca and K currents in vertebrate neurons will be to those described in snail neurons or the roles such processes may play in the functioning of neurons in the central nervous system (CNS). What we present here is a description of membrane characteristics that may provide a framework for additional complex interactions in multineuronal systems. We shall consider some points at which these properties may be important in the integrative functions of the CNS.

Assessing inward currents in the presence of large outward currents

The voltage clamp has proved a powerful technique for studying the fast inward Na current in axonal membranes. The method, however, cannot be expected to give unequivocal data on a slow inward current when outward currents occur simultaneously. During single voltage-clamp pulses in bursting pacemaker cells from the mollusc *Helix pomatia* (when identified neurons are found to have large slow inward currents; see Heyer and Lux, 1976a), the initial inward current typically turns rapidly into an outward current. It is unlikely that the true time course of the actual inward current with large depolarizations is reflected by this transient inward current; with low levels of depolarization a noninactivating inward current has been found in these neurons (Eckert and Lux, 1975, 1976). If a prolonged inward current is also activated by larger depolarizations, it is necessary to use additional techniques to differentiate it from changes in outward currents and to define its properties.

In many membranes opposing cationic currents can be separated either by selective block of one or more of the ionic conductances or by substitution of impermeant ion species (e.g., Cole, 1968). Unfortunately the use of such approaches to the study of persistent inward currents in snail neurons has not yet been successful. No pharmacological agent or combination of agents blocks all of the outward current without simultaneously abolishing the inward current (Heyer and Lux, 1976b; Thompson, 1977). While substances that normally block potassium currents in axonal membrane, such as tetraethylammonium (TEA) or cesium (Cs), leave the inward current,

they block only a portion of the outward current in snail neurons (Heyer and Lux, 1976b; Thompson, 1977; and unpublished observations). Eliminating the remaining (e.g., TEA-resistant) outward K current in these cells has thus far required procedures that would simultaneously block inward Ca currents. Promising techniques are being developed to allow better control of intracellular ion concentrations (Kostyuk, Krishtal, and Doroshenko, 1974; Lee, Akaike, and Brown, 1977); but there is as yet no evidence that, even under these conditions, K currents can be abolished without altering slow inward currents.

Since it is impossible with present pharmacological tools to isolate the slow inward current at moderate levels of depolarization, we questioned whether the persistent net inward current that appears during small depolarizations (Eckert and Lux, 1975, 1976) would at least represent the true amplitude and time course of the inward current at such potentials. Simultaneous and independent recording of K efflux shows, however, that even under these conditions the recorded inward current is actually contaminated by an outward current. Figure 1 shows the type of record obtained. Although in this example part of the outward current was abolished by Cs injections, a voltage-dependent K efflux remained at depolarizations that produced net inward currents. (Essentially similar recordings can be made from untreated cells; see, e.g., Figure 3 in Heyer and Lux, 1976a.) Indeed, the inward and outward currents may be of approximately the same magnitude (Heyer and Lux, 1976a), so the size of the recorded inward current represents only a fraction of its true magnitude.

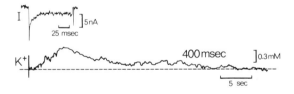

FIGURE 1 A persistent net inward current *I* is produced by small depolarizing voltage-clamp pulses. Simultaneously recorded increases in extracellular potassium activity *K* (note differences in time scales) show that there is a voltage-dependent K efflux at the same time. In net current measurements this outward K current is subtracted from the true inward current. Thus such results indicate that even when no outward current is recorded under voltage clamp, net current measurements alone are insufficient to determine the magnitude of the inward current. (Records are averaged responses to five trains of ten pulses each. Pulses from −50 mV to −35 mV were 100 msec in duration and repeated every 400 msec within each train.)

Because we cannot isolate the inward current either pharmacologically or at small depolarizations, and because opposing inward and outward currents can be of similar magnitudes, it is clearly necessary to use an independent measure for the movement of one or more of the ions in order to interpret changes in net currents under voltage clamp. For example, one of the classical approaches to this problem is measuring the movements of the radioactive isotopes of common ionic species (Cole, 1968). We have employed several techniques for separately assaying ion movements simultaneously with voltage-clamp currents. Changes in extracellular concentrations of specified ions can be monitored with high sensitivity and good time resolution during single trials by using ion-sensitive electrodes (see Lux, 1976). In much of our work we have measured increases in $[K]_0$ resulting from activation of outward K currents. These data can be used with measures of net currents under voltage clamp to detect slow inward currents even in the presence of large outward currents. The method has been discussed in detail (Neher and Lux, 1969, 1973; Lux and Eckert, 1974; Heyer and Lux, 1976a); here we need only briefly discuss the reasoning behind its use. If the net outward current were a pure K current, then measurements of K efflux (ΔK) and net current measurements (ΔI) would always agree. If an inward current were to partially short-circuit the outward K current, then absolute measures of ΔK and ΔI would differ. However, the value of $\Delta K/\Delta I$ would be constant if the relative proportions of inward and outward currents were the same. But if the inward current were to increase relative to the outward current, ΔI would decrease because of subtraction of the inward current, and ΔI would be less even for the same value of ΔK, resulting in an increase in the value of $\Delta K/\Delta I$. An apparent deficit in net charge transfer would be detected. This deficit is, then, a direct indication of a change in the relative magnitudes of the slow inward current and the outward K current. We have studied the variations in this "deficit current" as a function of voltage and time and its changes with pharmacological manipulation. An example is given in Figure 2A. In the upper records the net currents during repetitive depolarizations under voltage clamp and the simultaneously recorded changes in $[K]_0$ show that the net current decreases from pulse 1 to pulse 2 and from pulse 1 to pulse 3 are greater than corresponding decreases in K efflux. Deficits of 12% for the second pulse and 30% for the third pulse, compared with pulse 1, are calculated.

In addition to monitoring changes in $[K]_0$, we have used independent measures of Ca movements. Light emissions from neurons injected with the photoprotein aequorin increase with increasing $[Ca]_i$ (see Blinks, Pendergast, and Allen, 1976, for a recent discussion of the technique). We therefore used this technique (Lux and Heyer, 1977) to indicate increases in $[Ca]_i$. Examples of records of net currents under voltage clamp and simultaneously recorded light emissions are shown in Figure 2B. In addition, extracellular Ca-sensitive microelectrodes (Oehme, Kessler, and Simon, 1976; Nicholson et al., 1976; Heinemann, Lux, and Gutnick, 1977) were used to monitor decreases in $[Ca]_0$ caused by movement of that ion into cells during depolarizations. The decrease in $[Ca]_0$ during repetitive, short voltage-clamp pulses at two intervals is illustrated in Figure 2C.

THE SLOW INWARD CURRENT AND CALCIUM Changes in the deficit current in response to several experimental manipulations suggest that the inward current is carried predominantly by calcium ions (Lux and Eckert, 1974; Heyer and Lux, 1976a). The deficit is almost completely absent in the presence of typical blockers of Ca currents, such as Co, Mn, and La ions. Furthermore, with increasing depolarizations it does not decrease to a minimum until membrane potentials of +115 to +150 mV are reached. (The persistence of an inward current with such strong depolarizations also suggests that it is due to Ca influx.)

To confirm this prediction that the main inward current was carried by Ca, we used other measures for changes in Ca ions: Ca-sensitive microelectrodes and the Ca-sensitive photoprotein aequorin. In identified *Helix* neurons injected with aequorin, the voltage-dependent light signal is maximal at membrane potentials of +50 to +90 mV, that is, at levels where the absolute magnitude of the deficit is largest (Heyer and Lux, 1976a; Lux and Heyer, 1977). The increase in light emission with depolarization is abolished by extracellular cobalt (Lux and Heyer, 1977). As shown in Figure 2, changes in the magnitude of the deficit, decreases in $[Ca]_0$ measured with Ca-sensitive microelectrodes, and increases in light emission from aequorin-injected cells with repetitive depolarizations all showed similar patterns of changes with different experimental procedures. Such observations further demonstrate that the deficit current (representing the major component of the slow inward current) is a Ca current.

FREQUENCY DEPENDENCE OF THE CALCIUM CURRENT: FACILITATION Deficit measurements were useful because the ratio of K efflux to net outward current is not constant and varies with different voltage-pulse

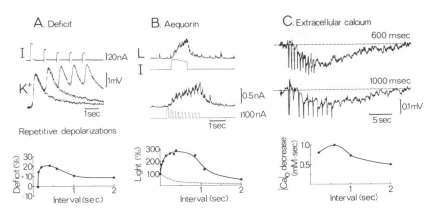

FIGURE 2 A summary of three methods for studying a persistent inward current in the presence of large outward currents. Use of the deficit measurement (A) does not require identification of the ion (or ions) carrying the inward current; methods B and C are quite specific for Ca currents. (A) A deficit in net charge transfer, reflecting changes in the short-circuiting effect of an outward current by an inward current, is calculated by comparing changes in the time integral of the net current I with changes in the time integral K of the increase in $[K]_0$. The use of this technique is discussed in the text. Compared with the first pulse, there are deficits of 12% for the second pulse and 30% for the third pulse in this example. (B) A voltage-sensitive increase in $[Ca]_i$ is indicated by increased light emissions from neurons injected with the Ca-sensitive photoprotein aequorin. These examples show the net currents I and light emissions L during a continuous 1 sec depolarization (from -50 mV to $+8$ mV, upper traces) and ten 100 msec pulses of the same magnitude repeated at 200 msec intervals (lower traces). (C) Changes in $[Ca]_0$ close to the neuron are measured with a Ca-sensitive microelectrode. Records showing the decrease in $[Ca]_0$ resulting from ten 100 msec pulses (from -50 mV to $+8$ mV) at 600 msec and 1,000 msec intervals are given.

The graph at the bottom of each column summarizes experiments in which the responses to ten 100 msec pulses (from -50 mV to 0 or $+8$ mV) are compared with responses to single 1 sec depolarizations of the same magnitude. The abscissa in each graph indicates the repolarization interval between the repeated short depolarizing pulses. In column A the $\Delta K/\Delta I$ values (see text) for continuous depolarizations have been normalized to 1.0, and the deficit measures the percentage change from this value for the ΔK and ΔI summed over the ten-pulse series. The values thus indicate the increased relative short-circuiting effect of an inward current. In B the time integral of the total light emission from aequorin-injected cells during ten pulses is compared with that during a continuous depolarization (normalized to 100%). The dashed line indicates total light output predicted from constant Ca influx during depolarizing pulses, light output which is a function of $[Ca]_i^2$, and $[Ca]_i$ removal during interpulse intervals, which depends linearly on concentration (see Lux and Heyer, 1977). In C the absolute magnitudes of decreases in $[Ca]_0$ near the neuron surface during trains of ten pulses are presented as a function of the repolarization interval.

patterns. The magnitude of Na currents in axon membranes is also clearly a function of the pattern of depolarization at a given command voltage (i.e., inactivation produced by sustained depolarization can be relieved by intermittent repolarization, etc.). We were therefore interested in determining whether or not changes in Ca currents could be described by similar activation and inactivation parameters. An increase in Ca current was originally found by comparing the K efflux and net outward currents during each of two voltage-clamp pulses of equal magnitude and duration; the deficit was larger during the second pulse (Lux and Eckert, 1974). In the case of a noninactivating current, this could be explained by incomplete activation of an inward current in the first pulse and more complete activation during the second pulse. If this were true, then simply prolonging the depolarization should produce a larger Ca current. However, the reverse was found: the total Ca current

is greater in the sum of a series of short depolarizing pulses than during continuous depolarizations of the same magnitude and total duration (Heyer and Lux, 1976a; Lux and Heyer, 1977). These results suggest that intermittent repolarization has an effect on this membrane current that has not been described previously in other systems.

To study this problem further we investigated the dependence of the inward current on the interval between successive depolarizations during repeated stimulation (Heyer and Lux, 1976a). (As a standard test we compared the inward current in a 1 sec continuous depolarization with the total deficit current during ten 100 msec pulses.) The observation of a small increase in total inward current calculated for widely spaced short pulses (e.g., intervals greater than about 2 sec: see lower curve, Figure 2A) suggests that depolarization can lead to some decrease in inward current and that repolarization can remove that inactivation. It is not clear whether this reflects only the sum of repeatedly activated fast inward currents (which do appear to inactivate during prolonged depolarization) or whether it implies, in addition, some inactivation of the persistent inward current during long pulses. In any event, the total increased inward current at long intervals is rather small and can be explained by normal activation-inactivation kinetics. However, if a removal of inactivation were the only effect evident, then the magnitude of inward current would be expected to decrease with decreasing repolarization intervals. This is clearly not the case, as shown by the lower graph in Figure 2A. With increasing stimulus frequencies (decreasing stimulus intervals) the total inward current actually increases to a maximum for repolarizations of 200–500 msec, depending on the neuron. Finally, these results cannot be due to variations in the clamp voltage during different tests. The series resistance is small ($<10^4$ Ω), giving no basis for such possible changes. We have also demonstrated that the Ca current and net voltage-clamp currents show distinctly different patterns of response to variations in the voltage and spacing of pulses within trains of depolarizations (Lux and Heyer, 1977). Because this pattern of frequency dependence cannot be explained by simple activation-inactivation models, we have suggested that the inward current facilitates with repetitive activation at intermediate frequencies.

To further substantiate our proposal that the Ca current facilitates, we recorded changes in extracellular and intracellular Ca ions with different repolarization intervals in the standard paradigm just described. The maximum decrease in $[Ca]_0$ occurred with repetitive depolarizations at about 500 msec intervals, suggesting a maximum Ca influx at intermediate intervals (lower graph, Figure 2C). In cells injected with aequorin, total light emissions were measured for different intervals between short pulses. The maximum increases in light emission, and therefore the maximum increase in $[Ca]_i$, occurred with repetitive depolarization at intermediate intervals (Figure 2B; for further discussion see Lux and Heyer, 1977). Thus three independent assessments of the inward current confirm that its behavior differs significantly from other known voltage-sensitive inward cationic currents and reveal a frequency-dependent facilitation of this current.

From our earlier work with net currents and K-efflux measurements, we suggested that facilitation is manifested as an increase in Ca influx per pulse during the trains of depolarizing voltage-clamp pulses (Heyer and Lux, 1976a). This was also dem-onstrated in aequorin-injected cells; light emission for the last two or three pulses of a series of ten could be several times greater than that for the first pulse (Lux and Heyer, 1977). The degree of facilitation depends on the magnitude of depolarization. Although total Ca influx was greater with depolarizations to potentials higher than +10 mV (Ca influx increases with increasing depolarization to about +50 to +100 mV) and the absolute increase in Ca influx with repetitive stimulation could be larger, there was a decreased facilitation (measured between pulse 1 and pulse 10 of a single train or between the total light emission from a series of pulses and a sustained depolarization). Depolarizations to less than 0 mV produced less total Ca influx as well as less facilitation.

Behavior of the outward currents

Experiments with various pharmacological agents failed to isolate the inward Ca current from outward K currents, but they did reveal two distinct components in delayed outward rectification (Heyer and Lux, 1976b). One part is only indirectly Ca-sensitive (see the definition in Reuter, 1973); the second is directly Ca-mediated and will be described below. The K current that depends on this rather unconventional Ca current may differ significantly from those previously described. To demonstrate the extent to which the Ca-mediated K (designated $I_{K(Ca)}$) differs from traditionally described membrane currents, we shall compare it with the other, primarily voltage-dependent component of delayed rectification (designated $I_{K(V)}$) in these same neurons.

DELAYED RECTIFICATION: $I_{K(V)}$ When current through the slow inward channel is blocked (e.g., in a bath of Co-Ringer's, made by substitution of Co^{++} for Ca^{++} and Mg^{++}; see Heyer and Lux, 1976a), a K current ($I_{K(V)}$; cf. I_{Co-res} of Heyer and Lux, 1976b) remains and displays many properties typical of other membrane currents. It is activated and inactivated by depolarizing voltage-clamp steps; $I_{K(V)}$ declines with continuous depolarization, and inactivation is removed as a function of the repolarization interval. Thus, with repetitive depolarizations $I_{K(V)}$ increases with increasing stimulus intervals (see Figure 3B). In some neurons there is relatively little Ca current, and the replacement of Ca by ions such as Co in the Ringer's removes correspondingly less of the total K current. The prediction is that this type of neuron should be dominated by $I_{K(V)}$; and indeed, even in normal Ringer's, its behavior is very similar to that of Co-treated cells (see Figures 5 and 11 in Heyer and

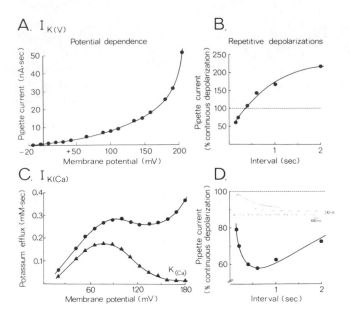

A. $I_{K(V)}$

Potential dependence

C. $I_{K(Ca)}$

B.

Repetitive depolarizations

D.

FIGURE 3 The responses of the voltage-dependent K ($I_{K(V)}$) and Ca-mediated K ($I_{K(Ca)}$) components of the outward K current in identified snail neurons are compared (see text for discussion of the definitions). (A) The potential dependence of the time integral of the net outward current of a neuron in Co-Ringer's is shown. (B) The net outward current at the end of ten 100 msec pulses (from −50 mV to 0 mV) is presented as the percentage of the current at the end of a continuous 1 sec depolarization of the same magnitude (ordinate) and as a function of the interval between the onset of the short pulses (abscissa). The neuron was in Ringer's in which Co replaced Ca and Mg. (C) The potential dependence of the K efflux (time integral of the K-sensitive electrode recording from very near the surface of the membrane) in an untreated neuron reveals a typical N-shape (filled circles). The bell-shaped curve for the voltage dependence of $K_{(Ca)}$ (triangles) results from subtracting for each voltage the K efflux attributable to the Co-resistive K current (latter not shown). (D) The dependence of net outward current on the interval between short depolarizing pulses is presented for an untreated neuron. An example of original current records is given in the inset, showing the responses to a 1 sec depolarization (upper, continuous trace) and ten 100 msec pulses originally separated by 400 msec intervals (lower, discontinuous trace; note that only portions of the intervals between pulses have been included).

Lux, 1976b). $I_{K(V)}$ therefore appears to be a normal constituent of the K current in these cells and not a result of some pharmacological action of Co-Ringer's. The plot of net outward current vs. voltage (I-V plot) for Co-treated cells shows a monotonically increasing outward current with increasing membrane depolarizations (Figure 3A). [Measurements with K electrodes indicate that changes in K efflux with different patterns of voltage pulses are very similar to the concomitant changes in net outward currents in cells in

Co-Ringer's (see Heyer and Lux, 1976b).] $I_{K(V)}$ is selectively blocked by TEA (Heyer and Lux, 1976b; Thompson, 1977) and at least partially by intracellular Cs ions (unpublished observations). Thus, in many respects it resembles the delayed rectifiers in such preparations as the squid giant axon (see Cole, 1968).

DELAYED RECTIFICATION: $I_{K(Ca)}$ As expected, the K current ($I_{K(Ca)}$) that is abolished by blocking the Ca current does have voltage- and frequency-dependent properties unlike those described for other K currents and can be contrasted with $I_{K(V)}$. The data suggest that the transient effect of Ca influx is to activate $I_{K(Ca)}$. For example, the voltage dependences of the slow Ca current and of $I_{K(Ca)}$ are similar. In voltage-clamp studies of many *Helix* neurons, there is a region of negative resistance (i.e., the net outward current decreases with increasing depolarization) at high membrane potentials. This results in an N-shaped *I*-*V* plot. We shall refer to this inclusion of a negative resistance region at high potentials as the *N-shaped characteristic* (see Meech and Standen, 1975; Heyer and Lux, 1976a,b). The hump of an N is even more pronounced in the relationship between K efflux and membrane potential (*K-V* relationship). Figure 3C shows an example of such a *K-V* plot (see also Figure 4 in Heyer and Lux, 1976a). Blocking the Ca current eliminates the component of K efflux responsible for this hump, suggesting that $I_{K(Ca)}$ increases to a maximum at potentials of about +50 to +70 mV and declines with further depolarization. An example of the computed potential dependence of $I_{K(Ca)}$ is shown in Figure 3C. It should be noted that the computed difference between *I-V* (or *K-V*) plots before and during treatment with Co-Ringer's declines rapidly with increasing depolarization but often does not go to zero at high potentials.

Another response evident in cells with large Ca currents is a long-lasting depression of the total outward K current (designated I_K), which is distinct from time- and voltage-dependent inactivations of other currents. This can be illustrated by comparing the outward current or K efflux resulting from repeated short pulses with that produced by a continuous depolarization of the same magnitude and total duration, as in the standard test procedure described earlier (cf. Figures 2 and 3A; an example of the current recorded during a continuous depolarization and repeated short pulses is shown in the inset to Figure 3D). As illustrated by the graph in Figure 3D, even when short pulses are separated by 2 sec, there is a long-lasting depression, and I_K at the end of the total of 1 sec of depolarization is actually less than it is at the end of a continuous 1 sec depolarization. The differences between this long-term depression and inactivation are obvious. Inactivation of $I_{K(V)}$ and other well-studied currents is removed by repolarization. As is evident from the frequency dependence of the responses shown in Figure 3D, the depression of I_K *increases* during repolarization with a maximum at about half-second intervals. (Of course, the decrease in net outward current is partially due to the increased short-circuiting effect of the inward Ca current, but measurements with K electrodes demonstrate that a true decrease in K efflux also occurs. When the contribution of $I_{K(V)}$ is subtracted, the percentage depression of the remaining I_K is even greater than indicated by the graph in Figure 3D.)

This long-term depression of I_K is caused by increased intracellular Ca. With repeated depolarizations, it occurs at frequencies near those producing the maximum Ca influx, whereas injection of the Ca-chelating agent ethylene glycol-*bis*-(β-aminoethyl-ether)-N,N'-tetraacetic acid (EGTA) to prevent an increase in $[Ca]_i$ greatly reduces the depression of I_K with repeated depolarizations. The effect of EGTA injection on this depression is shown by the data in Figure 4. Recordings from the extracellular K electrode in the first column of Figure 4 show that K efflux per pulse decreases during the ten-pulse series in the control condition; but after EGTA injection, repetitive depolarization produces far less depression. (Net currents for the first and last pulses in each train of ten are included in the second column of Figure 4 for comparison.) Finally, Ca injection (by pressure or iontophoresis, alone or with EGTA buffers) depresses I_K (see Figure 5).

Several observations suggest that increased $[Ca]_i$ selectively blocks $I_{K(Ca)}$. When Ca is injected into a neuron in which $I_{K(Ca)}$ has been abolished by substitution for external Ca, the Ca injection has no further depressing action (see Figure 5A). The voltage dependence of the current depressed by increased $[Ca]_i$ is also the voltage dependence of $I_{K(Ca)}$. In normal neurons with N-shaped *I-V* and *K-V* characteristics, Ca injection abolishes the hump in both the *I-V* and *K-V* relationships (Figure 5B); in addition, Ca entry during depolarization reduces the N-shape in the *I-V* plot even for pulses following a 1 sec repolarization (Eckert and Lux, 1977). It should be noted that EGTA injection can also reduce the N-shape of the *I-V* plot, but simultaneously monitored K efflux continues to provide an N-shaped *K-V* relationship, indicating that the primary change is an increased short-circuiting by the inward Ca current and that

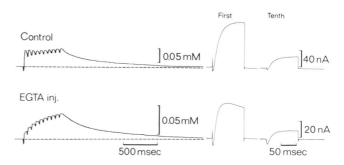

FIGURE 4 Repetitive voltage-clamp depolarizations produce depression in the K efflux per pulse (see continuous records, left) and net current per pulse (right, representing responses to the first and last pulses in the series) in an untreated (control) neuron. After EGTA injection (lower traces) the decrease in K efflux per pulse during the series of repeated depolarizations is largely eliminated. Current records still show a masked decrease in net outward current during the series after EGTA injection; together with the K record, this demonstrates that the short-circuiting effect of the inward Ca current has increased. In both sets of trials, ten 100 msec pulses for −50 mV to +12 mV were repeated at 600 msec intervals. (A 250 mM solution of EGTA was injected by pressure; injected volume was approximately 2.5% of soma volume.)

$I_{K(Ca)}$ is not abolished by such a treatment (see Figure 5C). It decreases with higher EGTA concentrations.

From the foregoing it appears that $I_{K(Ca)}$ is directly under the control of Ca: a transient action of Ca currents is to activate $I_{K(Ca)}$, but the effect of increased $[Ca]_i$ is to depress this current selectively.

CA-ACTIVATED LEAKAGE CONDUCTANCE   An increased K conductance and a hyperpolarization from resting potential following intracellular Ca injections into molluscan neurons has been described (Meech, 1972, 1974a; Brown and Brown, 1973; Parnas and Strumwasser, 1974). This effect of increased $[Ca]_i$ can be clearly differentiated from the Ca-mediated K current, $I_{K(Ca)}$, by a variety of tests. The increased instantaneous K conductance is activated by increased intracellular Ca, Ba, Sr, Pb, Hg, and Cd (Meech, 1974b; Meech and Standen, 1975). We have already described the blocking effect of increased $[Ca]_i$ on $I_{K(Ca)}$ (see also Heyer and Lux, 1976b); increased $[Ba]_i$, for example, blocks not only $I_{K(Ca)}$ but also $I_{K(V)}$ (Heyer and Lux, 1976b) and both resting and voltage-activated K conductances in other membranes (Sperelakis, Schneider, and Harris, 1967; Christ and Nishi, 1973; Hagiwara, Fukuda, and Eaton, 1974), and increased $[Cd]_i$ depresses K currents in squid axon (Begenisich and Lynch, 1974). Lanthanum injection strongly activates the K leakage conductance but has little effect on $I_{K(Ca)}$ (Hofmeier and Lux, un-

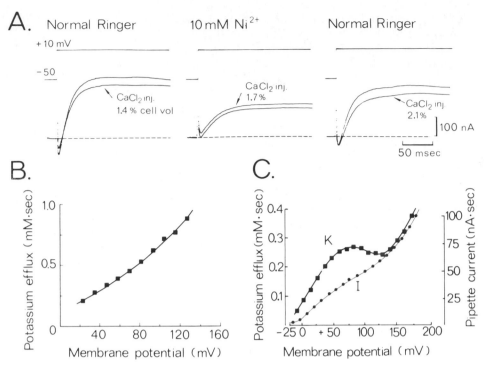

FIGURE 5   An increase in [Ca]$_i$ selectively decreases $I_{K(Ca)}$. (A) As shown in the first set of traces, measured volumes of a 10 mM Ca solution injected into an identified neuron bathed in normal Ringer's decreased the total net outward current. When the inward Ca current (and therefore $I_{K(Ca)}$) was blocked by bathing the cell in Ni-Ringer's (middle traces), a similar Ca injection did not cause a decrease in the measured current but produced only typical increased leakage conductance. The outward current, which can be depressed by increased [Ca]$_i$, recovered when the neuron was again bathed in normal Ringer's (right traces). (CaCl$_2$ pressure injected; G. Hofmeier, unpublished data.) (B) An example of the voltage dependence of K efflux in a Ca-injected neuron. The hump in the K-V plot, which was present before injection (not shown but similar to the one in Figure 3C), has been depressed (Ca injection by electrophoresis). (C) An injection of EGTA sufficient to greatly decrease the hump of the I-V plot (I) leaves a marked N-shape in the voltage dependence of K efflux (K). As in the experiment illustrated in Figure 4, this indicates an increased short-circuiting effect of the inward Ca current. (Pressure injection of a 250 mM EGTA solution totaling about 4% of soma volume.)

published observations). Intracellular (Parnas and Strumwasser, 1974) and extracellular TEA (Meech, 1972; Meech and Standen, 1975; Brown, Brodwick, and Eaton, 1977) block the K conductance activated by [Ca]$_i$, whereas intracellular (Heyer and Lux, 1976b) and extracellular TEA (Thompson, 1977) selectively block $I_{K(V)}$ but not $I_{K(Ca)}$. Finally, these two Ca-related K conductances respond to repetitive depolarization in opposite ways. The increased Ca influx during repeated depolarizations, either under voltage clamp or during spontaneous action potentials, increases the activation of the K leak (Meech, 1972, 1974a,b); the depression of $I_{K(Ca)}$ with repeated depolarizations was described above (see Figure 3D).

Under voltage clamp this effect of increased [Ca]$_i$ corresponds to an increased instantaneous conductance (Heyer and Lux, 1976b), but its high K selectivity (and the [Ca]$_i$ sensitivity) makes it different from

the leak conductance (g_L) of the squid axon (Hodgkin and Huxley, 1952a). The effect is generally small compared with the magnitude of $I_{K(Ca)}$, and we have not investigated the properties of this conductance change further.

A coupled calcium-potassium system

In preceding sections we have discussed some attributes of the slow inward Ca and Ca-mediated outward K currents in *Helix* neurons. These observations can be used as the basis for considering the mechanisms by which the ionic permeability of membranes are altered. As in most voltage-clamp studies, the original rationale of these experiments was a conceptualization of axonal membranes proposed by Hodgkin and Huxley (1952b). This formalization attributes ionic currents to a movement of ions down their electrochemical gradients following voltage-dependent increases in access to ion-selective membrane channels. Although some modifications have been required, this concept of basic mechanisms of membrane function has been extended with considerable success to a number of systems. But it appears unlikely that the slow voltage-sensitive Ca current and Ca-dependent K current in *Helix* neurons will fit easily into this pattern.

Mechanisms by which a current can facilitate have not been considered previously, and there is little concrete experimental data on which to base speculation. It seems reasonable to suppose that facilitation results either from a greater number of Ca channels or from an increased Ca conductivity of existing channels. Facilitation may arise from some property of the Ca-K coupling in the channel. The coupling of voltage- and time-dependent Ca and K currents implies, together with reasonable assumptions about ionic movements, that a Ca-K channel is, at a given moment, in either the Ca-conductive or the K-conductive state; flow of Ca and K as simultaneous and opposite charge movements in the same channel appears very unlikely. Measurements of instantaneous conductances provide additional evidence for the existence of singular states (unpublished observations). Thus facilitation could reflect an increasing number of Ca-conductive states. We also note that the inward flow of divalent ions appears to be much greater for neurons injected with EGTA (see Figures 4 and 5) or in Ba-substituted Ringer's. If this increased flow is not brought about by an increase in channel number, then the data suggest that the rate of movement through existing channels can be altered. The relation between these observations and facilitation needs to be clarified.

The conceptualization of relatively simple time- and voltage-dependent activation and inactivation parameters has remained basic to our understanding of K as well as Na currents. Attempts to isolate the slow inward current from outward currents in snail neurons failed, however, because a major component of the K current could not be separated from the Ca current. This meant, of course, that one of the major constituents of delayed outward rectification showed an unusual relationship with the rather unconventional slow Ca current. As we have already noted, this suggested that the capacity of the Ca current to influence electrical behavior was not limited to its role in depolarization, even in the complex temporal and voltage domain just described, but could be extended to a very direct relationship with another, opposing membrane current. We expected that the Ca-mediated K conductance would have unusual properties. The most outstanding feature of the control of $I_{K(Ca)}$ is its relationship with Ca ions. This K current is turned on by the transient effect of a voltage-activated Ca influx and is also turned off by an increase in $[Ca]_i$.

From available data a number of specific points can be established which must be accounted for by any formal model for the coupled Ca-K system. The behavior of the Ca-K system described here is consistent with a channel allowing the flow of both Ca and K and controlled by Ca at two sites. Ca interaction at one location activates the K current, and Ca interaction at the second site depresses the outward flow of K ions.

We propose that the Ca depression of K is due to binding at a site near the inner surface of the membrane, for we have detected no differences in the effectiveness of the depression of $I_{K(Ca)}$ by Ca, whether the Ca has entered during depolarization or has been injected. Although the frequency dependence of K depression (see Figure 3D) suggests that the interaction of Ca with this site is a relatively slow process, the question of time dependence is not yet resolved. Maximum decreases in K at intermediate intervals may simply reflect the greater influx of Ca at these frequencies. It appears—from current records such as those inset in Figure 3D and from the long-term depression represented in the graph in that figure—that continuous depolarization retards or prevents the blocking of $I_{K(Ca)}$ by $[Ca]_i$ and that in this type of test some minimal repolarization is required for blocking to become maximal.

A number of mechanisms would explain this property of depression: (1) the Ca-binding site could be directly voltage-sensitive in such a way that depolarization retards the ability of intracellular Ca to decrease the K current; (2) depolarization could change the channel configuration so that Ca binding is decreased; or (3) current flow through the channel could reduce binding. There is some evidence favoring the latter mechanism from experiments with large depolarizations. Our discussion of the N-shape in snail *I-V* plots has not, thus far, included possible effects of channel blocking. Indeed, previous investigators have suggested that the decline in $I_{K(Ca)}$ at high potentials results from the decreased electrochemical gradient for Ca (Meech and Standen, 1975), and the proposal that the normal voltage dependence of membrane currents might result from Ca blocking and unblocking channels (Heckmann, Lindemann, and Schnakenberg, 1972) has not been recognized as generally applicable to excitable membranes (see, e.g., French and Adelman, 1976). However, at high membrane potentials (e.g., above $+100$ mV) $I_{K(Ca)}$ decreases with increasing depolarization more rapidly than the rate at which the inward current declines with increasing membrane potential (see, e.g., records of net membrane currents and light emissions from neurons injected with aequorin: Lux and Heyer, 1977). Thus this decrease in outward current, which produces a region of negative resistance in the *I-V* plot, may in part be due to an increased depression of $I_{K(Ca)}$. This depression is persistently removed by extremely small inward Ca currents in contrast to intracellular Ca injections.

A remarkable feature of $I_{K(Ca)}$ is its almost exponentially increasing activation time with increasing depolarizing potentials. This slowing of activation is already obvious with relatively small depolarizations and continues within the region of the reduced K conductance at high potentials. Both the slowing of activation and the final depression of $I_{K(Ca)}$ appear to be consequences of progressively reduced Ca dissociation rates with increased inside positivity. Thus cleavage of bound Ca by activated Ca currents is likely to be a prerequisite for subsequent K conductivity. Instantaneous conductance measurements during the depression of $I_{K(Ca)}$ at higher depolarization reveal zero current potentials up to 120 mV more positive than the K equilibrium potential and indicate large Ca conductances. These observations support the view that the K-conductive site is first occupied by Ca and is Ca-conductive.

Transition to K conductivity as a consequence of inward Ca currents appears to occur with a potential-invariant time course on the order of 10 msec. This is observed with short preset or interposed pulses of millisecond duration, which elicit short-lasting Ca currents followed by smoothly rising and long-lasting K currents when we step back to a maintained test level (Hofmeier and Lux, unpublished observations). These extra K currents are up to four times the outward current during a maintained voltage step within the region of the depressed K conductivity and can nearly straighten the N-shaped *I-V* relation. The activation of $I_{K(Ca)}$ depends on actual inward current flow. If the Ca current turns off during progressively prolonged conditioning pulses (to resting or more negative potential levels), the subsequent activation becomes progressively less (Lux, unpublished observations). This fading of $I_{K(Ca)}$ activation starts within milliseconds, that is, at times when intracellular Ca would rather accumulate due to residual Ca currents, considering that removal of excess $[Ca]_i$ is a very slow process compared with the turning

on and off of Ca currents. These observations provide additional evidence against an activating role of intracellular Ca.

Our observations favor the interpretation that voltage-activated channels that are permeated by Ca ions transform with a characteristic time course into a more K-specific state. This intermediary state of transformation is obviously voltage-insensitive and separable by this and other properties from the initial Ca-conductive and late K-conductive state. The characteristic features of the transformation suggest a conformational change of the channel structure. There is the obvious possibility of describing this behavior by a model consisting of a linear array of three states with forward and backward transitions that are individual functions of time and voltage and, partially, of intracellular Ca activity (Hofmeier and Lux, unpublished observations). It is within the power of a simple chemical reaction model with four rate constants linking the states to approximate even such complex time-dependent behavior of $I_{K(Ca)}$ as was observed by Heyer and Lux (1976).

The requirement that divalent ions interact with sites in the channel and observations with Ba ions may perhaps suggest a reduced efficacy of more mobile ions (Sr^{++} and Ba^{++}; see Hagiwara, Fukuda, and Eaton, 1974) in activating $I_{K(Ca)}$. Indeed, Ba ions carry large inward currents but block rather than activate K currents. Mg produces a much smaller inward current than Ca but appears to be somewhat efficient in activating K currents. However, it is not yet possible to conclude that ionic mobility is the major determinant.

Individual characteristics of the unusual response patterns of $I_{K(Ca)}$ in snail neurons under ordinary voltage-clamp conditions can be mimicked by axonal membranes treated with various pharmacological agents. Studies on the interaction of these agents with membrane channels may be useful in unraveling the mechanisms by which channels in snail neurons are altered during normal activity. For example, the temporary blockage of the Ca-K channel by intracellular Ca is unidirectional; that is, the outward flow of K is occluded while the inward flow of Ca remains. (We have not tested the effects on outward Ca or inward K currents.) Similar blocking characteristics are found in axonal membranes. Although intracellular Ca is not an effective blocking agent in squid axons (Begenisich and Lynch, 1974), intracellular TEA and other quaternary ammonium (QA) ions and ions such as Cs specifically depress outward K currents in squid axons. Furthermore, several aspects of blocking of this type may be voltage-sensitive. For example, QA compounds cannot bind to produce blocking unless the channel has been opened by depolarization. Regions of negative resistance due to increased block at high membrane potentials are seen in *I-V* plots for axons with high internal Cs. In addition, increased inward current flow (e.g., of K ions in these examples of the axonal membrane) relieves the block of channels by QA or Cs ions. All of these are considered to be properties of a K pore with two distinct parts. The inner mouth of the channel is relatively nonspecific, and blocking ions can enter this portion; QA and Cs ions cannot pass through a second, more selective part of the pore (for discussions of this work with QA and Cs ions see Armstrong and Binstock, 1965; Armstrong, 1969, 1971; Bezanilla and Armstrong, 1972). It should be noted that intracellular Na acts very much like Cs in blocking currents (Bezanilla and Armstrong, 1972); but because $[Na]_i$ is ordinarily low in these axons, the depression of K currents is not usually recognized.

The type of block just discussed for K currents in squid axons has not been reported to show any properties that might be related to the long-term depression of $I_{K(Ca)}$. However, inward Na currents in squid axons treated with some lidocaine derivatives and strychnine do show a "use-dependent" block: that is, with repeated depolarizations, the drug-produced depression increases. The onset of and recovery from this type of block are complex functions of voltage and time. The mechanism may involve drug binding only to open channels and a binding that both blocks the channel and alters the voltage dependence of inactivation. Thus, with repeated depolarizations there is an accumulation of channels that have bound the drug and remain inactivated even at normal holding potentials (see Strichartz, 1973; Courtney, 1975; Cahalan and Shapiro, 1976; Shapiro, 1977).

The responses of axonal membranes treated with 2-, 3-, or 4-aminopyridine (AmP) are similar to yet other characteristics of $I_{K(Ca)}$. At high potentials, slowly rising outward currents are seen in both AmP-treated axons (Schauf et al., 1976) and snail neurons. The effects of AmP are interpreted as the result of voltage-dependent binding to the channel; but unlike the response to Cs, increased membrane potential decreases the blocking (Yeh et al., 1976a,b; Meves and Pichon, 1977). As mentioned earlier, even short pulses of increased depolarization can also alleviate the apparent depression of $I_{K(Ca)}$ that occurs at high membrane potentials. The AmP block is also relieved when voltage-clamp pulses are repeated at short intervals. This initially appears to be quite similar to the normal behavior of *Helix* neurons submitted to

the same patterns of voltage-clamp pulses. With *Helix* neurons, this augmentation at short intervals is specific to the Ca-mediated K current (Heyer and Lux, 1976b). As just discussed, the appearance of augmentation seems to depend on a second depolarization before the Ca current has been turned off and before the depression of $I_{K(Ca)}$ by increased $[Ca]_i$ can occur. As yet there has been no satisfactory explanation for the voltage and frequency dependence of the blocking by aminopyridines (see the discussion in Ulbricht and Wagner, 1976).

Slow calcium and calcium-potassium current in vertebrates

We have used our data on the slow Ca and Ca-mediated K currents in *Helix* neurons as a basis for describing the properties of a system underlying changes in the ionic permeabilities of membranes and to formulate some tentative ideas about the nature of interactions that appear to be responsible for these properties. This discussion indicated the extent to which these currents deviate from those normally studied in axonal membranes. It also served to illustrate characteristics by which these currents might be identified in other systems. Although the evidence is far from extensive, there are reasons to believe that slow inward Ca and Ca dependent K currents do occur in vertebrate neurons. The most thoroughly studied neuronal Ca currents in vertebrates are those mediating synaptic transmitter release (for review see Katz, 1969; Rubin, 1970). As far as data are available, synaptic currents resemble slow Ca currents in snail neurons in that they are blocked by such ions as Co, Mn, and La (see Rahamimoff, 1974), they persist after treatment with TTX and TEA (Katz and Miledi, 1971; Llinás and Nicholson, 1975), and they show a similar voltage dependence in voltage-clamp studies with single pulses (Llinás, Steinberg, and Walton, 1977).

Until recently there has been little evidence to suggest that Ca entry occurs through other vertebrate neuronal membranes, at least during normal function. Some of the effects of anoxia and even anesthesia have been attributed to increased $[Ca]_i$ but have not been related to any actual current (Krnjević, 1975). This lack of evidence may be due to the lack of experiments conducted to detect Ca currents. With the extension of voltage-clamp techniques to diverse types of neurons, slow inward currents (which are likely to be Ca currents) have been found in cultured neuroblastoma (Moolenaar and Spector, 1977) and in situ cat spinal motoneurons (Schwindt and Crill,

1976). A Ca-dependent K system has been reported for frog spinal motoneurons (Barrett and Barrett, 1976). The latter is TTX- and TEA-insensitive and is blocked by Co, Mn, or low $[Ca]_0$ but has not been studied under voltage clamp. Additional experiments are, of course, necessary to determine how similar the slow Ca and Ca-K systems reported for vertebrate cells are to those in snail neurons.

Since slow inward Ca currents have been found when experiments to detect them have been done, they may be present in many vertebrate neurons. It is not unreasonable to suppose that Ca-K systems similar to that in frog spinal motoneurons might also occur in other neurons. We should therefore ask what roles these currents could play in controlling neuron behavior. The activity endogenous in isolated somata from molluscan bursting pacemaker neurons (Alving, 1968) consists of complex patterns of bursts of action potentials and progressive changes in spike characteristics within the bursts (Strumwasser, 1968). The characteristics of facilitation of the Ca current and depression of the K current described here clearly provide mechanisms for patterned changes in neuronal behavior. A discussion of the relations between properties of soma membrane currents and patterns of burst activity in these molluscan cells is presented elsewhere (Lux and Heyer, 1975; Eckert and Lux, 1976; Heyer and Lux, 1978). We shall here consider briefly what the existence of these currents could mean to the function of a neuron in the vertebrate CNS.

Since Ca currents are normally necessary for synaptic transmission, the potential role of variations in these currents in mediating changes in presynaptic function is recognized. For example, it is clear that Ca is involved in facilitation (Katz and Miledi, 1968), although mechanisms have not yet been resolved. One recent study has suggested that explanations such as the residual Ca hypothesis are inadequate and that an actual facilitation of the Ca current is required (Zucker, 1974). Should this be true, the slow Ca current of *Helix* neurons would be an obvious model to investigate. Indeed, there are similarities between synaptic facilitation and the facilitation of the Ca current described here. For example, increasing Ca influx increases the release of transmitter but often decreases the degree of facilitation (Rahamimoff, 1968). This might be compared with the behavior of the *Helix* Ca current when depolarizations beyond levels for maximum facilitation produce even greater Ca influx but less facilitation (Heyer and Lux, 1976a; Lux and Heyer, 1977).

The slow inward Ca current does not inactivate completely with depolarization and is present at all potentials obtained during normal activity in some molluscan neurons (Eckert and Lux, 1975, 1976). Such a noninactivating inward Ca current might have many effects. It could produce inward-going (anomalous) rectification (an apparent increase in membrane resistance with depolarization) in molluscan neurons (see Lux and Schubert, 1975). Indeed, in cat spinal motoneurons (Liebl and Lux, 1975) and mammalian sympathetic ganglion cells (Christ and Nishi, 1973), an anomalous rectification has been found that is sensitive to manipulations that presumably alter Ca currents. At least in the latter, TEA does not block the inward-going rectification. A noninactivating Ca current also constitutes a continuous depolarizing drive that may help to sustain repetitive firing (see Schwindt and Crill, 1977). The presence of such a driving force at normal resting potentials may be suggested by the responses of frog motoneurons to hyperpolarizing current pulses. The observed increasing latency of the anode break spike with increasing hyperpolarization (Magherini, Precht, and Schwindt, 1976) is expected if increasing membrane potential inactivates a depolarizing current.

Inward-going rectification modifies synaptic efficacy by producing apparent changes in membrane resistance during changes in the membrane potential. Conductance changes during EPSPs and resultant shunting could be reduced; excitation could positively reinforce excitation in a limited voltage region. In the presence of a noninactivating Ca current, even small increases in tonic excitatory drive could produce large changes in activity. Of course, the strength of the effects on synaptic transmission would depend on the location of membranes with inward-going rectification. Comparisons of mammalian sympathetic ganglion cells (which show this rectification and possess dendrites) with frog ganglion cells (in which inward-going rectification and dendrites are absent) suggest a preferential dendritic location in vertebrate ganglion cells (Christ and Nishi, 1973). The presence of rectification could enhance dendritic electrotonic conduction of voltage transients such as EPSPs.

Graded responses to depolarization could be mediated by a Ca or Ca-K system. There is no evidence yet from vertebrate neurons, but synaptically induced postsynaptic Ca entry has been reported in an invertebrate preparation (Kusano, Miledi, and Stinnakre, 1975).

Finally, the slow Ca system could mediate action potentials. The slow Ca-K system in frog motoneurons produces spikelike responses after appropriate pharmacological manipulations (Barrett and Barrett,

1976). Evidence for the existence of TTX-insensitive action potentials abolished by treatments to block Ca currents in dendrites of vertebrate neurons has been presented (Llinás and Hess, 1976; Llinás, Sugimori, and Walton, 1977). Of course, the question of how Ca action potentials would relate to normal behavior remains. Synaptically activated dendritic action potentials may occur in a number of systems (axotomized·cat motoneuron, Purkinje cells, etc.: see Kuno and Llinás, 1970; Llinás and Nicholson, 1971) and serve to amplify the effectiveness of single synaptic inputs. Action potentials in dendrites could also produce short-term state changes in neurons; the responses of a neuron to injected current could be quite different in the presence or absence of dendritic action potentials. This could explain certain responses of cat spinal motoneurons: the sensitivity of these neurons to current injection (measured as an increase in firing frequency per nA injected current) suddenly increases at higher levels of depolarization (Kernell, 1966; Calvin and Schwindt, 1972). A level of responsiveness that is comparable to the highest obtained in normal motoneurons is seen at all levels of current injection in these neurons after axotomy (Heyer and Llinás, 1977), when the threshold for dendritic action potentials is presumably reduced. Consistent with this interpretation is the observation that the efficacy of synaptic input is suddenly decreased when a motoneuron is depolarized to the state more sensitive to current injection in the soma (Granit, Kernell, and Lamarre, 1966). The voltage and conductance changes associated with dendritic action potentials should decrease the effectiveness of summating synaptic inputs.

We have considered several mechanisms (facilitation of Ca currents, depression of a Ca-activated K conductance, anomalous rectification, and dendritic action potentials) by which Ca currents could produce short-term state changes in unit responsiveness. Further consideration of the role of Ca currents in controlling plasticity is beyond the scope of this paper. However, possible contributions from a Ca-K system such as that found in snail neurons to long-term information processing in the vertebrate brain are considered elsewhere in this volume by Wolf Singer.

REFERENCES

ALVING, B., 1968. Spontaneous activity in isolated somata of *Aplysia* pacemaker neurons. *J. Gen. Physiol.* 51:29–45.

ARMSTRONG, C. M., 1969. Inactivation of the potassium conductance and related phenomena caused by quaternary ammonium ion injection in squid axons. *J. Gen. Physiol.* 54:553–575.

ARMSTRONG, C. M., 1971. Interaction of tetraethylammonium ion derivatives with the potassium channels of giant axons. *J. Gen. Physiol.* 58:413–437.

ARMSTRONG, C. M., and L. BINSTOCK, 1965. Anomalous rectification in the squid giant axon injected with tetraethylammonium chloride. *J. Gen. Physiol.* 48:859–872.

BAKER, P. F., 1972. Transport and metabolism of calcium ions in nerve. *Prog. Biophys. Mol. Biol.* 24:177–223.

BAKER, P. F., and H. G. GLITSCH, 1975. Voltage dependent changes in the permeability of nerve membranes to calcium and other divalent cations. *Philos. Trans. R. Soc. Lond.* B270:389–409.

BAKER, P. F., A. L. HODGKIN, and E. B. RIDGWAY, 1971. Depolarization and calcium entry in squid giant axons. *J. Physiol.* 218:709–755.

BARRETT, E. F., and J. N. BARRETT, 1976. Separation of two voltage-sensitive potassium currents and demonstration of a tetrodotoxin-resistant calcium current in frog motoneurones. *J. Physiol.* 255:737–774.

BEGENISICH, T., and C. LYNCH, 1974. Effects of divalent cations on voltage clamped squid axons. *J. Gen. Physiol.* 63:675–689.

BEZANILLA, F., and C. M. ARMSTRONG, 1972. Negative conductance caused by the entry of sodium and cesium ions into the potassium channels of squid axons. *J. Gen. Physiol.* 60:588–608.

BLINKS, J. R., F. G. PENDERGAST, and D. G. ALLEN, 1976. Photoproteins as biological calcium indicators. *Pharmacol. Rev.* 28:1–93.

BROWN, A. M., M. J. BRODWICK, and D. C. EATON, 1977. Intracellular calcium and extra-retinal photoreception in *Aplysia* giant neurons. *J. Neurobiol.* 8:1–18.

BROWN, A. M., and H. M. BROWN, 1973. Light response of a giant *Aplysia* neuron. *J. Gen. Physiol.* 62:239–254.

CAHALAN, M. D., and B. I. SHAPIRO, 1976. Current and frequency dependent block of sodium channels by strychnine. *Biophys. J.* 16:76a.

CALVIN, W. H., and P. C. SCHWINDT, 1972. Steps in production of motoneuron spikes during rhythmic firing. *J. Neurophysiol.* 35:297–310.

CHRIST, D. D., and S. NISHI, 1973. Anomalous rectification of mammalian sympathetic ganglion cells. *Exp. Neurol.* 40:806–815.

COLE, K. S., 1968. *Membranes, Ions and Impulses.* Berkeley: Univ. California Press.

COURTNEY, K. R., 1975. Mechanism of frequency-dependent inhibition of sodium currents in frog myelinated nerve by the lidocaine derivative GEA 968. *J. Pharmacol. Exp. Ther.* 195:225–236.

ECKERT, R., and H. D. LUX, 1975. A non-inactivating inward current recorded during small depolarizing voltage steps in snail pacemaker neurons. *Brain Res.* 83:486–489.

ECKERT, R., and H. D. LUX, 1976. A voltage-sensitive persistent calcium conductance in neuronal somata of *Helix.* *J. Physiol.* 254:129–151.

ECKERT, R., and H. D. LUX, 1977. Calcium-dependent depression of a late outward current in snail neurons. *Science* 197:472–475.

FRENCH, R. J., and W. J. ADELMAN, 1976. Competition, saturation, and inhibition—ionic interactions shown by membrane ionic currents in nerve, muscle, and bilayer systems. *Curr. Top. Membr.* 8:161–207.

GRANIT, R., D. KERNELL, and Y. LAMARRE, 1966. Synaptic

stimulation superimposed on motoneurones firing in the "secondary range" to injected currents. *J. Physiol.* 187:401–415.

HAGIWARA, S., J. FUKUDA, and D. C. EATON, 1974. Membrane currents carried by Ca, Sr and Ba in barnacle muscle fiber during voltage clamp. *J. Gen. Physiol.* 63:564–578.

HECKMANN, K., B. LINDEMANN, and J. SCHNAKENBERG, 1972. Current-voltage curves of porous membranes in the presence of pore-blocking ions. I. Narrow pores containing no more than one moving ion. *Biophys. J.* 12:683–702.

HEINEMANN, U., H. D. LUX, and M. J. GUTNICK, 1977. Extracellular free calcium and potassium during paroxysmal activity in the cerebral cortex of the cat. *Exp. Brain Res.* 27:237–243.

HEYER, C. B., and R. LLINÁS, 1977. Control of rhythmic firing in normal and axotomized cat spinal motoneurons. *J. Neurophysiol.* 40:480–488.

HEYER, C. B., and H. D. LUX, 1976a. Properties of a facilitating calcium current in pace-maker neurones of the snail, *Helix pomatia. J. Physiol.* 262:319–348.

HEYER, C. B., and H. D. LUX, 1976b. Control of the delayed outward potassium currents in bursting pace-maker neurones of the snail, *Helix pomatia. J. Physiol.* 262:349–382.

HEYER, C. B., and H. D. LUX, 1978. Unusual properties of the Ca-K system responsible for prolonged action potentials in neurons from the snail *Helix pomatia.* In *Abnormal Neuronal Discharges,* N. Chalazonitis and M. Boisson, eds. New York: Raven Press, pp. 311–327.

HODGKIN, A. L., and A. F. HUXLEY, 1952a. The components of membrane conductance in the giant axon of *Loligo. J. Physiol.* 116:473–496.

HODGKIN, A. L., and A. F. HUXLEY, 1952b. A quantitative description of membrane current and its application to conduction and excitation in nerve. *J. Physiol.* 117:500–544.

HODGKIN, A. L., and R. D. KEYNES, 1957. Movements of labelled calcium in squid giant axon. *J. Physiol.* 138:253–281.

KATZ, B., 1969. *The Release of Neural Transmitter Substances.* Springfield, IL: Charles C Thomas.

KATZ, B., and R. MILEDI, 1968. The role of calcium in neuromuscular facilitation. *J. Physiol.* 195:481–492.

KATZ, B., and R. MILEDI, 1971. The effect of prolonged depolarization on synaptic transfer in the stellate ganglion of the squid. *J. Physiol.* 216:503–512.

KERNELL, D., 1966. High-frequency repetitive firing of cat lumbosacral motoneurones stimulated by long-lasting injected currents. *Acta Physiol. Scand.* 65:74–86.

KOSTYUK, P. G., O. A. KRISHTAL, and P. A. DOROSHENKO, 1974. Calcium currents in snail neurones. I. Identification of calcium current. *Pfluegers Arch.* 348:83–94.

KRNJEVIĆ, K., 1975. Is general anesthesia induced by neuronal asphyxia? In *Molecular Mechanisms of Anesthesia,* B. R. Fink, ed. New York: Raven Press.

KUNO, M., and R. LLINÁS, 1970. Enhancement of synaptic transmission by dendritic potentials in chromatolysed motoneurons of the cat. *J. Physiol.* 210:807–821.

KUSANO, K., R. MILEDI, and J. STINNAKRE, 1975. Postsynaptic entry of calcium induced by transmitter action. *Proc. R. Soc. Lond.* B189:49–56.

LEE, K. S., N. AKAIKE, and A. M. BROWN, 1977. Trypsin inhibits the action of tetrodotoxin on neurones. *Nature* 265:751–753.

LIEBL, L., and H. D. LUX, 1975. The action of Co^{++}, Ba^{++} and verapamil on "anomalous rectification" in cat spinal motoneurons. *Pfluegers Arch.* Suppl. 355:R80.

LLINÁS, R., and R. HESS, 1976. Tetrodotoxin-resistant dendritic spikes in avian Purkinje cells. *Proc. Natl. Acad. Sci. USA* 73:2520–2523.

LLINÁS, R., and C. NICHOLSON, 1971. Electrophysiological properties of dendrites and somata in alligator Purkinje cells. *J. Neurophysiol.* 34:532–551.

LLINÁS, R., and C. NICHOLSON, 1975. Calcium role in depolarization-secretion coupling: An aequorin study in squid giant synapse. *Proc. Natl. Acad. Sci. USA* 71:187–190.

LLINÁS, R., I. Z. STEINBERG, and K. WALTON, 1976. Presynaptic calcium currents and their relation to synaptic transmission: Voltage clamp study in squid giant synapse and theoretical model for the calcium gate. *Proc. Natl. Acad. Sci. USA* 73:2918–2922.

LLINÁS, R., M. SUGIMORI, and K. WALTON, 1977. Calcium dendritic spikes in the mammalian Purkinje cells. *Soc. Neurosci. Abstr.* 3:58.

LUX, H. D., 1976. Simultaneous measurements of extracellular potassium-ion activity and membrane currents in snail neurones. In *Ion and Enzyme Electrodes in Biology and Medicine,* M. Kessler, L. C. Clark, D. W. Luebbers, I. A. Silver, and W. Simon, eds. Munich: Urban and Schwarzenberg, pp. 302–310.

LUX, H. D., and R. ECKERT, 1974. Inferred slow inward current in neurones. *Nature* 250:574–576.

LUX, H. D., and C. B. HEYER, 1975. Fast K$^+$ activity determinations during outward currents of the neuronal membrane of *Helix pomatia. Bioelectrochem. Bioeng.* 3:169–182.

LUX, H. D., and C. B. HEYER, 1977. An aequorin study of a facilitating calcium current in bursting pacemaker neurons of *Helix. Neuroscience* 2:585–592.

LUX, H. D., and P. SCHUBERT, 1975. Some aspects of the electroanatomy of dendrites. *Adv. Neurol.* 12:29–44.

MAGHERINI, P. C., W. PRECHT, and P. C. SCHWINDT, 1976. Electrical properties of frog motoneurons in the *in situ* spinal cord. *J. Neurophysiol.* 39:459–473.

MEECH, R. W., 1972. Intracellular calcium injection causes increased potassium conductance in *Aplysia* nerve cells. *Comp. Biochem. Physiol.* 42A:493–499.

MEECH, R. W., 1974a. The sensitivity of *Helix aspersa* neurones to injected calcium ions. *J. Physiol.* 237:259–277.

MEECH, R. W., 1974b. Calcium influx induces a post-tetanic hyperpolarization in *Aplysia* neurones. *Comp. Biochem. Physiol.* 48A:387–395.

MEECH, R. W., and N. B. STANDEN, 1975. Potassium activation in *Helix aspersa* under voltage clamp: A component mediated by calcium influx. *J. Physiol.* 249:211–239.

MEVES, H., and Y. PICHON, 1977. The effect of internal and external 4-aminopyridine on the potassium currents in intracellularly perfused squid giant axons. *J. Physiol.* 268:511–532.

MOOLENAAR, W. H., and I. SPECTOR, 1977. Membrane currents examined under voltage clamp in cultured neuroblastoma cells. *Science* 196:331–333.

NEHER, E., and H. D. LUX, 1969. Voltage clamp on *Helix pomatia* neuronal membrane: Current measurements over a limited area of soma surface. *Pfluegers Arch.* 311:272–277.

NEHER, E., and H. D. LUX, 1973. Rapid changes of potassium concentration at the outer surface of exposed neurons during membrane current flow. *J. Gen. Physiol.* 61:385–399.

NICHOLSON, C., R. STEINBERG, H. STOECKLE, and G. TEN BRUGGENCATE, 1976. Calcium decrease associated with aminopyridine-induced potassium increase in cat cerebellum. *Neurosci. Lett.* 3:315–319.

NOBLE, D., 1966. Applications of Hodgkin-Huxley equations to excitable tissues. *Physiol. Rev.* 46:1–50.

OEHME, M., M. KESSLER, and W. SIMON, 1976. Neutral carrier Ca^{++}-mikroelektrode. *Chimia* 30:204–206.

PARNAS, I., and F. STRUMWASSER, 1974. Mechanisms of long-lasting inhibition of a bursting pacemaker neuron. *J. Neurophysiol.* 37:609–620.

RAHAMIMOFF, R., 1968. A dual effect of calcium ions on neuromuscular facilitation. *J. Physiol.* 195:471–480.

RAHAMIMOFF, R., 1974. Modulation of transmitter release at the neuromuscular junction. In *The Neurosciences: Third Study Program,* F. O. Schmitt and F. G. Worden, eds. Cambridge, MA: MIT Press, pp. 943–952.

REUTER, H., 1973. Divalent cations as charge carriers in excitable membranes. *Prog. Biophys. Mol. Biol.* 26:1–43.

RUBIN, R. P., 1970. The role of calcium in the release of neurotransmitter substances and hormones. *Pharmacol. Rev.* 22:389–428.

SCHAUF, C. L., C. A. COLTON, J. S. COLTON, and F. A. DAVIS, 1976. Aminopyridines and sparteine as inhibitors of membrane potassium conductance: Effects on *Myxicola* giant axons and the lobster neuromuscular junction. *J. Pharmacol. Exp. Ther.* 197:414–425.

SCHWINDT, P., and W. E. CRILL, 1977. A persistent negative resistance in cat lumbar motoneurons. *Brain Res.* 120:173–178.

SHAPIRO, B. I., 1977. Effects of strychnine on the sodium conductance of the frog node of Ranvier. *J. Gen. Physiol.* 69:915–926.

SPERELAKIS, N., M. F. SCHNEIDER, and E. J. HARRIS, 1967. Decreased K$^+$ conductance produced by Ba^{++} in frog sartorius fibers. *J. Gen. Physiol.* 50:1565–1583.

STRICHARTZ, G. R., 1973. The inhibition of sodium currents in myelinated nerve by quaternary derivatives of lidocaine. *J. Gen. Physiol.* 62:37–57.

STRUMWASSER, F., 1968. Membrane and intracellular mechanisms governing endogenous activity in neurons. In *Physiological and Biochemical Aspects of Nervous Integration,* F. D. Carlson, ed. Englewood Cliffs, NJ: Prentice-Hall, pp. 329–341.

THOMPSON, S. H., 1977. Three pharmacologically distinct potassium channels in molluscan neurones. *J. Physiol.* 265:465–488.

ULBRICHT, W., and H. H. WAGNER, 1976. Block of potassium channels of the nodal membrane by 4-aminopyridine and its partial removal by depolarization. *Pfluegers Arch.* 367:77–87.

YEH, J. Z., G. S. OXFORD, C. H. WU, and T. NARAHASHI, 1976a. Dynamics of aminopyridine block of potassium channels in squid axon membrane. *J. Gen. Physiol.* 68:519–535.

YEH, J. Z., G. S. OXFORD, C. H. WU, and T. NARAHASHI, 1976b. Interactions of aminopyridines with potassium channels of squid axon membranes. *Biophys. J.* 16:77–81.

ZUCKER, R. S., 1974. Characteristics of neuromuscular facilitation and their calcium dependence. *J. Physiol.* 241:91–110.

34 Calcium in Neurobiology: A General Theory of Its Function and Evolution

ROBERT H. KRETSINGER

ABSTRACT   The following postulates and summary statements constitute a general theory for the intracellular function of calcium in eukaryotes.

1. All resting eukaryotic cells maintain the concentration of free Ca^{2+} within the cytosol between 10^{-7} and 10^{-8} M. The extracellular concentration of free Ca^{2+} is much higher, 10^{-4} to 10^{-2} M.

2. The sole function of Ca^{2+} within the cytosol is to transmit information, that is, to function as a second messenger. Following a stimulus appropriate to that particular cell, the concentration of free Ca^{2+} rises temporarily within some region of the cytosol.

3. The target of Ca^{2+}, functioning as a second messenger, is a protein in the cytosol or on a membrane surface exposed to the cytosol; the Ca^{2+} target, or detector, is not a lipid or a carbohydrate. Of logical necessity, the Ca^{2+} dissociation constant of the calcium-modulated protein must lie between 10^{-7} and 10^{-4} M.

4. All calcium-modulated proteins are homologous. They contain one or several copies of the EF hand (helix/calcium-binding loop/helix) conformation seen in the crystal structure of muscle calcium-binding parvalbumin.

5. Cells initially evolved pumps to extrude Ca^{2+} in order to use (Mg^{2+}) HPO_4^{2-} as their basic energy currency. $Ca_3(PO_4)_2$ is insoluble. Having first developed a four-decade Ca^{2+} gradient, eukaryotic cells evolved the use of this Ca^{2+} gradient as an information potential.

Introduction

Many physiologists encounter calcium as a peripheral parameter to their main interest. Much of its early literature is anecdotal. Douglas (1963) and Rubin (1970) showed that Ca^{2+} couples stimulus to exocytosis. Sutherland (1972) first defined the concept of a second messenger during his pioneering studies on cyclic AMP. Rasmussen (1970) documented the generality of calcium's functioning as a second messenger. The first breakthrough in placing these phenomena on a molecular basis was the identification by

ROBERT H. KRETSINGER   Department of Biology, University of Virginia, Charlottesville, VA 22901

Ebashi (1963) of troponin as the protein that imparts Ca^{2+} sensitivity to skeletal muscle. The key advance in the study of cytosol levels of Ca^{2+} was the preparation and characterization of the luminescent protein, aequorin (Johnson and Shimomura, 1972).

In the last five years exciting advances related to calcium in numerous fields of biochemistry and physiology have made it possible to extend the ideas of these pioneers. As nerve cells and nervous tissue are subjected to detailed analysis, it becomes ever more apparent that many of the basic cellular mechanisms are common to all eukaryotic cells; they share a common origin and are evolutionarily related. In this paper I suggest five postulates to constitute a general theory for the intracellular function of Ca^{2+} in eukaryotes. The first three summarize and generalize a great number of commonly recognized and accepted results. The last two are somewhat more speculative and are becoming the targets of intensive research. I hope that this theory will serve the didactic and aesthetic function of ordering a mass of seemingly unrelated results. More important, it should focus future experiments on the critical points.

All resting eukaryotic cells maintain the concentration of free Ca^{2+} in the cytosol between 10^{-7} and 10^{-8} M

This generalization is now widely accepted, although it is based on a limited number of determinations. The volume of a 10 μm cell is less than 10^{-9} ml; and the concentration of calcium in double-distilled water is itself about 10^{-7} M. We must thus detect some 10^5 free Ca^{2+} ions in cells that have much larger quantities of complexed or sequestered calcium and that live in environments with near-ocean levels of calcium—over 10^{-3} M. The determination of cytosol- or organelle-free Ca^{2+} remains one of the outstanding technical challenges of contemporary cell biology.

Certainly the most reliable method used to date involves the injection of aequorin. Unfortunately the protein is precious, the light calibration is difficult, and the system is nonequilibratory. Various excitable tissues have been aequorin-injected—muscle, squid axon (Dipolo et al., 1976), *Helix* neuron (Meech and Standen, 1975) and *Limulus* photoreceptor (Brown and Blinks, 1974). All have less than 10^{-7} M resting free Ca^{2+}.

Several other methods have been tried:

1. Injection of Ca^{2+}-sensitive dyes such as murexide or arsenazo III. However, since the negative log of their Ca^{2+} dissociation constant, $pK_d(Ca^{2+})$, is about 5 or 6, they can provide only an upper limit to resting levels of free $[Ca^{2+}]$ in the cytosol. Moreover, neither their toxicity nor their effects on calcium stores have been fully explored.

2. Injection of known quantities of Ca^{2+} and/or Ca^{2+}-specific buffers such as ethylene glycol-*bis*-(β-amino-ethyl ether)-N,N'-tetraacetic acid (EGTA). One then monitors a response, such as a contraction, whose Ca^{2+} sensitivity has been determined by other means. However, since one does not know the Ca^{2+}-buffering capacity of the cell, one cannot determine the free $[Ca^{2+}]$ from a knowledge of the Ca^{2+} injected.

3. Insertion of a Ca^{2+} microelectrode. Recently Ammann et al. (1975) developed selective Ca^{2+} electrodes sensitive to pCa of 7, and within a few years similar microelectrodes should be available. Of course, any penetration method must be carefully controlled for cell damage and leakage.

4. Application of Ca^{2+}-specific ionophores such as A23187. The internal free Ca^{2+} can be equilibrated with the external free Ca^{2+}. These ionophores also interact with the membranes of various cell organelles such as mitochondria or endoplasmic reticulum, thereby releasing stored calcium.

5. Determination of free $[Ca^{2+}]$ in a cell lysate. The lysing process can release calcium and/or Ca^{2+}-sequestering molecules not actually present in the cytosol.

6. Determination of the Ca^{2+}-sequestering limit of an organelle such as the sarcoplasmic reticulum. One then infers that the free $[Ca^{2+}]$ of the resting cytosol is ultimately determined by the binding constants of these pumps.

Three corollaries are associated with this first postulate:

1. Eukaryotic cells usually live in an environment of about 10^{-3} M free Ca^{2+}, as in plasma or ocean.

2. Cells can control their cytosol-free Ca^{2+} by actively pumping Ca^{2+} into sequestering organelles and/or out to the extracellular environment and by allowing passive reentry.

3. Cytosol-free $[Mg^{2+}]$ is about 10^{-3} and does not vary greatly during an activation cycle.

The sole function of Ca^{2+} within the cytosol is to transmit information

The implication of these first two postulates is that for any eukaryotic cell at rest the cytosol concentration is pCa 7 to 8. Following an appropriate stimulus, Ca^{2+} enters from either the extracellular medium or from an internal store. This causes a transitory increase in Ca^{2+} to pCa 4 or 5, followed by a pumping down to pCa 8 or 7. Hence the target, the molecule with which Ca^{2+} interacts, has a $pK_d(Ca)$ between 7 and 5: if it bound more tightly than $pK_d \approx 7$, it could never release Ca^{2+} or relax; if it bound Ca^{2+} more weakly than $pK_d \approx 5$, it would never bind Ca^{2+} or activate.

Not only does the target of second-messenger calcium have a $pK_d(Ca)$ that lies between 5 and 7, but also any molecule in the cytosol whose $pK_d(Ca)$ lies between 5 and 7 is, by definition, modulated by Ca^{2+}.

If Ca^{2+} had any function in the cytosol other than serving as second messenger, then the entity that would bind calcium would have to have a $pK_d(Ca)$ greater than 7. I know of no evidence that any cytosol molecule can win a tug of war for Ca^{2+} with the calcium pumps. Further, I would argue that calcium does not function to transmit charge, as sodium does; calcium exerts its effect only through binding to a specific receptor.

This pulse of informational calcium may be restricted to a small fraction of the cytosol volume, as in *Chironomus* salivary gland (Rose, Simpson, and Loewenstein, 1977), in *Physarum* during contraction (Ridgway and Durham, 1976), or in *Medaka* egg cleavage furrow formation (Ridgway, Gilkey, and Jaffe, 1977).

The target of Ca^{2+}, functioning as a second messenger, is a protein in the cytosol

The validity of this postulate depends on the first postulate, that the resting cytosol concentration is low—pCa ≈ 7.5—and that the Ca^{2+} concentration rises to about 4.5 following a stimulus. The phospholipid, the nucleic acid, and the carbohydrate of the cytosol lack the combination of Ca^{2+} affinity and selectivity to bind Ca^{2+} at pCa ≈ 4.5 in the presence of cytosol levels of free Mg^{2+} of about 10^{-3} M. Proteins have evolved this affinity and selectivity simply because they can place 6–8 oxygen atoms, each carrying partial or full negative charge, in the exact position to form a cavity to accept a cation of crystal radius 0.99 Å, as opposed to the 0.65 Å of Mg^{2+}. Of course Ca^{2+}, as a second messenger, may modify a membrane via a membrane-bound protein. Specifically it may modify a protein associated with a membrane pore (Rose, Simpson, and Loewenstein, 1977) with membrane-bound adenylate cyclase (Lynch, Tallant, and Cheung, 1976), or with a membrane pump (Luthra, Au, and Hankan, 1977). As noted in the previous section, the $pK_d(Ca)$ for these calcium-modulated proteins must lie between 7 and 5—that is, between resting and excited levels of the free pCa.

Calcium-modulated proteins contain EF hands

The EF hand conformation, first observed in the crystal structure of carp muscle calcium-binding parvalbumin (Moews and Kretsinger, 1975), consists of two turns of α-helix, a twelve-residue loop containing six calcium-coordinating ligands, and two more turns of α-helix. The helix, loop, and helix are related to one another like the forefinger, middle finger, and thumb of a hand (Figure 1).

When I first presented this EF hand homology argument (Kretsinger, 1975), its appeal was primarily intuitive. It seemed to make evolutionary sense that once Nature had found a good target for Ca^{2+}, she would prefer to vary the basic theme than to start

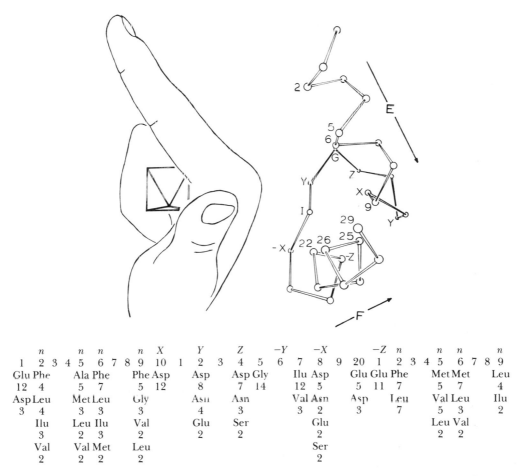

Frequency of occurrence at each conserved position (residue, frequency):

Label	Position	Residues (frequency)
n	1	Glu 12, Asp 3, Ilu 3, Val 2
	2	Phe 4, Leu 4
n	5	Ala 5, Met 3, Leu 2, Val 2
n	6	Phe 7, Leu 3, Ilu 3, Met 2
n	9	Phe 5, Gly 3, Val 2, Leu 2
X	10	Asp 12
Y	2	Asp 8, Asn 4, Glu 2
Z	4	Asp 7, Asn 3, Ser 2
	5	Gly 14
-Y	7	Ilu 12, Val 3, Glu 2, Ser 2
-X	8	Asp 5, Asn 2
-Z	20	Glu 5, Asp 3
n	22	Glu 11
	23	Phe 7, Leu 7
n	25	Met 5, Val 5, Leu 2
n	26	Met 7, Leu 3, Val 2
n	29	Leu 4, Ilu 2

FIGURE 1 The α-carbon drawing is from the crystal structure of carp muscle calcium-binding parvalbumin. The indicated positions are highly conserved in the two EF hands of parvalbumin, the four EF hands of TN-C, myosin light chains, and modulator protein, and the single EF hand of VitDCaBP. The frequency of occurrence, based on these 15 types of EF hands, are listed at each conserved position.

The inner residues (designated n) of both E and F α-helices tend to be hydrophobic. The Ca^{2+}-coordinating residues (X, Y, Z, $-X$, and $-Z$) have oxygen-containing side chains. At position 15, Gly usually occurs at a sharp turn. The Ilu, almost invariant at position 17, appears to hold the calcium-binding loop to the hydrophobic core of the molecule.

anew. That is, divergent rather than convergent evolution seemed more appealing; however, such an argument is not readily subjected to critical analysis. The following considerations and corollaries are associated with this homology postulate.

1. Nature has devised many ways of coiling a protein about a calcium ion. The various extracellular proteins—concanavalin A, thermolysin, *Staphylococcus* nuclease, trypsin, phospholipase A_2 and the γ-carboxyglutamic-acid-containing proteins—all bind calcium and are homologous neither to one another nor to the EF hand proteins. Their calcium affinities tend to be lower, pK_d(Ca) 3–5, and they function in extracellular environments having higher Ca^{2+} concentrations, pCa 3 to 2. However, their basic architectures could be used to achieve pK_d(Ca) values of 7. The EF hand conformation is certainly not required for high Ca^{2+} affinity or selectivity (review by Kretsinger, 1976).

2. In addition to affinity and selectivity, one might anticipate that Ca^{2+} should express its presence by inducing a significant conformational change in its target. This has been observed for parvalbumin, TN-C, and modulator protein (Liu and Cheung, 1976). Not only does the binding of Ca^{2+} alter the conformation of the protein, but changes in the protein conformation also alter the affinity of the protein for Ca^{2+}.

3. A calcium-modulated protein may be either an activator associated with an enzyme—as troponin and light chains are associated with myosin ATPase—or an enzyme itself—as is aequorin. This concept must

be broadened to include calcium buffer and/or transport proteins. The functions of parvalbumin and of the vitamin-D-induced calcium-binding protein are not yet established; however, they do not seem to be associated directly with enzyme activation.

4. In the course of evolution, an EF hand may have lost its ability to bind Ca^{2+} yet retained its conformation. The various myosin light chains consist of four EF hand regions; however, they bind only one or no Ca^{2+} ions. Skeletal TN-C consists of four EF-hands and binds four Ca^{2+} ions, but cardiac TN-C has lost two ligands in the first of its four EF hands and binds three Ca^{2+} ions (van Eerd and Takahashi, 1976). Relative to the "standard" EF hand of Figure 1, the first third of parvalbumin has two residues deleted, while the second EF hand, in sequence, of the alkali-extractable light chain has two residues inserted. The loop that connects the first pair of EF hands to the second pair is three residues shorter in modulator protein than in TN-C. The amino acid sequence of the calcium-binding protein from intestinal mucosa (Hofmann et al., 1977) indicates one EF hand. The other half of the molecule may have evolved from a different gene.

Several other proteins (Table I) of the cytosol, including membrane-associated proteins exposed to the cytosol surface, bind Ca^{2+} tightly—pK_d(Ca) > 5—and appear to be associated with a process involving Ca^{2+} as a second messenger. One might anticipate that they, too, contain EF hands.

In the evolutionary sense, cells first had to lower their intracellular free Ca^{2+} before they could use the

TABLE I
Possible calcium-modulated proteins

Protein	Function	pK_d (Ca)	n	$M_r \times 10^{-3}$	References
Phosphorylase b kinase (2.7.1.38)	phosphorylase b → a	6	1	55	Khoo (1976); Keppens, Vandenheede, and DeWolf (1977)
Tyrosine hydroxylase (1.14.16.2)	dopamine biosynthesis	5	?	40	Murrin and Roth (1976)
Aequorin	bioluminescence (?)	7	3	28	Cormier, Hori, and Anderson (1974)
Luciferin-binding protein	bioluminescence (?)	7	?	20	Cormier, Hori, and Anderson (1974)
ATPase (Ca^{2+})	calcium pump (SR)	7	1	102	
Spasmin	vorticellid contraction	7	2	20	Routledge et al. (1975)
Tubulin or associated proteins	spindles, cilia, etc.	4?	?	$110/\alpha\beta$	Solomon (1977); Schliwa (1976)
S-100	?	5	2	$21/\alpha_2\beta$	
L-1	?	5	2	14	Alema, Calissano, and Giuditta (1974)

pCa$_{out}$/pCa$_{in}$ gradient to transmit information. Certainly the most exciting prediction is that the calcium pump itself contains an EF hand.

Cells initially extruded calcium so they could use phosphate as their basic energy currency; Ca$_3$(PO$_4$)$_2$ is insoluble

Near pH 7, if [Ca^{2+}] were at ocean (or plasma) levels of 10^{-2} M, then [HPO$_4^{2-}$] + [H$_2$PO$_4^-$] could not exceed 10$^{-7.7}$ M. At physiological levels of phosphate, ~10^{-2} M, [Ca^{2+}] could not exceed 10$^{-5.2}$ (calculated from Sillén, 1961; see also Weber, 1976). Magnesium phosphate is soluble. Magnesium is the counterion associated with ATP and other biological phosphorylated compounds. Most enzymes dealing with phosphorylated substrates require magnesium; conversely, most magnesium-requiring enzymes have phosphorylated substrates. Williams (1974) realized that "the only general way to protect magnesium sites of this kind from calcium [whose affinity would be greater] is to pump calcium out." An interesting corollary to this Ca$_3$(PO$_4$)$_2$ postulate is that since prokaryotes also have phosphate-based energy systems, they too should actively extrude Ca^{2+}. This, in fact, appears to be true (Tsuchiya and Rosen, 1976; Silver, 1977). Whether this involves an ATPase (Ca) pump or an ATPase (Na) pump with subsequent Ca^{2+} for Na$^+$ or H$^+$ exchange is not definitely established. Nor is it known whether any prokaryotes have been clever enough to use their pCa$_{out}$/pCa$_{in}$ gradients for information transfer.

Discussion

The foregoing five postulates are appealing because of their simplicity and generality. Nonetheless I urge conceptual and experimental evaluation, not acceptance. To this end we might consider the following questions.

1. Somehow neurons must be different from other cells. Is their calcium physiology unique?

2. The cytoplasm is highly structured and varies enormously with cell type. Is the thermodynamic concept of free Ca^{2+} concentration valid in such a small and nonideal volume, touching so much surface?

3. The ion compositions and roles of various cell types are imperfectly known. Might not Ca^{2+} be sometimes used simply as a counterion or be seen in transit to sites of hydroxyapatite, Ca$_{10}$(PO$_4$)$_6$(OH$_2$), deposition?

4. Calcium at pCa ~ 3 does effect the fluidity of various synthetic lipid bilayers (Montal, 1973; Papa-

hadjopoulos and Poste, 1975). Do the lipids of cytosol-facing membranes never interact selectively with Ca^{2+}?

5. The EF hand has admittedly been found in several calcium-binding proteins of the cytosol. Is this mere coincidence? Could not Nature have easily evolved other conformations to perform these same functions?

6. Granted that Ca$_3$(PO$_4$)$_2$ is insoluble, the mitochondrion is able to function with inclusions of Ca$_3$(PO$_4$)$_2$ crystallites. Might there not be an inherent advantage to using Ca^{2+} as a second messenger, related perhaps to its coordination number, electronegativity (Williams, 1974), or rate of dehydration (Eigen and Winkler, 1970)?

Given the imperfect state of our present understanding of calcium physiology and its evolution, we must regard these five postulates as naive oversimplifications. I hope they will catalyze their own refutation and replacement by a more refined theory.

REFERENCES

ALEMA, S., P. CALISSANO, and A. GIUDITTA, 1974. Studies on a calcium binding, brain specific protein from the nervous system of cephalopods. In *Calcium Binding Proteins*, W. Drabikowski, H. Strzelecka-Golanszewska, and E. Carafoli, eds. Amsterdam: Elsevier, pp. 739–749.

AMMANN, D., M. GÜGGI, E. PRETSCH, and W. SIMON, 1975. Improved calcium ion-selective electrode based on a neutral carrier. *Anal. Lett.* 8:709–720.

BROWN, J. E., and J. R. BLINKS, 1974. Changes in intracellular free calcium during illumination of invertebrate photoreceptors. *J. Gen. Physiol.* 64:643–665.

CORMIER, M. J., K. HORI, and J. M. ANDERSON, 1974. Bioluminescence in coelenterates. *Biochim. Biophys. Acta* 346:137–164.

DIPOLO, R., J. REQUENA, F. J. BRINLEY, L. J. MULLINS, A. SCARPA, and T. TIFFERT, 1976. Ionized calcium concentrations in squid axons. *J. Gen. Physiol.* 67:433–467.

DOUGLAS, W. W., 1963. A possible mechanism of neurosecretion: Release of vasopressin by depolarization and its dependence on calcium. *Nature* 197:81–82.

EBASHI, S., 1963. Third component participating in the superprecipitation of "natural actomyosin." *Nature* 200:1000–1010.

EIGEN, M., and R. WINKLER, 1970. Alkali-ion carriers: Dynamics and selectivity. In *The Neurosciences: Second Study Program*, F. O. Schmitt, ed. New York: Rockefeller Univ. Press, pp. 685–696.

HOFMANN, T., M. KAWAKAMI, H. MORRIS, A. J. W. HITCHMAN, J. E. HARRISON, and K. J. DORRINGTON, 1977. The amino acid sequence of a calcium binding protein from pig intestinal mucosa. In *Calcium-Binding Proteins and Calcium Function*, R. Wasserman, R. Corradino, E. Carafoli, R. H. Kretsinger, D. MacLennan, and F. Siegel, eds. New York: Elsevier/North-Holland, pp. 373–375.

JOHNSON, F. H., and O. SHIMOMURA, 1972. Preparation and

use of aequorin for rapid microdetermination of Ca^{2+} in biological systems. *Nature New Biol.* 237:287–288.

KEPPENS, S., J. R. VANDENHEEDE, and H. DEWOLF, 1977. On the role of calcium as second messenger in liver for the hormonally induced activation of glycogen phosphorylase. *Biochim. Biophys. Acta* 496:448–457.

KHOO, J. C., 1976. Ca^{2+}-dependent activation of phosphorylase by phosphorylase kinase in adipose tissue. *Biochim. Biophys. Acta* 422:87–97.

KRETSINGER, R. H., 1975. Hypothesis: Calcium modulated proteins contain EF-hands. In *Calcium Transport in Contraction and Secretion*, E. Carafoli, ed. Amsterdam: North-Holland, pp. 469–478.

KRETSINGER, R. H., 1976. Calcium binding proteins. *Annu. Rev. Biochem.* 45:239–264.

LIU, Y. P., and W. Y. CHEUNG, 1976. Cyclic 3':5'-nucleotide phosphodiesterase: Ca^{2+} confers more helical conformation to the protein activator. *J. Biol. Chem.* 251:4193–4198.

LUTHRA, M. G., K. S. AU, and D. J. HANKAN, 1977. Purification of an activator of human erythocyte membrane (Ca^{2+} & Mg^{2+}) ATPase. *Biochem. Biophys. Res. Commun.* 77:678–687.

LYNCH, T. J., E. A. TALLANT, and W. Y. CHEUNG, 1976. Ca^{2+}-dependent formation of brain adenylate cyclase-protein activator complex. *Biochem. Biophys. Res. Commun.* 68:616–625.

MEECH, R. W., and N. B. STANDEN, 1975. Potassium activation in *Helix aspersa* neurones under voltage clamp: A component mediated by Ca influx. *J. Physiol.* 249:211–239.

MOEWS, P. C., and R. H. KRETSINGER, 1975. Refinement of the structure of carp muscle calcium-binding parvalbumin by model building and difference Fourier analysis. *J. Mol. Biol.* 91:201–228.

MONTAL, M., 1973. Asymmetric lipid bilayers: Response to multivalent ions. *Biochim. Biophys. Acta* 298:750–754.

MURRIN, L. C., and R. H. ROTH, 1976. Dopaminergic neurons: Effects of electrical stimulation on dopamine biosynthesis. *Mol. Pharmacol.* 12:463–475.

PAPAHADJOPOULOS, D., and G. POSTE, 1975. Calcium-induced phase separation and fusion in phospholipid membranes. *Biophys. J.* 15:945–948.

RASMUSSEN, H., 1970. Cell communication, calcium ion and cyclic adenosine monophosphate. *Science* 170:404–412.

RIDGWAY, E. B., and A. C. H. DURHAM, 1976. Oscillation of calcium ion concentrations in *Physarum polycephalum*. *J. Cell Biol.* 69:223–226.

RIDGWAY, E. B., J. C. GILKEY, and L. F. JAFFE, 1977. Free calcium increases explosively in activating *Medaka* eggs. *Proc. Natl. Acad. Sci. USA* 74:623–627.

ROSE, B., I. SIMPSON, and W. R. LOEWENSTEIN, 1977. Calcium ion produces graded changes in permeability of membrane channels in cell junction. *Nature* 267:625–627.

ROUTLEDGE, L. M., W. B. AMOS, G. L. GUPTA, T. A. HALL, and T. WEIS-FOGH, 1975. Microprobe measurements of calcium binding in the contractile spasmoneme of a vorticellid. *J. Cell Sci.* 19:195–201.

RUBIN, R. P., 1970. The role of calcium in the release of neurotransmitter substances and hormones. *Pharmacol. Rev.* 22:389–428.

SCHLIWA, M., 1976. The role of divalent cations in the regulation of microtubule assembly: In vivo studies on microtubules of the heliozoan axopodium using the ionophore A23187. *J. Cell Biol.* 70:527–540.

SILLÉN, L. G., 1961. The physical chemistry of sea water. In *Oceanography*, M. Sears, ed. Washington, D.C.: American Association for the Advancement of Science (pub. no. 67), pp. 549–581.

SILVER, S., 1977. Calcium transport in microorganisms. In *Microorganisms and Minerals*, E. D. Weinberg, ed. New York: Marcel Dekker, pp. 49–103.

SOLOMON, F., 1977. Binding sites for calcium on tubulin. *Biochemistry* 16:358–363.

SUTHERLAND, E. W., 1972. Studies on the mechanism of hormone action. *Science* 177:401–408.

TSUCHIYA, T., and B. P. ROSEN, 1976. Calcium transport driven by a proton gradient in inverted membrane vesicles of *Escherichia coli.* J. Biol. Chem. 251:962–967.

VAN EERD, J.-P., and K. TAKAHASHI, 1976. Determination of the complete amino acid sequence of bovine cardiac troponin C. *Biochemistry* 15:1171–1180.

WEBER, A., 1976. Synopsis of the presentations. *Symp. Soc. Exp. Biol.* 30:445–455.

WILLIAMS, R. J. P., 1974. Calcium ions: Their ligands and their functions. *Biochem. Soc. Symp.* 39:133–138.

35 Voltage-Driven Conformational Changes in Intrinsic Membrane Proteins

E. NEHER and C. F. STEVENS

ABSTRACT Underlying the nerve impulse are membrane permeability changes that most workers view as reflections of channel gating by macromolecules driven between closed and open conformational states by membrane voltage. To understand the physical basis of such gating, then, one must study the interaction of imposed electric fields with membrane macromolecules. Channels in certain postsynaptic membranes can be opened by application of acetylcholine, and the rate at which such channels then close can be easily measured. Because this closing rate is influenced by membrane voltage, the neurotransmitter-activated channels in postsynaptic membrane provide a good model system in which to study gate-electric field interactions. Such studies have shown that the electric field is coupled to the behavior of the gating molecule through the molecule's equivalent dipole moment, which is different for the open and closed conformations of the gate. Two simple cases are described to illustrate this concept. In the first, the dipole moment is independent of applied field, so the rate of conformational change depends exponentially on membrane voltage. In the second, the moment of the gate dipole is influenced by the field itself, so that transition rates between conformations depend on field strength in a more complicated way.

CONFORMATIONAL changes of intrinsic membrane proteins appear to play a central role in many processes that underlie nervous-system functioning; such conformational changes lie at the heart of the nerve impulse, excitation-secretion coupling, and postsynaptic changes induced by neurotransmitters. The transitions between various conformational states of the proteins in question serve a gating function; that is, the flow of specific ions through channels is controlled by the conformation of a molecule. Such a gating function is vital to the flow and processing of information because a small change in one variable—membrane voltage, for example—can give rise to a large change in another variable—calcium influx, for example. The energy stored in reservoirs (like concentration differences across cell membranes) can be spent in a finely controlled way. The controlled use of stored energy is necessary for the function of any information-processing machine.

In some cases, the variable that drives a gating molecule from one conformation to another is a voltage difference across the membrane containing the gate. In other instances, membrane voltage modulates the influences of other variables, such as neurotransmitter concentration, on protein conformation. A central question, therefore, is: How does the conformation of an intrinsic protein depend on membrane voltage? Our objective is to characterize the coupling between membrane voltage and protein conformation and to present some data relevant to this question from studies on a model system.

Theory

For simplicity, we shall restrict our attention to the special case of a protein with only two conformational states. If the protein were a gate, the two states would be *open* and *closed*. Doubtless most intrinsic proteins have more than two principal conformations, but generalizations from our simplified scheme are straightforward and involve no new principles of voltage-protein interaction.

Our system can be represented by the diagram

$$1 \underset{\alpha}{\overset{\beta}{\rightleftharpoons}} 0, \qquad (1)$$

where the two permitted conformations are 1 and 0 and the transition rate from 0 to 1 is α and from 1 to 0 is β. Because we have a gating molecule in mind, we shall say that conformation 0 is open and conformation 1 is closed.

E. NEHER and C. F. STEVENS Max Planck Institute for Biophysical Chemistry, 34 Göttingen-Nikolausberg, Federal Republic of Germany; Department of Physiology, Yale University School of Medicine, New Haven, CT 06510

A detailed treatment of scheme 1 requires a master-equation approach that specifies the conditional probability of having, say, state 0 at time t given state 1 at an initial time. For our present purposes, however, treatment of scheme 1 by standard chemical kinetics is completely equivalent. If $f(t)$ denotes the fraction of channels that are open at t, then scheme 1 is described by the usual loss-gain equation

$$\frac{df(t)}{dt} = -\alpha f(t) + \beta[1-f(t)] . \qquad (2)$$

According to this equation, the total rate at which $f(t)$ changes is made up of the loss from state 0 [loss rate $= -\alpha f(t)$] and the gain from state 1 (gain rate $= \beta[1-f(t)]$).

The equilibrium value of f is, according to equation 2 for $df/dt = 0$, given by

$$f(\infty) = \frac{1}{1 + (\alpha/\beta)} , \qquad (3)$$

and this equilibrium value is approached exponentially with a time constant

$$\tau = \frac{1}{\alpha + \beta} . \qquad (4)$$

From a functional point of view, we are interested in what fraction of the channels is finally open and in how rapidly they approach their equilibrium state. That is, we wish to know, for a voltage-driven conformation, how $f(\infty)$ and τ depend on voltage. From equations 3 and 4, it is clear that we must understand the voltage dependence of the basic rate constants α and β. We turn now to an examination of this question: How do rate constants depend on membrane voltage? The first step in answering it is to examine the general relation between energies associated with various conformational states of a protein and rates of transition between these states.

Each possible arrangement of atoms in a protein has associated with it a particular energy, made up of the various interaction energies of atoms with their neighbors and with the environment in which the protein is embedded. According to the Boltzmann relation, each configuration occurs at equilibrium with a probability that depends exponentially on the energy of that configuration. High-energy forms are therefore extremely rare, and a protein is usually found in configurations near those with the lowest energies. The energies associated with the various configurations of our two-state system are illustrated schematically in Figure 1. The two conformations 0 and 1 have the lowest energies and are thus most probable. Variations in structure from 0 and 1, rep-

resented by the points along the abscissa, are less probable.

The two energy minima, representing the open and closed conformations of our gate molecule, are separated by an energy barrier in Figure 1. The existence of such a barrier is implicit in the notion of distinct conformations. If no barrier were present, all possible intermediates in structure between 0 and 1 would occur as well. As long as the energy barrier separating the two states is significant—much larger than kT (where k is Boltzmann's constant and T is the temperature) the rate of transition depends exponentially on the height of the energy barrier. That is, the rate at which gates in the open state close is given by

$$\alpha = \nu e^{-U_{01}/kT} , \qquad (5)$$

where U_{01} is the height of the barrier going from 0 to 1 and ν is a constant, called the effective vibration frequency, with the units time^{-1}. A relationship with the same form specifies the opening rate of closed gates.

We now are in a position to examine the voltage dependence of the rate constants α and β. Because equation 5 is a general one, it is only necessary to determine the dependence of the energy barrier separating states on membrane voltage.

The details of the interaction between membrane voltage and intrinsic proteins are extremely complex. In an ideal case, the voltage would change linearly from V (the inside voltage) to zero (the outside voltage) through the membrane. In fact, the voltage changes widely from point to point because of complexities in membrane structure. Furthermore, the distribution of charges in this electric field is very complex, and their energies reflect not only local voltage but also such things as local dielectric prop-

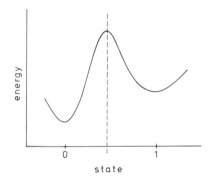

FIGURE 1 Schematic diagram of free energy associated with different states of a macromolecule, illustrating the concept of two principal conformations (0 and 1) separated by an energy maximum.

erties of neighboring molecules. Altogether, then, it would be very difficult to calculate the exact energy associated with a particular conformation as a function of voltage, even if the protein structure were known.

Fortunately the energy of a protein in an electric field can be characterized in a simple way, even though the detailed calculation of energies from a known structure is quite complicated. With any conformation of a protein one can associate a quantity μ called the effective dipole moment of the protein in that conformation. From physics it is known that the energy of such a dipole in an electric field is simply $\mu V/M$, where V is the membrane potential and M is the membrane thickness.

The dipole moments of proteins and other molecules have been measured, but it is important to emphasize that the quantity μ just described is not the same physical quantity as the usual dipole moment. First, μ is only the component of the total effective dipole moment that lies in the direction normal to the membrane surface. Second, μ incorporates all of the complexities in field structure and in molecular interactions (such as local dielectric saturation). The precise relation between μ and the dipole moment as measured by various physical techniques can be specified, but it is very complex. The advantages of using μ will become apparent in later discussion.

Generally each different conformation of a protein will have a different dipole moment μ. Not only does the distribution of bond dipoles and charged groups in hydrophilic regions depend on conformation, but the dissociation constants (and thus effective charge) of ionizable groups also vary with protein configuration. Because each state of a protein has, in general, a different value for μ, the energy associated with each state is differently affected by membrane voltage. The voltage effect on barrier height, and thus on transition rate, can be expressed by a modification of equation 5:

$$\alpha = \nu e^{-(U_{01} + \Delta\mu_{01}E)/kT}, \qquad (6)$$

where U_{01} is the energy barrier for gates closing at zero membrane voltage, E is the electric-field strength, and $\Delta\mu_{01}$ is the difference between the effective dipole moment of the gate in the open state and that of the transition state associated with the peak of the energy barrier. Let $A = -U_{01}$ and $B = -\Delta\mu_{01}/M$. Then

$$\alpha = \nu e^{(A+BV)/kT}. \qquad (7)$$

Equation 7 describes the voltage dependence of closing rate on membrane voltage, V. An expression of the same form, of course, holds for the opening rate β. Equation 5 seems, then, to answer the question posed earlier about how rates of conformational change depend on membrane voltage. There is a difficulty, however: B need not be constant, but may itself depend on V. This is so because the electric field can alter the charge distribution of the protein and the membrane matrix in which it is embedded and thereby change $\Delta\mu$. To some extent, bond dipole moments can be altered by the field, but probably the largest effect would be from electric-field influences on ionizable groups. Without a fuller knowledge of molecular structures, we cannot predict a priori the extent to which B would vary with voltage.

To examine the voltage dependence of B we now turn to studies on a system in which the electric-field effects on conformation transition rates can be approached experimentally.

The neuromuscular junction: A simple system for the study of voltage-dependent gating

In order to stay within the framework of our simple theory, we would like to have a system with a single conformational change that produces a measurable change in conductance. Any one of the known electrically excitable membrane channels obviously is more complicated than the ideal system since, in the framework of present theories, its description requires three or four voltage-dependent units.

A system that comes close to the required ideal is the acetylcholine (ACh)-activated channel at the neuromuscular junction. Although the general notion is that this channel is chemically excitable by binding a ligand such as ACh, it has been known for some time that the kinetics of the conductance changes involved are also dependent on voltage (Gage and Armstrong, 1968).

During transmission at the neuromuscular synapse, the following sequence of events is believed to occur. The nerve impulse arriving at the presynaptic terminal releases the neurotransmitter ACh, which diffuses across the synaptic cleft and binds to ACh receptors. Channels, with ACh bound, open transiently, thereby increasing ionic conductance. The experimentally observable signal is a rapidly (within 0.5 msec) rising membrane current (under voltage-clamp conditions), which then decays exponentially—the so-called endplate current (EPC). The feature most interesting in the context of this article is that the decaying phase of the EPC is voltage-dependent, that is, the time constant of decay is different when the experiment is performed at different membrane potentials.

It has been shown that this voltage-dependent decay is not determined by diffusion or degradation of the transmitter in the cleft (Magleby and Stevens, 1972; Anderson and Stevens, 1973). It reflects, rather, the closing of ionic channels. In other words, diffusion and the action of a powerful cholinesterase make the acetylcholine short-lived with respect to the mean open time of a channel, so that the rate-limiting step reflected in the EPC is the channel closing itself. About 0.5–1 msec after release, free transmitter has disappeared from the cleft. During the short lifetime of the released ACh molecules, however, they open several hundred thousand channels which then close during the following 1–5 msec. Thus the EPC decay reflects the closing rate of the channels, and the study of the EPC can tell us about molecular mechanisms of voltage-dependent gating.

The above mechanism of action can be illustrated in the following molecular scheme:

$$\begin{array}{c} \Big\downarrow \begin{array}{l} \text{transmitter} \\ \text{release} \end{array} \\ nT + R \underset{k_{-1}}{\overset{k_1}{\rightleftharpoons}} RT_n \underset{\alpha}{\overset{\beta}{\rightleftharpoons}} R^*T_n \qquad (8) \\ \Big\downarrow \begin{array}{l} \text{diffusion,} \\ \text{degradation} \end{array} \end{array}$$

where T stands for transmitter, R for the receptor or channel, RT_n for the receptor-transmitter complex in its closed conformation, R^*T_n for the open channel, and n for the number of transmitter molecules required to open a channel ($n \approx 2$; see Katz and Thesleff, 1957). Scheme 8 splits the total reaction into two steps—binding of the ligand followed by a conformational change. Since we see only one time constant of decay, one of the backward reaction rates in scheme 8 must be rate-limiting; we assume that it is the rate of conformational change α.

There are several experimental techniques with which this closing rate α can be measured.

1. *Decay rate of endplate currents.* Experimentally the most straightforward way to determine the channel closing rate α is to measure the time constant of decay of endplate current in a voltage-clamp experiment in which the motor nerve to the muscle is electrically stimulated to cause release of ACh. The rate α of the above scheme (measured in sec^{-1}) is the inverse of the time constant (see Figure 2A).

2. *Decay rate of miniature endplate currents.* This method is very similar to the one above; the only

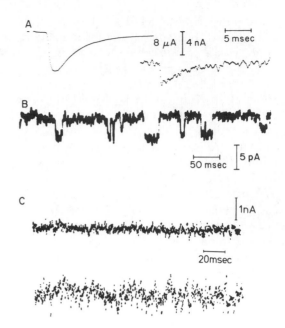

FIGURE 2 Recordings of membrane current suitable for analysis of channel closing rate. (A) Nerve-evoked endplate current (left) and miniature endplate current (right). (B) Single-channel recording from extrajunctional channels in the presence of the cholinergic agonist suberyldicholine at 10^{-7} M. (C) Typical current fluctuations in the presence (lower trace) of iontophoretically applied agonist. The upper trace gives a control record in the absence of agonist.

difference is that statistically occurring miniature endplate currents (MEPCs) are analyzed instead of nerve-evoked ones. MEPCs result from the spontaneous release of single transmitter packages, in contrast to the evoked release of about 100 such packages caused by nerve stimulation. MEPCs are very small in amplitude and difficult to analyze because of their limited signal-to-noise ratio. However, certain technical limitations of the voltage clamp impose less severe restrictions on recording of MEPCs than of EPCs. Therefore, MEPC decay can generally be regarded as a more faithful indicator of channel-switching kinetics than nerve-evoked EPC decay.

3. *Single-channel-open time distribution.* Conceptually the most straightforward way of measuring closing rates is to determine the open times of individual ionic channels and to calculate their mean. The closing rate α can be shown to be the inverse of this mean open time. This approach has recently become possible through the development of more sensitive recording techniques, which resolve discrete conductance steps connected to the opening and closing of individual channels (Neher and Sakmann, 1976). With this technique, randomly occurring square pulses of currents are observed as single channels

open and close (see Figure 2B). The square-pulse waveforms have statistically varying durations that are exponentially distributed. The channel closing rate α is obtained as the inverse of the mean value of open times from a long record during which transmitter is present at a very low concentration so that the probability that any given channel is open is extremely small. The results of this method will not be given, as it is applicable only under a very restricted set of optimal conditions. However, under these conditions the values obtained for α agree with those from other methods, which is evidence for the validity of the different techniques.

4. *Fluctuation analysis.* Consider using method 3 under the condition of an increased steady dose of transmitter so that many channels are open simultaneously. The open time of an individual channel will then no longer be measurable, and the number of open channels, although constant on average, will fluctuate around some mean value because of the statistically occurring opening and closing events. The resulting fluctuations in current are actually observed in standard voltage-clamp current records when transmitter is applied iontophoretically (Figure 2C). The time course of the fluctuations contains information about the mean channel open time, as can be shown quite generally by statistical theory. The mean channel open time is given by the time constant of the autocovariance function of the fluctuating record under the condition that only a small fraction of the total number of channels is open at a time (Stevens, 1972).

Thus the closing rate of channels can be determined under widely differing conditions of transmitter application (compare methods 1 and 4). The fact that similar results are obtained with all the methods proves that it is actually the channel gating, and not the kinetics of transmitter concentration changes, that is observed in the experiments.

Voltage dependence of the channel closing rate of frog neuromuscular junction

Anderson and Stevens (1973) measured the channel closing rate as a function of membrane voltage, employing three of the methods described above. The experiments were performed with cutaneous pectoralis muscles of the frog *Rana pipiens*. Their results are given in Figure 3A. The values from the three methods agree within experimental accuracy, and the data are very well approximated by a straight line in a plot of log (closing rate) vs. voltage.

Recently we performed a similar series of experi-

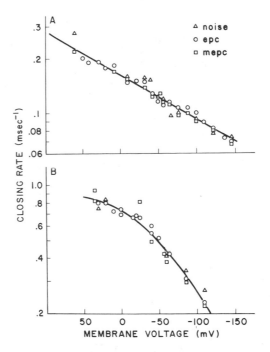

FIGURE 3 Dependence of the channel closing rate α on membrane voltage. (A) Experiments performed on muscles from the frog *Rana pipiens* at 8°C (after Anderson and Stevens, 1973). (B) Experiments on muscles from *Rana temporaria* at 13°C. There were no other differences in experimental procedures. The methods employed were fluctuation analysis (squares); analysis of EPC decay (circles); and analysis of MEPC decay (triangles). (For experimental details see Anderson and Stevens, 1973.)

ments in collaboration with Joseph H. Steinbach, now at the Salk Institute, San Diego. In this series, we compared the gating properties of channels from two different species of frog, *Rana pipiens* and *Rana temporaria*. Our experiments confirmed the earlier measurements of Anderson and Stevens for *Rana pipiens*. For *Rana temporaria*, we found higher absolute values of the rate constant α and an altered voltage sensitivity, which is of particular relevance to this discussion. The voltage dependence, which is about the same for both species of frogs at hyperpolarized voltages, levels off for *Rana temporaria* at depolarized voltages (see Figure 3B).

From the theoretical derivations above we deduce that the slope of the plots in Figure 3 should give the change in dipole moment during the closing reaction (equation 5) as a function of voltage. More specifically, the quantity B in equation 7 is $-\Delta\mu_{01}(V)/M$, where $\Delta\mu_{01}(V)$ is the difference in effective dipole moment between the open state and the activated state and M is the membrane thickness.

There are several molecular mechanisms by which an electric field can influence the dipole moment of a macromolecule, including bond polarization, field-dependent dissociation of an ionic bond, and rotation of the molecule.

Without specific knowledge of molecular details, the simplest approach is to expand the function $\Delta\mu(V)$ into a Taylor series:

$$\Delta\mu(V) = \Delta\mu_0 + V\frac{\partial\Delta\mu_0}{\partial V} + \cdots, \qquad (9)$$

where $\Delta\mu_0$ is the difference in dipole moment of the two states at zero voltage and $M\ \partial\Delta\mu/\partial V$ is the difference in polarizability. Truncation of the series in equation 9 after the second term will in general be a good approximation if the change in energy associated with polarization is small compared to kT over the voltage range studied. The approximation in that case is the same as Debye used in the low-field limit of his theory of dielectrics (Debye, 1929).

Considering the data in Figure 3A, it is obvious that we can neglect the second term in equation 9 in the case of *Rana pipiens*. The straight line was calculated assuming a value $\Delta\mu_0$ of 35 debye.

The data in Figure 3B, however, indicate that the polarizability terms in equation 9 are necessary in this case. The parabola in Figure 3B was calculated assuming a dipole-moment change of 33 debye and a polarizability change of 35^3Å^3. The literal interpretation of this result is that the channel protein in *Rana temporaria* is more polarizable, that is, more flexible in response to voltage changes, than the one in *Rana pipiens*. This flexibility, however, should not be considered to involve the basic structure of the protein. The difference between the two species might be explained by a small difference in pK value of an ionic bond. If, for instance, the pK, which generally should depend on both conformation and voltage, were around physiological pH in one species but different by 0.5 unit in the other species, the observed differences could be fully accounted for. Further characterization of such a mechanism would require experiments over a wider voltage range, or data would have to be obtained under a variety of ionic conditions.

Discussion

Our main conclusion is that the voltage dependence of transition rates should be described by an equation of the form

$$\alpha = \nu e^{a+bV+cV^2} \qquad (10)$$

where a, b, and c are all constants. The relative magnitudes of b and c appear to depend on the exact structure of the protein, but c is not always negligible. Over an appropriately restricted voltage range, the expression $\alpha = \nu e^{a+bV}$ should serve even for those cases where c cannot be neglected over the entire physiological range of voltages.

Although our experimental analysis has been fairly general, it is important to emphasize some of the limitations of our conclusions. First, of course, our measurements of α for the neuromuscular junction depend on the correctness of our conception of how ACh induces conductance increases; limitations in the analysis of endplate currents and alternative schemes for their interpretation have been discussed by Magleby and Stevens (1972), Anderson and Stevens (1973), Dionne and Stevens (1975), and others.

Second, even if our conclusions are accurate for the neuromuscular junction, extrapolation to other systems—the nerve membrane, for example—must be made carefully. Larger dipole moments may give field-molecule energies large compared to kT, so the Debye low-field limit would not hold. Further, differences in protein structure might alter the relative importance of b and c in equation 10; for example, b might vanish so that only the V^2 term would remain.

If our analysis can be extended without modification to nerve membrane, we should be able to account for the voltage dependence of conformational changes that underlie the nerve impulse. Currently, however, too little is known about the properties of the nerve gating molecules to decide the extent to which our conclusions are relevant to that system. The difficulty is that the activation and inactivation of channels in nerve membrane must, because a number of time constants appear, involve numerous conformational changes. Until methods are devised to study individual transitions in isolation, a direct comparison of experimentally derived rate constants as a function of voltage with equation 10 will not be possible.

To examine some of the implications of our conclusions for information transmission and processing by the nervous system, we return to equation 3 and rewrite it with the voltage dependence of rate constants explicitly included:

$$f(\infty) = \frac{1}{1 + e^{-m(V-V_0)}}, \qquad (11)$$

where $f(\infty)$ is the final (equilibrium) fraction of open gates. For simplicity, we have omitted the squared voltage term in the rate constants and have redefined constants to obtain the form shown. According to this equation, $f(\infty)$ is an S-shaped function of voltage. If the quadratic voltage term were not neglected, and if more complicated gating molecules with more than just two principal conformational states were considered, a more complicated expression for $f(\infty)$ would result. Nevertheless, the function would still have the same general S-shape, and the order-of-magnitude calculations to be presented would not be essentially changed.

We would like to examine one further question. How large a voltage change is required to open (or close) some particular fraction of channels, say 10%? Such an order-of-magnitude estimate might apply to synapses, retinal photoreceptors, or bipolar cells. We wish to estimate the receptor potential or the synaptic voltage change that would have a relatively marked effect on, for example, local calcium channels.

Realistic estimates for the gating dipole moment of calcium channels are, of course, not available from experimental studies on the molecules in question; but the order of magnitude of this quantity can be obtained from information on other proteins. Garden-variety proteins have dipole moments on the order of $10^2 D$, and from the range of values for various proteins it is not unreasonable to suppose that a molecule that has evolved for a gating function might have a dipole moment of $10^3 D$. This dipole moment—if it were substantially changed during the conformational transition—would imply that a tenfold change in number of channels open—between 0.01 and 0.1 for $f(\infty)$—would require a voltage change of only 14 mV.

What is the Ca^{++} flux through a single such channel? Single-channel conductance values for calcium channels have not yet been reported, but the values of 25 pS for endplate channels, 8 pS for frog node sodium channels and 4 pS for frog node potassium channels suggest the calcium channel to have a conductance on the order of 10 pS.[1] With a driving force on the order of 10^2 mV, 6.75×10^3 calcium ions would enter the cell per msec, or 675 calcium ions per msec average per channel if 10% of the channels were open. From these estimates it is clearly plausible

that according to the physical mechanisms discussed here, voltage changes in the millivolt range could well have quite substantial effects on a cell.

Another consequence of equation 11 relates to its S-shape. For voltages near V_0, $f(\infty)$ is nearly linearly related to membrane voltage V. The gain of this input-output relation is determined by m, and substantial changes in $f(\infty)$ can result from relatively small changes in V, as we have noted.

Systems for transmitting and processing information are always subject to noise, and some method of noise rejection must be used to achieve optimal performance. One technique is to use input-output relations that incorporate a threshold. In this way, subthreshold noise is rejected and becomes a negligible fraction of the total input once threshold is exceeded. The S-shape of the $f(\infty)$ curve provides just such a threshold effect. For appropriate values of m and V_0, then, the voltage dependence of channels can provide adequate sensitivity and rejection of noise.

ACKNOWLEDGMENTS The unpublished analysis of *Rana temporaria* discussed in this paper (see Figure 3B) was done in collaboration with Dr. J. H. Steinbach, to whom we are indebted. The work reported here was supported by NS Grant 12961.

REFERENCES

ANDERSON, C. R., and C. F. STEVENS, 1973. Voltage clamp analysis of acetylcholine produced end-plate current fluctuations at frog neuromuscular junction. *J. Physiol.* 235:655-691.

DEBYE, P., 1929. *Polar Molecules*. New York: Chem. Catalog Co.

DIONNE, V. E., and C. F. STEVENS, 1975. Voltage dependence of agonist effectiveness at the frog neuromuscular junction: Resolution of a paradox. *J. Physiol.* 251:245-270.

GAGE, P. W., and C. M. ARMSTRONG, 1968. Miniature endplate currents in voltage clamped muscle fibers. *Nature* 218:363-365.

KATZ, B., and S. THESLEFF, 1957. A study of "desensitivation" produced by acetylcholine at the motor endplate. *J. Physiol.* 138:63-80.

LLINÁS, R. R., and J. E. HEUSER, 1977. Depolarization-release coupling systems in neurons. *Neurosci. Res. Program Bull.* 15:557-687.

MAGLEBY, K. L., and C. F. STEVENS, 1972. A quantitative description of end-plate currents. *J. Physiol.* 223:173-197.

NEHER, E., and B. SAKMANN, 1976. Single-channel currents recorded from membrane of denervated frog muscle fibers. *Nature* 260:779-802.

STEVENS, C. F., 1972. Inferences about membrane properties from electrical noise measurements. *Biophys. J.* 12:1028-1047.

---

[1] Quite a different value for the conductance of a single Ca^{++} channel is obtained if the density of Ca^{++} channels is taken as the density of presynaptic intramembranous particles revealed by freeze-fracture electron microscopy and compared to the Ca^{++} current density of presynaptic membrane. Combining the available values from frog muscle endplate and squid giant synapse, a channel conductance of about 0.015 pS is obtained (Llinás and Heuser, 1977). Thus the estimates given might be lower by more than two orders of magnitude.

36 Electric-Field Effects on Macromolecules and the Mechanism of Voltage-Dependent Processes in Biological Membranes

GERHARD SCHWARZ

ABSTRACT Fundamental electric-field effects on macromolecular systems are examined with regard to the physicochemical nature of voltage-dependent biological processes. Particular stress is laid on the analysis of field-induced conformational changes of integral macromolecules in a membrane. Such phenomena prove to be appropriate means of controlling membrane properties through the difference of electric potential across the membrane.

Fairly high voltage changes are associated with the ionic gating of excitable membranes. So-called gating currents, which have recently been measured in squid axon, are quantitatively interpreted on the basis of independent structural transitions of individual macromolecules. However, macromolecules must interact cooperatively to produce the effects that have been observed in the nervous system at comparatively low fields.

Introduction

CERTAIN BIOLOGICAL functions associated with cell membranes can be controlled by the electric potential across the membrane. This is especially true in the nervous system, where the generation and transmission of action potentials (spikes) on nerve fibers have been shown to be based essentially on the pronounced voltage dependence of the passive permeabilities for the sodium and potassium ions (see, e.g., Cole, 1968; Kuffler and Nicholls, 1976).

Using the voltage-clamp technique—that is, electric measurements at stepwise changes of the membrane potential (Cole, 1949)—Hodgkin and Huxley (1952) derived a set of simple phenomenological equations for the conductances of sodium and potassium ions in the membrane:

$$g_{Na} = g_{Na}^0 m^3 h, \qquad g_K = g_K^0 n^4, \qquad (1)$$

GERHARD SCHWARZ Department of Biophysical Chemistry, Biocenter of the University, 4056 Basel, Switzerland

where m, h, and n are dimensionless, voltage-dependent functions of time that obey first-order rate laws (see Figure 1). The m and n functions, which describe the activation of sodium and potassium permeation, respectively, change from zero to unity following a sigmoidal course as the potential increases (the reference being the outside medium). The h function, which describes the eventual inactivation of sodium flux, displays an opposite behavior.

There is strong evidence that the effect is due to the voltage-induced opening and closing of channels for each kind of ion. The saturation effects observed at higher (and lower) voltage are then easily explained by envisioning a finite number of macromolecular structures all turned to states that form (or cannot form, respectively) such channels. The molecular mechanism of this voltage-dependent gating process is still unknown. It may be fairly complex, and it must involve at least one step that is sensitive to voltage changes. It will be pointed out in this article that these steps are most likely conformational changes of macromolecules in the membrane.

Fairly direct experimental access to any voltage-

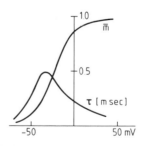

FIGURE 1 Typical dependences of the equilibrium value of the m function ($\bar{m}$) and the corresponding relaxation time τ on the membrane potential.

dependent property is provided by the inherent displacement current that occurs after a sufficiently fast voltage change. Use of this current allows evaluation of the overall charge transfer and the time course associated with the underlying mechanism. These can be analyzed with respect to a theoretical molecular model.

The existence of a displacement current caused by the gating effect was recognized by Hodgkin and Huxley. Unfortunately it was practically impossible to measure it as long as at least two other currents of much higher magnitude were superimposed on it. These currents are caused by the ion fluxes themselves and by the recharging of the overall membrane capacitance when the voltage is suddenly changed. Only recently have we been able to eliminate both of these effects. For the ion flux current this was done by substituting nonpermeable ions such as cesium or tetraethylammonium and by blocking channels with certain drugs. The recharging current, on the other hand, is a so-called symmetric displacement current (i.e., it is strictly proportional to the applied voltage pulse), and it can therefore be canceled by applying voltage pulses of exactly equal height and width but of opposite direction and adding the resulting currents on a signal averager. Actual gating currents are ordinarily asymmetric and consequently should give rise to a nonzero effect when this measuring technique is applied.

Such asymmetry currents have in fact been detected in excitable membranes of squid axon (Armstrong and Bezanilla, 1974; Meves, 1974; Keynes and Rojas, 1974) and frog nerves (Nonner, Rojas, and Stämpfli, 1975; Kniffki and Vogel, 1976). In some cases the underlying molecular process appears to be very simple, with only one relaxation time exhibited (see Figure 2); in others a more complex time course is found. It must be noted that the observed asymmetry currents are not *necessarily* a more or less direct manifestation of the gating; but it does seem quite likely. In any case, they must reflect some molecular event induced by comparatively strong variations of the electric field in the membrane.

These phenomena are by no means the only voltage-dependent processes of relevance to the nervous system. In fact, even fairly weak voltage changes are known to play a role. This is particularly striking with electric fish, which are ultrasensitive to electric fields. There is also the more generally important example of local circuits in brain cells responding to field variations that result from the flow of graded electrotonic currents generated mainly by dendritic sources (see Schmitt, this volume).

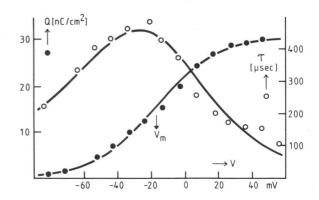

FIGURE 2   Measured charge transfer Q and relaxation time τ from asymmetry currents. The solid curves are calculated on the basis of the simple field-induced conformational transition discussed in this article. (After Rojas and Keynes, 1975; similar results have been reported by Meves, 1974.)

To approach an understanding of the molecular biophysics of such voltage dependences, we shall first analyze possible electric-field effects on macromolecular systems. Taking into account the structure of membranes, it will be shown that field-induced conformational transitions of integral proteins are the most likely causes for the processes under consideration. On this basis a straightforward quantitative interpretation of observed gating currents can be provided. Actual gating mechanisms, as well as weak-field-sensing effects, require more complex models.

Physical chemistry of field effects

Electric fields can affect molecular structures in various ways. The principal ones are associated with (1) the mechanical force exerted on electric charges, which leads to translational motion and/or internal charge separation and results in the formation of an induced dipole; (2) the torque on a molecular electric dipole tending to align it parallel to the field; and (3) the displacement of a chemical equilibrium toward the state of greatest overall dipole moment. The third possibility is less well known; it is not discussed in ordinary textbooks because it is usually thought to be negligible. We shall see, however, that it may be highly relevant to macromolecular reactions in a biological membrane.

Let us examine these effects from a quantitative point of view. Considering the case of translational motion we note that in general there exists an equilibrium distribution of charged bodies that obeys Boltzmann's law. Accordingly the number of bodies at a position i is given by

$$N_i = \frac{Nw_i \exp\{-q\phi_i/kT\}}{\sum_j w_j \exp\{-q\phi_j/kT\}}, \qquad (2a)$$

where N is the total number of equivalent bodies, q their individual electric charge, ϕ_i the electric potential at position i, and w_i the weight factor that determines the probability of finding the body at i if it were uncharged. The latter quantity can be expressed as

$$w_i = \exp\{-a_i/kT\}, \qquad (2b)$$

where a_i is the free energy of nonelectrical interaction with the surroundings.

In a homogeneous medium (e.g., in ordinary solution) the a_i would be independent of i, so that uniform distribution would occur at constant potential. This is no longer true in heterogeneous systems, such as biological membranes, in which the zero-field affinity to different positions can vary substantially.

In any event, it must be emphasized that these energetic conditions are decisive for the voltages required to induce displacements of charge. For a quantitative analysis, let us assume only two possible sites, $i = 1$ and 2. Applying equation 2a, the relative population of state 2 is then

$$\theta = e^x/(1 + e^x), \qquad x = -(\Delta a + qV)/kT, \qquad (3)$$

where $\Delta a = a_2 - a_1$ and $V = \phi_2 - \phi_1$ are the differences of the zero-field free energy and electric potential, respectively. If changes of the potential alone are to cause saturation of both states—that is, to drive most of the charges into either position—there must be an accessible voltage V_m associated with equal distribution (i.e., $\theta = 0.5$). Evidently we have

$$qV_m = -\Delta a. \qquad (4)$$

Going to $V = V_m \pm 3\,kT/q$ will practically lead to saturation (more precisely, $\theta \approx 0.05$ and 0.95). As can be readily evaluated, a voltage change of $3\,kT/q$ equals about 70 mV for one elementary charge (at room temperature). On the other hand, a Δa of ± 1 kcal/mol corresponds to $V_m = \pm 40$ mV.

The situation with regard to the rotational orientation of molecular dipoles is analogous. Considering N particles with a permanent dipole moment μ at equilibrium, the number falling in direction i is

$$N_i = \frac{Nw_i \exp\{\mu E_i/kT\}}{\sum_j w_j \exp\{\mu E_j/kT\}}, \qquad (5)$$

where E_i is the component of the field parallel to the direction i and w_i is the corresponding zero-field weight factor. The latter is again determined by a_i, the free energy of interaction with the surroundings.

In an isotropic system, where any direction is accessible and all a_i are equal, this immediately leads to the ordinary Debye theory of dipole orientation in an applied field. Saturation effects with field strengths on the order of 100 kV/cm (as is typical of a biological membrane) can be expected for dipole moments of some hundred debye units (1 D = 10^{-18} electrostatic units). Such values are indeed characteristic for protein molecules. In anisotropic media, however, differences in the nonelectrical interaction energies much greater than kT must be taken into account. These would have to be compensated for by the electrical energy difference $\mu\Delta E$ if saturation effects in the populations of the corresponding states are to be brought about. With the above values of μ and E, this does not yield much more than 1 kcal/mol.

Finally, we turn to the field effect on a general chemical equilibrium of the type

$$\nu'_1 B_1 + \nu'_2 B_2 + \ldots \rightleftharpoons \nu''_1 B_1 + \nu''_2 B_2 + \ldots, \qquad (6)$$

where the species B_i participate with stoichiometric coefficients ν'_i and ν''_i, depending on which side they occur. Generally such equilibrium can be displaced by an applied field E. The equilibrium "constant" in terms of equilibrium concentrations $\bar{c}_i$, namely

$$K = \bar{c}_1{}^{\nu_1}\bar{c}_2{}^{\nu_2} \ldots \qquad (\nu_i = \nu''_i - \nu'_i), \qquad (7)$$

is subject to the relation

$$\frac{\partial \ln K}{\partial E} = \frac{\Delta M}{RT}, \qquad (8)$$

where ΔM is the reaction-induced molar change of M, the overall dipole moment of the system parallel to the field.

This is exactly analogous to the well-known van't Hoff relation concerning the effect of temperature and follows directly from the first and second laws of thermodynamics. The increase in internal energy U upon a differential change of state is, accordingly,

$$dU = T\,dS - p\,dv + E\,dM - A\,d\xi^*, \qquad (9)$$

where the first term is the reversible heat influx (S is entropy), the second and third account for the volume and dipolar works, respectively, and the last refers to the energy balance of chemical conversion. The actual change in mole number of B_i is $dn_i = \nu_i\alpha\xi^*$ (ξ^* is the extent of reaction) as follows from mass conservation and stoichiometry. The affinity A, which is the negative free reaction enthalpy, is

$$A = -\Delta G = RT \left\{ \ln K - \sum_i \nu_i \ln c_i \right\}. \quad (10)$$

Now, if we introduce a specific free enthalpy, $G^* = U + pv - EM - TS$, equation 9 can be rewritten as

$$dG^* = -S\,dT + v\,dp - M\,dE - A\,d\xi^*. \quad (11)$$

Since G^* is a function of state, M and A are the negative partial derivatives with respect to E and ξ^*. Thus, because of independence of second derivatives relative to the order of differentiation,

$$\frac{\partial A}{\partial E} = \frac{\partial M}{\partial \xi^*} \equiv \Delta M, \quad (12)$$

which with equation 10 immediately leads to equation 8. A more detailed thermodynamic analysis has been given elsewhere (Schwarz, 1967).

To detect this effect experimentally, it is necessary to have either reaction-induced changes of macromolecular dipoles or extremely high field strengths. Under such circumstances the effect has indeed been measured by dielectric techniques (Schwarz and Seelig, 1968; Wada, Tanaka, and Kihara, 1972; Schwarz and Bauer, 1974) as well as by direct registration of the field-induced coil-to-helix transition of a polypeptide reflected in electric birefringence (Schwarz and Schrader, 1975).

Constraints of membrane structure

A discussion of voltage-dependent molecular processes in a biological membrane must take into account the fact that one deals with a peculiarly structured system that is neither homogeneous nor isotropic. The present state of our knowledge is effectively summarized in the fluid mosaic model of Singer and Nicolson (1972), based on a lipid bilayer matrix with an internal core of hydrophobic nonpolar hydrocarbon chains and interfaces with the outside aqueous regions composed of the hydrophilic polar head groups. Functional membrane proteins are incorporated in the bilayer and are stabilized by optimization of hydrophobic and hydrophilic interactions. For this reason, such integral proteins must have a pronounced amphiphilic nature, with a substantial hydrophobic part embedded in the nonpolar domain of the lipids and hydrophilic parts protruding into the polar membrane interfaces.

The electric potential V across the membrane is composed of $\Delta\psi$, the difference of the two interface potentials, and the voltage drop in the hydrophobic permeation barrier of the membrane. In this latter high-resistance domain, the inherent zero charge implies a constant field strength E, so that

$$V = \Delta\psi + Ed, \quad (13)$$

where d is the thickness of the hydrophobic core. External voltage changes have little effect on $\Delta\psi$, which is primarily determined by membrane surface charges and electrolyte concentrations. Thus they mainly control E. Accordingly voltage-dependent molecular structures must be located in the nonpolar domain. If they are responsible for a gating process, their function would naturally also require that they span hydrophobic and hydrophilic regions.

Field-induced rotations of integral macromolecules (particularly proteins) have been especially favored as the basic events of gating. First, we note that saturation effects with voltages on the order of 100 mV, or field strengths of about 100 kV/cm, can only occur when large angles of transverse rotation are involved, maybe even complete flip-flops. Small angles would be associated with unrealistically large dipole moments ($\gg$1,000 D). On the other hand, rotation about substantial angles necessarily implies the transfer of hydrophobic parts through hydrophilic ones and vice versa (see Figure 3). This is energetically highly unfavorable (Schwarz, 1978). To introduce only one methyl group into water or an appreciable dipole into a nonpolar medium (not to mention isolated charges) already requires the expenditure of 1–2 kcal/mol. Therefore the transverse rotation of an integral macromolecule in a membrane—which necessarily involves many such transfers—very likely requires much more energy than the 1 kcal/mol the field can contribute.

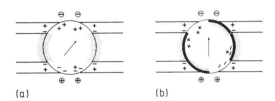

(a)   (b)

FIGURE 3 Schematic illustration of energetic implications upon transverse rotation of an integral macromolecule in the membrane. (a) Stable position at zero field: hydrophobic and hydrophilic areas of the particle in contact with like areas in the membrane and outside medium, respectively. (b) After appreciable rotation considerable areas of unlike nature come into contact (indicated by the thickened lines; shaded parts are hydrophobic).

Even if the equilibrium positions do not have appreciably different free energies, which is conceivable for a flip-flop, it is in any case the activation barrier of rotation that would be increased far beyond reasonable values. Macromolecules of roughly 50 Å extension are known to have a rotational relaxation time of some 10^{-8} sec in water. Since the viscosity in a membrane is greater by at least a factor of 100 (Edidin, 1974), the observed relaxation times of gating effects and asymmetry currents (around 1 msec) are consistent with an additional activation factor of only 10^{-3}, corresponding to 4 kcal/mol.

The actual activation energies of transverse rotation must be much higher. Indeed half-times of a few hours for flip-flops of certain phospholipids have been measured (Kornberg and McConnell, 1971) and are equivalent to an extra activation energy of 15 kcal/mol. Generally we can conclude that any amphiphilic molecular structure is practically fixed with its normal axis in the membrane. Fast lateral diffusion, as well as rotational motion around the normal axis, may still be possible and is in fact ordinarily encountered (Edidin, 1974; Cherry et al., 1976).

Analogous reasoning applies to the field-induced displacement of charged structures in the membrane. This, too, can be considered an unlikely mechanism for a voltage-dependent process that is fairly fast and/or displays saturation.

To avoid possible misunderstandings, it should be emphasized that the argument does not in any way imply that there can be no fast movement of charges in a membrane. Only the switching on and off of such events by a *direct* action of the available field is disqualified.

In principle, none of the shortcomings encountered for the purely electrical effects discussed above are associated with models based on conformational changes of intercalated macromolecules. As indicated in Figure 4, such transitions between different configurational states may in fact result in sufficiently large changes of dipole moments but little alteration of shape, so that hydrophobic and hydrophilic interactions are hardly affected.

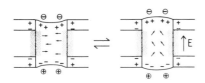

FIGURE 4 Schematic illustration of a field-induced conformational transition of an integral macromolecule spanning the membrane.

The basis of voltage-controlled conformational change

We propose a macromolecule P that is intercalated in the membrane with a fixed orientation parallel to the normal axis and that can exist in two conformational states—P_1 and P_2. The transition

$$P_1 \rightleftharpoons P_2 \tag{14}$$

is characterized by an equilibrium constant

$$K = \frac{\bar{\theta}}{1 - \bar{\theta}}, \tag{15}$$

where $\bar{\theta}$ is the equilibrium value of the degree of transition $\theta = [P_2]/[P]$, that is, the fraction of P in state P_2. If $\mu = \mu_2 - \mu_1$ is the change in dipole moment parallel to the membrane field associated with a molecular transition, we have $\Delta M = N_A \mu$ (N_A being Avogadro's number). Employing equation 8 we readily obtain the field dependence of K as

$$K = K_0 e^{(\mu/kT)E}, \tag{16}$$

where K_0 is the zero-field value of the equilibrium constant. Taking into account equations 13 and 15, this yields

$$\bar{\theta} = \exp \{b(V - V_m)\}/[1 + \exp \{b(V - V_m)\}], \tag{17}$$

where

$$b = \frac{\mu/d}{kT}, \qquad V_m = \Delta\psi - \frac{1}{b} \ln K_0. \tag{18}$$

Accordingly the voltage V_m, which determines the midpoint of the transition, is essentially controlled by the thermodynamic properties of the conformational states and can thus be shifted by external parameters such as temperature, pressure, pH, and interaction with certain ligands.

As far as the kinetics of the transition is concerned, we must consider a fairly large number of intermediate states through which the overall reaction proceeds. In the simplest case, one of the individual activation barriers is much higher than the others, so that the corresponding intermediate step becomes rate-limiting. Then the forward reaction can be written

$$P_1 \rightleftharpoons P^* \xrightarrow{k^*} P_2, \tag{19}$$

where P^*, the intermediate state associated with the rate-limiting elementary rate constant k^*, is in equilibrium with P_1. This implies a first-order rate law for $P_1 \rightarrow P_2$ and a rate constant $k' = K^* k^*$, where the equilibrium constant can be derived as

$$K^* = K_0^* \, e^{(\mu^*/kT)E} \qquad (20)$$

in analogy with equation 16. Since the field dependence of k^* may be neglected (because comparatively small dipole changes are to be expected in elementary reaction steps), the voltage dependence can be expressed as

$$k' = k_{\mathrm{m}} \, e^{b(V - V_{\mathrm{m}})} \qquad (21)$$

with the two new (kinetic) parameters $k_{\mathrm{m}} = k_0' K_0^{-\xi}$ and $\xi = \mu^*/\mu$. The reverse rate constant is then

$$k'' = k'/K = k_{\mathrm{m}} \, e^{-(1 - \xi)b(V - V_{\mathrm{m}})} . \qquad (22)$$

With such first-order rate laws, the time dependence of θ is readily formulated in terms of the relaxation equation

$$\frac{d\theta}{dt} = \frac{\bar{\theta} - \theta}{\tau} , \qquad (23)$$

involving the instantaneous equilibrium value of θ and the relaxation time τ, defined by

$$\frac{1}{\tau} = k' + k'' = k_{\mathrm{m}} \, (1 - \bar{\theta})^{-\xi} \, \bar{\theta}^{-(1-\xi)} . \qquad (24)$$

A graphic representation of $\bar{\theta}$ and τ vs. the membrane potential V is given in Figure 5.

Applying a voltage pulse to the system at time $t = 0$ will displace the original value $\bar{\theta}_0$ to the new equilibrium value $\bar{\theta} = \bar{\theta}_0 + \delta\bar{\theta}$. The actual time course of the transition follows from equation 23:

$$\theta = \bar{\theta} - \delta\bar{\theta} \, e^{-t/\tau} . \qquad (25)$$

The displacement current density j that results under these circumstances from the transition is determined by the time dependence of the contribution to the overall dipole moment:

$$M = M_1 + N\mu\theta , \qquad (26)$$

where M_1 is the dipole moment if all P are in state P_1 and N is the number of P-structures. Thus

$$j = \frac{1}{v} \frac{dM}{dt} = (\mu/d)c_{\mathrm{p}} \frac{\delta\bar{\theta}}{\tau} e^{-t/\tau} , \qquad (27)$$

where v is the volume of the membrane and c_{p} is the number of P per unit area.

As mentioned earlier, symmetric displacement currents are experimentally canceled out by successive depolarizing and hyperpolarizing voltage pulses. If the holding potential V_{h} (at which the pulses start) is chosen low enough so that $\bar{\theta}_0 = 0$ (i.e., all P are in state P_1), only the depolarizing step induces a contribution to the asymmetry current, and this is simply equal to the expression in equation 27 with $\delta\bar{\theta} = \bar{\theta}$ and τ taken at $V = V_{\mathrm{h}} + \delta V$. The charge Q transferred in sufficiently long pulses will then be directly proportional to $\bar{\theta}$; more precisely,

$$Q = \int_0^\infty j \, dt = (\mu/d)c_{\mathrm{p}} \, \bar{\theta}. \qquad (28)$$

At increasing pulse amplitudes, this apparently approaches an upper bound:

$$Q_\infty = (\mu/d)c_{\mathrm{p}}. \qquad (29)$$

This asymptotic behavior is indeed observed in gating-current experiments, as illustrated by the data in Figure 2.

Dipolar relaxation effects in the time domain, as reflected in asymmetry currents, must be accompanied by dielectric polarization to be registered in the frequency domain. In principle, there will be a complex dielectric increment,

$$\Delta\epsilon^* = \frac{1}{\epsilon_0} \frac{\partial(M/v)}{\partial E} , \qquad (30)$$

where ϵ_0 is the absolute permittivity of vacuum (Schwarz, 1967); this comprises a frequency-dependent dielectric constant and dielectric loss caused by the conformational transition of P. The increment of the real dielectric constant, $\Delta\epsilon'$ (Schwarz, 1977), implies a voltage-dependent capacitance increment of the membrane given by

$$\Delta C = \epsilon_0 \Delta\epsilon'/d = \bar{\theta}(1 - \bar{\theta}) \frac{(\mu/d)^2}{kT} c_{\mathrm{p}} \frac{1}{1 + \omega^2\tau^2} , \qquad (31)$$

where ω is angular frequency; this has a maximum at $\bar{\theta} = 0.5$ or $V = V_{\mathrm{m}}$, respectively.

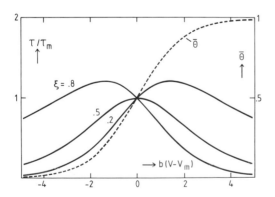

FIGURE 5 Theoretical course of $\bar{\theta}$ and τ vs. membrane potential according to the basic conformational model discussed in the text ($1/\tau_{\mathrm{m}} = 2 \, k_{\mathrm{m}}$).

Experimental results

Some gating-current experiments have resulted in asymmetry currents that exhibit only one relaxation time. We propose that these are due to single-step conformational changes. Examining the squid axon data of Rojas and Keynes (1975) as given in Figure 2 we find

$$Q_\infty = (\mu/d)c_p = 3.1 \times 10^{-8} \text{ C/cm}^2.$$

According to equations 17 and 28, $\ln \{Q/(Q_\infty - Q)\}$ must be a linear function of V. This is in close agreement with the measurements shown in Figure 6. One obtains

$$b = (\mu/d)/kT = 0.054 \text{ mV}^{-1},$$

so that by combination with Q_∞ it follows that

$$c_p = 2,000 \ \mu\text{m}^{-2}, \qquad \mu/d = 6 \text{ D/Å}.$$

In other words, the average distance between the P-structures is about 220 Å, whereas (with $d \approx 50$ Å) the dipole moment changes by roughly 300 D when P_1 turns to P_2.

Our assumed simple kinetics predicts that $\ln k'$ and $\ln k''$ are also linear functions of V. As shown by the plots in Figure 7, this is satisfactorily true for the special system in question. The corresponding parameter ξ is evaluated as 0.63. The theoretical courses of Q and τ are given as solid curves in Figure 2.

A frequency dispersion of the membrane capacitance, as predicted by equation 31, has been observed for a squid axon system by Takashima (1976). Using the above values of μ/d and c_p, the maximum value of ΔC (at $\omega \to 0$ and $\bar{\theta} = 0.5$) is about 0.5 μF/cm^2. This and the relaxation time of about 100 μsec agree fairly well with the measured data. Similar dielectric studies on muscle membranes (Adrian and Almers,

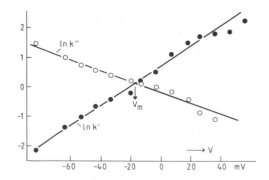

FIGURE 7   Linear plots of $\ln k'$ and $\ln k''$ vs. membrane potential, using data from Figure 2.

1976) have manifested the predicted maximum as a function of voltage.

Dependence on external parameters

Gating phenomena are generally affected by variations in external conditions, particularly temperature, pressure, and the concentrations of certain ligands. With our basic voltage dependent conformational transition in a membrane, this may be understood in terms of effects on the equilibrium constant and the kinetics of the transition. It becomes noticeable in a shift of the sigmoidal $\bar{\theta}$ curve toward higher or lower voltages.

Turning first to temperature effects we derive

$$\frac{\partial \bar{\theta}}{\partial T} = \frac{\partial \bar{\theta}}{\partial \ln K} \frac{\partial \ln K}{\partial T} = \bar{\theta} (1 - \bar{\theta}) \frac{\Delta H}{RT^2} \qquad (32)$$

if van't Hoff's relation is observed. In principle, one must take into consideration the fact that the reaction enthalpy ΔH still depends on the voltage. By differentiation of equation 16 with regard to T and use of equations 13 and 18, it follows that

$$\Delta H = \Delta H_0 - N_A \mu E = \Delta H_0 + RT \ln K_0 \\ - RTb (V - V_m). \quad (33)$$

The electrical contribution is, however, hardly more than 1–2 kcal/mol, as mentioned earlier. The displacement of V_m by changes in temperature can be expressed by

$$\frac{\partial V_m}{\partial T} = -\frac{(\partial \bar{\theta}/\partial T)_m}{(\partial \bar{\theta}/\partial V)_m} = -\frac{\Delta H_m}{b \, RT^2}$$

$$= -\frac{\Delta H_0 + RT \ln K_0}{N_A (\mu/d) \, T} . \quad (34)$$

Numerically this means that V_m is shifted by roughly 0.1 mV per degree and kcal/mol. Thus appreciable

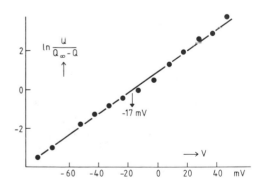

FIGURE 6   Linear plot of $\ln\{Q/(Q_\infty - Q)\}$ vs. membrane potential, using data from Figure 2.

shifts would first of all depend on a considerable zero-field (i.e., chemical) transition enthalpy ΔH_0.

The temperature dependence of measured relaxation times can be discussed analogously on the basis of chemical and electrical activation energies. In the framework of our kinetic model we obtain

$$\frac{\partial \ln \tau}{\partial T} = \{(1 - \bar{\theta})\Delta H - (E_a^* + \Delta H^*)\}/RT^2, \quad (35)$$

where E_a^* is the activation energy of the rate-limiting step in $P_1 \rightarrow P_2$ and ΔH^* is the reaction enthalpy for $P_1 \rightarrow P^*$. From the reported temperature dependence of τ for a squid-axon gating current (Keynes and Rojas, 1974), an overall activation energy of about 15 kcal/mol can be estimated.

The potential effect of certain ligands on the voltage-dependent transition will be a consequence of different binding affinities of the two conformational states. With A being the ligand, we have to consider the reaction system

$$\begin{array}{ccc} P_1 + A & \rightleftharpoons & P_1 A \\ \Updownarrow & & \Updownarrow \\ P_2 + A & \rightleftharpoons & P_2 A \end{array} \quad (36)$$

The total degree of transition from P_1 to P_2 (no matter in which binding state) can easily be calculated on the basis of the mass action laws. Generally we obtain

$$\frac{\partial \bar{\theta}}{\partial c_A} = \frac{K_2 - K_1}{(1 + K_1 c_A)(1 + K_2 c_A)}, \quad (37)$$

where K_1 and K_2 are the binding constants of the two states. Obviously the transition will be displaced toward the state of higher binding strength.

Outlook for more complex systems

Voltage-dependent processes in biological membranes must not generally be expected to result from such a simple transition. Even gating currents are by no means always of this type. Distinctly more complex behavior has indeed been observed, including the occurrence of more than one relaxation time, apparent differences in charge transfer after switching on and off a voltage pulse, and effects of temperature on the apparent value of Q_∞. However, such peculiarities can in principle be attributed to the existence of two or more (possibly coupled) conformational transitions.

Turning to an actual gating process, we note that the most straightforward mechanism consists of a single macromolecule existing in two states: one associated with a pore through the membrane to let the substrate pass, and another closing the pore. We cannot take this idea seriously because it does not agree with the Hodgkin-Huxley equations. To satisfy these, three different macromolecular species, corresponding to the m, h, and n functions, might be assumed to interact with each other in an adequate way. Attempts to interpret the reported asymmetry currents along these lines, as a direct manifestation of the m function, have been made. However, by measuring simultaneously asymmetry currents and the activation of sodium permeability on frog nerves, it was shown that there is no appropriate correlation between these properties (Neumcke, Nonner, and Stämpfli, 1976). This evidence points to a somewhat more sophisticated overall gating mechanism. Even so, the argument favoring conformational changes still applies to the decisive field-sensing step(s) in the mechanism. A reasonable gating model on this basis remains to be developed.

An important aspect of advanced concepts of voltage-dependent molecular systems will doubtless be that of cooperativity. Its potential may first be examined for the basic model used above in order to interpret measured asymmetry ("gating") currents of squid axon. Recall that the data could be fit by assuming independent conformational transitions of individual macromolecules with a change of dipole moment of a few hundred debye. In view of the known order of magnitude of protein dipole moments, this is not unreasonable. It should be emphasized, however, that much smaller changes would be required if an appropriate cooperative interaction occurred between two or more constituent macromolecules. In a fundamental all-or-none model of an aggregate of n strongly interacting macromolecular subunits, each would have to contribute only the nth part of the total dipole change.

In any event, schemes with interacting molecular structures will be indispensable in approaching the physicochemical nature of processes induced by weak electric fields. Transverse motion of dipoles and charges can be disregarded even more easily in these cases. Moreover, our basic conformational model becomes more and more unlikely because of the unreasonably large changes of dipole moments required. Small changes of the latter would be adequate, however, if there is a sufficient degree of cooperative interaction (which may include the cascade phenomena discussed by Stadtman in this volume). We must conclude that effects of weak voltage variations involve some kind of cooperativity in the membrane together with field-induced structural conversions.

ACKNOWLEDGMENTS Support by grants from the Swiss National Foundation (No. 3.487-0.75) and the National Institutes of Health (HL 1253-24) is gratefully acknowledged.

REFERENCES

ADRIAN, R. H., and W. ALMERS, 1976. The voltage dependence of membrane capacity. *J. Physiol.* 254:317–338.

ARMSTRONG, C. M., and F. BEZANILLA, 1974. Charge movements associated with the opening and closing of the activation gates of the Na channels. *J. Gen. Physiol.* 63:533–552.

CHERRY, R. J., A. BÜRKLI, M. BUSSLINGER, G. SCHNEIDER, and G. R. PARISH, 1976. Rotational diffusion of the band 3 proteins in the human erythrocyte membrane. *Nature* 263:389–393.

COLE, K. S., 1949. Dynamic electrical characteristics of the squid axon membrane. *Arch. Sci. Physiol.* 3:253–258.

COLE, K. S., 1968. *Membranes, Ions, and Impulses.* Berkeley: Univ. California Press.

EDIDIN, M., 1974. Rotational and translational diffusion in membranes. *Annu. Rev. Biophys. Bioeng.* 3:179–201.

HODGKIN, A. L., and A. F. HUXLEY, 1952. A quantitative description of membrane current and its application to conduction and excitation in nerve. *J. Physiol.* 117:500–544.

KEYNES, R. D., and E. ROJAS, 1974. Kinetics and steady-state properties of the charged system controlling sodium conductance in the squid giant axon. *J. Physiol.* 239:383–434.

KNIFFKI, K.-D., and W. VOGEL, 1976. Molecular concept of gating the ionic channels in the nerve membrane. *Proceedings of the Third Winter School on Biophysics of Membrane Transport,* vol. 2, J. Kuczera and S. Prestalski, eds. Wroclaw, Poland, pp. 71–116.

KORNBERG, R. D., and H. M. MCCONNELL, 1971. Inside-outside transitions of phospholipids in vesicle membranes. *Biochemistry* 10:1110–1120.

KUFFLER, S. W., and J. G. NICHOLLS, 1976. *From Neuron to Brain.* Sunderland, MA: Sinauer Associates.

MEVES, H., 1974. The effect of holding potential on the asymmetry currents in squid giant axons. *J. Physiol.* 243:847–867.

NEUMCKE, B., W. NONNER, and R. STÄMPFLI, 1976. Asymmetrical displacement current and its relation with activation of sodium current in the membrane of frog myelinated nerve. *Pfluegers Arch.* 363:193–203.

NONNER, W., E. ROJAS, and R. STÄMPFLI, 1975. Displacement currents in the node of Ranvier: Voltage and time dependence. *Pfluegers Arch.* 354:1–18.

ROJAS, E., and R. D. KEYNES, 1975. On the relation between displacement currents and activation of the sodium conductance in the squid giant axon. *Philos. Trans. R. Soc. Lond.* B270:459–482.

SCHWARZ, G., 1967. On dielectric relaxation due to chemical rate processes. *J. Phys. Chem.* 71:4021–4030.

SCHWARZ, G., 1977. Chemical transitions of biopolymers induced by an electric field and their effects in dielectrics and birefringence. *Ann. NY Acad. Sci.* 303:190–197.

SCHWARZ, G., 1978. On the physico-chemical basis of voltage dependent molecular gating mechanisms in biological membranes. *J. Membrane Biol.* 43:127–148.

SCHWARZ, G., and P.-J. BAUER, 1974. Structural flexibility and fast proton transfer reflected by the dielectric properties of poly-L-proline in aqueous solution. *Biophys. Chem.* 1:257–265.

SCHWARZ, G., and U. SCHRADER, 1975. The effects of cooperativity, finite change length, and field induced changes of the conformational equilibrium on the electric birefringence of polypeptides in the range of the helix-coil transition. *Biopolymers* 14:1181–1195.

SCHWARZ, G., and J. SEELIG, 1968. Kinetic properties and the electric field effect of the helix-coil transition of poly(γ-benzyl-L-glutamate) determined from dielectric relaxation measurements. *Biopolymers* 6:1263–1277.

SINGER, S. J., and G. L. NICOLSON, 1972. The fluid mosaic model of the structure of cell membranes. *Science* 175:720–731.

TAKASHIMA, S., 1976. Membrane capacity of squid giant axon during hyper- and depolarizations. *J. Membrane Biol.* 27:21–39.

WADA, A., T. TANAKA, and H. KIHARA, 1972. Dielectric dispersion of the α-helix at the transition region to random coil. *Biopolymers* 11:587–605.

37 The Mechanism of Electrical Excitation in Lipid Bilayers and Cell Membranes

PAUL MUELLER

ABSTRACT The conductance of excitable membranes is a sensitive function of the electrical potential, and kinetic current-voltage data suggest that a cooperative process is involved in the gating action. In principle, two different mechanisms could be operative: one involves an intramolecular configurational change within a permanent channel spanning the membrane; the other, the assembly of an open channel through the voltage-dependent aggregation of channel precursors. In biological membranes there is currently no compelling evidence favoring either alternative, but chemical and kinetic data from lipid bilayers rendered excitable by channel-forming compounds such as EIM, alamethicin, monazomycin, or DJ400 strongly indicate that these systems gate through an aggregation mechanism. The channels formed by these compounds exhibit the same voltage-dependent conductance changes as nerve, and the kinetic and steady-state aspects of the gating conform to the Hodgkin-Huxley scheme and can be described by the Hodgkin-Huxley equations. It is suggested that the gating process involves the voltage-dependent insertion of the channel-forming molecules into the hydrocarbon region and their subsequent aggregation by lateral diffusion into an open channel. The mathematical description of this process accounts quantitatively for the observed conductance kinetics, including inactivation as well as other kinetic features that lie outside the Hodgkin-Huxley domain but are also observed in nerve. For alamethicin, the single-channel conductance fluctuations are in agreement with this excitation model; and a complete set of the individual molecular insertion and aggregation rate constants has been derived from a combined analysis of single-channel statistics and multichannel, voltage-clamp kinetics in a lecithin bilayer. In this lipid most of the alamethicin exists as monomer, the dimer formation is rate-limiting, and there is a positive free-energy difference of approximately 4 kcal/mol between dimers and monomers. The relevance of this gating mechanism to cellular excitation is discussed.

Introduction

THERE IS A large body of evidence indicating that ions cross cell membranes through special pores or channels embedded in a lipid bilayer matrix and that, in many instances, the channels can be opened or closed by small changes of the membrane potential.

PAUL MUELLER Department of Molecular Biology, Eastern Pennsylvania Psychiatric Institute, Philadelphia, PA 19129

The structure of such channels and the mechanism by which the ion fluxes are gated by the electric field remain unknown; but the steady-state and kinetic relations between the potential and the ionic channels have been analyzed in great detail, first by Hodgkin and Huxley (1952a–d) for the squid axon membrane and subsequently by other investigators for many different cell membranes (see, e.g., Frankenhaeuser, 1960, 1963; Adrian, Chandler, and Hodgkin, 1970; Neher, 1971; Moolenaar and Spector, 1977). In all cases the basic aspects of these relations are essentially the same, suggesting that there may be a common gating mechanism, even though the channels may have different ion specificities.

Many current ideas about the existence, possible structure, and functions of membrane channels are based on experiments with lipid bilayers. Several compounds obtained from bacteria or fungi, when incorporated into bilayers, increase their ion permeability, apparently through the formation of channels (Mueller and Rudin, 1969; Cass, Finkelstein, and Krespi, 1970), and a few have been found to form channels that display voltage-dependent ion gating with steady-state and kinetic characteristics identical to excitable cell membranes (Mueller and Rudin, 1967, 1968a,b, 1969; Muller and Finkelstein, 1972). Although the ion specificities of these channels are limited to broad classes such as anions or cations, they are capable of generating typical action potentials under appropriate experimental conditions (Mueller and Rudin, 1968a). The chemical natures and molecular sizes of these compounds are rather diverse, ranging from a protein (EIM) and a polypeptide (alamethicin) to cyclic polyene (DJ400) and a polyene-like compound (monazomycin); but as in natural membranes, the similarities of the gating kinetics and other evidence point to a common gating mechanism.

For the cellular channels, it is commonly assumed that the gating mechanism involves a voltage-controlled configurational change of the channel structure and, more specifically, that there are well-defined parts of the channel, called gates, whose position or configuration can block the channel opening (Armstrong, 1975). In contrast, analysis of the bilayer channels has led to the conclusion that the gating process involves the formation of a channel through the field-dependent insertion of nonconducting channel precursors into the bilayer hydrocarbon region and their subsequent aggregation into an open channel (Mueller and Rudin, 1968b; Baumann and Mueller, 1974; Boheim, 1974; Mueller, 1975a, 1976). Whereas in the bilayers the evidence for an insertion-aggregation mechanism is rather compelling, the data currently available for nerve and other excitable tissues do not unequivocally support one or the other mechanism. The question of whether an aggregation mechanism applies also to biological membranes can only be resolved after chemical data similar to those available for the bilayers have been obtained.

Steady-state and kinetic aspects of the conductance-voltage relation

Examples of the principal relations between the average conductance of many channels and the potential are shown in Figure 1. Aside from the absolute values of the time constants, the following features appear identical in excitable cells and in bilayers.

1. The steady-state conductance is an exponential function of the membrane potential, with an e-fold change for 4–6 mV and a dynamic range of three to four orders of magnitude. The function saturates at higher potentials and can be shifted along the voltage axis by agents controlling the surface potential (such as divalent ions) and, in the bilayer case, by the lipid composition (Muller and Finkelstein, 1972). Potentials of only one sign increase the conductance. For the bilayers this is true only when the channel-forming molecules are added to one side and remain there.

2. The conductance rises with a sigmoidal time course after a sudden displacement of the membrane potential. The initial delay varies from system to system and can be controlled by the membrane potential and, in bilayers, by the lipid composition and the chemical nature of the channel former.

3. The transition from a high to a low conductance, following an appropriate potential change, is exponential with time constants that go through a maximum as a function of the potential.

4. In many instances the rising conductance goes through a maximum before reaching the steady-state level. This process, called inactivation, has been observed in varying degrees in all systems studied so far. It can be controlled experimentally and is most pronounced in the sodium channels of nerve.

Neglecting inactivation, the steep voltage dependence of the conductance, its delayed rise, and its exponential decay are accounted for by the Hodgkin-Huxley scheme, which can be summarized in simplified form as follows:

$$P_0 \underset{k_{10}}{\overset{k_{01}}{\rightleftarrows}} P_1; \qquad g \approx (P_1)^n, \qquad (1)$$

where the membrane potential controls the position or configuration of assumed gating particles between P_0 and P_1 through voltage-dependent rate constants k_{01} and k_{10}, and the conductance g is proportional to the nth power of P_1.

The long delays observed, for example, in the squid axon potassium system or with monazomycin in bilayers (Cole and Moore, 1960; Mueller, 1976) require values for n of up to 40; this makes a direct molecular interpretation of this scheme—in which n gating particles must be in a given position for the channel to open—rather awkward. Furthermore, more detailed kinetic experiments using more complex pulsing sequences have revealed that the opening and closing time constants depend not only on the membrane potential but also on the previous rate and direction of the conductance change. These and other observations have prompted consideration of alternative kinetic schemes (Goldman, 1975, 1976; Jakobsson and Scudiero, 1975; Jakobsson, 1976; Moore and Cox, 1976) that implicitly or explicitly assume a sequential configurational change of the channel in which the time constants of each step are voltage-controlled. For example:

$$P_0 \underset{k_{10}}{\overset{k_{01}}{\rightleftarrows}} P_1 \underset{k_{21}}{\overset{k_{12}}{\rightleftarrows}} P_2 \cdots P_n; \qquad g \approx P_n. \qquad (2)$$

In this case the conductance is proportional to the concentration of the channel molecules having the configuration P_n. Such schemes can account for some of the more complex kinetics lying outside the realm of the Hodgkin-Huxley equation. However, both the basic Hodgkin-Huxley scheme (Hodgkin and Huxley, 1952a–d) and the sequential models require additional, ad hoc assumptions about the inactivation process.

The insertion-aggregation mechanism

In the bilayer case additional data, not yet available for the cellular channels, strongly support an aggregation mechanisn. Much is known about the chemical structure of the channel-forming molecules, particularly alamethicin and its chemical analogs and

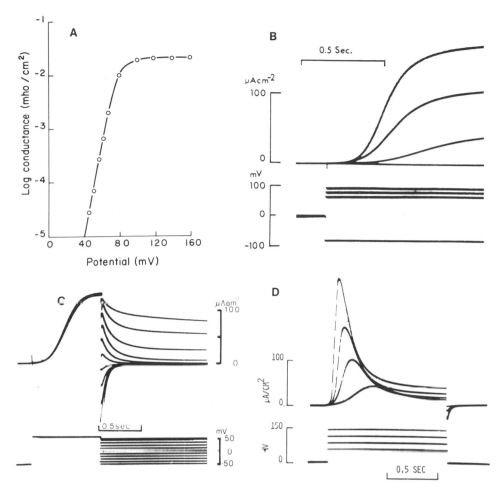

FIGURE 1   The primary aspects of the steady-state and kinetic relations between the potential and the currents in excitable membranes are illustrated by voltage-clamp records obtained from lipid bilayer membranes in the presence of monazomycin. (A) The relation between the steady-state conductance and the potential in a lecithin bilayer in the presence of 2×10^{-6} monazomycin on one side and 0.1 M KCl on both sides. The conductance-voltage curve can be shifted along the voltage axis by agents controlling the surface potential and in bilayers by the charge of the lipid head groups. (B) Membrane currents in response to applied potential steps of different amplitude and sign for a bilayer (oleyl phosphate-cholesterol) in the presence of 10^{-6} M monazomycin on one side and 0.01 M NaCl on both sides; temperature, 25°C. Several oscillograph sweeps are superimposed. Note the long delay of the current rise and the absence of measureable current for negative potential steps. (C) Membrane currents in response to applied po-

tential steps for a lecithin bilayer in the presence of 10^{-6} M monazomycin (one side) and 0.01 M KCl (both sides). Eleven records are superimposed. The voltage steps were applied at 20 sec intervals from a holding potential of -50 mV. Note that the time constants of the exponential conductance decays show a maximum near 35 mV (third trace from top in the current records). (D) Membrane currents (upper record) in response to applied potential steps (lower record) from a lecithin bilayer in the presence of 10^{-5} M monazomycin at a temperature of 38°C. At this concentration of monazomycin and at the elevated temperature, the currents show an early maximum and subsequent decline—that is, inactivation. The magnitude of inactivation—that is, the ratio of the steady state to the peak conductance   is a variable and depends in the bilayers on the nature and concentration of the translocator, the lipid composition, and external factors such as the ionic composition of the aqueous phase and temperature.

DJ400 (Bohlmann et al., 1970; Jung et al., 1976; Martin and Williams, 1976; Bukovsky, 1977; Gisin, Kabayashi, and Hall, 1977). The composition of the lipid phase, the concentration of channel formers, and their orientation can be controlled, and the arguments favoring aggregation rest primarily on the

observation that the steady-state conductance and the time constants of the voltage-controlled conductance change are high-order functions of the concentration of channel-forming compounds (see Figure 2).

Both results suggest that more than one molecule is involved in the formation of an open channel; but

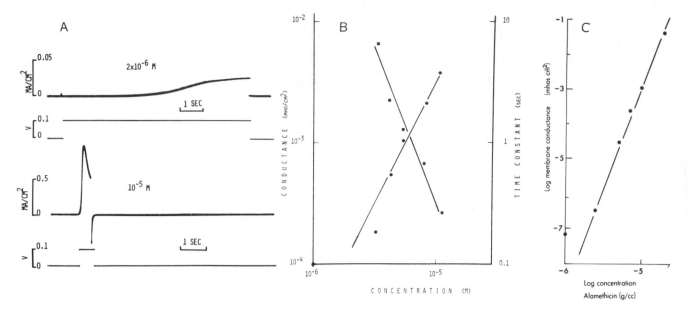

FIGURE 2 (A) Membrane currents in response to applied potential steps from a lecithin bilayer in the presence of different concentrations of monazomycin. A 5-fold increase in concentration causes a 25-fold decrease of the time constant and a 40-fold increase of the current amplitude. At the higher concentration the current inactivates. (From Mueller, 1976.) (B) The relation between the concentration of monazomycin in the aqueous phase, the time constant of the conductance rise (squares), and the peak conductance (circles) of a lecithin bilayer in response to a 100 mV potential step. The slope of the conductance-concentration curve increases at lower concentrations, and higher-order functions up to 8 have been observed between 10^{-7} and 10^{-6} M. (C) The relation between the membrane conductance and the concentration of alamethicin in the aqueous phase at constant ion concentration (0.01 M NaCl) and constant voltage (60 mV). (From Mueller and Rudin, 1968.) The slope of such curves varies with experimental conditions, but similar high-order functions with exponents between 2 and 10 have been observed with EIM, monazomycin, and DJ400.

more significantly, the relation between the gating time constants and concentration of channel formers indicates almost unequivocally that the gating process itself involves an association of several channel precursors to form an open channel.

In its simplest form the insertion-aggregation process may be illustrated by the scheme of Figure 3 and exemplified by the cyclic polyene DJ400 (Figure 4A). Many variants of this scheme involving more complex molecular structures can be realized, but the critical features would remain constant:

1. The channel-forming part of the molecule must be long enough to span the nonconducting region of the bilayer.

2. It must contain, at one end, a hydrophilic group that anchors that part of the molecule at the lipid-water interface.

3. Either the opposite end must contain a charged group or the channel-forming structure must have a large dipole moment.

4. The part of the molecule entering the hydrocarbon region must contain several polar groups facing one side; the other side should be predominantly hydrophobic.

If these conditions are fulfilled, the gating is assumed to proceed in the following way. At a potential where the membrane conductance is low, the molecules lie at the membrane surface. An applied field of appropriate sign pulls the charged end through the membrane toward the other side so that the molecules span the membrane. Aggregation of the monomers by lateral diffusion leads to the formation of dimers, trimers, and so on. Monomers and dimers do not form open channels, but higher oligomers do. In the open channels the polar groups face toward the center, forming a hydrophilic lining, while the nonpolar sides of the translocator face outward, interacting with the hydrocarbon chains. After removal of the field the molecules return to their original position at the membrane surface. The charge or dipole moment represents the gating charge, and its movement into and out of the membrane would generate a small displacement current also predicted by the Hodgkin-Huxley theory.

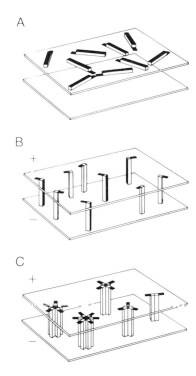

A

B

+

−

C

+

−

FIGURE 3   A model of the excitation process. (A) At rest, models of the translocator molecules lie flat on the membrane surface, represented by the upper plane. (B) An applied field has pulled the charged end of the translocator molecules into the membrane towards the trans surface. (C) Lateral diffusion within the membrane leads to aggregation of the monomers into oligomers. Trimers, tetramers, pentamers, and hexamers form a central opening, acting as a channel for the flow of ions. Dimers are not conductive. (From Baumann and Mueller, 1974.)

Although the cyclic polymers are ideally suited for this type of channel, the structural requirements for such a gating mechanism can also be met by peptide chains, either singly or in hairpin loops. For alamethicin a specific configuration had been suggested (Figure 4b), based on a cyclic structure in which the peptide is arranged into an ellipsoid with one side in β configuration and the other side forming a hydrophobic α-helix. Alamethicin is now known to be a linear peptide (Martin and Williams, 1970), but the proposed hairpin configuration could still be correct.

DJ400 has its own gating charge in the form of the amino group located at one end of the molecule. For alamethicin it had been suggested that a cation is coordinated in the hairpin loop (Baumann and Mueller, 1974) because the conductance is also a high-order function of the salt concentration. Although there is no direct evidence for cation binding, alamethicin does have a dipole moment of 70 debye units, which is sufficient to account for the steepness

of the conductance-voltage relation within the framework of the insertion-aggregation model (Yantorno, Takashima, and Mueller, 1977).

Mathematical description of the gating process

The formation of open channels through aggregation is assumed to proceed in two steps. The first is the insertion or orientation of precursor molecules from a position at the membrane surface into the membrane interior so that they span the hydrocarbon region. In the second step the inserted molecules aggregate through lateral diffusion and form open channels.

Formally the first step is described by

$$P_0 \underset{k_{10}}{\overset{k_{01}}{\rightleftharpoons}} P_1, \tag{3}$$

where P_0 represents the fraction of precursors at the membrane surface and P_1 that of inserted monomers.

The precursor molecules are assumed to have a large dipole moment, so that the insertion is voltage-dependent and equivalent to the motion of 1 or 2 electronic charges (gating charge) through the entire field, that is, through the hydrocarbon region. Thus the insertion rate constants have the following form:

$$k_{01} = A \exp\{-(E_{01} - 11.525zV/RT)\}, \tag{4}$$

$$k_{10} = A \exp\{-(E_{10} - 11.525zV/RT)\}. \tag{5}$$

These two first-order rate constants correspond to α and β in the Hodgkin-Huxley formulation; A is a constant determined by molecular parameters, E the activation energy, z the equivalent valency of the gating charge or the dipole moment, and V the membrane potential in electron volts. E and RT are expressed in kcal/mol, and a factor of 23.05 is used to convert electron volts into kcal/mol. An additional factor of 0.5 implies that the equivalent gating charge traverses the entire field.

During the second step the inserted monomers aggregate according to

$$P_1 + P_n \underset{k_{n+1,n}}{\overset{k_{n,n+1}}{\rightleftharpoons}} P_{n+1}, \tag{6}$$

$$P_1 + P_{m-1} \underset{k_{m,m-1}}{\overset{k_{m-1,m}}{\rightleftharpoons}} P_m, \tag{7}$$

where P_n varies from P_1 to P_m and represents the fraction of monomers, dimers, and higher oligomers, P_m being the largest oligomer formed.

The total concentration of channel formers, C, is then

$$C = P_0 + \sum_{n=1}^{m} nP_n. \tag{8}$$

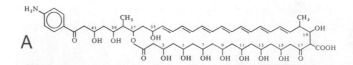

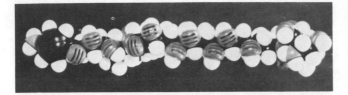

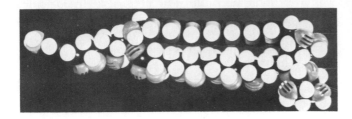

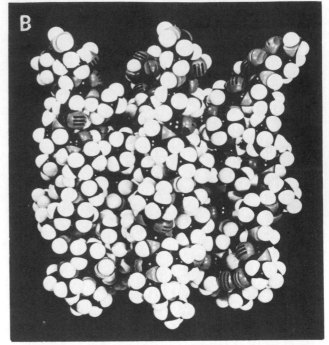

The differential rate equations describing this scheme have the following form:

$$\frac{dP_0}{dt} = P_1 k_{10} - P_0 k_{01} , \qquad (9)$$

$$\frac{dP_1}{dt} = P_0 k_{01} + 2P_2 k_{21} + \sum_{n=3}^{m} nP_n k_{n,n-1}$$

$$- \sum_{n=1}^{m-1} nP_1 P_n k_{n,n+1} - P_1 k_{10} , \qquad (10)$$

$$\frac{dP_n}{dt} = (n-1)P_1 P_{n-1} k_{n-1,n} + (n+1)P_{n+1} k_{n+1,n}$$

$$- nP_n k_{n,n-1} - nP_1 P_n k_{n,n+1} \qquad (n > 1), \quad (11)$$

$$\frac{dP_m}{dt} = mP_1 P_{m-1} k_{m-1,m} - mP_m k_{m,m-1} . \qquad (12)$$

In the calculations presented below it was assumed that the largest oligomer was a hexamer, so that $m = 6$.

In the simplest case one might assume that the aggregation rate constants k_{12} to k_{56} are independent of voltage and are of the general form

$$k_{n,n+1} = A \exp\left(-E_{n,n+1}/RT\right) , \qquad (13)$$

where A is again a constant expressing molecular parameters such as collision frequencies and steric factors. However, there is experimental evidence indicating that in the bilayer case the aggregation rates are dependent on the voltage, in the sense that the ratio of the aggregation rate constants to the dissociation constants increases with the applied potential in a manner that depends on experimental conditions such as lipid fluidity, translocator concentration, and temperature (Mueller, 1975b). Since this voltage de-

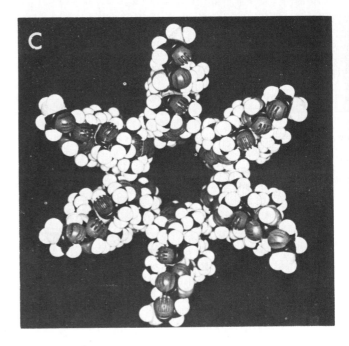

FIGURE 4   (A) The structure and a molecular model of the cyclic polyene DJ400. The formula (top) is that of the aglycone. The position of the sugar in the model is hypothetical but in agreement with the usual position of this residue in other polyenes. (From Mueller, 1975a.) (B, C) A molecular model of a hypothetical hexameric channel formed by the aggregation of six alamethicin molecules. (B) Side view. (C) Top view. (From Baumann and Mueller, 1974.)

pendence cannot be easily determined for the bilayer case and is certainly unknown for nerve, and since its physical origin is not fully understood, a more complex empirical expression allowing the adjustment of the voltage dependence of the rate constant has been used for some of the calculations.

For computational purposes the differential rate equations are solved by numerical methods. The computations are slow when the ratio of rate constants is greater than 10^2; and since most of the computations begin at a steady state corresponding to a holding potential, it was found useful to obtain the steady-state value of the individual oligomer concentrations from a polynomial expression, valid under conditions when

$$\frac{dP_n}{dt} = 0. \tag{14}$$

In this case

$$P_0 k_{01} = P_1 k_{10} \tag{15}$$

and

$$n P_1 P_n k_{n,n+1} = (n + 1) P_{n+1} k_{n+1,n}. \tag{16}$$

Substitution leads to the equations for P_n in terms of P_1:

$$P_0 = P_1 k_{10} / k_{01}, \tag{17}$$

$$P_1 = P_0 k_{01} / k_{10}, \tag{18}$$

$$P_n = (1/n) (P_1)^n \prod_{i=1}^{n} k_{i-1,i} \Big/ \prod_{i=1}^{n} k_{i,i-1} \quad (n > 1). \tag{19}$$

These equations are substituted into equation 16; the resulting polynomial is solved by numerical methods for P_1, and the individual values of P_0 and P_n are obtained by solving equations 17 and 19 for P_n.

Solution of equations 4–19 gives the concentrations of the individual oligomeric channels as a function of time and membrane potential in arbitrary units. To derive from this concentration the absolute values of the membrane conductance, the conductances of the individual oligomeric channels and the total surface concentrations of the channel precursors must be determined. For alamethicin the conductances of the individual oligomeric channels are known from single-channel data (Gordon and Haydon, 1972), and estimates are available for the concentrations of channel precursors. In this case, the membrane conductance in S/cm^2 is obtained from

$$g_m = \sum_{n=3}^{m} g_n \tag{20}$$

when C in equation 8 is expressed in molecules/cm^2 and the rate constants are expressed in cm^2/sec and molecule^{-1}. Equation 20 assumes that the monomers and dimers are not conductive.

Not only do solutions of these equations for different holding potentials and pulsing sequences conform to the basic conductance-voltage kinetics described by the Hodgkin-Huxley equations (see Figure 5), but, with appropriately chosen rate constants, they can also account for kinetic peculiarities that are not part of the Hodgkin-Huxley scheme. Such features appear in both the bilayer systems and, in almost identical form, the squid axon (W. Adelman, R. French, and P. Mueller, unpublished; G. S. Oxford, personal communication). Some examples are shown in Figure 6.

Within the framework of the aggregation model, these effects appear because dimers and higher oligomers cannot be pulled out of the membrane by the field before they have dissociated into monomers. For fast pulsing sequences these residual oligomers, especially the dimers, form a reservoir with which newly inserted monomers can react without going through the slow nucleation step of dimer formation.

The model can also account for the large variability of the delayed onset of the conductance increase observed in cell membranes and bilayers. With alamethicin the delay depends to a great extent on the lipid composition and viscosity; in lecithin membranes the conductance increase is almost exponential, with very short delays and disproportionately long time constants of the overall conductance increase; in bilayers containing monazomycin the delays are very large. In the Hodgkin-Huxley equations the delay after a voltage step is controlled by the exponent, n, in equation 1. Under the usual experimental conditions exponents between 3 and 6 fit the data. However, when the value of the holding potential is increased beyond 60 mV, the delay increases, and exponents up to 24 have been used to fit the curves for the squid axon potassium system (Cole and Moore, 1960). Even larger exponents are required to fit the monazomycin currents. Obviously such large values make little sense when they are interpreted as representing the molecularity of the gating reaction.

In the aggregation model the delay is controlled by the values of the individual rate constants. Short delays result when the formation of the smaller nonconducting oligomers has a higher activation energy than that of the larger oligomers; and very long delays can be obtained even for hexameric channels when the aggregation rates are assumed to become progressively lower with increasing channel size.

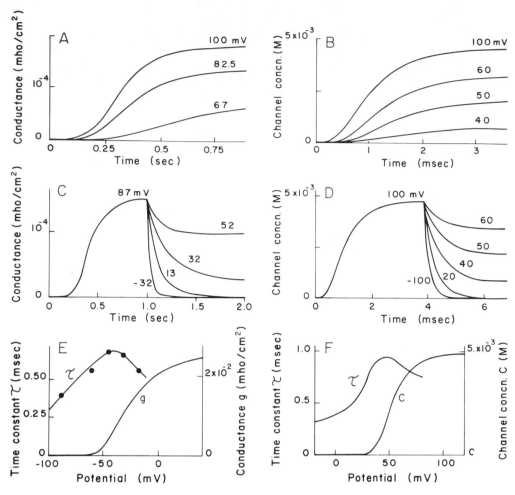

FIGURE 5 Comparison between recorded and calculated conductance changes. (A, C) Conductance changes in response to the indicated voltage-clamp pulses from a bilayer membrane in the presence of 10^{-6} M monazomycin. (B, D) Concentration of hexameric channels in response to similar voltage pulses, as calculated from equations 4–19 using the following constants: $C = 1$; $E_{01} = 3$; $E_{10} = 1$; all other Es are set equal to 2; $A = 100$. The time scale is arbitrarily adjusted by the choice of the frequency factor A, which causes merely a linear transformation of the current patterns. (E) Relations between peak sodium conductance, the time constants of the conductance changes, and the potential as an example of these relations (from data by Hodgkin and Huxley, 1952d). (F) The same relations as calculated using the constants from parts B and D.

Inactivation

Inactivation occurs to a variable degree in excitable bilayers and in cells. In order to account for it, Hodgkin and Huxley assumed a separate, voltage-dependent process and described it by separate equations. In recent years theoretical arguments and experimental data have been presented showing that inactivation is sequentially coupled to activation, that is, to the channel opening. Appropriate modifications of the Hodgkin-Huxley equations have been developed to take this fact into account (Hoyt, 1971; Goldman, 1976). These equations still assume a mechanism of inactivation that is physically separate from the activation process.

In the aggregation model inactivation is a direct consequence of the reaction, provided the rate constants are such that the nonconductive oligomers—for example, the dimers—have a lower free energy or are formed at a lower rate than the conducting oligomers. Under these conditions the concentration of higher oligomers, that is, of conducting channels, initially builds up very fast from the inserted monomers but then decays back into nonconductive dimers; in the inactivated state the majority of the translocators are in the form of dimers.

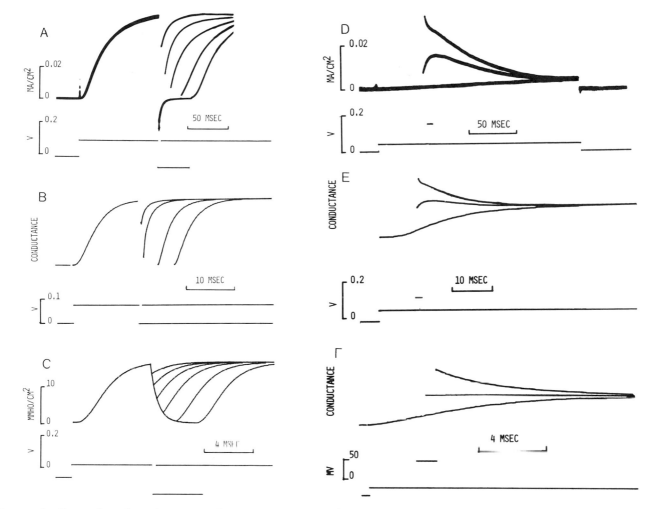

FIGURE 6 Examples of conductance voltage kinetics that are not in accordance with the Hodgkin-Huxley scheme, demonstrating that the time course of the conductance changes depends not only on the potential but also on the value and direction of change of the conductance itself. (A) Membrane currents in response to applied potential steps from a lecithin bilayer in the presence of 2×10^{-6} M alamethicin. Five records are superimposed on a storage scope. During each sweep the potential was raised first to 100 mV, then inverted to -50 mV for a variable time; it was then returned to 100 mV. The initial 100 mV pulse causes a delayed current rise; during the -50 mV pulse the current inverts and falls to zero. The membrane conductance also falls exponentially, as is evident from the instantaneous currents upon repolarizing to 100 mV. When the -50 mV pulse is short, the consequent current rise has a short time constant that increases with the duration of the -50 mV pulse and the decay of the conductance. (B) Conductance changes calculated from the aggregation model for the same pulse sequence as in part A but slightly different voltages. The curves were calculated from equations 4–20 using constants similar to those shown in Table I. For clarity, the conductance decay during the -10 mV pulse was not drawn. (C) The same pulse sequence as calculated from the Hodgkin-Huxley equations for the potassium conductance. In this case there is no shortening of the time constants. Instead the curves can be superimposed by simple displacement along the time axis—that is, the time constants do not change at all. (D) Membrane currents

in response to potential steps from a lipid bilayer (oleyl phosphate-cholesterol) in the presence of 10^{-6} M alamethicin. Three records are superimposed. During the first (lowest trace) the potential is stepped from 0 to 50 mV, causing a slowly rising current. During the next sweep a brief voltage pulse is superimposed on the 50 mV step. During this pulse the membrane current rises briefly (not visible in the record) and then continues to rise transiently after the end of the pulse (middle trace). During the continued rise the current overshoots the steady-state value. When the voltage pulse lasts longer, the current (top trace) starts from a higher level at the end of the pulse and falls monotonically to the steady-state level. (E) Conductance changes resulting from the voltage-pulse sequence shown in part D, as calculated from the aggregation model. The continued rise and overshoot of the conductance results in the model from the continued aggregation of the inserted monomers. The curves were calculated from numerical solutions of equations 4–20 as in part B. For clarity the conductance rise during the brief pulses was omitted from the tracings. (F) The same pulse sequence as in part D, calculated from the Hodgkin-Huxley equations for the potassium conductance. In the Hodgkin-Huxley scheme the currents do not exceed the steady-state value and do not show an early maximum; instead they approach the control current monotonically. These phenomena have also been observed with EIM, monazomycin, and DJ400 and in the potassium and sodium systems of nerve. (From Mueller, 1976.)

Calculations show that this process can account for all the kinetic phenomena related to inactivation, including not only the basic Hodgkin-Huxley kinetics (see Figures 7 and 8; but also deviations from this scheme—such as the variable degree of inactivation, the shifts of the inactivation curve along the voltage axis as a function of different test potentials, and the delayed onset of inactivation (Peller and Barnett, 1962). In this model inactivation is a polymerization overshoot, a phenomenon known to occur in linear polymerizations such as that of tobacco mosaic virus coat protein (Scheele and Schuster, 1974).

Gating currents

Gating currents have not yet been observed in the bilayer systems, primarily because there are no specific compounds available that block the channels without affecting the gating process. Nevertheless the dipole orientation or charge displacement associated with the insertion of the channel-forming monomers into the membrane should give rise to displacement currents similar to those observed in the squid axon (Armstrong and Bezanilla, 1973; Keynes and Rojas, 1974). Calculations show that such currents, which are time differentials of changes of monomer concentration, have a particular relation to the holding potential and the amplitude as well as to the direction of the applied potential changes.

Furthermore, the monomer aggregation has certain theoretical consequences for the time course and amplitude of these currents that are very similar to those observed in the squid axon, and again there are deviations from the basic Hodgkin-Huxley scheme. The time constants of the monomer removal connected with the closing of the gates become larger as more channels open, because the channels have to dissociate into monomers before they can be pulled back to the surface. This phenomenon becomes even more pronounced in the inactivated state because most of the monomers have formed dimers and, since a low free energy of the dimers is a prerequisite of inactivation, the dimer dissociation rate is low. Consequently, calculated gating currents associated with repolarizing pulses from the inactivated state have a small amplitude and two time constants—a fast one corresponding to the removal of still-existing monomers and a slower one that depends on the dissociation rate of dimers. The time constant of the slow phase is that of the recovery of inactivation, and gating currents associated with depolarizations at a time when the recovery from inactivation is incomplete have only a small amplitude because only a portion

of the monomers have returned to the membrane surface. The gating currents in the squid sodium system behave in this way (Armstrong and Bezanilla, 1977).

Single channels

In the bilayer systems the conductance fluctuations associated with the gating of a single channel provide further evidence for the aggregation model, and the fluctuation statistics can be used to derive the multi-channel kinetics.

The single channels of alamethicin have been studied in great detail (Gordon and Haydon, 1972; Eisenberg, Hall, and Mead, 1973; Boheim, 1974; Mueller, 1975b), and their kinetic properties can be summarized as follows:

1. At a constant voltage the conductance fluctuates among five or six well-defined levels.

2. The fluctuations occur sequentially between adjacent levels and never involve more than one level.

3. The spacing between the levels, that is, the amplitude of the conductance steps, increases in a systematic manner from the lower to the higher levels.

4. The frequencies of the transition from one level to the next follow a Poisson distribution.

5. The average lifetimes of the different levels have an approximate Gaussian distribution. The distribution maximum shifts from lower to higher levels with increasing membrane potential.

6. The individual transition rates, defined as the number of transitions from a given level to the next per unit lifetime of that level, depend on the voltage in the sense that the ratio of the upward transition rates to the downward transition rates increases with increasing voltage.

7. The individual transition frequencies increase with increasing voltage.

8. The transition frequencies at a fixed potential increase with increasing concentrations of alamethicin.

9. The lifetime distribution of the levels, measured at a fixed potential, is shifted to higher levels with increasing alamethicin concentrations.

10. The transition frequencies are an inverse function of the lipid viscosity.

The conductance values at the different levels can be derived quantitatively from the hypothetical channel dimensions, and the increase in level spacing is a direct consequence of the postulated channel enlargement by monomer interposition (Baumann and Mueller, 1974). The interlevel transition rates appear to be of first order because the concentration of mon-

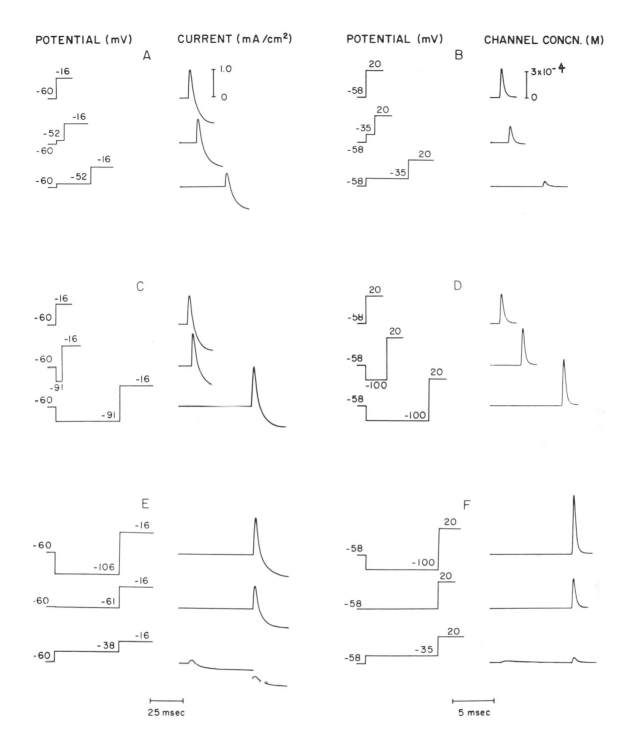

POTENTIAL (mV) · CURRENT (mA/cm²) · POTENTIAL (mV) · CHANNEL CONCN. (M)

25 msec

5 msec

FIGURE 7 Comparison between inactivation in nerve and in the aggregation model. Records A, C, and E are membrane currents in response to potential steps (replotted from Hodgkin and Huxley, 1952c). The upward peaks are primarily sodium currents, while the currents going below the baseline are potassium currents. Records B, D, and F represent the calculated channel concentrations in response to similar pulse patterns. They were obtained from numerical solutions of equations 4–19, assuming that only hexamers form a conductive channel and that they are the largest possible oligomers. The activation energies E of the rate constants (equations 4, 5, 13) had the following values (in kcal/mol): $E_1 = 0.9$; $E_{10} = 2.1$; $E_{12} = 0$; $E_{21} = 3.2$; E_{23} to E_{65} all 0. All pre-exponential factors (A) were set equal to 2×10^4, and $C = 1$ mol/l. With this set of rate constants, the dimers have a lower free energy, and in the inactivated state most of the inserted monomers have formed nonconducting dimers.

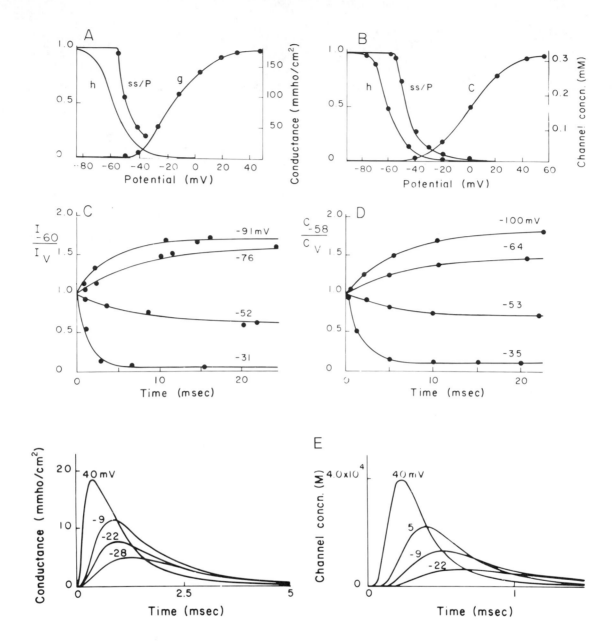

FIGURE 8 Summary of the data in Figure 7. (A) Relation between peak sodium conductance (curve g), inactivation (curves h and ss/P), and the membrane potential in the squid axon. Curve h represents the peak sodium currents in response to voltage steps from different holding potentials to a fixed test potential divided by the peak current in response to a voltage step from −80 mV to the test potential. Curve ss/P represents the ratio of the steady-state to the peak conductance for responses to voltage steps from a holding potential of −80 mV to different test potentials. (Replotted from data by Hodgkin and Huxley, 1952d.) (B) Relation between the peak hexameric channel concentration and the same voltage parameters as in part A, as calculated from the aggregation model. The rate constants were the same as in Figure 7. (From Mueller, 1975a.) (C) The time course of the inactivation at four different membrane potentials in the sodium system of the squid axon. The ordinate represents the ratio of the peak sodium currents in response to voltage steps from different holding potentials (I_V) to the peak current from a holding potential

of −60 mV (I_{-60}). The test potential was −16 mV, and the abscissa represents the time after application of the holding potential. (Replotted from Hodgkin and Huxley, 1952c.) (D) Relation between the peak channel concentration and similar voltage and time parameters as in part B, calculated from the aggregation model. The rate constants were as in part B. Note that there is a small delay at the onset and removal of inactivation and that the time constant does not decrease at the most negative potential, as it does in part C. (From Mueller, 1975a.) (E) The time course of inactivation. The curves on the left were plotted from data by Hodgkin and Huxley (1952) and represent the time course of the sodium conductance in the squid axon in response to voltage steps from a holding potential of −60 mV to the different potentials indicated above each curve. The curves on the right represent the concentration of hexameric channels as a function of time in response to voltage steps from a holding potential of −58 mV to the indicated values. Constants as in Figure 7.

omers is much higher than that of the open channels and thus stays constant during the observation time, as long as the potential is not changed.

The individual rate constants of the aggregation process for the conducting oligomers as a function of the membrane potential can be obtained directly from the statistics of the channel fluctuations at different applied voltages. However, the rate constants of the insertion and of the monomer-dimer transitions are not accessible to direct measurement. Approximate values can be obtained by fitting both the single-channel level distributions at different voltages and the multichannel kinetics by solving the differential equations 4–20. The fit of the level distributions illustrated in Figure 9 assumes the equivalence of the time and assembly averages and gives definite values of the free-energy difference between monomers and dimers and of the free-energy difference between inserted and surface monomers.

Using these values a fit of the multichannel kinetics, obtained at the same alamethicin concentration and from the same membrane, applying the pulsing sequence of Figure 6a and 6b, results in a unique set of rate constants for the entire reaction. The example summarized in Table I shows that in lecithin membranes the dimer formation is considerably slower and has a higher free energy than all other aggregation steps, a conclusion that is also supported by measurements of the latency distributions of the onset of channel fluctuations after voltage steps (Mueller, 1975b).

The reason for the voltage dependence of the aggregation rates has not yet been established, but there is some evidence that it may result from a voltage-induced lateral phase separation between lipids and inserted monomers (Mueller, 1975b). It should be emphasized that this particular set of rate constants holds only for this type of membrane and that even

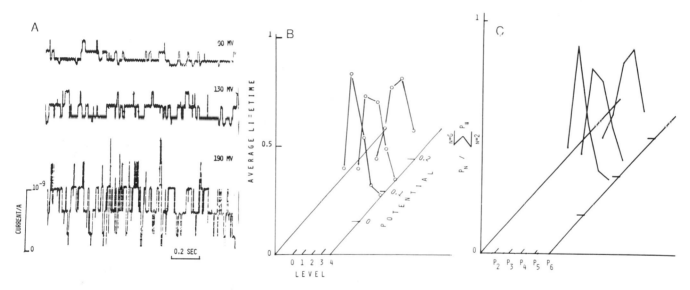

FIGURE 9   (A) Current fluctuations of a single alamethicin channel at three different potentials. Note that with increasing voltage the fluctuation frequencies increase and the conductance-level distribution shifts to higher values. Both effects may be caused by a lateral phase separation between lipid, solvent, and alamethicin. (Lecithin-octane membrane; temperature, 25°C.) Single channels were recorded from a 10 μm micropipette pressed against a preformed larger bilayer. In this way both the single-channel and multichannel kinetics can be recorded from the same membrane. (B) Distribution of average lifetimes among the single-alamethicin-channel conductance levels is plotted at three different membrane potentials. Each point represents the average level lifetime as a fraction of the sum of the lifetimes of levels 0–4 and corresponds in the model to the fractional average lifetime of a particular oligomer. These data were obtained from single-channel records, a portion of which is shown in part A. (C) Distribution of different

oligomers at the same potentials as in part B, calculated from equations 4–20. The rate constants k_{23} to k_{65} were obtained directly from the recorded level lifetimes and transitions shown in part A (as described by Mueller, 1975b). They are shown in Table I. The rate constants k_{01} to k_{12}, which cannot be measured directly from conductance fluctuations, were obtained by fitting the multichannel conductance data obtained from the same membrane to pulse patterns as shown in Figure 6, again using the directly measured rate constants for the higher oligomers. This procedure results in a set of rate constants for the entire insertion-aggregation process. It is valid only for a particular membrane. However, the fact that the electrically silent rate constants, k_{01} to k_{21}, as obtained from multichannel experiments, can be used together with single-channel rate constants for a sensitive fit of the single-channel data (B, C) indicates that the rate constants do not vary much for the different channels within one membrane.

TABLE I

Insertion and aggregation rate constants for alamethicin in a lecithin bilayer

Potential (mV)	k_{01}	k_{10}	k_{12}	k_{21}	k_{23}	k_{32}	k_{34}	k_{43}	k_{45}	k_{54}	k_{56}	k_{65}
90	5.6	0.94	0.035	5.3	19.3	3	5.3	9.1	3.5	15.6		
130	17.7	0.29	0.07	3.8	35	3	8.2	9	4.2	10		
190	38	0.14	0.14	3.8	115	13	45	14.5	25	22	11	35

$k = $ [transition rate]/[conductance-level lifetime $\times$ (level number + 2)] (sec^{-1}).
Constants k_{23} to k_{65} were obtained directly from the single-channel conductance-level transitions, constants k_{01} to k_{21} from fits of equations 4–20 to multichannel conductance data for various voltage-clamp pulsing sequences. The association rate constants increase with the potential, whereas the dissociation constants behave irregularly. Nevertheless the free energy of aggregation becomes more negative with higher potentials, resulting in a preference for the higher oligomers. The rate constants of the formation of dimers are 100- to 1,000-fold lower than those of the higher oligomers, a fact that can also be deduced directly from the single-channel data (Mueller, 1975b). All rate constants have units of sec^{-1} because the local concentration of alamethicin within the bilayer is not known and in the calculations was arbitrarily assumed to be 1.

the ratio of hydrocarbon solvent to lipids in the membrane-forming solution affects these constants.

Two additional points are of interest. Both the time constants of the multichannel conductance changes and the single-channel fluctuation rates depend to a very large extent on the lipid fluidity, the multichannel constants decreasing from a range of seconds in lecithin or oxidized cholesterol membranes to a few hundred microseconds in the very fluid glycerol diolein membranes; at the same time the single-channel fluctuation rates increase by factors between 10 and 100. It thus seems that in the more fluid membranes the dimer formation rate, which is slow and rate-limiting in the lecithin membranes, is disproportionately increased; this is also reflected in the qualitative appearance of the multichannel kinetics in terms of a definite delay followed by a fast conductance rise, instead of the almost exponential rise seen in the more viscous membranes. Why the dimer formation rate should be so slow in some membranes is not clear; nucleation steps are common in polymerization reactions, and it may be that the inserted monomers have a different configuration—their polar carbonyl groups might be shielded by nonpolar side chains—which must then change upon dimer formation. The apparent rate increase of dimer formation in the glycerol diolein membranes may also be a consequence of the different surface potential, and it is of interest in this respect that the kinetics of monazomycin, which are usually not dimer-limited, can become so in the presence of uranyl ions. Even more dramatic effects of the polar membrane surface on the gating kinetics are seen with EIM, where aggregation kinetics and efficient gating are only seen in sphingomyelin-tocopherol membranes.

It should also be kept in mind that the concentration dependence of the rate constant appears to be of high order only if the reactions between the higher aggregates are rate-limiting. Thus in the case of alamethicin in lecithin membranes, where the dimer formation is rate-limiting, the rate constant of the conductance increase is only modestly dependent on concentration.

Application to natural membranes

Because the kinetic aspects of the gating process are so similar in bilayers and in biological membranes, one may ask if the gating mechanisms are the same in both cases. Obviously arguments based on kinetics are by themselves not sufficient to establish a mechanism; only more direct chemical and structural data of the type available for bilayers can settle this question finally. Nevertheless it seems worthwhile to recount and emphasize the kinetic data, which eventually have to be accounted for by any valid model.

Aside from the Hodgkin-Huxley tetrad—the steep voltage dependence of the conductance, its delayed rise and exponential decay, the voltage dependence of the rate constants, and the inactivation—the following additional features have been observed in bilayers and nerve (for a summary see Goldman, 1976, and Mueller, 1976).

1. The gating time constants and, in some cases, the conductance time course depend on the holding potential and on the conductance history (as shown

in Figure 6). Such state-dependent conductance variations become most noticeable for particular pulsing sequences.

2. The inactivation can have a delayed onset, its voltage dependence can be shifted by the value of the test potential, and its time constants as measured by the conductance decay can differ from those measured by applying prepulses. In some membranes (see Goldman, 1976) the inactivation, as measured by the steady-state-to-peak ratio of the membrane current, can be larger or smaller than that measured with the prepulse technique.

The magnitude, time course, and time constants of the gating currents observed in nerve depend not only on the potential but also on the value and past history of the conductance.

All these effects are more or less pronounced in different preparations and under different circumstances, but they are sufficiently prominent to warrant the conclusion that a first-order process controlled by the membrane potential is not the only rate-limiting determinant of the gating process. The reaction or configurational change leading to the channel opening and closing must proceed through a number of sequential steps having separate rates. This would exclude any molecular model based strictly on the Hodgkin-Huxley equations. For example (see Llinas, Steinberg, and Walton, 1976), a channel consisting of several subunits capable of undergoing a voltage-controlled transition between two states—the channel being open when all subunits are in one state—will not show the observed gating kinetics if the subunits undergo their transitions independently of each other. In this case the number of subunits in one channel having the proper configuration depends only on statistical coincidence, and the gating kinetics are strictly voltage-determined.

The same model may, however, display at least some of the state-dependent conductance changes if the configurational changes are initiated by the potential step in one subunit and proceed sequentially from one subunit to the next, the reaction conforming to the scheme 2 above. Again, such a scheme would not show inactivation; but the same argument for the need of a sequentially coupled reaction would also apply to any postulated inactivation mechanism (Goldman, 1976).

Various kinetic schemes have been proposed to accommodate observed exceptions to the Hodgkin-Huxley kinetics (e.g., Hoyt, 1971; Goldman, 1975; Jakobsson and Scudiero, 1975; Moore and Cox, 1976). Most of these models do not attempt to describe a molecular mechanism, and none has been tested against the entire range of experimental data.

An aggregation model of the type described here for the bilayer systems does fulfill the requirement for a sequential coupled mechanism and can account for the more complex kinetics, especially when provisions are made for a voltage dependence of the aggregation rate constants. However, an extrapolation of this simple aggregation scheme to the gating process in biological membranes must take into account several features and observations that do not occur in the bilayer systems.

Most cellular channels show a high degree of cation selectivity, whereas the bilayer systems only distinguish between cations and anions. Certain toxins, such as tetrodotoxin, can block the channel without affecting the gating currents. Furthermore, tetrodotoxin blocks the channels from the outside without their previously having been opened by the potential, while pronase applied to the inside can block the inactivation (Armstrong, Bezanilla, and Rojas, 1973), indicating that parts of the channel are always accessible from both sides. These effects could be explained by the existence of a selectivity filter at the channel entrance. The selectivity filters may be either permanent parts of the channels, as is usually assumed, or separate entities at the membrane surface to which the gating structures link up after their insertion through the membrane. The selectivity conversion from cationic to anionic for EIM and alamethicin channels by externally applied protamine provides an example of a separate filter (Mueller and Rudin, 1968a,b). However, if the filter resides only at the membrane surface, there is no reason why those gating structures that do not link to the filter should not increase the conductance in an unspecific manner.

A specific model that avoids this difficulty is shown in Figure 10. It is assumed that the selectivity filter and the voltage-gated channel span opposite halves of the bilayer, but that the gating structures, after insertion and aggregation, link up with the filter, which itself is not voltage-dependent and is more or less static (although it might change configuration and conductance after linking). In this model the channel conductance would be determined only by the conductance of the filter channel and would be independent of the aggregation state and the channel diameter of the gating structure. This feature would result in only two conductance states (open or closed) for the single channel and would not show the multistate conductance fluctuations associated with an

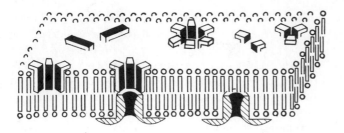

FIGURE 10 A modified insertion-aggregation model in which the aggregating gating parts of the channel are restricted to the upper half of the bilayer and must link up to ion selectors spanning the lower half before the ions can permeate the channel. The linkup may occur through lateral diffusion of the aggregated half-channels, or the inserted monomers may link individually to the selector. Half-channels of the fixed or aggregating type can be formed in bilayers by gramicidin, nystatin, or amphotericin. This model would maintain the aggregation kinetics but could also display some of the characteristics attributed to fixed channels usually assumed to exist in natural membranes.

aggregation process and seen in alamethicin. The model would thus be in agreement with results from noise analysis (Begenisich and Stevens, 1975), which suggest only two conductance states for the potassium channel.

In bilayers there are several examples of gating by the reversible linking of two half-channels. In these cases the channels are only long enough to span half of the bilayer, and a conductance appears only when two half-channels in the opposite faces of the bilayer link up end to end to form a channel. Gramicidin A, nystatin, and amphotericin seem to act in this manner. The process is particularly evident with nystatin and amphotericin (Finkelstein and Cass, 1968; Finkelstein and Holz, 1972), which do not seem to transfer easily from one bilayer half to the other; when used at low concentrations, they must therefore be added to both sides before the membrane conductance increases. In both compounds the half-channels are apparently aggregates, as deduced from the high-order concentration dependence of the conductances. The single-channel conductance fluctuations observed with amphotericin under these conditions show only a two-state behavior, most likely reflecting the half-channel linkup (Ermishkin, Kasumov, and Potseluyev, 1977). Gramicidin A seems to form a helical monomeric half-channel (Urry, 1971), which is able to cross over to the other side of the membrane. In this case the linkup mechanism has become evident only with a negatively charged analog containing three carbonyl groups at the terminal hydroxyl of the peptide (Appel et al., 1977). This form

cannot penetrate the bilayer and must be added from both sides.

It is interesting to note that in the gramicidin case the linkup mechanism seems to be weakly voltage-dependent, similar to the voltage dependence of the alamethicin aggregation-rate constants (see Figure 9 and Table I), and that, as suggested for alamethicin (Mueller, 1975b), this voltage dependence may be due to a voltage-induced lateral phase separation between gramicidin and lipid, leading to local clusters of gramicidin.

Another point deserving consideration is the relation between the integral of the gating currents and the conductance. In the aggregation scheme the insertion of the monomers would be the cause of the gating current, and the number of inserted monomers can be obtained from the integral of this current. If the single-channel conductance and the total conductance are also known, an estimate can be made of the ratio between free monomers and oligomeric channels. This ratio is determined by the free energies of monomers and oligomers and by the local concentrations of monomers. If the aggregates have a low free energy, most of the monomers will form oligomers. With alamethicin in lecithin membranes, this is not the case (see Figure 9 and Table I); only a fraction of the inserted monomers form dimers.

In nerve, estimates of the ratio between the number of available gating particles obtained from the integral of the maximal gating currents and the number of sodium channels, deduced from the peak conductance divided by the single-channel conductance, give values around three (Keynes and Rojas, 1974). Unfortunately the data are not good enough to exclude larger values; and in muscle, much larger values, up to 60, have been suggested for the potassium channel (Adrian and Peres, 1977). If the data from sodium channels are taken seriously, a large portion of the monomers would have to form higher oligomers. This would cause a problem if the aggregation overshoot were to account for inactivation, because if most of the inserted monomers aggregate transiently into higher oligomers, the dimer free energy must be negative with respect to that of the monomers by more than 5 kcal/mol. Such a large energy barrier would cause an extremely slow recovery from inactivation, which in the model depends on dimer dissociation. One way to overcome this difficulty is to assume a voltage dependence of the aggregation rate constants as outlined above, in the sense that the dimer association rate constants are more voltage-dependent than those of the higher oligomers. In this case the free energy of dimer formation increases with potentials that cause monomer insertion, and vice versa. Preliminary calculations have shown that under these conditions over 30% of the monomers can transiently form trimers and higher oligomers, of which more than 99% then dissociate into dimers. The quantitative limits of these ratios have not yet been explored, and at present the polymerization overshoot cannot be ruled out as a cause of inactivation. There may be, of course, other processes leading to inactivation—for example, blocking of the open channel by lipid or peptide groups (Armstrong, 1971) or the transfer of inserted monomers to the opposite membrane face—but if aggregation causes channel opening, then inactivation will be a very likely consequence.

It may be concluded that there can be many variations and elaborations of the basic aggregation scheme and that the process itself may not always be directly evident from multichannel or single-channel current-voltage data; whether the scheme is applicable to biological membranes remains to be seen. The far-reaching similarities between the data from bilayers and cells support such a notion, but they may be only a coincidence.

ACKNOWLEDGMENTS I appreciate the assistance of G. Baumann, H. Freifelder, P. Lewis, and S. Montimore. The work was supported by U.S. Public Health Service Grant GM 22655.

REFERENCES

ADRIAN, R. H., W. K. CHANDLER, and A. L. HODGKIN, 1970. Voltage clamp experiments in striated muscle fibers. *J. Physiol.* 208:607–644.

ADRIAN, R. H., and A. R. PERES, 1977. A gating signal for the potassium channel? *Nature* 267:800–804.

APPEL, H. J., E. BAMBERG, H. ALPES, and P. LAUGER, 1977. Formation of ion channels by a negatively charged analog of gramicidin A. *J. Membrane Biol.* 31:171–188.

ARMSTRONG, C. M., 1971. Interaction of tetraethylammonium ion derivatives with the potassium channels of giant axons. *J. Gen. Physiol.* 58:413–437.

ARMSTRONG, C. M., 1975. Ionic pores, gates and gating currents. *Q. Rev. Biophys.* 7:179–209.

ARMSTRONG, C. M., and F. BEZANILLA, 1973. Currents related to the movement of gating particles of the sodium channels. *Nature* 242:459–461.

ARMSTRONG, C. M., and F. BEZANILLA, 1977. Inactivation of the sodium conductance. II. Gating current experiments. *J. Gen. Physiol.* 70:567–591.

ARMSTRONG, C. M., F. BEZANILLA, and E. ROJAS, 1973. Destruction of sodium conductance inactivation in squid axons perfused with pronase. *J. Gen. Physiol.* 62:375–391.

BAUMANN, G., and P. MUELLER, 1974. A molecular model of membrane excitability. *J. Supramol. Struct.* 2:538–557.

BEGENISICH, T., and C. F. STEVENS, 1975. How many conductance states do potassium channels have? *Biophys. J.* 15:843–846.

BOHEIM, G., 1974. Statistical analysis of alamethicin channels in black lipid membranes. *J. Membrane Biol.* 19:277–302.

BOHLMANN, F., E. V. DEHMLOW, H. G. NEUHAHN, R. BRANDT, and H. BETHKE, 1970. Neue Heptaen Makrolide. II. Grundskelett, Stellung der Funktionellen Gruppen und Struktur der Aglykone. *Tetrahedron* 26:2199–2202.

BUKOVSKY, J., 1977. Production, purification and characterization of excitability inducing molecule. *J. Biol. Chem.* 252:8884–8889.

CASS, A., A. FINKELSTEIN, and V. KRESPI, 1970. The ion permeability induced in thin lipid membranes by the polyene antibiotics nystatin and amphotericin B. *J. Gen. Physiol.* 56:100–124.

COLE, K. S., and J. MOORE, 1960. Potassium ion current in the squid giant axon: Dynamic characteristics. *Biophys. J.* 1:1–14.

EISENBERG, J., J. E. HALL, and C. A. MEAD, 1973. The nature of the voltage dependent conductance induced by alamethicin in black lipid membranes. *J. Membrane Biol.* 14:143–157.

ERMISHKIN, L. N., KH. M. KASUMOV, and V. M. POTSELUYEV, 1977. Properties of amphotericin B channels in a lipid bilayer. *Biochim. Biophys. Acta* 470:357–367.

FINKELSTEIN, A., and A. CASS, 1968. Permeability and electrical properties of thin lipid membranes. *J. Gen. Physiol.* 52:145–172.

FINKELSTEIN, A., and R. HOLZ, 1972. Aqueous pores created in thin lipid membranes by the polyene antibiotics nystatin and amphotericin B. In *Membranes: A Series of Advances*, G. E. Eisenman, ed. New York: Dekker, pp. 377–406.

FRANKENHAEUSER, B., 1960. Quantitative description of sodium currents in myelinated nerve fibers of *Xenopus laevis*. *J. Physiol.* 151:491–501.

FRANKENHAEUSER, B., 1963. A quantitative description of potassium currents in myelinated nerve fibers of *Xenopus laevis*. *J. Physiol.* 169:424–430.

GISIN, B. F., S. KOBAYASHI, and J. E. HALL, 1977. Synthesis of a 19 residue peptide with alamethicin like activity. *Proc. Natl. Acad. Sci. USA* 74:115–119.

GOLDMAN, L., 1975. Quantitative description of the sodium conductance of *Myxicola* in terms of a generalized second order variable. *Biophys. J.* 15:119–136.

GOLDMAN, L., 1976. Kinetics of channel gating in excitable membranes. *Q. Rev. Biophys.* 9:491–526.

GORDON, L. G. M., and D. A. HAYDON, 1972. The unit conductance channel of alamethicin. *Biochim. Biophys. Acta* 255:1014–1018.

HODGKIN, A. L., and A. F. HUXLEY, 1952a. The components of membrane conductance in the giant axon of *Loligo*. *J. Physiol.* 116:473–496.

HODGKIN, A. L., and A. F. HUXLEY, 1952b. Currents carried by sodium and potassium ions through the membrane of the giant axon of *Loligo*. *J. Physiol.* 116:449–506.

HODGKIN, A. L., and A. F. HUXLEY, 1952c. The dual effect of membrane potential on sodium conductance in the giant axon of *Loligo*. *J. Physiol.* 116:494–448.

HODGKIN, A. L., and A. F. HUXLEY, 1952d. A quantitative description of membrane current and its application to conductance and excitation in nerve. *J. Physiol.* 117:507–544.

HOYT, R., 1971. Sodium activation in nerve fibers. *Biophys. J.* 8:1074–1097.

JAKOBSSON, E., 1976. An assessment of a coupled three-state kinetic model for sodium conductance changes. *Biophys. J.* 16:291–301.

JAKOBSSON, E., and C. SCUDIERO, 1975. A transient excited state model for sodium permeability changes in excitable membranes. *Biophys. J.* 15:577–589.

JUNG, K., D. SCIBPITZ, T. OOKA, W. A. KONIG, and G. BOHEIM, 1976. Structural and membrane modifying properties of Suzukacillin, a peptide antibiotic related to alamethicin. *Biochim. Biophys. Acta* 433:164–181.

KEYNES, R. D., and E. ROJAS, 1974. Kinetics and steady state properties of the charged system controlling sodium conductance in squid axon. *J. Physiol.* 239:393–434.

LLINÁS, R., I. Z. STEINBERG, and K. WALTON, 1976. Presynaptic calcium currents and their relation to synaptic transmission: Voltage clamp study in squid giant synapse and theoretical model for the calcium gate. *Proc. Natl. Acad. Sci. USA* 73:2918–2922.

MARTIN, D. R., and R. G. P. WILLIAMS, 1976. Chemical nature and sequence of alamethicin. *Biochem. J.* 153:181–190.

MOOLENAAR, W. H., and I. SPECTOR, 1977. Membrane currents examined under voltage clamp in cultured hemoblastoma cells. *Science* 196:331–333.

MOORE, G. W., and E. B. COX, 1976. A kinetic model for the sodium conductance system in squid axon. *Biophys. J.* 16:171–192.

MUELLER, P., 1975a. Electrical excitability in lipid bilayers and cell membranes. In *Energy Transducing Mechanisms* (International Review of Biochemistry, vol. 3), E. Racker, ed. London: Butterworths, pp. 75–120.

MUELLER, P., 1975b. Membrane excitation through voltage induced aggregation of channel precursors. *Ann. NY Acad. Sci.* 264:247–264.

MUELLER, P., 1976. Molecular aspects of electrical excitation in lipid bilayers and cell membranes. In *Horizons in Biochemistry and Biophysics*, vol. 2, E. Quagliariello, ed. Reading, MA: Addison-Wesley, pp. 230–284.

MUELLER, P., and D. O. RUDIN, 1967. Action potential phenomena in experimental bimolecular lipid membranes. *Nature* 213:603–605.

MUELLER, P., and D. O. RUDIN, 1968a. Resting and action potentials in experimental bimolecular lipid membranes. *J. Theoret. Biol.* 18:222–258.

MUELLER, P., and D. O. RUDIN, 1968b. Action potentials induced in bimolecular lipid membranes. *Nature* 217:713–719.

MUELLER, P., and D. O RUDIN, 1969. Translocators in bimolecular lipid membranes: Their role in dissipative and conservative bioenergy transductions. In *Current Topics in Bioenergetics*, vol. 3, D. R. Sanadi, ed. New York: Academic Press, pp. 157–249.

MULLER, R. U., and A. FINKELSTEIN, 1972. Voltage dependent conductance induced in thin lipid membranes by monazomycin. *J. Gen. Physiol.* 60:263–284.

NEHER, E., 1971. Two fast transient current components during voltage clamp on snail neurons. *J. Gen. Physiol.* 58:36–53.

PELLER, L., and L. BARNETT, 1962. On enzyme catalyzed polymerizations. I. Linear polymers by direct reaction and through primer initiation. *J. Phys. Chem.* 66:680–684.

SCHEELE, R. B., and T. M. SCHUSTER, 1974. Kinetics of protein subunit interactions. Simulation of a polymerization overshoot. *Biopolymers* 13:275–286.

URRY, D. W., 1971. The gramicidin A transmembrane channel; a proposed (L,D) helix. *Proc. Natl. Acad. Sci. USA* 68:1907–1911.

YANTORNO, R. E., S. I. TAKASHIMA, and P. MUELLER, 1977. The dipole moment of a voltage dependent conductance producing antibiotic—alamethicin. *Biophys. J.* 17:87a.

38 Action of Electric Fields on Biological Membranes: Photosynthesis as an Example of the Generation and Use of Electric Fields

P. GRÄBER and H. T. WITT

ABSTRACT The photosynthetic membrane is used as an example to study the principles of membrane processes on a molecular level. We describe briefly results on light reaction, electron transfer, and proton transport as a basis for the molecular concept of photosynthesis. The main part of the report is devoted to the electric events that occur within the membrane. First, an optical method that enables us to detect transmembrane electric fields without electrodes and without a time delay is described. Second, the light-driven electric generator discovered by this method is replaced by an external electric generator, which can be used for the generation of an artificial transmembrane field. In this way the action of the electric field can be investigated apart from electron transports, generation of pH gradients, and other events. The transmembrane field causes three reactions: (1) the field changes the conformation of the membrane-bound ATPase; (2) this conformational change induces a gating of a proton-conducting channel within the ATPase; and (3) the electric-field energy released by the proton efflux is used for the synthesis of ATP. The methods and results described may also be of interest for research on nerve membranes.

Introduction

Biological membranes are highly organized structures that allow reaction patterns of extraordinary specificity and efficiency. Table I lists events occurring in different types of biological membranes. Note that the functional membrane of photosynthesis performs all the operations realized in the other listed membranes. Photosynthesis, therefore, is not only interesting in itself but also provides a good model for studying general principles of molecular dynamics in

P. GRÄBER and H. T. WITT Max-Volmer-Institut für Physikalische Chemie und Molekularbiologie, Technische Universität Berlin, Strasse des 17. Juni 135, 1000 Berlin 12, Federal Republic of Germany

membranes. Furthermore, photosynthetic reactions have the unique advantage of being triggered by short light pulses (in the nanosecond range). Thus reactions can be studied in the whole range from excited singlet states down to the formation of end products.

The functional membrane of photosynthesis is discussed in this section of the ISP for several reasons:

1. For photosynthesis a new method (electrochromism) has been developed by which electric events can be measured without electrodes and with no time delay. This method may also be useful for investigations of nerves and vesicles produced from nerves when electrodes cannot be applied.

2. In photosynthesis the pathway can be described in terms of how electric fields are generated. This is one of the few relatively well-known electric generators operating in biological membranes.

3. Adenosine triphosphate (ATP) can be generated by using the energy of a transmembrane electric field. This is of interest because the reverse process is thought to generate the transmembrane field in the nerve membrane.

4. Evidence is presented that the transmembrane field induces conformational changes in the ATPase, coupled with the gating of ion fluxes through the enzyme. This mechanism may also operate during corresponding events in nerve membranes.

Light reactions and electron transport

Photosynthesis in green plants is based on a light-induced electron transport from H_2O via intermediates to $NADP^+$; the pathway of the electron is called an electron-transport chain. The electron transfer is accompanied by phosphorylation, that is, by the syn-

TABLE I

Events occurring in four types of biological membranes

	Light reaction	Electron transport	Electric potential difference	Ion flux	ATP synthesis
Photosynthesis	X	X	X	X	X
Respiration		X	X	X	X
Vision	X		X	X	X
Nerves			X	X	X

thesis of ATP from ADP and P_i. When NADPH and ATP are generated, CO_2 can be reduced by a subsequent dark reaction to energy-rich organic compounds. The reactions between the absorption of light quanta and the formation of NADPH and ATP occur in the membrane of so-called thylakoids. The latter are disc-shaped vesicles with diameters around 5,000 Å and are located within the chloroplasts (Figure 1). They are partially interconnected with each other. The membrane of one thylakoid contains about 200 electron-transport chains and 10^5 pigment molecules. Thus, on average, each electron-transport chain is surrounded by 500 chlorophyll and carotenoid molecules, which are the so-called antenna pigments (for references and details see Govindjee, 1975).

Light quanta absorbed by the antenna pigments are channeled by singlet-singlet energy migration to two photoactive centers of the electron-transport chain. These centers are Chlorophyll-a (Chl-a) molecules in a special environment (probably dimers bound to protein). One type of center, called Chl-a$_I$ (Kok, 1961), can be excited by light of wavelength up to 730 nm; the other type, Chl-a$_{II}$ (Gläser et al., 1974; Wolff, Gläser, and Witt, 1974), reacts to wavelengths up to 700 nm.

The photoactive chlorophylls Chl-a$_I$ and Chl-a$_{II}$ operate in series within the electron-transport chain (Hill and Bendall, 1960; Kok and Hoch, 1961; Duysens, Amesz, and Kamp, 1961; Witt, Müller, and Rumberg, 1961). The essential electronic link between the chlorophylls is a pool of plastoquinone (PQ) comprising perhaps five molecules (Stiehl and Witt, 1969). Both chlorophylls are oxidized in the light in less than 20 nsec (Witt and Wolff, 1970; Witt, 1975), thereby reducing $NADP^+$ and PQ. Chl-a$_I^+$ is rereduced by plastohydroquinone, and Chl-a$_{II}^+$ by H_2O.

The sum effect of these reactions is an electron transfer from H_2O to $NADP^+$. There are other electron carriers between $NADP^+$ and H_2O, such as plastocyanine, and cytochromes, which are necessary for

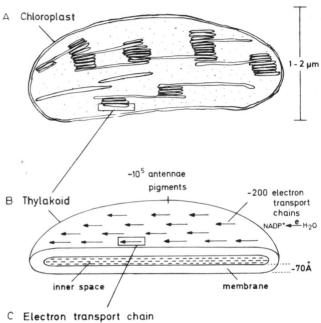

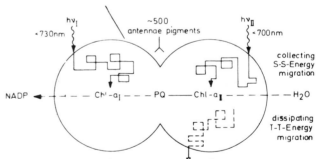

FIGURE 1 Scheme of the functional units of photosynthesis. *Top*: Chloroplast with thylakoids. *Center*: Thylakoid with electron-transport chains. *Bottom*: Simplified scheme of the electron-transport chain with the two photoactive chlorophylls and the area of antenna pigments.

the electron transport; they are omitted here because they are not necessary as building blocks of the concept to be outlined. The electron is transferred vectorially across the membrane from H_2O (inside) to

NADP+ (outside). In this way an electric field is generated across the photosynthetic membrane.

Generation of an electric field and its detection by electrochromism

Information on electric fields in the photosynthetic membrane was first obtained by Junge and Witt using absorption changes of membrane pigments due to electrochromism (Witt, 1967; Junge and Witt, 1968). Figure 2 (top) shows the underlying physical principle. On absorption of light quanta, an electron is raised from its ground state to an excited state. If an electric field is applied and if at least one state has a different dipole moment, the energy difference between these states depends on the magnitude of the field. Thus the absorption band of such a molecule is shifted. This shift causes a decrease of absorption below a certain wavelength and an increase above that wavelength, the magnitude of the change depending on the magnitude of the field. These field-indicating absorption changes are shown at the far right.

The lower section of Figure 2 shows the spectrum of such light-induced, field-indicating absorption changes for chloroplasts from green plants (Emrich, Junge, and Witt, 1969a) and for chromatophores from photosynthetic bacteria (Jackson and Crofts,

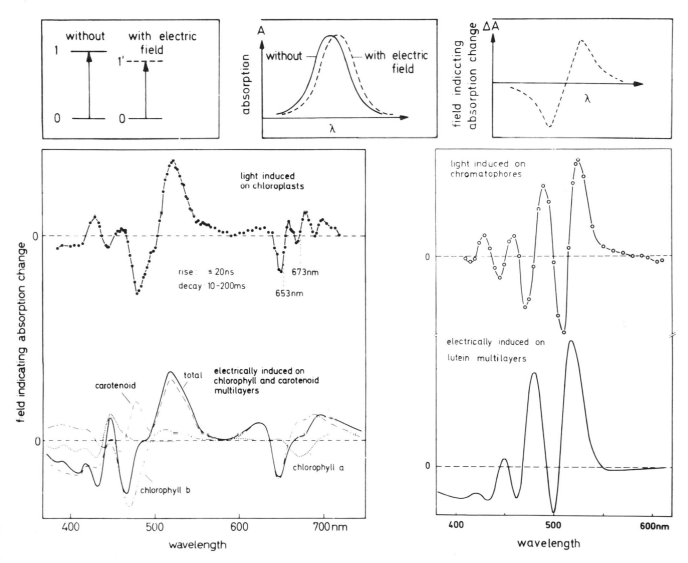

FIGURE 2   *Top*: Principal effects of an electric field on optical absorption bands (electrochromism). *Center*: Spectra of the field-indicating absorption changes induced by light in chloroplasts (left) and in chromatophores (right). *Bottom*: Spectra of absorption changes of the pigments of chloroplasts and chromatophores embedded in multilayers and induced in the dark by an electric field.

1969) Note that all absorption bands of all pigments present in the membrane respond to the electric field. For this reason these spectra are rather complicated compared to the schematic one shown at the top. The field-indicating absorption changes are characterized by a rise time faster than 20 nsec (Wolff et al., 1969) and a decay time in the range 0.01–1 sec, depending on membrane conductivity. That these absorption changes do indeed indicate transmembrane fields has been proven by kinetic (Junge and Witt, 1968), spectroscopic (Schmidt, Reich, and Witt, 1971), and electric (Witt and Zickler, 1973) experiments. At the bottom of Figure 2 the spectroscopic proof is presented. If the light-induced absorption changes in the center are indeed electrochromic shifts of the absorption bands of the pigments, it should be possible to induce such shifts in the dark in pigment layers by artificial electric fields. To test this the pigments of the photosynthetic membrane were embedded in 1,000-Å-thick multilayers between two transparent electrodes. A measuring light beam was directed through the electrodes. Application of 1–10 V between the electrodes resulted in an electric field of about 10^5–10^6 V/cm. This is approximately the order of magnitude estimated for the thylakoid membrane (and also for nerves). The difference spectra induced electrically on multilayers are shown at the bottom of Figure 2. They are in good agreement with the light-induced spectra in chloroplasts and chromatophores (Schmidt, Reich, and Witt, 1971).

Figure 3 (left) shows the kinetics of the light-induced, field-indicating absorption change. The height indicates the transmembrane voltage, the slope the current across the membrane. The fast rise of the signal represents field generation by a rapid shift of an electron across the membrane. The relatively slow decay represents the breakdown of the field by efflux of ions such as H^+ or K^+. The field is indicated by the electrochromism of the pigments embedded in the membrane. At the right an electric analog is shown. As outlined elsewhere (Witt, 1971; Witt, 1975), the absorption changes represent an intrinsic molecular voltmeter and ammeter with the following properties: (1) they respond in the range of nanoseconds to seconds; (2) they indicate an electric potential difference across the membrane; (3) they indicate the voltage linearly; (4) they have been calibrated in absolute values; and (5) the polarity has been measured.

Application of the electrochromic method to further events

Other data on membrane properties can be obtained by using the electrochromic method in the manner summarized in Figure 4.

The measurements of transmembrane voltages and currents depicted in parts A and B have already been discussed. If the membrane is discharged by protons, the rate of the potential decay depends on the internal proton concentration (at constant outside pH). Therefore, as in part C, the rate of the potential decay can be used as an indicator of the internal pH (Boeck and Witt, 1971; Gräber and Witt, 1978).

Alamethicin is known to form voltage-dependent pores in black lipid membranes (Mueller and Rudin, 1968). Incorporation of alamethicin in the chloroplast membrane leads to a sharp increase of the trans-

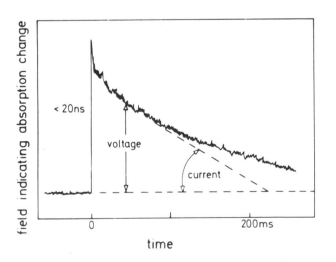 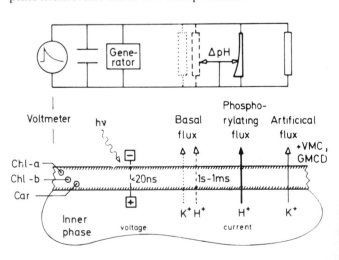

FIGURE 3 *Left*: Kinetics of the field-indicating absorption change. *Right*: Molecular events underlying the field changes and the corresponding electric analog.

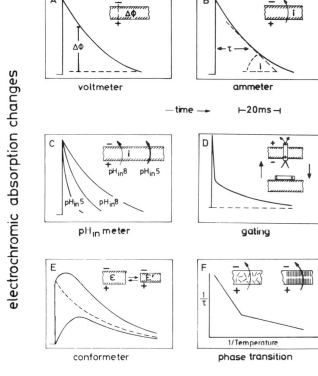

electrochromic absorption changes

voltmeter

ammeter

—time→ ⊢20ms⊣

pH$_{in}$ meter

gating

conformeter

phase transition

FIGURE 4 The electrochromic absorption change can be regarded as a "multimeter" for the measurement of the following events: (A) transmembrane voltage; (B) transmembrane currents; (C) internal pH; (D) gating processes; (E) conformational changes of the membrane; and (F) phase transition in the membrane.

membrane current above a critical voltage, which indicates a gating (part D). The relation between alamethicin concentration and the critical voltage found in black lipid membranes has been used as one of the four methods to calibrate the field-indicating absorption changes in chloroplasts in absolute transmembrane electric potentials (Zickler, Witt, and Boheim, 1976).

If changes of the membrane capacity are associated with changes of the dielectric constant ϵ (e.g., by conformational changes), it may be possible to monitor this effect by electrochromic shifts. The normal field-indicating absorption change is shown by the dotted curve in part E. This would be modulated by any change in the dielectric constant (upper curve). Thus the difference between the curves should indicate the time course of the conformational change (Witt, 1975). In bacteria such changes have been interpreted as indicating conformational changes of the ATPase (Baltscheffsky, 1976).

If a phase transition occurs within the lipids of the membrane, the activation energy of the ion transport

across the membrane should be influenced by the degree of order within the membrane. In this case an Arrhenius plot (rate constant vs. reciprocal absolute temperature) should reveal a break at the temperature where such a phase transition occurs (part F). Using this method a phase transition in the chloroplast membrane has been observed at about 18°C (Gräber and Witt, 1974b).

The electrochromic method is also useful for the analysis of electric phenomena in other biological membranes or interfaces in general. If these are not pigmented, they can be stained with dyes (Emrich, Junge, and Witt, 1969b). So far the method has been extended to bacteria (Jackson and Crofts, 1969) and to mitochondria (Akerman and Wikström, 1976); it would also be useful for electric measurements on vesicles of nerve membranes. Finally, as will be shown in more detail below, the electrochromic method is an ideal instrument for discriminating between the different hypotheses of phosphorylation.

Vectorial transport of electrons and protons and the sidedness of the membrane

The detection of a light-induced transmembrane electric field provided the first evidence that (1) the electron transport occurs vectorially across the membrane; (2) the membrane must therefore be built up asymmetrically; (3) the electron acceptors must be localized toward the outside and the electron donors toward the inside; and (4) the photoactive Chl-a$_I$ and Chl-a$_{II}$ must be localized toward the inside. (The last two points follow from the polarity of the field.)

Further studies on the correlation between the chlorophyll reactions, field generation, redox processes, and proton translocation lead to the following sequence of reactions (Figure 5, top): (1) excitation of Chl-a$_I$ and Chl-a$_{II}$; (2) photo-oxidation of Chl-a$_I$ and Chl-a$_{II}$; (3) vectorial transfer of the electrons from inside to outside the membrane; (4) oxidation of H$_2$O, reduction of NADP$^+$, and redox reaction of plastoquinone; (5) proton translocation into the inner phase through protolytic reactions with the charges at the outer and inner surfaces of the membranes; and (6) discharge of the energized membrane through efflux of ions, preferentially of protons. (For details see Witt, 1971, 1975.)

In a single turnover of this molecular machine, that is, when one electron is transferred through the chain, two protons are translocated from the outside to the inside and flow back out again (Schliephake, Junge, and Witt, 1968; Junge and Ausländer, 1974; Gräber and Witt, 1975; Ausländer and Junge, 1975).

To give a more realistic picture, the molecules of this scheme are shown in real dimensions at the bottom of Figure 5.

The generated transmembrane potential induced in a single turnover is about 50–100 mV (Junge and Witt, 1968; Zickler, Witt, and Boheim, 1976), but the transmembrane pH gradient is only about 0.2–0.6 pH units, because of the buffers in the inner thylakoid space. In continuous light, however—that is, after many turnovers of the molecular machine—large amounts of H⁺ are translocated to the inside. The corresponding charges are balanced by the flux of an equivalent number of counterions (e.g., K^+ or Cl^-). Under these conditions an electrochemical proton potential is built up that consists of a pH gradient of about 3 units (Rumberg and Siggel, 1969) and an

electric potential of about 100 mV (Gräber and Witt, 1974a).

Synthesis of ATP by the light-induced field

According to the chemiosmotic hypothesis of Mitchell (1966), the electrochemical proton potential can be used for ATP synthesis. This is realized by the potential-driven proton efflux via a special membrane-bound enzyme, the ATPase (see Figure 5). Other hypotheses of phosphorylation assume an energy transport between the electron-transport chain and the ATPase, either via (as-yet unknown) chemical intermediates or via protein-protein interactions (i.e., conformational changes). However, the action of the electrochemical proton potential can, of course,

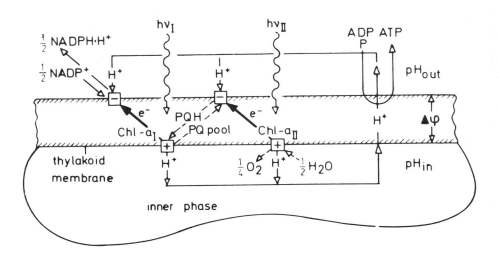

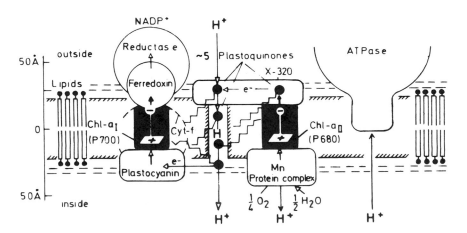

FIGURE 5 *Top*: Zigzag scheme with the vectorial pathway of electrons, protons, and hydrogens derived from pulse-spectroscopic studies. *Bottom*: Preliminary topography of the membrane of photosythesis based on functional exper-

iments. The two black "trunks" symbolize the two photoactive centers, consisting of Chl-a$_I$ and Chl-a$_{II}$, which are probably complexed with proteins.

induce secondary conformational changes in the ATPase.

The electrochromic method is an ideal instrument for discriminating between the different mechanisms. Several experimental findings accord with the proposals of the chemiosmotic hypothesis:

1. Field decay is accelerated during phosphorylation due to the additional proton flux via the ATPase. This is shown schematically in Figure 3 (Rumberg and Siggel, 1968; Junge, Rumberg, and Schröder, 1970).

2. The flux of protons occurs via a basal pathway and via the ATPase pathway. These fluxes depend on different powers of the electric potential difference, $\Delta\phi$, and the pH gradient, ΔpH (Gräber and Witt, 1976). This is reflected in the nonlinear resistance of the phosphorylating flux in Figure 3. The proton flux via the ATPase pathway is proportional to the rate of phosphorylation. The proportionality factor is $n \approx 2.5$; that is, about five protons are translocated via the ATPase to generate two ATP (Gräber and Witt, 1976).

3. If an artificial bypass is introduced parallel to the flux via the ATPase and the basal flux (see Figure 3), the decay of the field is accelerated. Such a bypass can be realized by gramicidin (GMCD), which is known to act in lipid membranes as an ionophore (e.g., for K^+). Figure 6 (left) shows that the half-life of the potential decay decreases as gramicidin concentration increases (Junge and Witt, 1968).

Because the bypass dissipates the electrochemical energy of the protons, the amount of ATP generated must decrease simultaneously (Figure 6, right). Half of both effects are observed at about 1 gramicidin molecule per 10^5 chlorophylls. Since each thylakoid contains about 10^5 chlorophylls, it follows that the

functional units of the electric potential and of phosphorylation are at least one thylakoid or a larger unit (perhaps several interconnected thylakoids); that is, the unit is a closed membrane vesicle (Boeck and Witt, 1971). As expected, in the same range the electron transport (demonstrated by the oxygen evolution in Figure 6) is not affected by the gramicidin concentration.

4. The electrochemical proton gradient in saturating continuous light ($\Delta\phi \approx 100$ mV, ΔpH ≈ 3.0) satisfies with $n \approx 2.5$ H$^+$ the energy requirement of ATP synthesis (Witt, 1975).

Synthesis of ATP by an external field

In light-induced phosphorylation an electric potential plus a pH gradient is always produced. To prove that ATP can be generated by the action of a transmembrane field alone, the light-driven electric potential generator was replaced by an external electric generator. Application of microelectrodes to one thylakoid does not allow detection of the ATP generated because the amount obtained from one vesicle is too small. However, electric fields can be induced at all vesicles, as shown schematically in Figure 7 (Witt, Schlodder, and Gräber, 1976). An aqueous solution is placed between two macroscopic electrodes with a distance of 1 mm (voltage, 200 V). Over a distance of 10^{-4} cm, 200 mV are present within the solution. If a nonconducting lipid sphere with a diameter of 10^{-4} cm is placed in the solution (center), the voltage across this sphere is increased because of the charge accumulation in the aqueous solution at the outer surface of the lipid. The voltage across the sphere can be calculated to be 300 mV if the conductivity λ_i of the lipid is small compared to the conductivity λ_a of the aqueous solution. If the inner space of the lipid sphere is replaced by an aqueous solution, this corresponds to a vesicle with a nonconducting membrane. The voltage across the whole sphere is still 300 mV, but now the voltage is restricted to the nonconducting shell, with 150 mV across the membrane at the upper half of the vesicle and 150 mV across the lower half. (There is in practice a constant electric potential within the vesicle because uncompensated ions compensate the external electric field in the aqueous solution at the inner surface of the sphere.)

The generated transmembrane field has in half the vesicle the same direction as the light-induced field, that is, it is positive inside and negative outside. (In the figure this is the left half.) For this reason the amount of ATP generated by two external voltage pulses must be compared with one light pulse. (ATP

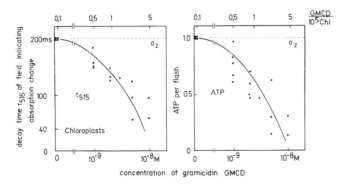

FIGURE 6 Titration of the functional unit of the electric events and ATP synthesis. *Left*: Effect of GMCD on the decay time of the field-indicating absorption change. *Right*: Effect of GMCD on the relative amount of ATP generated per flash.

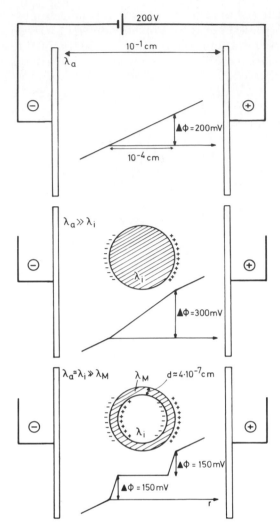

FIGURE 7 Principle of the external-field method. See text for details.

generated at the upper half cannot be hydrolyzed at the lower half because in this half the polarity is wrong with respect to the necessary activation of the ATPase; see Bakker-Grunwald and van Dam, 1974.)

We measured the amount of ATP generated in the dark by external voltage double pulses and found it almost the same as that generated by saturating light pulses of the same duration (see Table II). We concluded that phosphorylation generated by light is equivalent to phosphorylation generated by an external electric field in the dark. It was also shown that the amount of ATP generated increases linearly with the number of voltage pulses, indicating that the system is not deactivated and can work repetitively. Finally, it was demonstrated that electron-transport inhibitors such as DCMU have no influence on the ATP yield induced by external voltage pulses. On the other

hand, inhibitors of the ATPase such as phlorizin also completely inhibit ATP synthesis in the external voltage pulse.

In sum, these results indicate that the presence of an electric field alone is sufficient for synthesis of ATP.

Conformational change of the ATPase by an external field and its relation to ATP synthesis

It has been shown by different methods that conformational changes occur at the chloroplast ATPase on energization, that is, on illumination or after application of an artificial transmembrane pH gradient (Ryrie and Jagendorf, 1972; Kraayenhof and Slater, 1974; Harris and Slater, 1975). One method is based on the following effect. The ATPase contains tightly bound adenine nucleotides (AMP, ADP, and ATP), which are released only after energization. It is assumed that this release is caused by a conformational change of the ATPase. Thus the amount of nucleotide released is proportional to the number of ATPases that have changed their conformation. The latter are called "active" ATPases. To investigate the relation between the extent of the electric field, conformational changes, and ATP synthesis, we again applied external voltage pulses to a chloroplast suspension, as described above (Gräber, Schlodder, and Witt, 1977). Figure 8 (right) shows the result. The amount of nucleotide released, that is, the number of active ATPases, increases nonlinearly with the transmembrane potential. (The transmembrane potential is proportional to the external electric field strength. See the scale at the top.) The fraction of active ATPases (right) and the amount of ATP generated (left) were measured as functions of the electric potential under identical conditions (pulse duration, 30 msec). The amount of ATP generated is about six times larger than the fraction of active ATPases, independent of the transmembrane potential.

This result leads to several conclusions. If each active ATPase carries out six turnovers during a 30 msec pulse, the turnover time of the ATPase is $\tau_0 \approx 5$ msec, independent of the transmembrane potential. The average rate of ATP synthesis, $\langle ATP \rangle$, is proportional to the reciprocal turnover time of the ATPase, $1/\tau_0$, and to the number of active ATPases, N; that is,

$$\langle ATP \rangle \propto \frac{1}{\tau_0} N(\Delta\phi). \qquad (1)$$

Here τ_0 is constant and the dependence of N on $\Delta\phi$ is shown explicitly (see Figure 8).

TABLE II

Comparison of amounts of ATP generated by light pulses and by external voltage pulses

Material	Amount of ATP generated by five external voltage double pulses	Amount of ATP generated by five light pulses
Control	$3.8 \times 10^{-3} \dfrac{\text{Mol ATP}}{\text{Mol Chl}}$	$5.0 \times 10^{-3} \dfrac{\text{Mol ATP}}{\text{Mol Chl}}$
with DCMU (3×10^{-5} M) added	85% of control	0
with phlorizin (10^{-2} M) added	0	0

In Figure 9 (left) this result is depicted schematically. The particles with the transmembrane channels represent the ATPases within the membrane (total number, N_0). The active ones are white, the inactive ones are hatched. The lengths of the arrows indicate the turnover rates of individual ATPases. Scheme A corresponds to the results formulated in equation 1. Scheme B shows the other possible extreme: at low and high potentials, all ATPases are active, but the turnover rate depends on $\Delta\phi$:

$$\langle \text{ATP} \rangle \propto \frac{1}{\tau(\Delta\phi)} N_0. \tag{2}$$

The results discussed here show that mechanism A is realized.

Gating of the ATPase by the field-dependent conformational change

For the synthesis of one ATP molecule about 2.5 protons must be translocated via the ATPase. It is very likely that these protons pass only those ATPases that are active through a conformational change and that these changes open a gate for protons. Because the turnover time is 5 msec, the proton current through the active and opened ATPases should be 500 H$^+$ per active ATPase per second.

In Figure 10 the results are extrapolated to higher potentials. At the top the turnover time of the ATPase and the current per open channel are shown plotted against transmembrane potentials up to 200 mV (solid line). The extrapolation to voltages above 200 mV is in accordance with independent measurements (squares) (Smith and Boyer, 1976). At the bottom the fractions of active ATPases, N_A/N_0—that is, the relative numbers of open channels—are shown. The dotted part of the curve is extrapolated; it is likely, however, that this curve must end up at 1.0 at high potentials. Again the squares resulting from independent measurements (Smith and Boyer, 1976) are in accordance with our assumption. These results show that the chloroplast ATPase can work as an

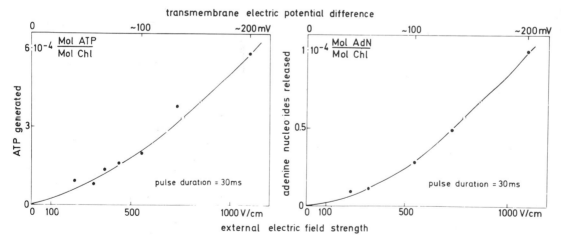

FIGURE 8 *Left*: Amount of ATP generated as a function of the transmembrane electric potential difference (scale at top) induced by an external electric field (scale at bottom). *Right*. Number of adenine nucleotides released as a function of the transmembrane electric potential difference (scale at top) induced by an external electric field (scale at bottom).

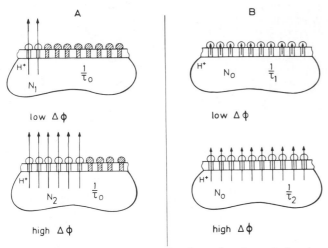

FIGURE 9 Two extreme mechanisms for the relation between the number of active ATPases, N, and the turnover rate, τ.

electrically gated enzyme. The number of active enzymes, or of open channels, increases with increasing potential. The turnover rate—the proton flux per open channel—is independent of the potential, presumably because of the coupled chemical reaction.

It should be mentioned that the fraction of active ATPases is not fixed to a special ensemble but migrates statistically between all ATPases within 3 sec (Gräber, Schlodder, and Witt, 1977).

Summarizing, we can say that some processes observed in photosynthetic membranes are strikingly

similar to processes that occur in the nerve membrane. In the thylakoid membrane the electric field has at least three different effects:

1. It changes the conformation of the APTase from an inactive to an active form.

2. The field-dependent conformational change is coupled with a gating for protons.

3. The energy necessary for ATP synthesis can be supplied by an electric field.

Thus, despite the differing functional behaviors of chloroplasts and nerves at the macroscopic level, surprising similarities are observed at the molecular level.

ACKNOWLEDGMENTS We would like to thank Mrs. Christel Proll for help in preparing the manuscript and Dipl.-Phys. E. Schlodder for helpful discussions. This work was supported by grants from the Deutsche Forschungsgemeinschaft and the Commission of the European Communities (Solar Energy Program).

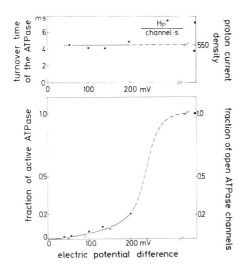

FIGURE 10 *Top*: Turnover time of the ATPase and the proton current per channel as a function of the transmembrane potential. *Bottom*: Fraction of active ATPases and number of open channels as a function of the transmembrane potential.

REFERENCES

AKERMAN, K. E., and M. K. F. WIKSTRÖM, 1976. Safranine as a probe of the mitochondrial membrane potential. *FEBS Lett.* 68:191–197.

AUSLÄNDER, W., and W. JUNGE, 1975. Neutral red, a rapid indicator for pH-changes in the inner phase of thylakoids. *FEBS Lett.* 59:310–315.

BAKKER-GRUNWALD, T., and K. VAN DAM, 1974. On the mechanism of activity of the ATPase in chloroplasts. *Biochim. Biophys. Acta* 347:290–298.

BALTSCHEFFSKY, M., 1976. Conversion of solar energy into energy-rich phosphate compounds. In *Living Systems as Energy Converters*, R. Buvet, M. J. Allen, and J. P. Massué, eds. Amsterdam, New York, Oxford: North-Holland Publishing Co., pp. 199–207.

BOECK, M., and H. T. WITT, 1971. Correlation between electrical events and ATP-generation in the functional membrane of photosynthesis. In *Proceedings of the 2nd International Congress on Photosynthesis Research*, Stresa, Italy, G. Forti, M. Avron, and A. Melandri, eds. The Hague: Dr. W. Junk N.V., pp. 903–911.

DUYSENS, L. N., J. AMESZ, and B. M. KAMP, 1961. Two photochemical systems in photosynthesis. *Nature* 190:510–511.

EMRICH, H. M., W. JUNGE, and H. T. WITT, 1969a. Further evidence for an optical response of chloroplast bulk pigments to a light-induced electrical field in photosynthesis. *Z. Naturforsch.* 24b:1144–1146.

EMRICH, H. M., W. JUNGE, and H. T. WITT, 1969b. An artificial indicator for electric phenomena in biological membranes and interfaces. *Naturwissenschaften* 56:514–515.

GLÄSER, M., CH. WOLFF, H. E. BUCHWALD, and H. T. WITT, 1974. On the photoactive chlorophyll reaction in system II of photosynthesis. Detection of a fast and large component. *FEBS Lett.* 42:81–85.

GOVINDJEE, ed., 1975. *Bioenergetics of Photosynthesis.* New York: Academic Press.

GRÄBER, P., E. SCHLODDER, and H. T. WITT, 1977. Conformational change of the chloroplast ATPase induced by a transmembrane electric field and its correlation to phosphorylation. *Biochim. Biophys. Acta* 461:426–440.

GRÄBER, P., and H. T. WITT, 1974a. On the extent of the electrical potential across the thylakoid membrane induced by continuous light in chlorella cells. *Biochim. Biophys. Acta* 333:389–392.

GRÄBER, P., and H. T. WITT, 1974b. The effect of temperature on flash-induced transmembrane currents in chloroplasts of spinach. In *Proceedings of the 3rd International Congress on Photosynthesis*, Rehovot, Israel, M. Avron, ed. Amsterdam: Elsevier, pp. 951–956.

GRÄBER, P., and H. T. WITT, 1975. Direct measurement of the protons pumped into the inner phase of the functional membrane of photosynthesis per electron transfer. *FEBS Lett.* 59:184–189.

GRÄBER, P., and H. T. WITT, 1976. Relations between the electrical potential, pH gradient, proton flux and phosphorylation in the photosynthetic membrane. *Biochim. Biophys. Acta* 423:141–163.

GRÄBER, P., and H. T. WITT, 1978. Analysis of the decay of the flash-induced electric potential difference across the photosynthetic membrane of chlorella cells. *Z. Naturforsch.* (in press).

HARRIS, D. A., and E. C. SLATER, 1975. Tightly bound nucleotides of the energy-transducing ATPase of chloroplasts and their role in photophosphorylation. *Biochim. Biophys. Acta* 387:335–348.

HILL, R., and D. S. BENDALL, 1960. Function of the two cytochrome components in chloroplasts: A working hypothesis. *Nature* 186:136–137.

JACKSON, J. B., and A. R. CROFTS, 1969. The high energy state in chromatophores from *Rhodopseudomonas spheroides*. *FEBS Lett.* 4:185–188.

JUNGE, W., and W. AUSLÄNDER, 1974. The electric generator in photosynthesis of green plants. I. Vectorial and protolytic properties of the electron transport chain. *Biochim. Biophys. Acta* 333:59–70.

JUNGE, W., B. RUMBERG, and H. SCHRÖDER, 1970. The necessity of an electric potential difference and its use for photophosphorylation in short flash groups. *Eur. J. Biochem.* 14:575–581.

JUNGE, W., and H. T. WITT, 1968. On the ion transport system of photosynthesis: Investigations on a molecular level. *Z. Naturforsch.* 23b:244–254.

KOK, B., 1961. Partial purification and determination of oxidation reduction potential of the photosynthetic chlorophyll complex absorbing at 700 nm. *Biochim. Biophys. Acta* 48:527–533.

KOK, B., and G. HOCH, 1961. Spectral changes in photosynthesis. In *Light and Life*, W. D. McElroy and B. Glass, eds. Baltimore: The Johns Hopkins Press, pp. 397–416.

KRAAYENHOF, R., and E. C. SLATER, 1974. Studies of chloroplast energy conservation with electrostatic and covalent fluorophores. In *Proceedings of the 3rd International Congress on Photosynthesis*, Rehovot, Israel, M. Avron, ed. Amsterdam: Elsevier, pp. 985–996.

MITCHELL, P., 1966. Chemiosmotic coupling in oxidative and photosynthetic phosphorylation. *J. Biol. Rev.* 41:445–502.

MUELLER, P., and D. D. RUDIN, 1968. Action potentials induced in biomolecular lipid membranes. *Nature* 217:713–719.

RUMBERG, B., and U. SIGGEL, 1968. Quantitative Zusammenhänge zwischen Chlorophyll-b-Reaktion, Elektronentransport und Phosphorylierung in der Photosynthese. *Z. Naturforsch.* 23b:239–244.

RUMBERG, B., and U. SIGGEL, 1969. pH-changes in the inner phase of the thylakoids during photosynthesis. *Naturwissenschaften* 56:130–132.

RYRIE, I. J., and A. T. JAGENDORF, 1972. Correlation between a conformational change in the coupling factor and the high energy state in chloroplasts. *J. Biol. Chem.* 247:4453–4459.

SCHLIEPHAKE, W., W. JUNGE, and H. T. WITT, 1968. Correlation between field formation, proton translocation and the light reactions in photosynthesis. *Z. Naturforsch.* 23b:1571–1578.

SCHMIDT, S., R. REICH, and H. T. WITT, 1971. Electrochromic measurements in vitro as a test for the interpretation of field-indicating absorption changes in photosynthesis. In *Proceedings of the 2nd International Congress on Photosynthesis Research*, Stresa, Italy, G. Forti, M. Avron, and A. Melandri, eds. The Hague: Dr. W. Junk N.V., pp. 1087–1095.

SMITH, D. J., and P. D. BOYER, 1976. Demonstration of a transitory tight binding of ATP and of committed P_i and ADP during ATP synthesis by chloroplasts. *Proc. Natl. Acad. Sci. USA* 73:4314–4318.

STIEHL, H. H., and H. T. WITT, 1969. Quantitative treatment of the function of plastoquinone in photosynthesis. *Z. Naturforsch.* 24b:1588–1598.

WITT, H. T., 1967. On the analysis of photosynthesis by the pulse techniques in the 10^{-1} to 10^{-8} second range. In *Fast Reactions and Primary Processes in Chemical Kinetics*. S. Claesson, ed. New York: Interscience, pp. 261–310.

WITT, H. T., 1971. Coupling of quanta, electrons, fields, ions and phosphorylation in the functional membrane of photosynthesis. *Q. Rev. Biophys.* 4:365–477.

WITT, H. T., 1975. Primary acts of energy conservation in the functional membrane of photosynthesis. In *Bioenergetics of Photosynthesis*, Govindjee, ed. New York: Academic Press, pp. 493–554.

WITT, H. T., A. MÜLLER, and B. RUMBERG, 1961. Experimental evidence for the mechanism of photosynthesis. *Nature* 191:194–195.

WITT, H. T., E. SCHLODDER, and P. GRÄBER, 1976. Membrane-bound ATP synthesis generated by an external electrical field. *FEBS Lett.* 69:272–276.

WITT, H. T., and A. ZICKLER, 1973. Electrical evidence for the field-indicating absorption change in bioenergetic membranes. *FEBS Lett.* 37:307–310.

WITT, K., and CH. WOLFF, 1970. Rise-time of the absorption changes of chlorophyll-a_I and carotenoids in photosynthesis. *Z. Naturforsch.* 25b:387–388.

WOLFF, CH., H.-E. BUCHWALD, H. RÜPPEL, K. WITT, and H. T. WITT, 1969. Rise time of the light-induced electrical field across the function membrane of photosynthesis. *Z. Naturforsch.* 24b:1038–1041.

WOLFF, CH., M. GLÄSER, and H. T. WITT, 1974. Studies on the photochemical active chlorophyll-a_{II} in system II of photosynthesis. In *Proceedings of the 3rd International Congress of Photosynthesis*, Rehovot, Israel, M. Avron, ed. Amsterdam: Elsevier, pp. 295–403.

ZICKLER, A., H. T. WITT, and G. BOHEIM, 1976. Estimation of the light-induced electrical potential of the functional membrane of photosynthesis using a voltage-dependent ionophore. *FEBS Lett.* 66:142–148.

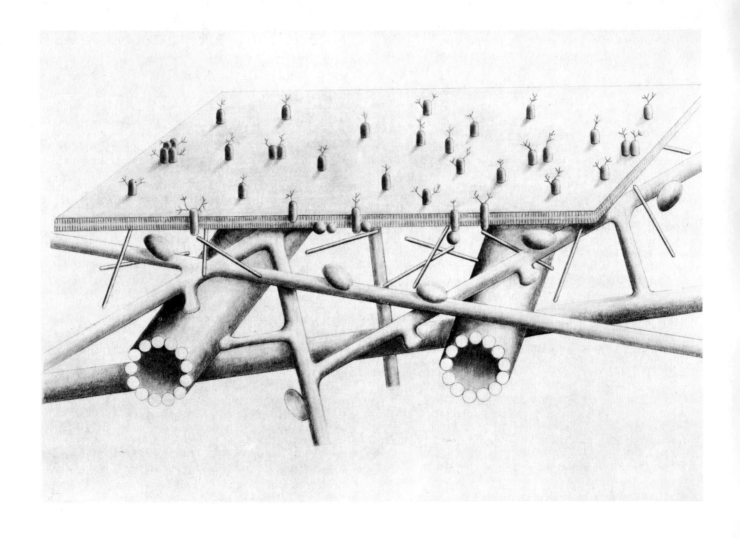

MEMBRANE
DYNAMICS
AND CELLULAR
INTERACTION

A schematic diagram (roughly in scale) illustrating the surface membrane bilayer. Integral and trans-membranous glycoproteins are shown as well as underlying cytoskeletal structures, which include microfilaments, microtubules, intermediate filaments, and their associated proteins.

Introduction

GERALD M. EDELMAN

OUR VIEW OF the cell surface has changed considerably in the last decade. The concepts that have emerged have a direct bearing on our understanding of the nature of signaling from inside or outside the cell, of cell-cell interactions in development, and of synapse formation. The papers in this session provide a view of these fields and relate it to major problems in developmental neurobiology and neurophysiology.

The key concepts underlying the new view of the cell surface-membrane complex are as follows: (1) The membrane bilayer is fluid. (2) The distribution of lipids and proteins in the bilayer is asymmetrical. (3) Surface proteins are mainly glycoproteins and are inserted into the membrane by special mechanisms involving amino acid sequences that act as signals for that insertion (signal hypothesis). (4) Some proteins are peripheral; others are either integral or transmembranous. (5) Most surface proteins and receptors have lateral mobility in the membrane and can exist in several mobility states. (6) Transmembranous proteins can interact with submembranous cytoskeletal structures. (7) There is evidence for transmembrane control and modulation of the mobility states of surface receptors and of cellular states via this control.

Clearly these ideas and facts provide a powerful basis for interpreting the mechanisms of cell interactions and understanding the role of intracellular structures in mediating surface events. As can be seen in the papers presented here, physicochemical studies correlated with cytological analyses and ultrastructural approaches have provided a comprehensive picture of the cytoskeleton and its possible functions. These developments suggest new models of signaling between the nucleus and the cytoplasm and between the cytoplasm and the surface of the cell. A beginning has also been made in the analysis of cell surface molecules that mediate adhesion in developing neural tissues. Moreover, chemical and functional analyses of surface receptors such as the acetylcholine receptor have led to new models of synaptic interaction.

These developments are of central significance for neurobiology and will undoubtedly lead to many new insights into synaptic function, tract formation, and cell communication. It may be useful to point out, however, that we still have much to learn in the area of cell surface dynamics. We need to know the detailed structure of more surface proteins, particularly transmembrane proteins. It would also be valuable to understand more exactly the function of bilayer lip-ids, especially their permissive and restrictive roles in lateral mobility. A related problem—the relative contributions of submembranous and external interactions to surface protein mobility—still has not been solved. Furthermore, we would like to know the rules for protein pairing or higher-order associations in the membrane. But perhaps the most challenging of all problems is to determine the exact linkage and order of interacting transmembranous proteins and cytoskeletal elements. A solution of this problem would enable us to specify more clearly the nature and pattern of signals controlling and coordinating the fundamental events of cell motion, division, and interaction. It is at this level that future neurobiological studies may benefit most from a more detailed understanding of surface and membrane dynamics.

39 The Dynamics of the Cell Surface: Modulation and Transmembrane Control

DONALD A. McCLAIN and GERALD M. EDELMAN

ABSTRACT The binding of multivalent lectins to local areas of cell surfaces induces a propagated, global reduction in the mobility of plasma membrane receptors. Low temperatures and antimitotic drugs reverse this so-called anchorage modulation, indicating that microtubles are involved in the restriction of receptor mobility. We have hypothesized that eukaryotic cells contain a surface-modulating assembly (SMA) consisting of membrane receptors and submembranous arrays of microfilaments, microtubules, and their associated proteins. Components of this assembly appear to play a role in growth control. In particular, intact microtubules are required at that stage of growth stimulation when previously resting cells become committed to reentering the cell cycle. Studies of cells transformed by oncogenic viruses support the postulated relationship between the state of the SMA and growth control. Some of these phenomena may be important in the disposition and functioning of the surface receptors of neurons.

THE CELL SURFACE plays a key role in neuronal and synaptic interactions. In the past, the main emphasis of neurobiological studies has been on the cell plasma membrane and ionic transport. Increasingly, however, interest has turned to macromolecules at the cell surface, including receptors for neurotransmitters, drug receptors, and surface glycoproteins. This interest reflects the realization that such proteins play a role in the ontogeny of the nervous system, in synaptic functions, and in a variety of specific interactions with molecules and other cells.

Along with increased interest in the specific structural and functional properties of particular receptors, there has been a renewed attack on the structural and functional properties of the entire cell surface-membrane complex. The current picture of the cell surface differs radically from that of a decade ago. It is now clear that the lipid bilayer is a fluid structure (Hubbell and McConnell, 1969) and that at least some of the proteins embedded in it can diffuse, independently of one another, in the plane of the membrane (Frye and Edidin, 1970; Poo and Cone, 1974). But the cell surface is not simply a fluid mosaic. There is now evidence that transmembranous proteins (Bretscher, 1971) can penetrate the bilayer and interact with submembranous structures in the cortex of the cell (Edelman, 1976), thus providing a basis for transmembrane control of various surface receptors. Such receptor-cytoplasm interactions may have an important role both in controlling recognition at the cell surface and in regulating major cell functions. This fact was first suggested after observations that certain surface receptor changes and alterations of growth control in lymphocytes were correlated (Edelman, Yahara, and Wang, 1973).

We have hypothesized (Edelman, Yahara, and Wang, 1973; Edelman, 1976) that surface-modulating assemblies composed of receptors, microfilaments, microtubules, and their associated proteins may provide a mechanism for coordinating cell-cell interaction, cell motion, and control of cell division. In the first part of this paper, we shall consider the evidence for surface modulation and provide evidence that perturbation of the cellular structures concerned with modulation can alter growth control in normal cells. We shall briefly consider the possible implications of this evidence for specific aspects of neuronal development and function.

Anchorage modulation

In analyzing the interaction of receptors with external ligands, as well as with cytoplasmic components, it is essential to consider certain properties of the cell membrane. The fluidity of the plasma membrane has been confirmed experimentally with respect to both membrane lipids (Hubbell and McConnell, 1969) and membrane proteins (Frye and Edidin, 1970; Poo and

DONALD A. McCLAIN and GERALD M. EDELMAN The Rockefeller University, New York, NY 10021

Cone, 1974). Recently a dramatic arrangement and redistribution of lymphocyte receptors has been studied by Taylor et al. (1971), whose work suggests that both local and global movement of receptors on the cell surface can be induced after binding of multivalent ligands to these receptors.

When multivalent ligands are added to cells, the receptors to which they bind can undergo patch formation and subsequent cap formation. For example, patch formation can be induced on lymphocytes by the binding of antibodies to immunoglobulin, resulting in cross-linking of the Ig receptors. This process depends on local diffusion of the receptors in the plane of the surface membrane and not on cellular metabolism (Taylor et al., 1971). Subsequent to patch formation, the cross-linked ligand-receptor complexes move toward one pole of the cell. This second process of cap formation does depend on cellular metabolism, for metabolic inhibitors such as sodium azide inhibit cap formation without restricting patch formation (Taylor et al., 1971; Yahara and Edelman, 1972).

Although the existence of capping implies that the cell possesses structures capable of inducing active movements of aggregates of receptors, it does not reveal much about the anchorage of individual receptors. The key observation on reversible anchorage of individual receptors was made when nonsaturating amounts of the plant lectin concanavalin A (Con A), which binds to the carbohydrate portion of various cell surface proteins, were added to lymphocytes (Yahara and Edelman, 1972, 1973a,b). Under these conditions, subsequent addition and binding of specific antibodies against various receptors failed to induce patches and therefore did not induce caps (see Figure 1). This restriction, which was called anchorage modulation, was reversed when the lectin was removed, and it therefore did not result from permanent interference with metabolism or from cell death. Electron-microscopic examination of lymphocytes treated with ferritin-labeled Con A indicated that this form of surface modulation acted to immobilize individual receptors (Yahara and Edelman, 1975a). Although anchorage modulation of a variety of receptors has been studied mainly in lymphocytes, it has also been observed for the surface H-2 antigen on several other cell types (Yahara and Edelman, 1975c).

An important property of anchorage modulation is that it is a propagated phenomenon; that is, binding of Con A to a well-defined, small region of the cell surface can induce a global modulation that alters the entire surface. To show this, we prepared Con A

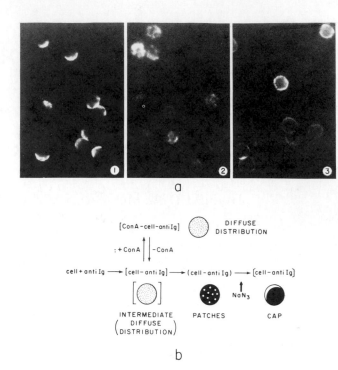

FIGURE 1   (a) Labeling patterns of surface immunoglobulin molecules or lymphocytes with fluorescein-conjugated anti-immunoglobulin antibodies. (1) Cap formation after incubation at 37°C. (2) Patch formation prior to cap formation or in the presence of 10 mM NaN₃. (3) Diffuse labeling pattern observed at 4°C or in the presence of Con A. (b) Schematic of events in patch and cap formation.

bound to platelets and latex beads and found that local attachment of these particles to a small fraction of Con A receptor sites on the cell surface inhibits the mobility of Ig and other receptors (Yahara and Edelman, 1974).

Perhaps the most direct evidence for the existence of a propagated effect of Con A on the mobility of membrane receptors comes from experiments using the fluorescence photobleaching recovery method (Schlessinger et al., 1977a). With this technique, the lateral diffusion of surface membrane components labeled with fluorescent antibodies can be measured quantitatively over distances of a few microns (Figure 2). Under these conditions, all of the surface receptors on 3T3 cells were found to be in one of two major states: anchored (A_1) or free (F). When Con A-coated platelets were used to cross-link glycoproteins in small localized regions of the cell surface, however, the diffusion coefficients of F-state receptors decreased; that is, they were converted to a less mobile state (A_2). The same result was obtained when soluble Con A was employed. The size of the immobile (A_1) fraction of the receptor population was not changed

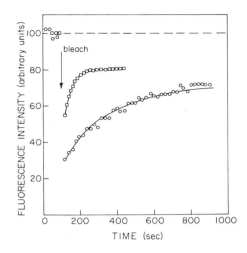

FIGURE 2 Fluorescence photobleaching recovery curves of two cells labeled with Fab fragments of rabbit antibodies to a variety of cell surface proteins. One cell had no Con A platelets (□), the other had approximately 60 platelets covering 13% of its area (○). Both recoveries fit the theory for a single diffusion coefficient within experimental error (superimposed curves). $D = 1.25 \times 10^{-10}$ cm²/sec and 1.8×10^{-11} cm²/sec, respectively.

by treatment with Con A platelets or with low doses (20 μg/ml) of soluble Con A.

The modulation effect exhibited a threshold and a plateau: occupancy of greater than 4% of the cell surface induced the effect, but larger occupancies did not increase it. Despite the fact that the platelets were localized on only a small region of the cell surface, the effect was seen in all regions of the surface. The propagated nature of the modulation of receptor mobility was confirmed by the position independence of the effect. The propagation time was faster than the relatively long periods required for measurement and has not yet been estimated.

These experiments eliminate two possible mechanisms of anchorage modulation: (1) that Con A modulates by trapping receptors in a meshwork of the cell surface glycoprotein receptors; and (2) that Con A modulates only by cross-linking the mobile glycoproteins directly to anchored or previously immobile membrane receptors. What properties of the lectin are responsible for these effects, and what structure in the cell mediates them? Experiments on the structure of Con A and on the effects of certain drugs have suggested some provisional answers.

It has been found that the valence of Con A can be changed by suitable chemical treatment and that this change in valence alters its modulating properties (Gunther et al., 1973). When Con A is succinylated, for example, it dissociates from a tetramer to a dimer, but its binding specificities for carbohydrates are un-

changed. Cells treated with succinyl-Con A show no alterations in their surface receptor mobility, and these receptors can undergo patch and cap formation. Treatment of the cells with divalent antibodies to Con A, however, cross-links the bound succinyl-Con A and induces anchorage modulation. Fab fragments of antibodies to Con A did not restore these phenomena (I. Yahara, G. M. Edelman, and J. Wang, unpublished observations), and anti-Con A alone had no effect. These observations suggest that cross-linking of cell surface glycoproteins is required to initiate anchorage modulation.

The effects of low temperature (4°C) and various antimitotic drugs indicate that certain cytoplasmic structures, particularly the cell's microtubular system, are concerned with Con A-induced anchorage modulation. If colchicine or various *Vinca* alkaloids are added to lymphocytes in concentrations ranging from 10^{-6} M to 10^{-4} M, anchorage modulation is reversed in many of the cells (Yahara and Edelman, 1973b); this effect is itself reversed by removal of the drugs. Inactive derivatives of colchicine such as lumicolchicine, which has no effect on microtubules, do not reverse anchorage modulation. Experiments with colchicine-resistant cell lines indicate that colchicine must enter the cytoplasm to affect anchorage modulation (Aubin, Carlsen, and Ling, 1975). Colchicine also partially reverses the Con A-induced inhibition of receptor mobility assayed by the fluorescence photobleaching recovery method (Schlessinger et al., 1977a). Treatment of modulated cells with a brief cold shock sufficient to depolymerize cellular microtubules (Behnke and Forer, 1967; Roth, 1967; Tilney and Porter, 1967) also releases the anchorage modulation (Yahara and Edelman, 1973a). The various properties of anchorage modulation are summarized in Table I.

What structural arrangement of submembranous components could account for these phenomena? Capping induced by Con A can also induce the re-

TABLE I

Properties of anchorage modulation

1. Modulation is induced by a cross-linkage of surface receptors.

2. The effect is propagated; that is, cross-linkage of receptors on a small area of the cell surface inhibits receptor mobility globally.

3. It is seen at the level of individual receptors.

4. It is seen in a variety of different cell types and different receptors.

5. Modulation is partially or completely reversed by treatments that disrupt microtubules

distribution of cytoplasmic microtubules (Albertini and Clark, 1975; Albertini and Andersson, 1977). Nevertheless, electron-microscopic studies (Yahara and Edelman, 1975a) suggest that, in lymphocytes, microtubules are not present at the inner lamella of the lipid bilayer. Therefore, even if cell surface glycoproteins penetrate the bilayer into the cytoplasm, some additional link between these receptors and the microtubules is required. Among the possible candidates for this role are certain microfilamentous structures found just under the membrane. It is likely that these actinlike molecules are involved in the capping of patched receptors, for it has been found that cytochalasin B, a drug that affects certain microfilaments, also inhibits capping (de Petris, 1975; Edelman, Yahara, and Wang, 1973). It has also been shown that in the presence of cytochalasin B, microfilaments can be induced to comigrate with surface receptors (Sundqvist and Ehrnst, 1976). The further observation that cytochalasin B and colchicine can act synergistically to inhibit capping (de Petris, 1975) argues that both microfilaments and microtubules are linked to the control of membrane receptor mobility.

It should be noted that cytochalasin B does not reverse anchorage modulation, and therefore some other link in addition to cytochalasin-sensitive microfilaments may be required for the proposed interaction between receptors and microtubules. Besides cytochalasin-resistant microfilaments, the linkage might consist of various assembly states of tubulin subunits (Edelman, Yahara, and Wang, 1973) or of additional proteins, possibly α-actinin or myosin (Ash and Singer, 1976).

On the basis of these observations, various models have been proposed to account for anchorage modulation (Edelman, Yahara, and Wang, 1973; Yahara and Edelman, 1975a; Berlin et al., 1975). A minimal model (Figure 3) suggests that the appropriate surface-modulating assembly (SMA) has a tripartite structure: (1) a subset of glycoprotein receptors that penetrate the membrane and confer specificity on the system; (2) various actinlike microfilaments and their associated proteins, such as myosin, conferring the properties of coordinated movement necessary for capping; and (3) dynamically assembling microtubules, both to provide anchorage of the receptors and to allow propagation and control of signals to and from the cell surface. High-voltage electron micrographs have provided evidence consistent with such a supramolecular structure consisting of interacting cytoskeletal and motility elements (Porter, 1977). These pictures show a system of microtrabeculae that exist throughout the cytoplasm and that

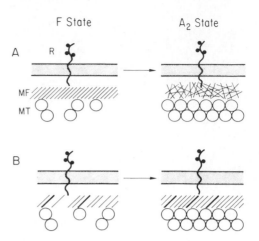

FIGURE 3 Schematic representation of different modes by which a surface-modulating assembly (SMA) might act to cause a change in receptor state from F to A_2. The various elements of the SMA have not been drawn to scale. (A) Modulation event induced by local cross-linkage of glycoprotein receptors, R, results in alteration of the submembranous components of the surface modulating assembly with gelatin of fibrils, MF, and restricted diffusion of the receptor. (B) Modulation results in enhanced binding of the cytoplasmic base of the receptor to submembranous structures. In either case, it is assumed that intact microtubules, MT, are essential for modulation.

appear to join to microtubules and actin-containing structures.

This model suggests that the receptors normally exist in two states, anchored and free. Cross-linking certain glycoprotein receptors alters the various equilibria between the microfilaments and microtubules and their subunits, thus inducing a propagated assembly of microtubules and fixation of microfilaments and increasing the proportion of anchored receptors. Conversely, changing the state of the cytoplasmic microfilaments and microtubules is supposed to alter the mobility and distribution of the surface receptors. Disruption of microtubules by drugs would still leave the microfilaments and their associated proteins free to induce capping.

The disorderly gelation of subunits of actin or tubulin in a submembranous location (Figure 3A) must be considered an alternative to specific interactions of receptors with cytoskeletal components. This mechanism can be reconciled with the observation that microtubule-disrupting agents partially reverse modulation if it is supposed that intact microtubules are necessary for formation of the postulated gel. The observation that cytochalasin B retards receptor diffusion but not lipid diffusion (Schlessinger et al., 1976a,b, 1977b) raises the possibility that it promotes disorder in submembranous microfilaments. According to the gelation model, the disassembled constituents of the SMA would form a submembranous layer that increases viscous drag on mobile receptors. As yet, however, a clear-cut choice cannot be made between the two models shown in Figure 3, nor can the possible involvement of other submembranous proteins be directly assessed.

Relation of the state of SMA components to the control of cell function

The facts reviewed above indicate that communication occurs between the cell surface and the cytoplasm, and they provide strong evidence for transmembrane control. Although a complete definition of the structures responsible for this effect is lacking, cytoskeletal and motility-related proteins appear to be involved. Given this system of cellular signaling mediated by such submembranous components, what might be its in vivo function?

One obvious possibility is in the control of cell motion. Certain surface glycoproteins are among the outermost macromolecules of the cell surface-membrane complex and are therefore likely to be in contact with solid substrates and other cells during movement. Anchorage modulation of such receptors would be expected to inhibit motions that lead to translocation of the cell as well as motions that lead to alterations in cell shape. Global modulation may, in fact, be the basis of the phenomenon of contact inhibition of cell movement (Abercrombie and Heaysman, 1954). A preliminary analysis of shape changes in lymphocytes (Rutishauser, Yahara, and Edelman, 1974) has emphasized the importance of microfilaments and microtubules and has indicated

that anchorage modulation is, in fact, accompanied by inhibition of cell movements.

Another cell function that appears to be altered by changes of state in the SMA is the control of cell division. Several types of experiments support the hypothesis that alterations in the state of SMA components affect the regulation of cell growth at crucial decision points in the G_1 phase of the cell cycle. One particularly useful experimental system is the mitogenic stimulation of lymphocytes by Con A and succinyl-Con A. The mitogenic dose-response curves for these two lectins are shown in Figure 4; the response measured is the synthesis of DNA as the stimulated cells enter the S phase. Whereas the curve for tetravalent Con A shows rising (stimulatory) and falling (inhibitory) limbs, divalent succinyl-Con A shows only stimulatory effects on mitogenesis. It appears, therefore, that the effect of Con A is the composite of two separate events, one stimulatory and the other inhibitory. Experiments on the modifications of the dose-response curve by phorbol esters and calcium ionophores (Wang, McClain, and Edelman, 1975) reinforce the idea of the independence of mitogenic stimulation and inhibition. The inhibitory limb is correlated with anchorage modulation, but their causal relationship has not yet been established. The correlation of the falling inhibitory portion of the Con A dose-response curve with anchorage modulation is based on two lines of evidence: (1) Con A, but not succinyl-Con A, is capable of inhibiting both mitogenesis and cell surface receptor mobility (Gunther et al., 1973); and (2) Con A inhibits receptor mobility with the same dose-response curve as it inhibits mitogenesis (Yahara and Edelman, 1972).

Further analysis of the inhibitory effects of Con A

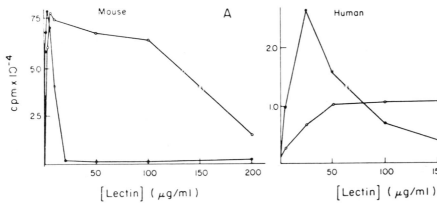

FIGURE 4 Stimulation of lymphocytes by Con A and succinyl-Con A. (A) Dose-response curves showing the incorporation of [³H]-thymidine after stimulation of mouse spleen cells by Con A (●————●) and succinyl-Con A (○————○). (B) Dose-response curves showing the incorporation of [³H]-thymidine after stimulation of human peripheral blood lymphocytes by Con A (●————●) and succinyl-Con A (○————○).

has shown that the high doses of Con A that appear to inhibit T-lymphocyte stimulation actually cause these lymphocytes to become commited to mitogenesis while also generating a dominant but reversible negative-growth signal (McClain and Edelman, 1976). The observed response to the stimulatory signal, as measured by the rate of commitment to enter the S phase, was found to increase with lectin concentration even in the inhibitory range. Cells that are committed but are simultaneously blocked from entering the S phase by the high doses of Con A can begin synthesizing DNA if the lectin is released through addition of a competitive inhibitor of binding. Experiments done in agarose cultures, in which lymphocytes are kept from contact with each other, suggest that the reversible inhibitory signal is mediated by structures in the individual cells rather than resulting from cellular agglutination. All of these experiments indicate that the inhibitory effects of Con A are not trivial: they are not due to nonspecific cell death but represent a "clamping" of otherwise stimulated cells. It should be emphasized, however, that the observations that Con A in high doses both modulates the surface and inhibits mitogenesis may be coincidental; the two events may in fact be causally related to some common prior signal resulting from the cross-linkage of surface glycoproteins by the lectin.

More persuasive evidence is available to implicate colchicine-sensitive structures (probably microtubules) in the crucial early commitment events of lymphocyte mitogenesis. We have, for example, observed that colchicine inhibits the incorporation of [^{3}H]-thymidine in mouse splenic lymphocytes stimulated by Con A (Wang, Gunther, and Edelman, 1975). Similar effects have been seen in PHA-stimulated lymphocytes (Medrano, Piras, and Mordoh, 1974) and Con A-stimulated thymocytes (Milner, 1977). Further analysis of this phenomenon has revealed that, in human lymphocytes, colchicine inhibited both lectin-induced blast transformation and entry into the S phase (Figure 5).

Mitogenesis was also blocked by vinblastine and vincristine but not by lumicolchicine, a photo-inactivated derivative of colchicine (Wilson and Friedkin, 1966). The effect of colchicine on mitogenesis could not be due to inhibition of nucleoside transport, since transport is also blocked by lumicolchicine but is not affected by vinblastine (Wilson et al., 1974). The inhibition of mitogenesis could not be attributed to effects on the mitotic spindle, because it occurred prior to the earliest evidence of cell division. Moreover, at the doses used, colchicine did not appear to

alter cell viabilities, and the effects of the drug were reversible. It was also found that colchicine did not affect DNA synthesis in cells synchronized by treatment with hydroxyurea after Con A stimulation. All of these observations prompted the inference that colchicine must inhibit stimulation prior to entry of the cell into the S phase.

To determine more precisely the stage of the cell cycle at which colchicine acts to inhibit stimulation and to determine whether all responding cells are susceptible to inhibition simultaneously, it is first necessary to consider the heterogeneity of the response of the cell population to Con A. The kinetics of cellular commitment have recently been analyzed for the stimulation by Con A of mouse splenocytes (Gunther, Wang, and Edelman, 1974) and human lymphocytes (Gunther, Wang, and Edelman, 1976). As used in these studies, the term "commitment" refers to the point at which a cell becomes irreversibly stimulated and no longer depends on the presence of the mitogenic agent. The kinetics of commitment for a cell population can be assayed by exposing the cells to Con A, removing the Con A at various times thereafter by treatment with the competitive binding sugar α-methyl-D-mannoside (αMM), and assaying the number of individual cells capable of synthesizing DNA 48 hours after the initial addition of the lectin. Under these conditions, cells become committed in an all-or-none fashion. Removal of Con A from the cell surface by αMM stops this recruitment of cells, thereby blocking a mitotic event that would otherwise occur some 20–48 hours later (Figure 6a). For mouse lymphocyte populations, the cells do not become committed simultaneously but rather respond at various times up to 20 hours after the addition of mitogen (Gunther, Wang, and Edelman, 1974). Similar results have been obtained by others for lymphocytes stimulated with PHA (Younkin, 1972) or Con A (Lindahl-Kiessling, 1972; Powell and Leon, 1970). In view of the complications introduced by daughter-cell proliferation, these conclusions concerning cellular commitment apply only to cells that have entered their initial S phase within 48 hours.

Once the kinetics of commitment were determined for human lymphocytes, colchicine was added at various times to human lymphocyte cultures containing Con A, the response was again measured in terms of total DNA synthesis, the percentage of blast transformation, and the percentage of the blast cells that synthesized DNA (Figure 6b; see also Gunther, Wang, and Edelman, 1976). As before, the later the colchicine was added, the greater the response observed in the culture. Furthermore, the shape of the curve was similar to that observed for inhibition by αMM. Blast-staining and autoradiographic procedures showed that an increasing number of cells respond to stimulation with later additions of colchicine. Furthermore, the average number of grains per labeled blast cell was constant. These results indicate, therefore, that with longer exposures to lectin, increasing numbers of cells become refractory to inhibition by colchicine. Colchicine does not bind to Con A, nor does it inhibit the cell-binding activity of the lectin (Edelman, Yahara, and Wang, 1973). Thus αMM and colchicine, two completely different reagents acting by different mechanisms, can block mitogenic stimulation with similar kinetics, as analyzed at the level of individual cells. The similarity in the kinetics of inhibition by colchicine and by αMM is consistent with the hypothesis that colchicine blocks stimulation near the time that a cell becomes committed to DNA synthesis and cell division.

If only uncommitted cells can be inhibited by col-

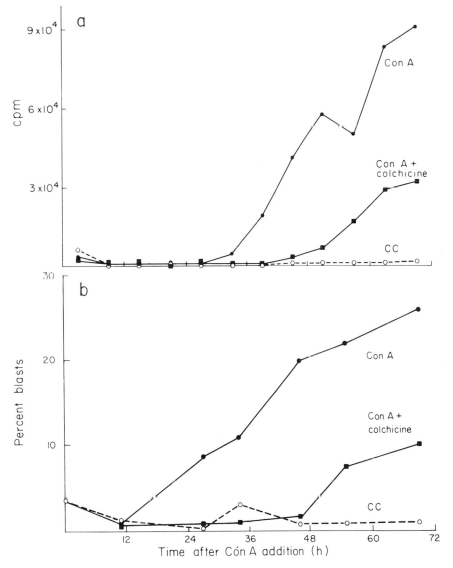

FIGURE 5 The effects of colchicine on the kinetics of appearance of blast cells and on the kinetics of [³H]-thymidine incorporation into human lymphocytes stimulated by Con A. Colchicine was present from the beginning of the experiment. At the indicated times, aliquots of cultures were removed and the total number of viable lymphocytes and blast cells were counted in a hemocytometer. The data are averages of determinations on duplicate cultures and are expressed as the percentage of blast cells present at various times after the addition of Con A (a). For measurements of DNA synthesis (b), parallel cultures were pulsed at various times with [³H]-thymidine for 6 hr. Data are plotted at the midpoint of this pulse. *Filled circles*: cultures containing Con A (20 μg/ml). *Filled squares*: cultures containing Con A (20 μg/ml) plus colchicine (10⁻⁶ M). *Open circles*: cell control (CC).

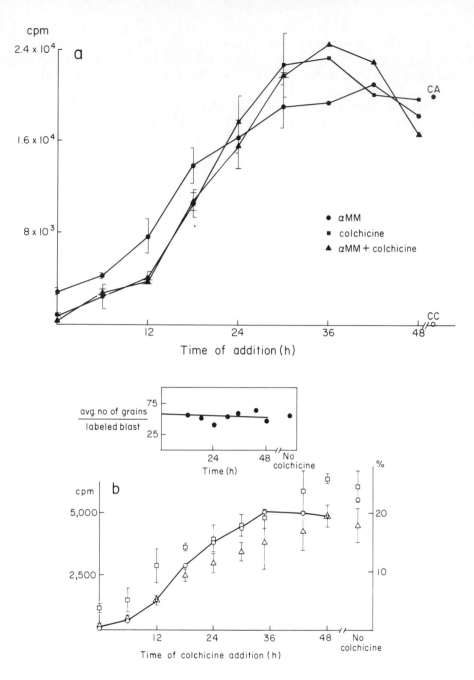

FIGURE 6   (a) Effect of simultaneous addition of αMM and colchicine on the stimulation of human lymphocytes by Con A. *Abscissa*: time after initiation of culture (hours). *Ordinate*: [³H]-thymidine incorporation expressed as percentage by the normalization procedure described below. Cultures initially contained 20 μg/ml Con A; at the indicated times parallel cultures received either αMM (●: 0.1 M final concentration), colchicine (■: 1 μM final concentration), or both reagents (▲). All cultures were assayed for [³H]-thymidine incorporation 48 hr after the initiation of the experiment. Three independent experiments were performed: two with triplicate cultures for each condition and one with duplicate cultures. Within each experiment, the counts per minute (cpm) for each condition were averaged,

and these values were normalized to the value for αMM added at 48 hr (100%). The normalized values from the three experiments were then averaged to give the points shown in the figure. The error bars represent ±1 S.D. of this final average. (b) The effect of colchicine added at various times on the stimulation of human lymphocytes by Con A. *Abscissa*: time after initiation of culture (hours). *Ordinate*: (inset) average number of autoradiographic grains per labeled blast; (left) [³H]-thymidine incorporation expressed as cmp (○); (right) percentage of cells present as blasts (□) or labeled blasts (△). Cultures initially contained 20 μg/ml Con A and were made 1 μM in colchicine at the times indicated. The error bars represent ±1 S.D. for triplicate counts of the same cell smear.

682   DONALD A. MCCLAIN AND GERALD M. EDELMAN

chicine, then the simultaneous addition of αMM and colchicine to cultures containing Con A should produce an effect equivalent to the addition of either reagent alone. To test this hypothesis, three series of parallel cultures received Con A at the same time. To one series αMM was added at various times thereafter; the second series received colchicine; and the third received both αMM and colchicine simultaneously. All three series of cultures produced similar rising curves for later times of addition of the reagents (Figure 6a). Most important, simultaneous addition of αMM and colchicine produced the same degree of inhibition as was observed when either reagent was added separately, a finding consistent with the hypothesis that both treatments affect the same cell population at a given time.

Modulation and growth control in normal and transformed fibroblasts

To determine whether the phenomena described above also occur in a different and more homogeneous cell type, we examined normal second-passage chicken embryo fibroblasts (CEFs) (McClain, D'Eustachio, and Edelman, 1977). CEFs were arrested in the G_1 phase of the cell cycle by incubation in a serum-free medium (Temin, 1972). Addition of serum to these starved fibroblasts resulted in a wave of DNA synthesis beginning at about the eighth hour (Figure 7a). Addition of colchicine to a final concentration of 1 μM at the same time as serum delayed the entry of cells into S-phase and reduced the number of cells entering S phase. Similar results were obtained with mouse 3T3 fibroblasts. The amount of label incorporated per cell in S phase (estimated from grain counts of autoradiograms) was not affected by colchicine; thus the effect of the drug did not appear to result from inhibition of [³H]-thymidine transport. Lumicolchicine, which does not dissociate microtubules, did not inhibit the entry of the CEFs into S phase. Other agents that disrupt microtubules—podophyllotoxin and vinblastine—had the same inhibitory effect at 1 μM as colchicine. The effect of colchicine was reversible: CEFs exposed to the drug but then washed free of it responded to serum as well as untreated cells.

Like lymphocytes stimulated by Con A, fibroblasts stimulated by serum did not become committed synchronously, and the kinetics of inhibition by colchicine closely paralleled the kinetics of commitment to serum stimulation (McClain, D'Eustachio, and Edelman, 1977). To study the kinetics of commitment, CEFs that had been arrested by serum starvation

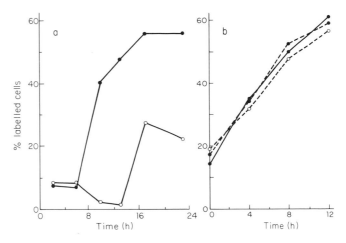

FIGURE 7 (a) Inhibition of DNA synthesis by colchicine after release of serum starvation in CEF. 2×10^5 cells were seeded into coverslips in 2 ml of medium with serum. After the cells settled, the coverslips were transferred to serum-free medium. After 60 hr, 0.22 ml of fetal calf serum was added (time 0 on abscissa) (●). Parallel cultures were also made 1 μM in colchicine (○). At various times, 6 μCi [³H]-thymidine were added to the cultures; after 2 hr the cultures were processed for autoradiography. (b) Effect of colchicine on commitment to serum stimulation. Serum-starved cells on coverslips were placed in medium containing 10% fetal calf serum at time 0. At the times indicated, coverslips were washed with buffered saline and put in serum-free medium (●———●), colchicine was added to 1 μM (○------○) or both (●------●). At 12 hr the cultures received 6 μCi [³H]-thymidine, and at 13 hr they were processed for autoradiography.

were exposed to serum. At various times thereafter, the serum was removed. Twelve hours after the initial exposure to serum, the number of cells in S phase was determined. In accord with previous observations (Temin, 1972), committed CEFs began appearing soon after serum was added, and the number of these cells increased for a period of at least 12 hours (Figure 7b). If, after serum addition, colchicine was added at various times, a reduced number of cells in S phase was observed 12 hours after the serum addition (Figure 7b). Less and less inhibition was seen the later the colchicine was added. When serum was removed at the same time that colchicine was added, the same amount of inhibition was observed as a function of time as with serum removal or colchicine addition alone. Thus both treatments of serum-stimulated CEFs appeared to affect the same subpopulations of cells at any given time.

The experiments on lymphocytes and fibroblasts suggest that microtubules or their interactions have a role in growth control. What can one say about modulation of the cell surface in these cells? It has been found that modulating doses of Con A inhibit the serum stimulation of resting fibroblasts (McClain, D'Eustachio, and Edelman, 1977). Autoradiographic analysis confirmed that this inhibition of growth reflected a restriction on the number of cells entering S phase. In contrast to tetravalent Con A, dimeric succinyl-Con A did not inhibit growth. Since the lectin and its derivative have similar binding specificities, this finding suggests that the inhibition by Con A is not due to competition for or interference with the binding of serum growth factors to the fibroblast surface. As is the case for lymphocytes, the doses of native Con A that prevent entry of the serum-stimulated cells into the S phase also cause anchorage modulation of the CEF surface.

If the state of components of the SMA is somehow related to growth control, one might expect components of the SMA to be altered in transformed cells. Pollack, Osborn, and Weber (1975), for example, have noted that the best in vitro correlate of in vivo tumorigenicity is the loss of anchorage-dependent growth control, which is correlated with the state of actin in the cell. A particularly valuable system in which to study this issue is provided by CEFs infected with Rous sarcoma virus (RSV) (Edelman and Yahara, 1976). It is known that several coordinated changes in growth control, cell shape, and cell matabolism occur upon transformation of chick fibroblasts by avian sarcoma virus (Kawai and Hanafusa, 1971). Inasmuch as a single viral gene (*src*) may be responsible for transformation (Stehelin et al., 1976), the site of action of this gene or its product attains cardinal significance.

The proposal that the SMA may be a central regulator of cell growth, shape, and interaction (Edelman, 1976) prompted the hypothesis that one or more of the components of the SMA may be targets of the *src* gene product. To test this hypothesis, we stained normal and transformed mouse and chick fibroblasts with fluorescent antibodies to visualize their microtubular and microfilamentous structures. In contrast to the orderly arrangements in untransformed cells (Lazarides, 1976; Weber, Bibring, and Osborn, 1975), the transformed cells of mouse and chick showed highly disordered patterns. There was a loss of the regular actin bundles making up stress filaments, with the concomitant appearance of a more diffuse pattern of staining. In addition, the normal tubulin pattern, consisting of a complex array of microtubules radiating from one or two central positions, was replaced by a fluffy pattern with multiple spots (SV 3T3 cells) or by a more diffuse pattern with a central concentration of stain (transformed chick

fibroblasts). This is in accord with results of other researchers who also used stains for tubulin, actin, and myosin (Brinkley, Fuller, and Highfield, 1976; Pollack, Osborn, and Weber, 1975; Ash, Vogt, and Singer, 1976).

The striking new observation was made that cells infected with an RSV having a temperature-sensitive mutation in its *src* gene (*ts*NY68) showed the normal pattern at the restrictive temperature and the disordered pattern at the permissive temperature (Figure 8). This was a reversible shift, and in a shift-down experiment the alteration took only about 1 hour to appear in the majority of cells. Comparisons of the normal and wild-type RSV-infected chick fibroblasts at both temperatures indicated that this early effect of expression of the *src* gene is not due to alteration of tubulin by the change in temperature itself.

It was also found that the capacity of Con A to induce cell surface modulation was markedly diminished in cells at the permissive temperature (Table II). Inasmuch as microtubules and associated structures are essential for anchorage modulation, it is reasonable to attribute this effect to the altered structure of the microtubules at the permissive temperature. This raises the possibility that the endogenous *src* gene product and the exogenous agent Con A may act ultimately on the same structures. If so, the addition of Con A might be expected to alter the expression of the transformed phenotype. When CEFs infected with the mutant virus and grown at 41° were shifted to 37° in the presence of Con A, the fraction of cells whose microtubular pattern was al-

TABLE II

Modulating effect of Con A on patch and cap formation in ts68-infected cells* as a function of temperature

Cell pattern		Distribution of fluorescence**		
		Cap	Patch	Diffuse
"Normal"				
(*ts*68 at 41°)	−Con A	83 (93)	6 (7)	0 (0)
	+Con A	24 (18)	36 (26)	76 (56)
"Transformed"				
(*ts*68 at 37°)	−Con A	41 (72)	16 (28)	0 (0)
	+Con A	68 (52)	44 (34)	19 (14)

* Fluorescein-labeled turkey antibodies (50 μg/ml) directed against cell surface antigens were used to induce cap and patch formation. When present, Con A was at 100 μg/ml.

** Number of stained cells; % stained cells is included in parentheses.

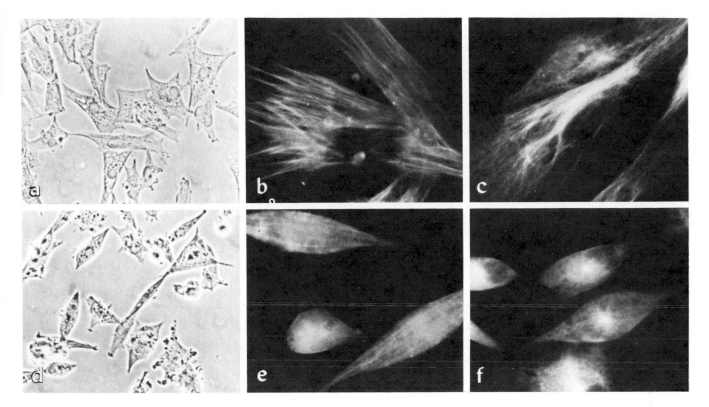

FIGURE 8   Comparison of *ts*68-infected cells at restrictive (41°C) and permissive (37°C) temperatures after binding of fluorescein-labeled antibodies to actin and tubulin: (a) 41°, phase contrast; (b) 41°, antiactin; (c) 41°, antitubulin; (d) 37°, phase contrast; (e) 37°, antiactin, (f) 37°, antitubulin. (Magnification: a and d, × 350; b, c, e, and f, × 900.)

tered was reduced (Figure 9). This inhibitory effect was not observed in cells treated with succinyl-Con A. Although definitive proof that the effects of transformation on the surface are directly attributable to microtubules has not been provided by these experiments, they do provide evidence for reciprocal effects in transmembrane control.

These experiments do not pinpoint the target of the *src* gene product, but they do suggest that components of the SMA are at least indirectly affected by this process. Preliminary studies (Edelman and Yahara, 1976) indicate that the capability of tubulin from transformed cells to polymerize in vitro is not impaired, suggesting that the *src* gene acts at a higher regulatory level than the tubulin itself to impair the SMA. This has recently been confirmed in another system (Wicke, Lundblad, and Cole, 1977). Moreover, there is evidence suggesting that whatever the causal connection between alterations in the SMA and the abrogation of growth control, the site of action of the *src* gene product is likely to be in the cytoplasm or at the cell surface (McClain, D'Eustachio, and Edelman, 1977).

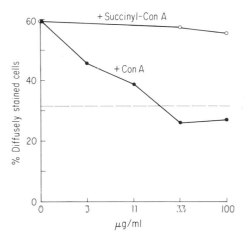

FIGURE 9   Inhibition by Con A of the conversion of cytoplasmic microtubules to a "transformed" pattern. CEF infected with *ts*NY68 virus and grown on coverslips for 36 hr at 40° were incubated for 15 min at 41° in the presence of various amounts of Con A (●) or succinyl-Con A (○), incubated with the lectin at 37° for 1 hr, then scored for microtubular morphology. The frequency of diffusely stained cells in a population grown continuously at 41° (no lectin) is shown by the dashed line.

Control points in cell proliferation

All of these observations provide evidence that the state of the SMA is well correlated with the growth-regulatory state of the cell for a variety of cell types, both resting and proliferating, normal and transformed. The data can be interpreted in terms of the schema of events leading to cell division given in Figure 10. Actions of any of a number of diverse stimuli at the cell surface probably initiate several biochemical events. Although the basis of stimulation remains unknown, a number of recent findings have suggested that calcium ion transport and increased levels of cyclic GMP both play prominent roles. It has been shown, for example, that intracellular levels of both calcium ions (Allwood et al., 1971; Whitney and Sutherland, 1972) cyclic GMP (Hadden et al., 1972; Watson, 1975) increase after mitogen binding. In addition, the ionophore A-23187, which mediates calcium ion transport, and TPA, which elevates cyclic GMP levels (Goldberg et al., 1974), are independently mitogenic for lymphocytes and are synergistic with lectins (Maino, Green, and Crumpton, 1974; Mastro and Mueller, 1974; Wang, McClain, and Edelman, 1975). Another early effect seen after mitogen binding is the increased metabolism of the phospholipids, particularly phosphatidylinositol (Fisher and Mueller, 1968), which may be controlled by changes in the intracellular concentration of free calcium (Allan and Michell, 1974). It is not clear which of these events are on the direct pathway required for initiation of DNA synthesis; some may reflect parallel effects of lectin binding that are not necessary to eventual replication.

It appears that high doses of Con A cause inhibi-

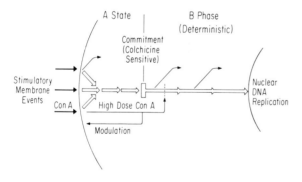

FIGURE 10 Schema of events and control points in mitogenic stimulation. "A state" refers to the stochastic period of commitment proposed by Smith and Martin (1973). Commitment appears to depend on the state of colchicine-sensitive elements, probably microtubules. After commitment occurs, events leading to surface modulation can block further transmission of stimulatory signals.

tion at some point in the pathway after the cell commitment event (McClain and Edelman, 1976). It is not known whether the surface modulation is causally related to the inhibition of mitogenesis or whether both events are independent results of some prior metabolic alteration.

In contrast, for both fibroblasts and lymphocytes, there is a colchicine-sensitive event in mitogenic stimulation that is so far kinetically indistinguishable from the commitment event itself. This commitment event represents the final integration of various stimulatory signals and is the point at which a cell becomes irrevocably fixed in a determined pathway leading to the S phase. Colchicine is also known to block entry of neuroblastoma cells (Baker, 1976) and insulin-stimulated mouse and human fibroblasts (Kamely, 1977) into S phase and to block the serum-induced increase of ornithine decarboxylase activity seen in the G_1 phase of fibroblasts (Chen, Heller, and Canellakis, 1976). All of these results suggest that colchicine blockage is a general effect observable in a variety of cells.

According to the scheme shown in Figure 10, only events that occur during or after commitment should be inhibited by colchicine. Thus the fact that colchicine inhibits phosphatidylinositol turnover (Schellenberg and Gillespie, 1977) but not calcium influx (Greene, Parker, and Parker, 1976) in stimulated lymphocytes places these events after and before the commitment point, respectively. There is some dispute about whether colchicine inhibits mitogen-induced increases in RNA synthesis, protein synthesis, lipid metabolism, and amino acid transport (Betel and Martijnse, 1976; Hauser et al., 1976; Resch et al., 1977; Vassalli and Silverstein, 1977). The resolution of these points of difference in either direction does not, however, directly challenge the now well-established phenomenon of the inhibition by colchicine of an early event in cell stimulation. The results only put restraints on the definition of precommitment and postcommitment events and of sequential versus parallel events in the stimulation pathway.

The body of evidence now at hand suggests that both cell surface interactions and alterations in microtubular states can affect the regulation of commitment to DNA synthesis. The nature of the commitment signal itself remains to be established. In the light of evidence suggesting the stochastic entry of cells into the S phase, it may be that colchicine perturbs the fluctuation or state of a key initiator of growth present in one or a few copies. Possible candidates include the centriole and the microtubule-organizing centers. Even after commitment mediated by such initiators of growth occurs, however, events leading to surface modulation can prevent further expression of mitogenic signaling. Thus the idea arises that growth regulation from within and without the cell may involve two factors: (1) a stochastically fluctuating initiating element present in small amounts; and (2) a regulated set of thresholds that determine the cellular response after a critical committing fluctuation has occurred.

Possible implications for neuronal interaction

At present, there are no reported experiments relating surface modulation to neuronal structure or function. A number of possible implications capable of experimental attack do come to mind, however. The most obvious is related to the observation that neurons in the CNS of mammals do not divide. The extensive connectivity of these neurons both synaptically and with glia may induce a block in the signal path for mitogenesis. One possible means of testing this hypothesis is to examine single neurons and neurons in contact in tissue culture for alterations in the mobility of their surface receptors. Surface modulation may also play a role in the development of the nervous system, particularly in the phenomena of contact guidance and neurite formation.

It is worth noting that because many neurons are polar structures with high degrees of local specialization, they may be particularly good objects for studies of the propagated nature of anchorage modulation. Another clear-cut problem at least superficially related to surface modulation is the localization of certain surface receptors in particular regions of the cell or synapse. Clear evidence exists for a major localization of acetylcholine receptors in the region of synaptic junctions and at the neuromuscular junction. Measurements of the mobility of such receptors (and of other surface proteins) before and after denervation of muscle or after sectioning of axons may reveal interesting propagated effects. A particularly pertinent question relates to receptors in the A_1 state: What is the nature of their anchorage and its relevance to microfilamentous and microtubular states?

Finally, one may speculate that a mode of metastable synaptic alteration that may have implications for memory storage is the modulation of the membrane at the synaptic junction of the dendritic spine. Analysis of this problem may depend on our finding native molecular species capable of inducing surface modulation. So far, such species have not been found. Until they are demonstrated, surface modulation must be considered a revealing effect induced by perturbation experiments; it cannot yet be adduced as a key functional event in any tissue. Nevertheless, the data do serve to focus attention on cell surface dynamics and the regulatory role of molecules and fibrillar elements in the submembranous cortex of the cell.

ACKNOWLEDGMENTS   We are grateful to Dr. Hidesaburo Hanafusa for his generous gift of the viruses used in this study and for his advice on their culture. This work was carried out under the support of U.S. Public Health Service grants AI-11378, AI-09273, and AM-04256 from the National Institutes of Health.

REFERENCES

ABERCROMBIE, M., and J. E. HEAYSMAN, 1954. Observation on the social behavior of cells in tissue culture. *Exp. Cell Res.* 6:293–306.

ALBERTINI, D. F., and E. ANDERSON, 1977. Microtubule and microfilament rearrangements during capping of concanavalin A receptors on cultured ovarian granulosa cells. *J. Cell Biol.* 73:111–127.

ALBERTINI, D. F., and J. I. CLARK, 1975. Membrane-microtubule interactions: Concanavalin A capping induced redistribution of cytoplasmic microtubule and colchicine binding proteins. *Proc. Natl. Acad. Sci. USA* 72:4976–4980.

ALLAN, D., and R. H. MICHELL, 1974. Phosphatidylinositol cleavage in lymphocytes: Requirement for calcium ions at a low concentration and effect of other cations. *Biochem. J.* 142:599–604.

ALLWOOD, G., G. L. ASHERSON, M. J. DAVEY, and P. J. GOODFORD, 1971. The early uptake of radioactive calcium by human lymphocytes treated with phytohemagglutinin. *Immunology* 21:509–516.

ASH, J. F., and S. J. SINGER, 1976. Concanavalin A-induced transmembrane linkage of concanavalin A surface receptors to intracellular myosin-containing filaments. *Proc. Natl. Acad. Sci. USA* 73:4575–4579.

ASH, J. F., P. K. VOGT, and S. J. SINGER, 1976. Reversion from transformed to normal phenotype by inhibition of protein synthesis in rat kidney cells infected with a temperature-sensitive mutant of Rous sarcoma virus. *Proc. Natl. Acad. Sci. USA* 73:3603–3607.

AUBIN, J. E., S. A. CARLSEN, and V. LING, 1975. Colchicine permeation is required for inhibition of concanavalin A capping in Chinese hamster ovary cells. *Proc. Natl. Acad. Sci. USA* 72:4516–4520.

BAKER, M. E., 1976. Colchicine inhibits mitogenisis in C1300 neuroblastoma cells that have been arrested in G_0. *Nature* 262:785–786.

BEHNKE, O., and A. FOREI, 1967. Evidence for four classes of microtubules in individual cells. *J. Cell Sci.* 2:169–192.

BERLIN, R. D., J. M. OLIVER, T. E. UKENA, and H. H. YIN, 1975. Control of cell surface topography. *Nature* 247:45–46.

BETEL, I., and J. MARTIJNSE, 1976. Drugs that disrupt microtubuli do not inhibit lymphocyte activation. *Nature* 261:318–319.

BRETSCHER, M., 1971. Major human erythrocyte glycoprotein spans the cell membrane. *Nature [New Biol.]* 23:229–231.

BRINKLEY, R. R., G. M. FULLER, and D. P. HIGHFIELD, 1976. Cytoplasmic microtubules in normal and transformed cells in culture. Analysis by tubulin antibody immunofluorescence. *Proc. Natl. Acad. Sci. USA* 72:4981–4985.

CHEN, K., J. HELLER, and E. S. CANELLAKIS, 1976. Studies on the regulation of ornithine decarboxylase activity by the microtubules. The effect of colchicine and vinblastine. *Biochem. Biophys. Res. Commun.* 68:401–408.

DE PETRIS, S., 1975. Concanavalin A receptors, immunoglobulins, and θ antigen of the lymphocyte surface: Interactions with concanavalin A and with cytoplasmic structures. *J. Cell Biol.* 65:123–146.

EDELMAN, G. M., 1976. Surface modulation in cell recognition and cell growth. *Science* 192:218–226.

EDELMAN, G. M., and I. YAHARA, 1976. Temperature-sensitive changes in surface modulating assemblies of fibroblasts transformed by mutants of Rous sarcoma virus. *Proc. Natl. Acad. Sci. USA* 73:2047–2051.

EDELMAN, G. M., I. YAHARA, and J. L. WANG, 1973. Receptor mobility and receptor-cytoplasmic interactions in lymphocytes. *Proc. Natl. Acad. Sci. USA* 70:1442–1446.

FISHER, D. B., and G. C. MUELLER, 1968. An early alteration in the phospholipid metabolism of lymphocytes by phytohemagglutinin. *Proc. Natl. Acad. Sci. USA* 60:1396–1402.

FRYE, C. D., and M. EDIDIN, 1970. The rapid intermixing of cell surface antigens after formation of mouse-human heterokaryons. *J. Cell Sci.* 70:319–335.

GOLDBERG, N. D., M. K. HADDOX, R. ESTENSEN, J. G. WHITE, C. LOPEZ, and J. W. HADDEN, 1974. In *Cyclic AMP Cell Growth and the Immune Response*, W. Braun, L. Lictenstein, and C. Parker, eds. New York: Academic Press, pp. 247–262.

GREENE, W. C., C. M. PARKER, and C. W. PARKER, 1976. Colchicine-sensitive structures and lymphocyte activation. *J. Immunol.* 117:1015–1022.

GUNTHER, G. R., J. L. WANG, I. YAHARA, B. A. CUNNINGHAM, and G. M. EDELMAN, 1973. Concanavalin A derivatives with altered biological activities. *Proc. Natl. Acad. Sci. USA* 70:1012–1016.

GUNTHER, G. R., J. L. WANG, and G. M. EDELMAN, 1974. The kinetics of cellular commitment during stimulation of lymphocytes by lectins. *J. Cell Biol.* 62:366–377.

GUNTHER, G. R., J. L. WANG, and G. M. EDELMAN, 1976. Kinetics of colchicine inhibition of mitogenesis in individual lymphocytes. *Exp. Cell Res.* 98:15–22.

HADDEN, J. W., E. M. HADDEN, M. K. HADDOX, and N. D. GOLDBERG, 1972. Guanosine 3′:5′-cyclic monophosphate: A possible intracellular mediator of mitogenic influences in lymphocytes. *Proc. Natl. Acad. Sci. USA* 69:3024–3027.

HAUSER, H., R. KNIPPERS, K. P. SCHÄFER, W. SONS, and H. J. UNSÖLD, 1976. Effects of colchicine on ribonucleic acid synthesis in concanavalin A-stimulated bovine lymphocytes. *Exp. Cell Res.* 102:79–84.

HUBBEL, W. L., and H. M. McCONNELL, 1969. Motion of steroid spin labels in membranes. *Proc. Natl. Acad. Sci. USA* 63:16–22.

KAMELY, D., 1977. Differential effects of inhibitors of cell division upon the growth stimulating activities of insulin and serum in nutritional depleted human and mouse cells. *J. Cell. Physiol.* 90:233–240.

KAWAI, S., and H. HANAFUSA, 1971. The effects of reciprocal changes in temperature on the transformed state of cells infected with a Rous sarcoma virus mutant. *Virology* 46:470–479.

LAZARIDES, E., 1976. Actin, α-actinin, and tropomyosin interaction in the structural organization in actin filaments in nonmuscle cells. *J. Cell Biol.* 68:202–219.

LINDAHL-KIESSLING, K., 1972. Mechanism of phytohemagglutinin (PHA) action. V. PHA compared with concanavalin A (Con A). *Exp. Cell Res.* 70:17–26.

MAINO, B. C., N. M. GREEN, and M. J. CRUMPTON, 1974. The role of calcium ions in initiating transformation of lymphocytes. *Nature* 251:324–327.

MASTRO, A. M., and G. C. MUELLER, 1974. Synergistic action of phorbol esters in mitogen-activated bovine lymphocytes. *Exp. Cell Res.* 88:40–46.

McCLAIN, D. A., P. D'EUSTACHIO, and G. M. EDELMAN, 1977. The role of surface modulating assemblies in growth control of normal and transformed fibroblasts. *Proc. Natl. Acad. Sci. USA* 74:666–670.

McCLAIN, D. A., and G. M. EDELMAN, 1976. Analysis of the stimulation-inhibition paradox exhibited by lymphocytes exposed to concanavalin A. *J. Exp. Med.* 144:1494–1506.

MEDRANO, E., R. PIRAS, and J. MORDOH, 1974. Effects of colchicine, vinblastine, and cytochalasin B on human lymphocyte transformation by phytohemagglutinin. *Exp. Cell Res.* 86:295–300.

MILNER, S. M., 1977. Activation of mouse spleen cells by a single short pulse of mitogen. *Nature* 268:441–442.

POLLACK, R., M. OSBORN, and K. WEBER, 1975. Patterns of organization of actin and myosin in normal and transformed cultured cells. *Proc. Natl. Acad. Sci. USA* 72:994–998.

POO, M. M., and R. A. CONE, 1974. Lateral diffusion of rhodopsin in photoreceptor membrane. *Nature* 247:438–441.

PORTER, K. R., 1977. Motility in cells. In *Cell Motility*, R. Goldman, T. Pollard, and J. Rosenbaum, eds. Cold Spring Harbor, NY: Cold Spring Harbor Laboratory, pp. 1–28.

POWELL, A. E., and M. A. LEON, 1970. Reversible interaction of human lymphocytes with the mitogen concanavalin A. *Exp. Cell Res.* 62:315–325.

RESCH, K., D. BOUILLON, D. GEMSA, and R. AVERDUNK, 1977. Drugs which disrupt microtubules do not inhibit the initiation of lymphocyte activation. *Nature* 265:349–351.

ROTH, L. E., 1967. Electron microscopy of mitosis in amebae. III. Cold and urea treatments. A basis for tests of direct effects of mitotic inhibitors on microtubule formation. *J. Cell Biol.* 34:4759.

RUTISHAUSER, U., I. YAHARA, and G. M. EDELMAN, 1974. Morphology, motility, and surface behavior of lymphocytes bound to nylon fibers. *Proc. Natl. Acad. Sci. USA* 71:1149–1153.

SCHELLENBERG, R. R., and E. GILLESPIE, 1977. Colchicine inhibits phosphatidylinositol turnover induced in lymphocytes by concanavalin A. *Nature* 265:741–742.

SCHLESSINGER, J., D. AXELROD, D. E. KOPPEL, W. W. WEBB, and E. L. ELSON, 1977a. Lateral transport of a lipid probe and labeled proteins on a cell membrane. *Science* 195:307–308.

SCHLESSINGER, J., E. L. ELSON, W. W. WEBB, and H. METZ-

GER, 1976a. Lateral motion and valence of Fc receptors on rat peritoneal mast cells. *Nature* 264:550–552.

SCHLESSINGER, J., E. L. ELSON, W. W. WEBB, I. YAHARA, U. RUTISHAUSER, and G. M. EDELMAN, 1977b. Receptor diffusion on cell surfaces modulated by locally-bound concanavalin A. *Proc. Natl. Acad. Sci. USA* 77:1110–1114.

SCHLESSINGER, J., D. E. KOPPEL, D. AXELROD, K. JACOBSON, W. W. WEBB, and E. L. ELSON, 1976b. Lateral transport on cell membranes: Mobility of concanavalin A receptors on myoblasts. *Proc. Natl. Acad. Sci. USA* 73:2409–2413.

SMITH, J. A., and L. MARTIN, 1973. Do cells cycle? *Proc. Natl. Acad. Sci. USA* 70:1263–1267.

STEHELIN, D., H. E. VARMUS, J. M. BISHOP, and P. K. VOGT, 1976. DNA related to the transforming gene(s) of avian sarcoma viruses is present in normal avian DNA. *Nature* 260:171–173.

SUNDQVIST, K. G., and A. EHRNST, 1976. Cytoskeletal control of surface membrane mobility. *Nature* 264:226–231.

TAYLOR, R. B., W. P. H. DUFFUS, M. C. RAFF, and S. DE PETRIS, 1971. Redistribution and pinocytosis of lymphocyte surface immunoglobulin molecules induced by anti-immunoglobulin antibody. *Nature* 233:225–229.

TEMIN, H. M., 1972. Stimulation by serum of multiplication of stationary chicken cells. *J. Cell. Physiol.* 78:161–170.

TILNEY, L. G., and K. R. PORTER, 1967. Studies on the microtubules in heliozoa. *J. Cell Biol.* 34:327–343.

VASSALLI, J. E., and S. C. SILVERSTEIN, 1977. Colccmid and related alkaloids inhibit lectin-mediated stimulation of RNA synthesis in human peripheral blood lymphocytes. *Exp. Cell Res.* 106:95–104.

WANG, J. L., G. R. GUNTHER, and G. M. EDELMAN, 1975. Inhibition by colchicine of the mitogenic stimulation of lymphocytes prior to the S phase. *J. Cell Biol.* 66:128–144.

WANG, J. L., D. A. MCCLAIN, and G. M. EDELMAN, 1975. Modulation of lymphocyte mitogenesis. *Proc. Natl. Acad. Sci. USA* 72:1917–1921.

WATSON, J., 1975. The influence of intracellular levels of cyclic nucleotides on cell proliferation and the induction of antibody synthesis. *J. Exp. Med.* 141:97–111.

WEBER, K., TH. BIBRING, and M. OSBORN, 1975. Specific visualization of tubulin-containing structures in tissue culture cells by immunofluorescence. *Exp. Cell Res.* 95:111–120.

WHITNEY, R. B., and R. M. SUTHERLAND, 1972. Enhanced uptake of calcium by transforming lymphocytes. *Cell. Immunol.* 5:137–147.

WICKE, G., V. J. LUNDBLAD, and R. D. COLE, 1977. Competence of soluble cell extracts as microtubule assembly systems. *J. Biol. Chem.* 252:794–796.

WILSON, L., J. R. BAMBURG, S. B. MIZEL, L. M. GRISHAM, and K. M. CRESWELL, 1974. Interaction of drugs with microtubule proteins. *Fed. Proc.* 33:158–166.

WILSON, L., and M. FRIEDKIN, 1966. The biochemical events of mitosis. I. Synthesis and properties of colchicine labeled with tritium in its acetyl moiety. *Biochemistry* 5:2463–2468.

YAHARA, I., and G. M. EDELMAN, 1972. Restriction of the mobility of lymphocyte immunoglobulin receptors by concanavalin A. *Proc. Natl. Acad. Sci. USA* 69:608–612.

YAHARA, I., and G. M. EDELMAN, 1973a. The effects of concanavalin A on the mobility of lymphocyte surface receptors. *Exp. Cell Res.* 81:143–155.

YAHARA, I., and G. M. EDELMAN, 1973b. Modulation of lymphocyte receptor redistribution by concanavalin A, anti-mitotic agents and alterations of pH. *Nature* 246:152–155.

YAHARA, I., and G. M. EDELMAN, 1975a. Electron microscopic analysis of the modulation of lymphocyte receptor mobility. *Exp. Cell Res.* 91:125–142.

YAHARA, I., and G. M. EDELMAN, 1975b. Modulation of lymphocyte receptor mobility by concanavalin A and colchicine. *Ann. NY Acad. Sci.* 253:455–469.

YAHARA, I., and G. M. EDELMAN, 1975c. Modulation of lymphocyte receptor mobility by locally bound concanavalin A. *Proc. Natl. Acad. Sci. USA* 72:1579–1583.

YOUNKIN, L. H., 1972. *In vitro* response of lymphocytes to phytohemagglutinin (PHA) as studied with antiserum to PHA. I. Initiation period, daughter-cell proliferation, and restimulation. *Exp. Cell Res.* 75:1–10.

40 Long-Range Motions on Cell Surfaces

E. L. ELSON and J. SCHLESSINGER

ABSTRACT Processes that control cell growth, metabolism, shape, and other important properties occur on the plasma membrane. Some of these involve changes in the patterns of arrangement of cell surface components, and direct measurement of the macroscopic lateral motions of specific membrane components provides the information needed for their analysis at a molecular level. A fluorescence photobleach method has recently been developed to carry out such measurements, and this paper summarizes and discusses results obtained with this method. These studies show that fluorescent lipid probes diffuse rapidly over large areas of the cell membrane. Labeled proteins, however, are divided into mobile and immobile states, and even mobile proteins move 10–50 times more slowly than the lipid probes. The forces constraining the motion of membrane proteins are unknown. Aggregation by antibodies and binding of the lectin concanavalin A to local regions of the cell surface provide apparently different ways of inhibiting the motion of particular cell surface proteins. Other proteins, such as the acetylcholine receptor and the CSP/LETS glycoprotein, form well-defined patterns of immobile molecules that are apparently required for their function.

Introduction

The cell surface participates in such important physiological functions as signal reception and transmission, endocytosis and exocytosis, locomotion, cellular recognition, adhesion, and control of morphology. Proteins and lipids of the plasma membrane must interact with each other and with molecules inside and outside the cell to carry out these functions. This often involves local or global reorganization of the membrane or of some of its components, so that at least some membrane molecules must move laterally over the cell surface as they take part in these events. One approach, then, to study the molecular mechanism of cell surface functions is to analyze directly the motions of these molecules. Such an analysis is the subject of this paper.

E. L. ELSON and J. SCHLESSINGER Department of Chemistry, Cornell University, Ithaca, NY 14853; Department of Applied and Engineering Physics, Cornell University, Ithaca, NY 14853, and Immunology Branch, National Cancer Institute, National Institutes of Health, Bethesda, MD 20014

Several examples can be used to illustrate the involvement of lateral movement in physiologically significant processes. One of these is the triggering of a cellular response by the association of a limited number of initially dispersed cell surface molecules. When IgE-receptor complexes on the surfaces of mast cells are cross-linked by antibodies against IgE or by multivalent antigens, a complex chain of events is initiated that results in exocytosis of basophilic granules and release of histamine and other active substances (Ishizaka and Ishizaka, 1971; Metzger, 1973). The IgE-Fc receptor complexes, which are initially randomly dispersed over the mast-cell surface, must move laterally to encounter one another in forming the requisite complexes. (Recent evidence indicates that aggregation to the level of dimers is sufficient for some degree of degranulation: see Siegel, Taurog, and Metzger, 1977.) Aggregation of surface immunoglobulin via anti-immunoglobulin antibody (Pernis, Forni, and Amante, 1970) and of concanavalin A (Con A) receptors via Con A (Rosenblith et al., 1973) are other instances in which molecules of similar specificities are bridged by multivalent ligands. Alternatively, the binding of a hormone may trigger the interaction of independent and different receptor and effector molecules. The activation of adenyl cyclase by the β-adrenergic receptor may be an example of this (Orly and Schramm, 1976). Lateral mobility of cell surface molecules is also necessary for changes in the distribution of membrane components associated with endocytosis and exocytosis. The clearing of intramembrane particles from the regions of plasma membrane through which exocytosis occurs has been observed by freeze-fracture electron microscopy in degranulation of mast cells (Chi, Lagunoff, and Koehler, 1976). Lateral transport is also seen at the site of release of synaptic vesicles at neuromuscular junctions (Heuser, this volume). A similar process in phagocytic leukocytes has been invoked to explain the retention of amino acid and nucleoside transport systems on the surface of cells that are rapidly internalizing substantial portions of their plasma membranes (Tsan and Berlin, 1971). Conversely, the enhanced loss of Con A receptors from the surfaces of these cells suggests that these molecules are selectively concentrated in regions of the plasma membrane engaged in endocytosis (Oliver, Ukena, and Berlin, 1974). Finally, the formation of viral buds in cells infected with enveloped viruses suggests lateral mobility of membrane-bound viral glycoproteins. The formation of buds seems to occur when initially dispersed glycoproteins are concentrated into small patches in the plasma membrane (Garoff and Simons, 1974). A similar lateral reorganization may be involved in the formation of patches of acetylcholine receptor in developing myotubes (Axelrod et al., 1976b).

Other surface molecules may be required by their physiological function to be immobile in the plasma membrane. For example, acetylcholine receptors remain confined to specialized postsynaptic regions (Fertuck and Salpeter, 1974). Another example is the large glycoprotein known as CSP (Yamada and Weston, 1974) or LETS (Hynes, 1976), which forms a fibrillar network over dense cell cultures and seems to be involved in adhesion of cells to each other and the substratum (Yamada, Yamada, and Pastan, 1976).

The aim of our work is to use direct measurements of the lateral mobility of specific cell surface components to characterize the range of dynamic phenomena that occur on the plasma membrane. These measurements provide information about the kinds and mechanisms of interaction of the components and should lead eventually to an analysis at the molecular level of the physiologically interesting behavior just discussed. In this paper we shall summarize some recent measurements that indicate the diversity of behavior of several membrane proteins and lipids and discuss current problems.

The method for determining lateral mobility is simple in concept and direct and flexible in application. A laser beam focused through the objective lens of a fluorescence microscope illuminates and defines a small ($\sim 3 \mu m^2$) region on the cell surface (Koppel et al., 1976). The amount of a labeled surface component in this region is proportional to the emitted fluorescence. The region is first exposed to a brief intense pulse of excitation light, which irreversibly destroys a portion of the fluorophore. This pulse establishes an initial concentration gradient of the fluorophore from the interior to the exterior of the region. If the labeled component is mobile, bleached molecules leave and unbleached molecules enter the region, causing an increase in the fluorescence measured through the microscope. During this observa-

tion phase of the experiment, the laser excitation intensity is highly attenuated to avoid further bleaching. The rate of increase of fluorescence depends on the speed of lateral motion of the mobile fluorophores and the size of the region. The larger the region, the longer the time required to reattain concentration equilibrium. Lateral transport can occur either by diffusion or by some directed process such as membrane flow. Once the size of the bleached region is known, the diffusion coefficient or flow velocity of the mobile fluorophores can be deduced from the observed rate of increase of fluorescence (Axelrod et al., 1976a). In principle, the rates of chemical reactions that change either the emitted fluorescence intensity or the lateral mobility of the labeled cell surface particles can also be measured (Elson et al., 1976). Typically these measurements are performed on living cells adhering to the tissue-culture dishes in which they have been grown.

This method derives from experiments in which Poo and Cone (1974) measured the lateral diffusion of rhodopsin in amphibian retinal disk membranes. The rhodopsin concentration was measured by its absorbance. A fluorescence photobleach experiment was first described by Peters et al. (1974) in a study of the lateral mobility of fluorescein-labeled proteins on red-cell membranes. The advantages of the current version of this approach include good spatial resolution, which permits measurements of mobility in several regions of the same cell; good sensitivity, to allow detection of relatively few fluorescent particles ($\sim 500/\mu m^2$) on the cell surface; capability of measuring a wide range of transport rates; and relatively little perturbation of the cell by the measurement.

Selected results and discussion

To establish a perspective for later studies we first compare the mobilities of a lipidlike molecule with a cross section of membrane components unselected for function or antigenic specificity (Schlessinger et al., 1977a). We have used 3,3'-dioctadecylindocarbocyanine iodide (diI) to indicate lipid behavior. The diI molecule has a positively charged fluorescent carbocyanine "head group" and two C_{18} hydrocarbon chains, which should intercalate into the membrane lipid bilayer. Although it is not derived from a biological lipid, diI does mimic the diffusion of phospholipids in model bilayers (Fahey et al., 1977). It may, however, differ from natural lipids in its interaction with membrane proteins. Figure 1a presents a typical fluorescence photobleach recovery (FPR)

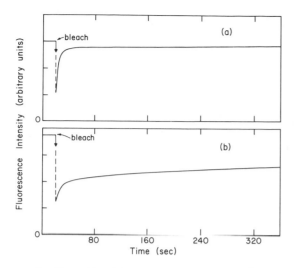

FIGURE 1 Photobleaching recovery curves of L6 myoblasts. (a) Myoblasts labeled with diI: $D = 9.2 \times 10^{-9}$ cm²/sec (for beam radius = 4 μm); 95% fluorescence recovery. (b) Myoblasts labeled with TNP and rhodamine-labeled antibodies against TNP: $D = 1.9 \times 10^{-10}$ cm²/sec (for beam radius = 1.1 μm); 54% fluorescence recovery. Note that the time for fluorescence recovery varies inversely as the square of the beam radius (Axelrod et al., 1976a). (Reprinted from Schlessinger et al., 1977a; copyright © 1977 by the American Association for the Advancement of Science.)

curve for diI in the plasma membrane of an L6 (rat myoblast) cell. The curve behaves according to theory (Axelrod et al., 1976a) for diffusion with a coefficient $D = 9.2 \times 10^{-9}$ cm²/sec. (Measurements on other cells—including rat peritoneal mast cells, chicken and rat embryo fibroblasts, chicken and rat embryo myoblasts and myotubes, mouse peritoneal macrophage, and 3T3 cells—also yield diffusion coefficients near 10^{-8} cm²/sec.) Measurements of diI diffusion in L6 and other types of cells usually show complete recovery of the fluorescence in the bleached region to the level prior to bleaching. Therefore, the lipid bilayer exists as a continuous membrane matrix over distances substantially greater than 1 μm (the largest beam radius used) without being significantly partitioned into closed regions. When incomplete recovery is observed in the first bleach, labeling of internal cell structures is also seen. This suggests that the immobile diI has been internalized. Cross-linking of membrane proteins does not effect the diI mobility, nor does treatment by azide (which poisons oxidative metabolism), by colchicine (which disrupts microtubule assembly), or by cytochalasin B (which, among other effects, disrupts some microfilaments).

The uniformity of the behavior observed for diI indicates that the factors controlling its lateral mobil-

ity vary little among cells of different types and under different conditions. Hence it appears that, to the extent that diI mobility measures a property which might be termed the "fluidity" of the membrane lipid bilayer, that fluidity is a fairly uniform property of cells. Other measures of membrane fluidity have been obtained by methods that detect microscopic rotational motions of spin-labeled (Hubbell and McConnell, 1969) or fluorescence-labeled (Shinitsky et al., 1971) probe molecules. In contrast to these methods, which primarily detect motions over ranges of molecular dimensions, FPR experiments observe lateral motions over macroscopic distances in the range of microns. The relationship between the membrane properties measured by microscopic and macroscopic transport is still unclear; for example, compartmentation could restrict the latter without affecting the former. Detailed experimental comparisons are needed to clarify this matter.

The lateral mobility of components of L6 plasma membranes labeled with fluorescein isothiocyanate or 2,4,6-trinitrobenzene sulfonate is both far slower and more heterogeneous than that of the lipid probe. Mostly these reagents label surface proteins (Edidin, Zagyansky, and Lardner, 1976; Comoglio et al., 1975), although membrane components other than proteins may also be labeled to some extent. Surface molecules labeled with trinitrophenol (TNP) groups were marked by rhodamine-labeled antibody directed against TNP. Diffusion coefficients of molecules marked in either way were close to 2×10^{-10} cm²/sec (Schlessinger et al., 1977a). Use of the antibody-labeling procedure verified that we were observing cell surface molecules, since the antibody molecules should not permeate the plasma membrane. Comparable results were previously obtained by Edidin, Zagyansky, and Lardner (1976) using a similar approach. The similarity in the diffusion coefficients measured for the two types of labels indicates that the hydrodynamic resistance to the motion of the antibody molecule had little effect on the mobility of the surface component to which it was bound. This is not surprising, since in free solution the mobility of an antibody molecule should be 100–1,000 times greater than that measured for the labeled surface components. Figure 1b presents a recovery curve from a cell labeled with TNP and anti-TNP antibodies. The measured diffusion coefficient is $D = 1.9 \times 10^{-10}$ cm²/sec. A noteworthy feature of this curve is that the fluorescence at long times recovered only to about 50% of its value before bleaching. This is in marked contrast to the behavior of diI and is most simply interpreted as an indication that a fraction of the fluorescence-labeled molecules are immobile on the time scale of our measurements. When these molecules are bleached, they cannot be replaced by exchange with unbleached molecules from other areas of the cell surface.

The existence of this immobile fraction prompted us to inquire into the structures and interactions that constrained the mobility of the labeled cell surface molecules. Neither colchicine nor azide affected the rate or extent of recovery; therefore, neither oxidative metabolism nor microtubules seem to be directly responsible for the constraint. Cytochalasin B, however, dramatically reduced the apparent diffusion coefficient of the labeled molecules (by about a factor of ten) without noticeably changing the extent of fluorescence recovery.

Since the labeling procedure used in this study should have marked a wide variety of membrane proteins and possibly also some nonprotein molecules, we have also measured the mobility of a well-defined surface protein, the Fc receptor for immunoglobulin E (IgE) on rat peritoneal mast cells (Schlessinger et al., 1976b). This receptor is highly specific for IgE and has been relatively well characterized (Newman, Rossi, and Metzger, 1977). The diffusion coefficient of the receptor marked with rhodamine-labeled IgE was 2×10^{-10} cm^2/sec; the extent of fluorescence recovery was incomplete—in the range 50–80%. Hence the distinction between mobile and immobile molecules is not based on biological function or specificity, since the specifically defined IgE-Fc receptors also divide into mobile and immobile classes. The effects of azide, colchicine, and cytochalasin B on the IgE-Fc receptor are as described for the fluorescein and TNP-labeled surface molecules. Similar results have been obtained for otherwise-defined collections of surface components, such as receptors of the lectin Con A (Schlessinger et al., 1976a) and antibodies directed against the mouse P388 lymphoid cell line (Schlessinger et al., 1977c). (The lateral mobility of Con A receptors seems to be somewhat slower than that of other surface components: see Schlessinger et al., 1976a.)

These results allow us to conclude that the lateral mobility of diI and labeled membrane proteins differ in two important respects: (1) the former diffuses about fifty times faster than the latter; and (2) the protein molecules are present in at least two classes, mobile and immobile, whereas all of the molecules of lipid probe are mobile. Although the existence of the immobile protein molecules suggests an interaction between them and some other molecules or supra-

molecular structures in the membrane or cytoplasm, we have as yet no notion of what these molecules may be. At this time we are unable to give a quantitative interpretation of the difference in diffusion coefficients of diI and the mobile labeled proteins. One possible interpretation is hydrodynamic: the proteins move more slowly because, being larger, they experience greater viscous drag. An analysis of this possibility could be carried out in principle using the theory of Saffman and Delbrück (1975). Supposing that membrane proteins have reasonable sizes (radii of 10–100 Å) and that the viscosity of the lipid bilayer is 1–10 poise, as expected from earlier measurements (Edidin, 1974), calculated diffusion coefficients are a minimum of tenfold greater than the values observed experimentally. This suggests that lipid viscosity does not control the lateral mobility of the labeled surface components.

The measurements of the lateral diffusion of rhodopsin in amphibian disk membranes may cast some further light on this hypothesis. In these membranes rhodopsin is the primary protein constituent and should not experience interactions with cytoskeletal structures. Poo and Cone (1974) determined the diffusion coefficient to be approximately 5×10^{-9} cm^2/sec; this is approximately twenty times faster than the value measured for nonselectively labeled L6 membrane proteins and for the IgE receptor on rat mast cells. If we suppose that retinal disks present an ideal fluid membrane in which the diffusion rate of the rhodopsin molecules is limited mainly by the viscosity of the lipid matrix, then the mobility of L6 membrane proteins seems to be limited by interactions in addition to viscous resistance. This comparison is somewhat weakened by the presence of relatively large amounts of highly unsaturated lipids in disk membranes (measured for bovine disks: see Nielsen, Fleischer, and McConnell, 1970), which could render them somewhat more fluid than myoblast or mast-cell plasma membranes. Direct comparisons of rotational and translational mobility, using photobleaching and fluorescence depolarization methods on disk membranes and plasma membranes, would clarify the validity of the comparison. Provisionally, however, we conclude that the viscous resistance of the fluid bilayer is insufficient to account for the measured mobility of plasma membrane proteins.

At this time we do not know what additional interactions are responsible for limiting the lateral mobility. Obvious possibilities include interactions with cytoskeletal structures that are independent of colchicine and cytochalasin B or with other proteins in the membrane. Membrane proteins are probably concentrated enough that some decrease in mobility might result from nonspecific collisions. This type of concentration-dependent behavior has been observed in a model system (Wolf et al., 1977). It does not seem likely, however, that this effect is sufficient to explain the twentyfold difference in diffusion coefficient between rhodopsin and L6 proteins. Further information about the behavior of membrane proteins in simple bilayers is clearly needed to confirm this hypothesis and, more important, to establish a baseline for the mobility of proteins in membranes in the absence of interactions with structures outside the membrane. Reconstitution experiments with well-characterized membrane proteins and lipid bilayers would best fill this need. This first analysis of membrane protein mobility already poses the challenge of explaining two seemingly different types of interactions: one causes a limited constraint on protein diffusion; the other seems to inhibit entirely the lateral motion of proteins within the limits of detection of the method. The structural basis and possible relationship, if any, of these two kinds of interactions remains to be discovered.

The studies just discussed have revealed constraints that appear to act commonly on different plasma membrane proteins in a variety of cultured animal cells. We now consider interactions that limit the mobility of specific membrane proteins in particular systems. The simplest and most directly demonstrable type of specific constraint results from the formation of aggregates due to external cross-linking reactions. For example, the complete immobilization of surface-bound Con A by anti-Con A antibodies (Schlessinger et al., 1976a) and of IgE bound to mast-cell Fc receptors by anti-IgE antibodies (Schlessinger et al., 1976b) have been experimentally demonstrated. The underlying reason for the lower mobility of the aggregates cannot yet be stated with certainty. It seems plausible that the viscous drag of the lipid bilayer could be large enough to decrease the mobility of very large aggregates. However, we do not yet know the dependence of diffusion in membranes on particle size. According to the theory of Saffman and Delbrück (1975), this dependence should be very weak and might not be strong enough to account for the observed effects. Nevertheless, the reduction of the mobility of synthetic lipopolysaccharides on black lipid model membranes by antibody cross-linking has been demonstrated (Wolf et al., 1977). It is also possible that the aggregation reaction enhances the interaction of the cross-linked molecules with stationary structures inside the cell or in the membrane. This mechanism seems to be involved, for example, in the global inhibition of membrane protein mobility by Con A discussed below.

An interesting apparent aggregation reaction was observed in a study of Con A bound to L6 myoblasts (Schlessinger et al., 1976a). Con A is a tetrameric molecule that binds as a tetravalent ligand to glycoproteins or glycolipids bearing glucose or mannose residues. It can be dissociated into two divalent dimers by succinylation. When the mobility of rhodamine-labeled Con A was measured on L6 plasma membranes, it was found that the diffusion rate varies with Con A dose, time of occupancy on the membrane, and valence. For a given dose, the recovery rate decreases with increasing time. The rate of decrease in mobility is faster at higher doses of Con A. Finally, the extent of decrease is far less for succinylated Con A. Similar behavior has also been observed on other cells (Zagyansky and Edidin, 1976). These results are expected for formation of a cross-linked aggregate of Con A-receptor complexes, which should be larger for tetravalent than for divalent ligands and which should form more rapidly at higher ligand concentrations. As before, this interpretation leaves open the question of the underlying cause of the reduced mobility of the aggregates; both hydrodynamic factors and enhanced interaction of aggregates with cytoskeletal structures could be involved. Alternatively, the reduction in mobility could result from the internalization of the aggregated Con A-receptor complexes into submembrane vesicles. Since these vesicles should be nearly immobile in our experiments, this mechanism might more plausibly be expected to lead to a systematic dependence of the fraction of fluorescence recovery rather than the diffusion coefficient on lectin dose and valence. Although an interpretation in terms of a progressive aggregation is consistent with the experimental results, other explanations are also possible; for example, there could be a valence and dose-dependent attachment of isolated, unaggregated Con A-receptor complexes to some intracellular anchoring structure. As discussed below, some cytoskeletal interaction with dispersed membrane components can be provoked by sufficient amounts of Con A cross-linking on the cell surface. It is doubtful, however, that this can account fully for the experimental results.

The cross-linking of cell surface receptors by Con A can also initiate a "global" inhibition of the mobility of other cell surface components, even when the latter do not directly interact with the bound Con A.

substantially after transformation (Hynes, 1976). Addition of exogenous CSP to transformed cells partially restores the morphology, adhesiveness, and parallel alignment typical of normal fibroblasts (Yamada, Yamada, and Pastan, 1976). These observations prompted us to study how CSP binds to cell surfaces, using fluorescence microscopy and photobleach methods.

In contrast to AChR, which resides in both diffuse (mobile) and patched (immobile) forms, CSP is detected only in a fibrillar, immobile state. Rhodamine-labeled anti-CSP antibody revealed the characteristic fibrillar pattern on primary chick embryo fibroblasts (Schlessinger et al., 1977b). Photobleach experiments detected no significant recovery on the time scale of the measurement. Motions of CSP fibrils, which are slow on the time scale of these experiments, have been observed by fluorescence photomicrography (unpublished observations). These motions seem to be associated with systematic movements of the cells to which the fibrils are attached.

The association of exogenous CSP to cells proceeds by attachment to regions already rich in CSP. This attachment can be demonstrated by comparing the fluorescent images produced by fluorescein-labeled exogenous CSP incubated with cultured fibroblasts to those produced by rhodamine-labeled anti-CSP antibody bound to the same cells. The images can be photographed independently because of the differences in the emission spectra of fluorescein and rhodamine. Apart from unavoidable differences in intensity, the two images seem identical. Therefore, within the sensitivity of the experiment, the fluorescein-labeled CSP does not appear to bind to regions of the cell surface that are free of preexisting CSP. Moreover, photobleaching measurements show that the adherent exogenous CSP is also immobile. The mechanism by which exogenous CSP is incorporated into fibrils may have no relevance for the process by which these structures are assembled from endogenous CSP. It may be significant, however, that neither endogenous nor exogenous CSP appears in a diffuse mobile form in detectable amounts on the cell surface. This in turn suggests that the mechanisms by which CSP fibrils and AChR patches are assembled may be quite different. This proposed mechanistic difference may reflect differences in the kinds of interactions that bind the two proteins to the membrane. AChR is a typical integral membrane protein that can be detached only by disruptive treatments with solubilizing agents such as detergents (Meunier et al., 1974). In contrast, CSP can be released from the cell surface without disrupting the membrane, for example by incubating with urea (Yamada and Weston, 1974).

The absence of a strong hydrophobic interaction between CSP and the membrane lipid bilayer was confirmed by the failure of fluorescein-labeled CSP to bind to synthetic black lipid membranes composed of oxidized cholesterol or phosphatidylcholine. The labeled CSP does, however, bind to black lipid membranes coated with a synthetic lipopolysaccharide, a stearoyl dextran derivative (Schlessinger et al., 1977b). In contrast to the fibrillar, immobile state of CSP on cells, the CSP bound to dextran-coated bilayers is diffuse and mobile, indicating that the CSP molecules do not interact strongly enough with each other to form large, immobile aggregates on the dextran-coated bilayers. It thus appears that CSP binds to regions of the cell surface rich in CSP but that the main energy of binding does not come from interactions with other CSP molecules or with the membrane lipid. This consideration, together with the difference between the diffuse and fibrillar patterns seen on the dextran-coated bilayers and cultured fibroblasts, respectively, suggests the existence of other membrane components that initiate or provide a framework for fibril formation and attachment to the cell surface. Furthermore, one might predict that erythrocytes, to which CSP binds weakly and diffusely, would lack these components but that transformed cells, to which exogenous CSP binds in an apparently normal pattern, would retain them. The development of patches of viral glycoproteins during the formation of buds on the plasma membranes of cells infected with enveloped viruses could provide a useful model for the study of pattern development on cell surfaces.

Summary and conclusions

Measurements of lateral mobility have revealed elements of both diversity and uniformity in the dynamic behavior of membrane components. Results obtained up to now are summarized in Table I. Observation of diI diffusion confirms the existence of a fluid membrane matrix in which lipid molecules are free to range over wide areas of the cell surface. The similarity of diI diffusion coefficients in different kinds of cells suggests that the "viscosity" that limits its lateral mobility does not depend sensitively on cell type. There may, however, be differences in diI mobility that are physiologically significant even though small compared to the precision of present measurements. The rough consistency of our direct measurements of macroscopic lateral diffusion with estimates

TABLE I
Lateral mobility of cell membrane components

Membrane component	Diffusion coefficient (cm²/sec)	Mobile fraction	References
Lipid probe (diI)	~10^{-8}	1.0	Schlessinger et al. (1977a)
Unselected surface "proteins" (labeled chemically)	~2×10^{-10}	0.3–0.8	Schlessinger et al. (1977a); Edidin, Zagyansky, and Lardner (1976)
Unselected surface antigens (labeled by anti-P388)	~2×10^{-10}	0.3–0.8	Schlessinger et al. (1977c)
Con A binding sites (S-Con A on Con A at low dose)	~4×10^{-11}	0.5–0.7	Schlessinger et al. (1976a); Jacobson, Wu, and Poste (1976)
Con A binding sites (high dose)	10^{-11}–3×10^{-12}	0.0–0.5	Schlessinger et al. (1976a); Zagyansky and Edidin (1976)
Acetylcholine receptor (diffuse)	~3×10^{-11}	0.8	Axelrod et al. (1976b)
Acetylcholine receptor (patch)	<10^{-12}	0.0	Axelrod et al. (1976b)
IgE-Fc receptor	~3×10^{-10}	0.5–0.8	Schlessinger et al. (1976b)
CSP/LETS	<3×10^{-12}	0.0	Schlessinger et al. (1977b)
Analog of ganglioside GMl	~5×10^{-9}	1.0	J. Reidler (personal communication)

derived from microscopic motions of lipids suggests that the same forces limit both. It may be misleading nevertheless to describe the factors limiting the mobility as a viscosity. It is not certain that fluid-dynamic factors limit the lateral mobility even of so relatively simple a molecule as diI. Interaction of authentic lipids and diI with hydrophobic membrane proteins could also limit their rate of motion.

Evidence for the immobilization of membrane lipids by hydrophobic proteins has been obtained in studies using spin-labeled fatty acids (Jost et al., 1973). The experimental results were interpreted in terms of a boundary layer of lipid strongly absorbed to the protein. The formation of a lipid boundary layer could influence the mobility of both the lipid and the protein. To study this phenomenon, it would be desirable to use fluorescence-labeled lipids that retain their capacity for binding to membrane proteins. Moreover, the diffusion of diI in black lipid model membranes is approximately tenfold faster than in plasma membranes (Fahey et al., 1977). This comparison is clouded, however, by doubts about the adequacy of black lipid membranes as models of biological membranes (P. Fahey and W. Webb, per-

sonal communication). It is also important to realize that diI may not participate in some interactions that involve biological lipids (e.g., interactions of glycolipids through their carbohydrate moieties).

Proteins present a more complex picture. They occur in both mobile and immobile states. We have considered two proteins that form specific structures on the cell surface in which the constituent molecules are essentially immobile. The mechanisms by which these structures develop and the forces that maintain them pose an interesting problem for further research. It seems likely that they are different for CSP and AChR. Furthermore, in contrast to CSP, AChR is also present on the cell surface in a diffuse patternless distribution that contains both mobile and immobile molecules. In this respect the diffuse AChR resembles other randomly distributed membrane proteins, even of defined specificity such as the IgE-Fc receptor, which are present in both mobile and immobile states. The physiological significance and structural explanation of these immobile proteins is now unknown, as are the forces that determine the diffusion rates of the mobile proteins. It seems that the apparent viscosity of the lipid bilayer may be too small to account for the measured diffusion coefficients. Measurements of the diffusion coefficients of assorted membrane proteins reincorporated into simplified model membranes should yield information on the dependence of lateral mobility on particle size that can be compared with theoretical work on this subject (Saffman and Delbrück, 1975). When this information is available, the need for additional factors—beyond simple bilayer viscosity—to explain the diffusion rates of individual proteins and aggregates will be clearer.

The studies of the modulation of membrane antigen mobility by locally bound Con A reveal the capability of membrane components for even greater diversity in dynamic behavior. These studies confirm the global inhibition of mobility and are generally consistent with the model proposed by Edelman (1976). Quantitative details of the results, such as the plateau/threshold, the retention of mobility in the A2 state, and the incomplete reversal of inhibition by microtubule-disrupting drugs, indicate that some further subtleties must be added to the interpretation.

The major goal of studies of the dynamic properties of membrane components should be a mechanistic interpretation of cellular physiological processes at the molecular level. Evidently far more than fluorescence microscopy and measurements of lateral mobility will be needed to achieve this goal. When interpreted in the context of ultrastructural, biochemical, and physiological studies, however, measurements of the kind described in this paper should be useful in deriving physiologically important mechanisms. At present we are still attempting to answer very elementary physicochemical questions about lateral mobility on membranes. When these answers are known, our attempts to study particular physiological phenomena should achieve sharper focus and more definite results.

ACKNOWLEDGMENTS We are especially grateful to W. W. Webb, who has participated with us in all of the work discussed in this article, and to our colleagues D. Axelrod, L. Barak, C. Eldridge, P. Fahey, D. Koppel, J. Reidler, and D. Wolf, who have worked with us on various phases of this project. We would also like to thank G. M. Edelman, U. Rutishauser, I. Yahara, H. Metzger, I. Pastan, and K. Yamada, without whom the studies on locally bound Con A, on mast cells, and on the CSP/LETS glycoprotein would not have been possible. Numerous conversations with K. Jacobson, P. Henkart, G. Hammes, and M. Edidin have been a source of enlightenment and pleasure.

This work was supported by NIH grants GM-21661 and CA-14454 and by NSF grant DMR 75-04509 (to W. W. Webb).

REFERENCES

AXELROD, D., D. E. KOPPEL, J. SCHLESSINGER, E. ELSON, and W. W. WEBB, 1976a. Mobility measurement by analysis of fluorescence photobleaching recovery kinetics. *Biophys. J.* 16:1055–1069.

AXELROD, D., P. RAVDIN, D. E. KOPPEL, J. SCHLESSINGER, W. W. WEBB, E. L. ELSON, and T. R. PODLESKI, 1976b. Lateral motion of fluorescently labeled acetylcholine. *Proc. Natl. Acad. Sci. USA* 73:4594–4598.

CHI, E. Y., D. LAGUNOFF, and J. K. KOEHLER, 1976. Freeze-fracture study of mast cell secretion. *Proc. Natl. Acad. Sci. USA* 73:2823–2827.

COMOGLIO, P. M., G. TARONE, M. PRAT, and M. BERTINI, 1975. Studies on the outer surface of normal and RSV-transformed BHK fibroblast plasma membrane. *Exp. Cell Res.* 93:402–410.

EDELMAN, G. M., 1976. Surface modulation in cell recognition and cell growth. *Science* 192:218–226.

EDIDIN, M., 1974. Rotational and translational diffusion in membranes. *Annu. Rev. Biophys. Bioeng.* 3:179–201.

EDIDIN, M., Y. ZAGYANSKY, and T. J. LARDNER, 1976. Measurement of membrane protein lateral diffusion in single cells. *Science* 191:466–468.

ELSON, E. L., J. SCHLESSINGER, D. E. KOPPEL, D. AXELROD, and W. W. WEBB, 1976. Measurement of lateral transport on cell surfaces. In *Membranes and Neoplasia: New Approaches and Strategies*, V. T. Marchesi, ed. New York: Alan R. Liss, pp. 137–147.

FAHEY, P. F., D. E. KOPPEL, L. S. BARAK, D. E. WOLF, E. L. ELSON, and W. W. WEBB, 1977. Lateral diffusion in planar lipid bilayers. *Science* 195:305–306.

FERTUCK, H. C., and M. M. SALPETER, 1974. Localization of acetylcholine receptor by ^{125}I-labeled α-bungarotoxin binding at mouse motor endplates. *Proc. Natl. Acad. Sci. USA* 71:1376–1378.

GAROFF, H., and K. SIMONS, 1974. Location of the spike glycoprotein in Semliki Forest virus membrane. *Proc. Natl. Acad. Sci. USA* 71:3988–3992.

HUBBELL, W. L., and H. M. McCONNELL, 1969. Motion of steroid spin labels in membranes. *Proc. Natl. Acad. Sci. USA* 63:16–22.

HYNES, R. O., 1976. Cell surface proteins and malignant transformation. *Biochim. Biophys. Acta* 458:73–107.

ISHIZAKA, K., and T. ISHIZAKA, 1971. IgE and reaginic hypersensitivity. *Ann. NY Acad. Sci.* 190:443–456.

JACOBSON, K., E. WU, and G. POSTE, 1976. Measurement of the translational mobility of Concanavalin A in glycerol-saline solutions and on the cell surface by fluorescence recovery after photobleaching. *Biochim. Biophys. Acta* 433:215–222.

JOST, P. C., O. H. GRIFFITH, R. A. CAPALDI, and G. VANDERKOOI, 1973. Evidence for boundary lipid in membranes. *Proc. Natl. Acad. Sci. USA* 70:480–484.

KOPPEL, D. E., D. AXELROD, J. SCHLESSINGER, E. L. ELSON, and W. W. WEBB, 1976. Dynamics of fluorescence marker concentration as a probe of mobility. *Biophys. J.* 16:1315–1329.

METZGER, H., 1973. The effect of antigen on antibody. In *Mechanisms in Allergy: Reagin-Mediated Hypersensitivity*, L. Goodfriend, A. H. Sehon, and R. P. Orange, eds. New York: Marcel Dekker, p. 301.

MEUNIER, J.-C., R. SEALOCK, R. OLSEN, and J.-P. CHANGEUX,

1974. Purification and properties of the cholinergic receptor protein from *Electrophorus electricus* electric tissue. *Eur. J. Biochem.* 45:371–394.

NEWMAN, S. A., G. ROSSI, and H. METZGER, 1977. Molecular weight and valence of the cell-surface receptor for immunoglobulin E. *Proc. Natl. Acad. Sci. USA* 74:869–872.

NIELSEN, N. C., S. FLEISCHER, and D. G. MCCONNELL, 1970. Lipid composition of bovine retinal outer segment fragments. *Biochim. Biophys. Acta* 211:10–19.

OLIVER, J. M., T. E. UKENA, and R. D. BERLIN, 1974. Effects of phagocytosis and colchicine on the distribution of lectin-binding sites on cell surfaces. *Proc. Natl. Acad. Sci. USA* 71:394–398.

ORLY, J., and M. SCHRAMM, 1976. Coupling of catecholamine receptor from one cell with adenylate cyclase from another cell by cell fusion. *Proc. Natl. Acad. Sci. USA* 73:4410–4414.

PERNIS, B., L. FORNI, and L. AMANTE, 1970. Immunoglobulin spots on the surface of rabbit lymphocytes. *J. Exp. Med.* 132:1001–1018.

PETERS. R., J. PETERS, K. H. TEWS, and W. BAHR, 1974. A microfluorimetric study of translational diffusion in erythrocyte membranes. *Biochim. Biophys. Acta* 367:282–294.

POO, M. M., and R. A. CONE, 1974. Lateral diffusion of rhodopsin in the photoreceptor membrane. *Nature* 247:438–440.

ROSENBLITH, J. Z., T. E. UKENA, H. H. YIN, R. D. BERLIN, and J. M. KARNOVSKY, 1973. A comparative evaluation of the distribution of Concanavalin A binding sites on the surfaces of normal, virally transformed, and protease-treated fibroblasts. *Proc. Natl. Acad. Sci. USA* 70:1625–1629.

SAFFMAN, P. G., and M. DELBRÜCK, 1975. Brownian motion in biological membranes. *Proc. Natl. Acad. Sci. USA* 72:3111–3113.

SCHLESSINGER, J., D. E. KOPPEL, D. AXELROD, K. JACOBSON, W. W. WEBB, and E. L. ELSON, 1976a. Lateral transport on cell membranes: Mobility of Concanavalin A receptors on myoblasts. *Proc. Natl. Acad. Sci. USA* 73:2409–2413.

SCHLESSINGER, J., W. W. WEBB, E. L. ELSON, and H. METZGER, 1976b. Lateral motion and valence of Fc receptors on rat peritoneal mast cells. *Nature* 264:550–552.

SCHLESSINGER, J., D. AXELROD, D. E. KOPPEL, W. W. WEBB, and E. L. ELSON, 1977a. Lateral transport of a lipid probe and labeled proteins on a cell membrane. *Science* 195:307–309.

SCHLESSINGER, J., L. S. BARAK, K. M. YAMADA, I. PASTAN, W. W. WEBB, and E. L. ELSON, 1977b. Mobility and distribution of a cell surface glycoprotein and its interaction with other membrane components. *Proc. Natl. Acad. Sci. USA* 74:2909–2913.

SCHLESSINGER, J., E. L. ELSON, W. W. WEBB, I. YAHARA, U. RUTISHAUSER, and G. M. EDELMAN, 1977c. Receptor diffusion on cell surfaces modulated by locally bound Concanavalin A. *Proc. Natl. Acad. Sci. USA* 74:1110–1114.

SHINITSKY, M., A.-C. DIANOUX, C. GITLER, and G. WEBER, 1971. Microviscosity and order in the hydrocarbon region of micelles and membranes determined with fluorescent probes. I. Synthetic micelles. *Biochemistry* 10:2106–2113.

SIEGEL, D. M., J. T. TAUROG, and H. METZGER, 1977. Dimeric immunoglobulin E serves as a unit signal for mast cell degranulation. *Proc. Natl. Acad. Sci. USA* 74.2993–2997.

TEICHBERG, V. I., A. SOBEL, and J.-P. CHANGEUX. 1977. In vitro phosphorylation of the acetylcholine receptor. *Nature* 267:540–542.

TSAN, M.-F., and R. D. BERLIN, 1971. Effect of phagocytosis on membrane transport in non-electrolytes. *J. Exp. Med.* 134:1016–1035.

WOLF, D. E., J. SCHLESSINGER, E. L. ELSON, W. W. WEBB, R. BLUMENTHAL, and P. HENKART, 1977. Diffusion and patching of macromolecules on planar lipid bilayer membranes. *Biochemistry* 16:3476–3483.

YAHARA, I., and G. M. EDELMAN, 1972. Restriction of the mobility of lymphocyte immunoglobulin receptors by Concanavalin A. *Proc. Natl. Acad. Sci. USA* 69:608–612.

YAHARA, I., and G. M. EDELMAN, 1975. Modulation of lymphocyte receptor mobility by locally bound Concanavalin A. *Proc. Natl. Acad. Sci. USA* 72:1579–1583.

YAMADA, K. M., and J. A. WESTON, 1974. Isolation of a major cell surface glycoprotein from fibroblasts. *Proc. Natl. Acad. Sci. USA* 71:3492–3496.

YAMADA, K. M., S. S. YAMADA, and I. PASTAN, 1976. Cell surface protein partially restores morphology, adhesiveness, and contact inhibition of movement to transformed fibroblasts. *Proc. Natl. Acad. Sci. USA* 73:1217–1221.

ZAGYANSKI, Y., and M. EDIDIN, 1976. Lateral diffusion of Concanavalin A receptors in the plasma membrane of mouse fibroblasts. *Biochim. Biophys. Acta* 433:209–214.

41 The Cytoskeleton

KEITH R. PORTER, H. RANDOLPH BYERS, and MARK H. ELLISMAN

ABSTRACT Three filament subclasses in cells are recognized as important components of the cytoskeleton: microtubules, 10 nm intermediate filaments, and 7 nm microfilaments. These function in one fashion or another as frameworks for the maintenance of cell anisometry, as directors of particle translocation, and as mediators of ameboid movement. There is accumulating evidence from electron microscopy of thin sections that these filaments and other organelles are suspended in a flocculent material termed the cytoplasmic ground substance (CGS). When the CGS is viewed stereoscopically, in high-voltage electron microscopy of whole cells, it presents itself as a three-dimensional lattice composed of slender strands from 4 nm to 10 nm (microtrabeculae). This system of microtrabeculae divides the cytoplasm into two phases: a protein-rich polymerized phase and a water-rich fluid phase. It is postulated that the microtrabeculae are responsible in part for the gel-like consistency of the cytoplasm and that they restrict Brownian motion of particles. Yet the microtrabeculae appear to be dynamic structures that participate in sol-gel transitions.

In fish erythrophores, the microtrabeculae show dramatic transformations as they mediate the displacement of pigment granules over a radially oriented framework of microtubules. Pigment aggregation involves a rapid and uniform withdrawal of granules into the cell center as part of the microtrabeculae are displaced into the center and another fraction is withdrawn into the cell cortices. Pigment dispersion (saltatory motion) appears to involve four events: an extension or reassembly of the microtrabeculae, local contractions, local withdrawal of the microtrabeculae, and a reattachment cycle between the microtubule framework and the granules via the microtrabeculae.

In the axoplasm, where similar saltatory and uniform motion is observed, albeit simultaneously bidirectional, a three-dimensional microtrabecular lattice is also seen but of necessity in thick sections. With the erythrophore as a model, various hypotheses for Ca^{++} control of macromolecular interactions in axoplasmic motility are discussed.

IN RECENT YEARS the cytoskeleton has graduated from a pure concept without visual evidence to a reality supported by micrographs and correlated functional and biochemical observations. Although some of this progress, as far as nerve cells are concerned, can be traced back earlier than the 1960s, when microtubules were first recognized as ubiquitous structures of the eukaryotic cells, the major developments are a product of the last fifteen years. It is now the consensus that one can expect to find in most cells the 240 Å microtubule (Figure 1), frequently focused on the centrioles, or some satellites of the centrioles recognizable as microtubule nucleating centers. These long unbranching rods vary in number depending on the cell type, but they are especially abundant in the more anisometric cells that make up the nervous system (Porter, 1966; Roberts, 1974). Besides these tubules, there are 100 Å filaments of unknown function, distributed in most instances without clear correlation to anything except perhaps the maintenance of established cell form. Finally, there is frequently a population of very fine, 70 Å filaments, usually aggregated into bundles that in turn occupy a position in the cell cortex or subcortical regions of the cytoplasm, including those of microvilli (Figure 1). These filaments have the capacity to change their position with cell motion and to shorten if the cell is appropriately stimulated (Buckley and Porter, 1967; Goldman et al., 1973).

It is generally conceded that the microtubules occupy a special place in this category of cell inclusions because they alone are clearly involved in shaping cells and giving direction to the translocation of cytoplasmic components. When the microtubules are disassembled by chilling or with colchicine, the anisometric cell or cell process they occupy collapses into a spherical form, only to regain its original asymmetry when the tubules reassemble (Tilney and Porter, 1965; Tilney, 1968). They are not essential to the development or maintenance of form in the smaller cell extensions such as microvilli (1,000 Å); but for whole cells or even cylindrical cell extensions such as cilia (2,000 Å), flagella, and axopods they appear to be indispensable skeletal structures (Tilney and Porter, 1965). They have no contractile properties as far as anyone has demonstrated but appear instead to act as a frame for the attachment of closely associated motile mechanisms, which will be discussed below (see also Byers and Porter, 1977). Microtubules are

KEITH R. PORTER, H. RANDOLPH BYERS, and MARK H. ELLISMAN Molecular, Cellular, and Developmental Biology, University of Colorado, Boulder, CO 80309; Department of Anatomy, Harvard Medical School, Boston, MA 02115; Department of Neurosciences, University of California at San Diego, School of Medicine, La Jolla, CA 92093

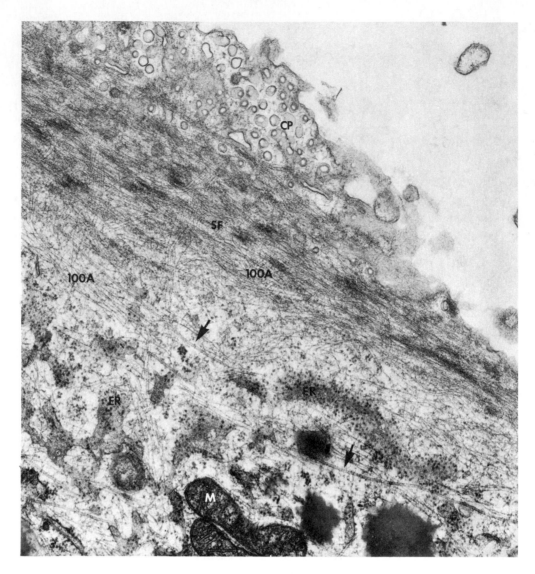

FIGURE 1 Margin of WI-38 cell in section cut parallel to surface. The section leaves the cell at the upper right and passes through several cortical pits (CP). Just inside this zone the section includes a stress fiber (SF) with a scattering of dense bodies. This SF represents a bundle of 60 Å actin filaments and associated matrix. Deeper into the cytoplast, and toward the lower left, the image shows random arrays of 100 Å filaments, which appear to blend into the stress fiber or underlie it. Deeper still are a few microtubules (arrows) oriented parallel to the long axis of the cell. Mitochondria (M) and elements of the endoplasmic reticulum (ER) are indicated.

also frequently observed in close association with the cell surface, and in this location they doubtless influence the distribution of membrane-integrated functions. This is especially true in plant cells, where the distribution and orientation of extracellular cellulose filaments coincides precisely with that of intracellular (cortical) microtubules (Brown and Willison, 1977). Whether microtubules in this association with the cytoplasmic cortex are functional in shaping cells and in cell motility remains to be determined, but the evidence suggests that they are.

The 100 Å filaments, termed *intermediate filaments* by Shelanski (Yen et al., 1976), although seemingly less sturdy than microtubules, are probably involved as structural elements. To arrive at this conclusion, it is assumed that all 100 Å filaments are similar in composition and function—an assumption that may well be erroneous. In epithelia, where they can be shown to span the cell from desmosome to desmosome, they are thought to strengthen the epithelial layer against lateral stretch. In nerve cells, where they are referred to as neurofilaments, the same role is not so readily assumed; also lacking, however, is any clear evidence that they are essential to the flow of axoplasm (Byers, 1974).

Bundles of 70 Å actin filaments are definitely contractile in nonmuscle cells. It is also evident from electron-microscopic observations that their presence and orientation give anisometric form to cell processes such as the microvilli on the apical surfaces of intestinal epithelial cells (Mooseker and Tilney, 1975). Here, as in other locations, their involvement in motility is patent.

In each instance of their occurrence these so-called cytoskeletal elements are suspended in a matrix usually referred to as the cytoplasmic ground substance (CGS), or hyaloplasm, in recognition of its unstructured appearance as viewed by light microscopy. This matrix has usually been regarded as a gel of uniform consistency and composition that has the capacity to transform into a sol when exposed to low temperatures, high hydrostatic pressure, or any condition that discourages oxidative phosphorylation. The behavior of the ground substance is consistent with the designation *thixtropic* (Marsland and Brown, 1936). There are, however, ample reasons for believing that the ground substance is neither homogeneous nor unstructured.

The gel-like consistency of the CGS has been recognized by a variety of techniques. Careful light microscopy has shown that the "gel" restrains the motion of the endoplasmic reticulum (ER) as though the latter were contained in a relatively fixed position within the matrix. When the gel is converted to a sol by exposing the cell to low temperatures, the ER is released and fragments into discrete vesicles. Thereafter the vesicles display a rapid Brownian motion that becomes especially noticeable in dark-field microscopy. These phenomena are reversed when the cell is returned to incubator temperatures.

The matrix has contractile properties that would be difficult to explain if the gel were not structured. For example, in the axopods of certain heliozoans there is obvious only an ordered array of microtubules, the axoneme, and a structured matrix showing bridges between the microtubules (Tilney and Byers, 1969; Roth, Pihlaja, and Shigenaka, 1970). When these axopods attach at their tips to a food organism, they immediately contract, in some instances so rapidly that the motion cannot be easily followed (Ockleford and Tucker, 1973). When the contracted axopod is examined by thin-section microscopy, it is found that the frame of microtubules has disassembled, apparently releasing an elasticity present in the ground substance.

The so-called bridges or links between the microtubules of the axoneme are repeated in several other locations. They appear as the spokes in the 9 + 2 complex of the cilium (Warner and Satir, 1974). They are present between the tubules in the axostyles of ciliates (McIntosh, Ogata, and Landis, 1973); and, most significantly for this review, they appear between the neurotubules of the axoplasm, although here they span greater distances than in the other examples (Burton and Fernandez, 1973). Indeed Yamada, Spooner, and Wessells (1971) described a whole reticular structure in the CGS of the growing processes of nerve cells in culture, especially in the growth cone; these investigators refer to it as a "complex three-dimensional lattice in which other structures are supported." A similar lattice was reported by Burton and Fernandez (1973) in the axoplasm of the crayfish ventral nerve cord, with the added observation that the filamentous elements stain with lanthanum. In thin sections of the presynaptic ending, Gray (1975) resolved the existence of a "cytonet," which coincides in its dimensions with that reported by Wessells and colleagues. Hinkley (1973) and Tani and Ametani (1970) added information suggesting that elements of the net include acid mucopolysaccharides; Samson (1971) interpreted these as having contractile properties that might operate to provide the motive force for the streaming in axoplasm.

Most compelling among the arguments in support of a structured ground substance are the polarity and other organizational features of cells (Figure 2). These features are expressed through the nonrandom distribution of cytoplasmic systems such as the Golgi complex and the ER, the nonrandom orientation of mitochondria, and constant positioning of the centrioles or their equivalents during interphase and in the differentiated cell (Figure 2). The centrioles and their satellites, which are structurally continuous with the CGS, function at one time or another as initiating sites for the assembly of microtubules. It is the patterned distribution of these cytoplasmic elements that influences, through the assembled microtubules, the shape the cell adopts. It is difficult to avoid the conclusion that information for the distribution of these initiating sites is built into the ground substance (see Berns et al., 1977).

With these and other observations as background, we began a few years ago to search the CGS for evidence of previously undetected structure (Buckley and Porter, 1973; Buckley, 1975; Wolosewick and Porter, 1976). This became feasible through the acquisition of a 1 MeV electron microscope. With the high-energy electrons it generates, one can penetrate

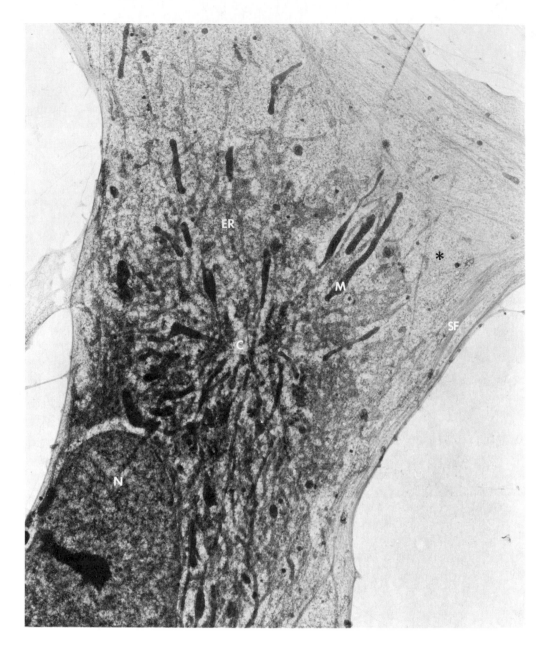

FIGURE 2 Part of a cultured chick fibroblast taken with the high-voltage microscope operated at 1 MeV. Besides illustrating the radial organization characteristic of eukaryotic cells from metazoa, the micrograph shows the capacity of high-energy electrons to penetrate relatively thick cells (1.5 μm) and provide high-resolution images. The centro-sphere (C), nucleus (N), mitochondrion (M), stress fibers (SF), and ER are indicated. The cytoplasmic matrix or ground substance, in which all organelles, etc. (except mitochondria), are anchored, is resolved (but barely visible; see Figure 3), especially in the thinner margins of the cell (∗). (Micrograph provided by John Wolosewick.)

the thickness of a whole, thinly spread cultured cell and obtain high-resolution images. The cells are fixed with glutaraldehyde plus OsO_4 and subsequently dried from liquid CO_2 using the critical-point method introduced to electron microscopy by Anderson (1951). This technique, which introduces few, if any, drying artifacts into the preparations, greatly im-proves on the early procedures of drying cells in air. With stereo views of a given field one can explore the depth dimension at magnifications as high as ×100,000. Similar studies can be made on thick (e.g., 0.5 μm) sections of fixed and embedded cells or tissues, although resins appear to have electron-scattering properties not dissimilar to those of the CGS.

706   K. R. PORTER, H. R. BYERS, AND M. H. ELLISMAN

As a consequence, some features of the ground substance are poorly imaged. A specific stain for these structures is being sought so that finer details can be observed even in stereo images of thick sections.

The image of the ground substance that emerges is unique to this region of the cell. It appears as a three-dimensional lattice of slender strands we call *microtrabeculae* (Figures 3 and 4), which range in diameter from 40 Å to 100 Å and in length from a few hundred to 1,000 Å. These broad dimensional ranges reflect substantial variations from cell type to cell type and from cell margin to cell center. The overall appearance is reminiscent of spongy bone, although several orders of magnitude smaller.

This network divides the ground substance into two phases: a protein-rich, polymerized phase comprising the microtrabecular lattice; and a water-rich, fluid phase that fills the intertrabecular spaces. The latter would seem to provide a medium for the diffusion of low-molecular-weight metabolites, whereas the former appears to be a complex polymer that gives the cytoplasm its gel-like properties. Most components of the cytoplasm are supported (i.e., contained) in the meshes of the lattice; the material of the lattice covers the surfaces of the ER cisternae, the ribosomes, and the microtubules (Figure 4). The lattice also extends to the undersurface of the cell membrane, where it becomes confluent with the cyto-

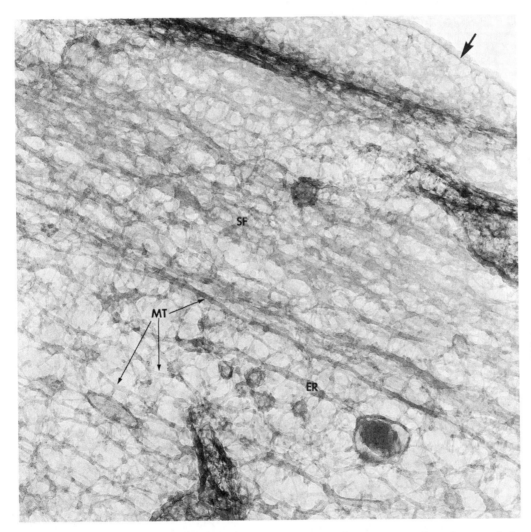

FIGURE 3 Margin of normal rat kidney (NRK) cell showing the structure of a stress fiber (after glutaraldehyde fixation and critical-point drying) and the CGS. The latter comprises a three-dimensional latticelike assemblage of microtrabeculae (30–60 Å) that interconnects microtubules (MT), ER, and the upper and lower cortices of the cytoplast. It appears to be the system that gives a gelatinous consistency to the cytoplasm, and it is the phase of the cytoplast engaged by the microtubules in their role as skeletal elements. The stress fibers (SF) appear as bundles of elongated trabeculae in which, presumably, the actin filaments assemble. (× 75,000.)

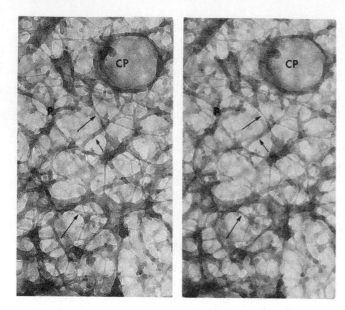

FIGURE 4 A small area of a thin NRK cell, showing (in stereo) the structure of the lattice in a small segment of a cell. The microtrabeculae stand out especially well (arrows), and when viewed stereoscopically they can be seen to run as bridges from one to another and also to join the upper and lower inner surfaces of the plasma membrane. The variations in density shown by the upper and lower cortices can only represent variations in thickness in these layers of the lattice material. Polysomes (P) populate the larger junction points in the lattice. A cortical pit (CP) or vesicle occupies the upper quarter of the image, and its surface is connected by trabeculae into the lattice. (× 70,000.)

plasmic cortex (Figure 4). Of the readily identified cellular structures, only the mitochondria seem to escape inclusion in the lattice (Porter, 1976; Wolosewick and Porter, 1976).

These features of the CGS are included in the model shown in Figure 5, which is a fair representation of the information gleaned from studying many electron micrographs in stereo and otherwise. It depicts a small rectangular block cut out of a thin margin of a cultured cell. The type of cell is not important; most of the observations have been made on human fibroblasts (WI-38) and normal rat kidney cells (NRK), which are probably endothelial rather than fibroblastic. These and other cells, particularly some endothelial units cultured from explants of chick embryo lung, all show the same features. Thus the model is really a synopsis of observations on a miscellany of cells.

The model shows the CGS as comprising a lattice of thin strands that support or contain the better-known components of the cytoplasm such as microtubules, microfilaments, cisternae of the ER, and polysomes. It essentially divides the ground substance into two phases, which we have referred to as protein-rich and water-rich. The material of the protein-rich phase, which probably includes more than proteins (see below), extends as a coating over the microtubules, the microfilaments, and the surfaces of the ER. It also contains the polysomes, which usually sit at the cross points where several trabeculae come together. The undersurfaces of the cell membranes are likewise coated with a thin layer (the cytoplasmic cortex) confluent with the trabeculae of the lattice. As mentioned before, the only surface in the cytoplasm that seems to be excluded from this association is that of the mitochondria. The so-called water-rich phase is also continuous throughout the cytoplasm and seemingly provides for the rapid diffusion of low-molecular-weight metabolites. This would seem to be especially significant for the polysomes and the functions they perform.

It is reasonable to assume that the structure depicted accounts for the gel-like consistency of the CGS and the general absence of Brownian motion. This is not to suggest that the structure is in any sense static. Rather it is assumed that it is constantly changing, displaying local "contractions" and even deformations of individual trabeculae with a consequent increase or decrease in the magnitude of intertrabecular spaces. Presumably such local alterations would account for the saltatory behavior occasionally displayed by cytoplasmic organelles in the living cell. The chromatophore we discuss below provides a particularly good example of the changes the system may undergo in its structural association with pigment motion.

To date the composition of this lattice material has not been studied sufficiently well to permit much in the way of comment. Since the actin filaments of the stress fibers appear to assemble within the lattice or the cytoplasmic cortex, it is reasonable to suppose that actin is one important ingredient. The same could be said of tubulin. It may follow that myosin and tropomyosin are present as well. A recent study from Stossel's laboratory on the composition of the ground substances of cell ruffles supports these conjectures and indicates that there are in addition a number of other unidentified proteins that will have to be sorted out according to their characteristics before we can provide a more precise description of composition (Hartwig, Davies, and Stossel, 1977). The demonstrated affinity of ruthenium red and lanthanum oxides for equivalents of the trabeculae in other preparations (see below) further suggests that they may contain an acid mucopolysaccharide. This possibility deserves further investigation.

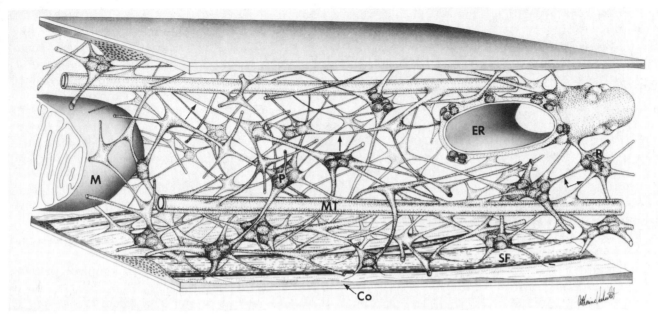

FIGURE 5 A model of the cytoplasmic matrix or ground substance. It depicts the current view that this part of the cell comprises a lattice of fine (30–60 Å) microtrabeculae (arrows), which can be supposed to give the CGS its gellike consistency. The lattice contains elements of the ER, microtubules (MT), and polysomes (P) and is confluent with continuous layers of lattice substance (cortices, CO) subjacent to the upper and lower membranes. The mitochondria (M) appear to be free. Stress fibers (SF), built into the cortices, are sometimes less closely related to the surfaces. The lattice obviously divides the CGS into two phases, one protein-rich (the lattice) and one water-rich (the intratrabecular spaces). This model, like all models, is subject to change with the acquisition of new information, but for working purposes it is presently valuable. (Reprinted from *Cell Motility*, Cold Spring Harbor Laboratory, 1976.)

There is no question but that the model reflects what has been observed with high-voltage microscopy. What it does not tell us is how much of the image is artifact or how closely the image coincides with what is actually present in the living cytoplast. The temptation, on the basis of its appearance, is to conclude that it is simply a condensation artifact of fixation and/or dehydration and to dismiss it from serious consideration. The problem is that such a conclusion is difficult to support in the face of evidence to the contrary. In an extensive study of this question, John Wolosewick has shown that the lattice is present in cells whether fixed by glutaraldehyde alone or by osmium tetroxide. These two reagents act quite differently in fixation and would not be expected to produce similar artifacts. He has shown further that cells fixed by instant freezing at liquid nitrogen temperatures and then dried from the frozen state display the same reticular structure. Erythrocytes and solutions of plasma proteins, as models of protein-rich systems, have been exposed to the same fixation and dehydration procedures without showing any evidence of a lattice structure. Recognizing these findings and the fact that the currently popular combination of glutaraldehyde and osmium fixes without evident distortion a wealth of other cell structures, we find it reasonable to conclude that the fixed image of the lattice is probably faithful to the original (Wolosewick and Porter, 1978).

Yet the evidence is not so conclusive as to dispel all doubts about the image or to tell us how faithful it is. The better position on the question of artifact is to remain flexible until further observations are available. What remains is the suggestion that what we are viewing is a condensation descriptive only of certain inhomogeneities in the CGS; that is, in fixation and dehydration the less-hydrated regions in a continuous ground substance, along with the formed structures such as microtubules and ER, serve as regions or surfaces upon which the more-hydrated materials condense. If true, however, it is difficult to see why the surfaces of the mitochondria should not be as useful for condensation as those of the ER. It is also hard to understand the configurations of structure that accompany the deformation of the lattice during the chilling of the cells and, more particularly, the rapid restucturing of the lattice when the cell is returned to incubator temperatures. Similarly, the form changes during pigment aggregation, and especially in dispersion, in chromatophores simply do not correlate easily with condensation phenomena (Byers and Porter, 1977).

If, in spite of evidence to the contrary, we concede that we are looking at a condensation artifact, are the observations without value? Obviously not, for at the very least the lattice describes, indeed exaggerates for observation purposes, a structural organization within the ground substance upon which the less-structured parts of the cytoplasm condense.

The problem becomes one of equivalence. Is the structure observed sufficiently equivalent to what was there before fixation to make it useful for understanding the role of the cytoplasm in the form and functional phenomena displayed by cells? We think it is. Obviously some way must eventually be found to resolve the structure of CGS in the living cell; but until then we are obliged to observe static images of the CGS in cells displaying cytoplasmic movements such as those discussed in the next sections of this paper or stages in the differentiation of cell structures that emerge from the CGS, such as myofibrils.

Dynamic changes in the ground substance associated with the motion of pigment in chromatophores

It has been our supposition for a number of years that if the movement of pigment in chromatophores were understood it would provide an explanation for the more limited cytoplasmic motions observed in other cells. For the present, the features of intracellular streaming common to pigment motion and axoplasmic transport deserve attention.

Chromatophores are neuroectodermal in origin, and the chromatophores of certain fish are heavily innervated. In response to appropriate stimuli, these fish will rapidly blanch as pigment granules of their chromatophores aggregate into small spherical masses surrounding the centrosphere of the cell. In response to other stimuli, the fish darkens as pigment granules are dispersed throughout the cell. The inward motion of pigment granules proceeds in a resolute fashion at a constant velocity until aggregation is complete. In erythrophores of *Holocentrus ascensionis*, granules aggregate at velocities of 15–20 μm/sec, and the entire process takes only 3–4 sec (Porter, 1973). In contrast, the dispersion of pigment granules proceeds at a slower rate, takes approximately twice as long as aggregation, and also involves saltatory motion. *This differential between the rates of aggregation and dispersion strongly recommends the chromatophore as a model system for studies of the translo-*

cation of particles and especially the involvement of the microtrabecular lattice. In addition, because the direction of migration can be controlled, the chromatophore system provides a unique opportunity to separate for study uniform as opposed to saltatory motion. This separation is difficult in the axoplasm as these movements occur simultaneously and bidirectionally.

Both the outward saltatory motions and the inward uniform motions of pigment granules in chromatophores are constrained to radial pathways in the cytoplasm. In ultrastructural studies of melanophores of *Fundulus heteroclitus*, Bikle, Tilney, and Porter (1966) and Green (1968) observed that microtubules are positioned parallel to the direction in which pigment migrates (Figure 6). These investigations suggested that microtubules are not only involved as an orienting framework for migration, but are also in some way intrinsic to the mechanism mediating this motion. Evidence in support of this hypothesis includes observations that migration of pigment is in-

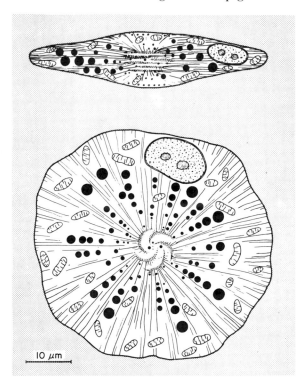

FIGURE 6 Diagram showing the usual distribution and orientation of microtubules (represented by lines) in an erythrophore. Pigment is distributed radially throughout the cell; mitochondria are scattered more randomly but tend to occupy the peripheral regions of the cytoplast. Part of the microtubules insert on dense elements in the centrosphere region of the cell; the balance seem to insert on the cell cortex. The top diagram depicts a vertical section.

hibited by vinblastine and colchicine with a concomitant disassembly of microtubules (Junqueira, Raker, and Porter, 1974; Wikswo and Novales, 1969, 1972).

Microtubules undoubtedly also play a major role in mediating the migration of pigment granules in amphibian chromatophores, for antimicrotubular agents disrupt the movement of pigment in these cells as well (Malawista, 1965). In addition, it appears that in amphibian melanophores 100 Å microfilaments may also help orient the motion of pigment granules. The slower migration of pigment granules in amphibian cells probably reflects only a slight variation from the motile mechanism in teleost chromatophores, as the general behaviors are similar.

Interest in the role of microfilaments in mediating pigment migration has led to experiments with cytochalasin B that have shown an inhibition of dispersion or an induction of aggregation (Malawista, 1971; McGuire and Moellmann, 1972). Cytochalasin B is known to disrupt microfilaments and to inhibit a variety of motile systems. There is some evidence that the drug affects glucose transport properties of the cell membrane and that it inhibits interactions between actin-binding protein and actin filaments (Hartwig and Stossel, 1976; Weihing, 1976). Thus the mechanism by which cytochalasin B inhibits the movements of pigment granules is unclear, and interpretations drawn from the use of the compound are still debated.

The motility mechanism

The relative contribution of microtubules, microfilaments, and other cytoplasmic compounds in mediating the differences between inward and outward migration of pigment granules has only begun to be answered in recent years. Green's observations (1968) on the behavior of pigment migration led her to speculate that the granules are embedded in a cytoplasmic continuum that expands during dispersion and contracts elastically on aggregation. Ultrastructural studies of thin sections, however, failed to identify any significant morphological connections between the pigment granules and microtubules. Porter (1973) suggested that the "flocculent" component that could be visualized throughout the cytoplasm in thin sections of erythrophores was the elastic continuum suggested by Green. He further postulated that this continuum expands by the assembly of microtubules and elastically contracts following the disassembly of microtubules. The elastic collapse of the continuum would thus be independent of microtu-

bules. Indeed, evidence for a microtubule-independent contractile system was reported by Schliwa and Bereiter-Hahn (1975) in melanophores of *Pterophyllum scalare*. Recent studies have shown that although many microtubules do in fact disassemble on aggregation, the majority remain assembled (Murphy and Tilney, 1974; Byers and Porter, 1977). It was thus necessary to search for an explanation of the expansion of the continuum other than one mediated by an assembly of microtubules.

Following a study that demonstrated a statistical association of granules with microtubules, Murphy and Tilney (1974) proposed a mechanism by which pigment granules slide upon the microtubules. But again no morphological connections could be consistently visualized between granules and microtubules. It was therefore still conceivable that granules were simply restricted to radial channels physically defined by microtubules.

Observations from whole erythrophores

In order to understand better the three-dimensional relationships among microtubules, granules, and other cytoplasmic components, we recently isolated erythrophores for the examination of whole cells in the high-voltage electron microscope (HVEM) (Byers and Porter, 1977).

Images of intact cells with dispersed pigment, obtained at relatively low magnification in the HVEM (Figure 7), reveal a basic cytoplasmic organization similar to that seen in thin sections from cells in situ. Microtubules and linear columns of pigment granules radiate outward from the centrosphere, which is usually obscured by pigment granules. Most important, however, is the obvious fine, three-dimensional lattice of the cytoplasmic ground substance similar to that described in the preceding section of this paper. At higher magnifications (Figure 8), and viewed stereoscopically, the dispersed pigment granules are seen to be embedded in a fine network of microfilaments, the so-called microtrabeculae. This alignment of granules along microtubules, in conjunction with observable cytoplasmic bridges, suggests a specialized interaction between granules and microtubules.

In erythrophores fixed during the process of aggregation, the HVEM images of the microtrabeculae are generally shorter and thicker than those of microtrabeculae seen in cells with dispersed granules. The once-fine network of the CGS is dramatically altered (Figure 9) and appears to be coarsened and disrupted. All internal surfaces of the cytoplasm, in-

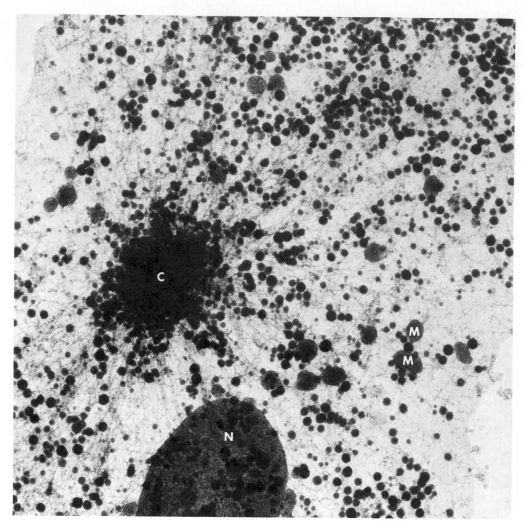

FIGURE 7   HVEM image of a whole-cell erythrophore with its pigment dispersed. Microtubules and aligned granules can be seen radiating outward from the pigment-obscured centrosphere (C). Mitochondria (M) and the cell nucleus (N) are excluded from the centrosphere. The CGS has a fine filamentous appearance that can just be detected at this relatively low magnification. (× 10,000.)

cluding the granules and cell cortices, are coated with a thickened, globular material. The magnitude of this transition in the organization of the CGS can best be appreciated in stereo images from the HVEM of erythrophores in which the pigment has completely aggregated following treatment with epinephrine (Figure 10). In such cells the fine microtrabecular lattice that once extended throughout the cytoplasm is largely absent. Only fragments of the microtrabeculae can be seen attached to microtubules and the cell cortices. The microtubules reside in the cell cortices, whereas in the dispersed cell the microtubules are at all levels of the cytoplasm and extend into the cortices only near the cell margin. In addition, the marginal regions of aggregated cells are frequently extremely attenuated, presumably because the micro-

trabeculae or the pigment granules are displaced into the cell's center.

Immediately after pigment dispersion begins, the microtrabeculae are again seen extending between the cell cortices (Figure 11). The microtrabeculae reappear ahead of the advancing front of pigment granules. In the zone between the microtrabeculae and the attenuated region, it appears that some of the thickened cortical material contributes to the re-structuring of the microtrabeculae.

Interpretation of erythrophore data

Recognizing the hazards of interpreting instantaneous images of a dynamic process, it is possible to describe a sequence of events that may explain the

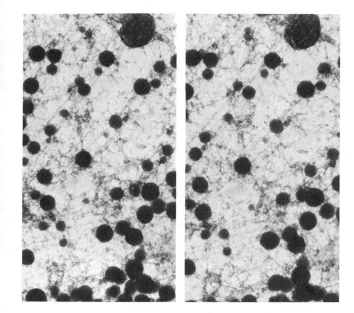

FIGURE 8 Stereo HVEM image of a dispersed erythrophore. The fine three-dimensional lattice, composed of microtrabeculae, can be seen interconnecting the granules, microtubules, and cortical surfaces of the cell. The granules are associated with the microtubules through microtrabecular bridges. 15° tilt. (× 20,000.) (Reprinted by permission of the *Journal of Cell Biology*.)

dramatic transformations seen in the organization of the CGS in the aggregated and dispersed state (Figure 12). Following an aggregating stimulus, the microtrabeculae shorten and, because of their connections with the granules, translocate the pigment granules toward the cell's center (Figure 12B). There also appears to be a separation of the continuum that yields two components of the microtrabeculae: one component is withdrawn into the cell cortices, displacing many of the microtubules with it; the other is withdrawn with the granules into the cell center (a deformation). As the granules disperse, there is a lengthening and restructuring (a re-formation) of the microtrabeculae outward from the cell cortices and the centrosphere. The reappearance of the lattice ahead of the advancing granules may reflect a restructuring of the microtrabeculae from the component withdrawn into the cell cortices. On dispersion, the pigment granules, suspended in the lattice, migrate relatively slowly and in saltatory fashion, reflecting, we feel, the re-formation of the microtrabeculae that had been withdrawn into the centrosphere with the granules (Figure 12A).

By now our supposition should be clear: namely, that the microtrabeculae represent the components of the "elastic" continuum postulated by Green as mediating the translocation of pigment granules. It

must be emphasized that the continuum is not simply a lattice with fixed intersecting components that expands and contracts, carrying the granules with it. To understand the hypothesized mechanism for translocation, the dynamic quality of each separate component of the continuum must be appreciated.

We propose that dispersion is the result of four simultaneous events: (1) a generalized extension of the microtrabeculae; (2) local contractions of the microtrabeculae, giving rise to small jumps in either direction; (3) local release or shearing of the microtrabeculae to allow jumps to occur; and (4) a reattachment process to allow the statistical cycle to continue. It has been shown that dispersion of granules is an energy-requiring process that is dependent on oxidative phosphorylation (Junqueira, Raker, and Porter, 1974; Saidel, 1977) and is induced with ATP and Mg^{++} in triton-X-treated cells (Miyashita, 1975). Hence any one or all of the four steps could require the hydrolysis of ATP. A greater affinity of the microtrabeculae between the granules and microtubules would orient the dispersion of granules and explain the intimate association of granules with microtu-

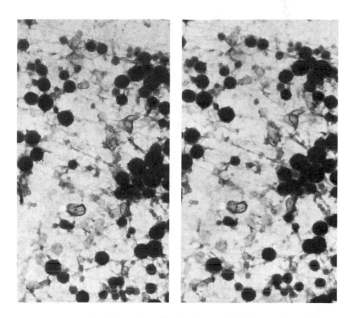

FIGURE 9 Following depolarization of the erythrophore membrane by increasing KCl in the perfusate, the erythrophore was fixed in the process of aggregation. It appears that a deformation of the fine three-dimensional lattice seen in the dispersed cell has taken place. The microtrabeculae between the granules have become shorter and thickened, and those attached to the cortices of the cytoplast have also become discontinuous and thickened. Some of the microtubules have disassembled. 12° tilt. (× 20,000.) (Reprinted by permission of the *Journal of Cell Biology*.)

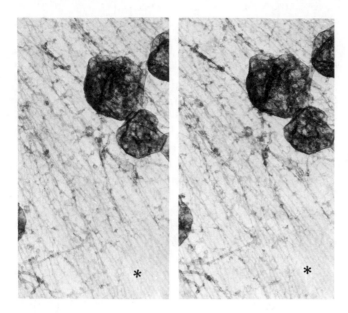

FIGURE 10   Stereo view of an erythrophore stimulated to aggregate its pigment by perfusion of the culture with 1-epinephrine. The dramatic transformation in the microtrabeculae is immediately apparent when the image is viewed stereoscopically. The microtrabeculae no longer extend throughout the cytoplasm, and the residual microtubules have relocated in the cell cortices, leaving the cytoplasm essentially free from structural components. An interesting interdigitation of dorsal and ventral populations of microtubules often occurs near the cell margin, where the cell attenuates during aggregation (∗). 8° tilt. (× 20,000.) (Reprinted by permission of the *Journal of Cell Biology*.)

bules. It must be stressed that this sequence of events would be a statistical effect of the extending microtrabeculae acting on a dispersing granule and that a smooth and unidirectional cycling mechanism does not operate; many microtrabeculae might at the same moment act so as to oppose each other. This might explain the striking saltatory feature of dispersion.

Aggregation is uniform in character and appears not to require oxidative phosphorylation (Junqueira, Raker, and Porter, 1974; Saidel, 1977), nor is it initiated by ATP and Mg^{++} (Miyashita, 1975). Aggregation may be looked upon as a release of stored elastic energy. The microtrabeculae, upon the appropriate stimulus, would suddenly contract into an energetically more stable conformation. A sudden decrease in the granule-to-microtubule affinity during the contraction of microtrabeculae would result in aggregation of granules into the centrosphere.

The specific macromolecules involved in aggregation and dispersion remain to be identified. For the moment, only slightly more is known about the cy-

toplasmic control of the elements that mediate the translocation of pigment granules. There is recent evidence that an elevation in the cytoplasmic concentration of Ca^{++} induces aggregation in chromatophores and that low Ca^{++} induces or is permissive for dispersion (Lambert and Fingerman, 1977).

It is possible that the energy-requiring step in dispersion is simply a Ca^{++} pump that eliminates Ca^{++} from the cell or sequesters it in the smooth endoplasmic reticulum (SER). The system of tubular surface invaginations observed in erythrophores (Figure 9) (Porter, 1973; Byers and Porter, 1977) may prove to be important for Ca^{++} influx during the depolarization of the cell membrane. That Ca^{++} induces an elasticlike aggregation of the pigment granules is reminiscent of the calcium-induced elastic contractions of the spasmoneme in the stalk of peritrich ciliates, which is also independent of ATP (Weis-Fogh and Amos, 1972).

But Ca^{++}-induced conformational changes need not be restricted to proteins. Mucopolysaccharides are also capable of dramatic shortening following a sudden rise in concentrations of divalent cations such as Ca^{++}. (For a detailed account of how conformational changes of polyelectrolytes transform chemical

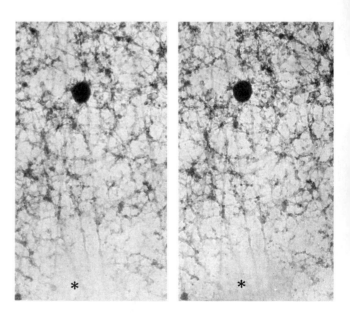

FIGURE 11   Fixed in the process of pigment dispersion, this image demonstrates that the microtrabeculae have already re-formed before the advancing front of pigment granules. In the upper third of the figure (∗), near the cell margin, it appears that the microtrabeculae are restructured in part from material stored in the cortical layer of the cytoplast. 9° tilt. (× 28,500.) (Reprinted by permission of the *Journal of Cell Biology*.)

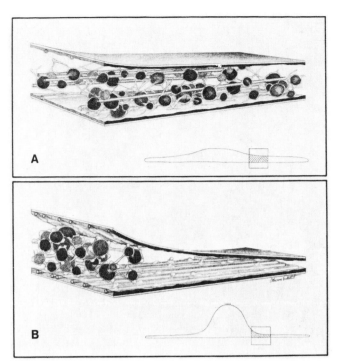

FIGURE 12 Schematic representation of the migration of pigment granules. (A) During dispersion the granules are suspended in a dynamic lattice composed of microtrabeculae undergoing regional extension, local contraction, release, and reattachment. Granules are associated with microtubules not by confinement to physical pathways but by microtrabecular bridges. (B) On aggregation the microtrabeculae suddenly contract into the cell center and cell cortices, displacing the granules into the centrosphere and the microtubules into the cortex. (Reprinted by permission of the *Journal of Cell Biology*.)

energy to mechanical work see Oosawa, 1971). The recognition of a mucopolysaccharide "fuzz" on neurotubules prompted the construction of a model for axoplasmic transport that involves these dynamic macromolecules as the motive force for the translocation of particles (Samson, 1971; Burton and Fernandez, 1973). This mucopolysaccharide model is consistent with the changes seen in the microtrabeculae; however, the validity of the model awaits a more detailed study of the composition of the microtrabeculae (see below).

It is possible that the microtrabeculae represent, at least in part, the filamentous coating seen on brain microtubules polymerized in vitro. When microtubule-associated proteins (MAPs) are removed before the polymerization procedure, the filamentous coating on the microtubules is lost (Dentler, Granett, and Rosenbaum, 1975). Recent evidence suggests that one of the MAPs that co-purifies with microtubules is a

cAMP-dependent kinase (Sloboda et al., 1975). This is of particular interest as elevations in the intracellular concentration of cAMP have long been known to induce prompt dispersion of pigment granules in chromatophores (for review see Novales, 1971). The possibility that a cAMP-dependent kinase catalyzes the attachment or lengthening of the microtrabeculae at the expense of ATP during dispersion deserves further investigation.

A discussion of a cytoplasmic motility system whose components have not yet been clearly defined would be incomplete without a consideration of the participation of actin and myosin. These contractile proteins are ubiquitous in nonmuscle cells (for review see Pollard and Weihing, 1974), and there is therefore reason to believe that they may compose, in part, the three-dimensional lattice seen in erythrophores. The energy-dependent lengthening and restructuring (polymerization?) of the microtrabeculae during dispersion may be analogous to the ATP- and Mg^{++}-requiring gelation of extracts of *Acanthamoeba* (Pollard, 1976). These extracts contain actin, myosin, an actin-binding protein, and several other proteins. The networks formed during the polymerization of the crude extracts can be induced to contract rapidly and to shear apart if the Ca^{++} concentration is significantly elevated. Likewise, this process might be occurring in the erythrophore as Ca^{++} apparently mediates the aggregation of pigment granules (Lambert and Fingerman, 1977). A Ca^{++}-regulated, actomyosin-mediated aggregation of pigment granules, in contrast to a spasmoneme-analogous protein or mucopolysaccharide-mediated model, would require the hydrolysis of ATP. Moreover, it should be repeated that the evidence thus far has suggested that aggregation is not energy-requiring, thus supporting the latter two models over the actomyosin-mediated model. However, we cannot confidently suggest one set of macromolecular interactions over another until the components of the microtrabeculae are more accurately characterized by biochemical or immunobiochemical techniques.

The model we have constructed for the transport of pigment granules is based on careful observations of pigment granules in motion, the controlling factors for aggregation and dispersion, the effect of antimicrotubular agents, and the ultrastructural transformations of the microtrabeculae as visualized in the HVEM. Testing the accuracy of the model and identifying the components of the microtrabeculae will provide a challenging task in the near future and will likely enhance our understanding of intracellular motility in the erythrophore's close relative, the neuron.

Axoplasmic motility

The streaming motion of the cytoplasm in nerve cells is one of the more dramatic examples of intracellular motility. Although the nerve cell is larger than the fibroblast or erythrophore, its cytoplasm must be differentiated to move formed components and metabolites from the perikaryon over much greater distances. In some ways the nerve cell resembles the plant cell, in that there are observable channels along which particulate components of the cytoplasm actively stream. Several investigators have recorded this phenomenon on motion picture film, and Pomerat and colleagues have perhaps made the best recordings from nerve cells maintained in vitro (Pomerat et al., 1967). Others have visualized similar streaming in axons and dendrites (Kirkpatrick, 1971; McMahan and Kuffler, 1971; Forman, Padjen, and Siggins, 1977a,b; see also the review by Wuerker and Kirkpatrick, 1972).

The rate of fast axonal transport is of the same order of magnitude as the rate of dispersion of erythrophore granules: 400 mm/day or about 5μm/sec, as compared with 6–8 μm/sec for the outward motion of pigment. Information obtained from observations of the dispersion of pigment granules along microtubules through the dynamic restructuring of the microtrabeculae of erythrophores is of value for consideration of the mechanisms of fast axonal transport.

THE STRUCTURE OF AXOPLASM Axoplasm contains its own complement of filamentous structures that presumably serve a guiding function similar to that of the tubules in the erythrophore. Their elements are remarkably similar to filaments found in other tissues: the 100 Å neurofilaments, the intermediate filament of Shelanski (Yen et al., 1976) and the 240 Å microtubule. The central regions of dendrites are especially rich in microtubules. In small or immature axons, neurofilaments are not as conspicuous as microtubules. Neurofilaments, however, are the most prominent fibrous elements in the large myelinated axons in which transport rates have been measured (Figure 13). In some species, neurofilaments are completely absent from axoplasm, as in the ventral nerve of the crayfish. This indicates that neurofilaments are not necessary for axonal transport. Moreover, the small numbers of microtubules in myelinated axons suggests that the tubule entity is not absolutely essential but that one or another of these fibrous elements

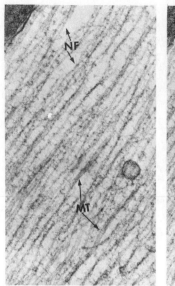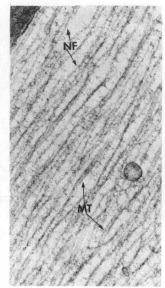

FIGURE 13 Stereo micrographs of axoplasm as preserved in an 0.5 μm section of a myelinated axon in the rat spinal cord. Microtubules (MT) and neurofilaments (NF) are readily identified. The wispy material associated with each, and in some instances cross-linking them, is regarded as equivalent to the microtrabeculae observed in similar relationships in cultured cells including erythrophores. Such trabeculae within axoplasm appear more prominently after staining with ruthenium red (Tani and Ametani, 1970).

will suffice. Many experiments have demonstrated the inhibition of axonal transport by colchicine and vinblastine (see review by Heslop, 1975). Since these drugs are known to act upon microtubules, most investigators have concluded, perhaps prematurely, that microtubules are indispensable to this motion. In this connection Byers has observed that inhibition of transport by colchicine is not complete at concentrations at which microtubules are completely disassembled (Byers, 1974). She also noted that rapid flow is peripheral to the major column of microtubules.

The zones of rapid streaming in time-lapse cinematographic recordings coincide with the distributions of microtubules in the perikaryon and dendrites and also with the neurofilaments and/or microtubules in the axoplasm. The motions of mitochondria within axoplasm are somewhat different from those of other particulate components of the stream. The mitochondrial motion is a snakelike undulation, along with intervals of saltatory movement, whereas other components visible at the light-microscopic level move with short, discontinuous jumps.

The ER in axoplasm is without attached ribosomes and forms a network of varicose, membrane-bound channels. Droz (1967) suggested that these cisternae, which appear as vesicles in thin sections, form a continuous channel from soma to terminal. We have not confirmed this supposition in our high-voltage images of thick sections of axoplasm. Most of the protein, moving rapidly within the axoplasm, is thought to be associated with these numerous vesicles or cisternae of the SER, since protein radioactively labeled and moving with fast flow is recovered in the particulate fraction (McEwen and Grafstein, 1968; Sjöstrand, 1970; Kirkpatrick, Bray, and Palmer, 1972). In addition, Byers (1974) was able to demonstrate by quantitative EM autoradiography that much of the labeled protein is associated with SER. Furthermore, there is a simultaneous accumulation of SER cisternae and radioactivity at distal ends of cut axons, demonstrating that the SER is part of the rapidly moving material. The transported compartments of SER in axoplasm may be considered similar in function to the erythrin granules of the erythrophore cytoplasm.

MICROTRABECULAR ELEMENTS IN AXOPLASM This analogy may be carried to the next level if we consider the ground substance of the nerve cell. In some instances "wispy" material appears to emanate from the surfaces of the neurofilaments and microtubules and to radiate laterally in continuity with similar wispy material in the neuroplasmic matrix, forming a three-dimensional latticework (Figure 13). These fine strands stain with ruthenium red (Tani and Ametani, 1970) or lanthanum (Lane and Treherne, 1970; Burton and Fernandez, 1973). Such staining is claimed to be specific for acid mucopolysaccharides or anionic sites that normally bind Ca^{++} (Overton, 1967). The lanthanum-staining material appears to be part of a three-dimensional mesh equivalent to the microtrabeculae seen in all cultured cells. Within the axon these trabecular elements interconnect microtubules and neurofilaments. Microtrabecular elements also link microtubules and neurofilaments with vesicles, plasma membrane, SER and multivesicular bodies (Droz, 1967; Metuzals, 1969; Smith, Järlfors, and Beranek, 1970; Smith, 1971; Weiss and Mayr, 1971; Yamada, Spooner, and Wessells, 1971; Burton and Fernandez, 1973; Holtzman, 1976). According to the EM images of axoplasm, tubules, filaments, and trabeculae compose a framework within which the large elements are suspended.

COMPOSITION OF AXOPLASM It may be instructive to review the composition of axoplasm—with particular attention to elements that move within the rapid system and elements that do not—in order to gain an understanding of how macromolecules interact within this transport framework.

Fast axonal transport is known to be bidirectional and energy-requiring. Most of our information about the velocity, metabolic requirements, and developmental aspects of rapid transport comes from studies in which protein is followed (Ochs, 1974a,b). Isotopically labeled amino acids injected into the spinal cord are picked up by neuronal somata, and labeled proteins soon appear in the axons. Rapid migration within axoplasm is an ATP-requiring process (Ochs and Hollingsworth, 1971). An Mg^{++}-Ca^{++}-activated ATPase has been demonstrated in nerves (Khan and Ochs, 1974). As yet, however, there seems to be no direct evidence for the involvement of this ATPase in the rapid transport system. Where this enzyme is located within the cytoplasmic matrix and whether it moves with the rapidly transported material or slowly remain unresolved questions.

Ca^{++} is needed for rapid transport (Kirkpatrick and Rose, 1972) and moves bidirectionally with the transported protein (Hammerschlag, Dravid, and Chiu, 1975a,b). A crucial requirement for Ca^{++} appears to be associated with transport functions occurring within the neuronal somata. Incubation of this portion of the nerve cell in Ca^{++}-free media decreases the amount of material transported, whereas similar treatment of the axon alone has no effect (Hammerschlag, Dravid, and Chiu, 1975a). Transport is also blocked by the substitution of Co^{++} for Ca^{++} in media surrounding somal regions but not when that substitution is made along axonal processes (Hammerschlag, Chiu, and Dravid, 1976; Hammerschlag et al., 1977). This inhibition of rapid transport by Co^{++} or low Ca^{++} is not mediated by a decrease in protein synthesis or a decrease in ATP levels (Hammerschlag, Chiu, and Dravid, 1976). Ca^{++} is clearly important in initiating movement of material contained in transport compartments of the SER through the axoplasm. It may well be that these compartments must be loaded with Ca^{++} at the outset of their transport, thereafter releasing and sequestering the ion in order to signal the axoplasmic matrix to act upon them. Support for such a hypothesis has recently been obtained through the localization of Ca^{++} concentrations to SER cisternae of axoplasm (Henkart, Reese, and Brinley, 1978), as well as the earlier isolation of two Ca^{++}-binding proteins from axoplasm (Iqbal and Ochs, 1975).

The rapid axonal transport of sulfated mucopolysaccharides and glycoproteins has also been demonstrated (Elam et al., 1970; Elam and Agranoff, 1971; Elam and Peterson, 1976). These sulfated macromolecules appear to be among the most rapidly transported components, along with Ca^{++}, protein, and SER. Their movement is likewise inhibited by low Ca^{++} and Co^{++} substitution (Hammerschlag et al., 1977). The fine, granular microtrabecular strands of material linking microtubules and neurofilaments are interpreted as being rich in acid mucopolysaccharide on the basis of their selective staining with ruthenium red (Tani and Ametani, 1970) and lanthanum (Lane and Treherne, 1970; Burton and Fernandez, 1973). If this identity is correct and these trabecular elements do move rapidly within the axon (as they do in the erythropore), we can reasonably ask whether they are moving with microtubules and neurofilaments or along them. If rapid axonal transport is similar to dispersion of pigment, these microtubules and neurofilaments should be relatively static, and Davison's (1975) studies of axons suggest that they are.

Another ubiquitous fibrous protein has been demonstrated in nerve cells. Microfilaments (70 Å) have been identified as actin in mouse neuroblastoma cells by HMM-binding (Burton and Kirkland, 1972) and in neurons of the CNS by similar procedures (LeBeux and Willemot, 1975). Similar actinlike proteins isolated from mammalian brain tissue (Berl, Puszkin and Niklas, 1973) and from cultured nerve cells (Fine and Bray, 1971) have been identified by gel electrophoresis. In addition, a tropomyosinlike protein has recently been isolated from brain and growing neurons (Fine et al., 1973). Thus there is no shortage of fibrous proteins in nerve cells from which to construct several transport systems. However, current concepts of the mechanisms responsible for fast axoplasmic transport do not disclose which particular macromolecules are interacting to convert chemical energy into motion. It is obvious from the foregoing discussion of relationships among macromolecular elements of axoplasm that there is at least no shortage of interacting components: the filamentous structures; microtubules, neurofilaments, and microfilaments (actin); a transport compartment (SER); sulfated mucopolysaccharides and glycoproteins (the wispy stuff); a Mg^{++}-Ca^{++}-activated ATPase; and Ca^{++}, possibly bound with a low-molecular-weight protein and/or contained within SER cisternae.

A few additional facts about neurofilaments, mucopolysaccharides, and actin should be noted in light of the suggestions here and those made earlier by Fernandez, Burton, and Samson (1971) and Samson (1971) that these components may interact. Three polypeptides—212,000, 160,000 and 68,000 daltons—appear to move together in the slow component of axoplasmic transport and thus may be associated with a single structure (Hoffman and Lasek, 1975). The 68,000 polypeptide has been labeled by antibodies specifically identifying it as a constituent subunit of neurofilaments in rat peripheral nerve (Schlaepfer, 1977). The 212,000 polypeptide, another suspected constituent of microfilaments, has been found to co-migrate in SDS gels with the heavy chain of chick myosin (Hoffman and Lasek, 1975). A potential myosinlike component of neurofilaments is exciting to those interested in explaining axoplasmic transport through an actin-myosin transaction. However, as with tubulin and neurofilament proteins, actin does not migrate with the fast axoplasmic transport components (Davison, 1975). Nonetheless, a stationary myosinlike molecule may interact with moving mucopolysaccharides by way of the Mg^{++}-Ca^{++} ATPase. This might provide the means for conversion of chemical into kinetic energy.

Mucopolysaccharides are polymers composed of alternating amino sugars and uronic acids. The chains are rich in carboxylic acid side groups and may be sulfated to varying degrees, conferring anionic polyelectrolytic properties. Such molecules are capable of rapid conformational changes in response to interactions between their polyanionic side groups and cations in their vicinity (Balazs and Laurent, 1951). Organic cations containing hydrophobic side chains are capable of precipitating these normally hydrophilic polyanionic macromolecules into a lipophilic phase; increasing the inorganic salt concentration will resolubilize the mucopolysaccharide (Laurent and Scott, 1964). Thus the conformations of polyelectrolytic mucopolysaccharides are very sensitive to concentrations of free cations or positively charged side groups on other molecules. In response to a slight increase in free Ca^{++}, for example, an elongated chain of an acid mucopolysaccharide can rapidly shorten to a small fraction of its original length; this shortening is accompanied by a large reduction in its viscosity (Katchalsky, 1964). The conformation of similar polyanionic macromolecular elements of the axoplasmic microtrabeculae may change systematically in response to controlled variation in their milieu—for example, the release of Ca^{++} from a transport compartment (SER). Such a polyelectrolyte gel can transform chemical energy to mechanical work through covalent linkages made between these macromolecules and protein (Oosawa, 1971). The suggestion by Burton and Fernandez (1973) and Samson (1971) that axoplasm contains a net of polyelectrolyte molecules attached to transported molecules or organelles that use microtubules as anchor points seems reasonable.

With this picture as a model, several basic questions arise. (1) Are there smoothly propagated viscosity changes moving through the network carrying material, or does the network alter conformation in isolated regions, responding to some sort of "move me" message from a transport granule? (One would suspect the latter on the basis of the irregular saltatory nature of the movement of particulate material visualized in the light microscope.) (2) Where is the ATP utilized in this process? (3) Is the Ca^{++} that moves with transported protein a signal for the trabecular links to change conformation (viscosity)? (4) Are the microtrabecular elements mainly attached to the transport compartments or to the fibrous proteins, or both? These are some of the many questions that will be investigated as cell biologists seek to understand the cytoskeleton and its associations with better-known components of the cell.

ACKNOWLEDGMENTS We are pleased to acknowledge the helpful interest of John Wolosewick and the use of some of his micrographs in the preparation of this manuscript. For technical assistance we are grateful to Karen Anderson, Judy Fleming, and Joyce Albersheim. Our work is supported by grants from NIH (Division of Research Resources, No. RR00592-07) and the Muscular Dystrophy Association of America.

REFERENCES

ANDERSON, T. F., 1951. Techniques for the preservation of three-dimensional structure in preparing specimens for the electron microscope. *Trans. NY Acad. Sci.* (Ser. 2) 13:130–134.

BALAZS, E. A., and T. C. LAURENT, 1951. Viscosity function of hyaluronic acid as a polyelectrolyte. *J. Polymer Sci.* 6:665–668.

BERL, S., S. PUSZKIN, and W. J. NICKLAS, 1973. Actomyosin-like protein in brain: Actomyosin-like protein may function in the release of transmitter material at synaptic endings. *Science* 179:441.

BERNS, M. W., J. B. RATTNER, S. BRENNER, and S. MEREDITH, 1977. The role of the centriolar region in animal cell mitosis. *J. Cell Biol.* 72:351–367.

BIKLE, D., L. G. TILNEY, and K. R. PORTER, 1966. Microtubules and pigment migration in the melanophores of *Fundulus heteroclitus* L. *Protoplasma* 61:322–345.

BLOODGOOD, R. A., and K. R. MILLER, 1974. Freeze-fracture of microtubules and bridges in motile axostyles. *J. Cell Biol.* 62:660.

BROWN, R. M., JR., and J. H. M. WILLISON, 1977. Golgi apparatus and plasma membrane involvement in secretion and cell surface deposition, with special emphasis on cellulose biogenesis. In *International Cell Biology, 1976–1977*, B. R. Brinkley and K. R. Porter, eds. New York: Rockefeller Univ. Press, pp. 267–283.

BUCKLEY, I. K., 1975. Three-dimensional fine structure of cultured cells: Possible implications of subcellular motility. *Tiss. Cell* 7:51.

BUCKLEY, I. K., and K. R. PORTER, 1967. Cytoplasmic fibrils in living cultured cells. *Protoplasma* 64:349.

BUCKLEY, I. K., and K. R. PORTER, 1973. Advances in electron microscopy of whole cells grown in vitro. *J. Cell Biol.* 59:37a.

BUCKLEY, I. K., and K. R. PORTER, 1975. Electron microscopy of critical point dried whole cultured cells. *J. Microsc.* (Oxford) 104:107.

BURTON, P. R., and H. L. FERNANDEZ, 1973. Delineation by lanthanum staining of filamentous elements associated with the surfaces of axonal microtubules. *J. Cell Sci.* 12:567.

BURTON, P. R., and W. L. KIRKLAND, 1972. Actin detected in mouse neuroblastoma cells by binding of heavy meromyosin. *Nature* [New Biol.] 239:244.

BYERS, H. R., and K. R. PORTER, 1977. Transformations in the structure of the cytoplasmic ground substance in erythrophores during pigment aggregation and dispersion. I. A study using whole-cell preparations in stereo high-voltage electron microscopy. *J. Cell Biol.* 75:541–558.

BYERS, M. R., 1974. Structural correlates of rapid axonal transport: Evidence that microtubules may not be directly involved. *Brain Res.* 75:97.

DAVISON, P. F., 1975. Neuronal fibrillar proteins and axoplasmic transport. *Brain Res.* 100:73–80.

DENTLER, W. L., S. GRANETT, and J. L. ROSENBAUM, 1975. Ultrastructural localization of the high molecular weight proteins associated with in vitro assembled brain microtubules. *J. Cell Biol.* 65:237–241.

DROZ, B., 1967. Synthèse et transfert des protéines cellulaires dans les neurons ganglionnaires: Etude radioautographique quantitative en microscopie électronique. *J. Microsc.* (Paris) 6:201–208.

ELAM, J. S., and B. W. AGRANOFF, 1971. Transport of proteins and sulfated mucopolysaccharides in the goldfish visual system. *J. Neurobiol.* 2:379–390.

ELAM, J. S., J. M. GOLDBERG, N. S. RADIN, and B. W. AGRANOFF, 1970. Rapid axonal transport of sulfated mucopolysaccharide proteins. *Science* 170:458–460.

ELAM, J. S., and N. W. PETERSON, 1976. Axonal transport of sulfated glycoproteins and mucopolysaccharides in the garfish olfactory nerve. *J. Neurochem.* 26:845–850.

FERNANDEZ, H. L., P. R. BURTON, and F. F. SAMSON, 1971. Axoplasmic transport in the crayfish nerve cord. *J. Cell Biol.* 51:176–192.

FINE, R. F., A. I. BLITZ, S. E. HITCHCOCK, and B. KAMINER, 1973. Tropomyosin in brain and growing neurones. *Nature* [New Biol.] 245:182.

FINE, R. E., and D. BRAY, 1971. Actin in growing nerve cells. *Nature* [New Biol.] 234:115.

FORMAN, D. S., A. L. PADJEN, and G. R. SIGGINS, 1977a. Axonal transport of organelles visualized by light microscopy: Cinemicrographic and computer analysis. *Brain Res.* 136:197–213.

FORMAN, D. S., A. L. PADJEN, and G. R. SIGGINS, 1977b. Effect of temperature on the retrograde transport of microscopically visible intraaxonal organelles. *Brain Res.* 136:215–226.

FREED, J. J., and M. M LEBOWITZ, 1970. The association of a class of saltatory movements with microtubules in cultured cells. *J. Cell Biol.* 45:334.

GOLDMAN, R. D., G. BERG, A. BUSHNELL, C.-M. CHANG, L. DICKERMAN, N. HOPKINS, M. L. MILLER, R. POLLACK, and E. WANG, 1973. Fibrillar systems in cell motility. In *Locomotion of Tissue Cells* (Ciba Foundation Symposium, vol. 14). New York: Associated Scientific Publishers, p. 83.

GOLDMAN, R. D., D. M. KNIPE, 1973. Functions of cytoplasmic fibers in non-muscle cell motility. *Cold Spring Harbor Symp. Quant. Biol.* 37:523.

GRAY, E. G., 1975. Synaptic fine structure and nuclear, cytoplasmic and extracellular networks. *J. Neurocytol.* 4:315–339.

GREEN, L., 1968. Mechanisms of movements of granules in melanocytes of *Fundulus heteroclitus*. *Proc. Natl. Acad. Sci. USA* 59:1179–1186.

HAMMERSCHLAG, R., C. BAKHIT, A. Y. CHIU, and A. R. DRAVID, 1977. Role of calcium in the initiation of fast axonal transport of protein: Effects of divalent cations. *J. Neurobiol.* 8:439–451.

HAMMERSCHLAG, R., A. Y. CHIU, and A. R. DRAVID, 1976. Inhibition of fast axonal transport of [³H] protein by cobalt ions. *Brain Res.* 114:353–358.

HAMMERSCHLAG, R., A. R. DRAVID, and A. Y. CHIU, 1975a. Mechanism of axonal transport: A proposed role of calcium ions. *Science* 188:273–275.

HAMMERSCHLAG, R., A. R. DRAVID, and A. Y. CHIU, 1975b. Inhibition of fast axonal transport of [³H]-proteins by cobalt ions. *Neurosci. Abstr.* 1:801.

HARTWIG, J. H., W. A. DAVIES, and T. P. STOSSEL, 1977. Evidence for contractile protein translocation in macrophage spreading, phagocytosis, and phagolysosome formation. *J. Cell Biol.* 75:956–967.

HARTWIG, J., and T. P. STOSSEL, 1976. Interactions of actin, myosin and actin-binding protein of rabbit pulmonary macrophages. III. Effects of cytochalasin B. *J. Cell Biol.* 71:295–303.

HENKART, M., T. S. REESE, and F. J. BRINLEY, 1978. Endoplasmic reticulum sequesters Ca++ in squid giant axon. *Science* (in press).

HESLOP, J. P., 1975. Axonal flow and fast transport in nerves. *Adv. Comp. Physiol. Biochem.* 6:75–163.

HINKLEY, R. E., 1973. Axonal microtubules and associated filaments strained by alcian blue. *J. Cell Sci.* 13:753–761.

HOFFMAN, P. N., and R. J. LASEK, 1975. The slow component of axonal transport: Identification of major structural polypeptides of the axon and their generality among mammalian neurons. *J. Cell Biol.* 66:351–366.

HOLTZMAN, E., 1976. *Lysosomes: A Survey.* Vienna: Springer-Verlag.

IQBAL, Z., and S. OCHS, 1975. Fast axoplasmic transport of calcium binding components in mammalian nerve. *Neurosci. Abstr.* 1:802.

JUNQUEIRA, L. C., E. RAKER, and K. R. PORTER, 1974. Studies on migration in the melanophores of the teleost *Fundulus heteroclitus* (L). *Arch. Histol. Jap.* 36:339–366.

KATCHALSKY, A., 1964. Polyelectrolytes and their biological interactions. In *Connective Tissue: Intercellular Macromolecules* (Proceedings of a symposium sponsored by the New

York Heart Association). Boston: Little, Brown, pp. 9–41.

KHAN, M. A., and S. OCHS, 1972. Mg²⁺-Ca²⁺-activated ATPase in mammalian nerves: Relation to fast axoplasmic transport and block with colchicine. *Amer. Soc. Neurochem.* (Abstr.) 3:93.

KHAN, M. A., and S. OCHS, 1974. Magnesium or calcium activated ATPase in mammalian nerve. *Brain Res.* 81:413–426.

KIRKPATRICK, J. B., 1971. Time-lapse cinematography of axoplasmic flow in peripheral nerves. In *Abstracts of the 11th Annual Meeting,* American Society for Cell Biology, New Orleans. Abstract 671.

KIRKPATRICK, J. B., J. J. BRAY, and S. M. PALMER, 1972. Visualization of axoplasmic flow in vitro by Nomarski microscopy: Comparison of rapid flow of radioactive proteins. *Brain Res.* 43:1–10.

KIRKPATRICK, J. B., and R. E. ROSE, 1972. Calcium requirements for axoplasmic flow. *Proc. Am. Soc. Neurosci.* 1972:225.

LAMBERT, D. T., and M. FINGERMAN, 1977. Calcium as the second messenger of the red pigment concentrating hormone (RPCH) in ovarian erythrophores of *Palaemonetes pugio*. *Yale J. Biol. Med.* 50 (abstract 68).

LANE, N. J., and J. E. TREHERNE, 1970. Lanthanum staining of neurotubules in axons from cockroach ganglia. *J. Cell Sci.* 7:217–231.

LAURENT, T. C., and J. E. SCOTT, 1964. Molecular weight fractionation of polyanions by cetylpyridium chloride in salt solutions. *Nature* 202:661–662.

LEBEUX, Y. J., and J. WILLEMOT, 1975. An ultrastructural study of the microfilaments in rat brain by means of E-PTA staining and heavy meromyosin labeling. II. The synapses. *Cell Tissue Res.* 160:37.

LUBINSKA, L., 1975. On axoplasmic flow. *Int. Rev. Neurobiol.* 17:241–296.

MALAWISTA, S. E., 1965. On the action of colchicine: The melanocyte model. *J. Exp. Med.* 122:361–384.

MALAWISTA, S. E., 1971. Cytochalasin B reversibly inhibits melanin granule movement in melanocytes. *Nature* 231:354–355.

MALAWISTA, S. E., 1971. The melanocyte model, colchicine-like effects of other antimitotic agents. *J. Cell Biol.* 49:848–855.

MARSLAND, D. A., and D. E. S. BROWN, 1936. Amoeboid movement at high hydrostatic pressure. *J. Cell. Comp. Physiol.* 8:167.

MCEWEN, B. S., and B. GRAFSTEIN, 1968. Fast and slow components in axonal transport of protein. *J. Cell Biol.* 38:494–508.

MCGUIRE, J., and G. MOELLMANN, 1972. Cytochalasin B: Effects on microfilaments and movements of melanin granules within melanocytes. *Science* 175:642–644.

MCINTOSH, J. R., E. S. OGATA, and S. C. LANDIS, 1973. The axostyles of *Saccino aculus*. *J. Cell Biol.* 56:304.

MCMAHAN, U. J., and S. W. KUFFLER, 1971. Visual identification of synaptic boutons on living ganglion cells and of varicosities in postganglionic axons in the heart of the frog. *Proc. R. Soc. Lond.* B177:485.

METUZALS, J., 1969. Configuration of a filamentous network in the axoplasm of the squid (Loligo pealii L.) giant nerve fibre. *J. Cell Biol.* 43:480–505.

MIYASHITA, Y., 1975. A preliminary report on the reactivation of pigment movements in Triton-treated model melanophores of fish. *J. Pre. Med. Course* (Sapporo Med. Coll.) 16:41–44.

MOOSEKER, M. S., and L. G. TILNEY, 1975. Organization of an actin filament-membrane complex. *J. Cell Biol.* 67: 725.

MURPHY, D. B., and L. G. TILNEY, 1974. The role of microtubules in the movement of pigment granules in teleost melanophores. *J. Cell Biol.* 61:757–779.

NOVALES, R. R., 1971. On the role of cyclic AMP in the function of skin melanophores. *Ann. NY Acad. Sci.* 85:494–506.

OCHS, S., 1974a. Axoplasmic transport. In *Peripheral Nervous System*, J. I. Hubbard, ed. New York: Plenum Press, pp. 47–72.

OCHS, S., 1974b. Systems of material transport in nerve fibers (axoplasmic transport) related to nerve function and trophic control. In *Trophic Function of the Neuron*, D. B. Drachman, ed. *Ann. NY Acad. Sci.* 228:202–223.

OCHS, S., and D. HOLLINGSWORTH, 1971. Dependence of fast axoplasmic transport in nerve on oxidative metabolism. *J. Neurochem.* 18:107–111.

OCKLEFORD, C. D., and J. B. TUCKER, 1973. Growth, breakdown, repair and rapid contraction of microtubular axopodia in the heliozoan *Actinophrys sol. J. Ultrastruct. Res.* 44:369.

OOSAWA, F., 1971. *Polyelectrolytes.* New York: Marcel Dekker.

OVERTON, J., 1967. Localized lanthanum staining of the intestinal brush border. *J. Cell Biol.* 35:100A.

POLLARD, T. D., 1976. The role of actin in the temperature dependent gelation and contraction of extracts of *Acanthamoeba. J. Cell Biol.* 68:579–601.

POLLARD, T. D., and R. R. WEIHING, 1974. Actin and myosin and cell movement. *CRC Crit. Rev. Biochem.* 2:1–65.

POMERAT, C. M., W. J. HENDELMAN, C. W. RAINBORN, JR., and J. F. MASSEY, 1967. Dynamic activities of nervous tissue in vitro. In *The Neuron*, H. Hyden, ed. Amsterdam: Elsevier, pp. 119–178.

PORTER, K. R., 1966. Cytoplasmic microtubules and their functions. In *Principles of Biomolecular Organization*, G. E. W. Wolstenholme and M. O'Connor, eds. London: J. & A. Churchill, pp. 308–345.

PORTER, K. R., 1973. Microtubules in intracellular locomotion. In *Locomotion of Tissue Cells* (Ciba Foundation Symposium, vol. 15). New York: Associated Scientific Publishers, p. 149.

PORTER, K. R., 1976. Introduction: Motility in cells. In *Cell Motility*, R. Goldman, T. Pollard and J. Rosenbaum, eds. Cold Spring Harbor Laboratory, pp. 1–28.

RAINE, C. S., B. GHETTI, and M. L. SHELANSKI, 1971. On the association between microtubules and mitochondria within axons. *Brain Res.* 34:389–393.

ROBERTS, K., 1974. Cytoplasmic microtubules and their functions. *Prog. Biophys. Mol. Biol.* 28:273.

ROTH, L. E., D. J. PIHLAJA, and Y. SHIGENAKA, 1970. Microtubules in the heliozoan axopodium. I. The gradion hypothesis of allosterism in structural proteins. *J. Ultrastruct. Res.* 30:7.

SAIDEL, W. M., 1977. Metabolic energy requirements during teleost melanophore adaptations. *Experientia.* 33:1573.

SAMSON, F., 1971. Mechanisms of axoplasmic transport. *J. Neurobiol.* 2:347–360.

SCHLAEPFER, W. W., 1977. Immunological and ultrastructural studies of neurofilaments isolated from rat peripheral nerve. *J. Cell Biol.* 74:226–240.

SCHLIWA, M., and J. BEREITER-HAHN, 1975. Pigment movements in fish melanophores: Morphological and physiological studies. V. Evidence for a microtubule-independent contractile system. *Cell Tissue Res.* 158:61–73.

SCHMITT, F. O., 1968. Fibrous proteins–neuronal organelles. *Proc. Natl. Acad. Sci. USA* 60:1092.

SJÖSTRAND, J., 1970. Fast and slow components of axoplasmic transport in the hypoglossal and vagus nerves of the rabbit. *Brain Res.* 18:461–467.

SLOBODA, R. D., S. A. RUDOLPH, J. L. ROSENBAUM, and P. GREENGARD, 1975. Cyclic AMP-dependent endogenous phosphorylation of a microtubule-associated protein. *Proc. Natl. Acad. Sci. USA* 72:177–181.

SMITH, D. S., 1971. On the significance of crossbridges between microtubules and synaptic vesicles. *Philos. Trans. R. Soc. Lond.* B261:395–405.

SMITH, D. S., U. JÄRLFORS, and R. BERANEK, 1970. The organisation of synaptic axoplasm in lamprey (*Petromyzon marinus*) central nervous system. *J. Cell Biol.* 46:199–219.

SPOONER, B. S., K. M. YAMADA, and N. K. WESSELLS, 1971. Microfilaments and cell locomotion. *J. Cell Biol.* 49:595.

TANI, E., and T. AMETANI, 1970. Substructure of microtubules in brain nerve cells as revealed by ruthenium red. *J. Cell Biol.* 46:159–165.

TILNEY, L. G., 1968. Studies on the microtubules in heliozoa. IV. The effect of colchicine on the formation and maintenance of the axopodia and the redevelopment of pattern in *Actinosphaerium nucleofilum* (Barrett). *J. Cell Sci.* 3:549.

TILNEY, L. G., and B. BYERS, 1969. Studies on the microtubules in heliozoa. V. Factors controlling the organization of microtubules in the Axonemal pattern in *Echinosphaerium* (*Actinosphaerium*) *nucleofilum. J. Cell Biol.* 43:148–165.

TILNEY, L. G., and K. R. PORTER, 1965. Studies on the microtubules in heliozoa. I. The fine structure of *Actinosphaerium nucleofilum* (Barrett) with particular reference to the axial rod structure. *Protoplasma* 60:317.

WARNER, F. D., and P. SATIR, 1974. The structural basis of ciliary bend formation. *J. Cell Biol.* 63:35–63.

WEIHING, R. R., 1976. Cytochalasin B inhibits actin-related gelation of HeLa cell extracts. *J. Cell Biol.* 71:303–307.

WEIS-FOGH, T., and W. B. AMOS, 1972. Evidence for a new mechanism of cell motility. *Nature* 236:301–304.

WEISS, P. A., and R. MAYR, 1971. Organelles in neuroplasmic (axonal) flow: Neurofilaments. *Proc. Natl. Acad. Sci. USA* 68:846–850.

WESSELLS, N. K., B. S. SPOONER, and M. A. LUDUENA. 1973. Surface movements, microfilaments and cell locomotion. In *Locomotion of Tissue Cells* (Ciba Foundation Symposium, vol. 14). New York: Associated Scientific Publishers, p. 53.

WIKSWO, M. A., and R. R. NOVALES, 1969. The effect of colchicine on migration of pigment granules in the melanophores of *Fundulus heteroclitus. Biol. Bull.* (Woods Hole) 137:228–237.

WIKSWO, M. A., and R. R. NOVALES, 1972. Effect of colchicine on microtubules in the melanophores of *Fundulus heteroclitus. J. Ultrastruct. Res.* 41:189–201.

WOLOSEWICK, J. J., and K. R. PORTER, 1976. Stereo high-voltage electron microscopy of whole cells of the human diploid cell line, WI-38. *Am. J. Anat.* 147:303–323.

WOLOSEWICK, J. J., and K. R. PORTER, 1978. The microtrabecular lattice of the cytoplasmic ground substance: Artifact or reality? *J. Cell Biol.* (in press).

WUERKER, R. B., and J. B. KIRKPATRICK, 1972. Neuronal microtubules, neurofilaments and microfilaments. *Int. Rev. Cytol.* 33:45.

WUERKER, R. B., and S. L. PALAY, 1969. Neurofilaments and microtubules in anterior horn cells of the rat. *Tissue and Cell* 1:387–402.

YAMADA, K. M., B. S. SPOONER, and N. K. WESSELLS, 1971. Ultrastructure and function of growth cones and axons of cultured nerve cells. *J. Cell Biol.* 49:614.

YEN, S.-H., D. DAHL, M. SCHACHNER, and M. L. SHELANSKI, 1976. Biochemistry of the filaments of brain. *Proc. Natl. Acad. Sci. USA* 73:529.

42 Microfilaments and Microtubules Studied by Indirect Immunofluorescence Microscopy in Tissue-Culture Cells

KLAUS WEBER and MARY OSBORN

ABSTRACT Microfilaments, microtubules, and intermediate filaments are fibrous structures in cells important for cellular organization, for the determination and maintenance of cell shape, and for cell movement. Specific antibodies allow the direct visualization of these structures in immunofluorescence microscopy. Here we review the biochemical anatomy of the microfilament bundles and of the ruffle and discuss the possible involvement of these structures in cell movement. We review the organization of microtubules in tissue-culture cells, where these structures run uninterrupted from the perinuclear area toward the plasma membrane. After depolymerization, microtubules regrow in an ordered unidirectional manner. Finally we discuss briefly the particular classes of intermediate filaments, with particular emphasis on tonofilaments.

Introduction

ELECTRON-MICROSCOPIC studies of numerous tissues and cells have documented three fibrous systems characteristic of higher cells. These are *microfilaments* (individual fibers 60 Å in diameter), *microtubules* (individual fibers 250 Å in diameter), and *intermediate filaments* (individual fibers 60–110 Å in diameter). These fibrous structures are thought to be involved in the determination of cell morphology, in cell locomotion, and in movements and organization within the cell (for a general review see Goldman, Pollard, and Rosenbaum, 1976).

Although the histochemical studies of Ishikawa, Bischoff, and Holtzer (1969) demonstrated that microfilaments contain F-actin and the reconstitution of microtubules in vitro from tubulin demonstrated that tubulin is the major structural protein of the microtubular system (Weisenberg, 1972), very little else has been learned about the biochemical anatomy of these structures from electron microscopy alone. Since antibodies can detect the intracellular organization of the antigen in immunofluorescence microscopy (Coons and Kaplan, 1950), it was tempting to see what antibodies against structural proteins could contribute to our knowledge of intracellular organization (Lazarides and Weber, 1974). Although limited in resolution, immunofluorescence microscopy offers several unique advantages. First, only the corresponding protein antigen will be specifically visualized. Second, if this protein is present in a supramolecular structure, the organization of this structure throughout the cell can be easily seen because of the overview provided. Third, numerous cells can be studied simultaneously, so that the unique features of the organization under different experimental conditions can be quickly discerned. Thus immunofluorescence microscopy can bridge the gap between classical electron microscopy and light microscopy (Weber, 1976a).

Here we would like to summarize the current state of the information obtained by studying tissue-culture cells by immunofluorescence methods. We shall concentrate on the structural and organizational aspect of the three fiber systems. The ultrastructure and the interaction with the cytoplasm were covered in the paper by Porter, Byers, and Ellisman. The question of membrane fluidity and surface-modulated assembly and disassembly of these structures is discussed by McClain and Edelman and by Elson and Schlessinger in this section. More biochemically oriented reviews are given, for example, by Pollard and Weihing (1974) and by Snyder and McIntosh (1976).

Microfilaments

DIFFERENT ACTIN ORGANIZATION Actin antibodies were first obtained in 1974 (Lazarides and Weber, 1974). They reveal two major types of actin organization in immunofluorescence microscopy of a variety

KLAUS WEBER and MARY OSBORN Max Planck Institute for Biophysical Chemistry, D-3400 Göttingen, Federal Republic of Germany

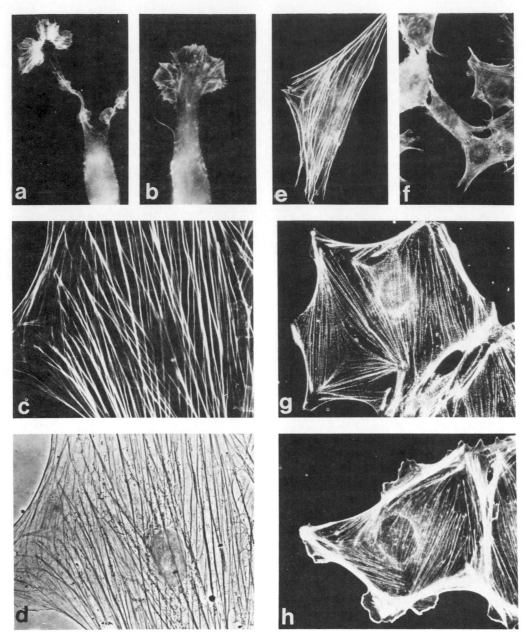

FIGURE 1   A ruffle (a), a cell process (b), and microfilament bundles (c, e, g, h) stained with antibodies to actin (a, b, c, e, f), myosin, (g) or filamin (h). Note the staining of the ruffle and the tip of the cell process by actin antibody, the striated staining with myosin antibody (g), and the 1:1 correspondence between the microfilament bundles in c and the stress fibers viewed in the same cell in phase microscopy in d. The cell types are mouse fibroblast (a, ×600), a neuroblastoma cell after induction (b, ×440), rat mammary cells (c and d, ×610), mouse 3T3 (e, ×390), SV40-transformed mouse 3T3 (f, ×390), rat kangaroo PtK2 cells (g and h, ×600). Note that some cell lines have almost no microfilament bundles (a, b, f) whereas other cell lines have very strong bundles.

of different tissue culture cells. The first is the unstructured bright fluorescence associated particularly with motile areas of the cell, including the ruffling membrane (Figure 1a, b), and probably also with microvilli. The second is a system of "actin cables"

(Lazarides and Weber, 1974; Goldman et al., 1975; Pollack, Osborn, and Weber, 1975), which is especially well developed in some strongly spread cell lines. These actin cables run for long distances parallel to the major axis of the cell and sometimes converge to focal points. The cables usually lie in a single focal plane just underneath the plasma membrane on the adhesive side of the cell. Cables run underneath the nucleus and do not enter into the ruffle. In nonruffling areas of the cell they are very close to the cell margin. During mitosis the actin cables are lost as the cell rounds up.

In well-spread cells, actin cables correspond to the stress fibers that are visible even in living cells by phase-contrast microscopy (Goldman et al., 1975). Figure 1c and d show the same cell after staining with actin antibody in fluorescence and in phase microscopy. The stress fibers in turn represent bundles of microfilaments (Buckley and Porter, 1967; Goldman et al., 1975), which because of their F-actin nature can be specifically decorated by heavy meromyosin in glycerinated cell models (Ishikawa, Bischoff, and Holtzer, 1969). The number, thickness, and arrangement of these structures vary in different cell types; and in some well-spread cells—for example, in human fibroblasts, rat mammary cells (Figure 1c), 3T3 cells (Figure 1e), and PtK2 cells—diameters of between 0.1 μm and 1 μm are found. Rat embryo cells at early passage numbers can contain actin fibers arranged in geodesic domes or polygonal nets. These are sometimes assumed to be intermediate stages during the cell-spreading process (Lazarides, 1976a), but they are also present in some established epithelial lines. Cells that are more rounded, such as Chinese hamster ovary cells and in particular fibroblasts transformed by certain DNA or RNA tumor viruses, have very few microfilament bundles; instead, the general fluorescence in the cytoplasm is stronger (Weber et al., 1974; Pollack, Osborn, and Weber, 1975; Ash, Vogt, and Singer, 1976; Edelman and Yahara, 1976; Wang and Goldberg, 1976). For example, well-developed actin cables are found in 3T3 cells (Figure 1e), but very few such cables are found in the same cells transformed by SV40 (Figure 1f). In some studies there is a good correlation between the presence of actin cables and "anchorage dependence"—that is, the requirement of a cell type for a solid substratum in order to show growth (Pollack, Osborn, and Weber, 1975). After induction neuroblastoma cells do not contain thick stress fibers, but they do have some thin fibers in their processes and also show a strong fluorescence at the tip of the process (Figure 1b).

General fluorescence is also seen in the cytoplasm of many types of cells and may represent other types of actin organization, including less highly polymerized forms of actin or perhaps even the microtrabec-

ulae described by Wolosewick and Porter (1976; see also Porter, Byers, and Ellisman, this volume).

BIOCHEMICAL ANATOMY OF THE STRESS FIBER Although bundles of microfilaments (actin cables) are not typical of all cell types, they have the advantage that, as illustrated in Figure 1c and d, the immunofluorescent image can be directly correlated with the phase-contrast pattern (Goldman et al., 1975). This relation allows the development of a "biochemical anatomy" of the thick microfilament bundles (Weber, 1976a) because it is possible to ask, with antibodies against other proteins, if they are accessory proteins of the stress fiber. Thus, for example, although myosin had been isolated from various eukaryotic cells by biochemical techniques (for a review see Pollard and Weihing, 1974), its intracellular localization in such cells had not been found by electron microscopy. Weber and Groeschel-Stewart (1974) used antibody against smooth-muscle myosin and found that in well-spread cells such as 3T3 or human fibroblasts it gave a striated or interrupted fiber pattern in immunofluorescence microscopy (see Figure 1g), which corresponded to the stress fibers in phase microscopy. The average length of the bright segment is around 5,000–6,000 Å. This finding led to the conclusion that at least part of the cellular myosin must be close to, or present in, the stress fiber, thus providing a possible basis for contractility in these cells. Decoration of fibers not visible by phase microscopy, as well as some general fluorescence in the cytoplasm, was also observed. Subsequent studies with different antibodies against myosin, including two monospecific preparations, have confirmed these results (see, e.g., Ash, Vogt, and Singer, 1976; Fujiwara and Pollard, 1976; Weber, 1976a).

Other studies have shown that tropomyosin and α-actinin, two proteins known to accompany actin filaments in muscle cells are also part of the microfilament bundles as revealed by immunofluorescence microscopy. Both give striated patterns of antibody decoration (Lazarides, 1975, 1976a; Lazarides and Burridge, 1975). Recently a new accessory protein of the microfilament bundles, filamin, was isolated (Wang, Ash, and Singer, 1975; Wang and Singer, 1977). This protein was purified originally from chicken gizzard and is especially interesting because it has been found in a variety of nonmuscle tissues, including brain, but seems to be conspicuously absent from skeletal muscle. Antibodies against filamin show that it gives uninterrupted staining of the stress fibers and of ruffles and that its cytoplasmic distribution parallels that of actin (Wang, Ash, and Singer, 1975; Wang and Singer, 1977; Figure 1h).

BIOCHEMICAL ANATOMY OF THE RUFFLE Immunofluorescence microscopy shows that the ruffling edge, an area of high cellular motility often found at the leading edge of the cell, is strongly stained by actin antibody (Lazarides, 1976b; Weber, 1976a) as well as by filamin antibody (Wang and Singer, 1977; Weber and Osborn, 1978). Staining with myosin antibody (Weber and Osborn, 1978), tropomyosin antibody, and α-actinin antibody (Lazarides, 1976b) shows that myosin and tropomyosin are conspicuously absent in the ruffling edge, whereas α-actinin is present. Studies on microtubules and tonofilaments indicate their absence from the direct ruffling area (see below and Weber and Osborn, 1978). Similar observations have been made on the growing tip of a neuroblastoma-cell process.

STRESS FIBERS, RUFFLES, AND CELL MOVEMENT Several points developed above show that the stress fiber is not simply F-actin in a storage form. The finding that stress fibers contain a variety of accessory proteins typical for muscle (myosin, tropomyosin, and α-actinin) suggests that they could indeed act as "cytomuscular structures." In agreement with such a model, and with the presence of myosin in the stress fiber, is the fact that in glycerinated models such fibers show an ATP-dependent contraction (Isenberg et al., 1976). The relatively short fluorescent segments detected by the myosin antibody (approximately 5,000–6,000 Å under optimal spreading conditions) could indicate that myosin is present in the form of short oligomers, which understandably could escape detection by electron microscopy against the complex background of F-actin fibers (Weber, 1976a). In this context it is interesting to note that myosin purified from nonmuscle tissues shows only 28 myosin molecules per in vitro formed filament (Pollard et al., 1976) and a total length of only 3,300 Å—a value not too far from that found by immunofluorescence microscopy. However, at this time we know neither the molecular details of membrane anchorage nor the direction of the individual F-actin fibers relative to each other and relative to the direction of cellular movement. Thus it is by no means proven that the stress fibers act in cellular movement as cytomuscular structures, and caution should also be used in extrapolating from our knowledge on the biochemical anatomy of the stress fiber to other microfilamentous arrangements. Experimentally it is clear that well-developed microfilament bundles are not obligatory for movement of cells in tissue culture, since cells such as SV101, which have few visible microfilament bundles (but which of course do contain microfilaments), move over the substratum at speeds of around 20 μm/hr. Other cells with highly developed systems of stress fibers (e.g., PtK2 and some lines of human fibroblasts) seem to have much slower rates of movement. In view of these results, it seems that stress fibers might have a dual function. They could provide structural support and confer rigidity on a system in which the cytoplasm is extremely well spread and stretched over the substratum, thus preventing the contraction of this cytoplasm into the round ball seen, for instance, when cells are released from their substratum. In addition, they could also, at appropriate times, permit the cell a major contraction event in order to allow the major cellular displacement necessary when a certain amount of cytoplasm has accumulated at the ruffling edge.

The absence of myosin and tropomyosin and the presence of actin and filamin in ruffles suggest a new possibility, since the actin organization of the ruffle, with its fine microfilamentous material, must differ from that of the stress fiber. The fact that F-actin and filamin form aggregates and gels in vitro and the finding that such gels can coagulate and contract clearly indicate gelation phenomena (Wang and Singer, 1977). Thus, under appropriate conditions, actin filaments can be condensed by filamin into a meshwork. Filamin might in this way regulate the ultrastructural state of F-actin organization, so that myosin-independent mechanochemical activities become a possibility—at least in some areas of the cell.

Finally, it is clear that the cell must be able to regulate, in a controlled reversible manner, the polymerization and depolymerization of actin from its soluble form into more highly ordered forms such as microfilaments and microfilament bundles. Although we do not understand the details of the equilibrium between these various forms of actin, they are likely to be important for cell division and for cell growth.

REARRANGEMENT OF MICROFILAMENT BUNDLES BY CYTOCHALASINS The cytochalasins are drugs that affect cell movement and cytoplasmic cleavage in cultured cells; at higher concentrations they can cause enucleation (Carter, 1967). The cytochalasins also interfere with microfilament structures and induce their rearrangement (for references see Weber et al., 1976). Although the molecular mechanisms by which they do so are still not determined, the final drug effects, even at 10^{-5} M, are dramatically obvious in immunofluorescence microscopy (Weber et al., 1976;

Weber, 1976a). Five minutes after the addition of cytochalasin B, the stress-fiber system of cells such as 3T3 or rat mammary cells breaks up into starlike "heaps" (Figure 2a). After 60 min the cells have contracted and show an arborized morphology, with several cytoplasmic processes extending out to the original attachment points, and a strongly fluorescent perinuclear area. Along these filopodia, actin is localized in strongly fluorescent starlike heaps, and even the finer secondary filopodia are characterized by this uneven distribution of actin (Figure 2b). The process of rearrangement is freely reversible; 60 min after removal of the cytochalasin, cells resume the original morphology and actin patterns. It is important to note that the cytoplasmic microtubule system is not disturbed. Microtubules traverse the cytoplasm of arborized cells, including the filopodia typical for this morphology. Cytochalasin C, D, and E have similar effects. Cytochalasin A, however, can also cause the formation of actin-containing rodlike elements (Rathke et al., 1977).

Microtubules

TUBULIN ANTIBODIES   Direct visualization of cytoplasmic microtubules in indirect immunofluorescence microscopy was found in tissue-culture cells with an antibody prepared against tubulin from the outer doublets of sea-urchin sperm flagella (Weber, Pollack, and Bibring, 1975). The expression of this complex system of fragile fibers (Figure 3a, b) was found to be sensitive to microtubule-depolymerizing agents such as colchicine and low temperature. These results have been confirmed by a variety of different antibody preparations, which in some cases were made monospecific by affinity chromatography (Brinkley, Fuller, and Highfield, 1975; Edelman and Yahara, 1976; Frankel, 1976; Osborn and Weber, 1976a; Weber, Wehland, and Herzog, 1976). In addition, it was found that tubulin antibodies also decorated other microtubule-containing structures such as mitotic spindles (Fuller, Brinkley, and Boughter, 1975; Weber, Bibring, and Osborn, 1975), vinblastin-induced paracrystals (Weber, Pollack, and Bibring, 1975), cilia (Osborn and Weber, 1976a), and flagella (Weber et al., 1977). (A metaphase spindle in a monkey kidney cell line is shown in Figure 3c.) In addition, reaction of cytoplasmic microtubules is observed in the electron microscope, using tubulin antibody in either the indirect peroxidase technique (DeMey et al., 1976) or with direct antibody decoration (Weber, Rathke, and Osborn, in preparation). Thus there would seem to be general agreement that tubulin antibodies do recognize microtubules when used in immunofluorescence microscopy.

CYTOPLASMIC MICROTUBULES   The majority of the microtubules in interphase cells traverse the cytoplasm from the perinuclear area toward the plasma membrane without interruption. They can be followed for very long distances as individual, fragile fluorescent fibers (Figure 3a, b). Depending on the cell type, microtubules with a total length of 20–60 μm can be found (Osborn and Weber, 1976a,b; Brinkley, Fuller, and Highfield, 1976). Very often the tubules come close to the membrane, and under certain circumstances they stop abruptly, seemingly at right angles to it. On other occasions, after reaching the membrane microtubules run parallel to it for

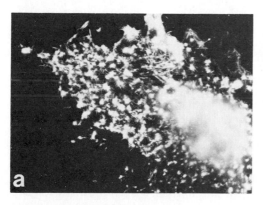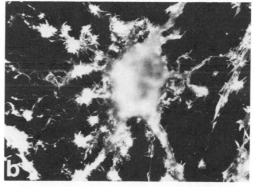

FIGURE 2   Cytochalasin B-induced contraction of 3T3 cells viewed by immunofluorescence microscopy with actin antibody, 5 min (a) and 60 min (b) after addition of the drug (10 μg/ml). The cell in a is moderately contracted, and the actin is located predominantly in starlike heaps ($\times$450).

The cell in b shows the typical appearance of the actin distribution in fully contracted cells ($\times$470). For the appearance of microfilament bundles in 3T3 cells without cytochalasin treatment see Figure 1e. (Reprinted by permission from Weber et al., 1976.)

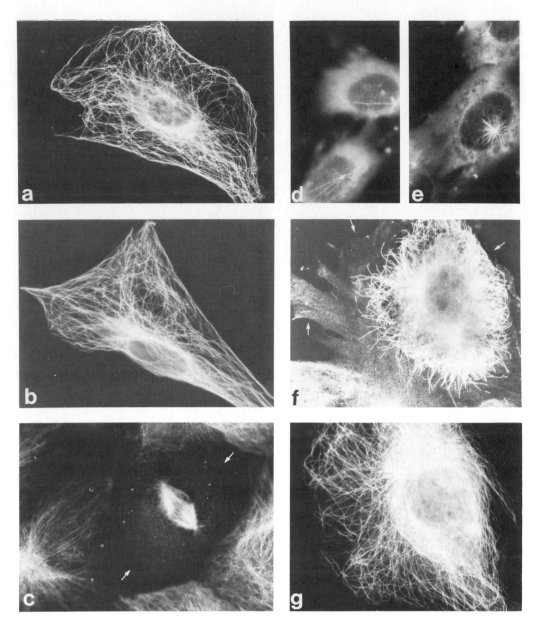

FIGURE 3 Decoration of cytoplasmic microtubules in mouse 3T3 cells (a, b) and of a metaphase spindle in monkey kidney TC7 cells (c) with monospecific tubulin antibody. The cytoplasmic microtubules are sensitive to colcemid (d: 0.5 μg/ml, 1 hr). Thirty minutes after removal of the drug, microtubules are seen reforming as a cytaster (e); 50 min after drug removal, microtubules can be seen to extend half way across the cytoplasm (f). At 75 min after drug removal, the microtubules reach the plasma membrane (g), and this distribution resembles that seen in untreated cells (a, b). The arrows in c and f indicate the position of the plasma membrane. Note the cilia visible in a, d, and e and that the apparent direction of growth of the microtubules is from the cytocenter toward the plasma membrane. (f, ×460; all others ×640.) (Part a reprinted with permission from Weber, 1976a; parts d–g from Osborn and Weber, 1976a.)

long distances (Figure 3a, b). Bends are frequently seen. We have argued elsewhere that in well-spread cells individual fluorescent fibers can correspond to individual microtubules (Weber, Pollack, and Bibring, 1975; Osborn and Weber, 1976a,b).

Because microtubules are present in more than one focal plane, it is sometimes difficult to document the whole complex system in a single photograph. In the well-stretched thin cytoplasm (ectoplasm) typical of tissue-culture cell lines such as mouse 3T3 cells and rat kangaroo PtK2 cells, the majority of microtubules are generally in one focal plane. In the thicker central endoplasm, microtubules often leave this focal plane and run around and above the nucleus. Some cell lines, noticeably virally transformed cells, have a very high ratio of endoplasm to ectoplasm, and in these cases it is more difficult to assess the complexity of the microtubular system. Improved technology and awareness of the fact that cytoplasmic microtubules are not displayed in the same focal plane—as, for example, stress fibers are (see above)—have also made it possible to document microtubules in these cells and to show that they form complex networks in these as in normal cells (Osborn and Weber, 1977b). Indeed all interphase cells attached to a substratum so far studied, including neuroblastoma cells, contain numerous microtubules. Asymmetric cells such as fibroblasts and neuroblastoma cells show that many microtubules follow the direction of the major axis of the cell. Depolymerization of the microtubular system by colcemid or other mitotic drugs gives rise to a more circular but still stretched cell morphology with an abundant undulating membrane. In this context it should be noted that in normal cells microtubules do not enter the ruffle and stop before they reach the very tip of a process of a neuroblastoma cell, again indicating the flexibility of these highly motile cell areas.

POLARITY OF GROWTH OF CYTOPLASMIC MICROTUBULES   Since microtubules can be followed under optimal conditions for very long distances, one can ask if they have the same directionality of assembly. To answer this question, mouse 3T3 cells were put under conditions that give rise to depolymerization of microtubules, for instance by addition of colcemid (Figure 3d). Then the drug was removed from the medium and the repolymerization of microtubules was followed as a function of time. Unidirectional assembly was observed with an apparent initial direction of growth from the cytocenter, acting as a microtubular organizing center, toward the plasma membrane (Osborn and Weber, 1976a). Thirty minutes after removal of the drug, very short microtubules formed a cytaster at the cytocenter (Figure 3e). At approximately 50 min numerous microtubules originating from the perinuclear area were seen stretching into the previously microtubule-free cytoplasm. They extended only part way across the cytoplasm, stopping at a point intermediate between the perinuclear space and the plasma membrane (Figure 3f). These "incomplete microtubules" became longer with increasing time; 2 hr after removal of the drug they reached the plasma membrane and reconstituted a normal pattern of cytoplasmic microtubules

(Figure 3g). Strikingly similar results were obtained with macrophages, where it was shown that the recovery is energy-dependent (Frankel, 1976); similar evidence for unidirectional assembly comes from studies on the recovery of cytoplasmic microtubules after cold treatment has been used as the depolymerizing treatment (Osborn and Weber, 1976a; Frankel, 1976). It is important to note that in these studies no evidence was found for assembly from the plasma membrane toward the cell center (i.e., for the plasma membrane acting as an initiator of microtubular polymerization or for a random polymerization within the cytoplasm). Thus our current view of microtubular assembly in vivo is that the cytocenter, which normally houses the centrioles, acts as an initial organizer and initiator of assembly and that the later elongation processes may be governed by the rules of self-assembly. How wrong assembly (e.g., in the cytoplasm or from the plasma membrane toward the nucleus) is suppressed in vivo is not known.

In a variety of cell types (e.g., PtK2, macrophages) the cytocenter is visible as a small dot or circle in the perinuclear space (Frankel, 1976; our unpublished data) and becomes more prominent after partial depolymerization of microtubules. In some fibroblasts and in a variety of established cell lines such as 3T3 cells, the cytocenter is more prominent because of the close proximity of a primary cilium, which is strongly stained by the tubulin antibody (see Figure 3a, d); this was originally documented electron-microscopically (Wheatley, 1972). The cilium is much more resistant to colcemid than the cytoplasmic microtubules and is therefore an excellent marker for the cytocenter. The cilium is lost some time prior to mitosis, and both electron-microscopic and fluorescence data of some cell lines indicate that almost all the cells in a given culture may have such a structure.

During the process of respreading of tissue-culture cells, drastic morphological changes occur as the rounded cell spreads and stretches on the substratum. During radial attachment of the cell, a ring of flattened cytoplasm is detected, and microtubules enter this spreading ring from the perinuclear area and elongate toward the plasma membrane (Figure 4a). In some cells microtubules appear to be nearly perpendicular to the membrane at some points in the respreading process, giving the impression of contacting the membrane (Figure 4b). In this figure several processes appear to lack microtubules.

The unidirectional assembly of microtubules, both during recovery from mitotic drugs and during respreading, suggests that the cell might use microtubules as direction markers in the cytoplasm and that

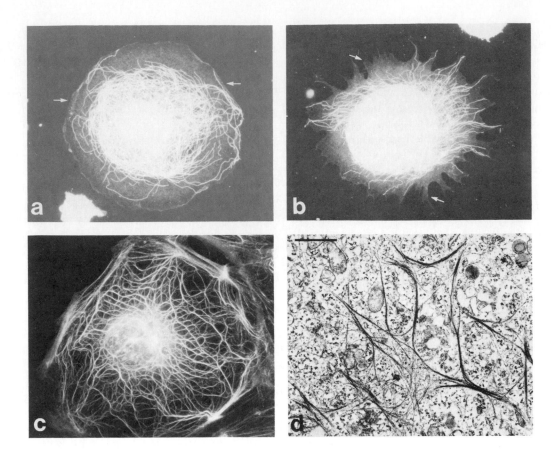

FIGURE 4   (a, b) Two 3T3 cells stained with tubulin antibody, 90 min after trypsinization and replating. In a, a ring of flattened cytoplasm, into which the microtubules are beginning to spread, can be seen. The arrows indicate the plasma membrane. Very occasionally, as shown in b, cells in which some cellular processes appear not to contain microtubules can be seen (arrows). (c, d) A comparison of the tonofilament system of PtK2 cells viewed in immuno-fluorescence microscopy after staining with an autoantibody (c, ×680) or by low-power electron microscopy (d, ×11,800). Note the characteristic wavy appearance of the tonofilaments in both micrographs. (Parts a and b reprinted with permission from Osborn and Weber, 1976b; parts c and d from Osborn, Franke, and Weber, 1977.)

these microtubules could be used for directed intra-cellular transport.

MITOSIS   With the onset of mitosis the pattern of cytoplasmic microtubules is lost; the different stages of the mitotic-spindle microtubule display have been recorded and correlated with corresponding results obtained by phase and by electron microscopy (Fuller, Brinkley, and Boughter, 1975; Weber, Bibring, and Osborn, 1975; Brinkley, Fuller, and High-field, 1975, 1976). In these cases the mass of microtubules in the spindle and the intercellular bridge (Flemming body) make it impossible to resolve individual fluorescent fibers or individual microtubules. Pictures such as Figure 3c, in which the metaphase spindle stains very strongly while the rest of the cell is dark, suggest that at this point in the cell cycle almost all the tubulin is present in the spindle. How the cell regulates this intriguing rearrangement of tubulin between cytoplasmic microtubules in interphase cells and the mitotic spindle in dividing cells is not known.

Intermediate filaments

The category of intermediate filaments includes by definition filamentous structures with diameters between 60 Å and 110 Å. In several studies of tissue-culture cells, they have been called 100 Å filaments; they can be seen in electron micrographs as individual fibers which, after treatment with microtubule-depolymerizing drugs, such as colchicine, reorganize into perinuclear caps and whirls of perinuclear fibers (Goldman and Knipe, 1973; Jorgensen et al., 1976). In brain, neurofilaments are abundant. They differ from microtubules and microfilaments (see, e.g., Yen

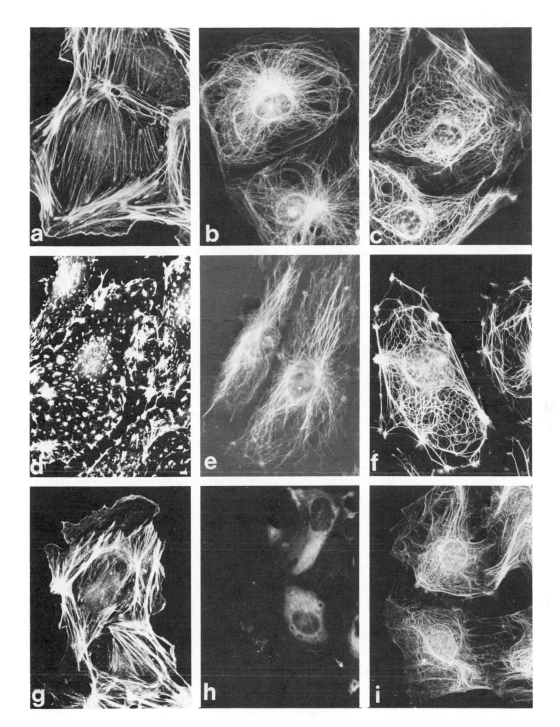

FIGURE 5   PtK2 cells stained directly (a–c) after treatment of cells with 10 μg of cytochalasin B for 30 min (d–f) or after treatment with 5 μg/ml of colcemid for 4 hr (g–i). Cells were stained with actin antibody (a, d, g), with microtubular antibody (b, e, h), or with an autoantibody (c, f, i). Note that cytochalasin B destroys the microfilament system, leaving the microtubules and tonofilaments intact, and that colcemid destroys the microtubules, leaving the microfilaments unaffected and the tonofilaments only slightly disturbed (×460). This figure shows that the three fibrous systems in PtK2 cells are different and can be distinguished by immunofluorescence microscopy. (Reprinted by permission from Osborn, Franke, and Weber, 1977.)

et al., 1976). In certain specialized cells, such as epidermal and epithelial cells, one finds wavy bundles of tonofilaments (Maltoltsy, 1975). Our knowledge of the function, distribution, organization, and potential interrelationship of these structures is still very spotty, for they have only recently begun to yield to biochemical and immunological techniques. We shall not go into this field in detail here, but it does seem appropriate to cite the results of some recent purification studies.

The major protein of the neurofilament can be isolated; it is a polypeptide of molecular weight 55,000 and is different from tubulin (Jorgensen et al., 1976; Yen et al., 1976). In neuroblastoma cells, antibodies against this protein stain, as expected, swirls of wavy perinuclear fibers, which seem to correspond to neurofilament-type fibers. They also stain the perinuclear ring of intermediate fibers in some endothelial cells and the perinuclear cap of intermediate fibers in colchicine-treated tissue-culture cells (Jorgensen et al., 1976; Blose, Shelanski, and Chacko, 1977). These results suggest an immunological and structural similarity between neurofilament protein, smooth-muscle fibers, and intermediate filaments of fibroblasts. In line with this possibility are several studies that have attempted to isolate the polypeptide of the intermediate-filament system from such sources. Pure protein from chicken-gizzard intermediate filaments has been called skeletin or desmin (Lazarides and Hubbard, 1976; Small and Sobieszek, 1977) and found to have a molecular weight of approximately 55,000. The protein of colchicine-induced caps of intermediate filaments isolated from BHK cells show two polypeptides, again with molecular weights of approximately 55,000 (Starger and Goldman, 1977); and intermediate filaments observed in cytoskeletons of chick embryo fibroblasts have a similar molecular weight (Brown, Levinson, and Spudich, 1976; Osborn and Weber, 1977a). Rigorous biochemical studies of these 55,000 dalton proteins from different sources are needed to prove or disprove their identity.

A different approach has been used to study the tonofilamentous 70–100-Å-thick wavy bundles of intermediate fibers typical of the epithelial cell line PtK2. Here rabbit sera containing autoantibodies can be used to specifically visualize this impressive system of fibers in PtK2 and in other cells and to document how similar the images of this structure are in immunofluorescence microscopy and in low-power electron microscopy (compare Figures 4c and d). Both methods indicate that the tonofilaments form a strong system of wavy, intermingled fibers of varying thickness, concentrated around the nucleus and at points close to the plasma membrane. The autoimmune sera that stain the tonofilaments in PtK2 cells also stain intermediate filaments in skin cells, whirls of intermediate fibers in Neuro 2a cells, and caps in colchicine-treated 3T3 cells. Unfortunately, until monospecific sera can be isolated from the pool, we will not know whether the decoration in these cases is caused by the same or by different autoantibodies. However, this study documents the degree of specificity that can currently be reached in immunofluorescence microscopy (Figure 5). Not only is the display and organization of the three fibrous systems different in normal PtK2 cells (Figure 5a, b, c), but they are also readily distinguished by their differential drug sensitivity as revealed by immunofluorescence microscopy. Thus cytochalasin B, a microfilament-"rearranging" drug does, as expected, break up the microfilament bundles into starlike heaps (see above and Figure 5d), but it does not change the display of microtubules or tonofilaments (Figure 5e,f). Furthermore, the microtubule-specific drug colcemid does depolymerize cytoplasmic microtubules as expected (see above and Figure 5h), but it does not change the display of the microfilament bundles. These data provide direct evidence that the three fibrous systems are different and that, at least in PtK2 cells, each individual system can be manipulated independently of the other two.

ACKNOWLEDGMENTS We thank H. J. Koitzsch for help with some of the experiments, T. Born for photography, and our colleagues for discussion.

REFERENCES

ASH, J. F., P. K. VOGT, and S. J. SINGER, 1976. Reversion from transformed to normal phenotype by inhibition of protein synthesis in rat kidney cells infected with a temperative sensitive mutant of Rous sarcoma virus. *Proc. Natl. Acad. Sci. USA* 73:3603–3607.

BLOSE, S. H., M. L. SHELANSKI, and S. CHACKO, 1977. Localization of bovine brain filament antibody of intermediate (100 Å) filaments in guinea pig vascular endothelial cells and chick cardiac muscle cells. *Proc. Natl. Acad. Sci. USA* 73:662–665.

BRINKLEY, B. R., G. M. FULLER, and D. P. HIGHFIELD, 1975. Cytoplasmic microtubules in normal and transformed cells in culture. Analysis by tubulin antibody immunofluorescence. *Proc. Natl. Acad. Sci. USA* 72:4981–4985.

BRINKLEY, B. R., G. M. FULLER, and D. P. HIGHFIELD, 1976. Tubulin antibodies as probes for microtubules in dividing and non-dividing mammalian cells. In *Cell Motility*, R. D. Goldman, T. D. Pollard, and J. Rosenbaum, eds. Cold Spring Harbor, NY: Cold Spring Harbor Laboratory, pp. 435–456.

BROWN, S., W. LEVINSON, and J. A. SPUDICH, 1976. Cyto-skeletal elements of chick embryo fibroblasts revealed by detergent extraction. *J. Supramol. Struct.* 5:119–130.

BUCKLEY, I. K., and K. R. PORTER, 1967. Cytoplasmic fibrils in living cultured cells. *Protoplasma* 64:349–380.

CARTER, S. B., 1967. Effects of cytochalasins on mammalian cells. *Nature* 213:256–261.

COONS, A. H., and M. H. KAPLAN, 1950. Localization of antigen in tissue culture cells. II. Improvements in a method for detection of antigen by means of fluorescent antibody. *J. Exp. Med.* 91:1–13.

DEMEY, J., I. HOEBEKE, M. DE BRABANDER, G. GEUENS, and M. JONIAU, 1976. Immunoperoxidase visualization of microtubules and microtubular proteins. *Nature* 264:273–275.

EDELMAN, G. M., and I. YAHARA, 1976. Temperature sen-sitive changes in surface modulating assemblies of fibro-blasts transformed by mutants of Rous sarcoma virus. *Proc. Natl. Acad. Sci. USA* 73:2047–2051.

FRANKEL, F. R., 1976. Organization and energy dependent growth of microtubules in cells. *Proc. Natl. Acad. Sci. USA* 73:2798–2802.

FULLER, G. M., B. R. BRINKLEY, and M. J. BOUGHTER, 1975. Immunofluorescence of mitotic spindles using monospe-cific antibody against bovine brain tubulin. *Science* 187:948–950.

FUJIWARA, K., and T. D. POLLARD, 1976. Fluorescent anti-body localization of myosin in the cytoplasm, cleavage furrow and mitotic spindle of human cells. *J. Cell Biol.* 71:848–875.

GOLDMAN, R. D., and D. M. KNIPE, 1973. Functions of cytoplasmic fibers in non-muscle cell motility. *Cold Spring Harbor Symp. Quant. Biol.* 37:523–534.

GOLDMAN, R. D., E. LAZARIDES, R. POLLACK, and K. WEBER, 1975. The distribution of actin in non-muscle cells. *Exp. Cell Res.* 90:333–344.

GOLDMAN, R. D., T. D. POLLARD, and J. ROSENBAUM, eds. 1976. *Cell Motility.* Cold Spring Harbor, NY: Cold Spring Harbor Laboratory.

ISENBERG, G., P. C. RATHKE, N. HUELSMANN, W. W. FRANKE, and K. E. WOHLFAHRT-BOTTERMANN, 1976. Cytoplasmic actomyosin fibrils in tissue culture cells: Direct proof of contractility by visualization of ATP-induced contractions on fibrils isolated by laser microbeam dissection. *Cell and Tissue Res.* 166:427–443.

ISHIKAWA, H. R., R. BISCHOFF, and H. HOLTZER, 1969. Formation of arrowhead complexes with heavy mero-myosin in a variety of cell types. *J. Cell Biol.* 43:312–328.

JORGENSEN, A. O., L. SUBRAHAMANYAN, C. TURNBULL, and V. I. KALNINS, 1976. Localization of the neurofilament protein in neuroblastoma cells by immunofluorescent staining. *Proc. Natl. Acad. Sci. USA* 73:3192–3196.

LAZARIDES, E., 1975. Tropomyosin antibody: The specific localization of tropomyosin in non-muscle cells. *J. Cell Biol.* 65:549–561.

LAZARIDES, E., 1976a. Actin, α-actinin and tropomyosin interaction in the structural organization of actin fila-ments in non-muscle cells. *J. Cell Biol.* 68:202–219.

LAZARIDES, E., 1976b. Two general classes of cytoplasmic actin filaments in tissue culture cells: The role of tropo-myosin. *J. Supramol. Struct.* 5:531–563.

LAZARIDES, E., and K. BURRIDGE, 1975. α-actinin: Immu-nofluorescent localization of a muscle structural protein in non-muscle cells. *Cell* 6:289–298.

LAZARIDES, E., and B. D. HUBBARD, 1976. Immunological characterization of the subunit of the 100 Å filaments of muscle cells. *Proc. Natl. Acad. Sci. USA* 73:4344–4348.

LAZARIDES, E., and K. WEBER, 1974. Actin antibody: The specific visualization of actin filaments in non-muscle cells. *Proc. Natl. Acad. Sci. USA* 71:2268–2272.

MALTOLTSY, A. G., 1975. Desmosomes, filaments and ker-atohyaline granules: Their role in the stabilization and keratinization of the epidermis. *J. Invest. Dermatol.* 65:127–142.

OSBORN, M., W. W. FRANKE, and K. WEBER, 1977. The visualization of a system of 7–10 mm thick filaments in cultured cells of an epitheloidal line (PtK2) by immuno-fluorescence microscopy. *Proc. Natl. Acad. Sci. USA* 74:2490–2494.

OSBORN, M., and K. WEBER, 1976a. Cytoplasmic microtu-bules in tissue culture cells appear to grow from an or-ganizing structure towards the plasma membrane. *Proc. Natl. Acad. Sci. USA* 73:867–871.

OSBORN, M., and K. WEBER, 1976b. Tubulin specific anti-body and the expression of microtubules in 3T3 cells after attachment to a substratum. *Exp. Cell Res.* 103:331–340.

OSBORN, M., and K. WEBER, 1977a. The detergent resistant cytoskeleton of tissue culture cells includes the nucleus and the microfilament bundles. *Exp. Cell Res.* 106:339–350.

OSBORN, M., and K. WEBER, 1977b. The display of micro-tubules in transformed cells. *Cell* 12:561–571.

POLLACK, R., M. OSBORN, and K. WEBER, 1975. Patterns of organization of actin and myosin in normal and trans-formed cultured cells. *Proc. Natl. Acad. Sci. USA* 72:994–998.

POLLARD, T. D., K. FUJIWARA, R. NIEDERMAN, and P. MAU-PIN SZAMIER, 1976. Evidence for the role of cytoplasmic actin and myosin in cellular structure and motility. In *Cell Motility*, R. D. Goldman, T. Pollard, and J. Rosen-baum, eds. Cold Spring Harbor, NY: Cold Spring Har-bor Laboratory, pp. 689–724.

POLLARD, T. D., and R. R. WEIHING, 1974. Cytoplasmic actin and myosin and cell movement. In *CRC Crit. Rev. Biochem.* 3:1–65.

RATHKE, P. C., E. SEIB, K. WEBER, M. OSBORN, and W. W. FRANKE, 1977. Rodlike elements from actin-containing microfilament bundles observed in cultured cells after treatment with cytochalasin A. *Exp. Cell Res.* 105:253–262.

SMALL, J. V., and A. SOBIESZEK, 1977. Studies on the func-tion and composition of the 10 nm (100 Å) filaments of vertebrate smooth muscle. *J. Cell Sci.* 23:243–268.

SNYDER, J. A., and J. R. MCINTOSH, 1976. Biochemistry and physiology of microtubules. *Annu. Rev. Biochem.* 45:699–720.

STARGER, J. M., and R. D. GOLDMAN, 1977. Isolation and preliminary characterization of 10 nm filaments from BHK cells. *Proc. Natl. Acad. Sci. USA* 74:2422–2426.

WANG, E., and A. R. GOLDBERG, 1976. Changes in micro-filament organization and suface topography upon trans-formation of chick embryo fibroblasts with Rous sarcoma virus. *Proc. Natl. Acad. Sci. USA* 73:4065–4069.

WANG, K., J. F. ASH, and S. J. SINGER, 1975. Filamin, a new high molecular-weight protein found in smooth muscle and non-muscle cells. *Proc. Natl. Acad. Sci. USA* 72:4483–4486.

WANG, K., and S. J. SINGER, 1977. Interaction of filamin with F-actin in solution. *Proc. Natl. Acad. Sci. USA* 74:2021–2025.

WEBER, K., 1976a. In *Contractile Systems in Non-Muscle Tissues*, S. V. Perry, A. Margreth, and R. S. Adelstein, eds. Amsterdam: North-Holland Publishing Co., pp. 51–66.

WEBER, K., 1976b. Visualization of tubulin containing structures by immunofluorescence microscopy. In *Cell Motility* (A), R. D. Goldman, T. Pollard, and J. Rosenbaum, eds. Cold Spring Harbor, NY: Cold Spring Harbor Laboratory, pp. 403–417.

WEBER, K., T. BIBRING, and M. OSBORN, 1975. Specific visualization of tubulin containing structures in tissue culture cells by immunofluorescence. *Exp. Cell Res.* 95:111–120.

WEBER, K., and U. GROESCHEL-STEWART, 1974. Myosin antibody: The specific visualization of myosin containing filaments in non-muscle cells. *Proc. Natl. Acad. Sci. USA* 71:4561–4564.

WEBER, K., E. LAZARIDES, R. D. GOLDMAN, A. VOGEL, and R. POLLACK, 1974. Localization and distribution of actin fibers in normal, transformed and revertant cells. *Cold Spring Harbor Symp. Quant. Biol.* 39:363–369.

WEBER, K., and M. OSBORN, 1978. Fibrous structures in cells as viewed by immunofluorescence microscopy. *Cell* 14:477–488.

WEBER, K., M. OSBORN, W. W. FRANKE, E. SEIB, U. SCHEER, and W. HERTH, 1977. Identification of microtubular structures in diverse plant and animal cells by immunological cross-reaction revealed in immunofluorescence microscopy. *Cytobiologie* 15:285–302.

WEBER, K., R. POLLACK, and T. BIBRING, 1975. Antibody against tubulin: The specific visualization of cytoplasmic microtubules in tissue culture cells. *Proc. Natl. Acad. Sci. USA* 72:459–463.

WEBER, K., P. C. RATHKE, M. OSBORN, and W. W. FRANKE, 1976. Distribution of actin and tubulin in cells and in glycerinated cell models after treatment with cytochalasin B. *Exp. Cell Res.* 102:285–287.

WEBER, K., J. WEHLAND, and W. HERZOG, 1976. Griseofulvin interacts with microtubules both *in vivo* and *in vitro*. *J. Mol. Biol.* 102:817–829.

WHEATLEY, D. N., 1972. Cilia in cell cultured fibroblasts. IV. Variation with the mouse 3T6 fibroblastic cell line. *J. Anat.* 113:83–93.

WEISENBERG, R. C., 1972. Microtubule formation *in vitro* in solutions containing low calcium concentrations. *Science* 177:1104–1105.

WOLOSEWICK, J. J., and K. R. PORTER, 1976. Stereo high voltage electron microscopy of whole cells of the human diploid line WI-38. *Am. J. Anat.* 147:303–324.

YEN, S., D. DAHL, M. SCHACHNER, and M. L. SHELANSKI, 1976. Biochemistry of filaments of brain. *Proc. Natl. Acad. Sci. USA* 73:529–533.

Note added in proof

This article was completed in September 1977. Since then a number of new aspects have been reported in the literature, and we would like to draw attention to some of these papers. It has been shown that intermediate filaments are cell type and tissue specific and that several classes can be distinguished immunologically (see, e.g., Franke et al., *Proc. Natl. Acad. Sci. USA* 75:5034–5038, 1978; Lazarides and Balzer, *Cell* 14:429–438, 1978; Bennett et al., *Proc. Natl. Acad. Sci. USA* 75:4364–4368, 1978). The intermediate filaments described here for PtK2 cells are of the prekeratin type since they are stained by monospecific antibodies to prekeratin (Franke et al., *Exp. Cell Res.* 116:429–446, 1978). Ferritin-conjugated antibodies have been introduced in the study of the cytoskeleton (Webster et al., *Proc. Natl. Acad. Sci. USA,* November 1978). In addition, a direct correlation by electron microscopy and immunofluorescence microscopy on a single specimen has shown that it is indeed possible to visualize an individual microtubule in the fluorescence microscope (Osborn, Webster, and Weber, *J. Cell Biol.* 77:R26–R34, 1978). It has also been suggested that the distribution of mitochondria in tissue-culture cells parallels that of microtubules (Heggeness, Simon, and Singer, *Proc. Natl. Acad. Sci. USA* 75:3863–3866, 1978). Immunofluorescence studies of neuroblastoma cells have been reported (Marchisio, Osborn, and Weber, *Brain Res.* 155:229–237, 1978; and *J. Neurocytol.* 7:571–582, 1978) as well as an interesting electron-microscopic study of cytoskeletons of these cells (Isenberg and Small, *Cytobiologie* 16:326–344, 1978). It has been suggested that some neuroblastoma clones may have multiple organizing centers for microtubules (Marchisio, Weber, and Osborn, manuscript submitted). Finally an easy stereo immunofluorescence procedure has been introduced, so that it is now possible to obtain three-dimensional fluorescence micrographs (Osborn et al., *Cell* 14:477–488, 1978).

43 Surface Molecules Mediating Interactions among Embryonic Neural Cells

URS RUTISHAUSER, JEAN-PAUL THIERY,
ROBERT BRACKENBURY, and GERALD M. EDELMAN

ABSTRACT   Interactions among the surfaces of embryonic neural cells are likely to be important in the formation of nervous tissue and neuronal tracts. To study these interactions, initial adhesion between individual cells has been analyzed in vitro. The experiments indicate that cells from different neural tissues adhere to each other through the same mechanism and that a 140,000 M_r cell surface protein is involved in the formation of cell-cell bonds. Specific antibodies have been used to demonstrate the presence of this molecule in intact tissue and on the surface of neuronal processes. They also have been used to perturb its function during the formation of neurite regions in aggregates of retinal cells and were found to alter the growth of neurites from dorsal-root ganglion cells. The results suggest that this protein is intimately involved in the development of cell and neurite patterns in the nervous system.

THE NERVOUS SYSTEM includes some of the most intricate tissue patterns to be found in multicellular organisms. The first step in the analysis of this complex structure has been to distinguish among the different levels at which organization and heterogeneity can be observed. The nervous system is unique in that these levels can be described not only in terms of the orientation and segregation of different cell types but also in terms of the specific short- and long-range interconnection of cells by networks of neuronal processes. At the macroscopic level, nervous tissue may be described in terms of (1) large functional compartments or regions and (2) the collection of individual neurites into nerve trunks that connect one region to another. At the cellular level, regions may be segregated into discrete layers containing different cell types (as in the cerebellum and retina), may be organized into groups of cells that are functionally integrated (such as columns in the somato-sensory and visual cortex), or may establish specific connections to other regions (as in the mapping of the visual field of the retina onto the visual cortex).

How is such a high degree of specific organization achieved? By examining the development of the nervous system, a number of parameters have been defined, including the migration of cells along defined routes, localized cell division, differentiation and death, the growth and branching of nerves along specific pathways, and synapse formation with subsequent stabilization or retraction. The mechanisms underlying these processes, however, have been described only in the most general terms. In particular, it is not clear how these events are coordinated so as to produce a precise tissue pattern. In other words, how does a cell receive the appropriate information so that it stops dividing at the right time, differentiates appropriately, and establishes interactions with the correct cells? The work of Holtfreter nearly four decades ago already suggested that this was in part a problem of cell recognition (Holtfreter, 1939; Townes and Holtfreter, 1955). He found that cells obtained from different tissues would stick together randomly and then sort themselves out to form separate regions containing structures characteristic of the parent tissues. These observations indicated that there is selective adherence among cells and suggested that this might be an important process in tissue formation.

Although Holtfreter's experiments provided a focus for later studies on cell recognition, the ensuing work has led to quite divergent hypotheses on the mechanism of cell adhesion. These hypotheses can be grouped into three classes. One position has been that differences in adhesiveness reflect the presence of different ligands on the cell surface (Moscona, 1962; Lilien, 1969). Alternatively, it is possible that aggregation of cells is governed not by particular

URS RUTISHAUSER, JEAN-PAUL THIERY, ROBERT BRACKENBURY, and GERALD M. EDELMAN   The Rockefeller University, New York, NY 10021

molecules but by differences in generalized interactions (hydrophobic, electrostatic, van der Waal's) between large areas of the cell surface (see Curtis, 1967). A third class of mechanisms is based on the assumption that cell adhesion is mediated by one or a few cell surface ligands and that adhesive specificity results from control of the amount of a ligand at the cellular level or of the ability of the ligand to form cell-cell bonds (Steinberg, 1963; Roseman, 1970; Shur and Roth, 1975; Rutishauser et al., 1976; Thiery et al., 1977). With respect to the latter two classes of models, it can be argued that cell recognition during development is too complex a phenomenon to be carried out by nonspecific forces or by a small set of ligands. It has been pointed out by Steinberg (1963), however, that the segregation of cells observed in the experiments of Holtfreter and in later studies could be accounted for by *quantitative* differences in adhesiveness rather than absolute binding specificities. That is not to deny, of course, that certain specialized cell interactions (e.g., graft rejection and sperm-egg fusion) employ specific recognition mechanisms.

A large number of the difficulties encountered in analyzing cell adhesion concern methodology. The major technical considerations are the design of an in vitro system for determining the magnitude and specificity of cell adhesiveness and the choice of criteria by which to detect molecules involved in cell-cell binding. Unfortunately there has been little uniformity in the approaches used, and it has therefore been difficult so far to compare results obtained in different laboratories. Recently improved methods have been introduced for measuring adhesion, and there is increasing agreement among the results—if not the interpretations—of different groups. The description of the molecular mechanism of adhesion, however, requires analysis of cell surface molecules by microchemical methods that are not as yet fully developed. As a result, a number of molecules that may be involved in adhesion have been reported (Balsamo and Lilien, 1974; Merrell, Gottlieb, and Glaser, 1975; Oppenheimer, 1975; Shur and Roth, 1975; Hausman and Moscona, 1976; Rutishauser et al., 1976; Thiery et al., 1977), but their precise relation to binding remains a matter of speculation.

Although the description of cell aggregation in vitro is at a rather preliminary stage, it is important to keep in mind that this process is only a model system for analyzing the role of cell adhesiveness in tissue formation. The physical conditions for cell aggregation—namely individual cells colliding in free solution—probably never exist in a developing embryo. In fact, the physiological correlate of aggregation may not resemble an adhesive event all. Therefore the ultimate goal of cell-aggregation studies should be to provide specific probes for cell-adhesion molecules and enough information about the chemistry of cell-cell binding to allow meaningful experimentation with intact tissues or with in vitro systems that more closely resemble physiological processes.

With this introduction as a background, the remainder of this text will focus on studies carried out in our laboratory on the relationship of cell adhesion to neuronal development. The studies have been carried out in three steps:

1. A quantitative description of neural cell aggregation in terms of specificity and developmental control (Rutishauser et al., 1976).

2. The identification, isolation, and characterization of a cell surface molecule involved in neural cell adhesion and the preparation of antibodies that react specifically with this molecule (Brackenbury et al., 1977; Thiery et al. 1977).

3. The use of the specific antibodies to localize the cell-adhesion molecule in tissues and to perturb the normal function of the molecule in development.

Aggregation of neural cells

As mentioned above, a variety of methods have been used to quantitate cell aggregation. An early method, comparison of aggregate size over a period of 24 hr (Moscona, 1962), has been useful for evaluation of histotypic development but cannot provide much information about individual cells or the specificity of binding between different cell types. To provide a more quantitative estimate of adhesiveness, assays were subsequently developed to determine the initial rate of binding by measuring the decrease in number of single cells that accompanies aggregation (Curtis and Greaves, 1965; Orr and Roseman, 1969). The problem of identifying binding events between *different* cell types was first attacked by preparing large aggregates of one cell type and then measuring the rate at which aggregates collect cells of the same or a different type (Roth, McGuire, and Roseman, 1971). More recently the aggregate has been replaced by cells attached to a surface in a monolayer, so that binding can be standardized in terms of cells bound per unit area of monolayer (Walther, Ohman, and Roseman, 1973; Rutishauser et al., 1976). In the assay developed in our laboratory, the lectin from wax-beans is used to immobilize the cells on a plastic dish, and the cells in suspension are internally labeled with fluorescein (Figure 1). Use of the lectin allows any cell type to be rapidly immobilized in a uniform mon-

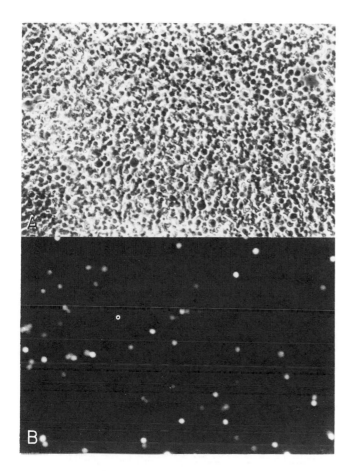

FIGURE 1 Cell-cell binding assay using cells immobilized on a wax bean agglutinin-coated petri dish. (A) Immobilized-cell monolayer as viewed by phase-contrast microscopy. (B) Cells containing fluorescein that have bound to the monolayer, as observed by fluorescence microscopy. (From Thiery et al., 1977.)

olayer, and the fluorescent label permits quantitation of individual binding events.

A second important technical consideration has been the method for preparing single cells from embryonic tissues. The most widely used procedure is trypsinization (Moscona, 1952), which often gives a high yield of single viable cells. Although the cells are not killed, their surface proteins are damaged or removed by the enzyme. This is an important problem because proteins are among the molecules most likely to be involved in formation of cell-cell bonds. Fortunately viable cells generally have the capacity to resynthesize their cell surface components, so that under appropriate conditions the damage caused by the trypsin can be repaired (Brackenbury et al., 1977). Unfortunately many measurements of cell adhesion have been made without a thorough evaluation of these conditions and are therefore difficult

to interpret. The recovery of cells obtained by treating retinal tissue with 0.5% crude trypsin (1-250, Nutritional Biochemicals) for 20 min at 37° is summarized in Figure 2. Cells trypsinized in this manner have diminished amounts of cell surface protein and aggregate poorly if at all. When these cells are cultured in 100 ml Bellco spinner flasks at 400 rpm, their surface proteins are gradually regenerated and their adhesiveness is increased, reaching a plateau after about 12 hr. We have therefore carried out all experiments with cells cultured in suspension for 18–24 hr.

Once these technical problems have been considered, it becomes possible to answer a central question about cell adhesion: How specific is the binding of cells from different tissues to each other? In contrast to earlier reports (Moscona, 1962; Lilien, 1969), we have found that there is no absolute specificity in the binding among cells from the retina and brain (Rutishauser et al., 1976) and from different regions of the brain (our unpublished results), although the adhesiveness of these cells does change during development (Rutishauser et al., 1976). The results with retinal and brain cells are shown in Table I. High levels of binding were obtained between pairs of cells from retinas of 8-day-old chick embryos and from brains of 6-day-old embryos. In both tissues, cells from older embryos were less adhesive, low levels of binding being obtained with 14-day retinal cells and 10-day brain cells. Although little binding occurred

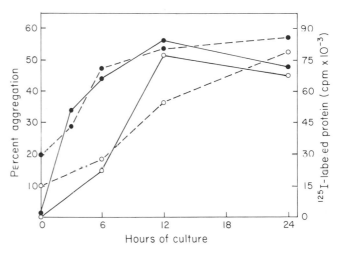

FIGURE 2 Aggregation of trypsinized retinal cells whose cell surface proteins have reappeared during culture in suspension. Percent aggregation (solid lines) and relative amount of total radioiodinated cell surface protein (dashed lines) are indicated as functions of culture time in two experiments (open and closed circles). (From Brackenbury et al., 1977.)

TABLE I

Binding among retinal and brain cells from embryos of different ages

| Cell-cell binding between:* | | |
Cell in monolayer	Cell in suspension	Cell-bound cells**
R_8	R_8	423
R_{14}	R_{14}	122
B_6	B_6	413
B_{10}	B_{10}	8
R_8	B_{10}	41
R_8	B_6	390

* R_8 and R_{14} are cells from retinas of 8-day-old and 14-day-old chick embryos; B_6 and B_{10} are cells from brains of 6-day-old and 10-day-old embryos.

** Expressed as the number of cells in suspension that bound to 1 mm² of cell monolayer.

Source: Data from Rutishauser et al. (1976).

between an 8-day retinal cell and a 10-day brain cell, an 8-day retinal and a 6-day brain cell bound just as well to each other as to themselves. This observation implied that the mechanism of adhesion is the same for most cells from nervous tissues. As we shall see, the variation in binding with developmental age suggests that adhesiveness may be important during a particular phase of nervous-tissue development. Moreover, it might be expected that some property of the molecules involved in adhesion would reflect this variation.

Identification and purification of a molecule involved in cell adhesion

A considerable effort has been made in several laboratories to identify the molecules that serve as ligands in cell adhesion. Many of these studies have focused on a search for endogenous substances that can either enhance or inhibit aggregation and that demonstrate tissue specificity (Balsamo and Lilien, 1974; Hausman and Moscona, 1976) or concentration gradients consistent with one of the mechanisms discussed above. Although in most cases the same cell types have been studied, little agreement has been reached as to the molecular basis of cell-cell binding.

We have developed a somewhat different approach to the identification of molecules involved in adhesion. These studies utilize an immunological assay for cell-adhesion molecules based on the inhibition of adhesion by antibodies prepared against whole cells (Brackenbury et al., 1977) and the identification of antigens recognized by these antibodies (Thiery et al., 1977). The advantages of this procedure are that

it does not require assumptions as to number, composition, or mode of action of these molecules; nor does it require that they retain their biological activity after having been removed from cells. The following sections describe the assay and its use in purifying from chick embryo retinal tissue a molecule associated with neural cell adhesion. Immunization of rabbits with the purified molecule has yielded a specific antiserum that inhibits cell adhesion. Immunoprecipitation with the specific antibodies has allowed detection and characterization of the molecule in membrane extracts of neural retinal cells.

An immunological assay for cell-adhesion molecules

The development of an assay for molecules involved in cell adhesion required the use of particle-counting methods for quantitating cell adhesiveness (Orr and Roseman, 1969), preparation of antibodies that specifically inhibit cell adhesion, and the preparation of antigens from retinal cells that can neutralize these antibodies.

Figure 3a and b show trypsin-dissociated retinal cells from 10-day-old chick embryos before and after rotation at 90 rpm in Dulbecco's Modified Eagle Medium for 30 min at 37°. Freshly trypsinized cells did not bind to each other, but cells that had been cultured after trypsinization aggregated rapidly. The retina at this stage of development contains several cell types. Nevertheless, in our experiments, essentially all the cells obtained from retinal tissue became associated with aggregates within 1 hr (see Figure 3b), which suggests that adhesiveness is a property of retinal cells in general.

As the retinal cells aggregate in suspension, the total number of particles in suspension decreases. As shown by other workers (Orr and Roseman, 1969), the rate of decrease in particle number is a convenient measure of aggregation and can be determined rapidly and precisely by use of a particle counter. To establish that aggregation could be used to quantitate the adhesiveness of single cells, results from this method were compared to those obtained using the monolayer assay for cell-cell binding. Aggregation of cells from 8-, 10-, 12-, and 14-day-old chick embryos was compared in the two assays; the results indicated that the decrease in particle number in the aggregation assay is proportional to the number of individual adhesive events in the monolayer assay (Table II).

A key step in our studies was to obtain antibodies that can inhibit cell adhesion. Such a reagent was produced by injecting rabbits with cells from retinas

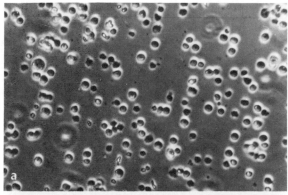
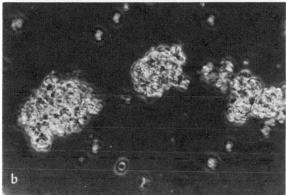
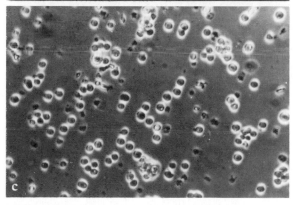

FIGURE 3 Aggregation of retinal cells from 10-day-old chick embryos. (a) Cells prior to aggregation. (b) Aggregates produced after incubation for 30 min at 37°. (c) Aggregation for 30 min at 37° in the presence of anti-R10 Fab'. (From Brackenbury et al., 1977.)

of 10-day-old chick embryos (anti-R10) and then preparing Fab' fragments from the antibodies. The Fab' fragments, being monovalent, did not cause agglutination; instead they inhibited the aggregation of the retinal cells (Figure 3c).

The immunological approach we have adopted is based on the assumption that cell-to-cell adhesion is mediated by *particular* cell surface molecules and that the inhibition of Fab' reflects a specific inactivation

TABLE II

Comparison of the cell-cell binding and reaggregation assays

Age of embryo (days)	Aggregation assay (Δ%)*	Cell-cell binding assay (cells/mm²)**
8	52 ± 2	450 ± 51
10	40 ± 2	363 ± 42
12	22 ± 1	179 ± 25
14	14 ± 1	105 ± 15

The standard deviation in triplicate assays is given.

* Expressed as the percentage decrease in particle number during a 20 min incubation.

** See Table I.

Source: Data from Brackenbury et al. (1977).

of these molecules. Alternatively it is possible that anti-R10 Fab' inhibits adhesion by nonspecifically coating the cell surface. Therefore two other surface-binding molecules—a lectin derivative (succinyl-concanavalin A) that binds to cell surface glycoproteins but does not agglutinate the cells (Gunther et al., 1973) and Fab' fragments of antibodies that bind to a variety of surface carbohydrates (Sela and Edelman, 1977)—were also assayed for inhibitory activity (Table III). Although all three reagents bound to the surface of retinal cells, giving bright staining when detected by immunofluorescence techniques, only anti-R10 Fab' caused a significant decrease in cell aggregation. This observation provided initial evidence that the inhibition of adhesion caused by anti-R10 Fab' does not result simply from a blockade of the cell surface as a whole.

The immunoassay for molecules involved in cell adhesion consists of measuring the ability of retinal-cell molecules to neutralize the adhesion-inhibiting activity of anti-R10 Fab', thus permitting aggregation to occur. Supernatants from 24 hr cultures of intact

TABLE III

Effect of molecules that bind to the cell surface on aggregation of retinal cells

Molecule	mg/assay	Aggregation (Δ%)*
Control	—	58 ± 2
Anti-R10 Fab'	1	5 to 25**
Succinyl-concanavalin A	0.2	57 ± 3
Anti–retinal cell surface carbohydrate Fab'	3	59 ± 2

* Percent decrease in particle number after 20 min.

** Range represents values obtained with antibodies from different rabbits. The standard deviation in triplicate assays is shown.

Source: Data from Brackenbury et al. (1977).

10-day retinal tissue (TCS) in serum-free medium were found to be a convenient source of such neutralizing antigens. Although the retinal-cell molecules present in the TCS did not by themselves block or enhance aggregation, they did reverse the inhibition by the anti-R10 Fab' (Table IV). The amount of neutralization, expressed as a percent decrease in inhibition, was nearly linear with respect to the logarithm of the supernatant volume added (Figure 4). It was therefore possible to estimate the relative amount of Fab'-neutralizing antigen in a sample by its effect on the aggregation of cells in the presence of a constant amount of Fab'. For purposes of quantitation, one unit of neutralizing activity was defined as the amount of antigen needed to cause a 25% decrease in the inhibition of adhesion produced by 1 mg of Fab' fragment.

Purification and characterization of a cell-adhesion molecule

Cell surface molecules recognized by adhesion-blocking antibodies were identified by a sequence of steps involving first the purification of neutralizing antigens from TCS, then immunization with the purified activity to produce a specific adhesion-blocking antibody, and finally the identification of the cell surface antigen recognized by this specific antibody.

To purify the molecules involved in the neutralization of anti-R10 Fab' by TCS, their presence was monitored throughout a fractionation of the TCS mixture by gel filtration and polyacrylamide gel electrophoresis. These fractionations resulted in a 500-

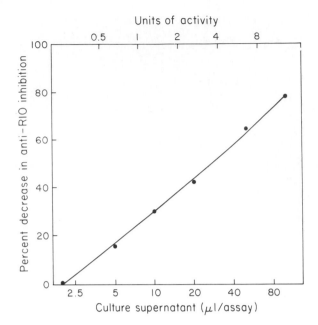

FIGURE 4 Neutralization of 1 mg of anti-R10 Fab' by tissue-culture supernatant (TCS). Neutralization is expressed as the percent decrease in the amount of inhibition of aggregation produced by the Fab' (see Table IV). One unit of activity is defined as the amount of the 50× concentrated TCS required to decrease the inhibition by 25%. (From Brackenbury et al., 1977.)

fold increase in specific neutralizing activity with a total yield of 50% (Table V).

The gel filtration of TCS on BioGel A0.5 is illustrated in Figure 5. Activity was found in a single region separated from the bulk of the protein and eluted before glutamic acid dehydrogenase (M_r = 320,000), near ferritin (M_r = 425,000), and after thyroglobulin (M_r = 670,000). This observation suggests that in PBS the molecules responsible for the activity have an apparent molecular weight of about 400,000; the exact molecular weight remains to be determined.

Further purification was achieved by electrophoresis on polyacrylamide gels in Tris-glycine buffer. The material in segments of the gel was eluted by electrophoresis, and the activity was found to be concentrated in a 1 cm region, again well-separated from most of the protein (Figure 6).

To obtain antibodies against the active antigen(s), rabbits were immunized with the active fraction from polyacrylamide gel electrophoresis (Figure 6). Each injection represented the material obtained from 200 retinas. After 6–10 intraperitoneal injections in complete Freund's adjuvant, antibodies were produced that strongly inhibited cell adhesion: 1 mg of Fab' caused a 90% decrease in retinal-cell or brain-cell aggregation.

TABLE IV

Effect of tissue-culture supernatant and anti-R10 Fab' on aggregation of cells from 10-day retinas

Assay	Anti-R10 Fab' (mg/assay)	Tissue culture supernatant (μl)	Aggregation (Δ%)*
Aggregation	0	0	41 ± 2
Effect of TCS	0	5–100	39 ± 2
Inhibition by Fab'**	1	0	18 ± 1
Neutralization of Fab' by TCS	1	50	33 ± 2

The standard deviation in triplicate assays is shown.

* Percent decrease in particle number after 20 min.

** Neutralizing activity is most reliably measured when the amount of Fab' added causes about a 50% inhibition of cell aggregation.

Source: Data from Brackenbury et al. (1977).

TABLE V

Fractionation of activity from tissue-culture supernatants

Fraction	Activity (units)	Protein* (μg)	Specific activity	Activity yield (%)
Total TCS (400 retinas)	1,622	30,000	0.054	100
Activity recovered following gel filtration (Figure 5)	1,151	2,600	0.44	71
Polyacrylamide gel electrophoresis (Figure 6)	811	29	28.0	50

* Based on optical absorbance, with 1 mg/ml protein equal to 1.0 absorbance at 280 nm.
Source: Data from Thiery et al. (1977).

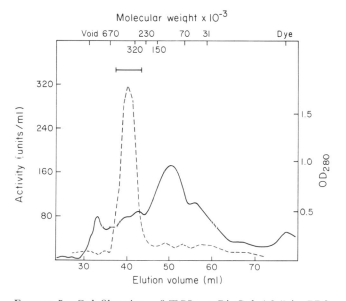

FIGURE 5   Gel filtration of TCS on BioGel A0.5 in PBS. The solid line represents optical density at 280 nm; the dashed line indicates Fab'-neutralizing activity. The fractions within the bar were pooled for further fractionation by polyacrylamide gel electrophoresis (see Figure 6). (From Thiery et al., 1977.)

The major purpose of these studies was to identify and characterize structures on the cell surface that are recognized by the antibodies that inhibit adhesion. To do this, molecules were extracted from cell membranes by nonionic detergents and then immunoprecipitated with the antibodies. Figure 7 shows proteins—labeled with [³H]-leucine and solubilized by treatment of retinal-cell membranes with Nonidet-P40 (Henning et al., 1976)—that could be immunoprecipitated (Brown et al., 1974) by anti-R10. A number of proteins were precipitated (Figure 7a), as would be expected with antibodies produced against whole retinal cells. In contrast, when antibodies to the purified activity were used, the precipitates contained two polypeptides—one with a molecular weight in SDS (Laemmli, 1970) of 140,000 and the other with an M_r of about 40,000 (Figure 7b). These two components were also detected when the specific antibodies were used to precipitate cell surface proteins that had been previously labeled with ^{125}I by the lactoperoxidase procedure (Marchalonis, Cone, and Sauter, 1971).

The 140,000 M_r component co-migrated with a molecule we had detected in earlier studies and had named cell-adhesion molecule or CAM (Rutishauser et al., 1976). The 40,000 M_r component, however, does not appear to be involved in adhesion, in that it could be precipitated by antibodies that did not inhibit cell adhesion and from Nonidet-P40 extracts of freshly trypsinized cells, which do not aggregate. This component probably represents actin that co-precipitates with antigen-antibody complexes: when, for example, anti-R10, antibodies to the purified activity, or antibodies from unimmunized rabbits were mixed with iodinated actin and then precipitated with goat anti-rabbit immunoglobulin, the precipitate con-

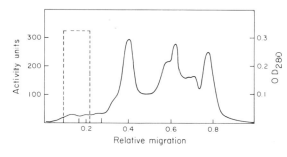

FIGURE 6   Preparative polyacrylamide gel electrophoresis in Tris-glycine buffer of the active fraction from gel filtration of TCS (Figure 5). The solid line represents a scan of optical density at 280 nm; the dashed line indicates the activity electro-eluted from gel slices. Active fractions were pooled and used to immunize rabbits. (Redrawn from Thiery et al., 1977.)

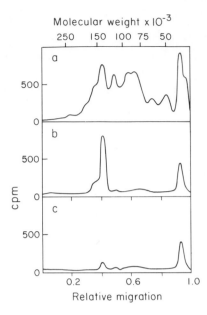

FIGURE 7 SDS-polyacrylamide gel electrophoresis of immunoprecipitated [³H]-labeled proteins extracted from membranes of retinal cells in 10-day-old chick embryos. (a) Immunoprecipitated with antibodies to whole retinal cells (anti-R10). (b) Immunoprecipitated with antibodies to the purified activity. (c) Immunoprecipitated with antibodies to purified activity in the presence of the active gel electrophoresis fraction (Figure 6). (Redrawn from Thiery et al., 1977.)

tained radioactive material that migrated in SDS gels at the same position as the 40,000 M_r component.

To establish the relationship between the 140,000 M_r cell surface molecule and the activity from TCS, unlabeled material from the active gel electrophoresis fraction (Figure 6) was added to the labeled membrane extract prior to immunoprecipitation. This resulted in an 80–90% decrease in the amount of the labeled 140,000 M_r cell surface protein precipitated (Figure 7) but did not affect the amount of actin.

Although the active antigen was purified 500-fold, it has not been shown that this material is homogeneous. It therefore remains a possibility that the 140,000 M_r component (CAM) was precipitated by antibodies against a minor TCS component unrelated to the neutralizing activity. We have also shown that the neutralizing activity found in deoxycholate extracts of retinal-cell membranes co-purifies with CAM in gel-filtration studies (our unpublished results). Although this result supports direct structural association of CAM with the activity, evidence will still be required to establish this relationship rigorously.

The major conclusion of these studies is that inhibition of cell adhesion by antibodies prepared against

whole retinal cells reflects the specific interaction of only a small subpopulation of these antibodies with a cell surface protein (CAM) having an M_r in SDS of 140,000. Purification of an antigen from TCS that is antigenically related to CAM has allowed the preparation of a specific adhesion-blocking antibody (anti-CAM). The 140,000 M_r polypeptide CAM exists as at least part of a membrane-bound molecule that, when released into culture supernatants, has a higher apparent molecular weight. Although these results might suggest that the TCS activity is composed of more than one polypeptide, it should be noted that molecular weight values obtained by gel filtration often cannot be compared directly to those determined from electrophoretic mobilities in SDS-polyacrylamide gels. Moreover, the present experiments do not exclude the possibility that the active components are associated with substances that were not radiolabeled.

The relationship of CAM to cell adhesion and to neural development

If inhibition of cell adhesion by Fab' fragments involves a direct inactivation of CAM by steric hindrance, then the simplest explanation would be that it is a ligand in the formation of cell-cell bonds. As yet, however, we have not demonstrated that solubilized CAM has a binding activity. We therefore cannot exclude the alternative that this polypeptide has an indirect influence on bond formation, either as a controlling element or as a structural component necessary for binding.

Direct involvement of CAM in cell adhesion is suggested by experiments indicating that the adhesiveness of cells from embryos of different ages is correlated with the amount of CAM on the cell surface. As discussed earlier, retinal cells from 8-day embryos aggregate three to four times more rapidly than cells from 14-day embryos (Table II). To estimate the relative amount of CAM on these two cell populations, a constant amount of anti-R10 Fab' was preincubated with increasing amounts of each cell type and then tested for its ability to inhibit aggregation of 10-day retinal cells (Figure 8). This procedure is analogous to the neutralization assay described above, except that cells are used instead of soluble antigens from tissue-culture supernatants. The results indicate that about three times more 14-day cells than 8-day cells are required to produce the same degree of neutralization. As shown in the studies on purification of neutralizing antigens, this difference should

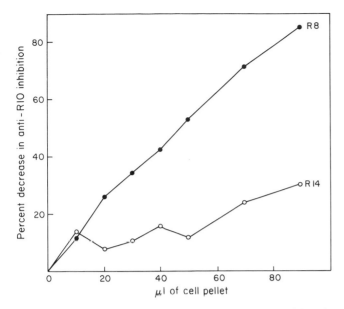

FIGURE 8 Neutralization of 1 mg of anti-R10 Fab' by absorption with increasing amounts of retinal cells from 8- and 14-day-old chick embryos. Neutralization is expressed as the percent decrease in the amount of inhibition of aggregation produced by the Fab' (see Table IV). The amount of cells used in each absorption is given in terms of the volume of packed cells.

reflect the amount of CAM added to the antibody and, therefore, the amount of CAM on the cell surface.

Adhesion of retinal cells to each other has also been compared with their ability to bind to nylon fibers coated with the antibodies against CAM. As shown in Figure 9, the aggregation of retinal cells from 5- to 14-day embryos is closely correlated with their binding to the fibers coated with anti-CAM. The results are consistent with the hypothesis that the amount of CAM on the cell surface is correlated with adhesiveness and also suggest that this molecule is capable of participation in the formation of bonds between the cell and another surface—in this case, a nylon fiber. All cell surface molecules do not display this property, in that cells having a high concentration of surface receptors for lectins are often unable to bind to lectin-coated fibers (Rutishauser and Sachs, 1975).

Although the experiments with cells from embryos of different ages provide indirect evidence that CAM is involved in cell adhesion in vitro, they do not necessarily indicate that the amount of CAM in retinal *tissue* varies as a function of developmental age. As described earlier, the cells used in aggregation studies have been obtained by trypsinization, and the CAM on their surfaces has appeared following dissociation.

For this reason differences in the amount of CAM on the cells may reflect not the amount of CAM in the tissue but rather the ability of the cell to re-express this molecule.

As shown in Figure 9, the number of cells in the chick retina varies as a function of developmental age. Although the retina is not uniformly developed during these stages of embryogenesis, the results suggest that the period during which dissociated retinal cells have the most cell surface CAM immediately follows the time of maximal increase in cell number. It is coincident with the time during which the plexiform layers appear (Coulombre, 1955) and precedes the formation of most synapses among retinal cells (Hughes and LaVelle, 1974).

Together, these observations suggest that CAM, a membrane-associated molecule involved in adhesion among dissociated cells, may play a strategic role in the development of neural tissue. They do not, however, specify what this role is or how it is carried out. Our initial studies on the possible function of CAM in developing tissue have included two types of experiments: (1) localization of the molecule in tissue, histotypic aggregates, and cell cultures; and (2) perturbation of CAM functions during development in vitro. Both localization and perturbation are carried out using the specific anti-CAM antibodies.

The distribution of CAM in the retinas of 14- and 7-day chick embryos is shown in Figure 10. At day

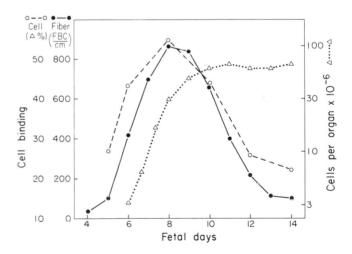

FIGURE 9 Age dependence of retinal-cell binding to nylon fibers coated with anti-CAM (filled circles), retinal-cell aggregation (open circles), and the number of cells obtained by dissociation of retinal tissue by trypsinization (triangles). Cell-fiber binding is expressed as the number of cells bound along one edge of a 1 cm fiber segment in 20 min; aggregation is expressed as the percent decrease in single cells after 20 min. (Redrawn from Rutishauser et al., 1976.)

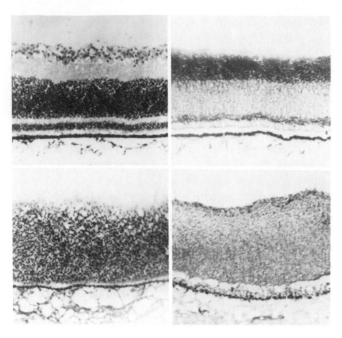

FIGURE 10 Distribution of CAM in frozen sections of retinas from chick embryos, as revealed by staining with anti-CAM, peroxidase-antiperoxidase complexes, and diaminobenzidine (Sternberger, 1973). *Left*: Hematoxylin-eosin staining of 14-day tissues (top) and 7-day tissues (bottom). *Right*: Anti-CAM staining (darker areas) of 14-day tissues (top) and 7-day tissues (bottom). (×150.)

14 most of the CAM is associated with regions almost entirely composed of neuronal processes—namely the two plexiform layers. At day 7, when these layers are not yet visible, CAM is uniformly distributed across the tissue, except for a higher concentration in the neurite bundles that will coalesce to form the optic nerve. Similar studies have indicated that, in addition to the retina, CAM is heavily concentrated in the brain, optic nerve, spinal cord, dorsal-root ganglia, and sympathetic ganglia. Other tissues in the embryo, such as muscle and liver, may contain small amounts of the molecule; but erythrocytes, thymocytes, and lymphocytes apparently do not have CAM on their surfaces (Rutishauser et al., 1976).

The results indicate that most of the CAM in a developing embryo is associated with nerve tissue. This does not necessarily mean that CAM is present in higher densities on nerve cells than on nonneuronal cells because of the large amount of plasma membrane in tissues containing neurites. However, other cell surface molecules, such as binding sites for the lectin concanavalin A, do not appear to be as heavily concentrated in nerve tissues.

The presence of a cell-adhesion molecule on nerve processes during the time when plexiform layers are being formed in the retina raises the possibility that it might function in the development of these layers. We have not yet explored this hypothesis in vivo, but we have carried out experiments in vitro using histotypic aggregates of retinal cells. If aggregates of 8-day-old cells are prepared and maintained in culture, large regions containing neurites and synapses are formed over an interval of 7–8 days in a manner that resembles the development of an intact retina (Vogel and Nirenberg, 1976; Vogel, Daniels, and Nirenberg, 1976). As in the retina, CAM is preferentially distributed in the neurite regions (Figure 11). When aggregates that have been cultured for one day are transferred to a medium containing anti-CAM Fab' fragments, however, the regions subsequently formed are smaller, are interspersed with cell bodies, and appear to be less densely packed with processes (Figure 12).

To examine the effects of anti-CAM Fab' in more detail, similar experiments have been carried out on the in vitro outgrowth of neuronal processes from intact dorsal-root ganglia. In the presence of nerve growth factor, a halo of processes and fascicles (bundles of processes) appears around each ganglion within 24 hr (Levi-Montalcini and Angeletti, 1968). Immunofluorescent staining techniques indicate that

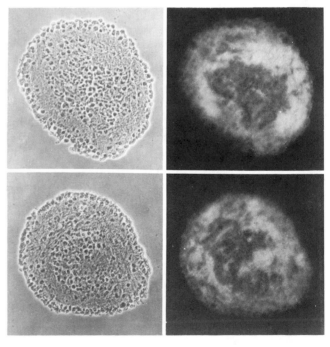

FIGURE 11 Distribution of CAM in frozen sections of retinal-cell aggregates, as revealed by fluoresence microscopy after staining with fluorescein-labeled anti-CAM. *Left*: unstained sections under phase contrast. *Right*: anti-CAM staining (light areas). (×190.)

744 URS RUTISHAUSER ET AL.

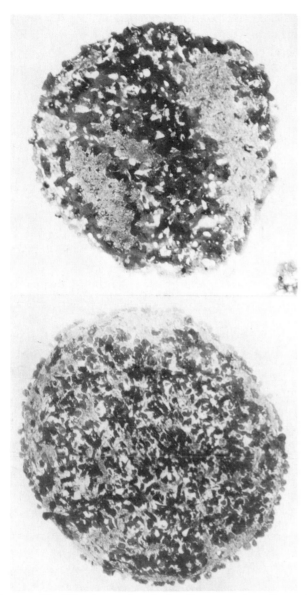

FIGURE 12 Histology of retinal cell aggregates after culture for 7–8 days. *Top*: Aggregates that have formed large neurite regions after culture in medium containing 1 mg/ml Fab′ from unimmunized rabbits. *Bottom*: Aggregates that have been cultured in 1 mg/ml anti-CAM Fab′. (×360.)

from rabbit antibodies against chick fibroblasts bound to the processes but did not affect their growth.

Considerably more investigation will be required to interpret these experiments at the molecular level. Nonetheless, we can now speculate about the possible action of anti-CAM Fab′. An intriguing possibility is that CAM is required for the formation of fascicles because it provides side-to-side adhesions between individual neurites. In this case the binding might have to be reversible to allow for modification of the route initially followed by a growing neurite. CAM might also mediate the interaction between a neuronal process and nonneuronal cells, which could be involved in nerve guidance or provide a foothold for

CAM is present on these processes and, within the resolution of light microscopy, appears to be uniformly distributed over their surfaces (Figure 13). Fibroblasts that were also present in these cultures were only weakly stained with anti-CAM antibody. The addition of anti-CAM Fab′ fragments to the ganglion cultures caused the morphology, but not the extent, of outgrowth to be altered; the major change being a relative abundance of thin processes and a paucity of thick fascicles. In contrast, Fab′ fragments

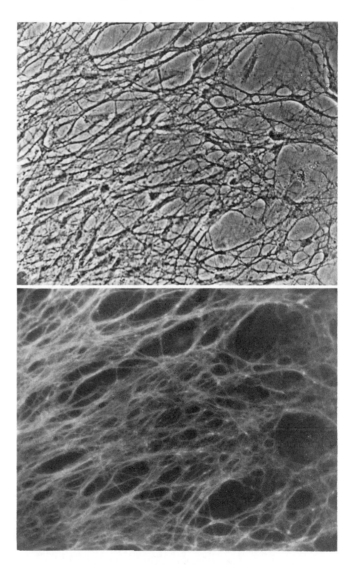

FIGURE 13 Presence of CAM on neurite outgrowth from a chick dorsal-root ganglion. *Top*: Phase contrast. *Bottom*: Fluorescence microscopy after staining with fluorescein-labeled anti-CAM. (×250.)

the tip of the neurite similar to the attachments that occur in vitro between the growth cone and a tissue-culture dish. With respect to the last point, anti-CAM Fab' does not appear to interfere with attachment of neural cells or tissues to plastic or collagen. These experiments, however, cannot exclude the possibility that adhesion of growth cones to a substrate is affected by the antibody. Alternatively it is possible that CAM is involved in maintaining membrane or cytoskeletal structures that are indirectly required for cell aggregation and fascicle formation and, therefore, that its function does not directly concern adhesion between membranes.

Prospective studies

The results and hypotheses described above point to the need for additional experimentation in several areas. Priority should be given to describing the chemical properties of CAM further, in particular to determining whether this molecule is a ligand in the formation of cell-cell bonds or whether it serves a controlling or supportive function in cell adhesion. These studies must include an analysis of the composition and structure of CAM and of possible interactions with other molecules, membrane components, or cytoplasmic structures that might affect its function. Such information is essential to further interpretation of the perturbation experiments that use anti-CAM Fab'.

The effects of anti-CAM Fab' on development must be examined in greater detail and in more systems, including nonneuronal tissues. With neural cells, the formation of side-to-side associations among neurites can be studied by cinematography at high magnification, and electron microscopy can be used to observe the location of CAM with respect to such specialized structures as junctions and synapses.

Another interesting line of investigation will be to determine if CAM is distributed in patterns within a tissue that might orient cells during development. For example, gradients of adhesive molecules have been suggested as a possible mechanism for organizing cells in the visual field of the retina and for connecting of retinal neurons with their appropriate target cells in the optic tectum (Sperry, 1963). Gradients have also been postulated to function in the development of limb buds (Summerbell, Lewis, and Wolpert, 1973) and as a potential factor in establishing or maintaining compartments derived from polyclones in early stages of embryogenesis (Crick and Lawrence, 1975).

At this stage, therefore, it seems possible that a number of well-defined experiments could provide information on important molecular mechanisms of pattern formation in developing tissues. The identification and purification of CAM and the preparation of specific antibodies to this molecule represent our initial steps in this approach. In addition, the immunological methods used in studying CAM may well be applicable in other systems and could lead to identification of other molecules involved in embryological development.

ACKNOWLEDGMENTS This work was supported by U.S. Public Health Service Grants HD-09635, AI-11378, and AM-04256.

REFERENCES

BALSAMO, J., and J. LILIEN, 1974. Functional identification of three components which mediate tissue-type specific embryonic cell adhesion. *Nature* 251:522–524.

BRACKENBURY, R., J.-P. THIERY, U. RUTISHAUSER, and G. M. EDELMAN, 1977. Adhesion among neural cells of the chick embryo. I. An immunological assay for molecules involved in cell-cell binding. *J. Biol. Chem.*, 252:6835–6840.

BROWN, J. L., K. KATO, J. SILVER, and S. G. NATHANSON, 1974. Notable diversity in peptide composition of murine H-2K and H-2D alloantigens. *Biochemistry* 13:3174–3178.

COULOMBRE, A. J., 1955. Correlations of structural and biochemical changes in the developing retina of the chick. *Am. J. Anat.* 96:153–190.

CRICK, F. H. C., and P. A. LAWRENCE, 1975. Compartments and polyclones in insect development. *Science* 189:340–347.

CURTIS, A. S. G., 1967. *The Cell Surface.* New York: Logos Academic Press, pp. 80–124.

CURTIS, A. S. G., and M. F. GREAVES, 1965. The inhibition of cell aggregation by a pure serum protein. *J. Embryol. Exp. Morphol.* 13:309–326.

GUNTHER, G. R., J. L. WANG, I. YAHARA, B. A. CUNNINGHAM, and G. M. EDELMAN, 1973. Concanavalin A derivatives with altered biological activities. *Proc. Natl. Acad. Sci. USA* 70:1012–1016.

HAUSMAN, R. E., and A. A. MOSCONA, 1976. Isolation of a retina-specific cell-aggregating factor from membranes of embryonic neural retina tissue. *Proc. Natl. Acad. Sci. USA* 73:3594–3598.

HENNING, R., R. J. MILNER, K. RESKE, B. A. CUNNINGHAM, and G. M. EDELMAN, 1976. Subunit structure, cell surface orientation and partial amino-acid sequences of murine histocompatibility antigens. *Proc. Natl. Acad. Sci. USA* 73:118–122.

HOLTFRETER, J., 1939. Tissue affinity, a means of embryological morphogenesis. Translated in *Foundations in Experimental Embryology,* B. Willier and J. Oppenheimer, eds. Englewood Cliffs, NJ: Prentice-Hall (1964), pp. 186–225.

HUGHES, W. F., and A. LAVELLE, 1974. On the synaptogenic sequence in the chick retina. *Anat. Rec.* 179:297–302.

LAEMMLI, U. K., 1970. Cleavage of structural proteins during the assembly of the head of bacteriophage T4. *Nature* 277:680–685.

LEVI-MONTALCINI, R., and P. U. ANGELETTI, 1968. Nerve growth factor. *Physiol. Rev.* 48:534–569.

LILIEN, J. E., 1969. Toward a molecular explanation for specific cell adhesion. In *Current Topics in Developmental Biology,* vol. 4, A. A. Moscona and A. Monroy, eds. New York: Academic Press, pp. 169–195.

MARCHALONIS, J. J., R. E. CONE, and V. SAUTER, 1971. Enzymatic iodination: A probe for accessible surface proteins of normal and neoplastic lymphocytes. *Biochem. J.* 124:921–927.

MERRELL, R., D. I. GOTTLIEB, and L. GLASER, 1975. Embryonal cell surface recognition. Extraction of an active plasma membrane component. *J. Biol. Chem.* 250:5655–5659.

MOSCONA, A. A., 1952. Cell suspensions from organ rudiments of chick embryos. *Exp. Cell Res.* 3:536–539.

MOSCONA, A. A., 1962. Analysis of cell recombinations in experimental synthesis of tissues *in vitro. J. Cell. Comp. Physiol.* 60 (Suppl. 1):65–80

OPPENHEIMER, S. B., 1975. Functional involvement of specific carbohydrate in teratoma cell adhesion factor. *Exp. Cell Res.* 92:122–126.

ORR, C. W., and S. ROSEMAN, 1969. Intercellular adhesion. 1. A quantitative assay for measuring the rate of adhesion. *J. Membr. Biol.* 1:109–124.

ROSEMAN, S., 1970. The synthesis of complex carbohydrates by multiglycosyltransferase systems and their potential function in intercellular adhesion. *Chem. Phys. Lipids* 5:270–297.

ROTH, S., E. J. McGUIRE, and S. ROSEMAN, 1971. An assay for intercellular adhesive specificity. *J. Cell Biol.* 51:525–535.

RUTISHAUSER, U., and L. SACHS, 1975. Receptor mobility and the binding of cells to lectin-coated fibers. *J. Cell Biol.* 66:76–85.

RUTISHAUSER, U., J.-P. THIERY, R. BRACKENBURY, B.-A. SELA, and G. M. EDELMAN, 1976. Mechanisms of adhesion among cells from neural tissues of the chick embryo. *Proc. Natl. Acad. Sci. USA* 73:577–581.

SELA, B.-A., and G. M. EDELMAN, 1977. Isolation by cell-column chromatography of immunoglobulins specific for cell surface carbohydrates. *J. Exp. Med.* 145:443–449.

SHUR, B. D., and S. ROTH, 1975. Cell surface glycosyltransferases. *Biochim. Biophys. Acta* 415:473–512.

SPERRY, R. W., 1963. Chemoaffinity in the orderly growth of nerve fiber patterns and connections. *Proc. Natl. Acad. Sci. USA* 50:703–710.

STEINBERG, M., 1963. Tissue reconstitution by dissociated cells. *Science* 141:401–408.

STERNBERGER, L. A., 1973. Enzyme immunocytochemistry. In *Electron Microscopy of Enzymes,* M. S. Hayat, ed. New York: Van Nostrand Reinhold, pp. 150–171.

SUMMERBELL, D., J. H. LEWIS, and L. WOLPERT, 1973. Positional information in chick limb morphogenesis. *Nature* 244:492–496.

THIERY, J.-P., R. BRACKENBURY, U. RUTISHAUSER, and G. M. EDELMAN, 1977. Adhesion among neural cells of the chick embryo. II. Purification and characterization of a cell adhesion molecule from neural retina. *J. Biol. Chem.* 252:6841–6845.

TOWNES, P. L., and J. HOLTFRETER, 1955. Directed movements and selective adhesion of embryonic amphibian cells. *J. Exp. Zool.* 128:53–120.

VOGEL, Z., M. P. DANIELS, and M. NIRENBERG, 1976. Synapse and acetylcholine receptor synthesis by neurons dissociated from retina. *Proc. Natl. Acad. Sci. USA* 73:2370–2374.

VOGEL, Z., and M. NIRENBERG, 1976. Localization of acetylcholine receptors during synaptogenesis in retina. *Proc. Natl. Acad. Sci. USA* 73:1806–1810.

WALTHER, B. T., R. OHMAN, and S. ROSEMAN, 1973. A quantitative assay for intercellular adhesion. *Proc. Natl. Acad. Sci. USA* 70:1569–1573.

44 Molecular Interactions in Adult and Developing Neuromuscular Junction

JEAN-PIERRE CHANGEUX

ABSTRACT Concepts of macromolecular interactions within the synaptic membranes and of their regulation by transsynaptic signaling during synapse formation are presented. The structural and functional properties of the acetylcholine (nicotinic) receptor from fish electric organ and vertebrate neuromuscular junction in its purified and membrane-bound states are reviewed. Special emphasis is placed on the regulation of the binding properties of the membrane-bound receptor and on its relevance to the changes of ionic permeability that take place during the activation and desensitization processes triggered by acetylcholine. The acetylcholine receptor protein is both a regulatory protein and a membrane-bound integral protein whose functional properties are conditioned by its lipid or protein environment in the membrane.

The dense accumulation of acetylcholine receptor in the subsynaptic membrane during development is viewed as a process of immobilization and protection against degradation of the receptor protein beneath the exploratory nerve terminal while the synthesis of receptor shuts off in the postsynaptic cell. On the presynaptic side, the elimination of redundant nerve endings appears linked with the activity of these terminals and with that of the postsynaptic cell. Such retrograde selective stabilization may, to some extent, account for the specification of neuronal networks.

"On ne saurait comprendre le fonctionnement du système nerveux central à moins de connaître celui de l'élément logique primaire que constitue la synapse."—Jacques Monod, *Le hasard et la nécessité* (1970), p. 163

Introduction

AMONG THE COMPLEX sequences of events that take place during the development of the nervous system one may distinguish two major steps. The first is the setting out of cell bodies—neuronal somas and glial cells—through cell proliferation, migration, and differentiation. This is a matter of embryonic development, and the mechanisms involved may be similar, if not identical, to those which account for the development of any organ of the body. The second step

is characteristic of the nervous system and of a higher degree of complexity; it concerns the establishment of a highly organized and complex network of interneuronal connections.

The extent to which the interaction of the organism with its environment regulates, or even modulates, neural development has long been debated. The schematic opposition between "empiricists" and "preformists" does not hold up under a close examination of the biological processes that occur during neurogenesis. For example, a neural organization or performance present at birth, prior to actual experience with the outside world, is often referred to as genetically determined. But we know that in ovo or in utero the vertebrate embryo experiences some behavior: after $3\frac{1}{2}$ days of incubation the chick embryo moves, and these movements are of neurogenic origin (Hamburger, 1970). In mammals, moreover, the cerebral cortex is electrically active days or even weeks before birth (Corner and Kwee, 1976; Adrien, 1976). At early stages of synapse formation, long before anatomical synapses become differentiated, signals are propagated in the developing neuronal network. The activity evoked by the interaction of the newborn with its environment may be viewed more as a modulation of this spontaneous activity than as an entirely de novo process. The genetic encoding of a protein sequence is indeed easier to define than that of a neuronal network.

If a neuronal network were genetically determined with the same rigidity as a protein sequence, its reproducibility would exhibit a similar degree of perfection. Detailed examination of the arborizations of a given neuron from brains of genetically identical individuals (parthenogenetic fish or crustaceans: see Levinthal, Macagno, and Levinthal, 1976) shows that these cells are almost superimposable but not exactly so. There are differences at the level of the precise number of synaptic contacts and the orientation of axons or dendrites. Often negligible in paucicellular invertebrates, these differences become more signif-

JEAN-PIERRE CHANGEUX Laboratoire Interactions Moléculaires et Cellulaires, associé au CNRS, Institut Pasteur, Collège de France, Paris, France

icant in the higher vertebrates. They may reflect an underlying fundamental process in neural development.

A classical paradox offered by the nervous system of the adult is the contrast between the complexity of its organization and the small number of genes available to program it in the fertilized egg. In fact, models have been proposed that can generate enormous complexity through the sequential expression of genes and their simple combination (see Wolpert and Lewis, 1975). The question, then, is, What are the signals responsible for differential gene expression? Regarding synapse formation three major categories of mechanisms have been suggested:

1. *Cell surface recognition.* As a result of the differentiation of neuronal somas during embryonic development, growing nerve fibers bear chemical labels complementary to those present on the target neurons. The selectivity of the assembly between pre- and postsynaptic partners depends on the affinity between cell surfaces. This chemoaffinity hypothesis is based on the postulate that a large repertoire of cell surface determinants exists in the embryo. This point has recently been challenged (see McClain and Edelman, this volume; Rutishauser et al., this volume), but a role for cell surface recognition between major classes of cells—rather than between particular nerve endings—might still deserve consideration.

2. *Timing.* The differential growth of the nerve terminals is instrumental in bringing about order. Reaching the target neurons at different moments they "number" them sequentially (Gaze, 1970; Jacobson, 1970). Such a timing hypothesis might indeed lead to a significant saving of genetic information (see Levinthal, Macagno, and Levinthal, 1976; Rutishauser et al., this volume).

3. *Transsynaptic exchange of diffusible signals.* Once formed, a developing synaptic contact need not be stable. A stabilization follows the early recognition between cell surfaces and is regulated by a reciprocal exchange of diffusible signals coupled directly or indirectly with the state of activity of the developing neuronal network. The selective-stabilization hypothesis (Figure 1) (Changeux, 1972; Changeux, Courrège, and Danchin, 1973; Changeux and Danchin, 1974, 1976) proposes that the proper interaction between main categories of neurons results only from autonomous embryonic development: the recognition between cell surfaces would therefore be categorical rather than punctual. As a consequence of the growth process and of the sprouting of the nerve terminals as they reach their targets, several contacts with the same specificity would thus form: the fields

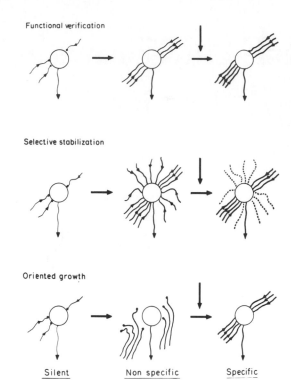

FIGURE 1   Three different hypotheses for the role of activity in the development of a neuronal network. According to the preformist view (functional-verification hypothesis) activity, spontaneous or evoked (vertical arrow), merely stabilizes the genetically specified synaptic organization. The oriented-growth hypothesis is a rather unplausible "instructive" mechanism. The selective-stabilization hypothesis is discussed in the text. (From Changeux and Danchin, 1976.)

of projection of neurons overlap, and a given neuron transiently innervates many more partners than in the final adult stage. At this critical stage a *limited redundancy* of connectivity therefore exists.

It is further postulated that the first synaptic contacts to form may exist under, at least, three states—labile (L), stable (S), and regressed (D)—the growth process being viewed as the emergence of labile states. The labile and stable states would transmit nerve impulses; the regressed state obviously would not.

The labile state may either become stabilized (L → S) or regress (L → D), regression being irreversible. An essential statement of the theory (Changeux, Courrège, and Danchin, 1973) is that the transitions of the labile state of the synapse (L → S and L → D) are regulated by the total activity of the postsynaptic cell, including the activity of the synapse itself. Accordingly the precocious activity of the developing network that is spontaneous in the embryo and/or evoked after birth would "selectively stabilize" particular synapses among the many equivalent contacts that emerge during growth; concomitantly, non-stabilized contacts would regress. By regulating the reduction of the transient redundancy of the developing network this early activity would create diversity and specificity and thereby bring additional order to the system. Thus a critical period exists in the development of a nerve terminal during which it requires a particular pattern of activity to become stable.

Because of its simplicity and its accessibility, the neuromuscular junction offers one of the most convenient systems in which to study synapse formation. This paper will be restricted to a discussion of the data available for this system. First, the cytoarchitecture of the adult neuromuscular junction will be described in terms of macromolecular assembly; then the structural and functional properties of one of its critical macromolecules—the acetylcholine regulator—will be briefly reviewed; finally, our current knowledge of its genesis during the development of the vertebrate embryo will be presented at length.

The adult cholinergic synapse in vertebrate skeletal muscle and fish electric organ

MORPHOLOGY As early as the mid-nineteenth century, it was observed that when the motor nerve fiber reaches the striated muscle fiber it loses its myelin sheath at the level of a granular thickening of the muscle surface that is particularly rich in nuclei (Doyère, 1840; Rouget, 1862); there it branches profusely into a terminal arborization (Krause, 1863; Kühne, 1887). Electron-microscopic observations of this highly differentiated structure, now referred to as the motor endplate, disclosed that its two basic components—the nerve and the muscle—are in close contact but separated by a space approximately 50 nm wide: the synaptic cleft. On one side lies the nerve ending, filled with numerous 30–60 nm vesicles and 10-nm-thick neurofilaments and limited by a membrane on which freeze-fracture reveals arrays of "pits," interpreted as release sites of the synaptic vesicles (see Heuser and Reese, this volume). On the other side, the subneural apparatus basically results from a dense folding of the cytoplasmic membrane, with marked membrane thickening at the level of the synaptic cleft. The outer surface of this postsynaptic membrane is covered by an electron-dense layer rich in mucopolysaccharides—the basal membrane or glycocalyx, which, at the edge of the cleft, appears to be continuous with collagen fibers. Between the folds,

but now on the sarcoplasmic side of the subneural apparatus, bundles of "subneural" filaments 5 nm in diameter are observed (Couteaux and Pécot-Dechavassine, 1968); these are possibly homologous to those present in the postsynaptic densities of central synapses (see references in Cohen et al., 1977; Blomberg, Cohen, and Siekevitz, 1977). On its two faces, the cytoplasmic membrane of the subneural apparatus is anchored to a complex network of filamentous material (for a general review see Couteaux, 1972).

CYTOCHEMISTRY Denervation experiments show that 80–90% of the muscle or electric-organ content in acetylcholine (ACh) and choline acetyltransferase belongs to the nerve terminals (Hebb, Krnjević, and Silver, 1964; Israel and Gautron, 1969; Rosenberg et al., 1964), whereas the enzyme acetylcholinesterase (AChE) revealed by the Koelle reaction and the acetylcholine receptor (AChR) remain attached to the muscle surface. These last two proteins may therefore be considered as markers of the postsynaptic membrane.

The distribution of the AChR site in the subsynaptic membrane has been quantitated by high-resolution autoradiography after labeling with radioactive snake α-toxins (for reviews see Fertuck and Salpeter, 1976; Bourgeois et al., 1978). More than 90%, if not all, of the AChR sites are located on the postsynaptic side of the endplate. In E. electricus electroplaque, the density of receptor sites is as high as 50,000 sites/μm^2 in the subsynaptic membrane; but it falls by a factor of 100 between the synapses and eventually reaches the background level on the noninnervated face of the electroplaque (Bourgeois et al., 1972, 1978). In the neuromuscular junction, the receptor protein (see references in Fertuck and Salpeter, 1976) appears unevenly distributed within the subsynaptic apparatus. The density is highest at the juxtaneural region of the folds where it reaches 30,000 ± 7,000 sites/μm^2, a value close to that found in E. electricus subsynaptic membrane. Outside the endplate, the density of AChR sites decreases sharply to about 4% of its maximal subsynaptic value within 1 μm to less than 0.2% beyond 7 μm from the nerve terminal. At the bottom of the junctional folds, the density of sites is of the same order of magnitude as that found on the sarcolemma at an equal distance from the synapse. In the juxtaneural region, the receptor molecules are densely packed, and there is little space available for another essential component of the subsynaptic apparatus, the enzyme AChE. Since the total number of its catalytic centers per endplate (measured with radioactive DFP) is close to that of α-toxin sites (about $3-8 \times 10^7$ sites in mouse endplates: see Barnard, Wieckowski, and Chiu, 1971), one is led to postulate that AChE is not integrated to the subsynaptic membrane in the same manner as AChR. Indeed:

1. AChE is released from the subsynaptic membrane in vitro by high ionic strength (Silman and Karlin, 1967) or in vivo by collagenase treatments (Hall and Kelly, 1971; Betz and Sakmann, 1971) under conditions in which the receptor protein remains membrane-bound.

2. Staining of thin sections by Karnovsky's reaction reveals AChE at the level of the basal membrane, both in the cleft and within the folds (Rash and Ellisman, 1974). On the other hand, freeze-fracture replicas of the electroplaque synapse and of the motor endplate disclose particles with the size and density expected for the receptor molecule deeply integrated within the subsynaptic membrane (Heuser, Reese, and Landis, 1974; Orci, Perrelet, and Dunant, 1974; Peper et al., 1974; Rash and Ellisman, 1974; Rosenbludt, 1974, 1975; Cartaud, 1975; Cartaud et al., 1977).

3. The concentration of AChE catalytic sites remains almost constant along the synaptic folds (Salpeter, 1967, 1969; Porter and Barnard, 1975), whereas there is a gradient of AChR such that at the receptive surface of the folds the density of α-toxin sites may exceed that of esterase sites by a factor of 5–10 (Fertuck and Salpeter, 1976).

In conclusion, AChE belongs to the so-called peripheral proteins and the AChR to the integral ones. Moreover, a close relationship seems to exist between the basal membrane and the esterase molecule, while the AChR protein is part of the cytoplasmic membrane *sensu stricto*.

The acetylcholine receptor protein in its purified and membrane-bound form

The most characteristic component of the subsynaptic membrane of the endplate, from both a functional and a structural point of view, is the macromolecular complex that accounts for the recognition of the neurotransmitter ACh and for its electrogenic action. A priori, this elementary functional unit, the *ACh regulator*, comprises two main categories of sites: (1) the AChR site that binds ACh (and related compounds) and snake venom α-toxins, and (2) the gate or channel involved in ion translocation. The macromolecular entities carrying those two categories of sites have been named, respectively, *AChR protein* and *ACh ionophore*.

The AChR protein has been extracted by nondenaturing detergents and purified from fish electric organ or vertebrate skeletal muscle in sizable amounts (for reviews see Changeux, 1975; Brockes, Berg, and Hall, 1976; Changeux et al., 1976; Fulpius, 1976; Lindstrom, 1976; Karlin, 1977; Heidmann and Changeux, 1978). It is an oligomer of 250,000–300,000 MW that splits in the presence of sodium dodecyl sulphate into a dominant component of apparent MW 40,000 labeled by MPTA, an affinity reagent of the AChR site (Karlin, 1977).

The protein MW per α-toxin site is close to 100,000, but the exact quaternary structure of the molecule is still not known. There are at least three, possibly more, α-toxin sites (and 40,000 chains) per oligomer.

The purified protein in detergent solution exhibits unusual hydrodynamic properties which are accounted for mostly by the abnormal density caused by the binding of significant amount of detergent (at least 10% of the total protein mass: see Meunier, Olsen, and Changeux, 1972). The hydrophobic character of the molecule is also manifested by its average amino acid composition (review in Changeux, 1975; Fulpius, 1976; Raftery et al., 1976), which lies between that of a peripheral protein, AChE, and that of an integral one, the Na^+-K^+ ATPase (Barrantes, 1975).

Like many membrane proteins, the AChR is a glycoprotein that reacts with concanavalin A and other plant lectins (Meunier et al., 1974; Brockes and Hall, 1975; Boulter and Patrick, 1977) and contains 3–5% neutral sugars (Raftery et al., 1976).

A particularly remarkable property of the isolated receptor protein is that it may exist under several states of affinity in both its membrane-bound and detergent-extracted forms (for review see Changeux et al., 1976); this has a more significant effect on the binding of agonists (several orders of magnitude) than on that of the antagonists d-tubocurarine and flaxedil (less than a factor of ten).

Fractionation of the electric organ from *Torpedo* yields membrane fragments that contain the AChR protein as approximately 40% of their proteins (Cohen et al., 1972; Duguid and Raftery, 1973; Nickel and Potter, 1973). The membrane fragments still respond in vitro to ACh by a change of ion permeability (Hazelbauer and Changeux, 1974; Popot, Sugiyama, and Changeux, 1976) and therefore contain the ACh ionophore. They constitute a particularly convenient material to study the functional properties of the ACh regulator in its membrane environment.

Local anesthetic amines and a number of toxins such as histrionicotoxin and derivatives (Daly et al., 1971; Albuquerque, Kuba, and Daly, 1974; Kato and Changeux, 1976; Dolly et al., 1977; Eldefrawi et al., 1977) and ceruleotoxin (Bon and Changeux, 1977) have been useful in investigating the regulation of ion translocation by ACh binding to its receptor site. These compounds block the pharmacological response to agonists in a noncompetitive manner and affect the all-or-none opening of the ACh ionophore as if they were interacting directly with the ion gate (Adams, 1977; Neher and Steinbach, 1978). In addition, they do not displace cholinergic ligands from the AChR sites in the membrane-bound and purified forms of AChR in the concentration range where they block the response (Kato and Changeux, 1976). Local anesthetics bind to a class of membranes sites (Weber and Changeux, 1974) distinct from the AChR site that might plausibly be part of the ACh ionophore. Direct evidence for the existence of these sites in AChR-rich membranes from *T. marmorata* was provided by spectroscopic methods, using fluorescent probes such as DNS-Chol (Cohen and Changeux, 1973; Cohen, Weber, and Changeux, 1974) and quinacrine (Grünhagen and Changeux, 1976) or binding studies with the radioactive local anesthetics quaternary dimethisoquin (Cohen, 1977) or a tritiated derivative of histrionicotoxin (Eldefrawi et al., 1977).

At physiological concentrations, local anesthetics cause an increase of the affinity of the membrane-bound AChR from *T. marmorata* for agonists and for some antagonists, as evidenced by enhanced binding of radioactive and fluorescent ligands (Cohen, Weber, and Changeux, 1974). Similarly, they cause a change of the ACh-binding curve from a sigmoid to a hyperbola (Cohen, Weber, and Changeux, 1974), an effect analogous to that reported for allosteric ligands in the case of regulatory enzymes (see references in Monod, Changeux, and Jacob, 1963; Monod, Wyman, and Changeux, 1965). Detergents such as Triton X-100, fatty acids at concentrations at which they do not release the AChR protein into solution (Brisson et al., 1975), and HTX (Kato and Changeux, 1976) have similar effects.

Conversely, agonists modify the binding of local anesthetics to the local anesthetic site (Grünhagen and Changeux, 1976; Cohen, 1977). All these effects are lost upon dissolution of the membrane fragments by detergents (Cohen, Weber, and Changeux, 1974; Briley and Changeux, 1977). In other words, allosteric interactions are established between the AChR site and the site for local anesthetics, and their actual functioning requires the integrity of the membrane structure.

The local anesthetic site (and therefore the ionophore) could be carried by the same polypeptide chain as the AChR site or by a distinct protein entity. Dissolution of the membrane by nondenaturing detergents followed by standard fractionation yields two components (Sobel, Heidmann, and Changeux, 1977; Sobel et al., 1978): (1) the AChR protein in a rather pure form that is not sensitive to local anesthetics, and (2) a high-molecular-weight aggregate that gives a single band of the approximate MW 43,000 on SDS gels. Freed from detergent, this "43K protein" gives a signal in the presence of quinacrine that histrionicotoxin reduces with the same apparent K_D as in the native membranes (8×10^{-7}M). The 43K protein therefore carries a site for HTX and local anesthetics and can be physically separated from the AChR site *sensu stricto*. The final demonstration that this component carries the actual site where the local anesthetics block ionic transport is still lacking; but a successful reassociation of the purified components into a functional ACh regulator might bring the final answer. The interaction of these two components in the native membrane would then strikingly resemble that observed between regulatory and catalytic subunits in the well-documented case of the regulatory enzyme aspartate transcarbamylase (Gerhart, 1970).[1]

The dynamic of the interaction between cholinergic ligands and local anesthetics at the level of the membrane-bound ACh regulator has been followed by fast mixing methods and spectroscopic recordings (Grünhagen and Changeux, 1976; Grünhagen, Iwatsubo, and Changeux, 1977). At least two kinetic processes have been distinguished: a fast transient one (in the msec–sec range), associated solely with the binding of agonists, and a slower one (in the sec–min range), observed with both agonists and antagonists. These spectral changes have been interpreted in terms of structural transitions of the ACh regulator between three discrete conformational states—resting (R), active (A), and desensitized (D)—which differ by their affinity for the agonists (which increases from R to A to D) and by the state of opening of the ionophore (open in A and closed in R and D).

The fast transition would then correspond to the activation R → A—that is, to the fast opening of the ionophore (which takes place during synaptic transmission)—and the slower one to the desensitization reactions R → D and/or A → D—that is, to the slow closing of the ion gate that takes place under prolonged exposure to the agonists. Thus the functional properties of the ACh regulator can be accounted for, at least in first approximation, by typical allosteric mechanisms (Figure 2).

The integration of the AChR protein into the cytoplasmic membrane has been investigated by various physical methods. Analysis of the X-ray diffraction images given by the AChR-rich membranes (Dupont, Cohen, and Changeux, 1974) suggests that a dense sheet of integral proteins spans the bilayer (indeed freeze-fracture reveals numerous "internal" particles; see Cartaud et al., 1977) and is responsible for the large effective thickness of the membrane (90–100 Å) calculated from weight measurements. Several sharp equatorial reflections indicate a regular organization of particles within the plane of the membrane and at the distance expected for an hexagonal arrangement (Dupont, Cohen, and Changeux, 1974). In these membrane fragments, the protein-lipid ratio is 1.5–2.0 and the buoyant density approximately 1.2 g/cm³ (Popot et al., 1978). The subsynaptic membrane, therefore, primarily consists of the dense semi-crystalline assembly of ACh regulator.

The rotational motion of AChR in AChR-rich membranes from *T. marmorata* has been followed by electron-paramagnetic-resonance spectroscopy with noncovalent doxyl palmitoyl cholines (Brisson et al., 1975; Bienvenue et al., 1977). A strong immobilization of the acylcholines takes place when they bind to the AChR site, although a significant motion is still detected (particularly when the paramagnetic probe is close to the methyl terminal of the fatty acid); the immobilization suggests that a fluid hydrophobic phase, possibly from a lipid bilayer, might be present in the vicinity of the AChR site (Bienvenue et al., 1977). Recent developments of the method of saturation transfer with covalent (maleimide) spin labels have made possible direct measurement of the mo-

tion of AChR protein. In fluid rod outer-segment membrane, the rotational correlation time of rhodopsin is $\tau = 20$ μsec (Baroin et al., 1977), but no motion is found in this time range with the maleimide derivative of AChR ($\tau \geq 1$ msec) (Rousselet and Devaux, 1977). The AChR protein is therefore strongly immobilized, presumably because protein-protein interactions exist in the subsynaptic membrane to restrict eventual motion in a fluid lipid bilayer.

Being an integral membrane protein, AChR can bind lipids. For instance, the purified AChR from *Torpedo* interacts with lipid monolayers, as shown from measurements of the surface tension or from the recovery of radioactive labels after film collection (Popot et al., 1977, 1978; Wiedmer et al., 1978). Incorporation into total erythrocyte lipids is enhanced at pH close to pI or by Ca⁺⁺ ions (Wiedmer et al., 1978). Pure lipids are distinguished only by their hydrophobic moiety (Popot et al., 1977, 1978). The purified AChR protein does not discriminate between phospholipids with different polar groups but does interact strongly with cholesterol (and some of its analogs) and long-chain phospholipids that are dominant components of the lipids present in the AChR-rich membranes (Figure 3).

Antibodies raised against purified AChR block the electrical response of *E. electricus* electroplaque to carbamylcholine (Patrick et al., 1973; Sugiyama et al., 1973) and impair neuromuscular transmission (see Lindstrom, 1976). Despite the fact that it is an integral membrane protein deeply imbedded in the lipid phase, the AChR molecule appears to be freely exposed to the outside surface of the membrane, as expected for a pharmacological receptor.

Thus, in sum, the subsynaptic membrane of the neuromuscular junction appears to be a compact and highly immobilized aggregation of ACh regulators and lipids that leaves enough freedom to the receptor and ionophore molecules for an "allosteric" regulation of membrane permeability.

Genesis of the subsynaptic membrane during embryonic development

STABILITY OF THE ADULT SUBSYNAPTIC MEMBRANE Sectioning the motor nerve causes degeneration of its distal segment within one week; this is manifested, for example, by the disappearance of the spontaneous miniature endplate potentials, the failure of evoked transmission, the disorganization of the ultrastructure, the fall in the content of choline acetyltransferase and acetylcholine, and, finally, the disappearance of the nerve endings (for detailed

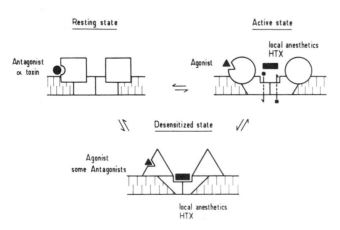

FIGURE 2 A model of the acetylcholine regulator and of its transconformations. (From Heidmann and Changeux, 1978.)

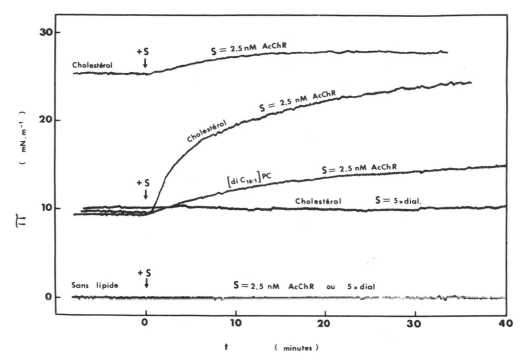

FIGURE 3 Incorporation of purified acetylcholine receptor protein into cholesterol and lecithin films. The surface pressure is measured as a function of time following the injection of receptor protein in the subphase. (From Popot et al., 1977.)

descriptions see, for frog, Birks, Katz, and Miledi, 1960; for rat, Miledi and Slater, 1970). In contrast, the postsynaptic structures survive strikingly well and for much longer periods (Tello, 1917; Tower, 1939). The former location of the endplate, revealed by the presence of AChE, and the accumulation of nuclei may persist for a year in man (Gutmann and Young, 1944; Filogamo and Gabella, 1967). The postsynaptic folds, thickenings, and particulate entities remain unaltered for several months in various frog muscles (Birks, Katz, and Miledi, 1960) and mammalian muscles (Reger, 1959; Bauer, Blumberg, and Zacks, 1962; Miledi and Slater, 1968, 1970; Nickel and Waser, 1968; Ellisman and Rash, 1977), as does the focal high sensitivity to iontophoretically applied ACh (Axelsson and Thesleff, 1969; Miledi, 1960a,b). In *Electrophorus* electroplaque the density of α-toxin sites in the subsynaptic membrane decreases by less than 50% after 52 days of denervation and is still present up to the 140th day (Bourgeois et al., 1972, 1978). Similar observations have been reported with rat soleus muscle (Frank, Gautvik, and Sommerschild, 1975, 1976), although 7 months after denervation the number of α-toxin binding sites at the endplate becomes reduced by as much as 60–70%, presumably as a consequence of muscle atrophy. No evidence

whatsoever exists that the development of extrasynaptic hypersensitivity following denervation results from the spread of subsynaptic receptors; on the contrary, no significant tendency for lateral diffusion of the receptor protein exists in the adult "uncovered" subsynaptic membrane (Bourgeois et al., 1973), an observation in agreement with the absence of rotational mobility of the receptor protein in vitro in isolated subsynaptic membrane fragments (Rousselet and Devaux, 1977).

The metabolic stability of the subsynaptic receptor protein in the adult synapse has been measured indirectly by following the fate of its complex with α-bungarotoxin. The half-life of the complex in vivo is 5–7 days (Chang and Huang, 1975; Berg and Hall, 1975), which is in the range of the spontaneous rate of dissociation of the toxin from the receptor site. The lifetime of the receptor protein might therefore be significantly longer than measured by this method. In any case, its turnover is strikingly slow. Thus in the adult subsynaptic membrane the receptor molecule is both *immobile* and *stable*.

EARLY EVENTS IN SYNAPSE FORMATION
Synthesis of the acetylcholine receptor In chick embryos, the receptor protein can be detected at very

early stages of development of skeletal muscles (Giacobini et al., 1973; Betz, Bourgeois, and Changeux, 1977; Burden, 1977), perhaps before the entry of exploratory motor fibers, although an unambiguous demonstration of this point has yet to be presented.

Upon fusion of myoblasts into myotubes, there is a several-fold increase in the number of AChR sites (as measured by α-toxin binding). This accumulation of receptor sites approximately parallels cell fusion (Patrick et al., 1972; Sytkowski, Vogel, and Nirenberg, 1973; Buckingham et al., 1974; Prives and Patterson, 1974; Merlie et al., 1975; Devreotes and Fambrough, 1975, 1976; Devreotes, Gardner, and Fambrough, 1977).

When cell fusion is inhibited by calcium deprivation in systems such as chick and veal, there is no change in the time course of appearance of AChR or in the final level of AChR sites in the culture (Patterson and Prives, 1973; Merlie and Gros, 1976; Teng and Fiszman, 1976; Patrick et al., 1977), indicating that fusion is not a necessary requirement for AChR accumulation. The increase in AChR observed both in the fused cells and in the calcium-deprived myoblasts could be due either to a neosynthesis of receptor molecules or to the unmasking of inactive molecules already present in the myoblasts. Evidence for the neosynthesis of AChR molecules has been demonstrated by the incorporation of radioactively labeled (Merlie et al., 1975; Merlie, Changeux, and Gros, 1978) or heavy-isotope-labeled (Devreotes and Fambrough, 1976; Devreotes, Gardner, and Fambrough, 1977) amino acids in the AChR protein. There is, however, a lag of about 3 hr between the moment the receptor molecules are synthesized and the time they appear on the cell surface (Devreotes, Gardner, and Fambrough, 1977; Patrick et al., 1977). About 18–22% (Devreotes, Gardner, and Fambrough, 1977) or 30–35% (Patrick et al., 1977) of the total number of receptor sites present in the cell are not accessible to the α-toxin without detergent extraction. About 40–50% (Patrick et al., 1977; Devreotes, Gardner, and Fambrough, 1977) of these "hidden" receptors subsequently appear on the cell surface and are considered as precursors for at least 50% of the surface receptors.

The accumulation of receptor molecules in the developing myotube is the net result of the incorporation of newly synthesized receptors into the cell surface and their degradation (see Devreotes and Fambrough, 1976). Incorporation into the cytoplasmic membrane proceeds at a rate of about 4% of the total surface receptors per hour (Devreotes, Gardner, and Fambrough, 1977). The rate of degradation found by following either the life-time of the α-toxin AChR complex (Devreotes and Fambrough, 1975) or the specific radioactivity of the [^{35}S]-methionine-labeled protein (Merlie, Changeux, and Gros, 1978) ranges between 16 and 28 hours (Devreotes and Fambrough, 1975; Merlie et al., 1975; Merlie, Changeux, and Gros, 1978). This value is similar to the rate of degradation of the extrasynaptic receptors that appear in adult skeletal muscle after denervation (Berg and Hall, 1974, 1975; Chang and Huang, 1975) but is strikingly different from that of the subsynaptic AChR at the adult endplate.

The embryonic nonsynaptic receptor molecule also exhibits significant lateral motion. The dynamic properties of the surface receptor were measured in primary cultures of rat myotubes in vitro after fluorescent labeling with tetramethyl-rhodamine-labeled α-bungarotoxin (Axelrod et al., 1976). Under these in vitro conditions, about 10% of the receptor molecules are aggregated into patches, the rest having a diffuse distribution. Recovery from photobleaching by a laser beam gives an average diffusion coefficient for the majority (75%) of the diffuse receptor molecule close to 7×10^{-11} cm^2/sec at 35°C (Axelrod et al., 1976; Elson and Schlessinger, this volume). Although similar measurements have not yet been carried out with embryonic myotubes in situ, it is likely that the conclusion of these experiments can be extended to the in vivo situation. The embryonic surface receptor protein therefore differs from the adult synaptic receptor by being both *labile* and *mobile*.

Arrival of the exploratory axons   In the chick embryo, the exploratory motor axons leave the anterior horns of the spinal cord around 46–48 hours after the start of incubation (Tello, 1923) and enter the myotome around the 56th hour (see Ramón y Cajal, 1929). Thanks to the motion of their growth cones, the motor fibers find their way to the target cells, and contacts are formed. The specificity of the formation of the early contact between growth cone and myotube has been investigated mainly in two ways:

1. *In vitro*: Functional contacts may be formed between explants of spinal cord and muscle (Crain and Peterson, 1971; Kano and Shimada, 1971; Robbins and Yonezawa, 1971; Cohen, 1972), dissociated cells in primary cultures (Fischbach, 1970, 1972; Fischbach et al., 1976), and even lines of nerve and muscle cells (Harris et al., 1971; Steinbach et al., 1973; Kidokoro et al., 1976; Puro and Nirenberg, 1976; Schubert, Heinemann, and Kidokoro, 1977).

2. *In vivo*: After section or crush of the motor nerve, functional reinnervation of the muscle may

take place (for a review see Fambrough, 1976). There are numerous examples showing that functional synapses may form between a wide spectrum of heterospecific and heterotypic partners: in vitro between fetal rodent cord and adult human muscle (Crain, Alfei, and Peterson, 1970), sympathetic neurons and skeletal myotubes (Nurse and O'Lague, 1975), chick ciliary ganglia and chick skeletal muscle (Hooisma et al., 1975; Betz, 1976); in vivo between fast nerve and slow muscle in the frog (Miledi and Stefani, 1969), vagus nerve and sartorius muscle in the frog (Landmesser, 1971, 1972), vagus nerve and diaphragm in the rat (Bennett, McLachlan, and Taylor, 1973), or the hypoglossal nerve and the nictitating-membrane smooth muscle (Koslow et al., 1972). Few specificity barriers seem to limit the establishment of a functional contact. Little, if any, complementarity between cell surfaces seems involved and, at most, some compatibility or loose adhesivity may be required (see papers by Rutishauser et al. and by McClain and Edelman, this volume).

LOCALIZATION OF THE ACETYLCHOLINE RECEPTOR AND OF ACETYLCHOLINESTERASE DURING NORMAL DEVELOPMENT   Only a limited set of results is available on the first stages of motor endplate development in the embryo (Diamond and Miledi, 1962; Bennett and Pettigrew, 1974a,b; Letinsky, 1974a,b; Dennis, 1975). Significant differences have already been noticed between synaptogenesis in situ and in vitro (e.g., the number and distribution of synapses formed per muscle fiber), and these limit the biological significance and generality of observations done under in vitro conditions.

Figure 4 outlines the stages of development of the neuromuscular junction. In rat embryos at 15 days in utero, exploratory motor axons enter the diaphragm and establish functional contacts (in 3 of 30 cells impaled) even before the presence of AChE can be detected by the Koelle method (Bennett and Pettigrew, 1974a,b). One day later a *single* localized spot of AChE is present in 30% of the myotubes, and in the majority of cells impaled evoked postsynaptic potentials are recorded. In the chick slow muscle anterior latissimus dorsi (ALD), a similar event takes place, except that several spots of cholinesterase are observed at regular intervals along the length of the developing muscle fiber and persist in the adult fiber. The postsynaptic localization process concerns both AChE and AChR protein.

Fetal-rat myotubes are sensitive to ionophoretically applied ACh over their entire length (Diamond and Miledi, 1962) but are more sensitive at the site where

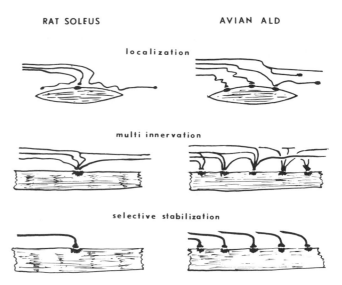

FIGURE 4   Development of the neuromuscular junction in focally innervated rat soleus and in avian anterior latissimus dorsi with distributed innervation.

spontaneous miniature endplate potentials are recorded (i.e., at the location of the nerve terminal). This localized increase of sensitivity at the postjunctional site follows within a day the onset of synaptic transmission (Bennett and Pettigrew, 1974a,b). In subsequent days the extrajunctional sensitivity to ACh gradually decreases but remains detectable through the first two weeks after birth (Diamond and Miledi, 1962). Quantitative autoradiographic studies on the distribution of AChR sites labeled with radioactive snake-venom α-toxin confirm the physiological measurements. In the embryonic myotube, the receptor sites are evenly distributed on the surface of the cell with a density of 160 sites/μm^2 in rat (Bevan and Steinbach, 1977) and 250 sites/μm^2 in chick (Burden, 1977). These values, assuming the calibration to be valid (see Land et al., 1977), are significantly lower than those found for diffuse receptors in cultured myotubes: rat, 1,500–2,000 sites/μm^2 (Hartzell and Fambrough, 1973), 1,000–2,000 sites/μm^2 (Axelrod et al., 1976), 54–900 sites/μm^2 (Land et al., 1977); L-6 clone, 400–500 sites/μm^2 (Land et al., 1977), 100 sites/μm^2 (Patrick et al., 1972). One day after the first functional contact becomes established (i.e., at 16 days in utero for rat diaphragm), the AChR accumulates at a single spot per muscle fiber, this being also the location of the AChE deposits. At this stage, the density of α-toxin sites at these dense patches would already be about 10,000 sites/μm^2, that is, 10–100 times more than the density of sites present when the motor axons contact the muscle fiber (Bevan and Steinbach, 1977; Burden, 1977; Bourgeois,

Betz, and Changeux, 1978). Once established, this elevated postjunctional density of receptor sites remains constant throughout the subsequent weeks (Burden, 1977), whereas the extrajunctional sites disappear at a fast rate (decreasing by half in about three days: see Betz, Bourgeois, and Changeux, 1977). The junctional area represents only a small fraction of the total area of the muscle fiber (50 μm^2 out of 50,000 μm^2 in chick posterior latissimus dorsi at 14 days). Thus a significant decrease in the total number of receptor sites per muscle accompanies the localization of the receptor protein (Betz, Bourgeois, and Changeux, 1977; Burden, 1977; Bourgeois, Betz, and Changeux, 1978). At least 95% of the total population of receptor molecules are lost during this process; the formation of the subsynaptic membrane thus takes place as the consequence of a severe molecular selection.

STRUCTURAL DIFFERENCES BETWEEN JUNCTIONAL AND EXTRAJUNCTIONAL ACETYLCHOLINE RECEPTORS One method of approach to the biochemistry of AChR localization during development is to compare the properties of the receptor proteins from junctional and extrajunctional areas in adult muscle. In many instances, the extrajunctional embryonic AChR resembles the extrajunctional AChR that appears outside the endplate after denervation of the adult muscle (this point requires further documentation: see Brockes, Berg, and Hall, 1976).

There are at least three mechanisms that can account for the striking metabolic differences already mentioned between extra- and subsynaptic receptors. (1) There could be a basic dissimilarity of primary structure; the two proteins could be coded for by distinct structural genes. (2) There may be a difference in the local environment of a single molecular species, resulting perhaps from interaction with other components (proteins or lipids) from the subsynaptic membrane, with the basal membrane on the outside surface, or with the cytoskeleton on its inside. (3) There could be a posttranscriptional covalent modification.

Pharmacological differences have been reported in vivo between the subsynaptic and the extrasynaptic receptors (Beranek and Vyskocil, 1967); in addition, noise measurements reveal that the opening time of the cholinergic ionophore increases after denervation (Katz and Miledi, 1972; Dreyer, Walther, and Peper, 1976; Neher and Sakmann, 1976); yet this may not indicate differences in the primary structure of the two classes of receptor molecules. In agreement with this interpretation are the following observations:

1. In vitro the binding constants for agonists and antagonists of the membrane-bound receptor do not change in chick embryo leg muscles from 8 days (extrasynaptic) before hatching until 70 days after hatching (subsynaptic) (G. Giacobini, unpublished data). The receptor proteins isolated from extra- and subsynaptic regions of rat diaphragm have been reported to show identical binding properties (Alper, Lowy, and Schmidt, 1974; Colquhoun and Rang, 1976; but see Brockes and Hall, 1975; Brockes, Berg, and Hall, 1976).

2. The equivalence points by immunoprecipitation seem to be identical for the two receptors (Brockes and Hall, 1975; G. Giacobini, unpublished data).

3. These two molecules have the same hydrodynamic properties (Brockes and Hall, 1975). Only isoelectric focusing unambiguously separates the two receptors, revealing a charge difference (Brockes and Hall, 1975; Brockes, Berg, and Hall, 1976).

Two isoelectric forms of the receptor protein have also been found in the electric organ of *Electrophorus* (Teichberg and Changeux, 1976), which offers a much more convenient material for biochemical studies than skeletal muscle. Interestingly these two forms can be interconverted in vitro. After incubation at 37°C of a crude extract in the presence of NaF, the more basic species disappears; in the absence of fluoride (i.e., with NaCl present), however, the opposite occurs. The interconversion between the two forms may therefore result from some covalent modification. A possible candidate for such a modification was a phosphorylation-dephosphorylation of the receptor protein by a protein kinase–phosphoprotein phosphatase present in the crude extract (Gordon, Davis, and Diamond, 1977; Teichberg and Changeux, 1977). The known inhibition of the phosphatase by fluoride ions would explain the differential effect of NaCl and NaF. Recently it has been shown by immunoelectrophoresis, with an antiserum directed against the receptor protein purified by affinity chromatography from either *E. electricus* or *T. californica* electric organ, that in the crude extracts, after incubation with $[^{32}P]$-γ-ATP, the immunoprecipitated receptor is $[^{32}P]$-labeled.

Without doubt, the receptor protein from fish electric organ can be covalently modified, but several questions remain about the biological significance of this modification:

1. The 48,000 dalton component of the receptor protein and not the 40,000 one that is labeled by $[^{3}H]$-MPTA seems to be the substrate of the phosphorylation reaction (Teichberg, Sobel, and Changeux, 1977).

2. There is no direct evidence yet that a phosphorylation of the receptor protein is indeed involved in its stablization during localization (the shift in isoelectric point can be taken only as indirect evidence).

3. If such modification is indeed important in the localization and stabilization of the receptor molecule, it might not be the only one.

FACTORS REGULATING ACETYLCHOLINE RECEPTOR METABOLISM, LOCALIZATION, AND STABILIZATION   Identification of the factors involved in the regulation of synapse formation is one of the most challenging problems of present-day neurobiology. One method of approach places emphasis on the activity (Changeux and Danchin, 1976) of the developing neuronal network (*activity* meaning both transmission of chemical signals at the synapse and propagation of spikes or of spikeless electric signals).

The spontaneous activity of the embryo   In the chick embryo, spontaneous movements begin as early as 3.5 days of incubation (for review see Hamburger, 1970) and are blocked by d-tubocurarine (Levi-Montalcini and Visintini, 1938; Kuo, 1939; Drachman, 1963), botulinum toxin (Drachman, 1968; Giacobini-Robecchi et al., 1975), or snake α-toxin (Giacobini et al., 1973). Spontaneous burst discharges are recorded in the spinal cord from day 4. A high correlation is found between visually observed movements and spinal-cord discharges until hatching. Moreover, the movements are completely absent when no burst activity is recorded (Ripley and Provine, 1972). The motility of chick embryo is neurogenic from the start. Spontaneous movements have also been observed

in all vertebrate embryos whose behavior has been studied: toadfish (Tracy, 1926), lizard (Hughes, Bellairs, and Bryant, 1967), turtle (Decker, 1967), and several mammals, including rat (Hamburger, 1970) and man (Hooker, 1952).

Finally, as we have already mentioned, the neuromuscular junctions in rat diaphragm transmit nerve impulses almost a day before localization of AChR and AChE. Sites of release have also been identified on restricted areas of outgrowing neurites from spinal-cord explant cell cultures in vitro (Fischbach et al., 1976). Thus there is good evidence that neuromuscular junctions are functional at very early stages of their formation (long before the differentiated synapses of the adult are formed) and also that they actively function during embryonic development. This spontaneous activity must have a biological significance.

The shutoff of acetylcholine receptor synthesis at the onset of muscle activity   At the time when synapses form, the total content of receptor molecules in the muscle starts to decline. This is particularly striking after the 14th day of incubation in the fast focally innervated posterior latissimus dorsi or in the breast muscle of chick embryo (Figure 5). There are two mechanisms that might account for this behavior. One possibility is that the rate of degradation of the receptor protein in the extrasynaptic areas increases, perhaps as a function of electrical activity; Stent (1973) proposed that the inversion of potential caused by the propagation of the action potential was responsible for the enhanced degradation of the extrasynaptic receptor. Alternatively, Changeux and Danchin (1976) hypoth-

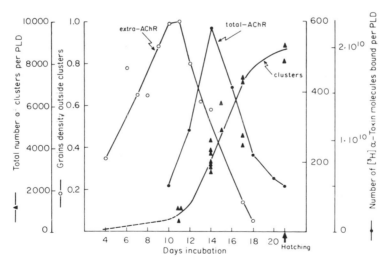

FIGURE 5   Evolution of the total content of nicotinic acetylcholine receptor ([³H]-α-toxin sites), the density of extrasynaptic receptor sites (measured by autoradiography), and the number of patches or clusters per muscle in chick embryo breast muscle during development. (From Betz, Bourgeois, and Changeux, 1977.)

esize that the synthesis of AChR stops, the receptor protein under the nerve terminals becomes stabilized, and the extrasynaptic molecules continue to be degraded at the same rate as in the embryonic, noninnervated myotube.

Four lines of experimental evidence support the second hypothesis:

1. In primary cultures of chick or mammalian myoblasts, the accumulation of receptor protein levels off; sometimes even the total content in receptor declines after about a week of culture (Patrick et al., 1972; Sytkowski, Vogel, and Nirenberg, 1973; Devreotes and Fambrough, 1975, 1976; Merlie et al., 1975; Prives, Silman, and Amsterdam, 1976; Shainberg, Cohen, and Nelson, 1976). Measurements of the rate of decay of the receptor molecule both indirectly by α-toxin binding (Devreotes and Fambrough, 1975, 1976) or directly after pulse-chase labeling by [^{35}S]-methionine (Merlie, Changeux, and Gros, 1978) unambiguously show that, from the start until the end of the culture, the degradation of the receptor protein proceeds at the same rate. In other words, regulation of receptor accumulation operates via changes in its rate of synthesis.

2. The number of AChR sites increases in extrajunctional areas of adult muscle after denervation as a result of de novo synthesis of receptor molecules (Fambrough, 1970; Grampp, Harris, and Thesleff, 1972; Brockes and Hall, 1975). Upon reinnervation, these extrasynaptic receptor molecules disappear. In many respects, this decrease in receptor concentration from extrajunctional areas reproduces that observed in the course of synapse formation in the embryo. After a long controversy, it is now widely accepted that the state of activity—mechanical and/or electrical—of the adult muscle regulates this evolution (Fischbach and Robbins, 1971; Lomo and Rosenthal, 1972; Drachman and Witzke, 1972; Lomo, Westgaard, and Dahl, 1974; Lomo and Westgaard, 1975, 1976; Lomo and Slater, 1976).

3. Under conditions of chronic electrical stimulation of either denervated muscle or myotubes in culture, the rate of receptor degradation either slightly decreases (Hogan, Marshall, and Hall, 1976) or does not change (Shainberg and Burstein, 1976; Shainberg, Cohen, and Nelson, 1976). Tetrodotoxin, which blocks both evoked or spontaneous activity of myotubes in culture, causes an increase of AChR content (Cohen and Fischbach, 1973), again without affecting the rate of receptor degradation (Shainberg and Burstein, 1976; Shainberg, Cohen, and Nelson, 1976). Finally, electrical stimulation of denervated adult muscle reduces incorporation of radioactive methionine into the receptor molecule (Hall and Reiness, 1977). In these systems, muscle activity shuts off AChR synthesis in extrajunctional areas.

4. In the chick embryo, when the total content of AChR in skeletal muscles declines (usually between days 10 and 19), the rate of receptor degradation measured with radiolabeled α-toxin again does not change (Burden, 1977; Bourgeois, Betz, and Changeux, 1978). Moreover, chronic blocking of embryonic muscle activity by the injection in ovo of botulinum toxin (Giacobini-Robecchi et al., 1975), d-tubocurarine (Burden, 1977), or flaxedil (Bourgeois, Betz, and Changeux, 1978) gives relatively higher content in muscle AChR sites. These observations strongly support the conclusion that in ovo the spontaneous activity of embryonic muscles shuts off the synthesis of the extrasynaptic receptor protein.

Most likely, the target of this regulation in the cell is gene transcription into mRNA (Shainberg, Cohen, and Nelson, 1976), but the chemical nature of the signal that accounts for the shutoff is not known. Possible candidates are the often-evoked Ca^{++} ions (Rasmussen, 1970) and cyclic nucleotides (Tomkins, 1975; Greengard, 1976). Ca^{++} would be a rather simple shutoff factor, since it might enter through the cholinergic ionophore (Takeuchi, 1963; Lièvremont, Czajka, and Tazieff-Dapierre, 1968; Kasai and Changeux, 1971; Evans, 1974) or the tetrodotoxin-sensitive ionic channels (Baker, Hodgkin, and Ridgway, 1971; Llinás, Blinks, and Nicholson, 1972; Stinnakre and Tauc, 1973) when they are activated. Signals directly coupled with the mechanical contraction of the muscle do not seem to have a role.[2] In any case, a first target for the regulation of AChR metabolism in the postsynaptic cell is the protein-synthetic machinery. It is worthwhile to note that the onset of activity has a negative effect on this synthesis.

Anterograde-factor regulation of localization of the acetylcholine receptor Another target for the regulation of receptor metabolism is the area of the cytoplasmic membrane that underlies the ingrowing nerve terminal.

Myotubes formed in vitro from chick, rat, or frog primary cultures of myoblasts show a nonrandom distribution of AChR in the absence of nerve. Regions of high sensitivity to iontophoretically applied ACh (Fischbach and Cohen 1973; Hartzell and Fambrough, 1973), called "hot spots," are observed and in several instances (Hartzell and Fambrough, 1973; Land et al., 1977) have been shown to coincide with clusters or patches of receptor sites labeled either with radioactive (Vogel, Sytkowski, and Nirenberg, 1972; Sytkowsky, Vogel, and Nirenberg, 1973; Hartzell and Fambrough, 1973; Land et al., 1977) or fluorescent (Axelrod et al., 1976; Anderson, Cohen, and Zorychta, 1977) α-bungarotoxin. The density of receptor sites in these patches is 6,000–8,000 (Axelrod et al., 1976) or 3,000–4,000 (Land et al., 1977) α-toxin sites/μm^2, which is close to the density found in the newly formed subsynaptic membrane under the nerve terminal (Bevan and Steinbach, 1977; Burden, 1977). In any case, it cannot be accounted for by a local folding of the membrane (Axelrod et al., 1976; Vogel and Daniels, 1976). These patches are about 10–60 μm in size, with distinct edges and a highly nonuniform speckle or strandlike internal structure on a micrometer scale (Axelrod et al., 1976; Anderson, Cohen, and Zorychta, 1977). They have an approximately constant average size, but several of them are present for each mature myotube with a random linear spacing (about 1 patch/400 μm of tube length: see Axelrod et al., 1976). They contain 10% (Axelrod et al., 1976) to 50% (Anderson, Cohen, and Zorychta, 1977) of the surface receptors but occupy only 3–4% of the cell area (Anderson, Cohen, and Zorychta, 1977). Most of the receptor molecules present in the patch exhibit little if any translational mobility, as measured by photobleaching recovery methods (diffusion coefficient, 10^{-12} cm^2/sec at 35°C). Once formed, these patches do not exchange the AChR with the surrounding areas of diffuse distribution. Moreover the patches are observed when staining is carried out after paraformaldehyde fixation, indicating that they are not induced by the dye-toxin conjugate (Anderson, Cohen, and Zorychta, 1977). To account for these observations and for the highly ordered structure with distinctive patterns of the AChR in the patches, it has been suggested that small clusters of receptor molecules are anchored to some intracytoplasmic (cytoskeleton) or extracellular (collagen, basal membrane) structure (Axelrod et al., 1976; Anderson, Cohen, and Zorychta, 1977). However, reagents known to disrupt cytoskeletal structure fail to convert the immobilized receptor in the patches to mobile, diffuse ones (Axelrod, unpublished data, quoted in Patrick et al., 1977).

The most evident difference between these "spontaneous" patches of receptor and those that are "induced" by the nerve terminal at the early stages of synapse formation in vivo is their distribution. In focally innervated muscle fibers, only *one* dense accumulation of AChR forms per myotube (counted on teased muscle fibers), and correlatively the total number of such patches per muscle equals the total number of muscle fibers in the muscle (Bourgeois, Betz, and Changeux, 1978). In muscles with distributed

innervation such as avian ALD, these subsynaptic patches (a few μm long) are regularly spaced along the developing muscle fiber. Outside of this subneural localization, no spontaneous patches appear during normal embryonic development in vivo, although the presence of such patches has been noticed in extrasynaptic areas of adult muscle after denervation (Ko, Anderson, and Cohen, 1977). Moreover, in vitro conditions have been defined in which spontaneous patches do not form (Slaaf et al., 1977; Slaaf, 1977).

In sum, the occurrence of spontaneous patching shows that all the components necessary for the assembly of receptor molecules into high-density patches are present in the developing myotube. The programmed localization of the receptor under normal conditions of embryonic development would then be regulated by a characteristic anterograde (or orthograde) signal emitted by the developing nerve terminal.

We have already noted that different isoelectric forms of the AChR are found in the junctional and extrajunctional regions of adult muscle and can be interconverted in vitro (Teichberg and Changeux, 1976; Teichberg, Sobel, and Changeux, 1977). The aggregation of the diffuse receptor under points of nerve-muscle contacts has been followed directly in primary cultures of myotomal muscle and neural tubes from *Xenopus laevis* morulae (Anderson and Cohen, 1977). The cultures of muscle cells were labeled with fluorescent α-bungarotoxin, and neural tube cells were added subsequently in the presence of unlabeled α-toxin. New areas of fluorescent stain develop at sites of nerve-muscle contacts; these are different from preexisting spontaneous patches. Nerve terminals can therefore induce the aggregation of preexisting diffuse receptor. But many questions are still unresolved. For example, how selective is this in vitro action of the nerve? Would a nylon string, for example, have the same effect? To what extent is such in vitro localization an image of the actual mechanism of subneural receptor localization in vivo?

Another point of controversy, related solely to in vitro nerve-muscle cultures, concerns the distribution of localized receptor under the nerve endings which, in these artificial conditions, run in an anarchic manner across the Petri dish. First of all, under these in vitro conditions, release of ACh can be elicited and synaptic currents recorded (for reviews see Fischbach et al., 1976; Kidokoro et al., 1976; Patrick et al., 1977). However, functional nerve muscle contacts may occur without localization of the receptor protein as long as the density of diffuse receptor on the surface of the myotube is large enough (Kidokoro et al., 1976).

At least with chick cells, however, accumulation of receptor protein as revealed by iontophoretic application of acetylcholine may take place under privileged sites of ACh release on the developing neurites (Fischbach et al., 1976). Again, it is not known whether or not this correlation is general (see Patrick et al., 1977) and what the actual sequence of events is in vivo.

Even if a causal relationship exists between sites of ACh release and postsynaptic areas of induced receptor localization, this does not mean that the neurotransmitter is the anterograde factor. Nerve-cell lines that make very low amounts of choline acetyltransferase, such as mouse C1300 and N13 (Steinbach et al., 1973; Steinbach and Heinemann, 1973), or cholinergic neurons in the presence of hemicholinium, an inhibitor of the transferase (Crain and Peterson, 1971), still cause receptor localization in spite of the fact that they do not release ACh. In culture, synapses may form in the presence of inhibitors of the action potential (Crain, Bornstein, and Peterson, 1968; Kidokoro et al., 1976; Obata, 1977) and in the presence of curare or snake α-toxins, which block the AChR site (Crain and Peterson, 1971; Cohen, 1972; Kidokoro et al., 1976; Obata, 1977; Anderson, Cohen, and Zorychta, 1977). However, one may argue that the localization of the receptor protein taking place under these in vitro conditions is not strictly identical with—or at least is not regulated in the same manner as—the first step of endplate formation in the embryo. However, chronic injection of the curarizing agent flaxedil in the yolk sac of chick embryos in ovo does not prevent the focal accumulation of AChR, even though it interferes with other events in endplate formation, such as the localization of AChE (Bourgeois, Betz, and Changeux, 1978). Furthermore, typical endplates are formed in muscular dysgenic mice, which are characterized by a failure to release ACh (Duchen, 1970). Thus the anterograde signal for localization cannot simply be ACh when it binds to the AChR site.

This does not exclude ACh from acting at a site distinct from the receptor site, such as a hypothetical ACh-sensitive adenylate cyclase or any regulatory protein, resistant to curare or flaxedil, that would possess a site for ACh. Factors other than ACh might also be considered: ATP (Hubbard, Musick, and Silinsky, 1972; Whittaker, 1973) might offer a convenient energy supply for reactions taking place on the external surface of the membrane; or proteins (Musick and Hubbard, 1972) that are known to be liberated by motor-nerve terminals.

Recently it has been shown that culture medium from a clone of hybrid nerve cells produces a marked increase (up to 3-4-fold) in the number of spontaneous patches of AChR appearing on myotubes in culture, without significantly changing the total number of receptor molecules per myotube (Christian et al., 1978; Podleski et al., 1978).

Ligand-induced patching of the receptor, analogous to that observed with lymphocytes and plant lectins (see McClain and Edelman, this volume), might also be suggested as an eventual mechanism for receptor localization. AChR is a glycoprotein (Meunier et al., 1974), and lectinlike agglutinins have been found in the electric organ (Teichberg et al., 1975) and in developing muscle (for reviews see Barondes and Rosen, 1976; Teichberg and Changeux, 1977). Ligand-induced patching caused by anti-AChR antibodies enhances AChR degradation (Heinemann et al., 1977; Kao and Drachman, 1977); on the other hand, the plant lectin concanavalin A has the opposite effect (Prives, 1977).

Finally, the simple adhesion of the nerve terminal to the surface of the myotube might cause a patching that would be protected against internalization by the presence of the nerve ending.

Formation of endplate patterns and receptor stabilization Two essential mechanisms in endplate formation are still not understood, even from a biological point of view. One is the focal versus distributed innervation of muscles such as avian PLD and ALD. Such patterns are not specified by the muscle but by the nerve (Hnik et al., 1967; Zelena and Jirmanova, 1973; Bennett, Pettigrew, and Taylor, 1973), and they disappear under in vitro culture conditions (Gutmann, Hanzlikova, and Holeckova, 1969). The PLD and ALD nerves show different programs of spontaneous activity in the embryo: in 16–18-day-old chick embryos, ALD fires continuously at a rate of 0.2–0.5 Hz, whereas PLD fires only occasionally at a rate of 4–8 Hz (Gordon, Purves, and Vrbová, 1977). Is, then, the activity of the muscle and of its innervation involved in the establishment of these endplate patterns? (See Gordon et al., 1974.)

Another unresolved question is the causal relationship between receptor localization and stabilization. Long-term measurements of the stability of the spontaneous patches of fluorescently labeled AChR reveal that in cultures of rat myotubes the patched receptor undergoes degradation at the same rate as the diffuse receptor (half-life on the order of 12–24 hr: see Axelrod et al., 1976). The receptor localized at nerve-muscle contacts in chick cell cultures also turns over rapidly (Fischbach et al., 1976). However, in chick subsynaptic membrane the degradation rate of the receptor protein does not change until several weeks after hatching (Burden, 1977; Bourgeois, Betz, and Changeux, 1978). Accordingly, at least in this system, localization would precede and be distinct from stabilization and would occur on a much shorter time scale (hours versus days or weeks).

The localization and stabilization of the receptor protein are only two steps in the complex chain of molecular interactions that lead to the adult synapse. A particularly important phenomenon in this late maturation is the increase in area of the subsynaptic membrane. For instance, in the chick embryo the surface of the junctional area labeled with α-bungarotoxin is about 50 μm^2 (approximately ten times less than a spontaneous patch formed in vitro: see Axelrod et al., 1976); but it increases to 2,200 μm^2 by five weeks after hatching (Burden, 1977). In 16-day rat fetuses the subsynaptic membrane is about 22.5 μm long; it decreases slightly in size around the 19th day, and increases to 30 μm in 3-week-old rats (60 μm in the adult). Subsynaptic folds appear in the rat 15 days after birth. A large increase in receptor molecules occurs in the postsynaptic membrane (Burden, 1977). Since at this stage little if any receptor protein persists in extrajunctional areas, a selective incorporation of receptor molecules into the endplate membrane must take place.

MODELS FOR THE LOCALIZATION AND STABILIZATION OF THE ACETYLCHOLINE RECEPTOR Three categories of events must therefore be distinguished: (1) the localization of the AChR protein; (2) its stabilization; and (3) the late maturation of the subsynaptic membrane. At present it is difficult to know whether steps 1 and 2 are entirely distinct or whether they are linked somehow. In any case, step 1 takes place within a much shorter span (hours) than steps 2 and 3 (days and/or weeks). Three categories of models can account for the available data (see Figure 6).

Model 1: Neurally induced aggregation and stabilization of the AChR protein (Changeux and Danchin, 1976; Courrège et al., 1979)

1. The receptor protein is inserted at random in the cytoplasmic membrane and may exist there in three interconvertible forms: (a) a labile and mobile form, L_d, which does not aggregate; (b) a labile and mobile form, L_a, which makes aggregates under

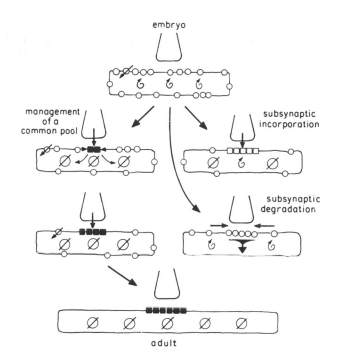

FIGURE 6 Three possible models for the metabolism of the acetylcholine receptor protein during localization of the endplate. Curved arrow means that the synthesis of the receptor protein is "on," $\varnothing$ that it is "off." The stabilization reaction is represented as $\bigcirc \rightarrow \blacksquare$.

which the receptor molecule becomes immobilized; and (c) a stable form, S, which is both immobilized and resistant to degradation. Thus

$$L_d \xrightarrow{(i)} L_a \xrightarrow{(ii)} (L_a)_n \xrightarrow{(iii)} S.$$

2. The transformation (i) is fast and regulated by an *anterograde factor* liberated by the nerve terminal during activity, and L_a aggregates (or crystallizes) into $(L_a)_n$ when its local concentration in the membrane reaches a finite threshold.

3. The synthesis of L_d slows down in the postsynaptic cell when activity starts in the myotube. An *internal shutoff factor* selectively blocks the expression of the receptor gene(s). In its aggregated form, the receptor protein becomes stable: $L_a \rightarrow S$. The same or a different anterograde factor as for (i) regulates this transformation. As a consequence, only the junctional receptor persists, and the extrajunctional, labile form disappears.

This model has been formalized and accounts for most of the known behavior of the receptor protein during endplate formation. It also accounts for the focal versus distributed pattern of endplates solely on the basis of different patterns of liberation of the anterograde factor and, as a consequence, of a competition between nerve endings for the aggregation of the receptor protein (see Courrège et al., 1979). The chemical reactions (i) and (iii) have not been identified but (i), for example a phosphorylation, might eventually take place in the postsynaptic cell in the absence of the anterograde factor and lead to spontaneous patch formation under in vitro culture conditions. In some systems L_a and S might be identical; in that case, aggregation would cause stabilization.

Model 2: Directional incorporation of AChR protein into the subneural areas   A neural anterograde factor triggers the local synthesis and incorporation of receptor molecules into the cytoplasmic membrane that underlies the nerve terminal. In the most extreme case, the junctional receptor would be determined by a structural gene different from the one that codes for the extrajunctional receptor. The two proteins might then have different aggregation and stability properties.

There is no evidence that such a mechanism accounts for the early state of endplate formation. However, it is likely that during the late maturation of the endplate, few if any molecules of receptor are present in extrajunctional areas, and the increase in size of the subsynaptic area must rely on directional incorporation of newly synthesized receptor molecules.

Model 3: Receptor flow (see, e.g., Edwards and Frisch, 1976)   At variance with model 2 and as in model 1, the receptor protein in model 3 is randomly incorporated into the membrane and flows continuously into a "sticky zone" under the nerve terminal, where it has a finite half-life, as in the extrajunctional areas. As a consequence of the steady-state flux of receptor, the density of receptor molecules increases under the nerve terminal.

This model does not deal with the stabilization of the receptor molecule. Moreover the photobleaching experiments with fluorescently labeled AChR indicate that, at least in the case of the spontaneous patches, little exchange exists between the diffuse and patched receptors (Axelrod et al., 1976). Finally, this model predicts that if the receptor molecules are "unstuck"—for example, as a consequence of denervation—the dense accumulation of receptor would disappear in less than an hour. This prediction is not experimentally fulfilled.

Localization of acetylcholinesterase

Accumulation of AChE in the subneural region of the endplate follows closely that of AChR, but different mechanisms are involved in its localization.

High ionic strength releases from *E. electricus* electric tissue several forms of AChE with sedimentation coefficients of 8S, 14S, and 18S (Massoulié and Riéger, 1969). When examined electron-microscopically, these forms appear as clusters of 4, 6–8, and 10 or more globular subunits, respectively, attached to an elongated tail (Riéger et al., 1973; Dudai, Herzberg, and Silman, 1973). Exposure to proteases (Massoulié, Riéger, and Tsuji, 1970, 1971) or collagenase converts all of these forms to a tetrameric 11S species (Dudai and Silman, 1974; Lwebuga-Musaka, Lappi, and Taylor, 1976). Current hypotheses hold that extensive intersubunit disulfide bonding contributes to the assembly of "catalytic subunits" with a tail that includes collagenlike subunits (containing about 30% glycine, 15% proline, 7% hydroxyproline, 7% hyroxylysine) of apparent MW 40,000 and 44,000 (Dudai and Silman, 1974; Anglister, Rogozinski, and Silman, 1976; McCann and Rosenberry, 1977; Rosenberry and Richardson, 1977).

Although less well understood, a comparable multiplicity of forms of AChE exist in striated muscle. Three forms, with sedimentation coefficients of 4S, 10S and 16S, have been identified in rat (Hall, 1973; Vigny, Koenig, and Riéger, 1976). The 4S and 10S forms are distributed throughout the muscle, but the 16S form is present only in the endplate region. This last species appears suddenly on day 14–15 of embryonic development in rat leg muscle, at the time endplates form. On the other hand, the 4S form seems a precursor of the 10S form (Riéger et al., 1976). A "junctional form" of AChE can therefore be distinguished from an extrajunctional one on the basis of striking differences of hydrodynamic behavior which, most likely, are relevant to the attachment of the enzyme to the basement membrane.

Different regulatory mechanisms command the localization and metabolism of AChE and AChR in muscle:

1. At the early stages of embryonic development in vivo, appearance of AChE in skeletal muscle closely parallels that of AChR (Giacobini et al., 1973; Betz, Bourgeois, and Changeux, 1977); and the same association is found with primary cultures of myotubes in vitro (Prives, Silman, and Amsterdam, 1976). On the other hand, the evolution of these two proteins diverges strikingly at later stages. As already mentioned, the total content of AChR starts to decline around day 14 in chick embryo (Burden, 1977; Betz, Bourgeois, and Changeux, 1977) as a consequence of a shutoff of its synthesis; the total content of AChE, however, continues to increase (Betz, Bourgeois, and Changeux, 1977). The same is true in vitro (Prives,

Silman, and Amsterdam, 1976). Also, clones of neuroblastoma cells have been selected that synthesize ratios of AChE to AChR with variations up to eightyfold (Simantov and Sachs, 1973).

2. Denervation does not cause a spread of AChE paralleling that of AChR but rather a decrease of AChE tested by both electrophysiological and biochemical techniques (Miledi, 1960a,b; Guth, Albers, and Brown, 1964; Guth and Brown, 1965; Crone and Freeman, 1972; Axelsson and Thesleff, 1959). The average specific activity of the enzyme in the muscle decreases by 50% by 15 days after denervation, but the 16S "endplate" form disappears almost completely (Hall, 1973; Vigny, Koenig, and Riéger, 1976).

3. Chronic blocking of neuromuscular transmission during development, for instance by botulinum toxin (Drachman, 1972; Giacobini-Robecchi et al., 1975), snake α-toxin (Giacobini et al., 1973), curare (Gordon et al., 1974), or flaxedil (Bourgeois, Betz, and Changeux, 1978), causes a marked decrease of endplate AChE (see also Filogamo and Gabella, 1966; Filogamo, 1969). At least in the case of flaxedil paralysis, however, the localization of AChR still takes place (Bourgeois, Betz, and Changeux, 1978). Rudimentary endplates are formed, which contain AChR but no AChE. Activity, therefore, regulates the localization of these two proteins by means of different mechanisms. This point has been further documented in the case of rat soleus muscle hyperinnervated by transplanted fibular nerve (Lomo and Slater, 1976). New endplates may be formed by the fibular nerve a few days outside the normal endplate region if the activity of the normal soleus nerve is blocked. Discrete spots of high ACh sensitivity appear at these new junctions (under the fibular nerve) and remain stable for days after section of the fibular nerve. A remarkable result of these experiments is that AChE appears at these spots of high ACh sensitivity with a delay of 6–8 days *even in the absence of nerve terminals.* Moreover AChE develops there only if the soleus muscle is chronically stimulated. Thus endplate AChE is synthesized by the muscle, and its appearance requires muscle activity. This behavior again strikingly differs from that of the AChR.

The mechanism of AChE localization most likely does not involve immobilization of a diffuse and mobile membrane molecule, as in the case of AChR. A possibility is that the protein is secreted (Gisiger and Vigny, unpublished data) in the extracellular space and hooked (e.g., via disulfide bonding) to the basement membrane at particular sites that underlie nerve terminals and remain stable after denervation.

Presynaptic stabilization of the motor nerve ending

CELL DEATH IN THE SPINAL CORD   It is an old observation (Collin, 1906) that at a critical stage of embryonic development a significant fraction of the motoneurons in the spinal cord die (see reviews by Hughes, 1968; Gaze, 1970; Prestige, 1970; Hamburger, 1976; Cowan, this volume). In the chick embryo, soon after the proliferation of neuroblasts has ceased—between days 6 and 10—the total number of cells per lateral motor column decreases from 20,000 to 12,000 (Hamburger, 1975). In *Xenopus* tadpoles, the total number of motoneurons may reach 5,000 or 6,000; but 60 days later, at the time of metamorphosis, only 1,200 (the adult number) persist. The total number of cells that disappear during this period could reach 10,000, even larger than the overall difference in total cell number (Hughes, 1961), since the periods of cell death and cell proliferation overlap. In the fetal mouse, similar events take place between days 10 and 15 of intrauterine life (Romanes, 1946; Harris-Flanagan, 1969). In all these instances neuronal death coincides with the entry of the exploratory motor fibers in their target muscle, which suggests an influence of the peripheral field of innervation on the cell death of central neurons.

This possibility was tested by following the consequences of limb-bud extirpation on motoneuron survival in the spinal cord (Harrison, 1908; Hamburger, 1958). Amputation at day $2\frac{1}{2}$ in chick embryos does not affect proliferation of the neuroblasts up to day 6; at that time they reach the same maximal number on both sides (9,000–10,000 per lateral motor column). By day $9\frac{1}{2}$, however, 92% of motoneurons have disappeared on the operated side (Hamburger, 1958). Early limb-bud extirpation causes a massive depletion of motoneurons, accompanied by a decrease of the enzyme choline acetyltransferase in the spinal cord (Burt and Narayanan, 1970). Removal of the peripheral target cells dramatically enhances the "normally occurring cell death"; enlargement of the periphery by implantation of a supernumerary leg reduces it (Hollyday and Hamburger, 1976).

Limb-bud extirpation carried out at various stages of development in *Xenopus* (Prestige, 1970) shows further that a critical period of lability exists during the life history of the motoneuron during which it becomes susceptible to death. At that stage, an interaction of the motoneuron with the periphery is required for the neuron to become stabilized and to continue its development. The stabilization of the motoneuron appears, therefore, to be regulated in a retrograde manner by the interaction of its axon with the target muscle cells. To test the possibility that the actual activity of the postsynaptic cell has any effect on this regulation, several cholinergic agents or toxins known to selectively block neuromuscular transmission were injected into developing chick embryos (Giacobini et al., 1973; Giacobini-Robecchi et al., 1975, 1976). These drugs stop the spontaneous movements of the embryo, which may nevertheless survive until hatching. Such treatments cause a marked atrophy of skeletal muscles, which show signs of delayed differentiation and regression (Drachman, 1967, 1968, 1971, 1972), and, as already mentioned, interfere with the localization of AChE. Interestingly, some of these pharmacological agents affect the motor innervation of the muscle, despite their almost exclusive postsynaptic site of action. The chronic injection of high doses of *Naja nigricollis* α-toxin (Giacobini et al., 1973, and unpublished data) or flaxedil (Betz, Bourgeois, and Changeux, submitted) causes a decrease of the content of the presynaptic enzyme choline acetyltransferase in the muscle and sciatic nerve and a dramatic reduction of the total number of myelinated and nonmyelinated axons in the ventral roots of the spinal nerves (in the dorsal roots no significant change takes place). Thus a selective loss of motor-nerve terminals and of motoneurons takes place.[3]

How, then, can an essentially postsynaptic block influence the motor-nerve terminal and its neuronal body? The possibility that α-toxin and d-tubocurarine interfere with the recognition step at the early stages of synapse formation is rendered unlikely by the observation that primitive junctions (as well as the content of choline acetyltransferase) in embryos injected at day 4 of incubation do not differ significantly from those of the noninjected control until day 12 of incubation. Similarly, d-tubocurarine or α-bungarotoxin do not prevent synapse formation in vitro or during reinnervation of adult rat diaphragm. At this early stage of development, therefore, the activity of the muscle exerts—in a direct or, most likely, indirect manner—a positive feedback on the stabilization of its motor innervation.

TRANSIENT POLYNEURONAL INNERVATION A second regressive phase occurs during the first weeks following hatching (chick) or birth (rat) and affects primarily motor-axon collaterals without making significant changes in cell number. For example, in fetal rat diaphragm at day 17, soon after the dense deposit of AChE and AChR appears in the middle of the muscle fiber, motor axons develop multiple branches and make, with a high degree of randomness, a complex network that increases in size until birth (Bennett and Pettigrew, 1974a). Observations of the endplate in the newborn cat (Riley, 1976) or rat (Brown, Jansen, and Van Essen, 1976) after silver-staining reveals several axon terminals converging to a single endplate. Also, electron microscopy confirms that several synaptic profiles are in contact with the same synaptic fold. The postsynaptic potentials of individual muscle fibers recorded with intracellular microelectrodes exhibit unusual features (Redfern, 1970; Bennett and Pettigrew, 1974a; Benoit and Changeux, 1975; Dennis, 1975; Brown, Jensen, and Van Essen, 1976): the amplitude increases discontinuously through successive steps (three or more) as a function of stimulus strength, instead of jumping in a single step as in adult muscle fibers. Analysis of this complex endplate potential shows that it is due not to electrical coupling between muscle fibers but to the presence of several functional axon terminals from different neurons at the same endplate; this explains the difference in threshold (Brown, Jansen, and Van Essen, 1976). A considerable redundancy therefore exists in the innervation of the muscle fiber. During the first postnatal week, the number of steps of the complex endplate potential progressively decreases: one of the endings finally dominates the others. At 3–5 weeks, all the synapses are innervated by a single nerve terminal, and noninnervated muscle fibers are not seen. More than 60% of the functional contacts have thus disappeared. The fine structure of the endplate does not in general reveal gross signs of degeneration of the axonal branches, and the number of axons in the ventral roots does not change significantly (Brown, Jansen, and Van Essen, 1976). A retraction of axon collaterals, rather than a degeneration, takes place. These observations have been repeated with various muscles, in particular, avian ALD (Bennett and Pettigrew, 1974a), in which each of the several endplates present per muscle fiber becomes innervated by several axon terminals. The transient polyneuronal innervation seems to be an obligatory step of endplate formation.

Since the number of muscle fibers and motor axons remains constant during this period (Sissons, 1963; Nystrom, 1968; Westerman et al., 1972), the number of muscle fibers innervated by a single motoneuron—that is, the size of the "motor unit"—should change (Bagust, Lewis, and Westerman, 1973, 1974; Brown, Jansen, and Van Essen, 1976; Jansen, Van Essen, and Brown, 1976). Indeed during postnatal development the average size of the motor unit decreases. In the 3-day-old rat soleus, single motor unit tension is about one-fourth of the total muscle tension. In the adult, the fields of innervation of the motoneurons no longer overlap, and a single motor fiber commands the contraction of a five times smaller set of fibers. The regressive process, which leads to the establishment of the "one motor terminal–one muscle fiber" relationship and the corollary decrease in size of the motor units, corresponds to an improvement in the motor command of the muscle. The elimination of redundant synapses increases the specificity of muscle innervation. Interestingly, it also coincides with the period when the baby rat learns to walk and acquires coordinated motor behavior.

To test the possibility that regression of polyneuronal innervation is regulated by the state of activity of the muscle, one of the tendons of the sartorius muscle was sectioned in infant rats (Figure 7). It is not yet known whether neonatal tenotomy modifies the chronic firing of the motoneurons, but it certainly changes the state of mechanical activity of the muscle. In any case, the regression of the polyneuronal innervation was significantly delayed.

A more direct test of the effect of nerve activity on the stabilization of motor terminals was carried out during reinnervation of the soleus muscle in adult rats (Benoit and Changeux, 1975). In the course of reinnervation following the crushing of the sciatic nerve, a transient multi-innervation of the muscle fibers takes place, although to a smaller extent than during development (MacArdle, 1975). Application of a cuff of local anesthetic (lidocaine) on the regenerating terminal immediately after the nerve has been crushed enhances the magnitude of the transient multi-innervation and delays its regression. The most likely interpretation of this effect is that the local anesthetic blocks the activity of the motor nerve and, as a consequence, slows down the regressive process. Accordingly, the elimination of redundant nerve terminals and the consequent selective stabilization of one motor axon per muscle fiber would be an "active" process, regulated by the activity of the motor nerve and of its postsynaptic target.

Another series of experiments, although relevant to a different paradigm, further suggest that the activity of the muscle is indeed sufficient to regulate the growth of its innervation. Botulinum toxin blocks ACh release from motor nerve terminals and subsequently causes extensive terminal sprouting. Inter-

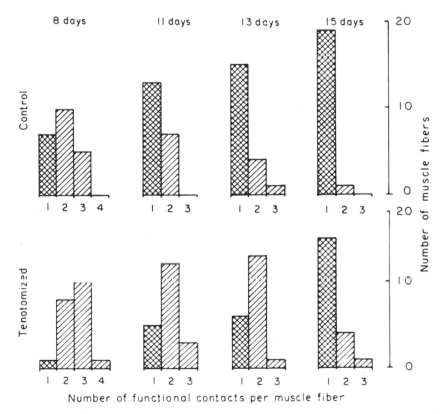

FIGURE 7 Effect of tenotomy on the postnatal evolution of polyneuronal innervation in rat soleus muscle. (From Benoit and Changeux, 1975.)

estingly, chronic electrical stimulation of poisoned muscles in mice prevents both the development of denervation hypersensitivity and nerve-terminal sprouting (Brown, Goodwin, and Ironton, 1977). The activity of the muscle commands in a retrograde manner the evolution of the motor-nerve endings.

RETROGRADE FACTORS At least two mechanisms may account for the retrograde action of the muscle on the nerve: (1) To become stable the nerve ending must occupy (or adhere to) a sufficient surface of the postsynaptic cell membrane (on which, for example, the density of AChR is large enough). (2) Diffusible "retrograde factors" are emitted by the muscle and affect in a transsynaptic manner the metabolism, growth, and/or stability of the nerve terminal.

At present it is difficult to decide among these and other possibilities. Perhaps the factors that regulate the levels of choline acetyltransferase in spinal-cord motoneurons (Giller et al., 1973, 1977) or sympathetic cells in culture (Patterson and Chun, 1974; Patterson, 1978, and this volume) are responsible for these retrograde effects. The factors secreted in a variety of cell types (including muscle cells) are heat-labile and have molecular weights greater than 50,000 daltons. They may cause a 10–20-fold increase of specific activity of choline acetyltransferase in spinal-cord cultures without affecting the level of AChE or glutamic acid decarboxylase activity (Giller et al., 1977). Yet the specificity of these factors is difficult to assess, since in several instances NGF or cAMP may produce similar effects (Schubert, Heinemann, and Kidokoro, 1977).

A MODEL FOR RETROGRADE SELECTIVE STABILIZATION The following model may account for the selective stabilization of one motor axon per muscle fiber (Changeux and Danchin, 1976). (1) All the motor-nerve terminals converging on a given endplate receive the same average number of impulses but in a random, nonsynchronous manner. (2) At the peak of the multi-innervation stage, all terminals share almost equivalent areas of the stabilized subsynaptic membrane surface and/or dispose of a limited stock of a postsynaptic "retrograde factor," x, the synthesis of which shuts off when the muscle becomes active. (3) At this critical stage, the arrival of impulses causes an increase of surface occupancy and/or utilization of x. (4) When the surface occupied by the nerve terminal and/or the amount of x utilized becomes lower than a critical value, this nerve terminal regresses.

This set of minimal assumptions may explain both the stabilization of a single nerve terminal and the constant size of the motor units. Accordingly, the size of the motor unit should be determined by the ratio of the number of muscle fibers to that of motoneurons, and this can be tested. An increase of surface occupancy by nerve terminals as a consequence of activity has been described; but the biochemical mechanisms by which a nerve terminal becomes stabilized once a critical surface of the postsynaptic membrane is occupied remains obscure. The postulated retrograde factor (substance x) has not been identified chemically; in the case of the neuromuscular junction, the concentration of calcium in the cleft or of macromolecular growth factor (different from NGF) are possible candidates. An interesting possibility would be that the retrograde effect consists of the covalent modification of presynaptic fibrillar or tubular proteins engaged in the maintenance of the shape of the nerve terminal by, for instance, regulating its internal cytoplasmic flow. A shutoff of the axoplasmic flow in a nerve terminal due to the lack of a retrograde factor would cause regression of the nerve terminal.

Conclusions

The main purpose of this review has been to present cellular and even molecular mechanisms that might account for the "specification" of the neuromuscular junction during development. Many elements are still missing, in particular the chemical identification of the diffusible signals involved. Nevertheless, these mechanisms make plausible the hypothesis that during development a selection of synapses takes place that is, directly or indirectly, regulated by the state of activity of the developing neuronal network.

Recent evidence indicates that the same hypothesis might be extended to systems other than the neuromuscular junction. For example, the development of hypersensitivity to ACh in extrasynaptic areas has been observed in a parasympathetic neuron as a consequence of denervation (Kuffler, Dennis, and Harris, 1971), but it is not known if the activity of the neuron per se is sufficient to regulate this evolution. A transient polyneuronal innervation has also been identified in rodent cerebellum (Crepel, Mariani, and Delhaye-Bouchaud, 1976; Crepel and Mariani, 1976; Mariani et al., 1977) during development of Purkinje-cell innervation by climbing fibers (Figure 8), in rat submandibular ganglion (Lichtman, 1977), and on spinal motoneurons (Conradi and Ronnevi, 1974, 1977). The restriction of the field of projection of geniculate neurons in mammalian visual cortex might

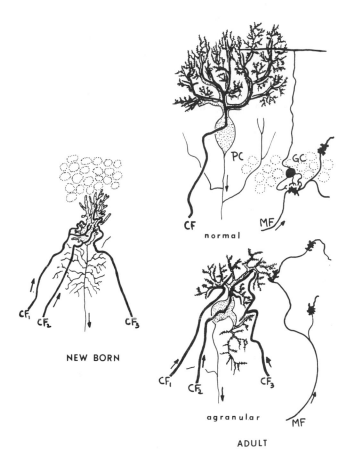

NEW BORN

normal

agranular

ADULT

FIGURE 8   Evolution of Purkinje-cell innervation by several climbing fibers in normal and agranular rodent cerebellum. In the agranular cerebellum the transient multi-innervation present in the newborn persists in the adult.

also be accounted for by similar mechanisms (Rakic, 1977; Hubel and Wiesel, 1977). The basic assumption of the theory that an increase of "specificity" accompanies the active stabilization of particular synapses and the regression of others remains to be tested at the cellular level.

One of the main advantages of this selective-stabilization hypothesis is that it affords an economy of genes. Some of the genes that dictate, for example, the general rules of growth, the stability properties of the immature synapses, the regulation of their stability by the activity of the immature synapse, and the integrative properties of the postsynaptic neuron may be shared by different categories of neurons or even be common to all neurons. The set of genes involved (the genetic envelope) should therefore be smaller than it would have to be if each synapse were determined individually.

Another advantage of the hypothesis is that it provides a plausible mechanism for learning. It illustrates

how a given temporal pattern of activity might be transcribed into a particular three-dimensional topology of synapses. It is radically different from so-called instructive theories, which postulate, for example, that a particular nervous activity directs the growth of nerve endings toward the suitable target or causes the appearance of new molecular species. According to our theory, "to learn" becomes "to eliminate."

An interesting prediction of the formalized model of selective synapse stabilization in a developing neuronal network is that the same final learned output might be achieved through stabilization of different synaptic pathways (Changeux, Courrège, and Danchin, 1973). In other words, it allows for what is referred to as a "variability" of the connectional organization, which is indeed observed in isogenic organisms. According to this view, the "degeneracy" of the code for behavior (see Edelman, this volume) appears as a consequence (and not as a prerequisite) of the selection.

For reasons that are not yet clear, the total stock of genes remains almost constant throughout the evolution of vertebrates (mammals in particular). Despite this the complexity of the nervous system and the correlative behavioral competences continue to increase. As the autonomous programming of the system becomes increasingly difficult, the genetic determinism must break down and the redundancy of the connectivity become amplified. The ability to learn might thus be viewed as the evolutionary result of an increased complexity of neuronal networks based on a constant number of genes.

ACKNOWLEDGMENTS This research was supported by grants from the Muscular Dystrophy Association of America, the Collège de France, the Délégation Générale à la Recherche Scientifique et Technique, the Centre National de la Recherche Scientifique, the Institut National de la Santé et de la Recherche Médicale, and the Commissariat à l'Energie Atomique.

REFERENCES

ADAMS, P. R., 1977. Relaxation experiments using bath-applied suberyldicholine. *J. Physiol.* 268:271–289.

ADAMS, P. R., 1977. Voltage jump analysis of procaine action at frog end-plate. *J. Physiol.* 268:291–318.

ADRIEN, J., 1976. Lesion of the anterior raphe nuclei in the newborn kitten and the effects on sleep. *Brain Res.* 103:579–583.

ALBUQUERQUE, E. X., K. KUBA, and J. DALY, 1974. Effect of histrionicotoxin on the ionic conductance modulator of the cholinergic receptor: A quantitative analysis of the end-plate current. *J. Pharmacol. Exp. Ther.* 189:513–524.

ALPER, R., J. LOWY, and J. SCHMIDT, 1974. Binding properties of acetylcholine receptors extracted from normal and from denervated rat diaphragm. *FEBS Lett.* 48:130–134.

ANDERSON, M. J., and M. W. COHEN, 1977. Nerve induced and spontaneous redistribution of acetylcholine receptors on cultured muscle cells. *J. Physiol.* 268:757–773.

ANDERSON, M. J., M. W. COHEN, and E. ZORYCHTA, 1977. Effects of innervation on the distribution of acetylcholine receptors on cultured muscle cells. *J. Physiol.* 268:731–756.

ANGLISTER, L., S. ROGOZINSKI, and I. SILMAN, 1976. Detection of hydroxyproline in preparations of acetylcholinesterase from the electric organ of the electric eel. *FEBS Lett.* 69:129–132.

AXELROD, D., P. RAVDIN, D. E. KOPPEL, J. SCHLESSINGER, W. W. WEBB, E. L. ELSON, and T. R. PODLESKI, 1976. Lateral motion of fluorescently labelled acetylcholine receptors in membranes of developing muscle fibers. *Proc. Natl. Acad. Sci. USA* 73:4594–4598.

AXELSSON, J., and S. THESLEFF, 1959. A study of supersensitivity in denervated mammalian skeletal muscle. *J. Physiol.* 147:178–193.

BAGUST, J., D. M. LEWIS, and R. A. WESTERMAN, 1973. Polyneural innervation of kitten skeletal muscle. *J. Physiol.* 229:241–255.

BAGUST, J., D. M. LEWIS, and R. A. WESTERMAN, 1974. The properties of motor units in a fast and a slow twitch muscle during post-natal development in the kitten. *J. Physiol.* 237:75–90.

BAKER, P. F., A. L. HODGKIN, and E. RIDGWAY, 1971. Depolarization and calcium entry in squid giant axons. *J. Physiol.* 218:709–755.

BARNARD, E. A., J. WIECKOWSKI, and T. H. CHIU, 1971. Cholinergic receptor molecules and cholinesterase molecules at mouse skeletal muscle junction. *Nature* 234:207–209.

BAROIN, A., D. D. THOMAS, B. OSBORNE, and P. F. DEVAUX, 1977. Saturation transfer electron paramagnetic resonance on membrane-bound proteins. I. Rotational diffusion of rhodopsin in the visual receptor membrane. *Biochem. Biophys. Res. Commun.* 78:442–447.

BARONDES, S., and S. D. ROSEN, 1976. Cell surface carbohydrate binding proteins: Role in cell recognition. In *Neuronal Recognition*, S. Barondes, ed. London: Chapman & Hall, pp. 331–356.

BARRANTES, F. J., 1975. The nicotinic cholinergic receptor: Different compositions evidenced by statistical analysis. *Biochem. Biophys. Res. Commun.* 62:407–414.

BAUER, W. C., J. M. BLUMBERG, and S. I. ZACKS, 1962. Short- and long-term ultrastructural changes in denervated mouse motor endplates. In *Proceedings of the Fourth International Congress on Neuropathology.* Stuttgart: G. Thieme, pp. 16–18.

BENNETT, M. R., E. M. MCLACHLAN, and R. S. TAYLOR, 1973. The formation of synapses in mammalian striated muscle reinnervated with autonomic preganglionic nerves. *J. Physiol.* 233:501–517.

BENNETT, M. R., and A. G. PETTIGREW, 1974a. The formation of synapses in striated muscle during development. *J. Physiol.* 241:515–545.

BENNETT, M. R., and A. G. PETTIGREW, 1974b. The formation of synapses in reinnervated and cross-reinnervated striated muscle during development. *J. Physiol.* 241:547–573.

BENNETT, M. R., A. G. PETTIGREW, and R. S. TAYLOR, 1973. The formation of synapses in reinnervated and cross-reinnervated adult avian muscle. *J. Physiol.* 230:331–357.

BENOIT, P., and J. P. CHANGEUX, 1975. Consequences of tenotomy on the evolution of multiinnervation in developing rat soleus muscle. *Brain Res.* 99:354–358.

BENOIT, P., and J. P. CHANGEUX, 1978. Consequences of blocking the nerve with a local anaesthetic on the evolution of multiinnervation at the regenerating neuromuscular junction of the rat. *Brain Res.* 149:89–96.

BERANEK, R., and F. VYSKOCIL, 1967. The action of tubocurarine and atropine on the normal and denervated rat diaphragm. *J. Physiol.* 188:53–66.

BERG, D. K., and Z. W. HALL, 1974. Fate of α-bungarotoxin bound to acetylcholine receptors of normal and denervated muscle. *Science* 184:473–475.

BERG, D.K., and Z. W. HALL, 1975. Loss of α-bungarotoxin from junctional and extrajunctional acetylcholine receptors in rat diaphragm *in vivo* and in organ culture. *J. Physiol.* 252:771–789.

BETZ, H., J. P. BOURGEOIS, and J. P. CHANGEUX, 1977. Evidence for degradation of the acetylcholine (nicotinic) receptor in skeletal muscle during the development of the chick embryo. *FEBS Lett.* 77:219–224.

BETZ, H., and J. P. CHANGEUX, 1979. Regulation of muscle acetylcholine receptor synthesis in vitro by derivatives of cyclic nucleotides. *Nature* (submitted).

BETZ, W., 1976. The formation of synapses between chick embryo skeletal muscle and ciliary ganglia grown *in vitro.* *J. Physiol.* 254:63–73.

BETZ, W., and B. SAKMAN, 1971. Effect of proteolytic enzymes on function and structure of frog neuromuscular junctions. *J. Physiol.* 230:673–688.

BEVAN, S., and J. H. STEINBACH, 1977. The distribution of α-bungarotoxin binding sites on mammalian skeletal muscle developing *in vivo. J. Physiol.* 267:195–213.

BIENVENUE, A., A. ROUSSELET, G. KATO, and P. F. DEVAUX, 1977. Fluidity of the lipids next to the acetylcholine receptor protein of *Torpedo* membrane fragments: Use of amphiphilic reversible spin-labels. *Biochemistry* 16:841–848.

BIRKS, R., B. KATZ, and R. MILEDI, 1960. Physiological and structural changes at the amphibian myoneural junction, in the course of nerve degeneration. *J. Physiol.* 150:145–168.

BLOMBERG, F., R. S. COHEN, and P. SIEKEVITZ, 1977. The structure of postsynaptic densities isolated from dog cerebral cortex. II. Characterization and arrangement of some of the major protein within the structure. *J. Cell Biol.* 74:204–225.

BON, C., and J. P. CHANGEUX, 1977. Chemical and pharmacological characterization of toxic polypeptides from the venom of *Bungarus caeruleus.* Ceruleotoxin: A possible marker of the cholinergic ionophore. *Eur. J. Biochem.* 74:31–51.

BOULTER, J., and J. PATRICK, 1977. Purification of an acetylcholine receptor from a nonfusing muscle cell line. *Biochemistry* 16:4900–4908.

BOURGEOIS, J. P., H. BETZ, and J. P. CHANGEUX, 1978. Effets de la paralysie chronique de l'embryon de poulet par le flaxédil sur le développement de la jonction neuromusculaire. *C.R. Acad. Sci. Paris* (D) 286:773–776.

BOURGEOIS, J. P., J. L. POPOT, A. RYTER, and J. P. CHANGEUX, 1973. Consequences of denervation on the distribution of the cholinergic (nicotinic) receptor sites from *Electrophorus electricus* revealed by high resolution autoradiography. *Brain Res.* 62:557-563.

BOURGEOIS, J. P., J. L. POPOT, A. RYTER, and J. P. CHANGEUX, 1978. Quantitative studies on the localisation of the cholinergic receptor protein in the normal and denervated electroplaque from *Electrophorus electricus. J. Cell Biol.* 79:200-216.

BOURGEOIS, J. P., A. RYTER, A. MENEZ, P. FROMAGEOT, P. BOQUET, and J. P. CHANGEUX, 1972. Localization of the cholinergic receptor protein in *Electrophorus* electroplax by high resolution autoradiography. *FEBS Lett.* 25:127-133.

BRILEY, M., and J. P. CHANGEUX, 1978. Recovery of some functional properties of the detergent-extracted cholinergic receptor protein from *Torpedo marmorata* after reintegration into a membrane environment. *Eur. J. Biochem.* 84:429-439.

BRISSON, A., P. DEVAUX, and J. P. CHANGEUX, 1975. Effet anesthésique local de plusieurs composés liposolubles sur la réponse de l'électroplaque de Gymnote à la carbamylcholine et sur la liaison de l'acétylcholine au récepteur cholinergique de Torpille. *C.R. Acad. Sci. Paris* (D) 280:2153-2156.

BRISSON A., C. J. SCANDELLA, A. BIENVENUE, P. DEVAUX, J. B. COHEN, and J. P. CHANGEUX, 1975. Interaction of a spin-labeled long chain acetylcholine with the cholinergic receptor protein in its membrane environment. *Proc. Natl. Acad. Sci. USA* 72:1087-1091.

BROCKES, J., D. BERG, and Z. W. HALL, 1976. The biochemical properties and regulation of acetylcholine receptor in normal and denervated muscle. *Cold Spring Harbor Symp. Quant. Biol.* 40:253-262.

BROCKES, J. P., and Z. W. HALL, 1975. Acetylcholine receptors in normal and denervated rat diaphragm muscle. I & II. *Biochemistry* 14:2092-2106.

BROWN, M. C., G. M. GOODWIN, and R. IRONTON, 1977. Prevention of motor nerve sprouting in botulinum toxin poisoned mouse soleus muscles by direct stimulation of the muscle. *J. Physiol.* 267:42P-43P.

BROWN, M. C., J. K. S. JANSEN, and D. VAN ESSEN, 1976. Polyneural innervation of skeletal muscle in newborn rats and its elimination during maturation. *J. Physiol.* 261:387-422.

BUCKINGHAM, M. E., D. CAPUT, A. COHEN, R. G. WHALEN, and F. GROS, 1974. The synthesis and stability of cytoplasmic messenger RNA during myoblast differentiation in culture. *Proc. Natl. Acad. Sci. USA* 71:1466-1470.

BURDEN, S., 1977. Development of the neuromuscular junction in the chick embryo: The number, distribution, and stability of acetylcholine receptor. *Dev. Biol.* 57:317-329.

BURT, A. M., and C. H. NARAYANAN, 1970. Effect of extrinsic neuronal connections on development of acetylcholinesterase and choline acetyltransferase activity in the ventral half of the chick spinal cord. *Exp. Neurol.* 29:201-210.

CARTAUD, J., 1975. Molecular organization of the excitable membrane of *Torpedo marmorata. Exp. Brain Res.* 23 (suppl.): 37.

CARTAUD, J., L. BENEDETTI, A. SOBEL, and J. P. CHANGEUX, 1978. A morphological study of the cholinergic receptor protein from *Torpedo marmorata* in its membrane environment and in its detergent extracted purified form. *J.*

Cell Sci. 29:313-337.

CHANG, C., and M. HUANG, 1975. Turnover of junctional and extrajunctional acetylcholine receptors of the rat diaphragm. *Nature* 253:643-644.

CHANGEUX, J. P., 1972. Le cerveau et l'évènement. *Communications* 18:37-47.

CHANGEUX, J. P., 1975. The cholinergic receptor protein from fish electric organ. In *Handbook of Psychopharmacology*, vol. 6, S. Snyder and L. Iversen, eds. New York: Plenum Pub., pp. 235-301.

CHANGEUX, J. P., L. BENEDETTI, J. P. BOURGEOIS, A. BRISSON, J. CARTAUD, P. DEVAUX, H. GRÜNHAGEN, M. MOREAU, J. L. POPOT, A. SOBEL, and M. WEBER, 1976. Some structural properties of the cholinergic receptor protein in its membrane environment relevant to its function as a pharmacological receptor. *Cold Spring Harbor Symp. Quant. Biol.* 40:203-210.

CHANGEUX, J. P., PH. COURRÈGE, and A. DANCHIN, 1973. A theory of the epigenesis of neuronal networks by selective stabilization of synapses. *Proc. Natl. Acad. Sci. USA* 70:2974-2978.

CHANGEUX, J. P., and A. DANCHIN, 1974. Apprendre par stabilisation sélective de synapses en cours de développement. In *L'Unité de l'homme*, E. Morin and M. Piatteli, eds. Paris: Le Seuil, pp. 320-357.

CHANGEUX, J. P., and A. DANCHIN, 1976. Selective stabilisation of developing synapses as a mechanism for the specification of neuronal networks. *Nature* 264:705-712.

CHANGEUX, J. P., M. HUCHET, and J. CARTAUD, 1972. Reconstitution partielle d'une membrane excitable après dissolution par le deoxycholate de sodium. *C.R. Acad. Sci. Paris* (D)274:122-125.

CHRISTIAN, C. N., M. DANIELS, H. SUGIYAMA, Z. VOGEL, L. JACQUES, and P. G. NELSON, 1978. A factor from neurons increases acetylcholine receptor aggregates on cultured muscle cells. *Proc. Natl. Acad. Sci. USA* 75:4011-4015.

COHEN, M. W., 1972. The development of neuromuscular connexions in the presence of d-tubocurarine. *Brain Res.* 41:457-463.

COHEN, J. B., 1977. Ligand-binding properties of membrane-bound cholinergic receptors of *Torpedo marmorata*. In *Molecular Specialization and Symmetry in Membranes*, A. K. Solomon, ed. Baltimore: University Park Press.

COHEN, J. B., and J. P. CHANGEUX, 1973. Interaction of a fluorescent ligand with membrane bound cholinergic receptor from *Torpedo marmorata. Biochemistry* 12:4855-4864.

COHEN, J. B., M. WEBER, and J. P. CHANGEUX, 1974. Effects of local anesthetics and calcium on the interaction of cholinergic ligands with the nicotinic receptor protein from *Torpedo marmorata. Mol. Pharmacol.* 10:904-932.

COHEN, J. B., M. WEBER, M. HUCHET, and J. P. CHANGEUX, 1972. Purification from *Torpedo marmorata* electric tissue of membrane fragments particularly rich in cholinergic receptor. *FEBS Lett.* 26:43-47.

COHEN, R. S., F. BLOMBERG, K. BERZINS, and P. SIEKEVITZ, 1977. The structure of postsynaptic densities isolated from dog cerebral cortex. I. Overall morphology and protein composition. *J. Cell Biol.* 74:181-203.

COHEN, S. A., and G. D. FISCHBACH, 1973. Regulation of muscle acetylcholine sensitivity by muscle activity in cell culture. *Science* 181:76-78.

COLLIN, R., 1906. Recherches cytologiques sur le développement de la cellule nerveuse. *Le Névraxe* 8:181-307.

COLQUHOUN, D., and H. RANG, 1976. Effects of inhibitors on the binding of iodinated α-bungarotoxin to acetylcholine receptors in rat muscle. *Mol. Pharmacol.* 12:519–535.

CONRADI, S., and L. O. RONNEVI, 1974. Ultrastructural evidence for spontaneous elimination of synaptic terminals on spinal motoneurons in the kitten. *Brain Res.* 80:335–339.

CONRADI, S., and L. O. RONNEVI, 1977. Ultrastructure and synaptology of the initial axon segment of cat spinal motoneurons during early postnatal development. *J. Neurocytol.* 6:195–210.

CORNER, M. A., and P. KWEE, 1976. Cyclic EEG and motility patterns during sleep in restrained infant rats. *Electroencephalogr. Clin. Neurophysiol.* 41:64–72.

COURRÈGE, P., J. M. LASRY, A. DANCHIN, and J. P. CHANGEUX, 1979. (Manuscript in preparation.)

COUTEAUX, R., 1972. Structure and cytochemical characteristics of the neuromuscular junction. In *Neuromuscular Blocking and Stimulating Agents* (IEPT, section 14), vol. 1, J. Cheymol, ed. New York: Pergamon, pp. 7–56.

COUTEAUX, R., and M. PÉCOT-DECHAVASSINE, 1968. Particularités structurales du sarcoplasme sous-neural. *C.R. Acad. Sci. Paris* (D) 266:8–10.

CRAIN, S. M., L. ALFEI, and E. R. PETERSON, 1970. Neurotransmission in cultures of adult human and rodent skeletal muscle after innervation *in vitro* by fetal rodent-spinal cord. *J. Neurobiol.* 1:471–489.

CRAIN, S. M., M. B. BORNSTEIN, and E. R. PETERSON, 1968. Maturation of cultured embryonic CNS tissue during chronic exposure to agents which prevent bioelectric activity. *Brain Res.* 8:363–372.

CRAIN, S. M., and E. R. PETERSON, 1971. Development of paired explants of fetal spinal cord and adult skeletal muscle during chronic exposure to curare and hemicholinium. *In Vitro* 6:373–389.

CREPEL, F., and J. MARIANI, 1976. Multiple innervation of Purkinje cells by climbing fibres in the cerebellum of the weaver mutant mouse. *J. Neurobiol.* 7:579–582.

CREPEL, F., J. MARIANI, and N. DELHAYE-BOUCHAUD, 1976. Evidence for a multiple innervation of Purkinje cells by climbing fibres in the immature rat cerebellum. *J. Neurobiol.* 7:567–578.

CRONE, H., and S. FREEMAN, 1972. The acetylcholinesterase activity of the denervated rat diaphragm. *J. Neurochem.* 19:1207–1208.

DALY, J. W., J. KARLE, C. W. MYERS, T. TOKUYAMA, J. A. WATERS, and B. WITKOP, 1971. Histrionicotoxins: Roentgen-ray analysis of the novel allenic and acetylenic spiro alkaloids isolated from a colombian frog, *Dendrobates histrionicus. Proc. Natl. Acad. Sci. USA* 68:1870–1875.

DECKER, J. D., 1967. Motility of the turtle embryo, *Chelydea serpentina* (Linné) *Science* 157:952–954.

DENNIS, M., 1975. Physiological properties of junctions between nerve and muscle developing during salamander limb regeneration. *J. Physiol.* 244:683–702.

DEVREOTES, P. N., and D. FAMBROUGH, 1975. Acetylcholine receptor turnover in membranes of developing muscle fibers. *J. Cell Biol.* 63:335–358.

DEVREOTES, P. N., and D. M. FAMBROUGH, 1976. Synthesis of acetylcholine receptors by cultured chick myotubes and denervated mouse extensor digitorum longus muscles. *Proc. Natl. Acad. Sci. USA* 73:161–164.

DEVREOTES, P. N., J. GARDNER, and D. FAMBROUGH, 1977. Kinetics of biosynthesis of acetylcholine receptor and subsequent incorporation into plasma membrane of cultured chick skeletal muscle. *Cell* 10:365–373.

DIAMOND, J., and R. MILEDI, 1962. A study of foetal and new-born rat muscle fibers. *J. Physiol.* 162:393–408.

DOLLY, J. O., E. X. ALBUQUERQUE, J. M. SARVEY, B. MALLICK, and E. A. BARNARD, 1977. Binding of perhydrohistrionicotoxin to the postsynaptic membrane of skeletal muscle in relation to its blockage of acetylcholine-induced depolarization. *Mol. Pharmacol.* 13:1–14.

DOYÈRE, L., 1840. Mémoire sur les tardigrades. *Ann. Sci. Nat.* (Ser. 2, Zoologie) 14:269–361.

DRACHMAN, D. B., 1963. The developing motor endplate: Pharmacological studies in the chick embryo. *J. Physiol.* 169:707–712.

DRACHMAN, D. B., 1967. Is acetylcholine the trophic neuromuscular transmitter? *Arch. Neurol.* 17:206–218.

DRACHMAN, D. B., 1968. The role of acetylcholine as a trophic neuromuscular transmitter. In *Growth of the Nervous System*, G. E. W. Wolstenholme and M. O'Connor, eds. London: J. & A. Churchill, pp. 251–273.

DRACHMAN, D. B., 1971. Neuromuscular transmission of trophic effects. *Ann. NY Acad. Sci.* 183:158–170.

DRACHMAN, D. B., 1972. Neurotrophic regulation of muscle cholinesterase: Effects of *Botulinum* toxin and denervation. *J. Physiol.* 226:619–627.

DRACHMAN, D. B., and F. WITZKE, 1972. Trophic regulation of acetylcholine sensitivity of muscle: Effect of electrical stimulation. *Science* 176:514–516.

DREYER, F., C. WALTHER, and K. PEPER, 1976. Junctional and extra-junctional receptors in normal and denervated frog muscle fibres. *Pflügers Arch.* 366:1–9.

DUCHEN, L. W., 1970. Hereditary motor end-plate disease in the mouse: A light and electron microscope study. *J. Neurol. Neurosurg. Psychiatr.* 33:238–250.

DUDAI, Y., M. HERZBERG, and I. SILMAN, 1973. Molecular structures of acetylcholinesterase from electric organ tissue of the electric eel. *Proc. Natl. Acad. Sci. USA* 70:2473–2476.

DUDAI, Y., and I. SILMAN, 1974. The effects of solubilization procedures on the release and molecular state of acetylcholinesterase from electric organ tissue. *J. Neurochem.* 23:1177–1187.

DUGUID, J. R., and M. A. RAFTERY, 1973. Fractionation and partial characterization of membrane particles from *Torpedo californica* electroplax. *Biochemistry* 12:3593–3597.

DUPONT, Y., J. COHEN, and J. P. CHANGEUX, 1974. X-ray diffraction study of membrane fragments rich in acetylcholine receptor protein prepared from the electric organ of *Torpedo marmorata. FEBS Lett.* 40:130–133.

EDWARDS, G., and H. L. FRISCH, 1976. A model for the localization of acetylcholine receptors at the muscle endplate. *J. Neurobiol.* 7:377–381.

ELDEFRAWI, A. T., M. E. ELDEFRAWI, E. X. ALBUQUERQUE, A. C. OLIVEIRA, N. MANSOUR, M. ADLER, J. W. DALY, G. B. BROWN, W. B. BURGERMEISTER, and B. WITKOP, 1977. Perhydrohistrionicotoxin: A potential ligand for the ion conductance modulator of the acetylcholine receptor. *Proc. Natl. Acad. Sci. USA* 74:2172–2176.

ELLISMAN, M., and T. RASH, 1977. Studies on excitable membranes. IV. Freeze-fracture examination of the membrane specialization at the neuromuscular junction and in the non-junctional sarcolemma after denervation. *Brain Res.* (in press).

EVANS, R. H., 1974. The entry of labelled calcium into the

innervated region of the mouse diaphragm muscle. *J. Physiol.* 240:517–533.

FAMBROUGH, D. M., 1970. Acetylcholine sensitivity of muscle fiber membranes: Mechanism of regulation by motoneurons. *Science* 168:372–373.

FAMBROUGH, D., 1976. Development of cholinergic innervation of skeletal, cardiac and smooth muscle. In *Biology of Cholinergic Function*, A. M. Goldberg and I. Hanin, eds. New York: Raven Press, pp. 101–160.

FERTUCK, H. C., and M. M. SALPETER, 1976. Quantitation of junctional and extrajunctional acetylcholine receptors by electron microscope autoradiography after ^{125}I α-bungarotoxin binding at mouse neuromuscular junction. *J. Cell Biol.* 69:144–158.

FILOGAMO, G., 1969. The normal regulation of the AChE activity of skeletal muscle and the influence of denervation and disease. *Excerpta Med. Int. Cong. Ser.* 199:709–713.

FILOGAMO, G., and G. GABELLA, 1966. Cholinesterase behavior in the denervated and reinnervated muscles. *Acta Anat.* 63:199–214.

FILOGAMO, G., and G. GABELLA, 1967. The development of neuromuscular correlations in vertebrates. *Arch. Biol. (Liège)* 78:9–60.

FISHBACH, G. D., 1970. Synaptic potentials recorded in cell cultures of nerve and muscle. *Science* 169:1331–1333.

FISHBACH, G. D., 1972. Synapse formation between dissociated nerve and muscle cells in low density cell cultures. *Dev. Biol.* 28:407–429.

FISCHBACH, G. D., D. K. BERG, S. A. COHEN, and E. FRANK, 1976. Enrichment of nerve-muscle synapses in spinal cord-muscle cultures and identification of relative peaks of ACh sensitivity at sites of transmitter release. *Cold Spring Harbor Symp. Quant. Biol.* 40:347–357.

FISCHBACH, G. D., and S. A. COHEN, 1973. The distribution of acetylcholine sensitivity over uninnervated and innervated muscle fibers grown in cell culture. *Dev. Biol.* 31:147.

FISCHBACH, G., and N. ROBBINS, 1971. Effect of chronic disuse of rat soleus neuromuscular junctions on postsynaptic membranes. *J. Neurophysiol.* 34:562–569.

FRANK, E., K. GAUTVIK, and H. SOMMERSCHILD, 1975. Cholinergic receptors at denervated mammalian endplates. *Acta Physiol. Scand.* 95:66.

FRANK, E., K. GAUTVIK, and H. SOMMERSCHILD, 1976. Persistence of junctional acetylcholine receptors following denervation. *Cold Spring Harbor Symp. Quant. Biol.* 40:275–281.

FREEMAN, J. A., 1977. Possible regulatory function of acetylcholine receptor in maintenance of retinotectal synapses. *Nature* 269:218–222.

FRIEDMAN, B. A., and J. A. POWELL, 1977. Method for maintenance of spontaneous membrane activity of cultured muscle. *J. Cell Biol.* 75:323a.

FULPIUS, B. W., 1976. Characterization, isolation and purification of cholinergic receptors. In *Motor Innervation of Muscle*, S. Thesleff, ed. London: Academic Press.

GAZE, R., 1970. *The Formation of Nerve Connections.* London and New York: Academic Press.

GERHART, J. C., 1970. A discussion of the regulatory properties of aspartate transcarbamylase from *Escherichia coli*. *Curr. Top. Cell. Reg.* 2:275–325.

GIACOBINI, G., G. FILOGAMO, M. WEBER, P. BOQUET, and J. P. CHANGEUX, 1973. Effects of a snake α-neurotoxin on the development of innervated motor muscles in chick embryo. *Proc. Natl. Acad. Sci. USA* 70:1708–1712.

GIACOBINI-ROBECCHI, M. G., G. GIACOBINI, G. FILOGAMO, and J. P. CHANGEUX, 1975. Effects of the type A toxin from *C. botulinum* on the development of skeletal muscles and of their innervation in chick embryo. *Brain Res.* 83:107–121.

GIACOBINI-ROBECCHI, M. G., G. GIACOBINI, G. FILOGAMO, and J. P. CHANGEUX, 1976. Effets comparés de l'injection chronique de toxine α de *Naja nigricollis* et de toxine botulinique A sur le développement des racines dorsales et ventrales de la moelle épinière d'embryons de poulet. *C.R. Acad. Sci. Paris* (D) 283:271–274.

GILLER, E. L., J. H. NEALE, P. N. BULLOCK, B. K. SCHRIER, and P. G. NELSON, 1977. Choline acetyltransferase activity of spinal cord cell cultures increased by co-culture with muscle and by muscle conditioned medium. *J. Cell Biol.* 74:16–29.

GILLER, E. L., B. K. SCHRIER, A. SHAINBERG, H. R. FISK, and P. G. NELSON, 1973. Choline acetyltransferase activity is increased in combined cultures of spinal cord and muscle cells from mice. *Science* 182:588–589.

GORDON, A. S., G. DAVIS, and I. DIAMOND, 1977. Phosphorylation of membrane proteins at a cholinergic synapse. *Proc. Natl. Acad. Sci. USA* 74:263–267.

GORDON, T., R. PERRY, A. R. TUFFERY, and G. VRBOVÁ, 1974. Possible mechanisms determining synapse formation in developing skeletal muscles of the chick. *Cell Tissue Res.* 115:13–25.

GORDON, T., R. PURVES, and G. VRBOVÁ, 1976. Nerve-muscle interaction: Differentiation of slow and fast chick muscle. In *Synaptogenesis*, L. Tauc, ed. Naturalia & Biologia Publishers, pp. 45–62.

GORDON, T., R. PURVES, and G. VRBOVÁ, 1977. Differentiation of electrical and contractile properties of slow and fast muscle fibres. *J. Physiol.* 269:535–547.

GRAMPP, W., J. B. HARRIS, and S. THESLEFF, 1972. Inhibition of denervation changes in skeletal muscle by blockers of protein synthesis. *J. Physiol.* 221:743–754.

GREENGARD, P., 1976. Possible role for cyclic nucleotides and phosphorylated membrane proteins in postsynaptic actions of neurotransmitters. *Nature* 260:101–108.

GRÜNHAGEN, H. H., and J. P. CHANGEUX, 1976. Studies on the electrogenic action of acetylcholine with *Torpedo marmorata* electric organ. 5. Qualitative kinetic study of the conformational transitions of the cholinergic receptor protein as revealed by quinacrine. *J. Mol. Biol.* 106:517–535.

GRÜNHAGEN, H., M. IWATSUBO, and J. P. CHANGEUX, 1977. Fast kinetic studies on the interaction of cholinergic agonists with the membrane-bound acetylcholine receptor from *Torpedo marmorata* as revealed by quinacrine fluorescence. *Eur. J. Biochem.* 80:225–242.

GUTH, L., R. W. ALBERS, and W. C. BROWN, 1964. Quantitative changes in cholinesterase activity of denervated muscle fibers and sole plates. *Exp. Neurol.* 10:236–250.

GUTH, L., and W. C. BROWN, 1965. Changes in cholinesterase activity following partial denervation, collateral reinnervation and hyperneurotization of muscle. *Exp. Neurol.* 13:198–205.

GUTMANN, E., V. HANZLIKOVA, and E. HOLECKOVA, 1969. Development of fast and slow muscles of the chicken *in vivo* and their latent period in tissue culture. *Exp. Cell Res.* 56:33–38.

GUTMANN, E., and J. Z. YOUNG, 1944. The reinnervation of muscle after various periods of atrophy. *J. Anat.* 78:15-43.

HALL, Z., 1973. Multiple forms of acetylcholinesterase and their distribution in endplate and non-endplate regions of rat diaphragm muscle. *J. Neurobiol.* 4:343-361.

HALL, Z., and R. KELLY, 1971. Enzymatic detachment of endplate acetylcholinesterase from muscle. *Nature [New Biol.]* 232:62-63.

HALL, Z., and C. G. REINESS, 1977. Electrical stimulation of denervated muscles reduces incorporation of methionine into the ACh receptor. *Nature* 268:655-657.

HAMBURGER, V., 1958. Regression versus peripheral control of differentiation in motor hypoplasia. *An. J. Anat.* 102:365-410.

HAMBURGER, V., 1970. Embryonic mobility in vertebrates. In *The Neurosciences: Second Study Program*, F. O. Schmitt, ed. New York: Rockefeller Univ. Press, pp. 141-151.

HAMBURGER, V., 1975. Cell death in the development of the lateral motor column of the chick embryo. *J. Comp. Neurol.* 160:535-546.

HAMBURGER, V., 1976. The developmental history of the motor neuron. The F. O. Schmitt Lecture in Neuroscience. *Neurosci. Res. Program Bull.* 15 (suppl.).

HARRIS, A. J., S. HEINEMANN, D. SCHUBERT, and H. TARAKIS, 1971. Trophic interaction between cloned tissue culture lines of nerve and muscle. *Nature* 231:296-301.

HARRIS-FLANAGAN, A. E., 1969. Differentiation and degeneration in the motor horn of the foetal mouse. *J. Morphol.* 129:281-305.

HARRISON, R. G., 1908. Embryonic transplantation and development of the nervous system. *Anat. Rec.* 2:367-410.

HARTZELL, C., and D. FAMBROUGH, 1973. Acetylcholine receptor production and incorporation into membranes of developing muscle fibers. *Dev. Biol.* 30:153-165.

HAZELBAUER, G. L., and J. P. CHANGEUX, 1974. Reconstitution of a chemically excitable membrane. *Proc. Natl. Acad. Sci. USA* 71:1479-1483.

HEBB, C., K. KRNJEVIĆ, and A. SILVER, 1964. Acetylcholine and choline acetyltransferase in the diaphragm of the rat. *J. Physiol.* 171:504-513.

HEIDMANN, T., and J. P. CHANGEUX, 1978. Structural and functional properties of the acetylcholine receptor protein in its purified and membrane-bound states. *Annu. Rev. Biochem.* 47:371-411.

HEINEMANN, S., S. BEVAN, R. KULLBERG, J. LINDSTROM, and J. RICE, 1977. Modulation of the acetylcholine receptor by anti-receptor antibody. *Proc. Natl. Acad. Sci. USA* 74:3090-3094.

HEUSER, J. E., T. S. REESE, and D. M. LANDIS, 1974. Functional changes in frog neuromuscular junction studied with freeze-fracture. *J. Neurocytol.* 3:108-131.

HNIK, P., I. JIRMANOVA, L. VYKLICKY, and J. ZEENA, 1967. Fast and slow muscles of the chick after nerve cross-union. *J. Physiol.* 193:309-325.

HOGAN, P. G., J. M. MARSHALL, and Z. HALL, 1976. Muscle activity decreases rate of degradation of α-bungarotoxin bound to extrajunctional acetylcholine receptors. *Nature* 261:328-330.

HOLLYDAY, M., and V. HAMBURGER, 1976. Reduction of the naturally occurring motor neuron loss by enlargement of the periphery. *J. Comp. Neurol.* 170:311-320.

HOOISMA, J., D. N. SLAAF, E. MEETER, and W. E. STEVENS, 1975. The innervation of chick striated muscle fibers by

the chick ciliary ganglion in tissue culture. *Brain Res.* 85:79-85.

HOOKER, D., 1952. *The Prenatal Origin of Behavior*. Lawrence: Univ. Kansas Press.

HUBBARD, J. I., J. MUSICK, and E. SILINSKY, 1972. Release of protein and ATP from stimulated myoneural junctions. In *Proc. INSERM Colloque: La transmission cholinergique de l'excitation*, pp. 187-195.

HUBEL, D. H., and T. N. WIESEL, 1977. Functional architecture of macaque monkey visual cortex. Ferrier Lecture. *Proc. R. Soc. Lond.* B 198:1-59.

HUGHES, A., 1961. Cell degeneration in the larval ventral horn of *Xenopus laevis* (Dandin). *J. Embryol. Exp. Morphol.* 9:269-284.

HUGHES, A., 1968. *Aspects of Neural Ontogeny*. London: Academic Press.

HUGHES, A., S. V. BRYANT, and A. BELLAIRS, 1967. Embryonic behavior in the lizard *Lacerta vivipara*. *J. Zool.* 153:139-152.

ISRAËL, M., and J. GAUTRON, 1969. Cellular and subcellular localization of acetylcholine in electric organs. *Symp. Int. Soc. Cell Biol.* 6.

ISRAËL, M., B. LESBATS, R. MANARANCHE, J. MARSAL, P. MASTOUR-FRACHON, and F. M. MEUNIER, 1977. Related changes in amounts of ACh and ATP in resting and active *Torpedo* nerve electroplaque synapses. *J. Neurochem.* 28:1259-1267.

JACOBSON, M., 1970. *Developmental Neurobiology*. New York: Holt, Rinehart & Winston.

JANSEN, J. K. S., D. C. VAN ESSEN, and M. C. BROWN, 1976. Formation and elimination of synapses in skeletal muscles of rat. *Cold Spring Harbor Symp. Quant. Biol.* 40:425-434.

KANO, M., and Y. SHIMADA, 1971. Innervation of skeletal muscle cells differentiated *in vitro* from chick embryo. *Brain Res.* 27:402-405.

KAO, I., and D. B. DRACHMAN, 1977. Myasthenic immunoglobulin accelerates acetylcholine receptor degradation. *Science* 196:527-529.

KARLIN, A., 1977. Current problems in acetylcholine receptor research. In *Parthogenesis of Human Muscular Dystrophies*, L. P. Rowland, ed. Amsterdam: Excerpta Medica.

KASAI, M., and J. P. CHANGEUX, 1971. *In vitro* excitation of purified membrane fragments by cholinergic agonists. I. Pharmacological properties of the excitable membrane fragments. II. The permeability change caused by cholinergic agonists. III. Comparison of the dose response curves to decamethonium with the corresponding binding curves of decamethonium to the cholinergic receptor. *J. Memb. Biol.* 6:1-80.

KATO, G., and J. P. CHANGEUX, 1976. Studies on the effect of histrionicotoxin on the monocellular electroplaque from *Electrophorus electricus* and on the binding of ^{3}H acetylcholine to membrane fragments from *Torpedo marmorata*. *Mol. Pharmacol.* 12:92-100.

KATZ, B., and R. MILEDI, 1972. The statistical nature of the acetylcholine potential and its molecular components. *J. Physiol.* 224:665-699.

KIDOKORO, Y., 1973. Development of action potentials in a clonal rat skeletal muscle cell line. *Nature [New Biol.]* 241:158-159.

KIDOKORO, Y., S. HEINEMANN, D. SCHUBERT, B. L. BRANDT, and F. G. KLIER, 1976. Synapse formation and neurotrophic effects on muscle cell lines. *Cold Spring Harbor Symp. Quant. Biol.* 40:373–388.

Ko, P. K., M. J. Anderson, and M. W. Cohen, 1977. Denervated skeletal muscle fibers develop discrete patches of high acetylcholine receptor density. *Science* 196:540–542.

Koslow, S. H., E. Giacobini, S. Kerpel-Fronius, and L. Olson, 1972. Cholinergic transmission in the hypoglossal reinnervated nictitating membrane of the cat: An enzymatic, histochemical and physiological study. *J. Pharmacol. Exp. Ther.* 180:664–671.

Krause, W., 1863. Uber die Endigung der Muskelnerven. *Z. Rationelle Med.* 18:136–140.

Kuffler, S. W., M. J. Dennis, and A. J. Harris, 1971. The development of chemosensitivity in extrasynaptic areas of the neuronal surface after denervation of parasympathetic ganglion cells in the heart of the frog. *Proc. R. Soc. Lond.* B177:555.

Kühne, W., 1887. Nene Untersuchungen über die motorische Nervendigungen. *Z. Biol.* 23:1–148.

Kuo, Z. Y., 1939. Studies in the physiology of the embryonic nervous system. I. Effect of curare on motor activity of the chick embryo. *J. Exp. Zool.* 82:371–396.

Laing, N., and M. Prestige, 1978. Prevention of spontaneous motor neurone death in chick embryos. *J. Physiol.* 282:33P–34P.

Land, B. R., T. R. Podleski, E. E. C. Salpeter, and M. M. Salpeter, 1977. Acetylcholine receptor distribution on myotubes in culture correlated to acetylcholine sensitivity. *J. Physiol.* 269:155–176.

Landmesser, L., 1971. Contractile and electrical responses of vagus-innervated frog sartorius muscles. *J. Physiol.* 213:707–725.

Landmesser, L., 1972. Pharmacological properties, cholinesterase activity and anatomy of nerve-muscle junctions in vagus-innervated frog sartorius. *J. Physiol.* 220:243–256.

Letinsky, M. S., 1974a. The development of nerve-muscle junctions in *Rana catesbeiana* tadpoles. *Dev. Biol.* 40:129–153.

Letinsky, M. S., 1974b. Physiological properties of developing frog tadpole nerve-muscle junctions during repetitive stimulation. *Dev. Biol.* 40:154–161.

Levi-Montalcini, R., and F. Visintini, 1938. Azione del curaro, della stricnina, dell'eserina, dell'acetilcolina sulla transmissione dell'influsso nell'embrione di pollo dal 4 all'8 giorno d'incubazione. *Boll. Soc. Ital. Biol. Sper.* 13:979–981.

Levinthal, F., E. Macagno, and C. Levinthal, 1976. Anatomy and development of identified cells in isogenic organisms. *Cold Spring Harbor Symp. Quant. Biol.* 40:321–332.

Lichtman, J. W., 1977. The reorganization of synaptic connexions in the rat submandibular ganglion during postnatal development. *J. Physiol.* 273:155–177.

Liévremont, M., M. Czajka, and M. Tazieff-Dapierre, 1968. Etude *in situ* d'une fixation de calcium et de sa libération à la jonction neuromusculaire. *C.R. Acad. Sci. Paris* [D] 267:1988–1991.

Lindstrom, J., 1976. Antibodies to receptors for acetylcholine and other hormones. In *Receptors and Recognition*, vol. 3, P. Cuatrecasas and M. F. Greaves, eds. New York: Halsted Press, pp. 1–45.

Llinás, R., J. R. Blinks, and C. Nicholson, 1972. Calcium transient in presynaptic terminal at squid giant synapses: Detection with aequorin. *Science* 176:1127.

Lomo, T., and J. Rosenthal, 1971. Development of acetylcholine sensitivity in muscle following blockage of nerve impulses. *J. Physiol.* 216:52P.

Lomo, T., and J. Rosenthal, 1972. Control of ACh sensitivity by muscle activity in the rat. *J. Physiol.* 221:493–513.

Lomo, T., and C. R. Slater, 1976. Control of neuromuscular synapse formation. In *Synaptogenesis*, L Tauc, ed. Naturalia & Biologia Publishers, pp. 9–31.

Lomo, T., and R. H. Westgaard, 1975. Further studies on the control of ACh sensitivity by activity in the rat. *J. Physiol.* 252:603–626.

Lomo, T., and R. H. Westgaard, 1976. Control of ACh sensitivity in rat muscle fibers. *Cold Spring Harbor Symp. Quant. Biol.* 40:263–274.

Lomo, T., R. H. Westgaard, and H. A. Dahl, 1974. Contractile properties of muscle: Control by pattern of muscle activity in the rat. *Proc. R. Soc. Lond.* B187:99–103.

Lwebuga-Musaka, J. S., S. Lappi, and P. Taylor, 1976. Molecular forms of acetylcholinesterase from *Torpedo californica*: Their relationship to synaptic membranes. *Biochemistry* 15:1425–1434.

McArdle, J. J., 1975. Complex endplate potentials at regenerating neuromuscular junction of the rat. *Exp. Neurol.* 49:629–638.

McCann, W. F. X., and T. L. Rosenberry, 1977. Identification of discrete disulfide linked oligomers which distinguish 18S from 14S acetylcholinesterase. *Arch. Biochem. Biophys.*

Mariani, J., F. Crepel, K. Mikoshiba, J. P. Changeux, and C. Sotelo, 1977. Anatomical, physiological and biochemical studies of the cerebellum from *reeler* mutant mouse. *Philos. Trans. R. Soc. Lond.* B281:1–28.

Massoulié, J., and F. Riéger, 1969. L'acétylcholinestérase des organes électriques de poissons, Torpille et Gymnote; complexes membranaires. *Eur. J. Biochem.* 11:441–455.

Massoulié, J., F. Riéger, and S. Tsuji, 1970. Solubilisation de l'acétylcholinestérase des organes électriques de Gymnote. Action de la trypsine. *Eur. J. Biochem.* 14:430–439.

Massoulié, J., F. Riéger, and S. Bon, 1971. Espéces acétylcholinestérasiques globulaires et allongées des organes électriques de poissons. *Eur. J. Biochem.* 21:542–551.

Merlie, J., J. P. Changeux, and F. Gros, 1978. Skeletal muscle acetylcholine receptor: Purification, characterization and turnover in muscle cell cultures. *J. Biol. Chem.* 253:2882–2891.

Merlie, J., and F. Gros, 1976. *In vitro* myogenesis, expression of muscle specific function in the absence of cell fusion. *Exp. Cell Res.* 97:406–412.

Merlie, J. P., A. Sobel, J. P. Changeux, and F. Gros, 1975. Synthesis of acetylcholine receptor during differentiation of cultured embryonic muscle cells. *Proc. Natl. Acad. Sci. USA* 72:4028–4032.

Meunier, J. C., R. W. Olsen, and J. P. Changeux, 1972. Studies on the cholinergic receptor protein from *Electrophorus electricus*. III. Effect of detergents on some hydrodynamic properties of the receptor protein in solution. *FEBS Lett.* 24:63–68.

Meunier, J. C., R. W. Olsen, A. Menez, P. Fromageot, P. Boquet, and J. P. Changeux, 1972. Studies on the cholinergic receptor protein of *Electrophorus electricus*. II. Some physical properties of the receptor protein revealed by a tritiated α-toxin from *Naja nigricollis* venom. *Biochemistry* 11:1200-1210.

MEUNIER, J. C., R. W. OLSEN, A. MENEZ, J. L. MORGAT, P. FROMAGEOT, A. M. RONSERAY, P. BOQUET, and J. P. CHANGEUX, 1971. Quelques propriétés physiques de la protéine réceptrice de l'acétylcholine étudiées à l'aide d'une neurotoxine radioactive. *C.R. Acad. Sci. Paris* [D] 273:595-598.

MEUNIER, J. C., R. SEALOCK, R. OLSEN, and J. P. CHANGEUX, 1974. Purification and properties of the cholinergic receptor from *Electrophorus electricus* electric tissue. *Eur. J. Biochem.* 45:371-394.

MICHAELSON, D. M., and M. A. RAFTERY, 1974. Purified acetylcholine receptor: Its reconstitution to a chemically excitable membrane. *Proc. Natl. Acad. Sci. USA* 71:4768-4772.

MILEDI, R., 1960a. The ACh sensitivity of frog muscle fibers after complete or partial denervation. *J. Physiol.* 151:1-23.

MILEDI, R., 1960b. Junctional and extrajunctional ACh receptors in skeletal muscle fibers. *J. Physiol.* 151:24-30.

MILEDI, R., and C. R. SLATER, 1968. Electrophysiology and electron microscopy of rat neuromuscular junctions after nerve degeneration. *Proc. R. Soc. Lond.* B169:289-306.

MILEDI, R., and C. R. SLATER, 1970. On the degeneration of rat neuromuscular junctions after nerve section. *J. Physiol.* 207:507-528.

MILEDI, R., and E. STEFANI, 1969. Non selective re-innervation of slow and fast muscle fibres in the rat. *Nature* 222:570-571.

MONOD, J., J. P. CHANGEUX, and F. JACOB, 1963. Allosteric proteins and cellular control systems. *J. Mol. Biol.* 6:306-328.

MONOD, J., J. WYMAN, and J. P. CHANGEUX, 1965. On the nature of allosteric transitions: A plausible model. *J. Mol. Biol.* 12:88-118.

MUSICK, J., and J. I. HUBBARD, 1972. Release of protein from mouse motor nerve terminals. *Nature* 237:279-281.

NEHER, E., and B. SAKMANN, 1976. Noise analysis of drug induced voltage clamps currents in denervated frog muscle fibres. *J. Physiol.* 258:705-729.

NEHER, E., and J. H. STEINBACH, 1978. Local anesthetics block currents through single acetylcholine-receptor channels. *J. Physiol.* 227:153-176.

NEUBIG, R. R., E. K. KRODEL, N. D. BOYD, and J. B. COHEN, 1979. Acetylcholine and local anesthetic binding to *Torpedo* nicotinic postsynaptic membranes after removal of nonreceptor peptides. *Proc. Natl. Acad. Sci. USA* (in press).

NICKEL, E., and L. T. POTTER, 1973. Ultrastructure of isolated membranes of *Torpedo* electric tissue. *Brain Res.* 57:508-517.

NICKEL, E., and P. G. WASER, 1968. Electronenmikroskopische interam diaphragma der maus nach einseitiger phrenikotomie. *Z. Zellforsch. Mikrosk. Anat.* 88:278-296.

NURSE, C. A., and P. H. O'LAGUE, 1975. Formation of cholinergic synapses between dissociated sympathetic neurons and skeletal myotubes of the rat in cell culture. *Proc. Natl. Acad. Sci. USA* 72:1955-1959.

NYSTRÖM, B., 1968. Post-natal development of motor nerve terminals in "slow-red" and "fast-white" cat muscles. *Acta Neurol. Scand.* 44:363-383.

OBATA, K., 1977. Development of neuromuscular transmission in culture with a variety of neurons and in the presence of cholinergic substances and tetrodotoxin. *Brain Res.* 119:141-153.

ORCI, L., A. PERRELET, and Y. DUNANT, 1974. A peculiar substructure in the postsynaptic membrane of *Torpedo* electroplaque. *Proc. Natl. Acad. Sci. USA* 71:307-310.

PATRICK, J., S. HEINEMANN, J. LINDSTROM, D. SCHUBERT, and J. STEINBACH, 1972. Appearance of acetylcholine receptors during differentiation of a myogenic cell line. *Proc. Natl. Acad. Sci. USA* 69:2762-2766.

PATRICK, J., S. HEINEMANN, and D. SCHUBERT, 1978. Biology of cultured nerve and muscle. Submitted for publication.

PATRICK, J., J. LINDSTROM, B. CULP, and J. McMILLAN, 1973. Studies on purified eel acetylcholine receptor and antiacetylcholine receptor antibody. *Proc. Natl. Acad. Sci. USA* 70:3334.

PATRICK, J., J. McMILLAN, H. WOLFSON, and J. O'BRIEN, 1977. Acetylcholine receptor metabolism in a non-fusing muscle cell line. *J. Biol. Chem.* 252:2143-2153.

PATTERSON, B., and J. PRIVES, 1973. Appearance of acetylcholine receptor in differentiating cultures of embryonic chick breast muscle. *J. Cell Biol.* 59:241-245.

PATTERSON, P., 1978. Environmental determination of autonomic neurotransmitter junctions. *Annu. Rev. Neurosci.* 1 (in press).

PATTERSON, P. H., and L. L. Y. CHUN, 1974. The influence of non-neuronal cells on catecholamine and acetylcholine synthesis and accumulation in cultures of dissociated sympathetic neurons. *Proc. Natl. Acad. Sci. USA* 71:3607-3610.

PEPER, K., E. DREYER, C. SANDRI, K. AKERT, and H. MOOR, 1974. Structure and ultrastructure of the frog motor endplate. A freeze-etching study. *Cell Tissue Res.* 149:347-455.

PITTMAN, R. H., and R. W. OPPENHEIM, 1978. *Nature* 271:364-365.

PODLESKI, T. R., D. AXELROD, P. RAVDIN, I. GREENBERG, M. JOHNSON, and M. SALPETER, 1978. Nerve extract induces increase and redistribution of acetylcholine receptors on cloned muscle cell. *Proc. Natl. Acad. Sci. USA* 75:2035-2039.

POPOT, J. L., R. A. DEMEL, A. SOBEL, L. VAN DEENEN, and J. P. CHANGEUX, 1977. Affinité préférentielle de la protéine réceptrice de l'acétylcholine pour certains lipides révélée par la méthode des monocouches. *C.R. Acad. Sci. Paris* [D] 285:1005-1008.

POPOT, J. L., P. A. DEMEL, A. SOBEL, L. VAN DEENEN, and J. P. CHANGEUX, 1978. Interaction of the acetylcholine (nicotinic) receptor protein from *Torpedo marmorata* electric organ with monolayers of pure lipids. *Eur. J. Biochem.* 85:27-42.

POPOT, J. L., H. SUGIYAMA, and J. P. CHANGEUX, 1976. Studies on the electrogenic action of acetylcholine with *Torpedo marmorata* electric organ. 2. The permeability response *in vitro* of the receptor-rich membrane fragments to cholinergic agonists. *J. Mol. Biol.* 106:469-483.

PORTER, C. W., and E. A. BARNARD, 1975. The density of cholinergic receptors at the endplate postsynaptic membrane: Ultrastructural studies in two mammalian species. *J. Membrane Biol.* 20:31-48.

POWELL, J. A., and B. A. FRIEDMAN, 1977. Electrical membrane activity: Effect on distribution, incorporation and degradation of acetylcholine receptors in the membranes of cultured muscle. *J. Cell. Biol.* 75:321a.

PRESTIGE, M. L., 1970. Differentiation, degeneration and the role of the periphery: Quantitative considerations. In *The Neurosciences: Second Study Program,* F. O. Schmitt, ed. New York: Rockefeller Univ. Press, pp. 73–82.

PRIVES, J. A., 1977. Biosynthesis of acetylcholine receptor during differentiation of embryonic muscle cells in culture. Institut Pasteur–Weizmann Institute Symposium on Structure and Development of the Nervous System. Abstract.

PRIVES, J. M., and B. M. PATTERSON, 1974. Differentiation of cell membranes in cultures of embryonic chick breast muscle. *Proc. Natl. Acad. Sci. USA* 71:3208–3211.

PRIVES, J., I. SILMAN, and A. AMSTERDAM, 1976. Appearance and disappearance of acetylcholine receptor during differentiation of chick skeletal muscle *in vitro. Cell* 7:543–550.

PURO, D., and M. NIRENBERG, 1976. On the specificity of synapse formation. *Proc. Natl. Acad. Sci. USA* 73:3544–3588.

RAFTERY, M. A., J. SCHMIDT, D. G. CLARK, and R. G. WOLCOTT, 1971. Demonstration of a specific α-bungarotoxin binding component in *Electrophorus electricus* electroplax membranes. *Biochem. Biophys. Res. Commun.* 45:1622–1629.

RAFTERY, M. A., R. L. VANDLEN, K. L. REED, and T. LEE, 1976. Characterization of *Torpedo californica* acetylcholine receptor: Its subunit composition and ligand-binding properties. *Cold Spring Harbor Symp. Quant. Biol.* 40:193–202.

RAKIC, P., 1977. Prenatal development of the visual system in the rhesus monkey. *Philos. Trans. R. Soc. Lond.* B278:245–260.

RAMÓN Y CAJAL, S., 1929. *Studies on Vertebrate Neurogenesis.* Springfield, IL: Charles C Thomas.

RASH, J. E., and M. H. ELLISMAN, 1974. Studies of excitable membranes. *J. Cell Biol.* 63:567–586.

RASMUSSEN, H., 1970. Cell communication, calcium ion and cyclic adenosine monophosphate. *Science* 190:101–108.

REDFERN, P. A., 1970. Neuromuscular transmission in newborn rats. *J. Physiol.* 209:701–709.

REGER, J. F., 1959. Studies on the fine structure of normal and denervated neuromuscular junctions from mouse gastrocnemius. *J. Ultrastruct. Res.* 2:269–282.

RIÉGER, F., S. BON, J. MASSOULIÉ, and J. CARTAUD, 1973. Observation par microscopie électronique des formes allongées et globulaires de l'acétylcholinestérase de Gymnote (*Electrophorus electricus*). *Eur. J. Biochem.* 34:539–547.

RIÉGER, F., A. FAIVRE-BAUMAN, P. BENDA, and M. VIGNY, 1976. Molecular forms of acetylcholinesterase: Their de novo synthesis in mouse neuroblastoma cells. *J. Neurochem.* 27:121–129.

RILEY, D. A., 1976. Multiple axon branches innervating single endplates of kitten soleus myofibers. *Brain Res.* 110:158–161.

RIPLEY, K. L., and R. R. PROVINE, 1972. Neural correlation of embryonic motility in the chick. *Brain Res.* 45:127–134.

ROBBINS, N., and T. YONEZAWA, 1971. Physiological studies during formation and development of rat neuromuscular junctions in tissue culture. *J. Gen. Physiol.* 58:467–481.

ROMANES, G. J., 1946. Motor localization and the effects of nerve injury on the ventral horn cells of the spinal cord. *J. Anat.* 80:117–131.

ROSENBERG, P., E. A. MACKEY, H. B. HIGMAN, and W. D. DETTBARN, 1964. Choline acetylase and cholinesterase activity in denervated electroplax. *Biochim. Biophys. Acta* 82:266–275.

ROSENBERRY, T. L., and J. N. RICHARDSON, 1977. Structure of 18S and 14S acetylcholinesterase. Identification of collagen-like subunits that are linked by disulfide bonds to catalytic subunits. *Biochemistry* 16:3550–3558.

ROSENBLUDT, J., 1974. Substructure of amphibian motor endplate. *J. Cell Biol.* 62:755–766.

ROSENBLUDT, J., 1975. Synaptic membrane structure in *Torpedo* electric organ. *J. Neurocytol.* 4:697–712.

ROSS, M. J., M. W. KLYMKOVSKY, D. A. AGARD, and R. M. STROUD, 1977. *J. Mol. Biol.* 116:635–659.

ROUGET, M., 1862. Note sur la terminaison des nerfs moteurs dans les muscles chez les reptiles, les oiseaux et les mammifères. *J. Physiol.* (Paris) 5:574–593.

ROUSSELET, A., and P. P. DEVAUX, 1977. Saturation transfer electron paramagnetic resonance on membrane-bound proteins. II. Absence of rotational diffusion of the cholinergic receptor protein in *Torpedo marmorata* membrane fragments. *Biochem. Biophys. Res. Comm.* 78:448–454.

SALPETER, M. M., 1967. Electron microscope radio autography as a quantitative tool in enzyme cytochemistry. I. The distribution of acetylcholinesterase at motor endplates of a vertebrate twitch muscle. *J. Cell Biol.* 32:379–389.

SALPETER, M. M., 1969. Electron microscope radio autography as a quantitative tool in enzyme cytochemistry. II. The distribution of DFP-reacting sites at motor endplates of a vertebrate twitch muscle. *J. Cell Biol.* 42:122–134.

SCHUBERT, D., S. HEINEMANN, and Y. KIDOKORO, 1977. Cholinergic metabolism and synapse formation by a rat nerve cell line. *Proc. Natl. Acad. Sci. USA* 74:2579–2583.

SHAINBERG, A., and M. BURSTEIN, 1976. Decrease of acetylcholine receptor synthesis in muscle culture by electrical stimulation. *Nature* 264:368–369.

SHAINBERG, A., S. A. COHEN, and P. NELSON, 1976. Induction of acetylcholine receptor in muscle cultures. *Pflüger's Arch.* 361:255–261.

SILMAN, H. I., and A. KARLIN, 1967. Effect of local pH changes caused by substrate hydrolysis on the activity of membrane-bound acetylcholinesterase. *Proc. Natl. Acad. Sci. USA* 58:1164.

SIMANTOV, R., and L. SACHS, 1973. Regulation of acetylcholine receptor in relation to acetylcholinesterase in neuroblastoma cells. *Proc. Natl. Acad. Sci. USA* 70:2902–2905.

SISSONS, H., 1963. In *Research in Muscular Dystrophy.* London: Pitman, pp. 88–98.

SLAAF, D., 1977. Electrophysiological characterization in tissue culture of striated muscle cells innervated by ciliary neurons. Ph.D. dissertation, Utrecht.

SLAAF, D. W., J. HOOISMA, R. VAN RULER, and W. F. STEVENS, 1977. Acetylcholine sensitivity of chick muscle cells innervated in tissue culture. Abstract.

SOBEL, A., A. HEIDMANN, and J. P. CHANGEUX, 1977. Purification d'une protéine liant la quinacrine et l'histrionicotoxine à partir de fragments de membranes riches en récepteur cholinergique de *Torpedo marmorata.* *C.R. Acad. Sci. Paris* 285D:1255–1258.

SOBEL, A., T. HEIDMANN, J. HOFLER, and J. P. CHANGEUX, 1978. Distinct protein components from *Torpedo marmorata* membranes carry the acetylcholine receptor site and the binding site for local anesthetics and histrionicotoxin. *Proc. Natl. Acad. Sci. USA* 75:510–514.

STEINBACH, J. H., A. J. HARRIS, J. PATRICK, D. SCHUBERT, and S. HEINEMANN, 1973. Nerve-muscle interaction *in vitro*: Role of acetylcholine. *J. Gen. Physiol.* 62:255–270.

STEINBACH, J. H., and S. HEINEMANN, 1973. Nerve-muscle interaction in clonal cell culture. In *Exploratory Concepts in Muscular Dystrophy*, vol. 2. Amsterdam: Excerpta Medica, pp. 161–169.

STENT, G., 1973. A physiological mechanism for Hebb's postulate of learning. *Proc. Natl. Acad. Sci. USA* 70:997–1001.

STINNAKRE, J., and L. TAUC, 1973. Calcium influx in active *Aplysia* neuron detected by injected aequorin. *Nature [New Biol.]* 242:113–115.

SUGIYAMA, H. P., P. BENDA, J. C. MEUNIER, and J. P. CHANGEUX, 1973. Immunological characterisation of the cholinergic receptor protein from *Electrophorus electricus*. *FEBS Lett.* 35:124–128.

SYTKOWSKI, A. J., Z. VOGEL, and M. W. NIRENBERG, 1973. Development of acetylcholine receptor clusters on cultured muscle cells. *Proc. Natl. Acad. Sci. USA* 70:270–274.

TAKEUCHI, N., 1963. Effects of calcium on the conductance change of the endplate membrane during the action of transmitter. *J. Physiol.* 167:141–155.

TEICHBERG, V., and J. P. CHANGEUX, 1976. Presence of two forms with different isoelectric points of the acetylcholine receptor in the electric organ of *Electrophorus electricus* and their catalytic interconversion *in vitro*. *FEBS Lett.* 67:264–268.

TEICHBERG, V., and J. P. CHANGEUX, 1977. Evidence for protein phosphorylation and dephosphorylation in membrane fragments isolated from the electric organ of *Electrophorus electricus*. *FEBS Lett.* 74:71–76.

TEICHBERG, V. I., I. SILMAN, D. BEITSCH, and D. RESHEFF, 1975. A β-D-galactoside binding protein from electric organ tissue of *Electrophorus electricus*. *Proc. Natl. Acad. Sci. USA* 72:1383.

TEICHBERG, V., A. SOBEL, and J. P. CHANGEUX, 1977. *In vitro* phosphorylation of acetylcholine receptor. *Nature* 267:540–542.

TELLO, F., 1917. Genesis de las terminaciones nerviosas motrices y sensitivas. *Trav. Lab. Invest. Biol. Univ. Mad.* 15:101.

TELLO, F., 1923. Les differenciations neuronales dans l'embryon du poulet pendant les premiers jours de l'incubation. *Trav. Lab. Rech. Biol. Univ. Madrid* 21:1–93.

TENG, N. N. H., and M. Y. FISZMAN, 1976. Appearance of acetylcholine receptors in cultured myoblasts prior to fusion. *J. Supramol. Struct.* 4:381–387.

TOMKINS, G., 1975. The metabolic code. *Science* 189:760–763.

TOWER, S., 1939. The reaction of muscle to denervation. *Physiol. Rev.* 19:1–48.

TRACY, H. C., 1926. The development of motility and behavior reactions in the toad fish (*Opsanus tau*). *J. Comp. Neurol.* 40:253–369.

VIGNY, M., J. KOENIG, and F. RIÉGER, 1976. The motor endplate specific form of acetylcholinesterase: Appearance during embryogenesis and re-innervation of rat muscle. *J. Neurochem.* 27:1347–1353.

VOGEL, Z., and M. P. DANIELS, 1976. Ultrastructure of acetylcholine receptor clusters on cultured muscle fibres. *J. Cell Biol.* 69:501–507.

VOGEL, Z., A. J. SYTKOWSKI, and M. W. NIRENBERG, 1972. Acetylcholine receptors of muscle cells grown *in vitro*. *Proc. Natl. Acad. Sci. USA* 69:3180–3184.

WEBER, M., and J. P. CHANGEUX, 1974. Binding of *Naja nigricollis* ³H-α-toxin to membrane fragments from *Electrophorus* and *Torpedo* electric organs. 1. Binding of the tritiated α-neurotoxin in the absence of effector. 2. Effect of the cholinergic agonists and antagonists on the binding of the tritiated α-neurotoxin. 3. Effects of local anaesthetics on the binding of the tritiated α-neurotoxin. *Mol. Pharmacol.* 10:1–40.

WESTERMAN, R. A., D. M. LEWIS, J. BAGUST, G. EDJEHADI, and D. PALLOT, 1972. Communication between nerves and muscles: Postnatal development in kitten hindlimb fast and slow twitch muscle. In *Memory and Transfer of Information*, H. P. Zippel, ed. New York: Plenum.

WHITTAKER, V. P., 1973. The biochemistry of synaptic transmission. *Naturwissenschaften* 60:281–289.

WIEDMER, T., V. BRODBECK, P. ZAHLER, and B. W. FULPIUS, 1978. *Biochim. Biophys. Acta* 506:161–172.

WOLPERT, L., and J. H. LEWIS, 1975. Towards a theory of development. *Fed. Proc.* 34:14–20.

ZELENA, J., and I. JIRMANOVA, 1973. Ultrastructure of chicken slow muscle after nerve cross union. *Exp. Neurol.* 38:272–285.

Notes added in proof

1 (p. 753). Recently Neubig et al. (1979) have reported that the 43K protein can be extracted from the AChR-rich membranes by treatment at pH 11, *in the absence of detergent*, and without loss of α-toxin binding sites. Interestingly, the alkaline-extracted membranes still bind a radioactive local anesthetic, [¹⁴C]-Meproadifen, in a manner similar to and with the same stoichiometry as the native membranes. Since in the alkali-treated membranes only the receptor peptides persist, the pharmacological action of local anesthetics must be carried out by one of these peptides rather than by the 43K protein.

2 (p. 760). Indeed, in cultures of muscles from a dystrophic strain of mouse, a similar regulation is observed in the absence of mechanical contraction (Powell and Friedman, 1977; Friedman and Powell, 1977). Finally, addition of dibutyryl cyclic GMP slows down AChR synthesis (Betz and Changeux, 1979), indicating that cyclic GMP might be one of the signals involved in the coupling between electrical activity and AChR synthesis.

3 (p. 766). The simplest interpretation of this result is that, since the skeletal muscles become atrophic and sometimes even disappear, a central hypoplasia or degeneration occurs which resembles that found after limb-bud extirpation (Hamburger, 1958). A rather different effect of chronic blocking of the neuromuscular junction in developing chick embryo has been observed when the total number of motoneuron cell bodies is counted in the lateral motor columns of the spinal cord. Prolonged paralysis does significantly prevent, or delay, the spontaneous death of the motoneurons (Pittman and Oppenheim, 1978; Laing and Prestige, 1978).

45 Synaptic-Membrane Differentiation

KARL H. PFENNINGER

ABSTRACT Comparison of synaptic membranes with axonal growth-cone and target-cell plasmalemma indicates that synaptogenesis is a process of localized membrane differentiation initiated by the recognition event. Current data suggest that recognition may occur by cell surface interaction involving carbohydrates. This appears all the more likely in view of the identification of a neuron-type-specific surface carbohydrate code. Maintenance of this code at the tip of the growing and advancing neurite is crucial to such a mechanism, and it may be achieved by localized insertion of patches of preassembled membrane carrying the full carbohydrate complement. Several possible mechanisms of membrane differentiation for synaptogenesis are considered. Although the factors controlling this process are not known, it seems likely that the future synaptic partners mutually influence one another's differentiation and that expression of specific synaptic-membrane properties may be the result of selective genome readout controlled by the recognition event.

Introduction

DURING BRAIN development and the formation of neuronal networks, nerve cells go through a series of differentiative steps (see Cowan, this volume). This chapter is concerned with the phase of differentiation during which an axon emerges from the neuron, finds its way to the proper target cell, recognizes it, and forms a synapse with it. This series of events appears to be quite complex, particularly when the following points are considered: (1) nerve outgrowth is a very rapid process; (2) the elongating axon is tipped with a unique structure, the growth cone; (3) synaptogenesis replaces the growth cone by an entirely different type of structure, the synaptic nerve terminal; and (4) recognition decides not only whether a synapse shall be made but also what type of synapse shall be formed. For analysis of this series of phenomena, it is essential to subdivide the different events into ever smaller, though still measurable, steps, to reach eventually the level of molecular mechanisms. While we are just barely able to recognize the molecular level as a distant, hazy shape, we can give—at best—only fragmentary answers to me-

chanistic questions. However, it is possible today to identify the important questions more clearly than before; as a consequence, we can postulate testable hypotheses.

From today's perspective, the important questions regarding synaptogenetic mechanisms may be grouped into three categories: (1) What kind of cellular event is synaptogenesis? (2) What types of mechanisms are involved in the formation of a synapse? (3) What controls synaptogenesis; that is, what kind of language do future synaptic partner cells use to interact with each other, and what type of additional controlling factors are involved?

Although the process of synaptogenesis can be described in fair detail as a morphological phenomenon, we still have great difficulty with questions of mechanism and control. Recent studies on the properties and dynamics of cell surface molecules in the growing neuron form an important background of this discussion, because they seem to open up new avenues that may well lead eventually to an understanding of at least some of the mechanisms of synaptogenesis. Currently available data characterizing plasma membranes in synapse formation deal primarily with the presynaptic element; accordingly, this chapter focuses on properties of the elongating neurite, the axonal growth cone, and the mature nerve ending.

The phenomenon of synaptogenesis

The membrane properties of mature synapses and axonal growth cones, as well as the morphological steps of the process of synapse formation, have been described in several recent reviews (Pfenninger, 1973, 1977, 1978; Elfvin, 1976; Pfenninger and Rees, 1976; Rees, 1978), so that we need deal with only the major points here.

SYNAPTIC MEMBRANES The synaptic nerve terminal is the distal secretory portion of the neuron (Figures 1A, 2A). It contains among its most prominent organelles synaptic vesicles for the storage of neurotransmitter (Geffen and Livett, 1971; Holtzman, 1977). Its plasmalemma exhibits nerve activity de

KARL H. PFENNINGER Department of Anatomy, Columbia University, College of Physicians and Surgeons, New York, NY 10032

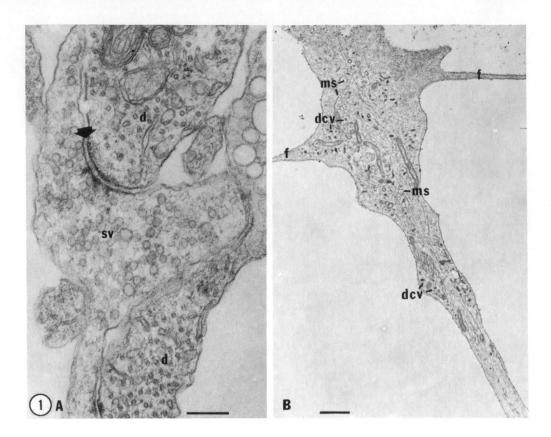

FIGURE 1 Two types of axonal ending, a synapse (A) and a growth cone (B), as seen in thin section. Whereas the synaptic terminal is characterized by electron-dense membrane specializations (arrow) and synaptic vesicles (sv), the nerve growth cone exhibits none of these structures. Instead, microfilament-filled filopodia (f), membrane sacs (ms) similar to smooth endoplasmic reticulum, and large, dense-core vesicles (dcv) are typical (this growth cone was labeled with ferritin–wheat-germ agglutinin prior to fixation, and some internalization of the label has occurred). From rat spinal cord (A) and superior cervical ganglion cultures (B). (d, dendritic profiles. Calibration, 0.2 μm for A and 1 μm for B.)

pendent sites for interaction with these vesicles and the concomitant release of transmitter (Pfenninger et al., 1972; Streit et al., 1972; Dreyer et al., 1973; Heuser, Reese, and Landis, 1974; Pfenninger and Rovainen, 1974; Wood, Pfenninger, and Cohen, 1977). These loci, termed *vesicle attachment sites*, are morphologically identifiable as small protuberances or pits in freeze-fracture replicas of presynaptic membranes (Figure 2A) and are found in close association with tuft- or bar-shaped cytoplasmic densities—the so-called dense projections (Figure 1A) or dense bars (Gray, 1963; Couteaux and Pécot-Dechavassine, 1970). The postsynaptic membrane is characterized, most importantly, by high content in transmitter receptors (which are difficult to identify morphologically; cf. Potter and Smith, 1977) and, most frequently, by a cytoplasmic electron-dense layer of varying width (Figures 1A, 3; Palay, 1958; for review

see Pfenninger, 1973, 1978). The two synaptic membranes are separated from each other by a cleft about 20 nm wide which can be divided into two layers: the presynaptic moiety and its postsynaptic counterpart. Each layer is probably composed of fibrillar protein and carbohydrate anchored in their respective plasma membrane (Figure 3; Pfenninger, 1971, 1973). The peripheries of these two layers of cleft material represent the actual areas of contact and interaction between the junctional partners. In modern terms, synaptic membranes are sites of massive development and high concentration of integral membrane proteins (and probably glycolipids) that extend far into the extracellular space and into the cytoplasm (Pfenninger, 1978). Not surprisingly, then, presynaptic membranes in general (Pfenninger et al., 1972; Venzin et al., 1977), and at least certain types of postsynaptic membranes (Sandri et al., 1972; Lan-

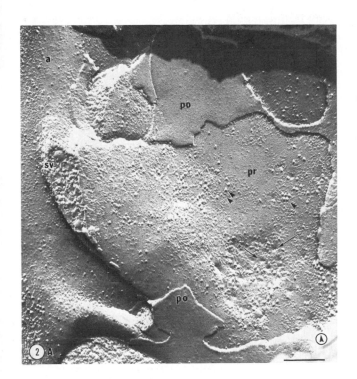

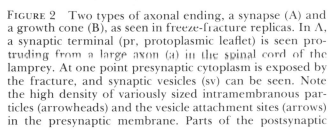

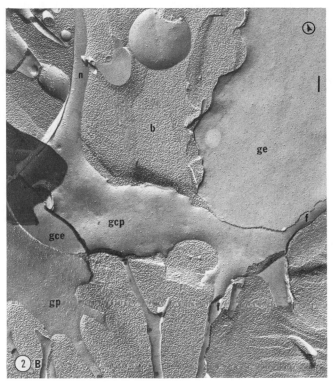

FIGURE 2 Two types of axonal ending, a synapse (A) and a growth cone (B), as seen in freeze-fracture replicas. In A, a synaptic terminal (pr, protoplasmic leaflet) is seen protruding from a large axon (a) in the spinal cord of the lamprey. At one point presynaptic cytoplasm is exposed by the fracture, and synaptic vesicles (sv) can be seen. Note the high density of variously sized intramembranous particles (arrowheads) and the vesicle attachment sites (arrows) in the presynaptic membrane. Parts of the postsynaptic membrane (po, external leaflet) are also visible. By contrast, the nerve growth cone in B is characterized by a particle-poor membrane without vesicle attachment sites. (gcp and gce, growth-cone plasmalemma, protoplasmic and external leaflets, respectively; n, neurite; f, filopodia; gp and ge, plasmalemma of glial processes, protoplasmic and external leaflets, respectively; b, vitrified glycerol buffer in the extracellular space. Circled arrow, shadowing direction. Calibration, 0.2 μm in both parts.)

dis and Reese, 1974), are rich in intramembranous particles, which are believed to be morphological correlates of at least certain integral membrane proteins.

RECOGNIZING MEMBRANES Whereas the future target site on the postsynaptic cell does not appear to exhibit specific properties, as compared to the membrane surrounding it (cf. Fambrough, 1976), the advancing axon forms a distinctive structure at its tip, the nerve growth cone (Figures 1B, 2B, 9A). This highly motile, palm-shaped distal structure contains a set of characteristic organelles (Tennyson, 1970; Yamada, Spooner, and Wessells, 1971; Bunge, 1973); these include an extensive submembranous microfilament network, a large number of smooth membrane cisternae similar to endoplasmic reticulum, clusters of large, clear vesicles (150 nm diameter), and numerous dense-core vesicles (120 nm). Growth-cone

plasma membrane, even if stained with bismuth iodide, does not exhibit any of the elaborate paramembranous densities that are characteristic of synapses (Pfenninger and Rees, 1976), nor does freeze-fracture reveal any vesicle attachment sites (Figure 2B; Pfenninger and Bunge, 1974). Moreover, in freeze-fracture replicas, growth-cone plasmalemma has an unusually low density of intramembranous particles (about 110/μm^2 for both leaflets)—a level approximately ten times lower than that of nonspecialized perikaryal plasma membrane of growing or mature neurons. Although an elaborate layer of cell surface material cannot be demonstrated, growth-cone plasmalemma does bear a substantial amount of carbohydrate on its surface.

MEMBRANE METAMORPHOSIS DURING SYNAPTOGENESIS Data on the crucial early events in synaptogen-

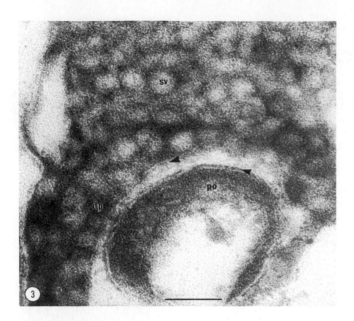

FIGURE 3 Synaptic contact opened by treatment with 1.5 M CaCl$_2$, aldehyde-fixed and impregnated with bismuth iodide. Trilaminar unit membrane structure cannot be seen, so that synaptic vesicles (sv) appear in negative contrast. However, presynaptic (dp) and postsynaptic (po) cytoplasmic densities, as well as cleft material (arrows), are densely stained. Note that pre- and postsynaptic moieties of the cleft material are separate structural entities. (Cat subfornical organ. Calibration, 0.1 μm. From Pfenninger, 1971.)

esis derive exclusively from observations of cultures in which growth cones approach and interact with putative target cells; the ensuing junctional development can be analyzed by both light and electron microscopy at timed intervals (Rees, Bunge, and Bunge, 1976). Various stages of synaptic development are schematically illustrated in Figure 4. The initial contact between axon and target prompts complete cessation of movement of the growth cone. If the contact is appropriate, close apposition of most growth-cone filopodia and lamellopodia to the target cell follows (Rees, Bunge, and Bunge, 1976). At many points of the contact region, the distance between the two interacting plasma membranes is only about 8 nm (Pfenninger and Rees, 1976). The cessation of growth and movement of the growth cone and its close conjunction with the future postsynaptic element are the first behavioral changes triggered by the encounter with the target cell. The initial phase of apposition is followed by a series of membrane-transformation steps. Coated vesicles appear near, and seem to fuse with, the future postsynaptic membrane, and the first postsynaptic cytoplasmic material becomes visible. Several hours later, signs of cyto-

plasmically oriented dense material appear on the presynaptic membrane. At about the same time, the first synaptic vesicles can be detected, and organelles typical of the growth cone are reduced in number (Rees, Bunge, and Bunge, 1976). During the process of accumulation of postsynaptic dense material and transformation of the growth cone into a presynaptic bouton, the synaptic cleft gradually widens until it reaches a width of about 20 nm at synaptic maturity (Figure 4; Pfenninger and Rees, 1976).

From the comparison of immature and established synaptic membranes, as well as from the course of synapse development, it is evident that synaptogenesis is a specific type of localized membrane differentiation involving both partner membranes of the junction, each in a characteristic way. Because it is believed that the junctional intramembranous particles, transmitter-receptor molecules, and at least some components contained in the pre- and postsynaptic densities are integral membrane proteins (and perhaps glycolipids; cf. Pfenninger, 1978), this process of membrane differentiation must result from insertion of new components into both plasmalemmas. (Naturally synapse formation also involves the onset of synaptic-vesicle synthesis by the presynaptic neuron.) In summary, then, synaptogenesis means localized insertion of synapse-specific membrane components as a consequence of recognition—that is, triggered by successful interaction between neurite and target cell.

Possible codes for recognition

In attempting to identify and analyze mechanisms involved in synaptogenesis, one of the first problems one must face is the definition of the code(s) that give developing cells recognition clues. Recognition and formation of a synapse seem to be dependent on the physical contact between the future partner membranes, except perhaps for the situation in the weaver mouse cerebellum. [In the cerebellum of the weaver mouse, spines on Purkinje dendrites exhibit postsynaptic membranes that are morphologically identical to those in normal synapses even though the appropriate afferent nerve fibers are absent (Hanna, Hirano, and Pappas, 1976).] In fact, even when a growth cone in culture reaches an inappropriate obstruction lying in its path of outgrowth, it will initially palpate it and dwell in contact with it for several minutes before retracting from it and altering its course (Rees, Bunge, and Bunge, 1976). If recognition depends solely on surface interaction, as this behavior sug-

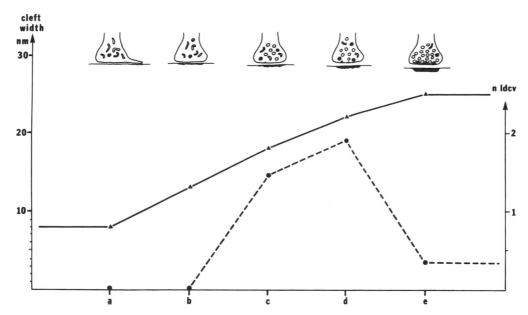

FIGURE 4 Schematic representation of synaptogenesis. Five steps can be distinguished morphologically (abscissa, a–e), but the duration of individual phases is not clear. The left ordinate indicates the width of the intercellular space at the contact site (filled triangles) as a function of synaptic maturation, whereas the right ordinate (filled circles) gives the average number of large, dense-core vesicles per section within 500 nm of the contact region. For further description see text (cf. Rees et al., 1976; Pfenninger and Rees, 1976).

gests, it still necessitates a mechanism by which the signal resulting from an encounter can travel from the cell surface across the membrane to the nucleus and other organelles. Signaling through transfer of substances from cell to cell—for example, via gap junctions—seems an unlikely mechanism for the following reasons: growth cones have not been seen to form gap junctions; gap-junction formation itself would necessitate a preceding recognition step; noncellular material is recognized as inappropriate. Yet we have no evidence to exclude either this or any other putative mechanism of "humoral" recognition (i.e., mechanisms involving transfer of free molecules versus interaction of membrane-bound components). Overall, our knowledge of the plasma membrane and of the influence of surface modification on cellular behavior (see, e.g., McClain and Edelman, this volume; Rutishauser et al., this volume; Barondes, 1976; Stallcup, 1977) strongly suggests that the plasmalemmal surface may contain the code as well as the sensing elements that permit cells to recognize each other. As previously mentioned, the true surface of cells and of their plasma membranes is formed by a layer of peptide and carbohydrate moieties that project for several nanometers from the lipid bilayer into the extracellular space and that are covalently linked to integral membrane proteins or lipids.

To test the hypothesis that surface carbohydrates

are involved in the process of neuronal recognition, we have first to deal with two questions: (1) Does the surface carbohydrate composition of the neuritic growth cone differ from that of its perikaryon? (2) Do growth cones originating from different types of neuron exhibit distinctive carbohydrate complements on their surfaces? We have attempted to answer these questions by labeling the surface of different types of growing neuron with lectins, covalently linked to the electron-optical marker ferritin (Figure 5A, C), and by subsequently quantifying the number of binding sites per unit area of membrane in electron micrographs of different neuronal regions (Pfenninger and Maylié-Pfenninger, 1975, 1976, 1978).

Such data can only be meaningful, however, if certain experimental conditions are met (see Maylié-Pfenninger, Palade, and Jamieson, 1975; Pfenninger and Maylié-Pfenninger, 1975; Maylié-Pfenninger and Jamieson, 1979):

1. The cell surfaces must be accessible to the marker; thus the labeling studies must be carried out on cultured neurons.

2. The cell surfaces must be free of adsorbed serum glycoproteins, which could feign the presence of certain carbohydrate residues. An extensive washing and desorption procedure is necessary to achieve uniformly clean cell surfaces.

3. The specificity and affinity of the lectin-ferritin

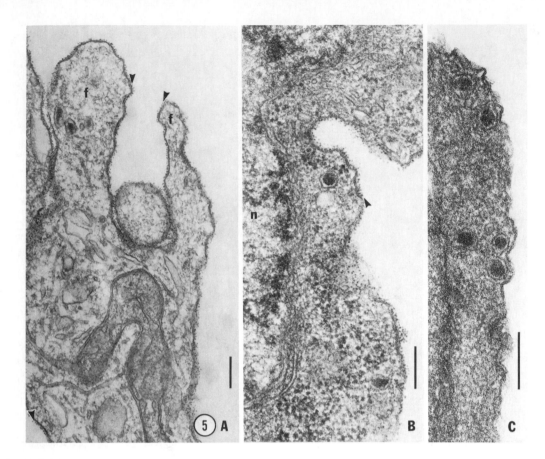

FIGURE 5   Labeling of the plasmalemma of the growing neuron with ferritin–wheat-germ agglutinin, specific for N-acetyl-glucosaminyl residues. The marker is used approximately at saturation level. (A) Part of a nerve growth cone from a superior-cervical-ganglion neuron. (B) Perikaryon of the same type of neuron. Note uniform distribution of the ferritin marker (arrows). (C) Control experiment; process of a superior-cervical-ganglion neuron labeled in the presence of 0.2 M N-acetyl-glucosamine. Absence of the ferritin marker in the control picture is evident. (f, filopodia; n, nucleus. Calibration: 0.2 μm in all parts. From Pfenninger and Maylié-Pfenninger, 1978.)

conjugates must be known. In our conjugate preparations these values are very close to the ones found for the native unconjugated lectins.

4. The ferritin-to-lectin ratio must be known, so that counting of ferritin particles can be used to determine the actual number of lectin-binding sites. The lectin-ferritin conjugates used for the present studies contained binding protein and marker in a ratio approximating 1:1.

Even if all these experimental criteria are met, steric hindrance may influence the measurement of very densely arranged carbohydrate moieties and, especially, of sugars that are contained more deeply inside the layer of membrane surface material.

When neurons, mechanically or enzymatically isolated from ventral regions of the spinal cord (rich in anterior-horn cells) or from superior cervical ganglia of embryonic rat, are grown for several days in vitro and labeled with a battery of lectins specific for the

sugars N-acetyl-glucosamine, galactose, fucose, and glucose/mannose, uniform binding across perikarya, neuritic shafts, and growth cones is observed (Figure 5A, B; Pfenninger and Maylié-Pfenninger, 1975, 1978). This uniform pattern seems to be independent of the age of the neurons as long as they exhibit neurite-forming capacity. Thus, at least in crude terms, plasmalemmal surface carbohydrate composition in the growth cone does not seem to differ from that in the perikaryon. This result, however, by no means indicates that the two membranes are identical. Indeed, the freeze-fracture studies mentioned previously have shown that the growth-cone plasmalemma is strikingly different from that in other parts of the neuron (Pfenninger and Bunge, 1974). The pronounced paucity of intramembranous particles in growth-cone plasmalemma—a total of $101/\mu m^2$ and $126/\mu m^2$ for both leaflets in neurons of rat spinal cord and olfactory bulb, respectively (Fig-

784   KARL H. PFENNINGER

ure 2B)—is even more intriguing when compared with the relatively high density of binding sites for certain lectins in the same membrane (approximately 2,000 binding sites for *Ricinus communis* agglutinin I after neuraminidase treatment; see Figure 6C and below). The large quantitative difference between particles and lectin-binding sites raises the question of whether most of these sugar moieties are linked to a protein or to a lipid backbone and may suggest that glycolipids (e.g., gangliosides) may be important determinants of growth-cone surface properties. In other words, the growth cone is enveloped by a rather unique plasma membrane. This notion is further enhanced by the fact that more distal portions of growing neurites are more sensitive to black-widow-spider venom. While leaving glia and neuronal perikarya intact, at very low concentration ($< 10^{-8}$M), this venom destroys growth cones and recently formed neurite segments within minutes of exposure (Rubin, Pfenninger, and Mauro, 1975).

The second and more important question concerns the comparison of carbohydrate contents on the surfaces of different types of growth cone. Application of lectin-ferritin conjugates to growth cones from rat embryonic superior cervical ganglion, dorsal-root ganglion, olfactory bulb (probably mainly from mitral cells), spinal cord (ventral region, probably mainly from motoneurons), and cerebellum (probably mainly from Purkinje cells) grown for several days in vitro yields the results illustrated in Figures 6A–C and the preliminary quantitative data in Table I (Pfenninger and Maylié-Pfenninger, 1976, 1978). It is evident that different types of growth cone exhibit clearly distinctive sugar complements on their surfaces (e.g., the variation in wheat-germ agglutinin

binding; see Hatten, Trenkner, and Sidman, 1976; McLaughlin and Wood, 1977; Trenkner et al., 1977). Not only is each growth cone characterized by its own *carbohydrate signature,* but there also seem to exist (at least) two classes of carbohydrate contents. In comparing the binding of *Ricinus communis* agglutinin I and wheat-germ agglutinin to the different membrane types, it becomes clear that the neurons of superior cervical and dorsal-root ganglia, both of which are neural-crest derivatives, carry many more lectin-binding sites than the three other types of growth cones, all of which are formed by neurons originating from the neural tube. However, treatment of aldehyde-prefixed, neural-tube-derived tissue with neuraminidase, followed by aldehyde inactivation and *Ricinus communis* agglutinin I binding, reveals a high density of previously inaccessible galactosyl residues (Figure 6B, C; Table I). Although further, direct proof is necessary, it seems likely that one of the major features distinguishing between neural-crest and neural-tube derivatives is the presence of substantial amounts of terminal sialic acid (masking galactosyl residues) on the plasmalemmal surface of neurons stemming from neural tube.

In contrast to its future presynaptic counterpart—the growth-cone plasmalemma—the future postsynaptic membrane site on the target cell does not appear to exhibit distinctive properties. As far as can be assessed today, the target-cell membrane seems to acquire specific synaptic properties only upon its interaction with an appropriate afferent nerve fiber (Fambrough, 1976; note the exception of the weaver mouse cerebellum mentioned above).

Even though we can detect only certain freely accessible sugar moieties, rather than specific glycopro-

TABLE I

Lectin receptor densities on developing neurites of different origin (Binding sites/μm^2 of plasma membrane)

	Con A glc/man	WGA glcNAc	RCA I gal	Neuramin. RCA I	SBA galNAc	LTA/UEA fucose
SCG	(1,400)	2,740	1,440	nd	(1,400)	0
DRG	(1,800)	2,220	(2,200)	nd	nd	0
SC	(800)	910	210	(2,200)	0	0
CBL	nd	530	560	2,210	0	0
OB	(600)	1,830	0	1,950	nd	0

Abbreviations: SCG, superior cervical ganglion; DRG, dorsal-root ganglion; SC, spinal cord; CBL, cerebellum; OB, olfactory bulb (fetal rat tissues); Con A, concanavalin A; WGA, wheat-germ agglutinin; RCA I, *Ricinus communis* agglutinin I; Neuramin., neuraminidase treatment before labeling; SBA, soybean agglutinin; UEA, *Ulex europeus* agglutinin; LTA, *Lotus tetragonolobus* agglutinin.

Source: Based on preliminary data; figures in parentheses are estimated values; nd, not done. (From Pfenninger and Maylié-Pfenninger, 1978.)

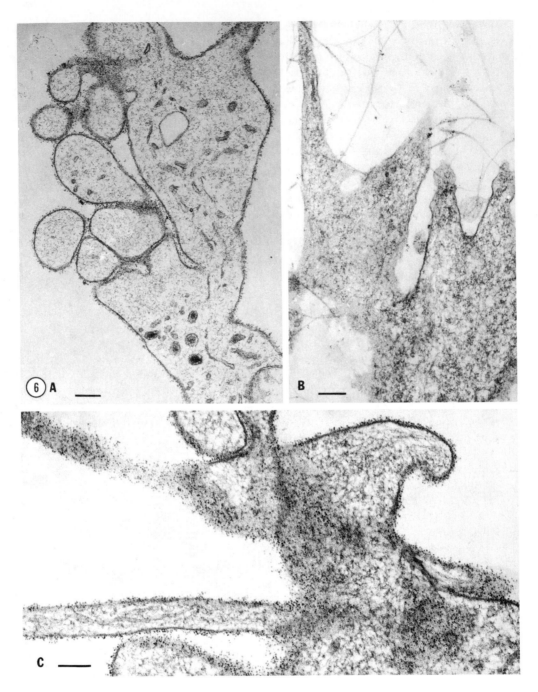

FIGURE 6 Differential labeling of cold- or aldehyde-immobilized distal parts of nerve growth cones with *Ricinus communis* agglutinin I, specific for galactosyl residues. Rat superior cervical ganglion (A); normal rat spinal cord (B); and rat spinal cord fixed with glutaraldehyde, neuraminidase-treated, and then labeled (C). Note the striking differences in labeling between superior cervical ganglion and spinal cord and between normal and neuraminidase-digested spinal cord. (Calibration: 0.2 μm in all parts. From Pfenninger and Maylié-Pfenninger, 1978.)

teins or glycolipids, by the lectin-mapping technique, the studies with this method have resulted in the determination of a cell surface signature (i.e., a carbohydrate code) which identifies neuronal types and classes. It is not clear, however, whether this code plays a role in tissue morphogenesis (i.e., in migration and aggregation of the neurons), whether it is of importance during synaptogenesis, or whether it serves cellular recognition in both situations. Yet the demonstration of this code proves the feasibility of a cell-surface-mediated mechanism for neuronal recognition. The finding of a cell surface carbohydrate code is in agreement with, and complementary to, the identification of membrane-bound lectins in a variety of developing tissues (Barondes and Rosen, 1976; Nowak, Haywood, and Barondes, 1976). These carbohydrate-binding proteins, or perhaps the postulated cell surface glycosyl-transferases (Roth, McGuire, and Roseman, 1971), might then represent the lock that recognizes and accepts a specific carbohydrate key. Such an interaction would then need to be transmitted across the plasma membrane for activation of the cellular processes that result from a successful recognition event.

Mechanisms of membrane growth and differentiation

The special membrane properties of the growth cone should not be considered from a purely static point of view. Indeed the outgrowing and rapidly advancing neurite is enlarging its surface at a fast rate. At the same time the growth cone must find its path to an appropriate target cell and be ready to recognize the future synaptic site. In this situation the appropriate membrane properties have to be maintained while the plasmalemma is being expanded. Later, when recognition has occurred and neuritic growth has stopped, the existing plasma membrane must be modified locally for synaptic function by a process of membrane differentiation. The two phenomena, plasmalemmal growth and differentiation, have in common the insertion of different components into the membrane and are the subject of the following paragraphs.

MEMBRANE EXPANSION   The mechanisms of membrane biogenesis are still very poorly understood; thus a series of theoretical possibilities must be considered (cf. Siekevitz, 1972; Singer and Rothfield, 1973; Malhorta, 1976). Plasmalemmal expansion could occur by insertion of preassembled membrane pieces or by intussusception of molecular units. Furthermore, both processes could occur in a random or in a localized fashion. None of these variants has been clearly established in the systems under investigation, except for the retinal rod, where an unknown, but localized, membrane-expansion mechanism occurs at the base of the outer segment for renewal of the photoreceptor disks (Hall, Bok, and Bacharach, 1969; Bibb and Young, 1974).

In growing neurites, it has been suggested, membrane expansion also occurs in localized form at or near the growing tip (Hughes, 1953; Bray, 1970, 1973). Freeze-fracture data (Pfenninger and Bunge, 1974; Pfenninger and Rees, 1976) as well as lectin pulse-chase experiments (Figure 7) seem to confirm this hypothesis (Pfenninger and Maylié-Pfenninger, 1975, 1977, 1978). When live nerve fibers are labeled with a lectin-ferritin conjugate, washed, and then allowed to survive for short periods (minutes), the originally homogeneous distribution of lectin receptor sites is no longer evident (cf. Figures 8A and 7A). Instead, label-free areas appear on the surface of moundlike protrusions that are filled with clear vesicles approximately 150 nm in diameter (Figure 8B; Pfenninger and Maylié-Pfenninger, 1975, 1978). These mounds (cf. Yamada, Spooner, and Wessells, 1971; Bunge, 1973; Wessels et al., 1976) are encountered particularly often on or near the growth cone (Figure 9A, B) but they are also seen on less distant portions of the neurite, especially near branch points. In addition, they occur in a great variety of proliferating nonneuronal cells. While this finding is compatible with the idea that pieces of membrane have been added to the surface of the mound during the chase period of the experiment, it could also be argued that receptor redistribution similar to patching or capping has occurred (although no rearrangement of lectin receptors can be seen in nonspecialized areas of neurite or perikaryon).

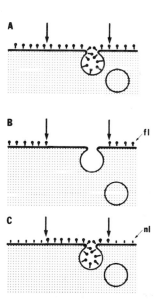

FIGURE 7   Schematic representation of the studies on lectin receptor dynamics during neuritic growth. The plasmalemmal region between the arrows is a hypothetical site of localized insertion of preassembled membrane by fusion of vesicles. (fl, ferritin-lectin conjugate; nl, native lectin. From Pfenninger and Maylié-Pfenninger, 1978.)

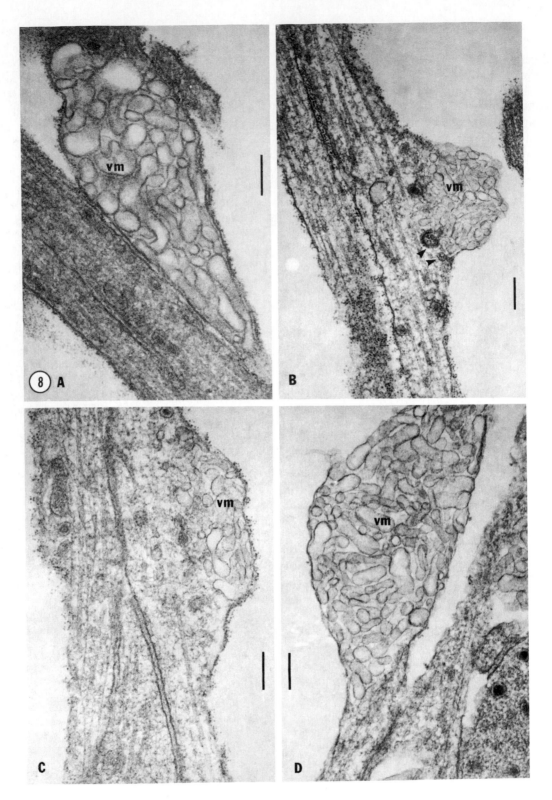

To resolve this problem, a double-label experiment (Figure 7C) is carried out; the mound surface is tested for the appearance of new lectin receptor sites, which would indicate the insertion of membrane components (Pfenninger and Maylié-Pfenninger, 1977, 1978). Live cultures are first labeled with native lectin, which is invisible in the electron microscope, then allowed to survive in the absence of the lectin before

FIGURE 8 Vesicle-filled mounds (vm) near nerve growth cones in lectin-label pulse-chase experiments. (A) Aldehyde-prefixed element labeled with ferritin–wheat-germ agglutinin. Note uniform labeling of mound surface and nerve fiber shafts. (B) Single-label pulse-chase experiment (15 min chase) with ferritin–*Ricinus communis* agglutinin I (RCA I). While nerve fiber shafts are still uniformly labeled, the mound surface is free of the marker. No internalization into mound vesicles has occurred. One of the basal, open cisternae, typical of the mounds, and a coated vesicle are labeled (arrows). (C) Double-label pulse-chase experiment with native RCA I, followed by 3 min chase, fixation, and postlabeling with ferritin–RCA I. Note the appearance of new lectin receptors mainly on the mound surface, less on nerve fiber shafts (compare perpendicularly sectioned membrane regions). (D) Double-label pulse-chase experiment at 0°C with ferritin–RCA II (specific for N-acetyl-galactosaminyl residues). Note the absence of ferritin label. Use of the different lectins yields comparable results in the various experiments. (Cultured rat superior cervical ganglion neurons. Calibration: 0.2 μm in all parts. From Pfenninger and Maylié-Pfenninger, 1978.)

being fixed with aldehydes. Subsequently, the cultures are relabeled with the ferritin conjugate of the previous lectin. Thus, only lectin receptors that have been newly added to the plasmalemmal surface should be labeled with the ferritin conjugate (Figure 7C). When the experiment is carried out in the cold (i.e., without membrane expansion occurring), very little ferritin is found randomly attached to the cell membrane (Figure 8D). However, if the experiment is carried out at 36°C under favorable growth conditions, a dense layer of ferritin-lectin label is found on the surface of the vesicle-filled mounds (Figure 8C). These preliminary results strongly suggest the localized appearance of new lectin receptors and are compatible with the freeze-fracture data (Figure 9B). Freeze-fractured mound plasmalemma is almost completely devoid of intramembranous particles, as is the membrane of the 150 nm vesicles underneath. These vesicles are also seen in groups in the neurite (Figure 9C) and in the perikaryon (Figure 9D), sometimes in association with the Golgi apparatus. Furthermore, continuity of the plasma membrane of the mound with the membrane of an underlying 150 nm vesicle has been observed.

Although further proof is necessary, these observations strongly support the following hypothesis for membrane expansion. The perikaryon, probably with involvement of the Golgi apparatus, produces membrane vesicles that are essentially devoid of intramembranous particles and that are transported down the neurite to the mound structures, where they fuse with, and are inserted into, the overlying plasma membrane. This addition of particle-free plasma membrane at or near the growth cone offers a good explanation for the density gradient of intramembranous particles found in the growing neurite (low density at the growth cone, high density at the perikaryon). The rate of membrane expansion in the advancing neurite is fast, estimated at 0.5 μm²/min. However, intramembranous particles appear more slowly, at a later stage of membrane development. From this it appears entirely possible that the expected equilibration of the density of particles by lateral diffusion lags behind. Thus, the particle density gradient would be maintained as long as the neurite is growing. The proposed hypothesis of membrane growth includes the notion of localized insertion of preassembled, but immature, plasma membrane (absence of intramembranous particles) by fusion of a special type of membrane-growth vesicle with the plasmalemma. Because the mound surface—that is, the site of insertion—has the same lectin-labeling properties as other plasmalemmal regions of the growing neuron, membrane-growth vesicles bring along the appropriate complement of cell surface carbohydrate, at least as far as this can be judged on the basis of lectin binding.

It follows from this hypothesis that the most recently synthesized membrane is inserted at or near the growing tip and, therefore, that growth-cone plasmalemma is under almost immediate control of perikaryal genetic and synthetic machinery. If the proposed mechanism of membrane expansion is correct, this last aspect of growth-cone membrane dynamics may be of great importance for the various mechanisms governing axonal pathfinding and the formation of synapses.

MEMBRANE DIFFERENTIATION In a fashion analogous to the membrane-expansion process, localized membrane differentiation (Figure 10) could occur either by insertion of patches of preassembled specialized membrane or by insertion of special molecules. Furthermore, enzymes located on the cell surface (e.g., transferases or hydrolases) could modify previously inserted membrane components. In either case, membrane differentiation could be a localized process; that is, insertion could occur at the site where specialized membrane is needed, or it could be a random process followed by redistribution and aggregation of the newly inserted (or modified) elements. Again, conclusive and decisive evidence is not yet available.

As explained before, synaptogenesis is, in essence, a process of localized membrane differentiation oc

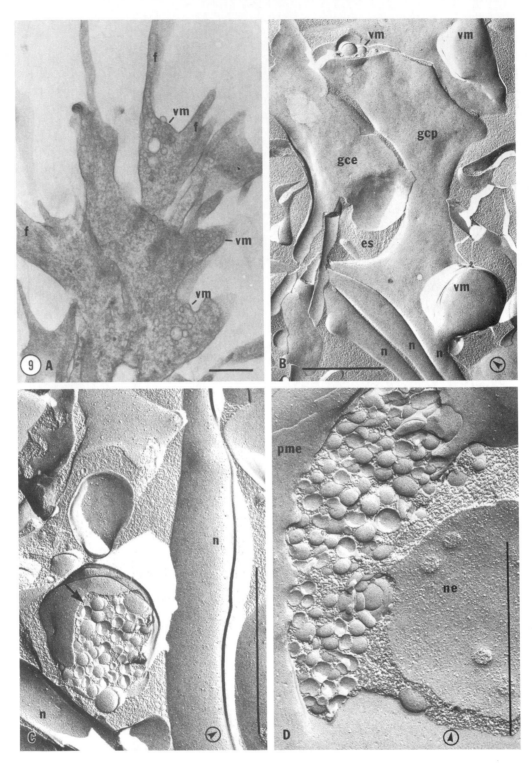

FIGURE 9 Micrographs of 150 nm clear vesicles in developing neurons. (A) Growth-cone filopodia and lamellopodia (f) in a rat spinal-cord culture. Note clusters of large, clear vesicles with an average diameter of about 150 nm (vm). (B) In a freeze-fracture preparation of a similar culture, mounds filled with clusters of the same vesicles (vm) can also be seen. The plasma membrane covering the mounds contains even fewer intramembranous particles than the surrounding growth-cone plasmalemma (gcp, protoplasmic leaflet; gce, external leaflet). (n, neurites; es, extracellular space.) (C) Developing neurites (n) in the fetal rat spinal cord (15 days gestation). Note the pocket of 150 nm vesicles (arrow) whose membranes are free of intramembranous particles. (D) Vesicle clusters (150 nm diameter) in the perikaryon of a neural cell in the same fetal spinal cord. The vesicles are unique among cytoplasmic organelles because of the almost complete absence of particles in their membranes. (ne, nuclear envelope with pores; pme, plasmalemma, external leaflet. Circled arrow, shadowing direction. Calibration: 1 μm in all parts.)

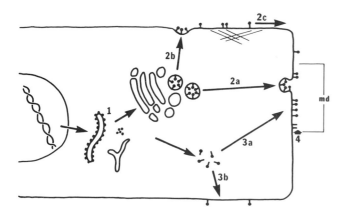

FIGURE 10 Schematic representation of possible mechanisms of membrane differentiation (md, area of specific differentiation). Genetic readout in the nucleus controls production of proteins (1), which are membrane-bound (involving rough endoplasmic reticulum) or free in the cytosol (involving free polyribosomes). Membrane-bound components may pass through the Golgi apparatus and reach the plasmalemma by fusion. This step could occur in a localized fashion—that is, at the site of differentiation (2a)—or randomly (2b), followed by diffusion or active transport (achieved by a submembranous contractile apparatus) to the appropriate area (2c). Components that are free in the cytosol could reach the plasma membrane by intussusception, again in a localized (3a) or a random (3b) manner. Lastly, enzymatic activities on the cell surface could modify already-inserted membrane components (4). Note that these different mechanisms are not mutually exclusive.

curring in both future synaptic partner membranes. In the case of the target-cell membrane, two obvious parameters are the aggregation of a large number of receptors at the junction and the formation of a postsynaptic density. With regard to receptor accumulation, studies on developing striated muscle and on the formation of neuromuscular junctions have produced data that are compatible with the idea that the acetylcholine receptor, which is randomly distributed in the myotube, becomes aggregated at the junctional site and is later modified to acquire the properties characteristic of the junctional receptor (Changeux, this volume; Fischbach and Cohen, 1973; Fambrough, 1976). The possibility that new and different receptor is inserted into the junctional sarcolemma upon interaction with the afferent nerve fiber has not been excluded, however. In the case of interneuronal synapse formation, the occurrence of coated vesicles at or near the future postsynaptic membrane has been known for some time (Altman, 1971; Stelzner, Martin, and Scott, 1973). It has been postulated recently (Rees, Bunge, and Bunge, 1976; Rees, 1978) that these vesicles are formed by the Golgi apparatus

and are then transported to the future junctional site, where they fuse with the plasmalemma for insertion of specific synaptic molecules. These vesicles may thus lay down their coats as the first detectable densities in the subsynaptic region. However, the similarity of vesicle coat and mature postsynaptic density is superficial at best and, therefore, does not provide evidence for the hypothesis that coated vesicles carry specific postsynaptic membrane elements to the junctional site. Should future results prove such a hypothesis correct, however, it might be an example of a mechanism of localized insertion of preassembled, specialized membrane.

The axonal growth-cone plasmalemma must also be equipped with a variety of specialized molecules in order to become a true presynaptic membrane. Comparison of the two stages of neuritic plasmalemma shows that densities in the cleft as well as on the cytoplasmic side of the membrane have to be formed and a large number of intramembranous particles inserted. The mechanisms by which this is achieved are completely unknown. In studies on growing neurites and on other elements of developing nerve tissue we have been unable to see vesicles that contain unusually high densities of intramembranous particles and thus could be carriers for these components to the plasma membrane. Nor is there any evidence for the existence of small, dense patches of intramembranous particles in the plasmalemma that could correspond to the sites of fusion of such vesicles. This negative evidence might seem to favor a mechanism of intussusception of intramembranous particles or their components. The possibility should not be overlooked, however, that intramembranous particles, which are probably composed of several integral membrane proteins of substantial size (see Pfenninger, 1978), could be formed by aggregation of previously invisible molecular subunits inserted into the membrane individually and considerably earlier. Frequent structures near the future presynaptic membrane during synaptogenesis (Figure 4) are large, dense-core vesicles, 120 nm in diameter, which are characteristic of a great variety of axonal growth cones, regardless of the type of neurotransmitter (Pfenninger and Rees, 1976). These vesicles contain cores with the same staining properties as the presynaptic densities, so that they might possibly serve as vehicles for specific presynaptic membrane components (see Pfenninger et al., 1969).

Synaptic-membrane differentiation clearly will remain a research topic for many years to come, and it will be necessary to draw on experience gained in studies of other systems of growing and developing membranes. Although the precise mechanisms are not known, it has been established in a variety of systems—including algae chloroplasts and mammalian liver endoplasmic reticulum—that membrane formation and maturation is a stepwise process; that is, different membrane components are inserted into the membrane sequentially rather than simultaneously (see, e.g., Siekevitz, 1972; Singer and Rothfield, 1973). Furthermore, it has been demonstrated in particularly revealing studies on viral membrane protein synthesis that different cellular pathways and transition times may exist for different types of plasmalemmal components (Grubman et al., 1975; Atkinson, Moyer, and Summers, 1976). Whereas certain membrane proteins are synthesized on free polyribosomes and reach the plasma membrane extremely rapidly, another membrane component, a glycoprotein, has been identified that is synthesized by rough endoplasmic reticulum and reaches the plasma membrane (probably already in membrane-bound form) after a considerably longer transition time. As mentioned earlier, preexisting membrane components could be modified by cell surface enzymes; in other words, membrane differentiation may be achieved by a multitude of coexisting mechanisms (see Figure 10). In fact, if the proposed theory of membrane expansion in the neuron proves to be correct, it represents the combination of at least two different mechanisms of membrane biogenesis: (1) insertion of preassembled, but incomplete, membrane patches; and (2) incorporation of additional membrane components, possibly by intussusception and/or modification of individual molecules. The diversity of the suggested insertion mechanisms is likely to be a function of the differing physicochemical properties of the various membrane components—lipids versus proteins versus protein or lipid backbones with large carbohydrate trees attached, whose passage through a lipid bilayer would pose great difficulty.

Control mechanisms in synaptogenesis

It has been pointed out that during development of neuronal networks the recognition event following an encounter of the future synaptic membranes tells the participating neuron and target cell not only that a synapse is to be made, but also what type of synapse is to be formed. This conclusion can be drawn from a well-known anatomical fact and from studies of synapse formation in vitro. Motor neurons (Figure 11A) of the spinal cord reach out into the periphery to skeletal muscle, where they form neuromuscular junctions. At the same time, motor axons form short

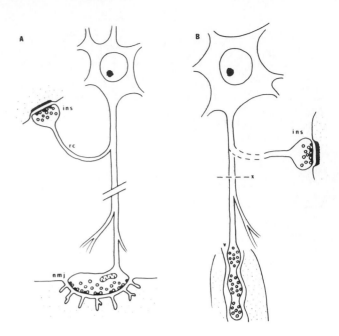

FIGURE 11   Differential response of presynaptic neuron to specific target cells. (A) Spinal-cord motor neuron with long, peripheral axon forming neuromusclar junction (nmj) and recurrent collateral (rc) forming interneuronal synapse (ins) in the spinal cord. (B) Principal neuron of the superior cervical ganglion forms "free" varicosities (v) in smooth muscle in vivo. In vitro, in the absence of physiological target cells (x), the same neurons form synapses (ins) with each other.

branches that remain within the spinal cord and form synapses with interneurons; these branches are the recurrent collaterals. In other words, the motor axon forms two distinctive types of synaptic nerve terminals on two different cells. The differences lie mainly in the arrangement of presynaptic cytoplasmic densities and in the composition of synaptic-cleft material. While the cytoplasmic dense material of the presynaptic membrane in interneuronal junctions is organized as a triagonal network of dense projections, it forms dense bars, separated by wide spaces, directly opposite the subneural folds of neuromuscular junctions (see, e.g., Pfenninger, 1977). Furthermore, the presynaptic membrane of interneuronal junctions exhibits highly developed, strongly bismuth-iodide-positive cell surface components in the synaptic clefts, whereas the axonal endings of neuromuscular junctions appear to be in direct contact with a weakly bismuth-iodide-stained basal lamina that occupies the cleft (see, e.g., Pfenninger, 1973). Postsynaptic sympathetic neurons in the superior cervical ganglion (Figure 11B) do not form true synapses in vivo, but rather send so-called free nerve terminals into the heart and into smooth muscle of vasculature and iris.

With the exception of the frog heart, where such nerve terminals contain cytoplasmic densities that are morphologically similar to those found in interneuronal synapses (McMahan and Kuffler, 1971), free nerve terminals have not been reported to contain synapse-typical presynaptic dense projections and have never been observed to form morphologically distinctive junctions. By contrast, if superior cervical-ganglion neurons are isolated and cultured in the absence of appropriate target cells, they start to form networks with morphologically and functionally competent synapses with each other (Rees and Bunge, 1974; Patterson, this volume). These synapses are indistinguishable from those built by physiological synaptic partners. In these two examples, the properties of the target cell seem to exert an influence on the differentiation of the presynaptic membrane. Conversely, the nature of the presynaptic terminal probably also plays a role in postsynaptic-membrane differentiation. An example of this phenomenon is the sharp plasmalemmal localization of the appropriate receptor type at synapses converging on the same neuron but utilizing different transmitters. Even more remarkably, the same neuron (in mollusc CNS) may be capable of forming and selectively localizing on its surface two types of acetylcholine receptors for two types of synapses receiving different cholinergic inputs (for review see Gerschenfeld, 1973).

It follows from these examples that interaction between pre- and postsynaptic membranes not only is required for the formation of a bilateral junction—that is, membrane differentiation in exactly juxtaposed membrane areas—but also critically influences the type of junctional membrane differentiation that is to occur. The example of the superior-cervical-ganglion neuron establishing a fully developed synapse in culture—a structure it never seems to form in vivo—is particularly striking in this sense. This de novo display of usually dormant cellular properties lends support to the hypothesis that the event of recognition is in some way linked to the genome (Figure 12). This hypothesis implies that recognition may trigger the expression of a particular set of genes for formation of a specific junction. However, control at the level of translation or posttranslational modification cannot be excluded at present. The hypothesis of a link between recognition and control of protein synthesis entails the existence of a mechanism that would transmit the information from the cell surface to the perikaryon (Figure 12; see also Edelman, this volume). It has been pointed out earlier that the onset of synaptic membrane differentiation

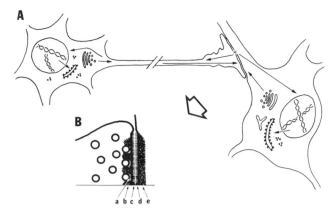

FIGURE 12 Hypothetical mechanisms involved in synaptic-membrane differentiation. (A) Contact (i.e., cell surface interaction) between growth cone and target cell may be the basis for recognition (asterisk), triggering, by means of intracellular messengers, specific genetic readout. Transcription and translation, in turn, may lead to the formation of the new synaptic-membrane components that are transported to, and inserted into, the future junctional membranes. (B) These components include presynaptic transmitter release sites (a), dense projection material (b), cleft moieties (c), and, on the postsynaptic side, cleft moieties (d) and postsynaptic density (e). These structural elements, which do not exist in growth cones or uncontacted target cells, are likely to be composed of a series of integral membrane proteins.

on the postsynaptic cell precedes that of the axonal growth-cone membrane (Rees et al., 1976). This time difference may be a consequence of the fact that, on the presynaptic side, signals from the cell surface usually have to travel over a far greater distance to reach the perikaryon than they do on the postsynaptic side.

During synaptic-membrane differentiation, stabilization of the recently established contact must occur. Functional validation of the synapse is necessary, as well as the expression of adhesive properties that link together the surface materials of pre- and postsynaptic membranes. The changes in membrane properties that lead to synaptic maturation (i.e., insertion of a variety of new membrane components) are likely to entail modification, masking, or even complete disappearance of the original recognition entities of growth-cone and target-cell plasmalemma. Could such a putative mechanism be part of a negative feedback system controlling synapse formation?

ACKNOWLEDGMENTS The work on lectin labeling of cell surfaces is the product of a collaborative effort with Dr. Marie-France Maylié-Pfenninger of the Memorial Sloan-Kettering Cancer Center, New York. Her contribution to this work and her generous permission to present some of the results of this effort are gratefully acknowledged. Many helpful suggestions for the improvement of the manuscript have been kindly offered by Dr. Julia Currie of this department. I would also like to thank Linda Siegel and Christine Wade for their skillful assistance in the preparation of this manuscript. This work is supported by USPHS grant NS-13466, by grant BNS-7618513 from the National Science Foundation, and by a Career Scientist Award from the I. T. Hirschl Trust Fund.

REFERENCES

ALTMAN, J., 1971. Coated vesicles and synaptogenesis: A developmental study in the cerebellar cortex of the rat. *Brain Res.* 30:311–322.

ATKINSON, P. H., S. A. MOYER, and D. F. SUMMERS, 1976. Assembly of vesicular stomatitis virus glycoprotein and matrix protein into HeLa cell plasma membranes. *J. Mol. Biol.* 102:613–631.

BARONDES, S. H., ed., 1976. *Neuronal Recognition.* New York: Plenum Press.

BARONDES, S. H., and S. D. ROSEN, 1976. Cell surface carbohydrate-binding proteins: Role in cell recognition. In *Neuronal Recognition*, S. H. Barondes, ed. New York: Plenum Press, pp. 331–356.

BIBB, C., and R. W. YOUNG, 1974. Renewal of fatty acids in the membranes of visual cell outer segments. *J. Cell Biol.* 61:327–343.

BRAY, D., 1970. Surface movements during the growth of single explanted neurons. *Proc. Natl. Acad. Sci. USA* 65:905–910.

BRAY, D., 1973. Branching patterns of isolated sympathetic neurons. *J. Cell Biol.* 56:702–712.

BUNGE, M. B., 1973. Fine structure of nerve fibers and growth cones of isolated sympathetic neurons in culture. *J. Cell Biol.* 56:713–735.

COUTEAUX, R., and M. PÉCOT-DECHAVASSINE, 1970. Vesicules synaptiques et poches au niveau des "zones actives" de la jonction neuromusculaire. *CR Acad. Sci. Paris [D]* 271:2346–2349.

DREYER, F., K. PEPER, K. AKERT, C. SANDRI, and H. MOOR, 1973. Ultrastructure of the "active zone" in the frog neuromuscular junction. *Brain Res.* 62:373–380.

ELFVIN, L.-G., 1976. The ultrastructure of neuronal contacts. *Prog. Neurobiol.* 8:45–79.

FAMBROUGH, D. M., 1976. Specificity of nerve-muscle interactions. In *Neuronal Recognition*, S. H. Barondes, ed. New York: Plenum Press, pp. 25–67.

FISCHBACH, G. D., and S. COHEN, 1973. The distribution of acetylcholine sensitivity over uninnervated and innervated muscle fibers grown in cell culture. *Dev. Biol.* 31:147–162.

GEFFEN, L. B., and B. G. LIVETT, 1971. Synaptic vesicles in sympathetic neurons. *Physiol. Rev.* 51:98–157.

GERSCHENFELD, H. M., 1973. Chemical transmission in invertebrate central nervous systems and neuromuscular junctions. *Physiol. Rev.* 53:1–119.

GRAY, E. G., 1963. Electron microscopy of presynaptic organelles of the spinal cord. *J. Anat.* 97:101–106.

GRUBMAN, M. J., S. A. MOYER, A. K. BANERJEE, and E. EHRENFELD, 1975. Sub-cellular localization of vesicular stomatitis virus messenger RNAs. *Biochem. Biophys. Res. Commun.* 62:531–538.

HALL, M. O., D. BOK, and A. D. E. BACHARACH, 1969.

Biosynthesis and assembly of the rod outer segment membrane system. Formation and fate of visual pigment in the frog retina. *J. Mol. Biol.* 45:397–406.

HANNA, R. B., A. HIRANO, and G. D. PAPPAS, 1976. Membrane specialization of dendritic spines and glia in the weaver mouse cerebellum: A freeze-fracture study. *J. Cell Biol.* 68:403–410.

HATTEN, M. E., E. TRENKNER, and R. L. SIDMAN, 1976. Cell migration and cell-cell interactions in primary cultures of embryonic mouse cerebellum. *Neurosci. Abstr.* 2:1023.

HEUSER, J. E., T. S. REESE, and D. M. D. LANDIS, 1974. Functional changes in frog neuromuscular junctions studied with freeze-fracture. *J. Neurocytol.* 3:109–131.

HOLTZMAN, E., 1977. The origin and fate of secretory packages, especially synaptic vesicles. *Neuroscience* 2:327–355.

HUGHES, A., 1953. The growth of embryonic neurites. A study on cultures of chick neural tissues. *J. Anat.* 87:150–163.

LANDIS, D. M. D., and T. S. REESE, 1974. Differences in membrane structure between excitatory and inhibitory synapses in the cerebellar cortex. *J. Comp. Neurol.* 155:93–126.

MALHORTA, S. K., 1976. Biogenesis of mammalian membranes. In *Mammalian Cell Membranes*, vol. 1: *General Considerations*, G. A. Jamieson and D. M. Robinson, eds. London: Butterworths, pp. 224–243.

MCLAUGHLIN, B. J., and J. G. WOOD, 1977. The localization of concanavalin A binding sites during photoreceptor synaptogenesis in the chick retina. *Brain Res.* 119:57–71.

MCMAHAN, U. J., and S. W. KUFFLER, 1971. Visual identification of synaptic boutons on living ganglion cells and of varicosities in postganglionic axons in the heart of the frog. *Proc. R. Soc. Lond.* B177:485–508.

MAYLIÉ-PFENNINGER, M.-F., and J. D. JAMIESON, 1979. Distribution of cell surface saccharides on pancreatic cells. I. General method for preparation and purification of lectins and lectin-ferritin conjugates. *J. Cell. Biol.* 80 (in press).

MAYLIÉ-PFENNINGER, M.-F., G. E. PALADE, and J. D. JAMIESON, 1975. Interaction of lectins with the surface of dispersed pancreatic cells. *J. Cell Biol.* 67:333a.

NOWAK, T. P., P. L. HAYWOOD, and S. H. BARONDES, 1976. Developmentally regulated lectin in embryonic chick muscle and a myogenic cell line. *Biochem. Biophys. Res. Commun.* 68:650–657.

PALAY, S. L., 1958. The morphology of synapses in the central nervous system. *Exp. Cell Res. (Suppl.)* 5:275–293.

PFENNINGER, K. H., 1971. The cytochemistry of synaptic densities. II. Proteinaceous components and mechanism of synaptic connectivity. *J. Ultrastruct. Res.* 35:451–475.

PFENNINGER, K. H., 1973. Synaptic morphology and cytochemistry. *Prog. Histochem. Cytochem.* 5:1–86.

PFENNINGER, K. H., 1977. Cytology of the chemical synapse: Morphological correlates of synaptic function. In *Neurotransmitter Function*, W. S. Fields, ed. Miami: Symposia Specialists, pp. 27–57.

PFENNINGER, K., 1978. Organization of neuronal membranes. *Annu. Rev. Neurosci.* 1:445–471.

PFENNINGER, K., K. AKERT, H. MOOR, and C. SANDRI, 1972. The fine structure of freeze-fractured presynaptic membranes. *J. Neurocytol.* 1:129–149.

PFENNINGER, K. H., and R. P. BUNGE, 1974. Freeze-fracturing of nerve growth cones and young fibers: A study of developing plasma membrane. *J. Cell Biol.* 63:180–196.

PFENNINGER, K. H., M.-F. MAYLIÉ-PFENNINGER, 1975. Distribution and fate of lectin binding sites on the surface of growing neuronal processes. *J. Cell Biol.* 67:322a.

PFENNINGER, K. H., and M.-F. MAYLIÉ-PFENNINGER, 1976. Differential lectin receptor content on the surface of nerve growth cones of different origin. *Neurosci. Abstr.* 2 (pt. 1):224.

PFENNINGER, K. H., and M.-F. MAYLIÉ-PFENNINGER, 1977. Localized appearance of new lectin receptors on the surface of growing neurites. *J. Cell Biol.* 75:54a.

PFENNINGER, K. H., and M.-F. MAYLIÉ-PFENNINGER, 1978. Distribution and appearance of surface carbohydrates on growing neurites. In *Neuronal Information Transfer (Proceedings of the P&S Biomedical Science Symposia)*, A. Karlin, H. J. Vogel, and V. M. Tennyson, eds. New York: Academic Press, pp. 373–386.

PFENNINGER, K. H., and R. P. REES, 1976. From the growth cone to the synapse: Properties of membranes involved in synapse formation. In *Neuronal Recognition*, S. H. Barondes, ed. New York: Plenum Press, pp. 131–178, 357–358.

PFENNINGER, K. H., and C. M. ROVAINEN, 1974. Stimulation- and calcium-dependence of vesicle attachment sites in the presynaptic membrane: A freeze-cleave study on the lamprey spinal cord. *Brain Res.* 72:1–23.

PFENNINGER, K., C. SANDRI, K. AKERT, and C. II. EUGSTER, 1969. Contribution to the problem of structural organization of the presynaptic area. *Brain Res.* 12:10–18.

POTTER, L. T., and D. S. SMITH, 1977. Postsynaptic membranes in the electric tissue of *Narcine*: 1. Organization and innervation of electric cells. Fine structure of nicotinic receptor-channel molecules revealed by transmission microscopy. *Tissue and Cell* 9:585–594.

REES, R. P., 1978. The morphology of interneuronal synaptogenesis: A review. *Fed. Proc.* 37:2000–2009.

REES, R. P., and R. P. BUNGE, 1974. Morphological and cytochemical studies of synapses formed in culture between isolated rat superior cervical ganglion neurons. *J. Comp. Neurol.* 157:1–12.

REES, R. P., M. B. BUNGE, and R. P. BUNGE, 1976. Morphological changes in the neuritic growth cone and target neuron during synaptic junction development in culture. *J. Cell Biol.* 68:240–263.

ROTH, S., E. J. MCGUIRE, and S. ROSEMAN, 1971. Evidence for cell-surface glycosyltransferases: Their potential role in cellular recognition. *J. Cell Biol.* 51:536–547.

RUBIN, L. L., K. H. PFENNINGER, and A. MAURO, 1975. Effect of black widow spider venom on neurons in tissue culture. *Neurosci. Abstr.* 1:623.

SANDRI, C., K. AKERT, R. B. LIVINGSTON, and H. MOOR, 1972. Particle aggregation in freeze-etched postsynaptic membranes. *Brain Res.* 41:1–16.

SIEKEVITZ, P., 1972. Biological membranes: The dynamics of their organization. *Annu. Rev. Physiol.* 34:117–140.

SINGER, S. J., and L. I. ROTHFIELD, 1973. Synthesis and turnover of cell membranes. *Neurosci. Res. Program Bull.* 11:1–86.

STALLCUP, W. B., 1977. Specificity of adhesion between cloned neural cell lines. *Brain Res.* 126:475–486.

STELZNER, D., A. MARTIN, and G. SCOTT, 1973. Early stages of synaptogenesis in the cervical spinal cord of the chick embryo. *Z. Zellforsch.* 138:475–488.

STREIT, P., K. AKERT, C. SANDRI, R. B. LIVINGSTON, and H. MOOR, 1972. Dynamic ultrastructure of presynaptic membranes at nerve terminals in the spinal cord of rats. Anesthetized and unanesthetized preparations compared. *Brain Res.* 48:11–26.

TENNYSON, V. M., 1970. The fine structure of the axon and growth cone of the dorsal root neuroblast of the rabbit embryo. *J. Cell Biol.* 44:62–79.

TRENKNER, E., K. HERRUP, M. E. HATTEN, and S. SARKAR, 1977. Staggerer mutant mice and normal littermates express different carbohydrates on potential cerebellar cells. *Neurosci. Abstr.* 3:62.

VENZIN, M., C. SANDRI, K. AKERT, and U. R. WYSS, 1977. Membrane associated particles of the presynaptic active zone in rat spinal cord: A morphometric analysis. *Brain Res.* 130.393–404.

WESSELLS, N. K., R. P. NUTTALL, J. T. WRENN, and S. JOHNSON, 1976. Differential labeling of the cell surface of single ciliary ganglion neurons *in vitro*. *Proc. Natl. Acad. Sci. USA* 73:4100–4104.

WOOD, M. R., K. H. PFENNINGER, and M. J. COHEN, 1977. Two types of presynaptic configurations in insect central synapses: An ultrastructural analysis. *Brain Res.* 130:25–45.

YAMADA, K. M., B. S. SPOONER, and N. K. WESSELLS, 1971. Ultrastructure and function of growth cones and axons of cultured nerve cells. *J. Cell Biol.* 49:614–635.

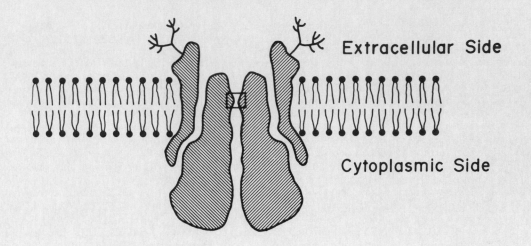

Extracellular Side

Cytoplasmic Side

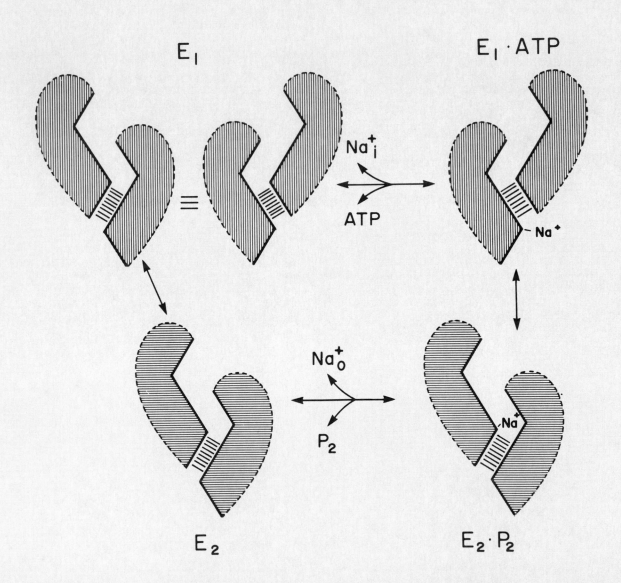

E_I

$E_I \cdot ATP$

Na^+_i

ATP

Na^+

Na^+_0

P_2

Na^+

E_2

$E_2 \cdot P_2$

CHEMICAL REGULATION AND TRANSDUCTION

Model for the transport of ions by the $(Na^+ + K^+)$ ATPase. The key feature in this model is the change in intersubunit contacts during turnover. (See the chapter by Guido Guidotti, this volume.)

Introduction

GORDON G. HAMMES

Two IMPORTANT aspects of neuronal interactions are the amplification of small signals into major responses and the coupling between chemical processes and ion transport. The theme of this section is how chemical processes can be used as a mode of communication and regulation in physiological systems. This includes consideration of the coupling of chemical processes with ion transport and the general implications of the results for neurosystems. Chemical regulation and transduction are of major importance in physiological systems, and a large variety of different mechanisms are utilized. A few relatively well-documented examples, which have obvious implications and applications to the nervous system, will be stressed, and emphasis will be placed on understanding the molecular bases of the underlying mechanisms.

First, E. R. Stadtman and P. B. Chock discuss cascade phenomena in enzyme regulation. Enzyme cascades feature a sequence of enzymatic processes, each one triggered by a prior reaction in the sequence. Examples are undirectional cascades, such as blood clotting, and cyclic cascades, such as are involved in metabolic regulation. The actual molecular mechanisms can involve proteolysis, enzyme-catalyzed covalent modification, and allosteric interactions. These cascades can produce a large amplification of small signals and can also provide delicately responsive regulation. A number of these mechanisms are now understood in considerable detail.

A. G. Gilman and E. M. Ross consider how communication occurs between the inside and outside of a cell in hormone-sensitive adenylate cyclase systems. While it is clear that hormone binding to a receptor on the outside of a cell membrane can stimulate adenylate cyclase bound to the inside of the cell, the molecular nature of the coupling is unknown. The hormone recognition sites and the adenylate cyclase are not covalently linked, and their coupling apparently involves several other components. Therefore, cascades and cooperativity may play an important functional role. Although a molecular description of this system is still not available, it represents an extremely important regulatory mechanism; a considerable amount of information and insight concerning the detailed mechanism is slowly emerging.

To conclude this section, G. Guidotti discusses the coupling of ion transport to enzymatic activity. The important role of ion fluxes in the operation of neurosystems is clear. More generally, ion gradients have been implicated in a variety of physiological mechanisms. The ion gradients are established by chemical energy obtained from membrane-bound enzymes. An understanding of the coupling between ion pumping and enzyme catalysis is of central importance. In recent years, several of the enzymes involved in ion pumping have been purified and reconstituted into phospholipid vesicles; this has provided a description of some of the molecular details of the coupling.

The dynamics of chemical processes are sufficiently rapid to regulate and to provide communication for virtually all physiological processes. The versatility of chemical reactions in regulation and transduction is apparent. Specific mechanisms used in neuronal systems may well be similar.

46 Advantages of Enzyme Cascades in the Regulation of Key Metabolic Processes

E. R. STADTMAN and P. B. CHOCK

ABSTRACT The important role of enzyme cascades in the regulation of numerous biological functions is suggested by the ever-increasing number of reports showing that the activities of key enzymes in metabolism are modulated by covalent modification reactions and by the fact that covalent modifications of membrane proteins (enzymes?) are associated with changes in exocytotic secretory processes, in bacterial chemotaxis, in membrane transport of electrolytes and metabolites, in muscle contractile processes, and in diverse neurochemical phenomena. Theoretical analysis of model systems and in vitro studies of mammalian pyruvate dehydrogenase and of *Escherichia coli* glutamine synthetase show that interconvertible enzyme cascades are endowed with extraordinary characteristics that make them uniquely effective for the regulation of key enzymic processes. Such cascades serve as amplifier systems with respect to both signal response and catalytic potential. By means of allosteric interactions, they serve as metabolic integration systems that continuously monitor the changes in many different metabolites and thus facilitate adjustments in the activities of key enzymes. In addition, enzyme cascades serve as multiplier systems with respect to rate functions and are therefore capable of generating an amplified response to primary stimuli within the millisecond time range.

Introduction

THE REGULATION of many important biochemical processes involves activation or inactivation of key enzymes by covalent modification reactions. Because these modification reactions are catalyzed by so-called converter enzymes, they involve the action of one enzyme upon another and are therefore referred to as cascade systems (MacFarlane, 1964; Stadtman and Chock, 1977a). Two types of covalent enzyme modification are illustrated in Figure 1. The one shown in Figure 1A involves proteolytic cleavage of a specific peptide bond, as occurs in the conversion of zymo-

E. R. STADTMAN and P. B. CHOCK Laboratory of Biochemistry, National Heart, Lung, and Blood Institute, National Institutes of Health, Bethesda, MD 20014

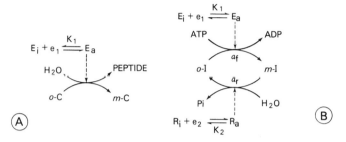

FIGURE 1 Schematic representation of a single-step unidirectional cascade (A) and a monocyclic cascade (B). The notation is as follows: K_1 and K_2 are dissociation constants for E_a and R_a, respectively; e_1 and e_2 are allosteric effectors; E_i and R_i are inactive converter enzymes; o-C and m-C are unmodified and modified protein (or enzyme), respectively; o-I and m-I are unmodified and modified interconvertible enzyme, respectively; $\alpha_f = k_f/K_f$ and $\alpha_r = k_r/K_r$, where k_f and k_r are specific rate constants for the forward and reverse reactions as designated and K_f and K_r are dissociation constants for the o-I·E_a and m-I·R_a complexes (not shown), respectively.

gens (pepsinogin, trypsinogen, etc.) to their activated forms (Neurath and Walsh, 1976); the other (Figure 1B) involves derivatization of a particular amino acid residue within the polypeptide chain, as occurs in the ATP-dependent phosphorylation of seryl hydroxyl groups of pyruvate dehydrogenase (Hucho et al., 1972) and in the ATP-dependent adenylylation of a tyrosyl hydroxyl group of *Escherichia coli* glutamine synthetase (Kingdon, Shapiro, and Stadtman, 1967; Wulff, Mecke, and Holzer, 1967). These two types of cascades are further distinguished by the fact that the proteolytic conversion of zymogens (proenzymes) to active enzymes is essentially irreversible, whereas enzyme derivatization is a cyclical process resulting from the coupling of two opposing cascades, one concerned with the covalent modification and the other with the demodification of an interconvertible enzyme.

More extended cascades are obtained when there is sequential modification of two or more convertible enzymes in a series such that the modified form of each successive enzyme in the series catalyzes the covalent modification of the next enzyme in the series (Figure 2). Multistep cascades involving a series of proteolytic events are concerned with blood clotting (Davie, Hougie, and Lundblad, 1969; Davie and Fujikawa, 1975) and complement fixation (Müller-Eberhard, 1975), whereas multicyclic cascades of interconvertible enzymes are involved in the regulation of glycogen phosphorylase (Fischer, Heilmeyer, and Haschke, 1971; Krebs, 1972), glutamine synthetase (Adler et al., 1974; Stadtman and Ginsburg, 1974), and polypeptide chain initiation factor eIF-2 (Datta et al., 1977).

General considerations

Cascade systems possess extraordinary regulatory characteristics because: (1) they serve as multiplier systems with respect to kinetic parameters; (2) they serve as amplifier systems with respect both to signal amplification and catalytic potential; (3) they are capable of responding to a multitude of allosteric interactions; (4) they are capable of generating a highly "cooperative" type of response to increasing concen-trations of allosteric effectors; and (5) they are highly flexible in their allosteric control patterns.

The multiplier effect derives from the fact that the rate of product formation in the last step (cycle) of the cascade is a multiplicative function of the rate constants of all the steps in the cascade. The capacity for signal amplification derives from the fact that, given sufficient time, any amount of the activated form of the first converter enzyme in the cascade can catalyze complete covalent modification of any amount of substrate enzyme. In this sense, the signal amplification of unidirectional cascades is infinite, whereas the signal-amplification potential of cyclic cascades is a finite variable function of many cascade parameters. Nevertheless, if the concentrations of positive effectors that control the activity of the first converter enzyme in the forward cascade are regulated reciprocally with respect to the concentrations of effectors that regulate the activity of the last converter enzyme in the regeneration cascade, the cyclic cascades will behave as open unidirectional cascade systems.

For quantitative comparative purposes the *signal-amplification potential* (*SA*) of a cyclic cascade is defined as the ratio of the concentration of effector, e_1, required to produce 50% activation of the first converter enzyme to the concentration of e_1 required to produce 50% modification of the last interconvertible

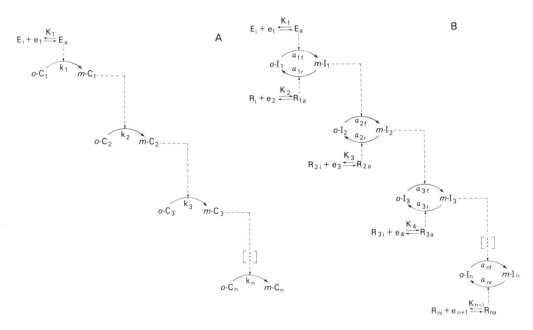

FIGURE 2 Schematic representation of a unidirectional cascade containing n steps (A) and a cyclic cascade consisting of n cycles (B). See Figure 1 for notation.

enzyme in the cascade:

$$SA = \frac{[e_1]_{0.5E}}{[e_1]_{0.5I_n}} .$$

The high *catalytic-amplification potential (CA)* of cascades is a consequence of the fact that in most cascades there is a pyramidal increase in the concentration of the convertible (interconvertible) enzymes with each successive step in the cascade. It follows that if the catalytic efficiencies of the first converter enzyme and the last interconvertible enzyme are the same, then *CA* is the ratio of the concentration of these enzymes:

$$CA = \frac{[I_n]}{[E]} = \frac{[C_n]}{[E]} .$$

For the blood-clotting system, in which there is a nearly tenfold increase in the concentration of convertible enzyme in each of six successive steps in the cascade (MacFarlane, 1964), $CA = 10^6$.

The ability of cascade systems to respond to a multiplicity of allosteric effectors is due to the fact that they are comprised of many different enzymes, each of which can be a separate target for allosteric interactions. Moreover, allosteric interactions at any step in the cascade will affect the rate and/or the extent of covalent modification of the last convertible or interconvertible enzyme in the cascade.

For situations in which a given effector can stimulate two or more steps in the cascade, the overall effect is to increase the apparent order of the activation process with respect to that effector. Thus, if a given ligand stimulates four separate steps in a multicyclic cascade, the overall effect of that ligand on the activity of the last enzyme in the cascade will be a sigmoidal function of the ligand concentration and, under ideal conditions, can yield a cooperativity index (Hill number) of 4. It is noteworthy that in cyclic cascades a cooperative response will be obtained if a given effector activates the forward converter enzymes and also inhibits the regeneration converter enzyme (Stadtman and Chock, 1977a). Cyclic cascades are therefore capable of generating higher degrees of cooperativity than are unidirectional cascades.

The unique regulatory capacities of cyclic cascades become apparent from detailed theoretical analyses of monocyclic, bicyclic, and multicyclic cascade models (Chock and Stadtman, 1977; Stadtman and Chock, 1977a,b) and also from detailed studies of allosteric effects on the phosphorylation and dephosphorylation of the mammalian pyruvate dehydrogen-

ase complex and on the adenylylation and deadenylylation of *E. coli* glutamine synthetase.

Monocyclic cascade systems

STEADY-STATE ANALYSIS The main features of a single interconvertible enzyme cascade system are shown in Figure 1B. The system consists of two essentially irreversible cascades. The *forward cascade* is triggered by the interaction of an allosteric effector e_1 with the inactive form of the converter enzyme E which converts it to the active form. This activated enzyme catalyzes the covalent modification (phosphorylation) of the original form o-I of the interconvertible enzyme I, which converts it to the modified form m-I. This cascade is opposed by the *regeneration cascade* triggered by the interaction of an allosteric effector e_2 with the inactive form of the converter enzyme R, which leads to its activated form. Dynamic coupling of the forward and regeneration cascades results in the cyclic interconversion of o-I and m-I and the concomitant conversion of ATP to ADP and Pi. With reasonable simplifying assumptions described elsewhere (Stadtman and Chock, 1977a,b), it can be shown that for any given metabolic situation, a steady state will be established in which the rate of m-I formation will be equal to the rate of o-I regeneration. For this situation the fraction of interconvertible enzyme in the modified form at steady state is given by

$$\frac{[m\text{-}I]}{[I]} = \left[\frac{\alpha_r[R][e_2](K_1 + [e_1])}{\alpha_f[E][e_1](K_2 + [e_2])} + 1 \right]^{-1}, \quad (1)$$

where [I], [E], and [R] represent the total concentrations of interconvertible enzyme, forward converter enzyme, and regeneration converter enzyme, respectively; $[e_1]$ and $[e_2]$ are the effector concentrations; K_1 and K_2 are the dissociation constants for reactions as indicated in Figure 1B; and $\alpha_f = k_f/K_f$ and $\alpha_r = k_r/K_r$, where k_f and k_r are specific rate constants for the forward and regeneration cascades, respectively, and K_f and K_r are dissociation constants for the converter enzyme–interconvertible enzyme complexes, o-I·E$_a$ and m-I·R$_a$, respectively (not shown).

Equation 1 shows that for any metabolic state the fraction of interconvertible enzyme in the modified form is a multiplicative function of ten different parameters (α_f and α_r are composed of two parameters each), each of which (except e_1 and e_2, which are needed to initiate the cascades) can be modulated by allosteric interactions of one or more of the cascade enzymes with one or more allosteric effectors. It is therefore evident that interconvertible enzyme cascades are endowed with extraordinary amplification potential and have a greater capacity for allosteric regulation than do other types of regulatory enzymes.

In the model depicted in Figure 1B, the interaction of effector e_1 with the E-converter enzyme ($e_1 + E_i \rightarrow E_a$) is the primary signal that triggers covalent modification of the interconvertible enzyme. The extraordinary ability of the cyclic cascade to amplify its response to this primary signal is illustrated by the curves in Figure 3, which are derived from equation 1. For each curve it was assumed that the dissociation constant K_1 for the allosteric reaction $E_a \rightarrow E_i + e_1$ is equal to 1.0 and that no cooperativity is involved in the binding of e_1 with E_i. With this assumption the dotted line in Figure 3 shows how the fractional saturation of E with e_1 (that is, the $[E_a]/[E]$ ratio) varies with the concentration of e_1. It is important to note that the binding of e_1 to E_i is the only step in the cascade in which e_1 is directly involved. Nevertheless, other curves in Figure 3 show that when the binding of e_1 to the converter enzyme is linked to the cascade via the catalytic action of E_a, the indirect effect of e_1 on fractional modification of the interconvertible enzyme can vary enormously, depending on the magnitudes of the other parameters

in the cascade cycle. Variations in these parameters have two effects on the interconvertible enzyme: (1) they determine the concentration of e_1 required to produce a given fractional modification of the interconvertible enzyme; (2) they determine the maximal level of modification that can be obtained with saturation concentrations of e_1 (i.e., when $[E_a]/[E] = 1.0$). In other words, both the amplification and the amplitude of the response to e_1 are affected.

Curve 1 in Figure 3 shows that when all parameters, except e_1, in equation 1 are assigned values of 1.0, a maximum of 67% of the interconvertible enzyme can be modified in the steady state obtained with saturating concentrations of e_1; moreover, the concentration of e_1 required to achieve a steady state in which 50% of the interconvertible enzyme is modified is the same (= 1.0) as that required to produce 50% saturation of the E-converter enzyme. Under these conditions, the amplitude of the e_1 response is 0.67 and, because $[e]_{0.5E}/[e]_{0.5I} = 1.0$, there is no signal amplification. However, other curves in Figure 3 show that as each of the six other parameters in equation 1 are varied by a factor of two, in a successively cumulative manner that favors modification of the interconvertible enzyme, there is a progressive increase in both the amplitude of the e_1 effect and in the signal-amplification potential (i.e., the $[e_1]_{0.5I}$ value decreases).

Since twofold changes in the cascade parameters are well within the range of allosteric effects, it appears highly significant that twofold changes in six parameters cause an eightyfold increase in the signal amplification and an increase in amplitude from 0.67 to 1.0 (compare curves 1 and 7 in Figure 3). Note also that as a consequence of the multiplicative effect obtained when several cascade parameters are varied simultaneously, interconvertible enzymes can respond to primary effector concentrations that are well below the dissociation constants of the effector-converter enzyme complexes. This is illustrated by a comparison of the dotted curve and curve 7 in Figure 3, which shows that with twofold changes in the six cascade parameters, a 2% activation of the converter enzyme leads to 90% activation of the interconvertible enzyme.

MULTIPLICITY OF REGULATORY PATTERNS If the binding of e_1 to the E-converter enzyme is always the primary signal that triggers the monocyclic cascade, then the four distinctly different allosteric control patterns illustrated in Figure 4 can be utilized to regulate the cascade. In case I, which is identical to that described in Figure 1B, effector e_1 activates the

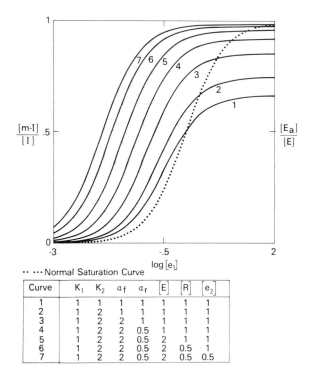

···· Normal Saturation Curve

Curve	K_1	K_2	a_f	a_r	[E]	[R]	e_2
1	1	1	1	1	1	1	1
2	1	2	1	1	1	1	1
3	1	2	2	1	1	1	1
4	1	2	2	0.5	1	1	1
5	1	2	2	0.5	2	1	1
6	1	2	2	0.5	2	0.5	1
7	1	2	2	0.5	2	0.5	0.5

FIGURE 3 Computer-simulated curves showing the effects of cumulative twofold changes in each cascade variable (except K_1) on the fractional modification of an interconvertible enzyme in a monocyclic cascade. (From Stadtman and Chock, 1977b, with the permission of Academic Press.)

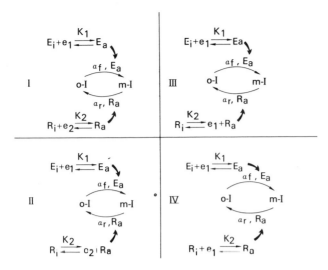

FIGURE 4 Four regulatory patterns derived from the monocyclic cascade system. Notation is as described in Figure 1, except that K_2 in II and III is a dissociation constant for R_i. (From Stadtman and Chock, 1977b, with the permission of Academic Press.)

E-converter enzyme and a different effector, c_2, activates the R-converter enzyme. Case II differs only in that e_2 inactivates rather than activates the R-enzyme. In case III, e_1 activates the E-enzyme and also inactivates the R-enzyme; and in case IV, e_1 is an activator of both converter enzymes.

The steady-state equations for each of these four

cases have been reported elsewhere (Stadtman and Chock, 1977a,b). Computer-simulated curves derived from these equations are shown in Figure 5. The curves show how the fractional modification of an interconvertible enzyme varies as a function of e_1 concentration in all four models when values of all other parameters in the steady-state equations are held constant. Note that a unique pattern of response to variations in the values of K_1 and α_f is obtained for each type of cascade control. These few examples do not begin to illustrate the enormous flexibility of the monocyclic cascade system with respect to allosteric control. Because each enzyme in the cascade can react with more than one positive or negative allosteric effector, it is evident that an almost unlimited number of allosteric control patterns can be elicited by extensions and combinations of the basic patterns illustrated in Figure 5.

REGULATION OF MAMMALIAN PYRUVATE DEHYDROGENASE Pyruvate dehydrogenase is a prototype for the kind of monocyclic cascade described above. As is shown in Figure 6, phosphorylation (inactivation) of the enzyme is catalyzed by a specific kinase, whereas dephosphorylation (activation) is catalyzed by a specific phosphatase (Hucho et al., 1972; Pettit, Pelley, and Reed, 1975; Reed et al., 1976); moreover, the kinase and phosphatase activities are controlled by numerous allosteric effectors. Figure 7 shows that for

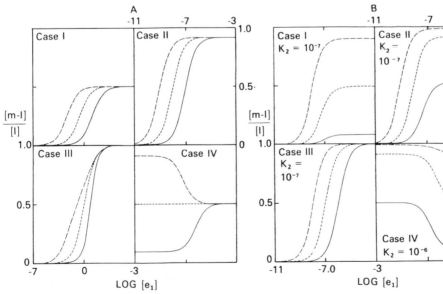

FIGURE 5 The effect of e_1 concentration on the fractional modification of an interconvertible enzyme as a function of K_1 (in A) and α_f (in B) for the four regulatory patterns depicted in Figure 4. The computer-simulated curves were obtained with the assumption that [E] = [R] and otherwise

as follows: (A) $\alpha_f = \alpha_r$ and $K_1 = 10^{-6}$ (———), 10^{-7} ($\cdot\cdot\cdot$), or 10^{-8} (---); (B) $K_1 = 10^{-7}$, K_2 is as shown, $\alpha_r = 10^{-5}$, and $\alpha_f = 10^{-4}$ (———), 10^5 ($\cdot\cdot\cdot$), or 10^6 (---). (From Stadtman and Chock, 1977b, with the permission of Academic Press.)

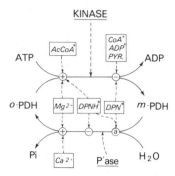

FIGURE 6 The role of some effectors in the interconversion of mammalian pyruvate dehydrogenase. * indicates that the effect is observed only in the presence of K^+ or NH_4^+; a indicates that DPN antagonizes the inhibition by DPNH; + and − indicate activation and inactivation, respectively.

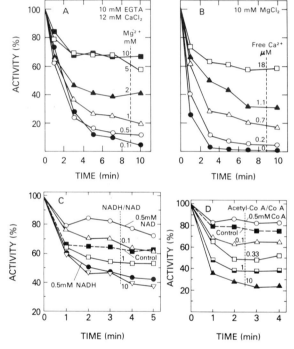

FIGURE 7 Steady-state levels of active mammalian pyruvate dehydrogenase (dephosphorylated form) as a function of allosteric effector concentrations. (Parts A and B from Reed et al., 1973. Parts C and D from Pettit, Pelley, and Reed, 1975.)

a given set of conditions, the fraction of phosphorylated dehydrogenase assumes a steady-state value that is determined by the relative concentrations of the effectors, Ca^{2+}, Mg^{2+}, DPNH, DPN, acetyl CoA, and CoA. These observations are therefore in qualitative agreement with predictions of the steady-state model described above. It is also noteworthy that three of the four regulatory patterns illustrated in Figure 4 are utilized in regulation of the pyruvate dehydro-

genase cascade. Thus acetyl CoA and Ca^{2+} have roles corresponding to e_1 and e_2 in case I; DPNH corresponds to e_1 in case III; and Mg^{2+} corresponds to e_1 in case IV.

IMPORTANCE OF ATP DECOMPOSITION IN CASCADE SYSTEMS It is evident from Figure 1B that each complete cycle in a phosphorylation-dephosphorylation cascade is associated with the net decomposition of ATP to ADP and Pi. In the steady-state analysis discussed here, the role of ATP has been disregarded since the concentration of ATP is maintained by metabolism at a nearly constant level several orders of magnitude greater than the cascade enzymes. Nevertheless, the decomposition of ATP is an essential feature of the interconvertible enzyme cascade; this decomposition provides the free energy that is needed to maintain a particular steady-state level of modified enzyme (Stadtman and Chock, 1977b). In the absence of a continuous supply of ATP, essentially all of the interconvertible enzyme would assume the thermodynamically most stable state, that is, the unmodified form (o-I). The consumption of ATP is the price that must be paid to support the cyclic cascade type of cellular regulation.

Bicyclic cascades

When the modified form of an interconvertible enzyme in one cycle catalyzes the covalent modification of an interconvertible enzyme in another cycle, the two cycles are coupled in such a way that the modification of the second interconvertible enzyme is a function of all the parameters in both cycles (Chock and Stadtman, 1977; Stadtman and Chock, 1977b). Figure 8 shows two types of bicyclic cascades that are involved in the regulation of key enzymes in metabolism. One of these, referred to as an "opened" bicyclic cascade, is utilized in the regulation of glycogen phosphorylase (Fischer, Heilmeyer, and Haschke, 1971; Krebs, 1972) and of the initiation factor eIF-2, which is involved in protein synthesis (Datta et al., 1977). The other, referred to as a "closed" bicyclic cascade, is utilized in the regulation of glutamine synthetase from gram-negative bacteria (Stadtman and Ginsburg, 1974; Adler et al., 1974).

THE OPENED BICYCLIC CASCADE As shown in Figure 8A, the glycogen phosphorylase cascade is initiated by the interaction of cAMP with the inactive protein kinase (PK_i), which is thereby converted to the active kinase (PK_a). Activated protein kinase then catalyzes the phosphorylation of inactive phosphorylase b kinase (o-PHOS b K) and thereby converts it to the active form (m-PHOS b K). Finally, the latter catalyzes the

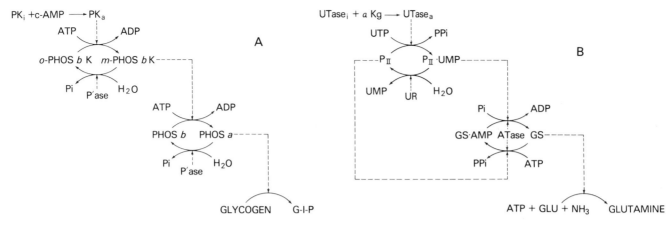

FIGURE 8 The glycogen phosphorylase cascade (A) and the glutamine synthetase cascade (B). Abbreviations are as follows: PK$_i$ and PK$_a$ are the inactive and active forms of cyclic AMP–dependent protein kinase; o-PHOS b K and m-PHOS b K, the unmodified and modified (active) forms of phosphorylase b kinase; PHOS b and PHOS a, the non-phosphorylated and phosphorylated (active) phosphoryl-ase; P′ase, phosphatase; α-KG, α-ketoglutarate; UTase and UTase$_a$, the inactive and active uridylyltransferase; UR, uridylyl-removing enzyme; P$_{II}$ and P$_{II}$·UMP, unmodified and uridylylated regulatory protein; ATase, adenylyltrans-ferase; GS·AMP and GS, adenylylated and unadenylylated glutamine synthetase.

phosphorylation of phosphorylase b to produce the active phosphorylase a. Note that this forward cas-cade is opposed by the action of two phosphatases that catalyze dephosphorylation of the activated forms of phosphorylase and phosphorylase b kinase.

Steady-state analysis of a bicyclic cascade model patterned after the glycogen phosphorylase system shows that fractional modification of the second in-terconvertible enzyme in the cascade is a multiplica-tive function of eighteen parameters, whereas only ten are involved in a monocyclic cascade (Chock and Stadtman, 1977). Since each parameter is susceptible to modulation by variations in the concentrations of allosteric effectors, bicyclic cascades are capable of achieving a much greater amplification of response to primary stimuli than are monocyclic cascades. In addition, the number of converter enzymes in a bi-cyclic cascade is greater than in a monocyclic cascade; bicyclic cascades can therefore assume a much greater number of unique regulatory patterns in response to positive and negative allosteric interactions. Further-more, four different steps in a bicyclic cascade can be regulated by one and the same allosteric effector; they are therefore capable of generating a highly "cooperative" response to increasing effector concen-trations (Chock and Stadtman, 1977; Stadtman and Chock, 1977b).

THE CLOSED BICYCLIC CASCADE THAT REGULATES E. COLI GLUTAMINE SYNTHETASE Figure 8B depicts the bicyclic cascade that regulates glutamine synthetase activity in E. coli and other gram-negative bacteria

(see Stadtman and Ginsburg, 1974). In this represen-tation, the cascade is initiated by the interaction of the allosteric effector α-ketoglutarate (αKg) with a uridylyltransferase (UTase) that catalyzes the UTP-dependent uridylylation of the hydroxyl group of a unique tyrosyl residue on each of four subunits of a regulatory protein, P$_{II}$. The uridylylation of P$_{II}$ is opposed by the action of a uridylyl-removing enzyme (UR) that catalyzes hydrolysis of the UMP-O-tyrosyl bond to form UMP and unmodified P$_{II}$.

The second cycle involves the adenylylation and deadenylylation of glutamine synthetase (GS), both of which are catalyzed by one and the same adeny-lyltransferase (ATase). Adenylylation involves trans-fer of the adenylyl group of ATP to the hydroxyl group of a particular tyrosyl residue in each subunit, whereas deadenylylation is by phosphorolysis of the AMP-O-tyrosyl bond to form ADP and unmodified glutamine synthetase. Because glutamine synthetase is composed of twelve identical subunits, up to twelve equivalents of AMP can be bound to each molecule. From the standpoint of cellular regulation, it is sig-nificant that under physiological conditions, the spe-cific activity of the enzyme is inversely proportional to the average number of adenylyl groups bound per molecule of enzyme. The adenylylation and dead-enylylation reactions are catalyzed by the same en-zyme (ATase); therefore the capacity of ATase to catalyze these opposing reactions must be strictly reg-ulated in order to avoid their indiscriminate coupling, which would lead to useless conversion of ATP and Pi to ADP and PPi. Indiscriminate cycling is prevented by the fact that the unmodified form of P_{II} is needed to activate the ATase for the adenylylation reaction, whereas the uridylylated form, $P_{II} \cdot UMP$, is required for ATase catalysis of the deadenylylation reaction. As shown by Figure 8B, the interactions of ATase with P_{II} on the one hand and with $P_{II} \cdot UMP$ on the other results in a "closed" coupling of the uridylylation and adenylylation cycles.

It follows from Figure 8B that for any metabolic situation, the specific activity of glutamine synthetase will be determined by the steady-state fraction of its subunits that are adenylylated and this will be specified by the relative activities of the converter enzymes, ATase, UR-enzyme, and UTase. Moreover, these activities will be functions of the various reaction constants and the relative concentrations of multiple allosteric effectors.

A steady-state analysis of a closed bicyclic cascade model of the glutamine synthetase type shows that the fractional modification (adenylylation) of the interconvertible enzyme in the second cycle is a multiplicative function of fourteen parameters, each of which can be modulated by variations in the concentrations of allosteric effectors (Chock and Stadtman, 1977; Stadtman and Chock, 1977b).

Glutamine occupies a central role in intermediary metabolism. It is a precursor in the biosynthesis of all amino acids, purine and pyrimidine nucleotides, and complex polysaccharides (Stadtman, 1973). The closed bicyclic cascade is therefore eminently suited for the regulation of glutamine synthetase, whose activity must be responsive to fluctuations in a huge number of metabolites. This need for rigorous control is evident from two facts: (1) in addition to its dependence of mono- and divalent cations, the activity of *E. coli* glutamine synthetase is susceptible to cumulative feedback inhibition by eight endproducts of glutamine metabolism (Woolfolk and Stadtman, 1967; Stadtman and Ginsburg, 1974); (2) collectively, activities of the three converter enzymes (ATase, UTase, and UR-enzyme) can be modulated by at least 27 different metabolites, the most important of which are ATP, UTP, CMP, glutamine, α-ketoglutarate, CoA, and orthophosphate (Stadtman, Chock, and Adler, 1976). It follows from a steady-state analysis of the closed bicyclic cascade that interactions of these several allosteric effectors with one or more of the glutamine synthetase cascade enzymes could lead to alterations in the effective enzyme concentrations and/or the kinetic constants of the modifying steps and could thereby influence the steady-state level of adenylylation (activity) of glutamine synthetase. Quantitative analysis of the glutamine synthetase cascade is not yet possible because we have insufficient knowledge of the specific rate constants of the individual steps in the cascade and of the stability constants of the various protein-protein intermediates and of the allosteric effector-enzyme complexes.

Nevertheless, preliminary in vivo and in vitro studies (Segal, Brown, and Stadtman, 1974; Senior, 1975; Rhee et al., 1977) have confirmed in principle the important features disclosed by the theoretical steady-state analysis (Chock and Stadtman, 1977; Stadtman and Chock, 1977b).

Multicyclic cascade systems

A better appreciation of the relationship between the number of cycles in a cascade and its regulatory characteristics is gained from a consideration of a cascade containing n cycles, as depicted in Figure 2B. In developing the steady-state analysis of this model it was assumed that the forward cascade is initiated by the binding of an allosteric effector e_1 to the first converter enzyme and that thereafter the modified form of an interconvertible enzyme in one cycle serves as the converter enzyme in the next cycle; also, the impact of effectors on the activities of the several regenerating enzymes was discounted to simplify the theoretical treatment. Otherwise the assumptions were the same as those made in deriving equation 1. Various interconvertible enzymes are identified by a numerical subscript corresponding to the order in which they appear in the cascade; thus the interconvertible enzyme in the first, second, $\ldots$, nth cycles are I_1, I_2, $\ldots$, I_n, respectively. The corresponding original and modified forms of these are identified as $o\text{-}I_1$, $o\text{-}I_2$, $\ldots$, $o\text{-}I_n$ and $m\text{-}I_1$, $m\text{-}I_2$, $\ldots$, $m\text{-}I_n$, respectively. Similarly, the R-converter enzymes in the first, second, $\ldots$, nth cycles are referred to as R_1, R_2, $\ldots$, R_n, respectively. The steady-state expression for fractional modification of the interconvertible enzyme in the nth cycle is (Chock and Stadtman, 1977):

$$\frac{[m\text{-}I_n]}{[I_n]} = \left[\frac{\alpha_{1r}\alpha_{2r}\alpha_{3r} \cdots \alpha_{nr}[R_1][R_2] \cdots [R_n][e_2][e_3] \cdots [e_{n+1}](K_1 + [e_1])}{\alpha_{1f}\alpha_{2f}\alpha_{3f} \cdots \alpha_{nf}[E][I_1][I_2] \cdots [I_{n-1}][e_1](K_2 + [e_2])(K_3 + [e_3]) \cdots (K_{n+1} + [e_{n+1}])} \right.$$

$$+ \frac{\alpha_{2r}\alpha_{3r} \cdots \alpha_{nr}[R_2][R_3] \cdots [R_n][e_3][e_4] \cdots [e_{n+1}]}{\alpha_{2f}\alpha_{3f} \cdots \alpha_{nf}[I_1][I_2] \cdots [I_{n-1}](K_3 + [e_3])(K_4 + [e_4]) \cdots (K_{n+1} + [e_{n+1}])}$$

$$+ \cdots + \left. \frac{\alpha_{nr}[R_n][e_{n+1}]}{\alpha_{nf}[I_{n-1}](K_{n+1} + [e_{n+1}])} + 1 \right]^{-1}.$$

$$(2)$$

Equation 2 shows that with each additional cycle in the cascade, the last interconvertible enzyme becomes dependent upon eight additional variables; moreover, the fractional modification of that enzyme is a multiplicative function of all these new parameters as well as all the ones involved in the preceding cycles. Therefore, the amplification potential and the allosteric-control potential increase enormously with each additional cycle in a cascade. The amplification effect is illustrated by the curves in Figure 9A. For reference, curve 0 shows the dependence of E activation on the concentration of e_1 when K_1 is 1.0. Other curves in Figure 9A show that if K_1 is held constant at 1.0 and all parameters that favor modification are assigned values of 2.0 while those that favor demodification are assigned values of 0.5, then the signal amplification $([e_1]_{0.5I_n})^{-1}$ is increased progressively by increasing the number of cycles in the cascade. It can be calculated from the data in Figure 9A that for 1-, 2-, 3-, and 4-cycle cascades, the amplification factors are 3.2×10^2, 1.02×10^5, 3.28×10^7, and 1.05×10^{10}, respectively. The inset in Figure 9A shows that the log of the amplification factor is proportional to the number of cycles in the cascade.

The exponential nature of signal amplification is more readily seen if it is assumed that the concentra-

tions of $R_1, R_2, \ldots, R_n$ are identical to those of $R_{1a}, R_{2a}, \ldots, R_{na}$ (i.e., that the roles of $e_2, e_3, \ldots, e_n$ are neglected) and also that

$$\frac{\alpha_{1r}[R_1]}{\alpha_{1f}[E]} = \frac{\alpha_{nr}[R_n]}{\alpha_{nf}[I_{n-1}]} = \frac{k'_r}{k_f}$$

for all values of n; then equation 2 reduces to

$$\frac{[m\text{-}I_n]}{[I_n]} = \left[\left(\frac{K_1}{[e_1]} + 1\right)\left(\frac{k'_r}{k'_f}\right)^n + \left(\frac{k'_r}{k'_f}\right)^{n-1}\right.$$
$$\left. + \ldots + \left(\frac{k'_r}{k'_f}\right) + 1\right]^{-1}. \quad (3)$$

Equation 3 illustrates more clearly the amplification capacity of multicyclic cascades, since the fractional modification of I_n is expressed as a function of k'_r/k'_f to the nth power, where n is the number of cycles in the cascade.

Data derived from this simplified equation with the assumptions $k'_f/k'_r = 10$ and $K_1 = 1.0$ are shown in Figure 9B. For these conditions, the amplification factors for 1-, 2-, 3-, and 4-cycle cascades are 9.1, 83, 833, and 8,333, respectively. The inset in Figure 9B shows that the log of the amplification factor is proportional to the number of cycles in the cascade.

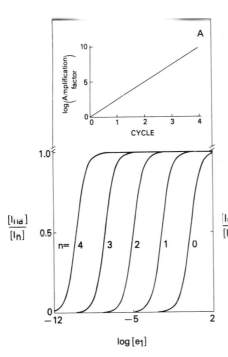 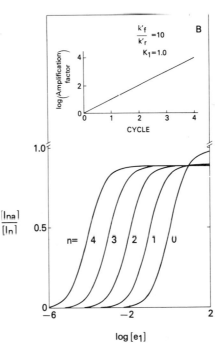

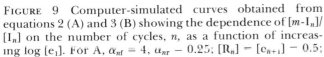

FIGURE 9 Computer-simulated curves obtained from equations 2 (A) and 3 (B) showing the dependence of $[m\text{-}I_n]/[I_n]$ on the number of cycles, n, as a function of increasing log $[e_1]$. For A, $\alpha_{nf} = 4$, $\alpha_{nr} = 0.25$; $[R_n] = [e_{n+1}] = 0.5$; $K_1 = 1$; $K_{n+1} = [E] = [I_{n-1}] = 2$. For B, $K_1 = 1$; $k'_f/k'_r = 10$. The insets in A and B show the linear relationship between the log of the amplification factor and n. (From Stadtman and Chock, 1977b, with the permission of Academic Press.)

With some extreme assumptions, Hemker and Hemker (1969) developed the following simple rate expression for unidirectional cascades of the type shown in Figure 2A:

$$[m\text{-}C_n] = (1/n!)t^n[E_a]k_1k_2 \cdots k_n, \qquad (4)$$

where t is time and k_n is the rate constant for the nth step in the cascade. In deriving equation 4 it was assumed that all the reactions proceed by a single step mechanism and that the activated forms of all converter enzymes are always saturated with their convertible enzyme substrates (e.g., $[E_a] \ll [o\text{-}C_1] \ll [o\text{-}C_2] \ll \ldots \ll [o\text{-}C_n]$). Although this assumption is probably not valid for most physiological situations, equation 4 is nevertheless very instructive. It shows that unidirectional cascades are multiplier systems with respect to time, because the concentration of modified convertible enzyme in the nth step, $m\text{-}C_n$, is a multiplicative function of the product of the rate constants of all steps in the cascade, the concentration of the first convertible enzyme E_a, and the reaction time raised to the nth power.

A more rigorous theoretical analysis of the model depicted in Figure 2A, involving no unreasonable assumptions, shows that the time course for a 1-, 2-, and 3-step unidirectional cascade can be determined by numerical integrations of the following equations (P. B. Chock, unpublished results):

$$\frac{d[m\text{-}C_1]}{dt} = \frac{k_1[E][e_1]}{K_{1f}(K_1 + [e_1])}\,([C_1] - [m\text{-}C_1]), \qquad (5)$$

$$\frac{d[m\text{-}C_2]}{dt} = \frac{k_2[m\text{-}C_1]}{K_{2f}}\,([C_2] - [m\text{-}C_2]), \qquad (6)$$

$$\frac{d[m\text{-}C_3]}{dt} = \frac{k_3[m\text{-}C_2]}{K_{3f}}\,([C_3] - [m\text{-}C_3]), \qquad (7)$$

where $[m\text{-}C_1]$, $[m\text{-}C_2]$, and $[m\text{-}C_3]$ are time-dependent variables; $[C_1]$, $[C_2]$, and $[C_3]$ are total concentrations; and K_{nf} is the dissociation constant for the converter–interconvertible enzyme complex in the nth step of the cascade.

Similarly, the rates of modified interconvertible enzyme formation in 1-, 2-, and 3-cycle cascades can be obtained from the following equations:

$$\frac{d[m\text{-}I_1]}{dt} = \frac{k_{1f}[E][e_1][I_1]}{K_{1f}(K_1 + [e_1])}$$
$$- [m\text{-}I_1]\left(\frac{k_{1f}[E][e_1]}{K_{1f}(K_1 + [e_1])} + \frac{k_{1r}[R_1][e_2]}{K_{1r}(K_2 + [e_2])}\right), \qquad (8)$$

$$\frac{d[m\text{-}I_2]}{dt} = \frac{k_{2f}[I_2][m\text{-}I_1]}{K_{2f}}$$
$$- [m\text{-}I_2]\left(\frac{k_{2f}[m\text{-}I_1]}{K_{2f}} + \frac{k_{2r}[R_2][e_3]}{K_{2r}(K_3 + [e_3])}\right), \qquad (9)$$

$$\frac{d[m\text{-}I_3]}{dt} = \frac{k_{3f}[I_3][m\text{-}I_2]}{K_{3f}}$$
$$- [m\text{-}I_3]\left(\frac{k_{3f}[m\text{-}I_2]}{K_{3f}} + \frac{k_{3r}[R_3][e_4]}{K_{3r}(K_4 + [e_4])}\right), \qquad (10)$$

where $[m\text{-}I_1]$, $[m\text{-}I_2]$, and $[m\text{-}I_3]$ are time-dependent variables.

Figure 10 shows the time courses for enzyme modifications calculated from equations 5–10 for situations in which the following assumptions can reasonably be made:

1. There is a tenfold increase in the concentration of convertible or interconvertible enzyme in each successive step (or cycle) in the cascade (as occurs in the blood-clotting cascade; see MacFarlane, 1964).

2. The specific rate constants k_n of all steps in the unidirectional cascade and all forward rate constants k_{nf} in the cyclic cascades are the same (1,000 sec^{-1}), whereas the rate constants of all reverse steps in the cyclic cascades (k_{nr}) are either 10 (solid lines) or 500 (dotted lines).

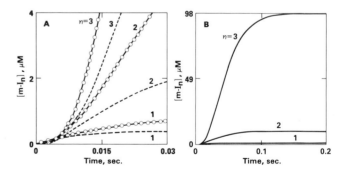

FIGURE 10 Computer-simulated time course for the cascade systems. Solid lines are obtained with a cyclic cascade system using equations 8, 9, and 10; n is the number of cycles (or steps for the unidirectional cascade). The parameters used are: $[e_1] = 10^{-7}$M; $[I_1] = 10^{-6}$M; $[I_2] = 10^{-5}$M; $[I_3] = 10^{-4}$M; $[E] = [R_1] = [e_2] = K_1 = K_2 = 5 \times 10^{-7}$M; $[e_3] = [R_2] = K_3 = 5 \times 10^{-6}$M; $[e_4] = [R_3] = K_4 = 5 \times 10^{-5}$M; $K_{1f} = K_{1r} = 2 \times 10^{-6}$M; $K_{2r} = K_{2f} = 2 \times 10^{-5}$M; $K_{3r} = K_{3f} = 2 \times 10^{-4}$M; $k_{nf} = 1,000$ sec^{-1}; and $k_{nr} = 10$ sec^{-1}. Open circles represent the unidirectional cascade obtained with equations 5, 6, and 7 with $[E] = K_1 = 5 \times 10^{-7}$M; $[e_1] = 10^{-7}$M; $K_{1f} = 2 \times 10^{-6}$M; $K_{2f} = 2 \times 10^{-5}$M; $K_{3f} = 2 \times 10^{-4}$M; $[C_1] = 10^{-6}$M; $[C_2] = 10^{-5}$M; $[C_3] = 10^{-4}$M; and $k_n = 1,000$ sec^{-1}. The dashed lines were obtained with the same parameter values used for the solid lines, except $k_{nr} = 500$ sec^{-1}. Graph A is the expansion of graph B.

3. The ratios of the dissociation constants for the enzyme-enzyme complexes to the concentrations of the interconvertible (convertible) enzymes for all forward steps in the cascade are the same (viz. $K_{1F}/[I_1] = K_{2f}/[I_2] = K_{3f}/[I_3] = 2.0$).

4. The concentrations of the allosteric effectors e_1, $e_2, \ldots, e_n$ are all maintained at a value equal to the dissociation constant of the effector-enzyme complex.

With these assumptions and the other conditions specified in the legend to Figure 10, it can be calculated from equations 8–10 that the time courses for modifications of interconvertible enzymes in the first three cycles of an opened cyclic cascade (solid line in Figure 10A) are almost identical to those calculated from equations 5–7 (open circles in Figure 10A) for the corresponding steps of a unidirectional cascade. Moreover, the time courses of unidirectional cascades calculated from equations 5–7 are qualitatively similar to those calculated from equation 4 (data not shown).

In addition, Figure 10A shows that for a one-step (or a one-cycle) cascade, the rate of modified enzyme (m-C_1 or m-I_1) formation is relatively slow and decreases exponentially with time. However, for cascades consisting of two or three steps (or cycles), there is a lag in the production of modified enzyme in the last cascade step, which increases with the number of steps in the cascade and is followed by an almost explosive burst of m-C_n or m-I_n formation.

Comparison of the solid and dotted lines in Figure 10A shows that changing the ratio k_{nf}/k_{nr} from 100 to 2 in cyclic cascades has relatively little effect on the rate of m-I_n formation, even though other studies (Chock and Stadtman, 1977) show that the steady-state level of m-I_n accumulation would be markedly shifted.

It is evident from Figure 10A that with assumed rate constants of 500–1,000 sec^{-1}, which are well within the range of enzyme-catalyzed reactions, multicyclic cascade systems can generate large biochemical responses to primary stimuli in the millisecond time range. For example, Figure 10B shows that within 100 msec, more than 95% of the interconvertible enzyme I_3 in a three-cycle cascade can be converted to its modified form, m-I_3. It should be emphasized that with these same kinetic constants, an even greater rate of response could be obtained by proper geographic positioning (immobilization) of the converter enzymes and interconvertible enzymes on membrane surfaces (Goldman and Katchalski, 1971) or in multienzyme complexes (Srere, Mattiasson, and Mosbach, 1973; Bouin, Attalah, and Hultin, 1976; Mosbach, 1976), as occurs in mammalian pyruvate dehydrogenase (Reed, 1969) and in the aro-

matic amino acid synthetase complex of *Neurospora* (Welch and Gaertner, 1975), or by assemblage of the cascade enzymes on a solid support, as occurs in the binding of glycogen phosphorylase cascade components on glycogen particles (Meyer et al., 1970). In fact, Cori and his associates (Danforth, Helmreich, and Cori, 1962) have shown that with electrical stimulation (1.5 msec duration, 30°C) of frog sartorius muscle, phosphorylase *b* is converted to phosphorylase *a* with a half-time of 700 msec.

Figure 11 illustrates that I_3 can be modified almost to completion prior to complete modification of I_1 and I_2. For the conditions described in Figure 11, 90% of I_3 is converted to m-I_3 within 60 msec, while only 35% of I_2 and 6% of I_1 is modified. The differences in time required for complete modification of interconvertible enzymes in various cycles of a cascade reflect the multiplier effects, with respect to specific rate constants, of a multistep system in which one catalyst acts upon another. This difference can vary enormously depending on the kinetic constants and concentrations of both effectors and enzymes.

The kinetic properties of this multiple-catalyst system are disclosed further in Figure 12, which shows how the relative rate of enzyme modification varies as a function of e_1 concentration. Data in Figure 12A2 show how the modification rate varies in a one-cycle ($\circ$), a two cycle ($\triangle$), and a three-cycle ($\square$) cascade when $[I_1] = [I_2] = [I_3]$ and the concentration of $[e_1]$ is varied from 3.5×10^{-11}M to 10^{-5}M. Similarly, the data in Figure 12B2 illustrate the relationship between modification rate and e_1 concentration when $[I_1] < [I_2] < [I_3]$ (e.g., 10^{-6}M, 10^{-5}M, 10^{-4}M, respectively).

It is evident from Figures 12A2 and 12B2 that at any low e_1 concentration, the rate of m-I_n formation

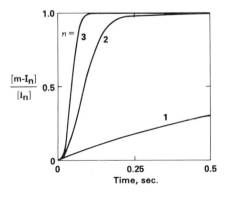

FIGURE 11 Computer-simulated time course for the cyclic cascade system with $[I_1] = [I_2] = [I_3] = 10^{-5}$M; $K_1 = K_2 = K_3 = K_4 = [e_2] = [e_3] = [e_4] = [E] = [R_1] = [R_2] = [R_3] = 5 \times 10^{-6}$M; $k_{nf} = 1,000$ sec^{-1}; $k_{nr} = 10$ sec^{-1}; $K_{nf} = K_{nr} = 4 \times 10^{-5}$M; $[e_1] = 3.5 \times 10^{-8}$M.

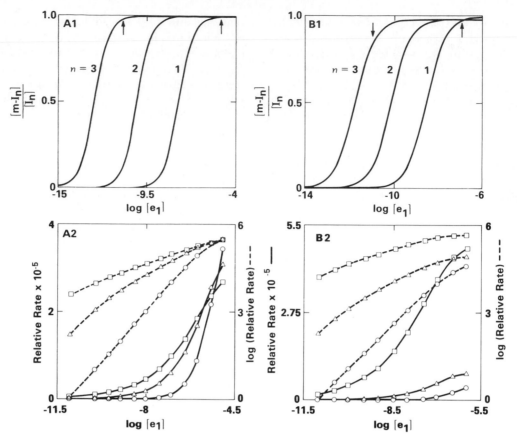

FIGURE 12 Relative rate as a function of $[e_1]$. The values of $[e_1]$ used to obtain A2 and B2 are between the two arrows in A1 and B1, respectively. The symbols ○, △, and □ represent $n = 1$, 2, and 3, respectively. The dashed lines are the log plot of the solid lines. The relative rate is defined as the inverse of the half-time for o-I to m-I conversion at the given $[e_1]$. System A is obtained with $[I_1] = [I_2] = [I_3] = 10^{-5}M$; $K_1 = K_2 = K_3 = K_4 = [e_2] = [e_3] = [e_4]$ $= [E] = [R_1] = [R_2] = [R_3] = 5 \times 10^{-6}M$; $k_{nf} = 1,000$ sec^{-1}; $k_{nr} = 10$ sec^{-1}; $K_{nf} = K_{nr} = 4 \times 10^{-5}M$. System B is obtained with $[I_1] = 10^{-6}M$, $[I_2] = 10^{-5}M$; $[I_3] = 10^{-4}M$; $[E] = [R_1] = [e_2] = K_1 = K_2 = 5 \times 10^{-7}M$; $[e_3] = [R_2] = K_3$ $= 5 \times 10^{-6}M$; $[e_4] = [R_3] = K_4 = 5 \times 10^{-5}M$; $K_{1f} = K_{1r} = 2 \times 10^{-6}M$; $K_{2f} = K_{2r} = 2 \times 10^{-5}M$; $K_{3f} = K_{3r} = 2 \times 10^{-4}M$; $k_{nf} = 1,000$ sec^{-1}; and $k_{nr} = 10$ sec^{-1}.

increases as n increases. The pronounced effect of increasing the number of cycles on the modification rate at low e_1 concentrations is more apparent from the dashed curves in Figures 12A2 and 12B2, which were obtained by plotting the log of the relative rate against the log of e_1. The dependence of rate amplification on the number of cycles is an intrinsic property of the multicatalyst cascade. It does not require the existence of a pyramidal increase in enzyme concentration with each successive cycle in the cascade since the data in Figure 12A2 are derived for the condition in which the concentrations of all interconvertible enzymes in the cascade are the same. Nevertheless, when $[I_1] < [I_2] < [I_3]$, amplification of the modification rate is more markedly dependent on the number of cycles involved (see Figure 12B2). Under this condition, even with relatively high concentra-

tions of e_1, a significant gain in conversion rate is achieved by increasing the number of steps in the cascade.

The relationship between effector concentration and rate of enzyme modification on the one hand and the steady-state level of enzyme modification on the other is evident from a comparison of the data in Figures 12A2 and 12B2 with the corresponding data (for the region between the two arrows) in Figures 12A1 and 12B1.

Biological functions of enzyme cascades

Unidirectional cascades of proteolytic enzymes of the blood-clotting type are clearly designed for the regulation of physiological functions that are fundamentally different from those regulated by cyclic cascades of interconvertible enzymes. When triggered by an appropriate alarm signal, the unidirectional cascades respond explosively to generate an avalanche of product required to meet specific biological challenges; when they have met the challenge, however, the cascades are terminated by a self-destructive process that is initiated by autoregulatory signals. Unidirectional cascades are therefore contingency systems which serve as biological switches that can be turned ON or OFF to meet occasional emergency situations.

In contrast, cyclic cascades are particularly well-designed for the regulation of key enzymes in metabolism. By means of allosteric-site and active-site interactions, the cascade enzymes can sense fluctuations in the concentrations of many different metabolites. These interactions lead to automatic adjustments in the activities of the converter enzymes and thereby determine the steady-state levels of covalent modification (specific activities) of the interconvertible enzymes. In essence, cyclic cascades serve as biological integration systems that can monitor the changes in a multitude of metabolites and modulate the activities of pertinent enzymes accordingly.

It is therefore not surprising that in recent years cyclic cascades have been demonstrated to be the basis of regulation of many enzymes that occupy strategic positions in metabolism. Multicyclic cascades are involved in the regulation of glycogen phosphorylase, glycogen synthase, peptide initiation factor eIF-2, and *E. coli* glutamine synthetase. Monocyclic cascades are involved in the regulation of adipose-tissue triglyceride lipase, pyruvate dehydrogenase, tyrosine-amino transferase, RNA-polymerase, phenylalanine hydroxylase, pyruvate kinase, and possibly fatty-acid synthetase, phosphofructokinase, acetyl CoA carboxylase (for a review and references see Stadtman and Chock, 1977b).

Whereas the extraordinary allosteric-control flexibility of cyclic cascades is of obvious advantage in the regulation of enzymes at metabolic crossroads, this flexibility and the enormous capacity cascades have for signal amplification should make cyclic cascades ideal for the regulation of other biological processes in which versatility and amplification of regulatory signals are important. In this respect the following facts are worthy of note:

1. The S-adenosylmethionine-dependent methylation of membrane proteins and the subsequent release of the methylated proteins into the cytosol might play an important role in the exocytotic secretion of catecholamines and other transportable products from chromaffin vesicles of adrenal medulla (Dilberto, Viveros, and Axelrod, 1976).

2. Methylation and dimethylation of membrane protein is involved in the chemotactic response of bacteria to exogenous metabolites (Kort et al., 1975; Springer and Koshland, 1977; Van der Werf and Koshland, 1977).

3. Phosphorylation and dephosphorylation (Sloboda et al., 1975) and peptidylylation and depeptidylylation of tyrosine by tubulin subunits (Hallek et al., 1977; Raybin and Flavin, 1975, 1977) might be important in the regulation of microtubule assembly or function.

4. Phosphorylation and dephosphorylation of troponin I (Lallemant et al., 1975), troponin T (Moir, Cole, and Perry, 1976), parvalbumin (Blum, Pocinwong, and Fischer, 1974), and the light chain of myosin (Perrie, Smillie, and Perry, 1973; Chacko, Conti, and Adelstein, 1977; Fraerson, Solaro, and Perry, 1976) are important in the regulation of muscle function.

5. The phosphorylation and dephosphorylation of a specific acidic protein component of brush-boarder membranes may be involved in the epinephrine and parathyroid hormone-dependent transport of amino acids in this tissue (Abou-Issa, Kratowich, and Mendicino, 1974).

6. Phosphorylation and dephosphorylation of membrane components of toad bladder epithelial cells may be related to the antidiuretic-hormone-induced Na^+ and water transport (Walton et al., 1975; Orloff and Handler, 1976).

7. Phosphorylation and dephosphorylation and/or ADP-ribosylation of RNA polymerase may be involved in DNA transcription (Bell, Valenzuela, and Rutter, 1977; Zillig et al., 1977).

POSSIBLE ROLE OF ENZYME CASCADES IN NEURAL FUNCTION More pertinent to the present discussion is the fact that various neuronal perturbations result in the phosphorylation and dephosphorylation of synaptic-membrane proteins (Goldstein, Anagnoste, and Shirron, 1973; Reddington, Rodnight, and Williams, 1973; Morgenroth et al., 1975; Gnegy, Costa, and Uzonov, 1976; Gnegy, Uzonov, and Costa, 1976; Williams and Rodnight, 1976; Gnegy, Nathanson, and Uzonov, 1977; Krueger, Forn, and Greengard, 1977; Reddington and Mehl, 1977; Teichberg and Changeux, 1977; Weller and Morgan, 1977). This suggests that cyclic cascades might have an important role in the regulation of nerve-terminal functions.

Indeed, the unusual signal-amplification capacity of cyclic cascades should make them particularly well-suited for the regulation of those nerve functions that are triggered by relatively minor physicochemical perturbations. However, in order to have an important role in several neurochemical processes—namely, neurotransmitter synthesis and/or release—and in postsynaptic events, a chemical cascade system must be able to function in the millisecond time range.

The kinetic analysis described above shows that monocyclic cascades might not meet the requirements, whereas multistep cascades can achieve a high degree of signal amplification in the millisecond range. It is not known whether the observed nerve-cell membrane protein phosphorylations are manifestations of mono- or multicyclic cascades. But even if they are monocyclic in nature, they may still be able to generate high rates of catalysis. If the modified forms of nerve membrane proteins are activated enzymes that catalyze conversions of substrates to products, then the number of coupled catalytic steps in the cascades is two, not one. Similarly, if formation of the effector (e_1) needed for activation of the first converter enzyme (E) in the cascade is modulated by an enzymic process, an additional catalytic step will be introduced at the top of the cascade. Thus a single interconvertible enzyme cascade can behave kinetically as a two- or three-step cascade with respect to overall catalytic activity.

This condition may, in fact, be realized in situations

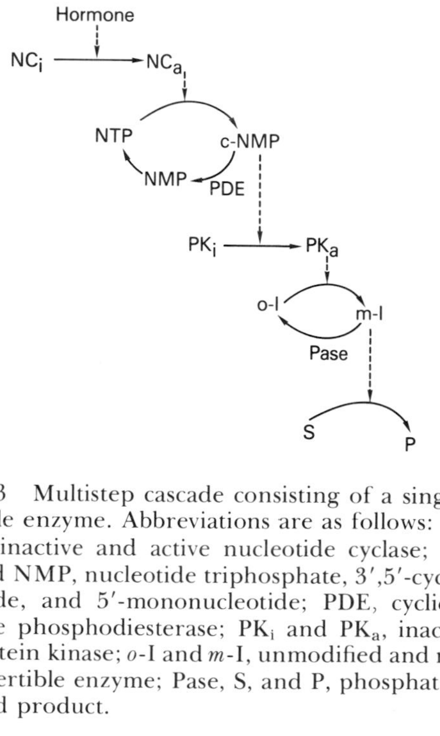

FIGURE 13   Multistep cascade consisting of a single interconvertible enzyme. Abbreviations are as follows: NC_i and NC_a are inactive and active nucleotide cyclase; NTP, c-NMP, and NMP, nucleotide triphosphate, $3',5'$-cyclic mononucleotide, and $5'$-mononucleotide; PDE, cyclic mononucleotide phosphodiesterase; PK_i and PK_a, inactive and active protein kinase; o-I and m-I, unmodified and modified interconvertible enzyme; Pase, S, and P, phosphatase, substrate, and product.

where the phosphorylation of an interconvertible enzyme is catalyzed by a cyclic-mononucleotide-dependent kinase. Such a cascade is illustrated in Figure 13. In this model, binding of a hormone to membrane receptor protein leads to activation of a nucleotide cyclase (conversion of NC_i to NC_a), which catalyzes the conversion of a nucleoside triphosphate (GTP or ATP) to the corresponding cyclic mononucleotide (cyclic NMP). Like effector e_1 in the previous cascade models, this cyclic nucleotide is needed to activate the protein kinase (conversion of PK_i to PK_a) that catalyzes phosphorylation of the interconvertible enzyme (conversion of o-I to m-I). Finally, the modified enzyme m-I catalyzes conversion of substrate to product (S to P). In this representation, the cascade consists of four coupled catalytic steps; $NC_i \rightarrow NC_a$, $NTP \rightarrow$ cyclic NMP, o-I $\rightarrow m$-I, and S $\rightarrow$ P. Therefore, from the kinetic point of view, this is a four-step cascade and under appropriate conditions should be capable of catalyzing considerable product formation in the millisecond time range.

Examination of Figure 13 shows that such cascades can function temporally as unidirectional cascades. Thus, in the absence of hormone stimulation and/or under conditions where activity of the cyclic mononucleotide phosphodiesterase (PDE) is high relative to the cyclase (NA_a) activity, the level of cyclic NMP may become vanishingly small, with the net effect that the protein kinase is not activated. Under these conditions, all of the interconvertible enzyme will assume the unmodified (inactive) form o-I. Similarly, any condition that leads to inactivation of the phosphatase catalyzing the conversion of m-I to o-I, without inactivation of the protein kinase, will result in complete conversion of o-I to m-I. Under these extreme, though feasible, conditions a cyclic cascade will operate as an ON-OFF switch with respect to the conversion of substrate to product.

Summary

The fact that nerve-cell membrane proteins are phosphorylated and dephosphorylated in response to electrical and hormonal stimuli suggests that interconvertible enzyme cascades play an active role in neurochemical events. Indeed, enzyme cascades possess many characteristics that make them attractive candidates for key roles in the regulation of neurochemical processes. Because they are multiplier systems with respect to rate functions and act as signal amplifiers with respect to biochemical and/or biophysical perturbations, they can generate an almost explosive increase in catalytic activity in response to minute stimuli. In addition, enzyme cascades can function as highly sophisticated metabolic integration systems; by means of allosteric interactions with one or more of the component enzymes, cascades can continuously monitor fluctuations in the concentrations of a multitude of allosteric effectors and adjust the specific activities of the ultimate interconvertible enzyme according to its biological necessity. Finally, cascades can, under extreme but physiologically feasible situations, serve as biological switches that can be turned on or off, intermittently, for temporal "all-or-none" control of key biological activities.

REFERENCES

ABOU-ISSA, H., N. KRATOWICH, and J. MENDICINO, 1974. Properties of soluble and bound protein kinases isolated from swine kidney. *Eur. J. Biochem.* 42:461–473.

ADLER, S. P., J. H. MANGUM, G. MAGNI, and E. R. STADTMAN, 1974. Uridylylation of the P_{II} regulatory protein in cascade control of *Escherichia coli* glutamine synthetase. In *Third International Symposium on Metabolic Interconversion of Enzymes*, E. H. Fischer, E. G. Krebs, and E. R. Stadtman, eds. New York: Springer-Verlag, pp. 221–233.

ASWAD, D., and D. E. KOSHLAND, JR., 1974. Role of methionine in bacterial chemotaxis. *J. Bacteriol.* 118:640–645.

BELL, G. I., P. VALENZUELA, and W. J. RUTTER, 1977. Phosphorylation of yeast DNA dependent RNA polymerases *in vivo* and *in vitro*. Isolation of enzymes and identification of phosphorylated subunits. *J. Biol. Chem.* 252:3082–3091.

BLUM, H. E., S. POCINWONG, and E. H. FISCHER, 1974. A phosphate-acceptor protein related to parvalbumins in dogfish skeletal muscle. *Proc. Natl. Acad. Sci. USA* 71:2198–2202.

BOUIN, J. C., M. T. ATALLAH, and H. O. HULTIN, 1976. Relative efficiencies of a soluble and immobilized two-enzyme system of glucose oxidase and catalase. *Biochim. Biophys. Acta* 438:23–36.

CHACKO, S., M. A. CONTI, and R. S. ADELSTEIN, 1977. Effect of phosphorylation of smooth muscle myosin on actin activation and Ca^{2+} regulation. *Proc. Natl. Acad. Sci. USA* 74:129–133.

CHOCK, P. B., and E. R. STADTMAN, 1977. Superiority of enzyme cascades in metabolic regulation: Analysis of multicyclic system. *Proc. Natl. Acad. Sci. USA* 74:2766–2770.

DANFORTH, W. H., E. HELMREICH, and C. F. CORI, 1962. The effect of contraction and of epinephrine on the phosphorylase activity of frog sartorius muscle. *Proc. Natl. Acad. Sci. USA* 48:1191–1199.

DATTA, A., C. DEHARO, J. M. SIERRA, and S. OCHOA, 1977. Role of 3':5'-cyclic AMP-dependent protein kinase in regulation of protein synthesis in reticulocyte lysates. *Proc. Natl. Acad. Sci. USA* 74:1463–1467.

DAVIE, E. W., and K. FUJIKAWA, 1975. Basic mechanisms in blood coagulation. *Annu. Rev. Biochem.* 44:799–829.

DAVIE, E. W., C. HOUGIE, and R. L. LUNDBLAD, 1969. Mechanisms of blood coagulation. In *Recent Advances in Blood*

Coagulation, L. Poler, ed. London: J. & A. Churchill, pp. 13–28.

DILBERTO, E. J., JR., O. H. VIVEROS, and J. AXELROD, 1976. Subcellular distribution of protein carboxymethylase and its endogenous substrates in the adrenal medulla: Possible role in excitation-secretion coupling. *Proc. Natl. Acad. Sci. USA* 73:4050–4054.

FISCHER, E. H., L. G. HEILMEYER, JR., and R. H. HASCHKE, 1971. Phosphorylase and the control of glycogen degradation. In *Current Topics in Cellular Regulation*, vol. 4, B. L. Horecker and E. R. Stadtman, eds. New York: Academic Press, pp. 211–251.

FRAERSON, N., R. J. SOLARO, and S. V. PERRY, 1976. Changes in phosphorylation of P light chain of myosin in perfused rabbit heart. *Nature* 264:801–802.

GNEGY, M. E., E. COSTA, and P. UZONOV, 1976. Regulation of transsynaptically elicited increase of 3':5'-cyclic AMP by endogenous phosphodiesterase activator. *Proc. Natl. Acad. Sci. USA* 73:352–355.

GNEGY, M. E., P. UZONOV, and E. COSTA, 1976. Regulation of dopamine stimulation of striatal adenyl cyclase by an endogenous Ca^{++}-binding protein. *Proc. Natl. Acad. Sci. USA* 73:3887–3890.

GNEGY, M. E., J. A. NATHANSON, and P. UZONOV, 1977. Release of the phosphodiesterase activator by cyclic AMP-dependent ATP: Protein phosphotransferase from subcellular fractions of rat brain. *Biochim. Biophys. Acta* 497:75–85.

GOLDMAN, R., and E. KATCHALSKI, 1971. Kinetic behavior of a two-enzyme membrane carrying out a consecutive set of reaction. *J. Theoret. Biol.* 32:243–257.

GOLDSTEIN, M., B. ANAGNOSTE, and C. SHIRRON, 1973. The effect of trivastal, haloperidol and dibutyryl cyclic AMP on [C] dopamine synthesis in rat striatum. *J. Pharm. Pharmacol.* 25:348–351.

HALLEK, M. E., J. A. RODRIGUEZ, H. S. BARA, and R. CAPUTTO, 1977. Release of tyrosine from tyrosinated tubulin. Some common factors that affect this process and the assembly of tubulin. *FEBS Lett.* 73:147–150.

HEMKER, H. C., and P. W. HEMKER, 1969. The kinetics of enzyme cascade systems. General kinetics of enzyme cascades. *Proc. R. Soc. Lond.* B173:411–420.

HUCHO, F., D. D. RANDALL, T. E. ROCHE, M. W. BURGETT, J. W. PELLEY, and L. J. REED, 1972. α-keto acid dehydrogenase complexes. XVII. Kinetic and regulatory properties of pyruvate dehydrogenase kinase and pyruvate dehydrogenase phosphatase from bovine kidney and heart. *Arch. Biochem. Biophys.* 151:328–340.

KINGDON, H. S., B. M. SHAPIRO, and E. R. STADTMAN, 1967. Regulation of glutamine synthetase, VIII. ATP: glutamine synthetase adenylyltransferase, an enzyme that catalyzes alterations in the regulatory properties of glutamine synthetase. *Proc. Natl. Acad. Sci. USA* 58:1703–1710.

KORT, E. N., M. F. GOY, S. H. LARSEN, and J. ADLER, 1975. Methylation of a membrane protein involved in bacterial chemotaxis. *Proc. Natl. Acad. Sci. USA* 72:3939–3943.

KREBS, E. G., 1972. Protein kinases. In *Current Topics in Cellular Regulation*, vol. 5, B. L. Horecker and E. R. Stadtman, eds. New York: Academic Press, pp. 99–133.

KRUEGER, B. K., J. FORN, and P. GREENGARD, 1977. Depolarization-induced phosphorylation of specific proteins, mediated by calcium ion influx, in rat brain synaptosomes. *J. Biol. Chem.* 252:2764–2773.

LALLEMANT, C., K. SERAYDARIAN, S. F. H. M. MOMMERTS, and M. SUH, 1975. A survey of the regulatory activity of some phosphorylated and dephosphorylated forms of troponin. *Arch. Biochem. Biophys.* 169:367–371.

MACFARLANE, R. G., 1964. An enzyme cascade in blood clotting mechanism, and its function as a biochemical amplifier. *Nature* 202:498–499.

MEYER, F., L. M. G. HEILMEYER, JR., R. H. HASCHKE, and E. H. FISCHER, 1970. Control of phosphorylase in a muscle glycogen particle. I. Isolation and characterization of the protein-glycogen complex. *J. Biol. Chem.* 245:6642–6648.

MOIR, A. J. G., H. A. COLE, and S. V. PERRY, 1976. The phosphorylation sites of troponin T from white skeletal muscle and the effect of interaction with troponin C on their phosphorylation by phosphorylase kinase. *Biochem. J.* 161:371–382.

MORGENROTH III, V. H., L. R. HEGSTRAND, R. H. ROTH, and P. GREENGARD, 1975. Evidence for involvement of protein kinase in the activation by adenosine 3′:5′-monophosphate of brain tyrosine 3-monooxygenase. *J. Biol. Chem.* 250:1946–1948.

MOSBACH, K., 1976. Immobilized enzymes. *FEBS Lett.* 62:E80–E95.

MÜLLER-EBERHARD, H. J., 1975. Complement. *Annu. Rev. Biochem.* 44:697–724.

NEURATH, H., and K. A. WALSH, 1976. The role of proteases in biological regulation. In *Proteolysis and Physiological Regulation*, E. W. Ribbons and K. Brew, eds. New York: Academic Press, pp. 29–40.

ORLOFF, J., and J. HANDLER, 1967. The role of adenosine 3′,5′-phosphate in the action of antidiuretic hormone. *Am. J. Med.* 42:757–768.

PERRIE, W. T., L. B. SMILLIE, and S. V. PERRY, 1973. A phosphorylated light-chain component of myosin from skeletal muscle. *Biochem. J.* 135:151–164.

PETTIT, F. H., J. W. PELLEY, and L. J. REED, 1975. Regulation of pyruvate dehydrogenase kinase and phosphatase by Acetyl-CoA/CoA and NADH/NAD ratios. *Biochem. Biophys. Res. Commun.* 65:575–582.

RAYBIN, D., and M. FLAVIN, 1975. An enzyme tyrosylating α-tubulin and its role in microtubule assembly. *Biochem. Biophys. Res. Commun.* 65:1088–1095.

RAYBIN, D., and M. FLAVIN, 1977. Enzyme which specifically adds tyrosine to the α chain of tubulin. *Biochemistry* 16:2189–2194.

REDDINGTON, M., and E. MEHL, 1977. Complexity of cyclic AMP-dependent phosphoproteins in membranes from brain tissue containing synapses. *FEBS Lett.* 75:61–64.

REDDINGTON, M., R. RODNIGHT, and M. WILLIAMS, 1973. Turnover of protein-bound serine phosphate in respiring slices of guinea-pig cerebral cortex. *Biochem. J.* 132:475–482.

REED, L. J., 1969. Pyruvate dehydrogenase complex. In *Current Topics in Cellular Regulation*, vol. 1, B. L. Horecker and E. R. Stadtman, eds. New York: Academic Press, pp. 233–251.

REED, L. J., F. H. PETTIT, T. E. ROCHE, and P. J. BUTTERWORTH, 1973. Regulation of the mammalian pyruvate dehydrogenase complex by phosphorylation and dephosphorylation. In *Protein Phosphorylation in Control Mechanisms*, F. Hujing and E. Y. C. Lee, eds. New York: Academic Press, pp. 83–97.

REED, L. J., F. H. PETTIT, T. E. ROCHE, J. W. PELLEY, and P. J. BUTTERWORTH, 1976. Structure and regulation of the mammalian pyruvate dehydrogenase. In *Metabolic Interconversion of Enzymes 1975*, S. Shaltiel, ed. New York: Springer-Verlag, pp. 121–124.

RHEE, S. G., R. PARK, P. B. CHOCK, and E. R. STADTMAN, 1977. The use of *E. coli* glutamine synthetase as a model to investigate the allosteric regulation of monocyclic interconvertible enzyme cascade systems. *Fed. Proc.* 36:777.

SEGAL, A., M. S. BROWN, and E. R. STADTMAN, 1974. Metabolite regulation of the state of adenylylation of glutamine synthetase. *Arch. Biochem. Biophys.* 161:319–327.

SENIOR, P. J., 1975. Regulation of nitrogen metabolism in *Escherichia coli* and *Klebsiella aerogenes*: Studies with the continuous-culture technique. *J. Bacteriol.* 123:407–418.

SLOBODA, R. D., S. A. RUDOLPH, J. L. ROSENBAUM, and P. GREENGARD, 1975. Cyclic AMP-dependent endogenous phosphorylation of a microtubule-associated protein. *Proc. Natl. Acad. Sci. USA* 72:177–181.

SPRINGER, W. R., and D. E. KOSHLAND, JR., 1977. Identification of a protein methyltransferase as the cheR gene product in the bacterial sensing system. *Proc. Natl. Acad. Sci. USA* 74:533–537.

SRERE, P. A., B. MATTIASSON, and K. MOSBACH, 1973. An immobilized three-enzyme system: A model for microenvironmental compartmentation in mitochondria. *Proc. Natl. Acad. Sci. USA* 70:2534–2538.

STADTMAN, E. R., 1973. A note on the significance of glutamine in intermediary metabolism. In *The Enzymes of Glutamine Metabolism*, S. Prusiner and E. R. Stadtman, eds. New York: Academic Press, pp. 1–6.

STADTMAN, E. R., and P. B. CHOCK, 1977a. Superiority of interconvertible enzyme cascades in metabolic regulation: Analysis of monocyclic systems. *Proc. Natl. Acad. Sci. USA* 74:2761–2765.

STADTMAN, E. R., and P. B. CHOCK, 1977b. Interconvertible enzyme cascades in metabolic regulation. In *Current Topics in Cellular Regulation*, vol. 13, B. L. Horecker and E. R. Stadtman, eds. New York: Academic Press, pp. 53–95.

STADTMAN, E. R., P. B. CHOCK, and S. ADLER, 1976. Metabolic regulation of coupled covalent modification cascade systems. In *Metabolic Interconversion of Enzymes 1975*, S. Shaltiel, ed. New York: Springer-Verlag, pp. 142–149.

STADTMAN, E. R., and A. GINSBURG, 1974. The glutamine synthetase of *Escherichia coli*: Structure and control. In *The Enzymes* (3rd ed.), vol. 10, P. D. Boyer, ed. New York: Academic Press, pp. 755–807.

TEICHBERG, V. I., and J. P. CHANGEUX, 1977. Evidence for protein phosphorylation and dephosphorylation in membrane fragments isolated from the electric organ of *Electrophorus electricus*. *FEBS Lett.* 74:71–76.

VAN DER WERF, P., and D. E. KOSHLAND, JR., 1977. Identification of α-glutamyl methyl ester in bacterial membrane protein induced in chemotaxis. *J. Biol. Chem.* 252:2793–2795.

WALTON, K. G., R. J. DELORENZO, P. F. CURRAN, and P. GREENGARD, 1975. Regulation of protein phosphorylation and sodium transport in toad bladder. *J. Gen. Physiol.* 65:153–177.

WELCH, G. R., and F. H. GAERTNER, 1975. Influence of an aggregated multienzyme system on transient time: Kinetic evidence for compartmentation by aromatic-amino-acid-synthesizing complex of *Neurospora crassa. Proc. Natl. Acad. Sci. USA* 72:4218-4222.

WELLER, M., and I. G. MORGAN, 1977. A possible role of phosphorylation of synaptic membrane proteins in the control of calcium ion permeability. *Biochim. Biophys. Acta* 465:527-534.

WILLIAMS, M., and R. RODNIGHT, 1976. Protein phosphorylation in respiring slices of guinea-pig cerebral cortex. Evidence for a role for noradrenaline and adenosine 3':5'-cyclic monophosphate in increased phosphorylation observed on application of electrical impulses. *Biochem. J.* 154:163-170.

WOOLFOLK, C. A., and E. R. STADTMAN, 1967. Regulation of glutamine synthetase. III. Cumulative feedback inhibition of glutamine synthetase from *Escherichia coli. Arch. Biochem. Biophys.* 118:736-755.

WULFF, K., D. MECKE, and H. HOLZER, 1967. Mechanism of the enzymatic inactivation of glutamine synthetase from *E. coli. Biochem. Biophys. Res. Commun.* 28:740-745.

ZILLIG, W., R. MAILHAMMER, R. SKORKO, and H. ROHRER, 1977. Covalent structural modification of DNA-dependent RNA polymerase as a means for transcriptional control. In *Current Topics in Cellular Regulation,* vol. 12, B. L. Horecker and E. R. Stadtman, eds. New York: Academic Press, pp. 263-271.

47 Regulation of Adenylate Cyclase Activity

ALFRED G. GILMAN and ELLIOTT M. ROSS

ABSTRACT Hormone-sensitive adenylate cyclase is responsible for the amplification and the transduction of certain information from the extracellular to the intracellular surface of the plasma membrane. The activity of the enzyme is under long-term and short-term control by hormones and neurotransmitters and by intracellular purine nucleotides; these two types of ligands interact in a complex and poorly understood fashion. We are attempting to resolve the components of a hormone-sensitive adenylate cyclase system by genetic and biochemical techniques. Responses to hormones can be restored to the solubilized, hormone-insensitive enzyme by the reassociation of the enzyme with membranes that contain hormone receptors. We have resolved at least two proteins that are necessary for the catalytic activity of adenylate cyclase and another that is probably involved in regulation by purine nucleotides. We are led to hypothesize the existence of at least five components of the hormone-sensitive enzyme system.

Introduction

The adenylate cyclase–catalyzed reaction—the formation of cyclic 3′,5′-adenosine monophosphate (cyclic AMP) and pyrophosphate from adenosine triphosphate—is of demonstrable importance in many bacteria and fungi and is essentially ubiquitous among animal cells. This reaction is the only known pathway for the synthesis of cyclic AMP; since the cyclic nucleotide is known to play a central role in the regulation of metabolic pathways and a large number of differentiated functions of specialized cells, it is appropriate that attention has been focused on the mechanisms of regulation of adenylate cyclase activity. Despite an extraordinary number of publications on this subject, concrete information is relatively limited. In this brief review we shall attempt to focus on these highlights.

With few exceptions, adenylate cyclase is a membrane-bound enzyme—the membrane in question usually being the plasma membrane. The catalytic site is presumably oriented to utilize intracellular substrate and to produce an intracellular reaction product. However, the enzyme is predominantly subject to regulation from without (by hormones, neurotransmitters, autacoids) by mechanisms that are poorly understood. Catalytic activity is also sensitive to influences from the interior of the cell, but the extent to which these influences vary or are regulated is, for the moment, almost entirely a subject for speculation.

A primary "job" of a hormone-sensitive adenylate cyclase complex is the transduction of information. Information inherent in the presence of hormone in the extracellular fluid becomes available to the interior of the cell, when appropriate; the appropriateness or selectivity of transduction is determined by the presence or absence of receptors for specific hormones or neurohormones in the plasma membrane. Many individual types of receptors, presumably oriented to bind extracellular regulatory ligands, function in tandem with the catalytic moiety of adenylate cyclase. The mechanism of this linkage will be a major subject of this discussion.

Another important role played by the system is amplification. There are many ways to express this fact, and some are more impressive than others. Simplistically, typical values for cellular receptor concentrations are about 10^{-14}-10^{-13} mol/mg protein (a few hundred or a few thousand receptors per cell); cyclic AMP concentrations generated in response to occupation of such receptors often approximate 10^{-9} mol/mg protein. (Basal concentrations of cyclic AMP are usually about 10^{-11} mol/mg protein.) The increment in the cellular concentration of the nucleotide is observed quickly—sometimes at a rate of 5×10^{-10} mol/min/mg protein. Since intracellular concentrations of ATP approximate 10^{-8} mol/mg protein, it is obvious that occupation of a few hundred receptors per cell can rapidly result in the conversion of a significant amount of total cellular ATP into cyclic AMP.

Additional mechanisms for amplification of the message occur subsequent to the stage of cyclic AMP

ALFRED G. GILMAN and ELLIOTT M. ROSS Department of Pharmacology, University of Virginia, Charlottesville, VA 22903

synthesis. It is perhaps more important that there are opportunities to recode the information in more permanent language. These subjects are discussed by other participants in the Study Program.

There are four primary reasons why progress in the elucidation of mechanisms of control of cyclic AMP synthesis has been unimpressive. First, the major components of the system are integral membrane proteins. Reproducible effects of hormones have never been observed in the absence of the membrane; evidence suggests that both the membrane lipids and an appropriate membrane structure are vital for the observation of regulation of enzymatic activity by hormones.

Second, some components of the system are present in trace quantities. Hormone-receptor concentrations may be only a few hundred per cell. If the turnover rate of adenylate cyclase is in the range of 10^4 molecules/min, an equivalent number of adenylate cyclase molecules is sufficient to account for the rates of enzymatic activity that are observed.

Third, some components of the system are labile. The half-life of adenylate cyclase activity in membranes incubated at 37° is measured in minutes.

Finally, the system is probably very complex. Our current working hypothesis includes five distinct functional components, and we have attempted to be conservative. This model makes no attempt to account for large numbers of descriptive observations of the system, and it is almost certainly simplistic.

Alterations of adenylate cyclase activity

A confusing array of compounds influence the rate of catalysis by adenylate cyclase. To a certain extent at least their number reflects the complexity of the system in terms of numbers of distinct macromolecular components.

Regulatory ligands of physiological significance include an impressive number of hormones, neurohormones and neurotransmitters, and autacoids. Included are several polypeptides (glucagon, the trophic hormones of the adenohypophysis, antidiuretic hormone), a variety of biogenic amines (catecholamines, 5-hydroxytryptamine, histamine), and certain of the prostaglandins, a group of potent acidic lipids. The ability of these agents to regulate adenylate cyclase activity is dependent on the presence in any given cell of a specific receptor for the compound under consideration. The receptor must not only interact with the ligand in question but must also be capable of functional interactions that result in an alteration of adenylate cyclase activity.

It may be noted at this point that the information-transduction systems in the membrane appear to be branched and complex, even when one considers those utilized by a single extracellular ligand. Consider the case of norepinephrine, the predominant neurotransmitter of the sympathetic nervous system. At least two types of receptors for norepinephrine can be distinguished (designated α and β). Occupation of β-adrenergic receptors is almost universally associated with stimulation of adenylate cyclase; α-adrenergic receptors occasionally appear to subserve this function, occasionally appear to cause inhibition of adenylate cyclase, and most commonly appear to function via mechanisms not mediated by cyclic AMP. Despite the fact that cyclic AMP concentrations almost always rise when β-adrenergic receptors are occupied by agonists, it is a matter of debate whether all β-adrenergic effects are mediated by the cyclic nucleotide (Figure 1).

In addition to complexities of hormone-receptor interactions, it is also clear that binding of appropriate ligands (hormones) to receptors that are linked to adenylate cyclase may not be sufficient to influence enzymatic activity. The two functions of hormone binding and enzyme activation may be readily uncoupled experimentally (see below). Furthermore, it appears that an additional regulatory ligand, a guanine or other purine nucleotide, is essential for normal coupling of hormone binding to enzyme activation. Credit for this discovery belongs to Rodbell and associates, who have extensively studied the effects of these nucleotides, particularly on hepatic glucagon-sensitive adenylate cyclase (Rodbell et al., 1975).

A confusing number of effects of GTP and other nucleotides have been noted in many laboratories. It is probable that much of the confusion derives from contamination of enzyme preparations (and substrates) with low concentrations of regulatory nucleotides. Since effects of GTP may be noted at 0.1 μM concentrations, a high level of contamination is not

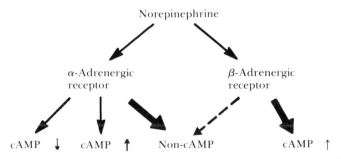

FIGURE 1 Effects of norepinephrine can be mediated by either α- or β-adrenergic receptors via cyclic AMP–mediated or cyclic AMP–independent pathways.

necessary. When membrane preparations are purified and when concentrations of ATP are not excessive, many hormone-sensitive adenylate cyclase systems are seen to have an absolute dependence on exogenous GTP (or other regulatory nucleotides) for the observation of effects of hormones (see Ross et al., 1977). There is no reason not to assume that this is a general phenomenon. The effect of GTP alone is usually minor; only when both GTP and hormone are added are significant stimulatory effects observed. Data illustrating this phenomenon, derived from the S49 lymphoma cell with which we work, are shown in Figure 2. The effect of addition of hormone plus GTP is essentially instantaneous, although transient lags have been observed and interpreted by Rodbell et al. (1975). Regulation of enzyme activity by hormones and GTP is readily reversible. The effect of hormone may be observed in both intact cells

and in membrane preparations; it is always lost when detergent-solubilized adenylate cyclase activity is examined.

In contrast to the cell-specific effects of various hormones, there are three essentially ubiquitous stimulators of adenylate cyclase activity: fluoride ion, certain guanine nucleotide analogs, and cholera toxin. The stimulatory effect of the fluoride ion was noted early. Despite this advantage, less is known about its effects than about those of other types of activators. High concentrations of F^- are required (1–10 mM), and the best data indicate that the activation is irreversible or only slowly reversible (Perkins and Moore, 1971). The effect is usually observed only with membranous or solubilized preparations; intact cells generally fail to respond.

Guanylyl imidodiphosphate (Gpp(NH)p), an analog of GTP that is resistant to hydrolysis at the β–γ phosphodiester bond, also stimulates adenylate cyclase from virtually all sources. Activation by Gpp(NH)p is observed with membrane preparations or in solubilized systems. The extent of activation is dependent on time and temperature and is reversible only under special conditions. GTP can prevent activation by Gpp(NH)p. The simplest hypothesis is that Gpp(NH)p and GTP bind to the same site; when nucleotide hydrolysis cannot occur, the enzyme becomes persistently activated. However, this is conjecture; the questions of mechanism and the role of nucleotide hydrolysis will be discussed below.

The third ubiquitous stimulator of adenylate cyclase is cholera toxin. Its action is normally manifest only on intact cells, but conditions have been found under which the toxin will activate the enzyme in homogenates (NAD, a reducing agent, and other factors are required: see Gill, 1977). The mechanism of toxin binding to the cell and certain steps that lead to irreversible activation of adenylate cyclase have been elucidated, but these subjects will not be discussed here.

Regulation of membrane-bound adenylate cyclase by hormones

The availability of radioactive ligands that bind specifically to hormone receptors has allowed the quantification of these binding sites, study of their ligand-binding properties, and examination of the relationship between hormone binding to receptors and activation of adenylate cyclase. We shall discuss only selected aspects of such studies on the relationship between the β-adrenergic receptor and adenylate cyclase. Considerable data also exist for the receptors

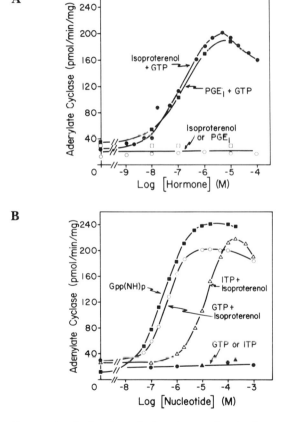

FIGURE 2 Activation of adenylate cyclase by hormones and purine nucleotides in purified plasma membranes of wild-type S49 lymphoma cells. (A) Circles indicate (−)-isoproterenol; squares, prostaglandin E_1; open symbols, no added nucleotide; filled symbols, 50 μM GTP present. (B) Circles indicate GTP; triangles, ITP; squares, Gpp(NH)p; filled symbols, no hormone present; open symbols, 1 μM isoproterenol present. (Data from Ross et al., 1977.)

for glucagon (Rodbell et al., 1975) and for antidiuretic hormone (Jard et al., 1975).

It proved to be difficult to find radioactive ligands that were suitable for assay of the β-adrenergic receptor. Numerous problems were encountered when the tritiated natural hormones were used, and the data that were acquired appeared to involve binding of the ligands to macromolecules other than the receptor (Maguire, Goldman, and Gilman, 1974; Maguire, Ross, and Gilman, 1977). Eventually, two suitable ligands were described; both were the result of clever experimental rationales. The two compounds in use are β-adrenergic antagonists (Aurbach et al., 1974; Lefkowitz et al., 1974). We have utilized [^{125}I]-iodohydroxybenzylpindolol (IHYP), originally described by Aurbach and co-workers (Brown et al., 1976a,b; Maguire et al., 1976). The ligand has a very high affinity for the receptor (K_D = 10–100 pM) and a very high specific activity (2,200 Ci/mmol). This combination of properties ensures great sensitivity in the receptor assay—a necessity when cultured cells are the source of the receptor of interest. The binding of [^{125}I]-IHYP to the β-adrenergic receptor can be studied directly—with intact cells, membrane preparations, or in solution—and the binding of other ligands to the receptor can be studied by virtue of their ability to compete with [^{125}I]-IHYP.

Purified plasma membranes from the S49 lymphoma cell contain β-adrenergic receptor sites at a concentration of approximately 300 fmol/mg protein (500–1,000 sites per cell) (Ross et al., 1977). Isoproterenol, a synthetic β-adrenergic agonist, binds to these sites with a K_D = 80 nM. The concentration dependence for isoproterenol to compete for [^{125}I]-IHYP binding sites does not describe a classical binding isotherm. Despite the fact that IHYP and other β-adrenergic antagonists bind to the receptor with a Hill coefficient near 1, isoproterenol and other agonists bind to the same sites with a Hill coefficient of approximately 0.6 (Figure 3). Furthermore, despite the fact that receptors can be saturated with isoproterenol, there is no effect of the drug on adenylate cyclase activity, since a regulatory purine nucleotide such as GTP has not been added. This is one example of uncoupling between receptor occupation and enzyme activation.

If minimal amounts of GTP are added—just sufficient to observe activation of adenylate cyclase by isoproterenol—the effect of the β-adrenergic agonist is characterized by K_{act} = 30 nM. Thus half-maximal activation of the enzyme is achieved at concentrations of isoproterenol that allow occupation of less than half of the receptor sites. As maximally effective concentrations of GTP are added, several changes are noted. The ability of isoproterenol to enhance enzymatic activity is increased (Figure 2), the affinity of isoproterenol for the receptor is decreased (Figure 3), the Hill coefficient for agonist binding increases toward a value of one (Figure 3), and a greater concentration of isoproterenol is necessary to stimulate the enzyme half-maximally. The GTP-induced alterations in binding to the receptor are specific for agonists; the binding characteristics of antagonists are not altered. In the presence of a maximal concentration of GTP, the K_D for isoproterenol is 500 nM, increased by a factor of six; the K_{act} is 100 nM—now even more discrepant from the K_D.

Other purine nucleotides also allow stimulation of adenylate cyclase by hormones. ITP, Gpp(NH)p, and Gpp(CH$_2$)p all alter the binding of isoproterenol to the receptor; the effects are indistinguishable except for the concentrations of nucleotide required (Figure 3). However, the potency of isoproterenol needed to activate adenylate cyclase does depend on the nucleotide. With ITP as the regulatory nucleotide, the K_{act} for isoproterenol is 50 nM, a full order of magnitude below its dissociation constant for the receptor. Activation of the enzyme by isoproterenol in the presence of Gpp(NH)p or Gpp(CH$_2$)p is complex and difficult to analyze, since the enzyme becomes irreversibly activated. Kinetic analysis suggests that the true K_{act} for isoproterenol in the presence of Gpp(NH)p is approximately 15 nM.

The role of guanine nucleotides in the interaction between hormone receptors and adenylate cyclase has been approached from an alternative path by Cassel and Selinger (1976), who have measured a catecholamine-stimulated GTPase activity in turkey erythrocyte membranes. Their data suggest that nucleotide hydrolysis may be involved in regulation of adenylate cyclase. If this is the case, the rate of hydrolysis of different nucleotides may dictate the differences in K_{act} observed for a single agonist (see Ross et al., 1977). This relationship is also supported by the fact that cholera toxin, which increases the potency of agonists without changing their binding affinities and also allows GTP to mimic Gpp(NH)p (Ross et al., 1977), has recently been shown to inhibit the membrane-bound GTPase activity (Cassel and Selinger, 1977).

The detailed hypotheses of receptor-enzyme interaction that can be drawn from these observations are complicated, and the conclusions are vague. It is clear that the relationship between occupation of receptors and activation of adenylate cyclase is a variable one. There appears to be no fixed stoichiometric relation-

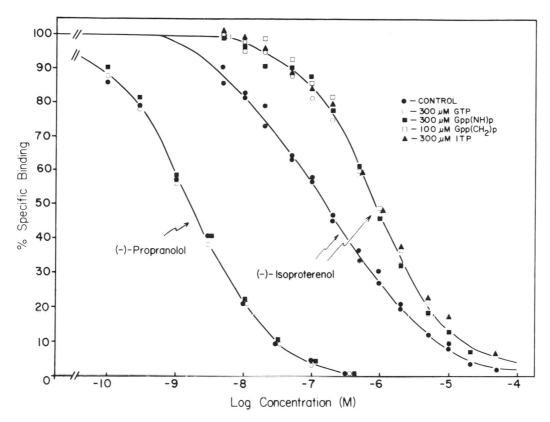

FIGURE 3   Effects of purine nucleotides on (−)-propranolol and (−)-isoproterenol binding to β-adrenergic receptors of S49 lymphoma plasma membranes. Specific binding of each ligand was assayed by competition for [125I]-IHYP binding sites. (Data from Ross et al., 1977.)

ship between agonist binding and enzyme activation. Thermodynamic (Biltonen, 1977) and kinetic (Rodbell et al., 1975) models have been constructed. Regulatory cascade mechanisms of the type discussed by Stadtman and Chock (this volume) might account for such variation in apparent stoichiometry and would also allow signal amplification within the membrane.

REFRACTORINESS AND POTENTIATION   Two additional phenomena that have been observed with hormone-sensitive adenylate cyclase systems are particularly pertinent to this discussion. Hormone-stimulated adenylate cyclase systems have a memory. Prolonged stimulation of the enzyme via certain receptors at least results in a subsequent diminution of hormone-stimulated enzyme activity—an inability to respond further to the agonist—a state of refractoriness. It is clear that multiple effects mediated by multiple mechanisms are involved. In some cases, stimulation via, for example, a β-adrenergic receptor results in a selective inability to respond to β-adrenergic agonists. If the system normally responds to other agents as well, it may continue to do so, despite the fact that the responses in question are properties of a single cell. This has been termed homologous refractoriness (Su et al., 1976a,b). In other cases, loss of the ability to respond to one agonist may result in the simultaneous loss of the ability to respond to agonists that function by means of distinct receptors (heterologous refractoriness).

Suggestions of further complexity come from studies that indicate distinct kinetic phases for the acquisition of refractoriness or the need, in certain cells, for protein synthesis in order for refractoriness to be observed (de Vellis and Brooker, 1974). Progress has been made in the elucidation of at least one possible mechanism of homologous refractoriness. The continued exposure of intact cells containing β-adrenergic receptors to appropriate agonists causes an apparent loss of these ligand-binding sites (Mukherjee, Caron, and Lefkowitz, 1975). It is not known if these sites are removed from the membrane or if they are in some way masked.

Another poorly understood but extremely interesting phenomenon is that of potentiative interactions between ligands that utilize distinct receptor systems. For example, the simultaneous application of norepinephrine and adenosine or norepinephrine and histamine to brain slices may result in accumulation of cyclic AMP greatly in excess of the amount observed with either agent alone (Sattin and Rall, 1970; Huang, Shimizu, and Daly, 1971). Observations of this type have largely been confined to experiments performed with intact cell preparations from brain; the effect is not observed in homogenates. It is not known if this is a single-cell phenomenon or if cellular interactions are required.

Resolution and reconstitution of hormone-sensitive adenylate cyclase

The obvious key to a mechanistic comprehension of the system lies in its biochemical dissection. Its components must be enumerated and resolved, and purified components must be reconstituted into a functional entity. How many components are involved in the pathway that starts with hormone and ends with the synthesis of cyclic AMP? Although early kinetic studies suggested that adenylate cyclase and the receptors for hormones were distinct molecular entities, thoroughly convincing data have been obtained only recently. Genetic and physical manipulations of the system have provided, in our opinion, the clearest picture.

The S49 murine lymphoma cell is killed when exposed to exogenous cyclic AMP or agents that cause elevation of intracellular cyclic AMP concentrations. This has allowed the selection of variants that are resistant to the lethal effects of β-adrenergic agonists or cholera toxin. The first variants of this type to be isolated (designated AC$^-$) lacked essentially all measurable adenylate cyclase activity (Bourne, Coffino, and Tomkins, 1975). However, wild-type and AC$^-$ clones both contain binding sites for [^{125}I]-IHYP with essentially identical capacities and affinities for the labeled ligand (Insel et al., 1976). Competition studies indicate that these sites are, in fact, β-adrenergic receptors and support the conclusion that the receptor and adenylate cyclase are distinct molecular entities under independent genetic control. Although several other studies noted chemical, developmental, or genetic properties of the system that are also consistent with this hypothesis, the clearest data demonstrate physical separation of ligand binding and catalytic sites following solubilization with nonionic detergents (Limbird and Lefkowitz, 1977; Haga, Haga, and Gilman, 1977). The β-adrenergic receptor and adenylate cyclase are readily separable by gel filtration or by sucrose density gradient centrifugation. Hydro-

dynamic properties of the receptor and the enzyme are noted in Table I.

Further genetic studies with the S49 lymphoma cell have suggested the possibility of a third component. In addition to the AC$^-$ variant just described, another variant with a second type of stable, inheritable defect in the hormone-sensitive adenylate cyclase has been isolated (Haga et al., 1977). These cells (designated UNC) are resistant to the cytocidal effect of β-adrenergic agonists (like the AC$^-$ variants), but they retain sensitivity to the killing effect of cholera toxin. Consistent with the latter fact, they have normal specific activities of basal and NaF-stimulated adenylate cyclase, and cholera toxin stimulates the accumulation of cyclic AMP in intact cells (Figure 4). By contrast, the responses of intact cells and membranes to both isoproterenol and PGE$_1$ are lost. The enzyme can, however, be stimulated by Gpp(NH)p. Binding studies with [^{125}I]-IHYP indicate that the cells do possess β-adrenergic receptors at a concentration slightly greater than that of the wild-type cells. The known components of the system thus appear to be present, and stimulation of the enzyme by the three ubiquitous stimulators is retained, but interaction between hormone-binding and catalytic sites is lost. The response system is permanently uncoupled. Several types of explanation are possible, and the molecular lesion is unknown. The major proteins of the membrane appear to be present; the gross lipid composition of the membrane is unaltered. It is conceivable that these cells lack a specific but as yet unknown coupling factor.

Attempts to reconstitute a hormone-sensitive adenylate cyclase system should go hand in hand with experiments designed to resolve its components. The separation of a component of the system may only be detectable by an inability to reconstitute activity. Conversely, the only assay for a resolved component may be its ability to reconstitute a depleted system. Reconstitution of hormone-sensitive adenylate cyclase has been achieved by two general techniques: by fusion of cells or membranes with complementary lesions or by the addition of soluble extracts containing necessary components to complementary acceptor membranes. Reconstitution of certain individual components necessary for basal or Gpp(NH)p- or NaF-stimulated adenylate cyclase activity has also been demonstrated in solution—in the absence of an organized membrane.

Initial success using the fusion approach was reported by Orly and Schramm (1976), who made heterokaryons by fusion of cells in the presence of Sendai virus. Cycloheximide was included, so that what

TABLE I

Hydrodynamic parameters of adenylate cyclase and the β-adrenergic receptor of S49 lymphoma cells

	Adenylate Cyclase	β-Adrenergic Receptor
Stokes radius	7.1 nm	6.4 nm
Partial specific volume	0.78 ml/g	0.83 ml/g
Sedimentation coefficient ($s_{20,w}$)	7.5 S	3.1 S
Molecular weight	2.7×10^5	1.3×10^5
Frictional ratio	1.6	1.8
Lubrol PX bound	0.2 mg/mg protein	0.7 mg/mg protein
Molecular weight of protein	2.2×10^5	7.5×10^4

The parameters shown were calculated from data on the gel filtration and sucrose density gradient centrifugation of these activities, which were solubilized with the nonionic detergent Lubrol PX. Data are from Haga, Haga, and Gilman (1977).

they studied was the interaction of proteins present prior to cell fusion. Two cell types were utilized: Friend erythroleukemia cells, which contain adenylate cyclase but no β adrenergic receptor, and turkey erythrocytes, which do contain the receptor. For these experiments, the adenylate cyclase activity of the turkey cell was inactivated, either with N-ethylmaleimide or by thermal denaturation. Fusion of these two cell types resulted in the prompt emergence of catecholamine-stimulated adenylate cyclase activity. These experiments suggest several important

conclusions. Necessary individual components of the system are apparently relatively free to diffuse, mix, and interact within the bilayer in a relatively short period of time (one hour or less). Furthermore, cellular and species barriers can be crossed: mouse cyclase can function in tandem with a turkey receptor.

To resolve the system into individual components prior to reconstitution, it is obviously necessary to solubilize them. Solubilization of adenylate cyclase has been possible for some time, and we have recently been able to reincorporate soluble enzyme activity

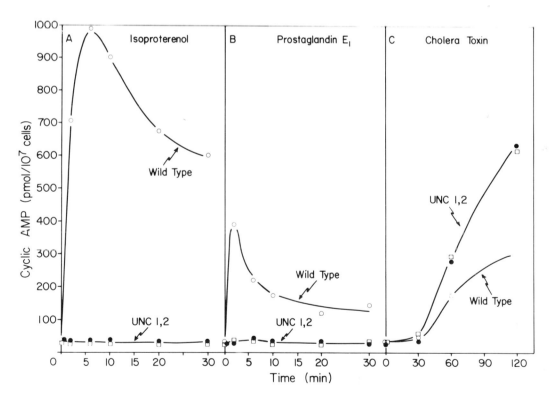

FIGURE 4   Cyclic AMP concentrations in intact S49 cells (wild type cells and UNC variants) following exposure to (A) (−)-isoproterenol, (B) prostaglandin E_1, or (C) cholera toxin. (Data from Haga et al., 1977.)

into receptor-replete AC⁻ membranes with concurrent reconstitution of catecholamine-stimulated enzymatic activity (Ross and Gilman, 1977a). This can be done with either the wild-type S49 cell as the donor of adenylate cyclase or with enzyme from a mouse L cell (B82), which contains no β-adrenergic receptors (Figure 5). Adenylate cyclase–containing donor extracts from UNC cells fail to restore catecholamine-stimulated enzyme activity to AC⁻ membranes, despite the fact that adenylate cyclase from UNC cells does respond to both Gpp(NH)p and NaF.

The UNC and AC⁻ variants of the S49 cell thus do not appear to be complementary. Hypothetically, AC⁻ and UNC share a common defect, and reconstitution of AC⁻ membranes with wild-type or B82 extracts may thus require factors in addition to those necessary for Gpp(NH)p- and NaF-stimulated adenylate cyclase activity.

In an attempt to resolve necessary components from the soluble-detergent extract of wild-type S49 cells, such extracts were incubated at 37°, since soluble (and membrane-bound) adenylate cyclase activity is known to be extremely labile to this treatment. After 30 min at 37°, no measurable adenylate cyclase activity remains. However, if such an incubated extract is combined with AC⁻ membranes or with detergent extracts of AC⁻ membranes, significant amounts of Gpp(NH)p- and NaF-stimulated enzyme activity appear (Figure 6). Our working hypothesis is that at least two components may be necessary before any adenylate cyclase activity is apparent; one component, which is presumably heat-labile, is still present in AC⁻. This clone is, however, deficient in certain factors that remain active in an incubated wild-type extract (Ross and Gilman, 1977b).

The thermal stabilities of the AC⁻ detergent extract and the incubated (37°, 30 min) wild-type extract have been examined. The AC⁻ extract loses its ability to complement with the incubated wild-type extract with

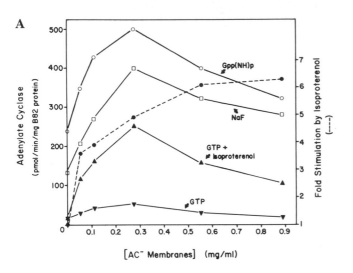

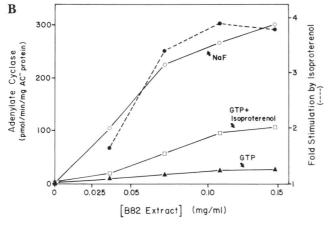

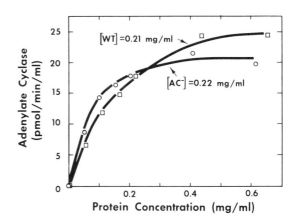

FIGURE 5 Reconstitution of catecholamine-sensitive adenylate cyclase activity. A detergent extract of B82 cell plasma membranes containing adenylate cyclase activity was added to plasma membranes of an adenylate cyclase–deficient S49 cell variant. Adenylate cyclase was assayed in the presence of NaF, Gpp(NH)p, GTP, or (−)-isoproterenol plus GTP. The dashed line shows the fold stimulation by isoproterenol. (A) An aliquot of the B82 membrane extract was added to suspensions of AC⁻ plasma membranes at increasing concentrations. (B) Increasing volumes of B82 membrane extract were added to a fixed amount of AC⁻ membranes. (Data from Ross and Gilman, 1977a.)

FIGURE 6 Reconstitution of Gpp(NH)p- and NaF-stimulated adenylate cyclase activity. Wild-type plasma membranes were solubilized with Lubrol PX, and the extract was then incubated at 37° for 30 min; such extracts then have no detectable adenylate cyclase activity. AC⁻ membranes were similarly solubilized with Lubrol PX, but the extract was not incubated. Addition of increasing amounts of AC⁻ extract to a fixed amount of incubated wild-type extract (square) or vice versa (circle) results in the reconstitution of Gpp(NH)p-stimulated enzyme activity. Similar curves are obtained if basal or NaF-stimulated activity are determined. (Data from Ross and Gilman, 1977b.)

a half-time of approximately 3 min at 30° (Figure 7). The decline in activity is a first-order process; NaF- and Gpp(NH)p-stimulated and basal activities all decline at the same rate. The more stable component(s) in the incubated wild-type extract are inactivated by exposure to 50° (Figure 8). Under this condition, Gpp(NH)p-stimulated reconstituted enzyme activity decays at about three times the rate of the NaF-stimulated enzyme activity, suggesting that independent components may be necessary for activation by these two ligands. The lability of the component presumed to be necessary for stimulation by Gpp(NH)p is decreased by the inclusion of the nucleotide in the 50° incubation.

These data are obviously incomplete. Components of the hormone-sensitive adenylate cyclase system that have been detected in other laboratories include the catecholamine-stimulated GTPase (Cassel and Selinger, 1976) and a guanine nucleotide-binding protein isolated by Pfeuffer and Helmreich (1975). It

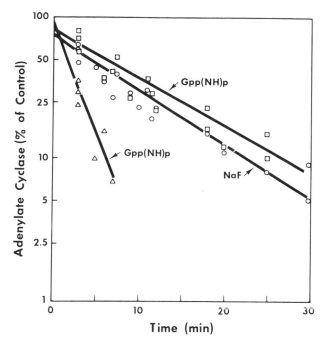

FIGURE 8 Inactivation at 50° of components of adenylate cyclase retained after mild heat treatment. An extract of wild-type S49 plasma membranes was first heated 30 min at 37° and then heated at 50° for the times shown. These extracts were mixed with an untreated AC⁻ extract, and adenylate cyclase activity was assayed in the presence of NaF (○) or Gpp(NH)p (△, □). The 50° incubation was performed in the absence (△, ○) or presence (□) of Gpp(NH)p. The data are from separate experiments, and activities are expressed as the percent of activity displayed by the sample that was not subjected to a 50° incubation. The lines are least-square fits of the data to a single exponential decay function. (Data from Ross and Gilman, 1977b.)

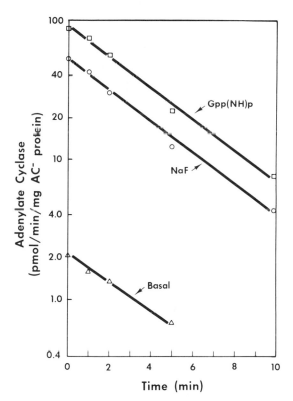

FIGURE 7 Inactivation at 30° of a component of adenylate cyclase that is retained in a phenotypically cyclase-deficient variant S49 clone (AC⁻). A Lubrol PX extract of AC⁻ plasma membranes was incubated for the times shown. A heat-inactivated extract of wild-type membranes was then added, and the adenylate cyclase of the reconstituted mixture was assayed in the presence of NaF or Gpp(NH)p or in the absence of effectors (basal). (Data from Ross and Gilman, 1977b.)

remains to be seen if the GTPase activity is related to this protein or if either or both are identical to the component we detected in the wild-type supernatant that is stabilized by Gpp(NH)p. We have also not yet begun to deal with the necessary lipid components of the system, although copious data argue that both the identity of the phospholipids present and their organization into a coherent bilayer are required for enzyme stimulation by hormone (see Maguire, Ross, and Gilman, 1977).

Figure 9 depicts our current thoughts on the number of essential components of a hormone-sensitive adenylate cyclase system. The AC⁻ cell is hypothesized to contain a protein that is necessary for any activity (perhaps the catalytic subunit). However, it is essentially devoid of enzyme activity in the absence of regulatory proteins that remain in the heated wild-type extract. It seems plausible that the hormone receptors and the hypothetical coupling factor (presumed to be missing from UNC) could act to control

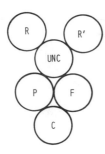

FIGURE 9 Current speculation on the protein components of a hormone-sensitive adenylate cyclase complex. One or more receptors (R) can influence the activity of an adenylate cyclase complex (PFC) in a manner that is dependent on a coupling factor (UNC). The labile catalytic unit (C) requires one protein (F) for basal, Gpp(NH)p-, or NaF-stimulated activity and another protein (P) for the effect of Gpp(NH)p.

enzyme activity by regulating the state of association between the catalytic unit and the regulatory proteins. This obviously remains to be seen. The crucial job for the immediate future will be to continue to resolve these factors, to purify them, and to study their ligand-binding properties and modes of interaction.

REFERENCES

AURBACH, G. D., S. A. FEDAK, C. J. WOODARD, J. S. PALMER, D. HAUSER, and F. TROXLER, 1974. β-Adrenergic receptor: Stereospecific interaction of iodinated β-blocking agent with high affinity site. *Science* 186:1223–1224.

BILTONEN, R. L., 1977. General thermodynamic considerations of receptor interactions. *Fed. Proc.* 36:2112–2114.

BOURNE, H. R., P. COFFINO, and G. M. TOMKINS, 1975. Selection of a variant lymphoma cell deficient in adenylate cyclase. *Science* 187:750–752.

BROWN, E. M., G. D. AURBACH, D. HAUSER, and F. TROXLER, 1976a. β-Adrenergic receptor interactions. Characterization of iodohydroxybenzylpindolol as a specific ligand. *J. Biol. Chem.* 251:1232–1238.

BROWN, E. M., S. A. FEDAK, C. J. WOODARD, G. D. AURBACH, and D. RODBARD, 1976b. β-Adrenergic receptor interactions. Direct comparison of receptor interaction and biological activity. *J. Biol. Chem.* 251:1239–1246.

CASSEL, D., and Z. SELINGER, 1976. Catecholamine-stimulated GTPase activity in turkey erythrocyte membranes. *Biochim. Biophys. Acta* 452:538–551.

CASSEL, D., and Z. SELINGER, 1977. Mechanism of adenylate cyclase activation by cholera toxin: Inhibition of GTP hydrolysis at the regulatory site. *Proc. Natl. Acad. Sci. USA* 74:3307–3311.

GILL, D. M., 1977. Mechanisms of action of cholera toxin. In *Advances in Cyclic Nucleotide Research,* vol. 8, P. Greengard and G. A. Robison, eds. New York: Raven Press, pp. 85–118.

HAGA, T., K. HAGA, and A. G. GILMAN, 1977. Hydrodynamic properties of the β-adrenergic receptor and aden-

ylate cyclase from wild-type and variant S49 lymphoma cells. *J. Biol. Chem.* 252:5776–5782.

HAGA, T., E. M. ROSS, H. J. ANDERSON, and A. G. GILMAN, 1977. Adenylate cyclase permanently uncoupled from hormone receptors in a novel variant of S49 mouse lymphoma cells. *Proc. Natl. Acad. Sci. USA* 74:2016–2020.

HUANG, M., H. SHIMIZU, and J. DALY, 1971. Regulation of adenosine cyclic 3',5'-phosphate formation in cerebral cortical slices: Interaction among norepinephrine, histamine, and serotonin. *Mol. Pharmacol.* 7:155–162.

INSEL, P. A., M. E. MAGUIRE, A. G. GILMAN, H. R. BOURNE, P. COFFINO, and K. L. MELMON, 1976. Beta-adrenergic receptors and adenylate cyclase: Products of separate genes? *Mol. Pharmacol.* 12:1062–1069.

JARD, S., C. ROY, T. BARTH, R. RAJERISON, and J. BOCKAERT, 1975. Antidiuretic hormone-sensitive kidney adenylate cyclase. In *Advances in Cyclic Nucleotide Research,* vol. 5, G. I. Drummond, P. Greengard, and G. A. Robison, eds. New York: Raven Press, pp. 31–52.

LEFKOWITZ, R. J., C. MUKHERJEE, M. COVERSTONE, and M. G. CARON, 1974. Stereospecific [³H](−)-alprenolol binding sites, β-adrenergic receptors and adenylate cyclase. *Biochem. Biophys. Res. Commun.* 60:703–709.

LIMBIRD, L. E., and R. J. LEFKOWITZ, 1977. Resolution of β-adrenergic receptor binding and adenylate cyclase activity by gel exclusion chromatography. *J. Biol. Chem.* 252:799–802.

MAGUIRE, M. E., P. H. GOLDMAN, and A. G. GILMAN, 1974. The reaction of [³H]norepinephrine with particulate fractions of cells responsive to catecholamines. *Mol. Pharmacol.* 10:563–581.

MAGUIRE, M. E., E. M. ROSS, and A. G. GILMAN, 1977. The β-adrenergic receptor: Ligand binding properties and the interaction with adenylyl cyclase. In *Advances in Cyclic Nucleotide Research,* vol. 8, P. Greengard and G. A. Robison, eds. New York: Raven Press, pp. 1–84.

MAGUIRE, M. E., R. A. WIKLUND, H. J. ANDERSON, and A. G. GILMAN, 1976. Binding of [¹²⁵I]iodohydroxybenzylpindolol to putative β-adrenergic receptors of rat glioma cells and other cell clones. *J. Biol. Chem.* 251:1221–1231.

MUKHERJEE, C., M. G. CARON, and R. J. LEFKOWITZ, 1975. Catecholamine-induced subsensitivity of adenylate cyclase associated with loss of β-adrenergic receptor binding sites. *Proc. Natl. Acad. Sci. USA* 72:1945–1949.

ORLY, J., and M. SCHRAMM, 1976. Coupling of catecholamine receptor from one cell with adenylate cyclase from another cell by cell fusion. *Proc. Natl. Acad. Sci. USA* 73:4410–4414.

PERKINS, J. P., and M. M. MOORE, 1971. Adenyl cyclase of rat cerebral cortex. Activation by fluoride and detergents. *J. Biol. Chem.* 246:62–68.

PFEUFFER, T., and E. J. M. HELMREICH, 1975. Activation of pigeon erythrocyte membrane adenylate cyclase by guanylnucleotide analogues and separation of a nucleotide binding protein. *J. Biol. Chem.* 250:867–876.

RODBELL, M., M. C. LIN, Y. SALOMON, C. LONDOS, J. P. HARWOOD, B. R. MARTIN, M. RENDELL, and M. BERMAN, 1975. Role of adenine and guanine nucleotides in the activity and response of adenylate cyclase systems to hormones: Evidence for multisite transition states. In *Advances in Cyclic Nucleotide Research,* vol. 5, G. I. Drummond, P. Greengard, and G. A. Robison, eds. New York: Raven Press, pp. 3–29.

Ross, E. M., and A. G. Gilman, 1977a. Reconstitution of catecholamine-sensitive adenylate cyclase activity: Interaction of solubilized components with receptor-replete membranes. *Proc. Natl. Acad. Sci. USA* 74:3715–3719.

Ross, E. M., and A. G. Gilman, 1977b. Resolution of some components of adenylate cyclase necessary for catalytic activity. *J. Biol. Chem.* 252:6966–6969.

Ross, E. M., M. E. Maguire, T. W. Sturgill, R. L. Biltonen, and A. G. Gilman, 1977. The relationship between the β-adrenergic receptor and adenylate cyclase. Studies of ligand binding and enzyme activity in purified membranes of S49 lymphoma cells. *J. Biol. Chem.* 252:5761–5775.

Sattin, A., and T. W. Rall, 1970. The effect of adenosine and adenine nucleotides on the cyclic adenosine 3′,5′-phosphate content of guinea pig cerebral cortex slices. *Mol. Pharmacol.* 6:13–23.

Su, Y.-F., L. X. Cubeddu, and J. P. Perkins, 1976a. Regulation of adenosine 3′:5′-monophosphate content of human astrocytoma cells: Desensitization to catecholamines and prostaglandins. *J. Cyclic Nucleotide Res.* 2:257–270.

Su, Y.-F., G. L. Johnson, L. X. Cubeddu, B. H. Leichtling, R. Ortmann, and J. P. Perkins, 1976b. Regulation of adenosine 3′:5′-monophosphate content of human astrocytoma cells: Mechanism of agonist-specific desensitization. *J. Cyclic Nucleotide Res.* 2:271–285.

de Vellis, J., and G. Brooker, 1974. Reversal of catecholamine refractoriness by inhibitors of RNA and protein synthesis. *Science* 186:1221–1223.

48 Coupling of Ion Transport to Enzyme Activity

GUIDO GUIDOTTI

ABSTRACT Osmotic gradients of ions across cell membranes are present in all cells, both prokaryotic and eukaryotic. Evidence for the existence of these gradients comes from the observation that the K^+ concentration is always higher inside cells than it is outside. These gradients can be set up by ion pumps, membrane-bound systems that use chemical energy to produce ion gradients. The ion gradients can be used for several purposes: to accumulate solutes in the cell against a concentration gradient; to set up a membrane potential; to activate intracellular enzymes; and to produce conditions for a sudden release of ions (as in sarcoplasmic reticulum and during the action potential in nerve cells). The central point is that the general reactions catalyzed by different ion pumps energized by chemical energy are basically similar. Thus the Na^+ pump, the Ca^{++} pump, and the H^+ pump (of mitochondria) can be envisaged as acting by a similar mechanism. This mechanism can be illustrated by looking in detail at the structure and function of the Na^+ pump, a membrane enzyme that has the structure $\alpha_2\beta_2$ (α having a molecular weight of 100,000; β, 50,000). The $\alpha_2\beta_2$ unit can be isolated, purified, and reconstituted into artificial lipid vesicles, where it pumps Na^+ and K^+ with the same stoichiometry as the native enzyme does: $Na^+/K^+/ATP = 3/2/1$. Several ion transport systems have similar structural features and may have arisen from a common ancestor.

Existence and use of osmotic gradients

IN ALL LIVING cells the concentration of many ions inside the cell is different from that in the extracellular fluid. This difference cannot be accounted for by the Donnan relationship, and it thus represents true osmotic gradients. Table I shows the situation for the distribution of ions across the membrane of the human erythrocyte and of the bacterium *E. coli*.

These ionic gradients have several uses. They are involved in solute transport, as in the intestine and in bacteria (Schultz and Curran, 1970; Harold, 1977). They are the source of the membrane potential, notably in nerves (Katz, 1966). Particular intracellular concentrations of some ions such as Ca^{++} and K^+ are required for the proper function of some enzymes (K^+ enzymes, muscle proteins) (Evans and Sorges, 1966; Ebashi, Endo and Ohtsuki, 1969). Moreover, the storage of ions in particular compartments can be used to bring about the sudden release of ions which can then affect intracellular functions. This happens, for example, in muscle sarcoplasmic reticulum (Ebashi, Endo, and Ohtsuki, 1969) and is thought to take place in retinal rods (Hagins and Yoshikami, 1974).

In any event, ion gradients are present in all living cells. These gradients are generated by membrane enzymes, so-called ion pumps, which utilize the energy stored in ATP or other chemicals to redistribute ions across a semipermeable barrier, the plasma or any other specialized membrane.

Ion pumps

Three ion pumps have been identified and extensively studied so far. These are the Na^+ pump of plasma membranes (Dahl and Hokin, 1974), the Ca^{++} pump of sarcoplasmic reticulum (MacLennan and Holland, 1975), and the H^+ pump of mitochondria, chloroplasts, and bacterial cells (Baird and Hammes, 1977). Some of the features of these systems are shown in Table II. Since the turnover number for all these enzymes for ATP is roughly 10^2 sec^{-1}, the ion-pumping power of the systems depends on the concentration of enzymes in the cell membrane. For example, there are less than 1,000 copies of the Na^+ pump per human erythrocyte membrane. This means that the maximum Na^+ pumping cannot exceed 3×10^5 Na^+ ions per cell per second. In other cells, however, such as the membrane of nerve axons and in the kidney medulla, the concentration of enzyme is at least 100 times greater (Bader, Post, and Bond, 1968). Thus the pumping ability can be at least 3×10^7 Na^+ ions per second per 100 μm^2 of membrane.

GUIDO GUIDOTTI The Biological Laboratories, Harvard University, Cambridge, MA 02138

TABLE I

TABLE I

Ionic composition of representative systems (mM)

	Plasma	Human Erythrocyte[1]	Growth Medium	*E. coli*[2]
Na^+	145	19	136	70
K^+	5	136	2.5	246
Cl^-	105	78	22.5	
HCO_3^-	30	18		
Mg^{++}	2	3.5	0.4	24
Ca^{++}	5	0.02		
$HPO_4^{--} + H_2PO_4^-$	2	0.36	70	10

[1] From J. C. Gamble, *Chemical Anatomy, Physiology and Extracellular Fluid* (6th ed.). Cambridge, MA: Harvard Univ. Press (1954).

[2] From W. Epstein and S. G. Schultz, Cation transport in *Escherichia coli*. V. Regulation of cation content. *J. Gen. Physiol.* 49:221–234 (1965).

TABLE II

Properties of ion pumps

	$(Na^+ + K^+)$ ATPase	Ca^{++} ATPase	H^+ ATPase (mitochondrial)
Molecular weight of native enzyme	300,000	(200,000?)	321,500
Molecular weights of component polypeptides	α–100,000 β–50,000	α–100,000	α–60,000 β–56,000 γ–34,000 δ–14,000 ϵ–7,500
Probable structure	$\alpha_2\beta_2$	α_2	$\alpha_2\beta_2\gamma_2\delta\epsilon$
Turnover number of ATP	50–100 sec^{-1}	50–100 sec^{-1}	500 sec^{-1}

General mechanism of reaction

In all three cases considered here—indeed in the general case—the reaction catalyzed by the transport enzyme can be written as follows:

$$Enz + nX_a + ATP \rightleftharpoons Enz + nX_b + ADP + Pi,$$

where Enz represents the membrane transport system, X_a and X_b stand for the transported ions on side a and b of the membrane, respectively, and n is the number of ions transported for each molecule of ATP hydrolyzed. It is obvious that the gradient of ions set up by the enzyme is limited by the free energy of hydrolysis of ATP. Furthermore, a sufficiently high gradient of ions (X_b/X_a) can lead to the synthesis of ATP. There is no obvious difference in the general reaction that can be written for any of these pumps.

Structure of the transport systems

There are two general types of intrinsic proteins that differ drastically in properties and arrangement in the membrane. They are called Type I and Type II proteins (Figure 1). Transport proteins appear to be Type II intrinsic membrane proteins.

Type I intrinsic proteins have most of their mass and all of their functional properties in the aqueous environment outside the cytoplasm. The intramembranous portion serves only to anchor the proteins to a particular membrane, and it consists of a short amino acid sequence sufficient to span the bilayer as an α helix. Type I proteins include the major sialoglycoprotein of the red-blood-cell membrane, several proteins of such enveloped viruses as Semliki forest virus and Sindbis virus, and the histocompatability antigens of human cells (HLA). The best-studied of these is the major sialoglycoprotein of the human erythrocyte (Marchesi, Furthmayr, and Tomita, 1976). This protein illustrates clearly the salient features of the intrinsic proteins of Type I: the proteins are basically aqueous with a hydrophobic anchor that attaches them to a membrane. The anchor comprises a small fraction of the polypeptide chain. All of the functional properties of the protein are in the aqueous compartments on the exterior of the membrane.

Type II intrinsic proteins have two major charac-

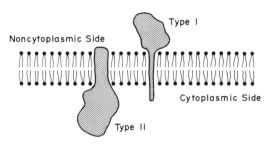

FIGURE 1 Arrangement in the membrane of the two types of intrinsic membrane proteins.

teristics: the major part of their polypeptide mass is in the cytoplasm and a very small fraction of their amino acid residues is exposed to the noncytoplasmic side of the bilayer. This means that over 90% of the amino acid residues are either in the bilayer or in the cytoplasm. Clearly, these proteins are drastically different in their membrane arrangement from the Type I proteins. It is also apparent that the mechanism by which the Type I proteins are inserted in the bilayer must differ from that used by Type II proteins. There appear to be two categories of Type II proteins. One group is represented by cytochrome b_5, cytochrome b_5 reductase, and stearyl-CoA desaturase (Enock, Catala, and Strittmatter, 1976). These proteins are similar to the Type I proteins in that their functional domains are entirely in the aqueous compartment, in this case in the cytoplasm. Cytochrome b_5 is attached to the membrane through a hydrophobic region of the molecule, which is COOH-terminal and contains 44 amino acids. It has not been established whether or not the intramembranous portion of this polypeptide transverses the bilayer entirely or is localized to the inner leaflet. The other proteins in this category resemble cytochrome b_5 in their arrangement on the membrane. One concludes that the attachment to the membrane of these proteins has the principal function of concentrating the enzymes on the endoplasmic reticulum.

The second category of Type II proteins is represented by proteins involved in transmembranous processes, for example, in transport. There are only a few well-characterized proteins in this group: the $(Na^+ + K^+)$ATPase (Dahl and Hokin, 1974), the Ca^{++}ATPase (MacLennan and Holland, 1975), band 3 of the human erythrocyte membrane, which is involved in anion exchange (Ho and Guidotti, 1975; Drickamer, 1976), vertebrate rhodopsin (Cone, 1976), and the acetylcholine receptor (Karlin, 1974). All of these intrinsic proteins have explicit or putative transport functions and thus are involved in the transfer of matter across the bilayer. It is likely that all transmembrane transport of matter is catalyzed by proteins that have properties similar to those of the proteins listed above. These proteins are all transmembranous oligomers, which are glycoproteins if attached to the plasma membrane (see Table III).

Structure of the $(Na^+ + K^+)$ATPase

The structure of the $(Na^+ + K^+)$ATPase is shown in Figure 2. The major components are two different polypeptide chains: α, with a molecular weight of about 100,000; and β, with a mass of about 50,000 daltons. Cross-linking studies done by Kyte (1975) and by Giotta (1976) show that two α chains can be cross-linked to an α_2 unit by oxidation of SH groups. Since an $\alpha\beta$ dimer can also be formed easily by imido esters (Kyte, 1972), one concludes that one form of the enzyme is an $\alpha_2\beta_2$ structure.

The β chain is a glycoprotein. While it is not clear

TABLE III

Properties of membrane transport systems

	$(Na^+ + K^+)$ ATPase	Ca^{++} ATPase	Anion-Exchange Protein	Acetylcholine Receptor	Rhodopsin
Molecular weights of component polypeptides	α–90,000 β–40,000	α–100,000	α–90,000	α–40,000 β–48,000 γ–58,000 δ–64,000 ϵ–105,000	α–38,000
Glycoproteins	β		α	$\alpha(\beta$–$\epsilon)$?	α
Probable structure and molecular weight of the protein part of the enzyme	$\alpha_2\beta_2$ 260,000	$(\alpha_2?)$ (200,000?)	α_2 180,000	ϵ_2 or $\alpha_2\beta_2$ 240,000	$(\alpha_2$ to $\alpha_4?)$ (76,000– 152,000?)
Transmembrane arrangement	α		α		α
Detergent binding (mg/mg of protein)	0.28	0.20	0.77	0.7	1.10
Relative hydrophobic surface area of subunit	0.20–0.24	0.2–0.25	0.5–0.65	0.5–0.6	0.54

Source: Guidotti (1976).

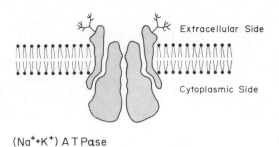

(Na⁺+K⁺) A T Pase

FIGURE 2 Oligomeric structure and arrangement in the membrane of the (Na⁺ + K⁺)ATPase (Na⁺ pump).

what the functional significance of glycosylation might be, it is a fact that all intrinsic proteins associated with the plasma membrane of eukaryotic cells are glycoproteins. Thus it is not surprising that one of the polypeptides of the Na⁺ pump is a glycoprotein. Indeed one wonders whether all intrinsic membrane proteins located in the plasma membrane must be glycoprotein, and thus whether the α and β chains might not have been synthesized as a single polypeptide, which was modified by proteolysis after synthesis. This could explain the lack of carbohydrate residues on the α chain.

The binding sites for ATP and for the cardiac glycosides are on the α chain. The α chain thus traverses the bilayer (Ruoho and Kyte, 1974). This observation is supported by the results of Clarke (1975) on the behavior of this enzyme in the detergent Triton X-100. At low concentrations, this detergent has no effect on the usual water-soluble enzymes, but it does bind to membrane proteins. The properties of the (Na⁺ + K⁺)ATPase in Triton X-100 are shown in Table IV. This enzyme binds a substantial amount of Triton X-100, a result that can be interpreted as indicating that about 20% of the surface of the enzyme is in the bilayer.

The arrangement of the major polypeptide with most of the mass on the inner surface of the bilayer is deduced from the following data. First, negative staining of the membrane fragments reveals a large particle on the inner surface of the membrane, in contrast to a smooth outer surface (Jorgensen, 1974). Second, proteolysis of intact red cells causes no change in (Na⁺ + K⁺)ATPase activity, while proteolysis of ghosts or of isolated enzyme causes rapid loss of activity and degradation of the peptide (Giotta, 1975).

An important question is whether these two polypeptides are responsible for Na⁺ and K⁺ transport. The answer to this question is given by the following experiments done by Goldin (1977). The purified enzyme, composed of the two polypeptide chains, can be reconstituted into artificial phosphatidyl choline vesicles with an average diameter of about 500 Å. Nearly 100% of the enzyme can be so reconstituted, and the resulting specific activity is about 40% of the unreconstituted enzyme. The permeabilities of vesicles containing the enzyme to Na⁺, K⁺, and Cl⁻ are shown in Figure 3. The Cl⁻ permeability is much greater than that of either Na⁺ or K⁺ (P_{Cl} = 4–8 × 10⁻¹⁰ cm/sec, $P_{Na,K}$ = 2–4 × 10⁻¹¹ cm/sec). When ATP is added to a suspension of vesicles containing the enzyme, the intravesicular Na⁺ concentration increases and the K⁺ concentration decreases dramatically (Figure 4). Figure 5 shows that the decrease in steady-state level of K⁺ relative to the steady-state increase in Na⁺ is independent of the initial intravesicular K⁺ concentration and corresponds to the movement of 3 Na⁺ for 2 K⁺. As shown in Figure 6, the initial rate of ATP-stimulated Na⁺ uptake is close to 3 Na⁺/ATP hydrolyzed. These results establish that the reconstituted enzyme, like the native enzyme in red blood cells and in axons, pumps 3 Na⁺ and 2 K⁺ for each ATP molecule hydrolyzed. Thus we are con-

TABLE IV

Properties of the (Na⁺ + K⁺)ATPase in Triton X-100

$s_{20,w}$	6.1 S	f/f_0	1.7
$\bar{v}$	0.76 cm³/g	g Triton/g protein	0.28
$D_{20,w}$	3.35 × 10⁻⁷ cm²/sec	g carbohydrate/g protein	0.05
M_r complex	185,000	M_r protein portion	140,000
Moles Triton/ mole protein	60	M_r protein (SDS)	95,000 45,000
Fraction of surface area covered by detergent	0.20–0.24	M_r (Triton)/M_r (SDS)	1

Source: Data from Clarke (1975).

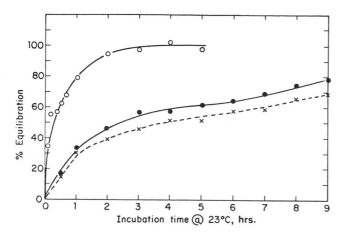

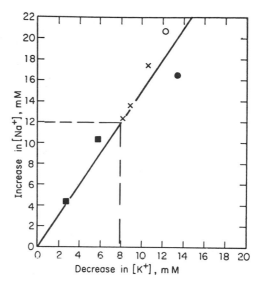

FIGURE 3 Permeability of reconstituted $(Na^+ + K^+)$ATPase vesicles to $^{22}Na^+$, $^{42}K^+$, and $^{36}Cl^-$. Vesicles were formed in 30 mM NaCl, 20 mM KCl. Radioisotopes were added to form radioisotopic but not concentration gradients of these ions. Entry of externally added ^{22}Na ($\times$), $^{42}K^+$ ($\bullet$), and $^{36}Cl^-$ ($\circ$) as percentages of equilibration of radioisotope with vesicles. (From Goldin, 1977.)

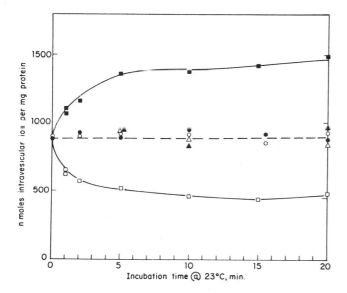

FIGURE 4 Double-label demonstration of nucleotide-stimulated changes in intravesicular content of Na^+ and K^+. $(Na^+ + K^+)$ATPase vesicles were formed in the presence of 30 mM $^{22}NaCl$ and 21 mM ^{42}KCl. Addition of 4 mM ATP increased ($\blacksquare$) Na^+ and decreased ($\square$) K^+ as compared with Na^+ ($\bullet$) and K ($\circ$) determined in the absence of any nucleotide additions. AMP-PNP (4 mM) showed no effect on levels of intravesicular Na^+ ($\blacktriangle$) or K^+ ($\triangle$). (From Goldin, 1977.)

fident that the two polypeptides shown here are the molecules responsible for the function of the enzyme: ATP hydrolysis and Na^+ and K^+ transport.

All these data suggest that the Na^+ pump has the structure $\alpha_2\beta_2$ and that it is a transmembranous oligomeric protein.

FIGURE 5 ATP-dependent increases on steady-state intravesicular $[Na^+]$ and decreases in steady-state $[K^+]$. All initial intravesicular Na^+ concentrations were 30 mM. Initial $[K^+]$ was 30 mM ($\circ$), 21 mM ($\times$), or 1 mM ($\blacksquare$). Steady-state intravesicular ion contents were determined as average levels between 10 min and 20 min of incubation with 4 mM ATP at 23°. (From Goldin, 1977.)

What is the structure of the oligomers? There are three areas of interest: the symmetry of the oligomer; the protein-protein interactions that stabilize the oligomers; and the structure of the intramembranous part.

The oligomeric arrangement of the subunits and the membrane asymmetry of polypeptide arrangement mean that the axis of symmetry of the oligomer must be perpendicular to the plane of the membrane. Since the oligomer is a dimer, homologous bonding between the subunits can satisfy this requirement. It should be emphasized that homologous bonding is the only arrangement that can close at a dimer stage. On the other hand, if the oligomer is larger than a dimer, say a tetramer or hexamer (the Ca^{++} ATPase of sarcoplasmic reticulum has been envisaged as a tetramer; see Murphy, 1976), then the requirements stated above can only be satisfied by heterologous bonding between the subunits. This means that an n-mer will have an n-fold axis of symmetry perpendicular to the bilayer. This also means, since heterologous bonding is less frequent than homologous bonding, that the most likely structure of membrane proteins is dimeric.

The possible interactions between subunits in this oligomeric membrane protein can involve the three parts of the polypeptide: that part outside the membrane, which is exposed to the extracellular fluid; the intramembranous part; and the major cytoplasmic

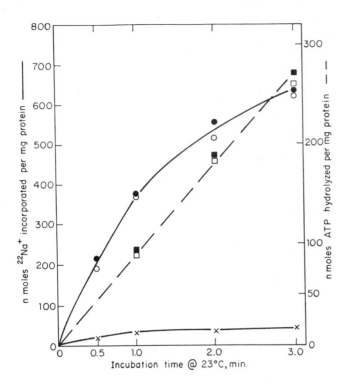

FIGURE 6 Determination of ATP hydrolysis in the absence (■) and in the presence (□) of 0.3 mM externally added ouabain in parallel with measurements of ATP-dependent $^{22}Na^+$ uptake in absence (●) and in presence (○) of 0.3 mM externally added ouabain. Crosses indicate control measurements of $^{22}Na^+$ uptake in the absence of ATP. The $(Na^+ + K^+)$ATPase vesicles were formed in 30 mM NaCl and 20 mM KCl. Carrier-free $^{22}NaCl$ was added externally. (From Goldin, 1977.)

component. Since evidence suggests that very little of the polypeptide is exposed to the outer environment, these interactions should be negligible. On the other hand, the intramembranous part and the cytoplasmic portion are likely to have major roles. The intramembranous piece of the polypeptide will interact with the lipid by nonpolar interactions but with other segments of the polypeptide and with other polypeptides by hydrogen bonds: these are clearly more stable in a nonpolar environment and will strongly stabilize protein-protein interactions. This means that the contact surface between two polypeptides will be stabilized by polar interactions: that is, there is likely to be a polar surface at the contact between membrane polypeptides. This is the surface that will probably interact with polar solutes. If the intramembranous segments of the polypeptide are the main ones involved in subunit-subunit interactions, and if these are necessarily polar interactions, they should vanish when these regions are exposed to water. Thus, un-

der conditions that eliminate the lipid bilayer, for example with detergents such as Triton X-100 or deoxycholate, transmembranous oligomers stabilized by the intramembranous segments should dissociate into proteins. This is the case with the Na^+ pump, as shown in Table IV. One might conclude that the major part of the stabilizing interactions between the monomers does involve the intramembranous portion.

Finally, the cytoplasmic portion of the protein, which is large for the α-chain polypeptide, can have a major role in the intersubunit interactions. These can be both polar and nonpolar interactions and can contribute the main stabilization for the oligomeric structure. Since the cytoplasmic portion of the protein is normally present in the aqueous environment, removal of the protein from the bilayer with detergents should have no effect on the oligomeric structure of the protein if the cytoplasmic portion is responsible for the association between subunits. However, this is not the case for the Na^+ pump (see Table IV).

Approximately 20% of the mass of the α chain is in the bilayer. Nothing is known about the structure of this segment nor has it been localized on the linear sequence of the α chain, as has been done for the band 3 polypeptide of the human erythrocyte membrane (Drickamer, 1976).

Mechanism of transport

Although the structure of the Na pump has been described and the stoichiometry of the reaction catalyzed by this enzyme ascertained by the reconstitution experiments, the mechanism of transport is still not obvious. A mechanism can, however, be suggested on the basis of the fact that there must be at least two conformations of the enzyme. The data of Karlish, Yates, and Glynn (1976) clearly show that the affinity of ATP for a form of the enzyme stabilized by Na^+ is greater than that for a form stabilized by K^+. This in itself is good evidence for the existence of two conformations of the enzyme.

Other evidence on the kinetics of ATP hydrolysis can be described by the scheme shown in Figure 7. The important feature of this scheme is that in one form (E_1) the enzyme has a high affinity for Na^+ and ATP (K_m values are 2 mM and 0.15 μM, respectively: see Taniguchi and Post, 1975), while in another form (E_2) the enzyme has a lower affinity for these ligands (K_m values of 0.5 M and 1 mM, respectively: see Karlish, Yates, and Glynn, 1975; Taniguchi and Post,

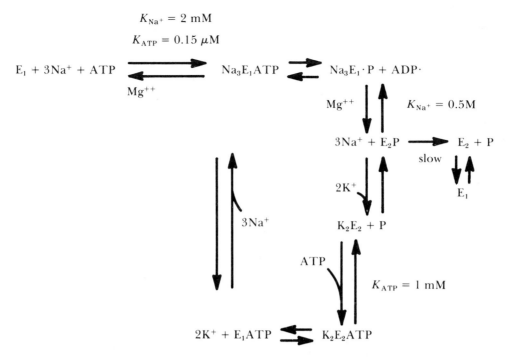

FIGURE 7 Reaction scheme for the Na⁺- and K⁺-dependent hydrolysis of ATP by the $(Na^+ + K^+)ATPase$.

1975; Cantley and Josephson, 1976). I wish to propose that the ability to undergo conformational changes is an absolute requirement for transport. If this hypothesis is correct, it would explain the transmembranous and oligomeric features of the enzyme.

The protein spans the bilayer (it is a transmembranous protein) because it catalyzes transport by undergoing small conformational changes rather than by diffusing backward and forward across the bilayer. It might be argued that a transmembranous protein could transport solutes by rotating through the bilayer around an axis parallel to the membrane. This is unlikely, however, because of the asymmetric arrangement of the transport systems $((Na^+ + K^+)ATPase$, anion exchange system, rhodopsin) with respect to the inner and outer surfaces of the membrane (Kyte, 1975; Cone, 1976). Therefore, the transport proteins are embedded in a fixed and time-independent asymmetric orientation in the bilayer. Accordingly, they catalyze transport through small conformational changes.

The protein is oligomeric either because the active site for transport is produced at the interfaces between subunits (much as the binding site for organic phosphates is at the adjacent surfaces between the β chains of hemoglobin) or because allosteric control is more easily realized in oligomeric proteins, or for both reasons. According to this view, the active site of the enzyme with respect to the solute to be transported is at the interface between the two subunits of the enzyme. This interface also provides the barrier to permeation and does not need to have the dimensions of the bilayer. Indeed, the barrier to solute movement at the points in the membrane where the transmembranous protein is located need be only a few angstroms thick. One can envisage a conformational change producing a sliding of the contact surfaces between the subunits one past the other, much as happens in the hemoglobin molecule when it changes from the oxygenated to the deoxygenated conformation (Figure 8). If the barrier to ion movement in the enzyme, which is at the subunit contact sites, were to move as shown in Figure 9, such a small sliding of one subunit relative to the other would be sufficient to transport ions across the barrier to movement. This is still a hypothesis, but it does allow one to devise experiments to disprove it.

Relationship between transport systems

I have noted that the three transport systems discussed here have certain structural similarities: they

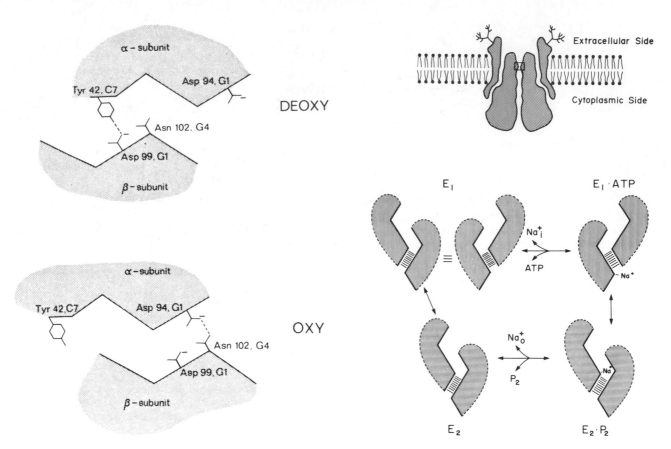

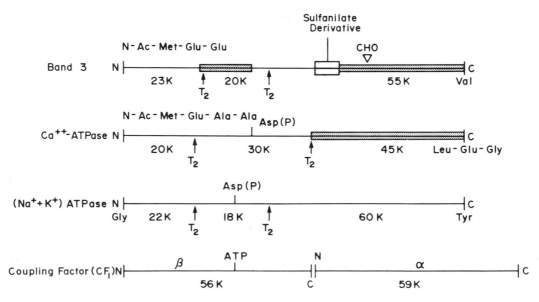

FIGURE 8 Change in $\alpha_1\beta_2$ contact of hemoglobin on oxygenation. The contact area clicks from one dove-tailed position to another, involving a switch of hydrogen bonding. Most of the other contacts are nonpolar. (From Morimoto, Lehmann, and Perutz, 1971.)

FIGURE 9 Model for the transport of ions by the $(Na^+ + K^+)$ATPase. The key feature of this model is the change in intersubunit contacts during turnover.

FIGURE 10 Schematic diagram of the main features of the structures of the anion exchange protein of human erythrocyte, the Ca^{++} pump, the Na^+ pump, and the H^+ pump of mitochondria. T_2 indicates a site of hydrolysis by trypsin.

all are transmembranous oligomeric protein complexes. Here I want to suggest that there may be even more striking similarities between these three transport systems, and also with the anion exchange system of human erythrocyte membranes (Figure 10).

The first point is that all four of these systems have as a major subunit either a polypeptide with a molecular weight of approximately 100,000 or a set of two polypeptides whose summed molecular weight is approximately 100,000. The second point is that the polypeptides with a molecular weight of 100,000 can be split by trypsin approximately into half-molecules that resemble in size the α and β polypeptides of the H^+ pump (Steck, Ramos, and Strapazon, 1976; Stewart, MacLennan, and Shamoo, 1976; Giotta, 1975). This trypsin-susceptible site is on the inner surface of the membrane, and proteolysis at this site does not necessarily cause loss of enzymatic activity. The third point is that all four systems can be lined up so that one of the active sites of the polypeptide (for example, the site that interacts with ATP) is located either on the NH_2-terminal tryptic polypeptide or on the smaller of the two natural polypeptides. The fourth point is that both the H^+ pump and the Na^+ pump can be inactivated by NBD-chloride (Cantley, Gells, and Josephson, 1977). In both cases this reagent reacts with one tyrosine residue per subunit and causes loss of enzymatic activity.

These similarities are striking. They support the hypothesis that all ion transport systems have similar structural features and thus may have arisen from a common ancestor. If this is so, substantial homology should exist in the detailed structure of these ion pumps. Furthermore, it would not be surprising if all the pumps operated by a similar mechanism.

REFERENCES

BADER, H., R. L. POST, and G. H. BOND, 1968. Comparison of sources of a phosphorylated intermediate in transport ATPase. *Biochim. Biophys. Acta* 150:41–46.

BAIRD, B. A., and G. G. HAMMES, 1977. Chemical cross-linking studies of beef heart mitochondrial coupling factor 1. *J. Biol. Chem.* 252:4743–4748.

CANTLEY, L. C., JR., J. GELLS, and L. JOSEPHSON, 1977. Reaction of (Na-K) ATPase with 7-chloro-4-nitobenzo-2-oxa-1,3-diazole: Evidence for essential tyrosine at the active site. *Biochemistry* 17:418–425.

CANTLEY, L. C., JR., and L. JOSEPHSON, 1976. A slow interconversion between active and inactive states of the (Na⁺ + K⁺)ATPase. *Biochemistry* 15:5280–5286.

CLARKE, S., 1975. The size and detergent binding of membrane proteins. *J. Biol. Chem.* 250:5459–5469.

CONE, R. A., 1976. Transductive coupling in the visual system. In *Functional Linkage in Biomolecular Systems*, F. O.

Schmitt, D. M. Schneider, and D. M. Crothers, eds. New York: Raven Press, pp. 234–246.

DAHL, J. L., and L. E. HOKIN, 1974. The sodium potassium adenosine triphosphatase. *Annu. Rev. Biochem.* 43:327–356.

DRICKAMER, L. K., 1976. Fragmentation of the 95,000-dalton transmembrane polypeptide in human erythrocyte membranes. *J. Biol. Chem.* 251:5115–5123.

EBASHI, S., M. ENDO, and I. OHTSUKI, 1969. Control of muscle contraction. *Q. Rev. Biophys.* 2:351–384.

ENOCK, H. G., A. CATALA, and P. STRITTMATTER, 1976. Mechanism of rat liver microsomal stearyl-CoA desaturase. *J. Biol. Chem.* 251:5095–5103.

EVANS, H. J., and G. J. SORGES, 1966. Role of mineral elements with emphasis on the univalent cations. *Annu. Rev. Plant Physiol.* 17:47–76.

GIOTTA, G. G., 1975. Native (Na⁺ + K⁺)-dependent ATPase has two trypsin-sensitive sites. *J. Biol. Chem.* 250:5159–5164.

GIOTTA, G. G., 1976. Quaternary structure of (Na⁺ + K⁺) adenosine triphosphatase. *J. Biol. Chem.* 251:1247–1252.

GOLDIN, S. M., 1977. Active transport of sodium and potassium ions by the sodium potassium ion activated adenosine triphosphatase from renal medulla. *J. Biol. Chem.* 252:5630–5642.

GUIDOTTI, G., 1976. The structure of membrane transport systems. *Trends Biochem. Sci.* 1:11–13.

HAGINS, W. A., and S. YOSHIKAMI, 1974. A role for Ca⁺⁺ in excitation of retinal rods and cones. *Exp. Eye Res.* 18:299–305.

HAROLD, F. M., 1977. Membranes and energy transduction in bacteria. *Curr. Top. Bioenergetics* 6:83–149.

HO, M. K., and G. GUIDOTTI, 1975. A membrane protein from human erythrocyte involved in anion exchange. *J. Biol. Chem.* 250:675–683.

JORGENSEN, P. C., 1974. Isolation and characterization of the sodium pump. *Q. Rev. Biophys.* 7:239–274.

KARLIN, A., 1974. The acetylcholine receptor: Progress report. *Life Sci.* 14:1385–1415.

KARLISH, S. J. D., D. W. YATES, and I. M. GLYNN, 1976. Transient kinetics of (Na⁺ + K⁺)-ATPase studied with a fluorescent substrate. *Nature* 263:251–253.

KATZ, B., 1966. *Nerve, Muscle and Synapse*. New York: McGraw-Hill, pp. 41–72.

KYTE, J., 1972. Properties of the two polypeptides of sodium- and potassium-dependent adenosine triphosphatase. *J. Biol. Chem.* 247:7642–7649.

KYTE, J., 1975. Structural studies of sodium and potassium ion-activated adenosine triphosphatase. *J. Biol. Chem.* 250:7443–7449.

MacLENNAN, D. H., and P. C. HOLLAND, 1975. Calcium transport in sarcoplasmic reticulum. *Annu. Rev. Biophys. Bioeng.* 4:377–404.

MARCHESI, V. T., H. FURTHMAYR, and M. TOMITA, 1976. The red cell membrane. *Annu. Rev. Biochem.* 45:667–698.

MORIMOTO, H., H. LEHMANN, and M. F. PERUTZ, 1971. Molecular pathology of human haemoglobin: Stereochemical interpretation of abnormal oxygen affinities. *Nature* 232:408–413.

MURPHY, A. J., 1976. Crosslinking of the sarcoplasmic reticulum ATPase protein. *Biochem. Biophys. Res. Commun.* 70:160–166.

RUOHO, A., and J. KYTE, 1974. Photoaffinity labeling of the

ouabain-binding site for (Na$^+$ + K$^+$)ATPase. *Proc. Natl. Acad. Sci. USA* 71:2352–2356.

SCHULTZ, S. G., and P. F. CURRAN, 1970. Coupled transport of sodium and organic solutes. *Physiol. Rev.* 50:637–720.

STECK, T. L., B. RAMOS, and E. STRAPAZON, 1976. Proteolytic dissection of band 3, the predominant transmembrane polypeptide of the human erythrocyte membrane. *Biochemistry* 15:1154–1161.

STEWART, P. S., D. H. MacLENNAN, and A. E. SHAMOO, 1976. Isolation and characterization of tryptic fragments of the ATPase of sarcoplasmic reticulum. *J. Biol. Chem.* 251:712–719.

TANIGUCHI, K., and R. L. POST, 1975. Synthesis of adenosine triphosphate and exchange between inorganic phosphate and adenosine triphosphate in sodium and potassium ion transport adenosine triphosphatase. *J. Biol. Chem.* 250:3010–3018.

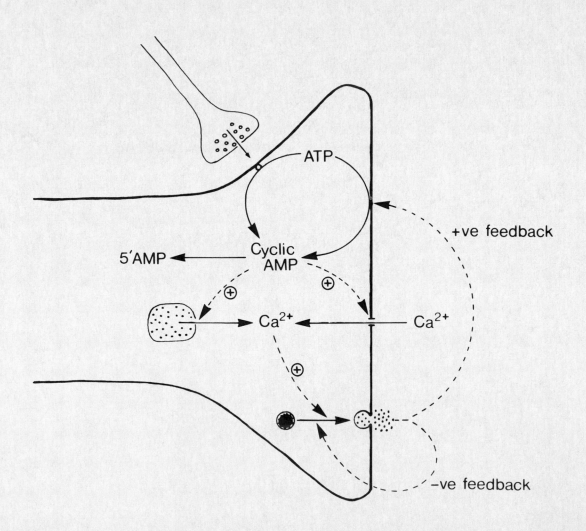

PHOSPHORYLATION
AND
ION TRANSPORT

Summary of some of the mechanisms that have been invoked to account for presynaptic modulation of transmitter release (see the chapter by M. J. Berridge, this volume).

Introduction

GORDON G. HAMMES

THIS SECTION will continue the theme developed in the last, namely, how chemical regulation and transduction are utilized in physiological systems, and how this may be relevant to understanding the mechanism of operation of neurosystems. Two specific types of systems will be considered: regulation by phosphorylation-dephosphorylation, as mediated by cyclic nucleotides, and the modulation of ion fluxes by direct and indirect mechanisms. The time required for the regulation of ion fluxes can range considerably: the action of acetylcholine is relatively rapid and direct, whereas phosphorylation mediated by nucleotides can produce relatively slow changes. Enzyme cascades and cooperative interactions can provide a modulation of the time over a wide range. This variation in response time may in itself be an important means of regulating physiological systems.

G. P. Hess discusses the control of Na^+/K^+ transport by acetylcholine, primarily in well-defined membrane vesicles. This contribution amplifies the earlier presentations of J.-P. Changeux concerning the acetylcholine receptor and of G. Guidotti concerning the coupling of chemical processes to ion pumping. Cyclic AMP plays a crucial role in the regulation of many cellular processes, including metabolism, membrane permeability, transport, and secretion. It also may be involved in neurohormone action. The regulatory role of cyclic AMP in hormone action is reviewed by T. W. Rall. A. M. Katz and his colleagues discuss the regulation of Ca^{2+} transport by phosphorylation of a single protein, phospholamban, in the sarcoplasmic reticulum and the important problem of the regulation of myocardial cell functions by cyclic nucleotides. Finally, M. J. Berridge considers the important coupling of cyclic nucleotides and calcium in regulation. Such interactions may be responsible for regulating both pacemaker and excitability activity.

49 Acetylcholine Receptor–Controlled Ion Fluxes in Microsacs (Membrane Vesicles) Obtained from the Electroplax of *Electrophorus electricus*

GEORGE P. HESS

ABSTRACT The combined action of diverse membrane-bound receptors determines whether or not a signal is propagated by a nerve cell. The conditions necessary for the propagation can be predicted if one can determine the relationship between ligand concentration and the rates at which a particular receptor allows a specific inorganic ion to move through the membrane. Investigations of this relationship with electroplax microsacs (membrane vesicles), which contain acetylcholine receptors and which respond to acetylcholine and its analogs, are described here. The experiments differ from previously reported investigations in that the effects of pH, temperature, and solution composition on both sides of the microsac membranes on the rate of movement of specific inorganic ions through the membrane are determined and the measurements are not obscured by passive or metabolically driven ion fluxes. New approaches for obtaining microsacs responsive to receptor ligands and the techniques developed to make the measurements are described. It was found that the concentration and type of inorganic ions on either side of the membrane determine the efflux kinetics of Na$^+$, K$^+$, and Rb$^+$ and that under appropriate experimental conditions, results obtained with microsacs can account, on the molecular level, for electrophysiological measurements with nerve or muscle cells.

Introduction

IN HIS PAPER, Guidotti discussed the role of a membrane-bound enzyme, the $(Na^+ + K^+)ATPase$, in establishing the electrical membrane potential of a cell. This chapter will focus on the role of membrane-bound proteins—in particular, the acetylcholine receptor—in abolishing the transmembrane potential

GEORGE P. HESS   Section of Biochemistry and Molecular Biology, Cornell University, Ithaca, NY 14853

of nerve and muscle cells and the way in which this process is used to transmit information between cells. Such receptor-mediated processes are of interest since they are believed to form the basis of integrated behavior in higher organisms.

At nerve terminals and in muscle cells there exist membrane-bound receptors which, on binding of appropriate ligands, modulate the flow of inorganic ions through the membrane and thereby change the transmembrane potential (Figure 1). The importance of these receptors in determining whether a nerve will propagate a signal has been deduced from electrophysiological measurements, particularly those made by Eccles (1964) and Katz (1969). When an electrical signal reaches a nerve terminal, small mol-

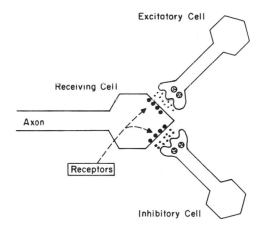

FIGURE 1 A diagrammatic synapse. (Redrawn from an article by Solomon Snyder in *Scientific American*, vol. 236 (March 1977), p. 56.)

ecules such as acetylcholine (ACh) are released. These compounds bind to receptors on the receiving cell, leading to changes in the permeability of the cell membrane to inorganic ions and thus in the transmembrane potential of the cell. Compounds released from inhibitory nerve cells make the transmembrane potential more negative (Figure 1). Excitatory nerve cells releasing ACh make the transmembrane potential more positive by increasing the permeability of the cell membrane to inorganic ions. When the combined action of these receptors results in a 20 mV increase in the transmembrane potential of the nerve terminal, the membrane potential all along the nerve axon, sometimes up to 1 m in length, collapses in an all-or-none process (Hodgkin and Huxley, 1952). Thus information is transmitted over some distance in a few milliseconds.

A quantitative description of the receptor-controlled changes in membrane potentials and an accurate prediction of the conditions necessary for the propagation of signals by nerve cells are not yet possible. Although one can in principle measure the relationship between ligand concentration and the transmembrane potential of a nerve cell for each of the different receptors separately, the combined action of the various receptors can not be predicted from such measurements. J. H. Freed and I are now developing a theory that relates the concentration of inorganic ions, the rate coefficients for the movement of specific ions through the membrane in the presence and absence of ligands, and the transmembrane potential of a cell.

The steady-state rate equation for the movement of inorganic ions through the cell membrane at constant transmembrane potential is given by

$$\phi_1 \{\alpha \, [Na^+]_i + \beta \, [K^+]_i + \ldots\}$$
$$= \phi_2 \{\alpha[Na^+]_o + \beta \, [K^+]_o + \ldots\}, \quad (1)$$

where

$$\alpha = k_{Na} + K_{Na(max)} \frac{L}{L + K_D} + \ldots,$$

$$\beta = Gk_K + K_{K(max)} \frac{L}{L + K_D} + \ldots,$$

$$\phi_1/\phi_2 = e^{V_m F / RT}.$$

The parameters ϕ_1 and ϕ_2 are the Nernst-Planck factors, which take into account the fact that some ions are accelerated and some retarded by the electric field. V_m is the membrane potential, and F is the Faraday constant. G indicates the stoichiometry of the Na^+-K^+ exchange by the $(Na^+ + K^+)$ATPase. This factor accounts for the action of the $(Na^+ + K^+)$

ATPase (see Guidotti, this volume), which maintains the steady-state concentration of inorganic ions inside the cell at the expense of externally supplied energy. The quantities inside the brackets—$[Na^+]$, $[K^+]$—represent the activities of the inorganic ions, and the subscripts "i" and "o" mean inside or outside the cell. k_{Na} and k_K are the rate coefficients associated with the movement of the respective inorganic ions through the cell membrane in absence of ligands. $K_{(max)}$ is the ligand-concentration-independent rate coefficient associated with the receptor-mediated movement of a particular inorganic ion through the cell membrane. L is the concentration of the receptor-ligand, and K_D is the dissociation constant of the receptor: ligand complex. If we omit from this equation all terms that refer to the function of the receptor and to the $(Na^+ + K^+)$ ATPase and multiply what remains by appropriate factors, it becomes the familiar Goldman-Hodgkin-Katz equation. Equation 1 allows us to predict whether a signal will be propagated by a nerve cell, providing we can determine the various constants.

Here I shall describe our investigations of the relationship between the concentration of ligands and the rate coefficients of the ACh receptor–mediated movement of specific inorganic ions across a membrane. I shall describe the preparation of the microsacs and the techniques we have developed to make the measurements. Our experiments differ from electrophysiological measurements in that we determine the rate coefficients for the movement of a particular inorganic ion in both directions across the membrane with well-defined and variable solution compositions both inside and outside the microsacs at defined pH and temperature.

The ACh receptor was chosen for these studies because the chemical and physical properties of this protein have been studied extensively. The results of such studies are summarized by Changeux (this volume) and in a recent review (Eldefrawi and Eldefrawi, 1977). Electroplax membrane preparations from *Electrophorus electricus* were chosen for the experiments because much biochemical work, including electrophysiological measurements, has already been done on this material (Nachmansohn, 1974) and because of the continuing interest of electrophysiologists in these cells (Sheridan and Lester, 1975). Seven years ago, Kasai and Changeux (1971a) showed that ACh receptor–rich microsacs could be obtained from homogenates of the electric organ. It was demonstrated that if the microsacs were incubated overnight with $^{22}Na^+$ and then diluted sevenfold into a solution containing nonradioactive sodium chloride, the exchange of hot and cold sodium could be measured by sampling the mixture at timed intervals, collecting the vesicles on Millipore filters, and determining the amount of $^{22}Na^+$ retained by the microsacs. This type of experiment is illustrated in Figure 2. The upper curve shows the efflux from the microsacs in the absence of ligand; the lower curve shows the efflux in presence of 0.1 mM carbamylcholine, an analog of ACh. If one considers the half-time of the efflux, τ, one notes that in the presence of carbamylcholine, it has been reduced by a factor of about two. This experiment by Kasai and Changeux (1971a) constituted the first proof that ACh receptor–mediated fluxes of inorganic ions through cell membranes could be investigated in a cell-free system. It was noted, however, by Katz and Miledi (1972) and by Rang (1974) that the number of ions that move per receptor site per unit time in the microsacs is about

five orders of magnitude less than that determined by electrophysiological measurements with whole cells. It seemed important to understand the reason for this discrepancy, and our first experiments were designed accordingly.

Results

ANALYSIS OF $^{22}Na^+$ EFFLUX FROM KASAI-CHANGEUX MICROSAC PREPARATION Three years ago, John Andrews, Gary Struve, Susan Coombs, and I decided to analyze the efflux curves shown in Figure 2. The first question we asked was: Do all microsacs in the preparation respond to carbamylcholine, or was the increased efflux due to only a small fraction of carbamylcholine-sensitive microsacs? The results of our kinetic analysis are given in Figure 3. At least three different processes can be detected, with half-times of 3, 35, and 330 minutes (Hess et al., 1975a). Assuming that these three processes are associated with different types of microsacs, only 15% of the microsacs—those that are very impermeable to Na^+—respond to carbamylcholine. On addition of carbamylcholine to these microsacs, the rate of efflux of $^{22}Na^+$ increases by a factor of sixty.

ISOLATION OF FUNCTIONAL MICROSACS John Andrews and I next considered the possibility of isolating these functional microsacs from the microsacs that do not respond to a receptor-ligand. The procedure we developed was based on the kinetic analysis shown in Figure 3. In particular, we took advantage of the impermeability of specific microsacs to inor-

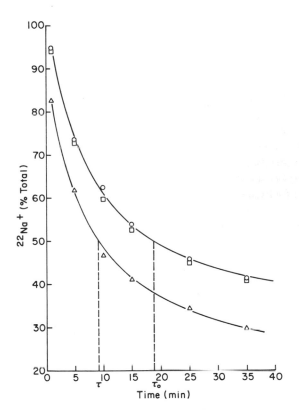

FIGURE 2 $^{22}Na^+$ efflux from *E. electricus* electroplax membrane vesicles, diluted 70-fold according to the procedure of Kasai and Changeux (1971a). Solution composition: 90 mM KCl, 10 mM NaCl, 0.4 M sucrose, 1 mM phosphate buffer, pH 7.0, 4°. The time for half-equilibration of the microsacs with the dilution buffer is given for the control curve (τ_0) and carbamylcholine-mediated flux curve (τ). Squares and circles show efflux in the absence of carbamylcholine (control); triangles, efflux in presence of 10^{-4} M carbamylcholine. (From Hess et al., 1975a.)

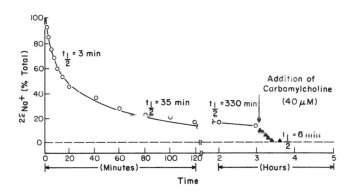

FIGURE 3 Kinetic analysis of $^{22}Na^+$ efflux from microsacs, pH 7.0, 4°. Experimental conditions as in Figure 2. The observed time course of the efflux in absence of carbamylcholine is fitted to the sum of three exponentials:

$$[^{22}Na^+]_t = [^{22}Na]_{t=0} \, (\alpha e^{-k_1 t} + \beta e^{-k_2 t} + \gamma e^{-k_3 t}).$$

The half-times of the three processes are given in the figure.

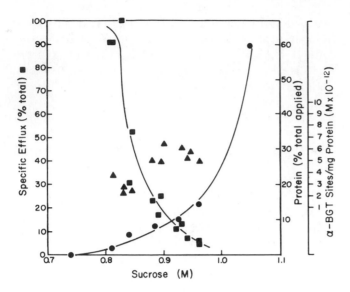

FIGURE 4a Purification of carbamylcholine-sensitive microsacs by sucrose–190 mM cesium chloride density gradient centrifugation. A population of microsacs rich in receptor sites and of similar density was collected by centrifugation on a discontinuous sucrose gradient. The material between layers of 0.9 M and 1.2 M sucrose was collected. The microsacs were then equilibrated with 190 mM NaCl for 24 hr, long enough for all microsacs to equilibrate with the outside solution (see Figure 3). The 190 mM NaCl in the external solution was exchanged for 190 mM CsCl using a Sephadex G-25 column. The microsacs were then allowed to reequilibrate for 2 hr. According to the analysis of the efflux data in Figure 3, this allows all the nonspecific microsacs to fill with CsCl ($t_{1/2}$ = 35 min) while the carbamylcholine-sensitive microsacs still retain most of their NaCl content.

Four milliliters of ACh receptor-rich microsacs (0.75 mg of membrane protein per ml, 1.1 M sucrose, 190 mM CsCl, 1 mM sodium phosphate buffer at pH 7.0) were placed on the bottom of a continuous gradient (32 ml, 0.7–1.1 M sucrose containing 190 mM CsCl, 1 mM sodium phosphate buffer, pH 7.0) and centrifuged in a Beckman SW-27 swinging bucket rotor for 2.5 hr at 4°. Two-milliliter fractions were collected and analyzed. The abscissa gives the molarity of sucrose in the fractions. The results of two experiments obtained with microsac preparations from different eels are shown. Circles show % of membrane protein; triangles, pM of α-bungarotoxin (α-BGT)-binding sites per mg of membrane protein; squares, carbamylcholine-sensitive efflux (% of total efflux). (From Hess and Andrews, 1977.)

ganic ions in the absence of ligand. We used this kinetic distinction to fill the functional microsacs with sodium chloride while the nonfunctional microsacs were filled with a cesium chloride solution (Hess and Andrews, 1977). The sodium chloride–filled microsacs were then separated from microsacs filled with heavier cesium chloride on the basis of their density in a continuous sucrose–190 mM cesium chloride density gradient. The results of such a density-gradient experiment are shown in Figure 4a. The abscissa of the graph gives the molarity of sucrose in various fractions collected from the continuous gradient. As indicated by the solid circles, most of the membrane protein was found in the denser portion of the gradient, that is, in the cesium chloride–filled, nonspecific microsacs. The squares indicate the percentage of sodium inside the microsacs whose flux rate is affected by ligands such as carbamylcholine. The fractions that were 0.8 M in sucrose contained only those microsacs that respond to ACh receptor-ligands. Therefore, as we expected from the kinetic measurements, we had succeeded in separating the microsacs that responded to carbamylcholine from those that did not. The data in Figure 4b indicate more clearly what the purification process accomplishes. The graph allows a comparison of ^{22}Na$^+$ efflux from the microsac preparation before and after purification. The dashed line represents the three processes observed before purification. The solid triangles represent the efflux from the purified preparation. In the absence of ligand, the purified microsacs were essentially impermeable to inorganic ions, and the half-equilibration time was more than six

hours. In the presence of 40 μM carbamylcholine, the ^{22}Na$^+$ efflux increased dramatically.

The number of receptor sites, as measured with an irreversible titrant, [^{125}I]-α-bungarotoxin, is about 2 pM per mg membrane protein in functional microsacs (Figure 4a). On the basis of preliminary estimates

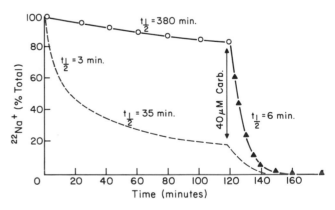

FIGURE 4b A comparison of ^{22}Na$^+$ efflux from a heterogeneous mixture of microsacs (dashed line) and after isolation of the carbamylcholine-sensitive microsacs (solid line), pH 7.0, 4°.

of the diameters of the microsacs (R. L. Noble, M. J. Cooper, and G. P. Hess, in preparation), the number of microsacs per mg membrane protein, and the number of receptor sites per ion channel, there may be only one channel per microsac. One can prepare microsacs from a *Torpedo* sp. in which the receptor density is several orders of magnitude higher than in *E. electricus* microsacs. The observed rate coefficients would be expected to increase, but not necessarily linearly, with increasing receptor sites. Both the flux measurements and the analysis of the data would, therefore, be much more difficult with such preparations.

KINETIC MEASUREMENTS OF RECEPTOR-MEDIATED ION FLUX IN MICROSACS

The kinetic method employed to make the flux measurements is based on the experiments I have already discussed. Accordingly, the receptor-mediated flux from an unfractionated microsac preparation can also be analyzed without the measurements being obscured by efflux from microsacs that do not respond to ACh: The radioactive inorganic ions in the nonspecific microsacs are first equilibrated with nonradioactive ions in the external solution in a time interval in which the functional microsacs retain most of their tracer. When ligand is subsequently added to the mixture of microsacs, efflux from only the functional microsacs is observed. John Andrews and I have shown that we obtain the same rate coefficient for $^{22}Na^+$ efflux whether we use this kinetic method for measuring receptor-mediated flux or make the measurements with the isolated functional microsacs (Hess and Andrews, 1977).

In subsequent experiments we used the kinetic techniques to determine the rate coefficients of the receptor-mediated flux of various inorganic ions and to investigate, in a systematic way, the effect of ligand concentration, pH, temperature, and solution composition on the flux parameters.

SYMMETRIC DISTRIBUTION OF INORGANIC IONS ON THE INSIDE AND THE OUTSIDE OF THE MICROSACS

The first question John Andrews, Gary Struve, and I asked was: Is the efflux of inorganic ions from functional microsacs as complex as it is from the unfractionated mixture? The data in Figure 5a indicate that the receptor-mediated $^{22}Na^+$ efflux follows a single exponential decay. In the figure $(cpm)_t$ is proportional to the concentration of the radioactive ion inside the microsacs at time t. From the slope of the line one can calculate an observed first-order rate constant, k_{obs}, for the receptor mediated flux of the

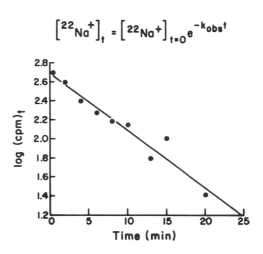

$$[^{22}Na^+]_t = [^{22}Na^+]_{t=0}\, e^{-k_{obs}t}$$

FIGURE 5a First-order plot of $^{22}Na^+$ efflux in presence of 0.2 mM carbamylcholine. Experimental conditions as in Figure 2 with pH 7.0, 4°. $[^{22}Na]_t$ represents the concentration of radioactive ion inside the microsacs at time t. k_{obs} was determined from the slope of the linear least square fit of the experimental points. $k_{obs} = 0.14 \pm 0.02$ min^{-1} (From Hess et al., 1975a.)

inorganic ion through the membrane of the microsacs.

In further experiments we determined the effect of the concentration of ACh analogs on k_{obs}. In the experiment shown in Figure 5b, line 1, the decamethonium-induced efflux of $^{22}Na^+$ was measured. The following information could be obtained from this experiment. The intercept of the ordinate by line 1 indicates that k_{obs} reaches a limiting value, k'_{max}, at high ligand concentrations. This ligand-independent value is given by the intercept ($k'_{max} = 0.15 \pm 0.01$ min^{-1}). The dissociation constant of the receptor:ligand complex, K_D, is obtained from the slope of the line ($K_D = 0.5 \pm 0.15$ μM). The same linear relationship between k_{obs} and k_{obs}/L was obtained in experiments with carbamylcholine, another analog of ACh. Evidence for cooperative effects was not found in these experiments. If in the same experiments we determine the half-times of the efflux from the mixture of microsacs in the absence of ligand, τ_0, and in its presence, τ, and plot $1/\tau - 1/\tau_0$ versus ligand concentration, apparent cooperativity is observed. These results are in excellent agreement with those of Kasai and Changeux (1971a). Gary Struve, John Andrews, and I have shown, however, that apparent cooperativity arises because τ is determined both by efflux from nonspecific microsacs and by ligand-induced efflux (Hess, Andrews, and Struve, 1976). Thus ligand-receptor interaction is much less effective in determining τ values at low ligand concentrations than at high concentrations. The resulting effect on

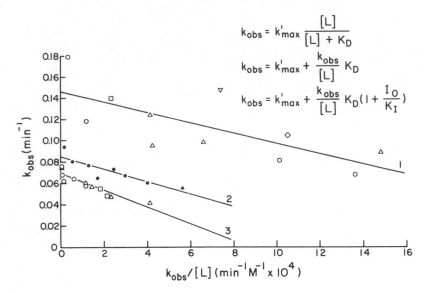

$$k_{obs} = k'_{max} \frac{[L]}{[L] + K_D}$$

$$k_{obs} = k'_{max} + \frac{k_{obs}}{[L]} K_D$$

$$k_{obs} = k'_{max} + \frac{k_{obs}}{[L]} K_D \left(1 + \frac{I_0}{K_I}\right)$$

FIGURE 5b The dependence of k_{obs} on decamethonium concentration in the absence (line 1) and presence of 0.2 μM (line 2) and 0.5 μM (line 3) d-tubocurarine. The data are plotted according to the equations shown. The slopes of the lines are proportional to K_D, the dissociation constant of the receptor:ligand complex, and the intercepts to k'_{max} in the absence of d-tubocurarine, and to $(k'_{max} K_I)(I_0 + K_I)^{-1}$ in the presence of a noncompetitive inhibitor. k'_{max} is the maximum rate coefficient obtainable for $^{22}Na^+$ efflux from the microsacs under specified conditions; the dissociation constant of the receptor:inhibitor complex is designated by K_I; I_0 is the molar concentration of the inhibitor. Line 1: $K_D = 0.5 \pm 0.15$ μM; $k'_{max} = 0.15 \pm 0.01$ min^{-1}. Line 2: $K_D = 0.6 \pm 0.1$ μM; $k'_{max}(obs) = 0.08 \pm 0.01$ min^{-1}. Line 3: $K_D = 0.8 \pm 0.1$ μM; $k'_{max}(obs) = 0.07 \pm 0.002$ min^{-1}; $K_I = 0.3$ μM. (From Hess et al., 1976.)

τ is similar to that observed when one determines the occupancy of binding sites when ligand binding is cooperative and the affinity of the ligand-binding sites increases with increasing ligand concentration.

In the next set of experiments, we determined the effect of a receptor inhibitor, d-tubocurarine, on decamethonium-induced $^{22}Na^+$ efflux. Lines 2 and 3 in Figure 5b represent experiments with different concentrations of curare. Similar results were obtained when carbamylcholine was used instead of decamethonium. If curare and decamethonium compete for the same receptor-binding site, one would expect line 1 (curare absent) and lines 2 and 3 (curare present) to have the same ordinate intercept. The different intercepts indicate noncompetitive inhibition and suggest separate receptor-binding sites for curare and receptor-ligand.

It is of interest to know whether these results are due to the molecular properties of the receptor or to properties of the microsacs unrelated to the receptor. There is independent evidence for separate receptor-binding sites for ACh and its analogs and for inhibitors such as d-tubocurarine and the snake neurotoxin, α-bungarotoxin (Fu, Donner, and Hess, 1974; Fu et al., 1977). In kinetic experiments with α-bungarotoxin, which is a specific irreversible inhibitor of the receptor (Lee, 1972), curare was found to be a competitive inhibitor of the slow phase of the reaction, while carbamylcholine and decamethonium were noncompetitive (Bulger and Hess, 1973; Bulger et al., 1977). In experiments performed by Helga Rübsamen, the Eldefrawis, and myself (Rübsamen et al., 1976), it was found that carbamylcholine displaces a fluorescent lanthanide, terbium, from the calcium-binding sites of the receptor, while curare does not. Similar results were obtained with ACh (Figure 6). In agreement with these experiments, Chang and Neumann (1976) found that ACh competes with calcium-binding sites of the receptor and can displace Ca^{2+}. α-Bungarotoxin causes an uptake of Ca^{2+} by the receptor. Recently it has been suggested (Maelicke et al., 1977) that cobra α-neurotoxin, a reversible inhibitor, and ACh or its analogs compete for the same binding site of the receptor. It was found that this toxin binds to the receptor to the same extent at high toxin concentrations, whether ACh or its analogs are absent or present. Indeed, if these data are plotted in the manner shown in Figure 5b, Y versus Y/L, where Y represents the fraction of receptor sites occupied, the lines representing toxin binding in presence or absence of ACh or its analogs have the same ordinate intercept. In equilibrium binding measure-

852   GEORGE P. HESS

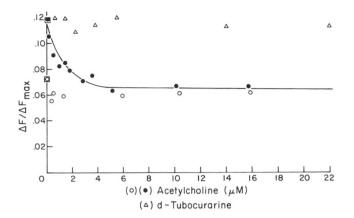

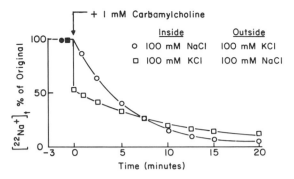

FIGURE 6 Displacement of Tb^{3+} from the purified ACh receptor by ACh (in 2 mM Pipes/Tris buffer, pH 6.5, 0.03% Triton X-100, 20°). ACh receptor (0.6 μM α-bungarotoxin binding sites), 3.3 μM $TbCl_3$. Filled circles indicate titration with ACh in the absence of $CaCl_2$; open circles, titration with ACh in the presence of 6 mM $CaCl_2$; triangles, titration with d-tubocurarine; square with filled circle, receptor: Tb^{3+} complex before addition of ligand; square with open circle, receptor:Tb^{3+} complex in the presence of 6 mM $CaCl_2$ before addition of ligand.

FIGURE 7 The effect of the asymmetrical distribution of KCl and NaCl across the microsac membrane on the efflux of $^{22}Na^+$ or $^{86}Rb^+$ from microsacs, pH 7.0, 4°. Circles indicate that the microsacs were equilibrated with 100 mM NaCl, 0.4 M sucrose, ^{22}NaCl, and efflux was measured in a solution of 100 mM KCl, 0.4 M sucrose; squares, that the microsacs were equilibrated with 100 mM KCl, 0.4 M sucrose, with the addition of either ^{22}NaCl or ^{86}RbCl as tracer, and efflux was measured in a solution of 100 mM NaCl, 0.4 M sucrose. Solid symbols indicate the $^{22}Na^+$ content of the microsacs before addition of carbamylcholine.

ments, in contrast to kinetic measurements, such results do not distinguish between competitive and noncompetitive interactions between two ligands.

In addition to curare, there are many interesting pharmacologically active compounds that are known to affect, in some way, receptor-mediated communication between nerve cells. Included among these compounds are cocaine, barbiturates, and anesthetics. Assessing the pharmacological properties of these compounds by determining their effect on the receptor-mediated flux in microsacs may prove convenient and may also yield information about the mechanism of action of these compounds that cannot be obtained from electrophysiological measurements with cells or from experiments with animals.

EFFECT OF AN ASYMMETRIC DISTRIBUTION OF INORGANIC IONS ON THE INSIDE AND THE OUTSIDE OF THE MICROSACS Experiments by Stanley Lipkowitz, Gary Struve, and myself (Figure 7) show that the asymmetric distribution of inorganic ions has a marked effect on the flux of such ions. The amount of $^{22}Na^+$ retained in specific microsacs as a function of time upon addition of carbamylcholine is given by the ordinate. The squares indicate efflux under conditions resembling those in nerve cells, that is, high potassium concentration inside and high sodium concentration outside the microsacs. We observed an initial, very fast flux rate followed by a slower, first-

order rate process. Before the first measurement could be made (in less than 10 sec), half the sodium originally present in the microsacs had already effluxed. When the solution compositions were reversed, with high sodium concentration inside the microsacs and high potassium on the outside (shown by the circles), a much slower single exponential decay without a fast initial flux rate was observed. The k_{obs} values are similar at the same carbamylcholine concentrations in this experiment and in the experiments described earlier in which the solutions on either side of the microsac membranes were identical (90 mM KCl, 10 mM NaCl).

Are other inorganic ions affected in the same way as sodium ions by an asymmetric distribution of NaCl and KCl inside and outside the microsacs? Our first experiments were done with Ca^{2+} because of its importance in affecting the electrical properties of nerve membranes and because it competes with ACh in binding to the receptor (Rübsamen et al., 1976; Chang and Neumann, 1976). The effect of carbamylcholine concentration on the k_{obs} of $^{45}Ca^{2+}$ efflux has been determined: we obtain similar results whether we have a symmetric or an asymmetric distribution of inorganic ions across the membrane. The k'_{max} and K_D values are similar to those obtained in $^{22}Na^+$ efflux experiments when the solution composition was the same inside and outside the microsacs. Carbamylcholine-induced $^{45}Ca^{2+}$ efflux is blocked by the same inhibitors as ligand-induced $^{22}Na^+$ and $^{86}Rb^+$

efflux. Nava Epstein, Gary Struve, Wasi Ahmed, and I have found, however, that at carbamylcholine concentrations at which the asymmetric distribution of inorganic ions across the microsacs membrane results in biphasic efflux kinetics of $^{22}Na^+$ and $^{86}Rb^+$ (triangles in Figure 8), $^{45}Ca^{2+}$ efflux (circles) follows a single exponential rate law and an initial fast phase could not be detected. The answer to the question asked is, therefore, that in these experiments $^{45}Ca^{2+}$ behaves differently from $^{22}Na^+$ and $^{86}Rb^+$. Another unusual property of $^{45}Ca^{2+}$ efflux, discovered by Nava Epstein, is that it requires Ca^{2+} in the external solutions, whereas $^{22}Na^+$ and $^{86}Rb^+$ effluxes do not.

In the next set of experiments (Figure 9a), Stanley Lipkowitz, Gary Struve, and I asked: What are the conditions necessary to change the mechanism from a slow exponential efflux to a biphasic efflux? The ordinate of the graph, α, indicates the fraction of the reaction that goes by an initial fast phase. The mole fraction of the sodium chloride in the external solution is given by the abscissa of the graph. The data show that when the mole fraction of Na^+ in the external solution is decreased, α also decreases. When the composition of the solution is the same on either side of the membrane ($[Na^+]/([Na^+] + [K^+]) = 0.1$), the measured values of the internal $^{22}Na^+$ content at zero time and the value calculated assuming efflux following a single exponential decay fall within the

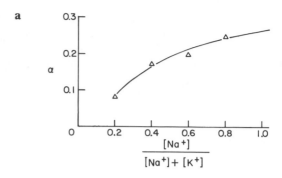

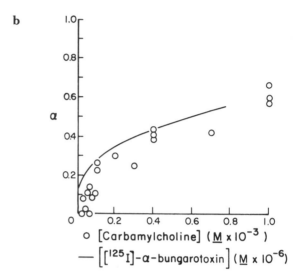

FIGURE 9   Fraction of carbamylcholine-induced $^{86}Rb^+$ efflux due to fast process (α). pH 7.0, 4°. Microsacs, incubated overnight with 100 mM KCl, 0.4 M sucrose, $^{86}RbCl$, were diluted into a medium containing 0.4 M sucrose, 1 mM phosphate, pH 7.0, and variable amounts of NaCl and KCl, with a total salt concentration of 100 mM (part a) and 100 mM NaCl (part b). (a) α versus mole fraction of NaCl in the external solution, 0.2 mM carbamylcholine. (b) α versus molar concentration of carbamylcholine. For comparative purposes, the solid line indicates the fraction of the fast phase of the reaction of $[^{125}I]$-monoiodo-α-bungarotoxin with the receptor of the microsacs. The experimental conditions are the same ones that lead to biphasic efflux of inorganic ions from the microsacs.

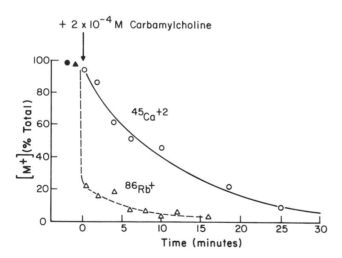

FIGURE 8   The effect of the asymmetrical distribution of KCl and NaCl across the microsac membrane on the efflux of $^{45}Ca^{2+}$ and of $^{86}Rb^+$, pH 7.0, 4°. Microsacs, incubated over night with 100 mM KCl, 1 mM $CaCl_2$, 0.4 M sucrose, and trace amounts of either $^{86}RbCl$ or $^{45}CaCl_2$, were diluted into 100 mM NaCl, 1 mM $CaCl_2$, 0.4 M sucrose, 1 mM phosphate, pH 7.0. Carbamylcholine was added to a final concentration of $2 \times 10^{-4}M$. Solid symbols refer to radioactive metal ion content of the microsacs before the addition of carbamylcholine.

estimated uncertainty of the measurements—about 15%.

We have investigated the effect of carbamylcholine concentration on α. The data in Figure 9b (open circles) indicate that α does depend on carbamylcholine concentration. At low carbamylcholine concentration ($<1.5 K_D$), one obtains a single exponential decrease of the $^{22}Na^+$ content of the microsacs and an initial fast phase could not be detected. At the highest carbamylcholine concentration used (1 mM), 60% of the reaction goes by an initial fast phase.

Some rather definite information can be obtained

from the concentration dependence of α. The biphasic efflux could be due to the presence of two types of microsacs or two types of receptors: one type responding to low concentrations of ligand and characterized by slow efflux of inorganic ions, the other responding only to high concentrations of carbamylcholine from which the efflux is fast. If this were the true situation, the total amount of radioactive ions involved in the efflux would depend on carbamylcholine concentration. We found, however, that the amount of radioactive ions involved is independent of carbamylcholine concentration.

An interpretation of the dependence of α on carbamylcholine concentration is that the receptor exists in two conformations and that ACh, or carbamylcholine, binding results in the conversion of one conformation into another. Independent evidence exists for this interpretation. The results of ligand-binding experiments of Changeux and others suggest the existence of at least two conformations of the receptor (Moore et al., 1974; Changeux et al., 1975; Hess et al., 1975b; Barrantes, 1976; Bonner, Barrantes, and Jovin, 1976; Cohen and Boyd, 1977; Fu et al., 1977; Maelicke et al., 1977).

The effect of ligand concentration on the interconversion of receptor conformations was determined (Hess et al., 1975b; Bulger et al., 1977) in investigations of the specific and irreversible reaction of α-bungarotoxin (Lee, 1972) with the membrane-bound receptor. These experiments employed the microsac preparation used in the flux experiments and the sodium chloride concentration that produces biphasic efflux. The results resemble those obtained in measurements of $^{22}Na^+$ efflux from the microsacs; the reaction is biphasic, the extent of the reaction is independent of toxin concentration, and α increases with increasing toxin concentration. The relationship between α and initial toxin concentration is given by the solid line in Figure 9b. It can be seen that α, whether measured in the reaction of receptor with toxin (solid line) or by flux measurements (open circles), depends on ligand concentration. These results are expected if the biphasic efflux of inorganic ions observed in the microsac experiments is due to the ligand-induced conversion of receptor conformations rather than to properties of the microsacs unrelated to the receptor. The ACh-induced interconversion of receptor conformations has recently been reported by Cohen and Boyd (1977) in experiments with *Torpedo* microsacs.

KINETIC MEASUREMENTS OF RECEPTOR-MEDIATED ION FLUX IN L6 MUSCLE CELLS The experiments with

muscle cells anticipate a final problem, namely expressing the regulation of the transmembrane potential in cells quantitatively, in terms of the activities of inorganic ions and the rate coefficients associated with the movement of individual ions. One of the reasons for choosing these particular cells is that they have been quite well characterized genetically by electron microscopy and by electrophysiological measurements (Land et al., 1977).

The L6 muscle cells were grown with tender loving care by Iris Greenberg in T. R. Podleski's laboratory. The experiments I shall discuss represent a collaborative effort between Podleski and his co-workers and Douglas Moore, John Andrews, and myself. From Figure 10 it can be seen that there are similarities in the ACh receptor-mediated efflux of ions from microsacs and from L6 muscle cells. The upper line represents $^{42}K^+$ efflux at the resting potential of these cells, approximately -40 mV (Sastre and Podleski, 1976). The lower line represents efflux in presence of 0.1 mM carbamylcholine. The latter efflux is biphasic, and the initial fast phase is over before one can make measurements using conventional techniques.

From the electrophysiological measurements of Land et al. (1977) one can calculate that at the concentration of carbamylcholine used, the resting membrane potential of the cell was reestablished before the slow phase of the $^{42}K^+$ efflux could be measured. Within 2 min of the addition of carbamylcholine, the

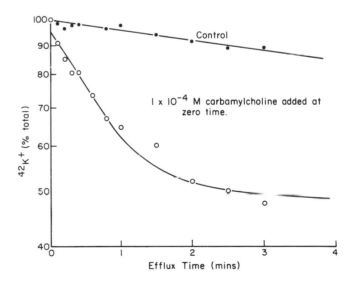

FIGURE 10 Efflux of $^{42}K^+$ from L6 muscle cells in the absence (upper line) and presence of 0.1 mM carbamylcholine (lower line), pH 7.4, 22°. External medium composition: 10 mM HEPES, 150 mM NaCl, 5.4 mM KCl, 1.8 mM CaCl$_2$, 0.8 mM MgCl$_2$, 5.5 mM glucose, 1.0 mM Na$_2$HPO$_4$.

efflux proceeds at apparently the same rate as the control, even though $^{42}K^+$ inside the cells has not yet equilibrated with potassium ions in the external solution. When carbamylcholine-induced $^{22}Na^+$ efflux is measured, only the initial fast phase of the efflux can be observed. The measurable efflux rate in presence of 0.1 mM carbamylcholine is identical to the control rate. This difference between carbamylcholine-induced $^{42}K^+$ efflux and $^{22}Na^+$ efflux is considered to be due to the $(Na^+ + K^+)$ ATPase, which actively moves Na^+ from the inside to the outside of the cell. The receptor-mediated rate of $^{22}Na^+$ efflux, therefore, reaches the $(Na^+ + K^+)$ ATPase-mediated rate within a short period of time, which can be prolonged by inhibiting the enzyme.

The influx of $^{22}Na^+$ from muscle cells, induced by ACh receptor-ligands has been observed by Stallcup and Cohn (1976), and by Catterall (1975), who analyzed his data in terms of receptor-mediated flux. Our data indicate that such an analysis may not be simple. The initial fast phase of the flux cannot be measured by conventional techniques; the slow phase reflects not only receptor-mediated processes but also the metabolically driven movement of inorganic ions. At least with L6 muscle cells, we have not yet succeeded in completely inhibiting the $(Na^+ + K^+)$ ATPase without altering other properties of the cell. Therefore, flux measurements of inorganic ions in muscle cells involve a number of interesting and unsolved intellectual problems. In addition, there are a number of challenging experimental problems to be solved, including the determination of the activities of the ions inside the cells.

Discussion

The experiments I have described were chosen to indicate the type of information one can obtain with the microsac preparation and the techniques we have developed. How relevant are these experiments to an understanding of ACh-induced changes in the transmembrane potential of nerve and muscle cells? One observation that was made in electrophysiological measurements with muscle cells but appears to be directly related to the results reported here is the phenomenon of desensitization. This concept was first treated quantitatively by Katz and Thesleff (1957) over 20 years ago and has been of considerable interest to electrophysiologists. The basic observation is that ACh-induced changes in transmembrane potential decrease with time, even though the ACh concentration remains at a constant level. Katz and Thesleff (1957) suggested that the receptor exists in two conformations, a reactive form that is converted to a nonreactive form.

Ideas about the molecular basis of the desensitization process obtained from our experiments are at present speculative but can be tested. The electrophysiological measurements can be related to the biphasic efflux of inorganic ions observed in the microsac experiments, since transmembrane potentials depend on the activities and rates of movement of inorganic ions through the membrane (equation 1). The initial fast flux of inorganic ions in the receptor-mediated process observed in our microsac experiments can be considered responsible for the observed changes in the transmembrane potential of cell. The return of the transmembrane potential to its resting value, in the presence of constant concentrations of ACh, can be considered to be due to the conversion of one receptor conformation to another. This second conformation is considered responsible for the slow single exponential efflux of inorganic ions from microsacs. The experiments with L6 muscle cells (Figure 10) suggest that the rate of movement of inorganic ions through the cell membrane associated with this second receptor conformation is comparable to that associated with the $(Na^+ + K^+)$ ATPase. Therefore, the inorganic ion flux mediated by this second conformation of the receptor is not expected to contribute to the transmembrane potential of the cell.

Although the restoration of the resting transmembrane voltages of muscle or nerve cells in the presence of a constant concentration of ligand is puzzling, in our view it is the consequence of a well-documented phenomenon in protein chemistry, namely the ligand-induced conversion of a protein conformation, which accounts for the ligand-binding mechanism of a number of well-characterized regulatory enzymes (Monod, Wyman, and Changeux, 1965; Koshland, Nemethy, and Filmer, 1966; Eigen, 1967; Hammes and Wu, 1974) and for the biphasic efflux of inorganic ions in our experiments with microsacs.

Another comparison between the experiments with microsacs and electrophysiological measurements requires a determination of the number of inorganic ions that pass through receptor-formed channels per unit time (Katz and Miledi, 1972; Rang, 1974). This number, calculated from the single slow exponential efflux of $^{22}Na^+$ from microsacs (Hess and Andrews, 1977), is about two orders of magnitude lower than the value determined in electrophysiological measurements with muscle cells (about 10^9 ions per min per receptor site: see Neher and Stevens, this volume; Katz and Miledi, 1972; Anderson and Stevens, 1973; Sheridan and Lester, 1975; Neher and Sakmann,

1976) but three orders of magnitude higher than the value calculated by Kasai and Changeux (1971b).

There are several outstanding problems to be solved before we can make a true comparison between flux measurements and electrophysiological experiments and before we can relate the concentration of ligand to changes in the transmembrane voltage of a cell. One of these is the development of techniques to measure the fast phase of the efflux of inorganic ions from microsacs.

Finally, I should mention that many neuronal cell lines have been developed, particularly by M. Nirenberg and his colleagues at NIH. Some of these cell lines have genetic defects in the communication process, many are sensitive to chemical transmitters other than ACh, some show decreases in membrane potential, and others show increases when the same transmitter is added to the cells. Methods for preparing and isolating microsacs that respond to specific receptor-ligands are currently being developed by Richard Noble and Mark Cooper. There is available, therefore, a wealth of interesting biological material with which to study receptor-mediated processes.

ACKNOWLEDGMENTS We are grateful for financial support from the National Institutes of Health: GM 04842 and NS 08527 (G. P. Hess); U.S. Public Health Service Fellowships NS 05107 (J. P. Andrews), NS 008527 (J. E. Bulger), GM 53965 (J.-J. L. Fu), and NS 05095 (G. E. Struve). Douglas E. Moore (on sabbatical leave from the University of Sydney, Australia) was supported in part by NIH grant CA 14454. Financial support also was provided by the National Science Foundation BMS 572-01908 (G. P. Hess), the Muscular Dystrophy Association (R. L. Noble), and the Max Kade Foundation (H. Rübsamen). Some of this work formed the bases for undergraduate Honors Theses at Cornell University (M. J. Cooper, S. Lipkowitz, R. Silberstein, and C. Zacharchuk).

We are grateful to M. McNamee (University of California, Davis) and A. Karlin (Columbia University College of Physicians and Surgeons, New York) for helping us in making the original electroplax membrane preparations.

REFERENCES

ANDERSON, C. R., and C. F. STEVENS, 1973. Voltage clamp analysis of acetylcholine produced end-plate current fluctuations at frog neuromuscular junction. *J. Physiol.* 235:655–691.

BARRANTES, F. J., 1976. Intrinsic fluorescence of the membrane-bound acetylcholine receptor: Its quenching by suberyldicholine. *Biochem. Biophys. Res. Commun.* 72:479–488.

BONNER, R., F. J. BARRANTES, and T. M. JOVIN, 1976. Kinetics of agonist-induced intrinsic fluorescence changes in membrane-bound acetylcholine receptor. *Nature* 263:429–431.

BULGER, J. E., J.-J. L. FU, E. F. HINDY, R. L. SILBERSTEIN, and G. P. HESS, 1977. Allosteric interactions between the membrane-bound acetylcholine receptor and chemical mediators. Kinetic studies. *Biochemistry* 16:684–692.

BULGER, J. E., and G. P. HESS, 1973. Evidence for separate initiation and inhibitory sites in the regulation of membrane potential of electroplax. I. Kinetic studies with α-bungarotoxin. *Biochem. Biophys. Res. Commun.* 54:677–684.

CATTERALL, W. A., 1975. Sodium transport by the acetylcholine receptor of cultured muscle cells. *J. Biol. Chem.* 250:1776–1781.

CHANG, H. W., and E. NEUMANN, 1976. Dynamic properties of isolated acetylcholine receptor protein: Release of calcium ions caused by acetylcholine binding. *Proc. Natl. Acad. Sci. USA* 73:3364–3368.

CHANGEUX, J.-P., L. BENEDETTI, J. P. BOURGEOIS, A. BRESSON, J. CARTAUD, P. DEVAUX, H. GRÜNHAGEN, M. MOREAU, J.-L. POPOT, A. SOBEL, and M. WEBER, 1975. Some structural properties of the cholinergic receptor protein in its membrane environment relevant to its function as a pharmacological receptor. *Cold Spring Harbor Symp. Quant. Biol.* 40:211–230.

COHEN, J. B., and N. D. BOYD, 1977. Kinetics of binding of cholinergic ligands to acetylcholine receptor–rich membranes. *Biophys. J.* 17:123a.

ECCLES, J. C., 1964. *The Physiology of Synapses.* Berlin: Springer-Verlag.

EIGEN, M., 1967. Kinetics of reaction controls and information transfer in enzymes and nucleic acids. *Nobel Symp.* 5:333–369.

ELDEFRAWI, M. E., and A. T. ELDEFRAWI, 1977. Acetylcholine receptors. In *Receptors and Recognition*, series A, vol. 4, P. Cuatrecasas and M. F. Greaves, eds. London: Chapman and Hall, pp. 197–258.

FU, J.-J. L., D. B. DONNER, and G. P. HESS, 1974. Half-of-the-sites reactivity of the membrane-bound *Electrophorus electricus* acetylcholine receptor. *Biochem. Biophys. Res. Commun.* 60:1072–1080.

FU, J.-J. L., D. B. DONNER, D. E. MOORE, and G. P. HESS, 1977. Allosteric interactions between the membrane-bound acetylcholine receptor and chemical mediators: Equilibrium measurements. *Biochemistry* 16:678–684.

HAMMES, G. G., and C.-W. WU, 1974. Kinetics of allosteric enzymes, *Annu. Rev. Biophys. Bioeng.* 3:1–33.

HESS, G. P., and J. P. ANDREWS, 1977. Functional acetylcholine receptor–electroplax membrane microsacs (vesicles): Purification and characterization. *Proc. Natl. Acad. Sci. USA* 74:482–486.

HESS, G. P., J. P. ANDREWS, and G. E. STRUVE, 1976. Apparent cooperative effects in acetylcholine receptor–mediated ion flux in electroplax membrane preparations. *Biochem. Biophys. Res. Commun.* 69:830–837.

HESS, G. P., J. P. ANDREWS, G. E. STRUVE, and S. E. COOMBS, 1975a. Acetylcholine receptor–mediated ion flux in electroplax membrane preparations. *Proc. Natl. Acad. Sci. USA* 72:4371–4375.

HESS, G. P., J. E. BULGER, J.-J. L. FU, E. F. HINDY, and R. J. SILBERSTEIN, 1975b. Allosteric interactions of the membrane-bound acetylcholine receptor: Kinetic studies with α-bungarotoxin. *Biochem. Biophys. Res. Commun.* 64:1018–1027.

HODGKIN, A. L., and A. F. HUXLEY, 1952. Quantitative

description of membrane current and its application to conduction and excitation in nerve. *J. Physiol.* 117:500–544.

KASAI, M., and J.-P. CHANGEUX, 1971a. *In vitro* excitation of purified membrane fragments by cholinergic agonists. I. Pharmacological properties of the excitable membrane. *J. Membrane Biol.* 6:1–23.

KASAI, M., and J.-P. CHANGEUX, 1971b. *In vitro* excitation of purified membrane fragments by cholinergic agonists. III. Comparison of the dose-response curves to decamethonium with the corresponding binding curves of decamethonium to the cholinergic receptor. *J. Membrane Biol.* 6:58–80.

KATZ, B., 1969. *The Release of Neural Transmitter Substances.* Liverpool: Liverpool Univ. Press.

KATZ, B., and R. MILEDI, 1972. The statistical nature of the acetylcholine potential and its molecular components. *J. Physiol.* 224:665–669.

KATZ, B., and S. THESLEFF, 1957. A study of the "desensitization" produced by acetylcholine at the motor endplate. *J. Physiol.* 138:63–80.

KOSHLAND, D. E., G. NEMETHY, and D. FILMER, 1966. Comparison of experimental binding data and theoretical models in proteins containing subunits. *Biochemistry* 5:365–385.

LAND, B. R., T. R. PODLESKI, E. E. SALPETER, and M. M. SALPETER, 1977. Acetylcholine receptor distribution in myotubes in culture correlated to acetylcholine sensitivity. *J. Physiol.* 269:155–176.

LEE, C. Y., 1972. Chemistry and pharmacology of polypeptide toxins in snake venoms. *Annu. Rev. Pharmacol.* 12:265–286.

MAELICKE, A., B. W. FULPIUS, R. P. KLETT, and E. REICH, 1977. Acetylcholine receptor. Responses to drug binding. *J. Biol. Chem.* 252:4811–4830.

MONOD, J., J. WYMAN, and J.-P. CHANGEUX, 1965. On the nature of allosteric transitions: A plausible model. *J. Mol. Biol.* 12:88–118.

MOORE, W. M., L. A. HOLLADAY, D. PRUETT, and R. N. BRADY, 1974. On the conformation of the acetylcholine receptor from *Torpedo nobiliana. FEBS Lett.* 45:145–149.

NACHMANSOHN, D., 1974. Biochemical foundation of an integral model of nerve excitability. In *Biochemistry of Sensory Functions*, I. Jaenicke, ed. Berlin: Springer-Verlag, pp. 431–464.

NEHER, E., and B. SAKMANN, 1976. Single-channel currents recorded from membrane of denervated frog muscle fibers. *Nature* 260:779–802.

RANG, H. P., 1974. Acetylcholine receptors. *Q. Rev. Biophys.* 7:283–399.

RÜBSAMEN, H., G. P. HESS, A. T. ELDEFRAWI, and M. E. ELDEFRAWI, 1976. Interaction between calcium and ligand-binding sites of the purified acetylcholine receptor studied by use of a fluorescent lanthanide. *Biochem. Biophys. Res. Commun.* 68:56–63.

SASTRE, A., and T. R. PODLESKI, 1976. Pharmacologic characterization of the Na^+ ionophores in L6 myotubes. *Proc. Natl. Acad. Sci. USA* 73:1355–1359.

SHERIDAN, R. E., and H. E. LESTER, 1975. Relaxation measurements on the acetylcholine receptor. *Proc. Natl. Acad. Sci. USA* 72:3496–3500.

STALLCUP, W. B., and M. COHN, 1976. Electrical properties of a clonal cell line as determined by measurement of ion fluxes. *Exp. Cell Res.* 98:277–284.

50 General Regulatory Role of Cyclic Nucleotides in Hormone and Neurohormone Action

THEODORE W. RALL

ABSTRACT Adenosine 3',5'-phosphate (cyclic AMP) and its synthesizing system (adenylate cyclase) are present in virtually all animal cells. Brain tissue contains the highest amount of this enzyme. The adenylate cyclase of animal cells is embedded in membranes, predominantly plasma membranes, where it is linked to various cell-specific receptors. Hormone-receptor interaction results in increased cyclic AMP synthesis, which in turn initiates a cascade of biochemical events beginning with the activation of a family of phosphotransferases. These enzymes and their protein substrates are distributed in both the soluble and membranous portions of cells. In various differentiated cells, cyclic AMP has been found to play crucial roles in the regulation of a variety of cellular processes, including metabolism, membrane permeability and transport, secretion, and processes leading to increased de novo synthesis of specific proteins. Evidence is beginning to accumulate that cyclic AMP functions in the generation of slow inhibitory potentials produced by catecholamines and in the regulation of transmitter release.

THIS ARTICLE is intended as an introduction to the presentations of others dealing with specific topics involving the metabolism and function of cyclic nucleotides. A comprehensive review emphasizing citations to the primary literature will not be attempted. Instead a summary of important background information and concepts will be provided and the interested reader will be directed principally to a number of excellent and current review articles and monographs.

Cyclic AMP metabolism

Adenosine 3',5'-phosphate (cyclic AMP) was discovered in 1957 during the course of investigations of the hyperglycemic effects of epinephrine and gluca-

THEODORE W. RALL Department of Pharmacology, University of Virginia, Charlottesville, VA 22903

gon (Rall, Sutherland, and Berthet, 1957; Sutherland and Rall, 1957). Initially it was found that the ability of the hormones to increase the accumulation of the active (and more phosphorylated) form of phosphorylase in liver homogenates involved the increased formation of a heat-stable "factor" (later identified as cyclic AMP) by particulate fractions of homogenates in the presence of ATP. Despite its relative chemical stability, cyclic AMP was found to be readily converted to 5' AMP enzymatically (Sutherland and Rall, 1958). This process was found to be inhibited by methylxanthines, substances that had accidentally been observed to potentiate glucagon effects in liver homogenates (Berthet, Sutherland, and Rall, 1957). Subsequent work in a number of laboratories has shown that peptide hormones of diverse origin, numerous biogenic amines, and certain prostaglandins influence the level to which cyclic AMP accumulates in either intact-cell or broken-cell preparations from a wide variety of animal tissues (Robison, Butcher, and Sutherland, 1971). There is also considerable evidence that alterations in the prevailing concentration of the nucleotide are capable of influencing the rate of various ongoing cellular processes. In a number of instances the production of hormone-induced alterations in tissue functions has been correlated with cyclic AMP accumulation both kinetically and pharmacologically, especially using agents that inhibit its degradation. These data have sometimes been supplemented by observations that the application of cyclic AMP or certain derivatives faithfully mimic some or all of the hormone actions in a particular tissue. This pattern of experimental results has been used to conclude that cyclic AMP functions as an intracellular mediator of a particular hormone action (Sutherland, Robison, and Butcher, 1968; Robison, Butcher, and Sutherland, 1971).

The second-messenger concept and cyclic GMP

Soon after the discovery of cyclic GMP in rat urine (Ashman et al., 1963), Sutherland and his co-workers put forth the generalized concept of "second messengers" in hormone action (Sutherland, Øye, and Butcher, 1965). It was proposed that nonpenetrating humoral regulating substances (first messengers) interacted with tissue-specific receptors, which in turn interacted with effector systems in the plasma membrane, resulting in the elaboration of intracellular mediators (second messengers) common perhaps to all cells. These mediators would then go on to alter the rate of certain processes characteristic of the particular differentiated cell, ultimately leading to the recognizable hormone-induced effects. Clearly, this concept was inspired by the observations dealing with cyclic AMP, including those showing that the enzyme system responsible for the formation of cyclic AMP from ATP (adenylate cyclase) was securely bound to membranous structures, particularly plasma membranes. When guanylate cyclase was discovered (Hardman and Sutherland, 1969; White and Aurbach, 1969), however, it was found largely in the cytosolic fractions of tissue homogenates. Further, no hormonal agent has been found to influence guanylate cyclase activity in broken-cell preparations, and only in relatively few instances have hormonal regulatory factors been observed to raise cyclic GMP in intact cells. In these instances, changes in cyclic GMP levels have been dependent on the presence of extracellular calcium ions, and calcium ionophores have also been effective. In addition, it has been difficult to identify specific, characteristic effects of exposure of most tissues to cyclic GMP or its derivatives. (One interesting exception is the depolarization produced by derivatives of cyclic GMP in rabbit cervical ganglia resembling the effects of muscarinic agonists: see McAfee and Greengard, 1972.) In general, the regulatory functions of cyclic GMP are much less well understood than are those of cyclic AMP, and the reader is referred to several reviews by Goldberg for more insight into this problem (Goldberg, O'Dea, and Haddox, 1973; Goldberg et al., 1975). Because of the relationship of calcium ions to regulation of cyclic GMP accumulation, it is possible that in some instances hormone-induced calcium influx represents the second messenger and that cyclic GMP functions as a "third messenger" in a sequence of events. It has also been pointed out that calcium ions may function as important intracellular mediators of hormone action in their own right (Rasmussen, 1970; Rasmussen et al., 1975). The complex interactions of calcium ions with cyclic nucleotide metabolism and function have been lucidly discussed by Berridge (1975), who also deals with certain aspects of this problem elsewhere in this volume. In addition, the mechanisms involved in hormonal stimulation of adenylate cyclase are also discussed elsewhere in this volume by Gilman and Ross.

Protein phosphorylation and cyclic AMP action

Initial studies using partially purified fractions of liver and muscle extracts showed that cyclic AMP promoted the accumulation of the more phosphorylated (and more active) species of glycogen phosphorylase. Subsequently it was found that cyclic AMP interacted with a protein phosphotransferase causing activation (Walsh, Perkins, and Krebs, 1968) by dissociation of a catalytic subunit from an inhibitory subunit (Reiman, Walsh, and Krebs, 1971). One substrate for this enzyme is the less phosphorylated (and less active) form of another protein phosphotransferase, phosphorylase b kinase. The active form of this enzyme in turn phosphorylates the less phosphorylated (and less active) species of glycogen phosphorylase. It is interesting to note that the reaction catalyzed by phosphorylase b kinase requires small quantities of calcium, in addition to Mg-ATP (Meyer, Fischer, and Krebs, 1964). This cascade of events is opposed and ultimately reversed by a family of phosphoprotein phosphatases. The phosphotransferase interacting with cyclic AMP (cyclic AMP–dependent protein kinase) also acts upon the less phosphorylated but more active species of glycogen synthase (Schlender, Wei, and Villar-Palasi, 1969), generating the inactive enzyme. Thus cyclic AMP mediates hormone-induced gylcogenolysis both by promoting glycogen breakdown and by reducing glycogen snythesis (see also Soderling and Park, 1974).

The mechanism of action of cyclic AMP in the regulation of glycogen metabolism is by far the best understood of all its functions. The crucial role of protein phosphorylation in this instance, as well as the widespread occurrence of cyclic AMP–dependent protein kinases in animal tissues, has led to the suggestion that all actions of cyclic AMP involve protein phosphorylation (Kuo and Greengard, 1969; see also Langan, 1973). Further support for this proposal comes from observations that a variety of cell proteins are substrates for cyclic AMP–dependent protein kinases, including f_1 histones (Langan, 1968, 1971), nuclear acidic proteins (Johnson and Allfrey, 1972), and microsomal proteins (Zahltan et al., 1972).

In addition, cyclic AMP–dependent protein kinases

and unidentified endogenous substrates have been found to be associated with particulate fractions of cell homogenates, including ribosomes (Fontana, Picciano, and Lovenberg, 1972) and fractions enriched in nerve endings and synaptic membranes (Weller and Rodnight, 1970; Maeno, Johnson, and Greengard, 1971; see also Greengard, 1975). However, in contrast to the enzymes of glycogen metabolism, it has not been possible to demonstrate discernible changes in functional properties of these proteins as a consequence of altered states of phosphorylation. On the other hand, it has been observed that the ability of cyclic AMP–dependent protein kinases to phosphorylate preparations of cardiac microsomes (sarcoplasmic reticulum) in vitro parallels stimulation of both calcium transport and calcium-activated ATPase in these preparations (see Katz, Tada, and Kirchberger, 1975). These observations as well as the characterization of the specific component undergoing phosphorylation are discussed further by Katz et al. elsewhere in this volume.

Cellular processes regulated by cyclic AMP

From early studies on the role of cyclic AMP in the actions of epinephrine and glucagon on hepatic tissue it was already apparent that a wide variety of cellular processes could be regulated with the aegis of cyclic AMP. In addition to glycogenolysis, these included gluconeogenesis, ketogenesis, and the release of potassium and calcium ions (see Robison, Butcher, and Sutherland, 1971). Besides these acute hormonal effects that could be generated rapidly in slices, perfused organ or dispersed cell preparations, glucagon and derivatives of cyclic AMP have been observed to bring about the increased synthesis and/or accumulation ("induction") of a number of hepatic enzymes either in vivo or in explants of fetal liver (see Wicks, 1974). These enzymes included tyrosine amino transferase, phosphoenolpyruvate carboxykinase, and serine dehydratase. The increased accumulation of these enzymes required de novo protein synthesis and several hours before becoming visible. This characteristic array of hormone-induced effects in liver implies that cyclic AMP can exert effects, either directly or indirectly, on a variety of cellular organelles in addition to cytosolic enzyme complexes, including mitochondria, ribosomes, nuclei, and cell membranes.

Further indication of the breadth of cellular processes and organelles influenced by cyclic AMP can be acquired by considering the evidence for its role in the actions of other hormones in other tissues. These include increased steroidogenesis by ACTH and LH in the adrenal cortex (see Halkerston, 1975) and corpus luteum (see Marsh, 1975), respectively, increased sodium transport by antidiuretic hormone in toad bladder (see Handler and Orloff, 1971), increased cardiac contractility by catecholamines (see Entman, 1974), and increased insulin secretion by glucagon in pancreatic islets (see Montague and Howell, 1975).

Of course, the demonstration that cyclic AMP can influence a given cellular process does not necessarily mean that regulation of this process occurs *exclusively* via cyclic AMP. For example, increases in active phosphorylase levels and glycogenolysis in skeletal muscle during repetitive muscular contraction do not appear to involve altered cyclic AMP metabolism or increases in the amount of the active species of phosphorylase *b* kinase (Mayer and Stull, 1971). Evidently, changes in cytosolic calcium ions can regulate the activity of a fixed amount of this enzyme. Another instructive example is provided by the observation that catecholamine-induced glycogenolysis and gluconeogenesis in rat liver is not abolished by β-adrenergic blocking agents, which abolish catecholamine-induced increases in cyclic AMP accumulation (see Exton and Harper, 1975). Evidently, there are mechanisms mediated by α-adrenergic receptors that coexist with those involving cyclic AMP but have not been elucidated as yet. It is also important to consider the possibility that not all hormone-induced effects in a given tissue are mediated by cyclic AMP, even though some actions appear to be so mediated. One clear and important example of this occurs in the insect salivary gland, where the transcellular potential changes induced by application of cyclic AMP derivatives are strikingly different from those produced by serotonin, even though the overall secretory response to the hormone is reproduced by exogenous cyclic AMP (see Berridge and Prince, 1972). Apparently, serotonin increases both the synthesis of cyclic AMP and the influx of calcium ions, which then go on to produce different changes in membrane permeability to ions.

Role of cyclic AMP in the nervous system

The role of cyclic AMP in the nervous system has been reviewed several times since 1970 (see Rall and Gilman, 1970; Bloom, 1975; Daly, 1977; Nathanson, 1977). Only a few important issues will be summarized here. To begin with, the nervous system has the highest capacity to synthesize and degrade cyclic AMP of all animal tissues. Despite the extreme cellular heterogeneity of brain tissue, it has sometimes been possible to observe quite large accumulations of cyclic AMP in slices from various brain regions exposed to a variety of biogenic amines. These have included norepinephrine, histamine, dopamine, and serotonin. Other putative neurotransmitters, such as acetylcholine, GABA, and glycine have been found not to influence cyclic AMP accumulation appreciably. The pattern of responses has been found to vary dramatically as a function of brain area, species, and developmental age. However, in all brain areas of all species examined, the metabolite adenosine has produced large increases in cyclic AMP accumulation that were specifically and competitively blocked by the methylxanthines (see Rall, 1971). Depending on the brain area and species, the combination of adenosine and either norepinephrine or histamine produced effects two to three times the sum of the individual effects. These actions of adenosine appear to be mediated by specific receptors on the cell surface (see Daly, 1977), and the methylxanthines appear to function as adenosine receptor blocking agents despite any inhibitory effects they might have on cyclic AMP degradation via phosphodiesterases. Depolarizing stimuli, such as those produced by electrical pulses, potassium ions, veratridine, batrachotoxin, and glutamate sometimes induce very large increases in cyclic AMP accumulation that can be only partially accounted for by the release and action of adenosine and other known substances.

Obviously a great deal is left to be learned about identity of endogenous humoral substances and the characteristics of corresponding receptors that influence cyclic AMP metabolism in the brain. It will be necessary to develop techniques that locate both the receptors and the relevant humoral agents on particular cell types and within synaptic regions. In addition, it will be necessary to understand both the mechanism and the functional meaning of potentiative interactions between dissimilar agonists. Finally, the regulatory role of adenosine and perhaps other metabolites acting as "local" hormones will have to be defined.

Cellular heterogeneity and the incompleteness of our knowledge concerning the regulation of cyclic AMP metabolism have made it difficult to identify the cellular processes regulated by cyclic AMP in the nervous system with the usual biochemical techniques. However, in view of the examples provided by the actions of cyclic AMP in other tissues, it seems safe to suggest that it ought to influence at least two important processes in synaptic transmission, namely secretion and membrane transport of ions. Cyclic AMP has been shown to augment the secretion of insulin induced by glucagon in pancreatic islets (see Montague and Howell, 1975), to inhibit the release of histamine, various vasokinins, and lysosomal enzymes from leucocytes and mast cells by antigenic stimuli (see Parker, Sullivan, and Wedner, 1974), and to mimic the release of anterior pituitary hormones by the various hypothalamic releasing factors (see Labrie et al., 1975). The modulation of transmitter release by cyclic AMP–mediated mechanisms is being actively investigated, and some observations have shown increased release of acetylcholine from neuromuscular preparations and of norepinephrine from sympathetic nerves produced by derivatives of cyclic AMP or by inhibitors of phosphodiesterase (see Daly, 1977). In view of the nonneural examples, it will be important not to assume that cyclic AMP should always be related in a positive fashion to transmitter release. In addition, care will be needed in order to distinguish actions of cyclic AMP from those of cyclic GMP. As for membrane transport of ions, cyclic AMP has been shown to be involved in the catecholamine-induced stimulation of bidirectional fluxes of both sodium and potassium ions in avian erythrocytes (see Aurbach 1975). Other relevant examples include the effects of cyclic AMP on potassium and calcium efflux in the liver and on sodium transport in toad bladder as cited above. Related observations have also been made with neural tissue and include the ability of cyclic AMP or its derivatives to hyperpolarize both sympathetic ganglion cells and cerebellar Purkinje cells (see Bloom, 1975). In the latter case, evidence has been presented for mediation of synaptic inhibition of cell firing by norepinephrine release and cyclic AMP formation and action. It appears that either sodium conductance is reduced or active sodium extrusion is stimulated, in contrast to the mechanisms operating in the generation of inhibitory postsynaptic potentials by substances such as GABA or glycine.

Conclusions

Despite the fragmentary information available and the inherent difficulties of investigating cellular chemistry in the nervous system, it seems clear that examination of cyclic AMP and cyclic GMP function in the brain will be profitable. Cyclic AMP metabolism is one useful index that can be exploited in the search for unidentified first messengers and in characterizing receptors. Cyclic AMP actions on cellular processes and organelles in neural tissue are apt to be as diverse as those already delineated in nonneural tissues and should provide an entrée to the characterization of processes important to brain function.

ACKNOWLEDGMENTS The author acknowledges support from U.S. Public Health Service grants NS 12764 and RR 05437.

REFERENCES

ASHMAN, D. F., R. LIPTON, M. M. MELICOW, and T. D. PRICE, 1963. Isolation of adenosine 3',5'-monophosphate and guanosine 3',5'-monophosphate from rat urine. *Biochem. Biophys. Res. Commun.* 11:330–334.

AURBACH, G. D., 1975. Beta-adrenergic receptors, cyclic AMP, and ion transport in the avian erythrocyte. In *Advances in Cyclic Nucleotide Research*, vol. 5, G. I. Drummond, P. Greengard, and G. A. Robison, eds. New York: Raven Press, pp. 117–132.

BERRIDGE, M. J., 1975. The interaction of cyclic nucleotides and calcium in the control of cellular activity. In *Advances in Cyclic Nucleotide Research*, vol. 6, P. Greengard and G. A. Robison, eds. New York: Raven Press, pp. 1–98.

BERRIDGE, M. J., and W. T. PRINCE, 1972. The role of cyclic AMP in the control of fluid secretion. In *Advances in Cyclic Nucleotide Research*, vol. 1, P. Greengard, R. Paoletti, and G. A. Robison, eds. New York: Raven Press, pp. 137–147.

BERTHET, J., E. W. SUTHERLAND, and T. W. RALL, 1957. The assay of glucagon and epinephrine with use of liver homogenates. *J. Biol. Chem.* 229:351–361.

BLOOM, F. E., 1975. The role of cyclic nucleotides in central synaptic function. *Rev. Physiol. Biochem. Pharmacol.* 74:1–103.

DALY, J., 1977. *Cyclic Nucleotides in the Nervous System.* New York: Plenum Press.

ENTMAN, M. L., 1974. The role of cyclic AMP in the modulation of cardiac contractility. In *Advances in Cyclic Nucleotide Research*, vol. 4, P. Greengard and G. A. Robison, eds. New York: Raven Press, pp. 163–193.

EXTON, J. H., and S. C. HARPER, 1975. Role of cyclic AMP in the actions of catecholamines on hepatic carbohydrate metabolism. In *Advances in Cyclic Nucleotide Research*, vol. 5, G. I. Drummond, P. Greengard, and G. A. Robison, eds. New York: Raven Press, pp. 519–532.

FONTANA, J. A., D. PICCIANO, and W. LOVENBERG, 1972. The identification and characterization of a cyclic AMP-dependent protein kinase on rabbit reticulocyte ribosomes. *Biochem. Biophys. Res. Commun.* 49:122–1232.

GOLDBERG, N. D., M. K. HADDOX, S. E. NICOL, D. B. GLASS, C. H. SANFORD, F. A. KUEHL, JR., and R. ESTENSEN, 1975. Biological regulation through opposing influences of cyclic GMP and cyclic AMP: The Yin Yang hypothesis. In *Advances in Cyclic Nucleotide Research*, vol. 5, G. I. Drummond, P. Greengard, and G. A. Robison, eds. New York: Raven Press, pp. 307–330.

GOLDBERG, N. D., R. F. O'DEA, and M. K. HADDOX, 1973. Cyclic GMP. In *Advances in Cyclic Nucleotide Research*, vol. 3, P. Greengard and G. A. Robison, eds. New York: Raven Press, pp. 155–223.

GREENGARD, P., 1975. Cyclic nucleotides, protein phosphorylation and neuronal function. In *Advances in Cyclic Nucleotide Research*, vol. 5, G. I. Drummond, P. Greengard,

and G. A. Robison, eds. New York: Raven Press, pp. 585–602.

HALKERSTON, I. D. K., 1975. Cyclic AMP and adrenocortical function. In *Advances in Cyclic Nucleotide Research*, vol. 6, P. Greengard and G. A. Robison, eds. New York: Raven Press, pp. 99–136.

HANDLER, J. S., and J. ORLOFF, 1971. Factors involved in the action of cyclic AMP on the permeability of mammalian kidney and toad urinary bladder. *Ann. NY Acad. Sci.* 185:345–350.

HARDMAN, J. G., and E. W. SUTHERLAND, 1969. Guanyl cyclase, an enzyme catalyzing the formation of guanosine 3',5'-monophosphate from guanosine triphosphate. *J. Biol. Chem.* 244:6363–6370.

JOHNSON, E. M., and V. G. ALLFREY, 1972. Differential effects of cyclic adenosine 3',5'-monophosphate on phosphorylation of nuclear acidic proteins. *Arch. Biochem. Biophys.* 152:786–794.

KATZ, A. M., M. TADA, and M. A. KIRCHBERGER, 1975. Control of calcium transport in the myocardium by the cyclic AMP–protein kinase system. In *Advances in Cyclic Nucleotide Research*, vol. 5, G. I. Drummond, P. Greengard, and G. A. Robison, eds. New York: Raven Press, pp. 453–472.

KUO, J. F., and P. GREENGARD, 1969. Cyclic nucleotide dependent protein kinases. IV. Widespread occurrence of adenosine 3',5'-monophosphate-dependent protein kinase in various tissues and phyla of the animal kingdom. *Proc. Natl. Acad. Sci. USA* 64:1349–1355.

LABRIE, F., P. BORGEAT, A. LEMAY, S. LEMAIRE, N. BARDEN, J. DROUIN, I. LEMAIRE, P. JOLICOEUR, and A. BELAMGER, 1975. Role of cyclic AMP in the action of hypothalamic regulatory hormones in the anterior pituitary gland. In *Advances in Cyclic Nucleotide Research*, vol. 5, G. I. Drummond, P. Greengard, and G. A. Robison, eds. New York: Raven Press, pp. 787–801.

LANGAN, T. A., 1968. Histone phosphorylation: Stimulation by adenosine 3',5'-monophosphate, *Science* 162:579–581.

LANGAN, T. A., 1971. Cyclic AMP and histone phosphorylation. *Ann. NY Acad. Sci.* 185:166–180.

LANGAN, T. A., 1973. Protein kinases and protein kinase substrates. In *Advances in Cyclic Nucleotide Research*, vol. 3, P. Greengard and G. A. Robison, eds. New York: Raven Press, pp. 99–153.

McAFEE, D. A., and P. GREENGARD, 1972. Adenosine 3',5'-monophosphate: Electrophysiological evidence for a role in synaptic transmission. *Science* 178:310–312.

MAENO, H., E. M. JOHNSON, and P. GREENGARD, 1971. Subcellular distribution of adenosine 3',5'-monophosphate-dependent protein kinase in rat brain. *J. Biol. Chem.* 246:134–142.

MARSH, J. M., 1975. The role of cyclic AMP in gonadal function. In *Advances in Cyclic Nucleotide Research*, vol. 6, P. Greengard and G. A. Robison, eds. New York: Raven Press, pp. 137–200.

MAYER, S. E., and J. T. STULL, 1971. Cyclic AMP in skeletal muscle. *Ann. NY Acad. Sci.* 185:433–448.

MEYER, W. L., E. H. FISCHER, and E. G. KREBS, 1964. Activation of skeletal muscle phosphorylase b kinase by Ca^{2+}. *Biochemistry* 3:1033–1039.

MONTAGUE, W., and S. L. HOWELL, 1975. Cyclic AMP and the physiology of the islets of Langerhans. In *Advances in Cyclic Nucleotide Research*, vol. 6, P. Greengard and

G. A. Robison, eds. New York: Raven Press, pp. 201–244.

NATHANSON, J. A., 1977. Cyclic nucleotides and nervous system function. *Physiol. Rev.* 57:157–256.

PARKER, C. W., T. J. SULLIVAN, and H. J. WEDNER, 1974. Cyclic AMP and the immune response. In *Advances in Cyclic Nucleotide Research*, vol. 4, P. Greengard and G. A. Robison, eds. New York: Raven Press, pp. 1–79.

RALL, T. W., 1971. Studies on the formation and metabolism of cyclic AMP in the mammalian central nervous system. *Ann. NY Acad. Sci.* 185:520–530.

RALL, T. W., and A. G. GILMAN, 1970. The role of cyclic AMP in the nervous system. *Neurosci. Res. Program Bull.* 8:221–323.

RALL, T. W., E. W. SUTHERLAND, and J. BERTHET, 1957. The relationship of epinephrine and glucagon to liver phosphorylase. IV. Effect of epinephrine and glucagon on the reactivation of phosphorylase in liver homogenates. *J. Biol. Chem.* 224:463–475.

RASMUSSEN, H., 1970. Cell communication, calcium ion, and cyclic adenosine monophosphate. *Science* 170:404–412.

RASMUSSEN, H., P. JENSEN, W. LAKE, N. FRIEDMANN, and D. B. P. GOODMAN, 1975. Cyclic nucleotides and cellular calcium metabolism. In *Advances in Cyclic Nucleotide Research*, vol. 5, G. I. Drummond, P. Greengard, and G. A. Robison, eds. New York: Raven Press, pp. 375–394.

REIMAN, E. M., D. A. WALSH, and E. G. KREBS, 1971. Purification and properties of rabbit skeletal muscle adenosine 3′,5′-monophosphate-dependent protein kinases. *J. Biol. Chem.* 246:1986–1995.

ROBISON, G. A., R. W. BUTCHER, and E. W. SUTHERLAND, 1971. *Cyclic AMP.* New York: Academic Press.

SCHLENDER, K. K., S. H. WEI, and C. VILLAR-PALASI, 1969. UDP-glucose: Glycogen-4-glucosyltransferase I kinase activity of purified muscle protein kinase. Cyclic nucleotide specificity. *Biochim. Biophys. Acta* 191:272–278.

SODERLING, T. R., and C. R. PARK, 1974. Recent advances in glycogen metabolism. In *Advances in Cyclic Nucleotide Research*, vol. 4, P. Greengard and G. A. Robison, eds. New York: Raven Press, pp. 283–333.

SUTHERLAND, E. W., I. ØYE, and R. W. BUTCHER, 1965. The action of epinephrine and the role of the adenyl cyclase system in hormone action. *Recent Prog. Horm. Res.* 21:623–646.

SUTHERLAND, E. W., and T. W. RALL, 1957. The properties of an adenine ribonucleotide produced with cellular particles, ATP, Mg^{++} and epinephrine or glucagon. *J. Am. Chem. Soc.* 79:3608.

SUTHERLAND, E. W., and T. W. RALL, 1958. Fractionation and characterization of a cyclic adenine ribonucleotide formed by tissue particles. *J. Biol. Chem.* 232:1077–1091.

SUTHERLAND, E. W., G. A. ROBISON, and R. W. BUTCHER, 1968. Some aspects of the biological role of adenosine 3′,5′-monophosphate (cyclic AMP). *Circulation* 3:279–306.

WALSH, D. A., J. P. PERKINS, and E. G. KREBS, 1968. An adenosine 3′,5′-monophosphate-dependent protein kinase from rabbit skeletal muscle. *J. Biol. Chem.* 243:3763–3765.

WELLER, M., and R. RODNIGHT, 1970. Stimulation by cyclic AMP of intrinsic protein kinase activity in ox brain membrane preparations. *Nature* 225:187–188.

WHITE, A. A., and G. D. AURBACH, 1969. Detection of guanyl cyclase in mammalian tissues. *Biochim. Biophys. Acta* 191:686–697.

WICKS, W. D., 1974. Regulation of protein synthesis by cyclic AMP. In *Advances in Cyclic Nucleotide Research*, vol. 4, P. Greengard and G. A. Robison, eds. New York: Raven Press, pp. 335–438.

ZAHLTAN, R. N., A. A. HOCHBERG, F. W. STRATMAN, and H. A. LARDY, 1972. Glucagon-stimulated phosphorylation of mitochondrial and lysosomal membranes of rat liver *in vivo*. *Proc. Natl. Acad. Sci. USA* 69:800–804.

51 Regulation of Cardiac Contractile Function by Cyclic AMP–Protein Kinase Catalyzed Protein Phosphorylation

ARNOLD M. KATZ, GARY BAILIN,
MADELEINE A. KIRCHBERGER, and MICHIHIKO TADA

ABSTRACT Phosphorylation of the cardiac sarcoplasmic reticulum by the cyclic AMP–protein kinase system has been shown to stimulate calcium transport by these membranes, possibly by increasing the Ca^{2+} affinity of the Ca-binding sites at the external surface of the membrane. This effect partly explains the ability of β adrenergic agonists to accelerate relaxation in the heart. The cyclic AMP–protein kinase system also facilitates relaxation by reducing the Ca^{2+} sensitivity of the troponin complex, which occurs when troponin I is phosphorylated. Phosphorylation of the cardiac sarcolemma by the cyclic AMP–protein kinase system might explain the increased Ca influx across this membrane that partly accounts for the positive inotropic effects of the β-agonists.

BOTH THE ELECTRICAL and the mechanical performance of the heart are controlled by changes in the intrinsic properties of the myocardial cells (Katz, 1977). Even though the heart is innervated by the autonomic nervous system, innervation is not essential for cardiac function. Instead, the electrical impulses that initiate and synchronize the pumping action of the heart arise in, and are conducted through, specialized muscle cells. The role of the nervous system, therefore, is to regulate the myocardial cellular processes responsible for impulse formation, impulse conduction, and contraction.

The sympathetic nervous system is one of the primary regulators of cardiac performance, and catecholamines have been shown to have profound effects on all aspects of myocardial cell function. These effects, which are mediated by the β-adrenergic receptors found in virtually every region of the heart, include an increased rate of spontaneous depolarization of cardiac pacemakers, accelerated impulse conduction, increased energy production, and enhanced contractility. All of these effects appear to be mediated by cyclic AMP, although in most cases the precise mechanism of action of this "second messenger" has not been completely described. From a biochemical standpoint, the best-characterized cardiac responses to catecholamines are those of the systems governing contraction and relaxation in the myocardial cell. These responses are described in the following section, after which our current understanding of the biochemical reactions that mediate these responses is examined in some detail. Finally, the prerequisites for an experimental approach to the analysis of similar control systems in other tissues are discussed.

Mechanical response of the heart to catecholamines

The typical response of the heart to agents that increase cyclic AMP production include an increased rate of tension rise, enhanced tension development, and an acceleration of relaxation (Table I). In view of the central role of Ca in activating the cardiac contractile proteins (Katz, 1970; Ebashi, 1976), these changes can be attributed to an accelerated rate of Ca delivery to the contractile proteins, an increase in the amount of Ca bound to the contractile proteins,

ARNOLD M. KATZ, GARY BAILIN, MADELEINE A. KIRCHBERGER, and MICHIHIKO TADA Division of Cardiology, Department of Medicine, University of Connecticut Health Center, Farmington, CT 06032; Department of Biochemistry, New Jersey School of Osteopathic Medicine, Piscataway, NJ 08854; Department of Physiology and Biophysics, Mount Sinai School of Medicine of the City of New York, NY 10029; First Department of Medicine, Osaka University Medical School, Fukushima-ku, Osaka 553, Japan

TABLE I
Mechanical responses to agents that increase cyclic AMP production in the heart

Mechanical Response	Probable Mechanism
Increased rate of tension rise	Increased rate of Ca delivery to the contractile proteins
Increased tension	Increased amount of Ca delivered to the contractile proteins
Increased rate of relaxation	Increased rate of Ca removal from the contractile proteins

and accelerated Ca removal from the contractile proteins, respectively.

INCREASED RATE OF TENSION RISE AND THE RATE OF CALCIUM RELEASE AT THE ONSET OF SYSTOLE In most adult mammalian hearts, as in skeletal muscle, most of the calcium that mediates the final step in excitation-contraction coupling is derived from stores within the sarcoplasmic reticulum. The mechanism by which the action potential causes calcium to be released from stores within this intracellular membrane system is controversial (see below), but it is generally agreed that an increase in the calcium permeability of the sarcoplasmic reticulum allows Ca^{2+} to flow down an electrochemical gradient from within the sarcoplasmic reticulum into the cytosol. For this reason, the increased rate of tension rise that characterizes the cardiac response to catecholamines probably results, at least in part, from an increase in the calcium permeability of the sarcoplasmic reticulum at the onset of systole. Whether this putative effect is due to a direct action on these membranes, to a change in the system that links depolarization of the sarcolemma to the proposed increase in the Ca^{2+} permeability of the sarcoplasmic reticulum, or to both, will be discussed later.

Two hypotheses have been advanced to explain the link between the passage of an action potential across the sarcolemma and the initiation of calcium release by the sarcoplasmic reticulum. The first hypothesis is that changes in an electrical potential across the membrane of the calcium-filled sarcoplasmic reticulum induces calcium release (Endo, 1977). The second hypothesis is that an increase in the level of ionized Ca^{2+} outside the sarcoplasmic reticulum, which itself is too small to initiate tension, causes a large but transient calcium release (Ford and Podolsky, 1972; Fabiato and Fabiato, 1977; Endo, 1977). Evidence that elevated Ca^{2+} outside sarcoplasmic re-

ticulum vesicles can induce a calcium release has been also provided by Katz and co-workers, who found that increasing Ca^{2+} concentrations in the medium surrounding calcium-filled sarcoplasmic reticulum vesicles increases their calcium permeability (Katz, Repke, and Hasselbach, 1977; Katz et al., 1977a). On the basis of our current knowledge, it is not possible to state with certainty which, if either, of these two hypotheses correctly explains this critical step in excitation-contraction coupling.

INCREASED TENSION AND THE AMOUNT OF CALCIUM RELEASED BY THE SARCOPLASMIC RETICULUM The ability of catecholamines to increase tension developed by cardiac muscle could be explained by an increase in the maximum calcium permeability of the sarcoplasmic reticulum during systole. This hypothesis, if correct, would provide a mechanism that supplements the well-documented ability of catecholamines to promote calcium influx across the sarcolemma, which allows calcium to enter the cell during the cardiac action potential by way of a slow inward current (Reuter, 1974). Although the amount of calcium entering the cell by way of the slow inward current during a single action potential is too small to contribute significantly to the tension developed in a given contraction (Bassingthwaite and Reuter, 1972), augmentation of this calcium influx can increase the calcium content of the sarcoplasmic reticulum during a series of contractions.

Perhaps the strongest evidence that cyclic AMP increases tension development through a direct effect on the cardiac sarcoplasmic reticulum comes from the experiments of Fabiato and Fabiato (1975), who found that cyclic AMP increased the tension developed by "skinned" cardiac muscle fibers in response to a calcium-triggered contraction.

INCREASED RATE OF FALL IN TENSION AND THE CALCIUM PUMP OF THE SARCOPLASMIC RETICULUM The sarcoplasmic reticulum plays a major role in reducing cytosolic Ca^{2+} concentration to levels sufficiently low to cause this cation to dissociate from its binding sites in the troponin complex (Ebashi, 1976). This is accomplished by an ATP-dependent calcium pump in these membranes. In view of the probable causal relationship between the rate of calcium transport by the sarcoplasmic reticulum and the rate at which a muscle relaxes, we (Kirchberger et al., 1972) and others (Wray, Gray, and Olsson, 1973; LaRaia and Morkin, 1974) investigated the possibility that the cyclic AMP–protein kinase system, previously shown in other reactions to mediate effects of catecholamines, might be able to stimulate the calcium pump of cardiac sarcoplasmic reticulum vesicles. The results of these studies are summarized in the following section.

Mechanism by which agents that increase myocardial cyclic AMP accelerate relaxation

Relaxation can be accelerated by any intervention that facilitates the removal of calcium from troponin—either increasing the rate of calcium transport into the sarcoplasmic reticulum or decreasing the Ca^{2+} affinity of troponin or both. It now appears that both mechanisms operate.

A number of early studies suggested that catecholamines or cyclic AMP could directly stimulate the calcium pump of the sarcoplasmic reticulum (Hess et al., 1968; Entman, Levey, and Epstein, 1969; Shinebourne and White, 1970). Several other groups, however, including our own (Katz and Repke, 1973), were unable to confirm these findings. The key to the mechanism by which catecholamines stimulate this calcium pump was provided by the discovery of the cyclic AMP–dependent protein kinases (Walsh, Perkins, and Krebs, 1968; Miyamoto, Kuo, and Greengard, 1969), which are stimulated by cyclic AMP to transfer the terminal phosphate of ATP to

form phosphoester bonds in proteins. When we included this enzyme in our studies of the calcium pump of the cardiac sarcoplasmic reticulum, we found a two- to threefold stimulation of the rate of calcium transport (Kirchberger et al., 1972). This led us to propose that the cascade of reactions shown in Figure 1 could explain the increased rate of cardiac relaxation in response to catecholamines (see Table I). Some of the findings that support this hypothesis are described in the following paragraphs, with the discussion focusing on the later reactions in the cascade (the initial steps in the cascade are discussed elsewhere in this volume).

PHOSPHORYLATION OF THE CARDIAC SARCOPLASMIC RETICULUM Cardiac sarcoplasmic reticulum vesicles serve as a substrate for both intrinsic and extrinsic cyclic AMP–dependent protein kinases (Wray, Gray, and Olsson, 1973; LaRaia and Morkin, 1974; Kirchberger, Tada, and Katz, 1974). The phosphoprotein formed in these reactions has the chemical characteristics of a phosphoester in which the phosphate is bound primarily as phosphoserine (Kirchberger, Tada, and Katz, 1974). The amount of phosphoester formed, approximately 1.5 nmol/mg protein, is similar to that incorporated into the calcium pump as the acyl phosphoprotein intermediate of the calcium-

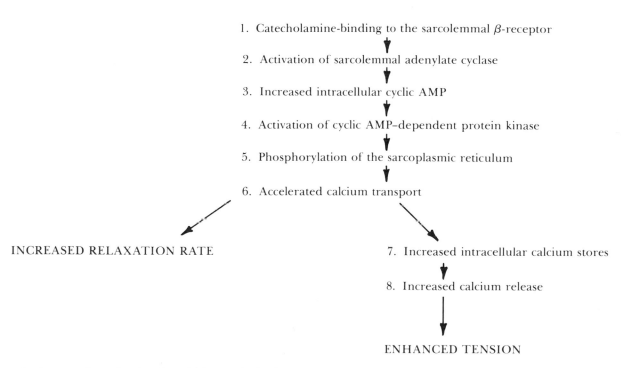

1. Catecholamine-binding to the sarcolemmal β-receptor

2. Activation of sarcolemmal adenylate cyclase

3. Increased intracellular cyclic AMP

4. Activation of cyclic AMP–dependent protein kinase

5. Phosphorylation of the sarcoplasmic reticulum

6. Accelerated calcium transport

INCREASED RELAXATION RATE

7. Increased intracellular calcium stores

8. Increased calcium release

ENHANCED TENSION

FIGURE 1 Proposed mechanism by which catecholamines modify the amount and rate of fall of tension in the myo-cardium. (Modified from Katz, Tada, and Kirchberger, 1975.)

pump ATPase (Shigekawa, Finegan, and Katz, 1976). This suggests that a 1:1 molar ratio exists between these two types of phosphoprotein.

The phosphoester formed by the action of cyclic AMP–dependent protein kinases in cardiac sarcoplasmic reticulum is dephosphorylated by phosphoprotein phosphatase (LaRaia and Morkin, 1974; Tada, Kirchberger, and Li, 1975; Kirchberger and Raffo, 1977), indicating that this phosphorylation can be reversed physiologically.

The protein that is phosphorylated by the cyclic AMP–dependent protein kinase can be shown by polyacrylamide gel electrophoresis to be distinct from the ATPase protein. The latter has a molecular weight of 90,000–100,000 (Fanburg and Matsushita, 1973; Suko and Hasselbach, 1976) whereas the protein phosphorylated by the cyclic AMP–protein kinase system (tentatively named "phospholamban") has an apparent molecular weight of approximately 22,000 (LaRaia and Morkin, 1974; Tada, Kirchberger, and Katz, 1975). Our inability to demonstrate phosphorylation of a protein corresponding to phospholamban in sarcoplasmic reticulum vesicles from rabbit fast skeletal muscle (Kirchberger and Tada, 1976) is in accord with the inability of catecholamines to stimulate relaxation in this muscle type (see Katz, Tada, and Kirchberger, 1975).

STIMULATION OF CALCIUM TRANSPORT IN THE CARDIAC SARCOPLASMIC RETICULUM Stimulation of calcium transport in cardiac sarcoplasmic reticulum vesicles by the cyclic AMP–protein kinase system (Kirchberger et al., 1972; LaRaia and Morkin, 1974; Tada et al., 1974; Will et al., 1976) suggested that phosphorylation of phospholamban accelerates calcium transport by the sarcoplasmic reticulum. Evidence for a causal link between membrane phosphorylation and stimulated calcium transport has been provided by Tada, Kirchberger, and Katz (1975), who found that brief, controlled, tryptic digestion of the sarcoplasmic reticulum caused proportionate decreases in the ability of the protein kinase to catalyze phosphate incorporation and to stimulate calcium transport. These findings suggest that a portion of the phospholamban molecule is located on the external surface of the vesicles, but it was found not to be iodinated by peroxidase in the presence or absence of Triton X-100 (Louis and Katz, 1977). Thus most of this protein may be located within the membrane of the sarcoplasmic reticulum, where it is tightly bound to membrane lipids.

Further evidence that phosphorylation of phospholamban is causally linked to stimulation of calcium transport was obtained by Tada, Kirchberger, and Katz (1975) and Kirchberger and Chu (1976), who found a close parallel between phosphoester formation and the degree to which calcium transport was stimulated by skeletal protein kinases. Kirchberger and Raffo (1977) also documented a parallel decrease in phospholamban phosphorylation and calcium transport stimulation when the phosphorylated cardiac sarcoplasmic reticulum was dephosphorylated by a phosphoprotein phosphatase associated with these membranes.

These experimental findings indicate that phosphorylation of phospholamban leads to a stimulation of the calcium pump of the cardiac sarcoplasmic reticulum. This evidence, however, cannot distinguish whether phosphorylated phospholamban is an activator of the calcium pump or whether, when dephosphorylated, phospholamban inhibits calcium transport. Evidence bearing on this question was reported by Tada et al. (1974), who found that the Ca^{2+} sensitivity of oxalate-supported calcium uptake rate increased when phospholamban was phosphorylated. These results cannot be interpreted with precision due to the complex Ca^{2+} kinetics (Li et al., 1974) of reactions carried out in the presence of oxalate, which is employed to stabilize the Ca^{2+} concentration inside the vesicles, but preliminary data of M. Shigekawa and co-workers indicate that the Ca^{2+} sensitivity of the ATPase reaction in the absence of this calcium-precipitating anion may be increased when phospholamban is phosphorylated. In view of the approximately threefold lower Ca^{2+} sensitivity of the calcium pump in cardiac sarcoplasmic reticulum vesicles, compared to those obtained from fast white skeletal muscle (Shigekawa, Finegan, and Katz, 1976), it is tempting to speculate that phosphorylation of phospholamban converts a low-sensitivity, "cardiac-type" calcium-pump enzyme to one with the higher Ca^{2+} sensitivity seen for the skeletal sarcoplasmic reticulum.

RELATIONSHIP BETWEEN STIMULATION OF CALCIUM TRANSPORT IN CARDIAC SARCOPLASMIC RETICULUM VESICLES AND THE INCREASED RATE OF RELAXATION IN THE HEART EXPOSED TO CATECHOLAMINES The causal relationships indicated by the arrows linking the first six steps in the cascade of Figure 1 have been described above, and there is substantial evidence that the increased rate of relaxation seen in the myocardium under the influence of catecholamines can be attributed, at least in part, to stimulation of the sarcoplasmic reticulum calcium pump. That phosphorylation of phospholamban, stimulation of calcium transport by the sarcoplasmic reticulum, and accelerated relaxation are causally related is suggested by the role played by this intracellular membrane structure in causing the heart to relax. Additional evidence for this view comes from the finding that the physiological ability of a muscle to respond to catecholamines with an increased rate of relaxation is correlated with the existence in the muscle of the phospholamban regulatory system.

Fast skeletal muscles are relatively insensitive to catecholamines, which act only to slightly prolong the active state without accelerating relaxation (Goffart and Ritchie, 1952; Bowman and Raper, 1967). We found that cyclic AMP–dependent protein kinases from both cardiac and skeletal muscle are unable either to phosphorylate a 22,000 dalton protein (phospholamban) or to stimulate calcium transport in rabbit fast skeletal muscle (Katz, Tada, and Kirchberger, 1975; Kirchberger and Tada, 1976). On the other hand, Schwartz et al. (1976) found significant stimulation of calcium transport by protein kinase in this type of muscle. This discrepancy may reflect the fact that most of the calcium transport measurements reported by Schwartz et al. (1976) were made at Ca^{2+} concentrations that were well above the physiological range where the change in Ca^{2+} sensitivity suggested by Tada et al. (1974) would stimulate calcium transport. The potential significance of the reported stimulation of calcium transport in fast-skeletal-muscle sarcoplasmic reticulum vesicles thus remains unclear.

In several slow skeletal muscles, in which relaxation is slightly enhanced by catecholamines (Bowman and Raper, 1967), Kirchberger and Tada (1976) documented both slight stimulation of calcium transport and phosphorylation of a 22,000 dalton protein in the sarcoplasmic reticulum. Phosphorylation of the sarcoplasmic reticulum thus appears to explain, at least in part, the ability of catecholamines to accelerate relaxation.

REDUCTION IN THE CALCIUM SENSITIVITY OF CARDIAC TROPONIN It has recently been reported that phosphorylation of troponin I, the inhibitory component of the troponin complex, by cyclic AMP–dependent protein kinases reduces the calcium affinity of the troponin complex (Ray and England, 1976; Reddy and Wyborny, 1976; Solaro, Moir, and Perry, 1976; Bailin, 1977). This shift in calcium sensitivity, which is opposite in direction to that caused by phosphorylation of the sarcoplasmic reticulum (Figure 2), could accelerate relaxation by facilitating the dissociation of Ca^{2+} from the troponin complex when cytosolic Ca^{2+} concentration is reduced by the sarco-

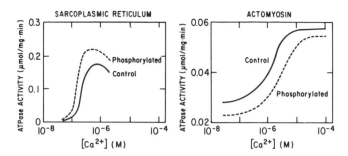

FIGURE 2 Effects of phosphorylation of the sarcoplasmic reticulum and troponin I on the Ca^{2+}-dependent ATPase activities of cardiac sarcoplasmic (left; data from Tada et al., 1974) and actomyosin (right; data from Bailin, 1977).

plasmic reticulum. This effect of the cyclic AMP–protein kinase system appears to be absent in fast-skeletal-muscle actomyosin. If the ability of cyclic AMP–dependent protein kinases to reduce the Ca^{2+} sensitivity of the cardiac troponin complex were the only response of the myocardial cell to an increased level of cyclic AMP, then elevation of cyclic AMP levels might be expected to reduce tension. The finding that the heart develops more tension under the influence of catecholamines must mean that the stimulation of calcium delivery to the contractile proteins described above provides enough of this activator to overcome the need for higher cytosolic Ca^{2+} levels to promote contraction.

Mechanism by which agents that increase myocardial cyclic AMP enhance tension and the rate of tension rise

Both the sarcolemma and the sarcoplasmic reticulum appear to participate in increasing the amount of calcium delivery to the contractile proteins of the heart in response to an elevation in cyclic AMP levels. The ability of both catecholamines and cyclic AMP to augment calcium influx across the sarcolemma has been extensively documented (Reuter, 1974). This sarcolemmal response alone could account for the ability of catecholamines to increase tension, but the finding that tension is also enhanced when skinned cardiac fibers are exposed to cyclic AMP (Fabiato and Fabiato, 1975) demonstrates that this mechanical response is not wholly dependent on an intact sarcolemma. The possibility that an increased release of calcium from stores within the sarcoplasmic reticulum contributes to this augmentation of tension was suggested by Katz, Tada, and Kirchberger (1975), who found that the rate of calcium efflux from cardiac sarcoplasmic reticulum vesicles increased after pretreatment with a cyclic AMP–dependent protein kinase.

The ability of phospholamban phosphorylation to increase calcium efflux from the cardiac sarcoplasmic reticulum, as well as to promote active calcium transport, is in accord with recent evidence that the calcium-pump ATPase protein can participate in the release of calcium from within the sarcoplasmic reticulum (Katz et al., 1977b). More recently, we have obtained evidence that the ability of the cyclic AMP–protein kinase system to accelerate calcium efflux from sarcoplasmic reticulum vesicles is due to an increased ability of external Ca^{2+} to promote Ca efflux (M. A. Kirchberger, D. Wong, and A. M. Katz, unpublished observations). This effect of phospholamban phosphorylation appears to result from an increase in the Ca^{2+} sensitivity of a site at the external surface of the membrane which, when bound to Ca^{2+}, increases calcium permeability (Katz et al., 1977b).

Possible actions of the cyclic AMP–protein kinase system on the cardiac sarcolemma

Catecholamines have been shown to increase the slow inward current. This effect appears to be mediated by cyclic AMP, but little is known of its biochemical mechanism. Wollenberger (1975) and Sulakhe, Leung, and St. Louis (1976) have suggested that the cardiac sarcolemma is a substrate for cyclic AMP–dependent protein kinase and that phosphorylation of a 24,000 dalton protein in this membrane is associated with increased calcium binding and transport in sarcolemmal vesicles. However, a causal relationship between these findings and the enhanced slow inward current remains to be documented.

Examination of the effects of the cyclic AMP–protein kinase system on ion fluxes in other membrane systems

The findings described in the article and summarized in Figure 1 provide strong evidence for a causal link between phosphorylation of the cardiac sarcoplasmic reticulum by the cyclic AMP–protein kinase system and both a functional change in an ion pump and the physiological response to catecholamines. For this reason, these studies may serve as a prototype for future investigations of the mechanisms by which catecholamines and the autonomic nervous system control other membrane pumps. It should be pointed out, however, that before such mechanisms can be demonstrated in other systems, a number of experimental requirements must be met. Unless all of these requirements are taken into consideration, actions such as those mediated by phospholamban phosphorylation in the cardiac sarcoplasmic reticulum may be overlooked, and false negative results obtained.

FAILURE OF CYCLIC AMP TO ACTIVATE THE PROTEIN KINASE   The demonstration of an effect of cyclic AMP on a membrane system in vitro requires that endogenous cyclic AMP levels be low. Some membrane preparations, however, contain endogenous adenylate cyclase activity, so that a stimulatory effect of cyclic AMP may be masked. In other cases, active phosphodiesterase activity might neutralize a potential cyclic AMP effect. For these reasons, it is advisable to confirm that the ability of the cyclic AMP–protein kinase system to phosphorylate substrate such as histone remains in the presence of the membrane system under study.

FAILURE OF THE ACTIVATED PROTEIN KINASE TO PHOSPHORYLATE THE MEMBRANE   Should the membrane system under study be isolated in a phosphorylated form, added cyclic AMP and protein kinase cannot induce either incorporation of phosphate or a functional change. Under such conditions, pretreatment with a phosphoprotein phosphatase may be necessary to unmask a cyclic AMP–protein kinase effect. Conversely, the presence in the membrane preparation of an active phosphoprotein phosphatase might dephosphorylate a phosphorylated regulatory protein more rapidly than it is phosphorylated. These possibilities, as well as the possible presence of a protein kinase inhibitor, must be excluded prior to accepting a negative result.

FAILURE OF A PHOSPHORYLATED MEMBRANE TO SHOW ALTERED FUNCTION   It is clear from our experience with the cardiac sarcoplasmic reticulum that had we not chosen the correct conditions to study the calcium pump in 1972, our work on this project would have been aborted. This is because there is little stimulation of calcium transport velocity at high Ca^{2+} concentrations (i.e., above 3–5 μM; see Figure 2). In addition, the calcium storage capacity of these membrane vesicles is only minimally stimulated under conditions where calcium transport rate is markedly enhanced (Kirchberger et al., 1972; Will et al., 1976). Yet the problem of a functional change in membrane properties is much simpler in the case of the sarcoplasmic reticulum, which is so specialized that it has only two functions: to pump and to release calcium. In contrast, studies of physiological changes associated with the phosphorylation of other membranes, which contain multiple functional components, may be much more difficult.

In view of these many potential problems in identifying mechanisms of action of the cyclic AMP–protein kinase system on cellular membranes, it is not surprising that progress in this area has been slow. For this reason, the experience with the cardiac sarcoplasmic reticulum described in this article may serve as a useful model for future studies of this potentially important control system.

ACKNOWLEDGMENTS Work reported in this paper was supported by Grants-in-Aid from the Connecticut Heart Association, the University of Connecticut Research Foundation, and U.S. Public Health Service Grants IIL-22135 01 and HL-21812-01.

REFERENCES

BAILIN, G., 1977. 3′:5′-Monophosphate-dependent protein kinase phosphorylation of a bovine cardiac actin complex. Biophys. J. 17:159a.

BASSINGTHWAITE, J. B., and H. REUTER, 1972. Calcium movements and excitation-contraction coupling in cardiac cells. In Electrical Phenomena in the Heart, W. C. DeMello, ed. New York: Academic Press, pp. 353–395.

BOWMAN, W. C., and C. RAPER, 1967. Adrenotropic receptors in skeletal muscle. Ann. NY Acad. Sci. 139:741–753.

EBASHI, S., 1976. Excitation-contraction coupling Annu. Rev. Physiol. 38:293–313.

ENDO, M., 1977. Calcium release from the sarcoplasmic reticulum. Physiol. Rev. 57:71–108.

ENTMAN, M. L., G. S. LEVEY, and S. E. EPSTEIN, 1969. Mechanism of action of epinephrine and glucagon on the canine heart. Evidence for increase in sarcotubular calcium stores mediated by cyclic 3′,5′-AMP. Circ. Res. 25:429–438.

FABIATO, A., and F. FABIATO, 1975. Relaxing and inotropic effects of cyclic AMP in skinned cardiac cells. Nature 253:556–558.

FABIATO, A., and F. FABIATO, 1977. Calcium release from the sarcoplasmic reticulum. Circ. Res. 40:119–129.

FANBURG, B. L., and S. MATSUSHITA, 1973. Phosphorylated intermediate of ATPase of isolated cardiac sarcoplasmic reticulum. J. Mol. Cell. Cardiol. 5:111–115.

FORD, R. E., and R. J. PODOLSKY, 1972. Intracellular calcium movements in skinned muscle fibres. J. Physiol. 223:21–33.

GOFFART, M., and J. M. RITCHIE, 1952. The effect of adrenaline on the contraction of mammalian skeletal muscle. J. Physiol. 116:357–371.

HESS, M. L., F. N. BRIGGS, E. SHINEBOURNE, and R. WHITE, 1968. Effect of adrenergic blocking agents on the calcium pump of the fragmented cardiac sarcoplasmic reticulum. Nature 220:79–80.

KATZ, A. M., 1970. Contractile proteins of the heart. Physiol. Rev. 50:58–163.

KATZ, A. M., 1977, Physiology of the Heart. New York: Raven Press.

KATZ, A. M., and D. I. REPKE, 1973. Calcium-membrane interactions in the myocardium: Effects of ouabain, epinephrine and 3′,5′-cyclic adenosine monophosphate. Am. J. Cardiol. 31:193–201.

KATZ, A. M., D. I. REPKE, J. DUNNETT, and W. HASSELBACH, 1977a. Dependence of calcium permeability of sarcoplasmic reticulum vesicles on external and internal calcium ion concentrations. J. Biol. Chem. 252:1950–1956.

KATZ, A. M., D. I. REPKE, G. FUDYMA, and M. SHIGEKAWA, 1977b. Control of calcium efflux from sarcoplasmic reticulum vesicles by external calcium. J. Biol. Chem. 252:4210–4214.

KATZ, A. M., D. I. REPKE, and W. HASSELBACH, 1977. Dependence of ionophore- and caffeine-induced calcium release from sarcoplasmic reticulum vesicles on external and internal calcium ion concentration. J. Biol. Chem. 252:1938–1949.

KATZ, A. M., M. TADA, and M. A. KIRCHBERGER, 1975. Control of calcium transport in the myocardium by the cyclic AMP-protein kinase system. In Advances in Cyclic Nucleotide Research, vol. 5, G. I. Drummond, P. Greengard, and G. A. Robison, eds. New York: Raven Press, pp. 453–472.

KIRCHBERGER, M. A., and G. CHU, 1976. Correlation between protein kinase-mediated stimulation of calcium transport by cardiac sarcoplasmic reticulum and phosphorylation of a 22,000 dalton protein. Biochim. Biophys. Acta 419:559–562.

KIRCHBERGER, M. A., and A. RAFFO, 1977. Decrease in calcium transport associated with phosphoprotein phosphatase-catalyzed dephosphorylation of cardiac sarcoplasmic reticulum. J. Cyclic Nuc. Res. 3:45–53.

KIRCHBERGER, M. A., and M. TADA, 1976. Effects of adenosine 3′,5′-monophosphate-dependent protein kinase on sarcoplasmic reticulum isolated from cardiac and slow and fast contracting skeletal muscles. J. Biol. Chem. 251:725–729.

KIRCHBERGER, M. A., M. TADA, and A. M. KATZ, 1974. Adenosine 3′,5′-monophosphate-dependent protein kinase-catalyzed phosphorylation reaction and its relationship to calcium transport in cardiac sarcoplasmic reticulum. J. Biol. Chem. 249:6166–6173.

KIRCHBERGER, M. A., M. TADA, D. I. REPKE, and A. M. KATZ, 1972. Cyclic adenosine 3′,5′-monophosphate-dependent protein kinase stimulation of calcium uptake by canine cardiac microsomes. J. Mol. Cell. Cardiol. 4:673–680.

LARAIA, P. J., and E. MORKIN, 1974. Adenosine 3′,5′-monophosphate dependent membrane phosphorylation; a possible mechanism for the control of microsomal calcium transport in heart muscle. Circ. Res. 35:298–306.

LI, H. C., A. M. KATZ, D. I. REPKE, and A. FAILOR, 1974. Oxalate dependence of calcium uptake kinetics of rabbit skeletal muscle microsomes (fragmented sarcoplasmic reticulum). Biochim. Biophys. Acta 367:385–389.

LOUIS, C. F., and A. M. KATZ, 1977. Lactoperoxidase coupled iodination of cardiac sarcoplasmic reticulum proteins. Biochim. Biophys. Acta (in press).

MIYAMOTO, E., J. F. KUO, and P. GREENGARD, 1969. Adenosine 3′,5′-monophosphate dependent protein kinase from brain. Science 165:63–65.

RAY, K. P., and P. ENGLAND, 1976. Phosphorylation of the inhibitory component of troponin and its effect on Ca²⁺

dependence of cardiac myofibril ATPase. *FEBS Lett.* 70:11–16.

REDDY, Y. S., and L. E. WYBORNY, 1976. Phosphorylation of guinea pig actomyosin and its effect on ATPase activity. *Biochem. Biophys. Res. Commun.* 73:703–709.

REUTER, H., 1974. Localization of beta adrenergic receptors and effects of non-adrenaline and cyclic nucleotides on action potentials, ionic currents and tension in mammalian cardiac muscle. *J. Physiol.* 242:429–451.

SCHWARTZ, A., M. L. ENTMAN, K. KANIIKE, L. K. LANE, W. B. VAN WINKLE, and E. P. BORNET, 1976. The rate of calcium uptake in sarcoplasmic reticulum of cardiac muscle and skeletal muscle. Effects of cyclic AMP-dependent protein kinase and phosphorylase *b* kinase. *Biochim. Biophys. Acta* 426:57–72.

SHIGEKAWA, M., J.-A. M. FINEGAN, and A. M. KATZ, 1976. Calcium transport ATPase of canine cardiac sarcoplasmic reticulum: A comparison with that of rabbit fast skeletal muscle sarcoplasmic reticulum. *J. Biol. Chem.* 251:6894–6900.

SHINEBOURNE, E., and R. WHITE, 1970. Cyclic AMP and calcium uptake of the sarcoplasmic reticulum in relation to increased rate of relaxation under the influence of catecholamines. *Cardiovasc. Res.* 4:194–200.

SOLARO, R. J., A. J. G. MOIR, and S. V. PERRY, 1976. Phosphorylation of the inhibitory component of troponin and the inotropic effect of adrenaline in perfused rabbit heart. *Nature* 262:615–616.

SUKO, J., and W. HASSELBACH, 1976. Characterization of cardiac sarcoplasmic reticulum ATP-ADP exchange and phosphorylation of the calcium transport adenosine triphosphatase. *Eur. J. Biochem.* 64:123–130.

SULAKHE, P. V., N. L. K. LEUNG, and P. ST. LOUIS, 1976. Stimulation of calcium accumulation in cardiac sarcolemma by protein kinase. *Can. J. Biochem.* 54:438–445.

TADA, M., M. A. KIRCHBERGER, and A. M. KATZ, 1975. Phosphorylation of a 22,000-dalton component of the cardiac sarcoplasmic reticulum by adenosine 3′,5′-monophosphate dependent protein kinase. *J. Biol. Chem.* 250:2640–2647.

TADA, M., M. A. KIRCHBERGER, and H.-C. LI, 1975. Phosphoprotein phosphatase-catalyzed dephosphorylation of the 22,000 dalton phosphoprotein of cardiac sarcoplasmic reticulum. *J. Cyclic Nuc. Res.* 1:329–338.

TADA, M., M. A. KIRCHBERGER, D. I. REPKE, and A. M. KATZ, 1974. The stimulation of calcium transport in cardiac sarcoplasmic reticulum by adenosine 3′,5′-monophosphate-dependent protein kinase. *J. Biol. Chem.* 249:385–389.

WALSH, D. A., J. P. PERKINS, and E. G. KREBS, 1968. An adenosine 3′,5′-monophosphate dependent protein kinase from rabbit skeletal muscle. *J. Biol. Chem.* 243:3763–3765.

WILL, H., J. BLANCK, G. SMETTAR, and A. WOLLENBERGER, 1976. A quench-flow kinetic investigation of calcium ion accumulation by isolated cardiac sarcoplasmic reticulum. Dependence of initial velocity on free calcium ion concentration and influence of preincubation with a protein kinase, MgATP and cyclic AMP. *Biochim. Biophys. Acta* 449:297–303.

WOLLENBERGER, A., 1975. The role of cyclic AMP in the adrenergic control of the heart. In *Contraction and Relaxation in the Myocardium*, W. G. Nayler, ed. New York: Academic Press, pp. 113–190.

WRAY, H. L., R. R. GRAY, and R. A. OLSSON, 1973. Cyclic adenosine 3′,5′-monophosphate-stimulated protein kinase and a substrate associated with cardiac sarcoplasmic reticulum. *J. Biol. Chem.* 248:1496–1498.

52 Modulation of Nervous Activity by Cyclic Nucleotides and Calcium

M. J. BERRIDGE

ABSTRACT A functional understanding of neuronal integration will depend on unraveling the complex mechanisms responsible for modulating the excitability of the individual units. Cyclic AMP, cyclic GMP, and calcium have all been implicated as second messengers in the nervous system. Apart from the role of calcium both in stimulus-secretion coupling and as a regulator of ionic permeability, we know very little about the mode of action of cyclic AMP or cyclic GMP even though these second messengers can yield marked changes in the activity of individual neurons. There is growing evidence from a wide variety of hormonal responses that second messengers can interact with each other to produce subtle modulations of cellular activity. In particular, the cyclic nucleotides are thought to alter calcium homeostasis. This paper will examine how some of these second messenger interactions may regulate both excitability and pacemaker activity.

"Judicious pursuit of the complicated interactions between cyclic nucleotide regulated events and Ca^{++}-regulated events within neurons and other cells seems clearly warranted."—F. E. Bloom (1975)

Introduction

NEURONS INTERACT with each other in many different ways. Information may be transmitted from one nerve to the next by an explosive release of neurotransmitter following each action potential or by small subtle alterations in the release rate from nonspiking neurons (Schmitt, Dev, and Smith, 1976). Despite the enormous and bewildering variability in the interactions that can occur between nerve cells, there are essentially two major questions we must consider in trying to understand how the individual units are regulated. First, what factors determine whether or not the nerve cell will release transmitter from its terminals? This problem concerns whether or not there will be a flow of information toward the terminals, either as action potentials or in the form of graded changes in membrane potential. Second, once

a signal arrives at the synapse, what factors modulate the amount of neurotransmitter that is released? In effect, we are dealing with a secretory cell, and we must consider those factors responsible not only for exciting the cell but also for modulating the amount of secretion released for any given stimulus.

The second messengers calcium, cyclic AMP, and cyclic GMP have a key role in regulating the activity of most cells, including nerve cells. An important feature of this second-messenger triumvirate is that they are linked together by means of feedback loops (Berridge, 1975), and their interactions may be essential for modulating neuronal activity. In describing the role of these second messengers, I shall begin with a general discussion of their metabolism and mode of action, with special emphasis on observations made on nerve cells. Some of these general features will be used to describe how second messengers may interact with each other to regulate a variety of postsynaptic and presynaptic events.

Some general aspects of calcium and cyclic nucleotide metabolism

CALCIUM HOMEOSTASIS A wide range of cellular processes are regulated by variations in the intracellular level of calcium. In the case of nerve cells, calcium regulates the release of synaptic vesicles at the terminals, and it can also regulate excitability in many nerves by controlling ionic permeabilities (e.g., changes in potassium and sodium conductance). Calcium may also have an important function in regulating cyclic nucleotide levels through a variety of feedback mechanisms, which will be described in more detail later. Considering this pleiotropic action of calcium, it is important to understand the factors responsible for regulating its intracellular level.

Cellular calcium homeostasis is complicated by the presence of both external and internal sources of calcium (Figure 1). The intracellular level of calcium can be varied by adjustments to any one of the many pathways concerned with either its entry or removal

M. J. BERRIDGE Unit of Invertebrate Chemistry and Physiology, Department of Zoology, University of Cambridge, Cambridge CB2 3EJ, England

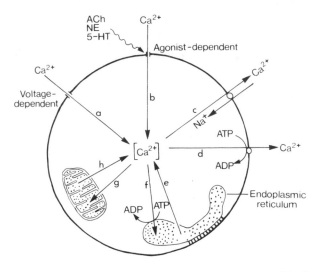

FIGURE 1 Summary of the major processes responsible for regulating the intracellular level of calcium.

from the cytoplasm. Since most of these mechanisms have been reviewed recently (Baker, 1976), I shall concentrate on aspects that seem to be particularly relevant to the control of calcium in nerve cells.

CALCIUM TRANSPORT ACROSS THE PLASMA MEMBRANE Under normal conditions the cell membrane is almost impermeable to calcium, which enables the cell to maintain very low internal calcium concentrations (0.1–1 μM or less). The intracellular level of calcium can be increased by opening up specific calcium channels, which seem to be of two main kinds. There are voltage-dependent channels that open when the membrane is depolarized (Figure 1a). The function of such channels in producing the intracellular calcium signal that triggers the release of neurotransmitters has been described in detail by Llinás (this volume) and will not be considered further. In addition to voltage-dependent channels, cells may also have agonist-dependent channels (Figure 1b). Specific agonist-receptor interactions are translated into an increase in the entry of calcium. Acetylcholine and α-adrenergic agents act in this way in the mammalian salivary gland (Selinger, Eimerl, and Schramm, 1974), while 5-hydroxytryptamine (5-HT) has a similar action in an insect salivary gland (Berridge and Lipke, 1979).

The way in which these neurotransmitters increase the influx of calcium has not been established. Michell and his colleagues have suggested that such agents may act by stimulating the turnover of phosphatidylinositol, which is then responsible for the opening of calcium "gates" (Michell, 1975; Michell, Jafferji, and

Jones, 1976). It is of some interest, therefore, that the activation of muscarinic receptors in the CNS leads to an increased turnover of phosphatidylinositol (de Scarnati, Sato, and de Robertis, 1976). When considering mechanisms of calcium entry it is relevant to consider the possible role of endoperoxides, which are formed during prostaglandin metabolism (see Samuelsson, this volume). It is, for example, conceivable that some of the endoperoxides, especially thromboxane A₂, may function as calcium ionophores. A number of mechanisms have been proposed to account for the extrusion of calcium across the surface membrane (Baker, 1976). Studies on the giant axon of the squid seemed to indicate that a sodium-calcium exchange mechanism might be the principal method of calcium extrusion (Figure 1c). However, more recent studies have shown that this sodium-calcium exchange mechanism may be less important than an ATP-dependent calcium pump (Figure 1d; see also Baker and McNaughton, 1978), similar to that originally described in red blood cells (Schatzmann, 1975). Duncan (1976) has now demonstrated that synaptosomal membranes have a high-affinity calcium transport system very similar to that found in the sarcoplasmic reticulum of muscle. The possible significance of this surface Ca-ATPase is highlighted by the observation that the membranes of seizure-prone mice have much less of this enzyme than is found in normal mice (Rosenblatt, Lauter, and Trams, 1976).

CALCIUM TRANSPORT ACROSS INTERNAL MEMBRANES In addition to entering from the outside, calcium may also be released into the cytoplasm from various intracellular reservoirs. The exact nature of these reservoirs is uncertain, but both the endoplasmic reticulum and the mitochondria are possible candidates. Henkart, Landis, and Reese (1976) have pointed out that many nerve cells have sacs of endoplasmic reticulum, which have many structural similarities to the sarcoplasmic reticulum of muscle. In particular, the flattened sacs lie very close to the neuronal plasmalemma, and there are periodic densities (similar to the SR feet in the muscle triad) spanning the 20 nm gap between the two membranes (Figure 1). These internal membranes, which are probably capable of storing calcium, may play an important role in homeostasis by releasing (Figure 1e) or sequestering calcium under different conditions (Henkart, Landis, and Reese, 1976). In muscle, methylxanthines such as caffeine and theophylline can release calcium from the sarcoplasmic reticulum. The ability of these agents to increase muscle end-

874   M. J. BERRIDGE

plate potentials (MEPP) (Ginsborg and Hirst, 1972), even in the absence of external calcium (Elmqvist and Feldman, 1965), could thus be explained by the release of calcium contained in membrane stores such as the endoplasmic reticulum.

The mitochondria also play a key role in calcium homeostasis. Using transmitter release as an indicator of the intracellular level of calcium, Alnaes and Rahamimoff (1975) have shown that a range of mitochondrial inhibitors (dicoumarol, DNP, antimycin, and cyanide) greatly enhance the frequency of MEPP and also lead to larger endplate potentials. By inhibiting the mitochondria, these agents divert energy away from the transport of calcium (Figure 1g), which then leaks out of the mitochondria, leading to an increase in its resting level. Similarly, the mitochondrial calcium uptake system is thought to be inhibited by lithium, which would account for the increase in MEPP when the frog neuromuscular junction is exposed to this cation (Crawford, 1975).

There is considerable evidence, therefore, to show that these internal reservoirs, especially the mitochondria, have more than enough calcium to produce a significant increase in the release of neurotransmitters. Alnaes and Rahamimoff (1975) calculate that the mitochondria occupy about 6.6% of the nerve terminal and store 1.9×10^{-15} M Ca/terminal, which is at least two orders of magnitude larger than the amount of calcium that enters each terminal during the course of an action potential. Since these large quantities of calcium contained in the mitochondria and perhaps also in the endoplasmic reticulum are labile and susceptible to agents such as lithium, metabolic inhibitors, or methylxanthines, it is important to consider whether there are any physiological mechanisms responsible for modulating the uptake or release of this stored calcium.

Before considering some of the mechanisms that may be responsible for releasing stored calcium, it is important to consider whether or not there is any evidence for a mobilization of internal calcium during normal cell activation. One way of monitoring the rate of mobilization of internal calcium is to study the rate of calcium efflux from cells that have been prelabeled with ^{45}Ca. The efflux of calcium from the cell will be determined by the rate at which it leaves the reservoirs (routes e and h, Figure 1) and is extruded from the cell via the surface pumps (routes c and d, Figure 1). Under normal conditions it is assumed that the rate at which calcium leaves these reservoirs is the limiting factor in the overall rate of efflux. For example, the efflux of calcium from guinea pig auricles is increased considerably after treatment with

caffeine, which stimulates the release of calcium from the sarcoplasmic reticulum (Jundt et al., 1975). Similar increases in calcium efflux have been reported during normal cell activation in liver cells (Friedmann, 1972), insulin-secreting β-cells (Brisson and Malaisse, 1973), and insect salivary gland (Prince, Berridge, and Rasmussen, 1972).

These experiments suggest that a mobilization of internal stored calcium may be a normal feature of cell activation in a wide range of cell types. However, the way in which hormones and neurotransmitters mobilize this internal calcium is still a matter of debate. The fact that cyclic AMP by itself is capable of increasing the efflux of calcium from the cells listed above has led to the suggestion that this nucleotide may mobilize calcium especially from the mitochondria. An earlier observation that cyclic AMP can induce the release of calcium from isolated mitochondria (Borle, 1974) cannot be repeated either by the original author (Borle, 1976) or by others (Scarpa et al., 1976).

It is important to point out that the total surface area of the inner mitochondrial membranes that face the cytoplasm is much larger than that of the plasma membrane. This implies that very small changes in the rates of calcium release or uptake across mitochondrial membranes are likely to have a profound effect on the intracellular level of calcium. It is conceivable, therefore, that cyclic AMP may exert small but significant effects on mitochondrial calcium transport that are difficult to detect by in vitro experiments. The possible involvement of cyclic AMP in the release of internal calcium remains an open question and will be considered further in the section on presynaptic facilitation.

The release of calcium from mitochondria may also be regulated by the intracellular level of sodium (Carafoli et al., 1975). Since calcium transport by isolated cardiac mitochondria seems to be sensitive to sodium, it has been proposed that an influx of sodium during the course of the action potential might be responsible for inducing the release of mitochondrial calcium. There is also some evidence from various secretory cells that an influx of sodium may release internal calcium (Williams, 1975; Lowe et al., 1976). The alkaloid veratridine, which increases sodium permeability, can increase the release of neurotransmitter from synaptosomes (Blaustein, 1975) and the hypogastric nerve (Thoa et al., 1975). This effect may not depend on the depolarizing action of veratridine because this agent can stimulate the release of insulin from β-cells in the complete absence of external calcium.

Likewise, ouabain, which leads to an increase in the intracellular level of sodium, can also stimulate the release of acetylcholine from neuromuscular end-plates (Baker and Crawford, 1975) and insulin from β-cells (Lowe et al., 1976) in the absence of external calcium. It is apparent from such experiments that an increase in the intracellular level of sodium induced by these drugs can stimulate the release of sufficient internal calcium to trigger these various secretory processes. It remains to be seen whether or not the intracellular level of sodium varies sufficiently under normal conditions to have a significant effect on mitochondrial calcium transport.

In addition to functioning as a source of activator calcium, these internal membranes are capable of sequestering calcium, thus functioning as internal buffers. The fact that the flattened sacs of endoplasmic reticulum are found in close juxtaposition to the surface membrane may be particularly significant (Henkart, Landis, and Reese, 1976). This endoplasmic reticulum, together with the mitochondria, constitutes a powerful buffering system that may function to confine "large calcium transients to a very narrow zone of axoplasm in the immediate vicinity of the plasma membrane" (Llinás, Blinks, and Nicholson, 1972). These authors have also pointed out that this buffering system would rapidly remove the transient increase in calcium concentration following an action potential. The fact that the iontophoretic application of calcium to presynaptic nerve terminals had no effect on transmitter release (Miledi and Slater, 1966) may have been due to the rapid removal of calcium by this internal buffering system.

Direct visualization of the action of this buffering system was obtained in the salivary-gland cells of an insect that had been injected with aequorin. When calcium was injected into these cells, there was a brief flash of light that rapidly waned as the calcium was removed by the mitochondria (Rose and Loewenstein, 1975). This rapid removal prevented the injected calcium from reaching the surface membrane and may help to restrict calcium signals to local synaptic regions. The potential of this buffering system to restrict calcium signals to small regions of cytoplasm may be particularly important in the functioning of local circuits.

In summary, this internal calcium storage system plays a key role in calcium homeostasis not only by being a potential source of activator calcium but also by functioning as a powerful buffering system that will rapidly terminate signals using calcium as an intermediary, thus helping to maintain a rapid processing of information.

CYCLIC NUCLEOTIDE-CALCIUM INTERACTIONS   In considering the role of second messengers in the control of cellular activity it is important to realize that these internal signals are not separate entities within the cell but are connected by a complex web of feedback interactions. The operation of such feedback mechanisms may form the basis of the subtle modulation of excitability and neurotransmitter release that plays such an essential role in both neural integration and plasticity. The details and full extent of these feedback interactions remain uncovered, but already it is clear from studies on many different cells that these interactions are of central importance in many cellular control mechanisms (Berridge, 1975). Those interactions which seem to be particularly relevant to nerve cells are illustrated in Figure 2.

There is increasing evidence that the intracellular level of calcium can play an important role in regulating the metabolism of cyclic nucleotides. The brain contains a specific calcium-binding protein that is capable of activating both adenylate cyclase and the nucleoside cyclic 3′,5′-monophosphate phosphodiesterases (Cheung et al., 1975). Although the modular protein was capable of activating both the cyclic AMP and the cyclic GMP phosphodiesterase, it seemed to be much more active against the latter. On the basis of these feedback relationships, an increase in the intracellular level of calcium would result in an increase in the intracellular level of cyclic AMP and a simultaneous fall in the level of cyclic GMP. Indeed, reciprocal changes in the level of these two nucleo-

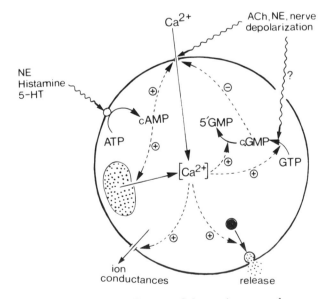

FIGURE 2   Summary of some of the major second-messenger feedback interactions that have been implicated in the control of nerve-cell activity.

tides have been measured after electroconvulsive shock in mice cerebellar tissue (Drummond and Ma, 1973).

It is still not clear whether such reciprocal changes in cyclic AMP and cyclic GMP levels are brought about through the activation of this modulator protein by calcium. The reason for this uncertainty stems from the fact that there is also evidence that calcium can bring about changes in cyclic AMP and cyclic GMP that are directly opposite to those mediated by the calcium–modulator protein complex. For example, there is considerable evidence that high intracellular levels of calcium inhibit adenylate cyclase, leading to a fall in the intracellular level of cyclic AMP. In the mammalian salivary gland, the ability of β-adrenergic agents to increase the intracellular level of cyclic AMP is markedly reduced in the presence of the calcium ionophore A 23187 (Butcher, 1975). α Adrenergic agents, which also act to increase the intracellular level of calcium, will also inhibit the increase in cyclic AMP levels induced by β-adrenergic agents. A similar phenomenon has been observed in brain slices, where the ability of various amines to elevate cyclic AMP levels is greatly enhanced if calcium is removed from the bathing medium (Schultz, 1975). Schultz argues that calcium may act by increasing phosphodiesterase activity, but the same effect could result from an inhibition of adenylate cyclase.

There is also considerable uncertainty concerning the effects of calcium on cyclic GMP metabolism. As mentioned earlier, the calcium-dependent modulator protein activates cyclic GMP phosphodiesterase. However, studies on intact cells clearly show a definite calcium requirement for the synthesis of cyclic GMP. The ability of cholinergic agents to increase the cyclic GMP levels in smooth muscle and mammalian salivary gland was abolished when calcium was withdrawn from the bathing medium (Schultz et al., 1973). Such observations have led to the suggestion that guanylate cyclase may be activated by an increase in the intracellular level of calcium (Figure 2). Some evidence for this has come from studies on membranous guanylate cyclase of fibroblasts that can be activated by calcium concentrations within the normal physiological range (Wallach and Pastan, 1976).

The importance of calcium in regulating the level of cyclic GMP has also been demonstrated in the brain (Ferrendelli, Kinscherf, and Chang, 1973; Ferrendelli, Rubin, and Kinscherf, 1976). Removal of calcium from the bathing medium completely abolished the ability of the depolarizing agents veratridine, ouabain, or elevated potassium concentrations to stimulate an increase in the cyclic GMP level. As mentioned earlier, veratridine and ouabain are capable of stimulating transmitter release by increasing the intracellular level of calcium. The fact that A 23187 can increase the level of cyclic GMP in cerebellar slices provides further evidence for the idea that calcium activates guanylate cyclase (Ferrendelli, Rubin, and Kinscherf, 1976).

The fact that calcium has been shown to activate both the synthesis and the hydrolysis of cyclic GMP would appear to be counterproductive (Figure 2). It is conceivable, however, that these two effects are sensitive to different calcium concentrations. A small increase in calcium may activate the phosphodiesterase, whereas higher concentrations may swamp this effect by stimulating the cyclase to bring about the large increase in cyclic GMP level, often with a parallel fall in the level of cyclic AMP. These reciprocal changes in cyclic AMP and cyclic GMP may play an important role in limiting further entry of calcium.

While there appears to be a strong link between calcium and the activation of guanylate cyclase, this does not preclude the possibility that certain neurotransmitters can activate the enzyme directly. We need to learn much more about cyclic GMP homeostasis, especially since this nucleotide seems to have such profound effects on the excitability of many nerve cells.

In nonnervous tissue there are strong indications that the mechanisms responsible for calcium entry across the plasma membrane might be modulated by the cyclic nucleotides (Figure 2). For example, there is good evidence from studies on the heart that cyclic AMP enhances the entry of calcium that takes place through the voltage-dependent calcium channels during the plateau phase of the action potential (Reuter, 1974). In contrast, cyclic AMP appears to inhibit the uptake of calcium that occurs when antigens interact with the surface antibodies of lymphocytes (Freedman, Raff, and Gomperts, 1975).

The possibility that cyclic GMP may play a role in inhibiting the entry of calcium has been raised by several authors (George, Wilkerson, and Kodowitz, 1973; Schultz et al., 1973; Schultz, Schultz, and Schultz, 1977). Some evidence for such an inhibitory effect of cyclic GMP on calcium entry has been obtained by studying calcium transport across the insect salivary gland (Figure 3). The entry of calcium across the basal (serosal) membrane appears to be the rate-limiting step in the net transport of calcium across the gland. When glands were treated with 8-bromo-cyclic GMP, the rate of calcium transport was greatly reduced as compared to the control glands treated with 5'GMP. This possible involvement of cyclic GMP

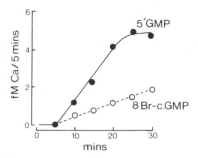

FIGURE 3 The effect of 8-bromo cyclic GMP (10 mM) on the rate of calcium transport across the salivary glands of a fly (Berridge, unpublished observations).

in regulating calcium entry into cells is potentially very important because it may explain why this nucleotide is capable of exciting a number of nerve cells, as will be described below.

In addition to modulating calcium entry across the plasma membrane, cyclic nucleotides may also effect calcium transport across internal membranes. The possible involvement of cyclic AMP in stimulating the release of calcium from the mitochondria has already been discussed. The role of cyclic AMP in modulating calcium transport across the sarcoplasmic reticulum of cardiac muscle is described by Katz et al. (this volume). At present, there is no indication of whether or not a similar control exists in nervous tissue.

THE MODE OF ACTION OF CYCLIC NUCLEOTIDES AND CALCIUM In considering how second messengers act it is important to remember that they may regulate more than one process within the cell. There may be a hierarchy of cellular events that are activated sequentially as the second-messenger level rises within the cell (Figure 4).

Such a hierarchy seems to exist for various cyclic AMP-dependent processes in liver. Half-maximal stimulation of glycogenolysis is present at 5×10^{-11} M glucagon, but higher doses—1×10^{-10}M and 5×10^{-8}M—are necessary to activate gluconeogenesis and ureogenesis, respectively (Park, Lewis, and Exton, 1972). Other studies have shown that as the glucagon concentration is increased, the cyclic AMP level rises far beyond what is required to maximally activate glycogenolysis (Exton et al., 1971). The higher concentration may thus function to activate subsequent processes in the hierarchy, such as gluconeogenesis and ureogenesis.

There appears to be a similar hierarchy for the various calcium-sensitive secretory events in insect salivary gland (Prince and Berridge, 1973; Hansen Bay, 1978). The most sensitive process appears to be

the release of amylase followed by the activation of the electrogenic potassium pump. Finally, the calcium-dependent increase in chloride permeability seems to require the highest levels of calcium. At an intermediate level of calcium, activation of the electrogenic potassium pump will hyperpolarize the apical membrane, whereas higher concentrations of calcium will open chloride channels, neutralizing the activity of this pump and causing the membrane to depolarize. Therefore, the same second messenger may cause the membrane potential either to depolarize or to hyperpolarize, depending on its concentration.

Another feature to emerge from these insect salivary gland studies is that amylase secretion, which is sensitive to low levels of calcium, may be inhibited if the concentration of calcium is too high (Hansen Bay, 1978). Excessive intracellular levels of calcium could also account for the inhibition of DNA synthesis in lymphocytes, which occurs at high A 23187 concentration or during administration of optimal doses of two mitogens (Wang, McClain, and Edelman, 1975).

Figure 4 shows another important aspect of second messengers, namely their resting levels, which may vary considerably and could be an important factor

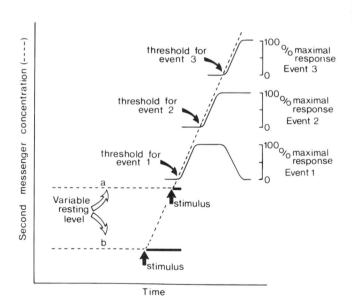

FIGURE 4 The hierarchical arrangement of different cellular events sensitive to varying second-messenger levels. Some of the early events in the hierarchy (e.g., event 1) may be inhibited at very high second-messenger levels. In a resting cell the second-messenger level may be close to the threshold for the first event (a) or it may lie at varying levels below this threshold (e.g., b). When the second messengers are set at a low level, the latency (represented by the solid bars) will be much longer than when the levels are close to threshold.

in adjusting the responsiveness of a cell to external stimuli, especially if these are close to threshold. For example, if the second-messenger level is close to threshold for event 1 (a, Figure 4), the cell is more likely to respond to low concentrations of an agonist than if the resting level is set at some lower level (b, Figure 4). Potentiation of the action of many hormones by methylxanthines seems to depend on their ability to inhibit phosphodiesterase, thus raising the resting level of cyclic AMP close to threshold for the hormonal response. There are also indirect observations indicating that the resting level of calcium can be varied to increase the responsiveness of cells to their normal agonists. In β-cells, for example, agents such as glucagon and methylxanthines, which increase intracellular levels of cyclic AMP, have no effect by themselves but can greatly potentiate the action of glucose on insulin release. It is proposed that the increase in cyclic AMP brings about a release of internal calcium, by a feedback mechanism similar to that described earlier, and that the subsequent increase in the resting level of calcium makes the cells much more sensitive to glucose (Brisson, Malaisse-Lagae, and Malaisse, 1972). Further evidence for a modulation of calcium levels in the subthreshold range has come from studies on calcium transport across the insect salivary gland. As discussed earlier, calcium entry across the basal membrane appears to be a rate-limiting step in calcium transport, which increases linearly with increasing 5-HT concentration (Berridge and Lipke, 1979). Of particular interest is the observation that 5-HT is capable of increasing calcium transport at concentrations considerably lower than those necessary to stimulate fluid secretion. Regulation of the resting level of second messengers may thus constitute an important mechanism for adjusting the sensitivity of cells to external stimuli and may be particularly important in considering the basis for presynaptic facilitation.

Furthermore, if the resting level is set somewhat below threshold, the long latencies that have sometimes been observed in the response of certain cells to external signals could be explained by the time taken for the relevant second messenger to reach an effective concentration (Figure 4).

It now remains to summarize current concepts concerning the specific mode of action of the various second messengers. Calcium not only plays an important role in regulating the release of neurotransmitters from axon terminals but can also modulate excitability by altering ion conductances (Figure 2). The ability of calcium to increase the potassium permeability of cell membranes seems to be widespread (Meech, 1976), and much of the work on this phenomenon has been done on nerve cells. If calcium is injected into the neurons of *Aplysia* or *Helix*, there is a rapid increase in potassium conductance resulting in membrane hyperpolarization and a decrease in excitability (Meech, 1972, 1974a). It is of considerable interest, therefore, that during normal neuronal activity there is a decrease in the level of calcium associated with an increase in the level of potassium in the extracellular space within the cerebellum (Nicholson et al., 1977). The decrease in calcium may arise as this ion enters the cells during neuronal activity, whereas the rise in potassium may depend, in part, on the subsequent calcium-dependent potassium efflux. In addition to affecting potassium conductance, calcium may also reduce sodium conductance, as it does in vertebrate photoreceptors. The effect of variations in the intracellular level of calcium on membrane potential will thus depend on the kinds of calcium-dependent ion conductances that are present in any given cell. Such variations might explain how in some cells calcium causes membrane hyperpolarization by an increase in conductance (potassium), whereas in others similar potential changes occur through a decrease in conductance (sodium).

While there is growing evidence for a role for cyclic nucleotides in both pre- and postsynaptic events (Drummond and Ma, 1973; Bloom, 1975; Greengard, 1976; Nathanson, 1977), there has been little progress in understanding how they might act. The ability of cyclic AMP to phosphorylate specific proteins in neuronal membranes has been advanced as one possible mechanism (Greengard, 1976). The extensive literature on protein phosphorylation in nervous tissue has been reviewed by Williams and Rodnight (1977), who point out that the precise function of the proteins that are phosphorylated has not been determined, so it is difficult to assess the functional significance of many of these observations. It is conceivable that some of the phosphorylated membrane components may be involved in some of the feedback mechanisms for modulating calcium homeostasis. The possibility that some of the effects of the cyclic nucleotides are mediated through their ability to modulate the level of calcium will be explored more extensively in the following section.

Control of postsynaptic events

The excitability of nerve cells depends on a variety of external and internal factors, most of which act by adjusting the membrane potential, usually by altering ionic permeabilities, although changes in ion pumping cannot be excluded. In the simplest case, we may consider a quiescent cell whose activity is regulated by excitatory and inhibitory inputs from other nerve cells (Figure 5). Excitation results in a depolarization of the membrane (an excitatory postsynaptic potential or EPSP), which may lead to the initiation of action potentials if the EPSP exceeds the threshold for spike initiation. On the other hand, input from the inhibitory neuron will hyperpolarize the membrane (creating an inhibitory postsynaptic potential or IPSP), thus reducing excitability. The ionic events associated with the EPSPs or IPSPs may be extremely fast or they may persist for long periods.

Weight (1974) has summarized the membrane conductance changes underlying fast EPSPs and IPSPs that result from direct effects of the neurotransmitters on membrane permeability. For example, acetylcholine acts on nicotinic receptors to produce a rapid but temporary increase in sodium permeability that results in a fast EPSP. Similarly, inhibitory neurotransmitters open up channels for chloride, and perhaps also potassium, to produce the fast IPSPs (Figure 5). Second messengers apparently do not participate directly in these fast potential changes, but there is growing evidence that calcium and the cyclic nucleotides may play an essential role in the postsynaptic events that generate the slow EPSPs and IPSPs. Since some of these potential changes persist for 30 sec or longer, these slow events are extremely important in modulating neuronal pathways. Such long-lasting changes in responsiveness could represent a mechanism for storing information (Libet, Kobayashi, and Tanaka, 1975; Schulman and Weight, 1976).

Slow EPSP   Most of the slow EPSPs that have been recorded in the central and peripheral nervous system seem to arise from the activation of muscarinic cholinergic receptors. The important differences between muscarinic and nicotinic acetylcholine receptors have been stressed by Purves (1976), who points out that nicotinic receptors usually produce a response of very short duration (10–100 msec), which gives rise to the fast EPSP and a one-to-one transmission between the communicating cells. Muscarinic receptors give rise to much longer responses (slow EPSPs), which allows for temporal summation and long-lasting changes in responsiveness. Schulman and Weight (1976) have shown that in the sympathetic ganglion of *Rana* the fast EPSPs have an increased amplitude and duration when they occur during a slow EPSP. In other words, the change in membrane properties that produce the slow EPSP seems to increase the efficacy of the postsynaptic events mediated by the nicotinic receptor. This effect seems to depend on the fact that the slow EPSP arises through a *decrease* in membrane conductance (Schulman and Weight, 1976). Similar decreases in conductance seem to be responsible for changes in membrane potential in several other nerves (Nathanson, 1977).

There is growing evidence that the slow EPSP in a number of nerve cells may be linked to an increase in the intracellular level of cyclic GMP (McAfee and Greengard, 1972; Kebabian, Steiner, and Greengard, 1975; Stone, Taylor, and Bloom, 1975; Hoffer et al., 1977; Stone and Taylor, 1977). The stimulation of muscarinic receptors in a variety of cells, including those in the nervous system, leads to an increase in the level of cyclic GMP (Lee, Kuo, and Greengard, 1972; Goldberg, O'Dea, and Haddox, 1973; Schultz et al., 1973). Moreover, cytochemical techniques have revealed that the increase in cyclic GMP level that occurs in peripheral ganglia takes place within the postganglionic neuron (Kebabian et al., 1975).

Further evidence for such a postsynaptic function has been obtained by studying the effects on membrane potential of adding this nucleotide or its analogs. The addition of dibutyryl cyclic GMP to postganglionic neurons in sympathetic ganglia resulted in a slow EPSP very similar to that produced by stimulating the preganglionic muscarinic fibers (McAfee and Greengard, 1972). Microiontophoretic application of cyclic GMP to pyramidal-tract neurons in the rat cerebral cortex increased the firing frequency of most of the neurons studied—an effect similar to that of acetylcholine (Stone, Taylor, and Bloom, 1975; Stone and Taylor, 1977). Similarly, microiontophor-

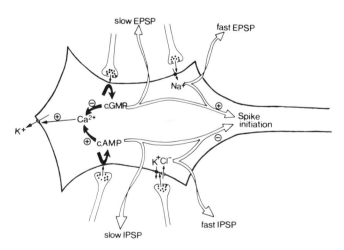

Figure 5   Summary of some of the mechanisms that have been proposed for regulating neuronal excitability.

etic application of acetylcholine or cyclic GMP to pyramidal neurons within the hippocampus also leads to a marked increase in excitability (Figure 6). The way in which cyclic GMP depolarizes the neuronal membrane and excites these pyramidal neurons in the cerebral cortex and hippocampus is unknown, but some possible mechanisms will be considered after we deal with slow IPSPs.

SLOW IPSP   In contrast to the excitation produced by cyclic GMP, cyclic AMP seems to play a role in mediating the action of inhibitory neurotransmitters such as norepinephrine (NE). The evidence pointing to a role for cyclic AMP in postsynaptic events has come mainly from studies on mammalian superior cervical ganglia (Greengard, 1976) and cerebellar Purkinje cells (Bloom et al., 1975).

In the superior cervical ganglion, dopamine released from an interneuron is responsible for elevating the intracellular level of cyclic AMP in the same postganglionic neuron in which there is an increase in cyclic GMP level during cholinergic stimulation (Kebabian et al., 1975). What is even more intriguing is that these two cyclic nucleotides exert opposite effects on membrane potential. While cyclic GMP was associated with the slow EPSP, cyclic AMP seems to mediate the slow IPSP. This membrane hyperpolarization can be potentiated by the phosphodiesterase inhibitor theophylline and mimicked by the addition of either mono- or dibutyryl cyclic AMP (McAfee and Greengard, 1972). Opposite effects of cyclic GMP and cyclic AMP on neuronal excitability have also been recorded in the pyramidal-tract neurons mentioned earlier (Stone, Taylor, and Bloom, 1975; Stone and Taylor, 1977). The firing rates of these neurons, which can be increased by acetylcholine and cyclic GMP, are markedly suppressed after application of NE or cyclic AMP (Figure 7).

In the case of the cerebellar Purkinje cells, the cyclic AMP level is elevated by NE released from the endings of nerves originating in the locus ceruleus (Bloom et al., 1975). Purkinje cells are spontaneously active, and the ability of NE to suppress this activity can be mimicked by cyclic AMP or dibutyryl cyclic AMP. The ability of a range of cyclic AMP analogs to depress the spontaneous activity of Purkinje cells is closely correlated with their ability to activate protein kinase (Siggins and Henriksen, 1975). The way in which cyclic AMP exerts its inhibitory effect in these examples has not been established.

THE MODE OF ACTION OF CYCLIC AMP AND CYCLIC GMP   On the basis of the studies described in the last two sections, it is clear that cyclic AMP and cyclic GMP exert opposite effects on certain nerve cells. Cyclic GMP seems to excite cells, whereas cyclic AMP is inhibitory. Similar antagonistic effects of these two nucleotides have been described on neuronal firing of blowfly chemoreceptors (Daley and Van de Berg, 1976) and on the beating rate of cultured mouse myocardial cells (Goshima, 1976). Similarly, the release of lysosomal enzymes from human neutrophils seems to be accelerated by cyclic GMP but inhibited by cyclic AMP (Ignarro, 1974). The antagonistic effects obtained with these two nucleotides may thus reflect a general cellular control mechanism that has been adopted by nerve cells to regulate excitability. A possible explanation for the antagonistic action of these cyclic nucleotides emerges from the feedback mechanisms discussed previously (Figure 5). It is proposed that in certain cells these nucleotides exert their effects indirectly by altering the level of calcium (Figure 2). Excitability may be set by the level of calcium, which is lowered by cyclic GMP but elevated by cyclic AMP.

The suggestion that the excitability of certain neurons might be set by the intracellular level of calcium is certainly consistent with numerous observations re-

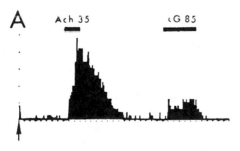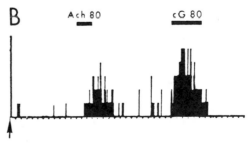

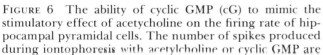

FIGURE 6   The ability of cyclic GMP (cG) to mimic the stimulatory effect of acetycholine on the firing rate of hippocampal pyramidal cells. The number of spikes produced during iontophoresis with acetylcholine or cyclic GMP are represented as histograms. Vertical axis: A = 15 counts; B = 4 counts. Horizontal axis: 10 sec in both cases. (From Hoffer et al., 1977.)

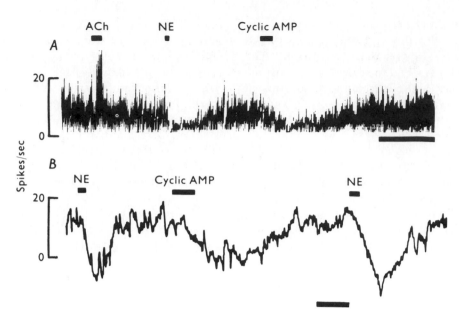

FIGURE 7   The ability of cyclic AMP to mimic the inhibitory effect of norepinephrine (NE) on the firing rate of cortical neurons. Horizontal bars = 1 min. (From Stone and Taylor, 1977.)

sulting from altering the internal or external level of calcium. The excitability of *Aplysia* neurons is increased by lowering the internal level of calcium by injecting the calcium-chelating agent ethylene glycol bis-(β-aminoethyl ether)-N,N'-tetraacetic acid (EGTA) (Meech, 1974b). On the other hand, when calcium is injected into neurons, the membrane hyperpolarizes (Meech, 1972, 1976). Lowering the external calcium concentration, which should lower the internal level, also leads to excitation of CNS neurons (Curtis, Perrin, and Watkins, 1960), mouse neuroblastoma cells (Tuttle and Richelson, 1975), and cultured tuberal neurons (Geller and Hoffer, 1977). Phillis, Lake, and Yarbrough (1973) have implicated an increase in calcium in the inhibitory effect of biogenic amines on cerebral cortical neurons.

Variations in calcium concentration could be translated into a change in membrane potential through alterations in calcium-sensitive ion conductances. For example, cyclic GMP may act by lowering the calcium level, thereby causing a decrease in potassium conductance and leading to membrane depolarization and increased excitability. Such a mechanism is consistent with the observation discussed earlier that slow EPSPs result from a decrease in membrane conductance (Schulman and Weight, 1976).

The inhibitory effect of cyclic AMP, especially in those cases where the two nucleotides are antagonistic to each other, may thus depend on an increase in the intracellular level of calcium. The hyperpolarization that develops in dorsal-root ganglion cells following a depolarizing current seems to depend on a calcium-induced increase in potassium conductance (Ransom, Barker, and Nelson, 1975). Similarly, the spike after-hyperpolarization of a sympathetic neuron may also arise from a calcium-dependent increase in potassium conductance (Busis and Weight, 1976). The after-hyperpolarization was abolished in calcium-free media but was considerably potentiated by theophylline, which may act by a direct effect on calcium permeability or by increasing the level of cyclic AMP (Busis and Weight, 1976). In the case of tuberal neurons, Geller and Hoffer (1977) have shown that the inhibitory effect of monamines is not dependent on external calcium, but they raised the possibility that calcium might be released from internal reservoirs. It is tempting, therefore, to suggest that the inhibitory effects in certain neurons might be mediated indirectly by increasing the intracellular level of calcium either by an effect on the internal reservoirs or by enhancing entry from the outside.

The hyperpolarization obtained in certain neurons cannot be explained on the basis of an increase in potassium conductance. For example, the cyclic AMP–dependent hyperpolarization of cerebellar Purkinje cells seem to arise from a *decrease* in conductance (Siggins et al., 1971), which implies that the ionic species involved must have equilibrium potentials more positive than the resting potential. On the basis of recent studies on paravertebral sympathetic ganglia, Smith and Weight (1977) favor the idea that hyperpolarization is caused by a decrease in sodium conductance. Another possibility is that the hyperpolarization develops through an increase in the electrogenic pumping of sodium. For example, in multipolar spinal-cord cells, the long-lasting hyperpolarization that follows a glutamate-induced burst of action potentials seems to depend on the active extrusion of the sodium that entered during the burst (Ransom, Barker, and Nelson, 1975). As yet there are no indications as to how cyclic AMP might effect such changes in sodium conductance or sodium pump rate.

SPONTANEOUS ACTIVITY   Many nerve cells are spontaneously active and will initiate regular trains or bursts of action potentials in the absence of any external input. The frequency of this rhythmical activity can usually be modulated by synaptic input. In some cases, the excitatory and inhibitory synaptic modulation of pacemaker activity can be long-lasting and may persist for as long as 4 hr (Parnas, Armstrong, and Strumwasser, 1974). Such long-lasting effects may be particularly important because in a recent study on the neural events underlying learning in insects, Woollacott and Hoyle (1977) have shown that there are marked shifts in pacemaker frequency. Using the same preparation as Woollacott and Hoyle, Nathanson (1977) has some evidence to suggest that cyclic AMP can interfere with this simple learning response. It is conceivable, therefore, that cyclic AMP exerts its effect by modulating this spontaneous activity. The ability of cyclic AMP to inhibit the spontaneous firing of cerebellar Purkinje cells was described earlier, and similar effects have been reported in burster cells of *Aplysia* (Triestman and Levitan 1976a,b). The mechanism of spontaneous activity, especially in mammalian neurons, is not fully understood, but there is considerable information on invertebrate burster neurons.

The large neurosecretory cells in the abdominal ganglion of *Aplysia* have an unstable membrane potential: there is a regular slow wave with bursts of action potentials on the crests (Figure 7). These action potentials are both sodium- and calcium-dependent. During the course of each burst there is a large increase in the intracellular level of calcium (Figure 8; see also Stinnakre and Tauc, 1973), which may be responsible for switching on the potassium channels that contribute to the membrane hyperpolarization that terminates the burst (Junge and Stephens, 1973). The existence of a calcium-dependent potassium conductance was previously demonstrated by injecting calcium into these neurons (Meech, 1972, 1976). After hyperpolarizing at the end of each burst, the

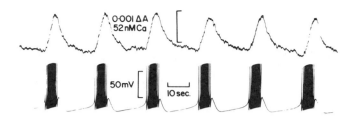

FIGURE 8   Changes in the intracellular level of calcium (upper trace) during spontaneous bursting pacemaker activity in the R15 neuron of *Aplysia*. The slow depolarization following the burst is illustrated in the lower trace. (From Thomas and Gorman, 1977.)

membrane gradually begins to depolarize (the pacemaker potential) until it reaches the threshold for the next burst of action potentials. This fluctuation in potassium conductance entrained to fluctuations in the intracellular level of calcium is a key feature of the oscillatory behavior of such burster cells (Eckert and Lux, 1976).

The picture is complicated by the existence of a slow background inward current (perhaps carried by calcium), which helps to depolarize the membrane during the pacemaker potential (Eckert and Lux, 1976). At the end of the burst, this slow inward current switches off and contributes, together with the calcium-induced increase in potassium conductance, to the rapid hyperpolarization that terminates the burst. It has not been established whether this slow inward current is separate from the fast inward current (calcium and sodium) responsible for the action potentials. It is also not clear how this slow current system is regulated.

An interesting feature of these burster cells is that the pacemaker rhythm persists even when the action potentials are abolished by adding TTX in a calcium-free medium (Junge and Stephens, 1973). In crustacean ganglia, there are oscillator neurons that do not have spikes even under normal conditions (Mendelson, 1971). The fact that oscillations persist in the absence of the large calcium input that occurs during the burst of action potentials suggests that this oscillator may not be driven solely by changes in the membrane but that there may be an interplay with underlying metabolic events.

Ionic fluxes induced by changes in the membrane may alter various cytoplasmic components, such as cyclic AMP and calcium, which in turn may feed back to affect the membrane. On the basis of our current information on the feedback interactions that exist between cyclic AMP and calcium, it is possible to construct a negative feedback oscillator that is theoretically capable of generating stable fluctuations of cyclic AMP and calcium that are 180° out of phase (Rapp and Berridge, 1977). It is interesting to speculate how such a cyclic AMP–calcium oscillator may function in concert with the membrane events described earlier to establish stable membrane fluctuations. The metabolic oscillator might be linked to the membrane through the effect of calcium on potassium conductance. The fluctuations in cyclic AMP level may also alter membrane potential if calcium entry in these nerve cells is sensitive to cyclic AMP, as is the case in the heart (Reuter, 1974). The main point to stress at this stage is that an understanding of oscillatory phenomena will develop not only from studying membrane events but also from considering how these events are integrated with underlying metabolic events.

Metabolic alterations brought about through the action of neurotransmitters may be particularly important in mediating long-lasting alterations in pacemaker activity. Parnas, Armstrong, and Strumwasser, (1974) found that exciting the cell with current did not duplicate the prolonged modulation of bursting activity normally elicited by synaptic activity. Therefore, in addition to mediating the short-term changes in ion conductance, the neurotransmitter was capable of inducing cellular changes of much longer duration. There are some indications that cyclic AMP may play a role in some of these long-lasting effects on burster activity (Triestman and Levitan, 1976a,b; see Levitan, this volume, for details on the role of neural peptides and cyclic AMP in the modulation of *Helix* and *Aplysia* neurons). The hyperpolarization that follows an increase in the intracellular level of cyclic AMP could develop through the positive feedback effect of this nucleotide that increases calcium to levels that induce longer-lasting increases in ion conductance. The time required to dissipate these much larger pulses of calcium will automatically lead to a slowing of the rhythm. Such a mechanism has been demonstrated by Thomas and Gorman (1977), who greatly increased the amount of calcium entering during a burst by passing current into the cell. The much larger increase in calcium concentration produced a much larger hyperpolarization, which led to a longer pacemaker potential. As noted above, such perturbations induced by current injection were short-lived and subsequent bursts were normal.

Control of release

Another way of regulating nerve function is to modulate, both positively and negatively, the amount of neurotransmitter released from the synaptic endings.

During synaptic depression there is a decline in the effectiveness of the synapse, which may account for the phenomenon of habituation that has been studied extensively in the gill-withdrawal reflex of *Aplysia* (Jacklet and Rine, 1977). The reason for this depression is not clear, but it most likely reflects a failure of the calcium-control mechanisms responsible for transmitter release. Since habituation can be reversed by cyclic AMP (Brunelli, Castellucci, and Kandel, 1976), it has been suggested that interactions between cyclic AMP and calcium play an important role in the facilitation of synaptic transmission.

Biogenic amines such as epinephrine and 5-HT can enhance transmission in both central and peripheral nerves. There are two major forms of control (Figure 9). First, the transmission at a synapse can be regulated by another nerve terminal. Second, the neurotransmitters released from the synapse can feed back to influence further release from that terminal. In addition, the synapse may be sensitive to agents that act as local hormones exerting global effects on large groups of nerve cells.

Starke (1977) has reviewed the presynaptic receptor systems responsible for regulating the release of norepinephrine. In general, α-adrenergic agents greatly reduce the stimulus-induced release of norepinephrine from a large number of tissues. This is surprising because in nonneuronal tissues, α-adrenergic agents usually act by increasing calcium entry. If activation of the α-receptor introduces large amounts of calcium into the terminal, it is conceivable

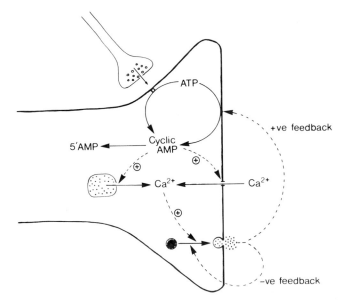

FIGURE 9 Summary of some of the mechanisms that have been invoked to account for presynaptic modulation of transmitter release.

that secretion may be blocked in the same way as amylase release from the insect salivary gland is inhibited by too much calcium. Activation of β-receptors seems to facilitate release, thus creating a positive feedback effect that seems to be mediated by cyclic AMP. It has been proposed that as norepinephrine is released, there is an initial positive feedback that facilitates further release until the transmitter level reaches the threshold concentration necessary to activate the α-receptors, which will then reduce release through their negative feedback effect (Adler-Graschinsky and Langer, 1975). Since little is known about the mechanism of the inhibitory effect exerted by adrenergic agents, attention will be focused on the possible role of cyclic AMP in mediating presynaptic facilitation produced by β-adrenergic agents and other amines such as 5-HT.

Exogenous cyclic AMP can increase transmitter release from neuromuscular junctions (Goldberg and Singer, 1969; Miyamoto and Breckenridge, 1974; Wilson, 1974; Dretchen et al., 1976; Standaert et al., 1976), sympathetic neurons (Wooten et al., 1973; Cubeddu, Barnes, and Weiner, 1975), rat striatal slices (Westfall, Kitay, and Wahl, 1976), and *Aplysia* neurons (Brunelli, Castellucci, and Kandel, 1976; Shimahara and Tauc, 1977). Cyclic AMP can increase the rate of spontaneous electrical activity in the neurohemal organ of an insect (Finlayson and Osborne, 1977). The physiological significance or the precise mode of action of cyclic AMP in many of these examples is still largely unknown. In their study on *Aplysia* neurons, Shimahara and Tauc (1977) noted that the ability of dibutyryl cyclic AMP to prolong facilitation was restricted to specific synapses and was not a general phenomenon common to all synaptic endings. This is an important point as it stresses the fact that facilitation may not be widespread but may be confined to specific synapses where it has a precise physiological role.

Since transmitter release is sensitive to the intracellular level of calcium, it is conceivable that cyclic AMP may act by somehow augmenting this calcium signal during stimulus-secretion coupling (Crain and Pollack, 1973; Wooten et al., 1973). Crain and Pollack (1973) proposed such an action in order to explain how cyclic AMP added to cultured CNS tissue was able to restore "complex bioelectric activities" in a low-calcium medium. They proposed that the calcium mobilized by cyclic AMP augments the small amount of calcium entering from outside to produce a calcium signal sufficient to trigger the synaptic events that mediate these bioelectric discharges (Figure 9). This may be an example of the threshold phenomenon discussed already (Figure 4). If the resting level of calcium falls during calcium deprivation, this might explain the very long stimulus-response latencies found in low-calcium media. When the resting level of calcium is set considerably below threshold, it will take much longer to develop an effective signal. The fact that normal latencies return after adding cyclic AMP lends support to the idea that it may raise the resting level of calcium. The restorative effect of cyclic AMP was not maintained, suggesting a depletion of the stores from which calcium was being released.

In *Aplysia*, there are 5-HT neurons that appear to facilitate the release of transmitter from a neighboring synapse (Brunelli, Castellucci, and Kandel, 1976; Shimahara and Tauc, 1977). In one case, the sensory neurons that innervate the gill motoneurons habituate during repetitive activity but can be sensitized if treated with 5-HT or with dibutyryl cyclic AMP (Brunelli, Castellucci, and Kandel, 1976). Brunelli, Castellucci, and Kandel (1976) propose that 5-HT released from the serotoninergic neurons act on the terminals of the sensory neurons to raise the intracellular level of cyclic AMP, which can then act to increase transmitter release either by increasing the level of free calcium or by enhancing the calcium conductance of the plasma membrane (Figure 9). Shimahara and Tauc (1977) favor the latter mechanism and have some evidence to suggest that cyclic AMP acts on the active channel for calcium in a manner similar to that described in the heart (Reuter, 1974). It should also be noted that 5-HT might have a direct effect on calcium entry, as occurs in the insect salivary gland (Berridge and Lipke, 1979), in addition to its indirect effects mediated by cyclic AMP.

It is important to stress that most of the evidence implicating an effect of cyclic AMP on calcium homeostasis is somewhat indirect. In the case of neurotransmitter release from the neuromuscular synapse, an early report that cyclic AMP can increase the frequency of MEPP (Goldberg and Singer, 1969) has not been supported by subsequent studies (Miyamoto and Breckenridge, 1974; Wilson, 1974). However, Miyamoto and Breckenridge (1974) did find that dibutyryl cyclic AMP was able to reverse neuromuscular fatigue that developed after prolonged stimulation. They suggested that cyclic AMP has an effect on calcium conductance that resembles the mechanism proposed by Shimahara and Tauc (1977). A similar mechanism may account for the "stimulus-bound repetitive activity" observed in mammalian motoneurons during stimulation with dibutyryl cyclic AMP (Dretchen et al., 1976).

While numerous attempts have been made to interpret the facilitation obtained with cyclic AMP in terms of effects on calcium homeostasis, it has also been suggested that cyclic AMP acts by stimulating the synthesis and availability of neurotransmitters (Wilson, 1974). The activity of tyrosine hydroxylase in rat striatal synaptosomes is markedly increased by dibutyryl cyclic AMP (Harris et al., 1975). It is clear that the control of transmitter release is complex and can involve short-term factors, perhaps using second messengers such as cyclic AMP and calcium, in addition to a number of long-term mechanisms (see Fillenz, 1977).

Conclusion

Cyclic nucleotides and calcium play a central role in the regulation and modulation of neuronal function. In addition to mediating the release of neurotransmitters from synaptic sites, calcium also regulates the excitability of many neurons through its ability to alter various ion conductances. While there is growing evidence that cyclic nucleotides are intimately involved in the modulation of various neuronal events, their precise mode of action is unknown. There is some evidence to suggest that they act indirectly by adjusting the level of calcium through a variety of second-messenger interactions. In general, cyclic AMP seems to augment the intracellular level of calcium, whereas cyclic GMP may act in the opposite way. Such antagonistic effects on the level of calcium is certainly compatible with the observation that these two nucleotides often exert opposite effects on neuronal excitability.

Another important feature of the action of cyclic nucleotides in the nervous system is that their effects are relatively long-lasting. For example, the inhibitory effect of cyclic AMP in burster cells can persist for many hours. Such long-lasting modulation of neuronal activity, which underlies a variety of higher brain functions, may thus depend on the action of cyclic nucleotides.

REFERENCES

ADLER-GRASCHINSKY, E., and S. Z. LANGER, 1975. Possible role of a β-adrenoceptor in the regulation of noradrenaline release by nerve stimulation through a positive feedback mechanism. *Br. J. Pharmacol.* 53:43–50.

ALNAES, E., and R. RAHAMIMOFF, 1975. On the role of mitochondria in transmitter release from motor nerve terminals. *J. Physiol.* 248:285–306.

BAKER, P. F., 1976. The regulation of intracellular calcium. *Symp. Soc. Exp. Biol.* 30:60–88.

BAKER, P. F., and A. C. CRAWFORD, 1975. A note on the mechanisms by which inhibitors of the sodium pump accelerate spontaneous release of transmitter from motor nerve terminals. *J. Physiol.* 247:209–226.

BAKER, P. F., and P. A. McNAUGHTON, 1978. The influence of extracellular calcium on the calcium efflux from squid axons. *J. Physiol.* 276:127–150.

BERRIDGE, M. J., 1975. The interaction of cyclic nucleotides and calcium in the control of cellular activity. *Adv. Cyclic Nucleotide Res.* 6:1–98.

BERRIDGE, M. J., and H. LIPKE, 1979. Changes in calcium transport across *Calliphora* salivary glands induced by 5-hydroxytryptamine and cyclic AMP. *J. Exp. Biol.* (in press).

BLAUSTEIN, M. P., 1975. Effects of potassium, veratridine and scorpion venom on calcium accumulation and transmitter release by nerve terminals *in vitro*. *J. Physiol.* 247:617–655.

BLOOM, F. E., 1975. The role of cyclic nucleotides in central synaptic function. *Rev. Physiol. Biochem. Pharmacol.* 74:1–103.

BLOOM, F. E., G. R. SIGGINS, B. J. HOFFER, M. SEGAL, and A. P. OLIVER, 1975. Cyclic nucleotides in the central synaptic actions of catecholamines. *Adv. Cyclic Nucleotide Res.* 5:603–618.

BORLE, A. B., 1974. Cyclic AMP stimulation of calcium efflux from kidney, liver and heart mitochondria. *J. Membr. Biol.* 16:221–236.

BORLE, A. B., 1976. Cyclic AMP stimulation of calcium efflux from isolated mitochondria: A negative report. *J. Membr. Biol.* 29:209–210.

BRISSON, G. R., and W. J. MALAISSE, 1973. The stimulus secretion coupling of glucose-induced insulin release. XI. Effects of theophylline and epinephrine on ^{45}Ca efflux from perifused islets. *Metabolism* 22:455–465.

BRISSON, G. R., F. MALAISSE-LAGAE, and W. J. MALAISSE, 1972. The stimulus-secretion coupling of glucose-induced insulin release. VII. A proposed site of action for adenosine 3′,5′-cyclic monophosphate. *J. Clin. Invest.* 51:232–241.

BRUNELLI, M., V. CASTELLUCCI, and E. R. KANDEL, 1976. Synaptic facilitation and behavioural sensitization in *Aplysia*: possible role of serotonin and cyclic AMP. *Science* 194:1178–1181.

BUSIS, N. A., and F. F. WEIGHT, 1976. Spike after-hyperpolarisation of a sympathetic neurone is calcium sensitive and is potentiated by theophylline. *Nature* 263:434–436.

BUTCHER, F. R., 1975. The role of calcium and cyclic nucleotides in α-amylase release from slices of rat parotid: Studies with divalent cation ionophore A-23187. *Metabolism* 24:409–418.

CARAFOLI, E., K. MALMSTRÖM, M. CAPANO, E. SIGEL, and M. CROMPTON, 1975. Mitochondria and the regulation of cell calcium. In *Calcium Transport in Contraction and Secretion*, E. Carafoli, F. Clementi, W. Drabikowski, and A. Margreth, eds. Amsterdam: North-Holland, pp. 53–64.

CHEUNG, W. Y., L. S. BRADHAM, T. J. LYNCH, Y. M. LIN, and E. A. TALLANT, 1975. Protein activator of cyclic 3′,5′-nucleotide phosphodiesterase of bovine or rat brain also activates its adenylate cyclase. *Biochem. Biophys. Res. Commun.* 66:1055–1062.

CRAIN, S. M., and E. D. POLLACK, 1973. Restorative effects of cyclic AMP on complex bioelectric activities of cultured fetal rodent CNS tissues after acute Ca⁺⁺ deprivation. *J. Neurobiol.* 4:321-342.

CRAWFORD, A. C., 1975. Lithium ions and the release of transmitter at the frog neuromuscular junction. *J. Physiol.* 246:109-142.

CUBEDDU, L. X., E. BARNES, and N. WEINER, 1975. Release of norepinephrine and dopamine-β-hydroxylase by nerve stimulation. IV. An evaluation of a role for cyclic adenosine monophosphate. *J. Pharmacol. Exp. Ther.* 193:105-127.

CURTIS, D. R., D. D. PERRIN, and J. C. WATKINS, 1960. The excitation of spinal neurones by the iontophoretic application of agents which chelate calcium. *J. Neurochem.* 6:1-20.

DALEY, D. L., and J. S. VAN DE BERG, 1976. Apparent apposing effects of cyclic AMP and dibutyryl cyclic GMP on the neuronal firing of the blowfly chemoreceptors. *Biochim. Biophys. Acta* 437:211-220.

DRETCHEN, K. L., F. G. STANDAERT, L. R. SKIRBOLL, and V. H. MORGENROTH, 1976. Evidence for a prejunctional role of cyclic nucleotides in neuromuscular transmission. *Nature* 264:79-81.

DRUMMOND, G. I., and Y. MA, 1973. Metabolism and functions of cyclic AMP in nerve. *Prog. Neurobiol.* 2:121-176.

DUNCAN, C. J., 1976. Properties of the Ca²⁺-ATPase activity of mammalian membrane preparations. *J. Neurochem.* 27:1277-1279.

ECKERT, R., and H. D. LUX, 1976. A voltage-sensitive persistent calcium conductance in neuronal somata of *Helix*. *J. Physiol.* 254:129-151.

ELMQVIST, D., and D. S. FELDMAN, 1965. Calcium dependence of spontaneous acetylcholine release at mammalian motor nerve terminals *J. Physiol.* 181:487-497.

EXTON, J. H., G. A. ROBISON, E. W. SUTHERLAND, and C. R. PARK, 1971. Studies on the role of adenosine 3',5'-monophosphate in the hepatic actions of glucagon and catecholamines. *J. Biol. Chem.* 246:6166-6177.

FERRENDELLI, J. A., D. A. KINSCHERF, and M. M. CHANG, 1973. Regulation of levels of guanosine cyclic 3',5'-monophosphate in the central nervous system: Effects of depolarising agents. *Mol. Pharmacol.* 9:445-454.

FERRENDELLI, J. A., E. H. RUBIN, and D. A. KINSCHERF, 1976. Influence of divalent cations on regulation of cyclic GMP and cyclic AMP levels in brain tissue. *J. Neurochem.* 26:741-748.

FILLENZ, M., 1977. The factors which provide short-term and long-term control of transmitter release. *Prog. Neurobiol.* 8:251-278.

FINLAYSON, L. H., and M. P. OSBORNE, 1977. Effect of cyclic AMP and other compounds on electrical activity of neurohaemal tissue in *Carausius*. *J. Insect Physiol.* 23:429-434.

FREEDMAN, M. H., M. C. RAFF, and B. GOMPERTS, 1975. Induction of increased calcium uptake in mouse T lymphocytes by concanavalin A and its modulation by cyclic nucleotides. *Nature* 255:378-382.

FRIEDMANN, N., 1972. Effects of glucagon and cyclic AMP on ion fluxes in the perfused liver. *Biochim. Biophys. Acta* 274:214-225.

GELLER, H. M., and B. J. HOFFER, 1977. Effect of calcium removal on monamine-elicited depressions of cultured tuberal neurons. *J. Neurobiol.* 8:43-55.

GEORGE, W. J., R. D. WILKERSON, and P. J. KODOWITZ, 1973. Influence of acetylcholine on contractile force and cyclic nucleotide levels in the isolated perfused rat heart. *J. Pharmacol. Exp. Ther.* 184:228-235.

GINSBORG, B. L., and G. D. S. HIRST, 1972. The effect of adenosine on the release of the transmitter from the phrenic nerve of the rat. *J. Physiol.* 224:629-645.

GOLDBERG, A. L., and J. J. SINGER, 1969. Evidence for the role of cyclic AMP in neuromuscular transmission. *Proc. Natl. Acad. Sci. USA* 64:134-141.

GOLDBERG, N. D., R. F. O'DEA, and M. K. HADDOX, 1973. Cyclic GMP. In *Advances in Cyclic Nucleotide Research*, vol. 3, P. Greengard and G. A. Robison, eds. New York: Raven Press, pp. 155-223.

GOSHIMA, K., 1976. Antagonistic influences of dibutyryl cyclic AMP and dibutyryl cyclic GMP on the beating rate of cultured mouse myocardial cells. *J. Mol. Cell. Cardiol.* 8:713-725.

GREENGARD, P., 1976. Possible role for cyclic nucleotides and phosphorylated membrane proteins in postsynaptic actions of neurotransmitters. *Nature* 260:101-108.

HANSEN BAY, C. M., 1978. The control of enzyme secretion from fly salivary glands. *J. Physiol.* 274:421-435.

HARRIS, J. E., R. J. BALDESSARINI, V. H. MORGENROTH, and R. H. ROTH, 1975. Activation by cyclic 3',5' adenosine monophosphate of tyrosine hydroxylase in the rat brain. *Proc. Natl. Acad. Sci. USA* 72:789-793.

HENKART, M., D. M. D. LANDIS, and T. S. REESE, 1976. Similarity of junctions between plasma membranes and endoplasmic reticulum in muscle and neurons. *J. Cell Biol.* 70:338-347.

HOFFER, B. J., Å. SEIGER, R. FREEDMAN, L. OLSON, and D. TAYLOR, 1977. Electrophysiology and cytology of hippocampal formation transplants in the anterior chamber of the eye. II Cholinergic mechanisms. *Brain Res.* 119:107-132.

IGNARRO, L. J., 1974. Nonphagocytic release of neutral protease and β-glucuronidase from human neutrophils. *Arthritis Rheum.* 17:25-36.

JACKLET, J. W., and J. RINE, 1977. Facilitation at neuromuscular junctions: Contribution to habituation and dishabituation of the *Aplysia* gill withdrawal reflex. *Proc. Natl. Acad. Sci. USA* 74:1267-1271.

JUNDT, H., H. PORZIG, H. REUTER, and J. W. STUCKI, 1975. The effect of substances releasing intracellular calcium ions on sodium-dependent calcium efflux from guinea-pig auricles. *J. Physiol.* 246:229-253.

JUNGE, D., and C. L. STEPHENS, 1973. Cyclic variation of potassium conductance in a burst-generating neurone in *Aplysia*. *J. Physiol.* 235:155-181.

KEBABIAN, J. W., F. E. BLOOM, A. L. STEINER, and P. GREENGARD, 1975. Neurotransmitters increase cyclic nucleotides in postganglionic neurons: Immunocytochemical demonstrations. *Science* 190:157-159.

KEBABIAN, J. W., A. L. STEINER, and P. GREENGARD, 1975. Muscarinic cholinergic regulation of cyclic guanosine 3',5'-monophosphate in autonomic ganglia: Possible role in synaptic transmission. *J. Pharmacol. Exp. Ther.* 193:474-488.

LEE, T.-P., J. F. KUO, and P. GREENGARD, 1972. Role of muscarinic cholinergic receptors in regulation of guanosine 3',5'-cyclic monophosphate content in mammalian brain, heart muscle, and intestinal smooth muscle. *Proc. Natl. Acad. Sci. USA* 69:3287-3291.

LIBET, B., H. KOBAYASHI, and T. TANAKA, 1975. Synaptic

coupling into the production and storage of a neuronal memory trace. *Nature* 258:155–157.

Llinás, R., J. R. Blinks, and C. Nicholson, 1972. Calcium transient in presynaptic terminal of squid giant synapse: Detection with aequorin. *Science* 176:1127–1129.

Lowe, D. A., B. P. Richardson, P. Taylor, and P. Donatsch, 1976. Increasing intracellular sodium triggers calcium release from bound pools. *Nature* 260:337–338.

McAfee, D. A., and P. Greengard, 1972. Adenosine 3′,5′-monophosphate: Electrophysiological evidence for a role in synaptic transmission. *Science* 178:310–312.

Meech, R. W., 1972. Intracellular calcium injection causes increased potassium conductance in *Aplysia* nerve cells. *Comp. Biochem. Physiol.* 42A:493–499.

Meech, R. W., 1974a. The sensitivity of *Helix aspersa* neurones to injected calcium ions. *J. Physiol.* 237:259–277.

Meech, R. W., 1974b. Prolonged action potentials in *Aplysia* neurones injected with EGTA. *Comp. Biochem. Physiol.* 48A:397–402.

Meech, R. W., 1976. Intracellular calcium and the control of membrane permeability. *Symp. Soc. Exp. Biol.* 30:161–191.

Mendelson, M., 1971. Oscillator neurons in crustacean ganglia. *Science* 171:1170–1173.

Michell, R. H., 1975. Inositol phospholipids and cell surface receptor function. *Biochim. Biophys. Acta* 415:81–147.

Michell, R. H., S. S. Jafferji, and L. M. Jones, 1976. Receptor occupancy dose-response curve suggests that phosphatidylinositol breakdown may be intrinsic to the mechanism of the muscarinic cholinergic receptor. *FEBS Lett.* 69:1–5.

Miledi, R., and C. R. Slater, 1966. The action of calcium on neuronal synapses in the squid. *J. Physiol.* 184:473–498.

Miyamoto, M. D., and B. McL. Breckenridge, 1974. A cyclic adenosine monophosphate link in the catecholamine enhancement of transmitter release at the neuromuscular junction. *J. Gen. Physiol.* 63:609–624.

Nathanson, J. A., 1977. Cyclic nucleotides and nervous system function. *Physiol. Rev.* 57:157–256.

Nicholson, C., G. ten Bruggencate, R. Steinberg, and H. Stöckle, 1977. Calcium modulation in brain extracellular microenvironment demonstrated with ion-selective micropipette. *Proc. Natl. Acad. Sci. USA* 74:1287–1290.

Park, C. R., S. B. Lewis, and J. H. Exton, 1972. Relationship of some hepatic actions of insulin to the intracellular level of cyclic adenylate. *Diabetes* 21:439–446.

Parnas, I., D. Armstrong, and F. Strumwasser, 1974. Prolonged excitatory and inhibitory synaptic modulation of a bursting pacemaker neuron. *J. Neurophysiol.* 37:594–608.

Phillis, J. W., N. Lake, and G. Yarbrough, 1973. Calcium mediation of the inhibitory effects of biogenic amines on cerebral cortical neurones. *Brain Res.* 53:465–469.

Prince, W. T., and M. J. Berridge, 1973. The role of calcium in the action of 5-hydroxytryptamine and cyclic AMP on salivary glands. *J. Exp. Biol.* 58:367–384.

Prince, W. T., M. J. Berridge, and H. Rasmussen, 1972. Role of calcium and adenosine-3′,5′-cyclic monophosphate in controlling fly salivary gland secretion. *Proc. Natl. Acad. Sci. USA* 69:553–557.

Purves, R. D., 1976. Function of muscarinic and nicotinic acetylcholine receptors. *Nature* 261:149–150.

Ransom, B. R., J. L. Barker, and P. G. Nelson, 1975. Two mechanisms for poststimulus hyperpolarisations in cultured mammalian neurones. *Nature* 256:424–425.

Rapp, P. E., and M. J. Berridge, 1977. Oscillations in calcium-cyclic AMP control loops form the basis of pacemaker activity and other high frequency biological rhythms. *J. Theoret. Biol.* 66:497–525.

Reuter, H., 1974. Exchange of calcium ions in the mammalian myocardium. *Circ. Res.* 34:599–605.

Rose, B., and W. R. Loewenstein, 1975. Calcium ion distribution in cytoplasm visualized by aequorin: Diffusion in cytosol restricted by energized sequestering. *Science* 190:1204–1206.

Rosenblatt, D. E., C. J. Lauter, and E. G. Trams, 1976. Deficiency of a Ca^{2+}-ATPase in brains of seizure prone mice. *J. Neurochem.* 27:1299–1304.

de Scarnati, O. C., M. Sato, and E. de Robertis, 1976. Muscarinic receptors and the ACh stimulated phosphatidylinositol effects in the CNS. *J. Neurochem.* 27:1575–1577.

Scarpa, A., K. Malmstrom, M. Chiesi, and E. Carafoli, 1976. On the problem of the release of mitochondrial calcium by cyclic AMP. *J. Membr. Biol.* 29:205–208.

Schatzmann, H. J., 1975. Active calcium transport across the plasma membrane of erythrocytes. In *Calcium Transport in Contraction and Secretion*, E. Carafoli, F. Clementi, W. Drabikowski, and A. Margreth, eds. Amsterdam: North-Holland, pp. 45–49.

Schmitt, F. O., P. Dev, and B. H. Smith, 1976. Electrotonic processing of information by brain cells. *Science* 193:114–120.

Schulman, J. A., and F. F. Weight, 1976. Synaptic transmission: Long-lasting potentiation by a postsynaptic mechanism. *Science* 194:1437–1439.

Schultz, G., J. G. Hardman, K. Schultz, C. E. Baird, and E. W. Sutherland, 1973. The importance of calcium ions for the regulation of guanosine 3′:5′-cyclic monophosphate levels. *Proc. Natl. Acad. Sci. USA* 70:3889–3893.

Schultz, J., 1975. Cyclic adenosine 3′,5′-monophosphate in guinea pig cerebral cortical slices: Possible regulation of phosphodiesterase activity by cyclic adenosine 3′,5′-monophosphate and calcium ions. *J. Neurochem.* 24:495–501.

Schultz, K.-D., K. Schultz, and G. Schultz, 1977. Sodium nitroprusside and other smooth muscle relaxants increase cyclic GMP levels in rat ductus deferens. *Nature* 265:750–751.

Selinger, Z., S. Eimerl, and M. Schramm, 1974. A calcium ionphore simulating the action of epinephrine on the α-adrenergic receptor. *Proc. Natl. Acad. Sci. USA* 71:128–131.

Shimahara, T., and L. Tauc, 1977. Cyclic AMP induced by serotonin modulates the activity of an identified synapse in *Aplysia* by facilitating the active permeability to calcium. *Brain Res.* 127:168–172.

Siggins, G. R., and S. J. Henriksen, 1975. Analogs of cyclic adenosine monophosphate: Correlation of inhibition of Purkinje neurons with protein kinase activation. *Science* 189:559–561.

Siggins, G. R., A. P. Oliver, B. J. Hoffer, and F. E. Bloom, 1971. Cyclic adenosine monophosphate and norepinephrine: Effects on transmembrane properties of cerebellar Purkinje cells. *Science* 171:192–194.

SMITH, P. A., and F. F. WEIGHT, 1977. Role of electrogenic sodium pump in slow synaptic inhibition is re-evaluated. *Nature* 267:68–70.

STANDAERT, F. G., K. L. DRETCHEN, L. R. SKIRBOLL, and V. H. MORGENROTH, 1976. Effects of cyclic nucleotides on mammalian terminals. *J. Pharmacol. Exp. Ther.* 199:544–552.

STARKE, K., 1977. Regulation of noradrenaline release by presynaptic receptor systems. *Rev. Physiol. Biochem. Pharmacol.* 77:1–124.

STINNAKRE, J., and L. TAUC, 1973. Calcium influx in active *Aplysia* neurones detected by injected aequorin. *Nature* [*New Biol.*] 242:113–115.

STONE, T. W., and D. A. TAYLOR, 1977. Microiontophoretic studies of the effects of cyclic nucleotides on excitability of neurones in the rat cerebral cortex. *J. Physiol.* 266:523–543.

STONE, T. W., D. A. TAYLOR, and F. E. BLOOM, 1975. Cyclic AMP and cyclic GMP may mediate opposite neuronal responses in the rat cerebral cortex. *Science* 187:845–846.

THOA, N. B., G. F. WOOTON, J. AXELROD, and I. J. KOPIN, 1975. On the mechanism of release of norepinephrine from sympathetic nerves induced by depolarizing agents and sympathomimetic drugs. *Mol. Pharmacol.* 11:10–18.

THOMAS, M. V., and A. L. F. GORMAN, 1977. Internal calcium changes in a bursting pacemaker neuron measured with arsenazo III. *Science* 196:531–533.

TRIESTMAN, S. N., and I. B. LEVITAN, 1976a. Alteration of electrical activity in molluscan neurones by cyclic nucleotides and peptide factors. *Nature* 261:62–64.

TRIESTMAN, S. N., and I. B. LEVITAN, 1976b. Intraneuronal guanylylimidodiphosphate injection mimics long-term synaptic hyperpolarization in *Aplysia*. *Proc. Natl. Acad. Sci. USA* 73:1689–1692.

TUTTLE, J. S., and E. RICHELSON, 1975. Ionic excitation of a clone of mouse neuroblastoma. *Brain Res.* 84:129–135.

WALLACH, D., and I. PASTAN, 1976. Stimulation of membranous guanylate cyclase by concentrations of calcium that are in the physiological range. *Bichem. Biophys. Res. Commun.* 72:859–865.

WANG, J. L., D. A. MCCLAIN, and G. M. EDELMAN, 1975. Modulation of lymphocyte mitogenesis. *Proc. Natl. Acad. Sci. USA* 72:1917–1921.

WEIGHT, F. F., 1974. Physiological mechanisms of synaptic modulation. In *The Neurosciences: Third Study Program*, F. O. Schmitt and F. G. Worden, eds. Cambridge, MA: MIT Press, pp. 929–941.

WESTFALL, T. C., D. KITAY, and G. WAHL, 1976. The effect of cyclic nucleotides on the release of ^{3}H-dopamine from rat striatal slices. *J. Pharmacol. Exp. Ther.* 199:149–157.

WILLIAMS, J. A., 1975. Na^+ dependence of in vitro pancreatic amylase release. *Am. J. Physiol.* 229:1023–1026.

WILLIAMS, M., and R. RODNIGHT, 1977. Protein phosphorylation in nervous tissue: Possible involvement in nervous tissue function and relationship to cyclic nucleotide metabolism. *Prog. Neurobiol.* 8:183–250.

WILSON, D. F., 1974. The effects of dibutyryl cyclic adenosine 3′,5′-monophosphate, theophylline and aminophylline on neuromuscular transmission in the rat. *J. Pharmacol. Exp. Ther.* 188:447–452.

WOOLLACOTT, M., and G. HOYLE, 1977. Neural events underlying learning in insects: Changes in pacemaker. *Proc. R. Soc. Lond.* B195:395–415.

WOOTEN, G. F., N. B. THOA, I. J. KOPIN, and J. AXELROD, 1973. Enhanced release of dopamine β-hydroxylase and norepinephrine from sympathetic nerves by dibutyryl cyclic adenosine 3′,5′-monophosphate and theophylline. *Mol. Pharmacol.* 9:178–183.

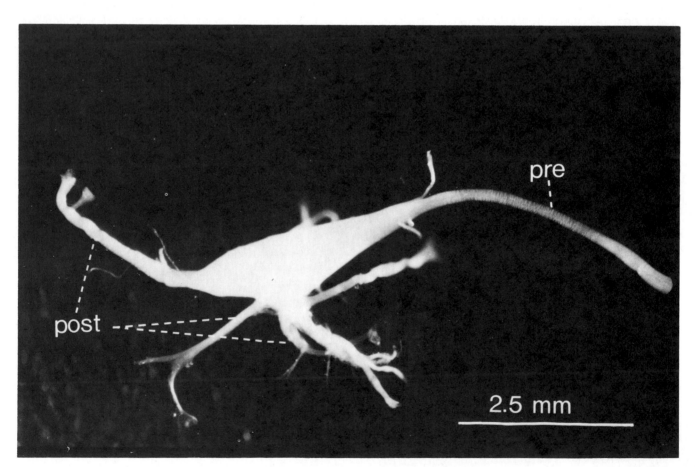

REGULATION OF GENE EXPRESSION IN THE NERVOUS SYSTEM

Organization of the peripheral sympathetic nervous system. The top part of the figure shows the scheme of preganglionic cholinergic and postganglionic adrenergic neurons with the pathway of synthesis of the adrenergic transmitter. The bottom shows a rat sympathetic ganglion with pre- and postganglionic fibers prepared for organ culture. (See the chapter by H. Thoenen, U. Otten, and M. Schwab, this volume.)

Introduction

HANS THOENEN

THIS SECTION compiles the essential information on the importance of the regulation of gene expression in the long-term modulation of neuronal function and structure. It will become clear that the interpretation of the topic has been handled liberally and that aspects have been included in which the regulation of gene expression is now only suspected of playing a causative role in conjunction with other processes such as the long term covalent modification of macromolecules, which was discussed in detail in the preceding section.

R. J. Wurtman, M. A. Moskowitz, and H. N. Munro set the framework for the discussion by summing up the present state of knowledge of eukaryotic protein synthesis and its regulation. They focus first on possible peculiarities of protein synthesis in neuronal systems, particularly the mammalian brain, and then characterize conditions under which the protein synthesis of the whole brain is affected by modifications of ribosomal function. These modifications are characterized by changes in the monopolymeric pattern of ribosomes, initiated either by direct actions on the ribosomes (as occurs, for instance, after administration of amphetamine) or by an indirect mechanism via membrane receptors (for example, by decarboxylation products of L-dopa). In addition to these general aspects of protein synthesis in neuronal systems, adrenal medullary phenylethanolamine N-methyltransferase is discussed as an example of a predominantly hormonally regulated synthesis of a neuronal macromolecule. This regulation is contrasted with the mainly transsynaptic transmitter-mediated synthesis of tyrosine hydroxylase.

Next, U. Otten, M. Schwab, and I discuss the peripheral sympathetic nervous system as a model for the regulation of the expression of genetic information by nerve impulses and by nerve growth factor. The latter reaches the perikaryon of the adrenergic neurons from their nerve terminals by retrograde axonal transport and so may act as a messenger between effector organs and the perikaryon of the innervating neurons. The selective transsynaptic induction of tyrosine hydroxylase and dopamine-β-hydroxylase is characterized as a special neuronal manifestation of a general phenomenon of cell function—namely, the regulation of gene expression in the cell nucleus as a result of functional changes in the cell membrane effected by exogenous factors. An additional subject is the modulatory role of glucocorticoids on both the selective enzyme induction by nerve growth factor and the transsynaptic induction mediated by acetylcholine. This modulatory role of glucocorticoids in differentiated neurons could be a correlate to the imprinting effect of sex steroids during critical periods of development. This latter aspect is discussed by R. A. Gorski at the end of the section.

Nerve growth factor, produced by nonneuronal cells, is essential for the survival, differentiation, and maintenance of function of sympathetic neurons. P. H. Patterson focuses on another aspect of the interaction between neuronal and nonneuronal cells, namely, how, where, and when the specific biochemical and morphological differentiation of neuronal cells migrating from the neural crest is determined. "Instructive" influences of the environment are well established and impressively demonstrated by transplantation experiments of neural-crest cells, showing that the environment and not the site of origin in the neural crest determines the fate of these neuroblasts. Patterson and his collaborators have developed an in vitro system allowing the analysis of the transformation of adrenergic neurons into cholinergic ones. In contrast to nerve growth factor, the protease-sensitive molecule responsible for this phenomenon is not essential for the survival of the sympathetic neurons. Instead, it carries instructive information, turning on and off the genetic information coding for enzymes synthesizing the corresponding transmitter substances. This instructive factor is formed by several nonneuronal cells such as Schwann cells and heart cells and, in contrast to nerve growth factor, seems to exhibit relatively strict species specificity.

Processes of development and axon regeneration in amphibia are presented by J. Diamond. Such systems proved to be particularly well suited for the study of another aspect of neuron-target interaction—namely, the determination of the density of innervation of a target organ and the delineation of the peripheral areas supplied by nerve fibers from corresponding spinal segments. Although the mechanisms of all these events are not yet understood, a clear descriptive characterization of them provides a solid basis for future studies aimed at the analysis of their underlying mechanisms.

In the subsequent contribution G. S. Lynch and R. M. Akers discuss the implications of "absolute specificity" operating during the formation of defined neuronal connections. They compare this factor with "the competitive growth of nerve fibers" into a given field of innervation, also taking into account the capacity for fiber production of the single neuron. The relatively simply organized mammalian hippocampus has proved a suitable object for such investigations. Here, as in the experiments described by Diamond, we are still in the stage of descriptive analysis, although the biological and biochemical characterization of factors that are released by glial cells and that influence the formation of processes in neuronal tumor cells may give a first insight into the underlying mechanisms. However, it seems too early to transfer the knowledge obtained in simple model systems directly to the interpretation of the mechanisms responsible for either the formation of complex neuronal connections during ontogenesis or their function-dependent modifications after differentiation.

In the last contribution, R. A. Gorski discusses a further aspect of gene regulation: the "imprinting" and "organizing" effects of sexual hormones during critical periods of ontogenesis. These imprinting effects are manifested by permanent changes in sexual behavior after modification of the endogenous hormone supply or hormone administration in the early postnatal period. The permanent behavioral changes are also reflected by marked morphological alterations in the hypothalamus. This imprinting effect of steroid hormones during critical periods of ontogenesis represents an impressive example of how the mosaic of our knowledge increases toward a comprehensive understanding of brain function, linking our knowledge of the molecular mechanism of steroid-hormone action with that of complex behavioral patterns.

The papers in this section suggest that the most promising approach to a comprehensive understanding of brain function—in our particular case of the implications of the regulation of gene expression—is the detailed analysis of simple model systems coupled with precise descriptive analysis of complex systems such as the mammalian brain. The relevance of information evolving from the analysis of model systems can then be verified in the integrated complex systems in a more selective manner, approaching as a final goal a molecular understanding of global functions.

53 Transsynaptic Control of Neuronal Protein Synthesis

RICHARD J. WURTMAN, MICHAEL A. MOSKOWITZ, and HAMISH N. MUNRO

ABSTRACT Some neurotransmitters, like certain hormones, can control the rates at which postsynaptic cells synthesize peptides and proteins. This article reviews the general mechanisms governing protein synthesis in all eukaryotic (nucleated) cells, describes some of the special characteristics of the formation of neuronal proteins, and presents evidence that three drugs that modify monoaminergic transmission—L-dopa, L-5-hydroxytryptophan, and d-amphetamine—can also affect brain protein synthesis. The decarboxylated products of L-dopa (dopamine) and L-5-hydroxytryptophan (serotonin) cause the disaggregation of polyribosomes (or polysomes)—the structures that actually carry out peptide synthesis. d-Amphetamine and related compounds may affect neuronal protein synthesis by a direct action on the protein-synthetic apparatus, that is, by suppressing the process of initiation instead of (or in addition to) acting on the plasma membranes of postsynaptic neurons and other brain cells. The transient polysome disaggregation and the consequent transient suppression of brain protein synthesis that these agents produce may provide useful experimental tools for examining the formation and kinetics of such particular brain proteins and peptides as substance P, a putative neurotransmitter.

Two of the enzymes in adrenomedullary chromaffin cells that catalyze steps in epinephrine biosynthesis are induced by neural or endocrine inputs to these cells. These are tyrosine hydroxylase, which is induced by the release of acetylcholine from the splanchnic nerves, and phenylethanolamine-N-methyl transferase, which is induced by high concentrations of glucocorticoid hormones delivered to the medulla through the intra-adrenal portal vascular system. Glucocorticoid hormones act at a translational level to control the state of polysome aggregation within the medulla; they may also affect protein synthesis at other loci. The mechanism by which cholinergic activation accelerates the synthesis of adrenal tyrosine hydroxylase remains controversial.

RICHARD J. WURTMAN, MICHAEL A. MOSKOWITZ, and HAMISH N. MUNRO Laboratories of Neuroendocrine Regulation and Physiological Chemistry, Department of Nutrition and Food Science, Massachusetts Institute of Technology, Cambridge, MA 02139; Section of Neurology, Department of Medicine, Peter Bent Brigham Hospital and Harvard Medical School, Boston, MA 02115

Introduction

IT IS WELL ESTABLISHED that hormones—particularly the steroids, which penetrate cells readily—can change the levels of proteins within their target organs by modifying the rates at which such proteins are synthesized or, less commonly, degraded (O'Malley and Means, 1974). Of particular interest to neuroscientists is the induction by certain adrenocortical hormones of an adrenomedullary enzyme, phenylethanolamine-N-methyl transferase (PNMT), that catalyzes the last step in epinephrine biosynthesis (Wurtman and Axelrod, 1966; Wurtman, Pohorecky, and Baliga, 1972). Recognition that neurotransmitters also can control protein synthesis has developed more slowly, probably because certain peculiarities of neurons and of the known neurotransmitters enormously complicate the design of experiments to examine this relationship. Chief among these difficulties have been the following:

1. the inability of neurotransmitters, as a group, to enter the cells upon which they act; and the consequent need for "second messengers"—yet to be positively identified (Guidotti and Costa, 1977; Thoenen and Otten, 1976)—to convey their instructions to the cell's nucleus;

2. the inability of neurotransmitters administered systemically even to enter the brain;

3. the fact that mature neurons—unlike the peripheral cells whose protein-synthetic mechanisms are most responsive to hormones—do not divide and probably do not even hypertrophy or shrink to a significant extent;

4. the paucity of well-characterized neuron-specific proteins that can be assayed;

5. the enormous cellular heterogeneity of the brain, which precludes examining the responses of distinct populations of cells without considerable background noise.

This review will summarize our knowledge of neurotransmitter control of neuronal protein synthesis. After a brief description of the steps and the components involved in protein synthesis by all eukaryotic (i.e., nucleated) cells, we shall consider the special characteristics of neuronal protein synthesis and the evidence that such synthesis is affected by neurotransmitters. This evidence derives largely from two kinds of experiments: (1) studies on the effects of various monoaminergic drugs on brain polyribosomes (the organelles that actually carry out the formation of peptide chains), and (2) the in vivo formation of proteins and studies on the effects of cholinergic stimulation on the production of adrenomedullary enzymes in postsynaptic chromaffin cells. (The latter topic is also discussed in this volume by Thoenen, Otten, and Schwab.)

Treatments that enhance the release of monoamine transmitters from neurons and drugs that stimulate pharmacologically defined receptors for these transmitters can affect the levels of proteins in neurons and related cells, probably by affecting the rates at which these proteins are synthesized. This can be shown experimentally by treating animals with drugs that act directly on the presynaptic neuron to enhance monoaminergic transmission (e.g., L-dopa; L-5-hydroxytryptophan; d-amphetamine) or with agents that facilitate neurotransmitter release by reflex mechanisms (e.g., insulin, which causes hypoglycemia, or peripheral 6-hydroxydopamine, which lowers blood pressure); we then measure the in vivo incorporation of isotopically labeled amino acids into proteins, tissue levels of particular proteins (assayed immunochemically), or changes in the extent to which the ribosomal RNA in brain homogenates is present as polyribosomal (or polysomal) aggregates. Only a very few specific proteins can conveniently be assayed in neural tissue; hence most studies on neurotransmitter-induced variations in protein synthesis have examined the changes that occur in proteins as a group. This approach suffers from the fact that brain proteins are highly heterogeneous with respect to turnover. For example, if a treatment doubles the synthesis rates of two brain proteins, one with a half-life of 2 days and the other with a half-life of 30 days, levels of the first protein would increase by almost half after one day, while levels of the second probably would not change detectably, even though its synthesis rate had doubled. Some of the studies described below have examined proteins as a group; others have measured specific proteins such as tubulin and tyrosine hydroxylase.

Mechanism of protein synthesis in eukaryotic cells

The synthesis of proteins involves two distinct phases: *transcription,* in which messenger RNA (mRNA) is copied from a DNA template in the nuclear chromatin, and *translation,* in which the ribosomes in the cytoplasm use the mRNA to direct the incorporation into peptide chains of amino acids bound to transfer RNA (tRNA) (see Figure 1). The two steps are often followed by enzyme-catalyzed (i.e., nonpolysomal) alterations in the newly synthesized peptides by posttranslational modification (e.g., the addition of sugars in the synthesis of glycoproteins; the methylation of histidine in actin; or the amidation of some brain peptides). Each of these processes is subject to regulation at one or more loci (Nowak and Munro, 1977).

TRANSCRIPTION, POSTTRANSCRIPTIONAL CHANGES, AND THEIR CONTROL The information stored in chromosomes is made available by transcribing chromosomal DNA into mRNA. In this process histones and other proteins that bind to chromatin regulate which portions of the encoded information are made available; the precise operation of this regulatory mechanism remains poorly understood. The nucleus

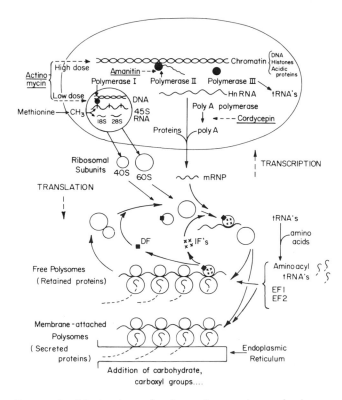

FIGURE 1 Mechanism of eukaryotic protein synthesis.

contains several forms of RNA, which can be separated on sucrose gradients. Ribosomal RNA (rRNA) is made in the nucleolus, initially as a single strand of 45S RNA; this strand undergoes fission to yield material of shorter lengths, ultimately the 28S and 18S RNA found in the 60S and 40S ribosomal subunits (Figure 1). Cleavage of the 45S RNA (maturation) is regulated by methylation of the ribose residues on certain strategic nucleotides. The other major species of RNA involved in protein synthesis—tRNA in the cytoplasm and mRNA within the nucleus—are also methylated. Thus catechols such as L-dopa (Wurtman et al., 1970) and drugs that affect the availability of the methyl donor S-adenosylmethionine could theoretically influence protein synthesis by a variety of mechanisms, provided they are able to enter cells.

Messenger RNA is first made as heterogeneous nuclear RNA (HnRNA) by transcription of the chromosomal DNA. It is subsequently cleaved, perhaps by a mechanism also involving methylation, to yield the mRNA species. Before most types of mRNA can be transferred from the nucleus to the cytoplasm, they must first become linked to polyadenylic acid, which is formed by the enzyme poly A polymerase. (Some messengers, such as those for histones, seem not to include poly A.) Then the mRNA becomes associated with several proteins to produce the particulate ribonucleoprotein *informosomes*, which pass into the cytoplasm. This formation of RNA from chromosomal DNA involves the action of several specific DNA-dependent RNA polymerases, which can be separated using DEAE-Sephadex. Polymerase I, which is present in the nucleolus, transcribes ribosomal RNA; polymerase II occurs in the nucleoplasm and transcribes HnRNA and the mRNA; polymerase III, also occurring in the nucleoplasm, transcribes transfer RNA (tRNA) and 5S RNA.

Inhibitors of these transcriptional processes constitute useful tools for exploring the control of protein synthesis (Figure 1). At low doses, *actinomycin D* inhibits only the synthesis of rRNA; larger doses also inhibit mRNA synthesis. Formation of mRNA is also inhibited by *amanitin*, which binds specifically to polymerase II rather than to the DNA template. Poly A polymerase can be inhibited by *cordycepin*. These three inhibitors can therefore be used to block the induction of proteins requiring additional mRNA synthesis and thus to determine whether treatment-induced changes in enzyme levels require the formation of additional mRNA.

A number of hormones stimulate RNA-synthesizing systems in their target organs. For example, systemic injection of a glucocorticoid hormone causes, after some hours, an increase in liver RNA content. This was initially shown to be associated with accelerated formation of 45S RNA within hepatic nucleoli and its more rapid processing into 28S and 18S ribosomal forms (Jacob, Sajdel, and Munro, 1969). Subsequent studies showed that these changes occurred not because more template DNA had been exposed to nucleolar polymerase but because of an increase in the activity of polymerase I (Sajdel and Jacob, 1971). Corticosteroid administration can also stimulate the formation of several specific types of hepatic mRNA, for example, those coded for synthesis of the enzymes tyrosine aminotransferase and tryptophan oxygenase (Kenney, 1970).

Changes in protein synthesis produced by lipid-soluble hormones are probably mediated by specific receptor proteins in the cells of the target organs. Thus, after estradiol enters the cells of its target organ (the uterus), it binds to a cytoplasmic receptor; the transformed receptor then enters the cell's nucleus and binds to the chromatin at specific acceptor sites. This binding activates transcription at that chromosomal site and, consequently, accelerates formation of new messenger and other species of RNA. The newly formed RNA passes into the cytoplasm, in some cases causing the synthesis of novel proteins (O'Malley, 1971) and in other cases increasing the amounts of existing proteins. Abundant evidence is available that particular brain neurons have the ability to take up and concentrate various circulating steroid hormones (McEwen, Magnus, and Wallach, 1972); this uptake might conceivably constitute binding to a cytoplasmic receptor that controls neuronal protein synthesis, especially in developing brain. To our knowledge, however, no present evidence indicates that such hormone binding does activate chromatin, accelerate mRNA synthesis, and so on. Cytoplasmic factors that are analogous to hormone "receptors" but do not require hormones may also participate in nucleic acid metabolism within brain cells. The addition of dialyzed brain cytosol to isolated brain nuclei influences their rate of RNA synthesis, their stability, and the amounts and the sizes of the RNA transcripts. One such cytoplasmic factor may be a catalytic form of protein kinase, generated by its phosphorylation, which in turn may phosphorylate chromosomal proteins (Guidotti and Costa, 1977).

TRANSLATION AND ITS CONTROL The process of RNA translation has been recently reviewed (Haselkorn and Rothman-Denes, 1973). Cytoplasmic protein synthesis occurs in three phases (Figure 1):

1. The initiation phase of peptide-chain formation, which requires the 60S and 40S ribosomal subunits; messenger RNA; several *initiation factors* (e.g., IF_1, IF_2); and a special type of tRNA known as initiator methionyl-tRNA. Phosphorylation of initiation factors transiently inactivates them; this process may allow cyclic AMP levels and phosphatase enzymes to couple neurotransmitter inputs to protein synthesis (Filipowicz et al., 1976).

2. Peptide-chain elongation through the sequential addition of particular amino acids. At each step in formation of the peptide, one of the sixty aminoacyl-tRNA species, charged with the twenty amino acids found in proteins, forms a complex with *elongation factor 1* (EF_1) and GTP. This complex then attaches to the ribosome and inserts the correct amino acid (as indicated by the codons of the mRNA). After each aminoacyl-tRNA has become bound to the ribosome, the growing peptide chain is translocated across the surface of the ribosome by the action of *elongation factor 2* (EF_2), which also requires GTP. During peptide-chain elongation, the ribosome undergoes conformational changes as amino acid–charged tRNAs and elongation factors bind and are released over and over again.

3. *Termination* of peptide-chain synthesis. This phase requires two additional protein factors (not shown in Figure 1). The ribosomal pair separates from the mRNA, becoming a *runoff ribosome,* and is dissociated into its two subunits by means of a *dissociation factor* (DF).

A given strand of mRNA tends to bind a number of ribosomal pairs simultaneously, thus forming a polyribosome (polysome). The proportion of the total ribosome population present as polysomes determines the efficiency with which existing mRNA is directing protein synthesis; that is, runoff ribosomes and ribosomal subunits (or messenger strands without ribosomes) are incapable of synthesizing protein. This proportion is determined by the balance between initiation, chain elongation, and the availability of the ribosome dissociation factor. Changes in the rate of translation are usually the result of changes in initiation. When initiation is slowed, the ribosomes accumulate as runoff ribosomes, and subunits and polysomes appear disaggregated in electron micrographs or in measurements of RNA separated by sucrose density gradients. The effects on polysome profiles of inhibiting chain elongation depend on the cause of inhibition. For example, the antibiotic cycloheximide interferes with the binding of EF_2 and GTP to polysomes, thus preventing translocation and causing the ribosomes to become frozen onto the mRNA; hence there is no disruption of polysomal aggregation. On the other hand, if a single amino acid (charged to tRNA) is not available in the cytoplasm in adequate amounts, chain elongation is blocked at those points where the amino acid is required for elongation of the peptide chain; nascent peptide chains are released prematurely, and polysomes tend to disaggregate by runoff beyond this point.

POSTRANSLATIONAL EVENTS AND THEIR CONTROL
The peptide chain often undergoes further change before becoming the final component of an enzyme or another cell protein. Proteins to be secreted from cells are often modified after their translation by the addition of carbohydrates, forming glycoproteins (see the review by Munro and Steinert, 1975). Such proteins are synthesized by polysomes, which are attached to the membranes of the endoplasmic reticulum (Figure 1): this organelle acts both as a conducting channel for secretion of the protein and as a locus for its postranslational modification.

Protein synthesis in the brain

COMPONENTS OF BRAIN PROTEIN-SYNTHESIZING SYSTEMS Various components of the protein-synthetic apparatus have been isolated from brain—for example, ribosomes, ribosomal subunits, free and membrane-bound polyribosomes, mRNA, and the crude pH5 enzyme fractions and ribosome-associated factors necessary for in vitro protein synthesis (Zomzely-Neurath and Roberts, 1972). These components do not appear to differ substantially from their counterparts in other tissues and can function in vitro when mixed with components from other tissues. A claim by Zomzely et al. (1966) of a special requirement for Mg^{2+} in the medium for the isolation of brain ribosomes has not been substantiated (see Fellous et al., 1973). The elongation factors EF_1 and EF_2 have been purified from brain, and it has been suggested that EF_1 is present in limiting concentrations (Girgis and Nicholls, 1972). One investigator (Gilbert, 1974) has claimed that a special initiation factor isolated from rat brain allowed a spectrum of proteins to be translated from brain RNA that is different from that generated by reticulocyte initiators. Messenger RNAs have been isolated from rat brain, and two subgroups with sedimentation coefficients of 8S and 16S have been described (Zomzely, Roberts, and Peache, 1970).

Although rapidly labeled RNA (considered to represent mRNA) obtained from polysomes of rat brain is heterogeneous in size, recent studies suggest that distinct broad classes of this RNA may characterize brain-cell fractions enriched with neurons or glia (Lovtrup-Rein and Grahn, 1974).

SYNTHESIS OF SPECIFIC PROTEINS BY BRAIN Marker proteins have been especially sought for the two major cell types in the brain—neurons and glia—and for the nerve endings. Cell-free synthesis of a neuronal protein designated 14-3-2 has been accomplished, as has that of protein S-100 (Zomzely-Neurath, York, and Moore, 1973), which is associated with (but not specific for) glia. The 14-3-2 protein, also called *neuron-specific protein* (NSP) represents a neuron-specific form of an enzyme, enolase, that converts 2-phosphoglycerate to phosphoenolpyruvate. In the rat this protein has been demonstrated within nerve terminals as well as in perikarya. In nerve terminals the major, and perhaps sole, locus of protein synthesis is the abundant mitochondria (Hernandez, 1974); such nonmitochondrial synthesis as occurs in synaptosomes may result from contamination with postsynaptic (dendritic) ribosomes. A distinct protein-synthesizing system prepared from synaptosomal fractions has been described; this may constitute polysomes bound to postsynaptic membranes (Morgan and Naismith, 1975).

Both membrane-bound and free ribosomes have been recovered from homogenates of brain tissue (Andrews and Tata, 1971), the ratio of bound to free being about 1:3 to 1:2. Membrane-bound brain ribosomes may secrete some proteins onto the cell surface, but most of this polyribosome population apparently discharges its products back into the cell cytosol (Andrews and Tata, 1971). Several specific brain proteins have been experimentally associated with membrane-bound or free polyribosomes. Preparations of mRNA produced from the bound and free polysomes of rat brain and translated in a cell-free system synthesized different spectra of proteins: protein S100 and protein 14-3-2 were both synthesized exclusively by the free ribosomes, whereas tubulin was made on both free and membrane-bound ribosomes (Floor, Gilbert, and Nowak, 1976). Tubulin subunits and actin have recently been synthesized in vitro by means of a partially purified fraction of poly A-rich brain mRNA (Gozes, Schmitt, and Littauer, 1975). Finally, mRNA extracted from rat brain has been shown to make myelin peptides in vitro; this mRNA is more abundant in membrane-bound than in free polyribosomes (Lim et al., 1974).

Effect of monoaminergic drugs on brain polysome profiles and protein synthesis

Administration of large doses of L-dopa (Weiss, Munro, and Wurtman, 1971), 5-hydroxytryptophan (5HT) (Weiss, Wurtman, and Munro, 1973), or *d*-amphetamine sulfate (Moskowitz et al., 1975) to rats causes brain polysomes to disaggregate (Figure 2) and slows the incorporation of radiolabeled amino acids such as [³H]-lysine into brain proteins in vivo (Figure 3) and in vitro (Roel et al., 1974). Inasmuch as L-dopa and L-5HT are converted by most brain cells to the monoamine neurotransmitters dopamine and serotonin, whereas *d*-amphetamine acts presynaptically to cause the release of catecholamines, it seemed likely that the effects of these agents on brain polysomes were also related to monoaminergic transmission. Studies were therefore performed to ex-

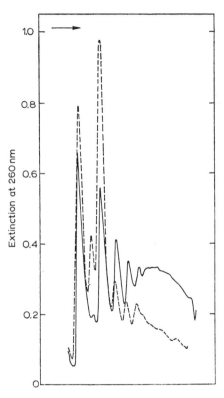

FIGURE 2 Brain polysome profile following L-dopa administration. 50 g male rats were injected intraperitoneally with L-dopa (500 mg/kg) or vehicle (0.05N HCl) and sacrificed 1 hr later. Brain polysomes were prepared as previously described (Weiss, Munro, and Wurtman, 1971). Polysome suspensions were then layered on a 10–40% linear sucrose gradient and centrifuged. Absorption profiles were recorded on a Gilford Spectrophotometer at 260 nM. The profiles prepared from the brains of the control and L-dopa-treated animals are represented by the solid and dashed lines, respectively.

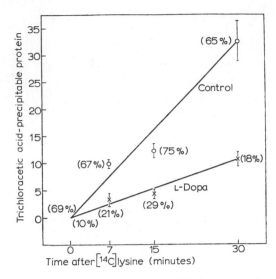

FIGURE 3 Radiolabeled amino acid incorporation into brain proteins in vivo following an injection of L-dopa. 50 g male rats received 1.5 μCi [^{14}C]-lysine intracisternally, 45 min after L-dopa (500 mg/kg) or the diluent alone (0.05 N HCl) had been injected intraperitoneally; animals were killed after 7, 15, or 30 min. The percentage of homogenate counts found in the protein fraction precipitable with trichloroacetic acid was compared for controls and L-dopa-treated rats, as was the percentage of rRNA present as polysomes (numbers in parentheses).

TABLE I

Effects of intraperitoneal administration of L-dopa and related drugs on brain polysome profiles

Treatment	Dose (mg/kg)	Time after Injection (min)	Polysome % Profile
Control	0	60	65
L-Dopa	500	60	43*
3-O-Methyldopa	500	60	60
		120	65
Control	0	60	65
L-Dopa	500	60	43*
D-Dopa	500	60	61
RO4-4602	800	90	65
RO4-4602	800	90 ⎫	60
plus L-Dopa	500	60 ⎭	
Control	0	60	73
L-Dopa	100	60	75
Pheniprazine	10	180	62
Pheniprazine	10	180 ⎫	32*
plus L-Dopa	100	60 ⎭	
Control	0	60	71
L-Dopa	500	60	32*
Pimozide	25	90 ⎫	66
plus L-dopa	500	60 ⎭	
Haloperidol	20	90 ⎫	65
plus L-dopa	500	60 ⎭	

* p < 0.001 differs from control group. Significance of differences was evaluated by Student's *t*-test.

amine the correlations between the drug-induced changes in polysome profiles, the levels of the monoamines in brain, and the activation of monoaminergic receptors.

In our initial experiments we investigated the correlations between the formation of particular dopa metabolites in whole rat brain and the disaggregation of polysomes (Weiss et al., 1972). Dopa can be decarboxylated to dopamine and subsequently β-hydroxylated to norepinephrine; these two monoamines can then be destroyed by monoamine oxidase. Alternatively, dopa (and its catecholamine derivatives) can be O-methylated to form 3-O-methyldopa and the corresponding methoxyamines. This process, catalyzed by catechol-O-methyltransferase, depletes the brain of S-adenosylmethionine. To identify which, if any, of these compounds mediates dopa's effect on polysome disaggregation, we examined polysomes in animals given 3-O-methyldopa (which cannot be converted to dopamine), *d*-dopa (which forms 3-O-methyldopa in brain but does not undergo decarboxylation to dopamine), or L-dopa, along with a drug (benzaseride, RO4-4602) that inhibits its decarboxylation (Weiss et al., 1972). Neither *d*-dopa nor 3-O-methyldopa affected polysome aggregation (Table I); hence dopa's effect did not result from the deple-

tion of S-adenosylmethionine or from the formation of O-methylated metabolites. Similarly, if we administered the decarboxylase inhibitor in doses sufficient to block decarboxylation in the brain, the effect of dopa on polysome disaggregation was also blocked (Weiss et al., 1972; see Table I). In contrast, if animals were pretreated with pheniprazine, an inhibitor of monoamine oxidase (MAO), prior to injection of L-dopa, L-dopa's effects on *both* brain dopamine and brain polysomes were potentiated (Table I). The decarboxylase inhibitor also blocked, and the MAO inhibitor also potentiated, the effect on polysomes of L-5HT (Weiss, Wurtman, and Munro, 1973).

Polysome disaggregation after L-dopa or 5-HT (or *d*-amphetamine, as described below) was observed in all brain regions and was always associated with parallel reductions of in vivo brain protein synthesis. Both particulate and soluble proteins were affected (including tubulin by L-dopa, but not by amphetamine). None of the drugs caused major changes in brain amino acid patterns. The specificity of the effects of dopamine and serotonin (formed from exogenous L-dopa and L-5HT) on brain polysomes was examined by using drugs that block receptors for these amines. Pretreatment of rats with pimozide or haloperidol, drugs known to block dopamine receptors, suppressed the effect of L-dopa on brain polysomes (Table I). In contrast, cyproheptadine or methysergide, drugs that block serotonin receptors, failed to modify L-dopa's effects on protein synthesis (Weiss et al., 1974). The latter drugs, unlike haloperidol or pimozide, did block the polysome disaggregation that follows L-5-HT administration (Weiss et al., 1974). The disaggregation of brain polysomes by systemically administered d-amphetamine could also be blocked by haloperidol or pimozide, implicating dopamine release, or at least dopamine receptors, in its effect (Moskowitz et al., 1975).

These observations suggest that pharmacologically defined central monoaminergic receptors mediate the effects of dopamine and serotonin on brain protein synthesis. One possible locus of these monoamine receptors might be the plasma membranes of brain cells. These would include—but not be limited to—the postsynaptic membranes of monoaminergic synapses; they would also include membranes of all cells that are capable of responding to monoamines (e.g., astrocytes: see Gilman and Nirenberg, 1971) and that also receive dopamine or serotonin after very large doses of their immediate precursors. [Although dopa decarboxylase is concentrated within monoaminergic cells, some of the enzyme apparently exists within most or all brain cells (Lytle et al., 1972); hence the two monoamines are probably present transiently throughout the brain.] The membrane receptors activated by d-amphetamine treatment would, in this explanation, be limited to those postsynaptic to monoaminergic neurons (Figure 4).

If the above schema were correct, it might be expected that pretreating animals with intracisternal 6-hydroxydopamine (which destroys many catecholaminergic neurons) would attenuate the disaggregation of brain polysomes by d-amphetamine. Similarly, systemic apomorphine, a dopaminergic agonist, would be expected to disaggregate brain polysomes. Neither of these predictions has been confirmed; thus the possibility must also be considered that the brain monoamines formed from exogenous dopa or 5-HT, or the amphetamine molecule itself, suppress brain protein synthesis by acting directly on receptors associated with the perikaryal organelles that control protein synthesis (Figure 4). This explanation would be compatible with the major disaggregation observed after administration of the drugs. The proportion of brain RNA present as polysomes falls by more than half (Table I and Figure 3); hence most brain cells—glia as well as neurons—must be affected, which implies either that a majority of brain cells can receive monoaminergic inputs—at synapses, or perhaps via the brain's extracellular space (Chan-Palay, 1975)—or that the effects of L-dopa, 5-HTP, and amphetamine on brain protein synthesis are not mediated through synapses but work directly on the

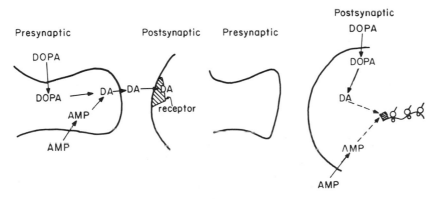

FIGURE 4   Loci at which L-dopa or d-amphetamine might act on polysomes. (A) Action via postsynaptic receptor. Evidence supporting this site includes the involvement of a "classical" dopamine receptor as shown by the blockade of dopa or amphetamine effects by haloperidol or pimozide (but not by 5-HT blockers); the transsynaptic control of neuronal polysomes (shown by suturing eyelids of kittens); and the potentiation of hyperthermia. Evidence opposing includes failure of i.c. 6-OHDA to block amphetamine effects; failure of apomorphine (1–20 mg/kg) to disaggregate; and the possibility that too few neurons and/or glia receive monoaminergic synapses. (B) Direct action on perikaryal contents. Evidence supporting this site includes the direct in vitro effects of amphetamine on protein synthesis. Evidence opposing includes the fact that there are no known monoamine receptors on the protein-synthesizing apparatus and the lack of effect of dopamine on in vitro protein synthesis. (AMP: amphetamine.)

TABLE II

Effect of amphetamine on [³H]-leucine incorporation into total protein in in vitro systems containing liver or brain polysomes and pH 5 enzymes (elongation) or mRNA with wheat-germ S30 fractions (initiation)

Incubation System	Deletion	d-Amphetamine (4 mM)	[³H]-Leucine Incorporated (pmol)	
			Liver	Brain
Polysome system	Ribosomes	−	0.14 ± 0.002	0.15 ± 0.01
	pH 5 enzyme	−	0.52 ± 0.02	0.40 ± 0.01
	None	−	17.00 ± 0.5	15.00 ± 0.6
	None	+	15.00 ± 0.2	16.00 ± 0.5
mRNA and wheat-germ S30 system	mRNA	−	1.9 ± 0.04	1.95 ± 0.03
	None	−	18.00 ± 0.04	7.00 ± 0.1
	None	+	9.65 ± 0.1	1.95 ± 0.05

protein-synthetic mechanisms of neurons and glia.

Recent in vitro studies with amphetamine confirm that this drug has a direct action on protein synthesis at the translational level (Baliga et al., 1976). Two cell-free systems were examined: in one, polyribosomes bearing nascent peptide chains were incubated in a medium that allowed elongation of preexisting chains; in the other, added mRNA plus amphetamine were incubated with ribosomal subunits and soluble factors from wheat germ. (This system displays both initiation and elongation.) *d*-Amphetamine inhibited protein synthesis only in the wheat-germ system, indicating that the drug blocks initiation but not elongation (Table II). Similar evidence that amphetamine affects initiation was obtained by using a fractionated reticulocyte lysate system. Moreover, studies employing radiolabeled amphetamine have shown that this drug apparently binds to the ribosome during initiation, and this binding is dependent on the presence of mRNA (Figure 5). Hence, it seems likely that amphetamine can act directly to prevent initiation, perhaps by binding to polysomes during or after its attachment to mRNA. (Numerous other lipid-soluble amines, such as parachloroamphetamine, share this effect.) Perhaps amphetamine affects protein synthesis by more than one mechanism. (See note, p. 909.)

As these monoaminergic drugs disaggregate brain polysomes, they must also induce a rise in body temperature (Table III; see Moskowitz et al., 1977). This, in turn, requires that animals be present in a relatively warm ambient temperature (26°C or warmer). An equivalent hyperthermia (created by keeping control rats at ambient temperatures of 40–44°C) does not by itself cause polysome disaggregation (Table IV); hence the hyperpyrexia is permissive, that is, necessary but not sufficient for suppressing protein

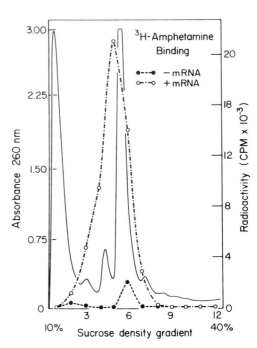

FIGURE 5 Binding of [³H]-amphetamine to mRNA-ribosome complex in vitro. Radiolabeled amphetamine was added to wheat-germ S30 fraction in the presence or absence of rat brain mRNA and incubated for 30 min. The mixture was then layered over a continuous sucrose gradient and the absorption profile recorded at 260 nM (represented by the continuous line). The gradient was then fractionated and radioactivity determined for each tendrop aliquot.

synthesis. The mechanism of this thermal effect awaits clarification.

That polysome disaggregation and aggregation occur normally within brain cells in response to transsynaptic signals has recently been shown by electronmicroscopic studies of the spiny stellate neurons in

TABLE III

Effects of varying ambient temperature on d-*amphetamine- and* L-*dopa-induced brain polysomal disaggregation*

| | Ambient Temperature | | | | | |
| | 26°C | | 18°C | | 10°C | |
Treatment	Rectal Temp.	Polysome % Profile	Rectal Temp.	Polysome % Profile	Rectal Temp.	Polysome % Profile
Vehicle	37.3 ± 0.1	73.8 ± 1.1	36.5 ± 0.2	70.9 ± 1.1	36.0 ± 0.2	71.7 ± 1.6
d-Amphetamine sulfate (40-day-old rats)	40.1 ± 0.2	42.6 ± 5.7	38.2 ± 0.3	69.3 ± 1.5	34.3 ± 0.5	68.8 ± 1.8
L-Dopa (20-day-old rats)	39.8 ± 1.7	40.0 ± 0.9	37.5 ± 0.5	75.0 ± 1.3	33.0 ± 0.6	73.4 ± 2.1

TABLE IV

Effect of hyperthermia on brain polysome profiles

Group	Ambient Temperature (°C)	Rectal Temperature (°C)	Polysomes % Profile
20-day-old rats	40–44	40.1 ± 0.1	68.0 ± 2.2
	20	37.2 ± 0.2	78.0 ± 1.9
40-day-old rats	40–44	40.2 ± 0.6	68.0 ± 1.4
	20	37.6 ± 0.2	74.0 ± 1.2

the fourth layer of the kitten's visual cortex (LeVay, 1977). These neurons normally exhibit polysome disaggregation and reaggregation during the second or third month of postnatal life, or shortly after synaptogenesis is complete (Figure 6). The physiological reaggregation of the RNA monomers into polysomes is reportedly suppressed in animals deprived of pattern vision; the process, therefore, appears to depend on neuronal activity within the geniculate afferents innervating the spiny stellate cells. Reaggregation is facilitated by subjecting animals to prolonged barbiturate anesthesia. These observations suggest that variations in neuronal activity can control protein-synthetic activity within postsynaptic cells. It seems likely that similar relationships will be observed in other brain neurons in animals exposed to appropriate experimental conditions.

The ability of monoaminergic drugs to transiently suppress translational processes within brain cells may provide the basis for an experimental tool to study the formation and turnover times of substance P and other peptides that are putative brain neurotransmitters. The cellular heterogeneity of the brain and the relative rarity of neurons that synthesize any particular peptide have precluded obtaining mRNA or polysomes coded for their synthesis—or even proving that such syntheses *are* polysomal. Similarly, antibiotics used successfully to suppress peptide and protein

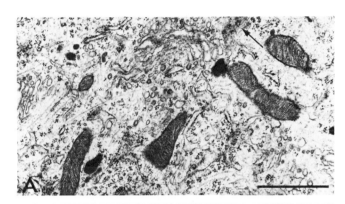

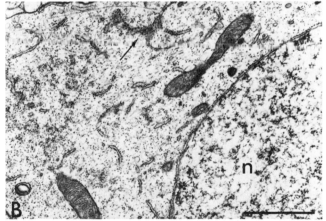

FIGURE 6 The disaggregation of polysomes within occipital cortical neurons taken from the fourth layer of area 17 in a binocularly deprived six-month-old kitten. Micrographs of two neurons show ribosomes that are predominantly clustered in polysomes (A) and ribosomes that are disaggregated (B). The arrows indicate where the membrane-bound ribosomes may be seen most clearly. (Bar: 1 µm.)

synthesis in other tissues have had very limited utility in brain studies, partly because few of these compounds seem to penetrate the blood-brain barrier well. We have recently found that doses of d-amphetamine that disaggregate brain polysomes also reduce the levels of substance P within the caudate nucleus, a brain region known to contain perikarya of substance P neurons (Pettibone, Wurtman, and Leeman, 1978). Perhaps this reduction is caused in part by a slowing of the formation of polysomes coded for substance P or a precursor peptide.

Potential sites of regulation of protein synthesis by neurotransmitters

The description given earlier of the mechanism of protein synthesis (see Figure 1) also suggests potential sites of action for neurotransmitters. These sites can be classified into those belonging to transcription and those belonging to translation. It will be noted that the former are likely to be much more sluggish than the latter. This implies that rapid changes are best effected at the translational level, while slower and longer-lasting changes could be brought about by altering nuclear control of the transcription process.

Thus transcription can be regulated by changes in: (1) availability of chromosomal template; (2) activity of RNA polymerases, particularly polymerase II, responsible for mRNA formation; (3) rates of maturation of HnRNA to provide mRNA; and (4) the packing of the mRNA, with the addition of polyadenylic acid and specific mRNP particle proteins, for transport to the cytoplasm.

Similarly, translation is affected by changes in: (1) the rate of initiation of new peptide chains and (2) the rate of elongation. A number of examples of both these actions have been described (see the review by Munro and Steinert, 1975). It has recently been shown that large doses of phenylalanine, which disaggregates brain polyribosomes, interfere with the charging of initiator met-tRNA in brain (Hughes and Johnson, 1977). This would imply a rather specific influence of phenylalanine excess on formation of the particular tRNA responsible for chain initiation. The initiation process can also be obstructed by a long series of chemical inhibitors, which probably act at a number of control sites. Full characterization of these control sites awaits a better understanding of the nature and identity of the initiation factors.

Neural and endocrine control of adrenomedullary enzyme synthesis

The chromaffin cells of the adrenal medulla provide an excellent experimental system for characterizing the mechanisms through which neural and endocrine inputs can affect the synthesis of specific proteins,

namely, enzymes that catalyze the formation of catecholamine neurotransmitters. These cells receive only a single neurotransmitter, acetylcholine released from the terminals of the splanchnic nerve—a preganglionic cholinergic sympathetic nerve. They also receive—through an intra-adrenal portal vascular system—very high concentrations of the steroid hormones secreted by the adrenal cortex. The major function of the chromaffin cells is to synthesize epinephrine from the circulating amino acid tyrosine; although the epinephrine they produce is released as a hormone into the blood stream, this catecholamine may also be utilized as a neurotransmitter by some brain cells. Its immediate precursor—norepinephrine—is, of course, a well-established neurotransmitter in the central and autonomic nervous systems.

The biosynthesis of epinephrine involves four enzymatic reactions. Initially, tyrosine is converted to dopa through the action of tyrosine hydroxylase, a cytoplasmic enzyme that contains iron and uses molecular oxygen and a reduced form of biopterin as a cofactor. The catechol amino acid is then immediately decarboxylated to form dopamine through the action of another cytoplasmic enzyme, dopa decarboxylase (aromatic l-amino acid decarboxylase). This enzyme is widely distributed and is generally present in excess quantities; it utilizes pyridoxal phosphate as a cofactor. Dopamine is taken up within a subcellular organelle, the chromaffin granule, and converted to norepinephrine through the action of dopamine-β-hydroxylase, a copper-containing, ascorbic-acid-dependent enzyme found only within norepinephrine- and epinephrine-producing cells. Finally, in most adrenal chromaffin cells and a few brain-stem neurons, the norepinephrine is converted to the secondary amine epinephrine by a cytoplasmic enzyme, phenylethanolamine-N-methyltransferase (PNMT), with S-adenosylmethionine as the source of the necessary methyl group. There is abundant evidence that the amount of tyrosine hydroxylase (e.g., both its activity, assayed in vitro, and the quantity of enzyme protein, assayed immunochemically) in chromaffin cells and in catecholaminergic neurons can be increased by treatments that enhance the cholinergic input to these cells. (As described in this volume by Thoenen, Otten, and Schwab, such treatments also increase dopamine-β-hydroxylase levels and may have a small effect on PNMT.) In contrast, the activity, levels, and synthesis of adrenal PNMT are all controlled by glucocorticoid hormones.

PNMT   Under normal conditions, the adrenal medulla is perfused with concentrations of glococorticoids that are several hundred times higher than those present in the systemic circulation. These high concentrations are necessary for the aggregation of adrenomedullary polyribosomes (Baliga et al., 1973) and specifically for synthesis of PNMT enzyme protein (Wurtman and Axelrod, 1966). When glucocorticoid secretion is diminished by treatments that deprive the adrenal cortex of ACTH, its physiological stimulus (e.g., hypophysectomy or the chronic administration of low "replacement" doses of glucocorticoids), PNMT activity falls, reaching levels only 15–20% of normal after a week (Wurtman and Axelrod, 1966). PNMT activity can be restored by treating animals with physiological doses of ACTH or with massive doses of a synthetic glucocorticoid, dexamethasone. The adrenal medulla is physiologically Cushingoid, by virtue of its special blood supply; hence, if systemic glucocorticoids are to be used to substitute for those normally received from the adrenal cortex, one side effect of the required doses is that they make the entire body Cushingoid. Treatments that increase the delivery of glucocorticoids to the normal adrenal fail to produce more than minimal further increases in PNMT activity, indicating that the steroid induction of PNMT is normally at the top of its dose-response curve. The suppression of glucocorticoid secretion has little effect on PNMT in brain neurons, which are normally at the bottom of this theoretical dose-response curve; however, brain PNMT may be elevated slightly by massive doses of glucocorticoids. The changes in adrenal PNMT activity caused by manipulating steroid availability are followed by parallel changes in the adrenal's content of epinephrine (Wurtman, Noble, and Axelrod, 1967) and, ultimately, in the quantities secreted basally and in response to stress (e.g., hypoglycemia: see Wurtman et al., 1968). It seems likely that the pronounced insulin sensitivity of people suffering from pituitary disease may result from impaired ability to secrete epinephrine when blood sugar falls.

Mammalian PNMT is biochemically heterogeneous; besides the steroid-inducible form, which is predominant in the adrenal, there is at least one isozyme that is not dependent on glucocorticoid availability. This form predominates in frog brain and heart, which lack an envelope of adrenal cortex, and also in some adrenomedullary tumors (pheochromocytomas) whose metastases continue to produce epinephrine.

Hypophysectomy also produces a decrease in the size of the adrenal medulla. No quantitative data are available on the number of chromaffin cells in the adrenal medullas of hypophysectomized animals; hence it is not possible to state whether glucocorticoid hormones control chromaffin-cell division (and/or life span) or only synthetic mechanisms within these cells. No data are available on the cytoplasmic receptors that presumably mediate chromaffin-cell responses to glucocorticoid hormones; in view of the very high hormone concentrations needed for such cell responses as polysome aggregation, it would be interesting to determine whether the kinetics governing the attachment of glucocorticoids to these receptors differ substantially from those characterizing glucocorticoid binding to hepatic receptors. One group of investigators has suggested that the fall in adrenal PNMT activity that follows hypophysectomy may also reflect accelerated degradation of the enzyme protein (Ciaranello, 1977).

Tyrosine Hydroxylase   There is general agreement that treatments that cause a sustained increase in the quantities of acetylcholine impinging on the nicotinic receptors located on chromaffin cells stimulate the synthesis of tyrosine hydroxylase (Thoenen and Otten, 1976; Guidotti and Costa, 1977). It has been difficult, however, to identify the process whereby activation of these receptors is transduced into a signal that changes the transcriptional or translational mechanisms responsible for the enzyme's synthesis. One group (Guidotti and Costa, 1977) proposes that the effects of cholinergic receptor activation are mediated by cAMP. The transient increase in intracellular levels of this nucleotide causes the activation of cytoplasmic protein kinases; the catalytic form of one of these kinases—PK_1—is then taken up by the cell nucleus, where, presumably, it phosphorylates acidic nuclear proteins, ultimately accelerating the synthesis of mRNA by polymerase II. Another group (Thoenen, Otten, and Schwab, this volume) fails to observe good correlations between treatment-induced increases in intracellular cAMP levels and tyrosine hydroxylase activity and concludes that the second messenger mediating the nuclear effects of cholinergic activation remains unknown. In any event, the necessary activation of cholinergic receptors can be produced by accelerating the firing rate of the splanchnic nerves (with insulin, drugs that induce hypotension, or hypothermia); by administering choline, which presumably increases the quantities of acetylcholine release per nerve firing (Ulus, Hirsch, and Wurtman, 1977); or by administering cholinergic agonists, which can act directly on the chromaffin cells.

ACKNOWLEDGMENTS Studies performed in the authors' laboratories were supported in part by grants from the U.S. Public Health Service (AM-14228) and the John A. Hartford Foundation. Dr. Moskowitz is the recipient of a teacher-investigator award (NS-11081) from the National Institute of Neurological and Communicative Disorders and Stroke and a fellowship in the neurosciences from the Sloan Foundation.

REFERENCES

ANDREWS, T. M., and J. R. TATA, 1971. Protein synthesis by membrane-bound and free ribosomes of secretory and non-secretory tissues. *Biochem. J.* 121:683-694.

BALIGA, B. S., L. A. POHORECKY, H. N. MUNRO, and R. J. WURTMAN, 1973. Control of adrenal medullary protein synthesis by corticosteroids. *Biochim. Biophys. Acta* 299: 337-343.

BALIGA, B. S., J. ZAHRINGER, M. TRACHTENBERG, M. A. MOSKOWITZ, and H. N. MUNRO, 1976. Mechanism of *d*-amphetamine inhibition of protein synthesis. *Biochim. Biophys. Acta* 442:239-250.

CHAN-PALAY, V., 1975. Fine structure of labelled axons in the cerebellar cortex and nuclei of rodents and primates after intraventricular infusions with tritiated serotonin. *Anat. Embryol.* 148:235-265.

CIARANELLO, R. D., 1977. Regulation of phenylethanolamine-N-methyl transferase synthesis and degradation. In *Structure and Function of Monoamine Enzymes*, E. Usdin, N. Weiner, and M. B. H. Youdim, eds. New York: Dekker, pp. 497-525.

FELLOUS, A., J. FRANCON, J. NUNEZ, and L. SOKOLOF, 1973. Protein synthesis by highly aggregated and purified polysomes from young and adult rat brain. *J. Neurochem.* 21:211-222.

FILIPOWICZ, W., J. M. SIERRA, C. NOMBELA, S. OCHOA, W. C. MERRICK, and W. F. ANDERSON, 1976. Polypeptide chain initiation in eukaryotes: Initiation factor requirements for translation of natural messengers. *Proc. Natl. Acad. Sci. USA* 73:44-48.

FLOOR, E. R., J. M. GILBERT, and T. S. NOWAK, JR., 1976. Evidence for the synthesis of tubulin on membrane-bound and free ribosomes from rat forebrain. *Biochim. Biophys. Acta* 442:285-296.

GILBERT, J. M., 1974. Differences in the translation of rat forebrain messenger RNA dependent on the source of protein synthesis factors. *Biochim. Biophys. Acta* 340:140-146.

GILMAN, A. G., and M. NIRENBERG, 1971. Effect of catecholamines on the adenosine 3':5'-cyclic monophosphate concentrations of clonal satellite cells of neurons. *Proc. Natl. Acad. Sci. USA* 68:2165-2168.

GIRGIS, G. R., and D. M. NICHOLLS, 1972. Protein synthesis limited by transferase I. *Biochim. Biophys. Acta* 269:465-476.

GOZES, I., H. SCHMITT, and U. Z. LITTAUER, 1975. Translation in vitro of rat brain messenger RNA coding for tubulin and actin. *Proc. Natl. Acad. Sci. USA* 72:701-705.

GUIDOTTI, A., and E. COSTA, 1977. Trans-synaptic regulation of tyrosine 3-monooxygenase biosynthesis in rat adrenal medulla. *Biochem. Pharmacol.* 26:817-823.

HASELKORN, R., and L. B. ROTHMAN-DENES, 1973. Protein synthesis. *Annu. Rev. Biochem.* 42:397-438.

HERNANDEZ, A. G., 1974. Protein synthesis by synaptosomes from rat brain: Contribution by the intraterminal mitochondria. *Biochem. J.* 142:7-17.

HUGHES, J. V., and T. C. JOHNSON, 1977. The effects of hyperphenylalaninaemia on the concentrations of aminoacyl-transfer ribonucleic acid *in vivo*. *Biochem. J.* 162:527-537.

JACOB, S. T., E. M. SAJDEL, and H. N. MUNRO, 1969. Regulation of nucleolar RNA metabolism by hydrocortisone. *Eur. J. Biochem.* 7:449-453.

KENNEY, F. T., 1970. Hormonal regulation of synthesis of liver enzymes. In *Mammalian Protein Metabolism*, vol. 4, H. N. Munro, ed. New York: Academic Press.

LEVAY, S., 1977. Effects of visual deprivation on polyribosome aggregation in visual cortex of the cat. *Brain Res.* 119:73-86.

LIM, L., J. O. WHITE, C. HALL, W. BERTHOLD, and A. N. DAVISON, 1974. Isolation of microsomal poly(A)-RNA from rat brain directing the synthesis of the myelin encephalitogenic protein in *Xenopus* oocytes. *Biochim. Biophys. Acta* 361:241-247.

LOVTRUP-REIN, H., and B. GRAHN, 1974. Polysomes and polysomal RNA from nerve and glial cell fractions. *Brain Res.* 72:123-136.

LYTLE, L. D., O. HURKO, J. A. ROMERO, K. COTTMAN, D. LEEHEY, and R. J. WURTMAN, 1972. The effects of 6-hydroxydopamine pretreatment on the accumulation of dopa and dopamine in brain and peripheral organs following L-dopa administration. *J. Neural Trans.* 33:63-71.

MCEWEN, B. S., C. MAGNUS, and G. WALLACH, 1972. Soluble corticosterone-binding macromolecules extracted from rat brain. *Endocrinol.* 90:217-226.

MORGAN, B. L. G., and D. J. NAISMITH, 1975. The effect of postnatal undernutrition on the activities of enzymes involved in the synthesis of brain lipids in the rat. *Nutr. Soc. Proc.* 34:40A-41A.

MOSKOWITZ, M. A., D. RUBIN, T. NOWAK, J. LIEBSCHUTZ, H. MUNRO, and R. J. WURTMAN, 1977. The permissive role of hyperthermia in the disaggregation of brain polysomes by L-dopa or *d*-amphetamine. *J. Neurochem.* 28:779-782.

MOSKOWITZ, M. A., B. F. WEISS, L. D. LYTLE, H. N. MUNRO, and R. J. WURTMAN, 1975. D-amphetamine disaggregates brain polysomes via a dopaminergic mechanism. *Proc. Natl. Acad. Sci. USA* 72:834-836.

MUNRO, H. N., and P. M. STEINERT, 1975. The intracellular organisation of protein synthesis. In *International Review of Science* (Biochemistry Series), vol. 7, H. R. V. Arnstein, ed. London: Butterworths.

NOWAK, T. S., JR., and H. N. MUNRO, 1977. Effects of protein-calorie malnutrition on biochemical aspects of brain development. In *Nutrition and the Brain*, R. J. Wurtman and J. J. Wurtman, eds. New York: Raven Press.

O'MALLEY, B. W., 1971. Mechanisms of action of steroid hormones. *N. Engl. J. Med.* 284:370-377.

O'MALLEY, B. W., and A. R. MEANS, 1974. Female steroid hormones and target cell nuclei. *Science* 183:610-620.

PETTIBONE, D. J., R. J. WURTMAN, and S. E. LEEMAN, 1978. *d*-Amphetamine administration reduces substance P concentration in the rat striatum. *Biochem. Pharmacol.* 27:839-842.

ROEL, L. E., S. A. SCHWARTZ, B. F. WEISS, H. N. MUNRO, and R. J. WURTMAN, 1974. *In vivo* inhibition of rat brain protein synthesis by L-dopa. *J. Neurochem.* 23:233–239.

SAJDEL, E. M., and S. T. JACOB, 1971. Mechanism of early effect of hydrocortisone on the transcriptional process: Stimulation of the activities of purified rat liver nucleolar RNA polymerase. *Biochem. Biophys. Res. Commun.* 45:707–715.

THOENEN, H., and U. OTTEN, 1976. Molecular events in trans-synaptic regulation of the synthesis of macromolecules. In *Essays in Neurochemistry and Neuropharmacology.* vol. 1, M. B. H. Youdim, W. Lovenberg, D. F. Sharman, and J. R. Lagnado, eds. New York: John Wiley, pp. 73–101.

ULUS, I., M. HIRSCH, and R. J. WURTMAN, 1977. Trans-synaptic induction of adrenomedullary tyrosine hydroxylase activity by choline: Evidence that choline administration increases cholinergic transmission. *Proc. Natl. Acad. Sci. USA* 74:798–800.

WEISS, B. F., H. N. MUNRO, L. A. ORDONEZ, and R. J. WURTMAN, 1972. Dopamine: Mediator of brain polysome disaggregation after L-dopa. *Science* 177:613–616.

WEISS, B. F., H. N. MUNRO, and R. J. WURTMAN, 1971. L dopa: Disaggregation of brain polysomes and elevation of brain tryptophan. *Science* 173:833–835.

WEISS, B. F., L. E. ROEL, H. N. MUNRO, and R. J. WURTMAN, 1974. L-Dopa, polysomal aggregation and cerebral synthesis of protein. In *Aromatic Amino Acids in the Brain* (Ciba Foundation Symposium), G. E. W. Wolstenholme and D. W. Fitzsimons, eds. Amsterdam: Elsevier.

WEISS, B. F., R. J. WURTMAN, and H. N. MUNRO, 1973. Disaggregation of brain polysomes by L 5 hydroxytryptophan: Mediation by serotonin. *Life Sci.* 13:411–416.

WURTMAN, R. J., and J. AXELROD, 1966. Control of enzymatic synthesis of adrenaline in the adrenal medulla by adrenal cortical steroids. *J. Biol. Chem.* 241:2301–2305.

WURTMAN, R. J., A. CASPER, L. A. POHORECKY, and F. C. BARTTER, 1968. Impaired secretion of epinephrine in response to insulin among hypophysectomized dogs. *Proc. Natl. Acad. Sci. USA* 61:522–528.

WURTMAN, R. J., E. P. NOBLE, and J. AXELROD, 1967. Inhibition of enzymatic synthesis of epinephrine by low doses of glucocorticoids. *Endocrinology* 80:825–828.

WURTMAN, R. J., L. A. POHORECKY, and B. S. BALIGA, 1972. Adrenocortical control of the biosynthesis of epinephrine and proteins in the adrenal medulla. *Pharmacol. Rev.* 24:411–426.

WURTMAN, R. J., C. M. ROSE, S. MATTHYSSE, J. STEPHENSON, and R. J. BALDESSARINI, 1970. L-Dihydroxyphenylalanine: Effect on S-adenosylmethionine in brain. *Science* 169:395–397.

ZOMZELY, C. E., S. ROBERTS, D. M. BROWN, and C. PROVOST, 1966. Cerebral protein synthesis. I. Physical properties of cerebral ribosomes and polyribosomes. *J. Mol. Biol.* 19:455–468.

ZOMZELY, C. E., S. ROBERTS, and S. PEACHE, 1970. Isolation of RNA with properties of messenger RNA from cerebral polyribosomes. *Proc. Natl. Acad. Sci. USA* 67:644–651.

ZOMZELY-NEURATH, C. E., and S. ROBERTS, 1972. Brain ribosomes. In *Research Methods in Neurochemistry*, vol. 1, N. Marks and R. Rodnight, eds. New York: Plenum Press.

ZOMZELY-NEURATH, C., C. YORK, and B. W. MOORE, 1973. In vitro synthesis of two brain-specific proteins (S100 and 14-3-2) by polyribosomes from rat brain. I. Site of synthesis and programming by polysome-derived messenger RNA. *Arch. Biochem. Biophys.* 155:58–69.

NOTE ADDED IN PROOF   For a report of evidence that amphetamine affects initiation obtained by using a fractionated reticulocyte lysate system, see M. A. Moskowitz, D. Rubin, T. Nowak, B. Baliga, and H. N. Munro, *Ann. NY Acad. Sci.* 305:96–106 (1978).

A direct effect of drugs on protein synthesis is also supported by amphetamine's ability to inhibit the formation of certain proteins in cultures of chick myotubes (see R. Salomon, *Life Sci.* 1941–1950, 1978).

SOURCE ACKNOWLEDGMENTS FOR FIGURES AND TABLES   Figure 1 is from Nowak and Munro (1977). Figure 2 and Table I are from Weiss, Munro, and Wurtman (1971), copyright © 1971 by the American Association for the Advancement of Science. Figure 3 and Tables III and IV are from Roel et al. (1974). Figure 5 and Table II are from Baliga et al. (1976). Figure 6 is from LeVay (1977).

54 Orthograde and Retrograde Signals for the Regulation of Neuronal Gene Expression: The Peripheral Sympathetic Nervous System as a Model

H. THOENEN, U. OTTEN, and M. SCHWAB

ABSTRACT   The peripheral sympathetic nervous system is presented as a model for the analysis of trophic interactions between neurons and other neurons or nonneuronal cells. It has been shown that nerve impulses can regulate transsynaptically the synthesis of specific neuronal enzymes and that nerve growth factor (NGF) acts as a macromolecular mediator of information between effector cells and innervating neurons. The transsynaptic regulation of the synthesis of specific macromolecules in postganglionic adrenergic neurons is discussed in connection with the question of the long-term modification of neuronal connectivity in response to changing functional requirements. The selective uptake of NGF by nerve terminals and its subsequent retrograde axonal transport to the perikaryon is taken as a model of a means by which effector organs can influence innervating neurons, in particular the regulation of the synthesis of macromolecules. Retrograde axonal transport is introduced as a tool to obtain information on the quality, quantity, and turnover of membrane constituents of nerve terminals.

Introduction

THE FUNCTIONAL capacity of integrated neuronal systems such as the mammalian brain is based not only on the large number of neurons and their complex synaptic connections but also on the ability of these neurons to adapt their long-term connectivity to changing functional requirements. This plasticity of adaptation which greatly expands the functional capacity of the brain, is a reflection of long-term covalent modifications (Stadtman and Chock, this volume) or changes in the de novo synthesis of specific neuronal macromolecules. These changes may even be-

come apparent in alterations of the morphological feature of neurons.

The same mechanisms that lead to reversible plastic modifications in fully differentiated neuronal systems elicit, during critical periods of ontogenetic development, irreversible (imprinting) effects (see Black, 1974; Thoenen, 1975), which are an integral part of the formation of the gross connections between single neurons and groups of neurons. These modifications are determined by epigenetic events such as cell migration, cell-cell recognition, and response to humoral (low and high molecular) factors originating from neuronal and nonneuronal cells (see also the papers by Changeux, Cowan, Gorski, Lynch and Akers, McClain and Edelman, Patterson, and Rutishauser et al. in this volume). The formation of the final outline of an integrated neuronal system requires not only the qualitative and quantitative characteristics of epigenetic functions mentioned above but also their well-orchestrated temporal sequence of occurrence.

It is evident that a highly complex neuronal system such as the mammalian brain is not a suitable object for studying the detailed molecular mechanisms of such processes. Investigations over the last few years, however, have shown that the peripheral sympathetic nervous system lends itself well to such studies. In addition to the relative simplicity of its organization (Figure 1), the biochemical and physiological analysis of this system is comparatively advanced, particularly with respect to the mechanism of synthesis, storage, release, and inactivation of transmitter substances (Geffen and Livett, 1971; Molinoff and Axelrod, 1971). Moreover, organ-culture methods have recently been developed that allow the study of single steps in the regulation of the synthesis of macro-

H. THOENEN, U. OTTEN, and M. SCHWAB   Department of Pharmacology, Biocenter of the University, Basel, Switzerland

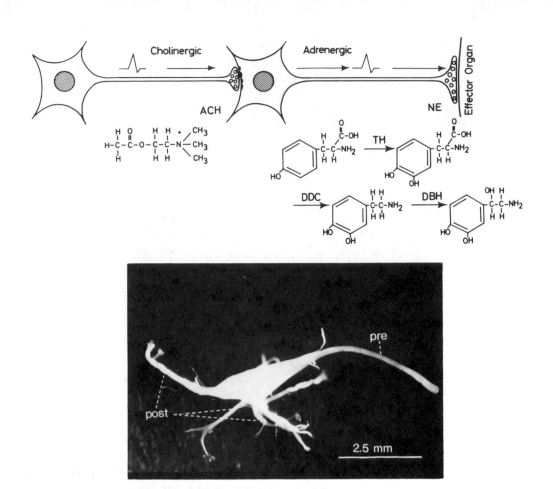

FIGURE 1 Organization of the peripheral sympathetic nervous system. *Top*: Scheme of preganglionic cholinergic and postganglionic adrenergic neurons with the pathway of synthesis of the adrenergic transmitter. *Bottom:* Rat sympathetic ganglion with pre- and postganglionic fibers prepared for organ culture.

molecules under well-controlled experimental conditions (Goodman, Otten, and Thoenen, 1975; Otten and Thoenen, 1976a). Extensive efforts are also being made to develop cell lines and clones from neuronal-crest tumors (Dichter, Tischler, and Green, 1977; Green and Rein, 1977; Green and Tischler, 1976; Tischler et al., 1977), in the hope that these may serve as representative models for the investigation of specific functional aspects of the peripheral sympathetic nervous system. Such cell-culture systems can provide the large amounts of homogeneous cells necessary for well-defined biological procedures and subsequent biochemical analysis, which would not be possible with the small samples of original tissue from sympathetic ganglia or adrenal medulla.

In addition to its usefulness for studying plastic neuron-neuron interaction, the peripheral sympathetic nervous system has also proven to be a good model for studies designed to investigate the "trophic" influences of effector organs on innervating neurons, that is, the mechanism of uptake of macromolecules by nerve terminals, the pathway of their axonal transport, their distribution and site of action in the perikaryon, and possibly their retrograde transsynaptic transfer to the proximal preganglionic nerve terminals (see Thoenen, Schwab, and Otten, 1978).

Regulation of the synthesis of specific macromolecules in the postganglionic adrenergic neurons by the activity of the preganglionic cholinergic nerve fibers

Since the original observation that selective destruction of adrenergic nerve terminals by 6-hydroxydopamine leads to augmented in vitro activity of tyrosine hydroxylase (TH) in rat adrenal medulla (Mueller, Thoenen, and Axelrod, 1969a), a great number of experimental conditions have been described that elicit a similar effect on TH in both sympathetic ganglia and adrenal medulla (e.g., Axelrod, 1971; Thoenen and Otten, 1976, 1978a). Although in this chapter we concentrate mainly on the sympathetic neurons, the adrenal medulla will be discussed in particular cases for reasons of comparison or complementation. The occasional inclusion of the adrenal medulla seems to be justified since sympathetic ganglia and adrenal medulla have the same ontogenetic origin, the neuronal crest (see Patterson, this volume). The adrenal medulla may be considered an aggregation of adrenergic neurons that lack neuronal processes and are exposed to high concentrations of glucocorticoids (Jones, Hillhouse, and Burden, 1977) via a capillary plexus from the adrenal cortex (Coupland, 1975).

The common denominator of all experimental conditions leading to augmented TH levels in terminal adrenergic neurons and adrenal medulla is enhanced activity of the corresponding preganglionic cholinergic nerves (Axelrod, 1971; Thoenen and Otten, 1976, 1978a). A causal relationship between this increased activity and the subsequent TH elevation can be deduced from the observation that transection of the preganglionic nerve fibers abolishes the effect on TH (Thoenen, Mueller, and Axelrod, 1969a,b). The augmented TH levels result from an enhanced synthesis of new enzyme protein rather than from the formation of an activator or a reduced production of an inhibitor. This fact is demonstrated by observations that enzyme activities of control and experimental samples are always additive, that the apparent K_m values for substrate and cofactors do not change, and that the increase in TH activity can be blocked by inhibitors of protein synthesis acting at the transcriptional and translational levels (Mueller, Thoenen, and Axelrod, 1969b,c). The most direct evidence for an augmented synthesis of new enzyme protein is provided by immunological procedures using monospecific antibodies against TH (Joh, Gegliman, and Reis, 1973; Chuang and Costa, 1974).

The enhanced synthesis of TH does not reflect a general increase in neuronal protein synthesis. Under experimental conditions that lead to a more than twofold increase in TH levels, the total protein content of the corresponding sympathetic ganglia—about 50% of their volume represents neuronal cells—is not augmented to a detectable extent (Mueller, Thoenen, and Axelrod, 1969b). Of all the enzymes studied so far, dopamine-β-hydroxylase (DBH) is the only one that has also been shown to be synthesized at an augmented rate (Molinoff et al., 1970; Gagnon, Otten, and Thoenen, 1976). Both TH and DBH are selectively located in adrenergic neurons and adrenal chromaffin cells and catalyze key steps in the biosynthesis of the adrenergic transmitter (Geffen and Livett, 1971; Molinoff and Axelrod, 1971). In contrast, the level of dopa decarboxylase (DDC), another enzyme involved in the formation of norepinephrine, is not affected by an augmented preganglionic cholinergic activity (Thoenen et al., 1971b), thus excluding the possibility that all the enzymes involved in the biosynthesis of norepinephrine are regulated as an operational unit, as is often the case for a given metabolic pathway in bacterial systems (Ames and Martin, 1964).

From a teleological point of view, the selective induction of TH and DBH can be considered a long-term adaptation to augmented transmitter utilization. Synthesis of the enzymes takes place in the perikaryon, whence they are transported by axoplasmic transport to the adrenergic nerve terminals (Brimijoin, 1972; Oesch, Otten, and Thoenen, 1973), the main sites of synthesis of the adrenergic transmitter (Geffen and Livett, 1971). However, the selectivity of the induction of these two enzymes is of more general interest if one considers the adrenergic neuron as a general model. The induction of TH and DBH may be analogous to the selective induction of specific membrane proteins, which may represent the biochemical basis for long-lasting changes in neuronal connectivity.

The fact that neuronally mediated TH and DBH induction can be abolished by ganglionic blocking agents (Mueller, Thoenen, and Axelrod, 1970) and can be mimicked both in vivo and in vitro by administration of actylcholine or other nicotinic cholinomimetics (Patrick and Kirshner, 1971; Otten and Thoenen, 1976a,b) demonstrates that the first messenger in this process is acetylcholine rather than other substances liberated from the preganglionic cholinergic fibers. Stimulation of the preganglionic cholinergic nerves in vivo for 30 min at a frequency of 10 Hz is sufficient to initiate the cascade of events that leads finally to maximal TH induction 48 hr later (Zigmond and Ben-Ari, 1977). In organ cultures of rat sympathetic ganglia the time of initiation is even shorter: a 5–10 min pulse of carbamylcholine, a cholinomimetic that activates nicotinic receptors (as does acetylcholine) but is not a substrate for acetylcholinesterase, is sufficient to trigger a selective TH and DBH induction if optimal culture conditions are provided (Thoenen and Otten, 1978a,b). This relatively short period of initiation is followed by a longer period of regulation at the transcriptional level, which overlaps with the enhanced synthesis of enzyme protein. Up to 6 hr after activation of the nicotinic receptors, the process of induction can be completely prevented by actinomycin D or α-amanitin. Thereafter, the impairing action of these inhibitors of RNA synthesis gradually decreases, and they become ineffective in 18–20 hr (Otten et al., 1973; Rohrer and Otten, in preparation). The cycloheximide-sensitive augmented synthesis of TH and DBH begins at about 6 hr and lasts up to about 40 hr.

The fact that transsynaptic induction of TH and DBH can be blocked by actinomycin D and α-amanitin implies that the primary regulation occurs at the transcriptional level. However, since direct evidence for an augmented formation of TH and DBH messenger RNA (mRNA) has not yet been provided, there remains the possibility that the selective TH and DBH induction depends on the formation of a factor that enhances the translation of these two mRNAs in a specific manner.

Although the mechanism of initiation and the temporal sequence of the following events have been characterized in a relatively detailed manner, it is not yet clear how the changes effected in the neuronal membrane by acetylcholine are transformed into a message that induces specific regulatory changes at the transcriptional level. Below, we summarize briefly the mechanisms that have been excluded and those that look promising for future studies.

1. There is general agreement that initial changes in cAMP and/or cGMP in postganglionic adrenergic neurons are not a prerequisite for the subsequent selective induction of TH and DBH (Hanbauer and Costa, 1975; Thoenen and Otten, 1976). In contrast, the role of cAMP as a second messenger in the adrenal medulla is a matter of controversy (cf. Costa et al., 1975; Thoenen and Otten, 1975, 1976; Guidotti and Costa, 1977). However, recent experiments have shown that the cyclic nucleotide changes in the adrenal medulla mainly reflect ACTH-mediated alterations in the adrenal cortex, which disappear after hypophysectomy or after the selective blockade of the activation of the pituitary-adrenocortical axis by high doses of glucocorticoids (Thoenen and Otten, 1976). Both hypophysectomy and glucocorticoids abolish the increases in cAMP and the cAMP/cGMP ratio that are often observed in the adrenal medulla under experimental conditions that lead to neuronally mediated TH and DBH induction (Figure 2). However, neither hypophysectomy nor glucocorticoids impair neuronally mediated TH and DBH induction, as demonstrated under various experimental conditions in vivo and in vitro (Ciaranello, Wooten, and Axelrod, 1976; Otten and Thoenen, 1976c; Thoenen and Otten, 1975, 1976). Thus it can be concluded that

the previously postulated lower-limit changes in overall levels of cAMP (a minimum rate of increase of 10 pmol cAMP/mg protein/min and a minimum duration of the cAMP increase above control of 60 min) and minimum fourfold increase in cAMP/cGMP ratio (Guidotti and Costa, 1973; Guidotti, Mao, and Costa, 1974; Hanbauer, Guidotti, and Costa, 1975) are not in fact necessary for subsequent TH induction. However, there remains the possibility that a small selective pool of one or both of these cyclic nucleotides plays an essential role that is not amenable to experimental verification because the changes are too small to be distinguished from the much larger, unchanging pool. This also seems improbable, however, since in organ cultures of sympathetic ganglia inhibitors of phosphodiesterase do not enhance the carbamylcholine-mediated selective enzyme induction (Otten, unpublished observations).

2. The depolarization of the neuronal membrane as such does not seem to be an essential mechanism for transmitting the acetylcholine-mediated signals from the cell membrane to the cell nucleus, since high potassium concentrations in the culture medium (Otten and Thoenen, 1976a), veratridine, and batrachotoxin (Otten and Thoenen, 1976b) do not mimic the effect of the activation of nicotinic receptors (Figure 3). The TH induction effected by high potassium concentrations in intact ganglia results from a release of acetylcholine from preganglionic nerve terminals. It can be blocked by ganglionic blocking agents (Otten and Thoenen, 1976a). Moreover, the initiation process is not impaired by concentrations of tetrodotoxin (TTX), which is known to suppress the formation of action potentials in rat sympathetic ganglia following activation of nicotinic receptors (Kao, 1966; Haefely, 1972).

3. Since the initiation of selective enzyme induction is possible in calcium-free medium supplied with 10 mM EGTA, the influx of calcium can be excluded as an essential event in transsynaptic enzyme induction (Figure 3). This is further supported by the fact that calcium ionophores cannot mimic the effect of acetylcholine in organ cultures of sympathetic ganglia (Otten, unpublished observations).

From all these experimental data it could be concluded that the initiation of transsynaptic enzyme induction is neither mediated by cyclic nucleotides nor related to changes in ionic membrane permeabilities effected by acetylcholine. However, in recent experiments we have shown that transsynaptic enzyme induction can be abolished by dopamine (Thoenen and Otten, 1978a), which is known to produce a hyperpolarization in rabbit sympathetic ganglia

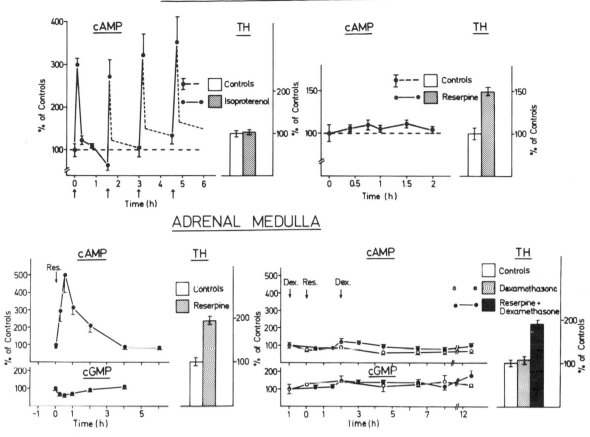

FIGURE 2 Relationship between changes in cyclic nucleotides and subsequent induction of TH in rat sympathetic ganglia and adrenal medulla. *Superior cervical ganglion*: Rats were injected with either a single 10 mg/kg dose of reserpine or four 0.4 mg/kg doses of isoproterenol at 90 min intervals. TH was determined 48 hr after reserpine or the first dose of isoproterenol. (From Otten, Oesch, and Thoenen, 1973, and Otten et al., 1974.) *Adrenal medulla*: Rats were injected either with 10 mg/kg of reserpine or the same dose of reserpine together with two 1.5 mg/kg doses of dexamethasone (sufficient to block the activation of the pituitary-adrenocortical axis). The first dose of dexamethasone was given 1 hr before reserpine, the second dose 2 hr after reserpine. cAMP and cGMP were determined at the given intervals, TH 48 hr after reserpine.

(Libet, 1970; Dun and Nishi, 1974). Although the ionic events underlying this hyperpolarization are not yet known, we investigated the possibility that this blocking effect might be related to the TTX-insensitive synaptic sodium channels. Such a relationship is supported by the observation that the replacement of sodium by Tris or lithium abolishes the acetylcholine-mediated TH induction (Thoenen and Otten, 1978a; Otten, unpublished observations). However, these experimental data do not yet allow definite conclusions. The experiments of Brown and Scholfield (1974a,b) showing that carbamylcholine (2×10^{-4}) produces a marked increase in intracellular sodium concentrations (from about 20 mM to 100 mM) in sympathetic ganglia within 5–10 min provide exper-

imental background for more direct studies of a possible relationship between changes in intracellular sodium concentrations and subsequent selective enzyme induction.

Furthermore, in recent experiments we have investigated the possible involvement of microfilaments and microtubules in transsynaptic induction. Neither colchicine, colcemid, and vinblastine, nor cytochalasins B and D interfered with the acetylcholine-mediated enzyme induction (Otten and Rohrer, unpublished observations). Thus the mechanism of transmission of acetylcholine-mediated changes in the neuronal membrane to the cell nucleus remains an open question, as is the case for antigen-mediated stimulation of antibody synthesis in lymphocytes and

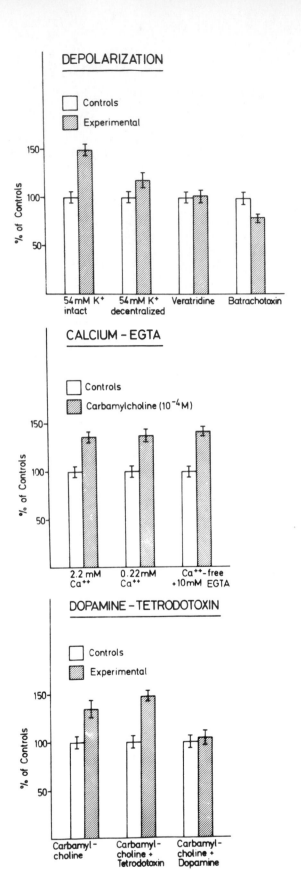

FIGURE 3 TH induction in sympathetic ganglia in organ culture. All the ganglia with the exception of "K⁺ intact" were decentralized 8–10 days before they were brought into organ culture according to Otten and Thoenen (1976a). All the ganglia were preincubated for 2 hr with 10^{-7}M dexamethasone (optimal concentration; see Figure 5) before the depolarizing agents or cholinomimetics were added for an additional hour to the corresponding medium. In some experiments, the ganglia were preincubated with tetrodotoxin or dopamine, together with dexamethasone or in a medium containing reduced concentrations of calcium with and without EGTA. After 3 hr of incubation in the presence of various drugs and ionic modifications of the media, the ganglia were rinsed and transferred to dishes containing normal media. Thereafter they were incubated for a further 47 hr before being homogenized; TH activity was then determined. The concentration of veratridine amounted to 10^{-6}M, batrachotoxin to 10^{-6}M, tetrodotoxin to 10^{-6}M, carbamylcholine to 10^{-4}M, dopamine to 10^{-4}M.

the initiation of histone synthesis in sea-urchin eggs by proteolytic enzymes or NH_3.

Modulatory role of glucocorticoids in transsynaptic enzyme induction

Wurtman, Moskowitz, and Munro (this volume) report on the central role of the pituitary-adrenocortical axis in the regulation of phenylethanolamine N-methyltransferase (PNMT) levels in the adrenal medulla. Although recent experiments of Ciaranello (1978) provide evidence that an intact cholinergic innervation is required for ACTH-mediated PNMT synthesis, the main regulatory factors for the level of this enzyme are the adrenocortical glucocorticoids. This is in distinct contrast to the predominant transsynaptic regulation of the synthesis of TH and DBH, which is also possible in hypophysectomized animals (Otten, Mueller, and Thoenen, 1975; Thoenen and Otten, 1975). Moreover, in organ cultures of sympathetic ganglia originating from animals adrenalectomized 10 days before, the activation of the nicotinic receptors by carbamylcholine still results in TH induction (Otten and Thoenen, 1976d). Thus transsynaptic induction does not depend on the presence of glucocorticoids. However, this finding does not preclude a modulatory role for glucocorticoids in this process; such a role has, indeed, been demonstrated both in vivo and in vitro. There is a causal relationship between the diurnal rhythm of the production of glucocorticoids by the adrenal cortex and the inducibility of TH by short-term increases in pregan-

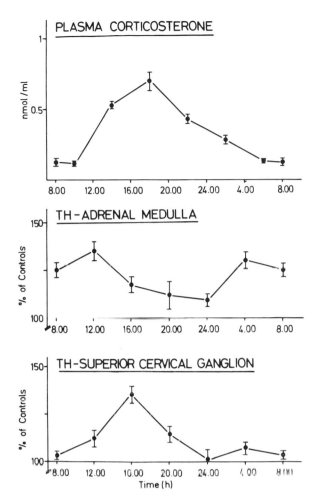

PLASMA CORTICOSTERONE

TH-ADRENAL MEDULLA

TH-SUPERIOR CERVICAL GANGLION

FIGURE 4 Circadian rhythm of plasma corticosterone levels and inducibility of TH in superior cervical ganglia. Seven groups of well-equilibrated (kept for at least 14 days in the same animal room at 21°C with a 12 hr light-dark cycle) male albino rats of 90–110 g body weight were exposed for 2 hr each to 4°C at different times of the day. The time of cold exposure began as indicated on the abscissa. Thereafter the animals were brought back to the animal room and killed 48 hr after the beginning of the cold exposure. TH was assayed in homogenates of superior cervical ganglia and adrenals. Plasma corticosterone levels were determined around the clock at the intervals shown. (From Otten and Thoenen, 1975.)

glionic nerve activity by cold stress (Figure 4). The optimal time for initiating transsynaptic enzyme induction in sympathetic ganglia coincides with the time of the highest steroid production in the adrenal cortex (Otten and Thoenen, 1975). In contrast, in the adrenal medulla, which is exposed to glucocorticoid concentrations two orders of magnitude higher than those of other organs due to its close relationship to the cortex (Ramaley, 1974; Jones, Hillhouse,

and Burden, 1977), the optimal time for the neuronally mediated enzyme induction is at the time of minimum glucocorticoid production. This concentration-dependent enhancing and inhibitory effect is also reflected in a bell-shaped concentration-response curve for the modulatory role of glucocorticoids in organ cultures of sympathetic ganglia (Figure 5). The optimal enhancing concentrations correspond to the maximum concentrations reached in vivo in the general circulation during the time of day of the highest production, whereas inhibitory concentrations are reached only in adrenal medulla during this time (Thoenen and Otten, 1978b). The modulatory role of the glucocorticoids in transsynaptic enzyme induction is also reflected by changes in the diurnal pattern of the neuronally mediated TH inducibility in the early postnatal period (Otten and Thoenen, 1975). Within the first two weeks after birth, the rat pituitary-adrenocortical axis is not yet fully functioning, and adrenocortical glucocorticoid production is not yet subjected to a diurnal rhythm (Ramaley, 1974). During this early postnatal period, short-term cold stress initiates TH induction in the adrenal medulla at any time of the day, whereas in the sympathetic ganglia an induction is not possible at any time of the day (Otten and Thoenen, 1975; Thoenen and Otten, 1978b). With the appearance of the diurnal rhythm of glucocorticoid production, induction in the ganglia becomes possible at the time of highest production in the late afternoon, whereas for the adrenal medulla this peak glucocorticoid production now causes inhibition of neuronally mediated enzyme production.

The modulatory role of glucocorticoids is most apparent during short-term enhancement of the activity of preganglionic cholinergic nerves. This fact was impressively demonstrated in organ-culture experiments with sympathetic ganglia. In the presence of optimal concentrations of glucocorticoids—a minimum preincubation of 60 min is necessary—a 10 min pulse of 10^{-4}M carbamylcholine is sufficient to initiate a maximum TH induction 48 hr later (Figure 5). In the absence of glucocorticoids, an exposure time of 4 hr is necessary to achieve a maximum response, which is still smaller than that initiated within 10 min in the presence of glucocorticoids.

Transfer of information from effector organs to innervating neurons by uptake and retrograde axonal transport of macromolecules

The marked influence of effector cells on innervating neurons is well established and has long been gen-

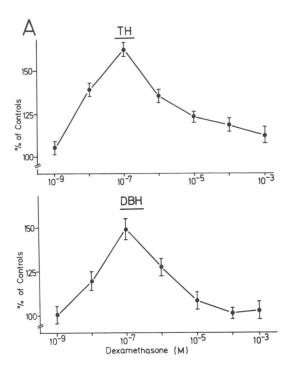

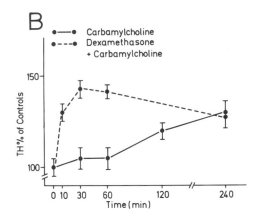

FIGURE 5 Modulatory role of gluococorticoids on TH induction mediated via nicotinic receptors. (A) Concentration-dependent modulation of TH induction mediated via nicotine receptors in rat sympathetic ganglia kept in organ culture. (From Otten and Thoenen, 1976d.) (B) Effect of glucocorticoids on the time required for initiation of TH induction in sympathetic ganglia in organ culture by carbamylcholine. In all experiments, the ganglia used had been decentralized in vivo 7–10 days before. A first series of ganglia was exposed to carbamylcholine (10^{-4}M) alone for up to 4 hr. The ganglia were then transferred to normal medium where they stayed until they were homogenized 48 hr after the beginning of the carbamylcholine pulse. A second series of ganglia was preincubated for 2 hr with 10^{-7}M dexamethasone before carbamylcholine was added for various time periods. Thereafter the same schedule was used as in the experiments with carbamylcholine alone.

erally acknowledged. In his classical experiments with chick embryos, Viktor Hamburger demonstrated that after amputation and/or transplantation of wing buds, the development of the spinal sensory and motor system corresponds to the volume of peripheral tissue to be innervated (Hamburger, 1934, 1939). Important information about the influence of effector cells on innervating neurons arose more recently from transplantation experiments with autonomically innervated peripheral organs (Burnstock, 1969, 1974; Olson and Malmfors, 1970; Chamley and Dowel, 1975), which showed that the transplanted tissue and not the site of transplantation determined both the quality and the quantity of reinnervation. Thus, if a piece of tissue is transplanted into the anterior eye chamber (a preferred site of transplantation), the reinnervating adrenergic and/or cholinergic nerve fibers originating from the iris restore the pattern and density of the original innervation. Björklund and collaborators supplemented these experiments by the important observation that the preincubation of the transplants in medium containing nerve growth factor (NGF) enhanced the rate and density of reinnervation. Conversely, preincubation with antibodies to NGF reduced and delayed the normally occurring reinnervation of the transplant by adrenergic nerve fibers (cf. Björklund, Bjerre, and Stenevi, 1974; Moore, Björklund, and Stenevi, 1974). These observations, together with the evidence that NGF is an absolute prerequisite for the normal development of sympathetic neurons and the maintenance of their function after differentiation (Levi-Montalcini and Angeletti, 1968; Hendry, 1976), led to the hypothesis that NGF might act as a messenger between effector organs and innervating adrenergic neurons (Hendry and Iversen, 1973).

Since several of the pleiotypic actions of NGF involve the synthesis of proteins, it was essential to evaluate whether NGF itself is transported to the perikaryon or whether a corresponding message is formed at the nerve terminal and is transferred indirectly to the cell body. In the following discussion we shall briefly summarize the evidence for NGF itself acting as mediator. Before doing so, however, we must state very clearly that we are referring only to regulation of the synthesis of specific macromolecules—TH and DBH in the perikaryon of adrenergic neurons—and not to the NGF-mediated stimulation of fiber outgrowth or its possible chemotactic guidance. There is evidence that the latter effects of NGF are mediated by a direct local action on the nerve fibers (see Patterson, this volume).

RETROGRADE AXONAL TRANSPORT OF NGF Investigations over the last few years have shown that NGF is taken up with high selectivity by adrenergic and sensory nerve terminals (see Figure 6) but not by motor cholinergic nerve terminals (Stöckel and Thoenen, 1975). After selective uptake by the nerve terminals, NGF is transported retrogradely to the perikaryon at a rate that is characteristic for a given species of neurons: 2–3 mm/hr for adrenergic neurons (Hendry et al., 1974); 10–13 mm/hr for sensory

neurons (Stöckel, Schwab, and Thoenen, 1975a,b). The retrograde axonal transport is sensitive to colchicine (Hendry et al., 1974; Stöckel, Schwab, and Thoenen, 1975a; Fillenz et al., 1976), as is the rapid orthograde axonal transport (Ochs, 1974). Interestingly, the retrograde transport of NGF does not seem to depend on neuronal activity: after decentralization of superior cervical ganglia, neither the rate nor the amount of retrogradely transported [125I]-NGF differed significantly from transport in neurons with

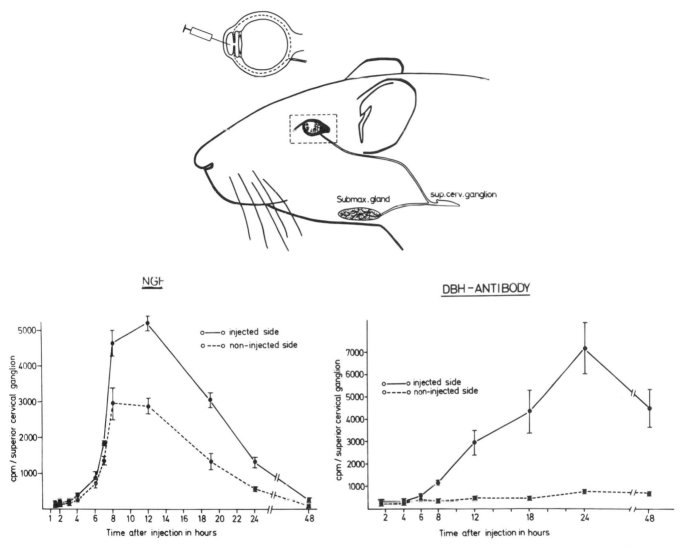

FIGURE 6 Retrograde axonal transport of NGF and antibodies to DBH in adrenergic neurons. [125I]-labeled NGF or antibodies to DBH were injected (unilaterally) into the anterior eye chamber (schematically shown at top). At the given time intervals after injection, the superior cervical ganglia were removed and their radioactivity was counted. This radioactivity proved to be more than 90% unchanged [125I]-NGF or [125I]-DBH-antibody (Stöckel et al., 1974; Fil-

lenz et al., 1976). The greater accumulation of [125I]-NGF as compared to [125I]-DBH-antibodies on the noninjected side reflects the larger proportion of the smaller molecules (NGF MW 26,500, DBH MW 150,000) that escape into the general circulation from the site of injection and reach the cell body of the contralateral side directly or by retrograde axonal transport. (From Stöckel et al., 1976.)

A

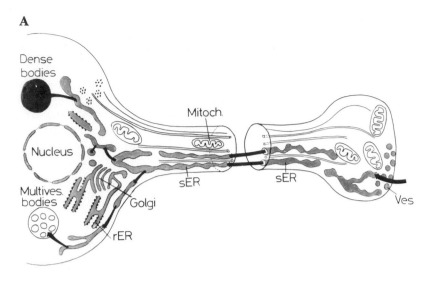

Dense bodies

Mitoch.

Nucleus

Multives. bodies

sER

sER

Golgi

rER

Ves

B

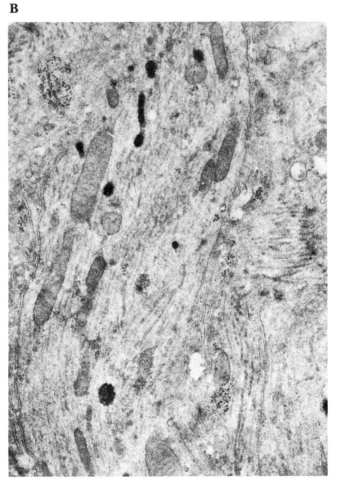

C

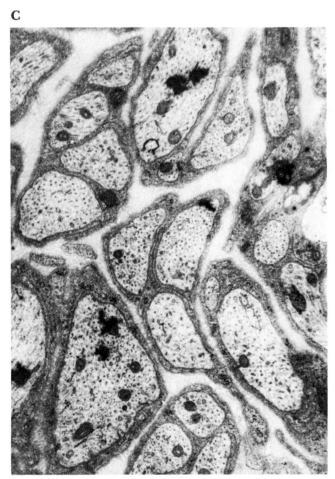

intact preganglionic nerve fibers. In addition, augmented activity of the peripheral sympathetic nervous system by cold stress or administration of reserpine enhanced neither the quantity nor the rate of

retrograde axonal transport of NGF (Stöckel and Thoenen, unpublished observations). Statistical evaluations of electron-microscopic autoradiographs (Schwab and Thoenen, 1977) and direct histochem-

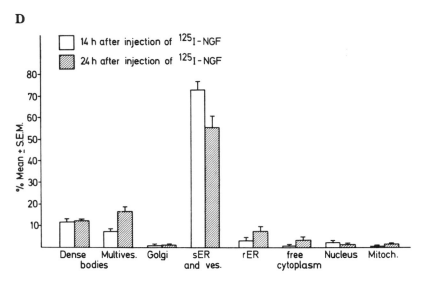

D

FIGURE 7 Pathway of retrograde axonal transport and subcellular distribution. (A) Schematic representation of the pathway of retrograde axonal transport of NGF. (B) Electron-microscopic histochemical localization of NGF covalently linked to horseradish peroxidase. The reaction product is confined to cisternae of the endoplasmic reticulum. (From Schwab, 1977). (C) Electron-microscopic autoradiograph of postganglionic adrenergic fibers originating from superior cervical ganglion after intraocular injection of [125I]-NFG. The label is exclusively located over axons. The resolution (~1,500 Å) of the autoradiography does not allow reliable direct localization of the individual silver grains over specific organelles. This is possible only on a statistical basis. (D) Statistical distribution of silver grains in electron-microscopic autoradiographs in the perikaryon of adrenergic neurons after retrograde axonal transport of [125I]-NGF. (After Schwab and Thoenen, 1977.)

ical localization of NGF coupled to horseradish peroxidase (Schwab, 1977) have shown that retrograde axonal transport is topographically linked to the same structures as orthograde transport (Droz, Rambourg, and Koenig, 1975)—that is, vesicles and cisternae of smooth endoplasmic reticulum (Figure 7).

Interestingly, neither electron-microscopic autoradiographic nor histochemical studies have provided evidence for an accumulation of NGF in the cell nucleus (Figure 7), thus demonstrating that a direct action of NGF on the cell nucleus is improbable or must occur at extremely low concentrations. In this context, a recent observation by Rohrer and Otten in organ cultures of sympathetic ganglia indicating that the regulation of the selective induction of TH and DBH by NGF occurs at the translational level is of particular interest. Although transsynaptic and NGF-mediated enzyme induction lead to very similar changes in the enzyme pattern—selective induction of TH and DBH (Thoenen et al., 1971 a,b)—the neuronally mediated induction can be abolished by α-amanitin and actinomycin D, whereas the NGF-mediated induction remains unchanged by the same concentrations of these two inhibitors of RNA synthesis. However, both transsynaptic and NGF-mediated enzyme induction can be abolished by the same concentrations of cycloheximide.

SPECIFICITY OF THE RETROGRADE AXONAL TRANSPORT OF NGF The retrograde axonal transport of NGF is of high specificity with respect to the neurons—peripheral adrenergic and sensory, but not motor, neurons—and also with respect to the molecules to be transported (cf. Stöckel and Thoenen, 1975). This high selectivity is not determined simply by the physicochemical properties of the protein, since a large number of macromolecules with molecular weights ranging from 6,000 to 500,000 and isoelectric points from 4 to 10 are not taken up and transported in adrenergic neurons when injected into the anterior eye chamber in similar molar concentrations and specific radioactivity as NGF (Hendry, Stach, and Herrup, 1974; Stöckel, Paravicini, and Thoenen, 1974). Of particular interest is the fact that cytochrome C, which has a nearly identical molecular weight as the monomer of B-NGF and also a virtually identical isoelectric point, was not transported to a detectable extent. The selectivity of the retrograde axonal transport of NGF is further emphasized by the fact that gradual oxidation of the tryptophan moieties of

B-NGF leads to a loss of its biological activity, as tested in chick dorsal-root ganglia, with a concomitant loss of its retrograde axonal transport (Stöckel, Paravicini, and Thoenen, 1974).

BIOLOGICAL SIGNIFICANCE OF RETROGRADELY TRANSPORTED NGF   That the moiety of NGF that reaches the cell body by retrograde axonal transport is of biological significance can be deduced from the fact that after unilateral injection of NGF into the anterior eye chamber, TH induction (Figure 8)—a characteristic biochemical response of the adrenergic cell body to NGF (Thoenen et al., 1971a)—is considerably greater in the superior cervical ganglion of the injected than of the noninjected side (Paravicini, Stöckel, and Thoenen, 1975). The smaller TH induction on the contralateral side has been shown to result from the escape of NGF from the injection site into the general circulation, so that it reaches the cell body both directly and, to a larger extent, via nerve terminals by retrograde axonal transport. Accordingly, the importance of the uptake by nerve terminals and the retrograde axonal transport has also been demonstrated for intravenously injected NGF (Stöckel et al., 1976b; Otten et al., 1977). Although NGF is taken up at the level of the cell body, the contribution of the retrogradely transported moiety is considerably greater. This may be based merely on the fact that the surface area of the axon terminals in an adrenergic neuron is much larger than that of the cell body.

So far no evidence has been provided for a relationship between the density of innervation of an organ and the quantity of NGF or NGF-like substances produced, activated, or accumulated. This gap in the chain of argument supporting the role of NGF as a mediator of information between effector cells and innervating neurons results from the insufficient sensitivity and reliability of the methods available for determining the presence of small amounts of NGF. The commonly used radioimmunoassays, which are based on the competition for monospecific NGF-antibody binding sites by defined quantities of labeled NGF and (unknown) endogenous NGF or NGF-like (cross-reacting) molecules, are complicated by the fact that both serum (of mice and rats) and tissue homogenates contain macromolecules that bind NGF with a sufficiently high affinity to compete with the binding sites of the antibodies. Consequently, erroneously high values for NGF are obtained that do not correspond to the results from "two-site" immunological or biological assays (Thoenen, Schwab, and Barde, 1978).

Evidence for the production or activation of NGF in effector organs and its physiological importance is entirely indirect. During the early postnatal period, the adrenergic neurons are very sensitive to interruption of the supply of NGF. General elimination of NGF by administration of NGF antibodies leads to destruction of the major part of the peripheral sympathetic neurons (Levi-Montalcini and Angeletti, 1968). At this stage of development, the same effect is produced by the interruption of the connections between the nerve terminals and the perikaryon (Figure 9). For example, surgical transection of postganglionic adrenergic fibers (Hendry, 1975a) or the destruction of the nerve terminals by 6-hydroxydopamine (Levi-Montalcini et al., 1975) leads to degeneration of the adrenergic cell body. In either case, however, the irreversible damaging effects can be prevented by exogenous administration of NGF (Hendry, 1975b; Levi-Montalcini et al., 1975), suggesting that both the effect of general antibody administration and the effect of surgical or chemical axotomy results from interruption of the normal supply of NGF to the perikaryon from the effector organ. In adult animals, transection of the postganglionic adrenergic nerve fibers and administration of monospecific antibodies to NGF has less dramatic but still distinct effects on the cell body, such as changes in the arrangement of the stacks of rough endoplasmic reticulum (chromatolysis); a transient decrease in TH activity (Figure 9); and detachment of the preganglionic cholinergic nerve terminals, leading to an impairment of ganglionic transmission (Matthews and Nelson, 1975; Purves, 1975, 1976).

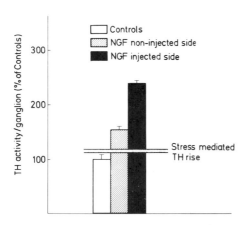

FIGURE 8   Effect of unilateral injection of 140 μg 2.5S NGF into the anterior eye chamber and the submaxillary gland (see scheme in Figure 6) on TH levels in the superior cervical ganglion of the injected and noninjected sides. The ganglia were removed 48 hr after NGF injection. (After Paravicini, Stöckel, and Thoenen, 1975.)

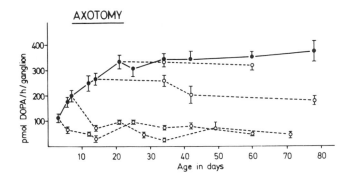

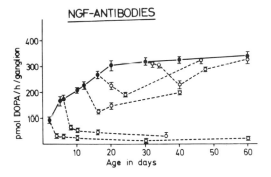

FIGURE 9 Comparison between the effect of axotomy and the administration of a single dose of antibody to NGF at different postnatal times. *Top*: Transection of the postganglionic fibers of the rat superior cervical ganglia was performed 3, 7, 14, and 21 days after birth; the subsequent development of the TH, which is an approximate measure of the number of surviving neurons, was determined up to 80 days. (From Hendry, 1975a.) *Bottom*: Rats were injected subcutaneously with single doses of 200 mg/kg of purified (Stöckel et al., 1976) monospecific antibodies to NGF 2, 6, 12, and 28 days after birth. TH was determined in a similar manner as after axotomy.

All these effects of axotomy can be prevented by administration of NGF (Purves and Nja, 1976), thus supporting the contention that retrogradely transported NGF is physiologically important in the fully differentiated system.

General aspects of retrograde axonal and transsynaptic transport of macromolecules

So far, evidence for the biological significance of the retrograde axonal transport of a macromolecule has been provided only for NGF. Indirect evidence, however, makes it reasonable to assume that the pathway of retrograde axonal transport, possibly followed by transfer across synapses to second-order neurons, could have more general implications with respect to the manner of ("trophic") communications between neurons and other neurons or nonneuronal cells (Cragg, 1970; see also Kreutzberg and Schubert, this

volume). A discussion of the general aspects of retrograde transport seems to be justified in this context, since it might be important to future investigations of macromolecules other than NGF that act as retrograde messengers.

We have already mentioned that retrograde axonal transport of NGF is highly specific with respect to both the structure of the molecule and the neurons by which it is transported. In principle, we can distinguish two groups of molecules that undergo retrograde axonal transport. For the majority of macromolecules (e.g., horseradish peroxidase, albumin, ferritin), retrograde axonal transport is only demonstrable if extremely high concentrations are brought into the vicinity of the nerve terminals in question (Kristensson, Olsson, and Sjöstrand, 1971; Nauta, Pritz, and Lasek, 1974). This nonspecific retrograde axonal transport, to which all macromolecules of a critical size are probably subject, is based on their being "trapped" in consequence of the release of transmitter by exocytosis (see also Heuser and Reese, this volume). This nonspecific retrograde axonal transport must be distinguished from the specific transport of NGF, which is independent of neuronal activity and occurs at much lower concentrations. This does not mean, however, that NGF is the only molecule transported in such a manner; indeed, recent experiments have shown that a series of toxins, lectins, and antibodies to specific macromolecules are taken up and transported in a similar manner (Table I; see Fillenz et al., 1976; Stöckel, Schwab, and Thoenen, 1975b, 1977; Ziegler, Thomas, and Jacobowitz, 1976). The high selectivity seems to support the notion that the prerequisite for this transport is high-affinity binding to specific receptors on the surface of the neuronal membrane. This ligand-receptor interaction initiates the endocytosis of the whole membrane complex through a sequence of events not yet understood in detail. A causal relationship between the high-affinity binding of the ligands and their subsequent internalization is supported by the fact that NGF is transported only in adrenergic and sensory neurons (Stöckel, Schwab, and Thoenen, 1975a), which, in contrast to other neurons, have been shown to bind NGF by high-affinity membrane receptors (Herrup, Stickgold, and Shooter, 1974; Snyder et al., 1974). The concept of high-affinity binding as a prerequisite for the initiation of retrograde axonal transport is also supported by the observation that horseradish peroxidase and monospecific antibodies to NGF are not taken up to a measurable extent by adrenergic nerve terminals if they are injected into the anterior eye chamber in low concentrations. How-

TABLE I
Selectivity and specificity of retrograde axonal transport

Ligand	Retrograde Axonal Transport		
	Adrenergic	Sensory	Motor
DBH antibody	+	−	−
NGF	+	+	−
Tetanus toxin	+	+	+
Cholera toxin	+	+	+
Wheat-germ agglutinin	+	+	+
Phytohaem-agglutinin	+	+	+
Ricin	+	+	+
Horseradish peroxidase	−	n.d.	n.d.
Horseradish peroxidase covalently linked to NGF	+	n.d.	n.d.
Antibody to NGF	−	n.d.	n.d.
Antibody to NGF "loaded" with NGF	+	n.d.	n.d.

All the [^{125}I]-labeled macromolecules were injected into the vicinity of adrenergic, sensory, and motor nerve terminals. The accumulation of radioactivity in the corresponding cell bodies was compared with that of the contralateral side. (n.d. = not determined.)

ever, if the horseradish peroxidase is covalently linked to NGF and the antibodies are "loaded" with NGF, then the two coupling products are transported as efficiently as NGF alone (Schwab, 1977; Dumas, Schwab, and Thoenen, unpublished observations). The most direct evidence for the importance of high-affinity binding to nerve terminals is derived from recent morphological studies in rat iris: colloidal gold particles coated with tetanus toxin become closely associated with the neuronal membrane of nerve terminals; this association is followed by their endocytosis and retrograde axonal transport in cisternae of smooth endoplasmic reticulum. In contrast, albumin-coated gold particles were neither associated with the neuronal membrane nor taken up into the nerve terminals (Figure 10).

The high-affinity binding of specific surface receptors can be used as a tool to characterize the properties of the surface of the cell membrane of the nerve terminals. Obtaining this information by a direct biochemical approach would involve barely surmountable technical difficulties. The macromolecules transported include specific antibodies (Fillenz et al., 1976), lectins that bind to specific sugar moieties of membrane constituents (Nicolson, 1974), and toxins that are known to have a high affinity for specific gangliosides (van Heyningen, 1974). Thus retrograde

axonal transport can be used to determine whether particular binding sites are present on the surface of the cell membrane of a particular type of nerve terminal. For example, transport of DBH antibodies exclusively in adrenergic neurons (Fillenz et al., 1976) provided indirect evidence that the storage vesicle membranes, which contain DBH as an integral part, are probably incorporated into the cell membrane as a consequence of exocytotic transmitter release. Moreover, it has been shown that retrograde axonal transport of tetanus toxin and cholera toxin can be blocked (Stöckel, Schwab, and Thoenen, 1977) by the simultaneous administration of those gangliosides that display a high affinity to these toxins (Heyningen, 1974).

Another aspect of the retrograde axonal transport was brought to light by recent studies showing that the transport of NGF, wheat-germ agglutinin, and tetanus toxin is saturable and that the binding and retrograde axonal transport of the single ligands do not interfere with each other. There is also evidence for consumption of the binding sites; rate of recovery of the binding sites allows an approximate determination of the turnover rate of the single species of receptors (Dumas, Schwab, and Thoenen, unpublished observation).

Lesion experiments in various neuronal systems have shown that the retrograde effect of axotomy is not confined to the perikaryon of the injured neuron but also involves second-order neurons transsynaptically (Cragg, 1970; Cowan, 1970). This might suggest, among other possibilities, that retrograde axonal transport of trophic substances is extended by transsynaptic transport. So far, such a transfer has not yet been shown for a defined endogenous macromolecule of known biological function. However, such a transsynaptic transfer has been demonstrated for tetanus toxin in both motor and adrenergic neurons (Schwab and Thoenen, 1976, 1977). This transsynaptic transfer of tetanus toxin following retrograde axonal transport answers the question of how the toxin, which cannot reach the spinal cord across the blood-brain barrier, reaches its site of action, namely the inhibitory nerve terminals ending on spinal motoneurons (Curtis and de Groat, 1968; Curtis et al., 1973). These observations demonstrate that mechanisms exist for selectively carrying macromolecules across synapses from post- to presynaptic structures. They are important for our understanding of the pathophysiological mechanism in tetanus, and they may also yield a base for further studies focusing on the general significance and requirements for transsynaptic transfer of macromolecules.

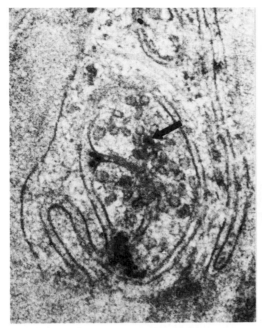 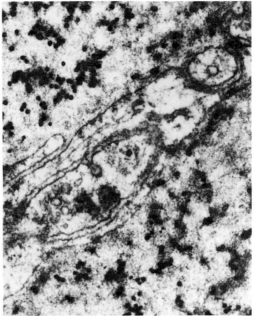

FIGURE 10 Electron-microscopic localization of gold particles coated with tetanus toxin or bovine serum albumin in the rat iris. Ten micrograms of colloidal gold was injected into the anterior eye chamber of a rat. The gold was coated either with tetanus toxin or with bovine serum albumin. *Left*: Gold particles coated with tetanus toxin adhere to the membrane of nerve terminals in the rat iris. Arrow points to a particle inside a nerve terminal. *Right*: Gold particles coated with bovine serum albumin. The lack of association between gold particles and neuronal membranes indicates no uptake into nerve terminals.

ACKNOWLEDGMENTS The authors are very grateful to Miss Vreni Forster for the careful preparation of the figures and the manuscript and to Mrs. Barbara Shomer and Dr. Stephen Max for linguistic revision. Our research group was supported by the Swiss National Foundation for Scientific Research (Grant No. 3.432.74).

REFERENCES

AMES, B. N., and R. G. MARTIN, 1964. Biochemical aspects of genetics: The operon. *Annu. Rev. Biochem.* 33:235–253.

AXELROD, J., 1971. Noradrenaline: Fate and control of its biosynthesis. *Science* 173:598–606.

BJÖRKLUND, A., B. BJERRE, and U. STENEVI, 1974. Has nerve growth factor a role in the regeneration of central and peripheral catecholamine neurons? In *Dynamics of Degeneration and Growth in Neurons*, K. Fuxe, L. Olson, and Y. Zotterman, eds. New York: Pergamon Press, pp. 389–409.

BLACK, I. B., 1974. Growth and development of cholinergic and adrenergic neurons in a sympathetic ganglion: Reciprocal regulation at the synapse. In *Dynamics of Degeneration and Growth in Neurons*, K. Fuxe, L. Olson, and Y. Zotterman, eds. New York: Pergamon Press, pp. 455–467.

BRIMIJOIN, S., 1972. Transport and turnover of dopamine β-hydroxylase (EC 1.14.2.1) in sympathetic nerves of the rat. *J. Neurochem.* 19:2183–2193.

BROWN, D. A., and C. N. SCHOLFIELD, 1974a. Changes of intracellular sodium and potassium ion concentrations in isolated rat superior cervical ganglia induced by depolarizing agents. *J. Physiol.* 242:307–319.

BROWN, D. A., and C. N. SCHOLFIELD, 1974b. Movements of labelled sodium ions in isolated rat superior cervical ganglia. *J. Physiol.* 242:321–351.

BURNSTOCK, G., 1969. Evolution of the autonomic innervation of visceral and cardiovascular systems in vertebrates. *Pharmacol. Rev.* 21:247–324.

BURNSTOCK, G., 1974. Degeneration and orientation of growth of autonomic nerves in relation to smooth muscle in joint tissue cultures and anterior eye chamber transplants. In *Dynamics of Degeneration and Growth in Neurons*, K. Fuxe, L. Olson, and Y. Zotterman, eds. New York: Pergamon Press, pp. 509–520.

CHAMLEY, J. H., and J. J. DOWEL, 1975. Specificity of nerve fiber "attraction" to autonomic effector organs in tissue culture. *Exp. Cell Res.* 90:1–7.

CHUANG, D. M., and E. COSTA. 1974. Biosynthesis of tyrosine hydroxylase in rat adrenal medulla after exposure to cold. *Proc. Natl. Acad. Sci. USA* 71:4570–4574.

CIARANELLO, R. D., 1978. Regulation of phenylethanolamine N-methyltransferase synthesis and degradation. In *Structure and Function of Monoamine Enzymes*, E. Usdin, N. Weiner, and M. B. Youdim, eds, New York: M. Dekker, pp. 497–525.

CIARANELLO, R. D., G. F. WOOTEN, and J. AXELROD, 1976. Regulation of rat adrenal dopamine β-hydroxylase. II. Receptor interaction in the regulation of enzyme synthesis and degradation. *Brain Res.* 113:349–362.

COSTA, E., D. M. CHUANG, A. GUIDOTTI, and P. UZUNOV, 1975. Cyclic 3′,5′-adenosine monophosphate dependent molecular mechanisms in the trans-synaptic induction of tyrosine hydroxylase in rat adrenal medulla. In *Chemical Tools in Cathecholamine Research*, vol. 2, O. A. Jonsson et al., eds. Amsterdam: North-Holland, pp. 283–292.

COUPLAND, R. F., 1975. Blood supply of the adrenal gland. In *Handbook of Physiology*, section 7: *Endocrinology*, vol. 6, R. O. Greep and E. B. Astwood, eds. Baltimore: Williams & Wilkins, pp. 283–294.

COWAN, W. M., 1970. Anterograde and retrograde trans-neuronal degeneration in the central and peripheral nervous system. In *Contemporary Research Methods in Neuroanatomy*, W. J. H. Nauta and S. O. E. Ebbesson, eds. Berlin: Springer-Verlag, pp. 217–251.

CRAGG, B. G., 1970. What is the signal for chromatolysis? *Brain Res.* 23:1–21.

CURTIS, D. R., and W. C. DE GROAT, 1968. Tetanus toxin and spinal inhibition. *Brain Res.* 10:208–212.

CURTIS, D. R., D. FELIX, C. J. A. GAME, and R. M. MC-CULLOCH, 1973. Tetanus toxin and the synaptic release of GABA. *Brain Res.* 51:358–362.

DICHTER, M. A., A. S. TISCHLER, and L. A. GREEN, 1977. Nerve growth factor–induced increase in electrical excitability and acetylcholine sensitivity of rat pheochromocytoma cell line. *Nature* 268:501–504.

DROZ, B., A. RAMBOURG, and H. L. KOENIG, 1975. The smooth endoplasmic reticulum: Structure and role in the renewal of axonal membrane and synaptic vesicles by fast axonal transport. *Brain Res.* 93:1–13.

DUN, N., and S. NISHI. 1974. Effects of dopamine on the superior cervical ganglion of the rabbit. *J. Physiol.* 239:155–164.

FILLENZ, M., C. GAGNON, K. STÖCKEL, and H. THOENEN, 1976. Selective uptake and retrograde axonal transport of dopamine β-hydrozylase antibodies in peripheral adrenergic neurons. *Brain Res.* 114:293–303.

GAGNON, C., U. OTTEN, and H. THOENEN, 1976. Increased synthesis of dopamine β-hydroxylase in cultured rat adrenal medullae after in vivo administration of reserpine. *J. Neurochem.* 27:259–265.

GEFFEN, L. B., and B. G. LIVETT, 1971. Synaptic vesicles in sympathetic neurons. *Physiol. Rev.* 51:98–157.

GOODMAN, R., U. OTTEN, and H. THOENEN, 1975. Organ culture of the rat adrenal medulla: A model system for the study of transsynaptic induction. *J. Neurochem.* 25:423–427.

GREEN, L. A., and G. REIN, 1977. Dopaminergic properties of a somatic cell hybrid line of mouse neuroblastoma X sympathetic ganglion cells. *J. Neurochem.* 29:141–150.

GREEN, L. A., and A. S. TISCHLER, 1976. Establishment of a noradrenergic clonal line of rat adrenal pheochromocytoma cells which respond to nerve growth factor. *Proc. Natl. Acad. Sci. USA* 73:2424–2428.

GUIDOTTI, A., and E. COSTA, 1973. Involvement of adenosine 3′,5′-monophosphate in the activation of tyrosine hydroxylase elicited by drugs. *Science* 179:902–904.

GUIDOTTI, A., and E. COSTA, 1977. Trans-synaptic regulation of tyrosine 3′-monooxygenase biosynthesis in rat adrenal medulla. *Biochem. Pharmacol.* 26:817–823.

GUIDOTTI, A., C. C. MAO, and E. COSTA, 1974. Trans-synaptic regulation of tyrosine hydrozylase in adrenal medulla: Possible role of cyclic nucleotides. In *Frontiers in Catecholamine Research*, E. Usdin and S. Snyder, eds. New York: Pergamon Press, pp. 231–236.

HAEFELY, W., 1972. Electrophysiology of the adrenergic neuron. In *Handbuch der Experimentallen Pharmakologie*, vol. 33, H. Blaschko and E. Muscholl, eds. Berlin: Springer-Verlag, pp. 661–725.

HAMBURGER, V., 1934. The effects of wing bud extirpation on the development of the central nervous system in chick embryos. *J. Exp. Zool.* 68:449–494.

HAMBURGER, V., 1939. Motor and sensory hyperplasia following limb bud transplantation in chick embryos. *Physiol. Zool.* 111:457–501.

HANBAUER, I., and E. COSTA, 1975. Trans-synaptic induction of tyrosine hydroxylase in superior cervical ganglia: Participation of postsynaptic and steroid receptors. In *Chemical Tools in Catecholamine Research*, vol. 2, O. A. Jonsson et al., eds. Amsterdam: North-Holland, pp. 175–182.

HANBAUER, I., A. GUIDOTTI, and E. COSTA, 1975. Involvement of cyclic nucleotides in the long term induction of tyrosine hydroxylase. *Excerpta Med. Int. Cong. Ser.* 359:935–943.

HENDRY, I. A., 1975a. The effects of axotomy on the development of the rat superior cervical ganglion. *Brain Res.* 90:235–244.

HENDRY, I. A., 1975b. The response of adrenergic neurones to axotomy and nerve growth factor. *Brain Res.* 94:87–97.

HENDRY, I. A., 1976. Control in the development of the vertebrate sympathetic nervous system. In *Reviews of Neuroscience*, vol. 2, S. Ehrenpreis and I. J. Kopin, eds. New York: Raven Press, pp. 149–194.

HENDRY, I. A., and L. L. IVERSEN, 1973. Reduction in the concentration of nerve growth factor in mice after sialectomy and castration. *Nature* 243:500–504.

HENDRY, I. A., R. STACH, and K. HERRUP, 1974. Characteristics of the retrograde axonal transport system for nerve growth factor in the sympathetic nervous system. *Brain Res.* 82:117–128.

HENDRY, I. A., K. STÖCKEL, H. THOENEN, and L. L. IVERSEN, 1974. Retrograde axonal transport of nerve growth factor. *Brain Res.* 68:103–121.

HERRUP, K., R. STICKGOLD, and E. M. SHOOTER, 1974. The role of nerve growth factor in the development of sensory and sympathetic ganglia. *Ann. NY Acad. Sci.* 228:381–392.

HEYNINGEN, W. E. VAN, 1974. Gangliosides as membrane receptors for tetanus toxin, cholera toxin and serotonin. *Nature* 249:415–417.

JOH, T. H., C. GEGLIMAN, and D. J. REIS, 1973. Immunochemical demonstration of increased accumulation of tyrosine hydroxylase protein in sympathetic ganglia and adrenal medulla elicited by reserpine. *Proc. Natl. Acad. Sci. USA* 70:2767–2771.

JONES, M. T., E. W. HILLHOUSE, and J. L. BURDEN, 1977. Dynamics and mechanics of corticosteroid feedback at the hypothalamus and anterior pituitary gland. *J. Endocrinol.* 73:405–417.

KAO, G. Y., 1966. Tetrodotoxin, saxitoxin and their significance in the study of excitation phenomena. *Pharamacol. Rev.* 18:997–1049.

KRISTENSSON, K., Y. OLSSON, and J. SJÖSTRAND, 1971. Axonal uptake and retrograde transport of exogenous protein in the hypoglossal nerve. *Brain Res.* 32:399–406.

LEVI-MONTALCINI, R., L. ALOE, E. MUGNAINI, F. OESCH, and H. THOENEN, 1975. Nerve growth factor induces volume increase and enhances tyrosine hydroxylase synthesis in chemically axotomized sympathetic ganglia of newborn rats. *Proc. Natl. Acad. Sci. USA* 72:595–599.

LEVI-MONTALCINI, R., and P. U. ANGELETTI, 1968. Nerve growth factor. *Physiol. Rev.* 48:534–569.

LIBET, B., 1970. Generation of slow inhibitory and excitatory postsynaptic potentials. *Fed. Proc.* 29:1945–1965.

MATTHEWS, M. R., and V. H. NELSON, 1975. Detachment of structurally intact nerve endings from chromatolytic neurones of rat superior cervical ganglion during the depression of synaptic transmission induced by post-ganglionic axotomy. *J. Physiol.* 245:91–135.

MOLINOFF, P. B., and J. AXELROD, 1971. Biochemistry of catecholamines. *Annu. Rev. Biochem.* 40:465–500.

MOLINOFF, P. B., S. BRIMIJOIN, R. WEINSHILBOUM, and J. AXELROD, 1970. Neuronally-mediated increase in dopamine β-hydroxylase activity. *Proc. Natl. Acad. Sci. USA* 66:453–458.

MOORE, Y. R., A. BJÖRKLUND, and U. STENEVI, 1974. Growth and plasticity of adrenergic neurons. In *The Neurosciences: Third Study Program*, F. O. Schmitt and F. G. Worden, eds. Cambridge, MA: MIT Press, pp. 961–977.

MUELLER, R. A., H. THOENEN, and J. AXELROD, 1969a. Adrenal tyrosine hydroxylase: Compensatory increase in activity after chemical sympathectomy. *Science* 158:468–469.

MUELLER, R. A., H. THOENEN, and J. AXELROD, 1969b. Increase in tyrosine hydroxylase activity after reserpine administration. *J. Pharmacol. Exp. Ther.* 169:74–79.

MUELLER, R. A., H. THOENEN, and J. AXELROD, 1969c. Inhibition of trans synaptically increased tyrosine hydroxylase activity by cycloheximide and actinomycin D. *Mol. Pharmacol.* 5:463–469.

MUELLER, R. A., H. THOENEN, and J. AXELROD, 1970. Inhibition of neuronally induced tyrosine hydroxylase by nicotinic receptor-blockade. *Eur. J. Pharmacol.* 10:51–56.

NAUTA, H. J. W., M. B. PRITZ, and R. J. LASEK, 1974. Afferents to the rat caudoputamen studied with horseradish peroxidase: An evaluation of a retrograde neuroanatomical research method. *Brain Res.* 67:219–238.

NICOLSON, G. L., 1974. The interactions of lectins with animal cell surfaces. *Int. Rev. Cytol.* 39:89–190.

OCHS, S., 1974. Systems of material transport in nerve fibers (axoplasmic transport) related to nerve function and trophic control. *Ann. NY Acad. Sci.* 228:202–223.

OESCH, F., U. OTTEN, and H. THOENEN, 1973. Relationship between the rate of axoplasmic transport and subcellular distribution of enzymes involved in the synthesis of norepinephrine. *J. Neurochem.* 20:1691–1706.

OLSSON, L., and T. MALMFORS, 1970. Growth characteristics of adrenergic nerves in the adult rat. *Acta Physiol. Scand.* (suppl. 348): 1–112.

OTTEN, U., R. A. MUELLER, F. OESCH, and H. THOENEN, 1974. Location of an isoproterenol-responsive cyclic amp pool in adrenergic nerve cell bodies and its relationship to tyrosine hydroxylase induction. *Proc. Natl. Acad. Sci. USA* 71:2217–2221.

OTTEN, U., R. A. MUELLER, and H. THOENEN, 1975. Effect of hypophysectomy on cAMP changes in rat adrenal medulla evoked by catecholamines and carbamylcholine.

Naunyn-Schmiedebergs Arch. Pharmakol. 289:157–170.

OTTEN, U., F. OESCH, and H. THOENEN, 1973. Dissociation between changes in cyclic AMP and subsequent induction of TH in the rat superior cervical ganglion and adrenal medulla. *Naunyn-Schmiedebergs Arch. Pharmakol.* 280:129–140.

OTTEN, U., U. PARAVICINI, F. OESCH, and H. THOENEN, 1973. Time requirement for the single steps in trans-synaptic induction of tyrosine hydroxylase in the peripheral sympathetic nervous system. *Naunyn-Schmiedebergs Arch. Pharmakol.* 280:117–127.

OTTEN, U., M. SCHWAB, C. GAGNON, and H. THOENEN, 1977. Selective induction of tyrosine hydroxylase and dopamine β-hydroxylase by nerve growth factor: Comparison between adrenal medulla and sympathetic ganglia of adult and newborn rats. *Brain Res.* 133:291–303.

OTTEN, U., and H. THOENEN, 1975. Circadian rhythm of tyrosine hydroxylase induction by short-term cold stress: Modulatory action of glucocorticoids in newborn and adult rats. *Proc. Natl. Acad. Sci. USA* 72:1415–1419.

OTTEN, U., and H. THOENEN, 1976a. Mechanisms of tyrosine hydroxylase and dopamine β-hydroxylase induction in organ cultures of rat sympathetic ganglia by potassium depolarization and cholinomimetics. *Naunyn-Schmiedebergs Arch. Pharmakol.* 292:153–159.

OTTEN, U., and H. THOENEN, 1976b. Role of membrane depolarization in trans-synaptic induction of tyrosine hydroxylase in organ cultures of sympathetic ganglia. *Neurosci. Lett.* 2:93–96.

OTTEN, U., and H. THOENEN, 1976c. Lack of correlation between changes in cyclic nucleotides and subsequent induction of tyrosine hydroxylase in the adrenal medulla. *Naunyn-Schmiedebergs Arch. Pharmakol.* 293:105–108.

OTTEN, U., and H. THOENEN, 1976d. Selective induction of tyrosine hydroxylase and dopamine β hydroxylase in sympathetic ganglia in organ culture: Role of glucocorticoids as modulators. *Mol. Pharmacol.* 12:353–361.

PARAVICINI, U., K. STÖCKEL, and H. THOENEN, 1975. Biological importance of retrograde axonal transport of nerve growth factor in adrenergic neurons. *Brain Res.* 84:279–291.

PATRICK, R. L., and N. KIRSHNER, 1971. Effect of stimulation on levels of tyrosine hydroxylase, dopamine β-hydroxylase and catecholamine in intact and denervated rat adrenal glands. *Mol. Pharmacol.* 7:87–96.

PURVES, D., 1975. Functional and structural changes in mammalian sympathetic neurones following interruption of their axons. *J. Physiol.* 252:429–463.

PURVES, D., 1976. Functional and structural changes in mammalian sympathetic neurones following colchicine application to postganglionic nerves. *J. Physiol.* 259:159–175.

PURVES, D., and A. NJA, 1976. Effect of nerve growth factor on synaptic depression after axotomy. *Nature* 260:535–536.

RAMALEY, J. A., 1974. The changes in basal corticosterone secretion in rats blinded at birth. *Experientia* 30:827.

SCHWAB, M. E., 1977. Ultrastructural localization of a nerve growth factor–horseradish peroxidase (NGF-HPR) coupling product after retrograde axonal transport in adrenergic neurons. *Brain Res.* 130:190–196.

SCHWAB, M. E., and H. THOENEN, 1976. Electron microscopic evidence for a trans-synaptic migration of tetanus toxin in spinal cord motoneurons: An autoradiographic and morphometric study. *Brain Res.* 105:213–227.

SCHWAB, M. E., and H. THOENEN, 1977. Selective trans-synaptic migration of tetanus toxin after retrograde axonal transport in peripheral sympathetic nerves: A comparison with nerve growth factor. *Brain Res.* 122:459–474.

SNYDER, S. H., S. P. BANERJEE, P. CUATRECASAS, and L. A. GREENE, 1974. The nerve growth factor receptor: Demonstration of specific binding in sympathetic ganglia. In *Dynamics of Degeneration and Growth in Neurons*, K. Fuxe, L. Olson, and Y. Zotterman, eds. New York: Pergamon Press, pp. 347–359.

STÖCKEL, K., C. GAGNON, G. GUROFF, and H. THOENEN, 1976a. Purification of nerve growth factor antibodies by affinity chromatography. *J. Neurochem.* 26:1207–1211.

STÖCKEL, K., G. GUROFF, M. SCHWAB, and H. THOENEN, 1976b. The significance of retrograde axonal transport for the accumulation of systemically administered nerve growth factor (NGF) in the rat superior cervical ganglion. *Brain Res.* 109:271–284.

STÖCKEL, K., U. PARAVICINI, and H. THOENEN, 1974. Specificity of the retrograde axonal transport of nerve growth factor. *Brain Res.* 76:413–421.

STÖCKEL, K., M. SCHWAB, and H. THOENEN, 1975a. Specificity of retrograde transport of nerve growth factor (NGF) in sensory neurons: A biochemical and morphological study. *Brain Res.* 89:1–14.

STÖCKEL, K., M. SCHWAB, and H. THOENEN, 1975b. Comparison between the retrograde axonal transport of nerve growth factor and tetanus toxin in motor, sensory and adrenergic neurons. *Brain Res.* 99:1–16.

STÖCKEL, K., M. SCHWAB, and H. THOENEN, 1977. Role of gangliosides in the uptake and retrograde axonal transport of choleratoxin and tetanus toxin as compared to nerve growth factor and wheat germ agglutinin. *Brain Res.* 132:273–285.

STÖCKEL, K., and H. THOENEN, 1975. Specificity and biological importance of retrograde axonal transport of nerve growth factor. In *Proceedings of the Sixth International Congress of Pharmacology, Helsinki, Finland*, J. Tuomisto and M. K. Paasonen, eds., vol. 2, pp. 285–296.

THOENEN, H., 1975. Trans-synaptic regulation of neuronal enzyme synthesis. In *Handbook of Psychopharmacology*, vol. 3, L. L. Iversen, S. D. Iversen, and S. H. Snyder, eds. New York: Plenum Publ., pp. 443–475.

THOENEN, H., P. U. ANGELETTI, R. LEVI-MONTALCINI, and R. KETTLER, 1971a. Selective induction of tyrosine hydroxylase and dopamine β-hydroxylase in the rat superior cervical ganglia by nerve growth factor. *Proc. Natl. Acad. Sci. USA* 68:1598–1602.

THOENEN, H., R. KETTLER, W. BURKHARD, and A. SANER, 1971b. Neuronally-mediated control of enzymes involved in the synthesis of norepinephrine: Are they regulated as an operational unit? *Naunyn-Schmiedebergs Arch. Pharmakol.* 270:146–160.

THOENEN, H., R. A. MUELLER, and J. AXELROD, 1969a. Increased tyrosine hydroxylase activity after drug-induced alteration of sympathetic transmission. *Nature* 221:1264.

THOENEN, H., R. A. MUELLER, and J. AXELROD, 1969b. Trans-synaptic induction of adrenal tyrosine hydroxylase. *J. Pharmacol. Exp. Ther.* 169:249–254.

THOENEN, H., and U. OTTEN, 1975. Cyclic nucleotides and trans-synaptic enzyme induction: Lack of correlation between initial cAMP increase, changes in cAMP/cGMP ratio and subsequent induction of tyrosine hydroxylase in the adrenal medulla. In *Chemical Tools in Catecholamine Research*, vol. 2, O. A. Jonsson et al., eds. Amsterdam: North-Holland, pp. 275–282.

THOENEN, H., and U. OTTEN, 1976. Molecular events in transsynaptic regulation of the synthesis of macromolecules. In *Essays in Neurochemistry and Neuropharmacology*, vol. 1, M. B. H. Youdim, W. Lovenberg, D. F. Sharman, and J. R. Lagnado, eds. New York: John Wiley, pp. 73–101.

THOENEN, H., and U. OTTEN, 1978a. Trans-synaptic enzyme induction: Ionic requirements and modulatory role of glucocorticoids. In *Structure and Function of Monoamine Enzymes*, E. Usdin, N. Weiner, M. B. H. Youdim, eds. New York: M. Dekker, pp. 439–464.

THOENEN, H., and U. OTTEN, 1978b. Role of adrenocortical hormones in the modulation of synthesis and degradation of enzymes involved in the formation of catecholamines. In *Frontiers in Neuroendocrinology*, vol. 5, W. F. Ganong and L. Martini, eds. New York: Raven Press, pp. 163–184.

THOENEN, H., M. SCHWAB and Y.-A. BARDE, 1978. Transfer of information from effector organs to innervating neurons by retrograde axonal transport of macromolecules. In *Neurobiologic Mechanisms in Manipulative Therapy*, I. Papaconstantinou and W. I. Rutter, eds. New York: Academic Press, pp. 101–118.

THOENEN, H., M. SCHWAB, and U. OTTEN, 1978. Nerve growth factor as a mediator of information between effector organs and innervating neurons. In *Molecular Control of Proliferation and Cytodifferentiation* (forthcoming).

TISCHLER, A. S., M. A. DICHTER, B. BIALES, and L. A. GREENE, 1977. Neuroendocrine neoplasms and their cells of origin. *N. Engl. J. Med.* 296:919–925.

ZIEGLER, M. G., J. A. THOMAS, and D. M. JACOBOWITZ, 1976. Retrograde axonal transport of antibody to dopamine β-hydroxylase. *Brain Res.* 104:390–395.

ZIGMOND, R. E., and Y. BEN-ARI, 1977. Electrical stimulation of preganglionic nerve increases tyrosine hydroxylase activity in sympathetic ganglia. *Proc. Natl. Acad. Sci. USA* 74:3078–3080.

55 Epigenetic Influences in Neuronal Development

PAUL H. PATTERSON

ABSTRACT Much of neuronal development depends on exogenous cues provided by the embryonic environment. Recent in vivo and in vitro studies have described the plasticity of developing autonomic neurons and how their differentiation can be influenced by other cell types. Nonneuronal cells can act through their surface membranes or through diffusible molecules to influence where neural-crest cells migrate, what type of neurotransmitter and synaptic function crest cells express, and in what direction crest derivatives grow their axons.

THE DEVELOPMENT of the nervous system is based on a sequential interplay of neuronal genes with the embryonic environment. The extracellular milieu can modulate the actions of previously translated neuronal proteins or it can regulate which genes are ultimately expressed. Here I shall briefly consider some examples of how nonneuronal cells can influence the development of neural-crest derivatives, including where crest cells migrate, the type of neurotransmitter and synaptic function they express, and the direction in which they grow their axons.

One of the most striking examples of embryonic cell migration is that of the neural crest. The crest is a transient embryonic structure whose cells lie on the dorsal margin of the neural tube (as illustrated in Figure 1). This seemingly homogeneous population of cells gives rise to an amazing variety of offspring, such as cartilage cells, pigment cells, gland cells, and the neurons and glia of the peripheral nervous system (Weston, 1970). Crest cells migrate out into the epithelial area to become melanocytes, into the ventrolateral mesenchyme to form sensory ganglia, ventrally to form chains of sympathetic ganglia, and into various target tissues to form parasympathetic (and enteric) ganglia. The neurons in the autonomic ganglia often innervate the same organs, such as blood vessels and the heart. However, sympathetic and parasympathetic neurons generally have opposite effects on their targets because they release different neurotransmitters. As a rule, sympathetic neurons release norepinephrine (NE), which accelerates the heart beat, while parasympathetic neurons release acetylcholine (ACh), which slows the heart beat. Thus crest cells migrate to different sites and are functionally distinct as well.

Actually Figure 1 is somewhat misleading because the neural-crest precursors of the sympathetic and parasympathetic ganglia do not migrate through the same areas of the embryo; rather they arise from different axial levels of the embryo (Figure 2). To define where crest cells at each axial level migrate, a number of different techniques have been used. The most recent and useful technique involves transplantation of quail crest cells into comparable sites of a chick host or vice versa (LeDouarin, 1969, 1974). Quail donor cells can be distinguished from the chick host cells by the differential staining properties of the interphase nuclei. Thus the fate of the cells of a donor graft can be followed in the presence of many host cells. Such transplantations have shown that sympathetic neurons and adrenal medullary cells arise from the trunk region of the crest, whereas neurons in the gut come from both the more rostral and the more caudal levels.

Regarding their differentiated fate, the question arises: Are crest cells at each axial level predetermined to become adrenergic or cholinergic regardless of their environment, or are they pluripotent and thus respond to local environmental cues at each axial level? Recent work by LeDouarin and colleagues has shown that the embryonic environment can influence the differentiated fate of crest cells. For instance, the rostral crest cells, which normally migrate to the gut and become cholinergic, can be transplanted to another embryo in the trunk region of the crest, which normally gives rise to adrenergic neurons. In such a transplantation, some of the donor crest cells do, in fact, migrate to the sympathetic chain and become adrenergic, as indicated by the formaldehyde-induced fluorescence technique (LeDouarin and Teillet, 1974). Thus at least some crest cells migrate to

PAUL H. PATTERSON Department of Neurobiology, Harvard Medical School, Boston, MA 02115

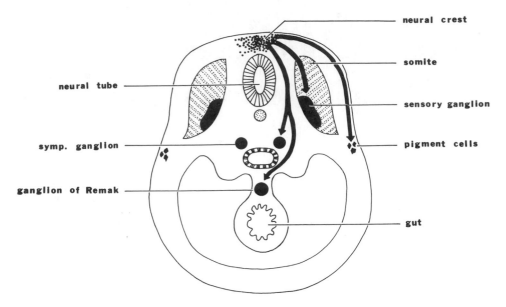

FIGURE 1　This cross section of the developing chick embryo illustrates the migration pathways of some neural-crest derivatives.

sites where they are not normally found, and they display a new phenotype as well. Similar conclusions were drawn from the reverse experiment: when trunk crest is transplanted to another embryo in the more rostral region, some of the donor crest cells populate the gut and may behave like cholinergic neurons when the vagus nerve is stimulated (Le-Douarin et al., 1975).

These experiments provided evidence that the embryonic environment of these neuronal precursor cells can influence their eventual phenotype—that is, in this case, the decision to become adrenergic or cholinergic. In fact, exogenous factors can influence this decision even after the crest cells have finished migrating and have formed a ganglion. This has been studied both in vivo with transplants and in cell culture. In the former experiment, LeDouarin and colleagues used the ganglion of Remak, sections of which contain cholinergic but not adrenergic neurons. They took a cholinergic region of this ganglion, just as it had formed in a quail embryo, and transplanted it to the neural-crest region of a younger chick embryo. The graft was placed in the trunk region of the crest, which normally gives rise to adrenergic neurons. The cells of the transplanted ganglion of Remak did not stay together as a cholinergic ganglion; instead they spread out and underwent a second migration, ending up in the sympathetic chain. Furthermore, some of these cells showed the fluorescence characteristic of adrenergic neurons

(LeDouarin, 1977). Similar results were obtained by transplanting the cholinergic ciliary ganglion to the trunk crest in the same manner (N. Le Douarin, personal communication). Thus cells that have already formed ganglia can be induced to migrate again and to differentiate along an alternate pathway. Of course, we cannot be sure in this experiment whether the cells that ended up becoming adrenergic had already begun differentiating into cholinergic neurons before the transplantation. Perhaps they were still neutral with respect to transmitters at the time they were transplanted. Another, perhaps related, question that arises concerning these transplantation experiments is that of selection versus induction. That is, did the environmental cues induce a new or different transmitter in pluripotent or reversibly committed cells, or did the environment select for survival among heterogeneous cells that were already irreversibly committed to one transmitter? The induction hypothesis implies that the choice of neurotransmitter is environmentally imposed on individual neurons, whereas the selection hypothesis supposes that the environment simply permits the expression of certain prior decisions but not others. Whichever is the case, the transplantation studies have clearly demonstrated the profound influence the embryonic environment can have on the expression of transmitter functions in vivo. These and related experiments have been discussed in more detail elsewhere (Patterson, 1978).

930　　PAUL H. PATTERSON

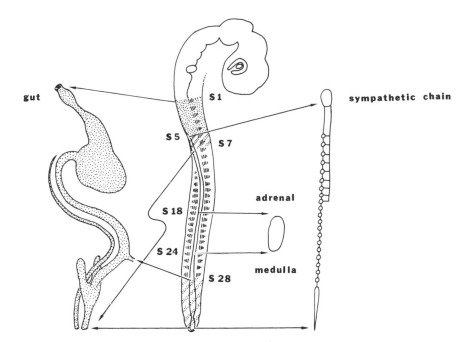

gut

S1

S5

S7

S18

S24

S28

sympathetic chain

adrenal

medulla

FIGURE 2 Sympathetic neurons (and adrenal medullary cells) arise from different axial levels of the neural crest than the cholinergic neurons of the gut. S1–S28 refer to somites. (Adapted from LeDouarin, 1977.)

A second series of experiments involves cultures of dissociated rat sympathetic neurons, and in this system questions similar to the ones just considered are being investigated on single cells as well as on populations of cells. Here again, even after the cells have formed a ganglion and, in fact, even after they have begun to express one set of transmitter functions, they can be induced to express an alternate set of functions. Sympathetic neurons, when grown in the absence of other cell types, can develop many of the properties expected of mature adrenergic neurons; they can synthesize, store, release, and take up NE and form adrenergic synapses (Claude, 1973; Mains and Patterson, 1973; Reese and Bunge, 1974; Burton and Bunge, 1975; Patterson, Reichardt, and Chun, 1975). However, if they are grown with certain types of nonneuronal cells or in tissue-culture medium previously conditioned by incubation with nonneuronal cells (CM), the neurons develop cholinergic functions; they synthesize, store, and release ACh and form cholinergic synapses (Patterson and Chun, 1974; O'Lague et al., 1974, 1975; Nurse and O'Lague, 1975; Ko et al., 1976). Furthermore, when grown with nonneuronal cells or in CM, they not only develop cholinergically, but their adrenergic properties are correspondingly reduced. These effects are graded: a higher proportion of CM (Landis et al., 1976; Patterson and Chun, 1977a) or a greater number of nonneuronal cells yields neurons with a higher

ratio of ACh to NE synthesis, a higher incidence of cholinergic transmission, and a higher proportion of synapses that lack small granular vesicles and thus appear cholinergic. Since the number of neurons surviving in culture is not affected by the CM treatments, the CM is not working by selectively allowing one or another population to survive. Similar conclusions come from the developmental time course of appearance of these properties (Johnson et al., 1976; Patterson and Chun, 1977b), as shown in Figure 3. Neurons grown in control medium develop adrenergic properties along a time course expected from in vivo studies and do not develop appreciable cholinergic properties. On the other hand, if grown in CM, their adrenergic properties initially increase but then decline while the cholinergic differentiation proceeds. Again, the same number of neurons survive in both cases.

Studies at the early stages, when both transmitters are being produced in equivalent amounts in the mass cultures, have also been done on single neurons in culture (Figure 4). The immature neuron pictured is growing on an island of heart cells. Furshpan and colleagues, using electrophysiological techniques, have found several cases of individual immature neurons simultaneously releasing both ACh and NE on the heart cells (Furshpan et al., 1976; see also Landis, 1976). However, our biochemical studies on mature single neurons have turned up few if any such dual-

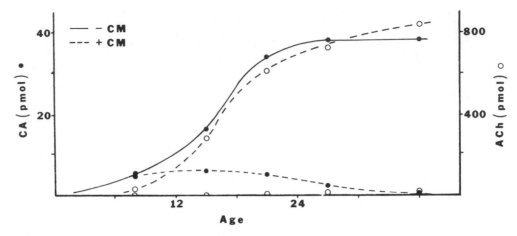

FIGURE 3 The development of adrenergic and cholinergic properties are shown for cultures of dissociated rat sympathetic neurons grown in the absence (solid line) or presence (broken line) of medium previously conditioned by incubation with heart-cell cultures. The ability to synthesize and accumulate catecholamines (filled circles) and acetylcholine (open circles) from [³H]-tyrosine and [³H]-choline, respectively, was determined in cultures of various ages. (From Patterson and Chun, 1977b.)

function cells (Reichardt and Patterson, 1977). Thus this dual functionality could be a transitory stage in neurons that eventually become either adrenergic or cholinergic. In addition, the neurons become less plastic as they mature. Recent work both in vivo (Hill and Hendry, 1977; Ross, Johnson, and Bunge, 1977) and in culture (Patterson and Chun, 1977b) has

shown that the neurons become increasingly less susceptible to cholinergic influences as they grow older; mature neurons do not respond nearly so dramatically as young ones to CM addition or withdrawal.

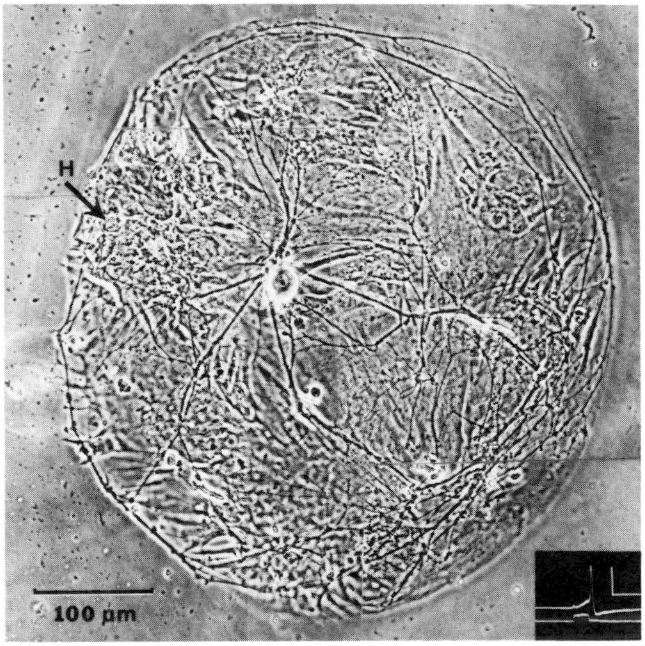

What is the role of nerve growth factor (NGF) in this development? NGF is a well-characterized protein that is required for survival of sympathetic neurons both in vivo and in vitro (Levi-Montalcini and Angeletti, 1968). Furthermore, it increases in a dose-dependent fashion both the growth and the differentiation of adrenergic sympathetic neurons (Chun and Patterson, 1977a). What is the role of NGF in the development of the cholinergic sympathetic neurons? We have found that NGF stimulates the survival and differentiation of these cholinergic neurons as well as the adrenergic neurons (Chun and Patterson, 1977b,c). In fact, NGF stimulates both adrenergic and cholinergic development to the same extent; that is, the ratio of ACh to NE, a reflection of the relative rates of synthesis of these transmitters, remains constant over a wide range of NGF concentration for both adrenergic (ACh/NE = 0.02) and cholinergic (ACh/NE = 200) cultures. Therefore, with respect to transmitter production, NGF is permissive rather than instructive, in that it is necessary for survival and stimulates growth and differentiation but does not tell the neurons which transmitter to produce.

Summarizing thus far (Figure 5), a number of exogenously supplied developmental cues are critical for the determination of synaptic functions of autonomic neurons. NGF enhances the differentiation of immature sympathetic neurons along either adrener-

FIGURE 4 A microculture containing a solitary sympathetic neuron, 19 days in vitro. The arrow at H indicates a cluster of myocytes. The inset shows an impulse in this neuron (scales are 50 mV and 20 msec for *y* and *x* axes, respectively). (From Furshpan et al., 1976.)

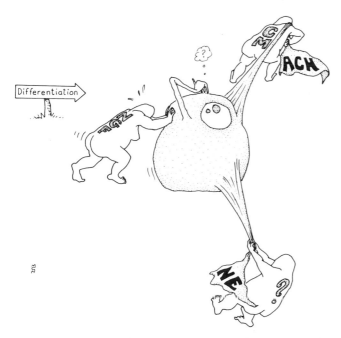

FIGURE 5 Some environmental signals influencing an immature sympathetic neuron.

gic or cholinergic paths. In fact, at least at young ages, some cultured neurons appear to secrete both transmitters simultaneously. The particular phenotype chosen depends on developmental cues other than NGF. CM produced by certain types of nonneuronal cells (as well as other components of the medium: see Ross and Bunge, 1976; Patterson and Chun, 1977a) can direct neurons to become cholinergic. CM is a qualitatively different developmental signal from NGF; it is not necessary for neuronal survival and does not stimulate growth (Patterson and Chun, 1977a). By analogy with the CM, there would be a similar cue for adrenergic function, which is not NGF. This factor may be produced by some part of the embryonic environment through which the crest cells migrate (for review see Patterson, 1978). However, even if the cells have been previously instructed as to transmitter synthesis, this order can be countermanded. As has been discussed, this reversal can occur after ganglion formation in vivo and after initial differentiation in vitro has begun. However, it does appear that after significant maturation has occurred, such reversal of function is not appreciable (Hill and Hendry, 1977; Patterson and Chun, 1977b; Ross, Johnson, and Bunge, 1977).

If sympathetic neurons do receive an early adrenergic influence, how is it possible to reverse this and obtain cultures with 80–90% cholinergic neurons? In vivo the vast majority of sympathetic neurons are adrenergic while only a few are cholinergic (Uvnäs, 1954; Sjöqvist, 1963; Aiken and Reit, 1969). We can speculate that only a small number of the neurons receive the countermanding cholinergic signal because it is selectively localized—perhaps in the target organs that receive cholinergic sympathetic innervation, such as the sweat glands (Sjöqvist, 1963; Aiden and Reit, 1969). Another possibility is that all of the neurons do receive the cholinergic signal but most are prevented from responding to it by factors that are not yet added to the cultures. Preganglionic innervation is not present in the cultures, and neuronal activity is known to be important in adrenergic development (see Thoenen, Otten, and Schwab, this volume). In fact, recent experiments indicate that one of the factors determining whether cultured sympathetic neurons become adrenergic or cholinergic is the level of their membrane potential (Walicke, Campenot, and Patterson, 1977). If the cultured neurons are treated with elevated K^+ or veratridine, which act as depolarizing agents, or stimulated directly with electrical current, either before or during CM additions, they display up to 300-fold lower ACh/CA ratios than they would have without depolarization, and thus they remain primarily adrenergic. Further results suggest Ca^{++} may be involved in the suppression of cholinergic differentiation by depolarization. Thus the developmental role of neuronal activity can be extended to that of a final determinant of transmitter function, ending the capacity to alter differentiated fate in response to developmental cues. If this effect of activity exists in other parts of the nervous system, the nature of the synaptic input on a cell—the balance between excitatory and inhibitory input—becomes even more critical than previously believed. Synaptic input not only establishes connectivity, but may also direct the developmental fate of its target.

Another aspect of neuronal development that appears not to be preprogrammed within individual neurons is the direction of outgrowth of axons. This is, of course, a critical aspect of setting up the appropriate wiring pattern in the nervous system: How do neurites find their targets? Much of the growth of axons appears to occur at their tips or growth cones (Bray, 1970). However, little is known of the mechanisms involved in the extension of growth cones. Neurons contain actinlike and myosinlike proteins, but it is not yet clear whether these are involved in the movements of neurites (Bray, 1977). There is evidence, however, that the direction the growth cone takes is sensitive both to the properties of the surface it moves over and to diffusible molecules. For instance, culture work has shown that growth cones adhere preferentially to plastic rather than to glass and prefer collagen-coated plastic to bare plastic. Examples of how such preferences can guide growth under controlled conditions have been provided by Letourneau (1975). For example, growth cones of sensory neurons follow pathways of polyornithine-coated plastic, while largely avoiding palladium-coated areas—at times turning at right angles to do so. Hierarchies of such affinities can be constructed for different types of neurons, and the goal is eventually to relate the molecular properties of the growth cone to various physical surfaces of known composition.

As one might predict, growing neurites show discrimination in contacting other cellular surfaces as well. For example, we can plate heart muscle cells and endothelial cells together and obtain islands of endothelial cells surrounded by a sea of muscle cells. If sympathetic neurons are plated on such cultures, the nerve processes almost completely avoid the islands (P. Patterson, unpublished). Similar neuronal growth patterns are seen on heat-killed endothelial-muscle cultures, suggesting that it is the surfaces of the nonneuronal cells that are important and not some poisonous material being emitted by the endothelial cells.

There is also good evidence that diffusible molecules can greatly influence the direction of neurite growth. One example is NGF. In addition to its previously described effects on survival, growth, and differentiation, NGF can influence the direction of neurite growth. Campenot (1977) devised a culture system in which neurons plated in one chamber send their neurites across a barrier into a second chamber. Although the barrier seal is permeable to the growing neurites, it is sufficiently impermeable to medium to hold a 5 mm hydrostatic head for at least four days without appreciable equalization. This culture system has made it possible to study the effects of chemical gradients on neurite growth and the effects of local application of substances to either the neurite endings or the somas. Neurites regularly crossed partitions into chambers containing NGF but did not grow into chambers containing little or no NGF. Furthermore, when NGF was removed from the local environment of the distal portions of the neurites, the growth of these portions stopped, and they appeared to degenerate. This degeneration occurred even though the somas and proximal portions of the neurites were exposed to a high NGF concentration. Thus NGF can act as a directional signal in the sense that even if the cell bodies of sympathetic neurons have direct access to it, NGF must also be present along the entire route the neurites travel to reach their targets or they will not go there. In addition, each individual growing tip must have its own *local* supply of NGF to survive. NGF has also been shown to influence the direction of neurite growth in vivo (Levi-Montalcini, 1976). These observations correlate well with the hypothesis, which has not yet been definitively proven, that the target organs of sympathetic neurons actually produce the NGF protein themselves and secrete it to attract their specific nerve fibers. In support of this notion are Hendry's results from cutting the axons of immature sympathetic neurons (Hendry, 1975). Young neurons are highly sensitive to NGF; if their growing axons are cut off (which by this hypothesis would remove their NGF supply), most of the neurons die very quickly. However, if NGF is added to these cut neurons, they survive.

Therefore, combining such a postulated gradient of NGF coming from the target tissues with judicious placement of surfaces for which the nerve fibers have differential affinities, one could explain, in theory at least, how these neurons find their targets. Furthermore, since NGF is necessary for survival and stimulates growth, it could be used to test speculations about competition between developing nerve terminals. If NGF were in limited supply, perhaps the largest or most active synapse, or the first synapse to form, would have a competitive advantage over other developing nerve terminals.

In sum, virtually every step of autonomic neuronal development examined has been shown to depend on specific signals provided by the embryonic environment. Purification of such factors may lead to a description at the molecular level of the various stages in neuronal development involving neuronal migration, determination of transmitter and synaptic function, and construction of the wiring of the nervous system. Such investigations may also reveal what role such developmental factors might continue to play in the modulation of function in the adult organism.

ACKNOWLEDGMENTS   I thank Margaret C. Nelson for the illustrations, Eleanor P. Livingston and Joe Gagliardi for help with the manuscript, several authors for supplying unpublished papers, my colleagues for advice, and the American and Massachusetts Heart Associations and the NINCDS for support.

REFERENCES

AIKEN, J., and E. REIT, 1969. A comparison of the sensitivity to chemical stimuli of adrenergic and cholinergic neurons in the cat stellate ganglion. *J. Pharmacol. Exp. Ther.* 169:211–223.

BRAY, D., 1970. Surface movements during the growth of

single explanted neurons. *Proc. Natl. Acad. Sci. USA* 65:905–910.

BRAY, D., 1977. Actin and myosin in neurons: A first review. *Biochemie* 59:1–6.

BURTON, H., and R. P. BUNGE, 1975. A comparison of the uptake and release of [³H] norepinephrine in rat autonomic and sensory ganglia in tissue culture. *Brain Res.* 97:157–162.

CAMPENOT, R. B., 1977. Local control of neurite development by nerve growth factor. *Proc. Natl. Acad. Sci. USA* 74:4516–4519.

CHUN, L. L. Y., and P. H. PATTERSON, 1977a. The role of nerve growth factor in the development of rat sympathetic neurons *in vitro*. I. Survival, growth and differentiation of catecholamine production. *J. Cell Biol.* 75:694–704.

CHUN, L. L. Y., and P. H. PATTERSON, 1977b. The role of nerve growth factor in the development of rat sympathetic neurons *in vitro*. II. Developmental studies. *J. Cell Biol.* 75:705–711.

CHUN, L. L. Y., and P. H. PATTERSON, 1977c. The role of nerve growth factor in the development of rat sympathetic neurons *in vitro*. III. Effect on acetylcholine production. *J. Cell Biol.* 75:712–718.

CLAUDE, P., 1973. Electron microscopy of dissociated rat sympathetic neurons *in vitro*. *J. Cell Biol.* 59:57a.

FURSHPAN, E. J., P. R. MACLEISH, P. H. O'LAGUE, and D. D. POTTER, 1976. Chemical transmission between rat sympathetic neurons and cardiac myocytes developing in microcultures: Evidence for cholinergic, adrenergic and dual-function neurons. *Proc. Natl. Acad. Sci. USA* 73:4225–4229.

HENDRY, I. A., 1975. The response of adrenergic neurons to axotomy and nerve growth factor. *Brain Res.* 94:87–97.

HILL, C. E., and I. A. HENDRY, 1977. Development of neurons synthesizing noradrenaline and acetylcholine in the superior cervical ganglion of the rat *in vivo* and *in vitro*. *Neuroscience* 2:741–749.

JOHNSON, M., D. ROSS, M. MYERS, R. REES, R. BUNGE, E. WAKSHULL, and H. BURTON, 1976. Synaptic vesicle cytochemistry changes when cultured sympathetic neurons develop cholinergic interactions. *Nature* 262:308–310.

KO, C.-P., H. BURTON, M. I. JOHNSON, and R. P. BUNGE, 1976. Synaptic transmission between rat superior cervical ganglion neurons in dissociated cell cultures. *Brain Res.* 177:461–485.

LANDIS, S. C., 1976. Rat sympathetic neurons and cardiac myocytes developing in microcultures: Correlation of the fine structure of endings with neurotransmitter function in single neurons. *Proc. Natl. Acad. Sci. USA* 73:4220–4224.

LANDIS, S. C., P. R. MACLEISH, D. D. POTTER, E. J. FURSHPAN, and P. H. PATTERSON, 1976. Synapses formed between dissociated neurons: The influence of conditioned medium. Sixth Annual Meeting, Society for Neurosciences, Abstract 280, p. 197.

LEDOUARIN, N., 1969. Particularités du noyau interphasique chez la Caille japonaise (*Coturnix coturnix* japonica). Utilisation de ces particularités comme "marquage biologique" dans des recherches sur les interactions tissulaires et les migrations cellulaires au cours de l'ontogènese. *Bull. Biol. Fr. Belg.* 103:435–452.

LEDOUARIN, N., 1974. Cell recognition based on natural morphological nuclear markers. *Med. Biol.* 52:281–319.

LEDOUARIN, N., 1977. The differentiation of the ganglioblasts of the autonomic nervous system studied in chimeric avian embryos. In *Cell Interactions in Differentiation,* M. Karkinen-Jääskeläinen, ed. London: Academic Press, pp. 171–190.

LEDOUARIN, N., D. RENAUD, M. TEILLET, and G. LEDOUARIN, 1975. Cholinergic differentiation of presumptive adrenergic neuroblasts in interspecific chimeras after heterotopic transplantation. *Proc. Natl. Acad. Sci. USA* 72:728–732.

LEDOUARIN, N. M., and M.-A. M. TEILLET, 1974. Experimental analysis of the migration and differentiation of neuroblasts of the autonomic nervous system and the neuroectodermal mesenchymal derivatives, using a biological cell marking technique. *Dev. Biol.* 41:162–184.

LETOURNEAU, P. C., 1975. Cell-to-substratum adhesion and guidance of axonal elogation. *Dev. Biol.* 44:92–101.

LEVI-MONTALCINI, R., 1976. The nerve growth factor: Its role in growth, differentiation and function of the sympathetic adrenergic neuron. *Prog. Brain Res.* 45:235–258.

LEVI-MONTALCINI, R., and P. U. ANGELETTI, 1968. Nerve growth factor. *Physiol. Rev.* 48:534–569.

MAINS, R. E., and P. H. PATTERSON, 1973. Primary cultures of dissociated sympathetic neurons. I. Establishment of long term growth in culture and studies of differentiated properties. *J. Cell Biol.* 59:329–345.

NURSE, C. A., and P. H. O'LAGUE, 1975. Formation of cholinergic synapses between dissociated sympathetic neurons and skeletal myotubes of the rat in cell culture. *Proc. Natl. Acad. Sci. USA* 72:1955–1959.

O'LAGUE, P. H., P. R. MACLEISH, C. A. NURSE, P. CLAUDE, E. J. FURSHPAN, and D. D. POTTER, 1975. Physiological and morphological studies on developing sympathetic neurons in dissociated cell culture. *Cold Spring Harbor Symp. Quant. Biol.* 40:399–407.

O'LAGUE, P. H., K. OBATA, P. CLAUDE, E. J. FURSHPAN, and D. D. POTTER, 1974. Evidence for cholinergic synapses between dissociated rat sympathetic neurons in cell culture. *Proc. Natl. Acad. Sci. USA* 71:3602–3606.

PATTERSON, P. H., 1978. Environmental determination of autonomic neurotransmitter function. *Annu. Rev. Neurosci.* 1:1–17.

PATTERSON, P. H. and L. L. Y. CHUN, 1974. The influence of non-neuronal cells on catecholamine and acetycholine synthesis and accumulation in cultures of dissociated sympathetic neurons. *Proc. Natl. Acad. Sci. USA* 71:3607–3610.

PATTERSON, P. H., and L. L. Y. CHUN, 1977a. The induction of acetylcholine snythesis in primary cultures of dissociated rat sympathetic neurons. I. Effects of conditioned medium. *Dev. Biol.* 56:263–280.

PATTERSON, P. H., and L. L. Y. CHUN, 1977b. The induction of acetylcholine synthesis in primary cultures of dissociated rat sympathetic neurons. II. Developmental aspects. *Dev. Biol.* 60:473–481.

PATTERSON, P. H., L. F. REICHARDT, and L. L. Y. CHUN, 1975. Biochemical studies on the development of primary sympathetic neurons in cell culture. *Cold Spring Harbor Symp. Quant. Biol.* 40:389–397.

REES, R., and R. P. BUNGE, 1974. Morphological and cytochemical studies of synapses formed in culture between isolated rat superior cervical ganglion neurons. *J. Comp. Neurol.* 157:1–11.

REICHARDT, L. F., and P. H. PATTERSON, 1977. Neurotransmitter synthesis and uptake by individual rat sympathetic neurons developing in microcultures. *Nature* 270:147–151.

ROSS, D., and R. P. BUNGE, 1976. Choline acetyltransferase in cultures of rat superior cervical ganglion. Sixth Annual Meeting. Society for Neurosciences, Abstract 1904, p. 769.

ROSS, D., M. JOHNSON, and R. BUNGE, 1977. Evidence that development of cholinergic characteristics in adrenergic neurons is age dependent. *Nature* 267:536–539.

SJÖQVIST, F., 1963. The correlation between the occurrence and localization of acetylcholinesterase-rich cell bodies in the stellate ganglion and the outflow of cholinergic sweat secretory fibres to the forepaw of the cat. *Acta Physiol. Scand.* 57:339–351.

UVNÄS, B., 1954. Sympathetic vasodilator outflow. *Physiol. Rev.* 34:608–618.

WALICKE, P. A., R. B. CAMPENOT, and P. H. PATTERSON, 1977. Determination of transmitter function by neuronal activity. *Proc. Natl. Acad. Sci. USA* 74:5767–5771.

WESTON, J. A., 1970. The migration and differentiation of neural crest cells. *Adv. Morphog.* 8:41–114.

56 The Regulation of Nerve Sprouting by Extrinsic Influences

J. DIAMOND

ABSTRACT   Nerves develop their terminal fields by collateral sprouting of their axons at the target tissue, followed by the functional maturation of terminals. The control of collateral sprouting, therefore, is the principal means by which the territory of a nerve is regulated. In the salamander, the density of the mechanosensory endings in the epidermis is determined by specific target cells—the Merkel cells. Merkel cells that appear in nerve-free, newly regenerated skin seem to evoke directional sprouting of fibers toward them, as do denervated Merkel cells in adult skin. After contact is established by the first endings to reach a Merkel cell, those of a second axon are no longer attracted to it, and sprouting eventually ceases as the available Merkel cells are innervated. This "neutralizing" effect of the nerve is dependent on continual axoplasmic transport of materials to the terminals; transient colchicine block, which leaves the sensory function of these axons unimpaired, leads to hyperinnervation of their target sites by newly sprouting endings from neighboring untreated axons; these extra terminals acquire normal function.

A separate mechanism limits the terminal-field areas of segmental nerves. This mechanism does not reside in the skin itself, and Merkel cells show no preference for the endings of one nerve over another. During development these nerves are seemingly allotted domains of body space whose coordinates relate to the limb as a whole. When adjacent skin is denervated, an intact nerve will not invade significantly beyond its domain frontier until about two months has elapsed; partial denervation within its domain, however, leads to sprouting of remaining fibers and occupation of vacated Merkel cells in less than three weeks.

The neuron-target interaction and the spatial-control mechanism probably operate in species other than salamander to regulate the density and area of peripheral and central nerve fields; such regulation could underlie some of the plasticity exhibited by both developing and mature nervous systems.

The establishment of nerve fields

THE WAY IN WHICH a neuron integrates and responds to the information it receives is a physiological characteristic of the cell. However, in any neural circuit

J. DIAMOND   Department of Neurosciences, McMaster University, Hamilton, Ontario, Canada

the influence of an individual neuron reflects both the distribution on it of the inputs arriving from other cells and the distribution of its own axonal endings on and among the other neurons. These distributions are the *terminal fields* that neurons, through their axonal arborizations, make upon their targets; their principal parameters are (1) the area of target tissue over which the axonal endings are distributed and (2) the density of the endings achieved within that area. In the central nervous system (CNS) a neuron with a concentrated and localized terminal field will have a very different influence from one whose field is relatively widespread over a large pool of neurons but is perhaps sparse in density. Although a great deal of investigation and discussion has centered on the ways by which axons are guided to make apparently preferential connections with their targets (Sperry, 1965), relatively little is known about how the sizes and dispositions of the terminal fields of axons are determined. Yet this is a point of particular interest, for in a mature nervous system characterized by an inability to make more neurons, one means of bringing about behavioral changes could be the modification of circuitry by appropriate adjustments in the areas and densities of terminal fields. Indeed the available evidence, which will be mentioned below, suggests that mechanisms that could make such adjustments do exist, and this could provide a means of conferring plasticity upon a neural system. This would be in contrast to, for example, alterations in conductivity within a morphologically rigidly determined and unchangeable array of nerve fields.

What are the mechanisms that regulate the establishment of nerve fields during development? The generally segmental nature of ontogeny (Balinsky, 1975) makes the peripheral nerves and their fields a favorable system for the study of this problem. The usual views about the way peripheral fields become established range from those bordering on dogma to altogether different ideas that, however, often suffer from ambiguities in the experimental data supporting them. The former extreme is nicely summarized in an authoritative textbook: "In general the pattern of distribution of the peripheral nervous system is due to an early and intimate association between the developing nerve fibre and the primordium of its terminal field. In vertebrates . . . the intrinsic distribution of the nerve in the limb is regulated by the segregation and the growth and positional changes of the limb tissues" (Hamilton and Mossman, 1972). However, information intrinsic to the neurons could cause axons themselves to become appropriately segregated and aligned with respect to each other, so that their ultimate projection onto the target tissue would determine the characteristic patterning of the nerve fields; in addition, the target tissue itself can have an important influence on the incoming nerves to develop their fields in specific regions and patterns (Detwiler, 1936; Piatt, 1942, 1952; Hughes, 1968).

These possibilities are not mutually exclusive, and all of them are almost certainly true to some extent; however, none satisfactorily explains exactly how terminal fields retain their characteristic identity and shape. Why do not the nerve terminals of one field freely intermingle with those of adjacent ones at the target tissues? The dermatomal patterning achieved by cutaneous nerves is a striking example of segmental field organization. The possibility that the absence of extensive overlapping between peripheral nerve fields depends simply on the attainment by nerves of an upper limit of growth (so that invasion of adjacent territory is not possible) seems untenable for a number of reasons, in particular because of the regenerative capacities of most nerves when they are sectioned (see below). Another possible explanation, which unfortunately begs the question, is that "competition" occurs: a nerve that has established its terminal field actively prevents other nerves from invading its territory. Since virtually all nerve fields are established consequent to the terminal branching of the axons, however, it would seem logical in considering these problems to look for mechanisms that can initiate and regulate collateral sprouting. In the final analysis, it is only by the regulation of axonal sprouting that the development of terminal fields can be controlled, both during early life and, as a possible mechanism of plasticity, in the mature organism (Diamond et al., 1976).

Sprouting of cutaneous nerves in the salamander

THE MERKEL CELL   We have some understanding of one peripheral system—the mechanosensory inner-

vation of salamander skin—which may offer clues concerning the general problems of the control of axonal sprouting and the establishment of terminal fields. The skin of the salamander (*Amblystoma tigrinum*) contains, near the basal layer of the epidermis, a specialized cell type, the Merkel cell, which occurs in the integument of most vertebrates (Winkelmann and Breathnach, 1973). The distinguishing characteristic of all Merkel cells is the presence of dense-core granules concentrated in the region of the cytoplasm closest to the dermis; on the deeper (dermal) surface of the cell one finds nerve terminations that in the salamander contain clear vesicles (Figure 1). In many vertebrate species Merkel cells occur as clusters in specialized, histologically identifiable structures such as the "touch domes" of the mammal (Iggo and Muir, 1969), and they are commonly regarded as sensory transducers, conferring upon the nerve endings the characteristics of mechanosensitivity and slow adaptation (e.g., Iggo, 1968; Düring and Andres, 1976). Salamander Merkel cells, however, are found singly, about one per thousand epidermal cells (Parducz et al., 1977). Histological examination of the salamander skin reveals no obvious sensory structures. We were naturally interested in the possibility that the Merkel cells are associated with the mechanosensory nerves, in which case their study in conditions of mechanosensory nerve sprouting could be revealing.

RECEPTIVE FIELDS OF MECHANORECEPTORS   Afferent impulses can be readily evoked by mechanical stimulation from any place on the salamander skin; but when excited by prodding with a controlled stimulator of about 200 μm diameter, the mechanoreceptors all seemed equally sensitive and, surprisingly, were all rapidly adapting (Cooper and Diamond, 1977). We have concentrated on the dorsal skin of the salamander hind limb. Since the Merkel cells occur only sparsely, we used a fine prodder of about

FIGURE 1   Merkel cells in salamander skin. (A) Light micrograph of skin. Merkel cells were always found near the basal layer of the epidermis. The one circled here was identified by electron-microscopic examination of an adjacent section, shown in B. (V, blood vessels; G, secretory glands.) (B) Electron micrograph of skin. The Merkel cell (M) from A above and its associated nerve endings (NE) are located near the basal lamina (BL). It can be distinguished from other epidermal cells (E) by the presence of dense-core granules in its cytoplasm. (D, dermis.) (C) Higher-power view of another Merkel cell and nerve endings, the former showing dense-core granules, the latter clear vesicles and mitochondria.

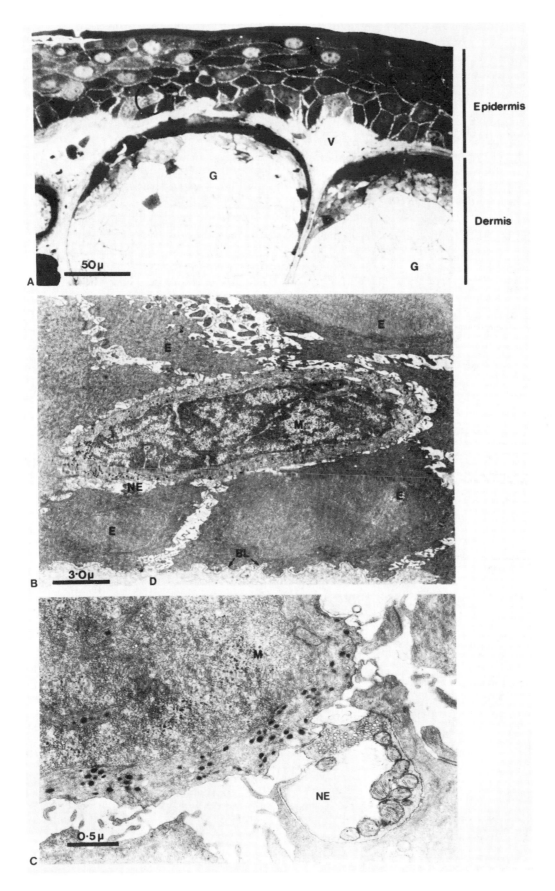

10 μm diameter to attempt a more detailed investigation (Figure 2). With this technique we found a continuous range of apparent sensitivities to mechanical stimulation, from low-threshold spots on the one extreme to totally insensitive spots on the other. Figure 2 shows the results from such experiments in the form of a frequency histogram of ranges of apparent thresholds; this histogram quantitatively describes the mechanosensitivity of the investigated skin. The histograms for any one animal were essentially the same, no matter what regions of skin were investigated, both on one limb and between the two hind limbs. The simplest interpretation of these results is that the salamander skin contains only one population of mechanoreceptors of fairly uniform threshold (corresponding to the lowest range of the histogram) and that they are spaced far enough apart so that a randomly located small prodder would frequently be situated between them and thus require larger stimuli to excite the nearest receptor. The approximate relationship between distance from the edge of a low-threshold site and the increase in stimulus required

to fire the same receptor was measured experimentally. From these results, assuming a single population, we estimated the average receptive-field size of the low-threshold receptors, (approximately 75 μm radius) and their mean distribution across the skin (150–250 μm apart) (Cooper and Diamond, 1977).

MECHANOSENSORY NERVE ENDINGS AND MERKEL CELLS   The apparent distribution of the mechanoreceptors based on this physiological analysis was certainly consistent with their having some relationship to the infrequently occurring Merkel cells; we therefore made a combined physiological and morphological study to investigate directly a possible correlation between the Merkel-cell locations and the prodder locations at which mechanosensitivity seemed highest (Parducz et al., 1977). By systematic physiological mapping of entire regions of skin we found that spots with sensitivities in the lowest threshold range, as defined from the frequency histogram, tended to occur in groups. In Figure 3 these highly sensitive areas are identified with contour lines drawn by eye; they are the presumed sites of the mechanosensory endings. We next examined these mapped skin regions systematically with the electron micro-

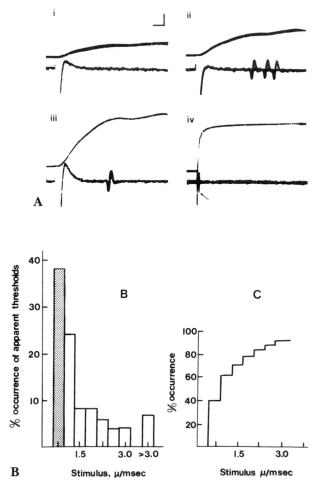

FIGURE 2   Characteristics of rapidly adapting cutaneous mechanoreceptors in the salamander. (A) The top trace of each pair shows the photocell output that monitors the prodder movement; the bottom trace shows the extracellular recording from the nerve trunk. (i) Subthreshold applied stimulus; three consecutive traces are superimposed. (ii) Stimulus intensity increased to threshold; one spike occurs in each of the three superimposed traces. The variation in the spike latencies is typical for a just-threshold stimulus. (iii) Response to a suprathreshold stimulus, which elicited one spike of constant latency in each of the three superimposed traces. (iv) Same as iii, but with the sweep speed slowed to show that these mechanoreceptors respond to a suprathreshold sustained stimulus with a single spike (arrow); that is, they are rapidly adapting. Horizontal calibration is 2 msec in i, ii, and iii and 50 msec in iv. Vertical calibration is 7 μm for prodder movement and 20 μV for extracellular records. (From Parducz et al., 1977.) (B) A prodder with a 10 μm tip was used to elicit impulses as in A. The total area of hind-limb skin surveyed was about 55 mm²; 75 points were tested, approximately 1 mm apart, and the percent occurrence of ranges of apparent thresholds is shown. The shaded column represents the low-threshold range of stimuli, which corresponds to prodder locations directly over touch spots (see text). (C) The results of B are replotted as a cumulative frequency curve. There are no threshold values shown corresponding to 100% occurrence, since at a number of locations no response was elicited with the maximum stimulus available (the >3.0 μm/msec column in B). (B and C from Cooper and Diamond, 1977.)

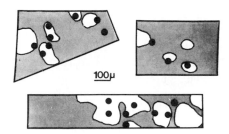

FIGURE 3 Relationship between low-threshold regions (white areas) determined in the physiological studies and Merkel cells (black spots), whose distribution was obtained by electron-microscopic examination of the same skins. The three skin samples are from three different animals. In each case the correlation between Merkel cells and sensitive areas is highly significant ($p < 0.001$, χ^2 test). (From Parducz et al., 1977.)

scope to determine the locations of the Merkel cells. After appropriate corrections for shrinkage we obtained maps of the Merkel cells across the skin of the investigated regions, which could then be superimposed on the corresponding physiological maps of the touch spots. Figure 3 shows that there is a significant correlation between the two maps for a given skin; we can assume, therefore, that the nerve endings associated with the Merkel cells are indeed the mechanosensory ones. In the salamander we rarely find epidermal nerve endings that are not associated with Merkel cells.

It seems, then, that salamander skin contains only rapidly adapting mechanoreceptors, each of which is associated with a single Merkel cell. The physiological finding that each low-threshold spot (the apparent receptive field of a single mechanoreceptor) is innervated almost always by only one axon was, therefore, of great significance (Cooper and Diamond, 1977). This means that each Merkel cell must be functionally innervated by the terminations of only one axon. Furthermore, our investigations of single axonal fields in the salamander skin—using two prodders in an occlusion technique—showed that these fields are organized essentially as a mosaic so that there is relatively little overlap between axonal fields. If each branch of a parent axon ends at a single low-threshold region on the skin, then the axons must divide from as few as four to as many as a hundred times, depending on the size of the field; each axon, therefore, contacts from four to a hundred Merkel cells.

Sprouting and the determination of axonal branching patterns

How does this pattern of terminations of the mechanosensory axons (i.e., the density of endings in their terminal fields) come about? Do the cutaneous nerves first branch and then induce the differentiation of Merkel cells in the skin? Or are these cells present in advance, the actual targets of the nerves? We studied newly regenerated skin in the hope that it would constitute a model system for primary development of the cutaneous innervation (Cooper, Scott, and Diamond, 1977). Portions of skin (up to 25 mm²) were removed from both normal and totally denervated hind limbs, and new skin allowed to regenerate in their place. Within 2–3 days a transparent sheet of epidermis formed: the dermis developed over the next few weeks, and, interestingly, the skin regenerated in the denervated limbs essentially as it did in the innervated ones. Subsequent ultrastructural studies of the skin in these denervated limbs provided a significant result: Merkel cells were indeed present, in about the number we find in normal skin; but of course these otherwise-typical Merkel cells had no nerves associated with them (Figure 4A). The immediate question then is, What happens when nerves are available?

The first experiments were physiological: regenerating nerves were allowed to grow into such newly formed skin, and the development of its mechanosensitivity was followed by the usual methods. Within a few weeks a fairly typical distribution of low-threshold spots was revealed (Figure 4B). Electron-microscopic examination showed that the Merkel cells of such mechanosensitive new skin were innervated normally along their dermal surface (Figure 4C). Recently we completed a correlative study of innervated, regenerated skin (Scott, Cooper, and Diamond, in preparation) which showed that the touch spots were indeed coincident with the locations of the Merkel cells (cf. Figure 3). We assume, then, that the innervation of newly regenerated skin is a useful model for the situation during primary development. We now know from the work of Tweedle (1978) that both early-developing and aneurogenic A. maculatum limbs contain normally differentiated but nerve-free Merkel cells in the epidermis; later the Merkel cells of the normal limbs are all innervated.

We conclude from all these findings that the Merkel cells constitute the true targets for the ingrowing axons that are destined to become mechanosensory in function. In the new skin, as in the embryonic limbs, the nerves could not have received any guidance from other nerve pathways, either normal or degenerated (cf. Weiss, 1941; Horch, 1976). We presume that the Merkel cells release a factor that attracts the nerves to them or that the ingrowing nerves are continually sampling their environment, ceasing

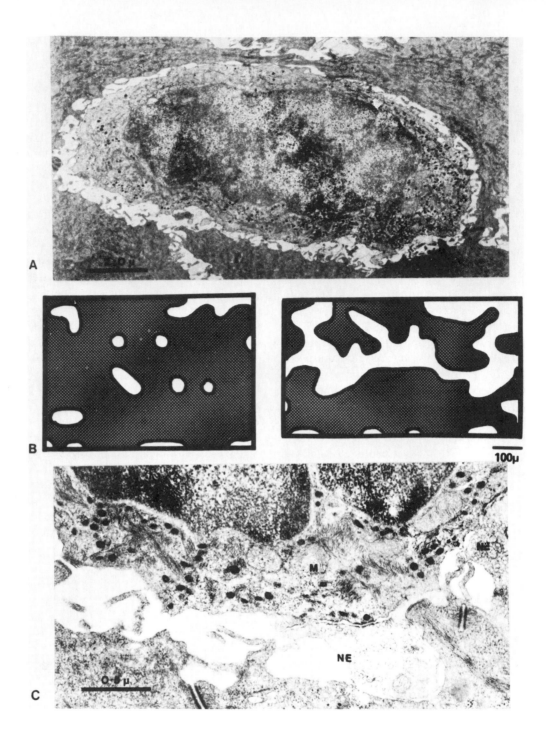

FIGURE 4 Merkel cells and mechanosensitivity of regenerated skin. (A) Merkel cell in skin that has regenerated for 6 months in a denervated hind limb. Note the absence of associated nerve endings (cf. Figure 1). (B) Distribution of low-threshold mechanosensitive areas in regenerated skin of two salamanders; nerves have been allowed to grow into the skin. The size and distribution of the sensitive areas are similar to those in normal animals (cf. Figure 3). (C) Merkel cell in regenerated, innervated skin (as in B). Nerve endings (NE) are found in association with the Merkel cells (M) in such preparations. (From Cooper, Scott, and Diamond, 1977.)

their search upon contacting the Merkel cells, which they "recognize" as their targets. The simplest hypothesis would seem to be that the Merkel cells release a growth-promoting substance whose concentration gradient leads to directional sprouting of the nerves. Moreover, in the newly regenerated skin, just as in normal skin, there is virtually no sharing of individual touch spots by different axons. Once it has become innervated, then, the trophic influence of the Merkel cell on other axons is switched off. It follows that the pattern of innervation normally established in the salamander epidermis must be a function of the distribution of the Merkel cells.

HYPERINNERVATION OF TARGET SITES? Both during primary development and in the mature organism, nerves freely sprout at uninnervated, or only partially innervated, target tissues (Ramón y Cajal, 1919; Diamond et al., 1976). As we have seen, in the salamander skin only those sprouts that successfully achieve an association with Merkel cells seem to become functional mechanosensory endings. What if there were unsuccessful ones, in excess of the number of available Merkel cells? It would hardly seem surprising for an axon to produce an initial excess of branches in response to some sprouting stimulus. It is interesting, therefore, that regression of nerve endings has been described in various developmental situations; Speidel (1942) in particular observed the phenomenon directly in living axons in the growing tadpole tail, and a transient hyperinnervation of other targets, in both the CNS (Crepel, Mariani, and Delhaye-Bouchaud, 1976) and the periphery (Fitzgerald, 1966; Redfern, 1970; Bennett and Pettigrew, 1974; Brown, Jansen, and Van Essen, 1976; Landmesser and Pilar, 1976), occurs in early life. Presumably endings that do not maintain successful relationships with appropriate target sites either degenerate or, as has been suggested for developing muscle and skin, regress (Korneliussen and Jansen, 1976; Fitzgerald, 1966). We have no data on this problem from the salamander skin experiments, but regression of excess endings certainly seems plausible.

COMPETITION The salamander findings provide a basis for understanding one form of apparent competition between nerves. It is a matter of timing. The axons whose endings first arrive at their targets (the Merkel cells) have the advantage; in some way they switch off the attractant influence of the cell, and the endings of other axons then fail to achieve a similar association with that target. A further experimental result indicates how this form of competition could operate during primary development. We partially denervated salamander hind limbs and created an opportunity for both regenerating and intact sprouting axons to compete for territory (Scott and Diamond, 1977). The results were quite clear. Some regenerating fibers were totally excluded *from regions of skin they had originally occupied* by collaterals sprouting from intact nerve branches; because of their proximity the latter were able to innervate these regions some weeks before the regenerating fibers could reach them (Figure 5). In the same limb, however, some of the regenerating fibers arrived at other regions of skin in advance of the sprouts from the intact fibers; then the latter were excluded. By this simple mechanism of timing of arrival, nerve axons were able to establish discrete areas of innervation and disallow other axons from invading them. Clearly such a mechanism of competition could operate during primary development, and so we must ask, What controls the timing of the arrival of nerves at target tissues? We shall return to this question later; first we must consider the mechanisms by which a successful innervation by one nerve disallows innervation by another.

Neuron-target interaction in the regulation of sprouting

We have summarized elsewhere the substantial evidence that target tissues produce sprouting stimuli (Diamond et al., 1976). In the salamander skin we can now point specifically to the Merkel cells as the targets of the mechanosensory nerves. Since we rarely find endings free and unassociated with Merkel cells, it seems probable, as noted above, that these cells are the source of a sprouting stimulus, whose concentration gradient attracts the nerves. A further finding is consistent with this conclusion. In a series of animals, we used the physiological analysis described above to measure quantitatively the sprouting of the remaining nerves that occurs after partial denervation of the salamander hind limb (Cooper, Diamond, and Turner, 1977). We found that there was apparently an exact restoration of innervation in the skin; that is, for every functional mechanosensory nerve ending lost, a new one appeared (Figure 6). This would be the expected result if (1) Merkel cells survived denervation in these circumstances and (2) these denervated Merkel cells resemble those in new skin and act as the true targets of the mechanosensory nerves. We therefore examined skin with the electron

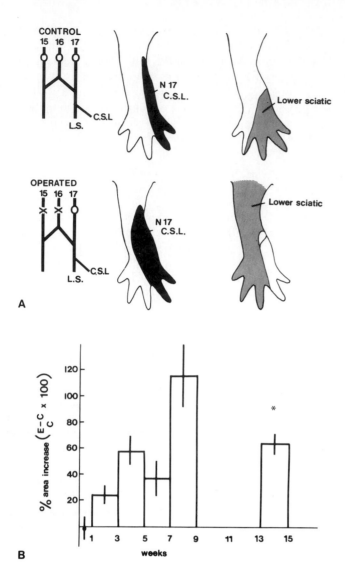

A

B

FIGURE 5 Simultaneous collateral sprouting and regeneration. (A) The top row shows the control mechanosensory fields of the two main divisions of the 17th spinal nerve, the CSL (cutaneous surae lateralis) and the lower sciatic (LS). The lower row shows, for the same animal, the extent to which these two N17 subfields enlarged following removal of the 15th and 16th dorsal-root ganglia and section of the lower sciatic some 14 weeks earlier. There was both sprouting of the CSL and extensive regeneration of the LS. Note, however, that the regenerated lower sciatic was apparently excluded from a portion of its original field. For convenience, in this and subsequent figures, the control and experimental limbs are represented with the same anteroposterior orientation. (B) Rate of sprouting of the CSL branch of N17. The experimental limbs were partially denervated in all animals as described in A. In one group of animals regeneration of the lower sciatic was prevented, and the sprouting of CSL was studied over 9 weeks. In a second group (*) the lower sciatic was allowed to regenerate freely; in these animals the CSL had sprouted much less by 13–15 weeks than it had by 9 weeks in the first group. Had there been no regeneration of the lower sciatic, the CSL field would have filled virtually the entire dorsal surface of the hind limb by 13 weeks (see Figure 10B). The regenerating fibers of the lower sciatic begin to reinnervate the limb at about 5–7 weeks after surgery and, apparently, are able to prevent the full sprouting of the CSL that would otherwise have occurred.

and O'Brien (1975) are of interest; they found that the epidermis of skin treated by a variety of physical and chemical methods became hyperplastic, and this hyperplasticity was associated with an extensive sensory-nerve ingrowth. The increased innervation, however, subsequently regressed as the epidermis reverted to its normal thickness.

That Merkel cells survive denervation and constitute the targets for incoming nerves is consistent with the results of the competition experiment described above; locally sprouting fibers were able to establish mechanosensory territory to the extent, in some regions of the skin, of totally excluding later-arriving ones. The implication again seems to be that skin with innervated Merkel cells no longer provides a stimulus for nerves to sprout into it; perhaps regression occurs of endings that have invaded but failed to contact Merkel cells.

THE ROLE OF NEURONAL TRANSPORT Why is the sprouting stimulus lost when the Merkel cell becomes innervated? Clearly the nerves themselves must be involved in changing the character of the Merkel cell. It follows that the nerves are involved in the regulation of the sprouting stimulus. This possibility was first suggested by Ramón y Cajal (1919), who commented on the fact that axonal sprouting appears to occur only at the target tissue and also, with extraor-

microscope at various intervals after nerve section (Cooper, Scott, and Diamond, 1977). Gratifyingly, we found typical Merkel cells, at about normal frequency, in skin that had been denervated for at least six months; the only difference between these Merkel cells and normal ones was the absence of associated nerve endings (cf. Figure 4A). Thus the simplest interpretation of the quantitative recovery of the density of endings after partial denervation is that sprouting continues until each denervated Merkel cell becomes reinnervated, at which time the stimulus to sprout disappears, endings are no longer attracted to the now-innervated Merkel cells, and (presumably) any excess endings regress, as mentioned earlier in relation to the transient hyperinnervation of targets during development. (In normal circumstances Merkel cells appear never to become hyperinnervated.) In this context the experiments of Fitzgerald, Folan,

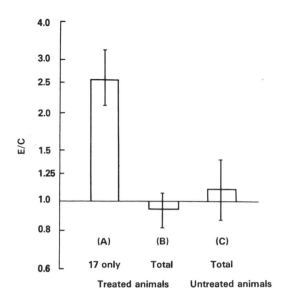

FIGURE 6 Quantitative sprouting after partial denervation. The percent occurrence of low-threshold receptors feeding into the 16th and 17th nerves from a shared region of skin was measured, and the values were compared between right and left limbs. Column A refers to a group of animals in which the right 16th nerve had been sectioned three weeks previously; it shows the right (E) to left (C) ratio for the 17th-nerve touch-receptor population only. An increase in 17th-nerve receptors is clearly seen. Column B shows, for the same group of animals, the right-left ratio for the total receptor population (i.e., the 17th on the treated side, the 16th plus the 17th on the control). Column C shows right-left ratios for the total population of touch receptors in a control group of animals, with 16th plus 17th nerves intact on both sides. There is no significant difference (p > 0.2) between columns B and C, indicating that the increase in 17th-nerve receptors on the right side of the experimental group had quantitatively made up the loss due to 16th-nerve section. Vertical bars give S.E. of mean; note that E/C is the "geometric mean." (From Cooper, Diamond, and Turner, 1977.)

dinary insight, on the implications of the apparent cessation of sprouting once an appropriate and uniform density of innervation has been achieved. Our denervation results indicate that the Merkel cell redevelops its trophic influence on nerves when its own axon is cut; this suggests the existence of an ongoing regulation. The specific possibility we investigated was that the influence of the nerve on the target depends on the continuous availability at the terminal of a factor that somehow reduces the effectiveness or production of the sprouting stimulus. This neural factor would disappear when the nerve is cut, leading to the reappearance of the sprouting stimulus, with consequent effects on intact nerves in the vicinity ("denervation sprouting"). We reasoned that the availability of this neural factor might also depend

on the supply of materials normally flowing down the nerve. We therefore investigated the effects on cutaneous mechanosensory nerve fields of interfering with neuronal transport, both by section of a nerve and by appropriate application of colchicine, a drug known to interfere with axoplasmic transport (Lubinska, 1975).

Utilizing histochemical, biochemical, and morphological techniques, we showed that external application of colchicine to a salamander nerve trunk, in appropriate dosage, interrupted fast axoplasmic transport without preventing slow flow or causing axonal degerneration (Aguilar et al., 1973; Holmes et al., 1977). When the 16th spinal nerve, which along with the 15th and the 17th supplies the salamander hind limb, was treated in this way, there was a sprouting of the untreated nerves, so that the 15th and 17th fields extended toward each other into the intervening region of skin (Figure 7). The result was essentially identical to that obtained after section of the 16th nerve, except in one important respect: the area of the mechanosensory field of the colchicine-treated 16th nerve was normal, so that the result was apparently not due to denervation per se (Aguilar et al., 1973). This finding and its interpretation were subsequently validated by a quantitative physiological

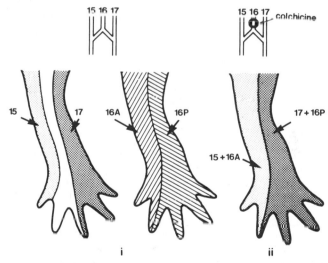

FIGURE 7 Collateral sprouting without denervation. Mechanosensory nerve fields in dorsal skin of the hind limb. (i) Control limb in which the fields of spinal nerves 15 and 17 do not abut. N16 innervates the whole dorsal surface; its two subfields, 16A and 16P, are shown separately for clarity. (ii) Experimental limb from the same salamander, investigated three weeks after N16 was treated with colchicine (100 mM for 30 min); the fields of N15 and N17 had enlarged to meet at the common border between 16A and 16P. (From Diamond et al., 1976. Copyright 1976 by the American Association for the Advancement of Science.)

study (Cooper, Diamond, and Turner, 1977), which showed that when the adjacent nerves were stimulated to sprout, the endings of the colchicine-treated nerves could be quite unchanged in distribution and in threshold (Figure 8). (The sensory threshold is an extremely sensitive indicator of the functional state of peripheral axons.) We have shown that colchicine-treated nerves do not themselves respond to the sprouting stimulus (Aguilar et al., 1973); the unchanged density of their endings, therefore, was not the result of degeneration of some made up by the sprouting of others. In addition, such degeneration would have occurred at the latest by about 10–12 days (Figure 8); it would have been detected physiologically well before the new sprouts could have matured to the normal low-threshold state (about three weeks: see Cooper, Diamond, and Turner, 1977). The sprouting stimulus thus was made available in the target tissue simply as a consequence of interference with neuronal transport in some of the nerves supplying it. It seems clear that Merkel cells innervated by the fibers whose axoplasmic transport had been reduced must have been involved in the appearance of the sprouting stimulus. Indeed our preliminary physiological findings suggest that the receptive fields of the individual newly sprouted endings overlap significantly with those of the colchicine-treated nerves (Figure 9); one obvious possibility, which we are now investigating, is that in such conditions individual Merkel cells become hyperinnervated.

These findings further support the Merkel cell as the source of the sprouting stimulus, and the conclusion seems inevitable that once a Merkel cell becomes innervated by a new sprout, a neural effect neutralizes the sprouting stimulus in some way or causes the Merkel cells to stop producing or releasing it. Denervation sprouting is a widespread phenomenon. (There may be a "critical period" for such sprouting in mammalian skin; see below.) It now seems justifi-

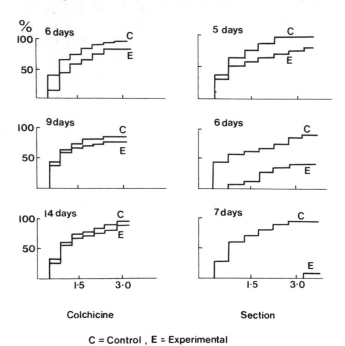

C = Control , E = Experimental

FIGURE 8 Comparison of the effects of nerve section and colchicine treatment on the density of mechanosensory endings of the treated nerve. *Left*: In three animals N16 was treated with colchicine, and the mechanosensitivity of both the experimental and control N16 fields was tested; each animal was examined at a different time after treatment. There was no significant difference ($p > 0.1$) between the results from the two sides in each of the animals. *Right*: The sensitivity of the control and experimental N16 fields was tested in three different animals, examined 5, 6, and 7 days after unilateral N16 section, respectively. There was no significant difference ($p > 0.2$) between the results on the two sides at 5 days after nerve section. On day 6, however, there was a significant change ($p < 0.005$) in the two distributions, and by day 7 only a few mechanoreceptors remained functional on the experimental side. This represents a true loss of sensory function at the endings, for at this time the distal nerve trunk was still excitable by direct electrical stimulation. Axes as in Figure 2. (From Cooper, Diamond, and Turner, 1977.)

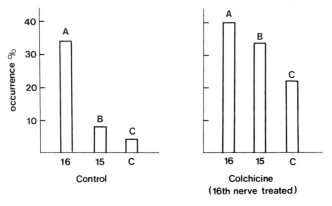

FIGURE 9 Sprouting *within* nerve fields. In a single animal the touch receptor density (i.e., the percent occurrence in the low-threshold range; cf. Figure 2B) in a region of skin shared by the 15th and 16th spinal nerves was investigated 3 weeks after the 16th nerve on one side was treated with colchicine. In this animal the number of touch receptors associated with the 15th nerve was only a small proportion of the total. There was no loss in mechanoreceptors of the treated nerve, compared to the control side (column A). On the treated side, however, the 15th nerve supplied an extra population of mechanoreceptors almost equal to the number associated with the 16th nerve (column B). Column C indicates the extent of the overlap between the individual fields of the low-threshold receptors, that is, the coincidence of 15th and 16th touch spots. (From Cooper, Diamond, and Turner, 1977.)

able to attribute this phenomenon to the elimination from target sites of an influence of the nerve endings that is itself dependent on materials normally supplied by neuronal transport; the reduction of the neural influence results in the appearance of the sprouting stimulus made by the target cells. Such an interaction between the target and the nerve could operate both in the mature organism and during development to regulate sprouting and could well be responsible for the achievement of an innervation of characteristic density for any given tissue (Olson and Malmfors, 1970; Diamond et al., 1976). Our colchicine evidence clearly points to axoplasmic transport as the means of supply of a neural agent involved in this regulation.

MECHANOSENSORY TRANSDUCTION AND THE MERKEL CELL The nerve-ending Merkel-cell complex in the salamander epidermis (and in other species: see Iggo and Muir, 1969; English, 1977; Düring and Andres, 1976) sometimes reveals suggestions of "synaptic" specializations (just-discernible synaptic thickenings, accumulations at the membrane of the nerve vesicles, and, more rarely, the dense-core granules). To date, however, there is no convincing indication of any sort of defined organization that suggests a physiological role for these ultrastructural features, even as to what is "presynaptic" and what is "postsynaptic," much less what is the nature and function of the vesicles and dense-core granules. Our own studies so far suggest that the Merkel cells do not contain monoamines, since they do not fluoresce when the Falck-Hillarp treatment is used; furthermore the sensory function of the touch domes in the cat was unchanged, and the osmiophilic granules of the Merkel cells did not disappear when the animal was given reserpine in doses that markedly affected the adrenergic function of the sympathetic supply to the nictitating membrane (Iggo and Muir, 1969). The origin of the Merkel cell is also unknown: some workers infer that it is a differentiated epidermal cell (English, 1977), others suggest that it migrates up from the dermis (Breathnach, 1971; Hashimoto, 1972). Our evidence that the Merkel cell has a trophic role in the establishment of the mechanosensory innervation does not, of course, exclude the possibility that it also contributes to sensory transduction. A point to keep in mind is that an afferent impulse set up at one mechanosensory ending might, by an "axon reflex," constitute an "efferent" input to another, and that a form of reciprocal synaptic function may exist at the nerve–Merkel-cell junction which involves both trophic and transducer mechanisms (Munger, 1977).

THE ROLE OF THE TARGET Possibly the sprouting stimulus acts directly at the level of the nerve endings, permitting the materials continually arriving by neuronal transport to be used for axonal elongation and branching. Indeed there is a problem in understanding how a nerve stops growing at all in the face of the constant movement of cytoskeletal elements and possibly membrane from the cell body to the terminals; this question has been discussed by Lasek and Hoffman (1976). It seems probable that mechanisms exist at the terminal level to bring about the disassembly of the axonal cytoskeleton and that these mechanisms (which are likely to be axoplasmic proteases) are activated when appropriate information is received from the target tissues. The target might thus have a role both as a source of a sprouting stimulus and as a source of information that stops growth of an ending when specific contact is made with the target site. Growth of other endings of the same axon need not be affected by such a local event. Later we shall return to this possibility of a dual role of the target in the regulation of sprouting.

In the light of these considerations, it would be interesting if specific target sites were always detectable before the arrival of nerves during development. In this regard we have the example of the Merkel cell not only in salamander skin but also in fetal sheep; here Merkel cells appear before the nerves are seen to contact them (Lyne and Hollis, 1971), and there is similar suggestive evidence for the human (Hashimoto, 1972). In mammalian tongue the gustatory nerves appear to arrive at characteristic basal cells (containing dense-core granules) at which sites the mature taste buds subsequently form (Farbman, 1965). In addition, there is now good evidence that in the Purkinje cell characteristic postsynaptic specializations can occur on dendritic spines that do not have a nerve supply (Herndon, Margolis, and Kilham, 1971; Rakic and Sidman, 1973; Aggerwal and Hendelman, 1975). Such target specializations thus may differentiate according to "intrinsic" instructions and not under the influence of the incoming nerve fibers; however, the fibers presumably cease to grow after they have made their specific contacts.

Of course, the occurrence of morphologically definable target sites is not always the rule, and there is undoubted evidence of the induction of characteristic junctional specializations (as in the case of muscle endplates; see Miledi, 1962) by the incoming nerves. The "hot spots" of acetylcholine sensitivity that develop on cultured nerve-free muscle fibers (Fischbach and Cohen, 1973; Bekoff and Betz, 1976) are probably not the sites at which motor nerves form synapses (Fischbach et al., 1976; Anderson, Cohen, and Zorychta, 1977; Anderson and Cohen, 1977). It is not known whether in the cat, as in the sheep, Merkel cells develop in the skin before the nerves reach them. However, there is evidence that the touch domes of cat skin, with their associated Merkel cells, disappear when the nerve is cut and subsequently reappear if the nerves are allowed to regenerate to the skin; the regenerating fibers appear to reach the original sites along the paths defined by the degenerated nerves and their associated Schwann cells (Burgess and Horch, 1973; English, 1977a; Burgess et al., 1974; Horch, 1976). This result is quite different from that in the salamander and, interestingly, from that in the rat (Smith, 1967). The problem is still not resolved, however, for a recent report claims that even in the cat Merkel cells do not degenerate or disappear when they are denervated (Hartschuh and Weihe, 1977). Possibly in some situations pioneering nerves (Weiss, 1941; LoPresti, Macagno, and Levinthal, 1973) first arrive at a target tissue and sprout there in response to a stimulus that also serves to guide them to specific target sites; subsequently these nerves and the others guided by them toward the same target tissue could induce the more readily observed specializations at the contact regions.

The spatial control of nerve fields

Our results indicate clearly that the nature of the neuron-target interactions that control the density of the nerve endings at the target tissue makes the timing of arrival of nerves a particularly important factor during development. If adjacent nerves were to grow out approximately at the same time to a developing target tissue such as skin, then the localized density of endings of one nerve would rapidly saturate the target-tissue sprouting stimulus immediately at hand and so prevent invasion of that territory by the adjacent nerves. (Whether such a process could adequately account for the relatively smooth borders and characteristic shapes attained by developing nerve fields is a moot point.)

These considerations seemed likely at first to explain our results with salamander preparations in which the 16th spinal nerve is cut. The 15th and 17th fields then enlarge only until they meet along a common frontier: they do not overlap (see Figure 7). If they are already at the common frontier, they do not invade each other's territory (Aguilar et al., 1973). Within their respective nerve fields, however, as indicated earlier (Figures 6 and 9), there is sprouting of the 15th and 17th nerves (Cooper, Diamond, and Turner, 1977) and presumed occupancy of the Merkel cells originally supplied by the 16th nerve endings. That neither of the two spinal nerves extends across the common frontier would be understandable if the endings of each nerve had readier access to the available sources of the sprouting stimulus within their respective territories, that is, to the denervated Merkel cells. Although the results were clear, the story turned out to be considerably more complex.

ANOTHER CONSTRAINT ON AXONAL SPROUTING? We were interested in a number of further questions: How much sprouting can a single nerve achieve? Is there exhaustion of the sprouting stimulus? What happens to the spinal reflex circuitry of a sensory nerve that is induced to sprout and take over the territory normally supplied by another (see Stirling, 1973)? With these questions in mind, we removed all but one of the three spinal nerves supplying the hind limb of a salamander and followed the sprouting of the remaining nerve physiologically. To our surprise, the field of the remaining 15th or 17th nerve was apparently contained, despite the presence of the immediately adjacent denervated skin and the sprouting stimulus that was presumably available within it (Diamond et al., 1976). The 17th nerve, for example, sprouted within its territory, as we have seen; but after an initial slight growth across the original frontier zone between the 15th and 17th nerve fields, it ceased to extend its field significantly for a period as long as two months (Figure 10A). Under these conditions there can be no question of competition between nerves; another explanation must be sought for this unexpected static period.

Interestingly, about two months after the initial partial denervation, sprouting of the 17th nerve resumed, although that of the 15th remained limited for as long as we followed it (about 3–4 months; Figure 10A). The 17th field eventually extended to fill the entire dorsal surface of the limb (Figure 10B; see also Macintyre and Diamond, 1977). Obviously the relative lack of sprouting during the static period was not due to the nerves reaching a ceiling in their growth capacity. (Other experimental findings also exclude this possibility; for example, after complete amputation of a hind limb—combined with ligation of selected nerves to hinder their regeneration—any remaining hind-limb nerve will grow continuously along with the regenerating limb and keep the skin's mechanosensitivity normal. The 17th nerve field, for example, could thus double in area within the critical two-month period.) A fortuitous finding excluded the possibility of a mechanical barrier to growth; in ex-

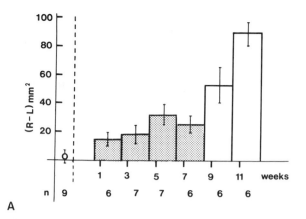

A

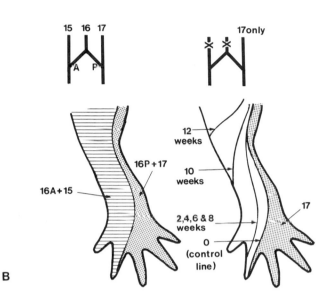

B

FIGURE 10 Increase in area of 17th nerve field after a partial denervation that left only N17 in the limb. (A) The data are grouped in 2-week time periods starting at 5 days; this is the earliest time at which mechanosensory area sprouting becomes readily detectable in these experiments (Aguilar et al., 1973). The number of animals in each bin is indicated below. There was a small but significant growth ($p < 0.025$) within the first 2 weeks, but then sprouting essentially ceased until a total postdenervation time of about 2 months had elapsed. At this time a significant ($p < 0.025$) field extension occurred (unhatched columns). (B) Diagrammatic representation of the data in A, indicating the portion of dorsal skin affected. On the left is a control limb in which the fields of spinal nerves 15 and 17 meet along a common frontier. On the right is a composite sketch of the results following a denervation of the limb that leaves only the 17th spinal nerve intact. By 12 weeks postoperative the 17th field usually extends to occupy almost the entire dorsal surface. 16A (P) = anterior (posterior) division of N16.

in the mechanically insensitive regions, nor were nerve fields surrounded by a fringe of "silent" endings that might eventually become functional when adjacent skin is denervated. Sprouting of axons is clearly a more plausible explanation of the field enlargement that occurs after partial denervation.

SPECIFICITY OF SPROUTING STIMULUS? Could there be a specific sprouting stimulus for each region of skin, appropriate only for the nerve normally supplying that region? The Merkel cells in the different regions would then make different sprouting stimuli, despite their morphological similarity. We tested this possibility in experiments involving skin rotation (Diamond et al., 1976). Areas of skin (dermis plus epidermis) extending across the 15th–17th border were removed and reimplanted, either in the original orientation, or after 180° rotation. The results were remarkable; the nerves reestablished their original field areas in the flap with reference to the limb coordinates, quite regardless of the orientation of the reimplanted skin flap or the original line of the 15th–17th frontier (Figure 11B). Most of the growth of nerves into the flap occurred from the edges, especially in the case of the 15th nerve; since the excised flap rarely included equal proportions of 15th and 17th territories, one set of fibers must have reached the frontier line, defined according to the spatial coordinates mentioned above, before the other.

In other animals the reimplantation of skin was done in a hind limb that had been partially denervated. In these experiments the 16th nerve usually sprouted uniformly across the limb, both within and outside the transplant, as in other experiments al-

periments in which one of the two major skin fields was completely denervated by cutting either the 15th nerve plus the anterior division of the 16th or the 17th plus the 16th posterior, the remaining 16th branch usually sprouted readily into the denervated territory, whereas the 15th or 17th remained at its original frontier location (see Figure 11C below). In the absence of a mechanical barrier to the sprouting fibers of the 16th nerve, it is difficult to suppose that there might be such a barrier to those of the 15th or 17th. Moreover, neither light- nor electron-microscopic examination of skin removed from the frontier zone has revealed any suggestion of a mechanical barrier.

Could the lack of detectable field enlargement during the first two months be due to a functional "invisibility" of new sprouts that do in fact exist but need that length of time to become mechanosensitive? This possibility was excluded by direct electrical stimulation of the skin: no electrically excitable fibers existed

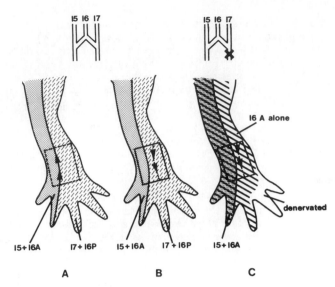

FIGURE 11 Evidence for nerve domains from skin-graft experiments. Hind limbs A and B show the spinal-nerve fields in the same animal, A being the control limb and B the experimental one. Limb C shows the fields in an experimental limb of another animal whose control limb was similar to A. (A) Control limb. The broken line indicates the original position, and the arrows the original orientation, of the skin that was rotated and grafted in the experimental limb. (B) Experimental limb. The skin flap had been rotated 180° six weeks earlier. Note that after the graft has been reinnervated, the 15th–17th boundary in it is reestablished according to the original location of this boundary with respect to the limb coordinates; the boundary bears no relation to its original position as defined on the skin itself, which is indicated by the arrowed line within the graft. (C) Experimental limb. The excised and reimplanted skin graft was rotated 180°; at the same time the combined trunk of N16P and N17 was cut and ligated. The control limb was similar to A above. The original 15th–17th line in the graft and its orientation are indicated by the broken line with arrows. Six weeks after the operation, N15 had sprouted a small amount, as would be expected at this time, and N16A had sprouted considerably more, again within the normal range for that nerve. Note that, within the graft, N15$_y$ had sprouted into skin originally supplied by N17 but had stopped along a frontier that was smoothly continuous with that of the N15 field outside the graft.

ready described; in the majority of these experiments, however, the 15th or 17th nerve sprouted essentially as it did in similar partial-denervation experiments done on limbs in which no skin transplantations had been made. The frontier finally established was located along a line normally reached within the two-month static period described above (see Figure 10A, B); this line was again related to the limb coordinates and not to the original (now-rotated) frontier line on the skin (Figure 11C; note that this "containment" of the 15th nerve's field also occurred

in experiments in which this was the only nerve remaining in the limb at the time of the skin rotation: see Diamond et al., 1976.)

DOMAINS   The conclusions from these experiments are that some mechanism operates to restrict (at least for a significant period) certain nerve fields to defined areas in the salamander skin and that this mechanism cannot reside in the skin itself. It appears that the nerves are contained in a domain whose coordinates are related to the limb as a whole (body-space) (Diamond et al., 1976).

Interestingly, regenerating nerves grow freely along pathways provided by degenerating nerve trunks and will readily innervate alien territory that intact sprouting nerves will not (at least for the two-month static period). Whatever the nature of the mechanism responsible for the constraint on the sprouting of the intact nerves, regenerating nerves do not seem susceptible to it, at least while they are en route to their eventual destination. We have other evidence that regenerating and intact fibers differ in regard to their sprouting (Diamond, 1976); it seems that, at least initially, regenerating nerves are under a "central drive" triggered by nerve section, in contrast to intact nerves, which are normally susceptible only to the influence of the target-tissue sprouting stimulus. However, both classes of nerves must interact with the latter at the target site, since neither normal nor regenerating fibers hyperinnervate touch spots.

It seems then that some mechanism acts to hinder collaterals of intact nerves from invading a foreign domain, at least for a period, and that this control relates to the spatial coordinates of the limb and not the skin itself. When the sprouting stimulus is located within a nerve domain, that nerve will respond to it; but for a significant period the sprouting stimulus is relatively ineffective on a nerve occupying an adjacent domain of body-space. There are no apparent differences among the sprouting stimuli provided by the different regions of the skin, and the spatial influence therefore operates separately from the sprouting stimulus.

Supporting this view of nerve domains is our finding that if all the nerves to the limb are cut except for a subdivision of the 17th spinal nerve, the CSL branch, the fibers of this nerve will readily sprout but, initially, entirely within the territory allotted to the parent nerve (Figure 12; note that in Figure 5 this sprouting of CSL would have initially filled the entire field of the lower sciatic, *had that nerve not itself regenerated*). The duration of the apparent constraint on sprouting into denervated territory of the adjacent

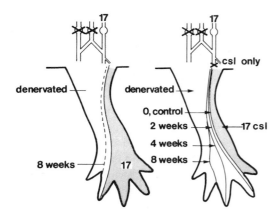

FIGURE 12   Pattern of sprouting when only a subpopulation of the fibers of a single "parent" spinal nerve remain in the limb. The left limb shows the extent of area enlargement of the entire 17th spinal nerve over the first 2 months after denervation of the adjacent "domain" (cf. Figure 10B). The limb on the right shows the pattern of sprouting of a subpopulation of the 17th-nerve fibers (the CSL branch), when all other nerves to the limb were eliminated. In this instance there was extensive and continuous sprouting during the first 8 weeks; note, however, that despite the nearness of the adjacent (and "foreign") denervated skin in the proximal and middle portions of the limb, the sprouting preferentially filled the domain of the parent 17th nerve. Only after 2 months did the sprouting extend to areas outside the parent domain (cf. Figure 10B at 10 and 12 weeks).

spinal nerve (two months for nerve 17 and certainly longer than three months for nerve 15; see Figure 10) is all the more remarkable when one considers the finding mentioned earlier, that during this same period, when the rate of regeneration of a hind limb after amputation reaches a maximum, the skin mechanosensitivity of such a regenerating limb is continually maintained at a normal level by a single remaining spinal nerve.

NEW FINDINGS IN THE MAMMAL   Recent findings suggest that denervation sprouting of low-threshold mechanosensory nerves in mammalian skin has a critical period, which in the rat ends at about 20 days of age (Diamond and Jackson, 1979). In addition, during the neonatal period when such sprouting occurs, a domain restriction appears to be present. The mechanosensory nerves of a fully innervated trunk dermatome do not sprout cranially or caudally into the skin of the adjacent dermatomes when these are denervated. However, when a *part* of the first dermatome is also denervated, it becomes rapidly invaded by mechanosensory sprouts from the remaining "island" of innervation. Even though there are no morphological features indicating where the skin of one

dermatome merges with that of its neighbors, the nerves appear to recognize a boundary and respect it.

We wonder if the domains suggested by our findings are related to the "compartments" described in insects (Garcia-Bellido, 1975). The operation of homeotic genes has been implicated in the development of these compartments (Morata and Lawrence, 1977), and their boundaries seem also to be respected by axons (Lawrence, 1975). If the ability of nerves at targets to extend their fields were differentially restricted by the appropriate operation of such control mechanisms, this would complement, or even substitute for, differences in the timing of arrival of the nerves during development. The kind of competition that depends on the nerve-target interaction described above could then operate to stabilize a territorial "claim" of a particular set of nerve fibers.

MECHANISMS OF SPATIAL CONSTRAINT   It is easier to consider the possible targets of the mechanism responsible for spatial control than the exact nature of that mechanism. If the nerves themselves were the targets, they would need to be labeled somehow during development, according to their allotted domain, so that they could be geographically distinguished one from another. Conceivably the spatial character of a nerve could be acquired as a consequence of the relative location of the neurons in the developing neural axis during embryogenesis, under the influence of appropriate craniocaudal chemical gradients (Sperry, 1965; Crick, 1970; Keating, 1976). Perhaps, too, the presence of a nerve (or its associated nonneural cells) specifies the spatial character of the domain itself, which then persists into maturity. This might explain the resumption of sprouting into a foreign domain after the static period: the loss of the particular spatial character of the foreign territory might depend on the total elimination from it of the influence originally provided by the axons or by their associated "supporting" cells.

Could nonneuronal cells be the target of the spatial influences? It is interesting that there are no reports of naked axons growing out in vivo more than a few hundred microns in the absence of accompanying cells (e.g., Harris, 1924). If, therefore, appropriate nonneuronal cells cannot accompany or become associated with naked nerve sprouts, then almost certainly the extension of these sprouts into foreign space would eventually cease. The in vitro situation certainly can differ in this regard, with quite extensive growth of naked axons (e.g., Mains and Patterson, 1973), and the culture may thus be substituting materials normally provided by nonneuronal cells in vivo. (By the same token, controls that develop in vivo may be absent from in vitro systems.) In one of his famous controversies with Ramón y Cajal, Held (1909) maintained that during embryogenesis a skeletal guideline of nonneuronal tissue develops, into which the outgrowing axons advance. His observations seem not to have been refuted (even by Ramón y Cajal). If Held was correct, nonneuronal cells would seem an attractive possibility as the target for the spatial control and as a useful means of containing sprouting axons within a domain. As before, it could be postulated that not until all Schwann cells, for example, have disappeared from a region of denervation, could those of a neighboring domain extend outwards to accompany nerve sprouts across the frontier.

Recent results from both in vivo and in vitro experiments point to important interactions between neurons and various types of nonneuronal tissues that influence the morphological and chemical characteristics of nerves (Aguayo, Charron, and Bray, 1976; Aguayo et al., 1977; Chun et al., 1977; Varon and Bunge, 1978). In our experiments, analogous interactions seem to play a large part in controlling the sprouting of axons and, consequently, the development of nerve fields. An interesting approach to the investigation of such interactions is the mouse chimera preparation, one animal composed of two genotypically distinct cell types (McLaren, 1976). This preparation has been used with great success to show that the dystrophic phenotype in murine dystrophy is not uniquely an expression of the muscle genotype and may in fact be imposed upon the muscle from an extramuscular source (Peterson, 1974, 1977). If the characteristics of nerve growth at a target are influenced by other tissues in the manner suggested above, then the chimera approach with appropriate animal models may be one way to determine the origin of the controlling influences.

SPROUTING AND SYNAPTOGENESIS The kind of question that can be usefully considered in the light of our findings is exemplified by the innervation of the Mauthner cell. Measurements in the goldfish Mauthner cell show that from an early age after hatching, the proportion of the lateral dendrite occupied by the proximal set of histologically identifiable nerve endings is always the same (~40%) relative to that occupied by a second, distal, set (~60%) (Bodian, 1942; Diamond, 1968, and unpublished observations). It seems that these two inputs apportion the territory between them at an early stage of develop-

ment and that the dendrite enlarges uniformly thereafter by interstitial growth, the proportion occupied by each nerve thus remaining constant. However, the dendrite must initially have grown out laterally from the soma region. One possibility is that the nerve input that arrives first establishes the proximal field and that for a short while thereafter, before the stage of uniform enlargement is reached, the increasing length of the dendrite is associated with the arrival of the second input. If so, then one wonders if a spatial control analogous to that described above operates to hinder the first input from sprouting over the newly developing dendritic surface, thus permitting the later arriving nerve to establish its territory.

In all these developmental situations, however, one must allow for the possible occurrence of specific sprouting factors localized to certain tissues. Such factors certainly exist, and in some circumstances nerves can be readily shown to innervate certain tissues in preference to others (cf. Taylor, 1944; Gutmann, 1945; Weiss and Edds, 1945). Also, a cell surface may be mosaic in nature (Singer and Nicholson, 1972), and this would provide another likely explanation of why incoming axons sometimes reveal a preference for one region of a neuron rather than another (Schwartz and Kane, 1977). Such membrane characteristics, however, seem unlikely to provide a means for controlling the sprouting of incoming axons. Could it be that a general sprouting stimulus is released from the target and that the actual association achieved by the nerve ending is more a function of the recognition by the ending of an appropriate surface region on the target cell?

The salamander Merkel cell seems most simply described as both the origin of the sprouting stimulus and the target of the nerve endings, but this description may not be generalizable to other systems. In the case of the Merkel cell, although it is probable that the nerve is attracted toward this small and infrequent target, the dermal surface of the cell is always the one innervated. Although this may be simply fortuitous, in that the dermal side of the cell may be the one first "seen" by the nerve endings, it is also possible that only this surface is appropriate and that it is therefore specialized to receive the nerve association. Thus a general description of targets as sources of sprouting stimuli may entail their having a specific mosaic character of membrane, so that arriving nerves can make selective attachments. It would appear to be economical for an organism to have targets able both to induce sprouting, and thus initiate the development of a terminal field, and at the same time to present appropriately organized surfaces to ensure both the specificity of connections and their density. As discussed earlier, the achievement of the association between a nerve ending and the target site could also provide the signal for cessation of growth of that ending, and it would be at this stage that the process of synaptogenesis characteristic for the particular tissue can be regarded as having begun.

Conclusion

These studies indicate the existence, in the mature organism, of mechanisms that could be used both to bring about modifications of terminal-field densities and possibly to regulate the areas of target tissue over which nerve fields can extend. During development, and perhaps also later in life, this ongoing regulation of collateral sprouting would afford a powerful mechanism for "plasticity" in the nervous system. Synapse "stabilization" consequent to repetitive activation of a circuit could also be involved in the expression of such a regulation (Young, 1951; Jacobson, 1970; Changeux and Danchin, 1976). A control of the spatial parameter of terminal fields, like that suggested by the salamander results and by other studies in which unexplained constraints on sprouting have been observed (see, e. g., Fitzgerald, 1963), would ensure that the gross distribution of nerve fields established during ontogeny need not be violated by "internal" adjustments of terminal densities. One wonders whether dendritic fields (Scheibel and Scheibel, 1967) are under an analogous control. Indeed, the now well-established existence in the brain of "columns" (Mountcastle, 1957; Hubel and Wiesel, 1963) and "barrels" (Woolsey and Van der Loos, 1970) suggests that the concept of domains as defined above may be applicable to the nervous system in a more generalized way than has been suggested for the more obvious dermatomal fields and that this aspect of genetic regulation (cf. Crick and Lawrence, 1975) may extend to the organization of circuitry in regions such as the cerebral cortex itself.

ACKNOWLEDGMENTS   I am extremely grateful to Mary Ban, Mike Holmes, Lynn Macintyre, Sheryl Scott, Ellis Cooper, and Anne Foerster, who willingly contributed help and criticism during preparation of this manuscript.

REFERENCES

AGGERWAL, A. S., and W. J. HENDELMAN, 1975. Electron microscopic study of Purkinje somatic spines in organotypic cultures. Anat. Rec. 181:298.

AGUAYO, A. J., L. CHARRON, and G. M. BRAY, 1976. Potential of Schwann cells from unmyelinated nerves to produce myelin: A quantitative ultrastructural and radiographic study. J. Neurocytol. 5:565–673.

AGUAYO, A. J., J. KASARJIAN, E. SKAMENE, P. KONGSHAVN, and G. M. BRAY, 1977. Myelination of mouse axons by Schwann cells transplanted from normal and abnormal human nerves. Nature 268:753–755.

AGUILAR, C. E., M. A. BISBY, E. COOPER, and J. DIAMOND, 1973. Evidence that axoplasmic transport of trophic factors is involved in the regulation of peripheral nerve fields in salamanders. J. Physiol. 234:449–464.

ANDERSON, M. J., and M. W. COHEN, 1977. Nerve-induced and spontaneous redistribution of acetylcholine receptors on cultured muscle cells. J. Physiol. 268:759–773.

ANDERSON, M. J., M. W. COHEN, and E. ZORYCHTA, 1977. Effects of innervation on the distribution of acetylcholine receptors on cultured muscle cells. J. Physiol. 268:731–756.

BALINSKY, B. I., 1975. An Introduction to Embryology, 4th ed. Philadelphia: W. B. Saunders.

BEKOFF, A., and W. J. BETZ, 1976. Acetylcholine hot spots: Development on myotubes cultured from aneural limb buds. Science 193:915–917.

BENNETT, M. R., and A. G. PETTIGREW, 1974. The formation of synapses in striated muscle during development. J. Physiol. 241:515–545.

BODIAN, D., 1942. Cytological aspects of synaptic function. Physiol. Rev. 22:146–169.

BREATHNACH, A. S., 1971. Embryology of human skin. A review of ultrastructural studies. J. Invest. Dermatol. 57:133–143.

BROWN, M. C., J. K. S. JANSEN, and D. VAN ESSEN, 1976. Polyneuronal innervation of skeletal muscle in new-born rats and its elimination during maturation. J. Physiol. 261:387–422.

BURGESS, P. R., K. B. ENGLISH, K. W. HORCH, and L. J. STENSAAS, 1974. Patterning in the regeneration of Type I cutaneous receptors. J. Physiol. 236:57–82.

BURGESS, P. R., and K. W. HORCH, 1973. Specific regeneration of cutaneous fibres in the cat. J. Neurophysiol. 36:101–115.

CHANGEUX, J. P., and A. DANCHIN, 1976. Selective stabilization of developing synapse as a mechanism for the specification of neuronal networks. Nature 264:705–712.

CHUN, L. L. Y., E. J. FURSHPAN, S. C. LANDIS, P. R. MACLEISH, C. A. NURSE, P. H. PATTERSON, D. D. POTTER, and L. F. REICHARDT, 1977. The role of non-neuronal cells in the development of rat sympathetic neurons in vitro. In Approaches to the Cell Biology of Neurons. (Society for Neuroscience Symposia, vol. 2), pp. 82–91.

COOPER, E., and J. DIAMOND, 1977. A quantitative study of the mechanosensory innervation of the salamander skin. J. Physiol. 264:695–723.

COOPER, E., J. DIAMOND, and C. TURNER, 1977. The effects of nerve section and of colchicine treatment on the density of mechanosensory nerve endings in salamander skin. J. Physiol. 264:725–749.

COOPER, E., S. A. SCOTT, and J. DIAMOND, 1977. The control of mechonsensory nerve sprouting in salamander skin. In Approaches to the Cell Biology of Neurons (Society for Neuroscience Symposia, vol. 2), pp. 120–138.

CREPEL, F., J. MARIANI, N. DELHAYE-BOUCHAUD, 1976. Evidence for a multiple innervation of Purkinje cells by climbing fibres in the immature rat cerebellum. *J. Neurobiol.* 7:567–578.

CRICK, F., 1970. Diffusion in embryogenesis. *Nature* 225:420–422.

CRICK, F., and P. A. LAWRENCE, 1975. Compartments and polyclones in insect development *Science* 189:340–347.

DETWILER, S. R., 1936. *Neuroembryology: An Experimental Study.* New York: Macmillan.

DIAMOND, J., 1968. The activation and distribution of GABA anL-glutamate receptors on goldfish Mauthner neurones: An analysis of dendritic remote inhibition. Appendix by A. F. Huxley: Effect of a local change of membrane resistance on the electrotonic potential recorded nearer to the source. *J. Physiol* 194:669–723.

DIAMOND, J., 1976. Target-cell innervation. *Neurosci. Res. Program Bull.* 14:337–346.

DIAMOND, J., and P. JACKSON, 1979. Regeneration and collateral sprouting of peripheral nerves. In *Nerve Repair: Its Clinical and Experimental Basis*, D. L. Jewett and H. R. McCarroll, eds. Saint Louis: C. V. Mosby.

DIAMOND, J., E. COOPER, C. TURNER, and L. MACINTYRE, 1976. Trophic regulation of nerve sprouting. *Science* 193:371–377.

DÜRING, M. VON, and K. H. ANDRES, 1976. The ultrastructure of taste and touch receptors of the frog's taste organ. *Cell Tiss. Res.* 165:185–198.

ENGLISH, K., 1977a. The ultrastructure of cutaneous Type I mechanoreceptors (Haarscheiben) in cats following denervation. *J. Comp. Neurol.* 172:137–164.

ENGLISH, K. B., 1977b. Morphogenesis of Haarscheiben in rats. *J. Invest. Dermatol.* 69:58–67.

FARBMAN, A. I., 1965. Electron microscope study of the developing taste bud in rat fungiform papillae. *Dev. Biol.* 11:110–135.

FISCHBACH, G. D., D. K. BERG, S. A. COHEN, and E. FRANK, 1976. Enrichment of nerve-muscle synapses in spinal cord–muscle cultures and identification of relative peaks of ACh sensitivity at sites of transmitter release. *Cold Spring Harbor Symp. Quant. Biol.* 40:347–357.

FISCHBACH, G. D., and S. A. COHEN, 1973. The distribution of acetylcholine sensitivity over uninnervated and innervated muscle fibres grown in cell culture. *Dev. Biol.* 31:147–162.

FITZGERALD, M. J. T., 1963. Transmedian cutaneous innervation. *J. Anat.* 97:313–322.

FITZGERALD, M. J. T., 1966. Perinatal changes in epidermal innervation in rat and mouse *J. Comp. Neurol.* 126:37–42.

FITZGERALD, M. J. T., J. C. FOLAN and T. M. O'BRIEN, 1975. The innervation of hyperplastic epidermis in the mouse: A light microscopic study. *J. Invest. Dermatol.* 64:169–174.

GARCIA-BELLIDO, A., 1975. Genetic control of wing disc development in *Drosophila*. In *Cell Patterning* (Ciba Foundation Symposium no. 29) New York: Elsevier, pp. 161–178.

GUTMANN, E., 1945. The reinnervation of muscle by sensory nerve fibres. *J. Anat.* 79:1–8.

HAMILTON, W. J., and H. W. MOSSMAN, 1972. In *Human Embryology*, 4th ed., W. J. Hamilton and H. W. Mossman, eds. Cambridge, England: W. Heffer, p. 49.

HARRIS, R., 1942. Neuroblast versus sheath cells in the development of peripheral nerves. *J. Comp. Neurol.* 37:123–205.

HARTSCHUH, W., and E. WEIHE, 1977. The effect of denervation on Merkel cells in cats. *Neurosci. Lett.* 5:327–332.

HASHIMOTO, K., 1972. The ultrastructure of the skin of human embryos. X. Merkel tactile cells in the finger and nail. *J. Anat.* 111:99–120.

HELD, H., 1909. *Die Entwicklung des Nervengewebes bei den Wirbeltieren.* Leipzig: von Johan Ambrosius Barth.

HERNDON, R. M., G. MARGOLIS, and L. KILHAM, 1971. The synaptic organization of the malformed cerebellum induced by prenatal infection with the feline leukopenia virus (PLV). II. The Purkinje cell and its afferents. *J. Neuropathol. Exp. Neurol.* 30:557–570.

HOLMES, M. J., C. TURNER, J. A. FRIED, E. COOPER, and J. DIAMOND, 1977. Neuronal transport in salamander nerves and its blockade by colchicine. *Brain Res.* 136:31–43.

HORCH, K. W., 1976. Specific conduit guidance after nerve crush and its absence after peripheral nerve transection in the cat. In *Society for Neuroscience 6th Annual Meeting* (Abstracts), vol. 2, part 2, p. 1042.

HUBEL, D. H., and T. N. WIESEL, 1963. Shape and arrangement of columns in cat's striate cortex. *J. Physiol.* 165:559–568.

HUGHES, A. F. W., 1968. *Aspects of Neural Ontogeny.* London: Logos Press, Elek Books Ltd.

IGGO, A., 1968. Electrophysiological and histological studies of cutaneous mechanoreceptors. In *The Skin Senses*, D. R. Kenshalo, ed. Springfield, IL: Charles C Thomas, pp. 84–111.

IGGO, A., and A. R. MUIR, 1969. The structure and function of a slowly adapting touch corpuscle in hairy skin. *J. Physiol.* 200:763–796.

JACOBSON, M., 1970. Development, specification, and diversification of neuronal connections. In *The Neurosciences: Second Study Program*, F. O. Schmitt, ed. New York: Rockefeller Univ. Press, pp. 116–129.

KEATING, J. J., 1976. The formation of visual neuronal connections: An appraisal of the present status of the theory of "neuronal specificity." In *Studies of the Development of Behavior and the Nervous System*, vol. 3: *Neural and Behavioral Specificity*, G. Gottlieb, ed. New York: Academic Press, pp. 59–110.

KORNELIUSSEN, H., and J. K. JANSEN, 1976. Morphological aspects of the elimination of polyneuronal innervation of skeletal muscle fibres in newborn rats. *J. Neurocytol.* 5:591–604.

LANDMESSER, L., and G. PILAR, 1976. Fate of ganglionic synapses and ganglion cell axons during normal and induced cell death. *J. Cell Biol.* 68:357–374.

LASEK, R. J., and P. N. HOFFMAN, 1976. The neuronal cytoskeleton, axonal transport and axonal growth. In *Cell Motility*, R. Goldman, T. Pollard, and J. Rosenbaum, eds. Cold Spring Harbor, NY: Cold Spring Harbor Laboratory.

LAWRENCE, P. A., 1975. The structure and properties of a compartment border: The intersegmental boundary in *Oncopeltus*. In *Cell Patterning* (Ciba Foundation Symposium no. 29). New York: Elsevier, pp. 3–23.

LOPRESTI, V., E. R. MACAGNO, and C. LEVINTHAL, 1973. Structure and development of neuronal connections in isogenic organisms: Cellular interactions in the development of the optic lamina of *Daphnia*. *Proc. Natl. Acad.*

Sci. USA 70:433–437.

LUBINSKA, L., 1975. On axoplasmic flow. *Int. Rev. Neurobiol.* 17:241–296.

LYNE, A. G., and D. E. HOLLIS, 1971. Merkel cells in sheep during fetal development. *J. Ultrastruct. Res.* 34:464–472.

MACINTYRE, L., and J. DIAMOND, 1977. Nerve domains and sprouting in salamander skin. *Society for Neuroscience 7th Annual Meeting* (Abstracts). In press.

MAINS, R. E., and P. H. PATTERSON, 1973. Primary cultures of dissociated sympathetic neurons. I. Establishment of long-term growth in culture and studies of differentiated properties. *J. Cell Biol.* 59:329–345.

McLAREN, A., 1976. Mammalian chimaeras. In *Developmental and Cell Biology Series*, vol. 4, M. Ambercrombie, D. R. Newth, and J. G. Torrey, eds. London: Cambridge Univ. Press.

MILEDI, R., 1962. Induced innervation of endplate free muscle segments. *Nature* 193:281–282.

MORATA, G., and P. A. LAWRENCE, 1977. Homeotic genes, compartments and cell determination in *Drosophila*. *Nature* 265:211–216.

MOUNTCASTLE, V. B., 1957. Modality and topographic properties of single neurons of cat's somatic sensory cortex. *J. Neurophysiol.* 20:408–434.

MUNGER, B. L., 1977. Neural-epithelial interactions in sensory receptors. *J. Invest. Dermatol.* 69:27–40.

OLSON, L., and T. MALFORS, 1970. Growth characteristics of adrenergic nerves in the adult rat. *Acta Physiol. Scand.* (Suppl. 348):1–112.

PARDUCZ, A., R. A. LESLIE, E. COOPER, C. J. TURNER, and J. DIAMOND, 1977. The Merkel cells and the rapidly adapting mechanoreceptors of the salamander skin. *Neuroscience* 2:511–521.

PETERSON, A. C., 1974. Chimaera mouse study shows absence of disease in genetically dystrophic muscle. *Nature* 248:561–564.

PETERSON, A. C., 1977. Complete rescue of genetically dystrophic muscle in mouse chimaeras. *Fed. Proc.* 36:555 (abstract).

PIATT, J., 1942. Transplantation of aneurogenic forelimbs in *Amblystoma tigrinum*. *J. Exp. Zool.* 91:79–101.

PIATT, J., 1952. Transplantation of aneurogenic forelimbs in place of the hindlimb in *Amblystoma*. *J. Exp. Zool.* 120:247–285.

RAKIC, P., and P. L. SIDMAN, 1973. Sequence of developmental abnormalities leading to granule cell deficit in cerebellar cortex of Weaver mutant mice. *J. Comp. Neurol.* 152:103–132.

RAMÓN Y CAJAL, S., 1919. Accion neurotropic de los epithelios (Algunos detalles solure el macanismo genetico de las laurificaciones nervioscis inuo epithcliales, sensitivas y sensoviales). *Trab. Lab. Invest. Biol. Univ. Madrid*

17:181–228. Reprinted in *Studies on Vertebrate Neurogenesis*, L. Guth, trans. Springfield, IL: Charles C Thomas (1960), pp. 149–200.

REDFERN, P. A., 1970. Neuromuscular transmission in newborn rats. *J. Physiol.* 209:701–709.

SCHEIBEL, M. E., and A. B. SCHEIBEL, 1967. Anatomical basis of attention mechanisms in vertebrate brains. In *The Neurosciences: A Study Program*, G. C. Quarton, T. Melnechuk, and F. O. Schmitt, eds. New York: Rockefeller Univ. Press, pp. 577–582.

SCHWARTZ, A. M., and E. S. KANE, 1977. Development of the octopus cell area in the cat ventral cochlear nucleus. *Am. J. Anat.* 148:1–18.

SCOTT, S. A., and J. DIAMOND, 1977. Neuron-target interactions explain competition between salamander mechanosensory axons. *Society for Neuroscience 7th Annual Meeting* (Abstracts).

SINGER, S. J., and G. L. NICHOLSON, 1972. The fluid mosaic model of the structure of cell membranes. *Science* 175:720–731.

SMITH, K. B., 1967. The structure and function of Haarscheibe. *J. Comp. Neurol.* 131:459–474.

SPEIDEL, C. C., 1942. Studies of living nerves. VII. Growth adjustments of cutaneous terminal arborizations. *J. Comp. Neurol.* 76:57–73.

SPERRY, R. W., 1965. Embryogenesis of behavioral nerve nets. In *Organogenesis*, R. L. DeHaan and H. Ursprung, eds. New York: Holt, Rinehart & Winston.

STIRLING, V., 1973. The effects of increasing the innervation field size of nerves on their reflex response time in salamanders. *J. Physiol.* 229:657–680.

TAYLOR, A. C., 1944. Selectivity of nerve fibres from the dorsal and ventral roots in the development of the frog limb. *J. Exp. Zool.* 96:159–185.

TWEEDLE, C. D., 1978. Ultrastructure of Merkel cell development in aneurogenic and control amphibian larvae (*Ambystoma*). *Neuroscience* 3:481–486.

VARON, S. S. and R. P. BUNGE, 1978. Trophic mechanisms in the peripheral nervous system. In *Annual Review of Neuroscience*, vol. 1, W. M. Cowan, ed. (in press).

WEISS, P., 1941. Nerve patterns: The mechanics of nerve growth. *Growth* 3:163–203.

WEISS, P., and M. V. EDDS, 1945. Sensory-motor nerve crosses in the rat. *J. Neurophysiol.* 8:173–193.

WINKELMANN, R. K., and A. S. BREATHNACH, 1973. The Merkel cell. *J. Invest. Dermatol.* 60:2–15.

WOOLSEY, T. A., and H. VAN DER LOOS, 1970. The structural organization of layer IV in the somatosensory region (SI) of mouse cerebral cortex. *Brain Res.* 17:205–242.

YOUNG, J. Z., 1951. Growth and plasticity in the nervous system. *Proc. R. Soc. Lond.* B139:18–37.

57 Extrinsic Influences on the Development of Afferent Topographies in Mammalian Brain

GARY LYNCH (with the collaboration of REBECCA M. AKERS)

ABSTRACT This paper reviews some of the extrinsic factors thought to be involved in governing the shape and size of the extensive axonal ramifications generated by developing neurons.

Some type of axoaxonic competition appears to play a major and perhaps primary role in dictating the distribution of terminal fields in mammalian brain. Evidence for several possible factors which might dictate the outcome of the competition between fibers are discussed. These include: (1) the orientation of the axons as they invade the developing target; (2) the timing between the arrival of afferents and the maturational status of the target; (3) the extent to which various afferents have innervated (or are innervating) other target areas; and (4) "usage" of the projection during development. At present almost nothing is known of the molecular processes that might mediate the competition, but several suggestions are briefly considered.

There is also a distinct possibility that nonneural factors participate in determining afferent topographies. Work with in vitro culture systems suggests that glial cells promote the biochemical and anatomical differentiation of neurons and possibly guide or influence the direction of growth by developing neurites in explants.

Introduction

PERHAPS THE MOST distinctive feature of the neuron is its extraordinary axonal arborization. This process can contain tens of thousands of terminals and a mass hundreds of times that of the cell that produced it. In the brain, axonal projections often extend for tremendous distances and then distribute themselves onto dendritic zones that are only a few microns high. How this is accomplished has been one of the fundamental issues in neurobiology and thus the subject of much speculation and experimentation. Understandably attention has focused on the contributions of neuroneuronal interactions in directing the distribution of developing afferent systems. One of the most influential ideas of this type to have emerged is that axons are chemically coded and, by a recognition process, are guided to and/or matched with their appropriate targets (Sperry, 1963). According to this hypothesis, the postsynaptic cell provides the primary source of extrinsic influence on the developing afferent as it enters the period of synaptogenesis. Somewhat in contrast to this model, an increasing body of data suggests that under some circumstances competitive or exclusionary interactions between developing afferents are responsible for the topography of terminal fields—a sort of blind, Darwinian competition between ingrowing fiber systems that determines their ultimate distribution. A number of excellent articles have reviewed the recognition model of afferent development (e.g., Gaze, 1974; Jacobson, 1976); the present chapter will therefore be concerned primarily with evidence relating to the competitive-interaction hypothesis. We shall also consider some of the mechanisms that might influence the outcome of such interactions.

In contrast to these purely neuronal accounts of how developing afferents achieve their ultimate distribution, several recent studies have called attention to the possibility that glial cells may play a modulatory role in this process. In view of the (still) indirect nature of the evidence, the subject will be reviewed only briefly; if nothing else, it should serve as a caveat to the purely "neuronal" hypotheses that will be our primary theme.

At the risk of being parochial, and except for a few excursions, the review will be restricted to mammalian brain and, for the most part, to only a few brain structures. Limiting the subject in this fashion permits a level of discussion that would not be possible in a more general review.

GARY LYNCH and REBECCA M. AKERS Department of Psychobiology, University of California, Irvine, CA 92717

Exclusionary (competitive) interactions between developing fiber systems

The idea that ingrowing fibers compete with one another for targets is an old one and has been extensively tested at the neuromuscular junction (for reviews see Edds, 1953; Fambrough, 1976). Attempts to demonstrate the operation of this principle in the brain have often centered around what might be called the *sprouting paradigm*. The rationale behind this strategy is that if fiber projections restrict the growth of their neighbors, then removal of one input should result in an expansion ("sprouting") of the terminal fields of the residual afferents. Examples of sprouting have been found throughout the neuroaxis of the developing mammalian brain (see, e.g., Lund and Lund, 1971; Lund, Cunningham, and Lund, 1973; Schneider, 1970; Devor and Schneider, 1975); in fact, entirely new fiber tracts have been generated in such experiments (Hicks and D'Amato, 1970; Leong and Lund, 1973).

A particularly apt example of the sprouting effect is provided by studies on the laminated afferents that innervate the granule cells of rat dentate gyrus (Figure 1). These fibers arrive in this dendritic field no later than the fourth or fifth postnatal day and quickly form segregated but contiguous terminal fields (Loy, Lynch, and Cotman, 1977). As the granule-cell dendrites extend themselves during subsequent development, this laminated pattern is retained, and the two inputs generate dense synaptic fields with essentially no overlap. What force causes these afferents to terminate in adjacent subregions of the dendrite and to maintain their isolation throughout the explosive synaptogenesis that occurs in the dentate gyrus during the postnatal period (Matthews, Cotman, and Lynch, 1976)? If it is some type of mutual exclusion (or competition), then removal of one input should cause an expansion of the remaining afferents. A number of experiments of this type have been carried out, and the results accord well with the competitive-interaction hypothesis. If the afferents to the outer 75% of the dendrites of the granule cells (i.e., the entorhinal fibers) are surgically eliminated up to 14 days after birth, then the commissural and associational fibers that innervate the inner dendritic field extend ("sprout") outwards and capture the vacated dendritic space (Figure 2; Lynch, Deadwyler, and Cotman, 1973; Lynch, Stanfield and Cotman, 1973; Zimmer, 1973, 1974). Recent autoradiographic tracing experiments (Gall and Lynch, 1978) have shown that in neonatal rats the commissural fibers extend throughout the denervated territory by 24 hours after a lesion of the entorhinal cortex. This extreme and rapid growth implies that the growth potential of these afferents is not fully utilized during normal development and is restricted by the presence of the entorhinal afferents.

An interesting problem posed by these results concerns the functional status of the terminal fields generated by sprouting fiber systems. An attempt was made, therefore, to establish whether the commissural fibers that reinnervate the middle and outer dendritic zones of the granule cells form functional contacts in those regions. Studies using laminar profile analysis have shown that the monosynaptic potentials recorded in the dentate gyrus of normal rats in response to stimulation of the commissural fibers are restricted to the inner molecular layer of the dentate gyrus—that is, to the zones in which these fibers establish synaptic contacts (see Deadwyler et al., 1975). In the case of the expanded projection,

FIGURE 1 These drawings summarize some of the anatomical features of the hippocampal formation discussed in the text. *Top left*: A horizontal section demonstrating the segregated and densely packed cell-body layers of the rat hippocampus (P, pyramidal-cell layer of the hippocampus proper; G, granule-cell layer of the dentate gyrus). *Top right*: A drawing of a comparable horizontal section that was well impregnated by the Golgi technique. This reveals the parallel orientation of the dendrites of the pyramidal cells. *Bottom left*: The distribution of entorhinal projections to the granule cells of the dentate gyrus, as shown by the Fink-Heimer method. These terminals (entor.) form a dense and very sharply defined layer, a feature characteristic of each of the major afferents of the dentate gyrus. The layer of granule-cell bodies runs horizontally across the bottom of the photomicrograph, and the clear zone immediately above it is innervated by the fibers of the commissural (comm.) and associational (assoc.) projections that originate in the pyramidal cells of the contralateral and ipsilateral hippocampus, respectively. (See Figure 2, top, for a photomicrograph of these projections.) The holes at the top of the figure are spaces occupied by vascular elements and mark the position of the hippocampal fissure, an obliterated cleft that separates the dentate gyrus from the hippocampus proper. *Bottom right*: Summary of the distribution of the three major afferents of the granule cells of the dentate gyrus. The inner 27% of the dendritic zone (i.e., the inner molecular layer) is occupied by the fibers and terminals originating from the pyramidal cells ipsilateral (associational) and contralateral (commissural) to the dentate gyrus. The remainder of the dendritic field (i.e., the middle and outer molecular layers) receives the great majority of its afferents from the ipsilateral entorhinal cortex. The two granule cells seen in the figure are camera lucida reconstructions from Golgi material. Note that the orientation and dimensions of the two bottom panels of this figure are essentially the same.

however, these potentials are readily recorded throughout the entire molecular layer, suggesting that the sprouted system has made functional contacts with its targets (Lynch, Deadwyler, and Cotman, 1973).

These results imply that the distribution of afferents is restricted by neighboring fiber projections and therefore that dendritic zones are not strictly specified to accept afferents from a single source. However, it is also possible that a weaker kind of specificity

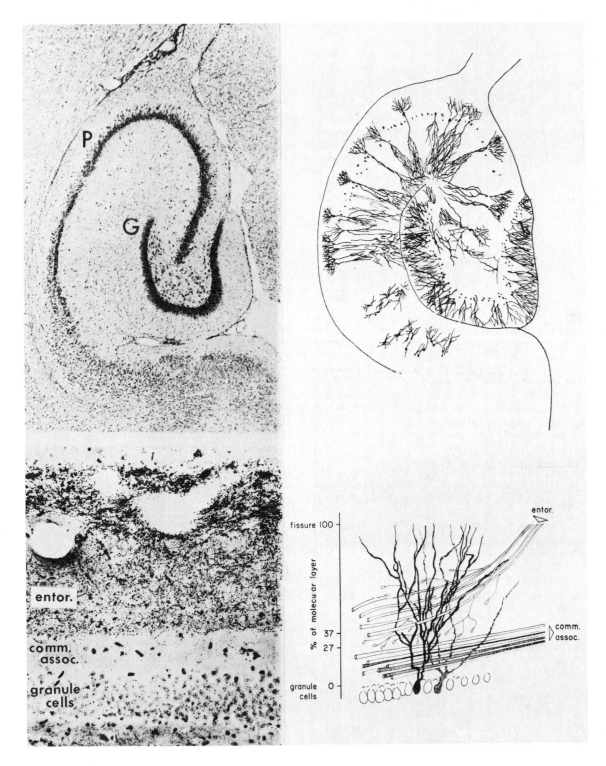

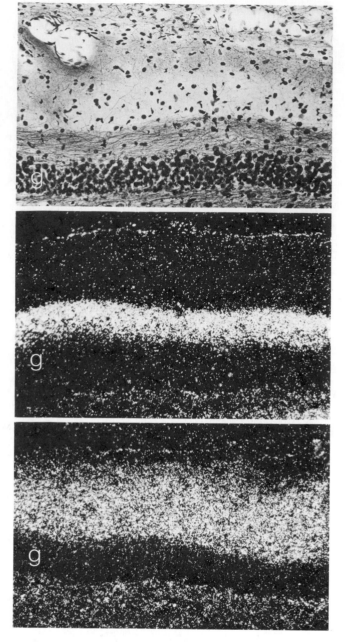

FIGURE 2   The distribution of the commissural projections to the normal (top two panels) and deafferented (bottom panel) dentate gyrus (g, granule-cell-body layer). The top panel is a photomicrograph of a Holmes-stained section and shows the axons of the commissural and associational projections; the blank region above these fibers is innervated by the entorhinal cortex (see Figure 1). The middle panel is a dark-field micrograph showing the terminals of the commissural system as revealed autoradiographically in a control rat. The bottom panel shows the results of an experiment in which this same procedure was used to identify the commissural terminal field in an animal that had received a complete lesion of the entorhinal cortex as a neonate. The commissural terminal field undergoes a marked expansion in the deafferented molecular layer.

exists, so that under normal conditions particular types of terminals are preferred and have a competitive advantage over ingrowing fibers from other sources. Thus sprouting studies (i.e., analysis of the growth of residual afferents following removal of a primary input) cannot provide information about possible interactions between competitive and specification mechanisms in controlling the distribution of developing axons. Furthermore, the sprouting experiments described above are open to the interpretation that deafferentation changes the target cells such that normally present specificities become lost, thereby opening the way for an expansion of residual inputs. In view of the dramatic anatomical adjustments that take place in deafferented neurons (e.g., loss of spines and generalized shrinkage), this possible disruption of normal matching mechanisms cannot be easily discounted. However, experiments of another type provide evidence that growing fiber projections can dramatically expand their terminal fields in target regions that have not been deafferented and that have a normal complement of afferents. In these studies (which will be discussed at greater length below) the target of a developing afferent is removed, and the distribution of that afferent in other brain areas is carefully measured. This work suggests that growing fibers compensate for the loss of their normal targets by developing extensive projections in other regions and, in some cases, by synapsing with cells they do not normally contact (Schneider, 1970; Lund and Lund, 1971; Devor and Schneider, 1975). Further studies have shown that in some cases aberrant development occurs at the expense of the normal inputs to these "secondary" regions; that is, the normally present afferents fail to gain the dendritic space they usually innervate. Thus target-removal experiments indicate that sprouting can occur in regions that have not been deafferented and that have their normal complement of projections. Sprouting phenomena under these conditions cannot result from a loss of specificity produced by deafferentation.

The experiments described in the preceding section reinforce the idea that competitive interactions play an important part in determining the distribution of afferents in the developing brain; but other work suggests that under certain circumstances some types of specificity help determine the distribution of fibers. Monoamine and cholinergic fiber projections have substantial regenerative properties, and recent evidence suggests that they may be biochemically coded to match their target cells. Implantation of the iris in the hypothalamus severs the ascending noradrenergic and dopaminergic projection systems; as these systems regenerate, they invade and terminate within the implant. The distribution pattern of these regenerating fibers is not random; it is, in fact, quite similar to the distribution of monoaminergic innervation of the iris in situ (for review see Svengaard, Björklund, and Stenevi, 1975). (The in situ innervation originates from the peripheral nervous system.) Furthermore, different target tissues will accept different monoaminergic inputs, suggesting that dopaminergic and noradrenergic fibers at least have biochemical markers that peripheral tissues can recognize.

Work with mutant (reeler) mice also suggests that some type of specific matching between afferents and targets occurs in cerebral cortex. In these animals the positions of the neurons in the cortex are reversed; that is, normally superficial cells are located deep in the cortex, and vice versa. Despite this inversion, callosal and thalamic afferents manage to distribute themselves to the appropriate cellular types. Furthermore, fibers from the misplaced neurons generate some of the normal intracortical circuits (Caviness, 1976). The afferents of the mutant cortex follow trajectories that are radically different from normal ones to reach their targets; this indicates that the matching mechanism between afferent fibers and cortical cells may be quite precise.

Is it possible that axodendritic affinities dictate organization in some circumstances, whereas competition is a dominant variable in others? One hypothesis that might be considered is that certain classes of axons possess specification mechanisms that are lacking in the remaining CNS fiber systems. It appears that monoamine systems have a number of characteristics that distinguish them from the majority of fiber systems in brain (e.g., they show vigorous regeneration); perhaps these systems are also highly specialized to form synapses only with certain types of neurons. Alternatively, classes of afferents might share specific matching properties. For example, the axons of pyramidal cells might have similar or identical surface chemistries quite distinct from those of interneurons or diffuse projection systems. In this case competition would dictate the distribution of fibers of the same class, while specificity would regulate the topographic arrangements in which different classes of fibers encounter each other. Finally, it is worth considering the possibility that specific affinities might exist between afferents and particular classes of cells but that there is no biochemical differentiation within the dendritic field of a particular type of neuron. According to this compromise hypothesis, interactions between fibers would govern afferent topographies within relatively homogeneous dendritic fields (as in hippocampus), while matching mechanisms would be influential in situations where axons are invading a diverse collection of cells (as in cerebral cortex).

In any event, several lines of evidence point to the conclusion that developing afferents compete with each other for dendritic space and that this provides a powerful, perhaps dominant, influence on the distribution of axonal and terminal-field topographies. If this is true, then two interrelated problems take on great significance for the understanding of brain development: First, what factors dictate the outcome of these competitive interactions? And second, what are the cellular processes by which competition is expressed? The following sections will deal with these problems.

Factors influencing the outcome of competitive interactions between developing afferents

ORIENTATION OF DEVELOPING AXONS Of the many factors that might be expected to influence the ultimate distribution of a terminal field, perhaps the most obvious is the orientation with which the parent fibers approach the target field. As will be seen, several examples of well-defined afferent topographies are readily explained by this factor. As in much of developmental anatomy, however, satisfactory experiments to test the operation of this variable are extremely difficult to perform; for example, one would like to explore the consequences of redirecting a fiber system for the ultimate distribution of its terminal fields. As it is, hypotheses about the processes leading to the organization of afferents must be inferred from the results of those processes, and this not uncommonly produces tautologies. Many ontogenetic theories thus resemble their evolutionary counterparts and suffer from the lack of reasonable experimental manipulations.

Several authors have proposed that the mutual orientation of retinal axons determines their distribution in the tectum (see Gaze, 1974; Lund and Lund, 1976). The trajectory of hippocampal fiber systems also suggests that the initial topography of their ingrowing axons plays a powerful role in shaping their terminal fields. The perforant-path fibers arise in the medial and lateral entorhinal cortices and swing around the edge of the lateral ventricle to enter the posterior aspect of the hippocampal formation. As they do so, their trajectory brings them into contact with the hippocampal fissure and the outer tips of the dendrites of the pyramidal and granule cells; it is in these distal regions that the entorhinal axons terminate. It appears, then, that the perforant path innervates the dendritic regions it first encounters during its invasion of the hippocampus. More detailed analysis provides additional evidence that initial orientation of the perforant path strongly influences the distribution of its terminal fields. The medial entorhinal fibers travel medially to those of the lateral cortex through the retrohippocampal area (Ramón y Cajal, 1909; Hjorth-Simonsen and Jeune, 1972a, b), a trajectory that brings them closer to the granule cells of the dentate gyrus than their lateral entorhinal counterparts (Figure 3). This could account for the fact that the medial entorhinal inputs gain the middle molecular layer, whereas the lateral cortical fibers are restricted to the outer zones (see Figure 2).

The commissural projections have a trajectory nearly opposite that of the entorhinal axons; that is, they penetrate the structure from its anterior and lateral aspects. They cross the pyramidal-cell layer near its lateral extension (CA3a) and then follow these cell layers medially and posteriorly. This trajectory causes them to encounter first the proximal aspects of the apical dendrites of the pyramidal cells, and these are the regions that become densely innervated by the commissural afferents. Again, it appears that the dendritic regions the developing afferent first contacts become the regions within which it terminates. The further growth of the commissural axons brings them into contact with the inner wing of dentate gyrus and, in particular, the inner molecular layer, the region in which they form their terminal fields. The outward expansion of the commissural

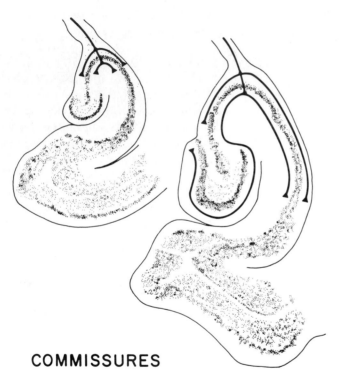

COMMISSURES

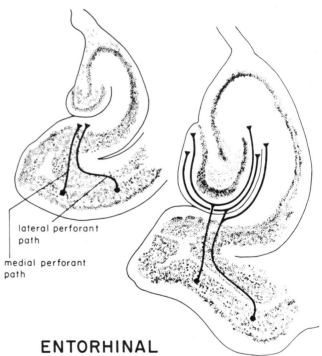

lateral perforant path

medial perforant path

ENTORHINAL

FIGURE 3 Schematic illustration emphasizing the possible contributions of the orientation of ingrowing commissural and entorhinal (perforant-path) fibers to their ultimate distribution within the hippocampus and dentate gyrus. The larger drawings are horizontal sections of the hippocampus and summarize the positions occupied by these two fiber systems as they are found in the adult. The smaller drawings are from neonatal rats and illustrate the suggested orientation of the commissures and perforant path as they invade the developing hippocampal formation. The trajectory of the commissural fibers as they enter the hippocampus brings them into immediate contact with the pyramidal-

cell-body layer, and it is proposed that they use this structural feature as a guide in their further extensions into the hippocampus. This course would carry them into the proximal dendritic regions of the pyramidal and granule cells; as shown by the larger drawings, these are the areas in which they ultimately terminate. The ingrowing perforant-path fibers, on the other hand, first encounter the hippocampal fissure, and as they follow it into the depths of the hippocampal formation, they are brought into contact with outer regions of the developing pyramidal-cell and granule-cell dendrites.

axons onto the distal dendrites of both pyramidal and granule cells is presumably checked by the entorhinal axons, which are growing inwards from the fissure (see above).

It must be appreciated that this analysis of the trajectories of the developing hippocampal afferents is based on the disposition of these projections in immature or adult animals. It is plausible to assume that this accurately reflects the situation when they first enter the hippocampal cell fields, but at present this assumption has not been validated by experimental evidence. Fortunately, the hippocampus also provides a case in which the afferents have assumed this topography before the target space has formed—namely, the development of the external (or infrapyramidal) wing of granule cells. The commissural and entorhinal fibers are present in the inner wing of granule cells by four days after birth (Loy, Lynch, and Cotman, 1977; Fricke and Cowan, 1977), at a time when the external blade of the dentate gyrus has only begun to be formed. The entorhinal and commissural projections form the same topographic distribution in the external as in the internal wing of granule cells, supporting the idea that the orientation of developing afferents as the target is being formed influences the distribution of the afferents within the target.

In sum, a reasonable case can be made that the afferents of the hippocampus innervate the first dendritic regions they encounter and thereafter are restricted to those regions by competitive interactions with projections terminating in contiguous zones.

TIMING   One factor that can be reasonably assumed to influence interactions between invading afferents is the timing of their arrival at the target sites and the maturational status of the dendrites they encounter there. Gottlieb and Cowan (1973) provided an interesting demonstration of this effect using the rat dentate gyrus system. Anatomical experiments have shown that the commissural axons arrive in the inner molecular layer during the first postnatal week, before the bulk of granule cells have formed. There are no comparable data on the arrival times of the associational fibers that share the inner molecular layer with the commissural fibers; but since they arise from the same collection of pyramidal cells as the commissural axons and are much closer to the granule cells, it is reasonable to assume that they arrive earlier. At the time of arrival of these projections, the inner wing of granule cells is much more complete than the outer wing. Using quantitative autoradiography, Gottlieb and Cowan found that the ratio of

associational to commissural terminals in the inner wing is 1:4 in the adult rat; in the outer wing the ratio is closer to 1:1. This can be interpreted as follows: the associational fibers, with their presumed earlier arrival time, take up most of the dendritic space that is available and developing in the inner wing of the granule cells; but the two afferents are both present while the outer wing of cells is still forming, and hence they gain roughly the same number of synaptic connections.

A second illustration of the possible significance of timing in determining the distribution of developing afferents can be found in the arrangement of basket-cell contacts on the somata of the granule cells. Ramón y Cajal (1909) noted that the outermost granule cells are more densely innervated by the basket cells than the inner neurons (Figure 4), and this has been recently confirmed by electron microscopy (Lee and Lynch, 1978). This pattern of innervation may reflect the unusual sequence and time course of the formation of the stratum granulosum. The granule cells are added to the stratum granulosum in an outside-in gradient; that is, the outermost cells are formed first and arrive in position before the innermost neurons. The interneurons, presumably including those that innervate the somata of these neurons, are formed prenatally, well in advance of the great majority of the granule cells (Angevine, 1975; Bayer and Altman, 1977). Consequently it can be anticipated that the axons of the interneurons will be in place as

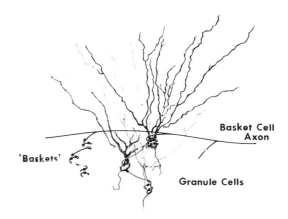

FIGURE 4   Schematic illustration of the organization of the basket complexes of the granule cells of the rat dentate gyrus. The neurons are camera lucida drawings from Golgi-impregnated material, and the distribution of the axon and its terminals is based on observations reported by Ramón y Cajal and on electron-microscopic material discussed in the text. Note the top-to-bottom change in the density of terminals on the cell bodies.

the granule cells are added over a three-week postnatal period. The oldest and most superficial granule cells therefore experience a period of synaptogenesis that begins much earlier and, in all likelihood, lasts much longer than that experienced by younger and deeper neurons. This would provide a reasonable explanation for the unequal distribution of the basket complexes across the depth of the granule-cell layer and illustrates the importance of time of arrival of afferent and target in determining the topography of a particular terminal population.

RESIDUAL GROWTH CAPACITY   Unused growth capacity is potentially a variable of great importance in determining the size and shape of axonal arborizations. Axons might be restricted to certain dendritic zones simply because they have exhausted their capacity to innervate new areas, or—more likely—the vigor with which fibers invade territory might depend on the extent to which they have begun to approach their genetic limitations for the synthesis of new branches and endings. A variable of this sort might play a major part in dictating the outcome of competitive interactions in brain in which relatively "committed" and relatively "uncommitted" projection systems come into contact.

There have been a number of attempts to measure the degree to which the extent of terminal field generated by an afferent at a particular site is influenced by the density of its connections elsewhere in brain. Schneider (1970) found that removal of one of the primary targets of the optic tract—the optic tectum— resulted in the generation by that fiber system of extensive terminal fields in areas where it typically provided few if any inputs (e.g., medial geniculate). He also found that projections that had lost targets extended branches into the contralateral tectum and captured considerable space, apparently at the expense of the fibers that normally innervate that region (see also Lund and Lund, 1971). A similar result was obtained in the hippocampus following destruction of 85% of the granule-cell population of the dentate gyrus by postnatal X-irradiation. This procedure has the advantage of not causing damage to the ingrowing afferents, thereby obviating complexities associated with the possibility that the systems under study are undergoing regeneration as well as normal developmental growth. As described above, the major input to the hippocampus is composed of fibers from the entorhinal cortex, and these terminate primarily on the granule cells and, to a lesser degree, on the pyramidal neurons. Removal of the granule cells therefore creates a situation in which

the primary afferent of the hippocampus develops in the absence of most of its normal target cells. Under these conditions the perforant-path axons invade dendritic territories they never reach under normal conditions (Laurberg and Hjorth-Simonsen, 1977). Furthermore, they expand their area of termination in those pyramidal-cell dendritic trees in which they are normally restricted to the outermost dendritic segments (Gerbrandt et al., 1978).

These results—using different brain systems, different manipulations, and different species—indicate that the success experienced by fiber systems in their competition is strongly influenced by the extent to which they have formed or are in the process of forming connections elsewhere. The obvious explanation of these findings is that the capacity of axons to generate collaterals and terminals is fixed and that the amount of territory gained at one site depends on the fraction of this capacity already committed.

USAGE   Several lines of evidence suggest that competition for postsynaptic space may be influenced by the relative functional states of the competing afferent fibers. This relationship has been demonstrated most clearly in the visual system of developing cats and monkeys. In these animals the visual cortex is composed of ocular-dominance columns, narrow strips of cortex that respond selectively to stimulation of a particular eye (Hubel and Wiesel, 1968). The thalamocortical projections to the visual cortex reflect this pattern of alternating left- and right-eye dominance; laminae of the lateral geniculate nucleus responsive to stimulation of one eye project to the cortex in a discontinuous fashion, and the resulting gaps in the terminal field are filled in by projections related to the other eye (Hubel and Wiesel, 1972; LeVay, Hubel, and Wiesel, 1974). If an animal is monocularly deprived of visual stimulation during the first few months of life, cortical cells become largely unresponsive to stimulation of the deprived eye (Wiesel and Hubel, 1965). Cortical ocular-dominance columns related to the deprived eye are reduced in size, while adjacent columns related to the normal eye are larger than those found in control animals. Anatomical evidence suggests that the terminal fields of lateral geniculate neurons responsive to the normal eye are expanded as a result of monocular deprivation and are actually redistributed to cortical cells that normally receive projections from the deprived eye (Hubel, Wiesel, and LeVay, 1975). (The effects of monocular deprivation are much more pronounced than those resulting from binocular deprivation, which suggests that the major deficit is not related so much to deprivation per se as to an alteration in competitive interactions between projections related to the two eyes: see Wiesel and Hubel, 1965.)

These experiments suggest that the success of a particular afferent in capturing synaptic space may be strongly influenced by its functional status during critical developmental periods. So far such demonstrations have been limited to competitive interactions between afferents arising from the same source; it remains to be seen whether usage may influence competition between different classes of afferent fibers.

Mechanisms by which competitive interactions might be achieved

"Competition" is a useful word to describe a set of interactions between afferents, but the observations so far discussed provide little insight into what this process actually is. What is needed is a more mechanistic, more cellular formulation of how developing afferents exclude one another from dendritic territory. It may be that the key step governing afferent topographies will be found in the postsynaptic cells; more specifically, a limited number of target sites may be produced, and if these become committed to one input or are filled as they become available, fibers arriving subsequently may find no place to terminate. This hypothesis implies that dendrites are genetically programmed to produce a fixed number of target sites, but this is not an easy implication to test. Quantitative electron-microscopic studies have shown that reinnervation of partially deafferented sites in the brain produces about the same density of synapses as are normally found at such sites (Raisman and Field, 1973; Matthews, Cotman, and Lynch, 1976); thus replacing one afferent with another does not change synaptic density. This finding provides indirect evidence that the target cells generate a given number of receptive sites and that the presynaptic elements simply grow until these sites are occupied.

Competition between afferents might also be achieved by a more direct mechanism—such as a direct inhibitory action of axons upon each other's growth. There is some evidence that negative neurotrophisms of this type do occur under some circumstances. For example, Aguilar et al. (1971) found that blocking axoplasmic transport in one set of peripheral fibers in the salamander resulted in an invasion of neighboring axons into the target territory of the blocked inputs. They suggest that nerves are constantly transporting and releasing materials that suppress their neighbors' growth. Tissue-culture experiments have also provided examples in which developing axons exert an exclusionary effect on the growth of nearby fibers (Dunn, 1971). Mechanisms of these types could clearly account for much of the competition observed in developing mammalian brain.

Nonneural influences on the development of afferent topographies

The above sections have dealt primarily with the possible role of axoaxonal interactions in the distribution of ingrowing fiber systems. We have also mentioned the hypothesis that the organizing principle lies in a specialized relationship between the developing axon and its dendritic targets. In both accounts, the extrinsic influences that regulate the development of afferent topographies arise from neural elements. The possibility that nonneural influences—for example, from glia cells—might participate in the process of organizing axonal and terminal fields has received much less attention. This is perhaps unfortunate since a growing body of literature has implicated a role for various types of glia in nearly every stage of development (e.g., Rakic, 1971a,b); it would hardly be surprising, then, if they were found to guide some aspects of axonal growth. In this section we shall very briefly consider recent evidence implying that glia have a modulatory role in axonal growth and arborization, and we shall mention some of the problems associated with testing for this in specific developmental situations.

It has frequently been observed that the behavior of neurons in culture is greatly influenced by the presence of glial cells; for example, the survival of dissociated sympathetic ganglion cells in the absence of nerve growth factor (NGF) requires the presence of glial cells. Several lines of eivdence indicate that the supportive function of glial cells is due to their production of NGF or some very similar material (Varon, 1975). Similarly, embryonic neurons from chick brains survive much better and undergo much more rapid differentiation when layered on top of "astroblasts" than when plated over other types of cells (Luduena, 1973; Sensenbrenner and Mandel, 1974). Experiments using well-studied tumor cell lines have also demonstrated that glial cells stimulate neurite extension from neurons. C-6 glioma cells release a material into the culture medium that induces differentiation of neuroblastoma cells (Monard et al., 1973); but subsequent experiments have pretty well eliminated the possibility that this substance is NGF (Monard et al., 1975).

Tissue-culture experiments using preparations

somewhat closer to normal developing tissue have also provided evidence linking glial cells to axonal growth. In explants taken from rodent spinal cord, astroglia have been observed to proliferate and migrate outwards, forming thin processes that cover much of the culture dish. Bundles of axons then emerge from the explant and establish close contacts with the sheets of astrocytic processes (Guillery, Sobkowicz, and Scott, 1970; Grainger and James, 1974); furthermore, glial processes are sometimes found to encircle the growth cones of the embryonic axons. On the basis of these results, it has been argued that glial cells form a favorable substratum for growth-cone adhesion and in this way promote and direct fiber growth.

A plausible, although still very indirect, case can thus be made for the hypothesis that axonal growth is regulated under many circumstances by glial cells. But is this also true of the mammalian brain, and, if so, at what points in development? One of the primary difficulties in evaluating this thesis is a lack of precise data on the arrival time and maturational status of various types of glial cells as afferents invade their targets and embark upon synaptogenesis. It is generally agreed that the bulk of the glial population is added postnatally; but this should not be taken to mean that glia are not present and active during even the earliest stages of neuronal development. Astrocytes are clearly evident in the molecular layer of the dentate gyrus of a five-day-old rat, at the time when the arriving afferents of these regions can first be detected.

Astroglia, then, may be situated in the right place and time to influence synaptogenesis, and from the tissue-culture experiments it appears that they influence axonal growth. In sum, the data reinforce the possibility that the distribution of terminal populations is not exclusively regulated by neuroneuronal interactions.

Comment

Theories about the factors that govern the development of neuronal connections are drawn from a diverse variety of preparations and methodologies; and hypotheses based on data from particular experimental arrangements understandably stress the developmental principles that arrangement is best suited to demonstrate. CNS structures such as the hippocampus provide opportunities to test for interactions between diverse populations of afferents that arrive in temporal and spatial proximity; and experiments in this area have indicated that these projections strongly influence each other with respect to their distribution on receptive cells. Tissue-culture studies, in which precise connnections are generally lost but in which cell-cell communication is apparent, have suggested an important role for the glial cells in directing the growth of afferent fibers. Put simply, developmental theories reflect the literatures from which they are evolved, and this should be borne in mind when considering the various models we have discussed.

With regard to the mammalian brain and the competition hypothesis, progress is contingent upon further advances in two areas: (1) detailed description of the development of afferents (and targets) that have been chosen for analysis; and (2) analysis of the cellular factors that mediate interactions between ingrowing fiber systems.

With few exceptions, developmental studies on particular brain regions have not been conducted with the express purpose of identifying variables that might govern the ultimate distributions of afferents. Consequently, information that could be important in evaluating hypotheses such as competition (e.g., the birth dates of the cells of origin, the trajectories followed by their growing axons, the relationship of these to glia and to axons arising from different sources) is usually not available. Normative data of this type about the development of specific connections would also allow stronger interpretations of the various experimental manipulations that have been conducted in developing brains (e.g., removal of particular afferents or target cells). The continuing development of new histological techniques and the increasingly routine use of some older ones make it likely that real progress will be made in this area.

Advances in the understanding of the cellular factors mediating interactions between developing afferents is more problematical. In addition to the absence of information about the site of the competition (axoaxonic, axodendritic; glial involvement?), almost nothing is known of the chemistries involved. It is likely that culture experiments will prove more useful than in vivo studies in resolving these types of questions (see, e.g., Dunn, 1971).

Finally, different brain structures follow very different developmental programs, and what might be a satisfactory description of the forces dictating afferent distribution for one region may prove inadequate elsewhere. We have made an effort to illustrate how different sequences or rates of development might influence the outcome of competitive interactions, but it is also possible that the significance of afferent competition in determining the final state might vary from system to system.

For the above reasons it is premature to seriously advocate universal explanations for the organization of afferent fields in mammalian brain; at this time we must be satisfied with demonstrating the existence of potent developmental forces and attempting to identify the circumstances under which they occur.

REFERENCES

AGUILAR, C. E., M. A. BISBY, E. COOPER, and J. DIAMOND, 1971. Evidence that axoplasmic transport of trophic factors is involved in the regulation of peripheral nerve fields in salamanders, *J. Physiol.* 234:449–464.

ANGEVINE, J. B., 1975. Development of the hippocampal region. In *The Hippocampus*, vol. 1, R. Isaacson and K. Pribram, eds. New York: Plenum Press, pp. 61–94.

BAYER, S. A., and J. ALTMAN, 1977. Radiation-induced interference with postnatal hippocampal cytogenesis in rats and its long-term effects on the acquisition of neurons and glia. *J. Comp. Neurol.* 163:1–20.

CAVINESS, V. W., 1976. Reeler mutant mice and laminar distribution of afferents in the neocortex. *Exp. Brain Res. Suppl.* 1:267–274.

DEADWYLER, S., J. R. WEST, C. W. COTMAN, and G. LYNCH, 1975. A neurophysiological analysis of the commissural projections to the dentate gyrus of the rat. *J. Neurophysiol.* 38:167–184.

DEVOR, M., and C. E. SCHNEIDER, 1975. Neuroanatomical plasticity: The principle of conservation of total axonal arborization. In *Aspects of Neuronal Plasticity/Plasticite Nerveuse, Inserm*, vol. 43, F. Vital-Demand and M. Jeaunerod, eds. pp. 191–200.

DUNN, G. A., 1971. Mutual contact inhibition of extension of chick sensory nerve fibers *in vitro. J. Comp. Neurol.* 143:491–508.

EDDS, M. V., JR., 1953. Collateral nerve regeneration. *Q. Rev. Biol.* 28:260–276.

FAMBROUGH, D., 1976. Specificity of nerve-muscle interactions. In *Neuronal Recognition*, S. Barondes, ed. New York: Plenum Press, pp. 25–67.

FRICKE, R., and W. M. COWAN, 1977. An autoradiographic study of the development of the entorhinal and commissural afferents to dentate gyrus of the rat. *J. Comp. Neurol.* 173:231–250.

GALL, C., and G. LYNCH, 1978. Rapid axon sprouting in the neonatal rat hippocampus. *Brain Res.* 153:357–362.

GAZE, R. M., 1974. Neuronal specificity. *Br. Med. Bull.* 30:116.

GERBRANDT, L. K., G. ROSE, R. WHEELER, and G. LYNCH, 1978. Distribution of the perforant path following selective elimination of granule cells. *Exp. Neurol.* 62:122–132.

GOTTLIEB, D. E., and W. M. COWAN, 1973. Autoradiographic studies of the commissural and ipsilateral association connections of the hippocampus and dentate gyrus of the rat: The commissural connections. *J. Comp. Neurol.* 149:393–422.

GRAINGER, F., and D. W. JAMES, 1974. Association of glial cells with the terminal parts of neurite bundles extending from chick spinal-cord *in vitro. Z. Zellforsch.* 108:93–104.

GUILLERY, R. W., H. M. SOBKOWICZ, and G. L. SCOTT, 1970. Relationships between glial and neuronal elements in the development of long term cultures of the spinal cord of the fetal mouse. *J. Comp. Neurol.* 140:134.

HICKS, S., and C. D'AMATO, 1970. Moto-sensory and visual behavior after hemispherectomy in newborn and mature rats. *Exp. Neurol.* 29:416–438.

HJORTH-SIMONSEN, A. M., and B. JEUNE, 1972a. Projection of the lateral part of the entorhinal area to the hippocampus and fascia dentate. *J. Comp. Neurol.* 146:219–232.

HJORTH-SIMONSEN, A., and B. JEUNE, 1972b. Origin and termination of the hippocampal perforant path in the rat studied by silver impregnation. *J. Comp. Neurol.* 144:215–232.

HUBEL, D. H., and T. N. WIESEL, 1968. Receptive fields and functional architecture of the monkey striate cortex. *J. Physiol.* 195:215.

HUBEL, D. H., and T. N. WIESEL, 1972. Laminar and columnar distribution of geniculocortical fibers in the macaque monkey. *J. Comp. Neurol.* 146:421–450.

HUBEL, D. N., T. N. WIESEL, and S. LeVAY, 1975. Functional architecture of area 17 in normal and monocularly deprived macaque monkeys. *Cold Spring Harbor Symp. Quant. Biol.* 40:581–589.

JACOBSON, M., 1976. Neuronal recognition in the retinotectal system. In *Neuronal Recognition*, J. Barondes, ed. New York: Plenum Press, pp. 3–24.

LAURBERG, S., and A. HJORTH-SIMONSEN, 1977. Growing central axons deprived of normal target neurones by neonatal X-ray irradiation still terminate in a precisely laminated fashion. *Nature* 261:158–160.

LEE, K. S., and G. LYNCH, 1978. The distribution of axosomatic synapses in the normal and x-irradiated dentate gyrus. American Association of Anatomists 91st Meeting.

LEONG, S. K., and R. D. LUND, 1973. Anomalous bilateral corticofugal pathways in albino rats after neonatal lesions. *Brain Res.* 62:218–221.

LeVAY, S., D. H. HUBEL, and T. N. WIESEL, 1974. The pattern of ocular dominance columns in macaque visual cortex revealed by a reduced silver stain. *J. Comp. Neurol.* 159:559–576.

LOY, R., G. LYNCH, and C. COTMAN, 1977. Development of afferent lamination in the fascia dentata of the rat. *Brain Res.* 121:229–243.

LUDUENA, M. A., 1973. Nerve cell differentiation *in vitro. Dev. Biol.* 33:268–284.

LUND, R. D., T. S. CUNNINGHAM, and J. W. LUND, 1973. Modified optic projections after unilateral eye removal in young rats. *Brain Behav. Evol.* 8:51–72.

LUND, R. D., and J. S. LUND, 1971. Synaptic adjustments after deafferentation of the superior colliculus of the rat. *Science* 171:804–807.

LUND, R. D., and J. S. LUND, 1976. Plasticity in the developing visual system: The effects of retinal lesions made in young rats. *J. Comp. Neurol.* 1969:133–154.

LYNCH, G., S. DEADWYLER, and C. W. COTMAN, 1973. Postlesion axonal growth produces permanent functional connections. *Science* 180:1364–1366.

LYNCH, G., B. STANFIELD, and C. W. COTMAN, 1973. Developmental differences in post-lesion axonal growth in the hippocampus. *Brain Res.* 59:155–168.

MATTHEWS, D. A., C. W. COTMAN, and G. LYNCH, 1976. An

electron microscopic study of lesion-induced synaptogenesis in the dentate gyrus of the adult rat. II. Reappearance of morphologically normal synaptic contacts. *Brain. Res.* 115:23–41.

McWILLIAMS, R., and G. LYNCH, 1978. Terminal proliferation and synaptogenesis following partial deafferentation: The reinnervation of the inner molecular layer of the dentate gyrus following removal of its commissural afferents. *J. Comp. Neurol.* 180:581–615.

MONARD, D., F. SOLOMON, M. RENTSCH, and R. GYSIN, 1973. Glia-induced morphological differentation in neuroblastoma cells. *Proc. Natl. Acad. Sci. USA* 70:1894–1897.

MONARD, D., K. STOCKEL, R. GOODMAN, and H. THOENEN, 1975. Distinction between nerve growth factor and glial factor. *Nature* 258:444–445.

RAKIC, P., 1971a. Guidance of neurons migrating to the fetal monkey cortex. *Brain Res.* 33:471–476.

RAKIC, P., 1971b. Neuron-glia relationship during granule cell migration in developing cerebellar cortex: A Golgi and electron microscopic study. *J. Comp. Neurol.* 141:283–312.

RAMÓN Y CAJAL, S., 1909. *Histologie du système nerveux de l'homme et des vertébrés*, vol. 2. Paris: Maloine.

RAISMAN, G., and P. A. FIELD, 1973. A quantitative investigation of the development of collateral regeneration after partial deafferentation of the septal nuclei. *Brain Res.* 50:241.

SCHNEIDER, G. E., 1970. Mechanisms of functional recovery following lesions of visual cortex or superior colliculus in neonate and adult hamsters. *Brain Behav. Evol.* 3:295–323.

SENSENBRENNER, M., and P. MANDEL, 1974. Behaviour of neuroblasts in the presence of glial cells, fibroblasts and meningeal cells in culture. *Exp. Cell Res.* 87:159–167.

SPERRY, R. W., 1963. Chemoaffinity in the orderly growth of nerve fiber patterns and connections. *Proc. Natl. Acad. Sci. USA* 50:703–710.

SVENDGAARD, N. A., A. BJÖRKLUND, and U. STENEVI, 1975. Regenerative properties of central noradrenaline, dopamine, and indoleamine neurones in adult rat brain using transplants of irides as target. *Adv. Anat. Embryol. Cell Biol.* 51(4):1–177.

VARON, S., 1975. Neurons and glia in neural cultures. *Exp. Neurol.* 48:93–134.

WIESEL, T. N., and D. N. HUBEL, 1965. Comparison of the effects of unilateral and bilateral eye closure on cortical unit responses in kittens. *J. Neurophysiol.* 28:1029–1040.

ZIMMER, J., 1973. Extended commissural and ipsilateral projections in postnatally de-entorhinated hippocampus and fascia dentata demonstrated in rats by silver impregnation. *Brain Res.* 64:293–311.

ZIMMER, J., 1974. Proximity as a factor in the regulation of aberrant growth in post-natally deafferented fascia dentate. *Brain Res.* 72:137–142.

58 Long-Term Hormonal Modulation of Neuronal Structure and Function

R. A. GORSKI

ABSTRACT That sex differences exist in brain function is illustrated particularly well in the rat by the regulation of pituitary secretory activity and female receptive behavior. These sex differences in neural function are established by the steroid-hormone environment during a specific stage of development which, in the rat, encompasses the perinatal period. Although the rat is frequently used as the experimental animal model, the sexual differentiation of the brain is not limited to this species or to the regulation of the pituitary gland or of sexual behavior. Although suggested mechanisms for this permanent or "organizing" action of gonadal steroids on the developing brain include an alteration in steroid-receptor interactions, or neurotransmitter function, the evidence reviewed here demonstrates that exposure to gonadal steroids at an appropriate stage in development produces morphological distinctions in the brain that range from subtle differences in the ultrastructural localization of dendritic terminals to gross differences visible to the naked eye. Although gonadal hormones may act during development, or perhaps under in vitro conditions, in a permissive way, the permanent morphological and functional consequences of early hormone exposure indicate that the hormonal environment plays an important, if not critical, role in determining neuronal differentiation, presumably by means of an alteration in neuronal genomic expression.

THE PROCESS of sexual differentiation of the brain is one of the more dramatic examples of the physiological modification of neuronal gene expression. Although this concept had its beginnings in purely functional terms, recent experimental evidence has begun to provide insight into a possible molecular basis for the permanent alterations in brain function induced by the hormone environment during development. Because of the past focus on function, and also because of the rather specific neuroendocrine nature of these functions, this discussion will first review and document at a general level the process of sexual differentiation of the brain. Possible mechanisms of differentiation will then be considered, particularly from the point of view of morphogenesis within the hypothalamus.

Sex differences in brain function

Although a detailed review of current concepts of neuroendocrinology would not be appropriate here, the understanding of a few fundamental principles is important to place the following experimental results in appropriate perspective. Although sexual differentiation of a number of functions has been documented or proposed, two examples will suffice for illustration: one is in the realm of animal behavior; the other concerns the pattern of gonadotropin secretion by the pituitary gland. With respect to the latter, it is well recognized that certain neurons of the hypothalamus terminate not in synapses or on muscles, but on the capillaries of the hypophyseal portal system. These nerves manufacture and release into the portal vessels small peptides that reach the pituitary gland and modify its synthetic and secretory activities (Harris, 1955; Szentágothai et al., 1968; Brawer and van Houten, 1976).

One such peptide, which regulates the secretion of hypophyseal luteinizing hormone (LH), is called luteinizing-hormone-releasing hormone (LH-RH) (Schally and Coy, 1977). This substance is also commonly called gonadotropin-releasing hormone (GnRH), since it also appears to bring about the release of the other hypophyseal gonadotropin, follicle-stimulating hormone. In the female rat (as in the females of many other species), a particular pattern of LH-RH secretion plays a critical role in ovulation. In fact, it is generally believed that rising plasma titers of estrogen, or perhaps the attainment of some threshold level, triggers neural processes that lead to an abrupt discharge of LH-RH and, subsequently, a tremendous surge of LH, which causes the rupture of mature ovarian follicles—that is, ovulation (Schwartz, 1973; Gorski, Mennin, and Kubo, 1975). In the rat, this surge of LH is followed by an increase in progesterone secretion and a few hours later, by

R. A. GORSKI Department of Anatomy and Brain Research Institute, UCLA School of Medicine, Los Angeles, CA 90024

sexual receptivity. Such dramatic neuroendocrine events are not characteristic of the intact male; moreover, even if the adult male is gonadectomized and primed with exogenous gonadal hormones at dosages very effective in the female, there is no surge of LH (Jackson, 1973; Harlan and Gorski, unpublished observations). Thus the ability of the hypothalamohypophyseal axis to support a surge of LH-RH (which normally occurs cyclically, every four or five days) is a sex characteristic of the female rat. Given this functional sexual difference, it is logical to ask, How is ovulation normally regulated in the female? or, Where might this sex difference reside?

Numerous studies of the neural regulation of ovulation in the normal adult female rat have provided evidence for a rather complex involvement of hypothalamic and extrahypothalamic systems in gonadal hormone feedback action and in ovulation (Figure 1). Although the preoptic area (POA) appears to play an important role in ovulation (Everett, 1964; Gorski, 1968a, 1971), the neural substrate involved in this one neuroendocrine event is diffuse and appears to be strongly dominated by limbic components (see Gorski, 1974a; Ellendorff, 1976). Direct retinohy-

pothalamic input may also be particularly important (Moore and Eichler, 1976). In addition, the aminergic systems have been implicated in this neuroendocrine process (Fuxe et al., 1976; Kordon et al., 1976; Kalra, 1976). Thus, to state simply that there is a sex difference in the complex neural regulation of ovulation hardly elucidates the question of the possible modification of neuronal gene expression. This problem must be approached with a much sharper focus.

With respect to the second example of functional sex differences in the brain, the regulation of sexual behavior in the female rat, once again much of the available experimental data serve to describe a phenomenon rather than to elucidate mechanisms. Nevertheless, evidence that the control system for this behavior undergoes sexual differentiation in the rat is convincing, and therefore it can serve as a useful model system. Although there are several components to sexual behavior, we shall focus on the fact that when the sexually receptive female is mounted by a male she displays a characteristic arching of the back, the lordosis reflex. Although it also appears to be regulated by a complex neural substrate (Gorski, 1976), lordosis behavior is a reliable and quantifiable

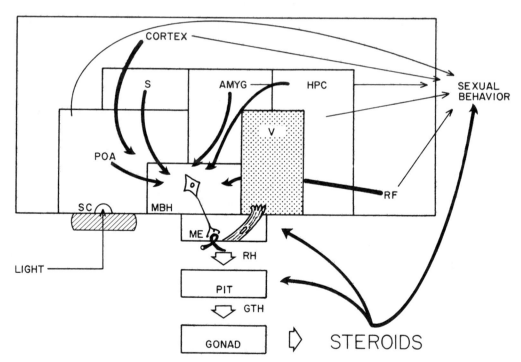

FIGURE 1 Highly schematic representation of the neural substrate that regulates hypophyseal activity (heavy arrows) and sexual behavior (thin arrows). The arrows signify functional influences and not neuroanatomical pathways. Based on experimental data reviewed in Gorski (1974a,b, 1976) and Ellendorff (1976). The cell passing from the median eminence (ME) to the ventricular system (V) represents the

ependymal tanacytes, which may play a role in neuroendocrine processes (Knigge et al., 1976). *Abbreviations*: Amyg, amygdala; GTH, gonadotropin; HPC, hippocampus; MBH, medial basal hypothalamus; PIT, pituitary; POA, preoptic area; RF, reticular formation; RH, releasing hormone; S, septum; SC, suprachiasmatic nucleus.

hormone-dependent index of sexual receptivity in the female (Gorski, 1974b). The intact adult male, even when he is gonadectomized and primed with a physiological regime of ovarian hormones adequate to facilitate lordosis behavior in the female, only rarely exhibits lordosis (see Gorski, 1974b). Thus there is a fundamental sex difference in the ability of the rat to display lordosis behavior in response to steroid-hormone priming within the physiological range.

Gonadal steroids as organizers of brain function

Although the existence of sex differences in these neuroendocrine functions of the brain might be assumed to be a natural consequence of differential neuronal gene expression in males and females, this is not the case. Rather, it has been extensively documented that the particular functional capacity of the adult brain depends on the steroid-hormone environment during a particular period of development—the period of sexual differentiation (see Gorski, 1971, 1974b; Gorski, Harlan, and Christensen, 1977). In the rat, the two functional systems we have considered as examples actually are organized shortly after birth; but other sexually dimorphic functions in the rat, and the entire process in other species, may take place prenatally. The basic evidence for the statement that hormones determine the functional capacity of the brain is dramatic and conclusive and is summarized in Figure 2. Although the dose of hormone and the age of the animal at hormonal exposure can alter the outcome (Gorski, 1968b; Harlan and Gorski, 1977), in general, when a neonatal female rat is exposed to exogenous gonadal steroids, either testosterone or estrogen, by a single injection (Barraclough, 1961; Gorski, 1963) or by direct application of the hormone to certain areas of the brain (Wagner, Erwin, and Critchlow, 1966; Nadler, 1968; Sutherland and Gorski, 1972; Hayashi and Gorski, 1974), that genetic female, when adult, does not ex-hibit lordosis behavior, nor can she secrete the surge of LH necessary for ovulation. She is, in fact, sterile. These are permanent deficits in neuroendocrine function. Similarly, a newborn male rat castrated within the first three days of postnatal life (the precise age is strain-specific), will, when adult and primed with exogenous steroids, display levels of lordosis behavior equivalent to those shown by the normal female (Grady, Phoenix, and Young, 1965; see also Gorski, 1974b). Moreover, he will respond to steroid feedback influences with a surge of LH, as judged by the luteinization of ovarian grafts (Pfeiffer, 1936; Gorski, 1971).

Observations of this nature support the concept originally proposed by Phoenix et al. (1959) that steroid hormones can have either organizational or activational effects on the brain, depending on the state of its development. In the adult, steroid hormones exert profound but transitory effects; conceptually, steroids activate or inhibit the function of existing neural circuits. During development, however, the same steroids have the capacity to influence the establishment (at least in functional terms) of the very neural circuits that will regulate neuroendocrine function in the adult. It is obvious from our two examples that neuronal genomic influences appear to be masked by the hormone environment.

It is important to stress that this concept of the sexual differentiation of the brain is not limited to the rat or to the expression of lordosis behavior or the cyclic surge of LH-RH. In addition to these brain functions, the regulation of masculine sexual behavior (Reinisch, 1974; Gorski, Harlan, and Christensen, 1977), food intake and body weight (Wade, 1972; Tarttelin, Shryne, and Gorski, 1975; Nance and Gorski, 1975), aggressive behavior (see Reinisch, 1974; Quadagno, Briscoe, and Quadagno, 1977), territorial marking (Turner, 1975), some aspects of maternal behavior (see Quadagno, Briscoe, and Quadagno, 1977), urination posturing (Beach, 1975), social and play behavior (Quadagno et al., 1972; Goy and Resko,

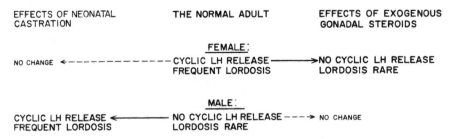

FIGURE 2 Schematic representation of the change from the normal neuroendocrine function of the adult rat produced by either neonatal castration or the perinatal injection of gonadal steroids.

1972), learning performance (Scouten, Grotelueschen, and Beatty, 1975; Stewart, Skvarenina, and Potter, 1975; see also Reinisch, 1974; Quadagno, Briscoe, and Quadagno, 1977), and even possibly gender identity (Money and Ehrhardt, 1972; Reinisch, 1974; Ehrhardt, 1975) may be subject to an organizing influence of gonadal steroids among the following mammalian species: rat, mouse, guinea pig, gerbil, hamster, ferret, monkey, and human. Moreover, the genetic male develops certain functional characteristics normally associated with the female if he is castrated before the period of sexual differentiation, whereas gonadectomy of the perinatal female is essentially without effect (see Figure 2); this suggests that the mammalian brain might be inherently female. At the very minimum, one is forced to conclude that the presence of testicular secretions (presumably testosterone) is essential to the normal functional development of the brain in the male.

Two additional questions must be discussed before the possible mechanisms of steroid-induced alteration in functional neuronal development can be considered: (1) Where in the brain does androgen act perinatally? (2) In general terms, what is the nature of that action? Since a complex neural substrate is apparently involved in the regulation of both ovulation and sexual receptivity—the two functions chosen as illustrative models—it is difficult to state definitively at which loci in these systems steroids act during development or in the adult. However, this question of the site(s) of action is critical, particularly for the application of sophisticated neurochemical, neuroanatomical, or molecular neurobiological techniques that will be required to establish the mechanisms involved. Although it has been suggested that steroids act perinatally in the mesencephalon (Gorski, 1976), or possibly in components of the limbic system (Kawakami and Terasawa, 1972), the localization of hormonal uptake systems in the adult and neonatal animal (Pfaff and Keiner, 1973; Stumpf, Sar, and Keefer, 1975; Sar and Stumpf, 1975; Sheridan, Sar, and Stumpf, 1975), plus the efficacy of local crystalline implants of steroids in the neonatal rat brain (see Gorski, Harlan, and Christensen, 1977), support the currently popular view that the POA is at least an important site for the organizing action of androgens (see Gorski, 1971). More recent evidence reviewed below supports this view rather dramatically.

With respect to the general nature of the perinatal action of steroid hormones, it should be stressed that sexually dimorphic functions are not necessarily exclusively present (or absent) in one sex or the other. For example, the normal male occasionally exhibits

lordosis behavior and can do so to a somewhat marked degree if primed with an excess of estrogen (Davidson, 1969; Whalen, Luttge, and Gorzalka, 1971). It is likely, therefore, at least as a general principle, that the perinatal steroid environment determines the ease with which sex-specific behavioral or functional patterns can be evoked in the adult. It would appear that the neural substrates for certain sex-specific functions are present in adults of both sexes, although they are very difficult to activate in one or the other sex.

Mechanisms of sexual differentiation

With respect to the ways in which androgen exposure could modify neuronal gene expression and thus alter neuronal differentiation, it must be stressed that we cannot at present speak in molecular terms. However, at the level of peripheral hormone target organs such as the uterus or oviduct, the molecular aspects of steroid action are much better understood (Jensen and De Sombre, 1973; Chan and O'Malley, 1976), and it may not be overly optimistic to look forward to significant progress in the near future in understanding how a steroid or the steroid-receptor complex might interact with the neuronal genome. In addition, it has been shown that several chemical-synthesis inhibitors such as cycloheximide (Gorski and Shryne, 1972) and hydroxyurea (Salaman, 1974) do interfere with the neonatal action of androgen. In spite of this limited understanding, it is possible to discuss the organizing actions of androgen at a level that is significantly more molecular than a discussion of the behavior of the rat or even of its pituitary gland.

Three not mutually exclusive possibilities can be proposed and will be presented in the order of their increasing general relevance to neuroscience.

ANDROGENS PRODUCE AN ALTERATION IN THE STEROID-RECEPTOR-EFFECTOR INTERACTION WITHIN HORMONE-RESPONSIVE NEURONS Many of the functions that are sexually dimorphic and undergo sexual differentiation depend on the activational actions of the same or similar steroids in the adult. For example, even the normal female rat, when gonadectomized, will not display lordosis behavior in response to the stimulus of the mounting male unless she is primed with ovarian hormones. (It has been reported, however, that lordosis can be evoked in the complete absence of ovarian hormones, provided a very intense stimulus is applied: see Komisaruk, 1974.) Arguing from current concepts of steroid action on peripheral tissues, one might hypothesize that steroid action on neurons involves an interaction between the steroid and a cytoplasmic "receptor" protein and that this activated steroid-receptor complex is then translocated into the nucleus where, in some way, it derepresses gene action. It has been shown, for example, that neurons that take up and retain labeled steroids do possess cytoplasmic receptors similar to those in peripheral target organs and that there is translocation of labeled steroid into the cell nucleus (McEwen, 1976; Kato, 1977). Presumably these receptor proteins must be continually renewed throughout life, and it may be that hormone exposure at a specific period of development alters the receptor synthesis or renewal process, interferes with steroid-receptor translocation, or perhaps disrupts the biochemical processes that lead to transcription and translation of the genomic information. Direct experimental support for this possibility is limited, but several investigators have reported sex differences in steroid-hormone uptake (see Gorski, 1971; Maurer and Woolley, 1975), in nuclear translocation (Vertes and King, 1971), and in cytoplasmic steroid-receptor repletion (Cidlowski and Muldoon, 1976). In contrast, under certain test conditions, the androgen-exposed female actually appears to be hyperresponsive to exogenous steroids (see Gorski, 1971). It is possible that because of compensatory processes and/or independent changes in functionally specific systems, it will be necessary to specify the system under study in great detail when specific mechanisms of early hormone action are postulated.

EARLY ANDROGEN EXPOSURE DISRUPTS NEUROTRANSMITTER PRODUCTION AND/OR RESPONSIVENESS WITHIN CERTAIN NEURONS OR NEURONAL SYSTEMS   Since the biogenic amines appear to be involved in normal neuroendocrine processes (Fuxe et al., 1976; Kordon et al., 1976; Kalra, 1977), it can be predicted that a direct action of steroids on the development of one or more of these neurotransmitter systems could have profound and permanent functional consequences. It has been reported that the cyclic changes in dopamine turnover that are characteristic of the adult female are eliminated by androgenization (Fuxe, Hökfelt, and Nilsson, 1972). Moreover, sex differences in amine content have been detected and found to be modified by perinatal hormone exposure (Ladosky and Gaziri, 1970; Hardin, 1973; Giulian, McEwen, and Pohorecky, 1974). In experiments of this type it is difficult to distinguish between primary and secondary or indirect effects of hormone action; however, Ladosky, Kesikowski, and Gaziri (1970) re-

port that an injection of chlorpromazine on day 10 can prevent masculinization of gonadotropin regulation and parallel changes in brain serotonin content. Moreover, the chemical destruction of serotoninergic neurons has been reported to induce ovulation in androgenized female rats (Ladosky and Noronha, 1974).

A recent study by Dyer, MacLeod, and Ellendorff (1976) provides experimental evidence that can be interpreted in terms of possible disturbances in unidentified neurotransmitter function. Using the technique of antidromic identification of POA neurons, which project to the medial basal hypothalamus, they reported the existence of a statistically significant sex difference in the responsiveness of these neurons to orthodromic input from the amygdala (Figure 3). Although these data were obtained in animals under different hormonal conditions, and thus could be complicated by the activational actions of steroids, it is possible that the effective connectivity between amygdaloid and POA neurons is altered by neonatal androgen exposure. The term "effective connectivity" is meant to imply disturbances in neurotransmit-

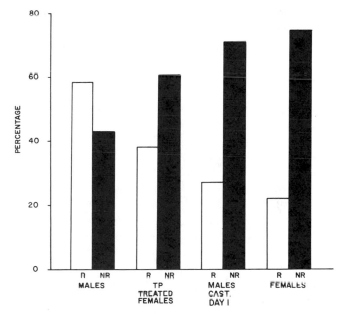

FIGURE 3   Histogram comparing the responses of preoptic neurons that project to the mediobasal hypothalamus to electrical stimulation of the corticomedial amygdala. The percentages of neurons that responded orthodromically to amygdala stimulation are indicated by the open bars; those that did not respond, by the solid bars. Note the reciprocal relationship in the series male, testosterone propionate (TP; 1.25 mg on day 3), treated females, males castrated (cast.) on day 1 of life, and females. (Modified with permission of the authors from Dyer, MacLeod, and Ellendorff, 1976.)

ter production or action in existing neural connections and is to be contrasted with another potential interpretation of these same data; that is, that actual morphological connectivity (presumably of the POA neurons) is altered by the neonatal hormone environment.

STEROID EXPOSURE PRODUCES MORPHOLOGICAL SEX DIFFERENCES IN THE BRAIN This third possibility has perhaps the most general relevance to neuroscience, since it suggests that a permanent structural alteration in the brain is imposed normally during development by the hormone environment. This hypothesis has received considerable experimental support. Several investigators have reported the existence of sex differences in neuronal nuclear and nucleolar size, which presumably could reflect metabolic and/or morphological differences (Ifft, 1964; Pfaff, 1966; Dörner and Staudt, 1968, 1969). However, in now-classic studies, Raisman and Field (1973) reported the existence of a significant sex difference in the rat brain at the ultrastructural level. After sectioning the stria terminalis in the rat, they counted the number of nondegenerating synapses on dendritic spines or shafts of POA neurons within a field of termination of the transected stria. Moreover, as illustrated in Figure 4, the significant sex difference was modified by neonatal hormone treatment in the direction predicted by the concept of sexual differentiation reviewed above. It is interesting that these two examples of sexual dimorphism—the electrophysiological studies of Dyer, MacLeod, and Ellendorff (1976) and the ultrastructural studies of Raisman and Field (1973)—involve the POA. However, in the morphological study, the stria terminalis was transected, so that the the sexual dimorphism is probably due to nonamygdaloid input to the POA. In the former study, the dimorphism was detected in the interaction between the amygdala and POA. Thus it is unlikely that the two observations have the same basis.

In a recent study, Greenough et al. (1977) added both another animal (the hamster) and another dimension to the possible morphological sex differences existing in the brain. They report a significant sex difference in the patterning of the dendritic branches of POA neurons. Adult gonadectomized hamsters were sacrificed following treatment with the same hormonal regime (so that they were exposed to similar "activational" influences) and Golgi-staining accomplished. Golgi-stained neurons in the dorsomedial POA were drawn at ×1,000 with a camera lucida, and the branching patterns of dendrites were quantified in terms of the number of intersections

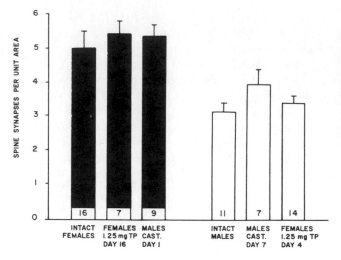

FIGURE 4   Influence of perinatal hormonal environment on the mean incidence of nonstrial synapses on dendritic spines of preoptic neurons. The number at the base of each bar indicates the number of rats in the group, and one standard error of the mean is indicated at the top of each bar. The solid bars represent animals in which gonadotropin secretory patterns were cyclic: the intact female, the male castrated (cast.) before the period of sexual differentiation, and the female exposed to testosterone propionate (TP) after this period. The open bars represent animals in which cyclic gonadotropin release was absent: intact males, androgenized females, or males castrated after the period of sexual differentiation. (Modified with permission of the authors from Raisman and Field, 1973.)

between dendritic branches and a standard grid overlay. These investigators report a statistically significant sex difference in the density of dendritic branching, particularly toward the center of this region (Figure 5). In general terms, dendrites of dorsomedial POA neurons in the female branch irregularly but tend to avoid the center of the region, whereas in the male the dendritic branching of Golgi-stained neurons is more uniform and focused toward the center. Interestingly, these investigators also report essentially similar results from an analysis of suprachiasmatic neurons (personal communication). At the present time, however, it is not known whether or not this sexual dimorphism is determined, or even influenced, by the prenatal steroid environment.

Recently there have been two reports of a rather gross morphological sexual dimorphism in the vertebrate brain. Nottebohm and Arnold (1976) have discovered that in the canary and the finch there is an obvious sex difference in the volume of the hyperstriatum ventrale pars caudale and the robust nucleus of the archistriatum. These two nuclei participate in the control of singing behavior, which is a

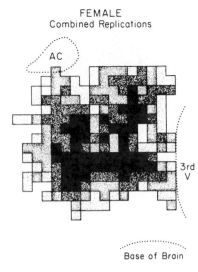

FEMALE
Combined Replications

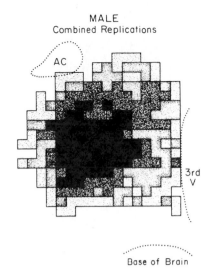

MALE
Combined Replications

FIGURE 5 Relative densities of dendrites from sampled Golgi-stained neurons in 100 μm^2 divisions of a coronal section of the dorsomedial preoptic area of the adult hamster. The darkest shaded areas indicate the highest 25%, the next darkest the next 25%, and so on. Each figure represents the quantitative evaluation of approximately 225 neurons from 15 male or 13 female animals. For orientation, AC is the anterior commissure, 3rd V the 3rd ventricle. (Reprinted with permission from Greenough et al., 1977.)

learned but hormone-dependent behavior in these species. Nuclear volume is greater in the male but is increased in the adult female canary upon testosterone treatment. Under testosterone treatment the female begins to sing, although her song is much more simple than that of the male. Thus in this case the gross volume of specific brain nuclei is both sexually dimorphic and also clearly dependent on the activational effects of gonadal steroids.

The second example comes from the rat and, in fact, from our own laboratory (Gorski, Harlan, and Christensen, 1977; Gorski et al., 1977). When the brain of the adult rat is sectioned at 60 μm and stained with thionin, it is actually possible to identify the sex of the animal by observation of brain sections through the POA with the naked eye (Figure 6). We performed a quantitative evaluation of the intensely staining component of the medial preoptic nucleus (ISC-MPON), upon which the identification of the sex of the animal is based, and found that its volume in the gonadectomized male can be up to eight times larger than that of the gonadectomized female (Figure 7). Moreover, this sexual dimorphism persists under widely different hormonal conditions in the adult, which suggests that it may be relatively independent of the activational effects of steroids. These results also suggest the existence of less-marked morphological sex differences in the suprachiasmatic nuclei and perhaps other areas (Figure 7).

It is of great significance to the topic under discussion that the volume of the ISC-MPON is clearly dependent on the perinatal hormone environment (Figure 8). Postnatal androgen injection significantly increases nuclear volume in the female, and neonatal castration of the male significantly decreases ISC-MPON volume in comparison to the male castrated at 21 days of age. The fact that perinatal hormone manipulation does not completely reverse the sex difference suggests either that the neuronal genome contributes to this sexual dimorphism or that some effects of gonadal steroids occur prenatally, or both.

It must be reemphasized that it is difficult to relate these morphological studies to each other. In the case of the studies on nuclear volume in songbird or rat, we have no information about dendritic branching patterns or the ultrastructural distribution of terminals on these neurons. Moreover, although the studies of the canary suggest a rather specific role for the sexually dimorphic areas in singing, the precise function of the sexually dimorphic ISC-MPON in the rat is unknown. Current evidence supports the possibility that these MPON neurons are involved in the regulation of masculine sexual behavior (Gorski et al., 1977); however, the precise sexually dimorphic function subserved by these neurons, if any, is unknown. Nevertheless, the obvious nature of this sex difference suggests that it may be a useful model for the study of hormone-induced alterations in brain morphology, neurochemistry, and/or function.

It should also be emphasized that the foregoing

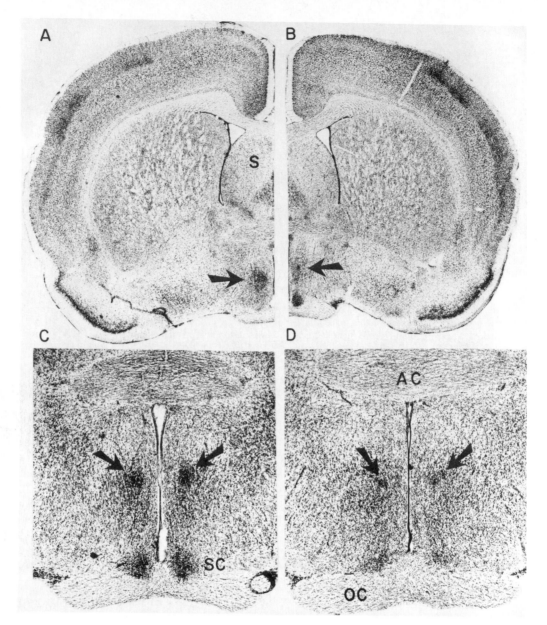

FIGURE 6 Thionin-stained histological sections (60 μm) through the point of maximum development of the sexually dimorphic intensely staining component (arrows) of the medial preoptic nucleus in two gonadectomized male (A, C) and two gonadectomized female (B, D) adult rats. Sections A and B are provided for orientation, with histological details more apparent in C and D. *Abbreviations*: AC, anterior commissure; OC, optic chiasm; S, septum; SC, suprachiasmatic nucleus. (Brain tissue from a study reported in Gorski, Harlan, and Christensen, 1977.)

data merely describe the adult condition following neonatal perturbations in the hormone environment. Very few studies of the possible morphological effects of early hormone injection have been performed on the perinatal animal (but see Matsumoto and Arai, 1976; Reier et al., 1977). Obviously the identification of even this one specific cerebral site in which dramatic changes in neuronal development occur could greatly facilitate attempts to unravel the molecular actions of hormones. However, another technique that should facilitate such studies is available and has already yielded data to support the view that gonadal steroids, particularly estrogen, exert a more general stimulatory influence on neural development than their action on the functional sexual differentiation of the brain. Toran-Allerand (1976) has studied the

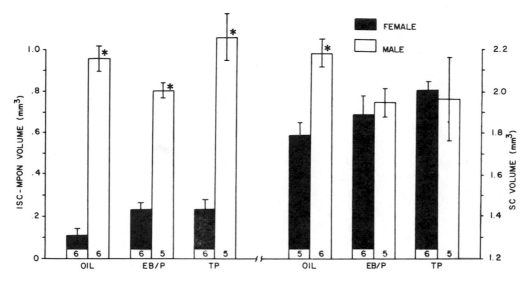

FIGURE 7 Influence of hormone treatment of the adult gonadectomized rat on the mean volume (plus standard error) of the intensely staining component of the medial preoptic nucleus (ISC-MPON, left half of figure) and of the suprachiasmatic nucleus (SC, right). The number at the base of each bar indicates the number of rats in the group. EB/P: 2 μg estradiol benzoate per day for 3 days, followed by 500 μg progesterone. TP: 500 μg testosterone propionate per day for 14 days. Oil: 0.05 ml sesame oil per day for 4 days. Asterisk indicates that nuclear volume in the male was significantly greater than that of the female under the same hormonal conditions; p values are not presented because these groups were only part of a larger study reported in Gorski et al. (1977).

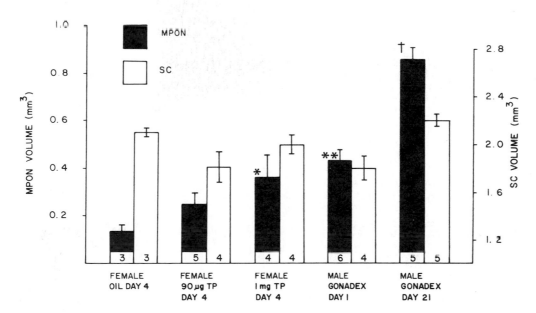

FIGURE 8 The influence of neonatal hormone treatment on the mean volume (plus standard error) of the intensely staining component of the medial preoptic nucleus (here labeled MPON) and of the suprachiasmatic nucleus (SC). Female rats were injected with 0.05 ml sesame oil on day 4 or with 90 μg or 1 mg testosterone propionate (TP) in oil and ovariectomized two weeks prior to sacrifice. Males were orchidectomized on day 1 or day 21 of life. The numbers of animals are indicated at the bases of the bars. There were no significant variations in SC volume. †Significantly (p < 0.01) larger than any other MPON group. **Significantly (p < 0.01) larger than oil-female. *Significantly (p < 0.05) larger than oil-female. (Reprinted from Gorski et al., 1977.)

influence of exogenous steroids on neurite outgrowths in tissue culture from explants of hormone-responsive hypothalamic tissue from the fetal or neonatal mouse of either sex. Steroid hormones in culture markedly stimulate or permit the formation of a very complex network of neurite branches (Figure 9). These studies are consistent with older reports that estrogen administration to young rats in vivo markedly stimulates myelinization and functional maturation of the brain (Heim and Timiras, 1963; Curry and Heim, 1966; Casper, Vernadakis, and Timiras, 1967).

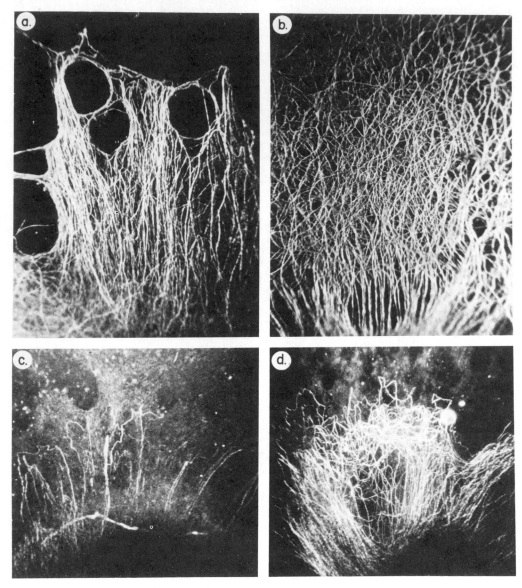

FIGURE 9   Photomicrographs (dark-field) of silver-impregnated (Holmes's) cultures (approximately 3 weeks in vitro) of newborn mouse brain. (a, b) Homologous (mirror-image) cultures of the premammillary region: a is a control, incubated with horse serum before extraction of endogenous steroids; b was incubated in a medium containing 100 ng estradiol/ml. Although photographed at the same magnification, neurite outgrowth in b in response to the estradiol extends for a distance 2.75 times that of a. (c, d) Homologous cultures of the preoptic area photographed at the same magnification: c was incubated in medium containing normal horse serum plus antibodies to estradiol and bovine serum albumin; d is a control, incubated with normal horse serum containing only antibodies to bovine serum albumin. Note the paucity of neurite outgrowth in the presence of antibodies to estradiol (c). In all four examples the explants were located just below the area of neurite outgrowth. (Modified from Toran-Allerand, 1976, and unpublished observations.)

Implications for neuroscience

Although the activational effects of steroid hormones on the adult brain represent an active area of neuroscientific investigation, this discussion has focused only on the ability of gonadal steroids to organize the developing brain. Such actions are not restricted to the gonadal steroids, however. It is well known that thyroid hormone is a prerequisite for normal brain development, and exogenous thyroxin produces marked neuroanatomical and functional changes in the brain (Grave, 1977). The general nature of thyroxin action, however, supports the view that this hormone acts in a "permissive" way, allowing or even interfering with the normal expression of the neuronal genome. The reported effects of estrogen on myelinization in vivo or on neurite outgrowth in vitro may also represent a permissive action of the hormone. Yet the fact that explants from all regions of the brain do not respond to estrogen (Toran-Allerand, 1976) suggests that the action of estrogen is specialized, in that it may be related to the presence of specific steroid receptors. Nevertheless, these permissive and perhaps (in some cases) pharmacologic effects of hormones can be contrasted with the special determinative action of steroids on the sexual differentiation of the brain.

During the process of sexual differentiation of the brain, neuronal gene expression is clearly and selectively altered toward one end of a sexually dimorphic functional (and apparently morphological) continuum by exposure (or lack of exposure) to gonadal hormones. It is difficult to conceive of these hormones merely playing a permissive role in neuronal differentiation, since they determine the direction of that differentiation. Given the complex processes that govern the development of the adult CNS, including programmed cell death, selective retention of neurons, cell surface recognition, chemotaxic and neurotropic influences, and a precise temporal requirement for development of interneuronal associations, it is obviously not possible at our current level of understanding to speculate on the precise mechanism of this hormonal "imprinting" action. Although study of this system is currently hampered by the need to evaluate and quantify complex processes at the level of the behaving organism or the integrative endocrine system, progress is being made in identifying brain areas that are particularly relevant to this process and in understanding hormone action at the molecular level. It may be that this dramatic process of sexual differentiation of the brain or the organizational action of gonadal steroids can serve as a valuable model of neuronal development and the modifications in that development that are environmentally determined.

As a final note, it is important to stress that the ability of steroid hormones to alter permanently neuronal function is not limited to the perinatal period. At this time the CNS is probably most sensitive to such hormonal influences, but in at least two specific situations, permanent and perhaps fundamentally similar effects from steroid hormones can take place in the adult brain. These two situations involve our two model systems, the control of the cyclic surge of LH-RH and of lordosis behavior. In the former case, when female rats are injected neonatally with a low dose of androgen, they appear to be unaffected by that treatment until weeks after puberty, when there is a rather abrupt cessation of ovulation (Gorski, 1968b). This loss of the surge mechanism for LH-RH release is attributable at least in part to a central and permanent effect of the postpubertal steroid environment, since early gonadectomy delays this loss of neuroendocrine function (Kikuyama and Kawashima, 1966; Arai, 1971; Harlan and Gorski, 1978). On the other hand, exogenous estrogen or androgen eliminates this delay (Harlan and Gorski, 1978). In the case of lordosis behavior, estrogen has been shown to exert an apparently permanent effect in promoting the display of this behavior in the adult *male* rat, provided it is administered during the period immediately following electrolytic destruction of the lateral septum (Nance, Shryne, and Gorski, 1975; Nance et al., 1977). This observation suggests that during recovery from central lesions, which process probably includes axonal sprouting and/or central reorganization, the steroid environment can have profound effects. Although the genomic basis for this reorganization and for the hormone action is unclear, it can be assumed that the neurons of the CNS retain their potential to respond to steroid hormones by means of a permanent alteration, at least in their function. It may be that the hormonal environment is an integral component not only of development but also of the processes we recognize as the plasticity of the brain.

ACKNOWLEDGMENTS The research from the author's laboratory is supported by U.S. Public Health Service grant HD-01182 and by the Ford Foundation. The author expresses his appreciation to J. Shryne, E. Freiberg, C. Kristensen, and L. Kelley for expert assistance and to his colleagues for their permission to reprint illustrations based on their work.

REFERENCES

ARAI, Y., 1971. A possible process of the secondary sterilization: Delayed anovulation syndrome. *Experientia* 27:463–464.

BARRACLOUGH, C. A., 1961. Production of anovulatory, sterile rats by single injections of testosterone propionate. *Endocrinology* 68:62–67.

BEACH, F. A., 1975. Hormonal modification of sexually dimorphic behavior. *Psychoeuroendocrinology* 1:3–23.

BRAWER, J. R., and M. VAN HOUTEN, 1976. Cellular organization of luteinizing hormone-releasing factor delivery systems. In *Subcellular Mechanisms in Reproductive Neuroendocrinology*, F. Naftolin, K. J. Ryan, and J. Davies, eds. Amsterdam: Elsevier, pp. 1–31.

CASPER, R., A. VERNADAKIS, and P. S. TIMIRAS, 1967. Influence of estradiol and cortisol on lipids and cerebrosides in the developing brain and spinal cord of the rat. *Brain Res.* 5:524–526.

CHAN, L., and B. W. O'MALLEY, 1976. Mechanism of action of the sex steroid hormones. *N. Engl. J. Med.* 294:1322–1328, 1372–1381, 1430–1437.

CIDLOWSKI, J. A., and T. G. MULDOON, 1976. Sex-related differences in the regulation of cytoplasmic estrogen receptor levels in responsive tissues of the rat. *Endocrinology* 98:833–841.

CURRY, J., and L. M. HEIM, 1966. Brain myelination after neonatal administration of oestradiol. *Nature* 209:915–916.

DAVIDSON, J. M., 1969. Effects of estrogen on the sexual behavior of male rats. *Endocrinology* 84:1365–1372.

DÖRNER, G., and J. STAUDT, 1968. Structural changes in the preoptic anterior hypothalamic area of the male rat, following neonatal castration and androgen substitution. *Neuroendocrinology* 3:136–140.

DÖRNER, G., and J. STAUDT, 1969. Structural changes in the hypothalamic ventromedial nucleus of the male rat, following neonatal castration and androgen treatment. *Neuroendocrinology* 4:278–281.

DYER, R. G., N. K. MACLEOD, and F. ELLENDORFF, 1976. Electrophysiological evidence for sexual dimorphism and synaptic convergence in the preoptic and anterior hypothalamic areas of the rat. *Proc. R. Soc. Lond.* B193:421–440.

EHRHARDT, A. A., 1975. Prenatal hormone exposure and psychosexual differentiation. In *Topics in Psychoneuroendocrinology*, E. J. Sachar, ed. New York: Grune & Stratton, pp. 67–82.

ELLENDORFF, F., 1976. Evaluation of extrahypothalamic control of reproductive physiology. *Rev. Physiol. Biochem. Pharmacol.* 76:103–127.

EVERETT, J. W., 1964. Preoptic stimulative lesions and ovulation in the rat: "Thresholds" and LH-release time in late diestrus and proestrus. In *Major Problems in Neuroendocrinology*, E. Bajusz and G. Jasmin, eds. Basel: S. Karger, pp. 346–366.

FUXE, K., T. HÖKFELT, L. AGNATI, A. LÖFSTROM, B. J. EVERITT, O. JOHANSSON, G. JONSSON, W. WUTTKE, and M. GOLDSTEIN, 1976. Role of monoamines in the control of gonadotrophin secretion. In *Neuroendocrine Regulation of Fertility* (International Symposium, Simla, 1974). Basel: S. Karger, pp. 124–140.

FUXE, K., T. HÖKFELT, and O. NILSSON, 1972. Effect of constant light and androgen-sterilization on the amine turnover of the tubero-infundibular dopamine neurons: Blockade of cyclic activity and induction of a persistent high dopamine turnover in the median eminence. *Acta Endocrinol. (Kbh)* 69:625–639.

GIULIAN, D., B. S. MCEWEN, and L. A. POHORECKY, 1974. Altered development of the rat brain serotonergic system after disruptive neonatal experience. *Proc. Natl. Acad. Sci. USA* 71:4106–4110.

GORSKI, R. A., 1963. Modification of ovulatory mechanisms by postnatal administration of estrogen to the rat. *Am. J. Physiol.* 205:842–844.

GORSKI, R. A., 1968a. The neural control of ovulation. In *Biology of Gestation*, vol. 1: *The Maternal Organism*, N. S. Assali, ed. New York: Academic Press, pp. 1–66.

GORSKI, R. A., 1968b. Influence of age on the response to paranatal administration of a low dose of androgen. *Endocrinology* 82:1001–1004.

GORSKI, R. A., 1971. Gonadal hormones and the perinatal development of neuroendocrine function. In *Frontiers in Neuroendocrinology, 1971*, L. Martini and W. F. Ganong, eds. New York: Oxford Univ. Press, pp. 237–290.

GORSKI, R. A., 1974a. Extrahypothalamic influences on gonadotropin regulation. In *The Control of the Onset of Puberty*, M. M. Grumbach, G. D. Grave, and F. E. Mayer, eds. New York: John Wiley, pp. 182–207.

GORSKI, R. A., 1974b. The neuroendocrine regulation of sexual behavior. In *Advances in Psychobiology*, vol. 2, G. Newton and A. H. Riesen, eds. New York: John Wiley, pp. 1–58.

GORSKI, R. A., 1976. The possible neural sites of hormonal facilitation of sexual behavior in the female rat. *Psychoneuroendocrinology*. 1:371–387.

GORSKI, R. A., J. H. GORDON, J. E. SHRYNE, and A. M. SOUTHAM, 1977. Evidence for a morphological sex difference within the medial preoptic area of the rat brain. *Brain Res.* 148:333–346.

GORSKI, R. A., R. E. HARLAN, and L. W. CHRISTENSEN, 1977. Perinatal hormonal exposure and the development of neuroendocrine processes. *J. Toxicol. Environm. Health* 3:97–121.

GORSKI, R. A., S. P. MENNIN, and K. KUBO, 1975. The neural and hormonal bases of the reproductive cycle of the rat. In *Biological Rhythms and Endocrine Function* (Advances in Experimental Medicine and Biology series, vol. 54), L. Hedlund, J. Franz, and A. Kenny, eds. New York: Plenum Press, pp. 115–146.

GORSKI, R. A., and J. SHRYNE, 1972. Intracerebral antibiotics and androgenization of the neonatal female rat. *Neuroendocrinology* 10:109–120.

GOY, R. W., and J. A. RESKO, 1972. Gonadal hormones and behavior of normal and pseudohermaphroditic nonhuman female primates. *Recent Prog. Horm. Res.* 28:707–733.

GRADY, K. L., C. H. PHOENIX, and W. C. YOUNG, 1965. Role of the developing rat testis in differentiation of the neural tissues mediating mating behavior. *J. Comp. Physiol. Psychol.* 59:176–182.

GRAVE, G. D., 1977. *Thyroid Hormones and Brain Development*. New York: Raven Press.

GREENOUGH, W. T., C. S. CARTER, C. STEERMAN, and T. J. DEVOOGD, 1977. Sex differences in dendritic patterns in hamster preoptic area. *Brain Res.* 126:63–72.

HARDIN, C. M., 1973. Sex differences and the effects of testosterone injections on biogenic amine levels of neonatal rat brain. *Brain Res.* 62:286–290.

HARLAN, R. E., and R. A. GORSKI, 1977. Steroid regulation of luteinizing hormone secretion in normal and androgenized rats at different ages. *Endocrinology* 101:741–749.

HARLAN, R. E., and R. A. GORSKI, 1978. Effects of postpubertal ovarian steroids on reproductive function and sexual differentiation of lightly androgenized rats. *Endocrinology* 102:1716–1724.

HARRIS, G. W., 1955. *Neural Control of the Pituitary Gland.* London: Edward Arnold, Ltd.

HAYASHI, S., and R. A. GORSKI, 1974. Critical exposure time for androgenization by intracranial crystals of testosterone propionate in neonatal female rats. *Endocrinology* 94:1161–1167.

HEIM, L. M., and P. S. TIMIRAS, 1963. Gonad-brain relationship: Precocious brain maturation after estradiol in rats. *Endocrinology* 72:598–606.

IFFT, J. D., 1964. The effect of endocrine gland extirpation on the size of nucleoli in rat hypothalamic neurons. *Anat. Rec.* 148:599–604.

JACKSON, G. L., 1973. Effect of progesterone on release of luteinizing hormone in gonadectomized adult and immature rats. *Biol. Reprod.* 8:58–61.

JENSEN, E. V., and E. R. DE SOMBRE, 1973. Estrogen-receptor interaction. *Science* 182:126–134.

KALRA, S. P., 1976. Neuroamines in gonadotropin secretion. In *Endocrinology,* vol. 1, V. H. T. James, ed. Amsterdam: Excerpta Medica, pp. 152–157.

KATO, J., 1977. Characterization and function of steroids receptors in the hypothalamus and hypophysis. In *Endocrinology,* vol. 1, V. H. T. James, ed. Amsterdam: Excerpta Medica, pp. 12–17.

KAWAKAMI, M., and E. TERASAWA, 1972. A possible role of the hippocampus and the amygdala in the androgenized rat: Effect of electrical or electrochemical stimulation of the brain on gonadotrophin secretion. *Endocrinol. Jap.* 19:349–358.

KIKUYAMA, S., and S. KAWASHIMA, 1966. Formation of corpora lutea in ovarian grafts in ovariectomized adult rats subjected to early postnatal treatment with androgen. *Sci. Papers Coll. Gen. Ed. Univ. Tokyo* 16:69–74.

KNIGGE, K. M., S. A. JOSEPH, J. R. SLADEK, M. F. NOTTER, M. MORRIS, D. K. SUNDBERG, M. A. HOLZWARTH, G. E. HOFFMAN, and L. O'BRIEN, 1976. Uptake and transport activity of the median eminence of the hypothalamus. *Int. Rev. Cytol.* 45:383–408.

KOMISARUK, B. R., 1974. Neural and hormonal interactions in the reproductive behavior of female rats. In *Reproductive Behavior,* W. Montagna and W. A. Sadler, eds. New York: Plenum Press, pp. 97–129.

KORDON, C., J. EPELBAUM, A. ENJALBERT, and J. MCKELVY, 1976. Neurotransmitter interactions with neuroendocrine tissue. In *Subcellular Mechanisms in Reproductive Neuroendocrinology,* F. Naftolin, K. J. Ryan, and J. Davies, eds. Amsterdam: Elsevier, pp. 167–184.

LADOSKY, W., and L. C. J. GAZIRI, 1970. Brain serotonin and sexual differentiation of the nervous system. *Neuroendocrinology* 6:168–174.

LADOSKY, W., W. M. KESIKOWSKI, and I. F. GAZIRI, 1970. Effect of a single injection of chlorpromazine into infant male rats on subsequent gonadotropin secretion. *J. Endocrinol.* 48:151–156.

LADOSKY, W., and J. G. L. NORONHA, 1974. Further evidence for an inhibitory role of serotonin in the control of ovulation. *J. Endocrinol.* 62:677–678.

MATSUMOTO, A., and Y. ARAI, 1976. Effect of estrogen on early postnatal development of synaptic formation in the hypothalamic arcuate nucleus of female rats. *Neurosci. Lett.* 2:79–82.

MAURER, R. A., and D. E. WOOLLEY, 1975. ^{3}H-estradiol distribution in female, androgenized female, and male rats at 100 and 200 days of age. *Endocrinology* 96:755–765.

McEWEN, B. S., 1976. Steroid receptors in neuroendocrine tissues: Topography, subcellular distribution, and functional implications. In *Subcellular Mechanisms in Reproductive Neuroendocrinology,* F. Naftolin, K. J. Ryan, and J. Davies, eds. Amsterdam: Elsevier, pp. 277–304.

MONEY, J., and A. A. EHRHARDT, 1972. *Man and Woman, Boy and Girl.* Baltimore: The Johns Hopkins Press.

MOORE, R. Y., and V. B. EICHLER, 1976. Central neural mechanisms in diurnal rhythm regulation and neuroendocrine responses to light. *Psychoneuroendocrinology* 1:265–279.

NADLER, R. D., 1968. Masculinization of female rats by intracranial implantation of androgen in infancy. *J. Comp. Physiol. Psychol.* 66:157–167.

NANCE, D. M., and R. A. GORSKI, 1975. Neurohormonal determinants of sex differences in the hypothalamic regulation of feeding behavior and body weight in the rat. *Pharmacol. Biochem. Behav.* 3 (Suppl. 1):155–162.

NANCE, D. M., C. PHELPS, J. E. SHRYNE, and R. A. GORSKI, 1977. Alterations by estrogen and hypothyroidism in the effects of septal lesions on lordosis behavior of male rats. *Brain Res. Bull.* 2:49–53.

NANCE, D. M., J. SHRYNE, and R. A. GORSKI, 1975. Facilitation of female sexual behavior in male rats by septal lesions: An interaction with estrogen. *Horm. Behav.* 6:289–299.

NOTTEBOHM, F., and A. P. ARNOLD, 1976. Sexual dimorphism in vocal control areas of the songbird brain. *Science* 194:211–213.

PFAFF, D. W., 1966. Morphological changes in the brain of adult male rats after neonatal castration. *J. Endocrinol.* 36:415–416.

PFAFF, D., and M. KEINER, 1973. Atlas of estradiol-concentrating cells in the central nervous system of the female rat. *J. Comp. Neurol.* 151:121–158.

PFEIFFER, C. A., 1936. Sexual differences of the hypophyses and their determination by the gonads. *Am. J. Anat.* 58:195–226.

PHOENIX, C. H., R. W. GOY, A. A. GERALL, and W. C. YOUNG, 1959. Organizing action of prenatally administered testosterone propionate on the tissues mediating mating behavior in the female guinea pig. *Endocrinology* 65:369–382.

QUADAGNO, D. M., R. BRISCOE, and J. S. QUADAGNO, 1977. The effect of perinatal gonadal hormones on selected nonsexual behavior patterns: A critical assessment of the nonhuman and human literature. *Psychol. Bull.* 84:62–80.

QUADAGNO, D. M., J. SHRYNE, C. ANDERSON, and R. A. GORSKI, 1972. Influence of gonadal hormones on social, sexual, emergence, and open field behaviour in the rat,

Rattus norvegicus. Anim. Behav. 20:732–740.

RAISMAN, G., and P. M. FIELD, 1973. Sexual dimorphism in the neuropil of the preoptic area of the rat and its dependence on neonatal androgen. *Brain Res.* 54:1–29.

REIER, P. J., M. J. CULLEN, J. S. FROELICH, and I. ROTHCHILD, 1977. The ultrastructure of the developing medial preoptic nucleus in the postnatal rat. *Brain Res.* 122:415–436.

REINISCH, J. M., 1974. Fetal hormones, the brain, and human sex differences: A heuristic, integrative review of the recent literature. *Arch. Sex. Behav.* 3:51–90.

SALAMAN, D. F., 1974. The role of DNA, RNA and protein synthesis in sexual differentiation of the brain. *Prog. Brain Res.* 41:349–362.

SAR, M., and W. E. STUMPF, 1975. Distribution of androgen-concentrating neurons in rat brain. In *Anatomical Neuroendocrinology,* W. E. Stumpf and L. D. Grant, eds. Basel: S. Karger, pp. 120–133.

SCHALLY, A. V., and D. H. COY, 1977. Stimulatory and inhibitory analogs of luteinizing hormone releasing hormone (LHRH). In *Hypothalamic Peptide Hormones and Pituitary Regulation* (Advances in Experimental Medicine and Biology series, vol. 87), J. C. Porter, ed. New York: Plenum Press, pp. 99–121.

SCHWARTZ, N. B., 1973. Mechanisms controlling ovulation in small mammals. In *Handbook of Physiology,* section 7, R. O. Greep and E. B. Astwood, eds., vol. 2, part 1. Washington, D.C.: American Physiological Society, pp. 125–141.

SCOUTEN, C. W., L. K. GROTELUESCHEN, and W. W. BEATTY, 1975. Androgens and the organization of sex differences in active avoidance behavior in the rat. *J. Comp. Physiol. Psychol.* 88:264–270.

SHERIDAN, P. J., M. SAR, and W. E. STUMPF, 1975. Estrogen and androgen distribution in the brain of neonatal rats. In *Anatomical Neuroendocrinology,* W. E. Stumpf and L. D. Grant, eds. Basel: S. Karger, pp. 134–141.

STEWART, J., A. SKVARENINA, and J. POTTER, 1975. Effects of neonatal androgens on open-field and maze learning in the prepubescent and adult rat. *Physiol. Behav.* 14:291–295.

STUMPF, W. E., M. SAR, and D. A. KEEFER, 1975. Atlas of estrogen target cells in rat brain. In *Anatomical Neuroendocrinology,* W. E. Stumpf and L. D. Grant, eds. Basel: S. Karger, pp. 134–141.

SUTHERLAND, S. D., and R. A. GORSKI, 1972. An evaluation of the inhibition of androgenization of the neonatal female rat brain by barbiturate. *Neuroendocrinology* 10:94–108.

SZENTÁGOTHAI, J., B. FLERKÓ, B. MESS, and B. HALÁSZ, 1968. *Hypothalamic Control of the Anterior Pituitary,* 3rd ed. Budapest: Akadémiai Kiadó.

TARTTELIN, M. F., J. E. SHRYNE, and R. A. GORSKI, 1975. Patterns of body weight change in rats following neonatal hormone manipulation: A "critical period" for androgen-induced growth increases. *Acta Endocrinol.* 79:177–191.

TORAN-ALLERAND, C. D., 1976. Sex steroids and the development of the newborn mouse hypothalamus and preoptic area *in vitro*: Implications for sexual differentiation. *Brain Res.* 106:407–412.

TURNER, J. W., 1975. Influence of neonatal androgen on the display of territorial marking in the gerbil. *Physiol. Behav.* 15:265–270.

VERTES, M., and R. J. B. KING, 1971. The mechanism of oestradiol binding in rat hypothalamus: Effect of androgenization. *J. Endocrinol.* 51:271–282.

WADE, G. N., 1972. Gonadal hormones and behavioral regulation of body weight. *Physiol. Behav.* 8:523–534.

WAGNER, J. W., W. ERWIN, and V. CRITCHLOW, 1966. Androgen sterilization produced by intracerebral implants of testosterone in neonatal female rats. *Endocrinology* 79:1135–1142.

WHALEN, R. E., W. G. LUTTGE, and B. B. GORZALKA, 1971. Neonatal androgenization and the development of estrogen responsivity in male and female rats. *Horm. Behav.* 2:83–90.

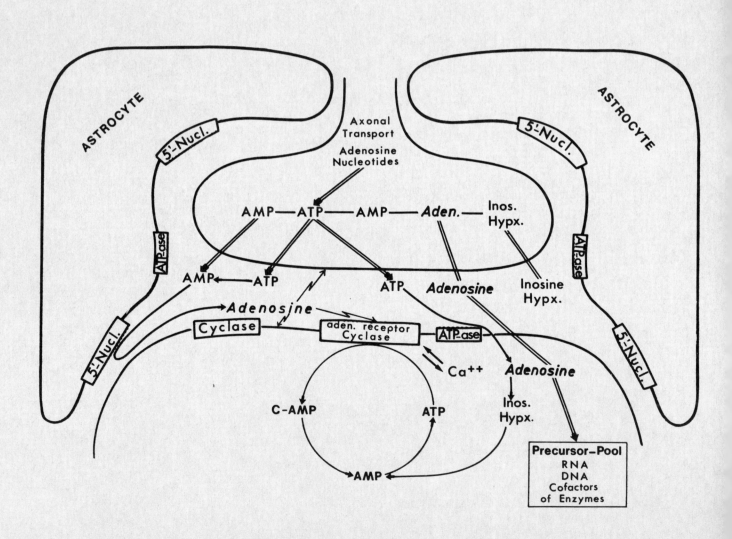

MODULATORS AND EFFECTORS OF NEURONAL INTERACTION

Scheme summarizing translocation, intra- and extracellular transformation, and some action of adenosine and its derivatives at the synapse. (See the chapter by G. W. Kreutzberg and P. Schubert, this volume.)

Introduction

LESLIE L. IVERSEN

THE PHENOMENON of chemical transmission at synapses in the mammalian CNS is well known and is believed to be the mode of information transfer employed at the great majority of such synapses. At least ten different chemical transmitters have been identified with some degree of certainty, and more probably remain to be discovered. It is now possible in some regions of CNS to fill in the blank Golgi maps with identified transmitters (M. Cuénod and P. Streit). The finding during the last few years that a variety of small neuroactive peptides exist in CNS may have added a whole new family of compounds to the list of possible neurotransmitters, and the chapters by W. Vale and M. Brown and by S. H. Snyder review this topic in detail. It remains unclear whether the neuroactive peptides should be regarded simply as a new category of neurotransmitters or whether their function is somehow different from that of previously known amine and amino acid transmitters. Perhaps the peptides are modulators of neuronal activity, in a manner similar to that proposed by W. Singer, who describes the modulatory actions of monoamines on the excitability of cortical neurons.

In this section emphasis is also placed on conventional modes of chemical signaling in the nervous system. Attention is given to various possible chemical mechanisms which may operate at a local level to modulate neuronal activity. In a previous Study Program (Iversen, 1974) I reviewed what was then known about the processes that can modulate the release of transmitters from chemical synapses locally at the nerve terminal level. Since then considerable progress has been made. There are now, for example, many more examples of presynaptic receptor mechanisms involved in regulating the amount of transmitter from presynaptic terminals. Many of these mechanisms involve specialized receptors on the surface of presynaptic terminals which recognize the transmitter released by that terminal (negative feedback by so-called autoreceptors: see Carlsson, 1975) or which recognize a variety of other transmitters (presynaptic inhibition or facilitation: see Langer, 1977; Starke, Taube, and Borowski, 1977).

Other chapters in this section, by G. W. Kreutzberg and P. Schubert and by B. Samuelsson, review the possible roles of adenosine and prostaglandins in the chemical modulation of neuronal activity by mechanisms possibly quite different from those involving conventional chemical transmitters. Adenosine seems to play a modulatory role in the responses of a number of peripheral tissues to endocrine hormones and may act similarly in the nervous system. The prostaglandins are the "local hormones" par excellence in peripheral tissues, and all of the components of the now exceedingly complex machinery of prostaglandin metabolism are present in the brain.

A further degree of complexity arises from the finding that conventional neurotransmitters sometimes exist in unconventional places. Thus there is now considerable evidence to suggest that in some neurons transmitter release may occur from dendritic processes as well as from the normal sites in the axon terminals. The dopaminergic neurons of substantia nigra in mammalian brain represent one such category of neuron, reviewed by L. L. Iversen and by J. Glowinski, who describes the first direct evidence for transmitter release from dendrites in the intact brain.

At the moment we have little understanding of the significance of these unconventional local circuit chemical interactions in nervous system function. However, it is clear that many mechanisms exist, particularly in neuropil regions of CNS, which potentially could allow local chemical signaling to occur. Furthermore, such interactions may well occur without the morphological specializations and point-to-point contacts normally associated with chemical synapses. Unraveling the complexities of such chemical modulation will be difficult, but it may represent one of the next big leaps forward in our understanding of neuronal signaling mechanisms.

REFERENCES

CARLSSON, A., 1975. Receptor-mediated control of dopamine metabolism. In *Pre- and Post-synaptic Receptors*, E. Usdin and W. E. Bunney, eds. New York: Marcel Dekker, pp. 49–63.

IVERSEN, L. L., 1974. Biochemical aspects of synaptic modulation. In *The Neurosciences: Third Study Program*, F. O. Schmitt and F. G. Worden, eds. Cambridge, MA: MIT Press, pp. 905–915.

LANGER, S. Z., 1977. Presynaptic receptors and their role in the regulation of transmitter release. *Br. J. Pharmacol.* 60:481–497.

STARKE, K., H. D. TAUBE, and E. BOROWSKI, 1977. Presynaptic receptor systems in catecholaminergic transmission. *Biochem. Pharmacol.* 26:259–268.

59 Amino Acid Transmitters and Local Circuitry in Optic Tectum

M. CUÉNOD and P. STREIT

ABSTRACT   Using the pigeon optic tectum as a model, the amino acid transmitter specificity in a neuronal network is examined. Evidence is presented that glutamate is involved in the tectal afferents from the retina. Certain types of neurons display an affinity for the inhibitory transmitter GABA, and others for glycine. When these tritiated amino acids are injected into the tectum, they label well-defined distant cell bodies, suggesting a specific uptake followed by somatopetal migration of the radioactivity. One glycine system shares its specificity with serine and alanine. A dendritic network of interneurons seems to operate with GABA. These observations may shed light on the functional role of the somatopetal axoplasmic transport in informing the cell body of events occurring at its periphery.

Introduction

AN UNDERSTANDING of the central nervous system requires characterization of its functional units and subunits at various levels of complexity. We must know not only the principles on which a model neuron operates, but also the peculiar morphological, biochemical, and physiological properties of each class of neurons in a network. In this paper we review an analysis of the optic tectum of the pigeon, emphasizing the particular transmitters involved.

Many aspects of neuronal cell biology are relevant to these studies. Besides its morphological characteristics, a neuron of a given class is likely to exhibit some biochemical specificity, related to functions such as the establishment of correct connections and intercellular communications (Smith and Kreutzberg, 1976). Synaptic transmission requires that the cell body supply to the nerve terminal the enzymes involved in the synthesis of both the transmitter and the membrane carrier systems that are responsible for the high-affinity uptake of the transmitter or its

M. CUÉNOD and P. STREIT   Brain Research Institute, University of Zurich, CH-8029 Zurich, Switzerland

metabolites (Snyder et al., 1973; Hökfelt and Ljungdahl, 1975; Iversen et al., 1975). These properties can be used to determine some of the biochemical specificities of a neuronal class. Somatofugal transport carries newly synthesized material from the cell body to the dendrites, the axon, and the terminals; somatopetal transport brings to the cell body material that originates in the neuronal expansions. Although we do not yet know whether the selection for this somatopetal transport of material takes place at the cell membrane or in the transport system itself, this mechanism would allow the cell body to be informed about events taking place at the terminals. Using both biochemical and morphological approaches, these general principles can be applied to the analysis of the biochemical specificities of neurons in a network such as the optic tectum. Needless to say, in the course of such a network analysis, new concepts may emerge that are pertinent to the cell biology of the neuron.

A brief description of the anatomical organization of the avian optic tectum will provide background information on the model used in this study. Then a search for the transmitter(s) of the retinotectal ganglion cells will be described followed by an analysis of some optic-lobe inhibitory systems that involve amino acids. Finally, the evidence for somatopetal migration of transmitter amino acids will be discussed.

Experimental model: Organization of the avian optic tectum

The visual system of the pigeon presents several advantages as a neurobiological model. Although the pigeon has a relatively small brain, its visual system is developed to a degree matched only by primates. The retinal input is almost completely crossed in the optic chiasm, allowing us to experiment on one side

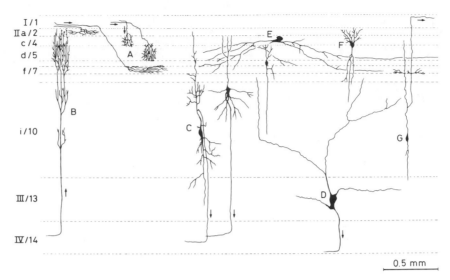

0.5 mm

FIGURE 1 Golgi pictures of some neuronal types described in the avian optic tectum by Ramón y Cajal (1891), van Gehuchten (1892), and Ris (1899). Layer nomenclature according to Cowan, Adamson, and Powell (1961) and Ramón y Cajal (1891). A, optic afferent fibers; B, Ipc afferent fiber; C, neuron projecting to Ipc; D, large efferent neuron; E, horizontal intrinsic neuron; F, radial intrinsic neuron; G, neuron with terminals in superficial tectum and in pretectum.

while using the other as a control. Moreover, the tectum is a highly organized laminated structure with clear landmarks, and tectal synaptosomes are easy to prepare. Finally, the avian visual system has been extensively investigated from morphological, physiological, biochemical, and behavioral points of view.

In order to place results presented below in proper perspective, a brief outline of the anatomical organization of the optic tectum, its inputs and outputs, and its synaptic contacts will be presented here (refer to Figures 1, 2, and 11). The optic tectum is quantitatively the most important first relay in the avian visual pathway; it connects the retina with the thalamus, pretectum, and lower brain stem. Besides the tectum, the retinal fibers are distributed to a series of contralateral mesodiencephalic nuclei, which will not be considered here. The tectal relay receives additional inputs from the telencephalon (Wulst), the nucleus spiriformis lateralis (SPL), and the contralateral tectum. There is a loop of reciprocal connections between the tectum and the subtectal nucleus isthmi, pars parvocellularis (Ipc nucleus). The tectum also projects to the isthmo-optic nucleus (ION), which in turn sends efferent fibers to the retina. Finally, many intrinsic neurons are present within the various tectal layers (Karten, 1969; Nauta and Karten, 1970; Repérant, 1973; Meier, Mihailovic, and Cuénod, 1974; Webster, 1974; Hunt and Webster, 1975; Hunt and Künzle, 1976a,b; Streit and Reubi, 1977a).

Cytoarchitectonically, the tectum is a well-laminated structure in which fifteen layers and sublayers can be distinguished. They were numbered by Ramón y Cajal (1891), from 1 at the surface to 15 in the depths. A second nomenclature, using roman numbers I to VI, with a further subdivision of lamina II into ten sublayers labeled IIa to IIj, was introduced by Cowan, Adamson, and Powell (1961). (See Repérant, 1973, for a comparison of the various nomenclatures in use.) The retinal afferent fibers run in layer I(1), then take a 90° turn to penetrate the superficial layers of the tectum. Six different types of terminal arborizations have been described, distributing to sublaminae IIa(2) through IIf(7) (Figure 1A; see Ramón y Cajal, 1891; van Gehuchten, 1892; Hirschberger, 1971; LaVail and Cowan, 1971a,b; Schonbach and Cuénod, 1971; Hunt and Webster, 1975; for review see Webster, 1974). Electron-microscopic observations indicate that these arborizations mainly make synaptic contacts with dendrites extending radially from neurons lying in the deeper layers of the tectum (Figure 6A). However, they also appear to contact horizontal dendrites, which most likely belong to intrinsic interneurons (Hayes and Webster, 1975; Angaut and Repérant, 1976). The efferent neurons have their cell bodies in layers IIg(8) to III(13); their dendritic arborization expands radially into the more superficial layers, and their axons leave the tectum in the depth, passing through layer IV(14) (Figure 1C, D). There is one exception to this pattern: one type of neuron with its perikaryon in sublamina IIi(10)

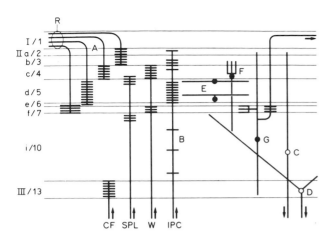

	AFFERENT	INTRINSIC	EFFERENT
TELENCEPHALON	Wulst (W)		—
DIENCEPHALON	Retina (R)		Rotundus DLL GL Pretectum
MESENCEPHALON	IPC SPL Contra-tectum (CF)		IPC ION
METENCEPHALON	—		Pons

FIGURE 2 Schematic representation of the input-output relationship in the avian optic tectum. Labels A–G refer to Figure 1. DLL, N. dorsolateralis anterior thalami, pars lateralis; GL, N. geniculatus; ION, N. isthmo-opticus, IPC, N. isthmi, pars parvocellularis, SPL, N. spiriformis lateralis.

and radial dendrites sends its axon to the superficial layer I(1), toward the pretectum (Figure 1G). The neurons projecting to nucleus Ipc have their cell bodies in sublamina IIi(10), while their radial dendrites reach the superficial layers (Figures 1C and 3); their axons project, in a point-to-point topographic manner, into Ipc. The loop is closed by neurons that lie in Ipc and project into the corresponding part of the tectum (Figures 1B and 4); their fibers start to branch in sublamina IIh(9) and terminate in diffuse cylindrical bushes, particularly in IId(5), but they reach as far as IIa(2) (Hunt et al., 1977). Their zone of termination thus overlaps extensively with that occupied by optic-nerve terminals. Their mode of termination, however, differs from that of optic-nerve afferents: Ipc fibers contact small dendritic elements mainly as *boutons en passage* (Figure 5), whereas retinal terminals appear mainly as clusters around similar postsynaptic structures. Many interneurons occupy layers IIc(4) and IId(5); some of them extend horizontally (Figure 1E) and apparently consist exclusively of dendrites (Hunt and Künzle, 1976b), which have been shown to be presynaptic to other neurons (Hayes and Webster, 1975; Angaut and Repérant, 1976).

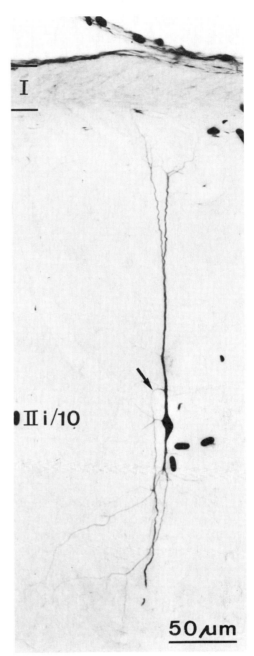

FIGURE 3 Homogeneously filled neuron projecting to Ipc with perikaryon in IIi(10) (see Figure 1C). Golgi-like staining following HRP injection into the Ipc nucleus. The axon (arrow) leaves the apical dendrite, which reaches with its uppermost arborization into sublayer IIa(2). (50 μm frozen section, diaminobenzidine [DAB] staining.)

Transmitter candidates in the avian optic tectum

To obtain indications about the transmitter(s) involved in the retinotectal neurons, the following approach was used. First, advantage was taken of the suggestion made by Logan and Snyder (1971) that

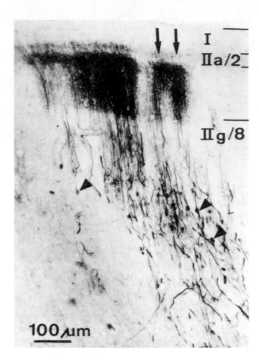

FIGURE 4 Light micrograph showing tectal region following HRP injection into the Ipc nucleus. Note the anterogradely filled terminal arborizations of Ipc afferent fibers (arrows) extending through most of layer II; they are most pronounced in sublayers IIb–f(3–7) (Figure 1B). Several nerve cell bodies (arrowheads) in IIi(10) (Figure 3) can be seen because of retrograde filling of these tectal efferents to Ipc. (50 μm frozen section, DAB staining.)

the presence of high-affinity uptake systems in synaptosomes for a particular substance correlates closely with a neurotransmitter function of that substance—as established by electrophysiological, pharmacological, and histochemical methods (Iversen, 1971; Snyder et al., 1973). Thus the uptake of various transmitter candidates was investigated in tectal fractions containing synaptosomes.

Both high- and low-affinity uptake have been reported for glutamate, aspartate, GABA, glycine, serine, proline, alanine, and choline (Henke, Schenker, and Cuénod, 1976a; Henke and Cuénod, 1978; Cuénod and Henke, 1978), most of which are well established as transmitters in the CNS. In contrast, the transmitter dopamine as well as leucine, an amino acid for which no indication of a transmitter function is available, were taken up by the low-affinity system only. The high-affinity uptake was temperature- and sodium-dependent. Hypo-osmotic shock released more than 95% of the substances taken up, indicating that they were trapped in organelles and not bound to membranes. In sucrose gradient, the organelles loaded by the uptake systems migrated to

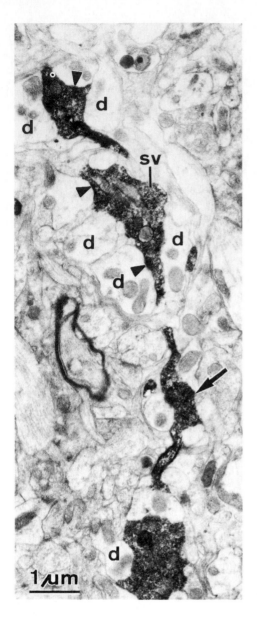

FIGURE 5 Electron micrograph showing HRP-filled Ipc terminals—partly as *boutons en passage* (arrow)—making asymmetric junctions (arrowheads) on clear dendritic elements (d). The synaptic vesicles (sv) are mainly spherical. (Sublayer IId(5), HRP injection in Ipc, DAB staining, uranyl block staining.)

the density characteristic of synaptosomes; although this suggests that the substances have been taken up in synaptosomes, it cannot be excluded that other organelles, originating from neurons or glial cells, might also contribute to the uptake compartment. Attempts to separate on sucrose density gradients the organelles taking up various transmitters at a given substrate concentration have been unsuccessful.

Beart (1976) observed high-affinity uptake of glutamate in synaptosomal fractions of pigeon optic tectum, with very similar K_m and V_{max}. He also reported the presence in the tectum of 1.38 μmoles/g wet wt of carnosine and a high-affinity uptake mechanism for norepinephrine. The results of Henke, Schenker, and Cuénod (1976a) were confirmed in the developing chick optic lobe by Bondy and Purdy (1977a), who added serotonin and dopamine to the list of substances taken up with high affinity. Their material, however, was not restricted to the tectal cortex, but included the whole optic lobe. In the adult pigeon tectum, H. Henke confirmed the presence of high-affinity uptake for serotonin (unpublished observations), but not for dopamine. Fuxe and Ljunggren (1965) demonstrated catecholamine terminals in the pigeon optic tectum by histofluorescence.

Therefore, based on high-affinity uptake studies, it appears that glutamate, aspartate, GABA, glycine, norepinephrine, serotonin, and acetylcholine are likely to be involved in synaptic transmission in the avian optic tectum; and there is some evidence that proline plays a role in the cerebellum as an inhibitory transmitter (Felix and Künzle, 1976). Serine and alanine, which do not have established neurotransmitter functions, will be discussed below.

Retinotectal neurons

Of the transmitter candidates that are taken up by high-affinity mechanisms in tectal homogenates, one or more may be concerned with synaptic transmission at the optic-nerve terminals. These terminals are labeled by fast axoplasmic transport of proteins after intravitreous injection of tritiated amino acids (Schonbach, Schonbach, and Cuénod, 1971; Schonbach and Cuénod, 1971). When tectal synaptosomal fractions are prepared under those conditions, they are preferentially labeled, which indicates that pinched-off terminals of the optic nerve contribute to the tectal synaptosomal population (Cuénod and Schonbach, 1971).

Retinal terminals are also selectively labeled following intravitreous injection of HRP (Figure 6A; Streit and Reubi, 1977a). The enzymatic reaction product is found in axonal tubular structures, which in terminals expand to form a network (Figure 6B, C). This system is reminiscent of the smooth endoplasmic reticulum, which was suggested as the intracellular compartment for material migrating under fast anterograde axoplasmic transport (Schonbach, Schonbach, and Cuénod, 1971; Droz, Rambourg, and Koenig, 1975; Markov, Rambourg, and Droz, 1976). The transport compartment outlined by HRP seems

to relate not only to the terminal area but also to the synaptic junction itself, as evidenced by the close apposition of certain vesicular structures (Figure 6D; Streit and Reubi, 1977b).

When the retina is removed, the optic-nerve fibers and terminals degenerate within 4–8 weeks, a relatively long period compared to other systems (Cuénod, Sandri, and Akert, 1970); thus the neuronal uptake compartment originating from the retinal ganglion cells should disappear within this period. The comparison of uptake in optic tecta deafferented of their retinal input and in control tecta should indicate some likely transmitter candidates for the optic nerve. Henke, Schenker, and Cuénod (1976b) observed that 4–8 weeks after retinal ablation, the high-affinity uptake in the whole tectum was decreased for glutamate by 60%, for GABA by 21%, and for proline by 14%; it was increased for glycine by 18% and for choline by 25%. The most striking decrease was for glutamate, where kinetic study revealed a 55% reduction in V_{max} without significant change in apparent K_m. This shows that the capacity of glutamate's high-affinity uptake system was diminished while the remaining uptake sites were unchanged.

These results were confirmed by Bondy and Purdy (1977b) in 23-day-old chicks enucleated at hatch. On the other hand, Beart (1976) detected no change in glutamate level and high-affinity uptake in the pigeon optic tectum 7 days after retinal ablation. Thus it appears that 2–3 weeks of optic-nerve degeneration are needed before a change can be detected in glutamate high-affinity uptake in the tectum. H. Henke and F. Fonnum (unpublished observations) also observed a 28% decrease in the glutamate pool in layer $IId(5)$ after retinal ablation, while the aspartate pool was not significantly altered. Looking at the pool of amino acids in the frog optic tectum, Yates and Roberts (1974) observed a 30% fall in glutamate 14 days after enucleation; for GABA the fall was 20% and 40% after 14 and 24 days, respectively.

Thus, in lower vertebrates, degeneration of the optic-nerve terminals is accompanied by a fall in the high-affinity uptake capacity and the levels of glutamate and, to a lesser extent, GABA. To interpret these results, it is important to estimate the extent to which the changes are related to (1) the degeneration of the optic-nerve fibers and terminals themselves and (2) the transneuronal consequences of this degeneration. Indeed, Hunt and Webster (1975) observed degenerating processes, radially oriented and extending to sublayer $IIh(9)$, 28 days after retinal ablation. Both possibilities might play a role for glu-

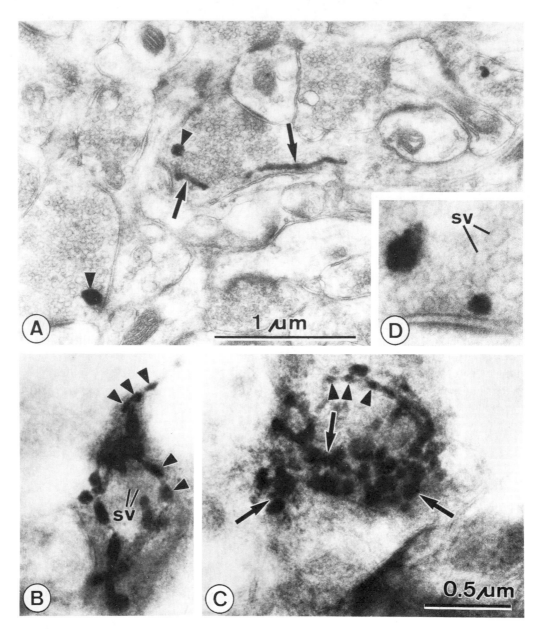

FIGURE 6 Electron micrographs from sublayer IId(5) two days after intraocular injection of HRP. (A) Terminals are labeled with reaction product in tubular (arrows) or vacuolar (arrowheads) structures. These optic endings contain spherical vesicles and make asymmetric synaptic contacts. (Thin section, DAB staining, uranyl block staining.) (B, C) In semithin sections, segmented, labeled profiles (arrowheads) are found to invade the terminal area (sv: synaptic vesicles) and to expand into a network (between the three arrows). (Sections not contrasted with heavy metals. Bar in C applies to B also.) (D) A labeled vesicular element is shown in close apposition with a synaptic junction. (Thin section, no contrast with heavy metals, ×120,000.)

tamate and GABA. However, since (1) glutamate acts as an excitatory and GABA as an inhibitory transmitter in the vertebrate CNS (Curtis and Johnston, 1974) and (2) the retinal input to the optic tectum is thought to be mainly excitatory, it may be assumed that the decrease in glutamate high-affinity uptake is mainly related to the degeneration of the optic-nerve terminals. Consequently, it appears that glutamate either is or mimics the physiological excitatory transmitter of at least part of the optic-nerve fibers. While the possibility that a population of these fibers are using GABA as transmitter cannot be excluded, it is also possible that transneuronal effects of optic-nerve degeneration would explain most of the GABA decrease. As we shall see later, the pigeon optic tectum contains at least three types of neurons that have a special affinity for GABA; however, none of these systems disappear after retinal ablation (Hunt and Künzle, 1976b). It should also be noted that Henke and Fonnum (1976) did not find changes in the laminar concentration of the GABA-synthesizing enzyme glutamic acid decarboxylase (GAD) 4–6 weeks after retinal ablation. Chakrabarti and Daginawala (1976), however, did observe a 12% decrease of GAD in the optic lobe 5–9 weeks after retinal ablation.

We have already mentioned that following intravitreous injection of radioactive leucine or proline, the proteins of the optic-nerve terminals are labeled by fast axoplasmic transport and that the radioactivity appears in synaptosomal fractions. When [^{14}C]-proline is injected into the vitreous body and, 24 hours later, when the endings are maximally labeled, the tectal crude mitochondrial fractions are incubated in [^{3}H]-glutamate, the two isotopes overlap perfectly in the sucrose density gradient region that is richest in synaptosomes. This indicates that glutamate is taken up by organelles having the same sedimentation characteristics as the optic-nerve synaptosomes (Henke, Schenker, and Cuénod, 1976a). Furthermore, using electron-microscopic autoradiography, Beart (1976) was able to show that a subpopulation of tectal synaptosome-like organelles is covered with silver grains after incubation in [^{3}H]-glutamate and that organelles having the same appearance are labeled following intravitreous injection of the precursor. This again suggests that some of the optic-nerve terminals possess a glutamate high-affinity mechanism. Unfortunately, double labeling of the same terminals has not yet succeeded; attempts by J. C. Reubi (unpublished data) to observe a stimulation-induced release of exogenous glutamate with the push-pull cannula technique were similarly inconclusive.

Felix and Frangi (1977) observed that a large number of tectal neurons are activated by microiontophoretic application of glutamate as well as aspartate. This effect was antagonized by L-nuciferine (10–100 nA) in 85% of the cells. Furthermore, the unit activity evoked in the optic tectum by electrical stimulation of the optic nerve was abolished by microiontophoretic application of L-nuciferine but not atropine or dihydro-β-erythroidine (D. Felix, personal communication). Since L-nuciferine has been shown to be a relatively specific blocker of the excitatory effect of glutamate and, to a lesser degree, of aspartate (Felix

and Frangi, 1977), these observations support the hypothesis that glutamate, or an unidentified substance, acts as an excitatory transmitter in the retinotectal pathway.

Could acetylcholine also be a transmitter in the avian optic nerve, as Gruberg and Freeman (1975) have proposed for the frog? This seems unlikely since optic-nerve degeneration does not induce a decrease in choline high-affinity uptake (Henke, Schenker, and Cuénod, 1976b; Bondy and Purdy, 1977b), in choline acetyltransferase levels (Marchisio, 1969; Henke and Fonnum, 1976), in acetylcholinesterase levels (Margolis and Bondy, 1969). Moreover, as mentioned above, microiontophoretic application of muscarinic and nicotinic receptor blockers did not affect the response of tectal neurons to optic-nerve stimulation.

In conclusion, then, we find that the biochemical, physiological, and pharmacological evidence favors glutamate (or a glutamate-like substance) as an excitatory transmitter in the avian retinotectal pathway.

Intratectal inhibitory neurons

GABA   The inhibitory neurotransmitter γ-aminobutyric acid (GABA) plays a prominent role in the avian optic tectum. We have seen that synaptosomes prepared from optic tectum take up GABA with high affinity (Henke, Schenker, and Cuénod, 1976a). The synthesizing enzyme glutamate decarboxylase (GAD) is present in the tectum, particularly in the superficial layers (Henke and Fonnum, 1976). Microiontophoretic application of GABA inhibits large numbers of neurons in the superficial half of the tectum (Barth and Felix, 1974). The intertectal inhibition (Robert and Cuénod, 1969) is antagonized by bicuculline, a specific blocker of GABA receptors (Barth and Felix, 1974).

Hunt and Künzle (1976b) investigated by light-microscopic autoradiography the distribution of [^{3}H]-GABA injected into the tectum. They observed four types of neurons that were labeled by GABA within 30 min. Two seem to be intrinsic tectal neurons, while the two others imply extratectal connections, one afferent, one efferent. This labeling was specific, as indicated by the fact that these neurons were not labeled by DABA or by glycine, alanine, serine, leucine, tyrosine, tryptophan, histidine, lysine, arginine, glutamate, or proline.

INTRINSIC GABA NEURONS   The GABA-labeled neurons of one type are localized in layer IId(5) and in the depth of IIc(6); their arborizations expand horizontally within these layers. At the border of the injection site, large perikarya (20–25µm) with processes extending for distances up to 2 mm are labeled (Figure 7). Golgi pictures of neurons in layer IId(5) reveal similar structures with long horizontal dendrites and very short axons, if any (Figure 1E).

At the electron-microscopic level, after injection of [³H]-GABA, silver grains are found over horizontal profiles characterized by a moderately clear cytoplasm, some axially running microtubules, and slight swellings containing clusters of pleomorphic vesicles at small, symmetric synaptic contacts (Figure 8). Hayes and Webster (1975) and Angaut and Repérant (1976) interpreted such profiles as presynaptic dendrites. Angaut and Repérant (1976) consider them to be the most common vesicle-containing profiles in the superficial tectum. Hayes and Webster (1975) observed triads of synapses in which an optic-nerve terminal is presynaptic to both a radial and a horizontal dendrite and the horizontal dendrite makes a synapse with the radial one (Figure 11). It would thus appear that in sublayers IIc(4) and IId(5) the elements labeled by GABA are long, horizontal dendrites of Golgi type II neurons and that these dendrites contain a large number of presynaptic profiles. By immunocytochemistry, presynaptic dendrites in the rat olfactory bulb have been demonstrated to contain glutamic acid decarboxylase (Ribak et al., 1977). If the membranes of presynaptic dendrites have the same properties as the axonal terminals, it can be assumed that specific uptake of transmitter takes place in such dendrites. Alternatively, the radioactivity could migrate along the dendrites from the neuronal soma. Such a system of horizontal inhibitory neurons—with dendrites both postsynaptic to optic-nerve terminals and presynaptic to radial dendrites (presumably leading to efferent neurons)—would play an essential role in the local circuits of the tectum, possibly for lateral inhibition. There is indeed a strong inhibition following an incoming volley in the optic nerve (Holden, 1968), and Stone and Freeman (1971) have recorded dendritic spikes in the neuropil of the pigeon's optic tectum.

The other intrinsic GABA-labeled neurons have their cell bodies in sublayer IIc(4), with short processes going radially into the depth of layer II (Figure 1F). Once again we find that there are Golgi profiles that correspond to this type of labeling (Hunt and Künzle, 1976b).

EXTRINSIC GABA NEURONS Following [³H]-GABA injections in the tectum, one pattern of silver grains

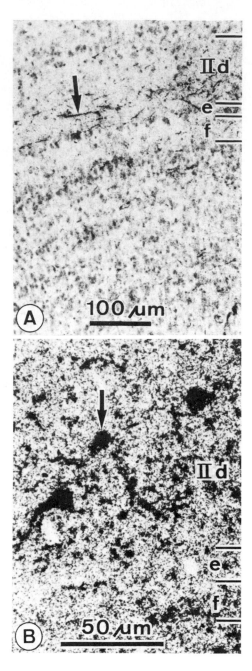

FIGURE 7 Light-field autoradiographs at the margins of an injection site after application of [³H]-GABA (50 µCi in 0.2 µl during 10 min); labeled processes (in A, arrow) and cell bodies (in B) appear in sublayer IId(5). The animal was perfused with 5% glutaraldehyde 20 min after the injection. (A) 50 µm Vibratome slice (cresylecht-violet staining). (B) 1 µm Epon section (no counterstaining; arrow indicates blood vessel).

observed by Hunt and Künzle (1976b) involved cell bodies in sublayer IIi(10) and radial processes in sublayer IIf(7) and layer I(1). Furthermore, the layer I(1) labeling extended rostrally into the pretectum

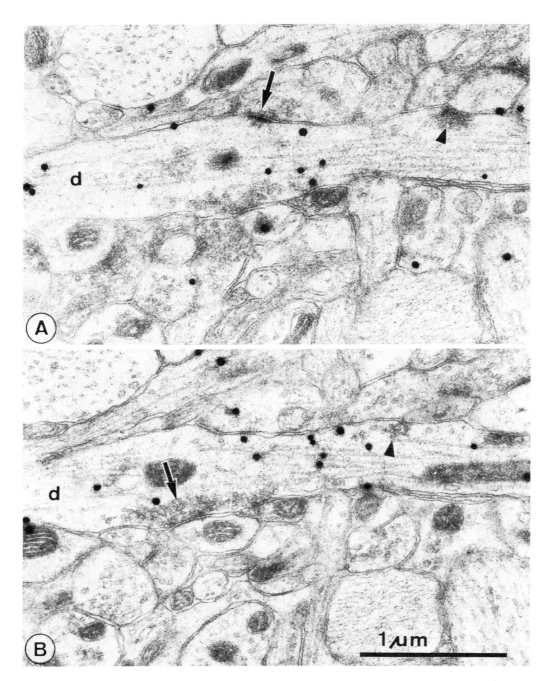

FIGURE 8 Electron micrographs from sublayer IId(5) adjacent to a [³H]-GABA injection. The horizontal profile, probably dendritic (d) and covered by silver grains, is postsynaptic in A (arrow) and presynaptic in B (arrow). Arrowheads indicate accumulations of vesicles. (Serial thin sections from the same material used for Figure 7. Autoradiographs poststained with heavy metals; Ilford L4 emulsion; phenidon physical development.) (From Streit et al., 1978.)

and ventral thalamus, indicating a projection area. When this zone of projection is injected, the same pattern of grains appears in the tectum (Figure 9A). This pattern can be explained by a type of neuron described by Ramón y Cajal (1891) and Ris (1899); its perikaryon lies in sublayer IIi(10), and it has apical and basal dendrites extending radially. The apical dendrite branches in sublayer IIf(7) and terminates in IIa(2); the axon extends from the apical dendrite, forms collaterals in sublayer IIf(7), and leaves the tectum through layer I, presumably reaching the pretectum and ventral thalamus (Figure 1G). Thus, after injection into the zone of termination, [³H]-GABA selectively labels the axons and terminals and mi-

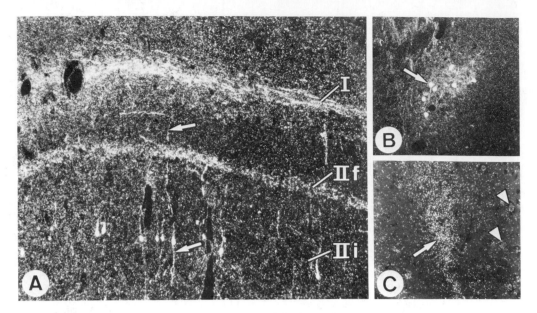

FIGURE 9 Dark-field photomicrograph of a horizontal section through the ventral tectum after injection of [³H]-GABA into the ventral thalamus, with some spread of activity into the underlying optic tract (30 min survival). Label has moved retrogradely to the cell bodies of origin of the layer I(1) pathway within IIi(10) and probably into both the dendrites and the axon collaterals of the system within IIf(7). ×110. (From Hunt and Künzle, 1976b.) (B, C) Dark-field autoradiographs of the Ipc nucleus following injections into the rostral tectum (OT). As shown in B (×60), injection of [³H]-GABA results in perikaryal (arrow) and neuropil labeling in Ipc (30 min survival). As shown in C (×125), injection of [³H]-glycine results in predominantly terminal labeling (arrow), with few grains lying over cells (arrowheads) (26 hr survival). (From Hunt et al., 1977.)

grates in a retrograde manner up to the cell body, filling axon collaterals and dendrites on its way.

It is worth noting that electrical stimulation of the ipsilateral or contralateral tectal surface inhibits the activity evoked in tectal neurons by optic-nerve stimulation. This inhibition is bicuculline-sensitive (Barth and Felix, 1974). It is probably mediated by antidromic or orthodromic activation of the GABA-specific neurons of sublamina IIi(10) that have their collaterals in IIf(7).

Following [³H]-GABA injection into the anterior part of the tectum, a group of intensely labeled cell bodies can be observed in the anterior portion of the Ipc nucleus (Figure 9B). This phenomenon is not observed after injection of [³H]-glycine (Figure 9C). The Ipc nucleus, which has a reciprocal connection with the tectum, sends axons with profuse terminal arborizations in bushes into sublayer IIb(3) and IId(5). Here again one may assume that [³H]-GABA is selectively taken up by the Ipc-tectal axons and terminals, then migrates in a retrograde, somatopetal manner toward the cell bodies in Ipc.

GLYCINE, SERINE, AND ALANINE In the pigeon optic tectum there is evidence that glycine, which is well established as an inhibitory transmitter in the vertebrate spinal cord, plays a special role. Glycine is taken up with high affinity by tectal synaptosomes (Henke, Schenker, and Cuénod, 1976a). Microiontophoretic application of glycine inhibits a large number of units throughout the tectum, and this effect is antagonized by strychnine (Barth and Felix, 1974). Strychnine binding displaced by glycine, as a measure of glycine receptors, is present in the chick optic lobe (Zukin, Young, and Snyder, 1975) and in the pigeon optic tectum (Le Fort, Henke, and Cuénod, 1978). Moreover, exogenous glycine is released in the tectum during electrical stimulation of an afferent pathway (Reubi and Cuénod, 1976).

Following injections of [³H]-glycine, [³H]-serine, or [³H]-α-alanine into the lateral region of the optic tectum, we find, in addition to some neuropil labeling, that the perikarya of neurons within the Ipc nucleus are thoroughly covered by silver grains (Figure 10A, B, C). The labeled zone is topographically related to the reciprocal tectal-Ipc connections, and the labeled perikarya are disposed in a row, forming a small column throughout the dorsoventral axis of the Ipc nucleus. This phenomenon has been observed to last for periods varying from 30 min to 24 hr. The Ipc

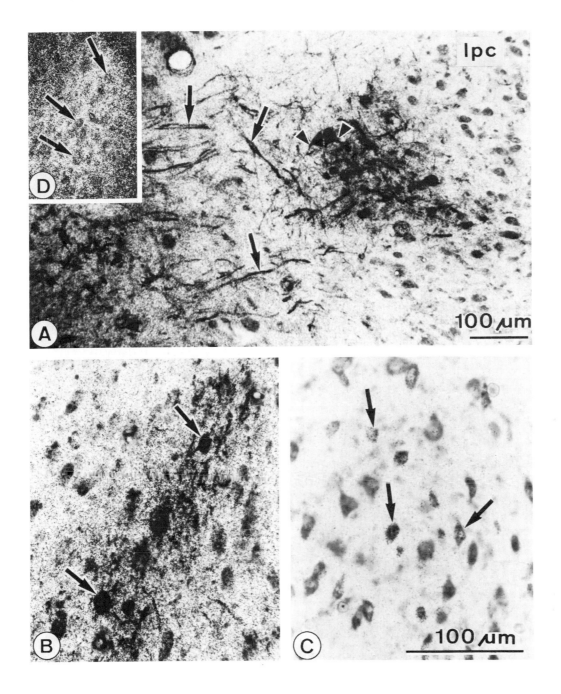

FIGURE 10 (A–C) Light-field autoradiographs of the Ipc nucleus following injections of [³H]-glycine (50 μCi in 0.2 μl during 10 min) into the lateral tectum. (A) Some heavily labeled perikarya are situated in a limited field of labeled neuropil. Note fibrous processes (arrowheads) arising from perikarya and labeled fibers (arrows) in the space between tectum and Ipc. (5% glutaraldehyde perfusion 20 min after injection, 50 μm slice, cresylecht-violet staining.) (B) Higher magnification of the labeled area in Ipc showing heavy perikaryal labeling (arrows) after glutaraldehyde fixation.

(C) After perfusion with 4% formaldchyde, the perikarya, but no fibrous elements, are slightly outlined by silver grains (arrows). The same amount of [³H]-glycine was injected with the same survival and injection times as in A and B. (D) Dark-field autoradiograph showing mainly neuropil labeling in Ipc after tectal injection of [³H]-proline. Note the low density of silver grains over perikarya (arrows) (24 hr survival). The bar in A applies to D also; the bar in C applies to B also. (D from Hunt et al., 1977.)

nucleus is located 3–4 mm from the tectum. By contrast, when tectal injections of tritiated leucine, proline, tyrosine, tryptophan, histidine, lysine, arginine, or glutamic acid are made, only the Ipc neuropil is labeled, not the cell bodies (Figure 10D). (This neuropil labeling with any precursor is probably due to axonal and terminal radioactivity transported in an anterograde, somatofugal manner within the tecto-Ipc neurons.) Injection of [³H]-GABA in the lateral part of the tectum does not lead to labeling of Ipc perikarya. Tectal injection of [³H]-choline, however, gave results very similar to those obtained with glycine, serine, and alanine.

After the glycine injection is given, how does the radioactivity reach the cell bodies in the nucleus Ipc? Diffusion of [³H]-glycine in the tissue followed by an uptake in Ipc neurons can be excluded since the sharp boundary of the population of labeled cell bodies is not compatible with extensive diffusion from the injection site. The radioactivity could be transported somatofugally in the tecto-Ipc pathway, however, and transferred transneuronally from the terminals to the Ipc neurons. Alternatively, it could be picked up by the axons and terminals of the Ipc-tectal pathway and from there migrate in a retrograde, somatopetal manner toward the cell bodies in the Ipc nucleus. To distinguish between these two possibilities, [³H]-glycine can be injected either into the deep tectal layers in the neighborhood of the cell of origin of the tecto-Ipc pathway or into the superficial layers, where the Ipc-tectal pathway terminates. With deep injection, only the Ipc neuropil is heavily labeled; as soon as the injected zone includes the more superficial tectal layers, the perikarya too are covered with silver grains. This suggests that [³H]-glycine is selectively taken up by the distal portions of the Ipc-tectal neurons and that the radioactivity then migrates 3–4 mm toward the cell bodies (Hunt et al., 1977).

Reubi and Cuénod (1976) showed that, after [¹⁴C]- or [³H]-glycine is injected in the superficial tectum, a push-pull cannula placed at the injection site collects radioactive glycine along with the perfusion solution. During electrical stimulation of the Ipc nucleus, the amount of radioactivity collected increases significantly over the resting situation. This suggests that glycine is taken up and then released during activation of the Ipc-tectal neurons, presumably from the loaded terminals. Thus glycine appears to be a transmitter within the Ipc-tectal pathway, or to mimic one. The Ipc-tectal loop could be responsible for delayed inhibition (Figure 11).

As we noted above, the retrograde labeling of Ipc

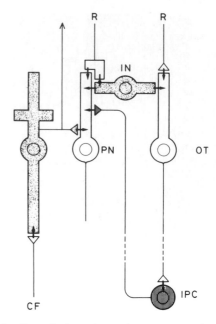

FIGURE 11   Speculative schematic representation of retinal afferents (R) and principal neurons (PN) in the avian optic tectum (OT). An interneuron (IN), GABA-ergic, connects horizontally the dendrites of principal neurons. The Ipc loop, glycine-ergic, and an extrinsic GABA neuron receiving commissural-fiber afferents (CF) are also represented.

neurons is observed after injection of [³H]-glycine, [³H]-serine, or [³H]-α-alanine. Reinvestigation of the uptake characteristics of these three amino acids confirmed that they are all taken up with high affinity by tectal synaptosomes. The serine or alanine uptake is competitively inhibited by glycine, but glycine uptake is only partially inhibited by serine or alanine; this suggests the existence of two glycine compartments: a mixed one, accessible to both serine and alanine, and one for glycine only. Furthermore, a differential distribution of these two compartments is observed in the pigeon CNS: in the spinal cord only the glycine compartment can be detected; in the telencephalon the glycine-serine-alanine compartment is mainly present; and the tectum possesses both compartments. Finally, some glycine derivatives inhibit glycine uptake more than serine or alanine, while cysteine has the opposite effect (Henke and Cuénod, 1978; Cuénod and Henke, 1978). The glycine compartment seems to correspond to nerve endings; we do not yet know the localization of the mixed compartments, but it is tempting to assume that it represents another population of nerve terminals to which the Ipc-tectal neurons would contribute, among others.

We have already noted that degeneration of the retinal afferents leads to a 25% increase in the V_{max}

of the high-affinity glycine uptake, suggesting a pre-synaptic glycinergic enhancement, whereas K_m remains constant. With the same delays, strychnine binding (B_{max}) is decreased by 22% with no change in K_D, indicating a drop in the amount of glycine receptors (Le Fort, Henke, and Cuénod, 1978). These two sets of observations could be explained as follows: A glycinergic input would impinge on retinal afferents or on neurons postsynaptic to retinal afferents. When the retinal afferents degenerate, or when their postsynaptic elements degenerate transneuronally (as suggested by Hunt and Webster, 1975), the glycine receptor would likewise be affected. Then the glycinergic terminals, missing their corresponding postsynaptic receptors, would tend to sprout, thus inducing an enhanced glycine high-affinity uptake.

In conclusion, there is good evidence favoring a specificity for glycine, serine, and alanine within part of the Ipc-tectal pathway.

Somatopetal migration of transmitter amino acids

Retrograde labeling of specific neurons has been described above both for GABA and for glycine, serine, and alanine. These observations suggest that an amino acid transmitter taken up specifically by the terminal axon migrates toward the cell body; there it could possibly deliver a message concerning the state of the ending. Although this suggestion is highly speculative, its potential significance makes it worth discussing briefly.

Where does the specific capture of GABA or glycine, serine, and α-alanine occur? At the moment it is difficult to give a clear-cut answer to this question. On the one hand, it is tempting to suggest the nerve terminals, which are known to be the seat of specific high-affinity uptake mechanisms. Synaptosomes prepared from the optic tectum take up GABA, glycine, serine, and α-alanine with high affinity, and there is good evidence that glycine is implied in the Ipc-tectal pathway. On the other hand, it is striking that application of the tritiated amino acids always implies a lesion in the tectum and consequently in the fibers that are selectively labeled. There is a rough correlation between the size of the lesion in the tectum and the population of labeled Ipc neurons; its columnar organization could reflect the tract of the injection needle. One wonders, therefore, whether a lesion is essential to reveal the specific uptake properties of the neuronal membrane: perhaps the membrane has to be freed from protecting glial cells, or

perhaps the membrane sealing off the cut end of an axon is particularly well-endowed with an uptake capacity. We should remember that the transmitter high-affinity uptake concept rests almost entirely on experiments with synaptosomes obtained by homogenization of the tissue (for the biochemical approach) and with autoradiographs of slices (for morphological localization). In both cases the axons are by definition disturbed. The uptake experiments made with tissue cultures also create an unphysiological situation. Only evidence coming from the retina in situ after intraocular injection of precursor is immune to this type of criticism. Nonetheless, whatever the site and mechanism of capture of the labeled amino acid, it remains evident that it has some specificity: in the case of the Ipc-tectal neuron, glycine, serine, and α-alanine are picked up only in the lateral tectum, whereas GABA is absorbed exclusively in the anterior tectum; in the case of the IIi(10) efferent neuron projecting to the pretectum, only GABA is labeling it after retrograde migration.

In what form is the radioactivity transported toward the cell body? Although no chemical analysis of the labeled material in the axons and cell bodies is available, the results after various types of fixation do give some definite indications. The silver-grain density is much higher when the animal is perfused with glutaraldehyde, which fixes the amino acids as well as the macromolecules, than with formaldehyde, which fixes macromolecules only (Figure 10B, C). Furthermore, with formaldehyde fixation, only the profiles of cell bodies are revealed by the silver grains, whereas the profiles of axons, dendrites, and cell bodies are disclosed by glutaraldehyde fixation (P. Streit, unpublished). Thus it is likely that the radioactivity taken up with amino acids in the distal part of the neuron remains in a soluble form during its somatopetal migration. Once in the perikaryon, it will label the pool of amino acids and appear later in the macromolecules.

Nothing is known about the mechanisms involved in this migration. The time period (30 min to travel 3–4 mm) is compatible with the speed reported for the retrograde transport. It should be noted that the length of the path in which migration has been observed never exceeds a few millimeters. This relatively short distance makes it difficult to exclude the possibility of diffusion. Subtectal injections of vinblastine, in doses known to block axoplasmic transport, prevented the labeling of Ipc perikarya after tectal application of [³H]-glycine (S. P. Hunt, unpublished). Although it suggests the existence of an active retrograde axoplasmic transport, this observation is not conclusive, for the drug itself may also have interfered with the uptake.

The finding of retrogradely labeled perikarya in the nucleus raphe dorsalis after [³H]-serotonin strial injection (Leger et al., 1977) suggests that retrograde labeling can be generalized to other transmitters. Künzle (1977) observed a retrograde labeling of cell bodies in the monkey nucleus ruber and cortex 3 days after [³H]-proline injection in the spinal cord, but not after [³H]-leucine application. Proline is by no means an established neurotransmitter, but there are indications in favor of such a role. Differential uptake of proline has been observed in the cat lateral reticular nucleus of the brain stem and in the cerebellar cortex (Künzle and Cuénod, 1973; Felix and Künzle, 1974); and microiontophoretic application of proline to Purkinje cerebellar cells has an inhibitory effect (Felix and Künzle, 1976). Thus Künzle's observation might belong to the category of phenomena in which small molecules are taken up in the distal part of a neuron and migrate toward the cell body.

Retrograde, somatopetal axoplasmic transport has been postulated for a long time (Morax and Marie, 1903; Lubińska, 1964), and it has been established by Kristensson (1970, 1975) for foreign substances such as Evans blue and horseradish peroxidase. Stöckel and Thoenen (1975) have shown that there is a retrograde somatopetal transport of nerve growth factor in adrenergic nerves from the terminal zone in the iris to the cell bodies in the superior cervical ganglion. Stöckel, Schwab, and Thoenen (1975) have established the retrograde transport of tetanus toxin from the neuromuscular junction to the motoneurons. Thus many macromolecules, once they are taken up in the axon, appear later on in the soma. Nerve growth factor is known to have an important functional role in adrenergic neurons, promoting the synthesis of specific enzymes such as tyrosine hydroxylase and dopamine-β-hydroxylase. The other macromolecules are nonfunctional or pathological. It might turn out to be highly significant if some of the transmitters or their metabolites specifically picked up in the terminal zone migrate back to the cell body, which would thus be informed about physiological events taking place at their endings.

ACKNOWLEDGMENTS The authors are grateful to Dr. H. Henke for valuable advice and to E. Knecht, D. Savini, E. Schneider, and M. Jäckli for excellent technical assistance. This work was supported by Grants 3.744.76 and 3.636.75 from the Swiss National Science Foundation, the Dr. Eric Slack-Gyr Foundation, the Emil Barrel Foundation, and the Stiftung für wissenschaftliche Forschung der Universität Zürich.

REFERENCES

ANGAUT, P., and J. REPÉRANT, 1976. Fine structure of the optic fibre termination layers in the pigeon optic tectum: A Golgi and electron microscope study. *Neuroscience* 1:93–105.

BARTH, R., and D. FELIX, 1974. Influence of GABA and glycine and their antagonists on inhibitory mechanisms of pigeon's optic tectum. *Brain Res.* 80:532–537.

BEART, P. M., 1976. An evaluation of L-glutamate as the transmitter release from optic nerve terminals of the pigeon. *Brain Res.* 110:99–114.

BONDY, S. C., and J. L. PURDY, 1977a. Development of neurotransmitter uptake in regions of the chick brain. *Brain Res.* 119:403–416.

BONDY, S. C., and J. L. PURDY, 1977b. Putative neurotransmitters of the avian visual pathway. *Brain Res.* 119:417–426.

CHAKRABARTI, T., and H. F. DAGINAWALA, 1976. Effect of unilateral visual deprivation and visual stimulation on the activities of glutamate decarboxylase, GABA-α ketoglutarate transaminase, aspartate aminotransferase and hexokinase of the optic lobe of the adult pigeon. *J. Neurochem.* 27:273–276.

COWAN, W. M., L. ADAMSON, and T. P. S. POWELL, 1961. An experimental study of the avian visual system. *J. Anat.* 95:545–563.

CUÉNOD, M., and H. HENKE, 1978. Neurotransmitters in the avian visual system. In *Amino Acids as Chemical Transmitters*, F. Fonnum, ed. New York: Plenum Press, pp. 221–239.

CUÉNOD, M., C. SANDRI, and K. AKERT, 1970. Enlarged synaptic vesicles as an early sign of secondary degeneration in the optic-nerve terminals of the pigeon. *J. Cell Sci.* 6:605–613.

CUÉNOD, M., and J. SCHONBACH, 1971. Synaptic proteins and axonal flow in the pigeon visual pathway. *J. Neurochem.* 18:809–816.

CURTIS, D. R., and G. A. JOHNSTON, 1974. Amino acid transmitters in the mammalian central nervous system. *Ergeb. Physiol.* 69:97–188.

DROZ, B., A. RAMBOURG, and H. L. KOENIG, 1975. The smooth endoplasmic reticulum: structure and role in the renewal of axonal membrane and synaptic vesicles by fast axonal transport. *Brain Res.* 93:1–13.

FELIX, D., and U. FRANGI, 1977. Dimethoxyaporphine as an antagonist of chemical excitation in the pigeon optic tectum. *Neurosci. Lett.* 4:347–350.

FELIX, D., and H. KÜNZLE, 1974. Iontophoretic and autoradiographic studies on the role of proline in nervous transmission. *Pflügers Arch.* 350:135–144.

FELIX, D., and H. KÜNZLE, 1976. The role of proline in nervous transmission. *Adv. Biochem. Psychopharmacol.* 15:165–173.

FUXE, K., and L. LJUNGGREN, 1965. Cellular localization of monoamines in the upper brain stem of the pigeon. *J. Comp. Neurol.* 125:355–382.

GRUBERG, E. R., and J. A. FREEMAN, 1975. Localization of acetylcholinesterase and synthesis of ACh in amphibian optic tectum. *Trans. Am. Soc. Neurochem.* 6:129.

HAYES, B. P., and K. E. WEBSTER, 1975. An electron microscope study of the retino-receptive layers of the pigeon optic tectum. *J. Comp. Neurol.* 162:447–466.

HENKE, H., and M. CUÉNOD, 1978. Uptake of L-alanine, glycine and L-serine in the pigeon central nervous system. *Brain Res.* 152:105–119.

HENKE, H., and F. FONNUM, 1976. Topographical and subcellular distribution of choline acetyltransferase and glutamate decarboxylase in pigeon optic tectum. *J. Neurochem.* 27:387–391.

HENKE, H., T. M. SCHENKER, and M. CUÉNOD, 1976a. Uptake of neurotransmitter candidates by pigeon optic tectum. *J. Neurochem.* 26:125–130.

HENKE, H., T. M. SCHENKER, and M. CUÉNOD, 1976b. Effects of retinal ablation on uptake of glutamate, glycine, GABA, proline and choline in pigeon tectum. *J. Neurochem.* 26:131–134.

HIRSCHBERGER, W., 1971. Vergleichend experimentell-histologische Untersuchung zur retinalen Repräsentation in den primären visuellen Zentren einiger Vogelarten. Thesis, J. W. Goethe-Universität, Frankfurt a.M.

HÖKFELT, T., and A. LJUNGDAHL, 1975. Uptake mechanisms as a basis for the histochemical identification and tracing of transmitter-specific neuron populations. In *The Use of Axonal Transport for Studies of Neuronal Connectivity*, W. M. Cowan and M. Cuénod, eds. Amsterdam: Elsevier, pp. 249–305.

HOLDEN, A. L., 1968. Types of unitary response and correlation with the field potential profile during activation of the avian optic tectum. *J. Physiol.* 194:91–104.

HUNT, S. P., and H. KÜNZLE, 1976a. Observations on the projections and intrinsic organization of the pigeon optic tectum: An autoradiographic study based on anterograde and retrograde, axonal and dendritic flow. *J. Comp. Neurol.* 170:153–172.

HUNT, S. P., and H. KÜNZLE, 1976b. Selective uptake and transport of label within three identified neuronal systems after injection of [³H]-GABA into the pigeon optic tectum: An autoradiographic and Golgi study. *J. Comp. Neurol.* 170:173–190.

HUNT, S. P., P. STREIT, H. KÜNZLE, and M. CUÉNOD, 1977. Characterization of the pigeon isthmo-tectal pathway by selective uptake and retrograde movement of radioactive compounds and by Golgi-like horseradish peroxidase labeling. *Brain Res.* 129:197–212.

HUNT, S. P., and K. E. WEBSTER, 1975. The projection of the retina upon the optic tectum of the pigeon. *J. Comp. Neurol.* 162:433–446.

IVERSEN, L. L., 1971. Role of transmitter uptake mechanisms in synaptic neurotransmission. *Br. J. Pharmacol.* 41:571–591.

IVERSEN, L. L., F. DICK, J. S. KELLY, and F. SCHON, 1975. Uptake and localisation of transmitter amino acids in the nervous system. In *Metabolic Compartmentation and Neurotransmission*, S. Berl, D. D. Clarke, and D. Schneider, eds. New York: Plenum Press, pp. 65–87.

KARTEN, H. J., 1969. The organization of the avian telencephalon and some speculations on the phylogeny of the amniote telencephalon. *Ann. NY Acad. Sci.* 167:164–179.

KRISTENSSON, K., 1970. Transport of fluorescent protein tracer in peripheral nerves. *Acta Neuropathol.* 16:293–300.

KRISTENSSON, K., 1975. Retrograde axonal transport of protein tracers. In *The Use of Axonal Transport for Studies of Neuronal Connectivity*, W. M. Cowan and M. Cuénod, eds. Amsterdam: Elsevier, pp. 70–82.

KÜNZLE, H., 1977. Evidence for selective axon-terminal uptake and retrograde transport of label in cortico- and rubrospinal systems after injection of [³H]-proline. *Exp. Brain Res.* 28:125–132.

KÜNZLE, H., and M. CUÉNOD, 1973. Differential uptake of [³H]-proline and [³H]-leucine by neurons: its importance for the autoradiographic tracing of pathways. *Brain Res.* 62:213–217.

LAVAIL, J. H., and W. M. COWAN, 1971a. The development of the chick optic tectum: I. Normal morphology and cytoarchitectonic development. *Brain Res.* 28:391–419.

LAVAIL, J. H., and W. M. COWAN, 1971b. The development of the chick optic tectum: II. Autoradiographic studies. *Brain Res.* 28:421–441.

LE FORT, D., H. HENKE, and M. CUÉNOD, 1978. Glycine specific [³H] strychnine binding in the pigeon CNS. *J. Neurochem.* 30:1287–1291.

LEGER, L., J. F. PUJOL, P. BOBILLIER, and M. JOUVET, 1977. Transport axoplasmique de la sérotonine par voie retrograde dans les neurones monoaminergiques centraux. *C. R. Acad. Sci. (Paris)* 285:1179–1182.

LOGAN, W. J., and S. H. SNYDER, 1971. Unique high affinity uptake systems for glycine, glutamic and aspartic acids in central nervous tissue of the rat. *Nature* 234:297–299.

LUBIŃSKA, L., 1964. Axoplasmic streaming in regenerating and in normal nerve fibres. In *Mechanisms of Neural Regeneration (Prog. Brain Res. 13)*, M. Singer and J. P. Schadé, eds. Amsterdam: Elsevier, pp. 1–71.

MARCHISIO, P. C., 1969. Choline acetyltransferase activity in developing chick optic centres and the effects of monolateral removal of retina to an early embryonic stage and at hatching. *J. Neurochem.* 16:665–671.

MARGOLIS, F. L., and S. C. BONDY, 1969. Unilateral visual deprivation and avian optic lobe development. *Life Sci.* 8:1195–1199.

MARKOV, D., A. RAMBOURG, and B. DROZ, 1976. Smooth endoplasmic reticulum and fast axonal transport of glycoproteins, an electron microscope radioautographic study of thick sections after heavy metals impregnation. *J. Microsc. Biol. Cell.* 25:57–60.

MEIER, R. E., J. MIHAILOVIC, and M. CUÉNOD, 1974. Thalamic organization of the retino-thalamo-hyperstriatal pathway in the pigeon (Columba livia). *Exp. Brain Res.* 19:351–364.

MORAX, V., and A. MARIE, 1903. Recherches sur l'absorption de la toxine tétanique. *Ann. Inst. Pasteur* 17:335–342.

NAUTA, W. J. H., and H. J. KARTEN, 1970. A general profile of the vertebrate brain with sidelights on the ancestry of cerebral cortex. In *The Neurosciences: Second Study Program*, F. O. Schmitt, ed. New York: Rockefeller Univ. Press, pp. 7–26.

RAMÓN Y CAJAL, S., 1891. Sur la fine structure du lobe optique des oiseaux et sur l'origine réelle des nerfs optiques. *Int. Mschr. Anat. Physiol.* 8:337–366.

REPÉRANT, J., 1973. Nouvelles données sur les projections visuelles chez le pigeon (Columba livia). *J. Hirnforsch.* 14:151–187.

REUBI, J. C., and M. CUÉNOD, 1976. Release of exogenous glycine in the pigeon optic tectum during stimulation of a midbrain nucleus. *Brain Res.* 112:347–361.

RIBAK, C. E., J. E. VAUGHN, K. SAITO, R. BARBER, and E. ROBERTS, 1977. Glutamate decarboxylase localization in neurons of the olfactory bulb. *Brain Res.* 126:1–18.

RIS, F., 1899. Ueber den Bau des Lobus opticus der Vögel. In *Archiv für Mikroskopische Anatomie une Entwicklungsgeschichte*, vol. 53, O. Hertwig, v. la Valette St. George, and W. Waldeyer, eds. Verlag von Friedrich Cohen, pp. 106–130.

ROBERT, F., and M. CUÉNOD, 1969. Electrophysiology of the intertectal commissures in the pigeon: II. Inhibitory interaction. *Exp. Brain Res.* 9:123–136.

SCHONBACH, J., and M. CUÉNOD, 1971. Axoplasmic migration of protein: A light microscopic autoradiographic study in the avian retino-tectal pathway. *Exp. Brain Res.* 12:275–282.

SCHONBACH, J., C. SCHONBACH, and M. CUÉNOD, 1971. Rapid phase of axoplasmic flow and synaptic proteins: An electron microscopical autoradiographic study. *J. Comp. Neurol.* 141:485–498.

SMITH, B. H., and G. W. KREUTZBERG, 1976. Neuron-target cell interactions. *Neurosci. Res. Program Bull.* 14:209–453.

SNYDER, S. H., H. I. YAMAMURA, C. B. PERT, W. J. LOGAN, and J. P. BENNETT, 1973. Neuronal uptake of neurotransmitters and their precursors in studies with "transmitter" amino acids and choline. In *New Concepts in Neurotransmitter Regulation*, A. J. Mandell, ed. New York: Plenum Press, pp. 195–222.

STÖCKEL, K., M. SCHWAB, and H. THOENEN, 1975. Comparison between the retrograde axonal transport of nerve growth factor and tetanus toxin in motor, sensory and adrenergic neurons. *Brain Res.* 99:1–16.

STÖCKEL, K., and H. THOENEN, 1975. Retrograde axonal transport of nerve growth factor: specificity and biological importance. *Brain Res.* 85:337–341.

STONE, J., and J. A. FREEMAN, 1971. Synaptic organisation of the pigeon's optic tectum; a Golgi and current source-density analysis. *Brain Res.* 27:203–221.

STREIT, P., and J. C. REUBI, 1977a. A new and sensitive staining method for axonally transported horseradish peroxidase (HRP) in the pigeon visual system. *Brain Res.* 126:530–537.

STREIT, P., and J. C. REUBI, 1977b. Synaptic localization of anterogradely transported horseradish peroxidase. *Experientia* 33:785.

STREIT, P., E. KNECHT, J.-C. REUBI, S. P. HUNT, and M. CUÉNOD, 1978. GABA-specific presynaptic dendrites in pigeon optic tectum: A high resolution autoradiographic study. *Brain Res.* 149:204–210.

VAN GEHUCHTEN, A., 1892. La structure des lobes optiques chez l'embryon du poulet. *Cellule* 8:1–43.

WEBSTER, K. E., 1974. Changing concepts of the organization of the central visual pathways in birds. In *Essays on the Nervous System*, R. Bellairs and E. G. Gray, eds. Oxford: Clarendon Press, pp. 258–298.

YATES, R. A., and P. J. ROBERTS, 1974. Effects of enucleation and intra-ocular colchicine on the amino acids of frog optic tectum. *J. Neurochem.* 23:891–893.

ZUKIN, S. R., A. B. YOUNG, and S. H. SNYDER, 1975. Development of the synaptic glycine receptor in chick embryo spinal cord. *Brain Res.* 83:525–530.

60 Adenosine Transport, Release, and Possible Action

G. W. KREUTZBERG and P. SCHUBERT

ABSTRACT Intraneuronal transport of adenosine or its TCA-soluble derivatives, as well as their release from axon terminals and transfer to postsynaptic cells, seems to be a rather general phenomenon in central neurons. Synaptic stimulation increases release and transfer, as demonstrated in the entorhinohippocampal projection. Adenine nucleotides released from terminals should undergo enzymatic degradation to yield the biologically active and membrane-permeable adenosine. A crucial enzyme in this process is 5′-nucleotidase. Cytochemically this enzyme is localized in plasma membranes of astrocytes in juxtasynaptic and perivascular positions.

The findings agree with the concept that adenosine is a neuronal modulator that is released in relation to nerve-cell activity along with the principal neurotransmitter. A broad range of actions of adenosine is seen in the CNS: stimulation of cAMP synthesis, depression of nerve-cell electrical activity, interference with Ca^{++} fluxes and with presynaptic transmitter release. By its vasodilatory action adenosine may regulate local blood supply. Since adenosine-induced cAMP increase is potentiated by monoamines, an integrated action with monoaminergic inputs from the central core seems possible.

Introduction

THERE IS GROWING evidence that transmission of the bioelectrical signal at the synapse is a highly complex event. It involves far more than changes in membrane conductance and ion fluxes induced by the release of a specific neurotransmitter. It is accompanied by the release of other molecular signals acting as cotransmitters, as modulators, or as neurohumoral agents. A considerable number of such substances belonging to the families of amino acids, amines, purines, or hormones have been identified as putative transmitters in recent years. Although we are far from understanding the complex action of these molecular signals, a few functions can already be delineated: tuning of neurons by changing the setting point; modulation of membrane properties leading to long-lasting effects; and alteration of the metabolism of the target cell, for instance, by enzyme induction, RNA and protein synthesis, or other changes commonly classified as trophic effects. Most frequently the effect on the neuronal target cell is mediated by second messengers, that is, cyclic nucleotides or Ca^{++}, and the modulator appears to act as a first messenger.

The formation of the second messenger seems to be a critical point at which different effects of neurotransmitters or modulators interfere with each other. Cooperative actions can potentiate or attenuate the effects leading to the amplification or depression of a transmitter action. In this connection there is increasing evidence that adenosine and other adenine derivatives may play an important role as molecular signals in intercellular communication in the nervous system (McIlwain, 1974).

This concept is based mainly on the following points: Like other neurohumoral agents (noradrenaline or histamine), adenosine increases cAMP formation in cerebral tissues (Sattin and Rall, 1970). Most likely an adenosine-activated adenylate cyclase is involved in this reaction, and it can be assumed that this effect is mediated by an adenosine receptor in the nerve-cell membrane (Shimizu and Daly, 1970; Sattin and Rall, 1970; Schultz and Daly, 1973). Adenosine-elicited effects on cAMP formation can be observed ubiquitously in the brain and even in cultures of nerve cells or glial cells (Clarke and Gross, 1974; Schultz and Hamprecht, 1973).

It seems clear that a substance such as adenosine, which increases cAMP very effectively, can be used to alter a variety of cellular processes. This includes metabolic changes ranging from enzyme induction to changes in membrane properties by the phosphorylation of appropriate proteins. The effects of a substance having such a powerful action are most probably dependent on its compartmentation. In particular, its formation by either de novo synthesis or by enzymatic degradation of nucleotides, its localization and translocation, and its release and inacti-

G. W. KREUTZBERG and P. SCHUBERT Max Planck Institute for Psychiatry, Kraepelinstrasse 2, 8000 Munich 40, Federal Republic of Germany

vation must be closely related to the structural components of the CNS. There is indeed a wealth of information on the distribution and concentration of adenosine and adenine nucleotides in the brain. K_m values of enzymes involved in adenosine metabolism are well known. They indicate the main routes that purine metabolism takes in the brain.

However, these quantitative data must be correlated with morphological data. From such studies an answer could be expected to questions as to how and where adenosine or its derivatives are formed and transported, released and transferred. Intracellular and intercellular translocation of these neurohumoral agents seems to be an important prerequisite to bringing the molecular signals into action. Therefore, one way to learn more about the functional dynamics of adenosine derivatives was to study their axonal, dendritic, and transneuronal transport.

Experimental evidence for transport and transfer of adenosine and derivatives

Most of our data concerning the intraneuronal transport and the release of [³H]-adenosine derivatives from neurons are derived from autoradiographic studies. Following the injection of [³H]-adenosine into brain tissue, the majority of nucleosides are found incorporated into TCA-soluble material, that is, ATP and its derivatives. When fresh tissue is analyzed, 92% of the radioactivity is recovered from the TCA-soluble fraction. Only about 8% of the radioactivity is TCA-insoluble; this represents mainly RNA. Tissue that has been processed through the histological procedure for autoradiography still contains a fraction of 10–20% of the TCA-soluble compounds (Schubert and Kreutzberg, 1975c). They can be visualized in the autoradiographs together with the macromolecular material.

TRANSPORT AND RELEASE FROM DENDRITES   Transport in and release from dendrites were studied on the cellular level in cat spinal motoneurons using the single-cell injection technique (Schubert and Kreutzberg, 1975b). Site and effect of injection were checked and recorded by electrophysiological methods. [³H]-adenosine derivatives are transported in dendrites at a fast rate of at least 3 mm per hour and also reach a high concentration in the peripheral branches of the dendritic tree (Figure 1B). In the same experiments a fast axonal transport of adenosine derivatives can also be observed (Figure 1C). A considerable amount of the transported material, probably the membrane-permeable nucleoside, is re-

leased from the dendrites as indicated by the presence of labeled glial cells (Figure 1B). Also the blood vessels within the extension area of the dendritic tree are reached by the released compounds. Adenosine accumulates here, as demonstrated after local injection and after blocking RNA synthesis.

In this context it is interesting to note that adenosine has been shown to influence the vascular tonus (Berne, Rubio, and Curnish, 1974; Berne et al., 1976). Vasodilatation is actually the longest-known effect of adenosine. It is assumed that vasodilatation is caused by a Ca^{++}-mediated effect on contractile elements of the vascular cells (Schrader, Rubio, and Berne, 1975). Through its release, the neurons may gain control of vascular function and thereby influence local blood supply (Schubert and Kreutzberg, 1976). A regulation of local blood flow related to nerve-cell function is indicated by clinical and experimental observations (Ingvar, 1973; Kato, Veno, and Black, 1974).

ORTHOGRADE TRANSPORT AND RELEASE FROM AXONS The transneuronal release of adenosine derivatives from axon terminals to target neurons has been studied in more detail in the rat entorhinohippocampal system (Schubert et al., 1976, 1977). The termination of entorhinal axons in a defined layer on the hippocampal granule-cell dendrites allows recognition of pre- and postsynaptic areas and quantitative analysis of the transfer. Within 18 hours after injection of [³H]-adenosine into the medial entorhinal cortex, radioactivity is found in both the area of axonal termination and the granule-cell layer (Figure 2). The fiber anatomy (one-way projection) rules out labeling by retrograde transport. Thus the findings strongly indicate that transported [³H]-adenosine derivatives are released from the entorhinal axon terminals, are taken up by the granule-cell dendrites, and accumulate in the soma of these hippocampal target neurons (see also Figures 3 and 4). There is also a minor but definite release from the axons all along the way from the originating neurons down to the target areas. This is indicated by the presence of labeled glial cells. But the amount released seems to be too low to be demonstrated in single axons after intracellular injection.

Adenosine transport and transfer has also been studied in an invertebrate preparation with electrotonic axoaxonal junctions (unpublished data by Rieske and Hermann). If [³H]-adenosine is injected into the lateral giant axon (LGA) of the crayfish, radioactivity spreads quickly in orthograde and retrograde direction within the axon. It also passes the

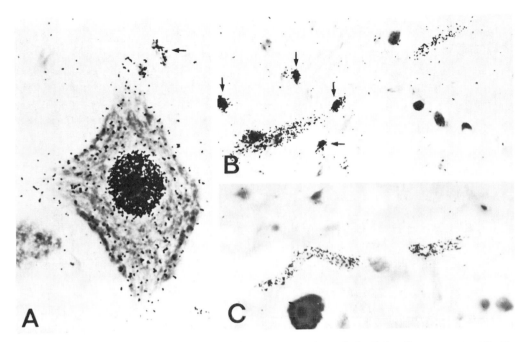

FIGURE 1 Intraneuronal transport of [³H]-adenosine derivatives in a cat spinal motoneuron after intracellular iontophoresis. (A) Somal injection site (×670). (B) Transport in a dendrite (×430); some of the transported radioactive nucleoside derivatives are released as indicated by the presence of labeled glial cells (arrows). (C) Transport in the axon (×430); no obvious release. Autoradiographs, counterstained with toluidine blue, 4 hr after injection. (From Schubert and Kreutzberg, 1975b.)

septate junction to the next segment of the LGA and reaches the nerve-cell perikaryon retrogradely. Interestingly, this axoaxonic transfer of adenosine at an electrotonic synapse depends on the presence of Ca⁺⁺. Experiments performed in a Ca⁺⁺-free, EGTA-containing bath demonstrate no transjunctional flux of radioactivity.

RETROGRADE AXONAL TRANSPORT In addition to an anterograde transneuronal transfer of adenosine derivatives, adenosine has been shown to be effectively taken up by central terminals and to be transported along to the neuronal perikaryon (Hunt and Künzle, 1976; Kruger and Sapporta, 1977; Wise and Jones, 1976).

Such an uptake and transport of adenosine also seems to exist at the neuromuscular junction and in mammalian motor nerve (Figure 5). Thus injection of [³H]-adenosine into the laryngical musculature results in a labeling of the motoneurons in the ambiguous nucleus (Jürgens and Schubert, in preparation).

Synaptic activity (stimulation) and release of adenosine derivatives

The recovery of adenosine derivatives from superfusates of brain slices after electrical stimulation was first demonstrated by Pull and McIlwain (1972). Later, a diffuse release from brain cortex previously exposed to [³H]-adenosine was shown to also occur in vivo (Sulakhe and Phillis, 1975). Yet it remained unclear from which structures this release might have occurred, and also what the target cells were for such molecular signals. These questions were approached by studying the effect of an electrophysiogically controlled synaptic stimulation on the release of adenosine derivatives from axon terminals to postsynaptic neurons (Schubert et al., 1976). Again using the entorhinohippocampal system of the rat, [³H]-adenosine was injected into the entorhinal cortex, a stimulation electrode was inserted, and the perforant axons were stimulated by suprathreshold current pulses of 1–8 Hz for 18 hours. During this period the postsynaptic potentials evoked in the hippocampal granule cells were continuously recorded in the awake and freely moving animal. Then the amount of radioactivity in the TCA-soluble material collected separately from the microdissected pre- and postsynaptic areas of the hippocampal dentate gyrus was measured in a scintillation counter. Stimulation of the perforant axons was found to increase the transfer of the TCA-soluble [³H]-adenosine derivatives from the axon terminals to the postsynaptic granule cells by some 40% as compared to unstimulated con-

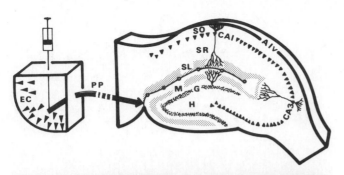

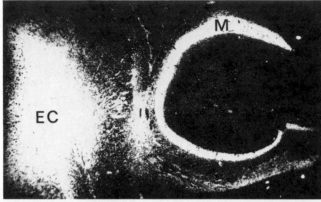

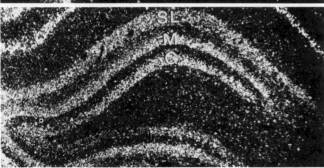

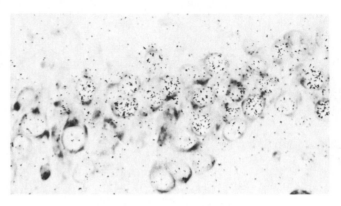

FIGURE 3 Selective accumulation of silver grains in the somas of the CA1 neurons following [³H]-adenosine injection into the entorhinal cortex indicates a transneuronal transfer to these hippocampal target neurons. (Autoradiograph, counterstained with toluidine blue, ×600. From Schubert et al., 1977.)

was found to be increased by about 300% in response to electrical stimulation (100 pulses), and the content of the preparations was diminished by 1.5% per minute (Barberis and McIlwain, 1976).

Specificity of adenosine derivatives

A purinergic system with ATP as an inhibitory transmitter has been described in the peripheral nervous system by Burnstock (1972). Is there any evidence for an analogous system in brain or spinal cord? This question is still open, but from transport studies it is suggested that nucleotide release occurs rather generally in functionally different tracts. Transport and release of adenosine derivatives from axon terminals is seen, for instance, in the afferent system to the rat hippocampus described above, in various pathways of the visual system such as the corticothalamic projection in the rabbit (Schubert and Kreutzberg, 1974, 1975a), in the retinotectal and tectothalamic fibers of the pigeon (Hunt and Künzle, 1976), and in pathways originating in the somatosensory cortex of the rat (Wise and Jones, 1976). A release of adenosine derivatives to target neurons was also found in the septal afferents to the hippocampus (Rose and Schubert, 1977). Since these septal fibers have been convincingly shown to be cholinergic, the finding indicates that the adenosine derivatives are released in addition to the principal transmitter, as is the case for monoaminergic and cholinergic peripheral nerves (Geffen and Livett, 1971; Silinsky and Hubbard, 1973). Thus the release of adenosine derivatives seems to be a rather general principle in the nervous system.

FIGURE 2 Transfer of adenosine derivatives in the entorhinohippocampal system. *Top*: The neurons of the medial entorhinal cortex (EC, injection site) send their axons via the perforant pathway (pp) to the hippocampus. They terminate within the shaded area on the dendrites of the target neurons, that is, in the middle molecular layer (M), on the granule cells (G), and in the stratum lacunosum moleculare (SL), on the CA1 and CA3 pyramidal cells. (H, hilus; SR, stratum radiatum; SO, stratum oriens; Alv, alveus. *Middle*: Control experiment: 24 hr after [³H]-leucine injection into EC, there is transport into axon terminals (M) but no label in the granule cells. *Bottom*: 24 hr after [³H]-adenosine injection into EC, labeling is seen in G, in addition to M and SL, indicating a release from the axon terminals to the granule cells. (Dark-field autoradiographs: B is a horizontal section, ×21; C is a frontal section, ×50. From Schubert et al., 1977.)

trols. The increase in the amount released is certainly higher, since reuptake into axon terminals and glial cells has to be taken into account. Thus the loss of adenine nucleotides from synaptosomal preparations

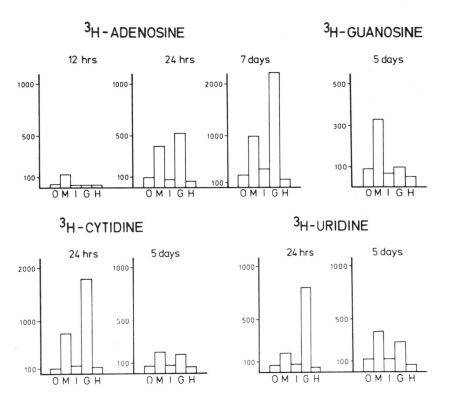

FIGURE 4 Dynamics of the transfer of the various nucleoside derivatives. The ordinate gives the analog values of the intensity of the autoradiographic label in the hippocampal target area after entorhinal injection at the times indicated. (O, outer; M, middle; I, inner molecular layer; G, granule-cell layer; H, hilus.)

Nature of the adenosine derivatives transported and released

More than 90% of the radioactive material recovered from the target area after axonal transport for 1–2 days were TCA-soluble compounds. Among these was ATP with all its derivatives, including cAMP and adenosine (Schubert and Kreutzberg, 1975c). Centrifugal separation of the cell components has also shown a movement of previously labeled nucleotides with time in favor of the synaptosomal fraction (Barberis and McIlwain, 1977). This strongly points to the nucleotides as the components that are intraneuronally transported. Since cAMP participates in the intraneuronal transport of nucleotides, McIlwain (1976, 1977) has considered this intraneuronal channeling of a second messenger as a possible mechanism of intracellular information processing.

Cyclic AMP is also clearly one of the major components released from the neuron in addition to ATP, ADP, and AMP. Up to 22% of the efflux of adenosine derivatives is reported to be derived from cAMP (Pull and McIlwain, 1977). An excitation-dependent release of ATP into the extracellular space has also been demonstrated very clearly in various systems that are generally accepted as models for synaptic-vesicle exocytosis. Its release has been shown to occur from chromaffin granules of the adrenal medulla (Douglas and Poisner, 1966; Smith and Winckler, 1972), from synaptosomes of the cholinergic *Torpedo* electric organ (Zimmermann and Whittaker, 1974), and from the mammalian neocortex in conjunction with other adenine nucleotides (Barberis and McIlwain, 1976). In the last instance, AMP was found to be the most prevalent compound among the nucleotides recovered from eluates of brain slices. It may be derived from ATP or ADP. When AMP appears in the extracellular space, it is rapidly broken down, yielding adenosine as the main product (Pull and McIlwain, 1977).

5'-Nucleotidase: The adenosine-producing enzyme

With adenosine emerging as an intercellular communication molecule, the crucial questions are where and how this substance is formed. Keeping in mind that most of the adenine derivatives in the brain are

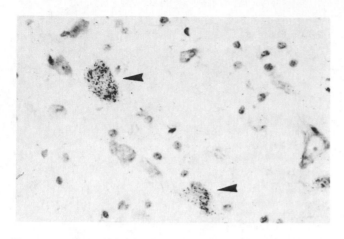

FIGURE 5 Retrograde transport. Selective labeling of motoneurons in the ambiguous nucleus (arrows) after injection of [³H]-adenosine into the cricothyroid muscle of a squirrel monkey. (Autoradiograph, counterstained with toluidine blue, ×300.)

nucleotides and also that nucleotides are released upon excitation, the adenosine-generating enzyme 5′-nucleotidase would be expected to be in a strategic position. In order to study the location of the enzyme by electron microscopy a cytochemical method was adapted for use in the nervous system (Barron, Kreutzberg, and Schubert, 1977). From light-microscopic histochemistry it is well known that the enzyme is located on myelinated nerve fibers of various parts of the brain (Naidoo, 1962). However, a finer localization of the enzyme activity is not possible at the light-microscopic level. Electron-microscopic cytochemistry now allows for a precise and reliable correlation of 5′-nucleotidase activity with cellular com-

ponents of the nervous system. We have investigated various parts of the brain in which histochemical methods had already revealed activity of the enzyme—for instance, the hippocampus, the caudate nucleus, the thalamus, cingulate cortex, neocortex, cerebellar cortex, and medulla oblongata.

In all these regions the most prominent and most frequent localization of the enzyme is on the plasma membranes of astrocytes (Figure 6). Lamellae-like processes of astrocytes can be seen in the neuropile surrounding synaptic complexes. These juxtasynaptic astrocytic lamellae are the main carriers of the enzyme (Figure 7). They are, of course, in an optimal location to catch any 5′-AMP that is released during synaptic activity or is formed after hydrolysis of ATP by extracellular ATPases. If adenosine is formed by 5′-nucleotidase activity in the extracellular space, this membrane-permeable molecule should have no problem entering the adjacent cellular processes, whether they are dendritic, axonal, or glial.

Perivascular astrocytic footplates also regularly show enzyme activity in their plasma membranes (Figure 8). In those locations where the endothelial basement lamina is in contact with a plasma membrane of an astrocyte process, enzyme activity is seen in the form of rather coarse deposits of the reaction product. In general, the enzyme is located more strongly on the astrocytic side than on the capillary side of the basement membrane. Plasma membranes of the endothelial cells do not show clear enzymatic activity. A reaction product that is frequently seen scattered over the capillary cells seems to represent nonspecific deposits, probably of lead precipitates.

Oligodendroglial cells were also found to demon-

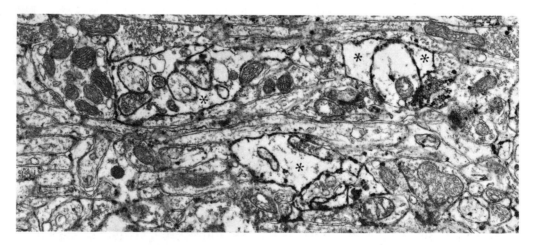

FIGURE 6 Rat cerebellar cortex. 5′-Nucleotidase activity can be recognized by the electron-dense reaction product deposited on astrocytic plasmalemma. Astrocytes have typical irregularly shaped profiles and very light cytoplasm (asterisks). (×18,750.)

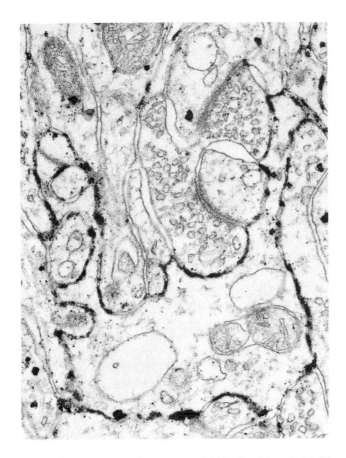

FIGURE 7 Rat cerebellar cortex. 5'-Nucleotidase is highly active in the plasma membrane of an astrocytic lamella covering a synaptic complex. Extracellular space is widened because of formalin fixation (×50,000.)

strate 5'-nucleotidase activity in their plasma membranes; compared to astrocytes, however, it is weak. Activity related to myelinated fibers is seen at the external surface of the myelin sheath and in the space between axolemma and the innermost lamella of the myelin sheath. Occasionally reaction product is demonstrated in the extracellular space of a mesaxon. The location of the myelinated fibers suggests that the enzyme is of oligodendroglial origin and not of neuronal origin. Since we were unable to demonstrate 5'-nucleotidase activity in nerve cells either in their perikarya or in plasma membranes of the soma or dendrites, we are tempted to suppose that neurons do not possess 5'-nucleotidase. This would mean that the neuron depends heavily on its satellite glial cells for the production of adenosine. The neuron may produce adenosine only by de novo synthesis. This is a rather complicated biosynthetic process, which is present to a particularly low extent in the nervous system. Instead, most of the adenosine seems to be constantly reutilized by a salvage pathway. Hypoxan-

thine phosphoribosyl transferase is the key enzyme of this pathway. Its activity in the brain is ten times higher than in other organs. If our interpretation of the 5'-nucleotidase localization is correct, it would mean that astrocytic plasma membranes are needed for production of adenosine from nucleotides. This production of the neurohumoral signal can only occur at synaptic sites accompanied by 5'-nucleotidase-carrying structures. Such a mechanism would add a certain degree of specificity or selectivity to the purinergic mechanisms.

As concluded from our transport data, adenosine derivatives (mainly ATP) are produced, transported, and released very generally in almost all systems tested. The actual amount of adenosine transported and released may be very small since little of the nucleoside will escape phosphorylation by the very active adenosine kinase. This means that during synaptic activity the postsynaptic neuron may not see much adenosine if the nucleotides are not enzymat-

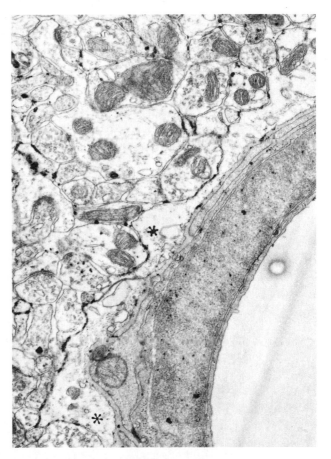

FIGURE 8 Rat dentate gyrus. Two astrocytic footplates (asterisks) are seen inserting on a capillary wall. 5'-Nucleotidase activity is present in the plasma membrane. (×25,000.)

ically converted into adenosine. The presence of ATPases and 5'-nucleotidase determines whether this conversion takes place. Areas of the forebrain that show no 5'-nucleotidase activity, such as parts of the parietal and temporal neocortex or certain brainstem areas, may not be able to produce adenosine. In such regions nucleotides released from terminals during excitation may not affect the postsynaptic neuron, but may travel in the extracellular space until they reach structures equipped with enzymes for adenosine production. This could be a perivascular site covered with astrocytic footplates, or a neighboring juxtasynaptic astrocyte lamella, or a bundle of myelinated fibers passing by. The same thing may happen in areas where 5'-nucleotidase is not present at every juxtasynaptic site. The distribution of the adenosine-producing enzymes on plasma membranes directed toward the extracellular space could determine how far adenosine as an intercellular communication molecule could spread.

In cases where the density of 5'-nucleotidase-carrying structures is high, such as in the cerebellum, adenosine should be produced close to the site of nucleotide release and must be taken up readily into the neuronal or glial processes bordering the releasing site. If 5'-nucleotidase activity is low and enzyme-carrying glial processes are scattered in the neuropil, adenosine formation is extended in both time and space. In this case the signal may reach many different cells as a more general messenger, whereas in the first case a target cell could be hit exclusively, precisely, and with a higher concentration. It would not

be surprising if the effect of a high local concentration of adenosine turned out to be different from a low and not locally accentuated concentration.

A very prominent increase in enzyme activity is seen during chromatolysis of the facial and hypoglossal nucleus. (Sjöstrand, 1966; Kreutzberg, 1968). EM cytochemistry has now revealed that enzyme activity is located on the plasma membranes of the proliferating microglial cells (Figure 9). These cells cover most of the surface of the chromatolytic motoneurons, thereby removing the presynaptic terminals (Blinzinger and Kreutzberg, 1968). The functional meaning of this is not clear, but we should realize that the brain obviously can produce within a short time mobile microglial cells having a high activity of an adenosine-producing enzyme. It is not unreasonable to assume that additional production of adenosine could be useful for increasing local blood supply during the pathological process of chromatolysis. The often close neighborhood of microglial cells and capillaries suggests such a relation (Figure 9).

Possible role of adenosine as molecular neuronal signal

Data accumulating from biochemical and electrophysiological experiments reveal a remarkable biological activity of adenosine in the brain. It leads to vasodilatation, stimulates cAMP synthesis, depresses nerve-cell bioelectrical activity, and seems to interfere with Ca^{++} fluxes and transmitter release. A substance

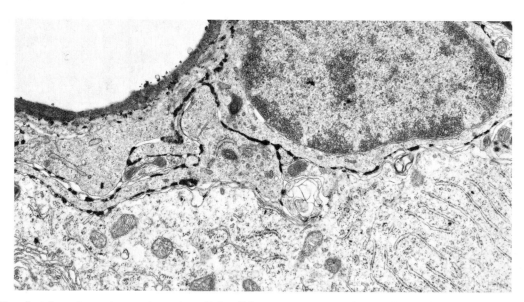

FIGURE 9 Rat facial nucleus. A reactive microglial cell is shown in contact with the surface of a chromatolytic motoneuron and a capillary. 5'-Nucleotidase activity is high in the plasma membrane of the microglial cell. ($\times 18,900$.)

with such properties may be acting as a molecular signal involved in intercellular communication. This proposed function would require a strict compartmentation and a control of the effective extracellular level of adenosine in the brain. The blood-brain barrier, which is rather impermeable for nucleotides (Berne, Rubio, and Curnish, 1974), protects the intracerebral nucleotide levels from being affected by the highly unstable blood levels. It makes the brain a nearly closed system in which the actual local concentration of nucleotides is predominantly determined by their intracerebral redistribution. In this respect, the intraneuronal transport and the activity-related release from neurons, as demonstrated, seem to be important for a controlled channeling of adenosine in the brain. Nucleotides represent a high proportion of the adenosine derivatives that are released from neurons. They are rapidly broken down in the extracellular space, yielding adenosine. Whereas the overall activity of these degrading enzymes seems to be rather high in the brain, they obviously show a very selective regional distribution, with the 5'-nucleotidase mainly associated with glial-cell membranes. The local level of adenosine that is found at a given point in the brain should therefore be determined by both the functionally related release of the nucleoside and nucleotides, and by the presence of the degrading enzymes. The presence of 5'-nucleotidase in the astrocyte processes engulfing the synaptic complexes ensures a rapid formation of adenosine in the vicinity of the postsynaptic membrane. The strategically optimal placing of this enzyme should also facilitate an uptake of adenosine into the astrocytes. They may serve as the preferential pathways in which adenosine, possibly in the form of nucleotides, is channeled from the site of release to a remote place of action such as the blood vessels.

The elevation of the adenosine level in the extracellular space in response to nerve-cell activation can also be reduced by its reuptake into axon terminals, nerve and glial cells, and by its further enzymatic breakdown to the inactive inosine and hypoxanthine.

So far the findings basically meet the criteria postulated for a substance that acts as a neuronal messenger: adenosine derivatives are released from nerve cells; their release is related to nerve-cell activity; enzymes are available to ensure the extracellular formation of adenosine; and mechanisms are present to terminate its action (see also Figure 10). On the other hand, a substance that is considered to be a

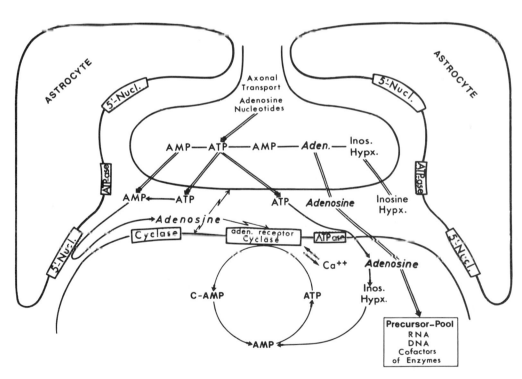

FIGURE 10 Scheme summarizing translocation, intra- and extracellular transformation, and some action of adenosine and its derivatives at the synapse.

candidate for a molecular messenger would be expected to show some kind of structural specificity, to be present only in a specific cell type, and to mediate a well-defined effect. Adenosine is certainly not such a specific substance. Therefore, one has to ask whether it can play a role in intercellular communication at all, and if so, what are the characteristics of its possible action. The finding that adenosine derivatives are released from a wide variety of central neuronal systems rules out the possibility that it acts like a classical transmitter—specific to a certain cell type. On the contrary, adenosine is better characterized as a universal signal that is commonly used by nerve cells and that can be received by a variety of targets eliciting quite heterogeneous effects. It carries the message that the nerve cells have been activated, and its function may be to evoke a coordinated (and functionally meaningful) reaction in the different elements of a functional unit in response to its activation.

By affecting the tonus and width of the cerebral vessels, adenosine may contribute to the regulation of the local blood flow and adjust it to the functional demand. This effect elicited at structures that are remote from the site of neuronal nucleotide release should be highly dependent on the parameters controlling the extraneuronal channeling of adenosine. Any change in the distribution of the 5′-nucleotidase—for example, by changing the number or location of its glial carriers—must be expected to modify the channeling of adenosine. This may be relevant under certain pathological conditions in which the activity of 5′-nucleotidase is known to increase dramatically.

Adenosine is also capable of exerting an electrophysiological modulatory effect on nerve-cell function. It has been shown to suppress spontaneous electrical activity in a variety of central systems (Phillis and Kostopoulos, 1975; Phillis and Edstrom, 1976) as well as the synaptically driven nerve-cell responses evoked by the stimulation of afferent fibers. The latter was seen in slice preparations of the olfactory cortex (Kuroda, Saito, and Kobayashi, 1976) and of the hippocampus (Schubert and Kreutzberg, 1977). This inhibitory effect of adenosine and of its even more potent analog chloroadenosine can be antagonized by theophylline, which is also known to block their stimulatory effect on cAMP synthesis. The mechanism of this adenosine action leading to a feedback inhibition of the synaptic transmission is unknown. It may be a presynaptic effect resulting from a suppression of transmitter release. Such a decrease in the release of acetylcholine has been observed in

the *Torpedo* electric organ elicited by a stimulation-induced, probably postsynaptic release of ATP (Israel and Meunier, 1977). Adenosine has also been shown to inhibit the transmitter release from adrenergic nerves (Clanachan, Johns, and Paton, 1977). Since transmitter release is known to be calcium-dependent, the recent observation of ten Bruggencate et al. (1977) may be of some relevance: they found that in the presence of adenosine the stimulation-induced drop of extracellular calcium level is diminished, suggesting that adenosine interferes with calcium fluxes (see also Schultz, 1976).

Considering the biochemically well-established stimulatory effect of adenosine on the synthesis of cAMP, adenosine must be expected to influence cell metabolism. Such a signal, which translates nerve-cell activation into defined metabolic changes, may be able to elicit a longer-lasting modulation of cell functions in response to nerve-cell activation. This may involve more general trophic processes and may even lead to specific functional changes, such as a conditioning of synaptic transmission. In speculating along this line the interaction of adenosine with monoamines leading to a potentiation of the reactive cAMP increase is of particular interest. A much greater than additive effect on the accumulation of cAMP was seen in cerebral cortical slices if adenosine was applied together with norepinephrine, histamine, or serotonin (Sattin and Rall, 1970; Schultz and Daly, 1973; see also Daly, 1975, and Rall, this volume). This offers a possible mechanism by which the inputs from adenosine-releasing specific afferents and from monoaminergic central-core neurons could be integrated. Thus a specific metabolic effect that is dependent on a particularly high cAMP level (see Berridge, this volume) may only be elicited if adenosine and norepinephrine are both present as first messengers, that is, if the activation of specific afferents and unspecific central-core systems occurs together. By such a mechanism, a metabolically linked and longer-lasting modulation of synaptic function could be elicited, depending on whether or not the monoaminergic central-core system is turned on. This could lead to an alteration of the subsequent signal transmission in that activated neuronal circuit. Such a modulatory effect is difficult to verify, since the electrophysiological techniques presently used are designed for the observation of rapid events on the order of milliseconds, neglecting or abolishing the slower changes in the baseline. Recording techniques are now required that will allow us to detect slow and minute changes in nerve-cell function.

REFERENCES

BARBERIS, C., and H. McILWAIN, 1976. 5-adenine mononucleotides in synaptosomal preparations from guinea pig neocortex: Their change on incubation, superfusion and stimulation. *J. Neurochem.* 26:1015-1021.

BARBERIS, C., and H. McILWAIN, 1977. Redistribution of adenine derivatives among subcellular fractions from guinea pig neocortical tissues, on incubation in vitro. *J. Neurochem.* 29:77-81.

BARRON, K. D., G. W. KREUTZBERG, and P. SCHUBERT, 1977. Histochemical demonstration of 5'-nucleotidase in normal and deafferented rat central nervous system. Seventh Ann. Meeting Soc. Neurosci. Abstract.

BERNE, R. M., R. RUBIO, and R. R. CURNISH, 1974. Release of adenosine from ischaemic brain. *Circ. Res.* 35:262-272.

BERNE, R. M., J. T. HERLIHY, J. SCHRADER, and R. RUBIO, 1976. Effect of adenosine on contraction of vascular smooth muscle. In *Ionic Actions on Vascular Smooth Muscle*, E. Betz, ed. Heidelberg, New York: Springer-Verlag, pp. 137-140.

BLINZINGER, K., and G. KREUTZBERG, 1968. Displacement of synaptic terminals from regenerating motoneurons by microglial cells. *Z. Zellforsch.* 85:145-157.

BURNSTOCK, G., 1972. Purinergic nerves. *Pharmacol. Rev.* 24:509-581.

CLANACHAN, A. S., A. JOHNS, and D. M. PATON, 1977. Presynaptic inhibitory actions of adenine nucleotides and adenosine on neurotransmission in the rat vas deferens. *Neuroscience* 2:597-602.

CLARK, R. B., and R. GROSS, 1974. Regulation of adenosine 3':5'-monophosphate content in human astrocytoma cells by adenosine and the adenine nucleotides. *J. Biol. Chem.* 249:5296-5303.

DALY, J., 1975. Role of cyclic nucleotides in the nervous system. In *Handbook of Psychopharmacology*, vol. 5, L. L. Iversen, S. D. Iversen, and S. H. Snyder, eds. New York: Plenum Press, pp. 47-130.

DOUGLAS, W. W., and A. M. POISNER, 1966. Extrusion of ATP (unhydrolysed) during release of catecholamines. *J. Physiol.* 183:249-256.

GEFFEN, L. B., and B. G. LIVETT, 1971. Synaptic vesicles in sympathetic neurons. *Physiol. Rev.* 51:98-157.

HUNT, S. P., and H. KÜNZLE, 1976. Bidirectional movement of label and transneuronal transport phenomena after injection of ³H-adenosine into the central nervous system. *Brain Res.* 112:127-132.

INGVAR, D. H., 1973. Cerebral blood flow metabolism in complete apallic syndromes, in states of severe dementia, and in akinetic mutism. *Acta Neurol. Scand.* 49:233-244.

ISRAEL, M. and F. MEUNIER, 1977. Postsynaptic release of adenosine triphosphate, induced by acetylcholine, a retroaction able to inhibit transmitter release. *Proc. Int. Soc. Neurochem.* 6:33.

KATO, M., H. UENO, and P. BLACK, 1974. Regional cerebral blood flow of the main visual pathways during photic stimulation of the retina in intact and split-brain monkeys. *Exp. Neurol.* 42:65-77.

KREUTZBERG, G. W., 1968. DNA metabolism in glial cells during retrograde changes. In *Macromolecules and the Function of the Neuron*, Z. Lodin and S. P. R. Rose, eds. Amsterdam: Excerpta Medica, pp. 51-57.

KREUTZBERG, G. W., K. D. BARRON, and P. SCHUBERT, 1978.

Cytochemical localisation of 5'-nucleotidase in glial plasma membranes. *Brain Res.* (in press).

KRUGER, L., and S. SAPORTA, 1977. Axonal transport of ³H-adenosine in visual somatosensory pathways. *Brain Res.* 122:132-136.

KURODA, Y., M. SAITO, and K. KOBAYASHI, 1976. Concomitant changes in cyclic AMP and postsynaptic potentials of olfactory cortex slices induced by adenosine derivatives. *Brain Res.* 109:196-201.

McILWAIN, H., 1974. Regulatory significance of the release and action of adenine derivatives in cerebral systems. *Biochem. Soc. Symp.* 36:69-85.

McILWAIN, H., 1976. Translocation of neural modulators: a second category of nerve signal. *Neurochem. Res.* 1:351-368.

McILWAIN, H., 1977. Extended roles in the brain for second-messenger systems. *Neuroscience* 2:357-372.

NAIDOO, D., 1962. The activity of 5'-nucleotidase determined histochemically in the developing rat brain. *J. Histochem. Cytochem.* 10:421-434.

PHILLIS, J. W., and J. P. EDSTROM, 1976. Effects of adenosine analogs on rat cerebral cortical neurons. *Life Sci.* 19:1041-1054.

PHILLIS, J. W., and G. K. KOSTOPOULOS, 1975. Adenosine as a putative transmitter in the cerebral cortex. Studies with potentiators and antagonists. *Life Sci.* 17:1085-1094.

PULL, I., and H. McILWAIN, 1972. Adenine derivatives as neurohumoral agents in the brain. *Biochem. J.* 130:975-981.

PULL, I., and H. McILWAIN, 1977. Adenine mononucleotides and their metabolites liberated from and applied to isolated tissues of the mammalian brain. *Neurochem. Res.* 2:203-216.

ROSE, G., and P. SCHUBERT, 1977. Release and transfer of ³H-adenosine derivatives in the cholinergic septal system. *Brain Res.* 121:353-357.

SATTIN, A., and T. W. RALL, 1970. Cyclic AMP content of guinea pig cerebral cortex slices. *Mol. Pharmacol.* 6:13-23.

SCHRADER, J., R. RUBIO, and R. M. BERNE, 1975. Inhibition of slow action potentials of guinea pig atrial muscle by adenosine: a possible effect on Ca⁺⁺ influx. *J. Mol. Cell. Cardiol.* 7:427-433.

SCHUBERT, P., and G. W. KREUTZBERG, 1974. Axonal transport of adenosine and uridine derivatives and transfer to postsynaptic neurons. *Brain Res.* 76:526-530.

SCHUBERT, P., and G. W. KREUTZBERG, 1975a. ³H-adenosine, a tracer for neuronal connectivity. *Brain Res.* 85:317-319.

SCHUBERT, P., and G. W. KREUTZBERG, 1975b. Dendritic and axonal transport of neucleoside derivatives in single motoneurons and release from dendrites. *Brain Res.* 90:319-323.

SCHUBERT, P., and G. W. KREUTZBERG, 1975c. Parameters of dendritic transport. In *Physiology and Pathology of Dendrites, Advances in Neurology*, vol. 12, G. W. Kreutzberg, ed. New York: Raven Press, pp. 255-268.

SCHUBERT, P., and G. W. KREUTZBERG, 1976. Communication between the neuron and the vessels. In *The Cerebral Vessel Wall*, J. Cervós-Navarro et al., eds. New York: Raven Press, pp. 207-213.

SCHUBERT, P., and G. W. KREUTZBERG, 1977. Adenosine in

the CNS: intraneuronal transport and release from neurons. In *Iontophoresis and Transmitter Mechanisms in the Mammalian Central Nervous System*, J. S. Kelly, ed. Amsterdam: Elsevier.

SCHUBERT, P., K. LEE, M. WEST, S. DEADWYLER, and G. LYNCH, 1976. Stimulation-dependent release of ³H-adenosine derivatives from central axon terminals to target neurones. *Nature* 260:541–542.

SCHUBERT, P., G. ROSE, K. LEE, G. LYNCH, and G. W. KREUTZBERG, 1977. Axonal release and transfer of nucleoside derivatives in the entorhinal-hippocampal system: An autoradiographic study. *Brain Res.* 134:347–352.

SCHULTZ, J., 1976. Calcium and the regulation of adenosine 3′,5′-monophosphate by neurotransmitters. In *Ionic Actions on Vascular Smooth Muscle*, E. Betz, ed. Heidelberg, New York: Springer-Verlag, pp. 39–43.

SCHULTZ, J., and J. W. DALY, 1973. Cyclic adenosine 3′,5′-monophosphate in guinea pig cerebral cortical slices. I. Formation of cyclic adenosine 3′,5′-monophosphate from endogenous adenosine triphosphate and from radioactive adenosine triphosphate formed during a prior incubation with radioactive adenine. *J. Biol. Chem.* 248:843–852.

SCHULTZ, J. and B. HAMPRECHT, 1973. Adenosine 3′,5′-monophosphate in cultured neuroblastoma cells: effect of adenosine phosphodiesterase inhibitors and benzazepines. *Naunyn-Schmiedeberg's Arch. Pharmacol.* 278:215–225.

SHIMIZU, H., and J. DALY, 1970. Formation of cyclic adenosine 3′,5′-monophosphate from adenosine in brain slices. *Biochim. Biophys. Acta* 222:465–473.

SILINSKY, E. M., and I. I. HUBBARD, 1973. Released ATP from rat motor nerve terminals. *Nature* 243:404–405.

SJÖSTRAND, J., 1966. Changes of nucleoside phosphatase activity in the hypoglossal nucleus during nerve regeneration. *Acta Physiol. Scand.* 67:219.

SMITH, A. D., and H. WINCKLER, 1972. Fundamental mechanisms in the release of catecholamines. In *Handbuch der experimentellen Pharmakologie*, vol. 33. Heidelberg: Springer-Verlag.

SULAKHE, P. V., and J. W. PHILLIS, 1975. The release of ³H-adenosine and its derivatives from the cat sensory motor cortex. *Life Sci.* 17:551–556.

TEN BRUGGENCATE, G., R. STEINBERG, H. STÖCKLE, and C. NICHOLSON, 1977. Modulation of extracellular Ca⁺⁺ and K⁺-levels in the mammalian cerebellar cortex. In *Iontophoresis and Transmitter Mechanisms in the Mammalian Central Nervous System*, J. S. Kelly, ed. Amsterdam: Elsevier.

WISE, S. P., and E. G. JONES, 1976. Transneuronal or retrograde transport of ³H-adenosine in the rat somatic sensory system. *Brain Res.* 107:127–131.

ZIMMERMANN, H., and V. P. WHITTAKER, 1974. Effect of electrical stimulation on the yield and composition of synaptic vesicles from the cholinergic synapses of the electric organ of *Torpedo*. *J. Neurochem.* 22:435–450.

61 Prostaglandin Endoperoxides and Thromboxanes: Role as Bioregulators

BENGT SAMUELSSON

ABSTRACT   Two groups of unstable endoperoxides, PGG and PGH compounds, have been isolated and shown to be precursors of the prostaglandins. The endoperoxides cause platelet aggregation and have unique actions on vascular and airway smooth muscle. The effects are not due to conversion to the stable prostaglandins (PGE, PGF, etc.). A new group of compounds derived from the endoperoxides—the thromboxanes—has been discovered. Thromboxanes have so far been found in platelets, leucocytes, lung tissue, spleen, kidney, umbilical artery, and brain. In some tissues the thromboxanes constitute the major products derived from the endoperoxides. A highly unstable intermediate between the endoperoxides and thromboxane B_2—called thromboxane A_2—has been detected. Structural work indicates that it has a bicyclic oxane-oxetane structure.

Thromboxane A_2 induces platelet aggregation and causes contraction of arteries. Endoperoxides and thromboxanes are essential for platelet aggregation. Platelet cyclo-oxygenase deficiency gives rise to a hemostatic defect due to an abnormal release mechanism. The aggregating effect of the endoperoxides and thromboxanes is mainly due to release of ADP and serotonin. Evidence is presented indicating that the decrease in cAMP concentration in platelet-rich plasma following addition of the endoperoxides is mediated by ADP.

The identification of thromboxane B_2 as a major metabolite of arachidonic acid in brain suggests that the thromboxanes may also have a regulatory function in the central nervous system.

Introduction

PROSTAGLANDINS have been found in the nervous system, and various biological effects of prostaglandins have been demonstrated. An extensive review on possible roles of prostaglandins in the nervous system has been published by Wolfe (1975), who also describes the general biosynthetic and catabolic pathways of the prostaglandins. (See also Samuelsson et al., 1971, 1975; Samuelsson, 1972.) The present review describes recent advances concerning endoperoxides, which are intermediates in the biosynthesis of prostaglandins, and thromboxanes, a new group of unstable compounds derived from the endoperoxides. Evidence will be presented indicating that the thromboxanes may have a regulatory function in the central nervous system.

Prostaglandin endoperoxides

During studies on the mechanism of formation of prostaglandins from polyunsaturated fatty acids (Figure 1) it was discovered that the oxygen atoms of the keto and hydroxyl groups in the five-member ring of PGE_1 originate in the same molecule of oxygen (Samuelsson, 1965). On the basis of this finding and other considerations it was proposed that an endoperoxide structure is formed as an intermediate in the biosynthesis of prostaglandins (Samuelsson, 1965).

Further studies on the mechanism of the transformation (for review see Samuelsson, 1972) showed that the initial step consists of a lipoxygenase-like reaction in which the pro-S hydrogen at C13 is re-

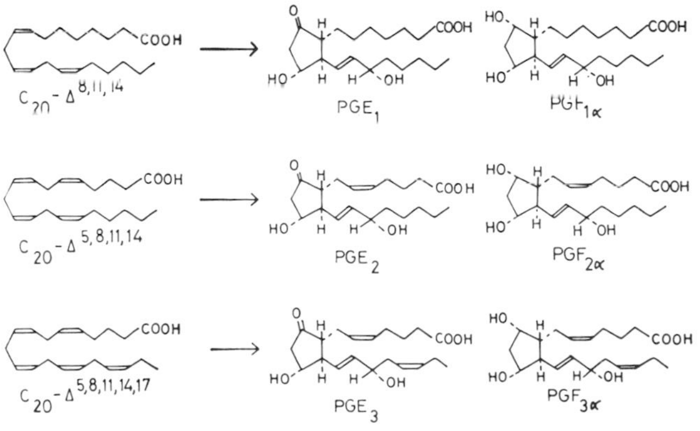

FIGURE 1   Biosynthesis of prostaglandins from polyunsaturated fatty acids.

BENGT SAMUELSSON   Department of Chemistry, Karolinska Institutet, s-104 01 Stockholm, Sweden

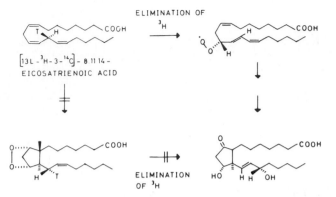

FIGURE 2 Two hypothetical pathways in the biosynthesis of prostaglandin E_1.

moved, the Δ^{11} double bond is isomerized into the Δ^{12} position, and oxygen is inserted at C11 (Figure 2). These experiments excluded an alternative pathway that was also in agreement with the isotopic oxygen experiment described above. The subsequent steps leading to the endoperoxide were visualized as consisting of attack by oxygen at C15, shift of the Δ^{12} double bond, and formation of a new bond between C8 and C12. In further studies, 12-hydroxy-8,10-heptadecadienoic acid and malonaldehyde were identified as by-products in the conversion of 8,11,14-dicosatrienoic acid into PGE_1 by microsomes from the vesicular gland of sheep (Hamberg and Samuelsson, 1966; Nugteren, Beerthuis, and van Dorp, 1966; Samuelsson, 1967; van Dorp, 1967). The formation of these compounds was considered to occur by fragmentation of an endoperoxide (Figure 3).

A few years ago we were able to isolate the methyl ester of an endoperoxide from short-time incubations of arachidonic acid with the microsomal fraction of homogenates of sheep vesicular glands (Hamberg and Samuelsson, 1973). In an extension of these studies, the endoperoxide was obtained as the free acid; in addition, an endoperoxide carrying a hydroperoxy group at C15 was isolated (Hamberg et al., 1974; Nugteren and Hazelhof, 1973). We suggested the trivial names PGG_2 for the less polar endoperoxide (15-hydroperoxy-9α-11α-peroxidoprosta-5,13-dienoic acid) and PGH_2 for the more polar endoperoxide (15 - hydroxy - 9α,11α - peroxidoprosta - 5,13 - dienoic acid). The structure of PGG_2 was established by three sets of experiments (Figure 4). Treatment of PGG_2 with mild reducing agents gave $PGF_{2\alpha}$ as the major product. This indicated the presence of a peroxide bridge between C9 and C11 but did not discriminate between a hydroxy and a hydroperoxy group at C15 since the agents used would reduce the latter group to the former. In a second experiment, PGG_2 was treated with lead tetra-acetate in benzene followed by triphenylphosphine. In this case 15-keto-$PGF_{2\alpha}$ was the major product. Lead tetra-acetate causes dehydration of hydroperoxides into ketones, so that formation of a 15-keto prostaglandin from PGG_2 by this treatment strongly indicated the presence of a hydroperoxy group at C15. The isomerization of PGG_2 into 15-hydroperoxy-PGE_2 in aqueous medium gave independent evidence for a peroxide group at C15. PGH_2 was found to be identical with the previously isolated 15-hydroxy prostaglandin endoperoxide by several criteria. It seems likely that PGG_2 is the first stable compound formed by the "prostaglandin synthetase" from arachidonic acid. The isolation of PGG_2

FIGURE 3 Formation of prostaglandins and by-products from an endoperoxide.

FIGURE 4 Reactions carried out on PGG_2 and PGH_2. $R_1 = CH_2CH{=}CH{-}(CH_2)_3{-}COOH$; $R_2 = (CH_2)_4{-}CH_3$; ϕ = phenyl.

demonstrated for the first time that introduction of the oxygen function at C15 of the prostaglandins occurs by a dioxygenase reaction.

Incubation of 1-[^{14}C]-PGG$_2$ and 1-[^{14}C]-PGH$_2$ with whole homogenates of sheep vesicular gland gave mainly PGE$_2$ (Nugteren and Hazelhof, 1973; Samuelsson and Hamberg, 1974). Two reactions are involved in the conversion of PGG$_2$ into PGE$_2$: isomerization of the endoperoxide structure into a β-hydroxyketone (endoperoxide isomerase), and reduction of the hydroperoxy group at C15 into a hydroxy group (peroxidase) (Figure 5). By incubation of 1-[^{14}C]-PGH$_2$ with different fractions of a homogenate of the sheep vesicular gland, the endoperoxide isomerase was shown to be almost entirely associated with the microsomal fraction. The enzymatic activity was stimulated by reduced glutathione and inhibited by p-mercuribenzoate and N-ethylmaleimide. Solubilization and partial separation of prostaglandin synthetase have been reported (Miyamoto et al., 1976; Hemler, Lands, and Smith, 1976).

Using in vitro preparations, it was found that the effects of the endoperoxides on gastrointestinal smooth muscle were comparable to those of PGE$_2$ and PGF$_{2\alpha}$ (Table I). On the other hand, the effects on vascular (rabbit aorta) and airway (guinea pig trachea) smooth muscle were considerably greater than those of PGE$_2$ and PGF$_{2\alpha}$, respectively (Hamberg et al., 1975). Both endoperoxides were potent contractors of the isolated human umbilical artery. The threshold concentrations were 3 (1–4) ng/ml for PGG$_2$ and 1 (1–12) ng/ml for PGH$_2$, compared with 200 (40–400) ng/ml for PGE$_2$ (Tuvemo et al., 1976). When given as intravenous injections to guinea pigs (Hamberg et al., 1975), PGG$_2$ and PGH$_2$ produced an increase in insufflation pressure more marked than that caused by corresponding doses of PGF$_{2\alpha}$.

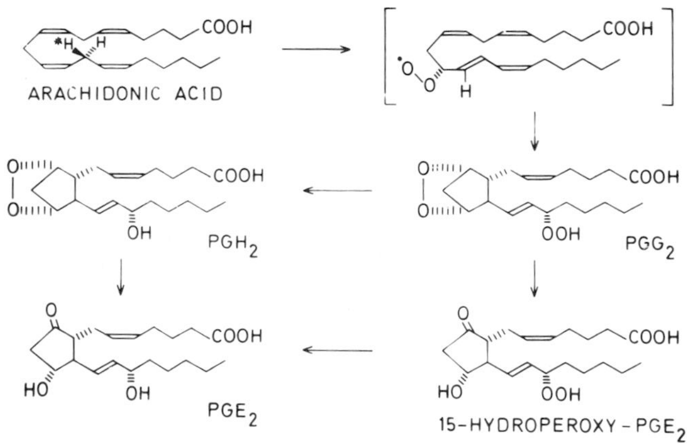

FIGURE 5 Pathways in the biosynthesis of PGE$_2$ from arachidonic acid.

The cardiovascular effects of the endoperoxides showed a complex pattern. The blood pressure response was triphasic: a transient fall was consistently followed by a short-lasting rise and then by a sustained reduction. Bradycardia was seen concomitantly with the initial fall in blood pressure. It seems likely that the long-lasting reduction in blood pressure is due to degradation of the endoperoxides, mainly into PGE$_2$. The preceding fall and rise in blood pressure might be caused by vasoconstriction, with the initial drop in blood pressure due to constriction of the pulmonary artery, leading to reduced venous return to the heart, and the subsequent rise due to constriction of vessels in the general circulation.

These studies on vascular and airway smooth muscle demonstrated that the endoperoxides had unique effects that could not be attributed to conversion into the stable prostaglandins. Additional work showed that the two endoperoxides also had unique effects

TABLE I

Relative contractile effects of various prostaglandins on some smooth muscle preparations

Prostaglandin	Gerbil Colon ($n = 5$)	Rat Stomach ($n = 5$)	Rabbit Aorta ($n = 5$)	Guinea Pig Trachea ($n = 7$)
PGG$_2$	1.5 ± 0.4 (n.s.)	1.9 ± 0.4 (n.s.)	80.4 ± 19.0 ($p < 0.05$)	7.5 ± 1.8 ($p < 0.05$)
PGH$_2$	1.2 ± 0.3 (n.s.)	3.3 ± 0.3 ($p < 0.01$)	210.4 ± 41.8 ($p < 0.01$)	9.3 ± 2.2 ($p < 0.01$)
PGD$_2$	0.3 ± 0.2 ($p < 0.05$)	1.4 ± 0.8 (n.s.)	—	5.2 ± 0.7 ($p < 0.01$)
PGE$_2$	2.9 ± 0.4 ($p < 0.05$)	5.7 ± 0.8 ($p < 0.01$)	1	relaxes
PGF$_{2\alpha}$	1	1	—	1

on platelets. Thus PGG$_2$ and PGH$_2$ induced rapid and irreversible aggregation of human platelets (Hamberg and Samuelsson, 1973; Hamberg et al., 1974; Samuelsson and Hamberg, 1974). Since aspirin, an inhibitor of endoperoxide formation, inhibits the second wave of aggregation, it was suggested that the endoperoxides play a role in the release reaction (Hamberg and Samuelsson, 1974a). The formation of material reducible with stannous chloride to PGF$_{2\alpha}$ during aggregation by various agents also supported this view (Hamberg and Samuelsson, 1974a; Smith et al., 1974). These findings with the pure endoperoxides were of particular interest in relation to other studies demonstrating that arachidonic acid causes aggregation when added to human platelets (Vargaftig and Zirinis, 1973; Silver et al., 1973) and that aggregating material (LASS) is formed when this acid is incubated with preparations of sheep vesicular gland (Willis, 1974a). LASS was considered to be due to endoperoxide but was not characterized in detail (Willis, 1974b; Willis et al., 1974).

Thromboxanes

The contracting effect of the endoperoxides on the isolated rabbit aorta was of particular interest in relation to the so-called rabbit aorta-contracting substance (RCS) (Piper and Vane, 1969). This was reported to be formed in guinea pig lung during anaphylaxis and was later suggested to be due to the endoperoxide intermediate in prostaglandin biosynthesis (Gryglewski and Vane, 1972). We found that material with similar biological properties was formed after addition of arachidonic acid to human platelets. However, with the pure endoperoxides (PGG$_2$ and PGH$_2$) available, we could demonstrate that the RCS from guinea pig lung and platelets consisted of a major component with $t_{1/2} \approx 30$ sec and a minor component of PGG$_2$ and/or PGH$_2$ with $t_{1/2} \approx 4$–5 min (Svensson, Hamberg, and Samuelsson, 1975).

The platelet system seemed attractive as an experimental model because we could generate the short-lived major component of RCS by addition of arachidonic acid. By incubating 1-[^{14}C]-arachidonic acid with suspensions of washed human platelets, we hoped to obtain structural information about RCS. Three major metabolites (I–III) could be demonstrated (Hamberg and Samuelsson, 1974a). Compound I was found to be 12L-hydroxy-5,8,10-eicosatetraenoic acid (HETE) (Figure 6). The corresponding hydroperoxide (HPETE) could be isolated following incubation of arachidonic acid with

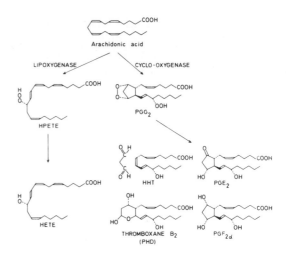

FIGURE 6   Transformation of arachidonic acid in human platelets.

sonicated plates. Formation of HETE from arachidonic acid in washed bovine platelets has also been reported (Nugteren, 1975).

Compound II was identified as 12L-hydroxy-5,8,10-heptadecatrienoic acid (HHT), and compound III was found to be the hemiacetal derivative of 8(1-hydroxy-3-oxopropyl)-9-12L-dihydroxy-5,10-heptadecadienoic acid (thromboxane B$_2$, PHD) (Figure 6). The structure of the latter compound was assigned mainly by mass-spectrometric analysis of a number of derivatives and by oxidative ozonolysis. 1-[^{14}C]-PGG$_2$ added to suspensions of human platelets was rapidly converted into HHT and thromboxane B$_2$. All of the identified products of arachidonic acid were stable compounds and so could not be identical with the very unstable RCS.

At this stage we continued the biological work with the platelets and characterized the material formed from arachidonic acid. When arachidonic acid was incubated with washed platelets and an aliquot of the incubate was transferred to a suspension of platelets preincubated with indomethacin, aggregation took place (Gryglewski and Vane, 1972). This was not due to PGG$_2$ or PGH$_2$ since the amounts found in two experiments were 1.2 and 0.4 ng of PGG$_2$/PGH$_2$ per 0.1 ml and the amounts required were 110 and 68 ng of PGG$_2$ per 0.1 ml, respectively. A more detailed analysis of the appearance of the aggregating factor and the endoperoxides PGG$_2$ and/or PGH$_2$ showed that the amount of endoperoxide was highest in the very early phase of the incubation period (maximum around 20 sec or earlier) whereas the aggregating factor had a maximum later (40–60 sec) (Figure 7; Samuelsson et al., 1976).

Similar results were obtained with filtrates of in-

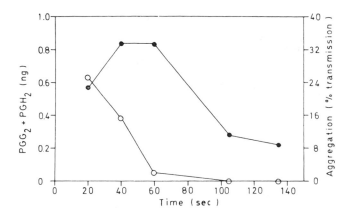

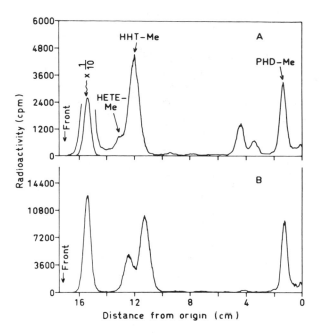

FIGURE 7 Maximum aggregation induced by 0.1 ml of suspensions of washed platelets incubated for different times with 120 ng of arachidonic acid (filled circles). The content of PGG$_2$/H$_2$ in these samples is also given (open circles). The platelet suspension in the aggregometer tube was preincubated for 2 min with 1.4×10^{-5}M indomethacin.

FIGURE 8 Thin-layer radiochromatograms of products isolated after incubation of 1-[^{14}C]-arachidonic acid (10 μg) with 1 ml of platelet suspension (10^6 platelets/μl) for 30 sec (upper) and 5 min (lower). The reactions were terminated by addition of 25 ml of methanol, and the esterified product was subjected to TLC (solvent system, organic layer of ethyl acetate-2,2,4-trimethyl-pentane-water 75:75:100, v/v/v).

cubates prepared as described above. In these experiments it was noted that the aggregating factor was very unstable. When the log dose (arbitrary units) was plotted against time of incubation at 37°C, a linear relationship was obtained. The half-life of the aggregating factor calculated from this plot was 43 sec. In two other experiments, half-lives of 33 and 46 sec were obtained. A factor with similar properties was also generated from PGG$_2$. In addition to inducing irreversible aggregation, the unstable factor also caused release of [^{14}C]-serotonin from platelets preincubated with [^{14}C]-serotonin. These results demonstrated that the factor was different from arachidonic acid, PGG$_2$, ADP, and serotonin and had practically the same $t_{1/2}$ as the major component of RCS.

At this stage we had obtained results from ^{18}O$_2$ experiments which suggested that thromboxane B$_2$ was formed from PGG$_2$ by rearrangement and subsequent incorporation of one molecule of H$_2$O (Hamberg and Samuelsson, 1974a). We reasoned that if the rearranged intermediate had an appreciable lifetime, it should be trapped in the presence of nucleophilic reagents (Hamberg, Svenson, and Samuelsson, 1975). As shown in Figure 8, addition of 25 volumes of methanol to washed platelets incubated with arachidonic acid at 37°C for 30 sec gave two derivatives that were less polar than thromboxane B$_2$. These derivatives were not present at longer incubation times, so that they could not have been formed by the action of methanol on one of the stable compounds in the incubation mixture (e.g., thromboxane B$_2$). The mass-spectrometric data indicated that the two compounds obtained by addition of methanol

were epimers of thromboxane B$_2$ methylated at the hemiacetal hydroxyl group. The two epimers also appeared when methanol was added to platelets incubated with PGG$_2$ for 30 sec. Addition of ethanol to platelets incubated with arachidonic acid for 30 sec similarly gave rise to epimers of thromboxane B$_2$ ethylated at the hemiacetal hydroxyl group. Finally, addition of 5 volumes of 5 M sodium azide to platelets incubated with arachidonic acid for 30 sec gave an azidoalcohol, a derivative of thromboxane B$_2$ in which the hemiacetal hydroxyl group is replaced by an azido group.

The trapping experiments described above revealed the existence of a very unstable intermediate in the conversion of PGG$_2$ into thromboxane B$_2$. In order to determine its half-life in aqueous medium, the platelet suspension was incubated with 1-[^{14}C]-arachidonic acid for 45 sec and the reaction was stopped by filtration. The clear, essentially platelet-free filtrate was kept at 37°C; aliquots were removed at different times and immediately added to 25 ml of methanol containing ^{3}H-labeled mono-O-methyl-thromboxane B$_2$. A linear relationship was obtained between the logarithms of the ^{14}C/^{3}H ratios of the purified methyl ester of mono-O-methyl-thromboxane B_2 and the times of incubation. The half-life was 32 ± 2 sec ($n = 3$).

The suggested structure of the unstable intermediate in the conversion of PGG$_2$ into thromboxane B_2 is given in Figure 9. The acetal carbon atom binding two oxygens should be susceptible to attack by nucleophils such as H$_2$O (giving thromboxane B_2) as well as CH$_3$OH, C$_2$H$_5$OH, and N$_3^-$ (giving derivatives of thromboxane B_2 as described above). This structure was also in agreement with the finding that the hydrogens at carbons 5, 6, 8, 9, 11, 12, 14, and 15 in arachidonic acid and PGG$_2$ were all retained in the conversion into thromboxane B_2. Addition of CH$_3$O^{2}H to platelets incubated with arachidonic acid led to formation of mono-O-methyl-thromboxane B_2 lacking carbon-bound ^{2}H. This finding excluded an alternate structure of the unstable intermediate—an unsaturated oxane (I in Figure 9). Furthermore, the $t_{1/2}$ of thromboxane A_2 seemed to exclude a carbonium ion structure (II in Figure 9), which in aqueous medium should be considerably less stable.

The RCS and the aggregating factor were both derived from arachidonic acid or PGG$_2$; their formation from arachidonic acid was blocked by indomethacin and their half-lives were similar, indicating that they were due to a single compound. It was proposed that this latter material is identical with the unstable intermediate detected chemically in platelets (Figure 9). This is also derived from arachidonic acid or PGG$_2$, its formation is blocked by indomethacin, and its half-life is close to that of the RCS and aggregating factors.

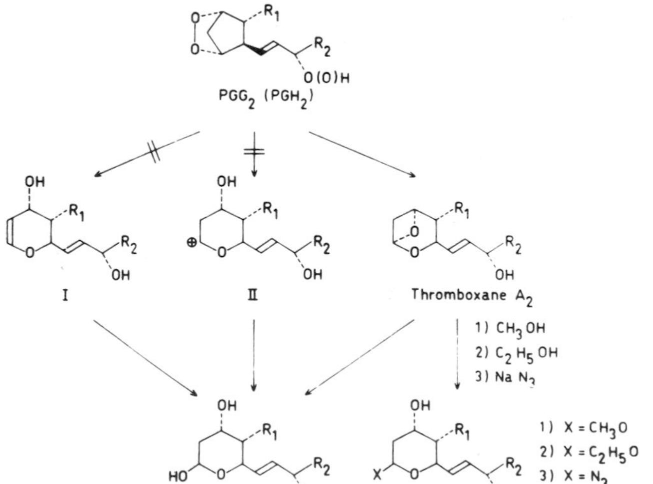

FIGURE 9 Scheme of transformations of endoperoxides into thromboxane derivatives.

The new oxane derivatives were named thromboxanes because of their structure and origin. Thromboxane A_2 is the highly unstable bicyclic compound, and thromboxane B_2 is the stable derivative provisionally named PHD. The subscript indicates the number of double bonds, as in the prostaglandin nomenclature.

The formation of thromboxanes is not limited to platelets. The transformation of arachidonic acid into thromboxane B_2 has also been observed in lung tissue (Hamberg and Samuelsson, 1974b), spleen, kidney, and leucocytes (Samuelsson, 1976), umbilical artery (Tuvemo et al., 1976), and brain (Wolfe, Rostworowski, and Marion, 1976). The structure of thromboxane B_2 has been confirmed by synthesis (Nelson and Jackson, 1976; Kelly, Schletter, and Stein, 1976; and Schneider and Morge, 1976).

Assay of thromboxanes

Methods have been developed for quantitative determination of thromboxane B_2. A mass-spectrometric method, based on multiple-ion analysis and the use of octadeuterated thromboxane B_2 as internal standard, has been employed in the analysis of platelets (Hamberg, Svensson, and Samuelsson, 1974), perfusate of guinea pig lung (Svensson, Hamberg, and Samuelsson, 1975), and bath medium of strips of the umbilical artery (Tuvemo et al., 1976). More recently a radioimmunoassay was developed for thromboxane B_2 (Granström, Kindahl, and Samuelsson, 1976a). The antisera were obtained by immunizing rabbits against a conjugate of thromboxane B_2 and bovine serum albumin. The method has high sensitivity (about 10 pg).

For assaying thromboxane A_2 a radioimmunoassay was developed for a mono-O-methyl derivative of thromboxane B_2 (Granström, Kindahl, and Samuelsson, 1976b). The samples to be analyzed were treated with a large volume of methanol, which converts thromboxane A_2 into the methyl acetal derivative of thromboxane B_2 (Figure 10). The antibodies showed high specificity for this compound and crossreacted only 1.2% with thromboxane B_2 and less than 0.1% with prostaglandins and prostaglandin metabolites. The method had a sensitivity of 7 pg. An application is shown in Figure 11.

Mode of action of prostaglandin endoperoxides and thromboxanes in platelets

The endoperoxide PGG$_2$ induced platelet aggregation and the platelet release reaction (release of ADP

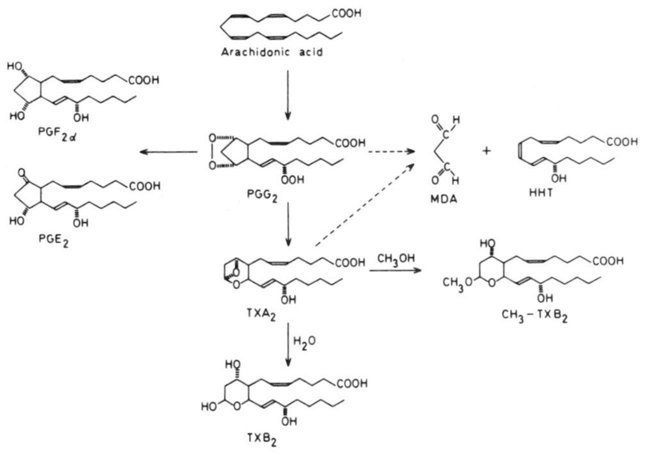

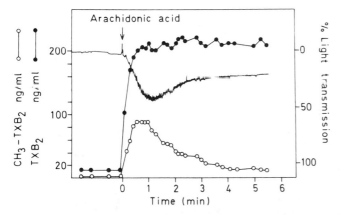

FIGURE 10 Transformation of arachidonic acid in platelets, and derivatization of thromboxane A_2 (TXA_2) into mono-O-methyl-thromboxane B_2 (TXB_2) by addition of methanol.

and serotonin) when added to human platelet-rich plasma (Malmsten et al., 1975). Formation of thromboxane B_2 accompanied the release reaction induced by aggregating agents such as collagen, ADP, epinephrine, and thrombin. Indomethacin inhibited the release reaction and PGG_2 and thromboxane B_2 formation caused by these agents but had no effect on the PGG_2 induced release reaction and aggregation.

A subject with a hemostatic defect due to an abnormal release mechanism was studied (Malmsten et al., 1975). Platelets from this subject did not aggregate on addition of collagen or arachidonate but did respond in a normal way to the endoperoxide PGG_2. The same was true for the release reaction; that is, there was a normal response to PGG_2 and a signifi-

cantly decreased release reaction on addition of ADP, collagen, or thrombin. This subject had a deficiency of platelet cyclo-oxygenase, which catalyzes the formation of PGG_2, but a normal content of the lipoxygenase. It was thus demonstrated that synthesis of PGG_2 is essential for normal hemostasis.

Recent studies from our laboratory (Claesson and Malmsten, 1977) indicate that the aggregation of platelets caused by PGG_2 in platelet-rich plasma is almost exclusively due to the release of ADP. This conclusion is based on the kinetics of the ADP release and the decrease in the aggregating effect of PGG_2 following enzymatic removal of ADP by phosphorylation. Furthermore, the aggregation calculated on the basis of the amount of ADP released by PGG_2 was essentially the same as the observed aggregation. Additional support for the essential role of ADP in PGG_2-induced aggregation was obtained from studies of platelet disorders (Malmsten et al., 1977). Platelets from a patient with the Hermansky-Pudlak syndrome (ADP deficiency) were almost refractory to PGG_2 but responded normally to ADP. Similarly, platelets from patients with Glanzmann's thrombasthenia (no aggregation with ADP) did not respond to PGG_2. In both disorders, addition of arachidonic acid resulted in normal synthesis of thromboxane B_2.

PGG_2 has been found to cause a decrease in the cAMP level of platelet-rich plasma when this level has been elevated by addition of PGE_1 (Claesson and Malmsten, 1977). Recent experiments indicate that this effect is also mediated through the released ADP instead of being a direct effect of PGG_2 on adenylate cyclase (Miller and Gorman, 1976). Further support for this mediator role of ADP was obtained from the observation that PGG_2 had only a decreasing effect on the cAMP level when ADP release was observed. The rapid release of ADP by PGG_2 and the kinetics of the effect of PGG_2 and ADP on the cAMP level also support this hypothesis. In addition, the decrease of the cAMP level caused by ADP was not abolished by such prostaglandin-synthesis inhibitors as indomethacin. The results are not consistent with a previous hypothesis (Salzman, 1976) involving prostaglandin biosynthesis as an essential step in the decrease of cAMP.

It was found earlier that increased concentration of endogenous cAMP or addition of dibutyryl cAMP was associated with decreased synthesis of PGG_2 in platelets (Willis et al., 1974; Malmsten et al., 1977). This finding, together with results showing that the endoperoxide did not cause aggregation when the cAMP level in platelet-rich plasma was elevated by preincubation with PGE_1, indicates that the regulat-

FIGURE 11 Mono-O-methyl-TXB_2 levels (open circles) and TXB_2 levels (filled circles) after addition of arachidonic acid to washed human platelets at 37°C. Light transmission was recorded simultaneously in an aggregometer. Arrow indicates addition of arachidonic acid.

TABLE II

Thromboxane B_2 and prostaglandin formation by various tissues

Tissue	AA added (μg)	TXB$_2$	PGF$_{2\alpha}$	PGE$_2$
		(μg/g/5 min incubation)		
Guinea pig				
Lung homogenate	10	5.729 (2)	—	—
Kidney homogenate	10	0.026 (2)	—	—
Cerebral-cortex homogenate	10	1.705 (2)	—	—
Cerebral-cortex homogenate	0	1.551 ± 0.203 (4)	0.286	0.074
Cerebral-cortex slices	0	0.555 (2)	0.170	—
Cerebral cortex + 1 mM NE	0	2.633 (2)	—	—
Cerebral cortex + 0.1 mM INDO	0	0.034 (2)	—	—
Cerebral cortex + 0.5 mM mercaptoethanol	0	0.019	—	—
Rat				
Cerebral-cortex homogenate	0	0.361 (2)	0.301	0.089

Abbreviations: AA, arachidonic acid; NE, norepinephrine; INDO, indomethacin; TXB$_2$, thromboxane B$_2$.

ing effect of cAMP on platelet aggregation is exerted not only on the cyclo-oxygenase reaction but also on the release reaction (Malmsten et al., 1977).

Formation of thromboxane B_2 by brain tissue

Wolfe, Rostworowski, and Marion (1976) reported that thromboxane B$_2$ is formed from endogenous precursors during short incubations of guinea pig and rat cerebral cortex. Thromboxane B$_2$ was identified by gas chromatography and mass spectrometry. In guinea pig cerebral-cortex homogenates, thromboxane B$_2$ synthesis was five to six times greater than the combined formation of prostaglandins F$_{2\alpha}$ and E$_2$ (Table II). The capacity of rat cerebral-cortex homogenate to synthesize thromboxane B$_2$ from endogenous precursor was less than that of guinea pig homogenate. The amounts of thromboxane B$_2$ were equivalent to the combined amounts of prostaglandins F$_{2\alpha}$ and E$_2$. The finding of thromboxane B$_2$ formation in brain suggests that the thromboxanes may have a role in neurotransmission in the central nervous system. Norepinephrine stimulated, and indomethacin and mercaptoethanol inhibited, thromboxane B$_2$ formation.

ACKNOWLEDGMENTS This work was supported by a grant from the Swedish Medical Research Council (project 03X–217).

REFERENCES

CLAESSON, H.-E., and C. MALMSTEN, 1977. On the interrelationship of prostaglandin endoperoxide G$_2$ and cyclic nucleotides in platelet function. *Eur. J. Biochem.* (in press).

GRANSTRÖM, E., H. KINDAHL, and B. SAMUELSSON, 1976a. Radioimmunoassay for thromboxane B$_2$. *Anal. Lett.* 9:611–627.

GRANSTRÖM, E., H. KINDAHL, and B. SAMUELSSON, 1976b. A method for measuring the unstable thromboxane A$_2$: Radioimmunoassay of the derived mono-O-methyl-thromboxane B$_2$. *Prostaglandins* 12:929–941.

GRYGLEWSKI, R., and J. R. VANE, 1972. The release of prostaglandins and rabbit aorta contracting substance (RCS) from rabbit spleen and its antagonism by anti-inflammatory drugs. *Br. J. Pharmacol.* 45:37–47.

HAMBERG, M., P. HEDQVIST, K. STRANDBERG, J. SVENSSON, and B. SAMUELSSON, 1975. Prostaglandin endoperoxides. IV. Effects on smooth muscle. *Life Sci.* 16:451–462.

HAMBERG, M., and B. SAMUELSSON, 1966. Novel biological transformations of 8,11,14-eicosatrienoic acid into prostaglandin E$_1$. *J. Am. Chem. Soc.* 88:2349–2350.

HAMBERG, M., and B. SAMUELSSON, 1973. Detection and isolation of an endoperoxide intermediate in prostaglandin biosynthesis. *Proc. Natl. Acad. Sci. USA* 70:899–903.

HAMBERG, M., and B. SAMUELSSON, 1974a. Prostaglandin endoperoxides. III. Novel transformations of arachidonic acid in human platelets. *Proc. Natl. Acad. Sci. USA* 71:3400–3404.

HAMBERG, M., and B. SAMUELSSON, 1974b. Prostaglandin endoperoxides. VII. Novel transformation of arachidonic acid in guinea-pig lung. *Biochem. Biophys. Res. Commun.* 61:942–949.

HAMBERG, M., J. SVENSSON, and B. SAMUELSSON, 1974. Prostaglandin endoperoxides. IV. A new concept concerning the mode of action and release of prostaglandins. *Proc. Natl. Acad. Sci. USA* 71:3824–3828.

HAMBERG, M., J. SVENSSON, and B. SAMUELSSON, 1975. Thromboxanes. A new group of biologically active compounds derived from prostaglandin endoperoxides. *Proc. Natl. Acad. Sci. USA* 72:2994–2998.

HAMBERG, M., J. SVENSSON, T. WAKABAYASHI, and B. SAMUELSSON, 1974. Isolation and structure of two prostaglandin endoperoxides which cause platelet aggregation. *Proc. Natl. Acad. Sci. USA* 71:345–349.

HEMLER, M., W. E. M. LANDS, and W. L. SMITH, 1976. Purification of the cyclo-oxygenase that forms prostaglandins. Demonstration of two forms of iron in the holo enzyme. *J. Biol. Chem.* 251:5575–5579.

KELLY, R. C., I. SCHLETTER, and S. J. STEIN, 1976. Synthesis of thromboxane B_2. *Tetrahedon Lett.* 37:3279–3289.

MALMSTEN, C., M. HAMBERG, J. SVENSSON, and B. SAMUELSSON, 1975. Physiological role of an endoperoxide in human platelets. VIII. Hemostatic defect due to platelet cyclo-oxygenase deficiency. *Proc. Natl. Acad. Sci. USA* 72:1446–1450.

MALMSTEN, C., H. KINDAHL, B. SAMUELSSON, S. LEVY-TOLEDANO, G. TOBELEM, and J. CAEN, 1977. Thromboxane synthesis and the platelet release reaction in Bernard-Soulier Syndrome, Thrombasthenia Glanzmann and Hermansky-Pudlak Syndrome. *Br. J. Haematol.* 35:511–520.

MILLER, O. V., and R. R. GORMAN, 1976. Modulation of platelet cyclic nucleotide content by PGE_1 and the prostaglandin endoperoxide PGG_2. *J. Cyclic Nucleotide Res.* 2:79–87.

MIYAMOTO, T., N. OGINO, S. YAMAMOTO, and O. HAYASHI, 1976. Purification of prostaglandin endoperoxide synthetase from bovine vesicular gland microsomes. *J. Biol. Chem.* 251:2629–2636.

NELSON, A. N., and R. W. JACKSON, 1976. Total synthesis of thromboxane B_2. *Tetrahedon Lett.* 37:3275–3278.

NUGTEREN, D. H., 1975. Arachidonate lipoxygenase in blood platelets. *Biochim. Biophys. Acta* 380:299–307.

NUGTEREN, D. H., R. K. BEERTHUIS, and D. A. VON DORP, 1966. The enzymatic conversion of all-cis 8,11,14-eicosatrienoic acid into prostaglandin E_1. *Recueil* 85:405–419.

NUGTEREN, D. H., and E. HAZELHOF, 1973. Isolation and properties of intermediates in prostaglandin biosynthesis. *Biochim. Biophys. Acta* 326:448–461.

PIPER, P. J., and J. R. VANE, 1969. Release of additional factors in an alphylaxis and its antagonism. *Nature* 223:29–35.

SALZMAN, F. W., 1976. Prostaglandins and platelet function. In *Advances in Prostaglandin and Thromboxane Research*, vol. 2, B. Samuelsson and R. Paoletti, eds. New York: Raven Press, pp. 767–780.

SAMUELSSON, B., 1965. On the incorporation of oxygen in the conversion of 8,11,14-eicosatrienoic acid to prostaglandin E_1. *J. Am. Chem. Soc.* 87:3011–3013.

SAMUELSSON, B., 1967. Biosynthesis and metabolism of prostaglandins. In *Progress in Biochemical Pharmacology*, vol. 3, D. Kritchevsky, R. Paoletti, and D. Steinberg, eds. Basel: S. Karger, pp. 50–70.

SAMUELSSON, B., 1972. Biosynthesis of prostaglandins. *Fed. Proc.* 31:1442–1450.

SAMUELSSON, B., 1976. Introduction: New trends in prostaglandin research. In *Advances in Prostaglandin and Thromboxane Research*, vol. 1, B. Samuelsson and R. Paoletti, eds. New York: Raven Press, pp. 1–6.

SAMUELSSON, B., E. GRANSTRÖM, K. GREEN, and M. HAMBERG, 1971. Metabolism of prostaglandins. *Ann. NY Acad. Sci.* 180:138–163.

SAMUELSSON, B., E. GRANSTRÖM, K. GREEN, M. HAMBERG, and S. HAMMARSTRÖM, 1975. Prostaglandins. *Annu. Rev. Biochem.* 44:669–695.

SAMUELSSON, B., and M. HAMBERG, 1974. The role of endoperoxides in the biosynthesis and action of prostaglandins. In *Prostaglandin Synthetase Inhibitors*, H. J. Robinson and J. R. Vane, eds. New York: Raven Press, pp. 107–120.

SAMUELSSON, B., M. HAMBERG, C. MALMSTEN, and J. SVENSSON, 1976. Role of prostaglandin endoperoxides and thromboxanes in platelet aggregation. In *Advances in Prostaglandin and Thromboxane Research*, vol. 2, B. Samuelsson and R. Paoletti, eds. New York: Raven Press, pp. 737–746.

SCHNEIDER, W. P., and R. A. MORGE, 1976. A synthesis of crystalline thromboxane B_2. *Tetrahedon Lett.* 37:3283–3286.

SILVER, M. J., J. B. SMITH, C. INGERMAN, and J. J. KOCSIS, 1973. Arachidonic acid induced human platelet aggregation and prostaglandin formation. *Prostaglandins* 4:863–875.

SMITH, J. B., C. INGERMAN, J. J. KOCSIS, and M. J. SILVER, 1974. Formation of an intermediate in prostaglandin biosynthesis and its association with the platelet release reaction. *J. Clin. Invest.* 53:1468–1472.

SVENSSON, J., M. HAMBERG, and B. SAMUELSSON, 1975. Prostaglandin endoperoxides. IV. Characterization of rabbit aorta contracting substance (RCS) from guinea-pig lung and human platelets. *Acta Physiol. Scand.* 94:222–228.

TUVEMO, T., K. STRANDBERG, M. HAMBERG, and B. SAMUELSSON, 1976. Formation and action of prostaglandin endoperoxides in the isolated human umbilical artery. *Acta Physiol. Scand.* 96:145–149.

VAN DORP, D. A., 1967. Aspects of the biosnythesis of prostaglandins. In *Progress in Biochemical Pharmacology*, vol. 3, D. Kritchevsky, R. Paoletti, and D. Steinberg, eds. Basel: S. Karger, pp. 71–82.

VARGAFTIG, B. B., and P. ZIRINIS, 1973. Platelet aggregation induced by arachidonic acid is accompanied by release of potential inflammatory mediators distinct from prostaglandin E_2 and prostaglandin F_2. *Nature [New Biol.]* 244:114–116.

WILLIS, A. W., 1974a. An enzymatic mechanism for the antithrombotic and antihemostatic actions of aspirin. *Science* 183:325–327.

WILLIS, A. W., 1974b. Isolation of chemical trigger for thrombosis. *Prostaglandins* 5:1–25.

WILLIS, A. W., F. M. VANE, D. C. KUHN, C. G. SCOTT, and M. PETRIN, 1974. An endoperoxide aggregator (LASS) formed in platelets in response to thrombotic stimuli. Purification, identification and unique biological significance. *Prostaglandins* 8:453–509.

WOLFE, L. S., 1975. Possible roles of prostaglandins in the nervous system. In *Advances in Neurochemistry*, vol. 1, B. W. Agranoff and M. H. Aprison, eds. New York: Plenum, pp. 1–49.

WOLFE, L. S., K. ROSTWOROWSKI, and J. MARION, 1976. Endogenous formation of the prostaglandin endoperoxide metabolite, thromboxane B_2, by brain tissue. *Biochem. Biophys. Res. Commun.* 70:909–913.

62 Neurobiology of Peptides

WYLIE VALE and MARVIN BROWN

ABSTRACT Secretory oligopeptides have been isolated from diverse biological sources based on various bioassays and have been shown to be present in the CNS by biological, immunological, and chemical methods. Subcellular distributions, specific high-affinity binding sites, enzymatic degradative systems, effects on neuronal membrane potentials and biochemical parameters, and numerous neuropharmacological and behavioral effects have been demonstrated for some of these peptides. Thus peptides, shown to possess various endocrine or paracrine actions on other organs, might play physiological roles as neuromodulators or neurotransmitters in the CNS.

Introduction

OVER THE PAST 25 years numerous oligopeptides with powerful biological actions have been identified in the CNS. In most cases the peptides were detected by virtue of non-CNS activities such as effects on the adenohypophysis (the hypophysiotropic peptides), the vascular system (neurotensin), or the gastrointestinal tract (bombesin). This essay will not attempt to cover the neurobiological aspects of all peptides but will discuss the natural history of some selected peptides (TRF, LRF, SS, neurotensin, and bombesin) and will highlight the types of available evidence supporting direct neurotropic roles for these peptides. Other equally interesting peptides, such as substance P and the opioid peptides, are described by Snyder and Iversen in this volume.

HYPOPHYSIOTROPIC NEUROPEPTIDES The hypophysiotropic neuropeptides (HNPs) were originally purified from hypothalamic extracts based on the peptides' abilities to modify the secretory rates of anterior pituitary hormones. According to the portal vessel chemotransmitter hypothesis, neurosecretory cells in the hypothalamus (including the preoptic regions) produce factors or hormones that reach the adenohypophysis by way of the hypothalamic-hypophyseal portal system. These neural factors act in concert with other blood-borne signals from the periphery to regulate the functions of the various anterior pituitary cells.

To date, three peptides have been characterized and shown to have unequivocal hypophysiotropic activities (Table I): thyrotropin-releasing factor (TRF), luteinizing hormone–releasing factor (LRF), and somatostatin (SS). Both active and passive immunoneutralization studies have provided evidence that LRF, TRF, and SS play physiological roles as regulators of pituitary function (Arimura and Schally, 1976; Koch et al., 1977). For example, the administration of anti-SS serum results in an elevation in basal and stimulated GH and TSH levels. Animals actively or passively immunized against LRF have nondetectable gonadotropin secretion. In addition to TRF, LRF, and SS, there is physiological evidence for the existence of the following putative hypophysiotropic factors: a growth-hormone-releasing factor (GRF), a prolactin (PRL) release–inhibiting factor (PIF), and an ACTH-releasing factor (CRF). It is also possible that known substances such as prostaglandins, dopamine, acetylcholine, and norepinephrine might reach the anterior pituitary from the CNS in biologically effective concentrations.

Pituitary cells possess functional receptors to a variety of naturally occurring substances including neurotransmitters, peptides, and peripheral hormones (for review see Vale, Rivier, and Brown, 1977). For instance, PRL secretion by mammotrophs is inhibited by dopamine, acetylcholine (muscarinic effect), SS (under some circumstances), thyroid hormones, and an uncharacterized peptidic release-inhibiting factor and is stimulated by TRF (which may be the PRL-releasing factor) and estrogens. The secretion of TSH by thyrotrophs is enhanced by TRF and estrogens and is inhibited by thyroid hormones and SS. The secretion of ACTH by adenohypophyseal corticotrophs is stimulated by CRF, vasopressin, and α-adrenergic agonists and is inhibited by prostaglandins and physiological concentrations of glucocorticoids and progesterone. Figure 1 illustrates the interaction between multiple concentrations of a glucocorticoid, dexamethasone, and a purified CRF preparation. Such results are a good example of the modulation of a peptide's action by nonpeptidic factors. In view

WYLIE VALE and MARVIN BROWN Peptide Biology Laboratory, The Salk Institute for Biological Studies, La Jolla, CA 92037

TABLE I

Sequences and direct hypophysiotropic activities of peptides

Peptide	Sequence	Hypophysiotropic Activity
TRF	pGlu-His-Pro-NH$_2$	TSH↑ PRL↑
LRF	pGlu-His-Trp-Ser-Tyr-Gly-Leu-Arg-Pro-Gly-NH$_2$	LH↑ FSH↑
SS	H-Ala-Gly-Cys-Lys-Asn-Phe-Phe-Trp-Lys-Thr-Phe-Thr-Ser-Cys-OH	GH↓ TSH↓
Neurotensin	pGlu-Leu-Thr-Glu-Asn-Lys-Pro-Arg-Arg-Pro-Tyr-Ile-Leu-OH	None
Bombesin	pGlu-Gln-Arg-Leu-Gly-Asn-Gln-Trp-Ala-Val-Gly-His-Leu-Met-NH$_2$	None

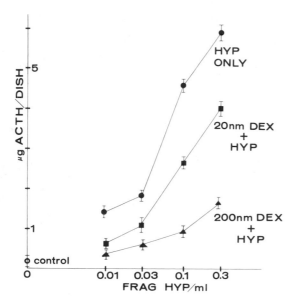

FIGURE 1   Effects of pretreatment for 16 hr with two doses of dexamethasone 21-PO$_4$ (DEX) on the secretion of ACTH due to an ovine hypothalamic corticotropin-releasing-factor preparation (HYP) by cultured adenohypophyseal cells. (From Vale and Rivier, 1977.)

of the numerous signals from neural and peripheral sources that are integrated by pituitary cells to determine their secretory patterns, this biological system could be an excellent model of neuronal integration.

Studies on various species suggest that blood, and therefore pituitary peptide hormones, can reach the hypothalamus directly via efferent pituitary portal vessels (Page and Bergland, 1976; Oliver, Mical, and Porter, 1977) or can have access to the CSF by means of an arachnoid channel continuous with the subdural and subarachnoid spaces (Boyd et al., 1976). Thus it is possible that peptides of pituitary origin that possess multiple CNS activities (e.g., α- and β-MSH and β-endorphin: see Kastin et al., 1975; Bloom et al., 1977b,c) could have access to, and exert physiological actions on, the CNS.

The direct role of the pituitary gland in the mod-ulation of brain function is particularly interesting in light of the revised view of the embryological origin of the adenohypophysis. Studies of Ballard (1964), Ferrand and Hraouri (1973), and Pearse and Takor (1976) suggest that the pituitary gland is not derived from an outpocketing of the stomodeum but, rather, arises from the ventral ridge and so shares a common origin with the hypothalamus. This controversial hypothesis would provide additional justification for regarding the hypothalamus and adenohypophysis as a single functional unit of a neural nature.

It is of particular interest that our most purified preparations of CRF stimulate the in vitro secretion not only of ACTH but also of β-endorphin by cultured anterior pituitary cells (Vale et al., 1978a). Furthermore, there is a good correlation between the in vivo secretion of immunoreactive ACTH and that of immunoreactive β-LPH and its probable derivatives, β-endorphin (β-LPH$_{61-91}$) and β-melanotropin (β-MSH$_{41-58}$), under circumstances such as surgical stress (Guillemin et al., 1977; for review see Vale, Rivier, and Brown, 1978). In view of suggestions that ACTH, β-LPH, and β-endorphin are produced by posttranslational processing of a 31,000 dalton glycoprotein precursor (Mains, Eipper, and Ling, 1977), such correspondence between the secretory rates of these peptides is not surprising. It might be proposed that CRF, presumably secreted during conditions such as stress, mediates the secretion of both ACTH and opioid peptides. These peptides might possibly have, besides their respective endocrine actions, gastrointestinal and CNS effects that could be of adaptive significance.

The HNPs have high potency to modify pituitary function in vitro (minimal effective dose, MED, 30–100 pmol; half-maximal response observed at 0.3–2.0 nmol) and in vivo (MED for LRF and TRF, 50–200 ng/kg body weight; MED for SS, 1–10 μg/kg). The effects of the HNPs on pituitary hormone secretion are immediate in onset and are rapidly reversed when they are removed. The HNPs act acutely to promote exocytotic release of previously synthesized pituitary hormones stored in secretory granules. Chronic exposure of pituitary cells to the stimulatory HRPs or to other secretagogues increases the rates of pituitary hormone snythesis (for review see Vale, Rivier, and Brown, 1977).

Pituitary cells have been shown to possess high-affinity specific binding sites (receptors?) for TRF and LRF. As is the case with brain tissues, changes in membrane ion permeability, ion distribution, and cyclic nucleotide levels are proposed to mediate the adenohypophyseal secretory processes. Kidokoro (1975) reported that adenohypophyseal GH-PRL-secreting tumor (GH_3) cells spontaneously depolarize and that the frequency of depolarization can be increased by adding TRF to the medium. It was shown years ago that elevating $[K^+]_0$ stimulates pituitary hormone secretion in vitro. The stimulated secretion of pituitary hormones is dependent upon $[Ca^{++}]_0$; furthermore, changes in calcium fluxes have been shown in response to various secretagogues. We have shown, for example, that TRF increases $^{45}Ca^{++}$ flux from GH_3 cells. Cyclic AMP derivatives and agents that increase adenohypophyseal cAMP levels, such as prostaglandins, cyclic nucleotide phosphodiesterase inhibitors, and cholera toxin, stimulate the secretion of some pituitary hormones. In addition, synthetic HNPs have been reported to modify intracellular cyclic nucleotide levels (for review see Boss et al., 1977).

Many neuropeptides are widely distributed throughout the gastrointestinal tract as well as the nervous system (Table II). SS-like peptides, for example, are found in nerve fibers or in endocrine-type D-cells in the stomach, duodenum, and small and large intestine. D-cells containing SS are found in particularly high concentrations in the islets of Langerhans of the pancreas. SS has a variety of effects on the gastrointestinal tract, inhibiting the secretion of enzymes, hormones, and ions. Of possible relevance to the theme of this study program is the anatomical and physiological relationships between peptide-secreting cells within the pancreatic islets of Langerhans. β-Cells secreting insulin, α-cells secreting glucagon, and D-cells secreting SS (Dubois, Barry, and Leonardelli, 1974; Hökfelt et al., 1975; Patton et al., 1976) are heterogeneously distributed but often situated within close proximity of one another within the islets. In some cases, tight junctions have been demonstrated between different cell types (Orci et al., 1976). Furthermore, each peptide has been shown to modify the secretory rates of the other two peptides under some circumstances. This morphological and functional arrangement illustrates two points: (1) The concept of paracrine mediation (Feyrter, 1953) whereby a cell modifies the function of its immediate neighbors in the absence of synaptic structures. This is an intermediate situation between transynaptic mediation (single cell to single cell) and endocrine mediation (cell to cells via bloodstream). (2) The endocrine pancreas may represent a model for cell-cell interactions involving both extracellular regulators and electrical coupling, analogous to those proposed to be involved in local circuit communication (Schmitt, Dev, and Smith, 1977)

NEUROTENSIN AND BOMBESIN Neurotensin was isolated from bovine hypothalamus by Leeman and associates during their search for the still-elusive corticotropin-releasing factor (Carraway and Leeman, 1973, 1975). The primary structure of hypothalamic

TABLE II

Anatomic distribution of peptides

	Hypothalamus	Brain (minus hypothalamus)	Spinal Cord	Peripheral Nerves	Gastrointestinal	Pancreas	Cutaneous	Pituitary
TRF	+	+	+		+		+	
LRF	+	+						
SS	+	+	+	+	+	+	+	+
Substance P	+	+	+	+	+		+	
Neurotensin	+	+	+		+	+		
Bombesin	+	+			+		+	
ACTH/β-LPH and related peptides	+	+	+	+	+			+
Glucagon					+	+		
VIP	+	+			+	+		
Gastrin	+				+	+		

bovine neurotensin has subsequently been shown to be identical to neurotensin isolated from bovine intestine. Neurotensin has a variety of pharmacological actions that resemble those of bradykinin: it produces hypotension, increases vascular permeability, and stimulates contraction of smooth muscle (Carraway and Leeman, 1973). Neurotensin also elevates blood glucose, probably by increasing endocrine pancreatic secretion of glucagon (Brown and Vale, 1976; Carraway and Leeman, 1976). Neurotensin given intravenously produces an insulin concentration gradient across the liver with normal or elevated plasma levels of insulin in the hepatic portal vein and decreased plasma insulin levels in the posthepatic circulation (Brown, Villarreal, and Vale, 1976).

Many of the actions of neurotensin are reversed by the H_1-histamine-receptor blocker diphenhydramine but not by the H_2-histamine-receptor blocker cimetidine (Brown, Villarreal, and Vale, 1976; Rivier, Brown, and Vale, 1977). Since many of the actions of neurotensin are mimicked by histamine, it is possible that neurotensin's various actions are mediated via histamine release. Such an action could result from neurotensin-induced mast-cell histamine release. It is interesting that the binding of neurotensin to mast cells has been reported (Lazarus, Perrin, and Brown, 1977).

Bombesin and a variety of closely related peptides have been isolated from frog skin (Erspamer and Melchiorri, 1973). When given to dogs and rats, bombesin increases blood pressure, stimulates the secretion of gastric acid, gastrin, and cholecystokinin, stimulates exocrine pancreatic secretion, and produces contraction of the gall bladder (Erspamer and Melchiorri, 1975).

Bombesin-like immunoactivity has been found in mammalian intestine and brain. We are currently isolating bombesin-like immunoactive material from ovine hypothalamus in quantities sufficient to allow its chemical characterization (Brown et al., 1977).

Neuropeptides in the CNS

Several criteria for the establishment of a substance as a neurotransmitter have been proposed (e.g., Mandel and Pasantes-Morales, 1976). Although nonsynaptic roles are also considered for neuropeptides, it is of heuristic value to evaluate a broad set of related topics with reference to selected peptides. Peptides have been shown to possess cellular and subcellular distributions, mechanisms, and locations of biosynthesis, secretion, and inactivation and a variety of biophysical, biochemical, and behavioral actions that would be consistent with their having functional neurotropic roles.

DISTRIBUTION OF NEUROPEPTIDES WITHIN THE CNS As shown in Tables II and III, several peptides are widely distributed throughout the CNS. Hökfelt and others have recognized peptides in nerve fibers and terminals in numerous regions, while the distribution of peptide-positive cell bodies has been more limited.

Somatostatin (SS) will be used as a model for the discussion of various aspects of the distribution of a neuropeptide. Although bioassays or chemical methods have sometimes been used to detect peptides in the CNS, reliance has been placed mainly on immunological methods. The ability of SS to inhibit the secretion of GH by anterior pituitary cell cultures is the basis of the principal bioassay applied to the detection of SS-like activity (SLA) of natural origin (Vale et al., 1975). Recently we have employed cultured primary anterior pituitary cells maintained in microwells in a volume of ≤ 60 μl for the measurement of small quantities of precious native SS-like substances purified in small amounts.

Radioimmunoassays (RIAs) of SS have been developed in several laboratories (Arimura et al., 1975; Patel, Rao, and Reichlin, 1976; Vale et al., 1976; Pimstone, Berelowitz, and Kronheim, 1976; Barden et al., 1977a; Brazeau and Epelbaum, 1977). Since SS

TABLE III

CNS distribution of peptides

Peptide-like Immuno-reactivity	Spinal Cord	Medulla Pons	Mesen-cepha-lon	Hypo-thala-mus	Median Eminence	Thalamus	Amyg-dala	Hippo-campus	Other Limbic Areas	Olfac-tory Bulb	Neo-cortex	Peripheral Nerves
TRF	+	+	+	++×	+++	0	(+)	0	0	0	0	0
LRF	0	0	(+)	+×	+++	0	(+)	0	0	0	0	0
SS	++	+×	+	+++×	++++	(+)	++×	+×	++×	0	+×	+

Subjective estimation of overall density of peptide-containing fibers: ++++, very high density; +++, high density; ++, moderate density; +, low density; (+), single occasional fibers; 0, no positive fibers observed; ×, peptide-containing cell bodies.
   Source: Based on immunocytochemical data and a table of Hökfelt et al. (1977).

does not contain histidine or tyrosine, SS analogs containing tyrosine (N-Tyr-SS, [Tyr^1]-SS, [Tyr^{11}]-SS) have been iodinated for use as tracers in RIAs. High-affinity anti-SS sera have been produced by many workers; reported minimal detectable SS doses range from 1.5 to 10 pg; half-maximal displacement is from 10 to 500 pg.

The specificities of four RIAs have been extensively characterized by Vale et al. (1976, 1978c). A101 (Arimura et al., 1975), R149 (Patel, Rao, and Reichlin, 1977), and S201 (Vale et al., 1976) are high-affinity sera that are directed toward the biologically important Phe^6 → Phe^{11} residues in SS. S39 was developed as an N-terminally directed antiserum using [Tyr^{11}]-SS coupled to human serum albumin by bisdiazotization (Vale et al., 1976).

Immunocytochemical techniques using various anti-SS sera have been employed for the cellular localization of SS. Each of the biological and immunological methods has advantages and drawbacks. Complementary results with multiple methods are needed to establish the presence of SS in any biological sample.

A variety of biological and immunological techniques have shown that high concentrations of SLA are present in the median eminence (Krulich et al., 1972; Pelletier et al., 1974; Vale et al., 1974; Arimura and Schally, 1975; Brownstein et al., 1975; Dube et al., 1975; Hökfelt et al., 1975; Alpert et al., 1976). The lateral external and medial internal layers of the median eminence are particularly rich in SLA. SS-positive granules within nerve fibers ending on portal capillaries in the zona externa (of the rat) have been demonstrated with electron-microscopic immunological methods; these are suggestive of a neurosecretory mechanism for the delivery of SS to the adenohypophysis (Pelletier, Dube, and Puviani, 1977).

Surgical isolation of the medial basal hypothalamus (Brownstein et al., 1977) and electrolytic destruction of the medial preoptic region (Critchlow et al., 1978) drastically reduce the concentrations of SLA in the median eminence. It is probable that axons of many of the abundant positive cell bodies in the preoptic and the periventricular region project to the median eminence.

In addition to the preventricular region, the arcuate, ventromedial, ventral premammillary, suprachiasmatic, and retrochiasmatic nuclei are high in SLA (Brownstein et al., 1975; Alpert et al., 1976; Kobayashi, Brown, and Vale, 1977). Of these, only the ventromedial nucleus was devoid of SS-like biological activity (Vale et al., 1975), perhaps due to the presence of a putative GRF (Krulich et al., 1972) in that area.

SS-like activity was first identified in the extrahypothalamic brain by bioassay (Vale et al., 1974); this was confirmed by RIA (Brownstein et al., 1975). Over ten times more SLA is found in the extrahypothalamic brain than in the hypothalamus (Brownstein et al., 1975; Vale et al., 1976). SLA is distributed generally throughout the CNS, with high concentrations in the preoptic region, amygdala, and circumventricular organs (Kizer et al., 1974; Brownstein et al., 1975; Dube et al., 1975; Pelletier et al., 1975; Alpert et al., 1976; Kobayashi, Brown, and Vale, 1977). Consistent with the finding of SLA in circumventricular organs, significant amounts of SLA have been detected in the CSF of rats and humans (Patel, Rao, and Reichlin, 1977). SLA has also been found in the spinal cord (Vale et al., 1975; Kobayashi, Brown, and Vale, 1977). Hökfelt et al. (1975) identified SLA by immunocytochemistry in the substantia gelatinosa of the dorsal horn and in the adjacent parts of the lateral funiculus as well as in spinal ganglion cell bodies. Since dorsal rhizotomy markedly reduces the levels of SLA in the dorsal horn, much of the SS in the spinal cord might be derived from cell bodies in the spinal ganglia.

SLA immunoreactivity has also been identified in principal ganglion cells of some sympathetic ganglia. Almost two-thirds of all principal ganglion cells of the guinea pig's superior celiac and inferior mesenteric ganglia are reported to contain SLA (Hökfelt et al., 1977). Since some neurons have been shown to contain both catecholamines and SLA, and both norepinephrine and SS might function as neurotransmitters or neuromodulators, these nerve cells might represent an example of mammalian neurons not conforming to Dale's "one neuron, one neurotransmitter" hypothesis.

SLA has been found in a variety of chordate species using immunocytochemical procedures (Dubois, Barry, and Leonardelli, 1974; Vale et al., 1976; Falkmer et al., 1977). Dubois, Barry, and Leonardelli (1974) found SLA in the median eminences of several mammals, a bird, and amphibian and teleost fish. In the trout, fibers containing SLA were observed to directly innervate the adenohypophysis, suggesting a direct neural control of adenohypophyseal hormone secretion in that species (Dubois, Barry, and Leonardelli, 1974). We have found SLA immunological activity in the brain and pancreas of the rat, pigeon, frog, catfish, electric ray, and hagfish (Vale, et al., 1976). SLA was detectable in the gastrointestinal tract of all of the above species except the hagfish. In the ray, SLA was detected in the stomach but not in the intestine (unpublished results).

Falkmer et al. (1977) detected SLA by RIA and immunocytochemistry in the gastrointestinal tract of a tunicate and cyclostome. In the latter species, *Myline glutinosa*, SLA was found in the bile duct and islet organ. As pointed out by Falkmer et al. (1977), SS-containing cells appear in the islets at an earlier evolutionary stage than the glucagon-storing cells, which in the cyclostomes are still in gastrointestinal mucosa.

SS and other peptides have been found in synaptosomal fractions (Barnea, Oliver, and Porter, 1977; Epelbaum et al., 1977; Styne et al., 1977). The peroxidase-antiperoxidase immunohistochemical technique has demonstrated the presence of peptide-containing granules in nerve terminals. Figure 2 depicts SS-positive immunofluorescence in numerous processes of a multipolar amygdaloid neuron. This observation, suggestive of the existence of SS in dendrites, is worthy of consideration in view of possible dendrodendritic communication. Peptides would be plausible candidates as extracellular mediators of local circuit interactions.

BIOSYNTHESIS AND SECRETION OF NEUROPEPTIDES
The mechanisms involved in the biosynthesis of the neuropeptides have not been rigorously established, but it is likely that the polypeptide chains of most CNS peptides are synthesized ribosomally. Controversies surrounding reports of a nonribosomal enzymatic synthesis of the tripeptide TRF have still not been resolved (McKelvy et al., 1975). Current views on the biosynthesis of peptides suggest that many are synthesized as part of larger precursor molecules (Gainer, Loh, and Sarne, 1977). Posttranslational processing involving enzymatic peptide-bond hydrolysis, C-terminal amidation, or N-terminal acetylation would be required to generate the known peptide. Larger (precursor?) peptides with immunological determinants for LRF and SS have been reported (Miller, Aehnelt, and Rossier, 1977; Spiess and Vale, 1978). We have evidence for a 12,000 dalton peptide with not only SS-like immunological activity but full biological activity as well, raising the possibility that larger species of some peptides might be functional forms.

In consideration of a ribosome-dependent biosynthetic mechanism, several distinctions can be made between peptide messengers and other neurotransmitters. Since the site of biosynthesis of peptides would be the perikaryon rather than nerve terminals, the secretory capacity of peptidergic neurons is dependent upon axonal flow and the presence of large pools near release sites rather than on local enzymatic synthesis. However, final processing could certainly occur at the terminals. The roles of uptake and local reutilization in the synthesis and termination of neural activities of peptides have not been established.

The probable mechanisms of synthesis of ACTH and the opioid peptides by pituitary cells may provide a dramatic model for the biosynthesis of CNS oligopeptides. Studies of Eipper, Mains, Lowry, Herbert, and their colleagues have suggested that a 31,000 dalton glycoprotein, 31K ACTH, is cleaved to 23K ACTH and β-LPH. The peptide β-LPH could be further processed to β-endorphin (β-LPH$_{61-91}$) and subsequently perhaps to [Met^5]-enkephalin (β-LPH$_{61-65}$) in certain tissues (Mains et al., 1977; for review see Vale, Rivier, and Brown, 1978). The glycopeptide 23K ACTH, on the other hand, can be converted to ACTH. In the intermediate lobe, the bulk of ACTH is probably further processed to α-MSH (acetyl-ACTH$_{1-13}$-NH$_2$) and CLIP (ACTH$_{17-39}$) (Lowry and Scott, 1975).

Although 31K ACTH is probably produced by cells in both the anterior and intermediate lobes of the pituitary, signals of secretory functions of these two cell types differ. Our purified CRF preparation, which stimulates ACTH and β-endorphin secretion by anterior-lobe cells, has no effect on intermediate-lobe β-endorphin secretion. Furthermore, dopamine markedly inhibits β-endorphin secretion by the intermediate lobe but has no effect on β-endorphin secretion from the anterior lobe (Vale et al., 1978b). Since both the posttranslational processing of pre-

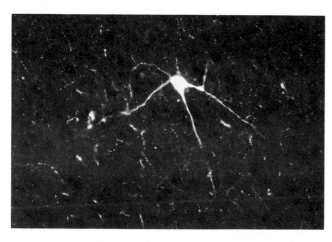

FIGURE 2 Immunofluorescence micrograph of the amygdaloid cortex of rat after incubation with antiserum to somatostatin. (From Hökfelt et al., 1977.)

cursors (31K ACTH) and the extracellular regulatory signals differ between these two pituitary cell types, it would not be surprising to find further differences in brain cells producing endorphins and enkephalins.

There is little doubt that neuropeptides are not only located in but also secreted from cells of the CNS. Porter, Iversen, and others have demonstrated the secretion of neuropeptides from a variety of preparations. Both TRF and LRF are released from hypothalamic synaptosomal fractions by a calcium-dependent depolarization (Porter et al., 1977). L. L. Iversen and co-workers (personal communication) have shown that SS and neurotensin are secreted by slices of the hypothalamus and amygdala; the depolarization-induced release of peptides was found to be calcium-dependent. As yet no in vivo studies have been reported, which could establish that the concentration of a peptide messenger within a discrete CNS region varies with the activities of effector cells.

DEGRADATION OF NEUROPEPTIDES   As is the case for other putative neuromediators, the neuropeptides are rapidly degraded by brain extracts and, in some cases, by blood (Marks, 1977). A variety of proteolytic enzymes may be involved in the breakdown of peptides. Endopeptidases such as cathepsin M cleave several peptides at internal peptide bonds. Peptides with free N- or C-termini can be substrates for exopeptidases. Other enzymes can hydrolyze peptides with blocked termini; for example, pyroglutamyl peptidases or carboxyamide peptidases can attack amidated N-termini. These degradative mechanisms may play a role in the removal of peptides from their target cells, thereby extinguishing past signals and permitting peptides to function as dynamic neuromodulators. The intermittent nature of signal exposure may be essential not only for moment-to-moment control, but also for the maintenance of full target-cell sensitivity. Constant exposure of responsive cells to peptides has been found to decrease sensitivity through a variety of mechanisms, including the loss of peptide receptors.

The importance of degradation to the termination of the (neuro) endocrine actions of the hypophysiotropic peptides has been confirmed by the prolonged actions and often high potencies of peptide analogs of LRF and SS that are resistant to enzymatic cleavage (Marks and Stern, 1974, 1975; Vale et al., 1976).

CNS BINDING OF NEUROPEPTIDES   The presence of cellular receptors capable of specific high-affinity binding of neuropeptides has been demonstrated.

Burt and Snyder (1975) have reported the presence of low- and high-affinity brain TRF receptors. The structural requirements for TRF to bind to these brain receptors are similar to the structure-activity relationships for TRF to bind to pituitary membranes of TSH. Veber et al. (1976) have demonstrated that some analogs of TRF exhibit selective CNS actions comparable to their pituitary effects. These results suggest that there are exploitable differences between the TRF receptors on different cell types. Alternatively, such differences in biological activity of TRF versus CNS parameters may result from differences in the distribution of these TRF analogs to their respective sites of action in the pituitary and brain.

The presence of specific high-affinity neurotensin receptors in rat and bovine brain has been demonstrated with values of K_d in the range 1–10 nM. The distribution density of these neurotensin receptors in rat brain closely parallels the concentrations of im-

TABLE IV

Distribution of neurotensin-like and somatostatin-like activities in rat brain regions (ng/mg protein)

Region	Neurotensin	Somatostatin
Forebrain		
Olfactory bulb	0.06 ± 0.04	0.5 ± 0.1
N. accumbens	1.37 ± 0.26	2.4 ± 0.5
Septal area	0.68 ± 0.09	1.9 ± 0.5
Caudate-putamen	0.03 ± 0.01	0.6 ± 0.2
Cingulate cortex	<0.02	0.7 ± 0.2
Hippocampus	<0.02	0.5 ± 0.1
Amygdala	0.65 ± 0.06	3.7 ± 0.4
Entorhinal cortex	0.06 ± 0.02	1.6 ± 0.3
Preoptic area	1.69 ± 0.43	4.3 ± 1.0
Anterior hypothalamus	0.36 ± 0.15	2.7 ± 0.5
Medial basal hypothalamus	0.92 ± 0.12	73.1 ± 26.6
Posterior hypothalamus	0.33 ± 0.16	2.5 ± 0.4
Thalamus	0.08 ± 0.04	0.5 ± 0.1
Pineal	<0.02	0.3 ± 0.1
Hindbrain		
Substantia nigra	0.29 ± 0.09	0.3 ± 0.1
Interpeduncular n.	0.85 ± 0.14	0.4 ± 0.1
Mesencephalon	0.14 ± 0.08	1.2 ± 0.3
Central gray of mesencephalon	0.75 ± 0.08	1.4 ± 0.3
Pons	0.10 ± 0.05	0.9 ± 0.2
Medulla	0.18 ± 0.07	2.4 ± 0.2
Cervical cord	0.14 ± 0.07	2.4 ± 0.3
Cerebellum	<0.02	0.4 ± 0.1

Source: Kobayashi, Brown, and Vale (1977).

munoassayable neurotensin in these same neuroanatomical areas (Lazarus, Brown, and Perrin, 1977; Kobayashi, Brown, and Vale, 1977).

Effects of peptides on the CNS

Neuropeptides have been demonstrated to exert numerous biophysical and biochemical effects on CNS cells that have pharmacological, physiological, and behavioral consequences.

Dyer and Dyball (1974), Renaud, Martin, and Brazeau (1975), Moss (1976), Nicoll (1976), Rezek et al. (1975), and others have demonstrated that the hypophysiotropic peptides modify membrane potentials of various neurons throughout the CNS. Studies suggest that surprisingly high fractions of central neurons can respond to TRF, LRF, or SS. However, since the concentration of peptides at the effector-cell receptors cannot be determined, the physiological significance of these observations is not established. Neuropeptides are also reported to modify biochemical parameters such as cyclic nucleotides, neurotransmitter turnover, and ion fluxes in the CNS. Finally, numerous neuropharmacological, hormonal, and behavioral manifestations of the effects of peptides on the CNS have been described and will be reviewed in this section.

The interpretation of these studies is difficult for several reasons. Observation of CNS effects often requires doses of peptides that are hundreds of times higher than those required to modify pituitary or peripheral functions. This may reflect rapid catabolism and/or poor distribution of peptides to the CNS. Furthermore, since remote administration of a peptide messenger cannot mimic local distribution patterns of an endogenous peptide, extraneous effects may be recruited, or physiological actions obscured. Several tests are apparently nonspecific in that multiple peptide classes have activity. These paradigms may be too inclusive to have value beyond simply indicating that a peptide can affect the CNS. The peptide actions do exhibit an aspect of specificity at the receptor level in that, within each class of peptide, neurotropic activities have strict structural requirements.

TRF   Reports of symptomatic improvement in clinically depressed humans following TRF administration suggested that TRF might have a direct effect on CNS actions (Kastin et al., 1972, 1975; Prange et al., 1972, 1977). Although considerable controversy exists over these human studies (Coppen et al., 1974;

Mountjoy et al., 1974), Prange and others have provided evidence that TRF does produce significant antidepressant activity in animal models independent of the pituitary thyroid axis (Kastin et al., 1975; Plotnikoff, Breese, and Prange, 1975; Prange et al., 1977). Other neuropharmacological studies have demonstrated that TRF reverses the duration of anesthesia and hypothermia induced by barbiturates, ethanol, chloral hydrate, chlorpromazine, and diazepam (Breese et al., 1974; Prange et al., 1975, 1977), lowers the ID_{50} for barbiturates (Brown and Vale, 1975), and potentiates behavioral changes following hydroxytryptamine accumulation in rats (Green and Grahame-Smith, 1974). TRF also potentiates the anticonvulsant activity of phenobarbitol (Nemeroff et al., 1975). High doses (100 μg/kg body weight) will inhibit morphine- or pentobarbital-stimulated GH secretion in the rat, most likely through a CNS-mediated mechanism (Brown and Vale, 1975; Chihara et al., 1976).

Wei et al. (1975) demonstrated motor activity similar to that observed in the morphine-abstinence syndrome following TRF microinjection into morphine-sensitive brain areas of rats addicted to morphine. We have also demonstrated the onset of rapid tail vibration in morphinized rats when TRF is administered (Brown and Vale, 1975).

TRF prevents growth-hormone secretion induced by morphine (Brown and Vale, 1976) or β-endorphin (Collu et al., 1977). TRF has also been reported to prevent β-endorphin-induced analgesia. In contrast, TRF does not significantly inhibit β-endorphin-induced hypothermia or hyperglycemia (M. Brown and W. Vale, unpublished observations).

Intraventricular administration of TRF elicits an increase in colonic intraluminal pressure in rabbits. This suggests that TRF may stimulate brain parasympathetic outflow by activity on the CNS (Smith et al., 1977). Abundant neuropharmacological data indicate an interaction of TRF with other CNS-acting drugs (for review see Prange et al., 1977).

TRF alone, given intracerebroventricularly (ic), increases spontaneous motor activity of freely moving rats (Segal and Mandel, 1974) and alters the sleep-awake pattern and rapid-eye-movement (REM) sleep in rats (King, 1975); given intraperitoneally (ip), it produces anorexia in rats (Barlow et al., 1975; Vijayan and McCann, 1977). TRF administered to sleeping humans results in production of a wakeful state and prevents the rise in GH associated with slow-wave sleep (Chihara et al., 1977). de Wied has reported inhibition of conditioned avoidance responses following TRF administration (de Wied, Witter, and Greven, 1975). TRF given ic produces hyperthermia in the rat and rabbit (Brown, Rivier, and Vale, 1977a; Carino et al., 1976) and hypothermia in the cat (Metcalf, 1974). The hyperthermia induced by TRF in the rat is reversed by the tetradecapeptide bombesin. We have suggested that TRF may be a modulator of both acute and chronic adaptation to cold by virtue of its ability to stimulate pituitary TSH secretion and to act directly on CNS thermoregulatory centers (Brown, Rivier, and Vale, 1977a).

Studies in which TRF was iontophoresed into selected populations of neurons throughout the CNS resulted in an overall suppression of the rate of discharge and of single-unit activity (Dyer and Dyball, 1974; Renaud, Martin, and Brazeau, 1975). TRF is released from synaptosomal structures following electrical stimulation and dopamine treatment, while 5-hydroxytryptamine (5 HT) inhibits this release (Bennett et al., 1975). Parker et al. (1977) have demonstrated that [³H]-TRH is not taken up by brain synaptosomes; however, the [³H]-TRH metabolite, [³H]-proline, is taken up by subneuronal organelles. An interaction of TRF with brain monoamines was first suggested by the ability of TRF to potentiate DOPA in pargyline-treated mice (Plotnikoff et al., 1972). TRF is reported to increase brain norepinephrine turnover (Keller, Barholini, and Fletscher, 1974), to release [³H]-dopamine from isolated synaptosomes (Horst and Spirt, 1974), and to enhance norepinephrine disappearance from nerve terminals as determined by amine fluorescence (Constantinidis et al., 1974). Generally, no increase in brain norepinephrine, dopamine, or 5-HT content has been observed following TRF administration (Prange et al., 1977). However, TRF does increase brain dopamine following DOPA-pargyline treatment. Although TRF does not alter the activity of brain tyrosine hydroxylase, it does inhibit the conversion of dopamine to norepinephrine (Stolk and Nisula, 1975). A role for the dopaminergic system in the CNS action of TRF has been suggested by Cohn, Cohn, and Taylor (1975), who reported head-to-tail rotation in rats given TRF ic, a behavioral pattern linked to alterations in central dopaminergic activity.

SS The first suggestion that SS might exert some neurotropic action was the tranquilizing effect exerted when large doses of the peptide were administered to monkeys (Yen et al., 1973). Segal and Mandell (1974) also observed that the ic injection of SS into rats resulted in a decrease in spontaneous motor activity (Segal and Mandell, 1974; Plotnikoff, Minard, and Kastin, 1974). In other studies, SS has been demonstrated to produce "barrel rotation," sedation, and hypothermia (Cohn and Cohn, 1975), to alter the sleep-awake cycle with a reduction of both slow-wave and REM sleep, to increase appetite, and to produce a partial ataxia or paraplegia-in-extension (Rezek et al., 1976). SS also alters the actions of various neuropharmacological substances; for example, it increases the LD_{50} of strychnine, decreases the LD_{50} of barbiturates (Brown and Vale, 1975), and potentiates the L-dopa-paragyline test (Plotnikoff, Minard, and Kastin, 1974).

SS acts within the CNS to prevent the hyperglycemia induced by the tetradecapeptide bombesin (Brown, Rivier, and Vale, 1978) or by stress (unpublished observations). The latter studies provide a model to study the role of the CNS in the control of glucose homeostasis.

It is interesting that several CNS and endocrine actions of SS are shared by nonpeptidic drugs—diphenylhydantoin (DPH) and the benzodiazepines—and result in lowering of both insulin and glucagon secretion (Gerich et al., 1972; Petrack and Czernik, 1976). Both diazepam (Valium) and DPH have been reported to inhibit the secretion of insulin and glucagon by the isolated perfused pancreas (Gerich et al., 1972; Petrack and Czernik, 1976). We have further shown that both DPH and diazepam inhibit the secretion of growth hormone by pituitary cells in vitro (Figure 3). Furthermore, several established CNS actions of DPH, diazepam, and SS are similar; for example, all three are anticonvulsant and sedative in some paradigms. It is possible that some of the effects of DPH and diazepam are mediated by an interaction with the SS receptor. The conformations of these substances may bear resemblance to that of the critical region of SS. Such a hypothesis becomes even more engaging in view of our finding of smaller cyclic analogs (8 versus 14 amino acids) of SS that are lipophylic and exhibit high biological potency, particularly on the CNS (Vale et al., 1977).

SS has been demonstrated to increase brain levels of cAMP both in vivo and in vitro (Enock and Cohn, 1975; Havlicek et al., 1976). Havlicek et al. (1976) reported an increase in brain cAMP in animals exhibiting barrel rotation following intracranial SS administration. Pretreatment of animals with a β-adrenergic blocking drug prevented the SS-associated rise in cAMP but did not prevent the onset of barrel rotation, suggesting that the changes in cyclic nucleotide concentration were not related to the behavioral

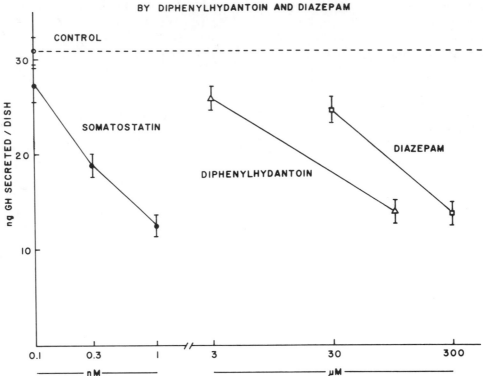

FIGURE 3   Inhibition of 3-isobutylmethylxanthine (IBMX)-induced growth-hormone (GH) secretion from cultured rat adenohypophyseal cells by somatostatin, diphenylhydantoin, or diazepam.

activity. Renaud, Martin, and Brazeau (1975) reported a decrease in the spontaneous firing of neurons in the hypothalamus, brain stem, cerebellum, and cerebral cortex following iontophoresis of SS.

LRF   Recent behavioral (Moss and McCann, 1973; Pfaff, 1973) and electrophysiological (Dyer and Dyball, 1974; Moss, 1976) studies have supported a possible direct action of LRF on the CNS that could modulate sexual behavior independently of sex steroid or pituitary gonadotropin status. Thus LRF may exert cooperative endocrine and behavioral actions.

BOMBESIN AND NEUROTENSIN   Bissette et al. (1976) have recently reported that intracisternal (cisterna magna) administration of neurotensin to cold-exposed rats or mice produced a dramatic reduction in core body temperature. The ED_{50} of neurotensin to produce this action is about 50–100 μg/kg. Inactive structural analogs of neurotensin do not lower body temperature in this paradigm, nor do a variety of other oligopeptides, such as substance P, bradykinin, LRF, TRF, SS, insulin, or glucagon.

Bombesin, when given intracisternally via the cis-terna magna, produces a dramatic acute reduction of body temperature in cold-exposed rats. The effect results from extremely low doses of peptide (MED ≤ 1 ng) and appears to be quite specific, since a variety of other oligopeptides and bombesin analogs fail to exert a similar action (Brown, Rivier, and Vale, 1977b).

TRF, prostaglandin E_2, and naloxone prevent bombesin-induced hypothermia (Brown, Rivier, and Vale, 1977b). Additionally, the hyperthermia induced by either TRF or prostaglandin E_2 is prevented by bombesin. These studies suggest that an endogenous mammalian bombesin-like peptide might be involved in thermoregulatory processes. Another potential action of bombesin on thermoregulation is based on the observation that bombesin prevents cold-induced TSH secretion (Brown, Rivier, and Vale, 1977b). Since TRF levels in pituitary portal blood are known to increase following cold exposure (Eskay et al., 1976), and bombesin does not prevent TRF-induced TSH secretion in vivo or in vitro, bombesin most likely inhibits brain secretion of TRF or delivery of TRF to the pituitary following cold exposure. Thus, in an integrated sense, bombesin and

TRF have opposite actions on body temperature and pituitary TSH secretion.

Bombesin also increases plasma levels of prolactin and growth hormone in rats. Since bombesin does not directly alter the secretion of prolactin or growth hormone in vitro, this action is most likely mediated via the CNS (Rivier, Rivier, and Vale, 1978.)

When given intracisternally, bombesin produces hyperglycemia lasting for several hours (Brown, Rivier, and Vale, 1977b). This hyperglycemia is prevented by acute adrenalectomy, suggesting that bombesin may act by altering brain sympathetic outflow resulting in an increased adrenomedullary release of catecholamine. Involvement of the adrenal cortex in this response is unlikely because of the magnitude of hyperglycemia and the inability of bombesin to increase plasma ACTH levels (Brown, Rivier, and Vale, 1977b). We have recently demonstrated that bombesin-induced hyperglycemia is prevented by intracisternal SS administration (Brown, Rivier, and Vale, 1978); thus, in addition to its glucoregulatory action on the gut, liver, pancreas, and pituitary, this peptide may also affect the brain to alter glucoregulation.

Conclusion

The neural distributions, metabolisms, and biological effects of several peptides are suggestive of their having physiological roles within the CNS. As is the case for other putative neurotransmitters, the elucidation of precise neurobiological functions of peptides is restricted by the complexity of the brain. In addition, neurobiological studies with peptides suffer from the absence of a fully developed pharmacology, since specific antagonists are not (yet) available for most peptides. It is reasonable at this time, however, to consider that peptides probably serve as extracellular brain messengers, and it is tempting to suggest that peptidergic neurons are key participants in brain physiology.

ACKNOWLEDGMENTS   Research in the authors' laboratory is supported by National Institutes of Health Grants HD 09690, AM-18811, and AM-20917, National Science Foundation Grant 411, and a Rockefeller Foundation Grant. We are grateful to Laurie Taylor for her assistance in the typing and editing of this paper.

REFERENCES

ALPERT, L. C., J. R. BREWER, Y. C. PATEL, and S. REICHLIN, 1976. Somatostatinergic neurons in anterior hypothalamus: Immunohistochemical localization. *Endocrinology* 98:225.

ARIMURA, A., H. SATO, D. H. COY, and A. V. SCHALLY, 1975. Radioimmunoassay for GH-releasing inhibiting hormone. *Proc. Soc. Exp. Biol. Med.* 148:784–789.

ARIMURA, A., and A. V. SCHALLY, 1975. Immunological studies on hypothalamic hormones. In *Hypothalamic Hormones: Chemistry, Physiology, Pharmacology and Clinical Uses*, M. Motta, P. G. Crosignani, and L. Martini, eds. New York: Academic Press, pp. 27–42.

ARIMURA, A., and A. V. SCHALLY, 1976. Increase in basal and thyrotropin releasing hormone (TRH)-stimulated secretion of thyrotropin (TSH) by passive immunization with antiserum to somatostatin in rats. *Endocrinology* 98:1069–1072.

BALLARD, W. W., 1964. *Comparative Anatomy and Embryology*, New York: Ronald Press, p. 158.

BARDEN, N., J.-P. COTE, M. LAVOIE, and A. DUPONT, 1977a. Secretion of somatostatin by rat islet of Langerhans and its role in the regulation of glucagon release. In *Proceedings of the International Symposium on Somatostatin, Freiburg, 1977*.

BARDEN, N., M. LAVOIE, A. DUPONT, J. COTE, and J.-P. COTE, 1977b. Stimulation of glucagon release by addition of anti-somatostatin serum to islets of Langerhans *in vitro*. *Endocrinology* 101:635–638.

BARLOW, T. S., B. R. COOPER, G. R. BREESE, A. J. PRANGE, JR., and M. A. LIPTON, 1975. Effects of thyrotropin releasing hormone (TRH) on behavior: Evidence for an anorexic-like substance. *Neuroscience* 1:59.

BARNEA, A., C. OLIVER, and J. C. PORTER, 1977. Subcellular compartmentalization of hypothalamic peptides: Characteristics and ontogeny. In *Hypothalamic Peptide Hormones and Pituitary Regulation*, J. C. Porter, ed. New York: Plenum Press, pp. 49–76.

BENNETT, G. W., J. A. EDWARDSON, D. HOLLARD, S. L. JEFFCOATE, and N. WHITE, 1975. Release of immunoreactive luteinizing hormone-releasing hormone and thyrotropin-releasing hormone from hypothalamic synaptosomes, *Nature* 257:232–234.

BISSETTE, B., C. B. NEMEROFF, P. T. LOOSEN, A. J. PRANGE, JR., and M. A. LIPTON, 1976. Hypothermia and intolerance to cold induced by intracisternal administration of the hypothalamic peptide neurotensin. *Nature* 262:607–609.

BLOOM, F., E. BATTENBERG, J. ROSSIER, N. LING, J. LEPPALUOTO, T. VARGO, and R. GUILLEMIN, 1977a. Endorphins are located in the intermediate and anterior lobes of the pituitary gland, not in the neurohypophysis. *Life Sci.* 20:43–47.

BLOOM, F., J. ROSSIER, E. BATTENBERG, and A. BAYON, 1977b. β-Endorphin: Cellular localization, electrophysiological and behavioral effects. In *Opioid Peptides*, E. Usdin and W. E. Bunney, Jr., eds. London: Macmillan.

BLOOM, F., D. SEGAL, N. LING, and R. GUILLEMIN, 1977c. Endorphins: Profound behavioral effects in rats suggest new etiological factors in mental illness. *Science* 194:630–632.

BOSS, B., W. VALE, P. LAD, and M. PERRIN, 1977. Hypothalamic hypophysiotropic hormones (HHH): Role of cyclic nucleotides in their mechanism of action. *Adv. Cyclic Nucleotide Res.* 2.

BOYD, A. E. III, E. SPENCER, I. M. D. JACKSON, and S. REICHLIN, 1976. Prolactin releasing factor (PRF) in porcine hypothalamic extract distinct from TRH. *Endocrinology* 99:861–871.

BRAZEAU, P., and J. EPELBAUM, 1977. Physiology of soma-tostatin secretion of rat cultured islets: Preliminary studies on the effect of glucose concentration, glucagon and insulin. In *Proceedings of the International Symposium on Somatostatin, Freiburg, 1977*.

BREESE, G. R., J. M. COTT, B. R. COOPER, A. J. PRANGE, JR., and M. A. LIPTON, 1974. Antagonism of ethanol narcosis by thyrotropin-releasing hormone. *Life Sci.* 14:1053–1063.

BROWN, M., J. RIVIER, R. KOBAYASHI, and W. VALE, 1977. Neurotensin-like and bombesin-like peptides: CNS distribution and actions. In *International Symposium on Gut Hormones*, S. Bloom and J. Polak, eds. New York: Churchill Livingstone.

BROWN, M., J. RIVIER, and W. VALE, 1977a. Actions of bombesin, thyrotropin releasing factor, prostaglandin E$_2$ and naloxone on thermoregulation in the rat. *Life Sci.* 22:1681–1688.

BROWN, M., J. RIVIER, and W. VALE, 1977b. Bombesin affects the central nervous system to produce hyperglycemia in rats. *Life Sci.* 21:1729–1734.

BROWN, M., J. RIVIER, and W. VALE, 1977c. Bombesin: Potent effects on thermoregulation in the rat. *Science* 196:998–1000.

BROWN, M., J. RIVIER, and W. VALE, 1978. Somatostatin: Central nervous system action on glucoregulation. *Metabolism* 27:1253–1256.

BROWN, M., and W. VALE, 1975. Central nervous system effects of hypothalamic peptides. *Endocrinology* 96:1333–1336.

BROWN, M., and W. VALE, 1976. Effects of neurotensin and substance P on glucoregulation. *Endocrinology* 98:819–822.

BROWN, M., J. VILLARREAL, and W. VALE, 1976. Neurotensin and substance P: Effects on plasma insulin and glucagon levels. *Metabolism* 25:1459–1461.

BROWNSTEIN, M. J., A. ARIMURA, R. FERNANDEZ-DURANGO, A. V. SCHALLY, M. PALKOVITS, and J. S. KIZER, 1977. The effect of hypothalamic deafferentation on somatostatin-like activity in the rat brain. *Endocrinology* 100:246.

BROWNSTEIN, M., A. ARIMURA, H. SATO, A. V. SCHALLY, and J. S. KIZER, 1975. The regional distribution of somatostatin in the rat brain. *Endocrinology* 96:1456–1461.

BURT, D. R., and S. H. SNYDER, 1975. Thyrotropin releasing hormone (TRH): Apparent receptor binding in rat brain membranes. *Brain Res.* 93:309–328.

CARINO, M. A., J. R. SMITH, B. G. WEICK, and A. HORITA, 1976. Effects of thyrotropin-releasing hormone (TRH) microinjected into various areas of conscious and pentobarbital-pre-treated rabbits. *Life Sci.* 19:1687–1692.

CARRAWAY, R. E., and S. E. LEEMAN, 1973. The isolation of a new hypotensive peptide neurotensin from bovine hypothalami. *J. Biol. Chem.* 248:6854–6861.

CARRAWAY, R. E. and S. E. LEEMAN, 1975. The amino acid sequence of a hypothalamic peptide, neurotensin. *J. Biol. Chem.* 250:1907–1911.

CARRAWAY, R. E., and S. E. LEEMAN, 1976. Characterization of radioimmunoassayable neurotensin in the rat. Its differential distribution in the central nervous system, small intestine and stomach. *J. Biol. Chem.* 251:7045–7052.

CHIHARA, K., Y. KATO, K. MAEDA, H. ABE, M. FURUMOTO, and H. IMURA, 1977. Effects of thyrotropin-releasing hormone on sleep and sleep-related growth hormone release in normal subjects. *J. Clin. Endocrinol. Metab.* 44:1094–1100.

CHIHARA, K., Y. KATO, S. OHTO, Y. IWASAKI, H. ABE, K. MAEDA, and H. IMURA, 1976. Stimulating and inhibiting effects of thyrotropin-releasing hormone on growth hormone release in rats. *Endocrinology* 98:1047–1453.

COHN, M. L., and M. COHN, 1975. 'Barrel rotation' induced by somatostatin in the non-lesioned rat. *Brain Res.* 96:138–141.

COHN, M. L., M. COHN, and F. H. TAYLOR, 1975. Thyrotropin releasing factor (TRF) regulation of rotation in the non-lesioned rat. *Brain Res.* 96:134–137.

COLLU, R., P. D. RUISSEAU, Y. TACHÉ, and J. R. DUCHARME, 1977. Thyrotropin releasing hormone in rat brain: Nyctohemeral variations. *Endocrinology* 100:1391–1393.

H. CONSTANTINIDIS, F. GEISSBUEHLER, J. M. GAILLARD, T. BOVAGUIMIAN, and R. TISSOT, 1974. Enhancement of cerebral noradrenaline turnover by thyrotropin-releasing hormone: Evidence by fluorescence histochemistry. *Experientia* 30:1182.

COPPEN, A., S. MONTGOMERY, M. PEET, et al., 1974. Thyrotropin-releasing hormone in the treatment of depression. *Lancet* 8:433–435.

CRITCHLOW, V., R. W. RICE, K. ABE, and W. VALE, 1978. Somatostatin content of the median eminence in female rats with elevated plasma growth hormone levels due to brain lesions. *Endocrinology* (submitted).

DE WIED, D., A. WITTER, and H. M. GREVEN, 1975. Behaviorally active ACTH analogues. *Biochem. Pharmacol.* 24:1463–1468.

DUBE, D., R. LECLERC, G. PELLETIER, A. ARIMURA, and A. V. SCHALLY, 1975. Immunohistochemical detection of growth hormone release inhibiting hormone (somatostatin) in the guinea pig brain. *Cell Tiss. Res.* 161:385–392.

DUBOIS, M. P., J. BARRY, and J. LEONARDELLI, 1974. Mise en evidence par immunofluorescence et repartition de la somatostatine (SRIF) dans l'eminence mediate des vertébrés (Mammifères, Oiseaux, Amphibiens, Poissons). *C.R. Acad. Sci. Paris* [D] 279:1899–1902.

DYER, R. G., and R. E. J. DYBALL, 1974. Evidence for a direct effect of LRF and TRF on single unit activity in the rostral hypothalamus. *Nature* 252:486–488.

ENOCK, D., and M. L. COHN, 1975. Somatostatin (SRIF) effects *in vivo* and *in vitro* on cyclic AMP concentrations in rat brain. *Neuroscience* 1:451A.

EPELBAUM, J., P. BRAZEAU, D. TSANG, J. BRAWER, and J. MARTIN, 1977. Subcellular distribution of radioimmunoassayable somatostatin in rat brain. *Brain Res.* 126:309–323.

ERSPAMER, V., and P. MELCHIORRI, 1973. Active polypeptides of the amphibian skin and their synthetic analogues. *Pure Appl. Chem.* 35:463.

ERSPAMER, V., and P. MELCHIORRI, 1975. Actions of bombesin on secretions and motility of the gastrointestinal tract. In *Gastrointestinal Hormones*, J. C. Thompson, ed. Austin: Univ. Texas Press.

ESKAY, R. L., C. OLIVER, J. WARBERG, et al., 1976. Inhibition of degradation and measurement of immunoreactive thyrotropin-releasing hormone in rat blood and plasma. *Endocrinology* 98:269–277.

FALKMER, S., R. P. ELDE, C. HELLERSTROM, and B. PETERSON, 1977. Phylogenetical aspects on the occurrence of somatostatin in the gastro-enteropancreatic endocrine system. In *Proceedings of the International Symposium on Somatostatin, Freiburg, 1977*.

FERRAND, R., and S. HRAOURI, 1973. Origine exclusivement ectodermique de l'adénohypophyse chez le Caille: Démonstration par la méthode des associations tissulaires interspécifiques. *C.R. Soc. Biol.* (Paris) 167:740–743.

FEYRTER, F., 1953. *Uber die Perpheren Endokrinen (Parakrinen) Drusen des Menchen*. Vienna and Dusseldorf: Maudrich, p. 2.

GAINER, H., Y. LOH, and Y. SARNE, 1977. Biosynthesis of neuronal peptides. In *Peptides in Neurobiology*, H. Gainer, ed. New York: Plenum Press, pp. 183–219.

GERICH, J. E., M. A. CHARLES, S. R. LEVIN, P. H. FORSHAM, and G. H. GRODSKY, 1972. In vitro inhibition of pancreatic glucagon secretion by dephenylhydantoin. *J. Clin. Endocrinol. Metab.* 35:823–824.

GREEN, A. R., and D. G. GRAHAME-SMITH, 1974. TRF potentiates behavioral changes following increased brain 5-hydroxytryptamine accumulation in rats. *Nature* 251:524–526.

GUILLEMIN, R., T. VARGO, J. ROSSIER, S. MINICK, N. LING, C. RIVIER, and F. BLOOM, 1977. β-Endorphin and adrenocorticotropin are selected concomitantly by the pituitary gland. *Science* 197:1367–1369.

HAVLICEK, V. et al., 1976. Somatostatin (SRIF) action on cyclic AMP in rat brain; role of central adrenergic mechanisms. *Fed. Proc.* 35:317A.

HÖKFELT, T., S. EFENDIC, C. HELLERSTROM, O. JOHANSSON, R. LUFT, and A. ARIMURA, 1975. Cellular localization of somatostatin in endocrine-like cells and neurons of the rat with special reference to the A1-cells of the pancreatic islets and to the hypothalamus. *Acta Endocrinol.* (Kbh) 80 (suppl. 200):5–41.

HÖKFELT, T., T. ELDE, O. JOHANSSON, A. LJUNGDAHL, M. SCHULTZBERG, K. FUXE, M. GOLDSTEIN, G. NILSSON, B. PERNOW, L. TERENIUS, D. GANTEN, S. L. JEFFCOATE, J. REHFELD, and S. SAID, 1978. Distribution of peptide-containing neurons. In *Psychopharmacology: A Generation of Progress*, M. A. Lipton, A. DiMascio, and K. F. Killam, eds. New York: Raven Press, pp. 39–66.

HÖKFELT, T., L. G. ELFVIN, R. ELDE, M. SCHULTZBERG, M. GOLDSTEIN, and R. LUFT, 1977. Occurrence of somatostatin-like immunoreactivity in some peripheral sympathetic noradrenergic neurons. *Proc. Natl. Acad. Sci. USA* 74:3587–3591.

HORST, W. D., and N. SPIRT, 1974. A possible mechanism for the antidepressant activity of thyrotropin releasing hormone. *Life Sci.* 15:1073–1082.

KASTIN, A. J., R. H. EHRENSING, D. S. SCHALCH, and M. S. ANDERSON, 1972. Improvement in mental depression with decreased thyrotropin response after administration of thyrotropin-releasing hormone. *Lancet* 10:740–742.

KASTIN, A. J., N. P. PLOTNIKOFF, R. HALL, and A. V. SCHALLY, 1975. Hypothalamic hormone and the central nervous system. In *Hypothalamic Hormones: Chemistry, Physiology, Pharmacology and Clinical Uses*, M. Motta, P. G. Crosignani, and L. Martini, eds. New York: Academic Press, pp. 261–268.

KELLER, H. H., G. BARHOLINI, and A. FLETSCHER, 1974. Enhancement of cerebral noradrenaline turnover by thyrotropin-releasing hormone. *Nature* 248:528–529.

KIDOKORO, Y., 1975. Spontaneous calcium action potentials in a clonal pituitary cell line and their relationships to prolactin secretion. *Nature* 258:741–742.

KING, C. D., 1975. Inhibition of slow wave sleep and rapid eye movement sleep by thyrotropin releasing hormone in cats. *Pharmacologist* 17:211.

KITABGI, P., R. CARRAWAY, and S. E. LEEMAN, 1976. Isolation of a tridecapeptide from bovine intestinal tissue and its partial characterization as neurotensin. *Biol. Chem.* 251:7053–7058.

KIZER, J. S., M. PALKOVITS, M. ZIVIN, JR., M. BROWNSTEIN, J. M. SAAVEDRA, and K. J. KOPIN, 1974. The effect of endocrinological manipulations on tyrosine hydroxylase and dopamine-beta-hydroxylase activities in individual hypothalamic nuclei of the adult male rat. *Endocrinology* 96:799–812.

KOBAYASHI, R. M., M. BROWN, and W. VALE, 1977. Regional distribution of neurotensin and somatostatin in rat brain. *Brain Res.* 126: 584–588.

KOCH, Y., G. GOLDHABER, Y. ZOR, J. SHANI, and E. TAL, 1977. Suppression of prolactin and thyrotropin secretion in the rat by anti-serum to thyrotropin-releasing hormone. *Endocrinology* 100:1476–1478.

KRAICER, J., and A. R. MORRIS, 1976. In vitro release of ACTH from dispersed rat pars intermedia cells. II. Effect of neurotransmitter substances. *Neuroendocrinology* 21:175–192.

KRIEGER, D. T., A. LIOTTA, and M. J. BROWNSTEIN, 1977. Corticotropin releasing factor distribution in normal and Brattleboro rat brain, and effect of deafferentation, hypophysectomy and steroid treatment in normal animals. *Endocrinology* 100:227–237.

KRULICH, L., P. ILLNER, C. P. FAWCETT, M. QUIJADA, and S. M. McCANN, 1972. Dual hypothalamic regulation of growth hormone secretion. In *Growth and Growth Hormones*, A. Pecile and E. E. Muller, eds. Amsterdam: Excerpta Medica, pp. 206–216.

LAZARUS, L. H., M. BROWN, and M. PERRIN, 1977. Distribution, localization and characteristics of neurotensin binding sites in the rat brain. *Neuropharmacology* 16:625–629.

LAZARUS, L. H., M. H. PERRIN, and M. R. BROWN, 1977. Mast cell binding of neurotensin. *J. Biol. Chem.* 252:7174–7179.

LEE, T. H., and M. S. LEE, 1977. Purification and characterization of high molecular weight forms of adrenocorticitropic hormones of ovine pituitary glands. *Biochemistry* 16:2824.

LOWRY, P. J., and A. P. SCOTT, 1975. The evolution of vertebrate corticotrophin and melanocyte stimulating hormone. *Gen. Comp. Endocrinol.* 26:16–23.

McKELVY, J. F., M. SHERIDAN, S. JOSEPH, et al., 1975. Biosynthesis of thyrotropin-releasing hormone in organ cultures of the guinea pig median eminence. *Endocrinology* 97:908–918.

MAINS, R. E., B. A. EIPPER, and N. LING, 1977. Common precursor to corticotropins and endorphins. *Proc. Natl. Acad. Sci. USA* 74:3014–3018.

MANDEL, P., and H. PASANTES-MORALES, 1976. Taurine: A putative neurotransmitter. In *First and Second Messengers—New Vistas*, E. Costa, E. Giacobini, and R. Paoletti, eds. New York: Raven Press, pp. 141–152.

MARKS, N., 1977. Conversion and inactivation of neuropeptides. In *Peptides in Neurobiology*, H. Gainer, ed. New

York: Plenum Press, pp. 221–250.

MARKS, N., and F. STERN, 1974. Enzymatic mechanisms for the inactivation of luteinizing hormone–releasing hormone (LH-RH). *Biochem. Biophys. Res. Commun.* 61:1458–1463.

MARKS, N., and F. STERN, 1975. Inactivation of somatostatin and its analogs by crude and partially purified rat brain extracts. *FEBS Lett.* 55:220–224.

METCALF, G., 1974. TRH: A possible mediator of thermoregulation. *Nature* 252:310–311.

MILLER, R. P., C. AEHNELT, and G. ROSSIER, 1977. Higher molecular weight immunoreactive species of luteinizing hormone releasing hormone: Possible precursors of the hormone. *Biochem. Biophys. Res. Commun.* 74:720.

MOSS, R. L., 1976. Unit responses in preoptic and arcuate neurons related to anterior pituitary function. In *Frontiers in Neuroendocrinology*, L. Martini and W. F. Ganong, eds. New York: Raven Press, pp. 95–128.

MOSS, R. L., and S. M. MCCANN, 1973. Induction of mating behavior in rats by luteinizing hormone–releasing factor. *Science* 181:177–179.

MOUNTJOY, C. Q., J. S. PRICE, M. WELLER, P. HUNTER, R. HALL, and J. H. DEWAR, 1974. A double-bind crossover sequential trial of oral thyrotropin-releasing hormone in depression. *Lancet* 5:958–960.

NEMEROFF, C. B., A. J. PRANGE, JR., C. BISSETTE, G. R. BREESE, and M. A. LIPTON, 1975. Thyrotropin-releasing hormone (TRH) and β-alanine analogue: Potentiation of the anticonvulsant potency of phenobarbital in mice. *Psychopharmacol. Commun.* 1:305–317.

NICOLL, R. A., 1976. Promising peptides. In *Neurotransmitters, Hormones and Receptors: Novel Approaches*. J. Ferrendilli, B. S. McEwen, S. H. Snyder, and G. Gurvitch, eds., Bethesda, MD: Society for Neuroscience, pp. 99–122.

OLIVER, C., R. MICAL, and J. PORTER, 1977. Hypothalamic-pituitary vasculature: Evidence for retrograde blood flow in the pituitary stock. *Endocrinology* 101:598–604.

ORCI, L., O. BAETENS, C. RUFENER, M. BROWN, W. VALE, and R. GUILLEMIN, 1976. Evidence for immunoreactive neurotensin in dog intestinal mucosa. *Life Sci.* 19:559–562.

PAGE, E., and R. BERGLAND, 1976. In *Fifth International Congress of Endocrinology*, Hamburg, July 18–24, Abstract 502.

PARKER, C. R., JR., W. B. NEAVES, A. BARNES, and J. C. PORTER, 1977. Studies on the uptake of [³H]-thyrotropin-releasing hormone and its metabolites by synaptosome preparations of the rat brain. *Endocrinology* 101:66–75.

PATEL, Y. C., K. RAO, and S. REICHLIN, 1977. Somatostatin in human cerebrospinal fluid. *N. Engl. J. Med.* 296:529–533.

PATTON, G. S., E. IPP, R. E. DOBBS, L. ORCI, W. VALE, and R. H. UNGER, 1976. Response of pancreatic immunoreactive somatostatin to arginine. *Life Sci.* 19:1957–1960.

PEARSE, A. G. E., and T. T. TAKOR, 1976. *Clin. Endocrinol.* 5:229–244.

PELLETIER, G., D. DUBE, and R. PUVIANI, 1977. Somatostatin: Electron microscope immunohistochemical localization in secretory neurones of rat hypothalamus. *Science* 196:1469–1470.

PELLETIER, G., F. LABRIE, A. ARIMURA, and A. V. SCHALLY, 1974. Electron microscopic immunohistochemical localization of growth hormone release inhibiting hormone (somatostatin) in the rat median eminence. *Am. J. Anat.* 14:445–450.

PELLETIER, G., F. LABRIE, R. PUVIANI, A. ARIMURA, and A. V. SCHALLY, 1974. Electron microscopic localization of luteinizing hormone releasing hormone in the rat median eminence. *Endocrinology* 95:314.

PELLETIER, G., R. LECLERC, A. ARIMURA, and A. V. SCHALLY, 1975. Immunohistochemical localization of somatostatin in the rat pancreas. *J. Histochem. Cytochem.* 21:699–701.

PELLETIER, G., R. LECLERC, F. LABRIE, J. COTE, M. CHRETIEN, and M. LIS, 1977. Immunohistochemical localization of β-lipotropic hormone in the pituitary gland. *Endocrinology* 100:770–776.

PETRACK, B., and A. J. CZERNIK, 1976. Inhibition of isoproterenol activation of adenylate cyclase by metoprolol, oxprenolol, and the para isomer of oxprenolol. *Mol. Pharmacol.* 12:203–207.

PFAFF, D. W., 1973. Luteinizing hormone–releasing factor potentiates lordosis behavior in hypophysectomized ovariectomixed female rats. *Science* 182:1148–1149.

PIMSTONE, B. L., M. BERELOWITZ, and S. KRONHEIM, 1976. Somatostatin. *S. Afr. Med. J.* 50:1471–1474.

PLOTNIKOFF, N. P., G. R. BREESE, and A. J. PRANGE, JR., 1975. Thyrotropin releasing hormone (TRH): DOPA potentiation and biogenic amine studies. *Pharmacol. Biochem. Behav.* 3:665–670.

PLOTNIKOFF, N. P., F. N. MINARD, and A. J. KASTIN, JR., 1974. DOPA potentiation in ablated animals and brain levels of biogenic amines in intact animals after prolyl-leucyl-glycinamide. *Neuroendocrinology* 14:271–279.

PLOTNIKOFF, N. P., A. J. PRANGE, JR., G. R. BREESE, M. S. ANDERSON, and I. C. WILSON, 1972. Thyrotropin releasing hormone: Enhancement of Dopa activity by a hypothalamic hormone. *Science* 178:417–418.

PORTER, J. C., R. ESKAY, C. OLIVER, N. BEN-JONATHON, J. WARBERG, C. PARKER, JR., and A. BARNEA, 1977. Release of hypothalamic hormones under *in vivo* and in *in vitro* conditions. In *Hypothalamic Peptide Hormones and Pituitary Regulation*, J. C. Porter, ed. New York: Plenum Press, pp. 181–202.

PRANGE, A. J., JR., G. R. BREESE, G. D. JAHNKE, B. R. MARTIN, B. R. COOPER, J. M. COTT, I. C. WILSON, L. B. ALLTOP, M. A. LIPTON, G. BISSETTE, C. B. NEMEROFF, and P. T. LOOSEN, 1975. *Life Sci.* 16:1907–1914.

PRANGE, A. J., JR., C. B. NEMEROFF, M. A. LIPTON, G. R. BREESE, and I. C. WILSON, 1977. In *Handbook of Psychopharmacology*, L. L. Iversen, S. D. Iversen, and S. H. Snyder, eds. New York: Plenum Press.

PRANGE, A. J., JR., I. C. WILSON, P. P. LARA, L. B. ALLTOP, and G. R. BREESE, 1972. Effects of thyrotropin-releasing hormone in depression. *Lancet* 11:999–1002.

RENAUD, L. P., J. B. MARTIN, and P. BRAZEAU, 1975. Depressant action of TRH, LH-RH and somatostatin on activity of central neurones. *Nature* 255:233–235.

REZĒK, M., V. HAVLICEK, K. R. HUGHES, and H. FRIESEN, 1976. Cortical administration of somatostatin (SRIF): Effect on sleep and motor behavior. *Pharmacol. Biochem. Behav.* 5:73–77.

RIVIER, C., M. BROWN, and W. VALE, 1977. Effect of neurotensin, substance P and morphine sulfate on the secretion of prolactin and growth hormone in the rat. *Endocrinology* 100:751–754.

RIVIER, C., J. RIVIER, and W. VALE, 1978. The effect of bombesin and related peptides on prolactin and growth hormone secretion in the rat. *Endocrinology* (in press).

SCHMITT, F. O., P. DEV, B. H. SMITH, 1977. Electronic processing of information by brain cells. *Science* 193:114–120.

SEGAL, D. S., and A. J. MANDELL, 1974. Differential behavioral effects of hypothalamic polypeptides. In *The Thyroid Axis Drugs and Behavior*, A. J. Prange, Jr., ed. New York: Raven Press, pp. 129–133.

SMITH, J. R., T. R. LA HANN, R. M. CHESNUT, M. A. CARINO, and A. HORITA, 1977. Thyrotropin-releasing hormone: Stimulation of colonic activity following intracerebroventricular administration. *Science* 196:660–661.

SPIESS, J., and W. VALE, 1978. Evidence for larger forms of somatostatin in pigeon pancreas and rat brain. *Metabolism* (in press).

STOLK, J. M., and B. C. NISULA, 1975. Interaction of the tripeptide pytoglutamyl-histidyl-proline amide (thyrotropin release factor) with brain norepinephrine metabolism: Evidence for an extra-hypophyseal action of TRH on central nervous system function. In *Hormones, Homeostasis and the Brain*, W. H. Gropen, T. B. van Wimersam Greidanus, B. Bohus, and D. de Wied, eds. Amsterdam: Elsevier, pp. 47–56.

STYNE, D. M., P. C. GOLDSMITH, S. R. BURSTEIN, S. L. KAPLAN, and M. M. GRUMBACH, 1977. Immunoreactive somatostatin and luteinizing hormone releasing hormone in median eminence synaptostomes of the rat: Detection by immunohistochemistry and quantification by radioimmunoassay. *Endocrinology* 101:1099–1103.

SWAN, H., and C. SCHÄTTE, 1977. Antimetabolic extract from the brain of the hibernating ground squirrel *Citellus tridecemlineatus* 195:84.

VALE, W., P. BRAZEAU, C. RIVIER, M. BROWN, B. BOSS, J. RIVIER, R. BURGUS, N. LING, and R. GUILLEMIN, 1975. Somatostatin. *Recent Prog. Horm. Res.* 31:365–397.

VALE, W., N. LING, C. RIVIER, J. RIVIER, J. VILLARREAL, and M. BROWN, 1976. Anatomic and phylogenetic distribution of somatostatin. *Metabolism* 25:1491–1494.

VALE, W., and C. RIVIER, 1977. Substances modulating the secretion of ACTH by cultured anterior pituitary cells. *Fed. Proc.* 36:2094–2099.

VALE, W., C. RIVIER, P. BRAZEAU, and R. GUILLEMIN, 1974. Effects of somatostatin on the secretion of thyrotropin and prolactin. *Endocrinology* 95:968–977.

VALE, W., C. RIVIER, and M. BROWN, 1977. Regulatory peptides of the hypothalamus. *Annu. Rev. Physiol.* 39:473–527.

VALE, W., C. RIVIER, and M. BROWN, 1978. In *Handbook of the Hypothalamus* (in press).

VALE, W., C. RIVIER, S. MINICK, and R. GUILLEMIN, 1978a. Concomitant secretion of ACTH, β-lipotropin and β-endorphin-like radioactivities by cultured adenohypophysial cells: Effects of purified CRF. *Endocrinology* (submitted).

VALE, W., C. RIVIER, S. MINICK, and R. GUILLEMIN, 1978b. Dopamine and purified CRF on secretion of β-endorphin-like radioimmunactivities by cultured pars intermedia cells. In preparation.

VALE, W., C. RIVIER, M. PALKOVITS, J. M. SAAVEDRA, and M. BROWNSTEIN, 1974. Ubiquitous brain distribution of inhibitors of adenohypophysial secretion. *Endocrinology* 94:A-78.

VALE, W., C. RIVIER, J. RIVIER, and M. BROWN, 1977. Pharmacology of thyrotropin-releasing factor (TRF), luteinizing hormone–releasing factor (LRF) and somatostatin. In *Hypothalamic Peptide Hormones and Pituitary Regulation*, J. C. Porter, ed. New York: Plenum Press, pp. 123–156.

VALE, W., J. RIVIER, L. YANG, B. BOSS, and M. BROWN, 1978c. Mode of action of somatostatin and somatostatin analogs. In *Proceedings of the International Symposium on Somatostatin, Freiburg, 1977*.

VEBER, D. F., F. H. HOLLY, S. L. VARGA, R. HIRSCHMANN, R. F. NUTT, V. J. LOTTI, and J. C. PORTER, 1976. The dissociation of hormonal and CNS effects in analogues of TRH. In *Peptides, 1976*, A. Loffet, ed. Brussels: Editions de l'Université de Bruxelles, pp. 453–462.

VIJAYAN, E., and S. McCANN, 1977. Suppression of feeding and drinking activity in rats following intraventricular injection of thyrotropin-releasing hormone. *Endocrinology* 100:1727–1730.

WEI, E., S. SEGAL, H. LOH, and E. L. WAY, 1975. Thyrotropin-releasing hormone and shaking behavior in rat. *Nature* 253:739–740.

YEN, S. S. C., et al., 1973. Effects of somatostatin on GH, TSH and insulin secretion in human subjects. In *Advances in Human Growth Hormone Research*, J. R. Gieger and S. Raiti, eds. Washington, D.C.: U.S. Government Printing Office, pp. 609–634.

63 Modulation of Neuronal Activity by Peptides and Cyclic Nucleotides

IRWIN B. LEVITAN

ABSTRACT The identified neurons R15 in *Aplysia californica* and F-1 in *Helix pomatia,* exhibit a characteristic "bursting" pattern of electrical activity. This endogenous rhythm can be modified for long periods (minutes to hours) by the vertebrate peptide hormones oxytocin and vasopressin, as well as by a peptide-containing extract from *Aplysia* or *Helix* nervous system. Extracellular or intracellular application of phosphodiesterase inhibitors and cAMP derivatives mimics this long-term response. The vertebrate peptides and the invertebrate peptide-containing extract cause an increase in cAMP and cGMP concentrations in *Helix* and *Aplysia* ganglia.

A long-lasting hyperpolarizing postsynaptic potential can be evoked in neurons R15 and F-1 by appropriate presynaptic stimulation. This long-term response is enhanced by application of phosphodiesterase inhibitors and can be mimicked by intraneuronal injection of an activator of adenylate cyclase. Both synaptic stimulation and treatment with neurotransmitters lead to increased cAMP production in *Aplysia* ganglia. The data are consistent with the possibility that cyclic nucleotides play a role in these long-lasting neuronal responses to hormonal and synaptic stimulation.

Introduction

IT IS WIDELY thought that relatively long-term changes in nervous-system function—those lasting for minutes, hours, and in some cases even longer—involve different intracellular mechanisms than the much shorter changes in neuronal activity usually associated with conventional neurotransmitters. In particular, the rapidly reversible fluctuations in ionic conductances, which give rise to fast postsynaptic potentials, may simply reflect rapidly reversible conformational changes in membrane components that control ionic permeability. Long-lasting modulations of neuronal function, on the other hand, may require more stable metabolic modification of the appropriate membrane components. I shall here attempt to demonstrate that two different effector agents—one a peptide hormone that may act as a long-term neuromodulator (Bloom, 1973), the other released by

IRWIN B. LEVITAN Friedrich Miescher-Institut, P.O. Box 273, CH-4002 Basel, Switzerland

presynaptic stimulation and possibly a classical neurotransmitter—have long-lasting effects on neuronal function that may be mediated by similar mechanisms. Such a conclusion suggests that it may not be appropriate to arbitrarily segregate classical neurotransmitters from other neuromodulators but, rather, that a distinction based on temporal or other aspects of the response of the target neuron might be more relevant.

Among the metabolic modifications that might give rise to altered neuronal function, phosphorylation of membrane proteins has received wide attention. The scheme in Figure 1 describes a hypothetical sequence of events that might lead to long-lasting changes in neuronal membrane permeability following interaction of an effector with its membrane receptor. The

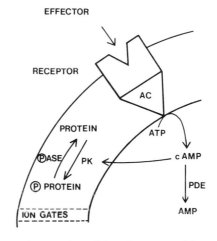

FIGURE 1 Scheme describing how peptide and neurotransmitter effector agents might modify neuronal electrical activity. Each effector interacts with its own specific membrane receptor, activating the adenylate cyclase coupled to that receptor. The cAMP so produced then activates a protein kinase, which in turn catalyzes phosphorylation of a membrane protein, leading to modification of ion gates and the subsequent physiological response. AC, adenylate cyclase; PDE, phosphodiesterase; PK, protein kinase; Ⓟase, phosphoprotein phosphatase. (Modified from Greengard, 1976.)

effector-receptor interaction activates a receptor-coupled adenylate cyclase, resulting in accumulation of adenosine-3′,5′-cyclic monophosphate (cAMP) and stimulation of cAMP-dependent protein kinase. The kinase catalyzes the phosphorylation of a specific membrane protein, which may directly or indirectly control membrane permeability to various ions. The protein can then be dephosphorylated by means of a phosphoprotein phosphatase, and the half-life of the functional alteration may reflect the half-life of the phosphorylated state of the protein.

Although certain aspects of this scheme have been intensively investigated (for reviews see Bloom, 1975; Greengard, 1976), large gaps remain in our knowledge, particularly with regard to the relationship between biochemical changes and modulation of neuronal function. We have studied this relationship in several of the large neurons found in the central ganglia of certain gastropod molluscs. Because of their size, and the fact that many of them can be reliably identified from one animal to the next on the basis of chemical, electrical, and morphological criteria, these neurons represent a model system in which one can simultaneously study biochemical and electrophysiological events.

Neuron R15 in the abdominal ganglion of *Aplysia californica*, and neuron F-1 in the right parietal ganglion of *Helix pomatia* (for nomenclature and criteria for identification see Frazier et al., 1967, for *Aplysia* and Kerkut et al., 1975, for *Helix*), share a number of common features and may be homologous. Both cells exhibit a characteristic "bursting" pattern of electrical activity (Figures 2 and 4), in which an oscillating membrane potential underlies alternating periods of action-potential bursts and interburst hyperpolarizations. This endogenous electrical rhythm can be modified for long periods by vertebrate (Barker and Gainer, 1974) and invertebrate (Ifshin, Gainer, and Barker, 1975; Mayeri and Simon, 1975) peptide hormones and also by synaptic stimulation (Waziri and Kandel, 1969; Parnas, Armstrong, and Strumwasser, 1974; Lambert, 1975). I here present evidence that both of these long-lasting alterations in neuronal function may be mediated by changes in intraneuronal cyclic nucleotide concentrations.

Peptide and cyclic nucleotide modulation of neuronal function

A variety of treatments that increase cAMP and cGMP levels in *Aplysia* and *Helix* nervous systems also modify the endogenous rhythm of electrical activity in neurons R15 and F-1 (Treistman and Levitan,

1976a,b; Levitan and Treistman, 1977). For example, certain 8-substituted cAMP derivatives, which are highly resistant to breakdown by phosphodiesterase and are potent activators of mammalian (Meyer and Miller, 1974) and invertebrate (I. Levitan and E. Bandle, unpublished) protein kinases, alter both the depolarizing and hyperpolarizing phases of the bursting rhythm. These derivatives, in addition to stimulating protein kinase by acting as cAMP analogs, also raise tissue cAMP and cGMP levels by inhibiting phosphodiesterases. When the derivatives are applied in the medium bathing an *Aplysia* abdominal ganglion, there is an increase in the frequency and number of action potentials within the burst, as well as an increase in the depth and duration of the interburst hyperpolarization (Figure 2A). The same result is obtained when the ganglion is bathed with the phosphodiesterase inhibitors isobutylmethylxanthine or papaverine, at concentrations sufficient to increase both cAMP and cGMP levels (Treistman and Levitan, 1976a). We cannot entirely rule out the possibility that these results are due to some side effects of the phosphodiesterase inhibitors that are not related to cyclic nucleotide metabolism. However, antagonism of adenosine receptors by methylxanthines (Rall, this volume) does not appear to be involved, since papaverine (which is not a methylxanthine) is highly effective in altering bursting rhythm. It is important to note that, although the bursting rhythm returns to normal when the drugs are washed from the bathing medium (Figure 2A), a rather prolonged recovery period (30–120 min) is often required—that is, the neuronal electrical response often long outlasts the stimulus.

In order to determine whether this response is due to a direct effect of these agents on R15, rather than on some presynaptic or nonneuronal element, we injected the cAMP derivatives intraneuronally (Figure 2B). Within 6 min the cell hyperpolarized to a level 23 mV below that of the preinjection interburst hyperpolarization and remained silent for several minutes. When bursting resumed, the pattern was similar to that observed after application of cAMP derivatives and phosphodiesterase inhibitors to the bath. It is probable that the apparent differences in response to extracellular (Figure 2A) and intracellular (Figure 2B) application of cAMP derivatives are simply quantitative. Although the derivatives are more lipid-soluble than cAMP itself, it is unlikely that their intracellular concentration following bath application will be as high as the approximately 5×10^{-5}M obtainable by injection.

Further evidence that phosphodiesterase inhibitors

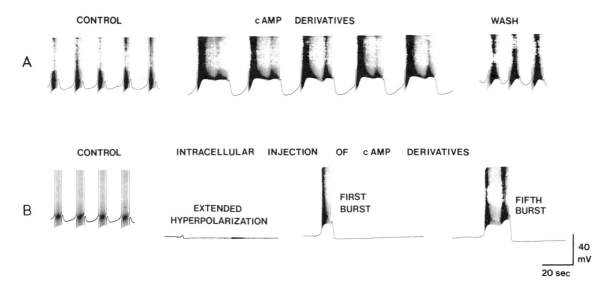

CONTROL   cAMP DERIVATIVES   WASH

A

CONTROL   INTRACELLULAR INJECTION OF cAMP DERIVATIVES

B   EXTENDED HYPERPOLARIZATION   FIRST BURST   FIFTH BURST

40 mV

20 sec

FIGURE 2 Effects of 8-substituted cAMP derivatives on electrical activity in *Aplysia* neuron R15. (A) Electrical activity was recorded in R15 during perfusion with normal medium (control), 45 min after addition of medium containing a mixture of 8-benzylthio cAMP and 8-(4-amino-butylamino) cAMP, and after a 90 min wash with normal medium. (B) Electrical activity in R15 before (control) and after intraneuronal injection of the mixture of cAMP derivatives. The first response of the cell was an extended hyperpolarization, followed by a bursting pattern similar to that produced by bath application of the cAMP derivatives (A). (Modified from Treistman and Levitan, 1976a.)

are acting directly on R15 comes from experiments using tetrodotoxin-treated *Aplysia* ganglia, in which action potentials are suppressed but slow oscillatory waves in R15 continue (Strumwasser, 1971). Under these conditions the durations of both the depolarizing and hyperpolarizing phases of the cycle were markedly enhanced following bath application of the phosphodiesterase inhibitor isobutylmethylxanthine (Figure 3). This suggests that the phosphodiesterase inhibitor–induced change in electrical rhythm (Treistman and Levitan, 1976a) does not result from an alteration in firing pattern of some presynaptic neuron and also does not require action potentials in R15.

The effect of cAMP derivatives on *Helix* neuron F-1 (Figure 4A) is identical to that on R15. These responses are similar to those produced in the same neurons by the vertebrate peptide hormones vasopressin and oxytocin (Barker and Gainer, 1974). Furthermore, a peptide-containing extract, prepared from either *Helix* or *Aplysia* ganglia, also modifies R15 and F-1 bursting rhythm in a remarkably similar way (Ifshin, Gainer, and Barker, 1975; Mayeri and Simon, 1975; Levitan and Treistman, 1977). The effect of a peptide-containing extract (PE) from *Helix* (prepared as described in Table I) on neuron F-1 is shown in Figure 4B. As in the case of the cAMP derivatives (Figure 4A), both the depolarizing and hyperpolarizing phases of the bursting rhythm are altered by

the PE. The effects of the PE can be reversed by washing (Figure 4B), but here again a prolonged recovery period is required. The vertebrate and invertebrate peptides alter the membrane characteristics of these neurons in a complex manner, several of the ionic conductances that underlie the bursting rhythm being affected (Barker and Smith, 1977).

Peptide modulation of cyclic nucleotide levels

Greengard (1976) has suggested a number of criteria that must be satisfied before a physiological response can be attributed to a cyclic nucleotide. One of the requirements is that the application of phosphodiesterase inhibitors or cyclic nucleotides must mimic the physiological response. Since this is clearly the case in the responses of R15 and F-1 to peptides, we further investigated the possibility that cAMP and/or cGMP might mediate this phenomenon. Treatment of *Aplysia* or *Helix* ganglia with vasopressin or oxytocin leads to a large increase in cAMP concentrations in the tissue (Levitan and Treistman, 1977). The response is half-maximal at a vasopressin concentration of approximately 5×10^{-8}M, in good agreement with the concentrations required to alter the bursting rhythm (Barker and Gainer, 1974). Furthermore the PE, at the same concentration that modifies electrical activity, also increases cAMP in *Helix* (Figure 5) and *Aplysia* (Table II) ganglia. The increase evoked by the

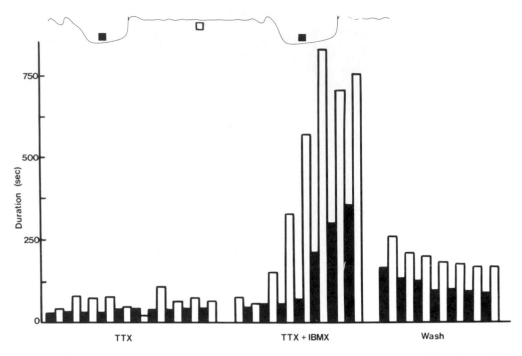

FIGURE 3 Alteration of electrical activity in R15 by iso-butylmethylxanthine (IBMX), in the presence of tetrodotoxin (TTX). The upper trace shows the oscillating membrane potential, with action potentials eliminated by TTX treatment. Plotted are the durations of the depolarizing (□) and hyperpolarizing (■) phases in the presence and absence of IBMX.

TABLE I

Preparation of peptide extract

1. Homogenize ganglia in 5% acetic acid
2. Centrifuge, then lyophilize supernatant
3. Resuspend dried supernatant in H_2O
4. Centrifuge, then lyophilize supernatant
5. Redissolve dried material in small volume of 5% acetic acid and pass over Sephadex G-10 column
6. Elute with 5% acetic acid; void (exclusion) volume is collected and lyophilized = peptide extract (PE)

Peptide extract was prepared from *Helix* or *Aplysia* ganglia, according to the scheme described above.

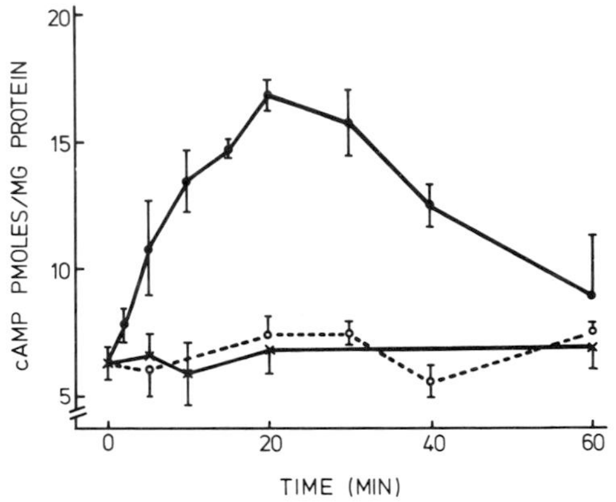

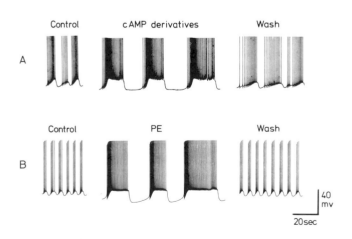

FIGURE 5 Effects of the PE on cAMP levels in *Helix* ganglia. Ganglia were incubated for varying periods of time in normal *Helix* medium (crosses) or in medium containing PE from *Helix* ganglia (filled circles) or *Helix* foot muscle (open circles), prior to measurement of cAMP concentrations. (From Levitan and Treistman, 1977.)

FIGURE 4 Effects of cAMP derivatives and PE on electrical activity in *Helix* neuron F-1. (A) Effects of a mixture of cAMP derivatives (details as in Figure 2A). (B) Effects of PE treatment and subsequent 60 min wash on electrical activity in F-1. Note the similarity of the responses in A and B. (Modified from Levitan and Treistman, 1977.)

TABLE II

Effect of Aplysia *PE on cAMP levels in various portions of* Aplysia *nervous system*

Tissue Fraction	Relative cAMP Concentration (PE-treated/control)
Neuron R2 cell body	0.87
Neuron R15 cell body	1.16
Neuron L10 cell body	1.08
Left pleural giant neuron cell body	0.96
Remainder of abdominal ganglion	2.51
Connective and peripheral nerves	0.89

Aplysia ganglia were incubated for 10 min in the presence or absence of PE, then were frozen for dissection of identified neuronal cell bodies and determination of cAMP levels. The neurons were identified on the basis of morphological criteria only. Modified from Treistman and Levitan (1976a).

PE is qualitatively similar to that evoked by vasopressin and oxytocin (Levitan and Treistman, 1977) but is considerably greater in amplitude and duration. Both the vertebrate peptides and the invertebrate PE cause an increase in cGMP in *Helix* and *Aplysia* nervous systems (I. Levitan and F. Bergström, unpublished). This response can be rather erratic and is occasionally difficult to reproduce, as are cGMP changes in several other systems, but we have observed it in a large number of experiments. The possible role of this cGMP increase in the generation of altered bursting rhythms will be discussed later.

We attempted to determine the cellular localization of the cAMP response by freezing *Aplysia* ganglia after treatment with the PE and keeping them frozen while identified neuronal cell bodies and other portions of the nervous system were dissected (Giller and Schwartz, 1971). As shown in Table II, there appeared to be no increase in cAMP following PE treatment in any of the four nerve-cell bodies (including R15) that we examined. Furthermore, no increase in cAMP was observed in connective nerves. In contrast, the PE did cause cAMP accumulation in that part of the ganglion remaining after removal of the various cell bodies (Table II). The lack of any cAMP response in the neuronal somata suggests that the increase is confined to the neuropil, which contains glia, neuronal processes (including those of R15), and all the synaptic contacts in the ganglion (Coggeshall, 1967). Although the connective nerves, which also contain glial cells (Coggeshall, 1967), do not accumulate

cAMP, the results of this experiment do not allow assignment of the PE response to neurons in general, and certainly not to any individual neuron in particular.

Peptide modulation of adenylate cyclase activity

Another of the Greengard criteria states that the physiological agent should stimulate nucleotide cyclase activity in cell-free membrane preparations from the target tissue. As shown in Figure 6, the PE markedly stimulates adenylate cyclase activity in a crude membrane preparation from *Helix* ganglia. Using this assay, which is simple and rapid, we have examined the effects of a number of treatments of the PE on its subsequent ability to stimulate adenylate cyclase activity. These results have been compared with the effects of the treated PE on bursting rhythm in neuron F-1 and on cAMP accumulation in intact ganglia. The results, summarized in Table III, demonstrate that the active factor in the PE is stable to boiling and treatment with acetic acid, is lost on dialysis, and is destroyed by treatment with pronase, pepsin, or carboxypeptidase A. All of these data suggest that the factor is a relatively small peptide. Furthermore, the various treatments affect the performance of the PE in all three assays in exactly the same way. In fact, in all the characteristics that we have investigated, we are unable to separate or distinguish between the factor that modulates neuronal electrical activity and the factor that alters cyclic nucleotide metabolism.

A pharmacological analysis of the adenylate cyclase and electrical responses to the PE would clearly be of interest. Unfortunately, specific peptide antagonists are not readily available, but there is a factor, extract-

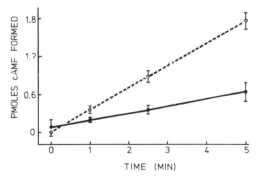

FIGURE 6   Effect of the PE on adenylate cyclase activity in membranes from *Helix* ganglia. Adenylate cyclase activity was measured using 10μg of membrane protein, in the absence (filled circles) or presence (open circles) of the PE. (From Levitan and Treistman, 1977.)

TABLE III

Effects of various treatments of the PE on its ability to modify cAMP metabolism and neuronal electrical activity

Pretreatment of PE	Subsequent Test Assay		
	cAMP Levels, Intact Ganglia	Adenylate Cyclase	R15 or F-1 Bursting Rhythm
Dialysis	−	−	−
Boiling	+	+	+
100% acetic acid	+	+	+
Pronase	−	NT	−
Pepsin	NT	−	−
Carboxypeptidase A	NT	−	−
RNAse	+	+	+

PE was treated as described above, then tested in each of three bioassays. + means treated PE was as active as control PE in that test assay; − means most or all of activity was lost. NT, not tested. Results taken from Levitan and Treistman (1977).

able from *Helix* and *Aplysia* ganglia, that inhibits the effects of the PE on neuronal electrical activity (Ifshin, Gainer, and Barker, 1975). We have found a factor prepared in the same way inhibits the effect of the PE on adenylate cyclase activity (Levitan and Treistman, 1977). This result conforms with another of the Greengard criteria, namely, that antagonists that block the physiological response should also block stimulation of adenylate cyclase activity by the effector. The nature of the endogenous blocking agent is at present unknown, but it may prove to be a useful pharmacological tool.

As another approach to the cellular localization of the cAMP response to the PE, we dissected identified neuronal cell bodies from *Aplysia* abdominal ganglia that had *not* previously been exposed to PE and looked at adenylate cyclase activity in crude membranes prepared from several pooled cell bodies. As shown in Table IV, the PE stimulated adenylate cyclase activity in membranes from all the cell bodies examined (including R15). In addition, membranes prepared from a region of neuropil largely devoid of neuronal somata also contain a PE-stimulated adenylate cyclase. Similar results were obtained with *Helix* tissue, although in this case the pooled cell bodies were from unidentified neurons. These data appear to conflict with those in Table II, which show that PE treatment of intact ganglia does not cause a cAMP increase in several neuronal cell bodies. One possible explanation of these results is that the cell bodies, as well as the neuropil, contain receptors for the active peptide, linked to adenylate cyclase, but that cAMP accumulates only in the neuropil region in the intact tissue.

In further experiments designed to investigate the

TABLE IV

Effect of Aplysia *PE on adenylate cyclase activity in membranes from neuronal cell bodies*

Source of Membranes	Relative Adenylate Cyclase Activity (PE-treated/control)
Neuron R2 cell body	1.79
Neuron R15 cell body	2.44
Neuron L10 cell body	1.53
Abdominal ganglion neuropil free of neuronal cell bodies	3.07
Unidentified *Helix* neuron cell bodies	2.11

Identified neuronal cell bodies, or a fraction of neuropil free of neuronal cell bodies, were dissected from *Aplysia*; unidentified neuronal cell bodies were obtained from *Helix*. Adenylate cyclase activity was measured in membranes prepared from 5–10 pooled neuronal cell bodies (or equivalent amount of neuropil) in the presence or absence of PE. Neurons were identified on the basis of morphological criteria only.

specificity of the adenylate cyclase response to PE, we prepared both PE and enzyme from several sources. Adenylate cyclase from *Helix* or *Aplysia* ganglia was stimulated by both *Helix* and *Aplysia* PE. Furthermore, a PE prepared from rat cerebral cortex also stimulates adenylate cyclase from *Helix* ganglia (I. Levitan, A. Drummond, and A. Harmar, unpublished). Our preliminary experiments suggest that the active factor in rat brain PE is different from that in *Helix* ganglion PE but that the two factors may be interacting with the same receptor. PE from *Helix* foot muscle affects neither foot muscle nor ganglion adenylate cyclase, and the ganglion PE does not stimulate the foot muscle enzyme (Levitan and Treistman, 1977). These results suggest that there may be tissue specificity for both the active factor in the PE and its membrane-bound receptor.

Synaptic modulation of neuronal function

Neuron R15 is postsynaptic to a number of neurons within the abdominal ganglion as well as to neurons in other parts of the nervous system. For example, stimulation of the right pleuroabdominal connective nerve gives rise to several different postsynaptic potentials in R15 (Figure 7), the nature of the response depending on the strength of stimulation (Parnas, Armstrong, and Strumwasser, 1974). One of these responses is a cholinergic fast excitatory postsynaptic potential, which is evoked at relatively low stimulus intensity and appears to be monosynaptic (Schlapfer et al., 1974). Stimulation of the right pleuroabdominal connective nerve at higher stimulus intensity gives rise to a complex postsynaptic potential, with a depolarizing component and one or two slower hyperpolarizing components (Parnas, Armstrong, and Strumwasser, 1974). This same response can be evoked by stimulation of the branchial nerve, indicating that it is mediated by an interneuron within the abdominal ganglion (Figure 7). This interneuron, designated interneuron II by Waziri and Kandel (1969), has not yet been identified. Although iontophoretic application of dopamine to R15 causes hy-

perpolarization (Ascher, Kehoe, and Tauc, 1967) similar to that evoked by branchial nerve stimulation, Ascher (1972) has concluded that dopamine is not the transmitter released by interneuron II, and this question remains open.

A similar complex postsynaptic potential can be evoked in *Helix* neuron F-1 by stimulation of the right pallial nerve (Lambert, 1975; Figure 8A). Using voltage clamping, we have investigated the ionic currents that give rise to this response in F-1 and found (Figure 8B,C) that two distinct outward currents with different time courses mediate the two phases of hyperpolarization. The faster current reverses to an inward current at approximately −80 mV (Figure 8C) and appears to be carried by potassium ions. The slower current does not reverse sign even at membrane potentials as large as −100 mV but does become very small in amplitude. Thus it may represent the turning off (by synaptic stimulation) of a normally flowing inward current carried by sodium or calcium ions. However, we cannot exclude the possibility that it is the turning on of an outward potassium current, as suggested by other workers using R15 (Ascher, 1972; Parnas and Strumwasser, 1974), and that it does not reverse at low membrane potential because the ionic gates involved are far from the cell body and cannot be effectively voltage-clamped. Thus this question also remains open.

Of particular interest is the fact that both R15 and F-1 may hyperpolarize for several minutes following

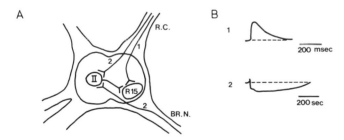

FIGURE 7 Organization of some of the synaptic inputs to neuron R15 from the right pleuroabdominal connective (R.C.) and the branchial nerve (BR.N). (A) A schematic view of the dorsal surface of the abdominal ganglion. Interneuron II is an unidentified interneuron that probably mediates the long-lasting complex postsynaptic potential (B₂) evoked by stimulation of R.C. or BR.N. Less intense stimulation of R.C. gives rise to a fast monosynaptic excitatory postsynaptic potential (B₁). Note the different time scales in B₁ and B₂. The numbers in A identify the pathways giving rise to the corresponding responses in B. Although interneuron II is shown in the left half of the abdominal ganglion, its position is not known, and in fact its cell body may not even lie within the ganglion. For convenience, the synapses are depicted as lying on the cell bodies, but they are almost certainly on processes in the neuropil.

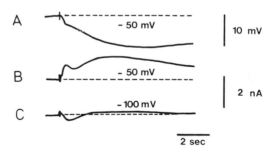

FIGURE 8 Membrane potential changes and ionic currents evoked in *Helix* neuron F-1 by stimulation of the right pallial nerve. F-1 was penetrated with a double-barreled microelectrode, one barrel of which was used to record potential and the other to pass current. The membrane potential was held at either −50 mV (close to normal resting potential) or −100 mV by conventional voltage-clamp techniques. (A) The complex change in membrane potential evoked by presynaptic stimulation. Note the two distinct hyperpolarizing phases, corresponding to the two distinct outward currents shown in B. (C) At −100 mV, the first current has reversed and flows inward. The second, longer-lasting current is much smaller in amplitude but has not reversed sign.

a single presynaptic stimulus, and after several stimuli the hyperpolarization may last for hours (Parnas, Armstrong, and Strumwasser, 1974; Lambert, 1975). That is, as in the case of application of peptide hormones, the response of the target neuron long outlasts the stimulus. We have investigated the possibility that cAMP may play a role in this long-term synaptic hyperpolarization.

Cyclic nucleotide modulation of synaptic response

If generation of cAMP in R15 is involved in the long-lasting hyperpolarization following branchial-nerve stimulation, then prevention of cAMP breakdown, by inhibiting phosphodiesterase, should alter the synaptic response. For these experiments we used theophylline, which is a less potent inhibitor of *Aplysia* abdominal ganglion phosphodiesterase than, for example, isobutylmethylxanthine or papaverine (I. Levitan and E. Bergström, unpublished). However, these latter drugs alter R15 bursting rhythm (Treistman and Levitan, 1976a), which interferes with a study of synaptic stimulation. Theophylline has little effect on the bursting rhythm but does modify the response to branchial-nerve stimulation (Figure 9). The stimulus parameters were adjusted to give a hyperpolarizing phase lasting approximately 30 sec, in order to allow a large number of test pulses to be given in a reasonable period of time. As shown in Figure 9A, the hyperpolarizing phase is considerably enhanced in the presence of theophylline. Note that the fast depolarizing component does not appear to be affected. The data from a number of stimuli are plotted in Figure 9B and demonstrate that the amplitude and

duration of the synaptic hyperpolarization are affected equally by theophylline.

Because methylxanthine phosphodiesterase inhibitors may act as antagonists at adenosine receptors (Rall, this volume) and may have other side effects not related to cyclic nucleotide metabolism, we attempted to increase cAMP levels in R15 by some mechanism other than phosphodiesterase inhibition. To this end we utilized the GTP analog guanylylimidodiphosphate (Gpp(NH)p), a potent activator of adenylate cyclase in cell-free membrane preparations (Lefkowitz, 1974; Schramm and Rodbell, 1975). Gpp(NH)p at high concentrations does not affect cAMP or cGMP phosphodiesterase activity in *Aplysia* abdominal ganglion, but at micromolar concentrations it does activate the adenylate cyclase (Figure 10). Activation of adenylate cyclase by Gpp(NH)p is also seen in homogenates of identified neuronal cell bodies, including that of R15 (Treistman and Levitan, 1976b).

We injected Gpp(NH)p directly into R15, to give an intraneuronal concentration between 10 μM and 100 μM, sufficient to fully activate adenylate cyclase (Figure 10). Following the injection, R15 abruptly hyperpolarized and remained silent for hours (Figure 11), with total abolition of burst activity. Periodic depolarization of the cell by current injection resulted in normal action potentials, indicating that the cell was not damaged. The membrane potential during the Gpp(NH)p-induced hyperpolarization of R15 was approximately -75 mV, similar to the potassium equilibrium potential for this neuron and also to the membrane potential observed during the synaptic hyperpolarization evoked by branchial-nerve stimu-

A
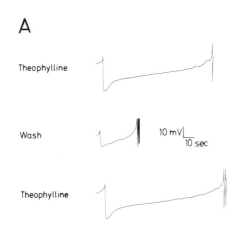

B
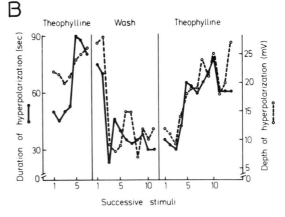

FIGURE 9 Effect of theophylline on synaptic potential recorded in R15 during branchial-nerve stimulation. (A) Examples of the complex potential recorded in R15 after single stimuli to the branchial nerve, in the presence or absence of theophylline. (B) Plot of duration (filled circles) and amplitude (open circles) of evoked potentials in R15 during theophylline exposure, wash, and reintroduction of theophylline. (From Treistman and Levitan, 1976b.)

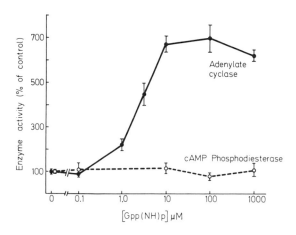

FIGURE 10 Effect of Gpp(NH)p on adenylate cyclase (filled circles) and cAMP phosphodiesterase (open circles) activities in *Aplysia* abdominal ganglion. (From Treistman and Levitan, 1976b.)

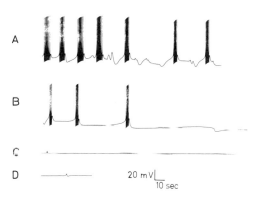

FIGURE 11 Response of R15 to intraneuronally injected Gpp(NH)p. (A) Baseline fluctuations caused by spurts of injected Gpp(NH)p are evident immediately prior to the fourth burst and continue for the duration of the trace. (B) Trace beginning 1.5 min after the end of A, illustrating abrupt hyperpolarization of R15. Trace C is 2 hr and trace D is 3.5 hr after Gpp(NH)p injection. (From Treistman and Levitan, 1976b.)

lation (Parnas, Armstrong, and Strumwasser, 1974). Thus this increase in intraneuronal cAMP, induced by activation of intraneuronal adenylate cyclase, produces a response in R15 that closely resembles long-lasting synaptic hyperpolarization. Brunelli, Castellucci, and Kandel (1976) and Shimahara and Tauc (1977) have recently described other *Aplysia* synapses that may also be mediated by cAMP.

Transmitter and synaptic modulation of cyclic nucleotide levels

Synaptic stimulation appears to alter cAMP metabolism in *Aplysia* abdominal ganglion. Cedar, Kandel,

and Schwartz (1972) found an increase in conversion of [3H]-adenine to [3H]-cAMP during stimulation of the pleuroabdominal connectives and peripheral nerves. However, no increase in total cAMP in the tissue was observed. This response appears to be due to synaptic activity, since it was blocked by incubating ganglia in high magnesium to prevent transmitter release. The cellular localization of this increased cAMP synthesis has not been established. It was not observed in connective nerves or in the cell bodies of neurons R2 or R15. Like the cAMP response to peptides (Table II), the synaptically induced increase in cAMP synthesis appears to be confined to the neuropil, but whether it occurs in neuronal processes or in nonneuronal elements remains to be determined.

Octopamine, dopamine, and serotonin, all of which are putative neurotransmitters in *Aplysia,* cause an increase in both [3H]-cAMP formation and in total cAMP in the abdominal ganglion (Levitan, Madsen, and Barondes, 1974; Cedar and Schwartz, 1972). On the other hand, several other neurotransmitter candidates (including acetylcholine and norepinephrine) are without effect (Cedar and Schwartz, 1972; I. Levitan and E. Bergström, unpublished). This cAMP response to putative transmitters was observed in the cell bodies of neurons R2 and R15 as well as in connective nerves (Cedar and Schwartz, 1972), in contrast to the response to synaptic stimulation (Cedar, Kandel, and Schwartz, 1972). The effects of octopamine and serotonin on cAMP levels are summarized in Table V. It can be seen that most of the stimulation by serotonin is antagonized by methysergide, which blocks serotonergic synaptic transmission in *Helix* (Cottrell, 1970).

It is difficult to relate these findings to specific physiological responses. The synapse studied by Brunelli, Castellucci, and Kandel (1976) may be mediated by serotonin, which does cause an increase in cAMP, but the evidence that serotonin is the transmitter is

TABLE V

Effects of octopamine and serotonin on cAMP levels in Aplysia abdominal ganglion

Treatment	Relative cAMP Concentration (treated/control)
Octopamine	3.7
Serotonin	5.9
Serotonin + methysergide	2.3

Abdominal ganglia were incubated for 10 min with the putative neurotransmitter, in the presence or absence of methysergide, prior to measurement of cAMP concentrations. Modified from Levitan, Madsen, and Barondes (1974).

not conclusive. Nor has it yet been established with certainty what neurotransmitter produces the long-lasting synaptic hyperpolarization in R15 and F-1, although, as discussed above, it may be dopamine, which also increases cAMP. Definitive information about the transmitters released at these synapses may have to await the identification of the presynaptic neuron in both cases.

The role of protein phosphorylation

If cAMP is indeed an intraneuronal second messenger for the peptide and neurotransmitter effector agents discussed above, how is the increase in cAMP transduced into the ultimate physiological response of the neuron? Certainly one possible participant in the transduction is Ca^{++}, which plays an important role in generation of endogenous bursting rhythms (Lux and Heyer, this volume) and may interact with cyclic nucleotides to produce a variety of physiological responses (Berridge, this volume). As described in Figure 1, another possibility for the transduction is phosphorylation of specific proteins, since cAMP-dependent protein kinases are so widely distributed in nervous system and other tissues (for review see Rubin and Rosen, 1975). Extensive phosphorylation is observed in synaptic membrane fractions from brain (Weller and Rodnight, 1970; Maeno, Johnson, and Greengard, 1971), and cAMP stimulation of phosphorylation of specific proteins has been reported in brain (Ueda, Maeno, and Greengard, 1973) and other tissues (Tada, Kirchberger, and Katz, 1975). Functional correlations have been investigated in only a few instances. The phosphorylation state of specific proteins may be associated with sodium permeability in toad bladder (DeLorenzo et al., 1973) and with calcium permeability in synaptic (Weller and Morgan, 1977) and sarcoplasmic reticulum (Kirchberger and Raffo, 1977) membrane preparations. However, no correlation of protein phosphorylation with a physiological response in intact neurons has yet been reported.

Williams and Rodnight (1976) found that norepinephrine stimulates total incorporation of phosphate into slices of rat brain. We demonstrated that octopamine and serotonin cause an increase in phosphorylation of a specific protein, of molecular weight 118,000 daltons, in *Aplysia* abdominal ganglion (Levitan and Barondes, 1974; Levitan, Madsen, and Barondes, 1974). This effect was not observed in several neuronal cell bodies; it appears to be confined to the ganglionic neuropil, like the cAMP increase induced by peptides (Table II; Treistman and Levitan, 1976a)

or synaptic stimulation (Cedar, Kandel, and Schwartz, 1972). Because of the complex time course of the phosphorylation response to octopamine and serotonin, it was not possible to determine whether this response is related to the increase in cAMP levels caused by these amines (Levitan, Madsen, and Barondes, 1974).

We have found that, in order to reliably reproduce these intact ganglion phosphorylation results, it is critical to control very carefully the physiological state of the *Aplysia* from which the ganglia are taken (I. Levitan and E. Bandle, unpublished). This fact and the complexity of the time course of the phosphorylation response in the intact ganglion have led us to question whether this phenomenon is in fact related to any physiological responses mediated by octopamine and serotonin. Accordingly, we have reexamined this problem in broken cell preparations, most recently from *Helix* ganglia, and have found that in such preparations, cAMP specifically stimulates the phosphorylation of a protein of approximate molecular weight 120,000 daltons (Bandle and Levitan, 1977). It is intriguing that the molecular weight of the protein phosphorylated in these short (0.5–5 min) incubations of *Helix* broken cell preparations so closely resembles that of the protein phosphorylated in the much longer (>15 hr) incubations of intact ganglia from *Aplysia* (Levitan and Barondes, 1974). Whether these two proteins are in any way related, and what role they may play in the control of neuronal membrane permeability to ions, remain to be determined.

Summary and conclusions

Cyclic nucleotides are known to influence neuronal activity in several systems, most notably superior cervical ganglion (Greengard, 1976) and cerebellar Purkinje cells (Bloom, 1975). It is now clear that changes in cyclic nucleotide metabolism modify electrical activity in several large identified molluscan neurons—neurons in which it may prove possible to ask direct questions about the relationship between biochemical and electrical events.

In order to assign cyclic nucleotides a role in the mediation of a physiological response, it is not sufficient simply to show that changes in cyclic nucleotide levels mimic that response; a number of additional criteria (Greengard, 1976) must be satisfied. Most of these criteria have been fulfilled for the two physiological responses described here: the long-term modulation of R15 and F-1 by peptide hormones and by synaptic stimulation. One major criterion that has not been satisfied for either response relates to the cellular localization of the cAMP increase. If, as the data seem to indicate, the cAMP increase is confined to the neuropil of the ganglion, it may be very difficult to definitively assign this response to either neuronal processes or glial cells. One possible approach might be intraneuronal injection of appropriate radioactive precursors into R15 and F-1, in order to directly measure formation of cAMP, and protein phosphorylation, in the processes of these neurons. Such experiments, which are not feasible in many other systems, are currently under way.

What are the functions of neurons R15 and F-1, and how are these functions modified by peptide and synaptic stimulation? Both of these neurons synthesize low-molecular-weight peptides, which are transported out of the cell bodies and may be released at nerve terminals (Strumwasser and Wilson, 1976; Loh, Barker, and Gainer, 1976). If these small peptides are indeed neurosecretory products, they may act as hormones influencing physiological functions in various parts of the animal. Kupfermann and Weiss (1976) have in fact demonstrated that a crude extract of R15 can affect water balance in *Aplysia*. The active factor in the PE, by increasing the net activity of R15 and F-1, would thus stimulate the release of neurosecretory peptides, analogous to the action of releasing factors on the anterior pituitary in higher organisms (Reichlin et al., 1976). Similarly, long lasting synaptic hyperpolarization may represent feedback inhibition of release of the peptides from the target tissues on which the peptides act. These ideas are highly speculative at present, but this model may prove to be a useful one for investigating control of release of neurosecretory products.

Finally, it is appropriate to ask how two distinct physiological processes, one resulting in inhibition of neuronal activity and the other producing excitation, may both be mediated by the same second messenger. Possible explanations include compartmentalization of receptor sites and ionic gates within the neuronal membrane, such that the intracellular second messenger can act only on those ionic gates adjacent to the site at which it is generated. Another possibility is that different concentrations of second messenger may produce different effects, as discussed by Berridge (this volume). However, the most likely explanation would appear to be that the electrical response to peptides cannot be explained by changes in cAMP alone. Our results indicate that peptide treatment increases not only cAMP but also cGMP in *Helix* and *Aplysia* ganglia. Furthermore, the agents that mimic the peptide effects, namely phosphodiesterase inhibitors and 8-substituted cAMP derivatives, also increase *both* cAMP and cGMP (as noted earlier, the cAMP derivatives act not only as cAMP analogs but also as phosphodiesterase inhibitors). Thus it is possible that cAMP and cGMP acting in concert produce a pattern of enhanced bursts and also enhanced interburst hyperpolarizations, the net effect of which is increased neuronal activity. In contrast, an increase in cAMP *without* an accompanying increase in cGMP, such as is produced by Gpp(NH)p treatment, leads only to hyperpolarization (see Figure 12). If this explanation is correct, it would suggest that synaptically induced hyperpolarization is a "pure" cAMP response, whereas the response to peptides is mediated jointly by cAMP and cGMP.

Determination of the precise role played by cyclic nucleotides in the control of neuronal membrane properties must await future investigation. What is clear is that cyclic nucleotides can produce long-last-

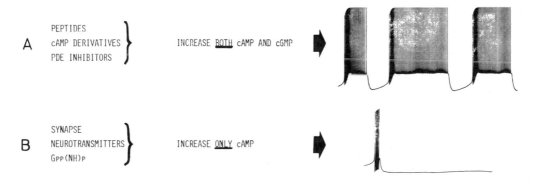

FIGURE 12 Hypothetical scheme describing how changes in intraneuronal cyclic nucleotide levels might produce both neuronal excitation and inhibition. Agents that lead to enhanced bursting appear to increase both cAMP and cGMP concentrations (A), whereas treatments that cause hyperpolarization seem to increase only cAMP levels (B). The details of this scheme are consistent with presently available data.

ing changes in neuronal electrical activity and may mediate certain long-term functional alterations induced by physiological stimulation.

ACKNOWLEDGMENTS   Dr. Steven N. Treistman was involved in the initiation of certain aspects of this work and collaborated in many of the experiments described here. Other experiments from my laboratory were done in collaboration with Drs. William Adams, Eric Bandle, Alan Drummond, and Anthony Harmar. I am grateful to Drs. Adams, Drummond, and Harmar for their critical comments on this manuscript and to Miss Eva Bergström for excellent technical assistance.

REFERENCES

ASCHER, P., 1972. Inhibitory and excitatory effects of dopamine on *Aplysia* neurones. *J. Physiol.* 225:173–209.

ASCHER, P., J. S. KEHOE, and L. TAUC, 1967. Effets d'injections électrophorétiques de dopamine sur les neurones d'Aplysie. *J. Physiol. (Paris)* 59:331–332.

BANDLE, E. F., and I. B. LEVITAN, 1977. Cyclic AMP–stimulated phosphorylation of a high molecular weight endogenous protein substrate in sub-cellular fractions of molluscan nervous system. *Brain Res.* 125:325–331.

BARKER, J. L., and H. GAINER, 1974. Peptide regulation of bursting pacemaker activity in molluscan neurosecretory cell. *Science* 184:1371–1373.

BARKER, J. L., and T. G. SMITH, JR., 1977. Peptides as neurohormones. *Neurosci. Symp.* 2:340–373.

BLOOM, F. E., 1973. Dynamic synaptic communication: Finding the vocabulary. *Brain Res.* 62:299–305.

BLOOM, F. E., 1975. The role of cyclic nucleotides in central synaptic function. *Rev. Physiol. Biochem. Pharmacol.* 74:1–103.

BRUNELLI, M., V. CASTELLUCCI, and E. KANDEL, 1976. Synaptic facilitation and behavioral sensitization in *Aplysia*. Possible role of serotonin and cyclic AMP. *Science* 194:1178–1181.

CEDAR, H., E. R. KANDEL, and J. H. SCHWARTZ, 1972. Cyclic adenosine monophosphate in the nervous system of *Aplysia californica*. I. Increased synthesis in response to synaptic stimulation. *J. Gen. Physiol.* 60:558–569.

CEDAR, H., and J. H. SCHWARTZ, 1972. Cyclic adenosine monophosphate in the nervous system of *Aplysia californica*. II. Effect of serotonin and dopamine. *J. Gen. Physiol.* 60:570–587.

COGGESHALL, R. E., 1967. A light and electron microscope study of the abdominal ganglion of *Aplysia californica*. *J. Neurophysiol* 30:1263–1287.

COTTRELL, G. A., 1970. Direct post-synaptic responses to stimulation of serotonin-containing neurones. *Nature* 225:1060–1062.

DELORENZO, R. J., K. G. WALTON, P. F. CURRAN, and P. GREENGARD, 1973. Regulation of phosphorylation of a specific protein in toad-bladder membrane by antidiuretic hormone and cAMP, and its possible relationship to membrane permeability changes. *Proc. Natl. Acad. Sci. USA* 70:880–884.

FRAZIER, W. T., E. R. KANDEL, I. KUPFERMANN, R. WAZIRI, and R. E. COGGESHALL, 1967. Morphological and functional properties of identified neurons in the abdominal ganglion of *Aplysia californica*. *J. Neurophysiol.* 30:1288–1351.

GILLER, E., JR., and J. H. SCHWARTZ, 1971. Choline acetyltransferase in identified neurons of abdominal ganglion of *Aplysia californica*. *J. Neurophysiol.* 34:93–107.

GREENGARD, P., 1976. Possible role for cyclic nucleotides and phosphorylated membrane proteins in postsynaptic actions of neurotransmitters. *Nature* 260:101–108.

IFSHIN, M. S., H. GAINER, and J. L. BARKER, 1975. Peptide factor extracted from molluscan ganglia that modulates bursting pacemaker activity. *Nature* 254:72–74.

KERKUT, G. A., J. D. C. LAMBERT, R. J. GAYTON, J. E. LOKER, and R. J. WALKER, 1975. Mapping of nerve cells in the subesophageal ganglia of *Helix aspersa*. *Comp. Biochem. Physiol.* 50A:1–25.

KIRCHBERGER, M. A., and A. RAFFO, 1977. Decrease in calcium transport associated with phosphoprotein phosphatase-catalyzed dephosphorylation of cardiac sarcoplasmic reticulum. *J. Cyclic Nucleotide Res.* 3:45–53.

KUPFERMANN, I., and K. R. WEISS, 1976. Water regulation by a presumptive hormone contained in identified neurosecretory cell R15 of *Aplysia*. *J. Gen. Physiol.* 67:113–123.

LAMBERT, J. D. C., 1975. A long-lasting hyperpolarization evoked in an identified neurone of *Helix aspersa*. *Brain Res.* 87:118–122.

LEFKOWITZ, R., 1974. Stimulation of catecholamine-sensitive adenylate cyclase by 5′-guanylyl imidodiphosphate. *J. Biol. Chem.* 249:6119–6124.

LEVITAN, I. B., and S. BARONDES, 1974. Octopamine and serotonin-stimulated phosphorylation of specific protein in the abdominal ganglion of *Aplysia californica*. *Proc. Natl. Acad. Sci. USA* 71:1145–1148.

LEVITAN, I. B., C. J. MADSEN, and S. H. BARONDES, 1974. Cyclic AMP and amine effects on phosphorylation of specific protein in abdominal ganglion of *Aplysia californica*; localization and kinetic analysis. *J. Neurobiol.* 5:511–525.

LEVITAN, I. B., and S. N. TREISTMAN, 1977. Modulation of electrical activity and cyclic nucleotide metabolism in molluscan nervous system by a peptide-containing nervous system extract. *Brain Res.* 136:307–317.

LOH, P. Y., J. L. BARKER, and H. GAINER, 1976. Neurosecretory cell protein metabolism in the land snail, *Otala lactea*. *J. Neurochem.* 26:25–30.

MAENO, H., E. JOHNSON, and P. GREENGARD, 1971. Subcellular distribution of adenosine 3′,5′-monophosphate–dependent protein kinase in rat brain. *J. Biol. Chem.* 246:134–142.

MAYERI, E., and S. SIMON, 1975. Modulation of synaptic transmission and burster neuron activity after release of a neurohormone in *Aplysia*. *Neurosci. Abstr.* 1:584.

MEYER, R. B., JR., and J. P. MILLER, 1974. Analogs of cyclic AMP and cyclic GMP: General methods of synthesis and the relationship of structure to enzymic activity. *Life Sci.* 14:1019–1040.

PARNAS, I., D. ARMSTRONG, and F. STRUMWASSER, 1974. Prolonged excitatory and inhibitory synaptic modulation of à bursting pacemaker neuron. *J. Neurophysiol.* 37:594–608.

PARNAS, I., and F. STRUMWASSER, 1974. Mechanism of long-lasting inhibition of a bursting pacemaker neuron. *J. Neurophysiol.* 37:609–620.

REICHLIN, S., R. SAPERSTEIN, I. M. D. JACKSON, A. E. BOYD, and Y. PATEL, 1976. Hypothalamic hormones. *Annu. Rev. Physiol.* 38:389–424.

RUBIN, C. S., and O. M. ROSEN, 1975. Protein phosphorylation. *Annu. Rev. Biochem.* 44:831–887.

SCHLAPFER, W. T., P. B. J. WOODSON, J. P. TREMBLAY, and S. H. BARONDES, 1974. Depression and frequency facilitation at a synapse in *Aplysia californica*: Evidence for regulation by availability of transmitter. *Brain Res.* 76:267–280.

SCHRAMM, M., and M. RODBELL, 1975. A persistent active state of the adenylate cyclase system produced by the combined actions of isoproterenol and guanylyl imidodiphosphate in frog erythrocyte membranes. *J. Biol. Chem.* 250:2232–2237.

SHIMAHARA, T., and L. TAUC, 1977. Cyclic AMP induced by serotonin modulates the activity of an identified synapse in *Aplysia* by facilitating the active permeability to calcium. *Brain Res.* 127:168–172.

STRUMWASSER, F., 1971. The cellular basis of behavior in *Aplysia*. *J. Psychiatr. Res.* 8:237–257.

STRUMWASSER, F., and D. L. WILSON, 1976. Patterns of proteins synthesized in the R15 neuron of *Aplysia*. Temporal studies and evidence for processing. *J. Gen. Physiol.* 67:691–702.

TADA, M., M. A. KIRCHBERGER, and A. M. KATZ, 1975. Phosphorylation of a 22,000 Dalton component of the cardiac sarcoplasmic reticulum by cAMP-dependent protein kinase. *J. Biol. Chem.* 250:2640–2647.

TREISTMAN, S. N., and I. B. LEVITAN, 1976a. Alteration of electrical activity in molluscan neurones by cyclic nucleotides and peptide factors. *Nature* 261:62–64.

TREISTMAN, S. N., and I. B. LEVITAN, 1976b. Intraneuronal guanylyl-imidodiphosphate injection mimics long-term synaptic hyperpolarization in *Aplysia*. *Proc. Natl. Acad. Sci. USA* 73:4689–4692.

UEDA, T., H. MAENO, and P. GREENGARD, 1973. Regulation of endogenous phosphorylation of specific proteins in synaptic membrane fractions from rat brain by adenosine 3′,5′-monophosphate, *J. Biol. Chem.* 248:8295–8305.

WAZIRI, R., and E. KANDEL, 1969. Organization of inhibition in abdominal ganglion of *Aplysia*. III. Interneurons mediating inhibition. *J. Neurophysiol.* 32:520–539.

WELLER, M., and I. G. MORGAN, 1977. A possible role of the phosphorylation of synaptic membrane proteins in the control of calcium ion permeability. *Biochim. Biophys. Acta* 465:527–534.

WELLER, M., and R. RODNIGHT, 1970. Stimulation by cyclic AMP of intrinsic protein kinase activity in ox brain membrane preparation. *Nature* 225:187–188.

WILLIAMS, M., and R. RODNIGHT, 1976. Protein phosphorylation in respiring slices of guinea-pig cerebral cortex. Evidence for a role for noradrenaline and adenosine 3′,5′-cyclic monophosphate in the increased phosphorylation observed on application of electrical pulses. *Biochem. J.* 154:163–170.

64 Opioid Peptides in the Brain

SOLOMON H. SNYDER

ABSTRACT Morphine-like "opioid" peptides were discovered as constituents of brain extracts that mimicked specific effects of opiates on smooth muscle or which competed for opiate-receptor binding. The two pentapeptide enkephalins appear to be the major brain opioid peptides. Endorphin designates "endogenous morphine-like substance" but is usually used to refer to opioid peptides isolated from the pituitary with longer amino acid sequences than enkephalin but comprising within them the enkephalin sequence. The 31-amino-acid peptide, β-endorphin, appears to be the major pituitary opioid peptide and has also been detected in the brain; hence it may be a precursor of methionine enkephalin. Immunohistochemical studies reveal the localization of enkephalin-containing neurons in similar areas as opiate receptors detected by autoradiography. Some of these discrete areas are also enriched with other neuropeptides such as neurotensin and substance P. Like other neuropeptides, enkephalin is localized in the central nervous system and intestine almost exclusively. Its synaptic actions, like those of opiates, seem to involve influences on sodium channels, paralleling the selective potent effects of sodium on opiate-receptor binding.

Introduction

RECENT AWARENESS that a variety of peptides might be neurotransmitters or neuromodulators has considerably augmented the number of possible neurotransmitters. Because many of these peptides were discovered as a result of their effects in other parts of the body, some quite fortuitously, one wonders whether the number of known peptide neuromodulators may be only the literal "tip of the iceberg." The discovery of the enkephalins and endorphins, the opioid peptides of the brain, provides a good example of the indirect means whereby these substances have come to the attention of brain researchers. Since the opioid peptides were discovered as the apparently normally occurring substrates for the opiate receptor, it is important first to review some of the major features of the opiate receptor.

For many years a variety of pharmacological data had suggested that opiate drugs act at highly selective sites in the brain. Some opiates are extraordinarily potent. Etorphine is an opiate that in intact animals and man can be up to 5,000–10,000 times more potent than morphine. Such a compound would be assumed to act at specific receptor sites. The pharmacological effects of opiates are generally stereospecific with the (−)-isomer being far more active than the (+)-isomer. Stereospecificity of action usually involves selective receptor sites. The existence of opiate antagonists also argues for specific receptors. A pure antagonist such as naloxone induces few if any pharmacological effects of itself, but in quite small doses it can fully antagonize the actions of drugs such as morphine and heroin.

Although many investigators acknowledged that opiates must act at specific receptor sites, demonstrating such sites biochemically proved to be a difficult task. The simplest paradigm for assaying hormone or neurotransmitter receptors would be to measure the binding of the radioactive transmitter substance, drug, or hormone to membranes from the appropriate target organ. However, nonspecific binding interactions would be expected to greatly exceed specific receptor binding. Successful identification of the opiate receptor involved the use of opiates of high specific radioactivity and measurements of binding under conditions in which nonspecific binding could be minimized by rapid washing after filtration (Pert and Snyder, 1973). Using filtration or centrifugation, stereospecific binding was also identified by Terenius (1973) and Simon, Hiller, and Edelman (1973). Employing the guinea pig intestine, in which influences of opiates on contraction involve receptor sites similar to those that mediate analgesia, we could show in a single tissue specimen that biological and binding potencies were very closely correlated (Creese and Snyder, 1975). This type of data establishes definitively that the pharmacologically relevant opiate receptors are being labeled.

Biochemical and autoradiographic studies established that the opiate receptor is distributed heterogeneously throughout the brain with high localized densities of opiate receptors in areas relating to functions influenced in vivo by opiates (Kuhar, Pert, and Snyder, 1973; Pert, Kuhar, and Snyder, 1976; Atweh

SOLOMON H. SNYDER Departments of Pharmacology and Experimental Therapeutics and Psychiatry and Behavioral Sciences, Johns Hopkins University School of Medicine, Baltimore, MD 21205

and Kuhar, 1977). For instance, laminae I and II in the dorsal gray matter of the spinal cord, well-known to be involved in integrating information about pain, contain high densities of opiate receptors.

The striking localizations of the opiate receptor suggested that it was not just an accident of evolution. Presumably it must serve some normal physiological function as a receptor for an endogenous opiate-like substance. Other evidence suggested the existence of an endogenous opiate. Akil, Mayer, and Liebeskind (1976) had shown that electrical stimulation in the brain stem could produce analgesia in rats that was blocked by the opiate antagonist naloxone. This strongly suggested that such stimulation evoked the release of an opiate-like substance.

Hughes (1975) endeavored to identify such a substance by determining whether brain extracts would mimic the ability of morphine to inhibit the electrically induced contractions of the mouse vas deferens and guinea pig intestine. He demonstrated the existence of such a substance whose effects were blocked by naloxone. In our own laboratory (Pasternak, Goodman, and Synder, 1975) and that of Terenius and Wahlstrom (1974), brain extracts were assayed for their ability to inhibit opiate-receptor binding. Such activity could be shown to be distributed among

brain regions in proportion to the relative densities of opiate receptors (Snyder, 1975). Hughes et al. (1975) isolated and identified a mixture of two morphine-like pentapeptides, methionine-enkephalin (m-enk) and leucine-enkephalin (l-enk) in pig brain with a ratio of about four parts of m-enk to one of l-enk. This finding was confirmed in our laboratory independently by identifying the two enkephalins in extracts of bovine brain with, however, a ratio of 4:1 of l-enk to m-enk (Simantov and Snyder, 1976a).

Since the enkephalins are endogenous opioid substances, they are also referred to generically as "endorphins," which designates any endogenous substance with morphine-like activity. Other opioid peptides have been identified in the pituitary and are referred to as α-, β-, and γ-endorphin, respectively. Even prior to the isolation of enkephalin, Cox et al. (1975) had found that pituitary extracts possess opiate-like activity. When the amino acid sequence of enkephalin was demonstrated, it became apparent that the amino acids contained in m-enk are also part of a 91-amino-acid peptide β-lipotropin identified some ten years earlier by C. H. Li (1964) (Table I). Soon after the publication of the amino acid sequence of enkephalins, Ling, Burgus, and Guillemin (1976) identified the 16- and 17-amino-acid peptides α-en-

TABLE I

Amino acid sequence of β-lipotropin and its biologically active constituent peptides

β-Lipotropin:
1
NH₂-GLU-LEU-ALA-GLY-ALA-PRO-PRO-GLU-PRO-ALA-ARG-ASP-PRO-GLU-ALA-PRO-ALA-GLU-
20
GLY-ALA-ALA-ALA-ARC-ALA-GLU-LEU-GLU-TYR-GLY-LEU-VAL-ALA-GLU-ALA-GLN-ALA-

β-Lipotropin (continued):
41   47
ALA-GLU-LYS-LYS-ASP-GLU-GLY-PRO-TYR-LYS-MET-GLU-HIS-PHE-ARG-TRY-GLY-SER-PRO-

β-MSH:
ASP-GLU-GLY-PRO-TYR-ARG-MET-GLU-HIS-PHE-ARG-TRY-GLY-SER-PRO-

ACTH₄₋₁₀:
MET-GLU-HIS-PHE-ARG-TRY-GLY

β-Lipotropin (continued):
61
PRO-LYS-ASP-LYS-ARG-TYR-GLY-GLY-PHE-MET-THR-SER-GLU-LYS-SER-GLN-THR-PRO-LEU-

β-MSH (continued):
PRO-LYS-ASP

α-Endorphin:
TYR-GLY-GLY-PHE-MET-THR-SER-GLU-LYS-SER-GLN-THR-PRO-LEU-

β-Endorphin:
TYR-GLY-GLY-PHE-MET-THR-SER-GLU-LYS-SER-GLN-THR-PRO-LEU-

Methionine enkephalin:
TYR-GLY-GLY-PHE-MET

β-Lipotropin (continued):
76   91
VAL-THR-LEU-PHE-LYS-ASN-ALA-ILE-VAL-LYS-ASN-ALA-HIS-LYS-LYS-GLY-GLN-OH

α-Endorphin (continued):
VAL-THR

β-Endorphin (continued):
VAL-THR-LEU-PHE-LYS-ASN-ALA-ILE-VAL-LYS-ASN-ALA-HIS-LYS-LYS-GLY-GLN-OH

dorphin and β-endorphin, whose amino terminal of 5 amino acids constitutes the sequence of m-enk. Li and Chung (1976) isolated β-endorphin, the 31-carboxyl-terminal amino acids of β-lipotropin, from pituitary extracts and showed that β-endorphin possesses a high degree of opiate-like activity upon smooth muscle. Independently, Bradbury et al. (1976) isolated the same 31-amino-acid peptide from the pituitary and showed that it possessed opiate-like activity in receptor-binding assays and upon smooth muscle. This latter group referred to this peptide as C fragment.

Recently Smyth and collaborators (personal communication) have obtained evidence that α- and γ-endorphins are formed in the process of extraction of pituitary extracts and may not be endogenous substances. Even if they are normally present in the pituitary, their concentrations are less than 5% of those of β endorphin. Thus the major opioid peptide of the pituitary is β-endorphin, since only negligible levels of enkephalins can be demonstrated in the pituitary. Specific radioimmunoassay reveals that endogenous β-endorphin does exist in the brain, although in concentrations only about 10% of those of the enkephalins (Rossier et al., 1977).

Since enkephalin constitutes part of the amino acid sequence of β-endorphin, one wonders whether it could have been formed during the extraction process and represent only an artifact. Experiments utilizing a variety of extraction techniques in animals killed by methods including microwave treatment (Simantov, Childers, and Snyder, 1977), as well as the immunohistochemical demonstration of enkephalins with antisera that do not recognize β-endorphin (Elde et al., 1976; Simantov et al., 1977), indicate that the enkephalins are not artifacts of the isolation procedure. Thus opioid peptides in the brain appear to consist entirely of the two pentapeptide enkephalins and β-endorphin. The pituitary contains very high levels of β-endorphin as apparently its only opioid peptide. The remainder of this chapter will evaluate the properties of these substances.

Metabolism

It is extraordinarily difficult to work out the pattern of the synthesis of endogenous peptides of any sort. Precedent with peptides such as insulin and angiotensin suggests that such compounds are usually formed by cleavage from larger peptides. Though peptide biochemistry is not sufficiently advanced that one can enunciate general rules with assurance, it appears likely that peptides with more than 3 amino

acids are not formed by enzymatic synthesis in which the individual amino acids are linked together. It is also generally felt that peptides containing fewer than 40 amino acids are not usually synthesized directly on ribosomes and hence must be formed as cleavage products of larger peptides, which are themselves manufactured on ribosomes. One strategy to study the biosynthesis of peptides is to label the tissue with radioactive precursor amino acids. After infusing 100 μCi of [³H]-tyrosine directly into the lateral ventricles of rats, H. Yang and E. Costa (personal communication) have recently demonstrated the formation of several nanocuries of [³H]-m-enk. Using a similar experimental procedure with strips of guinea pig intestine, J. T. Hughes (personal communication) has shown the incorporation of [³H]-tyrosine and [³H]-glycine into enkephalins. Of course, demonstrating the incorporation of an amino acid into enkephalin does not shed light on the mechanism of synthesis.

Greater success has been attained in studies of β-endorphin formation. Besides β-endorphin, the lipotropin sequence incorporates that of β-MSH as well as amino acids 4–10 of ACTH. Recently a 31,000 dalton precursor to ACTH (31K ACTH) had been demonstrated in pituitary tissue. Using an ACTH-secreting mouse pituitary tumor cell line, Mains, Eipper, and Ling (1977) showed that 31K ACTH contains within its sequence both ACTH and β-lipotropin, including the sequence of β-endorphin. This finding would indicate that β-endorphin and ACTH are stored and possibly released together. Such an assumption is consistent with findings that various physiological and pathological conditions alter ACTH and β-LPH release from the pituitary in a parallel fashion (Gilkes et al., 1975). Immunochemical studies have shown that β-LPH, β-endorphin, and ACTH occur in the same pituitary cells (Moriarty, 1973; Bloom et al., 1977); and Guillemin et al. (1977) have shown that when rats are stressed by having their legs broken, β-endorphin and ACTH are released into the circulation in parallel.

It is unclear whether or not β-endorphin is the physiological precursor of the enkephalins in the brain. Some observations seem to be inconsistent with such a possibility. First, one would expect that a leucine-containing analog of β-endorphin should exist in the brain. Extensive studies in the laboratories of Li, Guillemin, and Smyth (personal communications) have ruled out the possibility of a leucine analog of β-endorphin in the pituitary. It is still conceivable, however, that such a compound exists in the brain. Second, immunohistochemical studies (described below) show that β-endorphin in the brain is contained in different structures than enkephalin, arguing against a metabolic relationship between the two. However, it is still possible that in enkephalin-containing neurons, β-endorphin might exist as a rapidly turned-over precursor that would not be detected by normal assays. In other cells β-endorphin might be the only opioid peptide and might not be converted to enkephalins. This situation would be analogous to that of dopamine and norepinephrine. In norepinephrine neurons one cannot readily detect the existence of dopamine. Histochemical studies reveal dopamine-containing neurons that possess no norepinephrine. Third, large precursors of biologically active peptides are usually inactive, whereas β-endorphin possesses as much opioid peptide activity as the enkephalins.

If enkephalin were a neurotransmitter, one would expect a specific inactivating system to exist. Since the enkephalins are extremely labile, it is difficult to study their possible uptake into nerve terminals, inasmuch as the conditions under which synaptosomal uptake is usually examined will produce rapid degradation of enkephalins. Search for a selective "enkephalinase" proteolytic activity is equally difficult, since these small peptides can be degraded by a variety of peptidases that are abundant in most tissues, including the brain. Thus, at the present time, it is unclear how enkephalins are degraded or inactivated after their actions upon target cells. The extreme susceptibility of enkephalins to peptidases suggests that enzymatic hydrolysis might be involved in terminating their actions, much as in the case of acetylcholinesterase and acetylcholine. The relative stability of β-endorphin to such enzymes suggests that its effects on neuronal firing are considerably longer-lived than those of enkephalins. According to this reasoning, one might expect enkephalin to behave more like a rapidly acting neurotransmitter, whereas β-endorphin might exert a longer-term modulating effect on the firing of neurons.

Cellular localization

The major advances in our understanding of catecholamines in the brain during the past decade have been attributable in large part to the histochemical mapping of dopamine- and norepinephrine-containing neurons. The chemical identification of the enkephalins and β-endorphin enabled the preparation of specific antisera that have been used in immunohistochemical mapping studies (Elde et al., 1976; Simantov et al., 1977; Hökfelt et al., 1977; Watson et al., 1977; Uhl, Childers, and Snyder, 1978; Uhl et al.,

1978). Indirect immunofluorescence studies reveal the existence of enkephalin-containing fibers and terminals throughout the central nervous system (Figure 1). Vivid demonstration of enkephalin-containing cells with current antisera requires the pretreatment of rats with colchicine to block axonal flow so that the peptide will accumulate in proximal axons and cell bodies. β-Endorphin has been localized in cells and fiber terminals with the peroxidase-antiperoxidase method without colchicine pretreatment (F. Bloom and E. Battenberg, personal communication).

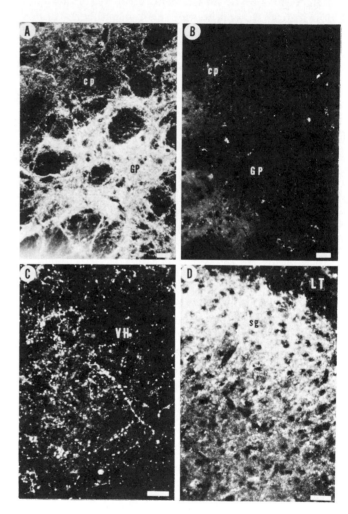

FIGURE 1 Immunofluorescence micrographs of (A and B) the globus pallidus (GP) and nucleus caudatus-putamen (cp) and of the cervical spinal cord showing (C) the ventral horn (VH) and (D) Lissauer's tract (LT) and substantia gelatinosa (sg). Micrographs A and B were taken from serial sections, but the primary serum used for staining in B was previously adsorbed overnight with 1 mM Leu-enk to establish a control. All sections were stained with rabbit antiserum against Leu-enk. Bars = 25 μM. (From Simantov et al., 1977.)

A close correspondence of enkephalin fluorescence and opiate-receptor density is revealed by autoradiography (Simantov et al., 1977; see Figures 2 and 3). This substantiates the assumption that enkephalin is the endogenous substance, presumably a neurotransmitter or neuromodulator, that interacts with opiate receptors.

In the spinal cord, enkephalin nerve fibers, terminals, and cells are highly concentrated in laminae I and II, in the substantia gelatinosa, and in the dorsal portion of the spinal cord (Figures 1 and 2). In the lower medulla oblongata, enkephalin cells and terminals, as well as opiate receptors, are localized to the substantia gelatinosa of the spinal tract of the trigeminal, which corresponds to the spinal cord's substantia gelatinosa (Figures 2 and 4). This structure in both spinal cord and brain stem is involved in pain perception. The close juxtaposition of enkephalin cells and terminals in such a narrow band of tissue suggests that in this region enkephalin may be contained in small interneurons. This supposition is supported by the observation that lesions of the dorsal root of the spinal cord fail to deplete enkephalin from the spinal cord (Elde et al, 1976; Uhl, Childers, and Snyder, 1978; Uhl et al., 1978). Moreover, enkephalin fluorescence is unaffected by knife cuts above or below the level examined.

One well-known function of interneurons in the dorsal gray matter of the spinal cord is presynaptic inhibition exerted upon excitatory nerve terminals of sensory afferents entering through the dorsal root. Classical instances of presynaptic inhibition are antagonized by drugs such as bicuculline and picrotoxin, blockers of GABA actions. Thus GABA is presumed to be one neurotransmitter of presynaptic inhibition. If enkephalin were also a transmitter of presynaptic inhibition, its receptors should be localized upon the nerve terminals of sensory afferents. In confirmation of this possibility, LaMotte, Pert, and Snyder (1976) found that lesions of the dorsal root deplete opiate-receptor binding in the dorsal part of the monkey spinal cord. Thus, by acting on nerve terminals of sensory afferents, enkephalin would be anticipated to alter the release of a sensory transmitter. Neurophysiological evidence indicates that the major sensory transmitters are excitatory and that sensory information, including that related to pain, involves an excitatory influence on spinal-cord cells. Thus if enkephalin does reduce painful stimulation, it should decrease the release of the sensory transmitter.

The identity of all sensory transmitters is not clear. Indirect evidence suggests that the larger-diameter sensory afferents may use an excitatory amino acid such as glutamate. Numerous small-diameter sensory fibers possess either substance P or somatostatin, but

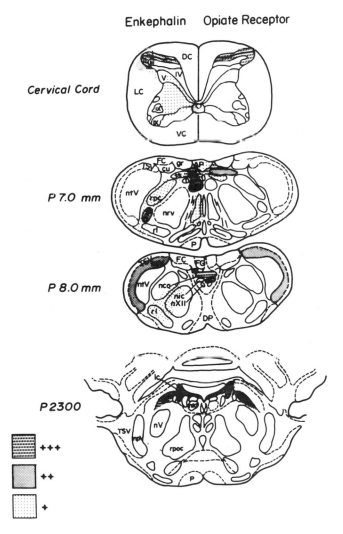

Enkephalin   Opiate Receptor

Cervical Cord

P 7.0 mm

P 8.0 mm

P 2300

+++
++
+

FIGURE 2 Distributions of enkephalin (left) and opiate receptors (right) at different levels of the spinal cord and medulla. *Abbreviations*: amb, nucleus ambiguus; AP, area postrema; cu, nucleus cuneatus; DC, dorsal column; DP, decussatio pyramidis; FC, fasciculus cuneatus; FG, fasciculus gracilis; gr, nucleus gracilis; io, nucleus olivaris inferior; LC, lateral column; lc, locus ceruleus; nco, nucleus commissuralis; nic, nucleus intercalatus; npV, nucleus principis nerve trigemenii; nrv, nucleus reticularis medullae oblongata pars ventralis; ntd, nucleus tegmenti dorsalis Gudden; nts, nucleus tractus solitarius; ntV, nucleus tractus spinalis nervi trigemini; nV, nucleus origini nerve trigemini; NX, nucleus originis dorsalis vagi; nXII, nucleus originis nervi hypoglossi; P, tractus corticospinalis; rl, nucleus reticularis parvocellularis; rpoc, nucleus reticularis pontis caudallis; sgV, substantia gelatinosa trigemini; ts, tractus solitarius; TSV, tractus spinalis nervi trigemini; VC, ventral column. (From Uhl, Childers, and Snyder, 1978.)

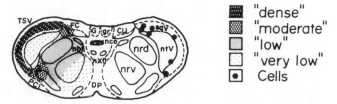

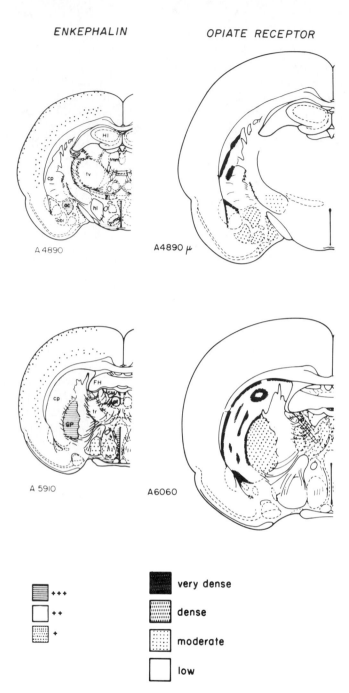

FIGURE 4 Enkephalin immunofluorescence at the decussation of the pyramids. *Abbreviations*: cu, cuneate nucleus; DP, decussation of the pyramids; FC, cuneate fasciculus; G, gracile fasciculus; gr, gracile nucleus; nbi, basilar internal nucleus of Cajal; nco, nucleus comissuralis; nrd, dorsal medullary reticular nucleus; nrv, ventral medullary reticular nucleus; ntv, nucleus of the spinal tract of the trigeminal; nXII, hypoglossal nucleus; PCI, inferior cerebellar peduncle; rl, lateral reticular nucleus; sgV, substantia gelatinosa of the trigeminal; TSV, spinal tract of the trigeminal. (From Uhl et al., 1978.)

not both (Hökfelt et al., 1975, 1976). Substance P- and somatostatin-containing sensory fibers each constitute about 15–25% of all sensory afferents. Substance P is well known to produce excitatory effects relatively selectively in spinal-cord cells that respond to noxious stimuli. The recent demonstration that opiates and opioid peptides inhibit release of substance P from the trigeminal nucleus of rat brain (Jessell and Iversen, 1977) is consistent with the suggestion that "presynaptic inhibition" mediates at least part of the analgesic effects of opiates. Only a portion of opiate analgesia occurs at a spinal-cord level. Besides substance P, it is conceivable that somatostatin plays a role in the analgesic effects of opiates.

Atweh, Murrin, and Kuhar (1978) found other sites where opiate receptors are located presynaptically. Lesions of the vagus nerve in the neck deplete autoradiographically detected opiate receptors in the nucleus of the solitary tract and the nucleus ambiguus, both vagal nuclei in the brain stem. Similarly, contralateral enucleation abolishes opiate receptors in the inferior accessory optic nuclei. In other areas it is likely that opiate receptors are localized to neuronal cells. Kainic acid administration in small quantities selectively destroys neuronal cells (Coyle and Schwarcz, 1976). In the corpus striatum, microinjection of kainic acid removes almost all neuronal cells, whereas glial nerve terminals and nerve fibers passing through the area are unaffected. Injections of kainic acid result in a loss of about 50% of opiate-receptor binding in the corpus striatum (Minneman, Quik, and Emson, 1978). The failure to attain a complete depletion of opiate receptors following kainic acid treatment suggests that some striatal opiate receptors are located presynaptically.

FIGURE 3 Distribution of enkephalin (left) and opiate receptors (right) at certain levels of the diencephalon and telencephalon. *Abbreviations*: abl, nucleus amygdaloideus basalis, pars lateralis; ac, nucleus amygdaloideus centralis; cp, nucleus caudatus putamen; ha, nucleus anterior (hypothalami); hl, nucleus lateralis (hypothalami); hvma, nucleus ventromedialis (hypothalami), pars anterior; pt, nucleus paratenialis; tmm, nucleus medialis thalami, pars medialis; tr, nucleus reticularis thalami; tv, nucleus ventralis thalami; FH, fimbria hyppocampi; GP, globus pallidus; HI, hippocampus; SM, stria medullaris thalami; ZI, zona incerta. (From Uhl, Childers, and Snyder, 1978.)

Yet another presynaptic localization of opiate receptors is suggested by the finding that destruction of dopamine nerve terminals in the corpus striatum elicits a 20% decrease in enkephalin binding to opiate receptors (Pollard, Llorens-Cortes, and Schwartz, 1977). These receptors might mediate locomotor influences of opiates and opioid peptides.

In the midbrain, enkephalin is contained in terminals and fibers but not in cells in the locus coeruleus (Figures 2 and 5). The nearby parabrachial nucleus is highly enriched in enkephalin-containing cells, with fibers emerging from the parabrachial nucleus and passing in the direction of the locus coeruleus. Enkephalin may therefore be contained in a pathway with cells in the parabrachial nucleus and terminals in the locus coeruleus. The locus coeruleus contains an extremely high density of opiate receptors (Pert, Kuhar, and Snyder, 1976), which respond selectively to the administration of opiates or enkephalin (Bird and Kuhar, 1977).

The locus coeruleus contains only about 1,400 cells, essentially all of which are noradrenergic; they send their axons and terminals to many distant parts of the brain including the cerebral cortex, hippocampus, and cerebellum. Since rats will press levers at high rates to obtain stimulation in this nucleus, it is possible that it is associated with pleasurable sensations. Thus the opiate receptors in the locus coeruleus might be involved in the euphoric effects produced by opiates. Moreover, the enkephalin neurons in this vicinity may play some role in normally modulating mood.

In the medulla and pons, high densities of enkeph-

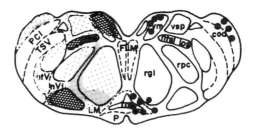

FIGURE 6   Enkephalin immunofluorescence at the level of the raphe magnus. *Abbreviations*: cod, dorsal cochlear nucleus; FLM, medial longitudinal fasciculus; LM, medial lemniscus; nts, nucleus of the solitary tract; ntV, nucleus of the spinal tract of the trigeminal; nVII, nucleus of the facial nerve; P, pyramid; PCI, inferior cerebellar peduncle; ps, parasolitary nucleus; rgi, gigantocellular reticular nucleus; rm, nucleus raphe magnus; rpc, parvocellular reticular nucleus; TSV, spinal tract of the trigeminal; vm, medial vestibular nucleus; vsp, spinal vestibular nucleus. See Figure 4 for key. (From Uhl, Childers, and Snyder, 1978.)

alin-containing cells and terminals, as well as opiate receptors, are observed in nuclei of the vagus, including the nucleus of the solitary tract, the nucleus ambiguus, and the nucleus commissuralis, formed by the confluence in the midline of the two nuclei of the solitary tract (Figures 2, 4, 6, and 7). These structures are known to be involved in various visceral reflexes. Thus they may mediate opiate influences on respiration, gastric emptying, and nausea and vomiting.

The periaqueductal gray of the midbrain contains moderate amounts of opiate receptors, enkephalin cells, and fibers. Since electrical stimulation in this region produces analgesia, this may be another site where enkephalin regulates pain perception.

The periaqueductal gray has fiber connections with

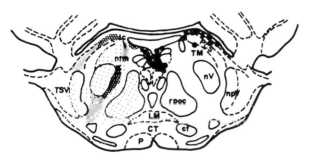

FIGURE 5   Enkephalin immunofluorescence at the level of the exit of the trigeminal. *Abbreviations*: CT, trapezoid body; ct, nucleus of the trapezoid body; lc, locus ceruleus; LM, medial lemniscus; npV, main nucleus of the trigeminal; ntm, nucleus of the mesencephalic tract of the trigeminal; nV, motor nucleus of the trigeminal; P, pyramid; PCS, superior cerebellar peduncle; rpoc, caudal pontine reticular nucleus; TM, mesencephalic tract of the trigeminal; TSV, spinal tract of the trigeminal. See Figure 4 for key. (From Uhl, Childers, and Snyder, 1978.)

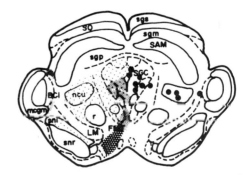

FIGURE 7   Enkephalin fluorescence at the level of the medial geniculate. *Abbreviations:* BCI, brachium of the inferior colliculus; FMT, mammillotegmental tract; LM, medial lemniscus; mcgm, medial geniculate; ncu, cuneiform nucleus; r, red nucleus; SAM, sgm, sgp, sgs, SO, superior colliculus layers; SGC, central gray; snl, lateral substantia nigra; sn, reticulata of substantia nigra. See Figure 4 for key. (From Uhl et al., 1978.)

the nucleus raphe magnus of the pons. Electrical stimulation in the raphe magnus elicits analgesia, as does stimulation in the nucleus gigantocellularis, located somewhat laterally to the raphe magnus. Hökfelt et al. (1977) reported enkephalin-containing cells in raphe magnus. We observed that enkephalin-containing cells are most highly concentrated between the raphe magnus and nucleus gigantocellularis, with a small number of cells overlapping into each of the nuclei (Figure 6). This suggests that electrical stimulation in the vicinity of the two nuclei elicits analgesia through a group of enkephalin cells located chiefly around the raphe magnus and between these nuclei. Conceivably, the enkephalin-containing cells at this level project to raphe magnus and gigantocellularis to influence the firing of neurons contained within these two areas, which in turn have analgesic effects. The raphe magnus, like other raphe nuclei, is enriched in serotonin and projects caudally to the spinal cord, with terminals in the substantia gelatinosa, where high concentrations of enkephalin exist (Basbaum, Clanton, and Fields, 1976).

The corpus striatum was the first brain structure shown to be highly enriched in opiate receptors (Pert and Snyder, 1973). Autoradiographic evidence confirmed that the caudate has a high density of opiate receptors (Figure 3). Enkephalin-containing terminals are more highly concentrated in the globus pallidus than in any other region of the brain, with much less enkephalin in the caudate (Figure 1). The density of enkephalin fluorescence in the globus pallidus is so great that it is difficult to differentiate cell bodies from terminals. Most structures of the corpus striatum are associated with regulation of locomotor activity. Morphine and β-endorphin do exert effects on locomotor behavior in rodents. Clinically, however, such effects are not pronounced. Neurologists, neurosurgeons, and neurophysiologists have speculated for many years that structures in the corpus striatum might also be involved in regulation of emotional behavior, since they are closely associated with limbic areas such as the amygdala.

The amygdala displays a high density of opiate receptors, enkephalin cells, and terminals (Figure 3). Whereas opiate receptors are highly concentrated in the lateral portions of the amygdala, enkephalin fluorescence is strikingly localized to the central nucleus.

The stria terminalis, a bundle of fibers that passes out of the amygdala, also appears to contain enkephalin fibers. The bed nucleus of the stria terminalis contains high concentrations of enkephalin cells and terminals. Within the stria terminalis itself, the fiber-like fluorescence of enkephalin is localized in the ventrolateral quadrant. DeOlmos (1972), in classic anatomic mapping studies, demonstrated a neuronal pathway connecting the central nucleus of the amygdala with the bed nucleus of the stria terminalis via fibers that passed through the ventrolateral portion of the stria terminalis (Figure 8). DeOlmos observed neuronal pathways passing between these two structures in both directions. Might an enkephalin-containing pathway be contained in the stria terminalis? We observed that electrolytic lesions of the central nucleus of the amygdala, but not of other portions of the amygdala, resulted in a depletion of enkephalin fluorescence within the stria terminalis (Figure 9B). Knife cuts of the stria terminalis elicited a buildup of fluorescence in the part of the stria terminalis closer to the amygdala (Figure 9D) and a diminution of fluorescence closer to the bed nucleus. These findings demonstrate that an amygdalofugal pathway passes from the central nucleus through the stria terminalis, with some terminals in the bed nucleus. Other projections of the stria terminalis include the hypothalamus, septum, nucleus accumbens, and preoptic area. Following stria terminalis or central amygdala lesions no diminution in enkephalin fluorescence is observed in any of these areas, suggesting that they do not receive terminals from the enkephalin cells of the amygdala. The demonstration of an amygdalofugal enkephalin pathway indicates that all enkephalin is not contained in interneurons.

Another potential pathway of enkephalin-containing neurons has been suggested by Cuello and Paxi-

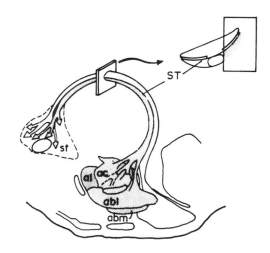

FIGURE 8 Origin course and termination of fibers running through the ventrolateral stria terminalis as determined by classical degeneration methods. Fibers arising from the central (ac), lateral (al), basolateral (abl), and basomedial (abm) amygdaloid nuclei pass through the ventrolateral stria terminalis (ST) and end in the interstitial nucleus of the stria terminalis (st). (Based on DeOlmos, 1972.)

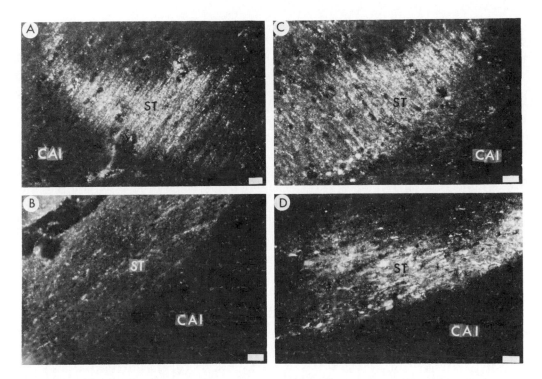

FIGURE 9 Photomicrographs of enkephalin immunofluorescence in the ventrolateral stria terminalis (ST) and internal capsule (CAI). (A) Normal. (B) Ipsilateral to electrolytic lesion destroying the central amygdala (10-day survival time). (C) Ipsilateral to electrolytic lesion sparing the central amygdala (10-day survival time). (D) Ipsilateral and posterior to knife cut of the stria terminalis (2-day survival time). Bars = 25 µm. (From Uhl, Kuhar, and Snyder, 1978.)

nos (1978), who found that knife cuts isolating the globus pallidus markedly reduced fluorescence within the globus pallidus. This suggests that caudate cells containing enkephalin give rise to terminals in the globus pallidus.

In summary, enkephalin is contained in cells and fibers in many different parts of the central nervous system. Their diverse localizations could explain the many and varied actions of opiate drugs. Enkephalin neurons presumably play a role in pain perception, but it should be emphasized that, as with the opiate drugs themselves, the functions of enkephalin may involve numerous other bodily activities.

In contrast to the widespread distribution of the enkephalins in the brain, β-endorphin appears to have a more restricted localization (Bloom et al., 1978). β-Endorphin-containing cells are localized to periventricular regions of the hypothalamus. β-Endorphin fibers appear to ascend and descend from this area, since knife cuts above and below the hypothalamus reduce the amount of β-endorphin fibers and terminals rostral and caudal to the hypothalamus. One β-endorphin-containing pathway appears to proceed from the hypothalamus to the periaqueductal gray of the midbrain. While enkephalin also occurs in the hypothalamus and the periaqueductal gray, in most of the brain the localizations of β-endorphin and enkephalin differ markedly. Thus the globus pallidus and substantia gelatinosa of the spinal cord, areas containing the highest densities of enkephalin in the central nervous system, display no β-endorphin fluorescence.

Release and postsynaptic actions of opioid peptides

If opioid peptides are neurotransmitters or neuromodulators, one would expect that depolarization of nervous tissue should result in their release. Preliminary experiments by Smith et al. (1976) demonstrated that depolarization of synaptosomal preparations by potassium lowered their enkephalin content. This effect was reduced when calcium was eliminated from the incubation medium, consistent with a depolarization-induced release of enkephalin. Electrical stimulation of guinea pig ileum strips also releases immunoreactive enkephalin (Schulz et al., 1977). Recently L. L. Iversen (personal communication) showed a calcium-dependent, potassium-depolarization-related release of enkephalin from slices of the globus pallidus.

What might be the mechanism of opiate and opioid peptide actions at opiate receptors? Many neurotransmitters act by changing ion permeability or by affecting some cyclic nucleotide which in turn influences ion conductance. Ion-specific actions of opiate, as well as effects on cyclic AMP, have been well documented. In low concentrations, sodium enhances opiate-receptor binding of antagonists while markedly lowering the binding of agonists (Pert and Snyder, 1974). This effect of sodium is exerted by concentrations as low as 1 mM and is selective, since it is not elicited by potassium, cesium, or rubidium and is elicited only to a limited extent by lithium.

The ability of sodium to differentiate the binding of agonists and antagonists to the opiate receptor suggests that the opiate receptor might function according to a two-state model analogous to the allosteric model of enzymes. According to this model, the opiate receptor would exist in two states, one favoring the binding of agonists and the other binding antagonists preferentially. Sodium would bind to and stabilize the antagonist state of the receptor. Opiates and enkephalins would elicit their synaptic actions only when they bound to the agonist state of the receptor. Since the two states of the receptor would be freely interconvertible, binding of an antagonist to the antagonist state could block the action of opiates, since it would shift the equilibrium between the two receptor conformations, making fewer agonist states available. By shifting this equilibrium, binding of the agonist would alter the ability of sodium to bind to the antagonist state of the receptor. In some unspecified fashion the changed binding of sodium would affect its conductance through the neuronal membrane.

This model of opiate-receptor functioning is supported by neurophysiological studies. Zieglgansberger and Fry (1976) has shown that opiates and enkephalin do not hyperpolarize cells. Instead they block the excitatory effects of both glutamate and acetylcholine. The actions of both acetylcholine and glutamate involve changes in sodium permeability, though the two transmitters act at different recognition sites. Thus Zieglgansberger and Fry (1976) concluded that opiates and enkephalin must act by interfering at the sodium conductance channel. Quite similar effects have been obtained on the firing of spinal-cord cells in culture (J. Barker, personal communication). In these cases enkephalin must be acting postsynaptically. Studies of the spinal cord and brain stem had suggested that at least some opiate receptors are located presynaptically on nerve terminals (LaMotte, Pert, and Snyder, 1976; Atweh, Murrin, and Kuhar, 1977). It is, of course, possible that enkephalin elicits both postsynaptic and presynaptic in-

hibition. GABA is well known to cause both types of neuronal inhibition. The ionic mechanism whereby enkephalin might elicit presynaptic inhibition is unclear. One would expect presynaptic inhibition to be involved in the actions of enkephalin in the dorsal spinal cord, as well as in the nucleus of the solitary tract and in the accessory optic nuclei, because in all of the locations opiate receptors are localized to nerve terminals.

Influences of divalent cations on opiate-receptor binding have also been described (Pasternak, Snowman, and Snyder, 1975; Simantov, Snowman, and Snyder, 1976). Low concentrations of manganese and magnesium selectively enhance the binding of opiate agonists with no influence on antagonist binding. This effect is virtually the opposite of the influence of sodium on receptor binding. Magnesium is less potent than manganese, but in both cases the concentrations that exert these effects are in the range of normal brain levels. Calcium fails to exert this effect. To determine whether the divalent-cation effect plays a normal regulatory role, influences of chelating agents were examined. EGTA is a relatively selective chelator of calcium, with negligible influences on manganese and magnesium, while EDTA influences all three cations. EDTA reduces the binding of opiate agonists selectively, an effect opposite to that of manganese, whereas EGTA has no influence. These observations suggest that manganese and magnesium normally regulate opiate-receptor functions.

Opiates also affect cyclic nucleotides. Opiates stereospecifically reduce the AMP concentrations of neuroblastoma-glioma cells in culture, an effect that is blocked by the opiate antagonist naloxone (Klee and Nirenberg, 1974). Opiates have also been reported to increase the cyclic GMP content of striatal slices (Minneman and Iversen, 1976).

Behavioral effects, including addiction

Numerous groups have shown that enkephalins and β-endorphin elicit analgesia when injected directly into the brain. After chronic administration, enkephalins and β-endorphin produce physical dependence, as evidenced by the appearance of tolerance and withdrawal symptoms upon termination of peptide administration. Though it is difficult to characterize addiction in animals with precision, there is no evidence that physical dependence on opioid peptides differs markedly from dependence on classical opiates.

The identification of the enkephalins provides new possibilities for an understanding of mechanisms that might result in addiction. One possibility is that changes in the firing rates of enkephalin neurons following opiate administration play some role. For instance, when opiates are administered chronically, bombarding the opiate receptors with levels of opiate-like material that they do not normally encounter, some feedback mechanism may cause enkephalin neurons to stop firing. Accordingly, opiate receptors would then be exposed to a lower total quantity of opiate-like substance than would occur at the initial administration of the opiate drug. Such an organism would be "tolerant" in that an additional amount of drug would be required to reach the degree of saturation of receptors obtained when the drug was first administered. Terminating administration of the drug would result in opiate receptors that possess neither enkephalin nor opiates; hence they are "abstinent." One prediction of this model is that chronic opiate administration should slow the firing of en kephalin neurons. In studies of biogenic amines such as dopamine and acetylcholine, numerous groups have found that a slowing of neuronal firing elevates transmitter levels. No consistent changes in brain levels of enkephalins have been reported after chronic treatment with opiates (Simantov and Snyder, 1976b; Childers, Simantov, and Snyder, 1977; Fratta et al., 1977).

ACKNOWLEDGMENTS   The work reported was supported by USPHS grants DA-00266 and DA-01645. Thanks to Susan M. Garonski for manuscript preparation.

REFERENCES

AKIL, H., D. J. MAYER, and J. C. LIEBESKIND, 1976. Antagonism of stimulation-produced analgesia by naloxone, a narcotic antagonist. *Science* 191:961–962.

ATWEH, S., and M. J. KUHAR, 1977. Autoradiographic localization of opiate receptors in rat brain, I. Spinal cord and lower medulla. *Brain Res.* 124:53–67.

ATWEH, S., L. C. MURRIN, and M. J. KUHAR, 1978. Presynaptic localization of opiate receptors in the vagal and accessory optic systems: An autoradiographic study. *Neuropharmacology* 17:65–71.

BASBAUM, A. I., C. H. CLANTON, and H. L. FIELDS, 1976. Opiate and stimulus-produced analgesia: Functional anatomy of a medullo-spinal pathway. *Proc. Natl. Acad. Sci. USA* 73:4685–4688.

BIRD, S. J., and M. J. KUHAR, 1977. Iontophoretic application of opiates to the locus coeruleus. *Brain Res.* 122:523–533.

BLOOM, F., E. BATTENBERG, J. ROSSIER, N. LING, J. LEPPAL-UOTO, T. M. VARGO, and R. GUILLEMIN, 1977. Endorphins are located in the intermediate and anterior lobes of the pituitary gland, not in the neurohypophysis. *Life Sci.* 20:43–48.

BLOOM, F., E. BATTENBERG, J. ROSSIER, N. LING, and R. GUILLEMIN, 1978. Neurons containing β-endorphin in rat brain exist separately from those containing enkephalin: Immunocytochemical studies. *Proc. Natl. Acad. Sci. USA* 75:1591–1595.

BRADBURY, A. F., D. G. SMYTH, C. R. SNELL, N. J. M. BIRDSALL, and E. C. HULME, 1976. C fragment of lipotropin has a high affinity for brain opiate receptors. *Nature* 260:793–795.

CHILDERS, S., R. SIMANTOV, and S. H. SNYDER, 1977. Enkephalin: Radioimmunoassay and radioreceptor assay in morphine dependent rats. *Eur. J. Pharmacol.* 46:289–293.

COX, B. M., K. E. OPHEIM, H. TESCHEMACHER, and A. GOLDSTEIN, 1975. A peptide-like substance from pituitary that acts like morphine. 2. Purification and properties. *Life Sci.* 16:1777–1782.

COYLE, J. T., and R. SCHWARCZ, 1976. Lesion of striatal neurons with kainic acid provides a model for Huntington's chorea. *Nature* 263:244–246.

CREESE, I., and S. H. SNYDER, 1975. Receptor binding and pharmacological activity of opiates in the guinea pig intestine. *J. Pharmacol. Exp. Ther.* 194:205–291.

CUELLO, A., and G. PAXINOS, 1978. Evidence for a long leu-enkephalin striopallidal pathway in rat brain. *Nature* 271:178–180.

DeOLMOS, J. S., 1972. The amygdaloid projection field in the rat as studied with the cupric-silver method. In *The Neurobiology of the Amygdala*, B. Eleftherious, ed. New York: Plenum Press, pp. 145–204.

ELDE, R., T. HÖKFELT, O. JOHANSSON, and L. TERENIUS, 1976. Immunohistochemical studies using antibodies to leu-enkephalin: initial observations on the nervous system of the rat. *Neuroscience* 1:349–355.

FRATTA, W., H.-Y. T. YANG, J. HONG, and F. COSTA, 1977. Stability of metenkephalin content in brain structures of morphine-dependent or foot-shock stressed rats. *Nature* 268:452–454.

GILKES, J. J. H., G. A. BLOOMFIELD, A. P. SCOTT, P. J. LOWRY, J. G. RATCLIFFE, J. LANDON, and L. H. REES, 1975. Development and validation of a radioimmunoassay for peptides related to β-melanocyte-stimulating hormone in human plasma: The lipotropins. *J. Clin. Endocrinol. Metabol.* 40:450–457.

GUILLEMIN, R., T. VARGO, J. ROSSIER, S. MINICK, N. LING, C. RIVIER, W. VALE, and F. BLOOM, 1977. β-Endorphin and adrenocorticotropin are secreted concomitantly by the pituitary. *Science* 197:1367–1369.

HÖKFELT, T., R. P. ELDE, O. JOHANSSON, R. LUFT, G. NILSSON, and A. ARIMURA, 1976. Immunohistochemical evidence for separate populations of somatostatin-containing and substance P-containing primary afferent neurons in the rat. *Neuroscience* 1:131–136.

HÖKFELT, T., J.-O. KELLERTH, G. NILSSON, and B. PERNOW, 1975. Experimental immunohistochemical studies on the localization and distribution of substance P in cat primary sensory neurons. *Brain Res.* 100:235–252.

HÖKFELT, T., A. LJUNGDAHL, L. TERENIUS, R. ELDE, and G. NILSSON, 1977. Immunohistochemical analysis of peptide pathways possibly related to pain and analgesia: Enkephalin and substance P. *Proc. Natl. Acad. Sci. USA* 74:3081–3085.

HUGHES, J. T., 1975. Isolation of an endogenous compound from the brain with the pharmacological properties similar to morphine. *Brain Res.* 88:295–398.

HUGHES, J. T., T. W. SMITH, H. W. KOSTERLITZ, L. FOTH-

ERGILL, B. A. MORGAN, and H. R. MORRIS, 1975. Identification of two related pentapeptides from the brain with potent opiate agonist activity. *Nature* 258:577–579.

JESSELL, T. W., and L. L. IVERSEN, 1977. Opiate analgesics inhibit substance P release from rat trigeminal nucleus. *Nature* 268:549–550.

KLEE, W. A., and M. NIRENBERG, 1974. A neuroblastoma-glioma hybrid cell line with morphine receptors. *Proc. Natl. Acad. Sci. USA* 71:3474–3477.

KUHAR, M. J., C. B. PERT, and S. H. SNYDER, 1972. Regional distribution of opiate receptor binding in monkey and human brain. *Nature* 245:447–450.

LaMOTTE, C., C. B. PERT, and S. H. SNYDER, 1976. Opiate receptor binding in primate spinal cord: Distribution and changes after dorsal root section. *Brain Res.* 112:407–412.

LI, C. H., 1964. Lipotropin, a new active peptide from pituitary glands. *Nature* 201:924.

LI, C. H., and D. CHUNG, 1976. Isolation and structure of an untriakontapeptide with opiate activity from camel pituitary glands. *Proc. Natl. Acad. Sci. USA* 73:1145–1148.

LING, N., R. BURGUS, and R. GUILLEMIN, 1976. Isolation, primary structure, and synthesis of α-endorphin and γ-endorphin, two peptides of hypothalamic-hypophysial origin with morphomimetic activity. *Proc. Natl. Acad. Sci. USA* 73:3942–3946.

MAINS, R., B. A. EIPPER, and N. LING, 1977. Common precursor to corticotropins and endorphins. *Proc. Natl. Acad. Sci. USA* 74:3014–3018.

MINNEMAN, K. P., and L. L. IVERSEN, 1976. Enkephalin and opiate narcotics increase cyclic GMP accumulation in slices of rat neostriatum. *Nature* 262:313–314.

MINNEMAN, K. P., M. QUIK, and P. C. EMSON, 1978. Receptor linked cyclic AMP systems in rat neostriatum: Differential localization revealed by kainic acid injection. *Brain Res.* 151:407–421.

MORIARTY, G. C., 1973. Adenohypophysis: ultrastructural cytochemistry. A review. *J. Histochem. Cytochem.* 21:855–894.

PASTERNAK, G. W., R. GOODMAN, and S. H. SNYDER, 1975. An endogenous morphine-like factor in mammalian brain. *Life Sci.* 16:1765–1769.

PASTERNAK, G. W., R. SIMANTOV, and S. H. SNYDER, 1975. Characterization of an endogenous morphine-like factor (enkephalin) in mammalian brain. *Mol. Pharmacol.* 12:504–513.

PASTERNAK, G. W., A. M. SNOWMAN, and S. H. SNYDER, 1975. Selective enhancement of ³H-opiate agonist binding by divalent cations. *Mol. Pharmacol.* 11:735–744.

PERT, C. B., M. J. KUHAR, and S. H. SNYDER, 1976. Opiate receptor: Autoradiographic localization in rat brain. *Proc. Natl. Acad. Sci. USA* 73:3729–3733.

PERT, C. B., and S. H. SNYDER, 1973. Opiate receptor: Demonstration in nervous tissue. *Science* 179:1011–1014.

PERT, C. B., and S. H. SNYDER, 1974. Opiate receptor binding of agonists and antagonists affected differentially by sodium. *Mol. Pharmacol.* 10:868–879.

POLLARD, H., C. LLORENS-CORTES, and J. C. SCHWARTZ, 1977. Enkephalin receptors on dopaminergic neurones in rat striatum. *Nature* 268:745–747.

ROSSIER, J., E. D. FRENCH, C. RIVIER, N. LING, R. GUILLEMIN, and F. BLOOM, 1977. Regional dissociation of β-endorphin and enkephalin contents in rat brain and pituitary. *Proc. Natl. Acad. Sci. USA* 74:5162–5165.

SCHULZ, R., M. WUSTER, R. SIMANTOV, S. H. SNYDER, and A. HERZ, 1977. Electrically stimulated release of opiate-like material from the myenteric plexus of the guinea pig ileum. *Eur. J. Pharmacol.* 41:347–348.

SIMANTOV, R., S. CHILDERS, and S. H. SNYDER, 1977. Opioid peptides: Differentiation by radioimmunoassay and radioreceptor assay. *Brain Res.* 135:358–367.

SIMANTOV, R., M. J. KUHAR, G. UHL, and S. H. SNYDER, 1977. Opioid peptide enkephalin: Immunohistochemical mapping in the rat central nervous system. *Proc. Natl. Acad. Sci. USA* 74:467–471.

SIMANTOV, R., A. M. SNOWMAN, and S. H. SNYDER, 1976. Temperature and ionic influences on opiate receptor binding. *Mol. Pharmacol.* 12:977–986.

SIMANTOV, R., and S. H. SNYDER, 1976. Morphine-like factors in mammalian brain: Structure-elucidation and interactions with the opiate receptor. *Proc. Natl. Acad. Sci. USA* 73:2515–2519.

SIMANTOV, R., and S. H. SNYDER, 1976b. Elevated levels of enkephalin in morphine-dependent rats. *Nature* 262:505–507.

SIMON, E. J., J. M. HILLER, and I. EDELMAN, 1973. Stereospecific binding of the potent narcotic analgesic ³H-etorphine to rat brain homogenate. *Proc. Natl. Acad. Sci. USA* 70:1947–1949.

SMITH, T. W., J. HUGHES, H. W. KOSTERLITZ, and R. P. SOSA, 1976. Enkephalins: Isolation, distribution and function. In *Opiates and Endogenous Opioid Peptides*, H. W. Kosterlitz, ed. Amsterdam: North-Holland, pp. 57–62.

SNYDER, S. H., 1975. The opiate receptor in normal and drug altered brain function. *Nature* 257:185–189.

TERENIUS, L., 1973. Characteristics of the "receptor" for narcotic analgesics in synaptic plasma membrane fractions from rat brain. *Acta Pharmacol. Toxicol.* 33:377–384.

TERENIUS, L., and A. WAHLSTROM, 1974. Inhibitor(s) of narcotic receptor binding in brain extracts and in cerebrospinal fluid. *Acta Pharmacol. (Kbh.)* 35(suppl. 1):55.

UHL, G. R., S. CHILDERS, and S. H. SNYDER, 1978. Opioid peptides and the opiate receptor. In *Frontiers of Neuroendocrinology*, W. Ganong and L. Martini, eds. New York: Raven Press.

UHL, G. R., R. R. GOODMAN, M. K. KUHAR, and S. H. SNYDER, 1978. Enkephalin and neurotensin: Immunohistochemical localization and identification of an amygdalofugal pathway. In *Endorphins*, E. Costa and M. Trabucchi, eds. New York: Raven Press, pp. 71–88.

UHL, G. R., M. J. KUHAR, and S. H. SNYDER, 1978. Enkephalin containing pathway: amygdaloid efferents in the stria terminalis. *Brain Res.* 149:223–228.

WATSON, S. J., H. AKIL, S. SULLIVAN, and J. D. BARCHAS, 1977. Immunocytochemical localization of methionine enkephalin: preliminary observations. *Life Sci.* 21:733–738.

WATSON, S. J., J. D. BARCHAS, and C. H. LI, 1977. β-Lipotropin: Localization of cells and axons in rat brain by immunocytochemistry. *Proc. Natl. Acad. Sci. USA* 74:5155–5158.

ZIEGLGANSBERGER, W., and J. P. FRY, 1976. Actions of enkephalin on cortical and striatal neurons of naive and morphine tolerant/dependent rats. In *Opiates and Endogenous Opioid Peptides*, H. W. Kosterlitz, ed. Amsterdam: North-Holland, pp. 231–238.

65 Some Properties of the Ascending Dopaminergic Pathways: Interactions of the Nigrostriatal Dopaminergic System with Other Neuronal Pathways

J. GLOWINSKI

ABSTRACT The substantia nigra (SN) and the ventrotegmental area contain the cell bodies of the three ascending dopaminergic (DA) systems: the nigrostriatal, mesolimbic, and mesocortical DA pathways, which are involved in motor and limbic functions. Unilateral destruction of DA neurons in the SN results in an asymmetric motor behavior. Bilateral destruction of the ventrotegmental area induces a permanent locomotor hyperactivity representing only one aspect of a more complex behavioral syndrome. Although little is known of the regulation of the mesolimbic and mesocortical DA neurons, major efforts have been made to analyze the interactions of the nigrostriatal DA pathway with other neuronal systems within the basal ganglia and with other structures involved in motor behavior. This DA pathway exerts a tonic inhibitory control upon striatal cholinergic neurons. It receives complex information from descending GABA-ergic and substance P neurons originating from the striatum and/or the pallidum. As revealed by recent in vivo release studies, a selective, experimentally induced decrease in the activity of one pathway is associated with an increased activity of the contralateral pathway. Such a balance can also be demonstrated by unilateral sensory stimuli or unilateral stimulation of some cerebellar nuclei. The unilateral stimulation of the motor cortex activates the release of DA from the terminals of the two pathways. In most cases, the increase in DA release from nerve terminals is associated with a parallel decrease of the transmitter release from dendrites within the SN, and vice versa. Thus the direct neurochemical monitoring of DA release can provide insight into some necessary functional operations underlying the behavioral role of this system.

Introduction

SEVERAL NEURONAL circuits connect the cerebral motor cortex, the cerebellum, and the basal ganglia, structures which are primarily involved in sensorimotor integration and the control of motor behavior (Poirier et al., 1975; Carpenter, 1976). The basal ganglia are essentially composed of the striatum (divided in most species into two nuclei: the caudate nucleus and the putamen), the pallidum, the subthalamic nuclei, and the mesencephalic substantia nigra (SN). Among the pathways that connect these different nuclei, one, the nigrostriatal dopaminergic (DA) system, has been the subject of extensive studies since its discovery (Anden et al., 1964). Several symptoms seen in patients with Parkinson's disease, particularly rigidity and akinesia, can be mainly attributed to the degeneration of the DA neurons (Hornykiewicz, 1966). In the rat, the unilateral destruction of the nigrostriatal DA pathway induces an asymmetric motor behavior. Drugs such as amphetamine, which enhance the release of DA from terminals of the contralateral unlesioned pathway, exacerbate this asymmetric motor behavior and cause rotatory movements toward the lesioned side (Ungerstedt, 1971a).

This article will analyze several interneuronal regulatory processes controlling the activity of the DA pathways, concentrating mainly on recent results obtained in our laboratory. We shall examine (1) the role of the nigrostriatal DA neurons in regulating the activity of the striatal cholinergic neurons; (2) the influence of descending striatonigral GABA and sub-

J. GLOWINSKI Groupe NB, INSERM U.114, Collège de France, Paris, France

stance P DA systems; (3) the functional significance of the recently discovered dendritic release of DA; (4) the effects of sensory messages and of messages originating from the cerebellum and the motor cortex on the activity of the two DA pathways; and (5) briefly, the characteristics of the mesolimbic and mesocortical DA neurons in comparison to the nigrostriatal DA neurons.

Some basic characteristics of the nigrostriatal dopaminergic neurons

A few thousand neurons constitute the two symmetric DA systems (Anden et al., 1964). Their cell bodies are mainly concentrated in the pars compacta of the SN; some of their dendrites extend to the pars reticulata and are surrounded with numerous nerve endings exhibiting synaptic contacts (Hassler et al., 1975). The DA fibers pass through the ventral tegmental area of Tsai and run with the medial forebrain bundle, reaching the striatum via the capsula interna (Moore, Bhatnagar, and Heller, 1971). The distribution of the DA terminals is much denser in the rostral than in the caudal part of the striatum in the rat (Tassin et al., 1976) and in the cat (Nieoullon, Chéramy, and Glowinski, 1977a).

It is well established that the activity of tyrosine hydroxylase, the rate-limiting enzyme of DA synthesis, is dependent on nerve impulse flow. When the neurons are activated by electrical stimulation or by neuroleptics, the affinity of the enzyme for its pteridine cofactor is enhanced, whereas its affinity for DA, its end product, is reduced (Zivkovic and Guidotti, 1974; Murrin, Morgenroth, and Roth, 1976). Curiously, a brief stimulation of DA synthesis is also observed shortly after the interruption of nerve firing (Carlsson et al., 1972; Agid, Javoy, and Glowinski, 1974). This may be related to the sudden disappearance of DA at presynaptic DA receptor sites.

In terminals, DA is stored in at least two compartments, which have been called the "functional" and "main" storage compartments. The former, small in size, contains the newly synthesized amine, which is preferentially released under nerve stimulation (Glowinski, 1975). The release of DA depends on nerve impulse flow, but it is also presynaptically controlled by receptors sensitive to the extraneuronal changes in amine levels (Westfall et al., 1976). Like other catecholamines, the released DA is mainly inactivated by reuptake into the terminals and by inactivating enzymes, catechol-O-methyltransferase and monoamine oxidase. The very efficient uptake

process can be specifically blocked by benztropine, an antiparkinsonian drug (Coyle and Snyder, 1969).

The DA postsynaptic receptors are associated with an adenylate cyclase (Greengard, 1976). The distribution of this DA-sensitive adenylate cyclase closely parallels the distribution of the DA terminals in the rat striatum (Bockaert et al., 1976). Binding studies with [³H]-DA or labeled neuroleptics have also been done to identify the DA postsynaptic receptors. In the cow, the number of binding sites is slightly higher in the caudal than in the rostral part of the structure (Burt, Creese, and Snyder, 1976). The apparent difference in the affinity of the DA-sensitive adenylate cyclase for DA and of the DA receptors for labeled ligands, as well as the difference in their distribution, suggests that not all the DA receptors are coupled to an adenylate cyclase. As indicated by behavioral responses to DA agonists, a supersensitivity develops after denervation of DA neurons or chronic neuroleptic treatments (Ungerstedt, 1971b). Changes in the sensitivity of the DA-sensitive adenylate cyclase after denervation have been found by some authors (Mishra et al., 1974) but not by others (Von Voigtlander, Boukma, and Johnson, 1973). The binding of [³H]-haloperidol to rat striatal DA receptors increases after degeneration of the DA neurons; this enhanced binding is associated with an increased number of receptor sites with no change in their affinity (Creese, Burt, and Snyder, 1977).

Several electrophysiological studies have been done to identify the nature of the influence of the DA neurons on striatal neurons. The majority of these cells are depressed by the iontophoretic application of DA; however, excitatory responses have also been observed (Bloom, Costa, and Salmoiraghi, 1965; McLennan and York, 1967; Connor, 1975). Earlier reports suggested that the nigrostriatal DA neurons exerted an inhibitory influence on striatal neurons; however, more recent results indicate that these neurons make excitatory synaptic contact with a population of striatal cells (Kitai, Sugimori, and Kocsis, 1976; Richardson, Miller, and McLennan, 1977). It cannot yet be excluded that the DA neurons exert opposite effects on distinct populations of striatal neurons.

Influence of the nigrostriatal dopaminergic neurons on the striatal cholinergic neurons

The caudate-putamen complex is particularly rich in acetylcholine (ACh) and choline acetyltransferase. ACh is mainly located in cholinergic neurons intrinsic to the structure (McGeer et al., 1971). Based on clinical observations and pharmacological studies, a relationship between the nigrostriatal DA neurons and the cholinergic intrastriatal neurons has been suspected for many years. Anticholinergic drugs are extensively used for the treatment of patients with Parkinson's disease or to correct some of the extrapyramidal side effects induced by neuroleptics.

Recent biochemical studies suggest that the DA neurons exert a tonic inhibitory influence on the activity of the striatal cholinergic neurons. As shown by the direct in vivo measurement of ACh release (Bartholini et al., 1976) or by changes in ACh turnover (Racagni et al., 1976) or ACh levels (Table I; Agid et al., 1975; Guyenet et al., 1975; Ladinsky et al., 1975),

TABLE I

Effects of various neuroleptics, some dopaminergic agonists, and an early lesion of the nigrostriatal dopaminergic neurons on the ACh content in the striatum of the rat

Treatment	ACh (nM/g)	
Saline	44.0 ± 2.2	
Chlorpromazine (15 mg/kg)	24.8 ± 2.8*	
Thioproperazine (5 mg/kg)	29.6 ± 4.5*	
Haloperidol (5 mg/kg)	28.2 ± 2.8*	
Pimozide (5 mg/kg)	23.6 ± 2.6*	
Apomorphine (10 mg/kg)	57.7 ± 2.6*	
	Unlesioned Side	Lesioned Side
Saline[a]	37.5 ± 1.3	38.6 ± 1.2
Chlorpromazine (10 mg/kg)[a]	26.2 ± 1.8*	24.8 ± 2.8*
Apomorphine (10 mg/kg)[a]	52.0 ± 1.6*	50.6 ± 3.8*
Saline[a]	40.0 ± 1.2	38.9 ± 1.7
Amphetamine (10 mg/kg)[a]	44.8 ± 1.5*	37.2 ± 1.9
Electrocoagulation:[b]		
10 min	49.5 ± 2.3	36.8 ± 2.2*
120 min	47.6 ± 3.0	34.4 ± 2.3*

The results are means ± S.E. of data obtained with groups of 7–10 rats. Saline and all drugs were injected intraperitoneally 1 hr before sacrifice by decapitation.

* p < 0.05 when compared to saline-treated rats (for drug-injected groups) or to the contralateral striatum (for electrocoagulated groups).

[a] Rats received a unilateral microinjection of 6-hydroxydopamine (4 μl, 8 μg) into the substantia nigra 10 days prior to the drug experiments.

[b] An electrolytic injection was performed unilaterally in the right substantia nigra. ACh levels were estimated in the striata corresponding to the unlesioned and lesioned sides 10 and 120 min after surgery.

the activity of cholinergic neurons is reduced when DA transmission is increased, and vice versa. For instance, by blocking DA receptors, neuroleptics stimulate the release of ACh in the cat caudate nucleus, accelerate ACh turnover, or reduce ACh levels in the rat striatum (the latter effect resulting from the enhanced utilization of the transmitter). Similar effects are induced by the blockade of DA synthesis with α-methylparatyrosine or the interruption of nerve firing in DA neurons. Opposite effects are seen with DA agonists such as apomorphine or piribedil, drugs that also antagonize the changes in ACh release induced by neuroleptics. Decreased activity of the cholinergic neurons is also observed after treatment with amphetamine or DOPA, or during electrical activation of the DA neurons.

Converging data suggest that some DA postsynaptic receptors are located on striatal cholinergic neurons. Thus changes in the activity of the cholinergic neurons induced by neuroleptics and apomorphine are still observed after degeneration of nigrostriatal DA neurons (Table I; Guyenet et al., 1975). The immunohistochemical visualization of the cholinergic neurons has revealed that these neurons are in contact with fibers *en passant* exhibiting the characteristics of the DA terminals (Hattori et al., 1976). Finally, the destruction of the cholinergic interneurons induced by the local injection of kainic acid is associated with a reduction of the DA-sensitive adenylate cyclase activity, that is, of postsynaptic DA-receptor sites (McGeer, Innanen, and McGeer, 1976).

From these biochemical results it is tempting to conclude that the DA neurons exert a direct inhibitory influence on the striatal cholinergic neurons. However, recent electrophysiological studies have revealed that some striatal cells are directly activated under stimulation of the DA neurons (Kitai, Sugimori, and Kocsis, 1976; Richardson, Miller, and McLennan, 1977). Further experiments are required to elucidate this discrepancy. In any case, the DA neurons are certainly not the only ones involved in the control of the activity of the cholinergic neurons; on the other hand, the DA neurons may influence other striatal neuronal populations besides the cholinergic neurons.

Control of the nigrostriatal dopaminergic neurons by identified neuronal pathways ending in the substantia nigra

Some of the pathways projecting into the pars compacta and the pars reticulata of the SN have already been identified. They may directly or indirectly regulate the activity of the nigrostriatal DA neurons. Combined lesion and biochemical studies (Hattori et al., 1973; Fonnum et al., 1974; Hong et al., 1977), and histochemical or autoradiographic studies (Bak et al., 1975; Ribak et al., 1976; Kanazawa, Emson, and Cuello, 1977), have revealed that the SN is innervated by both GABA-ergic and substance P-descending neurons, which originate mainly in the striatum and possibly (to a lesser extent) in the pallidum. As described in the rat, a distinct serotoninergic pathway emerging from the raphe nuclei also projects into the SN (Bunney and Aghajanian, 1976; Dray and Straughan, 1976). Although not wholly conclusive, some results suggest that some of the three types of neurons directly contact the dopaminergic neurons. The SN contains the highest concentration of GABA, substance P, and serotonin in the brain. It is also rich in other transmitters, such as ACh, glycine, histamine, enkephalin (Dray and Straughan, 1976). Some of these (ACh, glycine) may be located in interneurons; the others are contained in afferent fibers originating from still unidentified structures of the brain.

Since the release of DA is essentially dependent on nerve impulse flow, estimation of the in vivo transmitter release from nerve terminals allows detection of discrete changes in the activity of the DA neurons. Indirect information can also be obtained by measuring changes in the levels of DA metabolites or changes in DA turnover in the striatum. The most suitable approach for studying the in vivo release of transmitters is the use of push-pull cannulas that allow the superfusion of limited and deep areas of the brain. This technique has been used to study the release of endogenous DA in the cat caudate nucleus (McLennan, 1964; Riddell and Szerb, 1971). Some improved sensitivity for detecting DA released in superfusates can be obtained with a radioenzymatic assay (Chéramy et al., 1975; Bartholini et al., 1976). A still more sensitive and rapid method is to continuously deliver L-[^{3}H]-tyrosine of high specific activity and to measure [^{3}H]-DA released in serial superfusate fractions. The [^{3}H]-amine is endogenously formed in DA terminals, and quantities of [^{3}H]-DA as small as 3 pg can be detected and measured with great reproducibility. This isotopic method, initially developed in combination with a cup technique to superfuse the ventricular surface of the caudate nucleus (Besson et al., 1971), was recently adapted to use with push-pull cannulas (Nieoullon, Chéramy, and Glowinski, 1977a).

ROLE OF THE GABA-ergic NEURONS The activity of the cells in the pars compacta is reduced by the microiontophoretic application of GABA (Aghajanian and Bunney, 1975; Dray, Gonye, and Oakley, 1976) or during the electrical stimulation of the caudate nucleus (Precht and Yoshida, 1971), and these effects are antagonized by GABA-ergic antagonists such as picrotoxin or bicuculline. With the push-pull cannula method, we observed a stimulation of the release of newly formed [^{3}H]-DA in the cat caudate nucleus shortly after the peripheral injection or the nigral application of picrotoxin (Chéramy, Nieoullon, and Glowinski, 1977a). This effect was prevented or reversed by diazepam, a tranquilizing benzodiazepine (Chéramy, Nieoullon, and Glowinski, 1977b), which may act presynaptically and favor the release of GABA (Schaffner and Haefely, 1975). Moreover, a high concentration of GABA introduced into the SN reduced the rate of DA utilization in the rat striatum (Anden and Stock, 1973). Similar observations were made after the peripheral administration of large doses of γ-hydroxybutyrate, a general anesthetic which, like GABA, reduces the firing in nigral DA neurons activated by chloral hydrate anesthesia (Roth, Murrin, and Walters, 1976). Finally, muscimol, a potent GABA agonist, antagonized the increase of striatal tyrosine hydroxylase activity elicited by neuroleptics (Gale and Guidotti, 1976).

From these results it can be concluded that some descending GABA-ergic neurons inhibit the activity of the DA neurons. However, some of our experiments suggest that a contingent of the GABA-ergic fibers, possibly those projecting into the pars reticulata of the SN, facilitate DA transmission in the striatum. This could result from an indirect effect linked to the inhibition of intranigral inhibitory interneurons. To measure the changes in [^{3}H]-DA release in the cat caudate nucleus induced by the nigral application of GABA, GABA (10^{-5}M) was introduced through a second push-pull cannula inserted into the SN. GABA exerted a dual effect: an initial potent stimulation of [^{3}H]-DA release preceded a transient inhibition (Figure 1; Chéramy, Nieoullon, and Glowinski, 1978a,b). An activation of [^{3}H]-DA release was also seen with muscimol, GABA-choline or γ-hydroxybutyrate (Chéramy, Nieoullon, and Glowinski, 1978a,b). Furthermore, in the rat, Dray and Straughan (1976) observed that the unilateral nigral injection of ethanolamine-O-sulfate, a blocker of GABA transaminase, stimulated DA turnover in the ipsilateral striatum. Since GABA does not activate nigral cells, its stimulating effect on [^{3}H]-DA release

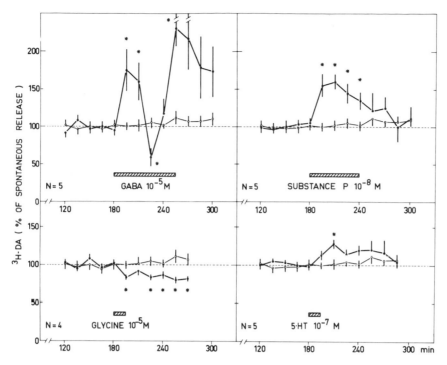

FIGURE 1   Effects of the introduction of various transmitters into the left substantia nigra on the release of dopamine in the ipsilateral caudate nucleus of the cat. The left caudate nucleus of "encéphale-isolé" or halothane-anesthetized cats was continuously superfused at a rate of 500 μl per 15 min with an artificial CSF containing L-3,5-[^{3}H]-tyrosine (20–25 μCi/15 min) using a push-pull cannula. The collection of superfusates for [^{3}H]-DA estimation in 15 min fractions started 105 min after the beginning of the superfusion. Three hours after the onset of the superfusion, GABA (10^{-5}M), substance P (10^{-8}M), glycine (10^{-5}M), or serotonin (5-HT) (10^{-7}M) was introduced for a brief period (15–75 min) into the superfusing fluid of a second push-pull cannula inserted into the left substantia nigra. In each animal, [^{3}H]-DA found in each fraction was expressed as a percentage of an average spontaneous release calculated from the five fractions collected before the drug application. Data are means ± S.E. of results obtained with groups of N animals. * $p < 0.05$ when compared to corresponding control values obtained in animals in which no compound was added into the superfusing fluid (open circles).

could be attributed to an inhibition of inhibitory interneurons in contact with the DA neurons. These inhibitory neurons could be glycinergic. Glycine, which is found in large amounts in the SN, inhibits numerous nigral cells when applied microiontophoretically (Dray and Straughan, 1976). Superfusion of the SN with glycine leads to a reduction in the release of [^{3}H]-DA in the ipsilateral caudate nucleus (Figure 1). Furthermore, this glycine-inhibiting effect is no longer seen in the presence of strychnine, a blocker of the glycinergic receptors (Chéramy, Nieoullon, and Glowinski, 1978c). The facilitation of [^{3}H]-DA release in the caudate nucleus induced by the nigral application of GABA could also be mediated by a polysynaptic pathway involving the nigrothalamic neurons and a thalamostriatal or corticostriatal projection that may regulate DA release by acting presynaptically on DA terminals.

ROLE OF THE SUBSTANCE P NEURONS   SN contains the highest concentration of substance P in the brain. The substance P nerve terminals, which have been visualized immunohistochemically, are primarily concentrated in the pars compacta. Their distribution closely parallels the immunohistochemical distribution of tyrosine hydroxylase (Hökfelt et al., 1975). Lesions made in the striatum and the pallidum of the rat reduced substance P levels in the SN, and substance P cell bodies have been identified in the striatum (Kanazawa, Emson, and Cuello, 1977; Hong et al., 1977).

A potassium-evoked release of substance P that is calcium-dependent has been found in slices of the SN (Jessel, 1977). Applied microiontophoretically, substance P induced a slow and small excitation of numerous nigral cells (Dray and Straughan, 1976). Finally, we recently reported that introduction of substance P (10^{-8}M) into the cat SN activated the release of [³H]-DA in the ipsilateral caudate nucleus (Chéramy et al., 1977; see Figure 1). All these observations suggest that a striatonigral and/or pallidonigral substance P pathway exerts a facilitory influence on the DA neurons.

ROLE OF THE SEROTONINERGIC NEURONS The predominant effect of 5-HT is to depress the activity of cells in the pars compacta of the rat SN (Aghajanian and Bunney, 1975; Dray and Straughan, 1976). Neurons located in the pars reticulata can be either inhibited or excited, or only activated. Similar effects are seen during the local stimulation of the median raphe (Dray and Straughan, 1976). These changes in activity of the nigral neurons can be antagonized by methiothepin, a serotoninergic blocker that can also act on DA receptors. These data suggest that the 5-HT neurons inhibit the activity of the DA neurons. However, results obtained in biochemical studies do not support this hypothesis. A lesion of the median raphe, which slightly decreased 5-HT levels in the rat SN, increased the levels of DA in the striatum (Dray and Straughan, 1976) and reduced those of homovanillic acid, the main metabolite of DA (Samanin et al., 1978). Furthermore, the local application of 5-HT in the SN activated the release of [³H]-DA in the ipsilateral caudate nucleus (Figure 1). As for the striatonigral descending GABA neurons, the 5-HT neurons may influence several mechanisms of DA transmission in the striatum.

Dendritic release of dopamine: Its role in the regulation of the activity of the dopaminergic neurons

Numerous dendrites of the DA neurons can be observed in the pars reticulata of the SN. On the basis of histochemical studies, Björklund and Lindvall (1975) proposed that DA could be released locally from dendrites. This hypothesis was strongly supported by Geffen et al. (1976), who observed that exogenous [³H]-DA, previously taken up in slices from the rat SN, was released by potassium in a calcium-dependent process. Korf, Zieleman, and Westerink (1976) detected an increased accumulation of dihydroxyphenylacetic and homovanillic acids in the rat SN following the electrical stimulation of the medial forebrain bundle. According to these authors, this resulted from an antidromic activation of DA release from DA dendrites.

In our laboratory, Nieoullon and Chéramy obtained direct evidence for the in vivo dendritic release

of DA in halothane-anesthesized cats (Nieoullon, Chéramy, and Glowinski, 1977b). Using the push-pull cannula method and the continuous labeling of the DA cell bodies and dendrites with L-[³H]-tyrosine, they observed that the quantity of [³H]-DA spontaneously released into the SN was just slightly lower than that observed in superfusates of a push-pull cannula introduced into the caudate nucleus. As observed in the caudate nucleus, the nigral release of [³H]-DA was significantly stimulated by potassium (30 mM) and by the addition of amphetamine or benztropine to the superfusion fluid. Furthermore, the unilateral electrical stimulation of the motor cerebral cortex activated the release of [³H]-DA in the ipsilateral SN (Nieoullon, Chéramy, and Glowinski, 1978a). This effect could be mediated by a direct corticonigral pathway (Rinvik, 1966).

These results raise two major questions: (1) How can we exclude the possibility that DA is released from axonal recurrent collaterals in the SN? (2) What is the function of DA released from dendrites?

Two observations, at least, suggest that DA is released from dendrites and not from collaterals. First, tetrodotoxin, which reduced the release of DA from nerve terminals in the caudate nucleus by blocking sodium channels, induced an opposite effect in the SN (Figure 2; Nieoullon, Chéramy, and Glowinski, 1977b). This suggests that DA is not released from terminals in the SN and that sodium channels are not

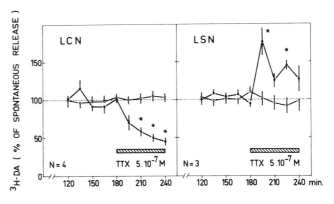

FIGURE 2 Effect of tetrodotoxin on dopamine release from the caudate nucleus and the substantia nigra of the cat. A discrete area of the left caudate nucleus (LCN) or of the left substantia nigra (LSN) of halothane-anesthetized cats was superfused continuously with L-3,5-[³H]-tyrosine using a push-pull cannula. [³H]-Dopamine was estimated in 15 min successive superfusate fractions. Tetrodotoxin (TTX, 5×10^{-7}M) was added for 1 hr to the superfusion fluid 180 min after the onset of the superfusion. Data are means ± S.E. of results obtained with groups of N animals. * $p < 0.05$ when compared to corresponding control values obtained in animals in which no TTX was added in the superfusing fluid (open circles).

involved in the release process of DA from dendrites. It also indicates that some neuronal afferent fibers exert an inhibitory effect on the dendritic release of DA. Furthermore, in several cases the changes in DA release from SN were the opposite of those detected in the ipsilateral caudate nucleus. In other words, activation of the DA neurons, which stimulated DA release from their striatal terminals, did not result in a parallel increase in the nigral release of DA.

The first evidence for a functional role of DA in the SN was obtained by Aghajanian and Bunney (1973). The iontophoretic application of DA inhibited the activity of the DA neurons in the SN, and this inhibition was antagonized by neuroleptics. It was thus proposed that DA was acting on dopaminergic receptors located on DA cells or their dendrites. A self-inhibition of the DA neurons was also suggested by Groves et al. (1975), who noted that neurons in the pars compacta were inhibited by the local application of amphetamine. This autoregulation of the activity of the DA neurons by DA released from dendrites is further supported by our experiments, in which the release of [³H]-DA in the caudate nucleus was reduced by the nigral application of DA (Chéramy et al., 1977) and also by the nigral introduction of amphetamine and benztropine (Chéramy, Nieoullon, and Glowinski, 1978a), two drugs that increase the dendritic release of DA. By contrast, haloperidol, a blocker of the DA receptor, stimulated the release of [³H]-DA in the caudate nucleus when introduced into the SN.

A DA-sensitive adenylate cyclase is present in the SN. This cyclase must be associated with DA receptors located on nigral afferent fibers because lesions that reduced GABA and substance P levels in the SN also decreased the activity of the DA-sensitive adenylate cyclase (Gale, Guidotti, and Costa, 1977). Furthermore, the DA-sensitive cyclase was still present after the destruction of the DA neurons induced by 6-hydroxydopamine (Premont et al., 1976). DA released from dendrites may, in the fashion of a local circuit neuron, exert a presynaptic control over the release of transmitters from nigral afferent projections and thus regulate the messages being delivered to the DA neurons. Indeed, DA has recently been shown to evoke the release of [³H]-GABA from rat SN slices (Reubi, Iversen, and Jessel, 1977).

Role of nigrostriatal dopaminergic neurons in sensorimotor integration

A recent study by Ljungberg and Ungerstedt (1976) emphasized the role of the nigrostriatal DA neurons in the control of sensorimotor integration. An unilateral 6-hydroxydopamine-induced degeneration of the DA pathway resulted in a profound deficiency in the ability of rats to orient themselves toward sensory stimuli presented on the contralateral side of the body. A contralateral inattention to olfactory, tactile, auditory, and visual stimuli was seen a few days after the lesion. Except for the tactile stimulus, this deficiency eventually disappeared, indicating that the deficit was not due to motor impairment.

EFFECTS OF SENSORY STIMULI ON THE ACTIVITY OF THE TWO DOPAMINERGIC PATHWAYS Some of our recent studies performed in the cat further support the role of the DA neurons in sensorimotor integration. We investigated the effects of a unilateral somatic sensory stimulus on the activity of both nigrostriatal DA pathways in animals slightly anesthetized with halothane (Nieoullon, Chéramy, and Glowinski, 1977c). The somatic stimulus consisted of a 10 min electrical stimulation of the paw of the right forelimb. A push-pull cannula was inserted into each caudate nucleus and the SN to study the release of [³H]-DA, which is continuously synthesized from L-[³H]-tyrosine in the terminals and dendrites of the two DA pathways. As indicated by the opposite changes in [³H]-DA release observed in the two caudate nuclei, the stimulus reduced the activity of the DA neurons in the contralateral side and activated the DA neurons in the ipsilateral side. Moreover, in contrast to the release observed in DA terminals, the dendritic release of [³H]-DA was enhanced on the contralateral side and reduced on the ipsilateral side (Figure 3).

These results suggest several comments: (1) As already discussed, the level of activity of the DA neurons seems to be inversely correlated to the extent of the dendritic release of DA in physiological states. (2) The asymmetric changes in the activity of the two DA pathways in response to unilateral sensory information provide further evidence for a specific role of the DA neurons in sensorimotor integration. (3) The marked opposite variations in the activities of the two DA systems could be initiated by messages preferentially delivered to one SN. In fact, a balance exists between the activities of the two DA pathways. Indeed, the electrocoagulation of one SN, which immediately interrupted the release of [³H]-DA in the ipsilateral caudate nucleus, surprisingly enhanced [³H]-DA release in the contralateral side (Nieoullon, Chéramy, and Glowinski, 1977d). Activation of the contralateral DA pathway was also seen after the local applications of DA, amphetamine, or benztropine in one SN—treatments that reduce the activity of the

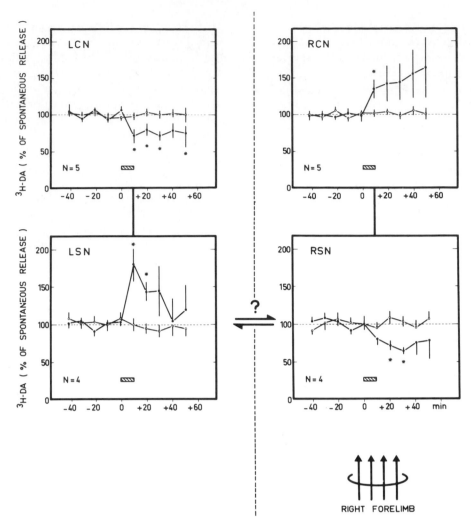

FIGURE 3   Effects of unliateral somatic electrical stimulation on the release of dopamine from the two caudate nuclei and the two substantiae nigrae in the cat. Four push-pull cannulas were simultaneously implanted in the left (LCN) and the right (RCN) caudate nuclei and in the left (LSN) and the right (RSN) substantiae nigrae. The four structures were superfused with an artificial CSF containing L-3,5-[³H]-tyrosine. [³H]-Dopamine was estimated in 10 min successive superfusate fractions. The paw of the right fore-limb was stimulated (hatched bars) for 10 min using a pair of electrodes (monophasic square pulses, 4–6 V, 0.5 msec, 0.25 Hz). In each animal and for each cannula, [³H]-dopamine in each successive fraction was expressed as a percentage of an average spontaneous release calculated from the five fractions collected before the stimulation. Data are means ± S.E. of results obtained with groups of N animals. * $p < 0.05$ when compared to corresponding control values (open circles) obtained in five nonstimulated animals.

DA neurons in the ipsilateral side. The connections involved in the reciprocal control of the two DA pathways have not yet been identified. In any case, this "balance" between the levels of activity of the two DA systems could contribute to the organization of postural adjustments and to motor coordination. This phenomenon should also be taken into consideration in explanations of the motor disorders induced by the unilateral degeneration of a nigrostriatal DA system.

ROLE OF THE CEREBELLUM IN THE CONTROL OF THE ACTIVITY OF THE NIGROSTRIATAL DOPAMINERGIC NEURONS   Like the basal ganglia, the cerebellum plays a critical role in sensorimotor integration. A major part of the information processed in the cerebellum reaches the cerebral motor cortex via the ventrolateral nucleus of the thalamus. It has generally been assumed that there was no relationship between the basal ganglia and the cerebellum and that these two structures independently influenced the cerebral cortex (Kemp and Powell, 1971). However, degeneration studies made by Snider, Maiti, and Snider (1976) have revealed that a pathway originating in the dentate and interpositate nuclei of the cerebellum projects into the pars compacta of the contralateral SN. Furthermore, these authors indicated that unilateral lesion of these two cerebellar nuclei reduced the turnover of DA in the contralateral forebrain of the rat (Snider and Snider, 1977).

We have explored the relationships between the cerebellum and nigrostriatal DA neurons in the cat (Nieoullon, Chéramy, and Glowinski, 1978b). The animals were implanted with four push-pull cannulas to continuously superfuse each caudate nucleus and SN with L-[³H]-tyrosine and to measure the release of [³H]-DA from terminals and dendrites. Unilateral electrical stimulation of the cerebellar dentate nucleus stimulated the release of [³H]-DA in the contralateral caudate nucleus. Activation of the DA neurons was associated with a reduction of the dendritic release of [³H]-DA. Furthermore, the interdependence of the two DA pathways was confirmed. The activity of the ipsilateral DA neurons was reduced, and corresponding to the decreased release of [³H]-DA in the caudate nucleus was an increased release of the [³H]-transmitter from dendrites.

This connection between the cerebellum and the DA neurons of the basal ganglia could explain some of the similarities between patients with Parkinson's disease and those affected by cerebellar disorders. In any case, these observations reveal once more the organized reactivity of the two DA pathways in situations affecting motor behavior and the multiplicity of events involved in the control of the activity of the DA neurons.

Interactions of striatal neurons or striatal neuronal afferent fibers with the terminals of the nigrostriatal dopaminergic neurons

The regulation of DA release from terminals of the nigrostriatal DA neurons may not depend solely on changes in nerve impulse flow triggered by inputs reaching the SN. The release of DA may also be presynaptically regulated, not only through presynaptic DA receptors, but also by striatal neurons or neuronal afferent fibers projecting into the striatum in connection with the DA terminals.

β-Endorphin has been shown to reduce the potassium-evoked release of [³H]-DA from striatal slices (Loh et al., 1976). Moreover, enkephalin receptors are located on striatal DA terminals (Pollard, Llorens-

Cortes, and Schwartz, 1977). This suggests that enkephalin-containing neurons interact with DA terminals, as may also be the case for the striatal cholinergic and GABA-ergic interneurons. GABA-ergic and substance P neurons may also be connected to the DA terminals by recurrent axonal collaterals. Finally, this type of regulation could also be exerted by thalamostriatal and corticostriatal neurons.

We have estimated the effects of several striatal transmitters on the release of [³H]-DA continuously formed from L-[³H]-tyrosine in striatal slices (Figure 4). Under these conditions, the spontaneous release of [³H]-DA is calcium-dependent. It is also reduced by tetrodotoxin, a neurotoxin that can be used to distinguish direct or indirect effects of transmitters on DA terminals (Giorguieff, Le Floc'h, Glowinski, and Besson, 1977). Indeed, by blocking sodium channels, the neurotoxin should interrupt firing in neurons connected to the DA terminals and thus protect them from interneuronal influences.

POSSIBLE ROLE OF CHOLINERGIC AND GABA-ERGIC INTRASTRIATAL NEURONS ACh, carbachol, and oxotremorine stimulated the release of [³H]-DA endogenously synthesized from L-[³H]-tyrosine in striatal slices. The preventive effects of various nicotinic and muscarinic blockers, such as pempidine, mecamylamine, or atropine, revealed that ACh was acting through both nicotinic and muscarinic receptors (Giorguieff et al., 1977). The involvement of cholinergic receptors in the control of DA release has also been postulated by Westfall (1974). Under our experimental conditions, GABA and several GABA agonists, or related compounds such as muscimol and γ-hydroxybutyrate, also stimulated the spontaneous release of [³H]-DA. The GABA-stimulating effect was partially prevented by picrotoxin, the GABA-ergic blocker (Figure 4; Giorguieff et al., 1978).

Both the ACh- and the GABA-stimulating effects on [³H]-DA release were calcium-dependent. While ACh or oxotremorine were still effective in the presence of tetrodotoxin, GABA was not (Figure 4). Under this condition, the ACh- and oxotremorine-stimulating effects on [³H]-DA release were still prevented by nicotinic and/or muscarinic blockers. We therefore concluded that nicotinic and muscarinic receptors located on DA terminals were involved in the control of DA release.

We cannot exclude the possibility that the striatal cholinergic interneurons presynaptically regulate the release of DA. Since most of them are under the control of the DA neurons, this presynaptic regula-

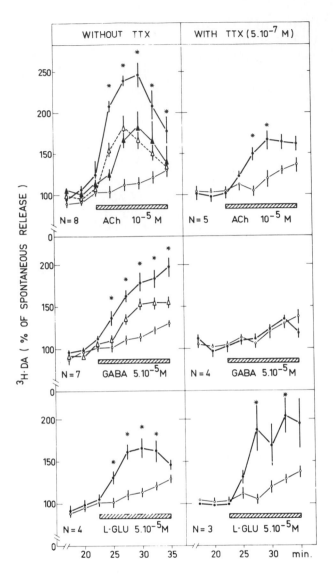

FIGURE 4 Effects of ACh, GABA, and L-glutamic acid on the spontaneous release of DA in striatal slices of the rat. Rat striatal slices were continuously superfused with an artificial CSF containing L-3,5-[³H]-tyrosine (25 μCi/500 ml) at a rate of 1 ml/5 min, and [³H]-dopamine was estimated in serial 2.5 min superfusate fractions. The different panels represent the effects of ACh (10^{-5}M), GABA (5×10^{-5}M) or L-glutamic acid (L-GLU) (5×10^{-5}M) on the spontaneous release of the [³H]-transmitters (black circles) in the presence or absence of tetrodotoxin (TTX) (5×10^{-7}M). The effect of atropine (10^{-6}M) (open triangles) and of pempidine (10^{-5}M) (black triangles) on the ACh-evoked release of [³H]-DA are illustrated in the upper left panel. The effect of picrotoxin (10^{-5}M) (open triangles) on the GABA-evoked release of [³H]-DA is illustrated in the center left panel. TTX and the blockers of the cholinergic and GABA-ergic receptors were added during the entire superfusion. In all cases the [³H]-DA content in each successive fraction was expressed as a percentage of an average release calculated in each experiment on the basis of the release of [³H]-DA between the fifteenth and the twentieth minute of the superfusion, that is, before the application of ACh, GABA, or L-glutamic acid. Data are means ± S.E. of results obtained with groups of N experiments. * $p < 0.05$ when compared to the corresponding control values (open circles).

tion could represent an efficient local interneuronal feedback regulatory process. If our hypothesis concerning the mechanism of action of tetrodotoxin is correct, the stimulating effect of GABA on the spontaneous release of [³H]-DA should not be mediated by GABA-ergic receptors located on the DA terminals. The GABA-ergic neurons that may be involved in the control of DA release from dopaminergic terminals should act indirectly.

POSSIBLE ROLE OF A CORTICOSTRIATAL GLUTAMATERGIC PATHWAY The striatum is densely innervated by neurons originating from the cerebral cortex. Those originating from the motor areas could be glutamatergic. In the rat, striatal neurons sensitive to L-glutamic acid were activated during the electrical stimulation of the motor cortex. This activation could

be prevented by the microiontophoretic application of glutamic-diethyl ester, an antagonist of glutamatergic receptors (Spencer, 1976). Furthermore, the high-affinity uptake process for glutamic acid was no longer detected in striatal synaptosomes of rats with lesions of the motor cerebral cortex (Divac, Fonnum, and Storm-Mathisen, 1977). Finally, binding studies made with [³H]-kainic acid, a rigid analog of L-glutamic acid, have suggested the presence of numerous glutamatergic receptors in the striatum (Simon, Contrera, and Kuhar, 1976).

These observations support the existence of an excitatory glutamatergic corticostriatal pathway. If this pathway is involved in the presynaptic control of DA release from DA terminals, its activation and the direct application of L-glutamic acid should stimulate DA release. The unilateral punctate electrical stimulation of the cortical motor area in the cat activated the release of endogenously formed [³H]-DA in both caudate nuclei. There is little doubt that these effects were mediated by the corticostriatal projection, since the contralateral activation of [³H]-DA release from terminals disappeared after the transection of the rostral corpus callosum (Nieoullon, Chéramy, and Glowinski, 1978a). Furthermore, L-glutamic acid activated the spontaneous release of newly formed [³H]-DA from rat striatal slices (Figure 4). This effect was not prevented by nicotinic or muscarinic antagonists, thereby excluding the intervention of cholinergic interneurons. The L-glutamic-acid-evoked release of [³H]-DA persisted in the presence of tetrodotoxin, suggesting the presence of presynaptic glutamatergic receptors on DA terminals (Giorguieff, Kemel, and Glowinski, 1977).

Some relationships between the nigrostriatal dopaminergic systems and the mesocortical and mesolimbic dopaminergic neurons

Two ascending DA pathways other than the nigrostriatal DA system have been identified. The mesolimbic DA pathway was discovered in earlier histochemical studies (Dahlström and Fuxe, 1964). The cell bodies (A10 group of DA neurons) are located in the ventral tegmental area, and the terminals project into various subcortical limbic nuclei. The presence of DA terminals in the cerebral cortex was first established with biochemical methods (Thierry et al., 1973). These terminals are essentially distributed in the frontal, cingular, and entorhinal cortices (Hökfelt et al., 1974; Lindvall and Björklund, 1974; Berger et al., 1974). They originate from cell bodies located both in the ventral tegmental area and in the SN (Lindvall et al., 1974; Simon et al., 1976). Some anatomical relationships exist between these systems and the nigrostriatal DA neurons. For many authors, the nucleus accumbens is part of the basal ganglia (Chung, Hassler, and Wagner, 1976). Like the caudate-putamen complex, it is connected to the pallidum by a pathway that could be GABA-ergic (Pycock and Horton, 1976); it also receives neuronal afferent fibers originating in the thalamus and the cerebral cortex (Powell and Leman, 1976). The striatum is innervated not only by the nigrostriatal DA neurons but also by a limited contingent of DA fibers originating in the A10 group of DA cell bodies and projecting into the rostral part of the head of the caudate-putamen complex (Tassin et al., 1977).

The extensive distribution of the cell bodies of the mesocortical DA neurons between the A10 group in the ventral tegmental area and the A9 group of nigral DA neurons may have several consequences. The nigrocortical DA neurons could be regulated like the nigrostriatal DA neurons, by the GABA-ergic, substance P, or 5-HT pathways innervating the SN. Furthermore, some of the behavioral disturbances induced by lesions of nigral DA neurons may be partly attributable to the destruction of the nigrocortical projection.

The mesocortical and mesolimbic DA neurons seem to play a critical role in limbic functions. The antipsychotic effects of neuroleptics could be me-diated by their interaction with DA receptors distributed in structures innervated by these neurons. The mesocortical DA neurons projecting into the frontal cortex are highly activated under stress; although less pronounced, a similar phenomenon is seen in DA neurons innervating the nucleus accumbens. In contrast, the nigrostriatal DA neurons are not affected (Thierry et al., 1976).

The mesolimbic and mesocortical DA neurons appear also to be implicated in motor function. An intense locomotor hyperactivity is induced by injections of DA or DA agonists into the nucleus accumbens (Kelly, Seviour, and Iversen, 1975). The changes in locomotor hyperactivity elicited by *d*-amphetamine are antagonized by neuroleptics introduced directly into the nucleus accumbens (Pijnenburg, Hönig, and Van Rossum, 1975) and are no longer seen after bilateral 6-hydroxydopamine lesions of the DA neurons projecting into this structure (Kelly, Seviour, and Iversen, 1975).

The destruction of the DA cells in the rat ventral tegmental area induces a more severe locomotor hyperactivity that lasts for several months and is associated with a complex syndrome characterized by a decrease in exploratory capacity, ongoing behavior, and attention span and a complete disruption of organized behavior reflecting a hypoarousal (LeMoal, Galey, and Cardo, 1975). The interruption of DA transmission in the frontal cortex seems to be largely responsible for this permanent disturbance in motor behavior (Tassin et al., 1977).

Conclusion

In summary, several tools are now available to map out the pathways involved in the control of the activity of the ascending DA systems in the brain. Besides classical electrophysiological approaches, the development of anatomical methods based on the use of the anterograde or retrograde axonal flows, or on the immunohistochemical localization of specific synthesizing enzymes of transmitters, will undoubtedly stimulate rapid progress. Even less is known about the interneuronal regulations of the mesocortical and mesolimbic DA systems. However, we are beginning to define the roles of several pathways originating from structures involved in sensorimotor functions in the regulation of DA transmission both in the SN and in the striatum.

The dynamic simultaneous monitoring of changes in DA release from dendrites and terminals of the two nigrostriatal DA pathways offers new possibilities in this field. This approach does present some limitations when compared to the electrophysiological recording of single cells: it only provides integrated responses, occurring in relatively long periods, of a large population of identified neurons. This may explain some of the discrepancy between the data obtained by the two approaches. Nevertheless, it now seems possible to monitor the reactivity of the two DA pathways in pharmacological as well as in physiological states. This should help to clarify the role of these pathways in the organization of sensorimotor behavior.

ACKNOWLEDGMENTS   I would like to thank Drs. A. Nieoullon and A. Chéramy for fruitful discussions and extensive help in the preparation of this review.

REFERENCES

AGHAJANIAN, G. K., and B. S. BUNNEY, 1973. Central dopaminergic neurons: Neurophysiological identification and responses to drugs. In *Frontiers in Catecholamine Research*, E. Usdin and S. Snyder, eds. London: Pergamon Press, pp. 643–648.

AGHAJANIAN, G. K., and B. S. BUNNEY, 1975. Dopaminergic and nondopaminergic neurons of the substantia nigra: Differential responses to putative transmitters. In *Neuropsychopharmacology*, J. R. Boissier, H. Hippius, and P. Pichot, eds. Amsterdam: Excerpta Medica, and New York: American Elsevier, pp. 444–452.

AGID, Y., P. GUYENET, J. GLOWINSKI, J. C. BEAUJOUAN, and F. JAVOY, 1975. Inhibitory influence of the nigrostriatal dopamine system on the striatal cholinergic neurons in the rat. *Brain Res.* 86:480–482.

AGID, Y., F. JAVOY, and J. GLOWINSKI, 1974. Chemical or electrolytic lesion of the substantia nigra: Early effects on neostriatal dopamine metabolism. *Brain Res.* 74:41–49.

ANDEN, N. E., A. CARLSSON, A. DAHLSTRÖM, K. FUXE, N. A. HILLARP, and K. LARSSON, 1964. Demonstration and mapping out of nigro-neostriatal dopamine neurons. *Life Sci.* 3:523–530.

ANDEN, N. E., and G. STOCK, 1973. Inhibitory effect of gammahydroxybutyric acid and gammaaminobutyric acid on the dopamine cells in the substantia nigra. *Naunyn-Schmiedeberg's Arch. Pharmakol.* 279:89–92.

BAK, I. J., W. B. CHOI, R. HASSLER, K. G. USUNOFF, and A. WAGNER, 1975. Fine structural synaptic organization of the corpus striatum and substantia nigra in rat and cat. In *Advances in Neurology*, vol. 9, D. B. Calne, T. N. Chase, and A. Barbeau, eds., New York: Raven Press, pp. 25–41.

BARTHOLINI, G., H. STADLER, M. GADEA-CIRIA, and K. G. LLOYD, 1976. The use of the push-pull cannula to estimate the dynamics of acetylcholine and catecholamines within various brain areas. *Neuropharmacology* 15:515–519.

BERGER, B., J. P. TASSIN, G. BLANC, M. A. MOYNE, and A. M. THIERRY, 1974. Histochemical confirmation for dopaminergic innervation of the rat cerebral cortex after destruction of the noradrenergic ascending pathways. *Brain Res.* 81:332–337.

BESSON, M. J., A. CHÉRAMY, P. FELTZ, and J. GLOWINSKI, 1971. Dopamine: Spontaneous and drug induced release from the caudate nucleus in the cat. *Brain Res.* 32:407–424.

BJÖRKLUND, A., and O. LINDVALL, 1975. Dopamine in dendrites of substantia nigra neurons: Suggestions for a role in dendritic terminals. *Brain Res.* 83:531–537.

BLOOM, F. E., E. COSTA, and G. G. SALMOIRAGHI, 1965. Anesthesia and the responsiveness of individual neurons of the caudate nucleus of the cat to acetylcholine, norepinephrine and dopamine administered by microelectrophoresis. *J. Pharmacol. Exp. Ther.* 150:244–252.

BOCKAERT, J., J. PRÉMONT, J. GLOWINSKI, A. M. THIERRY, and J. P. TASSIN, 1976. Topographical distribution of dopaminergic innervation and of dopaminergic receptors in the rat striatum. II. Distribution and characteristics of dopamine adenylate cyclase. Interaction of D-LSD with dopaminergic receptors. *Brain Res.* 107:303–315.

BUNNEY, B. S., and G. K. AGHAJANIAN, 1976. The precise localization of nigral afferents in the rat as determined by a retrograde tracing technique. *Brain Res.* 117:423–435.

BURT, D. R., I. CREESE, and S. H. SNYDER, 1976. Properties of [³H] haloperidol and [³H] dopamine binding associated with dopamine receptors in calf brain membranes. *Mol. Pharmacol.* 12:800–812.

CARLSSON, A., W. KEHR, M. LINDQVIST, T. MAGNUSSON, and C. ATACK, 1972. Regulation of monoamine metabolism in the central nervous system. *Pharmacol. Rev.* 24:371–384.

CARPENTER, M. B., 1976. Anatomy of the basal ganglia and related nuclei: A review. In *Advances in Neurology*, vol. 14, R. Eldridge and S. Fahn, eds. New York: Raven Press, pp. 7–48.

CHÉRAMY, A., B. BIOULAC, M. J. BESSON, J. D. VINCENT, J. GLOWINSKI, and C. GAUCHY, 1975. Radioenzymatic estimation of catecholamines released from the caudate nucleus in the cat and in the monkey. In *Neuropsychopharmacology*, J. R. Boissier, H. Hippius, and P. Pichot, eds. Amsterdam: Excerpta Medica, and New York: American Elsevier, pp. 493–498.

CHÉRAMY, A., A. NIEOULLON, and J. GLOWINSKI, 1977a. Effects of peripheral and local administration of picrotoxin on the release of newly synthesized ³H-dopamine in the caudate nucleus of the cat. *Naunyn-Schmiedeberg's Arch. Pharmakol.* 297:31–37.

CHÉRAMY, A., A. NIEOULLON, and J. GLOWINSKI, 1977b. Blockade of the picrotoxin-induced in vivo release of dopamine in the cat caudate nucleus by diazepam. *Life Sci.* 20:811–816.

CHÉRAMY, A., A. NIEOULLON, and J. GLOWINSKI, 1978a. In vivo changes in dopamine release in the caudate nucleus and the substantia nigra of the cat induced by nigral application of various drugs including GABA-ergic agonists and antagonists. In *Interactions among Putative Neurotransmitters in the Brain*, S. Garattini, J. F. Pujol, and R. Samanin, eds. New York: Raven Press, pp. 175–190.

CHÉRAMY, A., A. NIEOULLON, and J. GLOWINSKI, 1978b. GABA-ergic processes involved in the control of dopamine release from the terminals and the dendrites of the nigrostriatal dopaminergic neurons in the cat. *Eur. J. Pharmacol.* 48:281–296.

CHÉRAMY, A., A. NIEOULLON, and J. GLOWINSKI, 1978c. Inhibition of dopamine release in the cat caudate nucleus by nigral application of glycine. *Eur. J. Pharmacol.* 47: 141–147.

CHÉRAMY, A., A. NIEOULLON, R. MICHELOT, and J. GLOWINSKI, 1977. Effect of intranigral application of dopamine and substance P on the in vivo release of newly synthesized ³H-dopamine in the ipsilateral caudate nucleus of the cat. *Neurosci. Lett.* 4:105–109.

CHUNG, J. W., R. HASSLER, and A. WAGNER, 1976. Degenerated boutons in the fundus striati (nucleus accumbens septi) after lesion of the parafascicular nucleus in the cat. *Cell Tissue Res.* 172:1–14.

CONNOR, J. D., 1975. Electrophysiology of the nigro-caudate pathway. *Pharmacol. Ther.* 1:357–370.

COYLE, J. T., and S. H. SNYDER, 1969. Antiparkinsonian drugs: Inhibition of dopamine uptake in the corpus striatum as a possible mechanism of action. *Science* 166:899–901.

CREESE, I., D. R. BURT, and S. H. SNYDER, 1977. Dopamine receptor binding enhancement accompanies lesion-induced behavioral supersensitivity. *Science* 177:596–598.

DAHLSTRÖM, A., and K. FUXE, 1964. Existence of monoamine-containing neurons in the central nervous system. I. Demonstration of monoamines in the cell bodies of brain stem neurons. *Acta Physiol. Scand.* 62 (suppl. 232):1–55.

DIVAC, I., F. FONNUM, and J. STORM-MATHISEN, 1977. High affinity uptake of glutamate in terminals of corticostriatal axons. *Nature* 266:377–378.

DRAY, A., T. J. GONYE, and N. R. OAKLEY, 1976. Caudate stimulation and substantia nigra activity in the rat. *J. Physiol.* 259:825–849.

DRAY, A., and D. W. STRAUGHAN, 1976. Synaptic mechanisms in the substantia nigra. *J. Pharm. Pharmacol.* 28:400–405.

FONNUM, F., I. GROFOVA, E. RINVIK, J. STORM-MATHISEN, and F. WALBERG, 1974. Origin and distribution of glutamate decarboxylase in substantia nigra of the cat. *Brain Res.* 71:77–92.

GALE, K. N., and A. GUIDOTTI, 1976. GABA-mediated control of rat neostriatal tyrosine hydroxylase revealed by intranigral muscimol. *Nature* 263:691–693.

GALE, K., A. GUIDOTTI, and E. COSTA, 1977. Dopamine sensitive adenylate cyclase: Location in the substantia nigra. *Nature* 260:258–260.

GEFFEN, L. B., T. M. JESSEL, A. C. CUELLO, and L. L. IVERSEN, 1976. Release of dopamine from dendrites in rat substantia nigra. *Nature* 260:258–260.

GIORGUIEFF, M. F., M. L. KEMEL, J. GLOWINSKI, and M. J. BESSON, 1978. Stimulation of dopamine release by GABA in rat striatal slices. *Brain Res.* 139:115–130.

GIORGUIEFF, M. F., M. L. KEMEL, and J. GLOWINSKI, 1977. Presynaptic effect of L-glutamic acid on dopamine release in rat striatal slices. *Neurosci. Lett.* 6:73–77.

GIORGUIEFF, M. F., M. L. LE FLOC'H, J. GLOWINSKI, and M. J. BESSON, 1977. Involvement of cholinergic presynaptic receptors of nicotinic and muscarinic types in the control of the spontaneous release of dopamine from striatal dopaminergic terminals in the rat. *J. Pharmacol. Exp. Ther.* 200:535–540.

GLOWINSKI, J., 1975. Properties and functions of intraneuronal monoamine compartments in central aminergic neurons. In *Handbook of Psychopharmacology*, vol. 3, L. Iversen, S. Iversen, and S. Snyder, eds. New York: Plenum Press, pp. 139–167.

GREENGARD, P., 1976. Possible role for cyclic nucleotides and phosphorylated membrane proteins in postsynaptic actions of neurotransmitters. *Nature* 260:101–108.

GROVES, P. M., C. J. WILSON, S. J. YOUNG, and G. V. REBEC, 1975. Self-inhibition by dopaminergic neurons: An alternative to the "neuronal feedback loop" hypothesis for the mode of action of certain psychotropic drugs. *Science* 190:522–528.

GUYENET, P., Y. AGID, F. JAVOY, J. C. BEAUJOUAN, J. ROSSIER, and J. GLOWINSKI, 1975. Effect of dopaminergic receptor agonists and antagonists on the activity of the neostriatal cholinergic system. *Brain Res.* 84:227–244.

HASSLER, R., I. J. BAK, K. J. USUNOFF, and W. B. CHOI, 1975. Synaptic organization of the descending and ascending connections between the striatum and the substantia nigra in the cat. In *Neuropsychopharmacology*, J. R. Boissier, H. Hippius, and P. Pichot, eds. Amsterdam: Excerpta Medica, and New York: American Elsevier, pp. 397–411.

HATTORI, T., P. L. MCGEER, H. C. FIBIGER, and E. G. MCGEER, 1973. On the source of GABA-containing terminals in the substantia nigra. Electron microscopic autoradiography and biochemical studies. *Brain Res.* 54:103–114.

HATTORI, T., V. K. SINGH, E. G. MCGEER, and P. L. MCGEER, 1976. Immunohistochemical localization of choline acetyltransferase containing neostriatal neurons and their relationship with dopaminergic synapses. *Brain Res.* 102:164–173.

HÖKFELT, T., K. FUXE, O. JOHANSSON, and A. LJÜNGDAHL, 1974. Pharmaco-histochemical evidence of the existence of dopamine nerve terminals in the limbic cortex. *Eur. J. Pharmacol.* 25:108–112.

HÖKFELT, T., J. O. KELLERTH, G. NILSSON, and B. PERNON, 1975. Substance P: Localization in the central nervous system and in some primary sensorineurons. *Science* 190:889–890.

HONG, J. S., H. Y. T. YANG, G. RACAGNI, and E. COSTA, 1977. Projection of substance P containing neurons from neostriatum to substantia nigra. *Brain Res.* 122:541–544.

HORNYKIEWICZ, O., 1966. Dopamine (3-hydroxytyramine) and brain function. *Pharmacol. Rev.* 18:925–964.

JESSEL, T. M., 1977. Inhibition of substance P release from the isolated rat substantia nigra by GABA. *J. Pharmacol. Chemother.* 59:486p.

KANAZAWA, I., P. C. EMSON, and A. C. CUELLO, 1977. Evidence for the existence of substance P-containing fibresin striato-nigral and pallido-nigral pathways in rat brain. *Brain Res.* 119:447–453.

KELLY, P. H., P. W. SEVIOUR, and S. D. IVERSEN, 1975. Amphetamine and apomorphine responses in the rat following 6-OH-DA lesion of the nucleus accumbens septi and corpus striatum. *Brain Res.* 94:507–522.

KEMP, J. M., and T. P. S. POWELL, 1971. The connections of the striatum and globus pallidus: Synthesis and speculation. *Philos. Trans. R. Soc. Lond.* B262:441–457.

KITAI, S. T., B. M. SUGIMORI, and J. D. KOCSIS, 1976. Excitatory nature of dopamine in the nigrocaudate pathway. *Exp. Brain Res.* 24:351–363.

KORF, J., M. ZIELEMAN, and B. H. C. WESTERINK, 1976. Dopamine release in substantia nigra? *Nature* 260:257–258.

LADINSKY, H., S. CONSOLO, S. BIANCHI, R. SAMANIN, and D. GHEZZI, 1975. Cholinergic-dopaminergic interaction in the striatum: The effect of 6-hydroxydopamine or pimozide treatment on the increased striatal acetylcholine levels induced by apomorphine piribedil and d-amphetamine. *Brain Res.* 84:221–226.

LeMoal, M., D. Galey, and B. Cardo, 1975. Behavioral effects of local injection of 6-hydroxydopamine in the media ventral tegmentum in the rat. Possible role of the mesolimbic dopaminergic system. *Brain Res.* 88:190–194.

Lindvall, O., and A. Björklund, 1974. The organization of the ascending catecholamine neuron systems in the rat brain as revealed by the glyoxylic acid fluorescence method. *Acta Physiol. Scand.* (suppl. 412):1–48.

Lindvall, O., A. Björklund, R. Y. Moore, and U. Stenevi, 1974. Mesencephalic dopamine neurons projecting to neocortex. *Brain Res.* 81:325–331.

Ljungberg, T., and U. Ungerstedt, 1976. Sensory inattention produced by 6-hydroxydopamine induced degeneration of ascending dopamine neurons in the brain. *Exp. Neurol.* 53:585–600.

Loh, H. H., D. A. Brase, S. Sampath-Khanna, J. B. Mar, and E. L. Way, 1976. 3-Endorphin in vitro inhibition of striatal dopamine release. *Nature* 264:567–568.

McGeer, E. G., U. T. Innanen, and P. L. McGeer, 1976. Evidence on the cellular localization of adenylcyclase in the neostriatum. *Brain Res.* 118:356–358.

McGeer, P. L., E. G. McGeer, H. C. Fibiger, and V. Wickson, 1971. Neostriatal choline acetylase and acetylcholinesterase following selective brain lesions. *Brain Res.* 35:308–314.

McLennan, H., 1964. The release of acetylcholine and 3-hydroxytyramine from the caudate nucleus. *J. Physiol.* 174:152–161.

McLennan, H., and D. H. York, 1967. The action of dopamine on neurons of the caudate nucleus. *J. Physiol.* 189:393–402.

Mishra, R. K., E. L. Gardner, R. Katzman, and M. H. Makman, 1974. Enhancement of dopamine-stimulated adenylate cyclase activity in rat caudate after lesions in substantia nigra: Evidence for denervation supersensitivity. *Proc. Natl. Acad. Sci. USA* 71:3883–3887.

Moore, R. Y., R. K. Bhatnagar, and A. Heller, 1971. Anatomical and chemical studies of a nigro-neostriatal projection in the cat. *Brain Res.* 30:119–135.

Murrin, L. C., V. H. Morgenroth, and R. H. Roth, 1976. Dopaminergic neurons: Effects of electrical stimulation on tyrosine hydroxylase. *Mol. Pharmacol.* 12:1070–1081.

Nieoullon, A., A. Chéramy, and J. Glowinski, 1977a. An adaptation of the push-pull cannula method to study the in vivo release of ^{3}H-dopamine synthesized from ^{3}H-tyrosine in the cat caudate nucleus: Effects of various physical and pharmacological treatments. *J. Neurochem.* 28:819–828.

Nieoullon, A., A. Chéramy, and J. Glowinski, 1977b. Release of dopamine in vivo from cat substantia nigra. *Nature* 266:375–377.

Nieoullon, A., A. Chéramy, and J. Glowinski, 1977c. Release of dopamine from terminals and dendrites of the two nigrostriatal dopaminergic pathways in response to unilateral sensory stimuli in the cat. *Nature* 266:375–377.

Nieoullon, A., A. Chéramy, and J. Glowinski, 1977d. Interdependence of the two nigrostriatal dopaminergic systems in the cat. *Science* 198:416–418.

Nieoullon, A., A. Chéramy, and J. Glowinski, 1978a. Release of dopamine evoked under punctate electrical stimulations of the motor and associative visual areas of the cerebral cortex, in both caudate nucleus and in the substantia nigra in the cat. *Brain Res.* 145:69–83.

Nieoullon, A., A. Chéramy, and J. Glowinski, 1978b. Release of dopamine from terminals and dendrites of the two nigrostriatal dopaminergic pathways in response to unilateral cerebellar stimulation in the cat. *Brain Res.* 148:143–152.

Pijnenburg, A. J. J., W. M. M. Hönig, and J. M. Van Rossum, 1975. Inhibition of d-amphetamine induced locomotor activity by injection of haloperidol into the nucleus accumbens of the rat. *Psychopharmacologia (Berl.)*, 41:87–95.

Poirier, L., M. Filion, P. Langelier, and L. Larochelle, 1975. Brain nervous mechanisms involved in the so-called extrapyramidal motor and psychomotor disturbances. *Prog. Neurobiol.* 5:197–244.

Pollard, H., C. Llorens-Cortes, and J. C. Schwartz, 1977. Enkephalin receptors on dopaminergic neurons in rat striatum. *Nature* 268:745–747.

Powell, E. W., and R. B. Leman, 1976. Connections of the nucleus accumbens. *Brain Res.* 105:389–403.

Precht, W., and M. Yoshida, 1971. Blockade of caudate-evoked inhibition of neurons in the substantia nigra by picrotoxin. *Brain Res.* 32:229–233.

Premont, J., A. M. Thierry, J. P. Tassin, J. Glowinski, G. Blanc, and J. Bockaert, 1976. Is the dopamine-sensitive adenylate cyclase in the rat substantia nigra coupled with "autoreceptors"? *FEBS Lett.* 68:99–104.

Pycock, C., and R. Horton, 1976. Evidence for an accumbens-pallidal pathway in the rat and its possible gaba-minergic control. *Brain Res.* 110:629–634.

Racagni, G., D. L. Cheney, G. Zsilla, and E. Costa, 1976. The measurement of acetylcholine turnover rate in brain structures. *Neuropharmacology* 15:723–736.

Reubi, J. C., L. L. Iversen, and T. M. Jessel, 1977. Dopamine selectively increases ^{3}H-GABA release from slices of rat substantia nigra in vitro. *Nature* 268:652–654.

Ribak, C. E., I. E. Vauchn, K. Saito, R. Barber, and E. Roberts, 1976. Immunocytochemical localization of glutamate decarboxylase in rat substantia nigra. *Brain Res.* 116:287–298.

Richardson, T. L., J. J. Miller, and H. McLennan, 1977. Mechanisms of excitation and inhibition in the nigrostriatal system. *Brain Res.* 127:219–234.

Riddell, D., and J. C. Szerb, 1971. The release in vivo of dopamine synthesized from labelled precursors in the caudate nucleus of the cat. *J. Neurochem.* 18:989–1006.

Rinvik, E., 1966. The cortico-nigral projection in the cat. *J. Comp. Neurol.* 126:241–254.

Roth, R. H., L. C. Murrin, and J. R. Walters, 1976. Central dopaminergic neurons: Effects of alterations in impulse flow on the accumulation of dihydroxyphenylacetic acid. *Eur. J. Pharmacol.* 36:163–171.

Samanin, R., A. Quattrone, S. Consolo, H. Ladinsky, and S. Algeri, 1978. Biochemical and pharmacological evidence of the interaction of serotonin with other aminergic systems in the brain. In *Interactions among Putative Neurotransmitters in the Brain*, S. Garattini, J. F. Pujol, and R. Samanin, eds. New York: Raven Press, pp. 383–400.

Schaffner, R., and W. Haefely, 1975. The effects of diazepam and bicuculline on the strio-nigral evoked potential. *Experientia (Basel)* 31:732.

SIMON, H., M. LeMOAL, D. GALEY, and B. CARDO, 1976. Silver impregnation of dopaminergic systems after radiofrequency and 6-OH-DA lesions of the rat ventral tegmentum. *Brain Res.* 115:215–231.

SIMON, J. R., J. F. CONTRERA, and M. J. KUHAR, 1976. Binding of ^{3}H-kainic acid, an analog of L-glutamate, to brain membranes. *J. Neurochem.* 26:141–147.

SNIDER, R. S., A. MAITI, and S. R. SNIDER, 1976. Cerebellar pathways to ventral midbrain and nigra. *Exp. Neurol.* 53:714–728.

SNIDER, S. R., and R. S. SNIDER, 1977. Alterations in forebrain catecholamine metabolism produced by cerebellar lesions in the rat. *J. Neural Transmission* 40:115–128.

SPENCER, H. J., 1976. Antagonism of cortical excitation of striatal neurons by glutamic acid diethyl ester: Evidence for glutamic acid as an excitatory transmitter in the rat striatum. *Brain Res.* 102:91–101.

TASSIN, J. P., A. CHÉRAMY, G. BLANC, A. M. THIERRY, and J. GLOWINSKI, 1976. Topographical distribution of dopaminergic innervation and of dopaminergic receptors in the rat striatum. I. Microestimation of ^{3}H-dopamine uptake and dopamine content in microdiscs. *Brain Res.* 107:291–301.

TASSIN, J. P., L. STINUS, H. SIMON, G. BLANC, A. M. THIERRY, B. CARDO, and J. GLOWINSKI, 1977. Distribution of dopaminergic terminals in rat cerebral cortex. Role of dopaminergic mesocortical system in "ventral tegmental area syndrome." In *Nonstriatal Dopaminergic Neurons*, E. Costa and G. L. Gessa, eds. New York: Raven Press, pp. 21–28.

THIERRY, A. M., G. BLANC, A. SOBEL, L. STINUS, and J. GLOWINSKI, 1973. Dopaminergic terminals in the rat cortex. *Science* 182:499–501.

THIERRY, A. M., J. P. TASSIN, G. BLANC, and J. GLOWINSKI, 1976. Selective activation of the mesocortical dopaminergic system by stress. *Nature* 263:242–244.

UNGERSTEDT, U., 1971a. Striatal dopamine release after amphetamine or nerve degeneration revealed by rotational behavior. *Acta Physiol. Scand.* 82 (suppl. 367):49–68.

UNGERSTEDT, U., 1971b. Postsynaptic supersensitivity after 6-hydroxydopamine induced degeneration of the nigrostriatal dopamine system. *Acta Physiol. Scand.* 82 (suppl. 367):69–93.

VON VOIGTLANDER, P. F., S. J. BOUKMA, and G. A. JOHNSON, 1973. Dopaminergic denervation supersensitivity and dopamine stimulated adenyl cyclase activity. *Neuropharmacology* 12:1081–1086.

WESTFALL, T. C., 1974. Effect of nicotine and other drugs on the release of ^{3}H-norepinephrine and ^{3}H-dopamine from rat brain slices. *Neuropharmacology* 13:693–700.

WESTFALL, T. C., M. J. BESSON, M. F. GIORGUIEFF, and J. GLOWINSKI, 1976. The role of presynaptic receptors in the release and synthesis of ^{3}H-dopamine by slices of rat striatum. *Naunyn-Schmiedeberg's Arch. Pharmakol.* 292:279–287.

ZIVKOVIC, B., and A. GUIDOTTI, 1974. Changes of the kinetic constant of striatal tyrosine hydroxylase elicited by neuroleptics that impair the function of dopamine receptors. *Brain Res.* 79:505–509.

66 Neurotransmitter Interactions in the Substantia Nigra: A Model for Local Circuit Chemical Interactions

LESLIE L. IVERSEN

ABSTRACT This chapter briefly reviews the evidence for a dendritic release of dopamine from neurons in the mammalian substantia nigra and discusses the complex transmitter interactions that are now known to exist in the neuropil of this brain region. The substantia nigra offers a useful model for describing the chemical interactions that are possible within a small but well-defined area of CNS.

Anatomy of substantia nigra

The substantia nigra (s. nigra) is an important nucleus in the basal ganglia, associated with extrapyramidal motor function (Divac, 1977). Its name reflects its characteristic black pigmentation, which is due to the accumulation of neuromelanin in the dopaminergic neurons. The nucleus was first described by Vicq d'Azyr (1786), and its histological characteristics were defined by Ramón y Cajal (1904; see Figure 1). An excellent review of modern neuroanatomical knowledge of the neuronal connections of this area and of its relation to the extrapyramidal system has recently been published (Nieuwenhuys, 1977).

Histologically the s. nigra is divided into a narrow band of large, mainly pigmented neurons—the zona compacta—and a broader band of neuropil and small neurons—the zona reticulata. The dendrites of the large z. compacta neurons ramify throughout all parts of the nucleus. The s. nigra receives major and topographically organized inputs from neurons located in the striatum and globus pallidus and also from neurons in the subthalamic nucleus. The axons of z. compacta cells project to the striatum, and pro-

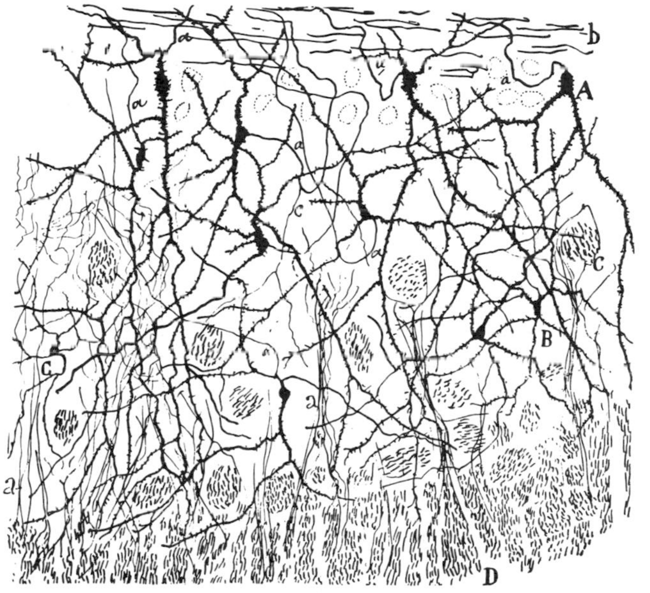

FIGURE 1 Ramón y Cajal's (1904) original drawing of Golgi staining from a coronal section of a cat substantia nigra. Among the features labeled are: A, superior cells (located in zona compacta of the modern terminology); B, inferior cells (neurons of the reticulata); C, short-axon corpuscle (interneuron); a, terminal branches from the crus cerebri.

jections from the z. reticulata are directed to various thalamic nuclei, the superior colliculus, and the reticular formation.

Neurotransmitters in substantia nigra

As in other regions of CNS, many different transmitters are involved in synaptic transmission within the s. nigra. The s. nigra is unusual, however, in that

LESLIE L. IVERSEN MRC Neurochemical Pharmacology Unit, Department of Pharmacology, Medical School, Cambridge, England

the identity of the transmitters used by many of the afferent and efferent pathways is known. The subject has been well reviewed by Dray and Straughan (1976).

The s. nigra has become a focus of research interest in CNS neuropharmacology because it represents one of the major catecholamine-containing nuclei in CNS. The majority of the pigmented "principal" neurons in the z. compacta are dopaminergic and give rise to an important projection of dopamine-containing nerve terminals in the caudate nucleus, putamen, and globus pallidus (Figure 2; Ungerstedt, 1971).

The s. nigra is also unique in containing the highest local concentrations in CNS of two other neurotrans-

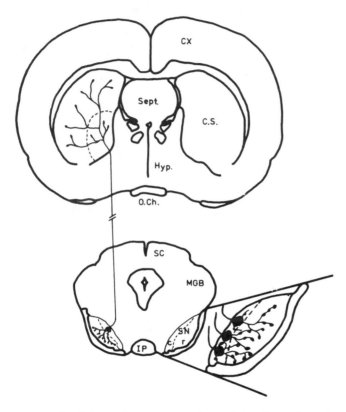

FIGURE 2 Schematic representation of the dopaminergic nigrostriatal pathway. The cell bodies of dopaminergic neurons are largely confined to the pars compacta of substantia nigra with a well-defined anatomical segregation of their axonal and dendritic processes. Within substantia nigra, the dendrites of these neurons radiate ventrolaterally into the pars reticulata, whereas the axons project rostromedially, ending mainly in the corpus striatum. Some dendrites are also present in the pars compacta. *Abbreviations*: CX, cerebral cortex; C.S., corpus striatum; Sept., septus pellucidum; Hyp., hypothalamus; O.Ch., optic chiasm; SC, superior colliculi; MGB, medial geniculate body; IP, nucleus interpeduncularis; SN, substantia nigra; c, pars compacta of the substantia nigra; r, pars reticulata of the substantia nigra. (From Geffen et al., 1976.)

mitters: the peptide substance P and the amino acid GABA. Substance P is largely contained within axon terminals in the z. reticulata and z. compacta that originate from neurons in the striatum and globus pallidus (Cuello et al., 1977). Similarly, the high GABA content of s. nigra is due to the presence of numerous GABA-containing nerve terminals, which also originate from a descending striatonigral pathway (Hattori et al., 1973; Fonnum et al., 1974). The actions of substance P within the s. nigra are predominantly excitatory, and those of GABA inhibitory (Dray and Straughan, 1976); thus they may represent the major excitatory and inhibitory inputs to nigral neurons.

There is also evidence for a 5-HT-containing population of nerve terminals in s. nigra, originating from neurons in the raphe nuclei (Kuhar, Aghajanian, and Rother, 1972; Dray et al., 1976). The s. nigra contains relatively low activity of the cholinergic marker enzyme, choline acetyltransferase (Fonnum et al., 1974), and only small amounts of norepinephrine. The identity of the transmitters contained within the neurons of the z. reticulata, which give rise to various efferent pathways, is unknown, although the possibility that glycine might be involved is a nigral transmitter has been considered (Dray and Straughan, 1976).

Dopamine release from substantia nigra dendrites

Interest in the possibility that dopamine might be released locally within the s. nigra from the dendrites of the dopaminergic neurons in the z. compacta was stimulated by a key paper published by Björklund and Lindvall (1975). They applied the recently developed glyoxylic acid histofluorescence method to s. nigra and showed that dopamine was present not only in the cell bodies of the dopaminergic neurons in the z. compacta, but also throughout the extensive dendritic network arising from these cells, with short-branched dendrites within the z. compacta and long and extensively branched processes extending throughout the z. reticulata (Figure 3). The dendritic dopamine histofluorescence reaction disappeared following treatment with reserpine in rats, but it could be reestablished by incubation of nigral tissue in vitro with dopamine.

Previous electron-microscopic evidence had also shown that labeled catecholamines could be selectively accumulated by the dendrites of z. compacta neurons when the catecholamines were injected into the s. nigra in vivo (Parizek, Hassler, and Bak, 1971;

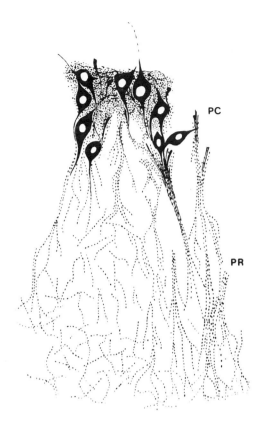

FIGURE 3   Diagrammatic representation of distribution of dopamine-induced glyoxylic acid histofluorescence in cell bodies and dendrites of neurons in zona compacta (PC) of rat s. nigra. Dopamine-containing varicosities in the dendritic field in PC and zona reticulata (PR) appear as dotlike structures. (From Björklund and Lindvall, 1975.)

Sotelo, 1971). Furthermore, immunocytochemical staining methods have shown that key biosynthetic enzymes for the synthesis of dopamine and other monoamine transmitters are present in the dendritic processes of these and other monoamine-containing neurons in CNS (Hökfelt, Fuxe, and Goldstein, 1973; Pickel, Joh, and Reis, 1975). Thus the dendrites of dopaminergic neurons in s. nigra contain dopamine and the enzymes needed for its synthesis, and like the axon terminals of these and other catecholamine neurons, they possess a specialized transport system for the uptake of dopamine from the extracellular space.

Because of this, and because the anatomical organization of the nigrostriatal dopaminergic neurons permits a simple physical separation of the cell bodies and dendrites from their axon terminals in the striatum, we and others have attempted to demonstrate that dopamine can be released locally within the s. nigra (Geffen et al., 1976). In most of our experiments we have made use of the specialized uptake properties of the dopamine-containing dendrites in s. nigra to prelabel these with [³H]-dopamine of high specific activity.

Using a microdissection technique developed by Zigmond and Ben-Ari (1976) in our laboratory, s. nigra tissue was carefully isolated from serial sections of fresh chilled rat brain (total wet weight from both sides of one brain about 5–6 mg), and incubated in vitro with [³H]-dopamine (1 μM). The labeled tissue fragments were then superfused with Krebs bicarbonate solution at 37°C, and the efflux of [³H]-dopamine was monitored in serial fractions collected at 2 min intervals. After a rapid initial efflux, [³H]-dopamine release (expressed as the fraction of total tissue content released per minute) became relatively stable, at approximately 0.5% per min, after 15–20 min of superfusion. At this time, brief exposure to a medium containing an elevated potassium chloride concentration (23.5 mM) evoked a large and consistent increase in [³H]-dopamine efflux, which was similar in magnitude to or somewhat larger than that observed in parallel experiments using fragments of tissue of similar size dissected from the striatum (Figure 4). In both striatal and nigral tissue, the potassium-evoked release of [³H]-dopamine was almost completely prevented if calcium ions were removed from the superfusing medium, and the potassium-evoked release was also markedly inhibited by elevating the magnesium ion concentration of the medium (Figure 4). The use of a high external potassium concentration to evoke release of putative transmitters from brain tissue in vitro through a calcium-dependent process is widely accepted as a useful model system for studying transmitter release from CNS neurons.

In further experiments, we were able to show that [³H]-dopamine uptake and potassium-evoked release occurred in both the z. compacta and the z. reticulata of rat s. nigra when these were separately dissected and incubated in vitro (Cuello and Iversen, 1977); this was expected because of the wide distribution of dopamine-containing dendrites in both of these regions. The fact that [³H]-dopamine uptake and release occurred in both regions of the tissue, however, ruled out the possibility that these phenomena reflected mainly uptake and release of the labeled catecholamine by the perikarya of the dopaminergic neurons, since these are almost entirely restricted to the z. compacta. In other experiments, using a sensitive radiochemical enzymatic assay method for dopamine, we were able to detect an increase in the rate of efflux of endogenous dopamine from s. nigra tissue exposed to high potassium concentration in vitro, con-

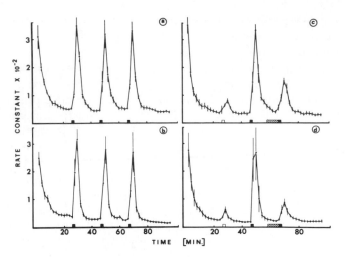

FIGURE 4   Release of [³H]-DA from superfused slices of rat substantia nigra (a, c) and corpus striatum (b, d). Tissues were superfused at a rate of 30 ml/hr with normal Krebs bicarbonate solution. At 20 min intervals, pulses of high potassium (23.5 mM) were given for 2 min. In a and b, potassium pulses were given during perfusion with normal Krebs (black bars); in c and d, superfusion throughout the experiment was with calcium-free Krebs. The first potassium pulse was applied in the continued absence of calcium (open bar). For the duration of the second (black bar) and third (black bar) potassium pulses, calcium was restored to normal. Four fractions before, and during the third potassium pulse, the magnesium concentration was raised to 24 mM (hatched bar); after the third potassium pulse, the magnesium concentration was restored to normal. Efflux of radioactivity was expressed as the fractional rate constant (d.p.m. released per min in superfusate/d.p.m. in tissue stores at time of collection). Each value is mean ± S.E.M. of four experiments. (From Geffen et al., 1976.)

firming the results obtained by the [³H]-dopamine prelabeling technique (Cuello and Iversen, 1977).

Support for the conclusion that dopamine release can occur from dendritic sites within s. nigra has come from other studies. Korf, Zieleman, and Westerink (1976) observed an increase in the concentration of the dopamine metabolite 3,4-dihydroxyphenylacetic acid (DOPAC) in rat s. nigra when the nigrostriatal pathway was antidromically stimulated through implanted electrodes in vivo, and they took this as evidence for a local release of dopamine within the s. nigra. Nieoullon, Chéramy, and Glowinski (1977a) also obtained direct evidence for a release of dopamine from s. nigra in vivo. They implanted a push-pull cannula into cat s. nigra and were able to superfuse the tissue locally with [³H]-tyrosine. The release of [³H]-dopamine formed within the s. nigra from the labeled precursor was monitored in the cannula effluent, and [³H]-dopamine efflux was

found to be markedly increased by elevated potassium concentration in the perfusing fluid or by addition of the drugs benztropine or d-amphetamine. They obtained the first indication that dopamine release from s. nigra may differ from that from axon terminals in striatum, since they found that the evoked release of [³H]-dopamine from cat s. nigra, unlike that from striatum, could not be blocked by addition of low concentrations of tetrodotoxin to the perfusing medium. In vitro experiments, using s. nigra tissue prelabeled in vitro with [³H]-dopamine, have also confirmed that the drug d-amphetamine, which displaces dopamine from nerve terminal stores, can cause a release of dopamine from dendrites in the s. nigra (Paden, Wilson, and Groves, 1976).

There is thus good evidence to support the hypothesis that dopamine can be released from its unconventional storage sites in dendrites within the s. nigra. The release process is similar in its dependence on external calcium and magnesium ions to the stimulus-secretion coupling process involved in the release of transmitters from nerve terminals or in other secretory processes. More detailed investigation, however, may reveal subtle differences between transmitter release from dendrites versus axon terminals.

One puzzling feature of the dendritic release mechanism in the s. nigra concerns the nature of the storage compartment from which endogenous or [³H]-dopamine is released. In electron-microscopic studies (Cuello and Iversen, 1977; and A. Cuello, unpublished results), we have been unable to identify any aggregations of synaptic vesicles within the dopamine-containing dendrites in rat s. nigra; this has also been the conclusion reached by others (Sotelo, 1971). Electron-microscopic studies of [³H]-dopamine localization in rat s. nigra and EM cytochemical studies following loading with the cytochemically reactive analog 5-hydroxydopamine suggest that the amine is stored mainly in cisterns of smooth endoplasmic reticulum, as suggested by Tranzer (1972) for amine storage in adrenergic axons.

A further and important conclusion from our electron-microscopic studies, and those of others, is that there is no evidence for the existence of morphologically specialized "dendritic synapses" within the neuropil of the s. nigra. Thus there is no morphological indication that dopamine is normally released within the s. nigra, nor is it clear which components within the s. nigra may be influenced by the dendritically released catecholamine.

Dopamine receptors in substantia nigra

There is considerable evidence that dopamine can influence neuronal activity in the s. nigra. Aghajanian and Bunney (1973, 1977) have carried out extensive neurophysiological studies of the effects of dopamine and dopamine-mimetic drugs, such as apomorphine, on the firing of single nigral cells. They find that direct microiontophoretic application of such drugs consistently inhibits the firing of the dopaminergic cells in the z. compacta and that this effect is blocked by various neuroleptic drugs, such as trifluoperazine; they have argued that this reflects the existence of inhibitory "autoreceptors" on the soma of these neurons.

Groves et al. (1975), in an important paper, also reported the inhibitory effects of microinfused dopamine on the firing of nigral neurons and the opposite effects elicited by infusion of neuroleptic drugs. They proposed that dopamine released within the s. nigra might act in a local circuit feedback loop. They attempted to explain the inhibitory effects of amphetamine on the firing of nigral neurons, and the opposite effect of neuroleptic drugs, in terms of the direct local actions of such drugs on this intranigral regulatory system, but this view has been challenged by Bunney and Aghajanian (1976).

Recent neurochemical evidence also suggests that dopamine receptors exist within the s. nigra, although these studies do not appear to support the localization of such receptors on the nigral dopaminergic neurons, as proposed by Aghajanian and Bunney (1973, 1977). Several laboratories independently discovered that a dopamine-stimulated adenylate cyclase could be detected in cell-free homogenates of rat s. nigra (Phillipson and Horn, 1976; Kebabian and Saavedra, 1976; Spano et al., 1976; Gale, Guidotti, and Costa, 1977). This biochemical system has been shown to occur in other dopamine-containing regions of CNS, and its pharmacological specificity for agonists and antagonists suggests that it reflects a CNS dopamine receptor (Iversen, 1975). However, this particular dopamine receptor (there may be more than one variety) does not correspond in cellular location to the proposed "autoreceptors" in the s. nigra.

The dopaminergic neurons in s. nigra can be largely destroyed by microinjection of the neurotoxin 6-hydroxydopamine in or near the s. nigra (Hökfelt and Ungerstedt, 1973). After such experimental lesions, however, the dopamine-stimulated adenylate cyclase persists unchanged in s. nigra homogenates, whereas lesions that interrupt and lead to degeneration of the striatonigral substance P and GABA-containing pathways lead to a virtually complete loss of the dopamine-stimulated adenylate cyclase from rat s. nigra (Premont et al., 1976; Gale, Guidotti, and Costa, 1977; Phillipson et al., 1977). So far it has proved impossible to cause selective experimental destruction of the GABA-containing or substance P striatonigral afferents by lesions, but these results strongly suggest that the dopamine-stimulated adenylate cyclase may be located presynaptically on one of these afferent terminals within the s. nigra.

With this in mind, we have recently tested the effects of dopamine on the release of GABA and substance P from nerve terminals in rat s. nigra, reasoning that if such terminals possess presynaptic dopamine receptors, it should be possible to demonstrate some effect of dopamine on the release of one or both transmitters. The results (Reubi, Iversen, and Jessell, 1977) showed that dopamine at a concentration of 50 μM had no effect on the spontaneous or potassium-evoked release of substance P from rat s. nigra tissue superfused in vitro, whereas dopamine at concentrations as low as 5 μM had a clear effect in stimulating the efflux of [^{3}H]-GABA from GABA-containing nerve terminals in s. nigra.

The stimulatory effect of dopamine on [^{3}H]-GABA release was dependent on the presence of calcium ions in the perfusing medium, and it could be mimicked by the dopamine-like drug 6,7-dihydroxy, 2-aminotetralin (ADTN) and blocked by the dopamine antagonists haloperidol and fluphenazine. It was, therefore, tentatively suggested that at least one target for locally released dopamine within the s. nigra might be to act on presynaptic receptors on GABA-containing terminals to promote GABA release. It is even conceivable that the inhibitory effects of locally applied dopamine on the firing of z. compacta cells observed in neurophysiological experiments might represent an indirect action, mediated through a release of the inhibitory substance GABA rather than by a direct effect on "autoreceptors" on the surface of the dopamine neurons themselves.

Further evidence for the existence of a cAMP-mediated presynaptic receptor mechanism in the s. nigra was provided by other recent studies from our laboratory. Minneman and Cuello (1978) found that cyclic nucleotide phosphodiesterase could be identified by an electron-microscopic cytochemical reaction within some nerve terminals in rat s. nigra. Parallel biochemical experiments showed that nigral phosphodiestrase activity was markedly reduced following lesions that interrupted the striatonigral projections, including that containing GABA.

Other transmitter interactions in substantia nigra

Although we have been unable to detect other effects of dopamine within the s. nigra, some other presynaptic local transmitter interactions seem to exist in this brain area. For example, GABA inhibits the potassium-evoked release of substance P from rat s. nigra (Jessell, 1977), and this effect can be mimicked by the GABA-like compound muscimol and antagonized by the GABA-blocking drugs picrotoxin and bicuculline.

Although GABA exerts direct inhibitory effects on the firing of cells in the z. compacta, there have been other reports which suggest that GABA also has paradoxical excitatory effects on the firing of the nigral dopaminergic neurons. The focal injection of ethanolamine-O-sulphate (EOS), an irreversible inhibitor of GABA-transaminase, into rat s. nigra resulted in behavioral and neurochemical changes suggestive of an increase in impulse traffic in the nigrostriatal dopaminergic neurons on the injected side (Dray, Oakley, and Simmonds, 1975). Furthermore, bilateral injections of EOS into rat s. nigra result in marked behavioral activation, including stereotyped behavior patterns, characteristic of activation rather than inhibition of nigrostriatal dopaminergic neurons (Koob, Del Fiacco, and Iversen, 1978). Chéramy, Nieoullon, and Glowinski (1977) also found complex effects following local perfusion of cat s. nigra with GABA-containing solutions. They observed an increase in the rate of release of [³H]-dopamine from ipsilateral striatum, suggesting activation of the nigrostriatal neurons.

It is possible that a projection of GABA-containing fibers to z. compacta cells mediates the direct inhibitory actions of GABA (Hattori, Fibiger, and McGeer, 1975), whereas GABA-containing fibers projecting to the z. reticulata might mediate the apparent excitatory effects, perhaps through an effect on local circuit inhibitory interneurons (Chéramy, Nieoullon, and Glowinski, 1977).

Functional implications

Studies of local transmitter interactions within the s. nigra are still in a very early stage of exploration. Furthermore, the exact function of this brain region in the overall control of extrapyramidal motor reg-

ulation is still unclear (Divac, 1977). It is thus impossible to construct even a preliminary model to explain the integrated working of the complex local chemical interactions that can occur in this nucleus. However, some useful information is beginning to emerge and there are some important implications for understanding similar phenomena in other regions of CNS.

In an important recent study, Nieoullon, Chéramy, and Glowinski (1977b) examined the effects of physiological sensory stimuli on the release of dopamine from the terminals and dendrites of nigrostriatal neurons in the intact cat brain. They achieved this remarkable tour de force by implanting four push-pull cannulas into the s. nigra and striatum on each side of the cat brain. Each cannula was perfused with a solution containing [³H]-tyrosine, and the release of newly synthesized [³H]-dopamine was continuously monitored. Electrical stimuli applied to a forepaw, or visual stimuli to one eye, caused a marked increase in the rate of [³H]-dopamine efflux from the contralateral s. nigra; at the same time there was a significant decrease in [³H]-dopamine release from the striatum on that side. On the side ipsilateral to the sensory stimuli, there were changes in the opposite direction.

The most important conclusion from these experiments is that changes in the rate of release of dopamine from the axon terminals and the dendrites of the same neurons in the s. nigra can occur in opposite directions; indeed the rate of firing of the dopamine neurons in the s. nigra, and hence the rate of release of dopamine from their axon terminals in striatum, seems to be inversely related to the rate of dendritic release of dopamine from these neurons. Furthermore, this complex interplay can readily be triggered by sensory information in different modalities.

The release of transmitter from the dendrites of neurons may be a widespread phenomenon in the CNS. It is notable that in the s. nigra this phenomenon appears not to involve any detectable morphologically specialized "dendritic synapses" such as have been described in other brain areas (Shepherd, 1974). This suggests that the release of transmitters from dendrites may occur in many areas of CNS even in the absence of morphological specializations. Similarly, interactions between neurotransmitters mediated by presynaptic receptors on nerve terminals, and leading to modulation of transmitter release, can occur without morphologically specialized synapses. The possibilities for local circuit chemical interactions is neuropil are, thus, perhaps even richer than might hitherto have been supposed.

REFERENCES

AGHAJANIAN, G. K., and B. S. BUNNEY, 1973. Central dopaminergic neurons: neurophysiological identification and responses to drugs. In *Frontiers in Catecholamine Research*, S. H. Snyder and E. Usdin, eds. New York: Pergamon, p. 643.

AGHAJANIAN, G. K., and B. S. BUNNEY, 1977. Dopamine "autoreceptors": Pharmacological characterization by microiontophoretic single cell recording studies. *Naunyn-Schmiedebergs Arch. Pharmakol.* 297:1–7.

BJÖRKLUND, A., and O. LINDVALL, 1975. Dopamine in dendrites of substantia nigra neurons: Suggestions for a role in dendritic terminals. *Brain Res.* 83:531–537.

BUNNEY, B. S., and G. K. AGHAJANIAN, 1976. d-Amphetamine-induced inhibition of central dopaminergic neurons: Mediation by a striato-nigral feedback pathway. *Science* 192:391–393.

CHÉRAMY, A., A. NIEOULLON, and J. GLOWINSKI, 1977. In vivo changes in dopamine release in the caudate nucleus and the substantia nigra of the cat induced by nigral application of various drugs including Gaba-ergic agonists and antagonists. In *Interactions Among Putative Transmitters in the Brain*, S. Garattini, J. F. Pujol, and R. Samanin, eds. New York: Raven Press.

CUELLO, A. C., P. EMSON, M. DEL FIACCO, J. GALE, L. L. IVERSEN, T. M. JESSELL, I. KANAZAWA, G. PAXINOS, and M. QUIK, 1977. Distribution and release of substance P in the central nervous system. In *Centrally Acting Peptides*, J. Hughes, ed. London: Macmillan.

CUELLO, A. C., and L. L. IVERSEN, 1977. Interactions of dopamine with other neurotransmitters in the rat substantia nigra: A possible role of dendritic dopamine. In *Interactions Among Putative Transmitters in the Brain*, S. Garattini, J. F. Pujol, and R. Samanin, eds. New York: Raven Press.

DIVAC, I., 1977. Does the neostriatum operate as a functional entity? In *Psychobiology of the Striatum*, A. R. Cools, A. H. M. Lohman, and J. H. L. van den Bercken, eds. Amsterdam: North-Holland, pp. 21–30.

DRAY, A., T. J. GONYE, N. R. OAKLEY, and T. TANNER, 1976. Evidence for the existence of a raphe projection to the substantia nigra in rat. *Brain Res.* 113:45–57.

DRAY, A., N. R. OAKLEY, and M. A. SIMMONDS, 1975. Rotational behaviour following inhibition of GABA metabolism unilaterally in the rat substantia nigra. *J. Pharm. Pharmacol.* 27:627–629.

DRAY, A., and D. W. STRAUGHAN, 1976. Synaptic mechanisms in the substantia nigra. *J. Pharm. Pharmacol.* 28:400–405.

FONNUM, F., I. GROFOVA, E. RINVIK, J. STORM-MATHISEN, and F. WALBERG, 1974. Origin and distribution of glutamate decarboxylase in substantia nigra of the cat. *Brain Res.* 71:77–92.

GALE, K., A. GUIDOTTI, and E. COSTA, 1977. Dopamine-sensitive adenylate cyclase: Location in substantia nigra. *Science* 195:503–505.

GEFFEN, L. B., T. M. JESSELL, A. C. CUELLO, and L. L. IVERSEN, 1976. Release of dopamine from dendrites in rat substantia nigra. *Nature* 260:258–260.

GROVES, P. M., C. J. WILSON, S. J. YOUNG, and G. V. REBEC, 1975. Self-inhibition by dopaminergic neurons. *Science* 190:522–529.

HATTORI, T., H. C. FIBIGER, and P. L. MCGEER, 1975. Demonstration of a pallido-nigral projection innervating dopamine neurons. *J. Comp. Neurol.* 162:487–504.

HATTORI, T., P. L. MCGEER, H. C. FIBIGER, and E. G. MCGEER, 1973. On the source of GABA containing terminals in the substantia nigra: Electron microscopic autoradiographic and biochemical studies. *Brain Res.* 54:103–114.

HÖKFELT, T., K. FUXE, and M. GOLDSTEIN, 1973. Immunohistochemical studies on monoamine-containing cell systems. *Brain Res.* 62:461–477.

HÖKFELT, T., and U. UNGERSTEDT, 1973. Specificity of 6-hydroxydopamine induced degeneration of central monoamine neurones: An electron and fluorescence microscopic study with special reference to intracerebral injection on the nigro-striatal dopamine system. *Brain Res.* 60:269–297.

IVERSEN, L. L., 1975. Dopamine receptors in the brain. *Science* 188:1084–1089.

JESSELL, T. M., 1977. Inhibition of substance P release from the isolated rat substantia nigra by GABA. *Br. J. Pharmacol.* 59:486P.

KEBABIAN, J. W., and J. M. SAAVEDRA, 1976. Dopamine-sensitive adenylate cyclase occurs in a region of substantia nigra containing dopaminergic dendrites. *Science* 193:683–685.

KOOB, G. F., M. DEL FIACCO, and S. D. IVERSEN, 1978. Spontaneous and amphetamine induced behaviour after bilateral injection of ethanolamine-O-sulphate into the substantia nigra. *Brain Res.* 146:313–323.

KORF, J., M. ZIELEMAN, and B. H. G. WESTFRINK, 1976. Dopamine release in substantia nigra? *Nature* 260:257–258.

KUHAR, M. J., G. K. AGHAJANIAN, and R. H. ROTHER, 1972. Trytophan hydroxylase activity and synaptosomal uptake of serotonin in discrete brain regions after midbrain raphe lesions: Correlations with serotonin levels and histochemical fluorescence. *Brain. Res.* 44:165–181.

MINNEMAN, K., and A. C. CUELLO, 1978. Cyclic nucleotide phosphodiesterase in nerve terminals of rat substantia nigra: Association with presynaptic receptors. *J. Neurochem.* (in press).

NIEOULLON, A., A. CHÉRAMY, and J. GLOWINSKI, 1977a. Release of dopamine from substantia nigra in vivo. *Nature* 266:375–377.

NIEOULLON, A., A. CHÉRAMY, and J. GLOWINSKI, 1977b. Release of dopamine from terminals and dendrites of the two nigrostriatal dopaminergic pathways in response to unilateral sensory stimuli in the cat. *Nature* 269:340–342.

NIEUWENHUYS, R., 1977. Aspects of the morphology of the striatum. In *Psychobiology of the Striatum*, A. R. Cools, A. H. M. Lohman, and J. H. L. van den Bercken, eds. Amsterdam: North-Holland, pp. 1–19.

PADEN, C., C. J. WILSON, and P. M. GROVES, 1976. Amphetamine-induced release of dopamine from the substantia nigra *in vitro*, *Life Sci.* 19:1499–1506.

PARIZEK, J., R. HASSLER, and I. J. BAK, 1971. Light and electron microscopic autoradiography of substantia nigra of rat after intraventricular administration of tritium labelled norepinephrine, dopamine, serotonin and precursors. *Z. Zellforsch. Mikrosk. Anat.* 115:137–158.

PHILLIPSON, O. T., P. C. EMSON, A. S. HORN, and T. M. JESSELL, 1977. Evidence concerning the anatomical localization of the dopamine stimulated adenylate cyclase in the substantia nigra. *Brain Res.* 136:45–58.

PHILLIPSON, O. T., and A. S. HORN, 1976. Substantia nigra of the rat contains a dopamine sensitive adenylate cyclase. *Nature* 261:418–420.

PICKEL, V., T. H. JOH, and D. REIS, 1975. Immunohistochemical localization of tyrosine hydroxylase in brain by light and electron microscopy. *Brain Res.* 85:295–309.

PREMONT, J., A. M. THIERRY, J. P. TASSIN, J. GLOWINSKI, G. BLANC, and J. BOCKAERT, 1976. Is the dopamine sensitive adenylate cyclase in the rat substantia nigra coupled with "autoreceptors"? *FEBS Lett.* 68:99–104.

RAMÓN Y CAJAL, S., 1904. *Textura del sistema nerviose del hombre y los vertebrados,* vol. 2. Madrid: Imprenta y Libreria de Nicolas Moya, pp. 553–556.

REUBI, J.-C., L. L. IVERSEN, and T. M. JESSELL, 1977. Dopamine selectively increases ³H-GABA release from slices of rat substantia nigra *in vitro. Nature* (in press).

SHEPHERD, G. M., 1974. *The Synaptic Organization of the Brain,* New York: Oxford Univ. Press.

SOTELO, C., 1971. The fine structural localization of norepinephrine-³H in the substantia nigra and area postrema of the rat. An autoradiographic study. *J. Ultrastruct. Res.* 36:824–841.

SPANO, P. F., G. DiCHIARA, G. C. TONON, and M. TRABUCCHI, 1976. A dopamine-stimulated adenylate cyclase in rat substantia nigra. *J. Neurochem.* 27:1565–1568.

TRANZER, J. P., 1972. A new amine storing compartment in adrenergic axons. *Nature [New Biol.]* 237:57–59.

UNGERSTEDT, U., 1971. Stereotaxic mapping of the monoamine pathways in the rat brain. *Acta Physiol. Scand.* 82 (suppl. 367):49–68.

VICQ D'AZYR, F., 1786. *Traité d'anatomie et de physiologie.* Paris, pp. 72–81.

ZIGMOND, R., and Y. BEN-ARI, 1976. A simple method for serial sectioning of fresh brain and the removal of identifiable nuclei from stained sections for biochemical analysis. *J. Neurochem.* 26:1285–1287.

67 Central-Core Control of Visual-Cortex Functions

WOLF SINGER

ABSTRACT Much work has been devoted to the analysis of local circuits in the visual cortex and to the description of functional properties of cortical units that result from the intracortical processing of specific sensory activity. Comparatively little, however, is known about the function of nonretinal pathways that ascend to the visual cortex. The purpose of this paper is to emphasize the important role these nonspecific projection systems might play in controlling the functional state of the visual cortex. Based on recent current-source and single-unit analysis, the flow of retinal activity through cortex will be briefly reviewed. Cortical excitability is markedly dependent on ascending reticular control. Several observations, especially those based on measurements of changes in extracellular potassium concentration, suggest that the connectivity of these nonspecific afferents differs from that of the specific input. Evidence from monocularly deprived cats characterizes nonspecific afferents as a deprivation-resistant input from the retina to cortex via subcortical stages other than the LGN. This parallel input alters the functional state of the cortex not only as a function of global changes in the animals' state of alertness but also in respect to more specific requirements of sensory processing.

Changes in synaptic efficiency during early postnatal development are also not solely dependent on local interaction between specific afferents and cortical target cells. These data lead me to postulate extrastriatal projection systems that gate changes in local circuits during the period of developmental plasticity.

The problem

The vertebrate brain is commonly subdivided into specific sensory and motor systems on one side and nonspecific modulatory systems on the other. This conceptual dichotomy seems to be well supported by structural and functional differences between specific and nonspecific systems. We have become impressed by the high degree of order and selectivity that governs the connectivity between specific afferents from the sense organs and the intrinsic circuits of thalamic and cortical processing areas. But we have also learned that this great precision in the specific sen-

W. SINGER Max Planck Institute for Psychiatry, Kraepelinstrasse 2, D-8000 Munich 40, Federal Republic of Germany

sory and motor circuits is in surprising contrast to the organization of nonspecific control systems, which ascend from the brain stem and diencephalon. Through extensive axonal branching, the latter seem capable of influencing many different structures in the brain simultaneously (Fuxe, 1965; Shute and Lewis, 1967; Lindvall and Björklund, 1974).

The terminals of the modulatory systems are apparently not connected to particular target cells as specifically as in classical sensory or motor pathways. On occasion, they seem to lack specialized synaptic contacts altogether and simply end in profuse varicosities that lie in intercellular space. Consequently they can exert only a rather global control of nervous functions. These striking differences in the organization of the two systems raise an intriguing question: How can such fundamentally different systems cooperate, and what could it mean for our models of rigidly wired hardware in sensory or motor systems if modulatory systems interfere in a global way with the thresholds of the elements therein.

We shall have to ask whether such modulatory influences can be accommodated within the framework of our current concepts of sensorimotor processes, or whether we must develop new ideas about the operations of local circuitry before we can assign a plausible functional role to the nonspecific modulatory systems. Because of personal bias, I shall approach these questions from the relatively safe ground of the rather thoroughly investigated visual system of mammals.

The processing of specific sensory activity in the visual system

Both the visual way station in the thalamus—the lateral geniculate nucleus (LGN)—and the visual cortex are commonly considered as neuronal nets with rather stationary properties, acting as passive filters for sensory activity. On their way through this cascade of serially aligned filters, retinal signals are supposed to be reshaped, with their redundancy reduced and particular features accentuated while others are suppressed. At the level of the LGN, the basic retinal properties of concentric receptive fields are maintained. As indicated in Figure 1, the local circuits in the LGN are exclusively inhibitory and derive from two different gating systems. One is intrinsic to the relay nucleus and mediates predominantly feedforward inhibition between adjacent retinocortical channels (Singer and Creutzfeldt, 1970; Singer, Pöppel, and Creutzfeldt, 1972; Singer and Bedworth, 1973). Because of its local action, it is assumed to gate transmission of retinal signals in a retinotopic and channel-specific way. This reduces redundancy, improves the signal-to-noise ratio, and develops bandpass responses for spatial and temporal patterns (for review see Singer, 1976a, 1977). The second inhibitory system is of the recurrent type and acts through interneurons that are located outside the LGN in nucleus reticularis thalami (Dubin and Cleland, 1977; Sumitomo, Nakamura, and Iwama, 1976). This second inhibitory pathway allows for widespread spatial interactions. Because it is recurrent, it may be regarded as the substrate for the characteristic synchronization of thalamic activity that occurs in drowsiness and slow-wave sleep (Andersen and Sears, 1964; Burke and Sefton, 1966). This recurrent inhibitory system controls transmission of visual information in a global way because it applies inhibition rather unselectively to all geniculocortical channels.

Like the LGN, the striate cortex is usually regarded

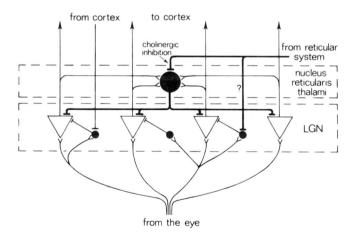

FIGURE 1 Simplified wiring diagram of inhibitory circuits in the LGN. The feedforward inhibition acts in a channel-specific way and is mediated by intrinsic inhibitory interneurons. The recurrent inhibition is conveyed by inhibitory cells located in nucleus reticularis thalami. The recurrent inhibition is gated by cholinergic reticular afferents. The intrinsic feedforward inhibition seems controlled by corticofugal fibers, but additional reticular control cannot yet be excluded.

as a passive, though much more complex, neuronal network that serves to increase the selectivity of neuronal responses to particular features of visual stimuli. As first described by Hubel and Wiesel (1962), cortical neurons no longer possess concentric fields but respond selectively to stimulus features such as orientation, direction of movement, and binocular image disparity. This increasing specificity of receptive-field properties is attributed to serial filter operations occurring repeatedly along the chain of intracortical polysynaptic pathways.

A comprehensive overview of the main streams of specific activity within the cortical network can be obtained by determining the latency and the laminar distribution of excitatory postsynaptic potentials (EPSPs) as they follow electrical stimulation of the specific afferents. Such a laminar profile of EPSP activity, elicited from the LGN, is shown in Figure 2. The traces were obtained by current-source-density analysis, a technique that has recently been adapted to the visual system (Mitzdorf and Singer, 1977, 1978).

A simplified circuit diagram that could account for this flow of specific activity is shown in Figure 3A. The specific afferents elicit monosynaptic EPSPs in layer IV and, to a much smaller extent, layer VI. From layer IV, activity is relayed through a monosynaptic link with a high safety factor to the apical dendrites of target cells in layer III. The axons of layer III cells in turn feed onto apical dendrites in layer II. A similar but somewhat more complicated picture emerges for the spread of activity toward the infragranular layers. Here also di- and trisynaptic responses can be identified in layers V and VI. Complementary single-unit analyses are compatible with this general scheme, but they also show that individual neurons, especially those below and within layer IV, quite commonly receive both direct thalamic input and additional polysynaptic afferents of intrinsic origin (Toyama et al., 1974; Singer, Tretter, and Cynader, 1975; Tretter, Cynader, and Singer, 1975).

The notion that pyramidal cells in supra- and infragranular layers are either driven exclusively through intrinsic connections or receive converging input from thalamic afferents and intrinsic sources is supported by the fact that their receptive fields are more complex than those of stellate cells in layer IV, which are driven mainly by thalamic afferents (Kelly and Van Essen, 1974; Singer, Tretter, and Cynader, 1975). In the present context, it is of particular importance that these excitatory pathways are paralleled by extremely efficient inhibitory circuits supplied by the same input (Watanabe, Konishi, and

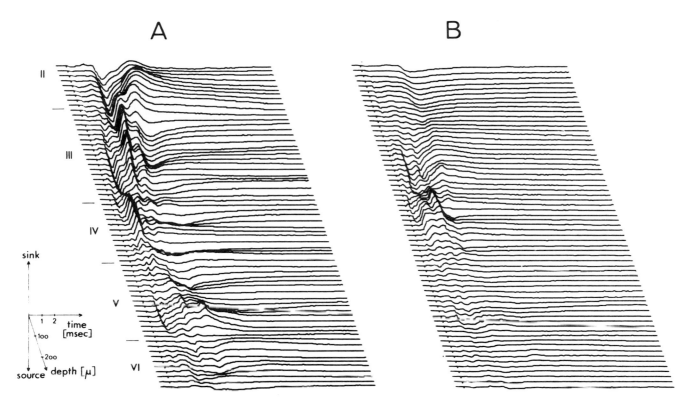

A   B

FIGURE 2 Current-source-density distributions measured in cat parastriate cortex after stimulation of LGN afferents. Parts A and B are the respective responses to two shock stimuli delivered with an interval of 20 msec. The numbers II–VI indicate the cortical layers. Upward deflections in the traces reflect EPSP activity; downward deflections correspond mainly to passive currents drawn from active sites of EPSP generation. Specific activity is relayed from the monosynaptic response in layer IV over two further synaptic steps, to both more superficial and deeper layers. The second of the two stimuli (B) elicits only the monosynaptic EPSPs in layer IV. The polysynaptic responses are missing because transmission from layer IV is blocked by inhibition. (Courtesy of U. Mitzdorf.)

Creutzfeldt, 1966; Toyama et al., 1974; Singer, Tretter, and Cynader, 1975; see Figure 3B).

Important also for later considerations is the abundant occurrence of recurrent axon collaterals. As indicated by the circuit diagram in Figure 3C, most, if not all, pyramidal-cell axons possess recurrent excitatory collaterals that ascend toward more superficial laminae (Szenthágothai, 1973; Lund and Boothe, 1975). These collaterals ramify and terminate mainly in the vicinity of neurons that send axons or axon collaterals back to the respective cells in deeper layers where the ascending collaterals originate. Such positive feedback loops are a characteristic feature of cortical circuitry. To complete this brief review of local circuitry in the visual cortex, the main efferent connections must also be considered. As shown in Figure 3D, efferent connections mainly originate from pyramidal cells in layers III, V, and VI, each layer projecting in a very specific way to particular subcortical and cortical visual centers (Holländer, 1974; Gilbert and Kelly, 1975). As predicted by the classical concept of serial processing, these output cells are either synaptically remote from specific input or, if they receive direct afferents, as is the case with layer V and VI cells, they receive additional input from intrinsic collaterals and from association fibers (Singer, Tretter, and Cynader, 1975; Tretter, Cynader, and Singer, 1975). It would be misleading, however, to assume that these pathways are only passive transmission links whose activity depends primarily or exclusively on the excitation from retinal afferents.

Evidence for nonretinal modulation of cortical activity

Apart from the retina, the most effective circumscribed site in the brain from which activity in the striate cortex can be influenced is the pontine and mesencephalic reticular core. It has been known for a long time that ascending pathways from the reticular core are involved in mediating arousal, which is

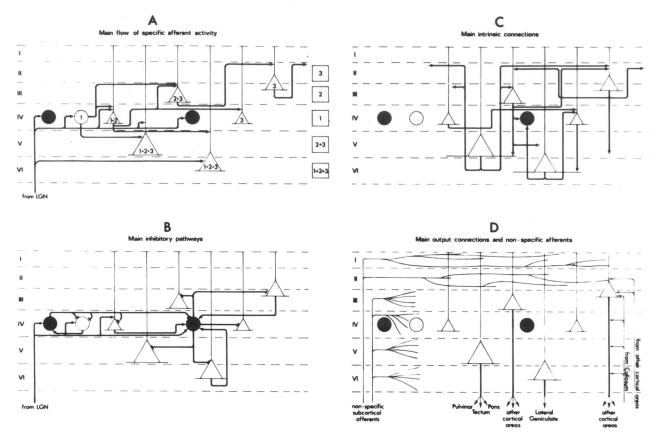

FIGURE 3   Schematic representation of afferent (A), intrinsic inhibitory (B), excitatory (C), and efferent (D) connections in cat striate cortex.

characterized by desynchronization of thalamic and cortical slow-wave activity (Moruzzi and Magoun, 1949) and by an increase in the resting discharge of cortical neurons (Murata and Kameda, 1963).

This effect of the ascending reticular arousal system (ARAS) is of a rather global nature and observable in most structures of the di- and telencephalon. Visual centers, however, and in particular the LGN and the visual cortex, seem to be controlled in a more specific way by activity from the brain stem. Rapid eye movements during paradoxical sleep are associated with characteristic negative field potentials, which first occur in the pontine and mesencephalic reticular core and subsequently in the LGN and visual cortex (Bizzi and Brooks, 1963; Mouret, Jeannerod, and Jouvet, 1963). Because of their topological distribution, these potentials are termed ponto-geniculo-occipital (PGO) waves. Slow potentials that seem to be conveyed by the same pathways as the PGO waves occur toward the end of voluntary saccadic eye movements and are termed eye-movement potentials

(EMPs) (Brooks, 1968; Brooks and Gershon, 1971; Munson and Schwartz, 1972; Sakai, Petitjean, and Jouvet, 1976).

Because both PGO waves and EMPs persist in darkness, even after enucleation of the eyes (Mouret, 1964; Jeannerod and Sakai, 1970), they are not merely a consequence of saccade-induced changes of retinal activity. Numerous studies suggest that both phenomena are generated by a pacemaker in the pontine reticular formation (Laurent, Cespuglio, and Jouvet, 1974; Sakai, Petitjean, and Jouvet, 1976; Hoshino et al., 1976). Consequently not only the arousal reaction but also the PGO waves can reliably be elicited by electrical stimulation of the pontine and mesencephalic reticular core (Bizzi and Brooks, 1963; Wilson, Pecci-Saavedra, and Doty, 1973; Singer and Bedworth, 1974; Sakai, Petitjean, and Jouvet, 1976; Singer, Tretter, and Cynader, 1976). This reproducibility of central-core effects by electrical stimulation has become very important for the analysis of underlying synaptic mechanisms.

Reticular control of thalamic transmission

Reticular influences on cortical functions cannot be interpreted without considering concomitant effects at the thalamic level. Only a brief account is given here (for a detailed review see Singer, 1977). As demonstrated with intracellular recordings from thalamic relay cells, reticular stimulation results in an inactivation of the local inhibitory circuits (Singer, 1973a,b). During the PGO wave, the inhibitory pathways are blocked completely and the pattern of LGN output activity is indistinguishable from the pattern of afferent retinal activity (Figure 4). A substantial increase in the concentration of extracellular potassium (up to 3–4 mM/ℓ above the resting level) is

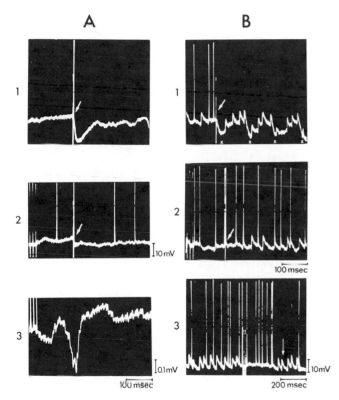

FIGURE 4 The disinhibitory effect of reticular stimulation in LGN relay cells. (A1, B1) Control IPSPs elicited in an LGN relay cell from the optic radiation (A1, recurrent IPSP) and the optic chiasm (B1, feedforward inhibition). (A2, B2) Traces obtained following conditioning reticular stimulation; the IPSPs are no longer visible. (A3) The corresponding MRF-induced negative field potential recorded in striate cortex. (B3) Trace showing the effect of reticular stimulation on spontaneous activity. For a period of about 200 msec after the reticular stimulus, all retinal EPSPs reach firing level; the LGN output is thus identical with the retinal input. This facilitatory period is followed by an interval of reduced responsiveness during which none of the EPSPs reach firing level (arrow).

associated with this facilitation of LGN transmission (Singer and Lux, 1973). Systemic application of atropine or scopolamine abolishes these effects of reticular stimulation (unpublished observations), which suggests the involvement of cholinergic mechanisms.

Recent pharmacological studies have provided direct evidence that the reticular inhibition of the inhibitory interneurons in nucleus reticularis thalami is mediated by acetylcholine, most likely through muscarinic receptors (Ben Ari et al., 1976). Comparative studies have shown that reticular stimulation has precisely the same effect on the cell groups in N. reticularis thalami as local iontophoretic application of acetylcholine (Godfraind, 1977; Dingledine and Kelly, 1978). We still do not know, however, whether the intrinsic inhibitory pathways are also blocked by direct action of cholinergic reticular afferents. It has been proposed that the inactivation of intrinsic inhibitory pathways is secondary to reticular activation of corticofugal neurons (Singer, 1977). A circuit diagram summarizing the interaction between reticular afferents and local thalamic circuits is shown in Figure 1.

In functional terms, the reticular afferents are thus capable of gating LGN transmission in a global but modality-specific way. This gating function is commonly related to the striking variations in sensory thresholds that occur with changes in alertness and shifts in selective attention (see Singer, 1977). A functional interpretation has also been given to the reticular volley that is associated with saccadic eye movements and that transiently erases intrinsic inhibition just before the eyes come to rest. It has been suggested that the eye-movement-related reticular volley resets the LGN relay characteristics to a neutral state whenever a change in retinal information can be anticipated (Jung 1972; Singer and Bedworth, 1974; Singer, 1976b).

The effect of reticular stimulation on cortical activity

At all levels of analysis, reticular activation has been shown to increase cortical excitability (Creutzfeldt, Spehlmann, and Lehmann, 1961; Bartlett and Doty, 1974; Kasamatsu, 1976; Singer, Tretter, and Cynader, 1976).

This facilitatory effect coincides in time precisely with the negative slow potential (PGO wave). It starts 40–50 msec after the mesencephalic-reticular-formation (MRF) stimulus, reaches its maximum at about 100 msec, and then decays over the next 100–200 msec. As in the LGN, the augmenting may be preceded by a slight reduction of cortical excitability when single shocks are applied to the MRF.

When the specific afferents (optic nerve or LGN) are stimulated during the PGO wave, the resulting cortical evoked potential is greatly enhanced. This increase in response amplitude is especially pronounced for the late components of the evoked potential (waves 3 and 4 in Figure 5). From current-source-density analysis (Mitzdorf and Singer, 1978) these late components can now be identified as reflecting mainly supragranular di- and trisynaptic responses. This indicates that transmission of signals from the specific afferents is facilitated along the intracortical polysynaptic circuits.

This conclusion from changes in bulk activity has been confirmed by single-unit analysis. In the large majority of units, conditioning MRF activation facilitates evoked responses to electrical stimulation of the specific afferent pathway and also of corticocortical association fibers. A marked facilitation is also observed for responses to light stimuli. MRF stimulation enhances the amplitude of light responses in most of the cells and brings out responses to stimuli that were ineffective without reticular activation. This facilitation also occurs in cells whose spontaneous discharge is not affected by reticular activation (see Figure 6). It is largest when the two stimuli are coincident and is then maintained over the whole duration of the light stimulus. As illustrated in Figure 6, the facilitation shows an interesting hysteresis. Delaying the

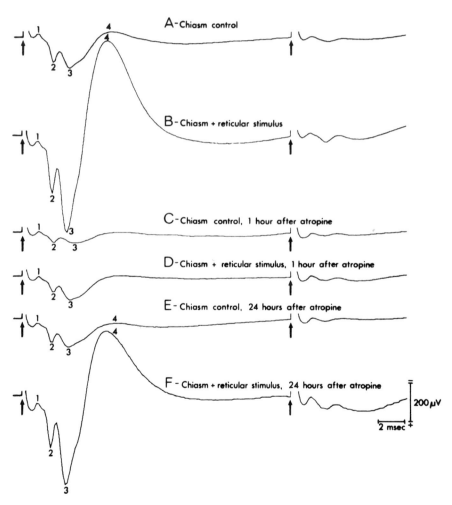

FIGURE 5   The effect of conditioning reticular stimulation on cortical evoked potentials elicited from the chiasm and the suppression of reticular facilitation by atropine. Reticular stimulation greatly enhances components 3 and 4 of the cortical evoked potential, which correspond to the di- and trisynaptic responses of supragranular cells shown in

Figure 2. Systemic application of atropine (2 mg/kg i.v.) reliably blocks this facilitation without substantially altering the control response. The consistently small responses to the second of the two shocks indicate that reticular stimulation had no effect on the cortical inhibitory mechanisms that are responsible for the suppression of these responses.

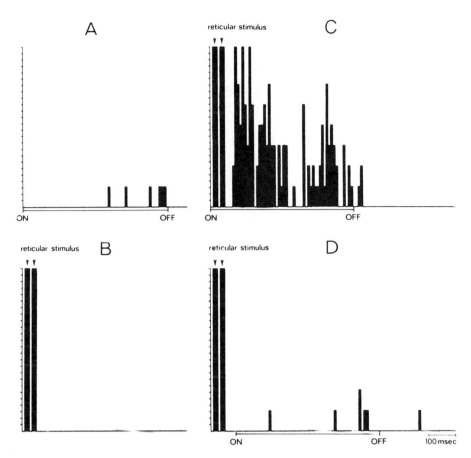

FIGURE 6 Reticular facilitation of responses to light stimulation. (A) Response of a simple cell in area 17 to a stationary flashed light slit positioned in the ON-band of the receptive field. (B) Response of the same cell to reticular stimulation. The stimulus elicits no action potentials. (C) Response to combined reticular and light stimulation with both stimuli delivered simultaneously. (D) Response to combined reticular and light stimulation with the light stimulus delayed by 100 msec. All histograms are compiled from responses to twenty stimulus sequences.

light stimulus by only 50 or 100 msec does not simply result—as one might expect—in a somewhat weaker facilitation of later components of the light response, but can lead to complete failure of the facilitatory effect. This suggests that cortical circuits tend to remain responsive and facilitated once they have been driven above threshold, this is most likely to occur when the phasic component of the light response in afferent LGN fibers coincides precisely with the reticular volley, that is, with the PGO wave.

A further consistent effect of MRF stimulation is the broadening of orientation tuning and the often complete abolition of direction selectivity (Singer, Tretter, and Cynader, 1976). These changes in response properties of cortical neurons can also be accounted for by increased cortical excitability. MRF stimulation unmasks subthreshold excitatory responses that occur to nonoptimally oriented stimuli or stimuli moving in the null direction (Creutzfeldt, Kuhnt, and Benevento, 1974).

In cats anesthetized with N_2O, MRF stimulation alters the resting discharge of about half of the cortical cells, increasing the spontaneous activity in 82% of these. These changes in resting activity are, however, moderate when compared to the marked facilitation of transsynaptically driven responses. The weak effect on resting activity is also reflected in the absence of major changes in the resting potential of intracellularly recorded cortical neurons. If there is a change at all, it consists of a slow depolarization of 1–2 mV that coincides in latency and duration with the negative field potential (Figure 8). Moreover, MRF stimulation appears to be particularly effective in increasing the resting activity of cortical output neurons.

In contrast to cells at the cortical input stage, these cells receive substantial excitatory drive even in the absence of retinal stimulation (Singer, Tretter, and Cynader, 1976). It thus appears that reticular stimulation is particularly effective in driving cells that already receive continuous EPSP bombardment under resting conditions.

The most striking effect of reticular stimulation, however, is the increase of extracellular potassium that occurs throughout all cortical layers and may far exceed the levels that can be obtained with appropriate light stimulation (Figure 7). We know that appropriately shaped light stimuli elicit vigorous responses in the thalamic afferents and in the large majority of cortical units within the respective orientation columns. As shown in Figure 7B, this evoked activity results in a transient increase in extracellular potassium (Singer and Lux, 1975), but its amplitude is much smaller than that observed after reticular stimulation, despite the fact that reticular activation causes only a moderate increase in the activity of afferent LGN fibers and cortical neurons. When many specific afferents are activated simultaneously and in an unstructured way by electrical stimulation of the optic nerve or by stroboscopic illumination of the eyes, extracellular potassium not only does not increase, but actually drops considerably below the resting level (Figure 7C). There is thus an interesting dissociation between specific and nonspecific afferents with respect to their influence on the extracellular ionic milieu.

The mechanisms of reticular activation

As demonstrated above, reticular activation results in a dramatic facilitation of transsynaptically evoked responses without substantially altering the neuron's resting discharge and membrane potential. The first question to be answered is whether these effects at the cortical level are merely secondary to the cholinergic disinhibition of thalamic transmission or whether they are caused by direct reticular control of cortical processes. Both thalamic disinhibition and cortical facilitation are suppressed by systemic application of muscarinic blocking agents such as atropine or scopolamine (Figure 5; Rinaldi and Himwich, 1955). This might suggest a single process. Moreover, effects similar to those observed after reticular stimulation can be obtained with cholinomimetic drugs

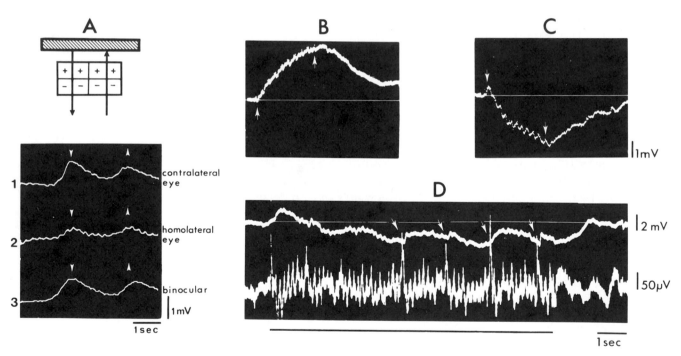

FIGURE 7 Variations of extracellular K^+ concentrations in striate cortex after activation of specific and nonspecific afferent pathways. (A) K^+ signals elicited with optimally oriented light bars moving in two directions over the receptive field of the projection column in which the ion-sensitive electrode was located. Upward deflections of the signal correspond to an increase in extracellular K^+. (B, C) K^+ signals after repetitive stimulation (between arrows) of the reticular formation and the optic radiation, respectively. While reticular stimulation leads to an increase in extracellular K^+, global activation of specific afferents leads to a decrease. The signals in A–C were averaged from ten stimulus sequences. (D) Potassium signals during stroboscopic illumination of the eyes (upper trace). After an initial rise there is a consistent decrease in extracellular K^+ below the resting level. Only when the flash elicits a large negative field potential (lower trace) does K^+ show a transient increase (arrows).

(Rinaldi and Himwich, 1955; Longo and Silvestrini, 1957).

Several independent observations suggest that there is direct reticular control of cortical excitability through pathways organized in parallel with the specific afferents. Disinhibition in the LGN merely causes an unstructured diffuse rise of background activity in relay cells. Because of the powerful inhibitory circuits at the cortical input stage (see Figure 3B), the net result of such an unstructured rise in specific afferent activity is a *decrease* in cortical excitability. Direct support for this conclusion comes from the opposite changes in extracellular potassium observed after stimulation of reticular and specific pathways, respectively. Direct reticular control of cortical activity is also suggested by the observation that cortical PGO waves persist during paradoxical sleep even after bilateral destruction of the LGN (Hobson, Alexander, and Frederickson, 1969).

Finally, a cholinergic innervation of cortex has been inferred from both histochemical and physiological experiments: high cortical levels of acetylcholinesterase (Shute and Lewis, 1967) and a five- to sixfold increase in the output of ACh from cerebral cortex after reticular stimulation (Szerb, 1967) have been presented as evidence for the presence of cholinergic mechanisms.

The reticular facilitation of cortical transmission could be achieved in three ways. Reticular afferents could (1) inactivate inhibitory mechanisms, as occurs at the thalamic level, (2) directly excite cortical cells, but sparing cells that feed to inhibitory circuits, or (3) selectively facilitate excitatory synaptic transmission. Intracellular measurements of IPSP changes after reticular stimulation as well as current-source-density analyses have failed to provide evidence for an extensive disinhibitory action (Singer, Tretter, and Cynader, 1976; Mitzdorf and Singer, 1978). Only very rarely were IPSP amplitudes found to decrease (Figure 8), although in most instances there was a moderate decrease in IPSP duration. Since the decrease in duration could be caused by facilitation of delayed, recycling excitation, a disinhibitory influence, if present at all, is certainly not as effective as in the thalamus.

The hypothesis of direct excitation of cortical neurons through reticular afferents is also unsatisfactory. It seems doubtful that the small measured depolarizations of individual neurons can account for the massive facilitation of transsynaptically evoked responses. Moreover, it is difficult to explain why direct excitation should have a differential effect on the resting activities of cells at the input and output stages

but nevertheless cause global facilitation of evoked responses throughout all layers.

The mechanism that would best account for all of the observed phenomena is heterosynaptic facilitation of transsynaptically induced responses. This could be achieved either presynaptically (e.g., by increasing the amount of transmitter released per action potential) or postsynaptically (e.g., by increasing the space and time constants of the dendrites). Given our present knowledge of the muscarinic actions of ACh, it is conceivable that a single primary mechanism might mediate both effects. The muscarinic depolarization of cortical neurons has been shown to be associated with an increase in membrane resistance (Krnjević, Pumain, and Renaud, 1971). In sympathetic ganglion cells such slow depolarization with concomitant increase in membrane resistance is due to synaptic inactivation of potassium conductance g_K (Weight and Votava, 1970; Kuba and Koketsu, 1976; for review see Weight, 1974).

A similar mechanism has been proposed for the increased membrane resistance of cortical cells (for review see Krnjević, 1975). Increased membrane resistance, however, leads to increased length constants and would therefore increase electrotonic propagation of postsynaptic potentials along the fairly long dendrites of cortical neurons. The same mechanism could, in addition, increase the amount of transmitter released. Reduced g_K results in prolonged action potentials; this should increase the influx of Ca^{++} ions into the presynaptic terminals and, consequently, the amount of transmitter released per action potential.

That such a process is involved is suggested by the finding that during iontophoretic application of ACh (Krnjević, Pumain, and Renaud, 1971) and after reticular stimulation (unpublished observations), delayed repolarization can increase the duration of intracellularly recorded action potentials. Moreover, selective facilitation of synaptic transmission can explain the dissociation between minor changes in resting potential and resting activity on the one hand, and the massive potentiation of synaptically evoked responses on the other. Such a mechanism can also account for the finding that reticular stimulation preferentially affects the resting activity of cells that are subject to permanent EPSP bombardment. As discussed in detail in Krnjević (1975), decreasing g_K should be particularly effective in depolarizing cells with high g_{Na}, that is, cells that are constantly receiving EPSPs.

Can a decrease in potassium conductance result in an increased extracellular accumulation of potassium ions? If ACh also reduces the g_K and thereby the K^+

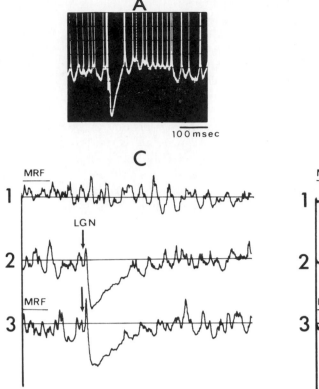

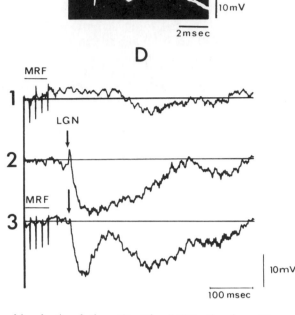

FIGURE 8 The effect of reticular stimulation on resting potentials and IPSPs in cortical cells. (A–C) Intracellularly recorded responses of a layer V corticotectal projection cell. A and B show responses to LGN stimuli at different time scales. The LGN stimulus elicits a large IPSP (A), the expected antidromic spike, and a mono- (2), di- (3), and trisynaptic (4) EPSP (B). C shows averaged membrane potential changes (ten stimulus sequences) of this cell following reticular stimulation (1), LGN stimulation (2), and com- bined stimulation (3). The MRF stimulus affects neither membrane potential nor IPSP amplitude. (D) Same stimulation procedure as in C applied to an intracellularly recorded complex cell in the infragranular layers. Here reticular stimulation leads to a small, slowly rising but long-lasting depolarization (1) and a transient reduction of IPSP duration (2, 3). The initial amplitude of the IPSP is unaltered.

buffering capacity of glial cells (Krnjević and Schwartz, 1967; Krnjević, Pumain, and Renaud, 1971), this would favor extracellular accumulation of K$^+$. Moreover, increased action-potential duration could greatly enhance the efflux of K$^+$ from neurons if there is a slow Ca^{++} current in cortical cells similar to that shown for snail neurons (see Lux and Heyer, this volume). A massive increase in extracellular potassium, associated with a negative field potential, has recently been observed in the cerebellar cortex after application of 3- and 4-aminopyridine substances that selectively reduce potassium conductance (Nicholson et al., 1976). It is possible that a similar effect may result in neocortex when g_K is reduced through the presumed action of ACh.

Clearly, specific experiments are needed at this stage to test these speculations. The proposed action of ACh seems attractive as a working hypothesis, however, since all the puzzling effects observed after reticular stimulation could then be accounted for by a single process, namely, heterosynaptic facilitation of synaptic transmission.

The role of modulatory systems in developmental plasticity

There is now some evidence suggesting that modulation of local circuit excitability through nonspecific pathways might play a role in gating circuit consolidation during early development. Monocular deprivation from contour vision during early postnatal life leads to functional disconnection of afferents from the deprived eye (Wiesel and Hubel, 1963). It has been inferred from more recent studies that this competition between afferents for effective connections with the respective cortical target cells is not solely dependent on differences in presynaptic activity (Singer, Rauschecker, and Werth, 1977). As proposed by Hebb (1949), it seems crucial that postsynaptic target cells be able to get into resonance with and respond to the presynaptic activity. When one eye is stimulated only with diffuse light flashes while the other eye is occluded, no ocular-dominance shift occurs (Figure 9 A, B); there are still large differences between the patterns of presynaptic activity in the afferents from the two eyes, but postsynaptic responses to diffuse stimulation are virtually absent. The importance of postsynaptic resonance for circuit consolidation has also been inferred from other ex-

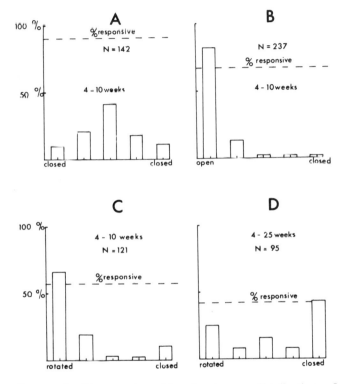

FIGURE 9 Changes in ocular-dominance distribution of cortical neurons in kittens following various raising conditions. All kittens were raised in the dark until the age of 4 weeks. (A) One eye closed, the other stimulated for 6 weeks with diffuse light flashes: the ocular-dominance distribution remains normal. (B) One eye closed, the other exposed to normal environment for 6 weeks: ocular dominance changes in the expected way. (C) One eye closed, the other rotated and exposed to normal environment for 6 weeks: the ocular dominance shift toward the open eye is apparent but less pronounced than in B; in addition, there is a decrease in responsiveness. (D) Same as in C but with an exposure time of 6 months: compared to B and C there is a marked decrease of responsiveness, and the ocular-dominance shift seen in C is no longer visible (N is the number of responsive cells shown in the graphs.)

periments in which ocular dominance and orientation selectivity were both modified through early visual experience (Singer, 1976b).

Related experiments have suggested that circuit consolidation and suppression of previously functional connections are not solely determined by such local interactions between retinal activity and cortical circuits. When retinal signals are manipulated in such a way that local responses to contours remain normal but no longer match the needs of more integral sensorimotor processes, ocular-dominance shifts may no longer occur and preexisting connections may become disrupted. This can be achieved by closing one eye and simultaneously fixing the open eye in a rotated position within the orbita. This manipulation does not affect the spatiotemporal pattern of retinal responses to contours. Nevertheless, the expected shift in ocular dominance is seen only during a transitional phase and is then followed by partial disconnection of the afferents from the open eye (Figure 9C, D; Singer, Yinon, and Tretter, 1979). One is led to postulate additional gating signals, coming from structures outside striate cortex, that determine whether activity in local circuits will induce long-lasting changes in synaptic transmission. In this particular case such a gating system must have access to information about the correspondence between retinal coordinates and the other sensorimotor maps because this has been the only altered parameter.

Since the regulation of synaptic efficiency during the critical period of early development seems to depend, at least initially, on the occurrence or failure of postsynaptic resonance with presynaptic activity, the postulated gating mechanism could very well act through feedback control of synaptic transmission between pre- and postsynaptic elements. It is, of course, premature to continue speculations along these lines, but there is at least some evidence that reticular activation might be one prerequisite for such early changes in connectivity.

Encouraged by the notion that ocular-dominance shifts can be induced with relatively brief exposure (Blakemore and Van Sluyters, 1974), we have attempted to induce these shifts with monocular light stimulation in anesthetized preparations that were kept alive over several days. These procedures failed consistently, although exposure times were considerably longer than those required in alert kittens. It was only after conditioning MRF stimulation was applied along with each of the structured moving light stimuli that ocular-dominance shifts became apparent in the evoked potential (Figure 10). We do not yet know which of the ascending modulatory systems

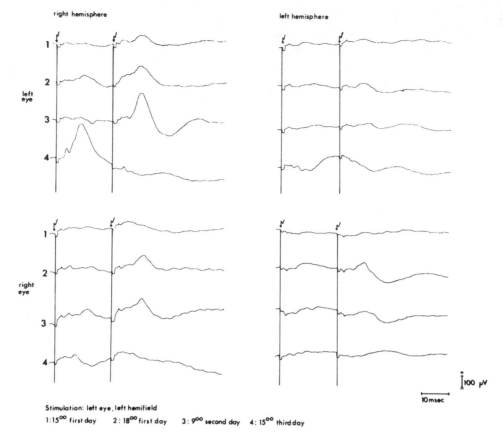

right hemisphere   left hemisphere

left eye

right eye

Stimulation: left eye, left hemifield

1:15°° first day   2:18°° first day   3:9°° second day   4:15°° third day

FIGURE 10 Evoked potential changes in a dark-raised, 4-week-old kitten monocularly stimulated over 4 days by a moving grating. The evoked potentials are elicited by electrical stimulation of the right and left optic nerve and recorded with bipolar electrodes from the right and left striate cortex. Each evoked potential is averaged from fifty stimulus presentations. The light stimulus was presented to the left eye and predominantly to the left visual field, thus stimulating mainly the right hemisphere. The numbers 1–4 in the four sets of crossed and uncrossed stimulation-recording conditions indicate the time of recording. Light stimuli were presented continuously and conditioned with reticular stimulation. At times 1 and 2, all responses are poorly structured, as is characteristic for inexperienced kit-tens of this age. The responses from the unstimulated eye and hemisphere remain rather unchanged over the next days. By contrast, the responses from the stimulated left eye and the hemisphere contralateral to the stimulated half-field show a clear enhancement. During the second day (trace 3), the response to the second of the double shocks increases in amplitude. This is still abnormal, indicating weak inhibition or protracted temporal facilitation. During the third day, however, the response changes to a normal pattern, differing from those in adult cats mainly by its long latency and less pronounced segregation into three distinct peaks. Such changes were only obtained when light stimulation was associated with conditioning reticular stimulation.

facilitated these changes in functional connections; specific experiments are required to answer this question. But heterosynaptic facilitation and concomitant control of postsynaptic resonance could very well be one way to gate the initial processes that eventually lead to circuit consolidation during early development.

The function of nonspecific modulation in sensory processing

Within our current concept of cortical operations and sensory processing it is rather difficult to assign a functional role to global modulatory influences. A solution to this problem seems to be relevant, however, since unselective modulation of general excitability levels and synaptic transmission appears to be a common feature of all ascending nonspecific systems. I shall therefore propose a slightly extended concept of cortical operations in which more emphasis is laid on dynamic properties of signal processing, such as state changes, resonance, hysteresis, and cooperativity.

Numerous observations, although never pursued in a systematic way, indicate that cortical processes may be highly dynamic and adaptive. Even in anesthetized animals the reproducibility of responses to light stimuli decreases as one moves away from the input stage, that is, from cells in layer IV to cells in the supra- and infragranular layers. There is some evidence, moreover, that this response variability is due not merely to global changes in arousal but also to local state changes in particular circuits. For example, the hysteresis effect that has been observed after reticular stimulation indicates that pathways can be opened by supracritical excitation and can then maintain a facilitated state over considerable periods of time. Stimulus-dependent state changes of neuronal subpopulations have also been demonstrated by recent studies on the corticothalamic feedback loop (Schmielau and Singer, 1977). From these and many other observations it can be inferred that the functional state of cortical neuronal populations is subject to permanent, partly stimulus-dependent, changes.

From our knowledge about thalamic and cortical circuits, in particular the inhibitory connections, it follows that: (1) each of these functional states consists of a balanced distribution of facilitated and inhibited subpopulations of neurons, and (2) any particular functional state tends to be stabilized by reverberation in positive feedback loops, aided by long time constants of inhibition.

These rather indirect conclusions from electrophysiological and anatomical evidence gain substantial support from numerous psychophysical data. The phenomenon of binocular rivalry, for example, indicates that visual information is selected in an alternating sequence from the right and left eyes when the two retinal patterns cannot be fused into one image.

State changes due to cooperative facilitation of neuronal arrays with particular properties are suggested by Julesz's experiments on stereoscopic vision. It takes a long time for depth planes to emerge from binocularly viewed Julesz stereograms, but once a depth plane has been "identified," its recognition is very stable. A possible mechanism for this convincing demonstration of hysteresis is the mutual facilitation of cortical-cell assemblies that have the same disparity selectivity (see Nelson, 1975). To account for the hysteresis, one must assume that once this cell assembly has reached a critical level of activity, it stabilizes and remains facilitated. State changes that presumably occur at higher levels of signal processing are evident during the perception of ambiguous figures. Here the system seems to be continuously testing hypotheses and apparently finding several stable states that match the pattern of afferent activity.

These and many other examples suggest that the visual system permanently alters strategies of analysis while it decodes the flow of retinal information. We have good reason to assume that such shifts in decoding strategy are not confined to some hitherto unknown central association area but are reflected in state changes of neuronal assemblies even at the level of striate cortex. Indeed, simple state changes such as those that occur with binocular rivalry are likely to affect visual centers as peripheral as the LGN (Schmielau and Singer, 1977). Moreover, if one admits that cortical areas dealing with higher levels of information processing are capable of such state changes, there seems to be no logical reason why this should not occur in the striate cortex. The intrinsic organizations of the various cortical areas are so strikingly similar that it is difficult to accept the possibility that they might differ in such fundamental properties.

In such dynamic processes, however, a nonspecific modulatory system that globally alters excitability levels could play a crucial role. It could determine the probability of occurrence of state transitions—in particular, from a given input pattern to a corresponding functional state. Moreover, the systematic variation of general excitability could provide a valuable indication of the stability or ambiguity of population responses. At high excitability levels, resonance to afferent activity is likely to occur in numerous circuits, and fluctuations between various states have a high probability. By subsequently reducing the unspecific drive, less stable constellations can be made to fade and the state with the highest stability can be identified. Setting the level of global excitability is thus equivalent to a scanning process in search of unambiguous output signals.

The continuous fluctuations of excitability, particularly those associated with eye movements, do in fact suggest the occurrence of such a scanning process. Predictable changes in the pattern of sensory signals, such as occur with eye movements, are associated with a brief and precisely timed volley in the reticular afferents. There is also evidence that externally produced changes in the flow of retinal activity can lead to secondary activation of the modulatory system (Singer, 1977). These transient reticular volleys enable maximal resonance and rapid state changes, which are prerequisites for the initial bias-free processing of unpredictable information. Because of their short duration, the most prominent or stable excitatory patterns can subsequently be selected by the decrease in excitability.

This model leads to several testable predictions

about the effect of eye movements on state changes. First, one expects that saccades should facilitate state transitions, such as shifts in ocular dominance during binocular rivalry, or changes in the perception of ambiguous figures. Psychophysical evidence indicates just this sort of correlation. Second, one would not be surprised by a transient interruption of visual perception during maximal reticular facilitation, since any coherent pattern in output activity might then be masked by noise. This idea seems to be supported by the fact that afterimages, which are purely retinal in origin, disappear briefly just after a saccade and then slowly reappear. Third, one might also expect that threshold elevations due to central adaptation could be reset by a saccadic eye movement, since this could bring corresponding circuits freshly into resonance. Several recent studies suggest that this seems to be the case (D. MacKay, personal communication; Singer, Zihl, and Pöppel, 1977). Of course, all these phenomena also occur independently of eye movements, which suggests that the "nonspecific" setting of excitability levels is a continuous process. It is tempting to speculate that the rhythms apparent in the EEG reflect such continuous modulation of synaptic transmission, especially since it seems well-established that the morphology of the EEG depends critically on activity in the ascending reticular pathways.

Long-term control of cortical excitability

So far I have dealt mainly with modulatory influences that induce fairly rapid state changes. But we have good reason to assume that there are also much slower modulatory systems that maintain particular excitability levels over minutes or even hours. Disre-garding any trophic effects for the moment, such long-term modulatory systems could determine the *range* within which excitability can be varied by the fast modulating cholinergic pathways.

A particularly nice example of a long-term change in human subjects is the diurnal variation of visual thresholds at the borders of scotomata due to cortical lesions (Zihl, Pöppel, and Cramon, 1977). These threshold changes probably directly reflect a diurnal variation of neuronal excitability in striate cortex (Figure 11).

The preceding arguments suggest that changes in the range of excitability should have effects beyond altered thresholds for simple detection tasks. When the upper limit of this range is lowered, resonance to particular input patterns should take longer to build up, especially when a high level of cooperativity is required, and state changes should occur at a slower rate. Such effects are indeed observed with fatigue: together with a rise in threshold there is also a marked prolongation of the time needed to analyze complex patterns such as Julesz stereograms. Disturbances of sensory processing should also appear when the lower boundary of the modulation range is permanently set too high: activity patterns should be less likely to stabilize in an unambiguous state. In hyperactive states such as alcoholic hallucinosis and various forms of deliria, disturbances of visual perception are a characteristic symptom, and one might speculate that these dysfunctions are also caused by distortions of the excitability range.

We know little about the mechanisms through which such long-term control of excitability ranges are achieved. The ascending monoamine pathways might be involved since there is good evidence that they play an essential role in controlling the sleep-

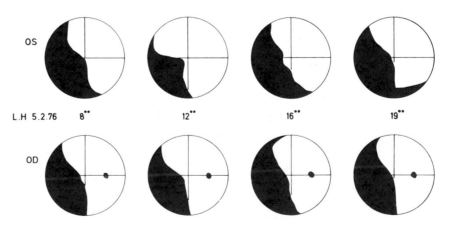

FIGURE 11 Diurnal variation of visual-field borders in a patient with partial destruction of the occipital lobe due to a vascular lesion. The visual field expands around noon and shrinks toward the evening. (Courtesy of J. Zihl.)

waking cycle (Jouvet, 1972, 1974). Moreover, at the mesencephalic level, the norepinephrine- and serotonin-containing neurons from locus coeruleus and raphe dorsalis have been shown to exert a gating function on the transmission of PGO activity (Jouvet, 1972; Simon, Gershon, and Brooks, 1973). Finally, also within the respective target areas, the monoamines could gate the facilitatory effects of ACh. Libet and Tosaka (1970) have shown that in sympathetic ganglia, dopamine can induce a long-lasting facilitation of the muscarinic ACh depolarization and thereby control the efficiency of the cholinergic mechanism. As suggested in Figure 12, one might think in terms of a hierarchy of mutually dependent control systems that differ in their degree of globality and, in particular, in the time constants of their influences.

The cholinergic reticular system seems to occupy an intermediate position between the specific sensory and motor centers on the one hand, and the monoaminergic pathways on the other. It has the characteristics of a modulatory system: the activity of reticular afferents is not fed directly into specific pathways but is used to gate transmission of specific signals within the latter. At the thalamic level, this is achieved through the control of inhibitory circuits. At the cortical level, modulation of intrinsic processes seems to be realized through heterosynaptic facilitation. These modulatory influences appear to be of crucial importance for the specific operations related to signal processing, for the initiation of the long-lasting changes in synaptic efficiency that occur in striate cortex during development, and probably in other areas during learning processes in adults. It may be questioned, therefore, whether we should maintain the conceptual dichotomy between specific sensory and nonspecific modulatory operations, at least with respect to the cholinergic reticular system. Its anatomical organization seems sufficiently differentiated, and its reciprocal connections with sensory areas sufficiently tight (Scheibel and Scheibel, 1967), that we should consider reticular control to be an integral feature of sensory processing. Such an approach will probably lead to an extension of our current concepts of cortical processing toward more dynamic, and perhaps even probabilistic, models in which rapid state changes in neuronal ensembles and active scanning processes will become as important as feature extraction by sequential filter operations. In such an extended concept, the antinomy between sophisticated local circuit operations and the global modulation of overall excitability will probably fade.

From the evidence to date, it appears that the

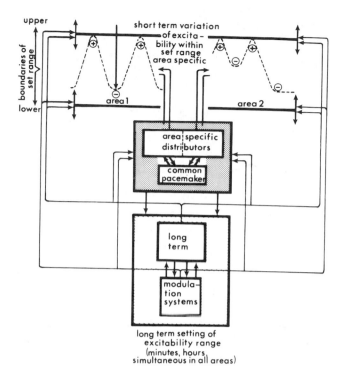

FIGURE 12 Block diagram of hierarchically organized modulatory control systems that differ in the time constants and the globality of their action. The hatched areas stand for control systems that set, in a rather global way and with long time constants, the boundaries within which short-term modulatory systems (stippled centers) can induce rapid and area-specific changes of neuronal excitability. The common pacemaker for the short-term modulatory system appears to be located in the pontine and mesencephalic reticular formation. The area-specific distribution of ascending activity is most likely accomplished at the diencephalic level by the nonspecific thalamic nuclear complex. This short-term modulatory system must contain cholinergic transmission links. The dashed curves indicate short-term variations of neuronal excitability in which peaks and troughs correspond to particular functional states of neuron ensembles. Peaks (+) are characterized by maximal resonance to specific input signals, high probability of transitions between functional states, and high ambiguity of output signals. At low excitability levels (−), only the most stable states persist, state transitions have low probability, and output signals from neuron populations have low ambiguity. The pharmacological nature of the range-setting, long-term modulatory systems is still hypothetical; the monoaminergic projection systems that arise from brain stem and control most of the forebrain centers through monosynaptic pathways are likely candidates.

monoamine pathways are less likely to be so intimately involved in information processing. Their anatomical organization excludes such sophisticated, area-specific gating operations as are needed for guiding selective attention or inducing modality-specific state changes. They do not seem to receive any refined feedback from sensory cortices. Activity in these pathways is low and subject only to slow modulations. All of these properties predispose these systems to set the working range for the faster, modulatory reticular system. Because of their direct action on cell metabolism, they might also act as gates for trophic processes that consolidate short-term changes in synaptic transmission. To my knowledge, we have not come across any phenomena in striate-cortex physiology that hint of other functions of the monoamine pathways in sensory systems.

REFERENCES

ANDERSEN, P., and T. A. SEARS, 1964. The role of inhibition in the phasing of spontaneous thalamo-cortical discharge. *J. Physiol.* 173:459–480.

BARTLETT, J. R., and R. W. DOTY, 1974. Influence of mesencephalic stimulation on unit activity in striate cortex of squirrel monkeys. *J. Neurophysiol.* 37:642–652.

BEN-ARI, Y., R. DINGLEDINE, J. KANAZAWA, and J. S. KELLY, 1976. Inhibitory effects of acetylcholine on neurones in the feline nucleus reticularis thalami. *J. Physiol.* 261:647–671.

BIZZI E., and D. C. BROOKS, 1963. Functional connections between pontine reticular formation and lateral geniculate nucleus during deep sleep. *Arch. Ital. Biol.* 101:666–681.

BLAKEMORE, C., and R. C. VAN SLUYTERS, 1974. Reversal of the physiological effects of monocular deprivation in kittens: Further evidence for a sensitive period. *J. Physiol.* 237:195–216.

BROOKS, D. C., 1968. Waves associated with eye movement in the awake and sleeping cat. *Electroencephalogr. Clin. Neurophysiol.* 24:532–541.

BROOKS, D. C., and M. D. GERSHON, 1971. Eye movement potentials in the oculomotor and visual systems of the cat: A comparison of reserpine induced waves with those present during wakefulness and rapid eye movement sleep. *Brain Res.* 27:223–239.

BURKE, W., and A. J. SEFTON, 1966. Inhibitory mechanisms in lateral geniculate nucleus of rat. *J. Physiol.* 187:231–246.

CREUTZFELDT, O. D., U. KUHNT, and L. A. BENEVENTO, 1974. An intracellular analysis of visual cortical neurones to moving stimuli: Responses in a co-operative neuronal network. *Exp. Brain Res.* 21:251–274.

CREUTZFELDT, O. D., R. SPEHLMANN, and D. LEHMANN, 1961. Veränderung der Neuronaktivität des visuellen Cortex durch Reizung der substantia reticularis mesencephali. In *Neurophysiologie und Psychophysik des visuellen Systems*, R. Jung and H. Kornhuber, eds. Berlin, Heidelberg, New York: Springer-Verlag, pp. 351–363.

DINGLEDINE, R., and J. S. KELLY, 1978. Brainstem stimulation and the acetylcholine-evoked inhibition of neurons in the feline nucleus reticularis thalami. *J. Physiol.* (in press).

DUBIN, M. W., and B. C. CLELAND, 1977. The organization of visual inputs to interneurons of the lateral geniculate nucleus of the cat. *J. Neurophysiol.* 40:410–427.

FUXE, K., 1965. Evidence for the existence of monoamine neurons in the central nervous system. IV. Distribution of monoamine nerve terminals in the central nervous system. *Acta Physiol. Scand.* 64 (suppl. 247):39–85.

GILBERT, C. D., and J. P. KELLY, 1975. The projections of cells in different layers of the cat's visual cortex. *J. Comp. Neurol.* 163:81–105.

GODFRAIND, J. M., 1977. Acetylcholine effects in the lateral geniculate nucleus region. In *Iontophoresis and Transmitter Mechanisms in the Mammalian CNS* (satellite symposium, 27th International Congress of Physiological Science). New York: Elsevier.

HEBB, D. O., 1949. New York: Wiley.

HOBSON, J. A., J. ALEXANDER, and C. J. FREDERICKSON, 1969. The effect of lateral geniculate lesions on phasic electrical activity of the cortex during desynchronized sleep in the cat. *Brain Res.* 14:607–621.

HOLLÄNDER, H., 1974. On the origin of the corticotectal projections in the cat. *Exp. Brain Res.* 21:433–439.

HOSHINO, K., O. POMPEIANO, P. C. MAGHERINI, and T. MERGNER, 1976. The oscillatory system responsible for the oculomotor activity during the bursts of REM. *Arch. Ital. Biol.* 114:278–309.

HUBEL, D. H., and T. N. WIESEL, 1962. Receptive fields, binocular interaction and functional architecture in the cat's visual cortex. *J. Physiol.* 160:106–154.

JEANNEROD, M., and K. SAKAI, 1970. Occipital and geniculate potentials related to eye movements in the unanaesthetized cat. *Brain Res.* 19:361–377.

JOUVET, M., 1972. The role of monoamines and acetylcholine-containing neurons in the regulation of the sleep. *Erg. Physiol.* 64:166–307.

JOUVET, M., 1974. Monoaminergic regulation of the sleep-waking cycle in the cat. In *The Neurosciences: Third Study Program*, F. O. Schmitt and F. G. Worden, eds. Cambridge, MA: MIT Press, pp. 499–508.

JUNG, R., 1972. Neurophysiological and psychophysical correlates in vision research. In *Brain and Human Behaviour*, A. G. Karczmar and J. C. Eccles, eds. Berlin, Heidelberg, New York: Springer-Verlag, pp. 209–258.

KASAMATSU, T., 1976. Visual cortical neurons influenced by the oculomotor input: Characterization of their receptive field properties. *Brain Res.* 113:271–292.

KELLY, J. P., and D. C. VAN ESSEN, 1974. Cell structure and function in the visual cortex of the cat. *J. Physiol.* 238:515–547.

KRNJEVIĆ, K., 1975. Acetylcholine receptors in vertebrate CNS. In *Handbook of Psychopharmacology*, vol. 6, L. L. Iversen, S. D. Iversen, and S. H. Snyder, eds. New York and London: Plenum Press, pp. 97–126.

KRNJEVIĆ, K., R. PUMAIN, and L. RENAUD, 1971. The mechanism of excitation by acetylcholine in the cerebral cortex. *J. Physiol.* 215:247–268.

KRNJEVIĆ, K., and S. SCHWARTZ, 1967. Some properties of unresponsive cells in the cerebral cortex. *Exp. Brain Res.* 3:306–319.

KUBA, K., and K. KOKETSU, 1976. Analysis of the slow excitatory postsynaptic potential in bullfrog sympathetic ganglion cells. *Jap. J. Physiol.* 26:651–669.

LAURENT, J. P., R. CESPUGLIO, and M. JOUVET, 1974. Delimitation des voies ascendantes de l'activité ponto-geniculo-occipitale chez le chat. *Brain Res.* 65:29–52.

LIBET, B., and T. TOSAKA, 1970. Dopamine as a synaptic transmitter and modulator in sympathetic ganglia: A different mode of synaptic action. *Proc. Natl. Acad. Sci. USA* 67:667–673.

LINDVALL, O., and A. BJÖRKLUND, 1974. The organization of the ascending catecholamine neuron system in the rat brain, as revealed by the glyoxylic acid fluorescence method. *Acta Physiol. Scand.* (suppl. 412), 48 pp.

LONGO, V. G., and B. SILVESTRINI, 1957. Action of eserine and amphetamine on the electrical activity of the rabbit brain. *J. Pharmacol.* 120:160–170.

LUND, J. S., and R. G. BOOTHE, 1975. Interlaminar connections and pyramidal neuron organisation in the visual cortex, area 17, of the macaque monkey. *J. Comp. Neurol.* 159:305–334.

MITZDORF, U., and W. SINGER, 1977. Laminar segregation of afferents to the lateral geniculate nucleus of the cat: An analysis of current source density. *J. Neurophysiol.* 40.1227–1244.

MITZDORF, U., and W. SINGER, 1978. Prominent excitatory pathways in the cat visual cortex (A17 and A18): A current source density analysis of electrically evoked potentials. *Exp. Brain Res.* 33:371–394.

MORUZZI, G., and H. W. MAGOUN, 1949. Brain stem reticular formation and activation of the EEG. *Electroencephalogr. Clin. Neurophysiol.* 1:455–473.

MOURET, J., 1964. Les mouvements oculaires au cours du sommeil paradoxal. Thesis, University of Lyon.

MOURET, J. M., M. JEANNEROD, and M. JOUVET, 1963. L'activité électrique due système visuel au cours de la phase paradoxale du sommeil chez le chat. *J. Physiol.* (Paris) 55:305–306.

MUNSON, J. B., and K. S. SCHWARTZ, 1972. Lateral geniculate and occipital cortex spikes with eye movements in awake and sleeping cats: Temporal and function correlations. *Exp. Neurol.* 35:300–304.

MURATA, K., and K. KAMEDA, 1963. The activity of single cortical neurones of unrestrained cats during sleep and wakefulness. *Arch. Ital. Biol.* 101:306–331.

NELSON, J. I., 1975. Globality and stereoscopic fusion in binocular vision. *J. Theoret. Biol.* 49:1–88.

NICHOLSON, C., R. STEINBERG, H. STÖCKLE, and G. TEN BRUGGENCATE, 1976. Calcium decrease associated with aminopyridine-induced potassium increase in cat cerebellum. *Neurosci. Lett.* 3:315–319.

RINALDI, F., and H. HIMWICH, 1955. Alerting responses and actions of atropine and cholinergic drugs. *Arch. Neurol. Psychiatr.* 73:387–395.

SAKAI, K., F. PETITJEAN, and M. JOUVET, 1976. Effects of ponto-mesencephalic lesions and electrical stimulation upon PGO waves and EMPs in unanaesthetized cats. *Electroencephalogr. Clin. Neurophysiol.* 41:49–63.

SCHEIBEL, M. E., and A. B. SCHEIBEL, 1967. Anatomical basis of attention mechanisms in vertebrate brains. In *The Neurosciences: A Study Program.* G. C. Quarton, T. Melnechuk, and F. O. Schmitt, eds. New York: Rockefeller Univ. Press, pp. 577–602.

SCHMIELAU, F., and W. SINGER, 1977. The role of visual cortex for binocular interactions in the cat lateral geniculate nucleus. *Brain Res.* 120:354–361.

SHUTE, C. C. D., and P. R. LEWIS, 1967. The ascending cholinergic reticular system: Neocortical, olfactory and subcortical projections. *Brain* 90:497–519.

SIMON, R. P., M. D. GERSHON, and D. C. BROOKS, 1973. The role of the raphe nuclei in the regulation of ponto-geniculo-occipital wave activity. *Brain Res.* 58:313–330.

SINGER, W., 1973a. The effect of mesencephalic reticular stimulation on intracellular potentials of cat lateral geniculate neurons. *Brain Res.* 61:35–54.

SINGER, W., 1973b. Brain stem stimulation and the hypothesis of presynaptic inhibition in cat lateral geniculate nucleus. *Brain Res.* 61:55–68.

SINGER, W., 1976a. Temporal aspects of subcortical contrast processing. *Neurosci. Res. Program Bull.* 15:358–369.

SINGER, W., 1976b. Modification of orientation and direction selectivity of cortical cells in kittens with monocular vision. *Brain Res.* 118:460–468.

SINGER, W., 1977. Control of thalamic transmission by corticofugal and ascending reticular pathways in the visual system. *Physiol. Rev.* 57.

SINGER, W., 1977. Effects of monocular deprivation on excitatory and inhibitory pathways in cat striate cortex. *Exp. Brain Res.* 30:25–41.

SINGER, W., and N. BEDWORTH, 1973. Inhibitory interaction between *x* and *y* units in the cat lateral geniculate nucleus. *Brain Res.* 49:291–307.

SINGER, W., and N. BEDWORTH, 1974. Correlation between the effects of brain stem stimulation and saccadic eye movements on transmission in the cat lateral geniculate nucleus. *Brain Res.* 72:185–202.

SINGER, W., and O. D. CREUTZFELDT, 1970. Reciprocal lateral inhibition of on- and off-center neurons in the lateral geniculate body of the cat. *Exp. Brain Res.* 10:311–330.

SINGER, W., and H. D. LUX, 1973. Presynaptic depolarization and extracellular potassium in the cat lateral geniculate nucleus. *Brain Res.* 64:17–33.

SINGER, W., and H. D. LUX, 1975. Extracellular potassium gradients and visual receptive fields in the cat striate cortex. *Brain Res.* 96:378–383.

SINGER, W., E. PÖPPEL, and O. D. CREUTZFELDT, 1972. Inhibitory interaction in the cat's lateral geniculate nucleus. *Exp. Brain Res.* 14:210–226.

SINGER, W., J. RAUSCHECKER, and R. WERTH, 1977. The effect of monocular exposure to temporal contrasts on ocular dominance in kittens. *Brain Res.* 134:568–572.

SINGER, W., F. TRETTER, and M. CYNADER, 1975. Organization of cat striate cortex: A correlation of receptive field properties with afferent and efferent connections. *J. Neurophysiol.* 38:1080–1098.

SINGER, W., F. TRETTER, and M. CYNADER, 1976. The effect of reticular stimulation on spontaneous and evoked activity in the cat visual cortex. *Brain Res.* 102:71–90.

SINGER, W., U. YINON, and F. TRETTER, 1979. Inverted monocular vision prevents ocular dominance shift in kittens and impairs the functional state of the visual cortex in adult cats. *Brain Res.* (in press).

SINGER, W., J. ZIHL, and E. PÖPPEL, 1977. Subcortical control of visual thresholds in humans: Evidence for modality specific and retinotopically organized mechanisms of selective attention. *Exp. Brain Res.* 29:173–190.

STONE, T. W., 1972. Cholinergic mechanisms in the rat somatosensory cerebral cortex. *J. Physiol.* 225:485–499.

SUMITOMO, I., M. NAKAMURA, and K. IWAMA, 1976. Location and function of the so-called interneurons of the rat lateral geniculate body. *Exp. Neurol.* 51:110–123.

SZENTÁGOTHAI, J., 1973. Synaptology of the visual cortex. In *Handbook of Sensory Physiology*, vol. VII/3B, R. Jung, ed. Berlin, Heidelberg, New York: Springer-Verlag, pp. 269–324.

SZERB, J. C., 1967. Cortical acetylcholine release and electroencephalic arousal. *J. Physiol.* 192:329–343.

TOYAMA, K., K. MATSUNAMI, T. OHNO, and S. TOKASHIKI, 1974. An intracellular study of neuronal organization in the visual cortex. *Brain Res.* 21:45–66.

TRETTER, F., M. CYNADER, and W. SINGER, 1975. Cat parastriate cortex: A primary or secondary visual area? *J. Neurophysiol.* 38:1098–1113.

WATANABE, S., M. KONISHI, and O. D. CREUTZFELDT, 1966. Postsynaptic potentials in the cat's visual cortex following electrical stimulation of afferent pathways. *Exp. Brain Res.* 1:272–283.

WEIGHT, F. F., 1974. Physiological mechanisms of synaptic modulation. In *The Neurosciences: Third Study Program*, F. O. Schmitt and F. G. Worden, eds. Cambridge, MA: MIT Press, pp. 929–941.

WEIGHT, F. F., and J. VOTAVA, 1970. Slow synaptic excitation in sympathetic ganglion cells: Evidence for synaptic inactivation of potassium conductance. *Science* 170:755–758.

WIESEL, T. N., and D. H. HUBEL, 1963. Single-cell responses in striate cortex of kittens deprived of vision in one eye. *J. Neurophysiol.* 26:1003–1017.

WILSON, P. D., J. PECCI-SAAVEDRA, and R. W. DOTY, 1973. Mesencephalic control of lateral geniculate nucleus in primates. II. Effective loci. *Exp. Brain Res.* 18:204–213.

ZIHL, J., E. PÖPPEL, and D. VON CRAMON, 1977. Diurnal variation of visual field size in patients with postretinal lesions. *Exp. Brain Res.* 27:245–249.

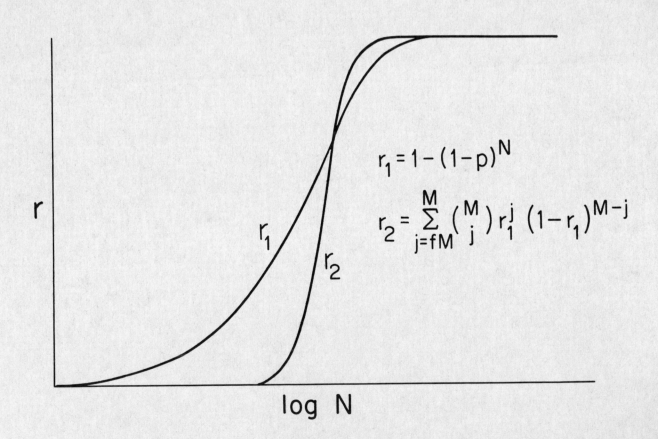

$$r_1 = 1 - (1-p)^N$$

$$r_2 = \sum_{j=fM}^{M} \binom{M}{j} r_1^j (1-r_1)^{M-j}$$

A THEORY OF

HIGHER BRAIN

FUNCTION

Dependency of two forms of recognition function on the number N *of elements in a repertoire, calculated according to a simple model. In this model, each element is assigned a constant a priori probability* p *of recognizing a randomly chosen signal. Here* r_1 *represents the expected fraction of all possible signals that will be recognized, and* r_2 *represents the probability that more than a fraction* f *(in this case 63%) of the* M *possible signals will be recognized. The shape of the curve is not sensitive to the value chosen for* M *if* M *is large. Similarly, if* p *is changed, the entire curve shifts left or right, reflecting the altered specificity of recognition, but the shapes of the curves do not change significantly. A more realistic model would assign different* p *values to different repertoire elements; this would increase the computational complexity, but the nature of the dependency of* r *upon* N *would not be fundamentally altered.*

68 Group Selection and Phasic Reentrant Signaling: A Theory of Higher Brain Function

GERALD M. EDELMAN

Introduction

THE REMARKABLE DIVERSITY of nervous systems in various animal species and their exquisite capacity for adaptive function are both intriguing and confounding to neurobiologists. Despite their complexity, however, all nervous systems appear to obey similar general principles at the level of morphological expression of neuronal structures and in their mechanisms of signal transmission. The recognition of these general principles and their application to the study of simple nervous systems as well as to subsystems in more complex brains have been among the greatest triumphs of neurobiology in this century (Quarton, Melnechuk, and Schmitt, 1967; Schmitt, 1970; Schmitt and Worden, 1974; Kuffler and Nicholls, 1977).

At the functional level, however, fundamental and methodological confusion still reigns. In many cases, the function of subsystems is only obscurely defined. Indeed, for higher brain functions expressed in perception, in awareness or consciousness, and in complex cognitive acts, the relation of nervous system structure and function has until recently (Eccles, 1966a) been a ground left mainly to philosophical speculation. At best, it has been the subject of psychological investigation under a variety of deliberately limited paradigms such as classical or instrumental conditioning, genetic epistemology, or linguistic analysis (Herrnstein and Bornig, 1965; Skinner, 1966; Piaget, 1950, 1954; Lenneberg, 1970). These efforts, while worthy, do not directly address the most challenging problem of neurobiology: the determination of the structural substrates and cellular mechanisms of higher brain functions, particularly those underlying consciousness.

Recent progress in the analysis of perception prompts the hope that the situation will improve in the next several decades. The pioneering studies of Mountcastle (1957, 1967) on sensory processing, of Hubel and Wiesel (1974) on visual processing, and of Sperry (1970a) on localization of brain function in the cerebral hemispheres are major developments relating cellular and neuronal activities to the performance of complex perceptual and conceptual tasks.

Despite these developments, the higher-order neural processing that leads to thinking, consciousness, and preparation for future acts has not been satisfactorily described in terms that explicitly take into account the details of brain structure. This is hardly surprising; the complexity of mammalian neuronal systems and their behavioral repertoires is enormous, and it would be premature to elaborate a detailed theory to account for their function. It may not be premature, however, to ask a more general question related to the evolution, development, and function of higher brain systems, particularly those in man: Does the brain operate according to a single principle in carrying out its higher-order cognitive functions? That is, despite the manifold differences in brain subsystems and the particularities of their connections, can one discern a general mechanism or principle that is required for the realization of cognitive faculties? If so, at what level does the mechanism operate—cells, molecules, or circuits of cells?

It is my purpose here to suggest such a principle on both theoretical and experimental grounds. After describing this principle and relating it to some of the available facts, I shall consider its application to an understanding of higher brain states with an emphasis on consciousness. The basic idea is that the

GERALD M. EDELMAN Rockefeller University, New York, NY 10021 brain is a *selective* system that processes sensorimotor information through the temporally coordinated interactions of collections or repertoires of functionally equivalent units each consisting of a small group of neurons. According to the model developed here, the brain processes sensory signals and its own stored information upon this selective base in a phasic (cyclic) and reentrant manner that is capable of generating the necessary conditions for conscious states.

In constructing a theory to account for higher brain function, several minimal criteria must be met:

1. The theory must be consistent with neuroanatomical, embryological, and neurophysiological information.

2. It must account for the distributive properties of memory and learning, for associative recall, as well as for the temporal properties and temporal "scale" of recall.

3. It must permit updating of memory to accord with current inputs.

4. It must reflect the main functions of higher brain systems as mediators between action and experience.

5. It must provide the necessary, if not the sufficient, conditions for awareness.

A number of theories meet some of these criteria but not all. Moreover, no current theory attempts to relate the embryonic development of the brain to its mature higher functions in any consistent fashion. This will be one of the major goals of the present formulation. At the same time, the theory will be couched in terms that are as general as possible. While this will result in a neuroanatomically impoverished model, in the sense that most circuit details will be left out, a deliberate effort will be made to avoid abstract model building that generates functional properties without reference to the nervous system.

Selection and its premises

In order to understand the idea of selection, it is useful to consider two extreme modes of possible brain function. In the first mode, the higher brain centers are connected in a rigorously defined and determinate fashion (Brodal, 1975), but they cannot function until properly transduced and processed sensory inputs instruct the circuitry to undergo stable changes in an equally unambiguous and determinate fashion. This instruction could operate at the level of molecules, synapses, cells (particularly cell membranes), or large groups of cells. The instructional mode has two characteristics: (1) the informational structure of the outside signal is primary and there-

fore necessary for the elaboration of the appropriately coded brain structure and for its function; and (2) there are no prior or preexisting states of the brain structure already capable of processing such a signal. Instruction implies that the interaction between brain structures and the first presentation of the signal is unique and determinate; that is, only following the signal input is a functioning brain structure or circuit formed that uniquely "corresponds" to sensory information of that kind.

Such an instructive model of higher brain function faces a number of difficulties. Instruction requires a precise mapping of corresponding information at either the molecular level (in terms of templates, for example) or the cellular level (in terms of an unambiguous and stable code). For instruction to occur, it would be necessary for each complex sensory event to result in storage of a particular *precise* complementary pattern that did not previously exist in the molecules or cells of the brain. New sensory events with some elements in common with previous events would have to share components of previous patterns or else lay down entirely new corresponding patterns. In the former case, successive experiences would require a higher-order mechanism for distinguishing old elements from new, and in the latter, the risk of exhausting the informational potential of the system would be great.

In general, the information that is processed in the brain arrives as a set of electrical or chemical signals whose molecular modes of production are already specified. It is difficult to understand on chemical grounds how either action potentials, graded potentials, or chemical transmitters could directly specify a stable pattern of complex coded information in macromolecules. Moreover, groups of cells cannot easily be "templated"—a variety of genetic, epigenetic, and transient alterations that are known to occur would threaten the stability of any unique circuit set up by outside instruction. Finally, an instructive theory of brain function would give no basis for understanding apparently autonomous higher activities such as conscious awareness and the creative programming of future events. In a sense, it puts the brain too much at the mercy of the outside world.

The alternative view is that the brain is a selective system, a proposal made by several authors, but without extensive elaboration (Jerne, 1967; Edelman, 1975; Young, 1975). Although the meaning of "selective" is best made clear by considering the detailed requirements of such a system, it may be useful to start off with a preliminary definition. "Selection" implies that after ontogeny and early development, the brain contains cellular configurations that can already respond discriminatingly to outside signals because of their genetically determined structures or because of epigenetic alterations that have occurred independently of the structure of outside signals. These signals serve merely to select among preexisting configurations of cells or cell groups in order to create an appropriate response.

Such selective notions have been prevalent in different forms in both evolutionary theory and immunology (Edelman, 1974a) and are understood in greater or lesser detail. The project I have set myself here, however, is not simply to make comparisons or analogies among these systems, but rather to explore whether a particular form of selection provides a basis for explaining higher brain function. A consideration of the general requirements and consequences of the operation of selective systems is nonetheless important, and in this context occasional comparisons with other systems may be useful.

Before discussing these requirements, it is necessary to specify briefly the level at which selection acts as well as to justify the theoretical need for selective mechanisms of brain function. Accordingly, the proposals made here rest on one experimental premise and one theoretical premise:

1. The main unit of function and selection in the higher brain is a group of cells (consisting of perhaps 50–10,000 neurons) connected in a large variety of ways but not necessarily in accord with the assumptions of the classical neuron doctrine (Bullock, 1959; Bodian, 1962). The grounds for altering these assumptions have been reviewed by Shepherd (1972) on the basis of work on the olfactory bulb and the retina. Additional evidence to support the cell group as the unit of selection comes from the work of Mountcastle (1957, 1967) and Hubel and Wiesel (1974), demonstrating both the existence and function of columns or slabs of cortical cells in sensory projection areas. A further (and so far hypothetical) assumption made here is that, in certain cortical areas, these groups of cells need not be connected in an absolutely fixed fashion from animal to animal and region to region; instead, local circuit neurons (LCNs) provide a very large variety of ways in which groups of cells may be connected both electrically and chemically (Schmitt, Dev, and Smith, 1976). A useful distinction can be made here. *Intrinsic connections* exist within a neuronal group and can involve a variety of modes of interaction within a local circuit, including all modes of nonsynaptic interaction. *Extrinsic connections* include all those outside a neuronal group, particularly those between groups. It is mainly

at the level of intrinsic connections that we assume great variability from group to group. Although some variability of extrinsic connections may exist, it is clear that at this level, the connectivity of the brain is quite specific and highly architectonic.

2. The nervous system of animals capable of carrying out complex sensorimotor acts can successfully adapt to complexes of informational input that have never before been encountered in the history of an individual or of its species. This premise is difficult to prove but is probably most defensible in man. Perhaps the most dramatic examples are the capacities of some individuals to solve highly abstract problems in mathematics, to generate new symbol structures of the complexity of a symphony, or to analyze such unique structures in a surprisingly efficient fashion upon seeing them for the first time.

This extraordinary capacity poses problems for both instructive and selective theories. On the surface, instructive theories can evade the problem by posing successive templates at higher and higher levels in the hierarchical organization of the brain; but this merely makes such theories seem all the more unlikely. On the other hand, to account for such grand feats of information processing, selective theories might be required to posit a very large repertoire of different preexisting functional units or neuronal groups. Is such a repertoire possible? In order to answer this question, we must extensively consider the nature and requirements of a selective theory of brain function.

The requirements of group selection and the need for degeneracy

It is clear from both evolutionary and immunological theory (Edelman, 1975) that in facing an unknown future the fundamental requirement for successful adaptation is preexisting diversity. This is achieved in evolution by mutation and gene flow and in immunological systems by a somatically generated antibody repertoire. For the nervous system, we may define a *primary repertoire* as a diverse collection of neuronal groups whose different functions are already prespecified during ontogeny and development. Without further specification at this point, we shall assume that if a neuronal group responds with characteristic output more or less specifically to an input consisting of a particular spatiotemporal configuration of signals, there is a "match" between that group and the signal configuration. In order to refine further the notion of selection from a repertoire of such neuronal groups, it is essential to consider the general requirements upon such a repertoire, particularly its diversity.

The first requirement is that this repertoire be sufficiently large; that is, it must contain enough diverse elements so that, given a wide range of different input signals, a finite probability exists of finding at least one matching element in the repertoire for each signal. Furthermore, for at least some elements of the repertoire, the match with input must be sufficiently specific to distinguish among different input signals (that is, to "recognize" them) with relatively low error. In the case of the immune system, this is accomplished by a repertoire of at least 10^6 different antibody molecules, each with a particular (or sterically defined) antigen-binding site, as well as by certain thresholding mechanisms controlling the immune response (Edelman, 1974b).

What are the general properties of such a large recognition repertoire that would render it capable of both a wide range of recognition and specificity for individual signals? First, for any arbitrarily chosen large number of different input signals, there must be a significantly larger number of components in the repertoire (Figure 1). Let a "match" be defined in terms of some threshold of recognition that gives the system the capacity to distinguish two closely related events within certain limits of error. If there

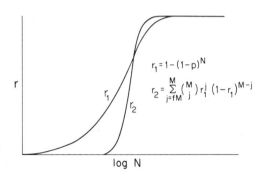

FIGURE 1   Dependency of two forms of recognition function on the number N of elements in a repertoire, calculated according to a simple model. In this model, each element is assigned a constant a priori probability p of recognizing a randomly chosen signal. Here r_1 represents the expected fraction of all possible signals that will be recognized, and r_2 represents the probability that more than a fraction f (in this case 63%) of the M possible signals will be recognized. The shape of the curve is not sensitive to the value chosen for M if M is large. Similarly, if p is changed, the entire curve shifts left or right, reflecting the altered specificity of recognition, but the shapes of the curves do not change significantly. A more realistic model would assign different p values to different repertoire elements; this would increase the computational complexity, but the nature of the dependency of r upon N would not be fundamentally altered.

are N elements in the repertoire and there is a probability p of a match between any such element and any signal, then we may define a recognition function $r = f(p, N)$ that measures the effectiveness of the system in recognizing a range of possible input signals. Several such functions can be defined, depending upon the particular measure of effectiveness chosen.

Now it is clear that if N is small, then for a large number of different inputs, r will be close to zero. For N above a certain number, r increases until, at some high value of N, a significant increase in the efficacy of matching under the threshold condition can no longer be achieved by a further increase in the size of the repertoire. This suggests that for the central nervous system, N must be large, but in itself it does not help us set any numerical limits. We may assume, however, that in a particular region of the human brain, a repertoire of 10^6 different cell groups, each consisting of 50–10,000 cells, would not exhaust the numbers of cells available.

A key consequence of this analysis is that the selective system for matching a signal or a configuration of signals to the repertoire must be degenerate. By *degeneracy* I mean that, in general, given a particular threshold condition, there must be more than one way of satisfactorily recognizing a given input signal. This implies the presence of multiple neuronal groups with different structures capable of carrying out the same function more or less well. I distinguish degeneracy from *redundancy*, which is used here strictly to imply the presence of repeated units or groups of *identical* structure.

The need for degeneracy is perhaps most easily seen by again assuming extreme cases, one without any degeneracy and the other with complete degeneracy (Figure 2). Consider a repertoire in which, for

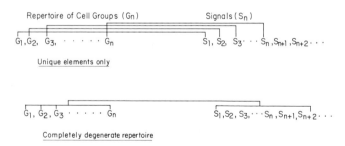

FIGURE 2   Two extreme cases of repertoires having unique (nondegenerate) and completely degenerate elements. In the first case, extension of the range of signals to be recognized (for example, beyond S_n) leads to a frequent failure of recognition. In the second, there is a loss of specificity and a frequent failure to distinguish different signals inasmuch as each G can respond to all signals.

any one arbitrarily chosen input signal, there is only one cell group capable of recognizing that signal. Under these conditions, in a system capable of recognizing previously unencountered signals, there must ensue a failure of range; that is, many inputs would go unrecognized. If we insist that a wide range of different previously unencountered signals be recognized and distinguished with high frequency by such a repertoire, then the fundamental requirement that there be no participation of the signal in forming the repertoire would have to be breached. Now consider the other extreme—that *every* element in the repertoire match *any* input signal. In this case, the range requirement would be satisfied, but there would be a severe loss of specificity and consequently of the capacity to distinguish between two different but closely related signal patterns. The composition of the repertoire must therefore be so constituted as to fall between these extremes, so that there are several (and possibly many) different cell groups capable of distinguishing a given input more or less well (that is, sufficiently above the threshold requirement for recognition).

The foregoing analysis suggests that degeneracy is a property fundamental to reconciling specificity of recognition with range of recognition. As we shall see, degeneracy is also consistent with a number of the observed properties of the central nervous systems of man and certain other animal species. As shown in Figure 3, degeneracy is different from strict redundancy but can include redundancy as a special case. Like redundancy, degeneracy can act to provide reliability in a system composed of unreliable components (von Neumann, 1956; Winograd and Cowan, 1963).

Besides these requirements on properties of the

Redundancy

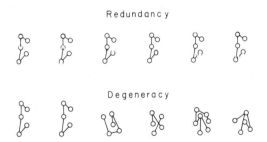

Degeneracy

FIGURE 3 Diagrams illustrating the distinction between redundancy and degeneracy. The structures of degenerate groups carrying out more or less the same function can differ in many respects, sharing only certain common features among their elements: degenerate groups are isofunctional but nonisomorphic. Redundancy is used here in the strict sense: redundant groups are isofunctional and isomorphic.

repertoire, there is another major requirement for the successful operation of a selective recognition system: a sufficiently large portion of the repertoire must be polled efficiently by various input signals. As in polling a network of computer terminals, the relevant signals must be able to encounter matching elements in the repertoire with a suitably high probability in a sufficiently short time. Moreover, the responses of such elements must be made available to higher-order elements for subsequent recognition events. Obviously this requirement must be met in the CNS by the various connections within and among cell groups. There is no dearth of such connections via either tracts or local circuit neurons, and the efficiency of signal transmission as well as its high signal-to-noise ratio would appear to allow the polling of large numbers of groups in short time periods (msec to sec). Furthermore, it is important to recognize that the total range of afferent inputs is not a random sample of all possible signals from the external world. At early levels of processing, a given input signal need not poll all neuron groups. The interface of sensory transducers with the world and the subsequent processing of their signals are themselves highly selective and thus enhance polling efficiency. We conclude that the CNS is highly efficient with respect to the polling and encounter requirement as compared to the immune system, in which encounter occurs by diffusion, flow, and cell movement.

In addition to the need for a large degenerate repertoire and high encounter probability, there is a third major requirement on a selective system. This is expressed in the need for *amplification* of a selective recognition event so that it can be stored, read out, and reflected stably in a favorable bias of the system for future recognition of the same event. At best, failure of amplification would result in only a transient match after encounter, with a small likelihood that the same selected cell group would be matched in future repetitions of the signal; at worst, it would result in a complete loss of matching in competition with other signals. In the immune system, amplification is achieved by maturation, cell division, and enhanced antibody synthesis by the progeny of selected cells. The net result is a gain of up to 10^5–10^6 in the production of the kind of antibody initially selected and an increase through cell division in the *repertoire frequency* of cells carrying antibodies of that type. In the nervous system, however, there is no neuronal cell division in the mature animal, and amplification presumably must be achieved by synaptic alterations that lead to facilitation of excitation or to suppression of particular pathways. For the present purposes, it is not important whether this occurs by formation of new synaptic contacts or by stable changes at already existing contacts (for example, by membrane changes at dendritic spines or by chemical alterations that change the thresholds of preexisting synaptic connections).

In accord with the amplification requirement, a central assumption in the present theory is that after initial selection, certain cell groups in the repertoire have a higher probability than others of being selected again by a similar or identical signal pattern. This can arise by synaptic facilitation or inhibition of pathways either within a cell group or between cell groups. This change in likelihood either enhances the probability of subsequent selection of some cell groups or reduces the probability that other cell groups will respond. In other words, selection can be either positive or negative. It is important to note, however, that after selection of groups in a degenerate primary repertoire of sufficient size, there would still remain other unselected cell groups of similar specificities. In general, these would have unchanged probabilities of being encountered and selected by repetition of some stimulus that had previously altered the probabilities of response of other cell groups.

Group-degenerate selection in the brain

With this background, we can now specify in more detail the system of group-degenerate selection that we suppose to have been evolved for higher brain functions. To begin with, the discussion will be limited to cortical areas, the thalamus, and the limbic system; the function of other parts of the neuraxis can then be considered in perspective.

The first question of importance is: What does the CNS recognize?—that is, what is the elementary substrate for higher brain function? Beyond the level of the interaction of an outside signal with sensory receptors, which can operate in a linear or nonlinear fashion (Mountcastle, 1957, 1967), the assumption here will be that the substrates for recognition are the spatiotemporal patterns of spikes and graded potentials (and their chemical concomitants) occurring in *groups of neurons*. By *recognition* I mean the selective and characteristic discriminative response of one or more groups of neurons to such patterns initiated or present in other groups to which they have access. The response of such recognizing groups is manifested in alterations in their further patterns of firing and in stable or metastable synaptic changes. A theoretical account of the possible internal properties of

neuronal groups, on which recognition between groups might be based, has been given by Wilson and Cowan (1973). It is important to stress that the present assumptions do not exclude recognition of the state of a single neuron in a hierarchy. In general, however, the patterns recognized by cell groups are assumed to be those generated by other groups. Some support for this position is obtained from the studies of Hubel and Wiesel (1974) on feature detection in the striate cortex and associated areas.

Although the neuroanatomical evidence for cell groups in other regions is sparse, it may be useful for clarity to review more extensively the notions of cell group, repertoire, and recognition against the background of previous analyses (Bullock, 1961). A cell group is considered to be a collection of contiguous neurons whose intrinsic connectivity is defined by events in ontogeny and development. The connections within a group are not random but are definite. Each such group may have divergent or convergent extrinsic connections to and from other such groups; these connections are also neuroanatomically defined and nonrandom. According to this notion, although a single neuron can rarely serve as a "group," randomly connected nets are excluded (Bullock, 1961). In accord with the distinctions made by Bullock (1961), a group could constitute a multiple-input metastable feedback loop consisting of a definitely specified meshwork of mutually interacting neurons. But several additional properties of groups are assumed here that have not been assumed by previous theorists (Bullock, 1961; Grüsser and Grüsser-Cornehls, 1976).

One of the most important is that groups form repertoires, that is, collections with diverse intrinsic connectivities but similar extrinsic connectivities. Such repertoires are prespecified during ontogeny and development and are degenerate with respect to recognition. Each group in a repertoire can act as a recognition unit carrying out one or more functions: encoding, decoding, identifying one of the lines of its extrinsic connectivity, timing signals, determining their strength or their rate of development or duration—all of which may be properties of signals from other cell groups. Of course, in most individual cases, the exact neural code is presently unknown.

If the extrinsic connectivity of a group is divergent, leading to many other groups, then the output of the group may poll the other groups more or less effectively depending upon a variety of factors such as signal pattern, signal strength, and local inhibition. As in the case of a jury, these groups may or may not respond characteristically to the input from the first group. If the extrinsic connectivity is convergent upon a group, a variety of responses may occur, including facilitation, differences in timing, or different response patterns, all depending upon the location and properties of the extrinsic connections. Thus a group can have different portals for input, and input to different combinations of these portals may or may not influence its response. Because of its patterns of intrinsic and extrinsic connectivity, a group has available to its neurons a variety of modes of interaction with external signals. In any event, each group is not pluripotent—rather, it has a limited set of characteristic spatiotemporal response patterns of firing as well as a characteristic set of connections to other groups.

Among the variabilities offered by such a set of connections, the most important in determining higher-order functions is that offered by the opportunity to alter intrinsic connectivity plastically at synapses ("commitment"), leading to stabilization of a particular output pattern. This will be discussed later in detail. The main point here is that alterations of this type, occurring mainly in the intrinsic synapses, would lead to favoring of certain intrinsic connectivities over others.

We may now consider a hierarchy of responses that, in its later stages, will be nonlinear because of the presence of feedback and feedforward loops with their associated alterations of temporal patterns and response times. Ignoring this nonlinearity for the moment, we consider the hierarchy

$$S \rightarrow R \rightarrow (R \text{ of } R)_n, \qquad n = 1, 2, 3, \ldots,$$

where S represents transduced sensory input from the environment (as but one example of input), R represents cortical cellular groups that can act as "recognizers" of that input (for example, groups of complex neurons in the striate cortex), and $(R \text{ of } R)$ represents groups of neurons in association cortex, or in temporal, frontal, or prefrontal cortex, that act as "recognizers of recognizers." According to this hierarchy, signals from neuronal groups of R (for example, a column) can be recognized by groups in $(R$ of $R)$. But it must be emphasized that at this higher level of recognition, the candidate neuronal groups in $(R \text{ of } R)$ form only a degenerate subset of all $(R$ of $R)$ cell groups (Figure 4a). That is, there is more than one group in $(R \text{ of } R)$ that can recognize a particular group in R; the response is based on the possibility of divergence and on multiple degenerate representation, providing together for the adequate recognition of R groups by the $(R$ of $R)$ repertoire. Note also that the arrows in this scheme do not necessarily imply unidirectional flow of information, but

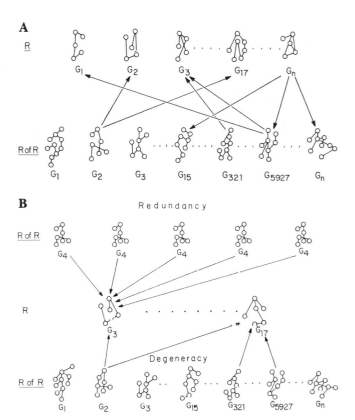

FIGURE 4   Interactions of degenerate groups in two repertoires, R and $(R$ of $R)$. Arrows connecting groups indicate recognition but do not necessarily imply unidirectional flow of information. (A) Degenerate recognition emphasizing bidirectional many–one relationships. (B) Contrast between redundancy and degeneracy in $(R$ of $R)$. Increase of redundant elements can only increase efficiency; for example, because of its structure and function, G_4, a strictly redundant group of $(R$ of $R)$, can never recognize G_{17} in R.

merely an initial sequence for recognition events. Indeed, the scheme must not be considered as strictly or exclusively hierarchical. Parallel organization is obviously of equal importance since it makes possible the output to action (motor response, neurohumoral response) from any level. The scheme also assumes that general properties of the input can be recognized early in the sequence $S \rightarrow R \rightarrow (R \text{ of } R)$.

We may summarize at this point by saying, somewhat loosely, that beyond the level of sensory transduction and sensory processing, the CNS recognizes *modes of itself* selectively and in a nonlinear and degenerate fashion. It is revealing to ask whether such degenerate recognition could be successfully accomplished by isomorphic or strictly redundant cell groups in $(R$ of $R)$. Provided that the threshold requirement for recognition does not imply absolute specificity, but only distinctions among classes of similar patterns, the answer is no, for the reasons adduced in the previous section (Figure 4b). Instead, a significant number of different but isofunctional cell groups, any one of which can respond to the class of patterns in R, is required. This implies that the same pattern can be recognized in more than one way and, indeed, that in successive presentations of the same pattern, different combinations of cell groups (R of R) would respond. Furthermore, there is no need to assume a priori that such groups necessarily have similar numbers or types of neurons.

Such a picture of neuronal groups selected from a degenerate repertoire must be distinguished from that of a fixed pattern of preprogrammed response that might occur in a single ganglion, and also from simple redundancy of neurons in subsystems such as the ganglia or nuclear cell masses in the brain. While these organizations are undoubtedly present in the brain, they cannot generate the kinds of responses produced by a degenerate repertoire.

So far I have only casually distinguished between the initial stable state and the ensuing responsive states of the subsets of cell groups in such a repertoire. According to the theory, the repertoire just described can be considered a *primary repertoire* formed during ontogeny and early development as a consequence of differentiation events leading to synaptic connectivity, both locally and in long pathways. As pointed out earlier, however, unless some form of stable amplification (or inhibition) of the responses of cell groups could occur in this repertoire, there would be no possibility for alteration of its properties as a result of experienced input. It would merely fluctuate reversibly in its selective response with varying relaxation times. It is at this point that we must suppose that the selection of certain subgroups results in an alteration of the probability that these subgroups will be selected again upon a repeated presentation of a similar stimulus pattern. As mentioned previously, this is assumed to occur as a result of synaptic alteration of some or all cells in a group so that intrinsic or extrinsic connectivity is functionally altered. This would be expected to occur mainly within the intrinsic connectivity of a group, with a concomitant change in its transfer functions, for example. The probability of selection could be decreased (inhibition) or increased (excitation, facilitation). In either case, a sufficient repetition of input within a given time is assumed to alter the likelihood of future selections of certain previously selected subgroups over their neighbors, a process that produces a *secondary repertoire*. Thus a secondary repertoire is a collection of different higher-order neuronal groups whose internal or external synaptic function has been altered by selection and commitment during experience. Moreover, repetition of input need not be confined to external signals, but may include reentrant inputs from the brain itself.

One might visualize such a nonlinear, many–one, time-dependent, and degenerate response in the fashion shown in Figure 5, where the superscripts refer to the successive patterned states and the subscripts refer to different cell groups in the repertoire. An enhanced probability of positive or negative selection is represented in the figure by a heavy arrow.

Alteration of this probability may also be connected with the threshold for recognition events. Cell groups with higher repetition rates of response may, because they have a better "fit" with input, be stabilized more effectively. This may be achieved intrinsically, but more likely by means of escape from inhibition. At the same time, an inhibitory signal that suppressed some recognizing cell groups having less response to the original input would effectively sharpen the specificity of the overall response and also enhance its stabilization. Thus cell group selection may occur in a filtered fashion—first by stimulation of groups that react more or less well and then by inhibition (or competitive exclusion) of those selected groups with an insufficient response in relation to some threshold (Figure 6).

We may now ask about the overall properties of such a system and then consider the evidence for the

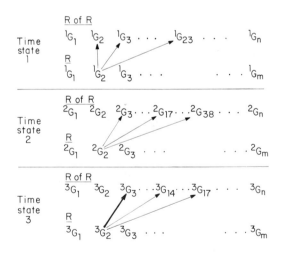

FIGURE 5 Variations of degenerate recognition with time depending upon polling and range of repertoires. Commitment or stable synaptic alteration of cells in (R of R) groups (indicated by a heavy arrow) occurs after repetition of recognition in different time states. Commitment is reflected in the increased probability of a subsequent response by certain groups in R. Superscripts on groups identify successive time states.

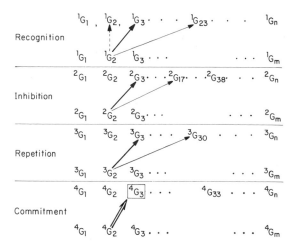

Recognition

Inhibition

Repetition

Commitment

FIGURE 6 Fixation of responses in a degenerate network by a combination of discriminatory inhibition and commitment, raising the probability of response and leading to entrance of $(R$ of $R)$ group G_3 into a secondary repertoire as marked by the box. Dashed line: weak recognition. Solid line: good recognition. Thick line: excellent recognition. Double line: commitment.

existence of candidate cell groups having such properties. Obviously the alterations of selective probabilities represent a memory phenomenon; what has not been emphasized in Figure 6 is the associative nature of this memory (Longuet-Higgins, Willshaw, and Berneman, 1970) that results from the properties of degenerate selection. In a later section, this will be extensively discussed in connection with the conditions for consciousness. A brief consideration of associative memory in degenerate systems may serve here to set the stage for that discussion.

Association involves an ordering such that presentation in input of various attributes of an object results in a linkage between these attributes in output (Figure 7). A whole group of such orderings in storage can form an associative memory if the means of access and readout are available. In the ideal case, presentation in the proper context of any one of a

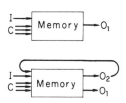

FIGURE 7 Representation of an associative memory in which input patterns I (for example, signals from cell groups) in a context C (representing background, inhibition, or other patterns) results in related output patterns O. Output patterns such as O_2 may be reentered as input in such a system.

set of stored items in an input should elicit recall of part or all of that set. Under certain conditions, related items not in that set should also be able to elicit that recall. In the brain, it is likely that this type of storage is content-addressable and that access is simultaneous and parallel.

A degenerate collection of cell groups has a number of features that could lead to association and yield a memory with such properties. Certain neuronal groups may recognize a given signal pattern only more or less well. Indeed, some of these groups may be capable of recognizing some other signal pattern better than the one to which they have responded in a particular event. This raises the possibility that two different events may elicit responses from the same group as well as simultaneously eliciting responses from completely different groups (Figure 8). Moreover, if the probability of response of all of these groups is altered by multiple presentations, there is an increased likelihood of their being excited together on future presentations of either signal event. Inasmuch as these groups may have different neuroanatomical connections, the association with other groups responding to additional signals would be further enhanced.

Presentation of two similar but not identical patterns to a degenerate collection of cell groups may stimulate a common subset of groups in that collection as well as different subsets unique to each pattern (Figure 9). If the common subset is connected to other neuronal groups, an association of the responses of those groups to that of the shared subset can be made. Moreover, sequential presentation of two related patterns can elicit the same responses by activating that subset, and $(R$ of $R)$ groups reading any of the subsets may thus become associated.

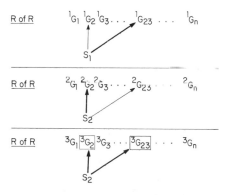

FIGURE 8 Association resulting from degenerate recognition and commitment for two unrelated signals S_1 and S_2. Heavy and light arrows indicate degree of recognition. Groups in squares are committed to secondary repertoire.

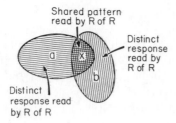

FIGURE 9 Reading, with association, of different collections of groups elicited by a structurally similar pair of input patterns, *a* and *b*. Collections of cell groups recognizing the patterns are marked by *a* and *b*; the shared subset of responding groups is marked by *x*. Different (*R* of *R*) groups reading these patterns may become associated in their responses.

There is the additional possibility that recognition of a cell group pattern requires only part of the intrinsically connected neuronal set within the recognizing group, leaving another part free for other recognitions. This is a special case akin to recognition by two spatially different groups. But because of local connectivity, it raises further opportunities for particular kinds of association by recombination of features within a group.

In discussing association, we must also consider the degree of hierarchical nesting possible in selective recognition events in associative systems of this kind. By *nesting* I mean the number of successive recognitions across different levels of organization such as *R* and (*R* of *R*). Although nested recognition can occur, the scheme has no implicit or necessary hierarchical restriction. An (*R* of *R*) subgroup can selectively "recognize" another (*R* of *R*) subgroup; recognition is not limited to cell groups of another level, such as *R*. This leads to the possibility of a reading *of* the states of cell groups whose probability of response has been stably altered in previous selections *by* cell groups that have not been so altered. In view of the degenerate nature of the repertoire, it also implies that a given pattern can be "stored" in the response of several, and perhaps many, isofunctional but not necessarily isomorphic groups. This provides ample opportunity for associative interactions in the reflexive recognition of (*R* of *R*) groups. At the same time, however, it must be stressed that certain neuronal groups must always remain in the primary repertoire. Indeed, there may have to be some neurons that are incapable of commitment so that groups of which they are composed do not become fixed to a given pattern of response.

Another important general feature of a system of group-degenerate selection is its *distributive property*.

A particular stable selected state or response to an input pattern is not likely to be uniquely represented in only one cell group in one place. Indeed, beyond particular neuroanatomical restrictions, there is no requirement that selected isofunctional cell groups be contiguous. This is in accord with the observations of Lashley (1950) on the failure of transection and ablation of cortical regions to impair learned behaviors, but it does not imply that his notion of equipotentiality is correct. Indeed, one can imagine that in some cases, particular recognizer properties are present only in certain larger *regions* of the brain as a result of evolutionary selection and requirements for efficiency of neuronal communication. This would appear to be reflected in the match that is found between the functional adaptation and density of peripheral innervation and the amount and sophistication of the central representation linked to that periphery. This qualified picture of distributed neuronal groups is consistent with evidence for gross localization of function but is still in accord with the distribution of both memory and learning patterns. It is also consistent with the functional interaction of distant groups to yield complex brain functions, as detected after brain lesions and ablation experiments (Luria, 1973). There is evidence for great variation in the threshold for tolerance of tissue destruction of different cell groups (Russell and Espir, 1961), a fact also in accord with group-degenerate selection.

It is important to emphasize that in a selective system, degeneracy and diversity are more important than absolute repertoire size. The requirement for limiting large numbers of diverse cell groups in a degenerate repertoire (see Figure 1) is nonetheless consistent with the failure to find neuronal types that are radically different from normal in nanocephalics (Seckel, 1950) and the failure to correlate higher function with gross estimates of brain size. Below a certain number of cells, however, and in the absence of the opportunity to make certain synaptic connections, the repertoire would fail either to contain sufficiently degenerate subsets or to be polled by input patterns in an efficient manner.

Neither the distributive nor the associative property is unique to selective systems; various instructive models that have these properties have been proposed (Longuet-Higgins, Willshaw, and Berneman, 1970; Cooper, 1973). The group-degenerate selection model places more emphasis on the features of cell groups and less on the general properties of an overall network, however. Thus it strongly emphasizes the role of neuroanatomy and development as fundamental in constructing particular primary repertoires and particular kinds of connected cell groups.

It is important to stress how the notion of memory is altered by the concept of group-degenerate selection. Fixation of the responses of a cell within a group or of the whole group via several cells can alter selective patterns at any level of recognition. In terms of group-degenerate selection, memory is not a localized property of any particular region of the nervous system. Rather, it is a general reflection of the enhanced interaction of cell groups that contain selectively committed cells and their synapses. If one adds to this the possibilities of long-tract connectivity, the notion of an active storage with high associative power, and the concept of reentrant signaling (to be discussed below), there is no need to posit memory as a property of a given region or as an exclusive emergent property of some particular higher brain function. Whatever the microscopic or molecular mechanism of memory or cell interaction (for example, new dendritic connections, metastable membrane and cell surface changes in dendritic spines, molecular alterations of synapses), this property is an obligate consequence of group-degenerate selection and must therefore be a property of neurons as they function in cell groups. Memory readout is not posed as a special problem; the *process* does not differ from other forms of neuronal communication in the group-degenerate system.

What can we say about the neuronal substrate for repertoire degeneracy? There is an emerging realization that in higher brain centers such as the olfactory bulb (Shepherd, 1972), the law of dynamic polarity associated with the classical neuron doctrine fails. Instead, the picture of a highly diverse set of dendritodendritic, axodendritic, axosomatic, and dendritosomatic connectivities emerges. This picture is likely to be seen in other cortical regions, and together with the evidence of Golgi II neuron interactions, and the impressive increase in the number of LCNs during phylogeny and in ascending the neuraxis (Rakic, 1975), it suggests an anatomical view entirely consistent with group-degenerate selection. The development of the neocortex appears to have been accomplished by a large increase in the number of cell columns or units as well as in their interconnections. In addition to the anatomy of cortical areas (Chow and Leiman, 1970; Peters, Paley, and Webster, 1976), that of certain limbic and reticular formation areas (Isaacson and Pribram, 1975a) is also consistent with the features of a degenerate repertoire.

While repertoires of cell groups are not random, there is a large opportunity for individual variation

in different regions and in different individual brains. Nevertheless, according to the theory, different brains should be able to carry out a particular recognition event with equal effectiveness even though, in their functional history, different isofunctional subgroups were selected (Figure 10). The consequence of the presence of degeneracy is therefore a high degree of diversity and individuality. This provides for rare or unusual fluctuations in the neural repertoires of certain individuals.

According to the present theory, embryogenesis and development provide a first repertoire; early learning and selective interactions lead to development of a second repertoire via chemical facilitation and memory processes. After several selective events, the statistics of the primary repertoire are altered so that a secondary repertoire of selected cell groups emerges. Although the statistics of repertoire response are thereby altered, a large number of possibilities still remain open. Cell groups in this secondary repertoire would, in general, have a higher likelihood of undergoing repeated selection by similar inputs than would isofunctional groups in the primary repertoire. It must be emphasized, however, that this is only a probabilistic statement; upon repeated presentation of a signal, groups in the primary repertoire could still undergo selection in preference to those in the secondary repertoire in response to a variety of circumstances. In any case, for a given input pattern at any time, primary repertoire groups capable of specific recognition of a given signal would still far outnumber those in the secondary repertoire. But because of the previous operation of commitment

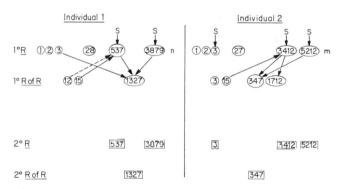

FIGURE 10 An illustration of the individuality of trace information during establishment of a secondary repertoire in different individuals given similar primary repertoires. Trace formation on differing neuroanatomical backgrounds could alter the encounter frequencies of cell groups represented by different numbers in different individuals. 1°R and 2°R denote primary and secondary recognizer repertoires; a similar notation is used for (R of R) repertoires.

and thresholding events, not many would be as "sharply tuned" to that signal.

The central neural construct is thus considered to be a result of two different selective processes: ontogenetic development of the first repertoire and selection by environmental interaction to form a second repertoire. The relationships of transition periods and critical periods in both processes—such as those explored by Blakemore (Blakemore and Van Sluyters, 1974) for Hubel and Wiesel neurons and by Piaget (1950, 1954) in the psychology of early growth and development—deserve extensive investigation in terms of these concepts.

Later I shall make some specific comments concerning the embryogenesis of the first repertoire. At this point, it may be more pertinent to summarize the process of second-repertoire formation. This process leads to formation of a unique trace of selection events, to an enhancement of the probability of reselection of elements of the second repertoire over those of the first, and to alterations of likelihoods of encounter thresholds, possibly at synapses. In such a system, the order of development of the second repertoire is very important. The number of cell groups, the number of cells, and the number of synapses possible in the CNS make for an extraordinarily large number of possibilities in forming a second repertoire. Regardless of the number of selective events, however, there would still remain a large, indeed a major, pool of uncommitted cell groups in the first repertoire.

The foregoing analysis bears on two key statements of Mountcastle (1976): "The central problem for brain physiology is how to understand the actions of large populations of neurons, actions that may not be wholly predictable from properties of subsets" and "The central problem of the intrinsic physiology of the cerebral cortex is to discover the nature of neuronal processing within the translaminar chains of interconnected cells (in columns)." In the light of the analysis so far, these statements might be transformed as follows: *The main problem of brain physiology is to understand the nature of repertoire building by populations of cell groups.* Of course, the solution of this problem requires a knowledge of transmission, polling, and encounter and of amplification and stabilization of synaptic events at the molecular level. The present theory is phenomenological in the sense that, at the level of description attempted here, it does not depend upon specification of these processes in great detail. This does not gainsay the need for an exact understanding of these processes; it simply stresses

that a variety of different solutions would be compatible with group-degenerate selection.

Reentrant selective signaling and the neural substrates for consciousness

So far this discussion of the degenerate selection of cell groups has ignored specific circuits of neuronal connections and their relation to particular higher brain functions. The task I shall undertake here is to consider the central problem of consciousness and to show how degenerate selection and cell-group signaling in a reentrant fashion can provide the necessary conditions for an explanation of this phenomenon at the cellular level. The problem of consciousness has resisted analysis in an experimental context until recently, and it still remains a formidable challenge. Perhaps no other subject has gathered around it so varied a set of speculations as consciousness: the mind-body problem (Campbell, 1970), the existence of spirits, the evaporation of the notion of "mind" by semantic analysis (Ryle, 1949), and the possibility of a pontifical neuron (Sherrington, 1941). Clearly there is a collective opinion that this brain function is somehow the central one that must be understood for a complete insight into learning and other higher functions.

Fortunately there are now some developments that allow us to narrow the issue. The experiments of Penfield (1975), Jasper (1966), and others (Isaacson and Pribram, 1975b) on the role of the reticular formation in arousal indicate that there are areas of the brain outside of the cortex that are necessary for consciousness. On the other hand, the experiments of Sperry (1970a) demonstrate that there are separate and specific hemispheric localizations of different brain functions related to consciousness. In addition, there is evidence that the hippocampal and limbic systems can function to distinguish novelty and read out short-term memory in a fashion that might modulate input to the conscious brain (Vinogradova, 1975). Perhaps the main impact of this and related work is that consciousness is *not* a property of the entire brain, but rather is a result of *processes* occurring in certain defined areas (admittedly gross), for example, the two cortical hemispheres, the thalamocortical radiations (Mountcastle, 1974), and the limbic and reticular systems. Nevertheless, the kinds of interactions that lead to consciousness remain unspecified.

The question therefore is: What are these interactions and what properties would they be expected to have? In attempting to answer this question, any proposed hypothesis obviously must not violate the laws of thermodynamics, posit entities that cannot be measured, or lead to an infinite regression of specified temporal recognition events. On the positive side, it must stress the main dynamic function of the brain in mediating between experience and action. In so doing, it must be able to account for updating of past storage and for the temporal properties of recall. Can any general model that includes group-degenerate selection be constructed that would meet these restrictions and account for a temporal sequence of conscious and recall states, the need for updating an informational store (MacKay, 1970), and the differentiation of immediate and long-term experience? And at its limit, could such a model be consistent with the distinction between self and non-self?

Among other things, such a model must specifically account for the continuity of perception, for temporal succession, and for the detection of novelty. The first decision to be made in building this model is whether to adopt a continuous or a discontinuous temporal mode of information processing. There are several reasons for choosing a discontinuous mode: (1) processing of any event must occur before awareness of it (that is, some output must be prepared before the outcome of a sensory input is decided); (2) there are stringent temporal constraints on recall that require the operation of a real-time clock; and (3) as discussed below, a discontinuous mode greatly simplifies our understanding of how coding for spatiotemporal continuity can occur in a degenerate selective system. These and other considerations to be discussed below suggest that the elementary processes leading to consciousness may be phasic, that is, they may require cyclic repetition of a sequence of neuronal events.

An approach to constructing a phasic model is illustrated in Figure 11. Suppose that some cell group in R receives sensory or sensorimotor information and that its action and storage are recognized by several cell groups in $(R$ of $R)$. At the same time, suppose that the same sensory input to the limbic and reticular centers is processed and relayed by the thalamus to the cortex to stabilize these particular $(R$ of $R)$ groups for several immediately subsequent events. By *stabilization* or *fixation* I mean in this context the continued firing of these groups in their typical patterns. This constitutes the first temporal phase of a cycle of input processing. Now suppose that in the succeeding phase, this processed signal is reentered

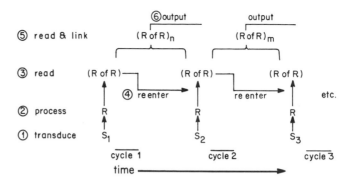

FIGURE 11 Reentrant signaling in the path from inputs S to recognizers R to "recognizers of recognizers" $(R$ of $R)$. The scheme indicates reentry in successive cycles; the temporal order of events within two successive cycles is indicated by numbers. The associative aspects of reentrant signaling are not indicated in this scheme (see Figure 12). $(R$ of $R)_n$ and $(R$ of $R)_m$ are higher-order associative neuronal groups whose output may reenter at later points, activate motor output, make associations, etc.

at a high level in the $S \rightarrow R \rightarrow (R$ of $R)$ information path of the next cycle. The reentered signal and new $(R$ of $R)$ signals from subsequent inputs are then read by $(R$ of $R)$ groups that make associations with stored patterns in $(R$ of $R)$ cell groups of the second repertoire as well as with groups in the first repertoire if there is any novelty. This constitutes the second or reentrant phase of input. Such a system is designed so that an internally generated signal is reentered *as if it were an external signal*. This is a key feature of the model, and it has two functions: to provide a means for dealing with novelty and to provide a match and a link between inner states and new sensory inputs of various modalities. In detail, it must be able to relate modalities as well as cross-correlate them. A possible means of accomplishing this will be described later.

As a result of reentry, this model assures that there will be continuity or linkage between successive phasic inputs. There is therefore no need for any higher-order recognition of the connection between states of objects as they are registered in time. This is an essential point: because of the degenerate nature of the selective system and its content-addressable nature, the absence of reentry might otherwise result in failure to associate successive properties as they are abstracted in time. Reentry guarantees that continuity in the neural construct is an obligate consequence of the spatiotemporal continuity of objects.

A second highly important property of this system is the capacity to assure the succession or order of associated $(R$ of $R)$ events for subsequent recall. Although orderly and precise sequencing is not an obligate condition for recall, it must be accounted for. We assume that the order of events in a context results in an order of association, so that recall of event 1 in (R of R) patterns is necessary for recall of event 2 and so on. The same "clock states" of the system required for the original integration and abstraction would then be used to call out this succession in the same measure and dimensions of real time. Obviously, however, the clock would only provide a real-time *base* for this process; recall need not take the same amount of time as the original events. The actual length of a reentrant cycle in real time will be discussed later.

Novelty of signals is dealt with in this system by comparison between reentrant and new signals in a cycle as well as by the fact that there are primary and secondary repertoires. Completely new information must activate primary repertoire. Match and mismatch of signal information may be accounted for by discriminating between activation of secondary repertoire and primary repertoire. The exact means by which the two repertoires are distinguished is not obvious, but frequency or latency properties may be sufficient to distinguish neuronal activity from each. The additional possibility that stored information in secondary repertoire is compared with new input in a highly efficient fashion to detect novelty cannot be neglected, however.

In the absence of a knowledge of the detailed anatomy, it is difficult to choose among the various circuits consistent with the scheme of reentrant signaling. But the theory does assume a certain minimal set of connections. Each afferent portal to the brain is linked first to a restricted set of R's located in the primary sensory cortex by connections that are mainly invariant. Divergence then occurs to (R of R) groups with greater or lesser specificity. The sensory signatures disappear at this point, and associative reentry leads to expression of higher functions by the many classes of (R of R) groups, which are no longer arranged sequentially. It is pertinent that the thalamocortical and corticothalamic radiations provide candidate circuits for portions of the reentry scheme (Mountcastle, 1974).

At this point, it is important to point out the conditions necessary for such a scheme to function and to describe some of its consequences. Assuming the proper anatomy for the moment, this scheme requires:

1. Recognition of R by (R of R) groups in temporal, frontal, and prefrontal regions. Under the scheme of selection, this is likely to involve neuronal divergence, rather than convergence, as a first step.

2. Pulsed states of input consistent with cerebral, thalamocortical, hippocampal, and limbic-reticular rhythms.

3. (R of R) subsets in secondary repertoire with stably altered synapses and transfer functions expressing committed patterns representing the storage of previous states.

4. Degenerate recognition of (R of R) cell groups by other (R of R) cell groups. At some level, convergence must also occur to provide an "abstract summary" or transform of complex patterns.

5. Stabilization of the selected (R of R) groups for at least one cycle (according to the present scheme, this is done via the limbic-reticular afferents in either a general or a specific fashion).

6. Short-term storage for holding patterns of "world inputs" (input state 1) and potentiality for storing reentrant "self inputs" (input state 2). Such storage allows for matching and association and is considered to be itself degenerate and widely distributed.

7. Linkage of (R of R) output to central states and to stored patterns concerned with the control of movement.

This model does not imply an infinite nest of recognizing neuronal groups. Indeed, since it depends upon comparisons between current input and stored states, and since associated degenerate groups are assumed to be available with similar recognition properties, it is not necessary that the same (R of R) cell group or groups recognize inputs in two successive cycles. The degeneracy of these groups would imply that the same input state could be recognized at different times by more than one such group. It is nevertheless important that *within* a cycle the same (R of R) groups be used, and a change of (R of R) groups must not interrupt the execution of a motor output pattern. As I shall describe in detail, awareness is considered to arise from the (R of R) repertoire having access to R and to stored multimodally generated states within itself. In turn, this access can lead to generation of associatively related signals, which are then processed again on the same input lines as an S signal; that is, the system is reentrant. The entire cycle provides for the possibility of modification by (R of R) output of the sensory input and its thresholds as well as for alteration of arousal and intentional or attentional states. The basic a priori condition for the conscious state is the ability to review the internal state by continual reentry of stored information. This review is obviously altered by the ability to recognize novelty and by states of arousal.

So far I have suggested that the conscious state requires the phasic recognition by degenerate (R of R) groups of signals representing the internal state of the organism and input. The discussion has centered on a rather artificial example of a single sensory signal of one modality. But it has not reemphasized a property of degenerate networks that is essential to their function in relation to conscious states: the associative nature of interactions among degenerate cell groups. Many of the neuronal cell groups called up by a given signal pattern match that pattern only more or less well. Moreover, these groups may contain neuronal configurations that can also recognize other, unrelated signal patterns more or less well; indeed, these other patterns might be recognized with even higher probabilities (or closer "fit") than the given pattern. This brings up the possibility that, because of their "unused" potential information, such cell groups have associative properties that allow them to interact with a variety of signals arising either from incoming information or from (R of R) store. Thus a cell group may be used more than once by different signals or may be used simultaneously by two signals. Evidence has in fact been obtained for multisensory input to a given cortical neuron (Eccles, 1966b), although this may be more concerned with level setting than with association.

The associative nature of the reentrant system would result in readout of groups of (R of R) neurons that represent past multimodal experiences. Indeed, one variant of the model (Figure 12) suggests that it is the readout of these groups in relation to current input that is essential for establishing the conscious state. Such associative properties raise the question of how the "correct" (R of R) groups in the store are made accessible for comparison with the output of R cell groups. One solution to this problem is to consider that the (R of R) groups that are in the secondary repertoire can recognize R states directly. This is possible if each such cell group has alternative configurations that allow responses to new signals in addition to those for which it was originally selected. A more specific (and I believe more attractive) alternative is that the (R of R) groups that recognize S via R also recognize the patterns of other (R of R) groups in storage. In any case, retrieval and comparison is not by means of random access; rather, it is related to a dense network of associative interactions that are enhanced in a degenerate system.

This associative potential may also be of impor-

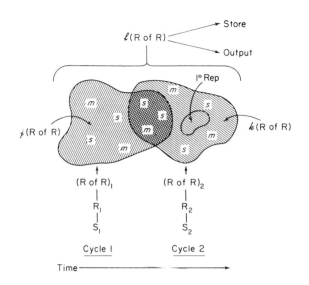

FIGURE 12 A diagram illustrating reentrant signals in two subsequent cycles to emphasize the associative multimodal readout of collections of groups containing stored patterns of past sensory inputs (s) or sensorimotor events (m). This readout is completed after the reentrant stage, thus linking the two successive patterns of (R of R) groups responding to R. Here $j(R$ of $R)$ and $k(R$ of $R)$ represent varying numbers of groups involved in the associative response to (R of R)_1 and (R of R)_2. The overlap of these groups (marked by the cross-hatched area) is related to similarities in S_1 and S_2. The area marked 1°Rep refers to the associative access to primary repertoire groups by new information contained in S_2. The $l(R$ of $R)$ neurons can store the result, output to other (R of R) groups, or call upon central routines for motor response. Continuity depends upon the linked reading of (R of R)_1 and (R of R)_2 and of the associative responses in $j(R$ of $R)$ and $k(R$ of $R)$. Novelty may be detected in part by differential response in the readout of neuronal groups in primary and secondary repertoires.

tance in considering another characteristic of the intact brain in relation to consciousness: the simultaneous *parallel processing* of a large variety of input signals of different modalities. One may imagine that when there are several inputs, S_1, S_2, S_3, . . . , each is handled in the fashion described for a single input. It is likely, however, that some inputs will overlap in time, albeit asynchronously. An important function of associative memory may involve recall of synesthetic components related to the simultaneous occurrence of associative signals arising from parallel and overlapping sensory inputs. Because of the associative property of degenerate networks, there is a high probability that numerous relationships are established between (R of R) groups in both the storage and readout modes. These relationships would result in a series of sampled associations between several different signals occurring at the same time. It is the relationship between these multimodal interactions and the multimodal abstract patterns that have been stored that is supposed to be important in generating the conscious state.

Output to motor systems and reentrant input from store would provide continuous confirmation or alteration of this relationship. The presence of abstract representation, perhaps arising from convergence of afferent pathways on cell groups in those areas of cortex carrying out linguistic functions, would serve both to condense and to integrate past experiences. The cell groups serving such a function could be called upon to integrate conscious states arising from current input by associative interaction. All of these factors would tend to make the transient, probabilistic, parallel, and phasically distinct processes described previously connect in a richly associated network of interactions that is constantly changing under changes of input. In effect, this would smooth out and connect responses and patterns of awareness resulting from the activity of different $(R \text{ of } R)$ groups. It would also provide for rapid variable access to large portions of storage with new associations at each cycle. Moreover, as pointed out above, because the access to storage also depends on a cycle and "clock state," the formidable problem of generating a memory of the time duration of a given set of recalled events is mitigated: the same time base is used for both recall and awareness.

If this analysis is correct, a subject would be aware of duration but would not be aware of alternate states in the cycle, because memory states, parallel processing of other signals, and asynchrony would lead to a smoothing of various inputs over longer time periods than a single reentrant cycle. This touches upon the critical question of the time period assumed for the phasic states. Hippocampal rhythms with frequencies of 3–8 Hz have been detected, and it is conceivable that cycles could be as long as 300 msec. There is, however, no clear-cut correlation between informational processing and θ rhythms (Bennett, 1975). Perhaps more detailed information on the temporal interactions of the thalamic pacemaker with the ascending reticular system will provide the most relevant information (Mountcastle, 1974). The evidence for a minimal "activation period" of about 200–500 msec for awareness of a near-threshold stimulus is also pertinent (Libet, 1966). I would suspect that much faster entry is possible; work in experimental psychology suggests that a full perception requires no more than 100 msec of intracortical processing time. One calculation that might be valuable would be to estimate the transmission time and delay expected in all parts of the cycle postulated here, but at present, in the absence of detailed anatomical information, this calculation is not possible. It is worth noting, however, that after periods of time of this order of magnitude, the hippocampus experiences inhibitory signals and "wipeout" (Pribram and Isaacson, 1975). This is just what would be required in portions of a phasic reentrant scheme. Moreover, the existence of a short-term memory of the kind known to be related to hippocampal transactions (Vinogradova, 1975) may also be essential to "sample and hold" phasic input for the high-level processing described here.

In dealing with novelty, the brain is centrally concerned with mediating between experience and action. Because the brain functions for action, it may seem strange that the discussion here has not centered upon motor output or function. Evaluation of the evidence (Evarts et al., 1971) that central programming of motor patterns is apparently predominant over simple reflex patterns enables us, however, to look upon motor repertoire in much the same fashion as sensory repertoire. An important feature to be stressed is that central states can selectively call for whole patterns of motor activity that have been previously shaped by selective processes. Furthermore, there is evidence (Vanderwolf et al., 1975) that hippocampal function in attentional states is related to the performance of motor acts.

There is one particularly important feature of sensorimotor interaction that focuses on the input to a selective system: the motor repertoire further channels, restricts, and helps to program encounters in the sensory domain. Carrying out certain motor acts may therefore alter the density and nature of input signals and help to refine selection in ways that would otherwise not be very probable. The influence of motor functions on the paradigms for conscious behavior has been discussed penetratingly by MacKay (1966).

To summarize, it may be valuable to reconsider, at a naive level, the minimal set of features that are absolutely required for awareness according to the reentrant-signal model. There must be degenerate selection, reflexive recognition of $(R \text{ of } R)$ neuronal groups by each other, $(R \text{ of } R)$ storage, processing of activation and S signals in a coordinate fashion, rhythmic activity with phased states, and appropriate signal-holding networks to allow reentrant processing and coordination with external sensory input for at least some short period of time. Removal of higher midbrain input, removal of $(R \text{ of } R)$ storage, and removal of sensory input would each be expected to cause vast disturbances in consciousness. Clearly, however, after some time, this system would not be rigorously stimulus-bound: memory states and proprioceptive inputs could keep it functioning, if only in a deranged fashion (Jasper, 1966). One must conceive of $(R \text{ of } R)$ store as being kept in a continuously active state. Of course, alteration or obliteration of the phasic excitatory and inhibitory signals for alternate reentrant processing would also have massive effects. Indeed, one amusing prediction of this model is that consciousness is "digitized" and lagged: input state 1 is a period in which *no* consciousness of the signal state is yet possible. A test within the time period of this state, if feasible, would reveal no awareness of signal content. Only in input state 2 is there the possibility of "consciousness."

The sufficient conditions for conscious awareness

The discussion has not yet dealt with all of the sufficient conditions for awareness, nor has it considered the related problem of the quality of sensory modalities. At a certain point, the problem of quality is private and not scientifically testable. At best, public verifications can occur by means of reports, but the direct comparison of sensory qualities identically reported by two individuals still cannot verify their qualitative similarity or difference. This is all the more true if one takes into account the richly different present phenomenal states of two conscious reporters. But there is some profit in considering certain aspects of sensory quality in the light of a selective theory of brain function.

To begin with, it is useful to note that, because sensory modalities are mediated by signals on "labeled lines," there is no problem in principle of identifying *different* modalities. Their recognition by R and $(R \text{ of } R)$ groups proceeds, however, through a series of hierarchically ordered abstract transforms that result from the activity of these groups. According to the selective theory, simultaneity of inputs S_1, $S_2, \ldots, S_n$ is sufficient to raise the possibility of higher-order associations among their respective transforms; it is not necessary that these S's be causally connected.

With this in mind, it is likely that the sufficient conditions for awareness arise from a historical process in each individual whereby increasingly abstract routines are placed in the secondary repertoire. The additional possibility must be entertained, however, that *early* associations with those areas of the brain

concerned with affective states are critical in distributing into storage a series of response patterns that are sampled frequently later in life. These distributed "primitives" may consist of modally related patterns of motor and sensory responses that have been initially mediated, for example, by hypothalamic areas and the medial forebrain bundle. Such patterns may lead to chemically mediated changes in a variety of somatic responses. Although their "quality" is not discussable in scientific terms because the only possible access to these responses is indirect (behavioral observation) or verbal (possibly at a time when verbal communication has not developed), later verbally reportable "qualities" may be tied to their responses by abstraction through $(R \text{ of } R)$ groups. The capacity to distinguish modalities may play a major role in this process inasmuch as associative cross-correlations of modalities are made by the simultaneity of different S inputs. In any event, the expression of sensory quality is a highly abstract process, as pointed out by Miller and Johnson-Laird (1976). In view of the evidence from a variety of studies (Piaget, 1950, 1954; Miller and Johnson-Laird, 1976), this also implies that *awareness* of quality is a historically developed process.

Figure 13 illustrates the later access to various $(R \text{ of } R)$ hierarchies via cross-correlation of S's and interaction with primitives in the repertoire. Because of the complexity of these interactions, this diagram and the assumptions upon which it is based must both be taken as skeletal and highly provisional.

From this discussion, it is clear that if one insists that the sufficient conditions for consciousness must include an explanation of quality in the sense that it is experienced by an individual through direct acquaintance, then no scientific theory can be constructed that is satisfactory. The present theory has therefore not provided a definition of consciousness that would meet sufficiency conditions of the kind prescribed by philosophers. It can be said, however, that several previously annoying conditions have been removed by the present model:

1. The need for a "thinking homunculus" is removed by the ties between phasic reentrant processing and abstract multidimensional store, defining "self" and a world model in terms of past sensory and motor experience. In their most sophisticated forms, such models are likely to require the existence of elements capable of language (Miller and Johnson-Laird, 1976), but language is probably not generally necessary for their manifestation.

2. The need for an infinite regress or hierarchy is removed by the degeneracy and associative proper-

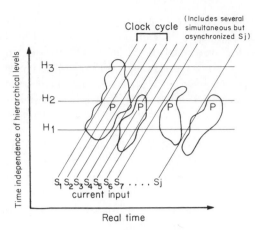

FIGURE 13 An attempt to illustrate how successive cycles of phasic reentry with associative readout may call upon hierarchical levels of (R of R) neurons of increasing degrees of abstract coding. "Primitives" (P), consisting of distributed stored patterns of early experiences associated to various extents with different hierarchical levels H_1–H_3, have a high likelihood of interaction with current input and of being read by (R of R) neurons. The three arbitrarily chosen hierarchical levels of storage consist of (R of R) neuronal groups that contain increasingly abstract information, and they therefore represent a variety of routines accumulated during experience. The higher levels contain more abstract stable representations that do not depend as much on immediate temporal change. For example, H_1 might represent instantaneous feature detection and pattern recognition; H_2, associative and perceptual routines; and H_3, internal models or "theories" of self, possibly based in linguistic routines. Association of current input S_j at H_1 and H_2 leading to modality correlation may be read by groups that associate with H_3. Time relations, modality, and affective connections may lead to different motor responses dependent upon access to primitives.

ties of cell groups. It is further relieved by the phasic reentrant nature of signaling, which allows "restarts" to occur without loss of reference to long-term memory. The divergent (degenerate) and convergent (abstracting) properties of (R of R) ensembles suggest that a *sequential* process can deal with nests of higher-order abstractions. Furthermore, because of the associative properties of group-degenerate selection, the need for a program or a "programmer" is mitigated. In this sense, the analogy between the higher nervous system and computers fails, although at higher levels such a system is capable of carrying out routines (Miller and Johnson-Laird, 1976).

3. No causal requirements are placed on input signals: simultaneity is sufficient, provided the time constants of cerebral, reticular, and limbic responses are met.

According to this view, conscious awareness re-quires temporal processes that are both parallel and sequential. There is a constant shuttling among cross-correlated multimodal signals, phasically accessing a historically developed storage. In the operational sense, this view states that if a machine with these properties were built, it would report conscious states (or reveal them under test). But the quality "by acquaintance" of its sensation or perception would be neither directly accessible nor operationally definable, unless the machine could be connected to a human nervous system, an even more unlikely event than the construction of the machine itself. About such qualities the machine might say, "If they were not this way, they would be that way." The main requirement for adequate functioning is that, having once labeled modalities, the machine must not confuse them.

Some implications and comparisons with alternative views

Some of the general implications of this model need to be stressed. First, there is no need to postulate that the molecules of the brain are *directly* influenced by conscious processes, as specified by Sperry (1969, 1970b) in his proposals for modified mentalism. Besides being stated in terms that are thermodynamically unclear or dubious, such assumptions are unnecessary, as are emphases on emergent properties of "the brain" and holistic explanations without mechanistic detail. Under the present scheme, there is also no need to assume dualistic or pluralistic models (Eccles, 1974; Popper, 1974) or to rely upon determinate sequential states with psychophysical parallelism. Instead, the position taken here is consistent in the main with that of so-called central-state materialism (Campbell, 1970) or the more sophisticated versions of the "identity" hypothesis (Feigl, 1967). But as a scientific theory, the present argument proposes a particular set of mechanisms to account for higher brain function, and it must stand or fall on their verifiability, not upon its philosophical alliances.

It would be a mistake to conclude from the present description that a system of group-degenerate selection with reentry of signals operates in clockwork fashion. Slight fluctuations in the outside S signal, in activating systems, or in (R of R) would yield very large numbers of isofunctional but nonidentical (R of R) responses generating states from which further selective responses can occur. Selection can occur from cell groups participating in these states without "telling molecules what to do." At this level of description, the essential units of the conscious process are the cell groups, their connectivity, and the diverse repertoire they generate. Inasmuch as an enormous set of possibilities exists in comparing the states of such groups to successive states, particularly upon slight biasing of outside signals, there is no need to invoke determinate "mechanical" sequences of responses. This is all the more true if one considers that two equivalent states of consciousness may represent entirely different subsets of (R of R) repertoire. More important, recombination of such states would generate an almost limitless set of possibilities of association.

Given long-term memory in (R of R) and the ability to change the degree of processing of S and of activating signals, it is not particularly difficult to see how such a system could be modulated for planning and programming, for limiting S signals to proprioceptive inputs, or for emphasizing (R of R) interactions in altered attentional states (Vinogradova, 1975). In this connection, it is worth stressing again that the outcome at any time of the process occurring in a group-degenerate system with phasic reentry is probabilistically determined. For example, competitive selection between or among groups in the primary and secondary repertoires would be determined by (1) the polling process, that is, which cell group or groups of sufficient "fit" were first encountered by a given signal; (2) the presence of inhibitory processes that remove the responses of cell groups having lesser degrees of recognition; and (3) the degree of commitment and recognizing efficiency of a previously selected group in the secondary repertoire. This does not rule out the possibility in a mature system that S can be internally generated. Indeed, the replacement of or competition with an "external" S by an internally generated S would be essential for central planning and programming. But I suspect that this would require considerable prior selective experience and a higher-order processing that is related, in its most sophisticated forms, to the acquisition of language (Miller and Johnson-Laird, 1976). This holds a fortiori for refined distinctions between self and nonself (Piaget, 1950, 1954).

The main point in any case is that consciousness involves selective phasic interactions with both storage and external input, and that it depends absolutely upon both past and present experience. There is freedom ("free will" or "free agency") in such a system—the freedom is in the selective grammar of the neuronal groups—but this freedom is not limitless and is bound by a variety of constraints implicit in the properties of the neuronal groups.

Ontogeny and the development of a first repertoire

One of the major assumptions of the present theory is that prior to the development of conscious awareness (and essential for it) is the formation of a degenerate primary repertoire of recognizer cell groups. It is therefore essential to ask how such a first repertoire can develop during ontogeny and how its specific properties arose during evolution. At this point, I consider briefly the problem of ontogeny; in a later section, I shall make some comparative observations on the phylogeny of selective recognition systems.

The problem of embryogenesis, particularly of histotypic interactions, is at present far from solution at the molecular level. It is exquisitely posed by the development of higher nervous systems: for example, the "wiring problem" in developing a system such as the retinotectal projection is a formidable one (Barondes, 1976). One method of solving this problem essentially begs the question, namely, positing for each pair of cells a set of specific complementary recognizer molecules appearing under gene programming at the appropriate time of development (Moscona, 1974). An increasing body of evidence suggests, however, that such a prior repertoire of fixed gene products will not suffice. Both embryological (Hamburger, 1970) and regeneration (Weiss, 1970) experiments indicate, for example, that neuromuscular interactions are not prespecified but are modeled with time.

The data indicate that competitive exclusion of synapses occurs after initial multiple synapse formation, generally leading to 1:1 axon-to-muscle endplate ratios. Moreover, there is evidence that in the formation of some limb nerve plexuses, branching occurs before neuromuscular interaction (Landmesser and Pilar, 1970, 1972). In the optic tectum, removal of part of the tectum still allows formation of the proper gross projections (Yoon, 1975), suggesting that there is no prefixed code for *individual* cell–nerve fiber interaction. Finally, chemical analyses of retinal cell adhesion (Brackenbury et al., 1977; Thiery et al., 1977) implicate one or a few surface protein molecules but no extensive retina-specific or neuron-specific molecular repertoire.

The question therefore remains: How can a primary repertoire be formed? I shall suggest here the elements of a provisional hypothesis for the development of a primary repertoire whose properties are consistent with later group-degenerate selection to form a secondary repertoire.

1. Early in development, cell groups or polyclones are determined by gene expression and programming.

2. A large degeneracy is built into this system, there being many more cell groups than are ultimately used to make projections and connections. Many of the "unused" cells die (Prestige, 1970; Cowan, 1973).

3. A hierarchy of interactions occurs, with early decisions (such as branching of limb plexus neurons) being relatively few in number and decided by the gene program.

4. Interactions between cell groups are sequential, selective, and determined by mutual influence. For example, innervation of a limb by a portion of the spinal cord involves neuromuscular interactions and synapse formation, which depends upon anterograde and retrograde signals. Of the several synapses formed initially, usually only one survives. This selective survival of certain synapses is in accord with suggestions made by Weiss (1970) and by Changeux and Danchin (1976). The end result of such selective interaction is the loss of synaptic connections and the death of many CNS neurons during development. Nevertheless, after such selective stabilization (Changeux and Danchin, 1976), there remains a high degree of redundancy and degeneracy of specific isofunctional cell groups.

5. The major shaping of final connections at the level of synapses is therefore considered to be a selective interaction based on certain aspects of function. Once formed, these connections are in general not remade. Despite its selective nature, however, much in this system is still genetically predetermined, such as the position of nuclei, their particular differentiation path, and their gross location. For example, ocular dominance columns are in general prespecified, but they can be committed during the critical period (Blakemore and Van Sluyters, 1974), and right and left eyes compete finally at the level of forming synapses with individual striate cortical neurons.

According to the present hypothesis, the first repertoire, like the second, is selectively formed at the level of its fine structure. But even if this view is correct, much has first to be done by gene programming, and the sequences of development are particularly critical (Bodian, 1970). The distinctive element in the hypothesis is that there is enormous degeneracy and selection early in the system, even before primary repertoire formation is complete. Later developments, such as those in critical periods, may reduce this degeneracy by selective synaptic stabilization (Changeux and Danchin, 1976). In ascending the neuraxis, one might expect later and later effects of critical selection and more and more evidence for degeneracy. There is very little need for degeneracy in certain subsystems, and evolutionary selection as well as critical-period shaping may remove it almost completely. But the need to develop a second repertoire in higher brain function requires that most of the degeneracy must remain in cortical and limbic-reticular areas. Under this view, the prefrontal, frontal, and temporal cortexes have a constantly extended critical period which in fortunate individuals may be delayed until death.

Evolution of degenerate systems, cortex, and local circuit neurons

There is ample evidence to indicate that in many nervous systems, no large need exists for degenerate repertoires. In insects (Bullock and Horridge, 1965) and molluscs (Kandel, 1976), for example, it is likely that the combination of fixed central pattern generators, unique but non-necessary neurons, compensatory behavioral options, and autonomous reflexes (Wilson, 1970) could all give rise to highly adaptive and complex forms of behavior without the kind of system discussed here. At some time during evolution, however, a new pattern of more plastic behavior must have had selective advantage. It is difficult to identify the origins of nervous systems capable of more refined learning, but it is likely (with the exception of highly developed marine organisms such as the octopus and the shark) that the major continuing developments occurred upon the assumption of terrestrial life by backboned organisms.

For certain species, survival under these conditions obviously involved a gradual shaping of eye, limb, and brain for the performance of complex sensorimotor acts. A more rapid change is seen in comparing the avian brain with that of mammals and primates: the shaping of cortical regions from external striatum (Nauta and Karten, 1970). And by the time of primate and hominid evolution, an extraordinarily rapid change occurred in the assumption of predominance of other neocortical regions over olfactory cortex. Consistent with the present theory, it appears likely that early awareness developed in step with both limbic (Vinogradova, 1975) and cortical change. The case for animal awareness in more modern forms has recently been eloquently made (Griffin, 1977); but the most striking case is still that of hominid development with its associated emergence of language and symbolic representation.

At the cellular level, neocortical development

brought with it a large increase in the number of LCNs (Rakic, 1975; Schmitt, Dev, and Smith, 1976). An emphasis on number alone (for example, a tenfold increase) does not serve, however, to suggest the massive increase in possible degenerate connectivity allowed by this development. According to the present theory, this and the associated increase in numbers of cell groups are the fundamental roots of higher-order consciousness with symbolic representation and awareness. While limbic-cortical and thalamocortical interactions and reentrant signaling may have already been developing slowly for purposes of behavioral advantages in mating, defense, or other fundamental mechanisms of survival, the emergence of a degenerate cortical repertoire mediated by extensive LCN connections was probably relatively explosive and marked a large selective advantage in CNS function.

If we assume, for the moment, that such developments in the CNS of "higher" mammals define a selective system, it is illuminating to compare its properties with those of two other biological systems known to involve selection: evolution and the immune system. Evolution is, of course, at the basis of all of biology, and the immune system is a special development in the vertebrate species. If the present theory is correct, the cognitive systems that are realized most extensively in hominid brains constitute a third and most recent development (Table I).

The first difference to note is the time scale of the selective operation: years to millions of years for natural selection, hours and days for immune selection, seconds and milliseconds for neural selection. The most "complicated" system is evolution, with hosts of conditions, species, and variations, among which is the appearance of the brain itself. The next most complicated is the nervous system, with enormous numbers of cell types, abstract hierarchies, and selective interactions. The least complex is the immune system, with only one kind of target molecule (antibodies) and relatively few cell types.

In both the nervous system and immune systems, it is possible to have unused variants, and degeneracy in such somatic systems does in fact require the presence of many irrelevant neutral variants that will never be used. In the natural selection of organisms,

TABLE I
Some characteristics of selective systems

	Evolution	Immune Response	Group Selection in CNS
Time scale for fixation of selective unit	Years to 10^6 years	Hours, days	Milliseconds, seconds, hours
Recency	3×10^9 years	600×10^6 years	?Birds (160×10^6 years) ?Mammals (200×10^6 years)
Overall system complexity	Greatest	Least	Median
Basis of variational process	Germ-line mutation	Somatic mutation	Somatic combination
Level of repertoire diversification	Mutation, gene flow	Somatic mutation of V genes	Embryogenesis, cell-group recombination
Unit of selection	Phenotype	Individual lymphocyte	Neuron and neuron group
Selective interactions	Environment (general) on phenotype by natural selection	Antigen and cell–cell interaction	Environment (sensory) via cell group–cell group interaction
Neutrality (neutral variants)	No	Yes	Yes
Renewal	Yes	Yes	No for cells Yes for synapses
Novelty	Yes	Rare or absent	Yes

however, there are few or no neutral mutations. Thus, although most surviving genomes are adaptively useful and viable in natural selection, in the CNS and in the immune system the patterns of selection are not necessarily adaptive.

What about "creativity" in such systems? Because of the limitation on input, clonal selection in immunity is a fixed system with variations on a theme; in natural selection and group-degenerate selection, completely new themes are possible. The immune system and evolution are renewable systems: new variants are always generated in the primary repertoire. In the CNS, this may not be true for cells but it may be true for synapses. From a methodological point of view, the problem of analysis of the two somatic systems of selection is different: in the immune system, much more is known about repertoire than about regulation; in the CNS, it is the other way around.

One final comment: If the higher brain is a selective system, it must be about as efficient a selective system as can be evolved, given the nature of the molecules that must be used. That is to say, the time constants of ionic fluxes and of impulse conduction and the neuronal packing are as efficient as can be arranged, and they result in a high signal-to-noise ratio and error-free propagation at extremely low thresholds. Encounter in the selective higher CNS is no problem; the problem is the development of powerful primary and secondary repertoires.

Some predictions and consequences

The main predictions of the theory of group-degenerate selection are as follows:

1. Groups of cells, not single cells, are the main units of selection in higher brain function.

2. Such groups will be found to be multiply represented, degenerate, and isofunctionally overlapping. Many–one interactions via LCNs as well as via connecting axons will be found, with extensive divergence as a sign of degeneracy.

3. At the same time, multiple inputs from R and $(R \text{ of } R)$ neurons will be found to converge to the same $(R \text{ of } R)$ cell group, leading to abstract cell-group codes.

4. Although single neurons may occasionally function as a group, no pontifical neuron or single-neuron "decision unit" (Bullock, 1961) will ever be found at the highest levels of a system of any large degree of plasticity.

5. Selection will be found to play a large, but not exclusive, role in forming a first repertoire during embryogenesis. The position and occurrence of synapses is not determined by complementary interactions among surface proteins specific for each particular synapse. Thus, no sizable precommitted molecular repertoire will be found to explain cell–cell interaction in the developing nervous system.

6. Correlations will be found that suggest phased reentrant signaling on degenerate neuronal groups with periods of 50–200 msec. The most likely correlations will be found between cortical, thalamocortical, and limbic-reticular signals.

The theory will be falsified if any of the following conditions are found to hold:

1. Single cells are capable alone of "abstracting" sensory input in temporal or frontal cortex.

2. Removal of any single cell or distant combination of single cells relevant to a higher function results in loss of that function.

3. CNS cell groups are merely isomorphically and isofunctionally redundant but not degenerate.

4. Degenerate cell groups are found, but in such small numbers or restricted locales that their presence cannot account for a repertoire having both range and specificity. For example, if a total of only 10^3 groups were present for higher-order $(R \text{ of } R)$ processing of sensory modalities, it would be highly unlikely that they could carry out a wide range of different recognition functions.

5. The function of intrinsic connectivity within cell groups in the cortex and limbic areas (and possibly thalamic areas) is found to be completely fixed and determinate.

6. Evidence is obtained to rule out the presence of phasic reentrant signaling.

Summary

A review of the properties of the central nervous system in higher mammals and particularly in man suggests that an adequate brain theory must account for the distributed nature of learning, the associative nature of recall, the adaptive reaction to novelty, and the capacity to make highly abstract representations in a world model. A selective theory of brain function in which the unit of selection is a neuronal group appears to account satisfactorily for these properties.

In the theory, it is assumed that structured neuronal groups containing up to 10,000 neurons are formed during embryogenesis and development. The intrinsic connections within a group and extrinsic connections among groups are specified by gene programming and synaptic selection. Upon completion of this process, primary repertoires are formed from neuronal groups of different structures and connectivity, more than one of which can respond to or recognize a particular signal pattern. This many-one response implies that each repertoire is degenerate. The polling of such degenerate primary repertoires by signals leads to associative recognition. Moreover, repetition of signals interacting with selected neuronal groups results in the emergence of secondary repertoires of groups with a higher likelihood of response. Such a process is selective in the sense that the signals play no role in the formation of anatomical connections within groups of the primary repertoire but only select appropriate groups from the preformed repertoire.

This selective theory of higher brain function requires no special thermodynamic assumptions and is free of mentalistic notions. Because the proposed system is selective and degenerate, however, it is not mechanistically determined in the sense that a clockwork machine is determined. On the basis of group-degenerate selection, an effort is made to account for the properties of consciousness by a phenomenological theory consistent with neuroanatomy and neurophysiology. The properties of consciousness to be accounted for include (1) the ability to appreciate or distinguish different events; (2) the capacity to react critically to inner or outer states and to update information; (3) the ability to accumulate memories and to recall them associatively in temporal sequences; and (4) the capacity to distinguish self from nonself (self-awareness). A satisfactory hypothesis accounting for these properties must avoid an infinite regression of hierarchical states and must provide for anticipatory planning and motor output without a programmer; that is, it must mitigate the need for programming.

The hypothesis advanced here is that the conscious state results from phasic reentrant signaling occurring in parallel processes that involve associations between stored patterns and current sensory or internal input. Each phasic process has two stages. The first stage consists of entry of processed input and holding of the resultant and associated signals for reentry into the second stage. In this stage, a subsequent processed input signal is linked with the reentrant signals and associated with the responses of groups in both primary and secondary repertoires. This cycle is completed in periods of milliseconds. Awareness is assumed to arise as a result of the access by groups of higher-order neurons to rich multimodal associative patterns stored in long-term memory as a result of past experience.

In this theory, the time base of reentry and that of recall are assumed to involve the same clock cycles.

In concert with the sequential tagging of stored events, this allows for recall in a proper time scale and order. Because of the selective, group-degenerate, and phasic nature of reentrant cycles and the capacity of higher-order neurons to abstract sequences of events, a continuous shifting pattern of associations can be made. After sufficient development and experience, such a system can become capable of distinguishing abstract complexes such as the "self" from environmental input. Although this system is not dependent upon a fixed program or programmer, its properties are consistent with the ability of the brain to carry out complex routines.

According to this view, consciousness is considered to be a form of associative recollection with updating, based on present reentrant input, that continually confirms or alters a "world model" or "self theory" by means of parallel motor or sensory outputs. The entire process depends upon the properties of group selection and reentrant signaling in a nervous system that is already specified by embryological, developmental, and evolutionary events.

ACKNOWLEDGMENTS I am grateful to Francis O. Schmitt for his generous encouragement and valuable criticism, without which this paper would not have been written. My thanks are also due to Vernon Mountcastle whose expertise and judgment were invaluable during its preparation. The main argument of this paper remains my responsibility, however, and I assume the burden of any faults that may have escaped their notice.

REFERENCES

BARONDES, S., ed., 1976. *Neuronal Recognition.* New York: Plenum Press.

BENNETT, T. L., 1975. The electrical activity of the hippocampus and the process of attention. In *The Hippocampus: Neurophysiology and Behavior,* vol. 2, R. L. Isaacson and K. H. Pribram, eds. New York: Plenum Press.

BLAKEMORE, C., and R. C. VAN SLUYTERS, 1974. Reversal of the physiological effects of monocular deprivation in kittens: Further evidence for a sensitive period. *J. Physiol.* 237:195–216.

BODIAN, D., 1970. A model of synaptic and behavioral ontogeny. In *The Neurosciences: Second Study Program,* F. O. Schmitt, ed. New York: Rockefeller Univ. Press, pp. 129–140.

BODIAN, D., 1962. The generalized vertebrate neuron. *Science* 137:323–326.

BRACKENBURY, R., J.-P. THIERY, U. RUTISHAUSER, and G. M. EDELMAN, 1977. Adhesion among neural cells of the chick embryo. I. An immunological assay for molecules involved in cell-cell binding. *J. Biol. Chem.* 252:6835–6840.

BRODAL, A., 1975. The "wiring patterns" of the brain: Neuroanatomical experiences and their implications for general views of the organization of the brain. In *The Neu-*

rosciences: Paths of Discovery, F. G. Worden, J. P. Swazey, and G. Adelman, eds. Cambridge, MA: MIT Press, pp. 123–140.

BULLOCK, T. H., 1959. Neuron doctrine and electrophysiology. *Science* 129:997–1002.

BULLOCK, T. H., 1961. The problem of recognition in an analyzer made of neurons. In *Sensory Communication*, W. A. Rosenblith, ed. Cambridge, MA: MIT Press, pp. 717–724.

BULLOCK, T. H., and G. A. HORRIDGE, 1965. *Structure and Function in the Nervous Systems of Invertebrates*, vols. I and II. San Francisco: W. H. Freeman.

CAMPBELL, K., 1970. *Body and Mind*. New York: Anchor Books, Doubleday and Co.

CHANGEUX, J.-P., and A. DANCHIN, 1976. Selective stabilization of developing synapses as a mechanism for the specification of neuronal networks. *Nature* 264:705–712.

CHOW, K. L., and A. L. LEIMAN, 1970. The structural and functional organization of the neocortex. *Neurosci. Res. Program Bull.* 8, No. 2.

COOPER, L. N., 1973. A possible organization of animal memory and learning. *Nobel Symp.* 24:252–264.

COWAN, W. M., 1973. Neuronal death as a regulative mechanism in the control of cell number in the nervous system. In *Development and Aging in the Nervous System*, M. Rockstein and M. L. Sussman, eds. New York: Academic Press, pp. 19–41.

ECCLES, J. C., ed., 1966a. *Brain and Conscious Experience*. New York: Springer-Verlag.

ECCLES, J. C., 1966b. Cerebral synaptic mechanisms. In *Brain and Conscious Experience*, J. C. Eccles, ed. New York: Springer-Verlag, pp. 24–50.

ECCLES, J. C., 1974. Cerebral activity and consciousness. In *Studies in the Philosophy of Biology—Reduction and Related Problems*, F. J. Ayala and T. Dobzhansky, eds. London: Macmillan, pp. 87–105.

EDELMAN, G. M., 1974a. The problem of molecular recognition by a selective system. In *Studies in the Philosophy of Biology—Reduction and Related Problems*, F. J. Ayala and T. Dobzhansky, eds. London: Macmillan, pp. 45–56.

EDELMAN, G. M., 1974b. Origins and mechanisms of specificity in clonal selection. In *Cellular Selection and Regulation in the Immune Response*, G. M. Edelman, ed. New York: Raven Press.

EDELMAN, G. M., 1975. Molecular recognition in the immune and nervous systems. In *The Neurosciences: Paths of Discovery*, F. G. Worden, J. P. Swazey, and G. Adelman, eds. Cambridge, MA: MIT Press, pp. 65–74.

EVARTS, V., E. BIZZI, R. E. BURKE, M. DELONG, and W. T. THACH, JR., 1971. Central control of movement. *Neurosci. Res. Program Bull.* 9, No. 1.

FEIGL, H., 1967. *The "Mental" and the "Physical": The Essay and a Postscript*. Minneapolis: Univ. Minnesota Press.

GRIFFIN, D., 1977. *The Question of Animal Awareness*. New York: Rockefeller Univ. Press.

GRÜSSER, O.-J., and U. GRÜSSER-CORNEHLS, 1976. Neurophysiology of anuran visual system. In *Frog Neurobiology, A Handbook*, R. Llinás and W. Precht, eds. Berlin: Springer-Verlag, pp. 297–385.

HAMBURGER, V., 1970. Embryonic motility in vertebrates. In *The Neurosciences: Second Study Program*, F. O. Schmitt, ed. New York: Rockefeller Univ. Press, pp. 141–151.

HERRNSTEIN, R. J., and E. G. BORNIG, 1965. *A Source Book in the History of Psychology*. Cambridge, MA: Harvard Univ. Press.

HUBEL, D. H., and T. N. WIESEL, 1974. Sequence regularity and geometry of orientation columns in the monkey striate cortex. *J. Comp. Neurol.* 158:267–294.

ISAACSON, R. L., and K. H. PRIBRAM, eds., 1975a. *The Hippocampus: Structure and Development*, Vol. 1. New York: Plenum Press.

ISAACSON, R. L., and K. H. PRIBRAM, eds., 1975b. *The Hippocampus: Structure and Development*, Vol. 2, New York: Plenum Press.

JASPER, H. H., 1966. Pathophysiological studies of brain mechanisms in different states of consciousness. In *Brain and Conscious Experience*, J. C. Eccles, ed. New York: Springer-Verlag, pp. 256–282.

JERNE, N. K., 1967. Antibodies and learning: Selection versus instruction. In *The Neurosciences: A Study Program*, G. C. Quarton, T. Melnechuk, and F. O. Schmitt, eds. New York: Rockefeller Univ. Press, pp. 200–208.

KANDEL, E., 1976. *Cellular Basis of Behavior*. San Francisco: W. H. Freeman.

KUFFLER, S. W., and J. G. NICHOLLS, 1977. *From Neuron to Brain*. Sunderland, MA: Sinauer Associates.

LANDMESSER, L., and G. PILAR, 1970. Selective reinnervation of two cell populations in the adult pigeon ciliary ganglion. *J. Physiol.* 211:203–216.

LANDMESSER, L., and G. PILAR, 1972. The onset and development of transmission in the chick ciliary ganglion. *J. Physiol.* 222:691–713.

LASHLEY, K., 1950. In search of the engram. In *Physiological Mechanisms in Animal Behavior* (Society of Experimental Biology Symposium, No. 4). New York: Academic Press, pp. 454–482.

LENNEBERG, E. H., 1970. Brain correlates of language. In *The Neurosciences: Second Study Program*, F. O. Schmitt, ed. New York: Rockefeller Univ. Press, pp. 361–371.

LIBET, B., 1966. Brain stimulation and the threshold of conscious experience. In *Brain and Conscious Experience*, J. C. Eccles, ed. New York: Springer-Verlag, pp. 165–176.

LONGUET-HIGGINS, H. C., D. J. WILLSHAW, and O. P. BERNEMAN, 1970. Theories of associative recall. *Q. Rev. Biophys.* 3, No. 2.

LURIA, A. R., 1973. *The Working Brain: An Introduction to Neuropsychology*. New York: Basic Books.

MACKAY, D. M., 1966. Cerebral organization and the conscious control of action. In *Brain and Conscious Experience*, J. C. Eccles, ed. New York: Springer-Verlag, pp. 422–445.

MACKAY, D. M., 1970. Perception and brain function. In *The Neurosciences: Second Study Program*, F. O. Schmitt, ed. New York: Rockefeller Univ. Press, pp. 303–316.

MILLER, G. A., and P. N. JOHNSON-LAIRD, 1976. *Language and Perception*. Cambridge, MA: Harvard Univ. Press.

MOSCONA, A., 1974. Surface specification of embryonic cells: Lectin receptors, cell recognition and specific cell ligands. In *The Cell Surface in Development*, A. Moscona, ed. New York: John Wiley.

MOUNTCASTLE, V. B., 1957. Modality and topographic properties of single neurons of cat's somatic sensory cortex. *J. Neurophysiol.* 20:408–434.

MOUNTCASTLE, V. B., 1967. The problems of sensing and the neural coding of sensory events. In *The Neurosciences:*

A Study Program, G. C. Quarton, T. Melnechuk, and F. O. Schmitt; eds. New York: Rockefeller Univ. Press, pp. 393–408.

MOUNTCASTLE, V. B., 1974. Sleep, wakefulness, and the conscious state: Intrinsic regulatory mechanisms of the brain. In *Medical Physiology*, vol. 1, V. B. Mountcastle, ed. St. Louis: C. V. Mosby Co., pp. 254–281.

MOUNTCASTLE, V. B., 1976. The world around us: Neural command functions for selective attention. *Neurosci. Res. Program Bull.* 14, Supplement.

NAUTA, W. J. H., and H. J. KARTEN, 1970. A general profile of the vertebrate brain with sidelights on the ancestry of the cerebral cortex. In *The Neurosciences: Second Study Program*, F. O. Schmitt, ed. New York: Rockefeller Univ. Press, pp. 7–26.

PENFIELD, W., 1975. The mind and the brain. In *The Neurosciences: Paths of Discovery*, F. G. Worden, J. P. Swazey, and G. Adelman, eds. Cambridge, MA: MIT Press, pp. 437–454.

PETERS, A., S. L. PALAY, and H. DE F. WEBSTER, 1976. *The Fine Structure of the Nervous System*. Philadelphia: Saunders.

PIAGET, J., 1950. *Psychology of Intelligence*, New York: Harcourt, Brace and World.

PIAGET, J., 1954. *The Construction of Reality in the Child*. New York: Basic Books.

POPPER, K. R., 1974. Scientific reduction and the essential incompleteness of all science. In *Studies in Philosophy of Biology—Reduction and Related Problems*, F. J. Ayala and T. Dobzhansky, eds. London: Macmillan, pp. 259–283.

PRESTIGE, H. C., 1970. Differentiation, degeneration, and the role of the periphery. In *The Neurosciences: Second Study Program*, F. O. Schmitt, ed. New York: Rockefeller Univ. Press, pp. 73–82.

PRIBRAM, K. H., and R. L. ISAACSON, 1975. Summary. In *The Hippocampus: Neurophysiology and Behavior*, Vol. 2, R. L. Isaacson and K. H. Pribram, eds. New York: Plenum Press, pp. 429–441.

QUARTON, G. C., T. MELNECHUK, and F. O. SCHMITT, eds., 1967. *The Neurosciences: A Study Program*. New York: Rockefeller Univ. Press.

RAKIC, P., 1975. Local circuit neurons. *Neurosci. Res. Program Bull.* 13, No. 2.

RUSSELL, W. R., and M. L. E. ESPIR, 1961. *Traumatic Aphasia*. London: Oxford Univ. Press.

RYLE, G., 1949. *The Concept of Mind*. New York: Barnes and Noble.

SCHMITT, F. O., ed., 1970. *The Neurosciences: Second Study Program*. New York: Rockefeller Univ. Press,

SCHMITT, F. O., and F. G. WORDEN, eds., 1974. *The Neurosciences: Third Study Program*. Cambridge, MA: MIT Press.

SCHMITT, F. O., P. DEV, and B. H. SMITH, 1976. Electrotonic processing of information by brain cells. *Science* 193:114–120.

SECKEL, H. P. G., 1950. *Bird Headed Dwarfs*. Springfield, IL: Charles C Thomas.

SHEPHERD, G. M., 1972. The neuron doctrine: A revision of functional concepts. *Yale J. Biol. Med.* 45:584–599.

SHERRINGTON, C. S., 1941. *Man on His Nature*. Cambridge, England: Cambridge Univ. Press.

SKINNER, B. F., 1966. The phylogeny and ontogeny of behavior. *Science* 153:1205–1213.

SPERRY, R. W., 1969. A modified concept of consciousness. *Psychol. Rev.* 76: 532–536.

SPERRY, R. W., 1970a. Perception in the absence of the neocortical commissures. In *Perception and Its Disorders*, D. A. Hamburg, K. H. Pribram, and A. J. Stunkard, eds. Baltimore: Williams & Wilkins, pp. 123–138.

SPERRY, R. W., 1970b. An objective approach to subjective experience. *Psychol. Rev.* 77:585–590.

THIERY, J.-P., R. BRACKENBURY, U. RUTISHAUSER, and G. M. EDELMAN, 1977. Adhesion among neural cells of the chick embryo. II. Purification and characterization of a cell adhesion molecule from neural retina. *J. Biol. Chem.* 252:6841–6845.

VANDERWOLF, C. H., R. KRASSIES, L. A. GILLESPIE, and B. H. BLOND, 1975. Hippocampal rhythmic slow activity and neocortical low voltage fast activity: Relations to behavior. In *The Hippocampus: Neurophysiology and Behavior*, vol. 2, R. L. Isaacson and K. H. Pribram, eds. New York: Plenum Press, pp. 101–128.

VINOGRADOVA, O. S., 1975. Functional organization of the limbic system in the process of the registration of information: Facts and hypotheses. In *The Hippocampus: Neurophysiology and Behavior*, vol. 2, R. L. Isaacson and K. H. Pribram, eds. New York: Plenum Press, pp. 3–69.

VON NEUMANN, J., 1956. Probabilistic logics and the synthesis of reliable organisms from unreliable components. In *Automata Studies*, C. Shannon and J. McCarthy, eds. Princeton: Princeton Univ. Press, pp. 43–98.

WEISS, P., 1970. Neural development in biological perspective. In *The Neurosciences: Second Study Program*, F. O. Schmitt, ed. New York: Rockefeller Univ. Press, pp. 53–61.

WILSON, D. M., 1970. Neural operations in arthropod ganglia. In *The Neurosciences: Second Study Program*, F. O. Schmitt, ed. New York: Rockefeller Univ. Press, pp. 397–409.

WILSON, H. R., and J. D. COWAN, 1973. A mathematical theory of the functional dynamics of cortical and thalamic nervous tissue. *Kyternetik* 13:55–80.

WINOGRAD, S., and J. D. COWAN, 1963. *Reliable Computations in the Presence of Noise*. Cambridge, MA: MIT Press.

YOON, M. G., 1975. Topographic polarity of the optic tectum studied by reimplantation of the tectal tissue in adult goldfish. *Cold Spring Harbor Symp. Quant. Biol.* 40:503–519. New York: Cold Spring Harbor Laboratory.

YOUNG, J. Z., 1975. Sources of discovery in neuroscience. In *The Neurosciences: Paths of Discovery*, F. G. Worden, J. P. Swazey, and G. Adelman, eds. Cambridge, MA: MIT Press, pp. 15–46.

LIST OF AUTHORS

PARTICIPANTS, INTENSIVE STUDY PROGRAM, 1977

ADELMAN, GEORGE   Neurosciences Research Program

ADEY, W. ROSS   Jerry L. Pettis Memorial Veterans Hospital, Loma Linda, CA

BERRIDGE, MICHAEL J.   Unit of Invertebrate Chemistry and Physiology, Department of Zoology, Agricultural Research Council, Cambridge, England

BIVENS, LYLE W.   Behavioral Science Research Branch, National Institute of Mental Health

BLOOM, FLOYD E.   The Arthur Vining Davis Center for Behavioral Neurobiology, Salk Institute for Biological Studies

BRANDT, BRUCE L.   Neurosciences Research Program

BROWN, GENE   Department of Biology, Massachusetts Institute of Technology

BROWN, JAMES H.   Division of Behavioral and Neural Sciences, National Science Foundation

BROWNSTEIN, MICHAEL J.   National Institute of Mental Health

BULLOCK, THEODORE H.   Department of Neurosciences, University of California, San Diego, School of Medicine

BURKE, NANCY   Neurosciences Research Program

BURMAN, NELLIE RAE   Neurosciences Research Program

BURROWS, MALCOLM   Department of Zoology, University of Cambridge

CALVIN, WILLIAM H.   Department of Neurological Surgery, University of Washington School of Medicine

CHANGEUX, JEAN-PIERRE   Neurobiologie Moléculaire, Institut Pasteur

CHUBB, IAN W.   Department of Pharmacology, Oxford University

COWAN, W. MAXWELL   Departments of Anatomy and Neurobiology, Washington University School of Medicine

CREPEL, FRANCIS   Laboratoire de Physiologie Comparée, Université Pierre et Marie Curie

CUÉNOD, MICHEL   Brain Research Institute, University of Zurich

CUSICK, KATHERYN   Neurosciences Research Program

CUSICK, PAUL V.   Massachusetts Institute of Technology

DEV, PARVATI   Neurosciences Research Program

DIAMOND, JACK   Department of Neurosciences, McMaster University Medical Center

DINGLEDINE, RAYMOND   Medical Research Council Neurochemical Pharmacology Unit, Department of Pharmacology, University of Cambridge

DISMUKES, R. KEY   Neurosciences Research Program

DODGE, FREDERICK A.   Mathematical Sciences Department, IBM Thomas J. Watson Research Center

DOWLING, JOHN E.   The Biological Laboratories, Harvard University

EDELMAN, GERALD M.   The Rockefeller University

ELSON, ELLIOT L.   Department of Chemistry, Cornell University

EVARTS, EDWARD V.   Laboratory of Neurophysiology, National Institute of Mental Health

EYSEL, ULF   Institut für Physiologie, Universitätsklinikum der Universität Essen

FAIN, GORDON L.   Department of Ophthalmology, University of California, Los Angeles, School of Medicine

FRANK, KARL   Fundamental Neurosciences Program, National Institute of Neurological and Communicative Disorders and Stroke

GALAMBOS, ROBERT   Department of Neuroscience, University of California, San Diego, School of Medicine

GERSCHENFELD, HERSCH M.   CNRS Laboratoire de Neurobiologie, École Normale Supérieure

GILMAN, ALFRED G.   Department of Pharmacology, University of Virginia School of Medicine

GILULA, NORTON B.   The Rockefeller University

GLOWINSKI, J.   INSERM, Groupe de Neuropharmacologie Biochimique, Collège de France

GOODMAN, COREY S.   Department of Biology, University of California, San Diego

GORSKI, ROGER A.   Department of Anatomy, University of California, Los Angeles, School of Medicine

GRÄBER, PETER   Max-Volmer-Institut für Physikalische Chemie und Molekularbiologie, Technische Universität Berlin

GRAUBARD, KATHERINE   Department of Zoology, University of Washington

GRUNHAGEN, HANS-HEINRICH   Institut für Physiologische Chemie, Universität des Saarlandes, Homburg/Saar

GRÜSSER, OTTO-JOACHIM   Department of Physiology, Freie Universität Berlin

GUIDOTTI, GUIDO   The Biological Laboratories, Harvard University

HAGINS, WILLIAM A.   Section of Membrane Biophysics, Laboratory of Chemical Physics, National Institute of Arthritis, Metabolism, and Digestive Diseases

HAMMES, GORDON G. Department of Chemistry, Cornell University

HENNERICI, MICHAEL Neurologische Universitätsklinik mit Abteilung für Neurophysiologie, Freiburg i. Br.

HESS, GEORGE P. Section of Biochemistry, Cornell University

HEUSER, JOHN E. Department of Physiology, University of California, San Francisco, School of Medicine

HILLMAN, DEAN E. Department of Physiology, New York University Medical Center

HÖKFELT, TOMAS Department of Histology, Karolinska Institutet, Stockholm

HOMSY, YVONNE M. Neurosciences Research Program

ILES, JOHN F. University Laboratory of Physiology, Oxford

IRWIN, LOUIS N. Neurosciences Research Program

IVERSEN, LESLIE L. Medical Research Council Neurochemical Pharmacology Unit, Department of Pharmacology, Medical School, Cambridge

JACK, JULIAN University Laboratory of Physiology, Oxford

JOHNSON, HOWARD W. Massachusetts Institute of Technology

JONAS, GERALD *The New Yorker*

KALDERON, NURIT The Rockefeller University

KATZ, ARNOLD M. Department of Medicine (Cardiology), University of Connecticut Health Center

KELLY, JAMES P. Department of Anatomy, College of Physicians and Surgeons, Columbia University

KIRSCHFELD, KUNO Max-Planck-Institut für Biologische Kybernetik, Tübingen

KOESTER, JOHN Division of Neurobiology and Behavior, College of Physicians and Surgeons, Columbia University

KORN, HENRI INSERM U3, Laboratoire de Physiologie, CHU Pitié-Salpêtrière, Paris

KRETSINGER, ROBERT H. Department of Biology, University of Virginia

KREUTZBERG, GEORG W. Department of Neuropathology, Max-Planck-Institut für Psychiatrie, Munich

LESTER, HENRY A. Division of Biology, California Institute of Technology

LEVITAN, IRWIN B. Friedrich Miescher Institute, Basel

LJUNGDAHL, ÅKE Department of Histology, Karolinska Institutet, Stockholm

LLINÁS, RODOLFO R. Department of Physiology and Biophysics, New York University Medical Center

LOEB, GERALD E. Laboratory of Neural Control, National Institute for Neurological and Communicative Diseases and Stroke

LUX, HANS DIETER Max-Planck-Institut für Psychiatrie, Munich

LYNCH, GARY S. Department of Psychobiology, University of California, Irvine

McCLAIN, DONALD M. Research Department of Communication, University of Keele

MALLET, JACQUES Institut Pasteur

MASON, CAROL ANN Department of Anatomy, Bardeen Medical Laboratories, University of Wisconsin

MILLER, JAMES JACKSON Department of Physiology, University of British Columbia

MILLER, JULIE ANN *Science News*

MILLER, ROBERT F. Department of Ophthalmology, Washington University School of Medicine

MOOLENAAR, WOUTER H. Department of Physiology, University of Leiden

MOORE, ROBERT Y. Department of Neurosciences, University of California, San Diego, School of Medicine

MOSKOWITZ, MICHAEL A. Department of Nutrition and Food Science, Laboratory of Neuroendocrine Regulation, Massachusetts Institute of Technology

MOUNTCASTLE, VERNON B. Department of Physiology, The Johns Hopkins University School of Medicine

MUELLER, PAUL Department of Molecular Biology, Eastern Pennsylvania Psychiatric Institute

MULLONEY, BRIAN Department of Zoology, University of California, Davis

NEHER, ERWIN Max-Planck-Institut für Biophysikalische Chemie, Göttingen

NICHOLSON, CHARLES Department of Physiology and Biophysics, New York University Medical Center

PALAY, SANFORD L. Department of Anatomy, Harvard Medical School

PARNAS, ITZCHAK Neurobiology Unit, Institute of Life Sciences, The Hebrew University, Jerusalem

PATTERSON, PAUL H. Department of Neurobiology, Harvard Medical School

PEARSON, KEIR G. Department of Physiology, University of Alberta

PELLIONISZ, ANDRÁS First Department of Anatomy, Semmelweis University Medical School, Budapest

PFENNINGER, KARL H. Department of Anatomy, Columbia University

PLOOG, DETLEV Max-Planck-Institut für Psychiatrie, Munich

PORSCHKE, DIETMAR Max-Planck-Institut für Biophysikalische Chemie, Göttingen

PORTER, KEITH R. Department of Molecular, Cellular, and Developmental Biology, University of Colorado

PROCHIANTZ, ALAIN Groupe NB, Collège de France

PUJOL, JEAN-FRANCOIS INSERM U52, Laboratoire de Médecine Expérimentale, Lyon

QUARTON, GARDNER C. Mental Health Research Institute

and Neuroscience Laboratories, University of Michigan

RALL, THEODORE W. Department of Pharmacology, University of Virginia School of Medicine

RALL, WILFRID Mathematical Research Branch, National Institute of Arthritis, Metabolism, and Digestive Diseases

RALSTON, HENRY J., III Department of Anatomy, University of California, San Francisco, School of Medicine

READER, TOMAS A. Département de Physiologie, Faculté de Médecine, Université de Montréal

REICHARDT, WERNER E. Max-Planck-Institut für Biologische Kybernetik, Tübingen

RUBIN, ALBERT L. Cornell University Medical College

RUTISHAUSER, URS The Rockefeller University

SAMUELSSON, BENGT Department of Chemistry, Karolinska Institutet, Stockholm

SAMSON, FRED E., JR. Ralph L. Smith Research Center, Department of Physiology, University of Kansas Medical Center

SCHEIBEL, ARNOLD B. Departments of Anatomy and Psychiatry and Brain Research Institute, University of California Medical Center, Los Angeles

SCHLESSINGER, JOSEPH School of Applied and Engineering Physics, Cornell University

SCHMITT, FRANCIS O. Neurosciences Research Program

SCHMITT, OTTO H. Biophysics Group, University of Minnesota

SCHUBERT, PETER Max-Planck-Institut für Psychiatrie, Munich

SCHWARTZKROIN, PHILIP A. Department of Neurology, Stanford University Medical Center

SCHWARZ, GERHARD Department of Biophysical Chemistry, Biocenter of the University of Basel

SHAMOO, ADIL E. Department of Radiation Biology and Biophysics, University of Rochester, School of Medicine and Dentistry

SHAW, STEPHEN R. Department of Neurobiology, Research School of Biological Sciences, Australian National University

SHEPHERD, GORDON M. Department of Physiology, Yale University School of Medicine

SHINODA, YOSHIKAZU Department of Neurophysiology, Institute of Brain Research, University of Tokyo School of Medicine

SHOULSON, IRA Departments of Neurology, Medicine, Pharmacology, and Toxicology, University of Rochester Medical Center

SILLITO, ADAM M. Department of Physiology, The Medical School, University of Birmingham

SINGER, WOLF Max-Planck-Institut für Psychiatrie, Munich

SIZER, IRWIN W. Health Sciences Fund, Massachusetts Institute of Technology

SMITH, BARRY H. Neurosciences Research Program

SNYDER, SOLOMON H. Departments of Pharmacology and Psychiatry, The Johns Hopkins University School of Medicine

SPERK, GUNTHER Psychiatric Research Laboratories, Massachusetts General Hospital

STADTMAN, EARL R. Laboratory of Biochemistry, National Heart, Lung, and Blood Institute

STEINBERG, IZCHAK Z. Department of Chemical Physics, The Weizmann Institute of Science

STEVENS, CHARLES F. Department of Physiology, Yale University School of Medicine

SWEET, WILLIAM H. Neurosurgical Service, Massachusetts General Hospital

SZENTÁGOTHAI, JOHN First Department of Anatomy, Semmelweis University Medical School, Budapest

TASSIN, JEAN-POL Groupe NB/INSERM U144, Laboratoire de Neurobiologie Moléculaire, Collège de France

THOENEN, HANS Department of Pharmacology, Biocenter of the University of Basel

TIEMAN, SUZANNAH BLISS Department of Anatomy, University of California, San Francisco, School of Medicine

TORRE, VINCENT Laboratorio de Neurofisiologia del CNR, Pisa

UNSICKER, KLAUS Department of Anatomy, University of Kiel

UYLINGS, HARRY B. M. Netherlands Institute for Brain Research of the Royal Netherlands Academy of Sciences, Amsterdam

VALE, WYLIE Peptide Biology Laboratory, The Salk Institute for Biological Studies

VOGEL, ZVI Neurobiology Department, The Weizmann Institute of Science

WALTON, KERRY Department of Physiology, New York University Medical Center

WEBER, KLAUS Karl-Friedrick-Bonhoeffer-Institut, Max-Planck-Institut für Biophysikalische Chemie, Göttingen

WEHRHAHN, CHRISTIAN Max-Planck-Institut für Biologische Kybernetik, Tübingen

WERBLIN, FRANK S. Department of Electrical Engineering, Neurobiology Group, University of California, Berkeley

WHITE, EDWARD L. Department of Anatomy, Boston University School of Medicine

WILSON, MARTIN Department of Neurobiology, Research School of Biological Sciences, Australian National University

WONG, BONNIE M. Neurosciences Research Program

WOOD, JOHN GRADY Department of Anatomy, University of Tennessee Center for Health Sciences

WOOLLACOTT, MARJORIE H. Department of Biology, Virginia Polytechnic Institute and State University

WOOTEN, GEORGE FREDERICK, JR. Department of Neurology, Baines Hospital, Washington University

WORDEN, FREDERIC G. Neurosciences Research Program

WURTMAN, RICHARD J. Department of Nutrition and Food Science, Massachusetts Institute of Technology

ASSOCIATES, NEUROSCIENCES RESEARCH PROGRAM

Julius Axelrod   National Institute of Mental Health

Floyd E. Bloom   The Salk Institute for Biological Studies

Jean-Pierre Changeux   Collège de France

W. Maxwell Cowan   Washington University

John E. Dowling   Harvard University

Gerald M. Edelman   The Rockefeller University

Manfred Eigen   Max Planck Institute for Biophysical Chemistry, Göttingen

Edward V. Evarts   National Institute of Mental Health

Ann M. Graybiel   Massachusetts Institute of Technology

Paul Greengard   Yale University

Roger C. L. Guillemin   The Salk Institute for Biological Studies

Richard M. Held   Massachusetts Institute of Technology

Tomas Hökfelt   Karolinska Institutet, Stockholm

John J. Hopfield   Princeton University

David H. Hubel   Harvard Medical School

Leslie L. Iversen   Medical School, Cambridge

Eric R. Kandel   Columbia University, College of Physicians and Surgeons

Ephraim Katzir-Katchalski (on leave)   The Weizmann Institute of Science

Seymour S. Kety   McLean Hospital, Harvard Medical School

Richard D. Keynes   University of Cambridge

Masakazu Konishi   California Institute of Technology

Daniel E. Koshland, Jr.   University of California, Berkeley

Alvin M. Liberman   Haskins Laboratory, New Haven

Rodolfo R. Llinás   New York University

Robert Y. Moore   University of California, San Diego

Paul Mueller   Eastern Pennsylvania Psychiatric Institute

Walle J. H. Nauta   Massachusetts Institute of Technology

Detlev Ploog   Max Planck Institute for Psychiatry, Munich

Fred Plum   New York Hospital–Cornell Medical Center

Werner E. Reichardt   Max Planck Institute for Biological Cybernetics, Tübingen

Francis O. Schmitt   Neurosciences Research Program, Massachusetts Institute of Technology

Richard L. Sidman   Harvard Medical School, Children's Hospital Medical Center

Solomon H. Snyder   The Johns Hopkins University

John Szentágothai   Semmelweis University, Budapest

Hans Thoenen   Biocenter of the University, Basel

Frederic G. Worden   Neurosciences Research Program, Massachusetts Institute of Technology

Richard J. Wurtman   Massachusetts Institute of Technology

HONORARY ASSOCIATES

W. Ross Adey

David Bodian

Theodore H. Bullock

Melvin Calvin

Leo C. M. De Maeyer

Humberto Fernández-Morán

Robert Galambos

Donald A. Glaser

John B. Goodenough

Holger V. Hydén

Marc Kac

Michael Kasha

Heinrich Klüver

Albert L. Lehninger

Robert B. Livingston

Christopher Longuet-Higgins

Harden M. McConnell

Donald M. MacKay

Neal E. Miller

Frank Morrell

Vernon B. Mountcastle

Marshall W. Nirenberg

Severo Ochoa

Sanford L. Palay

Gardner C. Quarton

Richard B. Roberts

William T. Simpson

William H. Sweet

Paul A. Weiss

NAME INDEX

(Chapters in this volume are indicated by inclusive page references.)

Clusin, W., 564
Coffino, P., 824
Coggeshall, R. E., 146, 152, 1047
Coghill, G. E., 388
Cohen, A. I., 185
Cohen, A. M., 68
Cohen, I. S., 425, 583
Cohen, J. B., 752, 753, 754, 855
Cohen, L. B., 471
Cohen, M. J., 70, 152
Cohen, M. W., 756, 761, 762, 948
Cohen, R. S., 751
Cohen, S., 791
Cohen, S. A., 760, 947
Cohn, M., 856, 1035
Cole, H. A., 813
Cole, K. S., 423, 424, 428, 526, 528, 529,
    601, 602, 603, 606, 631, 642, 647
Cole, R. D., 685
Coleman, P. D., 479, 480, 486
Collette, T. S., 82, 84, 85, 87
Collier, H., 1067
Collin, R., 65, 765
Collins, C. C., 541
Collins, G. H., 459, 469
Collins, R. C., 138
Colon, E. J., 479
Colonnier, M., 33, 122, 374, 400, 404, 486
Colquhoun, D., 758
Comoglio, P., 693
Cone, R. A., 186, 188, 281, 594, 675, 676,
    692, 694, 837
Cone, R. E., 741
Conel, J. L., 393
Conradi, S., 328, 768
Constantinidis, H., 1035
Conti, M. A., 813
Contrera, J. F., 1078
Cook, J., 63, 73
Cooley, J. W., 441, 442, 443, 450, 502,
    503, 529
Coombs, J. S., 499
Coombs, S., 849
Coons, A. H., 723
Cooper, E., 938, 940, 941, 942, 943, 944,
    945, 946, 948
Cooper, L. N., 1124
Cooper, M., 857
Cooper, P. D., 13
Cooper, R. L., 851
Copenhagen, D. R., 197, 209, 219, 286
Cori, C. F., 811
Corner, M. A., 749
Costa, E., 566, 813, 897, 899, 907, 913,
    914, 1059, 1070, 1075, 1089
Cotman, C. W., 75, 958, 959, 963, 965
Cottrell, G. A., 215, 1051
Couineau, S., 12
Coulombre, A. J., 743
Coupland, R. F., 913
Courrège, P., 750, 763, 764, 769
Courtney, K. R., 611
Couteaux, R., 560, 573, 579, 580, 581,
    582, 751, 780
Cowan, J. D., 1119, 1120
Cowan, W. M., 59–79; 7, 9, 60, 62, 63, 65,
    66, 67, 68, 70, 71, 72, 75, 117, 376,
    390, 765, 779, 911, 924, 963, 990, 1134
Cox, B. M., 1058

Cox, E. B., 642, 655
Coy, D. H., 969
Coyle, J. T., 1062, 1070
Cragg, B. G., 413, 923, 924
Crain, S. M., 756, 757, 762, 885
Crank, J., 185
Crawford, A. C., 875, 876
Creese, I., 1057, 1070
Crelin, E. S., 473
Crepel, F., 116, 340, 343, 346, 348, 349,
    768, 943
Creutzfeldt, O.-D., 25, 251, 1094, 1095,
    1097, 1099
Crick, F. H. C., 746, 951, 953
Crill, W. E., 326, 327, 428, 434, 440, 446,
    481, 482, 483, 490, 491, 492, 531, 534,
    611, 612
Critchlow, V., 971, 1031
Crofts, A. R., 661, 663, 664
Crone, H., 765
Cronly-Dillon, J. R., 62, 73
Crothers, D. M., 12
Crow, T. J., 56
Crowell, J., 573
Crowther, R. J., 592
Crumpton, M. J., 686
Cubeddu, L. X., 885
Cuello, A. C., 1064, 1072, 1073, 1086,
    1087, 1088, 1089
Cuénod, M., 989–1004; 141, 328, 987,
    990, 992, 993, 995, 998, 1000, 1001,
    1002
Culvenor, J. G., 363
Cunningham, T. S., 958
Curnish, R. R., 1006, 1013
Curran, P. F., 831
Currie, J., 63, 65, 794
Curry, J., 978
Curtis, A. S. G., 736
Curtis, D. R., 441, 442, 499, 882, 924, 994
Curtis, H. J., 428
Cusick, K., vii
Custer, N. V., 177
Cuthbert, A. W., 555
Cutting, J. A., 588
Cynader, M., 1094, 1095, 1096, 1097,
    1099, 1101
Czajka, M., 760
Czéh, G., 532, 542, 543
Czernik, A. J., 1035

D

Dacheux, R. F., 201, 204, 205, 206, 209,
    210, 214, 227, 228, 229, 230, 231, 232,
    233, 234, 235, 236, 237, 238, 241, 243
Daemen, F. J. M., 188
Daginawala, H. F., 995
Dahl, H. A., 760
Dahl, J. L., 831, 833
Dahlström, A., 1079
Daley, D. L., 881
Daly, J., 13, 755, 824, 861, 862, 1005,
    1014
Damassa, D. A., 594
D'Amato, C., 958
Danchin, A., 75, 109, 116, 750, 759, 763,
    768, 769, 953, 1134
Danforth, W. H., 811
Danielli, J. F., 551

Daniels, M. P., 744, 761
Dartnall, H. J. A., 281
Das, G. D., 63
Datta, A., 802, 806
Davidson, J. M., 972
Davie, E. W., 802
Davies, T. L., 376, 383, 384, 385, 390
Davies, W. A., 708
Davis, G., 758
Davis, H., 137
Davis, L., 424
Davson, H., 459, 460, 551
Daw, N. W., 242, 243, 248, 250, 265
Deadwyler, S., 958, 959
Debbage, P., 153
Debye, P., 552, 628, 633
Decker, J. D., 759
Decker, R. S., 361
de Groat, W. C., 924
Deiters, O., 477
Delbrück, M., 694, 695
Del Castillo, J., 173, 446
Delhaye-Bouchard, N., 116, 768, 943
De Long, G. R., 63, 65, 68
DeLorenzo, R. J., 1052
Dembitzer, A., 114
De Mello, W. C., 362
DeMey, J., 727
Dennis, M., 574, 575
Dennis, M. J., 757, 766, 768
Dentler, W. L., 715
DeOlmos, J. S., 1064
dePetris, S., 678
de Robertis, E., 874
de Scarnati, O. C., 874
Descarries, L., 16
Deschenes, M., 466
De Sombre, E. R., 972
Detwiler, S. R., 874, 938
Detzer, K., 12
D'Eustachio, P., 683, 684, 685
Dev, P., vi, 5, 9, 10, 34, 54, 109, 145, 151,
    247, 395, 413, 430, 551, 873, 1029,
    1117, 1135
Devaux, P. P., 754, 755
de Vellis, J., 824
DeVoe, R. D., 303
Devor, M., 958, 960
Devreotes, P. N., 566, 756, 760
DeWeer, P., 470, 471
Dewey, M. M., 359, 361
de Wied, D., 1034, 1035
DeWolf, H., 620
Diamond, J., 937–955; 757, 894, 938, 940,
    941, 942, 943, 944, 945, 946, 948, 949,
    950, 951, 952
Diamond, M. C., 70
Dichter, M. A., 454, 563, 912
Didio, J., 12
Dilberto, E. J., Jr., 813
Dingledine, R., 1107
Dionne, V. E., 628
Di Polo, R., 562, 618
Divac, I., 1078, 1085, 1090
Dixon, J. S., 62, 73
Dodge, F. A., 439–455; 282, 420, 441,
    442, 443, 448, 450, 454, 499, 502, 503,
    529, 533, 564
Dodt, E., 250
Doetsch, G. S., 31

Fischbach, G. D., 114, 364, 454, 563, 756, 759, 760, 761, 762, 763, 791, 947, 948
Fischer, E. H., 802, 806, 813, 860
Fisher, B., 25, 28, 29
Fisher, D. B., 686
Fisher, R. S., 460, 464, 466
Fisher, S. K., 249, 266
Fisken, R. A., 28
Fiszman, M. Y., 756
Fitzgerald, M. J. T., 943, 944, 953
FitzHugh, R., 250, 251, 529
Flavin, M., 813
Fleischer, S., 694
Fleischauer, K., 12, 385, 395
Fletscher, A., 1035
Flinn, R. M., 479
Flock, A., 562
Floor, E. R., 901
Foerster, M. H., 253, 257, 262, 263, 264, 265, 268
Folan, J. C., 944
Fonnum, F., 993, 995, 1072, 1078, 1086
Fontana, J. A., 861
Foote, S., 55
Ford, R. E., 866
Forei, A., 677
Forman, D. S., 13, 716
Forn, J., 813
Forni, L., 691
Forssman, W. G., 361
Foster, D. H., 94, 95
Fourtner, C. R., 11, 45, 147, 148, 149, 150, 151, 304, 305, 318
Fox, C. A., 382, 486, 493
Fox, M. R., 388
Fraerson, N., 813
Franceschini, N., 93, 278, 298, 300, 306
Frangi, U., 995
Frank, E., 755
Franke, W. W., 730, 732
Frankel, F. R., 727, 729
Frankenhaeuser, B., 441, 442, 454, 465, 466, 467, 500, 501, 507, 508, 529, 555, 641
Franklin, G. G., 528
Fratta, W., 1067
Frazier, W. T., 1044
Frederickson, C. J., 1101
Freed, J. H., 848
Freedman, M. H., 877
Freedman, R., 55
Freeman, J. A., 460, 461, 533, 995, 996
Freeman, R. B., Jr., 250
Freeman, S., 765
Freifelder, H., 657
French, A. S., 280, 287
French, J. H., 114
French, R., 647
French, R. J., 610
Frenk, S., 168
Freund, H.-J., 250
Fricke, R., 963
Friede, R. L., 488
Friedkin, M., 680
Friedman, K., 562
Friedmann, N., 875
Friend, D. S., 360, 361
Friesen, O. W., 499
Frisch, H. L., 764
Frontali, N., 567

Frost, D. O., 120
Frumkes, T., 236, 243
Fry, F. J., 60
Fry, J. P., 1066
Frye, C. D., 675
Fu, J.-J., 852, 855
Fujikawa, K., 802
Fujita, S., 61, 62
Fujiwara, K., 725
Fukuda, J., 562, 607, 610
Fukuda, Y., 250, 251
Fuller, G. M., 684, 727, 730
Fulpius, B. W., 279, 281, 752
Fuortes, M. G. F., 167, 169, 184, 189, 201, 219, 220, 222, 232, 276, 280, 281
Furman, G. G., 255
Furshpan, E. J., 44, 223, 334, 335, 336, 338, 339, 350, 361, 597, 931, 932
Furthmayr, H., 832
Furukawa, T., 223, 334, 335, 336, 338
Futamachi, K. J., 463, 466, 469
Fuxe, K., 970, 973, 993, 1079, 1087, 1093

G

Gabella, G., 755, 765
Gaertner, F. H., 811
Gage, P. W., 625
Gagnon, C., 913
Gainer, H., 1032, 1044, 1045, 1048, 1053
Galambos, R., 136
Gale, K. N., 1072, 1075, 1089
Galey, D., 1079
Gall, C., 958
Gallego, A., 175, 262
Gamble, J. C., 832
Garcia-Bellido, A., 951
Gardner, E. B., 31
Gardner, J., 756
Gardner-Medwin, A. R., 464
Garey, L. J., 28, 33, 400
Garoff, H., 692
Garvey, C. F., 480
Gatter, K. C., 23
Gautron, J., 751
Gautvik, K., 755
Gaze, R. M., 60, 62, 72, 74, 750, 765, 957, 961
Gaziri, I. F., 973
Geduldig, D., 562
Geffen, L. B., 779, 911, 913, 1008, 1086, 1087, 1088
Gegliman, C., 913
Geiger, G., 89, 92, 93, 96
Gelbfish, J., 488, 491, 495
Gelfan, S., 485, 486, 488
Geller, H. M., 882
Gells, J., 839
Gemperlein, R., 283
Gennaro, J. F., 587
Gentschev, T., 346
George, W. J., 877
Geren, B. B., 488
Gerhart, J. C., 753
Gerich, J. E., 1035
Gerschenfeld, H. M., 213-226; 162, 167, 171, 174, 175, 178, 197, 201, 215, 216, 219, 220, 222, 223, 229, 247, 793
Gershon, M. D., 1096, 1107
Getchell, T. V., 130, 131, 134, 135, 136

Giacobini, G., 758, 759, 764, 765, 766
Giacobini-Robecchi, M., 759, 760, 765, 766
Gilbert, Ch. D., 33, 250, 1095
Gilbert, J. M., 900, 901
Gilkes, J. J. H., 1059
Gilkey, J. C., 618
Gill, M., 821
Giller, E., Jr., 1047
Giller, E. L., 768
Gillespie, E., 686
Gillette, R., 146
Gilman, A. G., 819-829; 12, 53, 799, 822, 824, 825, 826, 827, 860, 861, 903
Gilula, N. B., 359-366; 8, 166, 219, 248, 316, 360, 361, 362, 363, 364, 591
Ginsborg, B. L., 562, 875
Ginsburg, A., 802, 806, 807, 808
Giorguieff, M. F., 1077, 1079
Giotta, G. G., 833, 834
Girardier, L., 361
Girgis, G. R., 900
Gisin, B. F., 643
Giuditta, A., 620
Giulian, D., 973
Gjedde, A., 138
Glagoleva, I. M., 557
Glaser, E. M., 478, 479, 480, 486
Glaser, L., 69, 736
Gläser, M., 660
Glasser, S. M. W., 326, 480
Glickstein, M., 33
Glitsch, H. G., 558, 601
Globus, A., 71, 382, 400
Glowinski, J., 1069-1083; 565, 988, 1070, 1072, 1073, 1074, 1075, 1077, 1078, 1079, 1088, 1090
Glynn, I. M., 470, 836
Gnegy, M. E., 813
Godfraind, J. M., 1097
Goffart, M., 869
Gogala, M., 299
Gogan, P., 345
Gold, G. H., 166, 169, 174, 177, 197, 219
Goldberg, A. L., 885
Goldberg, A. R., 725
Goldberg, N. D., 13, 686, 860, 880
Goldin, S. M., 834, 835, 836, 839
Goldman, L. G. M., 642, 647, 650, 654, 655
Goldman, P. H., 822
Goldman, P. S., 33, 35, 117, 399
Goldman, R., 811
Goldman, R. D., 703, 723, 724, 725, 730, 731
Goldsmith, T. H., 275, 278, 299
Goldstein, A., 502, 511
Goldstein, J. L., 588
Goldstein, M., 813, 1087
Goldstein, M. H., Jr., 30
Goldstein, S. S., 132, 426, 434
Golgi, C., 477, 478
Gomperts, B., 877
Gonye, T. J., 1072
Goodenough, D. A., 8, 360, 361, 363
Goodman, C. S., 148
Goodman, D. B. P., 189, 566
Goodman, H., 27
Goodman, L. J., 286
Goodman, R., 912, 1058

Held, H., 952
Heller, A., 1070
Heller, J., 189, 686
Helmholtz, H., 526
Helmreich, E., 811, 827
Hemker, H. C., 810
Hemker, P. W., 810
Hendelman, W. J., 947
Hendrickson, A., 119
Hendriks, Th., 188
Hendrix, C. E., 12
Hendry, I. A., 918, 919, 921, 922, 923, 932, 933, 934
Hengstenberg, R., 93, 150, 305, 307, 308
Henkart, M., 717, 874, 876
Henkart, P., 700
Henke, H., 992, 993, 995, 998, 1000, 1001
Henn, F. A., 464
Henneman, E., 447, 448
Hennerici, M., 250
Henning, R., 741
Henriksen, S. J., 881
Henrikson, C. K., 492, 493
Herbert, E., 1032
Hering, E., 262
Herman, M. M., 374, 377
Herman, W. S., 360, 362
Hermann, A., 14
Hernandez, A. G., 901
Herndon, R. M., 71, 114, 947
Herrick, C. J., 381
Herrnstein, R. J., 1115
Herrup, K., 114, 921, 923
Hertz, L., 464, 465, 470
Herz, A., 463
Herzberg, M., 764
Herzog, W., 727
Heslop, J. P., 716
Hess, G. P., 847–858; 845, 848, 849, 850, 851, 852, 853, 854, 855, 856
Hess, M. L., 867
Hess, R., 463, 467, 470, 532, 564, 613
Heuser, J. E., 573–599; 11, 552, 555, 560, 567, 574, 575, 576, 577, 578, 579, 580, 581, 582, 583, 586, 588, 590, 591, 592, 593, 594, 595, 596, 597, 629, 691, 751, 752, 780, 923
Heyer, C. B., 601–615; 467, 470, 507, 510, 519, 552, 564, 602, 603, 604, 605, 606, 607, 608, 610, 611, 612, 613, 1052, 1102
Hibbard, E., 74
Hicks, S., 958
Highfield, D. P., 684, 727, 730
Highstein, S. M., 587
Hill, A. V., 528
Hill, C. E., 932, 933
Hill, R., 660
Hill, R. M., 227, 241, 243
Hillarp, N.-A., 14
Hille, B., 453, 454, 471
Hiller, J. M., 1057
Hillhouse, E. W., 913, 917
Hillman, D. E., 477–498; 114, 382, 420, 426, 480, 482, 488, 491, 530, 531, 532, 534, 535, 537, 538, 539
Himwich, H., 1100, 1101
Himwich, W. A., 388
Hinds, J. W., 61, 71

Hinds, P. L., 71
Hinkley, R. D., 705
Hinojosa, R., 340, 350
Hinrichsen, C. F., 345
Hiorns, R. W., 6, 23, 36, 400, 412
Hirano, A., 114, 782
Hirata, Y., 129
Hirsch, M., 907
Hirschberger, W., 990
Hirst, G. D. S., 563, 875
Hiscoe, H. B., 13
Hjorth-Simonsen, A. M., 962, 964
Hnik, P., 762
Ho, M. K., 833
Hobson, J. A., 56, 1101
Hoch, G., 660
Hodgkin, A. L., 43, 177, 189, 219, 224, 280, 283, 424, 425, 428, 432, 434, 435, 441, 465, 466, 467, 500, 501, 503, 508, 510, 528, 551, 555, 558, 560, 561, 562, 563, 567, 601, 608, 631, 632, 638, 641, 642, 644, 647, 648, 649, 650, 651, 652, 654, 655, 760, 848
Hodos, W., 22
Hoffer, B. J., 16, 52, 55, 116, 880, 882
Hoffman, P. N., 718, 947
Hoffmann, K. P., 249, 250, 252
Hofmann, T., 620
Hofmeier, G., 608, 610
Hogan, P. G., 760
Hohberg, E., 488, 491
Hökfelt, T., 52, 56, 139, 140, 973, 989, 1029, 1030, 1031, 1032, 1060, 1062, 1064, 1073, 1079, 1087, 1089
Hokin, L. E., 831, 833
Holden, A. L., 996
Holeckova, E., 762
Holland, P. C., 831, 833, 837
Holländer, H., 250, 264, 1095
Hollingsworth, D., 717
Hollingworth, T., 71, 479
Hollis, D. E., 947
Hollyday, M., 66, 765
Holmes, M. J. 945
Holtfreter, J., 69, 735, 736
Holtzer, H., 723, 725, 801
Holtzman, E., 779
Holz, R., 656
Hong, J. S., 1072, 1073
Hönig, W. M. M., 1079
Hooisma, J., 757
Hooker, D., 759
Horch, K. W., 941, 948
Hore, J., 55
Horn, A. S., 1089
Horn, R., 562, 563
Hornykiewicz, O., 1069
Horridge, G. A., 46, 146, 147, 152, 153, 275, 462, 1134
Horst, W. D., 1035
Horton, R., 1079
Hoshino, K., 1096
Hougie, C., 802
Howell, S. L., 861, 862
Howse, P. E., 146, 151
Hoyle, G., 883
Hoyt, R., 648, 655
Hraoui, S., 1028
Hu, K. G., 306
Huang, M., 755, 756, 824, 825

Hubbard, B. D., 731
Hubbard, I. I., 1008
Hubbard, J. J., 340, 762
Hubbell, W. L., 188, 675, 693
Hubel, D. H., 6, 25, 28, 29, 33, 35, 74, 117, 118, 120, 122, 123, 167, 248, 251, 385, 399, 517, 769, 953, 964, 965, 1094, 1102, 1115, 1117, 1120, 1126
Hucho, F., 805
Hughes, A., 116, 250, 251, 759, 765, 787
Hughes, A. F. W., 60, 75, 938
Hughes, G. M., 499
Hughes, J. T., 1058, 1059
Hughes, J. V., 906
Hughes, W. S., 743
Hultin, H. O., 811
Humphrey, D. R., 33
Hunt, R. K., 60, 63, 72, 73
Hunt, S. P., 990, 991, 993, 995, 996, 998, 999, 1001, 1007, 1008
Hunter, P. J., 432
Hurlbut, W. P., 581, 587
Huxley, A. F., 441, 501, 507, 528, 529, 551, 558, 560, 561, 608, 631, 632, 638, 641, 644, 647, 648, 649, 651, 652, 654, 655, 848
Hyde, A., 360, 362
Hyde, J. E., 541
Hynes, R. O., 692, 697
Hyvärinen, J., 25

I

Iansek, R., 427, 433, 434
Iberall, A., 482, 486, 491, 495, 566
Ifft, J. D., 974
Ifshin, M. S., 1044, 1045, 1048
Iggo, A., 518, 938, 947
Ignarro, L. J., 881
Ikeda, H., 250, 251, 253
Iles, J. F., 429, 433, 434, 436, 448
Imamoto, K., 345
Imig, T. J., 30
Ingvar, D. H., 470, 1006
Innanen, U. T., 1071
Insel, P. A., 824
Ioannides, A. C., 283
Iqbal, Z., 717
Irman, O. R., 388
Ironton, R., 768
Isaacson, R. L., 1125, 1126, 1130
Ishida, A. T., 166, 174
Ishikawa, H. R., 723, 725
Ishikawa, T., 166
Ishizaka, K., 691
Ishizaka, T., 691
Israël, M., 751, 1014
Ito, H., 184
Ito, M., 112, 530, 534, 536, 543
Ito, S., 395
Ivanyshyn, A. M., 306
Iversen, L. L., 987–988, 1085–1092; vi, 15, 564, 918, 988, 989, 992, 1027, 1033, 1062, 1065, 1066, 1067, 1075, 1087, 1089
Iversen, S. D., 56, 1079
Iwama, K., 131, 1094
Iwatsubo, M., 753

Klee, W. A., 1066
Kleene, S. C., 527
Kleinhaus, A. L., 562
Kleinschmidt, J., 169, 196
Klingman, A. D., 284, 291
Kniffki, K.-D., 632
Knigge, K. M., 970
Knight, B. W., 282
Knight, P. L., 30
Knipe, D. M., 730
Ko, C.-P., 931
Ko, P. K., 761
Kobayashi, H., 54, 880
Kobayashi, K., 1014
Kobayashi, R. M., 1031, 1034
Kobayashi, S., 643
Kocsis, J. D., 1070, 1071
Koda, L., 55
Kodowitz, P. J., 877
Koehler, J. K., 691
Koenderink, J. J., 94
Koenig, H. L., 567, 921, 993
Koenig, J., 764, 765
Koike, H., 45, 519
Kok, B., 660
Koketsu, K., 135, 563, 1101
Kolb, H., 166, 174, 176, 243, 248, 266
Koles, Z. J., 13, 14
Kölliker, A. V., 477, 478
Kollros, J. J., 63
Komisaruk, B. R., 972
Konishi, M., 1086
Koppel, D., 692, 700
Kordon, C., 970, 973
Korf, J., 1074, 1088
Korn, H., 333–358; 8, 223, 315, 316, 334,
    335, 336, 337, 338, 339, 340, 341, 342,
    343, 344, 345, 346, 348, 349, 350, 361,
    462
Kornberg, R. D., 635
Korneliussen, H., 943
Kornguth, S. E., 112, 493
Kort, E. N., 813
Koshland, D. E., Jr., 813, 856
Koslow, S. H., 757
Kosterlitz, H. W., 56
Kostopoulos, G. K., 1014
Kostyuk, P. G., 558, 562, 602
Kraayenhof, R., 666
Kraig, R. P., 468, 469, 472
Kratowich, N., 813
Krause, W., 751
Kravitz, E. A., 215
Krebs, E. G., 802, 806, 860, 867
Krespi, V., 641
Kretsinger, R. H., 617–622; 53, 552, 565,
    566, 619, 620
Kreutzberg, G. W., 1005–1016; 14, 15, 16,
    53, 362, 395, 434, 440, 441, 445, 481,
    482, 483, 486, 491, 492, 565, 566, 923,
    988, 989, 1006, 1007, 1008, 1009, 1010,
    1012, 1014
Kriebel, M. E., 343
Krishtal, O. A., 558, 562, 563, 602
Kristensson, K., 923, 1002
Křivánek, J., 468, 469, 470
Kříž, N., 463, 464, 466, 469
Krnjević, K., 214, 464, 466, 468, 469, 564,
    611, 751, 1101, 1102
Kronheim, S., 1030

Krueger, B. K., 813
Kruger, L., 1007
Krulich, L., 1031
Kuba, K., 755, 1093
Kubo, K., 969
Kuffler, S. W., 44, 136, 167, 227, 243,
    250, 251, 460, 464, 499, 631, 716, 768,
    793, 1115
Kuhar, M. J., 291, 1057, 1058, 1062,
    1063, 1065, 1066, 1078, 1086
Kühne, W., 751
Kuhnt, U., 1091
Kuiper, J. W., 288, 299, 301, 306
Kung, C., 562
Kuno, M., 431, 435, 446, 448, 450, 451,
    453, 517, 520, 613
Kunze, P. L., 94, 278, 306
Künzle, H., 35, 990, 991, 995, 996, 998,
    1002, 1007, 1008
Kuo, J. F., 860, 867, 880
Kuo, Z. Y., 759
Kupfermann, I., 1053
Kuroda, Y., 1014
Kusano, K., 174, 465, 467, 556, 557, 612
Kuypers, H. G. J. M., 24, 33
Kwee, P., 749
Kyte, J., 833, 834

L

Labeyrie, E., 350
Labrie, F., 862
Lacey, P. L., 248, 264
Ladinsky, H., 1071
Ladosky, W., 973
Laemmli, U. K., 741
Lagunoff, D., 691
Lake, N., 882
Lallemant, C., 813
Lam, D. M. K., 117, 175, 200, 216
LaManna, J. C., 470
Lamarre, Y., 519, 613
Lamb, T. D., 170, 177, 186, 189, 197, 224
Lambert, D. T., 714, 715
Lambert, J. D. C., 1044, 1049, 1050
LaMotte, C., 1061, 1066
LaMotte, H., 25, 26
Lance, J. W., 250
Land, B. R., 757, 760, 761, 855
Land, M. F., 82, 84, 85, 87
Landau, W. U., 250
Landgren, S., 35, 399
Landis, D. M. D., 114, 115, 130, 346, 573,
    575, 576, 577, 580, 582, 595, 752, 780,
    874, 876
Landis, S. C., 705, 931
Landmesser, L., 943, 1133
Landowne, D., 565
Lands, W. E. M., 1019
Lane, N. J., 717, 718
Lane, P., 114
Langan, T. A., 860
Langer, H., 278
Langer, S. Z., 885, 988
Langer, T. P., 328, 329, 330
Langworthy, O. R., 388
Lapham, L. W., 61
Lappi, S., 764
LaRaia, P. J., 866, 867, 868
Lardner, T. J., 693, 699

Larramendi, L. M. H., 74, 112, 345
Larsen, W. J., 360, 362
Laruelle, L., 385
Lasansky, A., 166, 194, 199, 201, 222, 281
Lasek, R. J., 718, 923, 947
Lash, J. W., 492
Lashley, K. S., 22, 24, 1124
Lassek, A. M., 391, 392, 394
Lassignal, N. L., 588, 592
Lasson, N. A., 470
Laties, A. M., 175
Lauffer, M., 247
Laughlin, S. B., 278, 280, 282, 284, 285,
    286, 287, 288, 289, 290, 291, 303
Laurberg, S., 964
Laurent, J. P., 1096
Laurent, T. C., 718
Lauter, C. J., 874
LaVail, J. H., 62, 990
LaVelle, A., 743
Lawrence, P. A., 364, 746, 951, 953
Lazarides, E., 684, 723, 724, 725, 726,
    731
Lazarus, L. H., 1030, 1034
Leaf, A., 470
Leao, A. A. P., 468
LeBeux, Y. J., 718
Leblond, C. P., 395
Lebovitz, R. M., 465
LeDouarin, N. M., 929, 930, 931
Lee, C. Y., 852, 855
Lee, K. S., 560, 602, 963
Lee, T.-P., 880
Leeman, S., 906
Leeman, S. E., 1029, 1030
Lefkowitz, R. J., 822, 824, 1050
Le Floc'h, M. L., 1077
Le Fort, D., 998, 1001
Leger, L., 16
Lehmann, D., 1097
Lehmann, H., 838
Lehninger, A. L., 395
Leicester, J., 250
Leiman, A. L., 1125
Leman, R. B., 1079
LeMoal, M., 1079
Lenneberg, E. H., 1115
Lennie, P., 250
Lenon, R. N., 31
Leon, M. A., 680
Leonardelli, J., 1029, 1031
Leong, S. K., 958
Lester, H. A., 560
Lester, H. E., 848, 856
Letinsky, M. S., 757
Letourneau, P. C., 934
Lettvin, J. Y., 227, 243, 391, 499
Leung, N. L. K., 870
Leutscher-Hazelhoff, J. T., 288
LeVay, S., 33, 74, 117, 118, 120, 122, 123,
    399, 905, 964
Levey, G. S., 867
Levick, W. R., 94, 95, 172, 227, 241, 242,
    243, 249, 250, 251, 252
Levi-Montalcini, R., 64, 65, 744, 759, 918,
    922, 932, 934
Levine, R., 73
Levinson, W., 731
Levinthal, C., 70, 480, 749, 750, 948
Levinthal, F., 749, 750

Williams, R. G. P., 643, 645
Williams, R. J. P., 621
Williams, R. S., 114
Williams, V., 385
Willis, A. W., 1020, 1023
Willis, W. D., 385
Willison, J. H. M., 704
Willmer, E. N., 248, 250
Willshaw, D. J., 1123
Wilson, B. D., 61
Wilson, C. J., 1088
Wilson, D. F., 885, 886
Wilson, D. L., 1053
Wilson, D. M., 1134
Wilson, H. R., 1120
Wilson, L., 680
Wilson, M., 284, 285, 287, 288, 292
Wilson, P. D., 1096
Wilson, V. J., 340
Winckler, H., 1009
Windle, W. F., 388
Wine, J. J., 152, 520
Winfield, D. A., 23, 33
Winkelmann, R. K., 938
Winkler, B. S., 229
Winkler, R., 621
Winlow, W., 146
Winograd, S., 1119
Winson, J., 56
Wise, S. P., 25, 33, 1007, 1008
Witkovsky, P., 166, 171
Witt, H. T., 659–669; 552, 553, 660, 661, 662, 663, 664, 665, 666
Witter, A., 1035
Wittkowski, W., 385, 395
Witzke, F., 760
Wolf, D., 579, 695, 700
Wolf, M. K., 494
Wolfe, L. S., 1017, 1022, 1024
Wolff, Ch., 660, 662
Wolff, J. R., 399
Wollenberger, A., 870
Wolosewick, J. J., 705, 706, 708, 709, 719, 725
Wolpert, L., 746, 750
Wong, D., 870
Wong, K. S., 151
Wong, M. T. T., 374
Wong, R. K. S., 564
Wong, W. C., 486
Wong-Riley, M. T. T., 194, 203
Wood, J. G., 567, 785
Wood, M. R., 152, 780
Wood, P. M., 65
Woodward, D. J., 116

Woody, C. D., 1101
Woolfolk, C. A., 808
Woolacott, M., 883
Woolley, D. E., 973
Woolsey, C. N., 24, 25, 27, 29
Woolsey, T. A., 27, 953
Wooten, G. F., 885, 914
Worden, F. G., v–vii
Worth, R. M., 566
Wray, H. L., 866, 867
Wright, K. A., 64
Wright, M. J., 250, 251, 253
Wright, W. E., vii
Wu, C.-W., 856
Wu, E., 699
Wuerker, R. B., 488, 716
Wulff, K., 801
Wunk, D. F., 204, 209, 210
Wurtman, R. J., 897–909; vi, 15, 893, 899, 901, 902, 906, 907, 916
Wyatt, H. J., 242, 243
Wyborny, L. E., 869
Wylie, R. M., 340
Wyman, J., 753, 856
Wyss, R., 480
Wyzinski, P. W., 56, 383

Y

Yahara, I., 675, 676, 677, 678, 679, 681, 684, 685, 696, 700, 725, 727
Yamada, E., 166
Yamada, K. M., 488, 493, 692, 697, 698, 700, 705, 717, 781, 787
Yamada, S. S., 692, 697, 698
Yamamoto, C., 131
Yamamoto, M., 250
Yamamoto, T., 131
Yang, H., 1059
Yantorno, R. E., 645
Yarbrough, G., 882
Yarom, Y., 499, 500, 501, 502, 510, 511
Yates, D. W., 836
Yates, R. A., 993
Yau, K.-W., 511
Yazulla, S., 216
Yeandle, S., 280, 281
Yedlin, M., 460
Yeh, J. Z., 469, 611
Yeh, T. A., 575
Yen, S., 730, 731
Yen, S.-H., 704, 716
Yen, S. S. C., 1035
Yingling, C. D., 384

Yinon, U., 1103
Yip, P., 361
Yonezawa, T., 756
Yoon, M. G., 73, 1133
York, C., 901
York, D. H., 1070
Yoshida, M., 1072
Yoshii, M., 562
Yoshikama, S., 184, 185, 186, 187, 188, 189, 284, 287, 288, 831
Young, A. B., 998
Young, D., 59
Young, J. Z., 146, 147, 151, 527, 556, 755, 953, 1116
Young, R. R., 131, 443, 450, 451
Young, R. W., 787
Young, W. C., 971
Younkin, L. H., 680

Z

Záborszky, L., 399
Zacks, S. I., 755
Zagyansky, Y., 693, 695, 699
Zahltan, R. N., 860
Zamora, A. J., 346
Zantema, A., 299, 301, 306
Zawarzin, A., 147, 148
Zecevic, N., 114
Zeeman, W. P. C., 117
Zeevi, Y. Y., 507
Zeki, S. M., 29, 248
Zelena, J., 762
Zenker, W., 488, 491
Zettler, F., 283, 284, 285, 287, 288, 289, 302, 303, 318
Zickler, A., 662, 663, 664
Ziegler, M. G., 923
Zieglgänsberger, W., 463, 1066
Zieleman, M., 1074, 1088
Zigmond, R. E., 913, 1087
Zihl, J., 1106
Zillig, W., 813
Zimmer, J., 958
Zimmerman, R. P., 285, 287
Zimmermann, G., 94
Zimmermann, H., 1009
Zirinis, P., 1020
Zivkovic, B., 1070
Zomzely-Neurath, C. E., 900, 901
Zonana, H. V., 281
Zorychta, E., 761, 762, 948
Zucker, R. S., 583, 612
Zukin, S. R., 998

SUBJECT INDEX

(Page references to figures and tables appear in italics.)

Circuits (continued)
defined, 107, 109, 146
distribution in mammalian brain, 9
electrotonic mechanisms in, 9ff, 338ff
functional analysis of, 129–142
genetic and epigenetic determinants in
development of, 72, 109ff
information processing by, 163–179
larger cell sets in, 47–48
in lateral geniculate nucleus, 318, 1094,
1094
mapping by 2-deoxyglucose, 138, 139,
996
model systems, 132–136, 163–179
in neocortex, 399–413
in neuropil of s. nigra, 1085ff
in olfactory bulb, 9, *10*, 129–142
progressive remodeling of, 110
regional independence, 145, 149, 291,
373, 378, 499
replicated modules in brain entities, 22,
36–37
in retina, 9, *10*, 163–179, 193–211
in retina, pharmacology of, 218–224
structural aspects of, 7–9, 371ff
tracing techniques, 14
in visual cortex of rhesus, *118*
see also Local circuit neurons
Climbing fibers
Purkinje-cell system and, 116, 530ff
synaptic development of, 111–112, *113*
CNS. *See* Central nervous system
Cobalt, 447
in giant axon, 500, *500*
ion conductance and, 606, *606*, 612
in retina, 230, 232, *233*
Cockroach
axonal geometry of, 510
giant axon, conduction in, 465, 499ff
giant fiber systems in, 152
nonspiking neurons in, 304
thoracic ganglia, local neurons in, 148,
148, 152
walking system of, 151
Coeruleocerebellar fibers, 55
Colcemid, effect on microtubules, *731*,
732
Colchicine, 493, 677ff
cell dynamics and, 693–694, 703, 730
microtubules and, 493, 727
mitogenesis and, 680ff, *681*ff
neuronal transport and, 945, *945*
pigment migration and, 710
Columns, cortical, 25ff
in auditory cortex, 29–30
Golgi types I and II neurons in, 6
individuality of size and shape, 399
as input-output devices, 25, 31
in lobuli of fly, 298
macrocolumn, 28
in medulla of fly, 298
minicolumn, 9–10, 36, 37, 1117
in motor cortex, 30–31
in parietal homotypical cortex, 32
as processing and distributing units, 37,
1117
selection mechanism for output, 406–
409, *408*
in somatic sensory cortex, 26–29
as units of higher brain function, 1117

vertical organization of, 26, 399ff, 403
in visual cortex, 117, 120, *120*, 122,
123, 964, 1134
see also Cerebral cortex; Cortex;
Neocortex
Compound eye. *See* Eye, compound
Computer models
action potential train, *503–505*
dendrodendritic circuit, 134, *135*
granule cell, 132–134, *132, 133*
mitral cell, 132–134, *132, 133*
neurons and neuronal network, 477–
494, 501ff, 525–543
olfactory bulb, 132ff, *132–135*
Purkinje cell, 530ff, *531*ff
Concanavalin A, effects on cell surface,
620, 676ff, *679*, 691ff
Conduction, differential, of action
potentials in axons, 499ff
Cone transmitter, 213–214, *214*
Consciousness
and higher brain function, 18, 1126ff
motor function influence on, 1130
neural substrates for, 1126ff
phasic reentry and, 1126ff, *1127*
sufficient conditions for, 1130–1132,
1132
Cordycepin, effect on RNA synthesis,
899
Cortex
architecture of, 412
cell orientation in, 23
cholinergic innervation of, 1101
columnar organization of, 25ff
cytoarchitectural differences among
regions of, 24
excitatory neuron circuit in, 400–403,
403
fields in, definition of, 24–25
functional organization of, 24–25, 37–
38
immature, *391*
inhibitory mechanisms in, 403ff, *404,
406*
intracortical connections, 412
local neurons in, 5, 109, 410, *410* (*see
also* Local circuit neurons)
mature, *392*
modular design of, 407–409, *408*, 412
neuronal connectivity in, 72
neuropil in, 411, *411*
selection mechanism for output, 406–
409
see also specific areas
Crab
axonal innervation in, 511
oculomotor system of, 152
Crayfish
abdominal ganglia, local neurons in,
148
adenosine in giant axon of, 1006
axonal innervation in, 511
giant fiber systems, 152
local chemical circuits in, 14
nerve cord, microtubular lattice, 705
neuromuscular system, 154
ommatidia of, 282
CRF (ACTH-releasing factor), 1027ff
Critical period
for afferent systems, 964–965

for denervation sprouting in
mammalian skin, 951
for functional capacity of adult brain,
971
for lability in motoneurons, 765
for laterogeniculate body in primates,
124
for nerve terminal development, 751
for neuronal systems, 61, 911
for regenerative proliferation, 64
in retinal ganglion cells, 72
Crustacean visual receptors, 152
CSF. *See* Cerebrospinal fluid
Current-source-density analysis, for visual
system, 1094, *1095*, 1098
Cyclic adenosine monophosphate (cAMP)
adenosine and, 862, 1005, 1009, 1014,
1023
in *Aplysia* burster cells, 883
calcium and, 882–883
cell processes regulated by, 861–862
in cortical neurons, 881, *882*
endoperoxides and, 1023
hormone-induced glycogenesis and, 860
intracellular information processing
and, 1009
ion flux and, 862
metabolism of, 859–860
in myocardial function, 865–871, *866*
in nervous system, 861–862
norepinephrine and, 820, *820*, 862,
881, *882*
pituitary hormones and, 1029
protein phosphorylation and, 860–861,
865–871, *1043*
somatostatin effect on, 1035
protein phosphorylation and, 860–861,
865–870, 877
in Purkinje-cell firing, 883
in S49 lymphoma cell, 824, *825*
s. nigra presynaptic receptor and, 1089
synthesis pathway, 819
transmitter release and, 862
see also Cyclic nucleotides; Second
messengers
Cyclic guanosine monophosphate (cGMP)
acetylcholine and, 881, *882*
calcium interaction with, 877–878, *878*
in pyramid cells, 881, *881*
second-messenger concept and, 860
see also Cyclic nucleotides; Second
messengers
Cyclic nucleotides, 53
ACTH and, 914
in biosystems, 12–13, *13*
calcium interaction with, 876–879, *876,
878*
dopamine-β-hydroxylase and, 914
in hormone action, 859–863
metabolism of, 873–879, *876*
neuronal activity and, 873–886, 1043–
1054
opiates and, 1066
peptide modification of, 1034, 1045–
1047
pituitary hormones and, 1029
synaptic response and, 879, 1050–1052,
1050
tyrosine hydroxylase and, 914, *915*
see also specific names

Cyclic nucleotide phosphates, in retina, 189
Cycloheximide
  enzyme induction and, 921
  neonatal action of androgen and, 972
Cytidine, and transfer dynamics, *1009*
Cytoarchitecture, 23–25
  functional significance in brain, 457ff
Cytochalasins
  cell dynamics and, 678, 693–694, 711
  microfilament bundles and, 726–727, *727, 732*
Cytodifferentiation, in neurogenesis, 59
Cytokinesis, in cell proliferation, 61
Cytoplasm
  filament systems in, 678, 703ff, *707*ff
  saltatory behavior of, 708
  translocation in, hypothesis, 710ff
Cytoplasmic ground substance (CGS), 705ff, *706, 709*
  protein-rich phase, 708, *709*
  water-rich phase, 708, *709*
Cytoskeleton, 12–13, 703–719

D

Death, neuronal, 65–67, 765–766
Debye theory of dipole orientation, 628, 633
Degeneracy, as a principle of brain function, 1117ff
Deiters nucleus of rat, electrotonic coupling in, 346
Dendrites
  action potentials in, *450–452,* 451–452, 563, *564*
  adenosine transport and release in, 1006, *1007*
  in chromatolytic neurons, 450, *450,* 453
  concept of, revised, 419
  developmental plasticity in organization of, 70
  dopamine release from, 1074–1075, 1086–1088, *1087*
  electrotonic activity in, 12, 483
  equivalent-cylinder model of, 426, 440, *441,* 445, 483, 529, 530, 532
  filaments in, *490,* 491
  form of, and synaptic efficacy, 325–326, *326*
  geometry of, 317–330, 482
  growth mechanism of, 71
  integrated receptive region of, 43
  mitral, 373
  morphology, 70
  in motoneurons, 386, *386,* 442–452, *443, 445, 447, 452,* 478
  myelination of, 131
  in olfactory bulb, 129, 373
  parallelization, 12
  plasticity of, 71
  presynaptic, 317–330, 373–378
  processes of, 7, *8,* 46, 47, 69–71, 112, 114
  of Purkinje cells, 111
  of retinal ganglion cells, 168
  sexual dimorphism in, *975*
  synapses, and hormones, *974*
  synaptic connections, 145 (*see also* Synapses)

synaptic efficacy, 325, *326,* 327
  transmitter released from, 16
Dendritic branches, 70
  density of, in cytoskeletal structures, 484, *484*
  geometrical model of, 317–330
  independent action of, 373, 378
  orientation of, *487*
  regional computation of, 321, 329, 330
Dendritic bundles, 383–413, 462
  development of, and behavior, 387
  maturation of reciprocal activity in, 387–389, *388*
  modes of operation, 394–396, *395*
  in olfactory bulb, 390
Dendritic inhibition, in retinal information processing, 241–242
Dendritic spikes
  in amacrine cells, 237, 238, *238*
  calcium-dependent, 564–565, *565*
  in optic tectum of pigeon, 996
Dendritic tree
  branch-power rules, 482, *483*
  daughter-branch ratio, 484ff, *485*
  postsynaptic potentials in, 323, 328, *328, 329*
  sculpting process, 71
  size determination, 479ff
  topological types, 487
Dendrodendritic circuit, compartmental model, *134, 135*
Dendrodendritic inhibition, 390
Dendrodendritic synapses, 7–10, 317–330
  neurotransmitters at, 140–141
  in olfactory bulb, *10,* 129–130, 136
  spikes not necessary for function of, 329
Dendrogenesis, 70
Dentate gyrus (hippocampal)
  adenosine derivatives and, 1007
  astrocytes in, 966
  axonal connectivity in, 75
  cell generation in, 62, 65
  commissural projections, 958, *960, 962*
  laminar profile analysis, 958
  neurogenesis of, 62
  5′-nucleotidase activity in, *1011*
  synaptogenesis, 958
2-Deoxyglucose mapping, 1³8, 139, 996
Diencephalon, cell proliferation in, 62
diI (3,3′-dioctadecylindocarbocyanine iodide), mobility in cell membrane, 692–693, 698
Diptera, gap junctions in salivary gland cells of, 362. *See also* Insects
Disfacilitation mechanism, 232, *233*
Distributed systems in higher brain function, 22, 37, 38, 1124
DJ400B (cyclic polyene)
  insertion-aggregation process and, 644ff, *645, 649*
  structure and molecular model of, *646*
DNA
  chromosomal, and mRNA, 899
  gene expression control by, 898
DNA synthesis, 679ff, *679*
  in neuronal cell cycle, 61, 65
  sequential cessation, 64
L-Dopa, and protein synthesis, 15, 898, 901–903, *901–903, 905*

Dopamine
  adenylate cyclase and, 1070, 1075, 1089
  androgenization effect on, 973
  cAMP and, 862, 1051
  dendritic release of, 1074–1075
  in dorsal hypothalamus, 54
  in endoplasmic reticulum, 1088
  β-endorphin secretion and, 1032
  in molluscan CNS, 215
  at nerve terminals, 1070, 1077
  in periglomerular cells, 139–140
  potassium-evoked release of, 1087, *1088*
  prolactin secretion and, 1027
  in retina, 175–176, *176–177*
  sensorimotor integration and, 1075–1077
  in s. nigra, 16, 54, 1075, 1089–1090
  systems, 52
  transsynaptic enzyme induction and, 914
  TRF release and, 1035
  in tufted cells, 140
  in ventral tegmentum, 54
Dopamine-β-hydroxylase
  in adrenal medulla, 913ff
  and NGF, 1002
  selective induction of, 913
Dopaminergic pathways, ascending nigrostriatal, 1069–1080, *1086*
Dragonfly
  local neurons in larval thoracic ganglia, 148, *148,* 149
  visual system of, 279, 283–284, *286–287,* 291 (*see also* Insect vision)
Drosophila, 82
  diurnal rhythms in, 302
  flight system, 152, 154
  mutants, 298, 306
  visual system, 93, *93,* 298
  see also Fly

E

Ectodermal placodes, 59
Ectopic cells, in chick spinal cord, 67–68
Efferent systems
  of chemically coded neurons, 52, 53
  from locus coeruleus, 55
EF hand
  in calcium-modulated proteins, 619–621, *619*
  conformation, 619, *619,* 620
EGTA [ethylene glycol-*bis*-(β-aminoethyl-ether)-N,N′-tetracetic acid]
  adenosine at synapse and, 1007
  Aplysia neurons and, 882
  ion conductance and, 607, *607, 608,* 609, 618
  in retina, 186–187, *187–188*
Electrical circuitry in brain, overview, 9–12
Electric fields
  effects on macromolecular systems, 631–638
  electrochromism and, 661, *661,* 662
  in photosynthetic membrane, 659–668
  physical chemistry of effects of, 632–634
Electric organ, of *Electrophorus* and ATP release, 1009

Filaments, 703ff, 723ff
  intermediate (100 Å), 703–704, 730–731
  tonofilaments, 731, *732*
  see also Microfilaments; Microtubules;
    Microtrabeculae
Filamin, 725–726
Finch, sexual dimorphism in brain of,
  974
Fish
  chromatophore, pigment motion in,
    708–711, *710*
  electroreceptor synapse of, 286
  erythrophore, cytoplasmic matrix of,
    710ff, *710*ff
  see also Electric organ
Fluorescence photobleach technique, 676,
  677, 692, *693*
Fluoride ions, and adenylate cyclase, 821ff
Fly
  behavioral model for, 7, 81–102
  direction-sensitive turning response,
    306
  landing response, 306–307
  lift response, 306–307
  nonspiking neurons in, 304–306
  ommatidium, 297ff, *301* (*see also*
    Ommatidium)
  optic cartridge, 149, 278–279, *279*
  optomotor turning response, 89ff, 277,
    306–307, *307*
  pattern-induced fixation response,
    306
  polarized light, response to, 306
  rhabdomeres of, 282, 298
  salivary gland of, 877, *878–879*
  simuliid (*see* Simuliid fly)
  torque response, 83ff, *84*ff
  tracking behavior, *88*
  visual system, 81–102, 275ff, 297–308
  see also Insect vision
Follicle-stimulating hormone (FSH), and
  studies of cell communication, 364
Food intake
  gonadal steroids and, 971
  TRF and, 1034
Forebrain, cell proliferation in, 62
Fourier analysis, of nonlinear components
  in visual system, 91, 263
Frog
  cell proliferation in tectum, 63
  cerebellar calcium and synaptic
    transmission in, 467
  cerebellar cortex, model of, 537, *538*
  channel gating in two species of, 627–
    628
  electrotonic transmission in brain,
    340
  neuromuscular junction, aminopyridine
    and, *576*
  optic tectum of, 993
  photoreceptors of, 184, *184*
  Purkinje cell of, *531*
  quick-freezing of muscles of, *574*
  retina, *165*, 168, 185, *185*, 248, *250*
  skeleton, computer model of, 541–542,
    542
  spinal motoneuron, calcium/potassium
    system in, 612–613
  sympathetic ganglion, EPSPs in, 880
FSH. *See* Follicle-stimulating hormone

G

GABA (gamma-aminobutyric acid)
  in amacrine cells, 236, 243
  in avian optic tectum, 992–998
  modulatory role of, 15
  in olfactory bulb, 139
  in periglomerular cells, 140
  presynaptic inhibition by, 465, 1061
  in retina, 175
  in s. nigra, 1072–1073, *1073*, 1075,
    1077, *1078*, 1086, 1089
Ganglia, basal, anatomy of, 1069
Ganglia, metathoracic, action potentials in,
  500, *502*
Ganglia, of Remak, transplantation study
  in, 930
Ganglia, retinal
  cell adhesiveness in, 737ff
  chloride-free medium in study of,
    227ff, *228*, *230*
  excitation of, *248*, *252*, 253–259, *256–*
    257
  inhibition of, *252*, 253–259, *256–257*
  mechanisms of, 233, *234*
  on-off amacrine cells in, 231
  pathways in receptive field of, *248*, *252*,
    252, *253*
  receptive-field organization in, 227ff,
    *228*ff, 247–268, *252*ff
  spatial summation in, 253–260, *254*
  synaptic inputs, 204–208, *204–207*
  types of, 250–251
Ganglia, spinal, neuronal processes in
  vitro, 744–745, *745*
Ganglia, stomatogastric, of lobster, 152,
  153, 318ff, *327*
Ganglia, superior cervical, *784*, *786*, *788*
  cyclic nucleotides in, 881, *915*, 1052
Ganglia, sympathetic
  cAMP and, 862
  tyrosine hydroxylase in, 912ff, *915–916*
Gap junctions, 8, *8*, 14, 338ff, 359–365
  biochemical characterization, 363–364
  calcium and, 362
  communication specificity of, 362
  in differentiating systems, 364
  distribution of, 359–360
  in excitable tissues, 361
  formation and turnover, 361
  glial cells and, 278
  between horizontal cells, 262
  hormonal influence on, 360–361, 364
  intracellular pH and, 362
  isolation of, 363–364
  in mammalian CNS, 345–349, *347–349*
  in neuroepithelium, 62
  in nonexcitable tissues, 361–362
  in opossum brain, 346
  pathway for electrotonic coupling, 362
    (*see also* Electrotonic coupling)
  physiological properties of, 361–362
  protein synthesis and, 361
  in retina, *165*, 166
  selective permeability of, 362
  separation with hypertonic sucrose, 361
  structure of, 359–360, 362
  turnover rate in, 360
Gating mechanisms
  behavioral changes via, 56

in ionic channels, 11, 425
  mathematical description of, 645–648
  membrane proteins and, 623–629
  in membranes, 632, 638, 641ff, *656*
Gene expression
  in nervous system, 893ff, 911–925
  neuronal, *14*, 15, 969–970, 972
  sexual differentiation in brain and,
    969ff
  synapse formation and, 750–751
Gene mutation, in cerebellar Purkinje
  cells, 110
Genome
  cell shape and, 492
  communication with cell membrane
    and, 12, 13, *13*
  expression, 53, *54*
Geometry of cells, 326–329
GH. *See* Growth hormone
Glanzmann's thrombasthenia, ADP and,
  1023
Glial cells
  adenosine derivative transport and, *1007*
  adenosine production by, 1011
  and axonal growth, 965–966
  cortical orientation of, 23
  in extracellular space, 458ff
  influence on afferent topographies, 957,
    965–966
  interaction with neurons, 492
  ionic control by, 460
  and locust receptor axons, 278
  microglia, 1012
  Müller cells, in retina, 163, *164*, 169
  neuronal migration guided by, 67
  5′-nucleotidase and, 1013
  oligodendroglia, 1011
  potassium and, 464, 465
  proliferation of, 59, 61, 65
  Schwann cells, 65, 948, 952
  supportive function of, 965
  in sympathetic ganglion cell survival,
    965
  in visual system, 117
Glial sheath, 501, 510
  of ommatidium, 277
Gliogenesis, afferent deprivation and, 63
Glucocorticoids
  as ACTH inhibitors, 1027, *1028*
  effect on tyrosine hydroxylase
    induction, 917, *918*
  modulatory role in transsynaptic
    enzyme induction, 916–917, *917–918*
  role in adrenal medulla, 906–907, 913–
    914
Glucose homeostasis, role of CNS in, 1035
Glutamate
  in avian optic tectum, 992–995
  opioid peptides and, 1066
  in retina, 175, *213*, 215ff, *216*, *221*,
    993ff
Glutamic acid
  effect on release of dopamine in
    striatum, 1078, *1078*
  modulatory role of, 15
Glutamine synthetase cascade, 807–808,
  807
Glycine
  in avian optic tectum, 992–993, 998ff,
    999

Information processing
  bidirectional transport, 12, *13-14*
  in extracellular space, 459ff
  in fly visual system, 81ff
  by sensory transduction, 11, *11*
Inhibition
  chemical, in CNS, 336
  dendrodendritic, 390
  electrical, 334, *334*, 335, *335*, 338
  intracortical, 27
  lateral (*see* Lateral inhibition)
  mixed synaptic action, 336, *337*
  pericolumnar, 37
  presynaptic, 374
  putative mechanisms of, in neocortex,
    403ff
  recurrent, 336
Inhibitory postsynaptic potential (IPSP),
    130, *131*, 133, 135, *135*
  in amacrine cells, 231ff
  chloride conductance and, 233
  in ganglion cells, 205, *206-207*, 233
  ionic events and, 880, *880*, 881
  in mammalian thalamus, 378
  reticular stimulation and, 1101, *1102*
Insects
  calcium in salivary gland, 875ff
  local neurons in thoracic ganglia of,
    148, *148*
  nonspiking interneurons in, 149-151,
    150
  nonspiking neurons in, 304-306
Insect vision
  graded slow potentials in, 275-292
  neural interactions in, 81-102
  see also Eye, compound
Insulin
  ouabain effect on release of, 876
  protein synthesis and, 898
Integration, neuronal
  chemical, in CNS, 51-56
  local, evolving concepts of, 43-48
  local, nonanatomical factors affecting,
    44
Intercellular space, 12. *See also*
    Microenvironment
Interneurons
  axoaxonic, 406, *406*
  GABA-ergic, *1000*
  Golgi type II, 405, *406*
  granule cells, 134
  membrane potential, graded, 149
  neocortical, 402ff, *410*
  neurogenesis of, in cortex, 62
  nonspiking, 149-151, *150*
  periglomerular, 134-136, *136*, 140
  see also Local circuit neurons
Interneuronal associations
  ionic influence, 465
  temporal requirement, 979
Interplexiform-layer cells, pharmacology
    of, 174-176, *176*
Invertebrates
  local neurons in, 145-155, *147-148*
  synapses, reciprocal and serial, 151-155,
    153-154
  visual pigments of, 299
  see also Arthropods; Insects; Insect
    vision; *specific names*
Ion flux
  drug effects on, 849ff, *850*ff

IPSPs and, 849ff, *850*ff
  peptide modification of, 1034
  receptor-mediated, 847-857
  spikeless membrane potential and, 53
Ionic channels, 425, 439ff
  gating mechanism in, 11, 623-629, 631-
    638, 641-642
  in membrane of nerve axons, 11
Ionic milieu, of extracellular space, 12,
    459ff, *471*
Iontophoresis
  mapping techniques, 113
  of somatostatin, 1036
  of TRF, 1035
Ion pumps, chemical processes and, 831-
    836, *832*ff. *See also* Calcium ion
    pump; Hydrogen ion pump; Sodium-
    potassium pump
Ion transport
  deficit measurement, 603, *604*
  enzyme activity coupling to, 831-839
  in mitochondrial membrane, 621, 874-
    876
  transmembrane, 425
IPSP. *See* Inhibitory postsynaptic potential
Islets of Langerhans, peptide-secreting
    cells in, 1029
Isthmo-optic nucleus
  ectopic neurons and, 68
  neuronal death and, 66

K

Kirchoff's law, 424
Kitten
  cortex, immature, *391*
  motoneuron dendrites, 453
  ocular-dominance changes in, *1103-
    1104*
  spinal cord, dendrite bundles in, 387-
    389, *388*

L

Lambert-Beers absorption law, 300
Lamina monopolar cells, in arthropod
    visual system, 275ff, *276*
  lateral inhibition in, 289
  light adaptation to, 290-291, *291*
  postsynaptic responses of, 284-288,
    286-287
  potassium in, 290
  slow potentials, 277, 288-291, *289*
Laminar analysis, of calcium and
    potassium in cortex, 466, *467*
Lamprey
  dual synaptic transmission in, 351, *352*
  gap junctions in, 340
  giant synapse of, 318
  spinal cord, synaptic terminal of, *781*
Lateral geniculate nucleus
  connectivity patterns in, 74
  cortical development and, 23
  EPSP profile, 1094, *1095*
  Golgi type II neurons in, *318*
  inhibitory circuits in, 1094, *1094*
  lesions of, 402, *402*
  in visual system, *117*
Lateral inhibition
  in auditory cortex, 29-30
  in lamina monopolar cells, 289

in optic tectum, 996
  in retinal ganglion cells, *252*, *253*, *259*
Lectin, receptor density, 785, 787
Leech
  branching neurons of, 511
  local circuit, chemical, 14
  potassium in ganglia, 465
  Retzius cell, 14
  rhabdomeres of, 281
  touch cells of, 511
Lemniscal afferents, development of, 383-
    384
LH. *See* Luteinizing hormone
LH-RF. *See* Luteinizing-hormone-
    releasing factor
Ligands
  for β-adrenergic receptors, 822
  ion flux effect of, 848ff
  in regulation of adenylate cyclase
    activity, 820
Limbic system, consciousness and, 1126,
    1130, 1131, 1134
Limulus, lateral eye of, 276ff, 308
Lipid bilayers, 430, 440, *458*, 459, 551,
    634, 692
  alamethicin and, 647ff, *649*, *653-654*
  in biological membranes, 654
  channel-forming molecules in, 642-644
  continuous matrix of, 693, 695
  drug effects on conductance in, 641-
    644, *643-644*, *648*, 655
  electrical excitation mechanism of, 641-
    675
  fluidity and calcium currents in, 560,
    621
  fluid structure of, 675
  gating in, 641ff
  hydrocarbon region of, 642, 644-645
  inactivation in, 648, *651-652*
  insertion-aggregation process, 642ff,
    *642*ff
  proteins in, 675, 837
  viscosity of, 694
Lipolysis, and cardiac catecholamines, 55
β-Lipoprotein, amino acid sequence of,
    1058, *1058*
Lizard (*Lacerta viridis*)
  electrotonic transmission in, 340, *341*
  retinal cones of, 186
Lobster
  axonal action potentials, 504-506, 511
  axonal geometry, 510
  postsynaptic potentials, *327*
  stomatogastric ganglion of, 152, *153*,
    318ff, *327*
Local circuit neurons (LCNs)
  and amino acid transmitters, 989-1002
  in annelids, 146
  chemical, in leech, 14
  chemical integration of, 14
  chemically coded, *52*
  connectivity, 22, 1117, 1121, 1135
  in cortex, 5, 109, 410, *410*
  in crayfish abdominal ganglia, 148
  dendrites of, 145
  development of, 62, 72, 109
  electrical properties, 149-151
  in evolution of neocortex, 1134-1135
  in invertebrate nervous systems, 145-
    155, *147*, *148*
  in invertebrate thoracic ganglia, *148*

Local circuit neurons (continued)
  in lateral geniculate, *318*
  in locust thoracic ganglion, 148
  in molluscs, 146, 148
  in octopus brain, 146
  in olfactory bulb, 61, 129–142
  proliferation of, 62
  regional independence of, 145, 149,
    291–292, 373, 378, 499
  in retina, 163–179, 193
  in worm segmental ganglia, 148
Local neuronal circuits. *See* Circuits, local
  neuronal
Locus coeruleus
  axonal innervation patterns, 55
  biasing function, 55
  efferent systems of, 55
  intranuclear feedback inhibition by, 55
  noradrenergic system from, to CNS, 32
  opiate receptors in, 1063
  transmitter action by, 16
Locust
  nonspiking neurons of, 304
  thoracic ganglia, local neurons in, 148,
    148
  visual system of, 277, *277*, *280*, 281ff,
    285, *287*, *290*
Lordosis behavior, 970ff
LRF. *See* Luteinizing-hormone-releasing
  factor
Luteinizing hormone (LH), surge of, 969,
  971
Luteinizing-hormone-releasing factor
  (LRF), 531, 1027, *1028*, 1029, 1036
Luteinizing-hormone-releasing hormone
  (LH-RH), 969
  cyclic surge of, 970, 971, 979
  see also Luteinizing-hormone-releasing
  factor
Lymphocytes, and cell surface dynamics,
  676–687, *679*ff
Lymphoma cells, adenylate cyclase in,
  821ff

M

Macaque, cerebral cortex of, *112*. *See also*
  Monkey
Macromolecules
  channel gating by, 623–627, *624*
  electric field effects in, 631–638
Magnesium
  effect on dopamine in s. nigra, 1087,
    1088
  effect on exocytosis, 577
  effect on horizontal cells, 173, *173*
  effect on opiate-receptor binding, 1066
  phosphorylation and, 621
Mammals, electrotonic coupling in CNS
  of, 345
Manganese
  effect on opiate-receptor binding, 1066
  as synaptic blocker, *461*, 463, 467, 558,
    612
Mast cells
  immunoglobulin receptor on, 694
  neurotensin binding to, 1030
  surface receptors, 691
Matrix, of cells. *See* Cytoplasmic ground
  substance

Mauthner cells, 223
  in axolotl, 71
  chemical inhibition in, 336–338, *337*
  dual synaptic action in, 336–338, *337*,
    350, *351*
  electrical inhibition in, 334–338, *334–
    335*
  in goldfish, 334ff, *351*, 359
Mauthner fibers, gap junctions in, 359
Membranes
  calcium transport in, 874–876
  carbohydrate code of, 786
  carbohydrate moiety of, 783ff
  current-voltage relations, 441
  electrical excitation mechanism, 641–
    657, *645*
  electric-field effects, 631–638, 659–668
  of erythrocyte, human, 831, *832*, *838*
  of erythrophore, *713*
  fluidity of, 654, 675, 693, 698
  fluid mosaic model of, 634
  gene linkage, *13*
  glycocalyx, 457, 459
  of growth cones, 781, 784
  hydrophobic areas, 634, *634*
  ionic channels in, 425
  ionic theory of, 430
  ion pumps in, 831ff
  lateral mobility in, 692–693, *699*
  lipid bilayers (*see* Lipid bilayers)
  mitochondrial, 875ff
  molecular dynamics in, 659ff
  neuronal, compartmentalization, 1053
  peptide moiety, 783
  permeability of, 460–461, 528, 558, 848,
    1043, *1043*, 1044
  phosphorylation in, 13, 1005, 1043ff,
    1043
  photosynthetic, 659–668
  plasma, 566, 567 (*see also* Plasma
    membranes)
  postsynaptic, 780, *781*
  potential (*see* Membrane potential)
  presynaptic, and aminopyridine, 575,
    575, 593
  presynaptic, and exocytosis, 573, 577,
    578, 593
  proteins in, *458*, 459, 623–629, 693–
    695, 832ff, *832–833*
  recognition and, 781–787
  resistivity of, 516
  subsynaptic, 752ff
  synaptic, differentiation of, 779–793,
    *780*ff
  trypsin-susceptible, 839
  vectorial transport across, 663–664
  vesicles of, ion flux in, 847–857
Membrane potential
  in abdominal ganglion, 883
  acetylcholine receptor role in, 847–
    857
  in amacrine cells, 235
  calcium and, 879
  concept of revised, 419
  cyclic nucleotides and, 881
  vs. electric-field effects, *636–637*
  gating current of, 425
  peptide modification of, 1034
  sodium pump and, 833–839, *833*ff
  spikeless, 53
  waveforms of, 531ff, *531*ff

Memory
  associative, 1123ff, *1123*ff
  group-degenerate selection and, 1125
  long-term, 1133
  short-term, 1126, 1130
Menkes's disease, polydendritic Purkinje-
  cell somas in, 114
Merkel cells
  in cat skin touch domes, 948
  mechanosensory nerves and, 938ff,
    *940*ff
  in salamander skin, 938ff, *939*
Metabolic mapping, by 2-deoxyglucose,
  138
Metabolic pools, and spikeless membrane
  potential, 53
Metathoracic ganglia, action potentials in,
  500, 502
Methodology
  cell-cell binding assay, 736, *737*
  2-deoxyglucose mapping, 138, 139, 996
  electrochromism, 659ff
  fluorescence photobleaching, 676, *692*,
    698
  high-voltage electron microscope,
    cytoskeletal application, 705ff
  immunofluorescence microscopy, 723ff
  immunological assay, for cell-adhesion
    molecule, 738ff
  microdissection, to isolate s. nigra tissue,
    1087
  for olfactory receptor stimulation, 137,
    137
  for peptide extract preparation, *1046*
  quick-freezing, 573ff, *574*
  spherical coordinates, for describing
    neuronal form, 486–487, *487*
  trypsinization, of single cells, 737, *737*
  see also Autoradiography; Computer
    models
Microcircuits, information processing by,
  9. *See also* Circuits, local neuronal
Microenvironment
  of brain cell, 457–472, *458*ff
  in dendrites, *490*, 491
  electric fields in, 461–463, 466
  energy and, 470–471
  ionic milieu of, 12, 459–470, *461*ff
  see also Extracellular space
Microfilaments
  cytochalasins and, 678, 711, 726–727
  filamin as accessory protein in, 725
  proteins in, 725
  in tissue-culture cells, 723–727
Microglia. *See* Glial cells
Microtrabeculae
  in axoplasm, 717
  in cytoplasmic system, 678, 703ff,
    *707*ff
Microtubules
  cell growth control and, 683
  cell shape and, 703–705
  cell surface dynamics and, 677–678,
    684, *685*, 696, 703ff, 727–730, *728*
  dendritic, *489–491*
  drug effects on, 493, 696
  in erythrophore, *710*
  in fibroblasts, 729
  in neuroblastoma, 729
  pigment migration and, 711ff
  receptor mobility and, 677ff

Microtubules (continued)
  tubulin antibodies and, 727, *730*
  see also Microfilaments
Minicolumns. *See* Columns, cortical
Mitochondria
  ATP production site, 470
  in axoplasm, motions of, 716
  calcium storage and release and, 621,
    874-876
  cytoplasmic, 705ff, 708, *709-710*
  hydrogen ion pump in, 831, *832, 838*
  protein synthesis in, 901
Mitogenesis
  control points in, *686*
  drug effects on, 679, *680, 682*
Mitosis, sequence in precursors, 64
Mitral cells, 108
  antidromic criteria, 131
  computer model, 132-134, *132-133*
  dendrites of, 129ff, 373
  dendritic bundles of, 389-391, *389*
  electrotonic potentials in, 9
  excitatory-suppressive sequence, 138
  hyperpolarization in, 130, *131*
  lateral inhibition in, 134, *135*
  in olfactory bulb, 61, 129ff
  periglomerular, 9, 135
  self-inhibition of, 134, *135*
Models
  of branching dendrite, 445ff
  of cerebellum, 528, 530ff
  of formal neurons, 527.
  of motoneurons, 444, 445
  of neuronal electrical phenomena, 528
  of neuronal networks, 525-543
  olfactory bulb as local circuit model,
    132-136
  of *on-off* cells, 240
  pancreas as cell-cell interaction model,
    1029
  pigeon visual system, 989ff
  Purkinje-cell computer model, 530-536
  Rall's, of nerve cell, 421, 433
  retina as local circuit model, 163ff
  single cell, 530-536
Mollusks, local neurons in, 146, 148
Monazomycin, lipid bilayers and, 642ff,
    *643*ff
Monkey
  amacrine cells of, *235*
  axoaxonic cells of, 406
  fetal visual cortex, *121*
  gap junctions in, 346
  myelinated dendrites of, 131
  olfactory bulb, dendrite bundles in, *390*
  parietal cortex of, 32, *410*
  presynaptic dendrites in, 374-377
  retinal receptive field of, 29, 168
  somatic sensory cortex of, 26
  star pyramids in central sulcus of, 71
Monoamines
  activation of, 53, 55
  adenosine interaction with, 1014
  see also Adenylate cyclase; Biogenic
    amines; Catecholamines; *specific names*
Monoaminergic drugs, effects on protein
    synthesis, 901-906, *901-905*
Morphology, neuronal, 478-488
  local environmental factors in, 70
  mechanical factors in, 70-71

Mossy-fiber system, 382, 530
Motoneuron
  of *Aplysia*, 354, *354*
  calcium-dependent potassium system in,
    611-612
  cat spinal, 322, 327-328, 386, *386*, 447,
    447, 1006, *1007*
  chromatolytic, 450-453, *450, 1012*
  dendrites in, 327, 386, *386*, 445-452,
    *445*ff, *478*, 489-491, *489-490*
  excitability of, 439-445, *443*
  form, determinants of, *481, 484*
  maturation of, *385, 388*
  model, 444, 445
  nonspiking interneurons in, 149, *150*
  retrograde stabilization of, 765-766
  squirrel monkey, retrograde transport
    in, *1010*
Motor cortex
  columnar organization of, 30-31
  development of pyramidal cells in, 391-
    394, *391-392*
Mouse
  gap junctions in, 345-346, *359*, 363-364
  steroid hormones in brain of, *978*
Mouse mutants
  behavioral abnormalities, 114
  neuronal cell cycle in, 61
  perisomatic spines in, 114
  synaptic abnormalities in, 114
  ultrastructural characteristics of, 114
  see also Nervous mouse; Reeler mouse;
    Staggerer mouse; Weaver mouse
Mudpuppy (*Necturus maculosus*)
  amacrine cells of, 229ff
  eyecup preparation, 227ff
  ganglion cells of, *196*
  retina of, 163ff, *164, 194, 204*
Müller cells, in retina, 163, *164*, 169
Musca. See Fly
Muscle cells, ion flux in, 855-856, *855*
Myelin sheath, axolemma contact with,
    1011
Myocardial cells
  cAMP in, 865-871
  catecholamines in, 865-868
Myosin, and cytoplasmic motility, 12, *13*,
    715
Myostatin, and lipid bilayers, 656

N

Necturus maculosus. See Mudpuppy
Neocortex
  ATP release from, 1009
  cell proliferation in, 62
  central-core system of, 32
  columnar organization of, 36-37
  cytoarchitecture of, 23-25
  distinctive functions of, 24
  evolution of, 22-25
  extrinsic connectivity of, 24-25, 34-35
  inhibitory mechanisms in, 403-407, *404,
    408*
  internal connectivity, 33-34, 37, *408,
    412*
  as large processing unit, 36-37
  local neuron circuits in, 399-413
  morphological differentiation of, 24
  neurogenesis of, 62

  ontogenetic development of, 23-24
  phylogeny of, 22-23, 400
  progression indices, 22
  see also Cortex
Nernst equation, 460, 507
Nerve cells. *See* Neurons
Nerve domains, 950, *950, 951*, 953
Nerve fibers
  afferent-systems, 957ff
  associational, 958, 963
  biochemical coding of, 961
  commissural, 958ff
  monoamine systems and, 960-961
  myelinated, and 5'-nucleotidase, 1010-
    1011
  in optic tract, 964
  peptides in, 1030
  preganglionic cholinergic, 912-916, *912*
  regeneration of, 960-961
  sprouting, 958ff
  see also Axons; Dendrites
Nerve field
  establishment of, 937-938
  of mechanoreceptors, 938-939
  spatial control of, 948-949, 951
Nerve growth factor (NGF), 61, 64, 965
  acetylcholine/norepinephrine ratio and,
    932-933
  direction of neurite growth and, 934
  in dorsal-root ganglia, 744
  neuron plasticity and, 932-934
  retrograde transport of, 14-15, 919-
    924, *919, 921*, 1002
  tyrosin hydroxylase and, 922, *922*, 923
Nerve membrane
  vs. photosynthetic membrane, 668
  transmembrane field, generation of,
    659
  see also Membranes
Nerve processes
  connectivity of, 109-110
  regeneration of, 943, *944*
Nerve sprouting
  axonal branching and, 941-943
  in brain fibers, 958, 960
  extrinsic regulation of, 937-953
  in mammals, 951
  neuronal transport and, 944-947
  neuron-target interaction and, 943-948
  in salamander skin, 938ff
  synaptogenesis and, 952
Nerve terminals
  dopamine storage in, 1070
  motor, presynaptic stabilization of, 765-
    768
  peptides in, 1030, 1032
  protein synthesis in, 901
  synaptic, 779, *780*, 781, 993
  synaptic vesicles in, *578*
  transmembrane potential and, 848
  see also Synapses
Nervous mouse, Purkinje-cell dendrites
  of, 114
Nervous system
  modular construction of, 35-36
  peripheral sympathetic, 911-925, *912*
  see also Central nervous system
Network
  brain as, 457
  cerebellar, 536

Neuropil (continued)
   ganglionic, cAMP in, 1047, 1051
   ganglionic, protein phosphorylation in,
      1052
   of insect medulla, 279
   lamina synaptic, 275
   in olfactory bulb, 138, 389ff
   optic, 298, *299*
   in primate neocortex, 117
   specific patterns in, 381–382
   of s. nigra, dopamine and, 1085ff
   synaptic connections in, 108
   thalamic, 382–383
   thoracic, 299
Neurotensin, 53, *1028*, 1030, 1033, *1033*,
   1036
Neurotransmitters
   adrenergic, 929ff, *930, 932*
   androgenization effects on, 973
   calcium influx and, 874
   cholinergic, 929ff, *930, 932*
   embryonic environment and, 930
   metabolic alterations via, 884
   neuronal protein synthesis and, 897ff
   in olfactory bulb, 138–141, *140*
   peptides and turnover of, 1034
   pituitary cells and, 1027
   release, presynaptic, 884ff, *884*
   see also Transmitters; *specific names*
Nexus. *See* Gap junctions
NGF. *See* Nerve growth factor
Nigrostriatal dopaminergic neurons. *See*
      Neurons, nigrostriatal dopaminergic
Nodes of Ranvier, *441, 442,* 453
Nonspiking neurons, in insects, 149–151,
      150, 304–306. *See also* Spikeless
      neuronal communication; Synaptic
      transmission
Noradrenaline. *See* Norepinephrine
Noradrenergic action
   central integrative, 53–54
   firing, sleep cycles and, 56
Noradrenergic projections
   divergent anatomy of, 54
   latencies and duration of effects, 55
Noradrenergic systems, 52
   collateral arborization in, 55
   sleep cycles and, 56
Norepinephrine
   adenylate cyclase and, 55, 820, *820*
   biosynthesis of, 881, *882,* 913
   effect on cAMP accumulation, 1014
   gap junctions and, 364
   as modulatory transmitter, 15, *16*
   in optic tectum, 993
   release, regulation of, 884
   thromboxane B₂ and, 1024
   tyrosine hydroxylase and, 15
Novelty detection, 1126–1129
5′-Nucleotidase
   adenosine-producing enzyme, 1009–
      1014, *1010–1012*
   glial-cell membrane and, 1013
Nystagmus, vestibular, 343, *344–345,* 542

O

Ocellus, 275ff, 298
   L-cells of, 284–288, *287*
Octopus, local neurons in brain of, 146

Ocular dominance, 117–124
   changes in kitten, 1103–1104, *1104*
   cortical columns and, 964, 1134
Olfactory bulb, 52, 108
   anatomical studies of, 129–130, *130*
   cell proliferation in, 61
   dendritic bundles in, 387, 389–391,
      389–390
   dendrodenritic synapses in, *10*
   GABA in, 139
   inhibition in, 131, 133–134
   local circuit neurons in, 61
   local circuits in, 129–142
   metabolic mapping of, 138, *139*
   mitral cells of, 61, 373, 389–391, *389*
   morphology of synapses in, 130
   as neuronal local circuit prototype, 9
   neurotransmitters in, 138–141, *140,* 373
   periglomerular cells in, 129ff
   physiological studies of, 130–132, *131*
   potential divider model of, 133
   presynaptic dendrites in, 996
   rabbit, *130*
   reciprocal synapses in, 129
   synaptic circuits, glomerular, *136,* 137
   synaptic connections, *130*
   synaptic organization, *389*
   theoretical models of, 132–134, *132–136*
Olfactory cortex, electrophysiological
      modulation by adenosine, 1014
Olfactory nerves, biochemistry of, 140
Oligodendroglia. *See* Glial cells
Ommatidium
   cartridge processes in, 149, 278–279,
      279 (see also Optic cartridge)
   of fly, 297ff
   of grasshopper, *278*
   photoreceptors in, 90, 277ff, *277, 282–
      284, 283, 285, 289*
   receptor axons of, 302
On-off cells, *196*
   in chloride-free medium, 231, *232*
   cobalt effect on, 232, *233*
   EPSP-IPSP sequence, 233–234, 241,
      241
   functional model of, 240, *240*
On-off mechanisms, 170, *171, 172,* 178,
      178, 206, *207,* 227ff
Opiate receptors
   in brain, 1057ff
   and enkephalin, *1061*
   in guinea pig intestine, 1059
   in mouse vas deferens, 1059
Opioid peptides. *See* Peptides, opioid
Opossum, gap junctions in brain of, 346
Optic cartridge, 278–279, *279*
   in fly lamina, 298, 302
Optic chiasm, *117, 976*
   of pigeon, 989
Optic lobe, of insect, 275, *276*
Optic tectum, 1133
   amino acid transmitters in, 989–1002
   anatomical organization of, 989–991,
      990–991, 1000
   cell proliferation in, 62–63
   cell reaggregation in, 69
   GABA-labeled neurons in, 995–998
   neuronal migration in, 67
   neuronal types in, *990*
   norepinephrine in, 993

retinal axon distribution in, 961
   and retinal connections, 993ff
Optomotor response
   of beetle, 94
   of fly, 89ff, 306, *307*
Orthodromic activation, model, 533, *533–
      534*
Ouabain, 185, *836,* 876, 877
   sodium-potassium pump and, 470, 510,
      876
Ovulation, sexual specificity in triggering
      of, 969–970
Oxytocin, effect on cAMP levels, 1045

P

Pacemaker cells
   calcium in, 601ff, 866, 883, *883*
   cardiac, catecholamines and, 56
   cAMP in, 883–884
   neurotransmitters and, 884
   spike trains and, 519
Pancreas, as cell-cell interaction model,
      1029
Paracrine mediation, 1029
Parallel fibers
   in cerebellar cortex, 71, 114
   in molecular layer, 70
   Purkinje cells and, 71, 382, 461, *461,*
      530
Parietal cortex, columnar organization of,
      32
Passive potential, vs. active propagation,
      431–433
Peptide bonds, proteolytic cleavage of,
      801, *801*
Peptide extracts
   adenylate cyclase and, 1047, *1047,* 1048
   cAMP levels and, 1045, *1046–1047,*
      1048
   cerebral cortex from, 1048
Peptides, 15, 52–53
   in amygdaloid cortex, 1032
   anatomical distribution of, *1029–1030*
   biosynthesis and secretion of, 1032
   chain-synthesis of, 900
   in CNS, 1030, *1030,* 1033–1037
   cyclic nucleotides and, 1034, 1045–1047
   degradation of, 1033
   effect on adenylate cyclase activity,
      1047–1049, *1047*
   effect on neuronal activity, 1043–1054
   hypophysiotropic activities, *1028*
   modulation by nonpeptidic factors,
      1027
   neurobiology of, 1027–1037
   neurotransmitter function of, 15, 1032,
      1034
   pituitary function and, 1027, 1028
   systems mediated by, 56
   see also specific names
Peptides, opioid, 17, 1032, 1057–1067
   cellular localization of, 1060–1065,
      1060–1065
   metabolism of, 1059–1060
   receptors for, 1057ff, *1061–1062*
   release and postsynaptic actions of,
      1065–1066
   synthesis of, 1032

Periglomerular (PG) cells
dopamine as transmitter in, 140
impulse activity effects of, 134–136,
136, 140
mitral-cell responses and, 9, 135
in olfactory bulb, 129ff
Peripheral nervous system (PNS)
cell proliferation in, 64
purinergic system in, and ATP, 1008
synaptic remodeling in, 113
Phasic reentry, 38, 1116, 1127ff
Phospholamban, 13, 868–870
Phosphoprotein, in sarcoplasmic
reticulum, 867–868
Phosphorylation
ADP removal by, 1023
by calcium, 566, 865ff
enzyme cascades and, 803, 805ff, *805–
806*
field decay during, *662*
of proteins, 865–871, 1043, *1043*, 1044
Photoreceptors
calcium effect on, 879
excitation in, 183–189
in insect eye, *276–277, 279–284, 279–
285, 290, 299*
postreceptor neurons and, 229
vertebrate, rhodopsin in, *299*
Photosynthesis, 659–668
electrochromism in, 659ff, *661*
electron-transport chains, 658–661, *660*,
663
electron-transport inhibitors, 666, *667*
functional units, scheme of, *660*
pathway of, 659
Pigeon
adenosine derivatives, specificity in,
1008
electrotonic transmission in, 340
retina, receptive field in, 168
visual system, as neurobiological model,
989ff
Pigment granules, transport of, 710–718,
*710*ff
Pituitary
binding sites for TRF and CRF in, 1029
β-endorphin in, 1059
functional receptors in, 1027
role in modulation of brain function,
1028
sexual differentiation in, 969
Plasmalemma. *See* Membranes
Plasma membranes, 566, 567
calcium channels in, 580
composition of, 783, *832*
differentiation and, 782
endocytosis and, 692
exocytosis and, 579, 594
Plasticity
of nervous system, 911–912, 937
of neuronal connectivity, 75
role in modulatory systems, 1102–1104
of synapses, 513
Platelets
aggregation of, and endoperoxides,
1020ff, *1021–1022*
thromboxane and endoperoxides in,
1022–1024
PNMT (phenylethanolamine-N-
methyltransferase), 897, 906–907

ACTH and, 916
glucocorticoids and, 916
PNS. *See* Peripheral nervous system
Polypeptides
adenylate cyclase and, 820
in gap junctions, 363
Polyribosomes (polysomes), 708, *708–709*,
900ff
monoaminergic drugs and, 901–906,
901–905
temperature effect on, 904, *905*
Postsynaptic potential (PSP), *244*, 317ff,
319
amacrine-cell response and, 203, *203*
in dendritic tree, 323ff
in ganglion cell, 206, *206*
geometric vs. cable factors in, 326
input, 519
size profiles of, 324–325, *324–325*
weighting of, 516
see also Excitatory postsynaptic potential;
Inhibitory postsynaptic potential
Potassium
aequorin and, 610
aminopyridine and, 575
current, calcium-mediated, 601ff
dendrites, slow channels in, 445
dopamine release and, 1087, *1088*
intracellular charge carrier, 425
in lamina monopolar cells, 290
in brain-cell microenvironment, 460–
466, *462–463, 467, 469, 508, 508*
nonlinear conductance, 440–441
outward currents, 605–608, *606–607*
in periaxonal space, 500ff
reticular stimulation and, 1100, *1100*
seizure activity and, 466
voltage-clamp pulses and, 602, *602, 608*
Preoptic area
role in sexual behavior, 970ff, *970*
sexual dimorphism of, 975, *976–977*
steroid hormones and, 972ff, *973*ff
Presynaptic dendrites, in vertebrate CNS,
373–378
Presynaptic facilitation, 520
Presynaptic inhibition, 44, 374, 520
enkephalin and, 1061–1062, 1066
Presynaptic interaction, electrical and
chemical, *44*, 45
Presynaptic structures, dendritic origin of,
374, *375*
Prolactin, 1027
Progesterone
as ACTH inhibitor, 1027
in adult gonadectomized rat, *977*
secretion of, 969
Projection neurons, 108, 373, 439
Prokaryotes, calcium extrusion and, 621
Proline, as neurotransmitter, 1002
Prostaglandins
biosynthetic pathways of, *1018*
in cellular events, 15, 53–54
effect on ACTH secretion, 1027
effect on adenylate cyclase activity, 820
endoperoxides and, 1017–1024
and pituitary hormone secretion, 1029
from polyunsaturated fatty acids, 1017,
1017
Protein 14-3-2 (neuron-specific protein),
901

Protein S100, 901
Protein kinase
calcium activation of, 566
cAMP and, 860–861, 865–871, 1043
Proteins
anion-exchange, *833, 838*
calcium-modulated, 618–621, *619–620*
conformational changes in, 623–629,
635
energy of, characterized, 625
in eukaryotic cells, 898ff, *898*
intrinsic, types I and II, 832ff, *832*
membrane, voltage-driven gating of,
623–629
phosphorylation of, and cAMP, 860–
861, 865–870, 879
Protein synthesis
in adrenal medulla, 906–907
in brain, 900ff, *901*ff
cycloheximide inhibition of, 900
cytoplasmic, *898*, 900
dissociation factor, 900
hormone stimulation of, 899
initiation factors in, 900
mitochondrial, 901
monoaminergic drugs and, 901–906,
901–905
neuronal, 897–907
neurotransmitter control of, 897, 906
ribosomal, 898ff
temperature and, 904, *905*
transcription, 898, *898*
transsynaptic control of, 897–907
Pseudemys. See Turtle
PSP. *See* Postsynaptic potential
Psychoneural Identity, 21
Puffer fish (*Spheroides maculatus*),
electrotonic coupling in, 343, *344–345*
Purine, 53
metabolism in brain, 1006
Purine nucleotide
as adenylate cyclase regulator, 820, *821*,
822
β-adrenergic receptors and, 822, *823*
Purinergic system, ATP as inhibitor of,
1008
Purkinje-cell dendrites, *461*
branching, human, *478*
branch power, 71, *484*, 490, *490*
calcium spikes, 565
fibers, cardiac, 56
Purkinje cells, 56
action potentials in, 531, *535, 564*
calcium-dependent spikes in, 564
cerebellar, development of synaptic
input to, 111ff, *112–113, 115, 769*,
883
climbing fibers, 74, 530ff
complex spike of, 531, 534–535, *535*
computer model of, 530–536, *531*ff
cyclic nucleotides and, 862, 881, 1052
morphology of, 111–112, *112*
in mouse mutants, 114, 782, 785
neuronal cycle and, 62
orthodromic stimulation in, 533, *533–
534*
parallel fibers of, 71, 461, 530ff
postsynaptic specialization in, 947
soma of, 531
waveform in, 531

Steroids
  behavior regulation by, 971–972
  cytoplasmic receptors for, 973
  morphological sex differences and,
    974–978
  mRNA synthesis and, 889
  neural circuits and, 971
  sexual behavior and, 970ff, 970
  translocation to cell nucleus, 973
  see also specific names
Stomatogastric ganglia, in lobster, 152,
    318ff, 327
Stress fibers, 704, 706–707, 708
  biochemical anatomy of, 725
Striate cortex
  diurnal change in, 1106
  isolation of processing function of, 28
  mapping of visual space on, 28
  nonretinal modulation of activity in,
    1095–1097
  reticular control of, 1100–1101
  specific activity in, 1094, 1095–1096
Structural circuitry in brain, overview,
    7–9
Suberyldicholine, membrane current and,
    626
Substance P, 53
  monoaminergic drugs and, 905
  opiates on release of, 1067
  in sensory fibers, 1061–1062
  in s. nigra, 1072–1075, 1073, 1086,
    1089
Substantia nigra, 16, 54
  anatomy of, 1085, 1085
  dopamine in, 1069–1080, 1086–1090,
    1087
  GABA in, 1072–1073, 1073, 1075,
    1086, 1089–1090
  glycine in, 1073, 1073
  serotonin in, 1072, 1073, 1074, 1086
  substance P in, 1072–1075, 1073, 1086,
    1089–1090
Superior cervical ganglia, 784, 786, 788
  cyclic nucleotides in, 881, 915, 1052
Superior colliculus
  gliogenesis in, 63
  horizontal cells in, 328–329, 328
  see also Optic tectum
Sympathetic ganglia
  cAMP and, 862
  tyrosine hydroxylase in, 912ff, 915–916
Sympathetic nervous system
  gene expression in, 911–924
  neuronal interaction in, 929, 933
  organization of, 912
Synapse formation
  in embryo, 755ff
  genetically perturbed, 114, 115, 116
  mechanisms of, 750
  in neuromuscular junction, 751ff, 757
  selective-stabilization hypothesis, 750ff,
    750
  see also Synaptogenesis
Synapses, 780–781
  axoaxonic, 405
  cholinergic, 751
  conventional, basal, 164, 165, 166
  cyclic nucleotides and, 879
  dendrodendritic, 12, 136, 317–330
  diagrammatic, 847

dual action at, 336–338, 337, 349–351,
    351–352
electroreceptor of, in fish, 286
excitatory, 129–130
giant, 151, 317–319, 321, 556
gain properties, 561–562, 563
inhibitory, 129–130
input-output properties, 317–321, 517,
    520
in invertebrates, 146ff, 151–155, 153–
    154
molecular signals at, 1005
of motor system in squid, 286
in olfactory bulb, 129–130
pharmacology of, 52
phasic, 193, 213
plasticity of, 513
in plexiform layers of retina, 163
in retina, interactions, 194, 194, 197,
    198
ribbon, 11, 164, 165, 177, 249
site redistribution of, 113–114
somatic, 518
synchronizing, 343
tonic, 193, 214
Synaptic activity
  action potentials and, 502
  adenosine derivative release and, 1007–
    1008, 1008
  mixed chemical and electrical, 336, 337
Synaptic circuitry
  binocular vision in monkey and, 117
  multidisciplinary approach to, 129ff
Synaptic cleft, 751, 780, 782
  neurotransmitter in, 16
Synaptic connections
  functional validation of, 75
  genetics and environment of, 111
  learning and memory related to, 110
Synaptic delay, 558–560, 559
Synaptic discs. See Gap junctions
Synaptic function, developmental cues
    for, 929ff, 931–933
Synaptic inhibition
  mixed chemical and electrical, 336, 337
  without concurrent impulse activity, 131
Synaptic membrane, differentiation of,
    779–793, 780ff
Synaptic operations
  domains of, 52ff, 52, 54
  nonconforming, 52
Synaptic potentials, dendritic geometry
    and, 321–326
Synaptic transmission
  adenosine and, 1014
  calcium effect on, 466–467, 555ff
  electrical, 338–355, 1005
  electrotonic, 339–340, 341
  mathematical model of, 560, 561
  in optic tectum, 993
  requirements for, 989
  spikeless, 317–330, 319, 513
  see also Spike trains; Spike transmission
Synaptic transport, 14
Synaptic vesicles
  acetylcholine in, 574–579
  aminopyridine effect in, 574ff, 574ff
  axonal, 779ff, 780ff
  calcium in, 582
  clear, 789, 791

coated, 588–595, 592–593, 782
exocytosis in, 573–598, 1009
in optic tectum, 992, 994
quick-freezing visualization method,
    573–598
in thalamic relay nuclei, 378
Synaptogenesis, 779–782, 783
  control mechanisms in, 791, 792–793,
    793
  recognition codes, 782–787
  see also Synapse formation
Synaptosomes
  axonal, 1001
  calcium transport in, 874
  cAMP and, 886
  glutamate in, 993
  protein synthesis in, 901
  transmitter uptake in, 992–993, 1000
  veratridine and, 877

T

TEA (tetraethylammonium)
  endplate potential and, 575
  ion conductance and, 470, 557, 557,
    602, 606ff
  neuromuscular junction and, 575, 581
Tectum. See Optic tectum
Temperature, and cell dynamics, 684,
    684–685
Terminal fields
  commissural, 959, 960, 962
  of lateral geniculate nucleus, 964
  in mammalian brain, 957ff
  of neurons, 937ff
  topography of, 957, 960, 961
Testosterone
  adult gonadectomized rat and, 977
  avian singing behavior and, 974
  brain development and, 972, 973
  neonatal influence of, 977
Tetanus toxin, retrograde transport of,
    14, 1002
Tetrodotoxin, 463, 467, 469
  dopamine release and, 1074, 1074,
    1077, 1079, 1088
  ion conductance and, 556–557, 557,
    564, 601, 612–613
  ocellar receptors and, 283
  pre- and postsynaptic effects of, 319,
    319, 320, 321
  in retina, 9, 204, 235, 237, 238
  spreading depression and, 469
  in squid axon, 601
Thalamocortical relay cells, 375–376
Thalamus
  cell proliferation in, 62–63
  dendrite bundles in, 385–413
  ^{3}H-leucine in, 376, 376, 377
  neuropil in, 381–413
  presynaptic dendrites in, 373–378
  relay nuclei in, 374ff, 382, 400
  ventrobasal, 340, 340, 373ff, 375–377,
    382ff, 383, 385, 400
Thromboxane, 1017–1024
  A$_2$, 1022, 1022
  B$_2$, 1020–1023, 1020, 1022
  B$_2$, formation in brain tissue, 1024,
    1024
Thylakoids, in photosynthesis, 660ff, 660

Thyroid hormones, prolactin secretion and, 1027. *See also* Hormones; TRF; TSH

Thyroid-stimulating hormone. *See* TSH

Thyrotropin-releasing factor. *See* TRF

Toadfish (*Opsanus tau*), electrotonic transmission in, 340, *341-342*, 343

Transmembrane properties, 55

Transmitters
active vs. passive, 53
chemical ontology of, 51
modulatory action of, 15, *16*
nonspecific action of, 45
release from dendrites, 16, 377-378
synthesis of, 53, 70
see also Neurotransmitters

Transneuronal input-output curves, 320, *320*, 321, *321*

Transport
anterograde, 13
bidirectional, 13
fast, mediators of, 12-13
fast, therapeutic value of, 14
intracellular via neurites, 13, *14*
retrograde, 13-14, 917-924, *919, 921, 924*
see also Axonal transport; Axoplasmic transport; Ion transport

TRF (thyrotropin-releasing factor), 1027ff, *1028*, 1034

Troponin
effects on calcium and skeletal muscle, 617
in sarcoplasmic reticulum, 867, 869, *869*

TSH (thyroid-stimulating hormone), 1027

Tubulin
bidirectional transport of, 12, *13*
synthesis of, 898, 901

Tufted cells
in cortex, *404*, 405
dopamine in, 140
in olfactory bulb, 129

Turtle
cone, pharmacology of, 220-222, *200, 221*
retina, 189, *189*, 215ff

Tyrosine hydroxylase
in adrenal medulla, 912ff, *915*
in chromaffin cells, 906, 907

cyclic nucleotides and, 914, *915*
glucocorticoids and, 917, *918*
NGF and, 922, *922-923*, 1002
and norepinephrine synthesis, 15
selective induction of, 913
in sympathetic ganglia, 912ff, *915-916*
in synaptosomes, 886

U

Uridine, transfer dynamics of, *1009*

V

van't Hoff relation, 633, 637

Vasodilatation
adenosine and, 1006
calcium-mediated, 1006

Vasopressin
ACTH secretion and, 1027
cAMP levels and, 1045

Veratridine, effect on neurotransmitter release, 875, 877

Vertebrates
electrotonic transmission, 339ff
neurogenesis in, 59
neurons of, electrical interactions, 333-356
retina studies in, 163-179, 183-189
see also specific names

Vesicles
membrane, ion flux in, 847-857
synaptic (*see* Synaptic vesicles)
transmitter release from, 11

Vestibular nystagmus, 343-345, 542

Vestibular stimulation
electrical transmission and, 340ff
in frog, model of, 536-537, *540*
and nystagmus, 542

Vision, insect. *See* Insect vision

Visual cortex
binocular rivalry in, 1105
central-core control of, 1093-1108
cholinergic pathways in, 1106-1107
circuit consolidation in, 1103-1104
columnar organization of, 28-29, 117, 120, *120*, 122, 123
diurnal variation in, human, 1106, *1106*
excitability, control of, 1106-1108, *1107*

in fetal monkey, *121*
gating signals in postulated, 1103
monoaminergic pathways in, 1106-1107
monocular deprivation in, 964, 1102
ocular-dominance shift in, 1103, *1103-1104*
orientation selectivity of, 1103
receptive-field disparity in, 29
stereopsis, 29

Visual function, synaptic mechanisms of, 208-210, *208-209*

Visual processing, 194-197, 1115

Visual system
arthropod peripheral, 275-292
binocular, 108, 117, *117*
current-source-density analysis, 1094, *1095*, 1098
crustacean visual receptors, *152*
of dragonfly, 279, 283-284, *286-287*, 291
of *Drosophila*, 93, *93*, 298
of fly, 81-102, 297-308, *298*ff
Fourier analysis, 91, 263
genesis of, 116ff
of insects, 81-102, 275-292, 298, *298*, 299
of locust, 277, *280*, 281ff, *285*, 287, *290*
ocular dominance in, 117-124
ommatidia of crayfish, 282
plasticity of, 1102-1104
primate, 74, 116
single-unit analysis of, 1098
specific sensory activity in, 1093-1095

Voltage attenuation in neurons, *322*, 323-324

Voltage-dependent processes, mechanisms in membrane, 623ff

W

Weaver mouse
cerebellum of, 782
glial process breakdown in, 67
morphology of Purkinje cells in, 114, *115*
see also Mouse mutants

Weber-Fechner relation, 291

Worm, local neurons in segmental ganglia of, 148